ALPHABETICAL LIST OF NANDA-ACCEPTED DIAGNOSES

Activity intolerance
Activity intolerance, potential
Adjustment, impaired
Airway clearance, ineffective
Anxiety
Aspiration, potential for
Body image disturbance
Body temperature, altered, potential
Breastfeeding, ineffective
Breathing pattern, ineffective
Cardiac output, decreased
Communication, impaired verbal
Constipation
Constipation, colonic
Constipation, perceived
Coping, defensive
Coping, family: potential for growth
Coping, ineffective family: compromised
Coping, ineffective family: disabling
Coping, ineffective individual
Decisional conflict (specify)
Denial, ineffective
Diarrhea
Disuse syndrome, potential for
Diversional activity deficit
Dysreflexia
Family processes, altered
Fatigue
Fear
Fluid volume deficit (1)
Fluid volume deficit (2)
Fluid volume deficit, potential
Fluid volume excess
Gas exchange, impaired
Grieving, anticipatory
Grieving, dysfunctional
Growth and development, altered
Health maintenance, altered
Health seeking behaviors (specify)
Home maintenance management, impaired
Hopelessness
Hyperthermia
Hypothermia
Incontinence, bowel
Incontinence, functional
Incontinence, reflex
Incontinence, stress
Incontinence, total
Incontinence, urge
Infection, potential for
Injury, potential for

Knowledge deficit (specify)
Mobility, impaired physical
Noncompliance (specify)
Nutrition, altered: less than body requirements
Nutrition, altered: more than body requirements
Nutrition, altered: potential for more than body requirements
Oral mucous membrane, altered
Pain
Pain, chronic
Parental role conflict
Parenting, altered
Parenting, altered, potential
Personal identity disturbance
Poisoning, potential for
Post-trauma response
Powerlessness
Rape-trauma syndrome
Rape-trauma syndrome: compound reaction
Rape-trauma syndrome: silent reaction
Role performance, altered
Self care deficit, bathing/hygiene
Self care deficit, dressing/grooming
Self care deficit, feeding
Self care deficit, toileting
Self-esteem disturbance
Self-esteem, chronic low
Self-esteem, situational low
Sensory/perceptual alterations (specify) (visual, auditory, kinesthetic, gustatory, tactile, olfactory)
Sexual dysfunction
Sexuality patterns, altered
Skin integrity, impaired
Skin integrity, impaired, potential
Sleep pattern disturbance
Social interaction, impaired
Social isolation
Spiritual distress (distress of the human spirit)
Suffocation, potential for
Swallowing, impaired
Thermoregulation, ineffective
Thought processes, altered
Tissue integrity, impaired
Tissue perfusion, altered (specify type) (renal, cerebral; cardiopulmonary, gastrointestinal, peripheral)
Trauma, potential for
Unilateral neglect
Urinary elimination, altered patterns
Urinary retention
Violence, potential for: self-directed or directed at others

From the Proceedings of the Eighth National Conference of the North American Nursing Diagnosis Association held in St. Louis, Missouri, March 13-16, 1988. Reflects revised taxonomy, Fall 1988.

MEDICAL-SURGICAL NURSING

A Nursing Process Approach

MEDICAL-SURGICAL NURSING

A Nursing Process Approach

Edited by

BARBARA C. LONG, M.S.N., R.N.

Associate Professor Emerita of Medical-Surgical Nursing
Frances Payne Bolton School of Nursing
Case Western Reserve University
Cleveland, Ohio

WILMA J. PHIPPS, Ph.D., R.N., F.A.A.N.

Professor Emerita of Medical-Surgical Nursing
Frances Payne Bolton School of Nursing
Case Western Reserve University
Cleveland, Ohio

SECOND EDITION

with 740 illustrations

THE C. V. MOSBY COMPANY

ST. LOUIS • BALTIMORE • TORONTO   1989

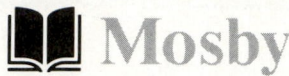

Editor: Linda L. Duncan
Assistant editor: Joanna May
Project manager: Suzanne Seeley
Production editors: Mary G. Stueck, Kathy Burmann
Book and cover designer: Gail Morey Hudson

SECOND EDITION

Copyright © 1989 by The C.V. Mosby Company

Printed in the United States of America

The C.V. Mosby Company
11830 Westline Industrial Drive, St. Louis, Missouri 63146

Library of Congress Cataloging in Publication Data

Medical-surgical nursing.

  Rev. ed. of: Essentials of medical-surgical nursing. 1985.
  Includes bibliographies and index.
  1. Nursing. 2. Surgical nursing. I. Long,
Barbara C. II. Phipps, Wilma J.
III. Essentials of medical-surgical
nursing. [DNLM: 1. Nursing Care. 2. Nursing Process.
3. Surgical Nursing.   WY 150 M48933]
RT41.E87 1989   610.73   88-13257
ISBN 0-8016-3246-3

GW/VH/VH 9 8 7 6 5 4 3

Contributors

DOROTHY O. DLEVINS, M.S N , R.N.

Associate Professor of Nursing, Kent State University, Kent, Ohio

LINDA ANNE BROSEMAN, M.S.N., R.N.

Head Nurse, University Hospitals of Cleveland; Clinical Instructor in Medical-Surgical Nursing, Frances Payne Bolton School of Nursing, Case Western Reserve University, Cleveland, Ohio

PATRICIA BUERGIN, B.S.N., R.N.

Head Nurse, University Hospitals of Cleveland; Clinical Instructor in Medical-Surgical Nursing, Frances Payne Bolton School of Nursing, Case Western Reserve University, Cleveland, Ohio

VIRGINIA L. CASSMEYER, Ph.D., R.N.

Associate Professor of Medical-Surgical Nursing, University of Kansas, Kansas City, Kansas

ELIZABETH CAMERON ECKSTEIN, M.S.N., R.N.

Formerly Infection Control Nurse, University Hospitals of Cleveland, Cleveland, Ohio

H. FRED FARLEY, M.S.N., R.N.

Assistant Director of Medical-Surgical Nursing, University Hospitals of Cleveland; Clinical Instructor in Medical-Surgical Nursing, Frances Payne Bolton School of Nursing, Case Western Reserve University, Cleveland, Ohio

GREER GLAZER, Ph.D., R.N.

Associate Professor of Nursing, Kent State University, Kent, Ohio

JUDITH L. GREIG, M.S.N., R.N.

Associate Professor of Nursing, Lakeland Community College, Mentor, Ohio

GRACE McCARTHY HARLAN, M.S.N., R.N.

Formerly Associate Professor of Medical-Surgical Nursing, Cleveland State University, Cleveland, Ohio

ROSEMARIE HOGAN, M.S.N., R.N.

Associate Professor of Nursing, Kent State University, Kent, Ohio

MAURA A. HOPKINS, M.S.N., R.N., CCRN

Head Nurse, Intensive Care Unit, University of California San Francisco Medical Center, San Francisco, California

DEBORAH GOLDENBERG KLEIN, M.S.N., R.N., CCRN

Clinical Nurse Specialist, Cleveland Metropolitan General Hospital/Highland View Hospital; Clinical Instructor in Medical-Surgical Nursing, Frances Payne Bolton School of Nursing, Case Western Reserve University, Cleveland, Ohio

MARY KAY LEHMAN, M.S.N., R.N.

Instructor in Medical-Surgical Nursing, Frances Payne Bolton School of Nursing, Case Western Reserve University; Associate in Nursing, University Hospitals of Cleveland, Cleveland, Ohio

RUTH LINCOLN, M.S.N., R.N.

Clinical Nurse Specialist in Gerontology, University Hospitals of Cleveland; Clinical Instructor in Medical-Surgical Nursing, Frances Payne Bolton School of Nursing, Case Western Reserve University, Cleveland, Ohio

*BENITA C. MARTOCCHIO, Ph.D., R.N.

Associate Professor of Medical-Surgical Nursing, American Cancer Society Professor of Oncology, Frances Payne Bolton School of Nursing, Case Western Reserve University, Cleveland, Ohio

---

* Deceased 1987.

MARY LOU MONAHAN, M.S.N., M.B.A., R.N.

Director of Trauma and Critical Care Services, Cleveland Metropolitan General Hospital/Highland View Hospital, Cleveland, Ohio

ELLEN F. OLSHANSKY, D.N.S., R.N.

Assistant Professor, University of Washington, Seattle, Washington

GAIL OSTERFIELD, M.S.N., R.N.

Assistant Professor of Nursing, Kent State University, Kent, Ohio

DORA RICE, M.S.N., R.N.

Infection Control Nurse, Cleveland Veterans Administration Medical Center, Cleveland, Ohio

GRACE A. ROTTER, M.S.N., R.N.

Infection Control Nurse, Cleveland Veterans Administration Medical Center; Clinical Instructor in Community Health Nursing, Frances Payne Bolton School of Nursing, Case Western Reserve University, Cleveland, Ohio

ELIZABETH SCHENK, M.S.N., R.N.

Director of Nursing, Heather Hill Rehabilitation Hospital, Chardon, Ohio; Clinical Instructor in Medical-Surgical Nursing, Frances Payne Bolton School of Nursing, Case Western Reserve University, Cleveland, Ohio

SUSAN M. SCHNEIDER, M.S.N., R.N.

Clinical Nurse Specialist in Oncology, University Hospitals of Cleveland; Clinical Instructor in Medical-Surgical Nursing, Frances Payne Bolton School of Nursing, Case Western Reserve University, Cleveland, Ohio

BARBARA SOLTIS, M.S.N., R.N.

Formerly Clinical Nurse Specialist, Cleveland Metropolitan General Hospital/Highland View Hospital, Cleveland, Ohio

EILEEN WALSH, M.S.N., R.N.

Assistant Professor of Nursing, Medical College of Ohio; Program Coordinator, Henry L. Morse Physical Health Research Center, Toledo, Ohio

NANCY FUGATE WOODS, Ph.D., R.N., F.A.A.N.

Professor and Chair, Parent and Child Nursing, University of Washington, Seattle, Washington

E. RONALD WRIGHT, Ph.D.

Associate Professor of Microbiology, Frances Payne Bolton School of Nursing, Case Western Reserve University, Cleveland, Ohio

MARY A. (SANDY) WYPER, Ph.D., R.N.

Assistant Professor of Nursing, Kent State University, Kent, Ohio

MARGARET VETTESE ZACK, M.S.N., R.N.

Ph.D. Candidate; Clinical Specialist in Medical-Surgical Nursing, University Hospitals of Cleveland; Clinical Instructor in Medical-Surgical Nursing, Frances Payne Bolton School of Nursing, Case Western Reserve University, Cleveland, Ohio

Preface

Medical-surgical nursing continues to expand, with increased promotion of health care and technological advances. Of particular note is the refining of accepted nursing diagnoses and beginning developments toward a taxonomy of nursing diagnoses by the North American Nursing Diagnosis Association (NANDA). The purpose of this book is to present information on the care of adult persons with common medical-surgical disorders. Content specific to other nursing fields, such as pediatric or maternity nursing, has not been included.

OVERVIEW

The approach used in the first edition was favorably received and thus is continued in this edition. Some of the changes are as follows.

The first two units present a summary of the bases of medical-surgical nursing practice (Unit I) and health promotion (Unit II). It is expected that students will have had at least one introductory course in nursing before beginning to use this text, therefore much of the information in the first two units is provided for its usefulness in medical-surgical nursing practice, for student review, and for a reference source as students study subsequent chapters.

Units III and IV focus on common problems or situations (surgery) experienced by many persons with medical-surgical disorders. The chapter on stress has been rewritten to include both physiologic and psychologic responses to stress in addition to stress management techniques. A new chapter on substance abuse has been added. The chapter on dying and death includes a new section on ethical dimensions.

The next six units follow the same format as in the first edition. Discussion centers on problem areas: sensorimotor (Unit V), gas transport (Unit VI), endocrine and metabolic (Unit VII), digestion and elimination (Unit VIII), sexual and reproductive (Unit IX), and physiologic defense mechanisms (Unit X). Medical disorders are grouped according to similar nursing interventions. A nursing process approach is used, and the implementation section clearly identifies nursing activities that (1) assist with achievement of therapeutic goals, (2) assist with comfort and activities of daily living, and (3) counseling and teaching. A new chapter, The Patient with a Sexually Transmitted Disease, has been added to Unit IX. Chapter 37, Biologic Defense Mechanisms, has been moved from the early part of the book and placed immediately before Chapter 38, The Patient with Immunologic Problems, to facilitate student understanding of the immunologic concepts in Chapter 38.

The last unit (XI) summarizes care required in emergencies and disasters and care of critically ill persons. The last chapter provides an overview and understanding of what the patient experiences in critical care units.

Throughout the book the recipients of the services of nurses are referred to as *patients* rather than as *clients*. Although client is widely used in the nursing community, the article "Complexities and Clarity in Nurse-Client and Nurse-Patient Relationships" by L. Nowakowski, which appeared in the July-August 1985 issue of the *Journal of Professional Nursing*, makes a real distinction between who is a client and who is a patient. Using her framework, we decided that patient was a better term to use in this book. We found Nowakowski's criteria for differentiating between clients and patients to be thought provoking and helpful, and we recommend the article to the reader.

FEATURES

We have endeavored in the second edition to maintain essentially the same **five-step nursing process approach.** The most recent **NANDA-approved nursing diagnoses** (at the time of publication, including the revised taxonomy, Fall 1988) have been incorporated in this edition. New listings of some possible pertinent **etiologies** have been added to the lists of nursing diagnoses. Selected **Nursing Care Plans** have been included in most "problem" chapters to provide students with some examples. More **pathophysiology** has been added as well as more explanations for the **rationales of nursing interventions.**

The use of boxes for highlighting important information was well-received in the first edition and has been continued here. We have been more selective in this edition, and at times have placed the information as lists within the text to ensure the reader noting the information. Citations of boxed materials have also been included in the text to direct the reader. The tables of medical information, providing a quick reference source, have been continued.

New to the second edition are the list of **Objectives** at the beginning and the **Summary** (list of important points) at the end of each chapter. The section **Putting Knowledge to Practice** is also new and incorporates some of the study questions from the first edition. This latter section provides some suggested student activities to aid in application of the knowledge and to prepare students for care of patients with medical-surgical disorders.

To enable instructors and students to easily access select topics, nursing diagnoses, and care plans, we have included a **Quick Reference Guide,** which may be found on the inside of the front and back covers.

TEACHING-LEARNING PACKAGE

For the second edition of our text we are pleased to offer an extensive number of ancillary products for instructors and students to use in class and clinical settings.

Instructor's manual. Includes topical outlines for each chapter and suggested ways of presenting content. Also features tips for special class and clinical activities. An extensive Test Bank with an answer key assists instructors in formulating test questions.

MicroTest II. Computerized Test Bank for use with IBM PC and Apple IIe, II+, and IIc. Includes multiple-choice questions and a user's manual so that you can add, delete, or rearrange test items from any part of the text.

CAI software. These four unique interactive disks covering pain, shock, fluids and electrolytes, and cancer feature 1 hour of instruction for students. Each disk presents self-assessment questions, a review of concepts, clinical simulations, and a posttest.

Study guide. Developed by Mary Nichols, this study guide enables students to make maximum use of review time by presenting objectives, outlines, self-assessment activities and checklists, and decision-making tools.

Clinical manual of medical-surgical nursing. Practical clinical references and study tool that enforces a systematic approach to nursing care. Provides quick information for over 275 common disorders and procedures.

ACKNOWLEDGMENTS

We are grateful for the expert contributions by our chapter authors. We thank the readers who wrote to us with ideas or suggestions and trust that they will be pleased with changes that have been made. New illustrations are the work of Nancy Burgard of Cleveland. The preparation of parts of the manuscript was by Sondra Patrizi.

We greatly appreciate the strong support we have received from editors and project managers at The C.V. Mosby Company, particularly Linda Duncan, Suzanne Seeley, Joanna May, Susie Baxter, and Don Ladig. We could not have completed this second edition without them.

Barbara C. Long
Wilma J. Phipps

Contents

Detailed Contents

20 The Patient with Eye Problems, 515

BARBARA C. LONG

30 The Patient with Hepatic, Biliary, and Pancreatic Problems, 991

DOROTHY R. BLEVINS and VIRGINIA L. CASSMEYER

UNIT VIII

PROBLEMS OF DIGESTION OR ELIMINATION

31 The Patient with Gastrointestinal Problems, 1047

BARBARA C. LONG and REBECCA ROBERTS

32 The Patient with Urinary Problems, 1123

H. FRED FARLEY

UNIT I
Medical-Surgical Nursing Practice

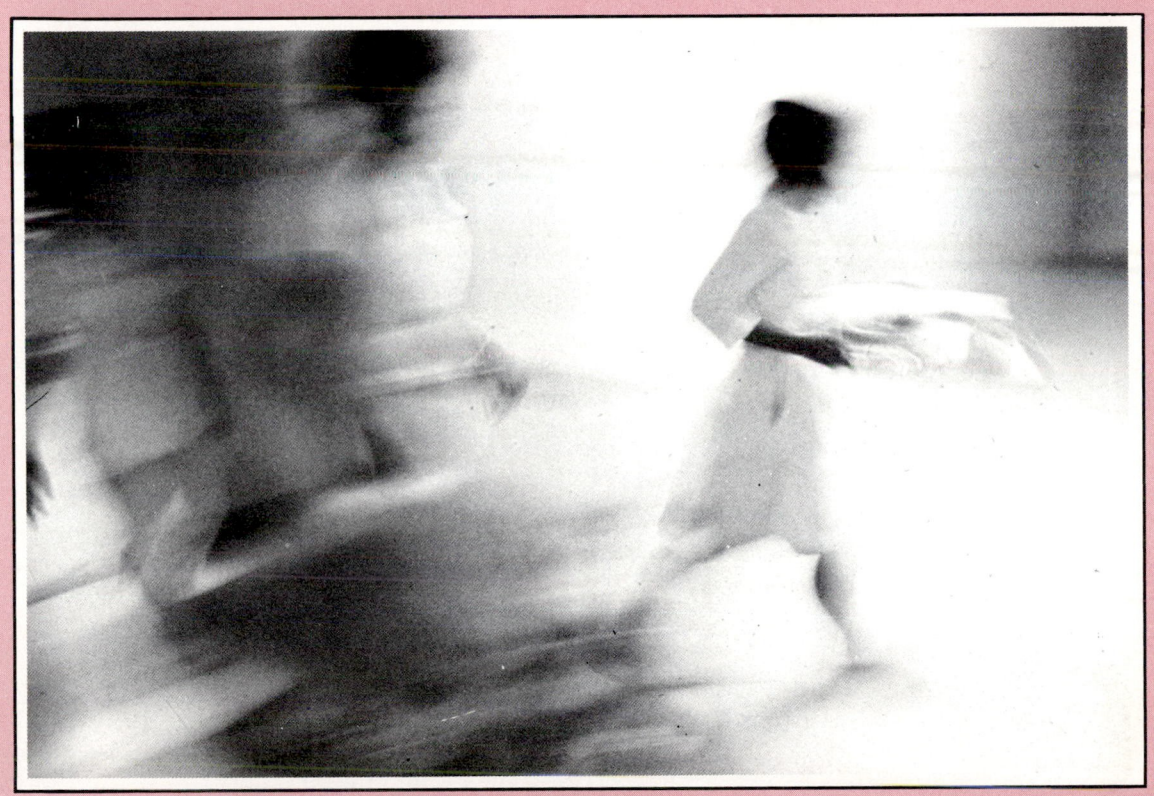

1

Perspectives of Medical-Surgical Nursing

BARBARA C. LONG

CHAPTER OBJECTIVES

After studying this chapter, the student should be able to:

- Differentiate the practice of medical-surgical nursing from the other disciplines (for example, pediatric, psychiatric).

- Differentiate between health promotion and prevention of illness and describe the three levels of prevention.

- Define "at risk" status and explain the relevance for nursing practice.

- Differentiate between illness and disease and identify stages of disease development.

- Identify actions people take when illness is perceived.

- Describe the "sick role."

- Describe the scope of medical-surgical nursing practice: independent and interdependent functions, use of specific knowledge (pathophysiology, signs and symptoms, medical therapies), and types of nursing interventions.

■ SCOPE OF MEDICAL-SURGICAL NURSING

Medical-surgical nursing practice encompasses the nursing care of persons who are at risk for or who are experiencing pathophysiologic disorders. In most health care centers children are separated from adults because of their different needs, and the specialty practice of pediatric nursing has developed with the focus on the nursing care of children. Thus medical-surgical nursing practice has developed primarily as the nursing care of persons (1) who have attained physical/developmental maturity, (2) who are at risk for or who have expressed variations in their personal norms of physical functioning, and (3) who may require therapeutic medical or surgical intervention.

In the past *medical care* was the general term for the care given sick persons by professionals; it is now used to denote the care given by members of the medical profession (physicians). The trend in American society is toward a health orientation; therefore, *health care* is the more acceptable term for the care provided by all health care professionals. The term *health care* is broader in that it includes assisting people to stay well in addition to providing care when they are ill. The care of the sick remains a primary responsibility of health care professionals, and this care is still provided primarily in health care institutions such as acute care hospitals or long-term care centers. There is an increased use, however, of ambulatory care, primary care, and family care centers as well as other types of health care services, in part because it is more economic to keep people well than to provide care when they are sick.[3]

Nurses are one group of health care professionals. In addition to participating in health promotion, nurses are becoming more actively involved in prevention of disease and health education for persons who are at high risk for acquiring specific diseases. Health promotion, disease prevention, and care of persons with specific pathophysiologic disorders require a knowledge base of the following:

1. Health and illness
2. Factors influencing the occurrence and course of specific disorders
3. Common responses to the disorders
4. Nursing interventions that assist the person to achieve optimal health or to die with maximum comfort and dignity

■ HEALTH AND ILLNESS

Health and illness are complex concepts, and they are interpreted in different ways by different individuals or groups. Both health and illness are multidimensional concepts; that is to say, there are multiple aspects to be considered and multiple factors that may be of influence.

■ Definitions of health

During the early centuries health was defined in terms of that which was normal or natural. Therefore, anything abnormal or against nature was considered not healthy and to be avoided; for example, lepers were called "unclean." Treatment of diseases consisted of amulets or spells to drive out the evil or unnatural spirits causing the abnormality. "Leeching" was a popular treatment and consisted of applying leeches (blood-sucking worms) to suck out the tainted blood. Wounds were treated by cautery to burn out the evil forces that would prevent healing. Even in more modern times, "tonics," which often included a laxative, were taken frequently by people to stay healthy.

In later years health was defined primarily as freedom from disease. During the middle of the 20th century the concept of *mental health* was introduced, meaning the ability of the individual to cope successfully with stress in a functional manner. In 1974 the World Health Organization (WHO) defined health more broadly: complete physical, mental, and social well-being and not merely the absence of disease and infirmity. This definition introduced the concept of the subjective as well as the objective physical or behavioral responses.

The various views about health usually contain one or more of the following perspectives:

Biologic or clinical: absence of pathologic condition
Psychologic: well-being and self-actualization
Sociologic: ability to meet social responsibilities and role functions
Adaptive: adaptation to a changing environment

Patients and health care providers may have different views of health and may therefore be working toward different goals that may or may not be in conflict. For example, people who "feel well" and who hold the view that health is a sense of well-being may not be willing to follow-up on screening tests even when a disease may be suspected by the clinician.

Health is a dynamic, ever-changing state. It reflects the person's level of functioning in various physiologic, psychologic, and sociocultural dimensions. People can simultaneously be functioning at a high level in one aspect, such as nutrition, but at a low level in another aspect, such as oxygenation or self-esteem. Nursing is concerned with holistic health, the effect of functioning of the subcomponents on total functioning. Thus each patient is assessed in various dimensions, with consideration given for the person's overall functioning and sense of well-being. Each person presents different genetic factors and is exposed to different environmental factors. There is therefore *no one* nursing approach for all persons who are at risk for or who have a specific illness, disease, or injury. The approach used by nurses to provide care to a specific patient will depend on the pertinent factors unique to that patient.

■ Health promotion and prevention

The goal of nursing is to assist people to achieve optimal health, the highest level of functioning that is achievable for each person. This includes activities that promote health and prevent illness.

■ HEALTH PROMOTION

Health promotion refers to activities directed toward helping persons maintain or achieve a high level of functioning and feeling of well-being. The nursing activities include teaching, counseling, and motivating persons to develop life-styles that include adequate nutrition, exercise, and rest or relaxation. Persons functioning at a high level have an increased capacity to withstand physical and emotional stressors.[19] (See Chapter 6 for further information on health promotion.)

Health promotion activities are carried out whenever the opportunities occur. Thus health teaching and counseling are instituted not only with well persons but also when persons are hospitalized. For example, teaching about adequate nutrition can be done while assisting a patient to select items from a hospital menu.

■ PREVENTION

Prevention refers to activities directed toward protecting persons from potential or actual threats to health and the subsequent consequences.[17] In other words, prevention means inhibiting the development of disease, slowing down the progression of disease, and protecting the body from further harmful effects. There are three different levels of protection: primary, secondary, and tertiary (Table 1-1).

□ Primary prevention

Primary prevention includes specific protective measures against disease or trauma, such as immunizations against diphtheria or measles, environmental sanitation, and protection against occupational hazards (for example, wearing safety glasses to prevent eye injuries). Early successes in primary prevention have been the result of activities directed at preventing the occurrence of infectious diseases such as polio or smallpox through immunization and typhoid fever through purification of water. More recently dental caries have been prevented by fluoridation of water supplies.

The major health problems today are chronic diseases and accidental injuries and their sequelae, both of which require modification of deeply rooted behaviors such as the use of alcohol, tobacco and drugs, and poor nutritional and exercise patterns. Health promotion activities are considered a form of primary prevention.

□ Secondary prevention

Secondary prevention includes early detection and prompt intervention to stop the disease at an early stage, decrease the intensity, or prevent complications. This is accomplished by screening for diseases such as diabetes, carcinoma in situ, tuberculosis, or glaucoma. The purpose is to detect early symptoms about which the patient is unaware or lacks knowledge, so that prompt intervention is effective for control or cure. Screening for contacts of persons with sexually transmitted diseases and treating the infected person to prevent spread of the disease are other examples of secondary prevention.

□ Tertiary prevention

Tertiary prevention consists of activities that prevent or limit disabilities and help restore the person with a disability to an optimal level of functioning (that is, rehabilitation). Tertiary prevention begins in the early period of recovery from an illness and includes activities such as moving and turning immobile patients to prevent respiratory complications or decubiti, encouraging leg exercises to prevent muscle weakness, and encouraging or assisting with range of motion exercises to prevent contractures.

Rehabilitation programs for persons with cardiac disease or with disabilities resulting from a cerebral vascular accident (stroke) are initiated before the patient is discharged from the hospital. Chapter 14 discusses the concept of rehabilitation in more detail. Preventive measures for specific disorders are described in the appropriate chapters of this text.

■ At risk status

Some persons are considered to have a greater possibility of becoming ill or acquiring a specific disease because of the presence of certain factors. These persons are considered to be *at risk* and the specific factors are termed *risk factors*. For example, a woman over age 35 with a family history of breast cancer who had her first menstrual period before age 12 and who has never had a child would be

Table 1-1 Levels of prevention

Level	Definition	Examples
Primary	Prevention of disease	Immunization, environmental sanitation, accident prevention, anticipatory counseling and guidance (for example, premarital counseling)
Secondary	Early detection and treatment of disease	Screening for tuberculosis, diabetes, glaucoma Breast or testes self-examination Outpatient mental health programs
Tertiary	Prevention of disabilities, rehabilitation	Prevention of complications of immobility Cardiac rehabilitation programs

considered at high risk for developing breast cancer because several of the known risk factors for breast cancer are present. This woman may not develop breast cancer, but there is a greater than normal probability that she might.

Some risk factors, such as age and genetic factors, cannot be altered, whereas other factors, such as smoking or diet, are under the control of the person. To alter the risk factor, persons need to receive information related to the specific health threats. People frequently test the validity of health information by asking laypersons and professionals about the specific risks. Knowing about the risks does not always result in altered behavior, since some people receive satisfaction from the risk behaviors and deny the risk for themselves, even in the presence of contradictory information, saying, in effect, "It won't happen to me." Frequently there is no direct causal relationship, therefore the behaviors are easy for some persons to dismiss. There are also no immediate tangible rewards for engaging in the desired behaviors. Some persons therefore deliberately choose to continue engaging in the risk behaviors.

To promote health behaviors that decrease the at risk status, people first have to receive the information. Then positive reinforcement for altering behavior is more effective than negative comments about the at risk behaviors. Group sessions (such as weight loss groups or smoker's groups) may be helpful when participants reinforce each other's positive behaviors. Finally, health care professionals should be *role models,* demonstrating the desired health behaviors.

■ Illness

Although the terms *illness* and *disease* are sometimes used interchangeably, the terms do not relate to the same concepts. A person with a chronic disease such as diabetes may say, "I feel well." Illness is a more abstract term than disease and is essentially the opposite of wellness. Both illness and wellness have a strong subjective component, that of feeling ill or that of feeling well. Illness implies malfunctioning, a lower level of functioning.

Humans are constantly responding and adapting to changes in the external and internal (body) environments. There are a variety of chemical, physical, biologic, and psychosocial factors in the external environment that can influence a person's functioning (Table 1-2). Defense mechanisms, either biologic (Chapter 37) or psychologic (Chapter 7), serve to protect the person from environmental factors that may cause harm. Illness results when defense mechanisms become inadequate or inappropriate.

A relatively stable internal environment is necessary for cellular growth and functioning. The process of maintaining this relatively constant environment is the process of *homeostasis* or *dynamic equilibrium.* The term *dynamic equilibrium* is more descriptive, because it implies fluctuations within a normal range rather than a static condition. Maintaining a dynamic equilibrium involves an adequate exchange of oxygen and carbon dioxide through respiration, an adequate nutrient supply to meet basal metabolic needs,

Table 1-2 Environmental factors affecting health

Type	Examples	Possible effects
Chemical	Lead, arsenic	Poisoning
	Cholesterol	Myocardial infarction
Physical	Automobiles	Accidents
	High noise level	Deafness
	Heat	Burns, heatstroke
	Cold	Frostbite, hypothermia
	Radiation	Cancer
Biologic	Bacteria, virus, fungi	Infections
Psychosocial	Stress	Ulcers, hypertension

and a normal balance of fluids and electrolytes. Variations above or below normal ranges lead to illness and disease.

■ Disease

Diseases are specific pathologic conditions with characteristic signs and symptoms. Diseases may involve a specific organ or body part or may affect the body as a whole. Functioning of the part or body system may be impaired. The body has many integrated defense mechanisms and compensatory responses that maintain functioning for a period of time when a threat to the system occurs, but if the causative factors or stressors persist, altered structure or functioning results. Terms commonly used when discussing specific diseases are listed in the box on p. 7.

Diseases have a natural life history, usually progressing through stages. The time factor varies; acute diseases have a sudden onset and are usually of short duration, whereas chronic diseases often have a gradual or indefinite onset and have a longer duration. In the first stage of development of a disease, the *presymptomatic* or *subclinical stage,* the pathogenic changes have started to occur but there are no detectable signs or symptoms. Examples of this stage are the formation of atheromatous plaques in the coronary vessel or early malignant growth.[15] The second stage, the *clinical stage,* is characterized by the presence of signs and symptoms. It is at this stage that the person seeks help. The third stage, the *rehabilitation stage,* occurs with chronic diseases and is characterized by residual disabilities. During this stage the person must learn how to adapt to changes in life-style that result from the disability and learn how to prevent further disability.

■ Illness behavior and sick role

When people perceive that they are ill, they may take action for relief of symptoms; they may decide to take no action; or they may vacillate between action and no action. Persons who decide to take action may seek help from a friend or family member, from a "folk-specialist" (someone of their cultural group who is frequently consulted about illness), from a professional such as a minister, or from a

---

Terminology used with disease

Acute	Disease with sudden onset and short duration
Chronic	Disease of long duration
Signs	Observable changes in body function (objective)
Symptoms	Changes in body function, usually expressed by the patient (subjective)
Syndrome	Cluster of signs and symptoms that collectively indicate altered functioning
Incidence	Frequency of occurrence of a disease
Onset	Beginning of a disease
Course	Pattern of development of a disease
Duration	Length of time disease is present
Prognosis	Ultimate outcome
Morbidity	Number of persons having the disease in a given population
Mortality	Number of persons who die from the disease
Spontaneous resolution	Healing occurs with little or no treatment
Therapeutic intervention	Treatment directed toward a cure or alleviation of signs and symptoms

---

health care professional. Non-health care persons may either deal with the problems themselves or refer the patient to someone else. Often these people act as gatekeeper in helping make the decision when and from whom the sick person should seek help. Persons who perceive they are ill but take no action do so for a variety of reasons (see the box above). Low income persons are more apt to seek assistance when they are ill if the health care provider or agency is within the community. Some persons know they should take action but some reason holds them back and thus they vacillate between action and no action.

Some persons are labeled as "noncompliant" because they do not follow the directions of the health care provider. Noncompliance may be defined as the failure of the person to participate in carrying out the plan of care after initially indicating the intention to comply or because of the presence of factors that prevent action.[10] Failure to carry out an action may result from some of the same reasons as failure to seek health care rather than a deliberate action of noncompliance.

When illness becomes legitimized by the physician during the clinical stage, the patient assumes the *sick role* and is exempted from normal social roles and responsibilities as required by the type and severity of the illness. The social expectation is that the sick person will seek help and wants to get well. The sick role permits the patient to assume a dependent relationship that facilitates receiving the required health care. Many persons find the sick role undesirable and have difficulty with the enforced dependency, although they see it as necessary to achieve the desired end, that is, wellness. They find it helpful if they are kept informed and allowed to make decisions if they are able and desire to do so. The patient is expected to relinquish the sick role and assume increasing independence during the recovery and rehabilitation stage.

Selected reasons for not seeking health care

Denial that symptoms are present
Symptoms not viewed as important
Fear of consequences (for example, pain, cancer, death)
Fear of health care professionals or health care agencies
Lack of knowledge concerning which symptoms require medical care
Lack of availability of transportation
Lack of money for transportation or health care
Disabilities that hinder getting to health care agency

■ MEDICAL-SURGICAL NURSING PRACTICE

Nursing actions can be divided into two types—independent and interdependent. *Independent* nursing actions are those which the nurse takes after analysis of data pertaining to those aspects of the patient's health that are amenable to nursing intervention. Providing quality care for persons at risk for or experiencing pathophysiologic disorders requires a systematic approach. In recent years the term *nursing process* has become synonymous with the systematic approach used in providing nursing care (Chapter 2).

Interdependent or collaborative nursing actions are those taken by the nurse in assisting other health care profes-

---

Definitions of the nature and treatment of disease

Epidemiology	The study of rate and influencing factors of disease occurrence in given populations
Etiology	The study of the cause of disease
Pathophysiology	The study of mechanisms and physiologic effects of disease processes
Signs and symptoms	Objective and subjective evidence of disease, including significant results of diagnostic tests
Medical therapy/treatment	Commonly used interventions by physicians directed toward cure/control of diseases, such as pharmacologic and dietary prescriptions, surgery, or radiation treatments

---

sionals. Nurses are the health care professionals who have the greatest patient contact. They are therefore in a position to assist other professionals by providing additional data through monitoring and by carrying out prescribed treatments patients are unable to do for themselves. As patients are able to assume greater responsibility for their own care, *self-care activities* are promoted.

The ability to plan and implement nursing care, monitor the patient's condition, and carry out treatments effectively requires a sound knowledge base not only about people and factors pertaining to their health but also about the pathophysiologic disorders per se. The following types of knowledge about diseases can be useful in planning and providing patient care: epidemiology and etiology, pathophysiology, signs and symptoms of disease, and medical therapy.

Knowledge of epidemiologic and etiologic factors helps to identify the populations at risk. *Epidemiology* is the study of the incidence, distribution, and determinants of diseases and injuries in human populations. In other words, epidemiology is concerned with the extent of specific diseases or injuries in specific groups of people and the factors that influence that distribution.[15] *Etiology* refers to the specific causes of a disease. Most diseases have *multiple causality;* that is, there are multiple factors working and interacting together that lead to disease occurrence. This is an important point when teaching about prevention of disease, since avoidance of only one factor may not prevent disease occurrence.

Pathophysiology is the study of the effect of disease (pathology) on body organs and systems and on total body functioning. A *pathophysiologic* disorder is one in which there is altered physiologic functioning, as differentiated from a *pathopsychologic* disorder in which there is altered mental functioning. Knowledge of the physiologic effects of pathology and the nature of the compensatory or adaptive responses facilitates understanding of patient responses for the purposes of monitoring the patient's status for maladaptive responses and teaching the patient about the disease.

Knowledge of the signs and symptoms and medical therapies of common diseases facilitates monitoring for presence and course of diseases, supporting and teaching the patient, and carrying out therapies patients cannot do for themselves.

Nursing care of patients at risk for or who have a pathophysiologic disorder

Health restoration

Assisting with achievement of therapeutic goals
   Monitoring for signs of healing or complications
   Carrying out prescribed medical therapies that the patient is unable to do for self
   Promoting functioning of those mechanisms necessary for optimal health, for example, oxygenation, nutrition, elimination
Promoting comfort and activities of daily living (ADL)
   Promoting physical and psychologic comfort
   Assisting with ADL as necessary until self-care is possible
Modifying the environment to enhance healing and wellness
Counseling and teaching
   Promoting coping and adaptation to changes in health care
   Teaching the patient to care for self

Health maintenance

Monitoring for changes in health status
Teaching the patient and family or friends
   The nature of the illness or disease
   Signs and symptoms indicating presence of disease or complications to be reported to physician
   Health promotion activities (nutrition, activity, etc.)
   Specific preventive measures
   Rationale for medical therapies
   Name, dosage, actions, and side effects of prescribed medications
   Availability of community resources
   Need for continual monitoring or follow-up care, as necessary

---

Putting knowledge to practice

- Describe in your own words the difference between being "ill" and having a disease.
- Ask five of your patients how they feel in terms of being "ill." Compare their responses.
- Think of some practices you follow to promote health or prevent disease. Now think of any practices that are deterrents to health. How difficult would it be for you to change your behavior?
- What effect do you think there would be if the nurse smoked a cigarette when teaching a patient the ill effects of smoking?

■ Nursing interventions

Nursing interventions for persons who are at risk for or who have pathophysiologic disorders are directed toward *restoring* optimal health and *maintaining* optimal health (see the box on p. 8). Although the major focus of the care of the person who is ill may be health restoration, health maintenance interventions may be carried on concurrently to help the person maintain optimal functioning wherever possible. The interventions selected for a specific patient will be determined by the identified nursing diagnoses and the specific pathophysiologic disorders present or for which the person is at risk. Possible nursing interventions are described in appropriate chapters in this text.

■ SUMMARY

1. Medical-surgical nursing focuses on the care of adults who are at risk for or who have medical-surgical disorders.
2. Health promotion refers to activities directed toward helping persons to maintain or achieve a high level of functioning and feeling of well-being.
3. Prevention refers to activities directed toward protecting persons from potential or actual threats to health and the subsequent consequences.
4. Primary prevention includes protective measures against disease or trauma. Secondary prevention includes early detection and treatment to decrease the intensity or to prevent complications. Tertiary prevention consists of activities that prevent or limit disabilities and help promote rehabilitation.
5. Persons at risk as those considered to have a greater possibility of becoming ill or acquiring a certain disease. Factors that place the person at risk are termed risk factors.
6. Illness can be considered the opposite of wellness and implies a lower level of functioning. Disease is a pathologic process having a characteristic set of signs and symptoms. Diseases may be acute or chronic.
7. The stages of disease progression are (1) presymptomatic or subclinical stage in which changes are occurring but no signs or symptoms are present; (2) the clinical stage, characterized by signs and symptoms; and (3) the rehabilitation stage (in chronic diseases), characterized by residual disabilities.
8. People may take a variety of actions when they perceive they are ill and for a variety of reasons.
9. The sick role exempts the person from normal social roles and responsibilities and permits the person to assume a dependent relationship that facilitates receiving the required health care.
10. Independent nursing actions are those which the nurse takes after analysis of data pertaining to those aspects of the person's health that are amenable to nursing intervention. Interdependent or collaborative nursing actions are those taken by the nurse in assisting other health care professionals.
11. Epidemiology is the study of the incidence, distribution, and determinants of diseases and injuries in human populations. Etiology refers to the study of specific causes of diseases.
12. Pathophysiology is the study of the effect of disease on body organs and systems and on total body functioning.
13. Signs are objective evidence and symptoms are subjective evidence of disease or dysfunction.
14. Nursing interventions are directed either to restoring or maintaining optimal health.

REFERENCES AND SELECTED READINGS
Contemporary

1. Alan, DK, and Boldt, J: A study of preventive health attitudes and behaviors in a family practice setting, J Fam Prac 11:77-84, 1980.
2. Alonzo, AA: Acute illness behavior: a conceptual exploration and specification, Soc Sci Med 14A:515-526, 1980.
3. *American Nurses Association: Nursing: a social policy statement, No NP-63, Kansas City, Mo, 1980, The Association.
4. Demers, RW, and others: An explanation of the dimensions of illness behavior, J Fam Pract 11:1085-1092, 1980.
5. *Diekelmann, N: Wellness: approaches and resources, Nurse Pract 5:41-44, 1980.

---

*References preceded by an asterisk are particularly well suited for student reading.

6. Edelman, C, and Mandle, CL: Health promotion throughout the life span, St. Louis, 1986, The CV Mosby Co.
7. Flynn, PR: Holistic health: the art and science of care, Bowie, Md, 1980, Robert J Brady Co.
8. George, JB (editor): Nursing theories: the base for professional nursing practice, ed 2, Englewood Cliffs, NJ, 1985, Prentice-Hall, Inc.
9. Gillick, MR: Common-sense models of health and disease, N Engl J Med 313(11):700-703, 1985.
10. *Gordon, M: Nursing diagnosis: process and application, ed 2, New York, 1987, McGraw-Hill Book Co.
11. *Greenberg, JS: Health and wellness: a conceptual differentiation, J Sch Health 55:403-406, 1985.
12. Groer, MW, and Shekleton, ME: Basic pathophysiology: a conceptual approach, ed 2, St. Louis, 1983, The CV Mosby Co.
13. Houston, TP: Priorities in health promotion, Postgrad Med 76:223-230, 1984.
14. *Keller, MJ: Toward a definition of health, Adv Nurs Sci 4:43-64, 1980.
15. Mausner, JS, and Kramer, S: Epidemiology: an introductory text, ed 2, Philadelphia, 1985, WB Saunders Co.
16. Najam, JM: Theories of disease causation and the concept of a general susceptibility: a review, Soc Sci Med 14A:231-237, 1980.
17. *Pender, NJ: Health promotion in nursing practice, ed. 2, New York, 1982, Appleton-Century-Crofts.
18. *Prohaska, TR, and others: Health practices and illness cognition in young, middle aged, and elderly adults, J Gerontol 40:569-578, 1985.
19. *Shamansky, SL, and Clausen, CL: Levels of prevention: examination of the concept, Nurs Outlook 28:104-108, 1980.
20. Smith, JA: The idea of health: a philosophical inquiry, Adv Nurs Sci 3:42-50, 1981.
21. *Webster, JA: The wellness mode: feeling good about you, AORN J 41:713-718, 1985.

Classic

22. Alonzo, AA: Everyday illness: a situational approach to health status deviation, Soc Sci Med 13A:397-404, 1979.
23. Dougherty, CJ, and Walker, VR: Scientific medicine, technology, and concept of health, Ethics Sci Med 5:75-81, 1978.
24. Dunn, HL: What high-level wellness means, Health Values: Achieving High Level Wellness 1:9-16, 1977.
25. French, RM: Dynamics of health care, ed 3, New York, 1979, McGraw-Hill Book Co.
26. Segall, A: The sick role concept: understanding illness behavior, J Health Soc Behav 17:163-170, 1976.

2

Nursing Process:
A Systematic Approach

BARBARA C. LONG

CHAPTER OBJECTIVES

After studying this chapter, the student should be able to:

- Describe five steps of nursing process.

- Describe at least one framework that can be used for data collection and analysis.

- State four general conclusions that can be drawn from analysis of patient data.

- Define nursing diagnosis and describe the component parts.

- State five reasons for standardizing and classifying nursing diagnoses.

- Explain at least one method for setting priorities.

- Write goals in terms of observable patient behaviors.

- Describe five different action strategies for providing nursing care.

- Describe different methods of documentation.

- Identify the source of evaluation criteria.

■ INTRODUCTION TO NURSING PROCESS

■ Characteristics and steps

The systematic approach used to carry out nursing's independent functions (p. 7) is frequently termed *nursing process*. It is a way of thinking and acting based on the scientific method rather than on intuition. It provides organization and direction of nursing activities, a means for predicting outcomes and evaluating results, and a method for establishing standards of nursing care. The characteristics of nursing process are listed in the box at right.

Nursing process provides a framework for (1) identification of health care needs amenable to nursing care, (2) determination of patient goals (outcomes) and nursing actions, (3) implementation of nursing actions, and (4) evaluation of results of nursing actions. This systematic process is usually divided into either four or five steps; the overall process is the same regardless of the number of steps. The five-step process is as follows:

1. Assessment: collecting patient data of pertinence to nursing
2. Data analysis: using the collected data to identify the patient's health care needs that can be influenced by nursing care (nursing diagnoses)
3. Planning: determining priorities, expected patient outcomes, and specific nursing actions
4. Implementation: carrying out the planned nursing actions necessary to accomplish the defined goals
5. Evaluation: determining the extent to which the goals have been achieved

Nurses who use a four-step approach include data analysis as part of assessment; thus the four steps become assessment, planning, implementation, and evaluation.

■ Frameworks for nursing practice

The focus of nursing practice depends on the nurse's philosophical framework. In earlier years of professional nursing, the medical model was the primary approach. Thus when a systematic approach to data collection was first initiated, *body systems* was a framework that was commonly used. For example, data that pertained specifically to the respiratory system were collected, then analyzed to identify respiratory problems.

■ HUMAN NEEDS FRAMEWORK

Another framework that has been used in the practice of medical-surgical nursing is *human needs*. Maslow describes a hierarchy of needs in which physiologic needs are the most basic, followed by safety, love and belonging, self-esteem, and self-actualization (Fig. 2-1). The needs are ranked in ascending order from the needs that are basic to survival to those that focus on development of self (growth-motivated needs). In principle, the more basic needs are satisfied first. For example, a person who is

Characteristics of nursing process	
Systematic	Consists of an organized series of steps
Purposeful	Has as its aim the meeting of nursing needs of the patient
Interac-tional	Involves interaction among nurse, patient, and significant others
Dynamic	Involves continued action and evaluation until nurse-patient relationship is terminated
Scientific	Is based on a scientific problem-solving approach; provides for identification of recurrent problems, which then initiates nursing research

having difficulty breathing (physiologic need for oxygen) will attend to that need before dealing with a feeling of loss of worth as a person (self-esteem). In most situations, however, the needs in the hierarchy exist simultaneously to different extents. Lower level needs have to be met, at least partially, before seeking gratification of higher order needs. For example, a person may omit a meal to carry out an activity that increases self-esteem. New needs usually emerge gradually except when danger is present or when the person is acutely ill.

Physiologic needs include oxygen, nutrition, elimination, activity, comfort, rest and sleep, and reproduction. All are vital for existence or survival. (Reproduction is vital for survival of the human race.) *Oxygen* needs include everything that influences (1) taking in oxygen and eliminating carbon dioxide as carried out by the respiratory system and (2) transportation of the gases to and from the tissues as carried out by the circulatory system and its components. *Safety* (security) needs include both protection of self from psychologic threats and protection of self from the physical environment. This requires ability to see and to hear, to activate the body if threatened (neuroendocrine response),

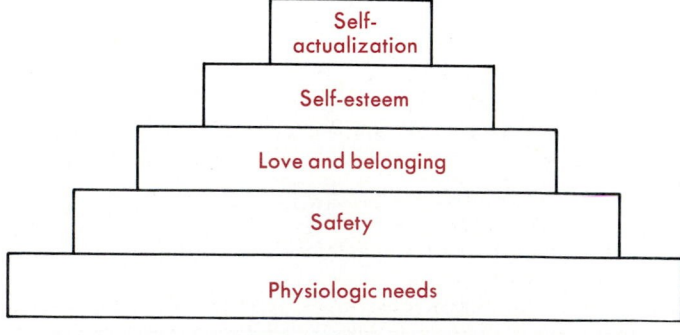

Fig. 2-1 Maslow's hierarchy of needs.

and to protect the body from invading microorganisms (immune response and intact skin).

Persons with medical-surgical disorders may also experience threats to the higher order needs of love and self-esteem. Humans have a need to relate to others in a meaningful way (*love and belonging* or *affiliation needs*). Most persons affiliate by means of long-term relationships with one or more persons (family members, close friends). A few persons can meet their belonging needs by indirect approaches, such as through creative endeavors (for example, an artist).

Self-esteem refers to the need to feel good or satisfied with oneself. This includes a feeling of confidence in oneself, of valuing oneself, and of being valued by others. Self-esteem needs are influenced by the person's ability to perceive and cope with changes in the environment. Persons with changes in their appearance (for example, facial disfigurement or amputation) or in body functions (for example, colostomy) are at higher risk of developing problems with affiliation or self-esteem. These changes can influence conscious or unconscious feelings, thoughts, and perceptions of one's body (body image).

The need for *self-actualization* (realizing one's full potential) is one that most individuals are seeking to reach throughout their lives. The need gratification is seldom reached until older age. The need to grow and develop in a meaningful way, however, is always present.

The use of human needs as a framework for nursing care consists of collecting and analyzing data that pertain to each of the need categories. The concept of hierarchy of needs is useful during planning of care by helping to set priorities; for example, survival needs would usually take priority over growth needs.

■ CONCEPTUAL FRAMEWORKS FOR NURSING PRACTICE

Several nurses in recent years have offered unique conceptual frameworks to serve as a reference to guide nurses in assessment and implementation of nursing care. The concepts are abstract to allow for broad application. All the frameworks are applicable to the care of patients with medical-surgical disorders. Some of the more commonly used frameworks include those of Dorothea Orem, Martha Rogers, Sister Callista Roy, and Dorothy Johnson. A very brief description of these models follows; see the references at the end of the chapter for sources of in-depth discussions of these models.

The *Orem self-care agency model*[27] is based on the concept of self-care. Within this frame of reference, nurses provide a helping system to facilitate self-care (the ability to engage in self-care for meeting activities of daily living). The focus of assessment is on eight universal, two developmental, and six health deviation self-care categories. Nursing actions toward promoting self-care depend on one of three systems of care: wholly compensatory, partly compensatory, or supportive-educative.

The *Rogers life-process model*[30] focuses on "unitary man" or a human being's "wholeness." Persons are considered as more than the sum of their parts and are continually

---

Gordon's Functional Health Patterns

Health perception—Health management
Nutritional—Metabolic
Elimination
Activity—Exercise
Cognitive—Perceptual
Sleep—Rest
Self-perception—Self-concept
Role relationship
Sexuality—Reproductive
Coping—Stress tolerance
Value—Belief

From Gordon, M: Manual of nursing diagnosis 1986-1987, New York, 1987, McGraw-Hill Book Co.

---

evolving and changing. Persons are viewed as influenced by energy fields, both human and environmental. The goal of nursing is to help the person achieve a maximal level of wellness. The approach used with this model is in recognizing patterns and organization of human-environmental relationships.

The *Roy adaptation model*[31] also views person-environment interaction, specifically the adaptation of the person to the internal/external environment. The goal is directing the person toward wellness, and the nurse determines the degree of assistance with adaptation required by the person. The four identified adaptation modes are physiologic, self-concept, role function, and interdependence.

The *Johnson behavioral systems model*[17] focuses on behavior that is at variance with the system. Identified subsystems include affiliative, dependency, ingestive, eliminative, sexual, aggressive, and achievement. The goal of nursing is the protection, nurturing, and stimulation of the subsystems.

The way in which data are used and organized differs with the conceptual frameworks. There is, however, basic data that are collected for all persons; a sample nursing history and physical examination are described in Chapter 3. Gordon[13] has identified 11 *functional health patterns* (see the box above) that contribute to health, quality of life, and achievement of human potential. These patterns are interrelated, interactive, and interdependent; thus all patterns need to be assessed for function or dysfunction. The health patterns can be used as a guiding framework for data collection, regardless of the conceptual framework for nursing practice used by the practitioner.

⬛ ASSESSMENT

The assessment process consists of collecting data about the patient that are pertinent for providing nursing care. Some of the data may be the same as those collected by

Table 2-1 Methods of data collection from specific sources

Source	Method
Primary	
Patient	Interview (formal, informal), physical examination, general observations
Secondary	
Family or friends	Interactions
Patient records	Written notes of other health care professionals, nurses's notes, diagnostic reports (laboratory, x-ray films, etc.), admission record
Health team members	Interaction with other nurses, physicians, physical therapist, occupational therapist, social worker, dietitian, respiratory therapist
Literature	Consultation of textbooks (nursing, medical, pharmacologic, nutrition) and journals (nursing, medical)

other health care professionals but different use is made of the data. The sources and methods of data collection in nursing are listed in Table 2-1.

■ Initial assessment

Patient data are obtained by a nurse when the patient first enters the hospital or other health care agency. This initial data base provides a basis for planning nursing care. Specific information that may be collected by patient interview or physical examination is described in Chapter 3. The extent of patient data collected initially depends on the specific circumstances. For example, fewer data would be required for a patient being admitted for a 2-day hospital stay for a hernia repair than for a patient being admitted for an expected longer hospital stay for diagnosis and treatment of a probable malignancy. Many hospitals develop an admission patient data form identifying the data pertinent to their specific patient population.

Data collected from the patient may be *subjective* or *objective* (Table 2-2). The differentiation is important. Subjective data are necessary for providing understanding of the patient's experience and sense of illness or well-being, but since they cannot be validated, they are subject to wide interpretation. For example, one person may describe a specific pain intensity as "severe," while another person may describe the same pain intensity as "mild." Objective data are verifiable; for example, each person palpating the same lymph node can describe it as 2 × 3 cm in size, oval

shaped, and freely movable. Subjective and objective data are separated in the problem-oriented method of recording (p. 21).

■ Ongoing assessment

Since health is a dynamic, ever-changing state, assessment must be a continuous process; thus assessment does not end with the data collected on admission. During every nurse-patient interaction, additional data are gathered. These data are used for evaluation of already identified problems and for identification of new problems. A planned, organized approach is as important for ongoing assessment as it is for the initial assessment.

Observations are made of the patient and the patient's environment. *Baseline observations* establish where a patient is at any point in time and serve as a basis for future comparison. For example, an observation of warm, dry skin made in the morning is useful as a comparison when cold, moist skin is observed later in the day. Baseline observations are made early in the person's admission to the hospital, at the beginning of a time period when a particular nurse will be providing care, and whenever changes occur in the patient's condition or environmnent, such as a transfer to or from a special care unit.

The ability to make specific pertinent observations depends on knowledge and past experiences. A sound knowledge base facilitates making comprehensive and pertinent observations. Included in the knowledge base is informa-

Table 2-2 Types of data

Type	Definition	Methods	Examples
Subjective	Statements by the person concerning thoughts or feelings (psychologic, physical) that cannot be validated	Interview, interaction	Statements about pain, nausea, itching Statements about fears, desires, beliefs, attitudes, values
Objective	Data perceptible by the external senses that can be validated by others	Inspection, auscultation, palpation, percussion, olfaction	Vomiting, scratching, auditory breath sounds, palpable lymph nodes, breath odor

tion about the patient's medical diagnosis (usual cause, risk factors, usual symptoms and course, and usual medical treatment).

■ Recording patient data

Patient data must be recorded promptly to ensure accuracy and usefulness. The initial patient data include information from the nursing history and physical examination and are recorded and used in analysis and planning of care and to provide a baseline for comparison. The method of recording the data varies with the institution and with the framework used by the nurse for collecting the data. Many hospitals place portions of the patient's chart in or immediately outside the patient's room so that ongoing observations and subsequent actions can be recorded promptly.

➡ DATA ANALYSIS: NURSING DIAGNOSIS

The second step of nursing process is making conclusions from the collected data. The process of data analysis may be referred to as *diagnosis*; however, so as not to confuse the process with the end product, the term *nursing diagnosis* in this discussion will be limited to the end product of data analysis. A framework, such as one of those described earlier as frameworks for nursing practice (p. 12), is especially helpful for grouping the data for analysis to facilitate arriving at sound conclusions from the data base. It is extremely difficult to deal with a large amount of data unless it is grouped in some manner.

The seventh conference of the North American Nursing Diagnosis Association (NANDA) in 1986 developed a taxonomy for nursing diagnoses that groups the NANDA nursing diagnoses under the nine headings of exchanging, communicating, relating, valuing, choosing, moving, perceiving, knowing, and feeling. This taxonomy may be used by the nurse as a framework for organizing patient data in practice.

■ General conclusions

Four general conclusions can be drawn from analysis of patient data (Fig. 2-2):

1. Data is insufficient; more data must be gathered before conclusions can be made.
2. The person or family is functioning at optimal level and is not at high risk; no interventions are required.
3. The person or family is functioning well, but health risk factors are high; a "potential" dysfunction is present, such as "Infection, potential for."
4. The person or family is functioning inadequately and actions are desirable.

When dysfunctions are identified, one of three approaches may be taken. First, the person or family may

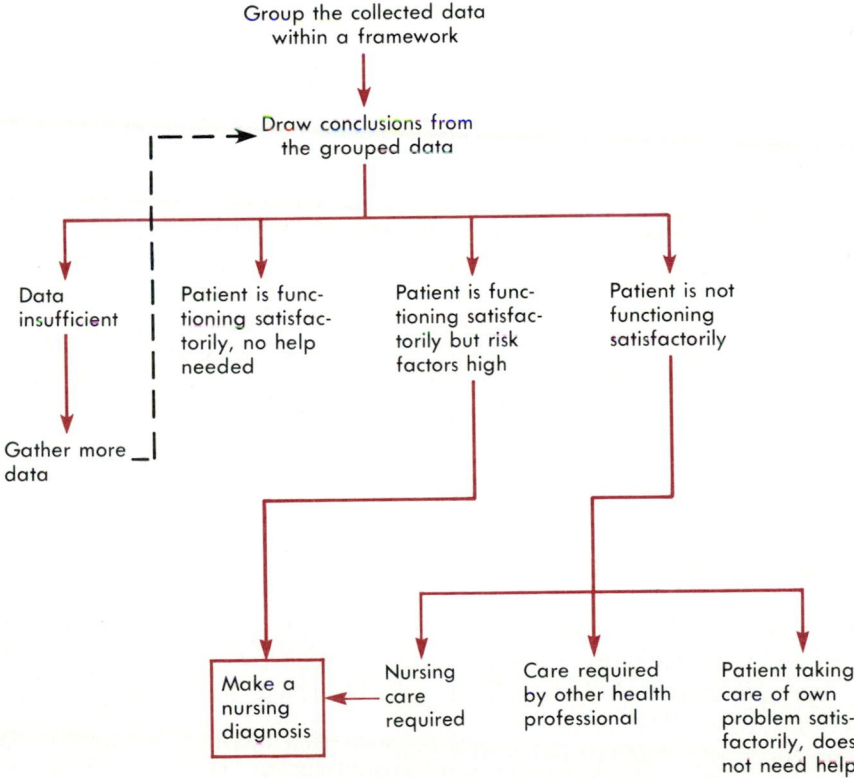

Fig. 2-2 Process of data analysis.

have already identified the dysfunction and be taking appropriate actions; therefore, no further help is needed. Second, action is needed that is better carried out by another health professional; the nurse makes the appropriate referral. In the third option, nursing interventions are indicated and the nurse then makes nursing diagnosis statements.

■ Nursing diagnosis

■ DEFINITION

Definitions of nursing diagnosis by various nurse authors are listed in the box below. Common ideas described in the definitions include the following:

1. A statement or conclusion
2. An actual or potential health problem
3. Identified from a nursing assessment
4. The legal and educational domain of nursing

Nursing diagnoses are therefore different from medical diagnoses. The domain of medical practice is the identification of disease (medical diagnosis) and the treatment of these diseases. In 1980, the Congress of Nursing Practice of the American Nurses' Association defined nursing as "the diagnosis and treatment of *human responses to actual or potential health problems.*"[2] Thus a disease cannot be considered a nursing diagnosis, but how a person *responds* to dysfunction, such as by activity intolerance, anxiety, incontinence, and so forth, is the domain of nursing.

Definitions of nursing diagnosis

Gebbie: The judgment or conclusion that occurs as a result of nursing assessment.

Bircher: An independent nursing function; an evaluation of a client's personal responses to his human experiences throughout the life cycle, be they developmental or accidental crises, illness, hardships, or other stresses.

Gordon: Actual or potential health problems which nurses, by virtue or their education and experience, are capable and licensed to treat.

Moritz: Responses to actual or potential health problems which nurses by virtue of their education are able, licensed, and legally responsible and accountable to treat.

Carpenito: A statement that describes the human response (health state or an actual/potential altered interaction pattern) of an individual or group which the nurse can legally identify and for which the nurse can order the definitive interventions to maintain the health state or to reduce, eliminate, or prevent alterations.

From Carpenito, LJ: Nursing diagnosis: application to clinical practice, ed 2, Philadelphia, 1987, JB Lippincott Co, pp 4-5.

Some nursing actions, however, do *not* ensue from nursing diagnoses. Recall that nursing actions may be of two types, independent and interdependent or collaborative (Chapter 1). Making a nursing diagnosis and carrying out actions appropriate for the identified nursing diagnoses are nursing's independent actions. Monitoring activities to collect data for the physician (collaborative action) is not an action that ensues from nursing diagnoses.

Nursing diagnoses statements are not limited to dysfunction (patient problems). The goal of nursing is optimal health of the person/family; support and assistance may be needed to help persons *maintain* certain health practices. For example, one woman sought assistance from a nurse to help her work through her feelings about caring for her dying mother. The woman was coping satisfactorily but needed support from the nurse to maintain coping. Most accepted nursing diagnoses identified to date relate primarily to problems or potential problems. It is anticipated that in the future more diagnoses will be developed that are intended to help persons move toward optimal levels of health.

■ STRUCTURE

A nursing diagnosis statement consists of two parts: (1) a pattern of functioning or health problem, and (2) the factors that influence or are related to the functioning (etiologic or related factors). In addition, each diagnosis has defining characteristics, such as a cluster of signs and symptoms, that serve as criteria for diagnostic judgment. Gordon[13] refers to the three components as the *PES* format: health problem (P), etiologic or related factors (E), and defining characteristics or cluster of signs and symptoms (S). The third component (S) is not listed in the diagnosis statement but can be found in reference materials.

An example of a nursing diagnosis is as follows:

Alteration in bowel elimination: constipation related to decreased activity following surgery and to low fluid intake

The phrase "related to" is used to cite the etiologic factors rather than "due to," as an indication of relatedness but not necessarily to show cause and effect.

To make this nursing diagnosis, data would have been collected that supported both the problem statement *and* the etiology. The defining characteristics for the problem (or potential problem) statement serve as a guide for data that need to be collected. Thus for the preceding diagnosis, the following data were collected:

Hard formed stool ×2 in past 7 days
Report of feelings of pressure and fullness in rectum
Report of straining when passing stool
Surgery 1 week ago (ambulation to be encouraged)
Spends most of day sitting at bedside
Fluid intake for past 3 days: 750 ml, 850 ml, 900 ml

Note that the first four items support the problem statement and the last three items support the etiology. The etiologic factors provide direction for nursing actions; in the preceding example, activities would be planned to assist the person to be more active and to drink more fluids.

North American Nursing Diagnosis Association (NANDA) approved nursing diagnoses, 1988

Activity intolerance
Activity intolerance, potential
Adjustment, impaired
Airway clearance, ineffective
Anxiety
Aspiration, potential for
Body image disturbance
Body temperature, altered: potential
Breastfeeding, ineffective
Breathing pattern, ineffective
Cardiac output, decreased
Communication, impaired verbal
Constipation
Constipation, colonic
Constipation, perceived
Coping, family: potential for growth
Coping, ineffective family: compromised
Coping, ineffective family: disabling
Coping, ineffective individual
Decisional conflict (specify)
Denial, ineffective
Diarrhea
Disuse syndrome, potential for
Diversional activity deficit
Dysreflexia
Family processes, altered
Fatigue
Fear
Fluid volume deficit (1)
Fluid volume deficit (2)
Fluid volume deficit, potential
Fluid volume excess
Gas exchange, impaired
Grieving, anticipatory
Grieving, dysfunctional
Growth and development, altered
Health maintenance, altered
Health seeking behaviors (specify)
Home maintenance management, impaired
Hopelessness
Hyperthermia
Hypothermia
Incontinence, bowel
Incontinence, functional
Incontinence, reflex
Incontinence, stress
Incontinence, total
Incontinence, urge
Infection, potential for
Injury, potential for

Knowledge deficit (specify)
Mobility, impaired physical
Noncompliance (specify)
Nutrition, altered: less than body requirements
Nutrition, altered: more than body requirements
Nutrition, altered: potential for more than body requirements
Oral mucous membrane, altered
Pain
Pain, chronic
Parental role conflict
Parenting, altered
Parenting, altered, potential
Personal identity disturbance
Poisoning, potential for
Post-trauma response
Powerlessness
Rape-trauma syndrome
Rape-trauma syndrome: compound reaction
Rape-trauma syndrome: silent reaction
Role performance, altered
Self care deficit, bathing/hygiene
Self care deficit, dressing/grooming
Self care deficit, feeding
Self care deficit, toileting
Self-esteem disturbance
Self-esteem, chronic low
Self-esteem, situational low
Sensory/perceptual alterations (specify) (visual, auditory, kinesthetic, gustatory, tactile, olfactory)
Sexual dysfunction
Sexuality patterns, altered
Skin integrity, impaired
Skin integrity, impaired, potential
Sleep pattern disturbance
Social interaction, impaired
Social isolation
Spiritual distress (distress of the human spirit)
Suffocation, potential for
Swallowing, impaired
Thermoregulation, ineffective
Thought processes, altered
Tissue integrity, impaired
Tissue perfusion, altered (specify type) (renal, cerebral, cardiopulmonary, gastrointestinal, peripheral)
Trauma, potential for
Unilateral neglect
Urinary elimination, altered patterns
Urinary retention
Violence, potential for: self-directed or directed at others

■ CLASSIFICATION OF NURSING DIAGNOSES

Nursing does not yet have a firm classification of nursing diagnoses that are accepted by all nurses. The first national conference on the classification of nursing diagnoses was held in 1973, the eighth such conference in 1988. The group that is continuing the development of the diagnostic classification system is now called the North American Nursing Diagnosis Association (NANDA). The list of nursing diagnoses as accepted in 1988 can be noted in the box on p. 17. These diagnoses have been selected for use in later chapters of this text.

Why is a classification system necessary? Webster[33] has identified five major reasons for standardization of nomenclature and classification of nursing diagnoses: (1) facilitation of communication, (2) computer stores and access of information, (3) political and legal needs, (4) advancement of nursing theory and science, and (5) education. Nursing care is facilitated when all nurses are familiar with and use the same system.

Development of a classification system takes many years; however, practice must continue during the developmental phase. It is therefore important to remember that the diagnostic categories are in the *process of evolving* and that changes can be anticipated with research and further development. New diagnoses are being developed and some of the earlier diagnoses are being reworded or changed in substance. Some of the newer diagnoses have been accepted in concept but have not yet been defined. Development is progressing in the identification of defining characteristics and etiologies of the newer diagnoses.

An organizing framework for nursing diagnoses is also in the process of development. The NANDA list of nursing diagnoses had been issued alphabetically until formation by the group of an organizing framework. The seventh NANDA conference led to development of the NANDA Taxonomy I (p. 15).

A different organizing framework for organizing nursing diagnoses is Gordon's Functional Health Patterns (p. 12). The list of NANDA nursing diagnoses can be subsumed within this framework.

⊔ PLANNING

Planning nursing care involves several steps:
1. Setting priorities when several nursing diagnoses have been identified
2. Determining goals (outcomes) of care for each nursing diagnosis
3. Selecting specific nursing actions

■ Setting priorities

When several nursing diagnoses have been identified, it must be determined which diagnoses take priority. One approach is the basic needs approach. Nursing diagnoses that pertain to physiologic and safety needs usually take precedence over love and belonging or self-esteem needs.

Priorities can also be determined by considering threats to the integrity of the individual. The following priority system can be used:

First   Immediate life-threatening problems (for example, lack of oxygen)
Second   Threats to physiologic or psychologic integrity for which the person is at *high risk*
Third   Threats to physiologic or psychologic integrity for which the person is at *low risk* (but which may occur if action is not taken)
Fourth   Health maintenance

This system does not deny the importance of health maintenance but emphasizes that when health problems are present, these problems are attended to first.

Setting of priorities does not mean numbering each nursing diagnosis from 1 to N in order of importance. It means that when a large number of nursing diagnoses have been identified, the most important diagnoses are selected to be principally addressed.

■ Goal setting

The next step in planning is to determine the goals or desired patient outcomes to be achieved. There should be *mutual nurse-patient goal setting* whenever possible so that there is congruency between what both the nurse and the patient expect as a result of nursing interventions. The role of the nurse is to facilitate the patient's recovery and future health maintenance; thus both must be moving toward the same goals.

Goals (expected patient outcomes) are stated as *observable patient behaviors,* that is, behavior (or signs) that can be observed in the patient if the goal is met. For example, the statement "prevent skin breakdown" is a poor goal, since it indicates nursing action and does not indicate a patient outcome to be met. The same idea stated in observable patient-outcome terms would be "skin on sacral area remains intact, no redness is observed." To evaluate whether this goal had been met, the sacral area would be inspected for signs of redness or breakdown in skin integrity.

Patient outcomes are written according to the following criteria: have measurable verbs, be specific in content and time, and be attainable.[8] Examples of verbs that are *not* measurable are "understands," "knows," or "appreciates." Time is included when appropriate; for example, "Walks around room 6/24, to nurses station 6/25, and to lounge 6/26." The more specifically the expected outcomes are written, the easier is the evaluation. The expected patient outcomes serve as the criteria for evaluation.

Health care agencies participate in quality assurance review (see Chapter 4). During the process of quality assurance review, *standards* are developed and outcome criteria are identified. Some of these outcome criteria are useful guidelines in determining expected patient outcomes.

Goals are derived primarily from the first part (the pattern of functioning) of the nursing diagnosis statement.

Example:

Nursing diagnosis	Activity intolerance: decreased muscle strength (legs) related to decreased activity
Long-term goal	Leg muscles return to full baseline strength
Short-term goal	Patient raises legs 2 inches above bed against resistance within 3 days

Long-term goals describe what patient behaviors are expected for resolution of the nursing diagnosis. Short-term goals describe expected patient behaviors indicating that action is headed in the right direction toward resolution, that is, they are short steps to be achieved toward reaching the long-term goal.

■ Selection of nursing actions

There are usually several alternative actions that can be chosen to reach a desired outcome or goal. Selection of actions is usually guided by the second part (etiologic factors) of the nursing diagnosis. For example, different nursing actions would be selected for a nursing diagnosis of "Sleep pattern disturbance: insomnia related to fear of surgery" than would be selected for a nursing diagnosis of "Sleep pattern disturbance: insomnia related to persistent cough."

The action alternatives are identified and choices are made depending on the specific patient situation. Patient input is sought when feasible. When a nurse follows a preset plan of action for any given nursing diagnosis, patient care is not individualized and there is less potential for accomplishment of the desired outcomes. The determination of action alternatives is based on knowledge from experts, suggestions from the patient, observations of actions of others, suggestions from other health care providers, and the nurse's own creativity. Actions are based on scientific principles.

Selection of action is based on the following guidelines:
- The greatest possibility of success
- The least risk
- The least discomfort
- The least intrusiveness for the patient

Once the course of action has been selected, the *frequency* of action must also be determined. For example, the frequency of deep breathing and coughing exercises selected as an activity would be planned at different time intervals for different patients based on risk factors such as obesity and smoking habits identified through analysis of the data.

Plans for selected actions are *recorded* so that other persons providing nursing care may follow through, thus providing continuity of care. The nursing care plan may be placed in a Kardex or on the patient's chart. The plan includes the nursing diagnoses, expected patient outcomes and nursing actions. The actions are often termed "nursing orders" and provide explicit directions for care.

▨ IMPLEMENTATION

■ Action strategies

The nurse can assist the patient to meet the goals in a number of ways (Table 2-3). The goal of nursing care is the patient's optimal health; therefore self-care is stressed to the extent possible, since it is the patient who is usually ultimately responsible for on-going health maintenance. Thus teaching, supporting, and motivating are major nursing strategies. If self-care is impossible or inappropriate, the nurse then compensates for the patient's inability by performing the actions. Monitoring is an ongoing strategy; the type and degree usually depend on the illness or disease.

Nursing activities can be directed toward different ends.

Table 2-3 Action strategies for providing nursing care

Strategy	Definition	Examples of activities
Monitoring	Collecting data on an ongoing basis	Vital signs, intake and output, cardiac monitoring, assessing level of consciousness, skin turgor, urine tests
Compensating (partially or wholly)	Performing or assisting patient to perform necessary activities that patient is unable to or has difficulty performing	Assisting patient with comfort measures, ADL, carrying out prescriptive activities (medication, treatments)
Teaching	Helping patients learn what they can do to maintain or restore optimal health	Health education, methods of disease prevention, teaching skills such as dressing changes, injections, taking vital signs
Supporting	Helping patients cope with changes in life-style, environment, or new experiences	Use of empathy skills to help patient explore feelings, assistance with problem solving, facilitation of coping skills
Motivating	Providing an environment that facilitates achieving optimal health	Encouragement to carry out difficult or painful actions, health maintenance activities

Flow sheet

Name: Ms. Smith
Date:

Parameter observed	Third hospital day		Fourth hospital day		Fifth hospital day
	Hour				
	9 PM	11 PM	1 AM	3 AM	4 PM
Vital signs					
Blood pressure	140/100	130/100	128/98	130/100	110/80
Pulse	126	120	118	122	80
Respirations	26	24	24	22	16
Fluid intake					
Oral	Refused	120 ml OJ	Refused	150 ml	240 ml OJ
IV	—	—	—		—
Protein snacks	Nauseated	Nauseated		One cheese cracker	Peanut butter crackers
Fluid output					
Urine	—	100 ml	—	200 ml	400 ml
Emesis	50 ml	—	—	100 ml	—
Other	—	—	—	—	—
Patient's behavior state	Hearing voices; moving nervously about in bed	Somewhat calmer; still having auditory hallucinations	Unchanged	Increased restlessness; visual hallucinations	Some tremulousness; embarrassed
Activity	Position changed	Up with assistance to bathroom	Turned	Turned	Up walking and in chair
Sedation	Chlordiazepoxide, 100 mg IM	—		—	—
Mouth care	Done	Done	Done	Done	Self-care
	P. Craig, R.N.	P. Craig, R.N.	J. Fugate, R.N.	N. Yates, R.N.	J. Gelein, R.N.

Example of a SOAP format for recording

Problem: Constipation: related to inadequate fluid intake

S	"I never have problems at home; my BM is usually soft. It was OK 4 days ago."
O	Small hard stool past 2 days. Fluid intake averaging 900 ml/day past 3 days. Taking fluids mostly with meals.
A	Constipation is temporary. Fluid intake needs to be increased to at least 2000 ml/day
P	Evaluate patient's understanding of adequate hydration to promote normal stool. Give 240 ml fruit juice mid-AM, mid-PM, and at bedtime. Encourage patient to drink full glass of water with medications.

One categorization that will be followed in this text is as follows:

1. *Assisting with achievement of therapeutic goals.* This category includes those activities directed toward restoration of optimal health. It includes such activities as assisting the person to carry out medical prescriptions (for example, medications, treatments), promoting nutrition and elimination, and maintaining fluid balance.
2. *Assisting with comfort and ADL.* Promotion of comfort is a major nursing activity in the care of patients with pathophysiologic disorders. In addition, some disorders limit the patient's ability to carry out ADL.
3. *Control of environment.* Some pathophysiologic conditions, such as allergies, infections, or immunosuppression, require control of environmental factors such as humidity, dust, or pathogenic organisms.
4. *Counseling and teaching.* Providing patients with support in dealing with their psychosocial needs and teaching the patient are major nursing activities for persons with pathophysiologic disorders.

Not all of the planned care is provided by the professional nurse. Some of the care may be delegated to other health-care providers working in a collegial relationship with the nurse.

■ Recording (documentation)

Actions that have been taken and the patient's response to the actions need to be documented. Responses to monitoring activities are most easily recorded on *flow sheets.* The flow sheets provide a means of quick comparison of a specific monitoring parameter over time. Data such as vital signs, fluid intake and output, activity, and urine tests are recorded as they are gathered. In some institutions these sheets subsequently become part of the patient's permanent record. In others the data are recopied onto other sheets in the permanent record. Flow sheets are used extensively in special care areas such as intensive care units, where continual monitoring of several parameters is necessary.

■ PROBLEM-ORIENTED RECORD

The problem-oriented system provides a means of following the progress of each identified nursing diagnosis and the patient's response to the planned interventions.

In this approach, baseline data are collected and recorded (the *database*), and a *master problem list* is developed and placed in the front of the patient's record. Each problem is numbered, and subsequent charting identifies the problem being charted by number or name. When there are data suggesting a problem but inadequate data to draw a conclusion, the symptoms are listed as the "problem" until a conclusion can be reached. Each problem is dated when identified and again when resolved. This method of documentation provides easy access to the identification, progress, and resolution of patient problems.

Narrative notes may be used for charting significant data pertaining to each problem, or a *SOAP format* may be used.

In the SOAP format, the first two letters, S and O, refer to sources of the data, that is, subjective and objective data. The last two letters, *A* and *P,* refer to analysis or assessment and to plans for further action. The SOAP format can be used to record the *initial* plan and to record subsequent progress notes.

⊞ EVALUATION

The last step of nursing process consists of determining whether the desired outcomes were met, analyzing the effectiveness of nursing interventions, and planning for subsequent care. The method of evaluation consists of collecting data from the patient based on the criteria established as patient goals (outcomes). Thus the more specifically the goals were stated in observable patient behaviors, the easier the task of evaluation. For example, a nursing diagnosis of "Constipation: related to inadequate fluid intake" could have a goal of "Stool soft and formed." Evaluation would then consist of inspecting the stool. If it were soft and formed, the goal would be achieved and the patient's constipation would be corrected.

Some of the reasons why goals are not achieved are listed in the box below.

Once the possible reason for the lack of goal achievement is identified, revisions are made and the process is repeated. As can be noted, nursing care is an ongoing and dynamic process that requires constant assessment and evaluation.

■ SUMMARY

1. The five steps of nursing process are assessment, data analysis, planning, implementation, and evaluation.
2. Maslow's hierarchy of needs include physiologic, safety, love and belonging, self-esteem, and self-actualization. This framework is useful in setting priorities of care.

Possible reasons for not achieving patient goals

Database	Incomplete; changes in data
Nursing diagnosis	Inaccurate data analysis; inaccurate statement
Goals	Unrelated to nursing diagnosis; nonspecific; unrealistic
Nursing actions	Unrelated to nursing diagnosis or goal(s); nonspecific, therefore poorly implemented; inadequate in degree of action taken

---

Putting knowledge to practice

- What are some frameworks that can be used in medical-surgical nursing for data analysis? What framework do you now use? Is this framework adaptable for patients with medical-surgical conditions?
- Differentiate between baseline and ongoing assessment; between subjective and objective data.
- How do the different parts of a nursing diagnosis assist you in planning nursing care?
- Examine the list of nursing diagnoses identified by the North American Nursing Diagnosis Association (NANDA). What use could you make of this list?
- Define what is meant by *observable patient behaviors*. Write some examples of goals written in terms of observable patient behaviors.
- Analyze the nursing activities that you carried out in your last three patient assignments in terms of action strategies (Table 2-3). Which strategies did you use? Could you have used any of the remaining strategies?

---

3. Four commonly used frameworks for nursing practice are Orem's self-care agency model, Roger's life-process model, Roy's adaptation model, and Johnson's behavioral systems model.

4. Gordon's 11 functional health patterns are useful for data collection and analysis regardless of the conceptual model.

5. Two types of assessment are initial and ongoing; baseline observations are those that are made initially for future comparison.

6. Four general conclusions from analysis of patient data are: data is insufficient, person is functioning optimally, person is at high risk, person is functioning inadequately.

7. Nursing diagnosis is a statement of an actual or potential health problem identified from nursing assessment and which is the legal and educational domain of nursing.

8. Nursing diagnosis statements consist of two parts: pattern of functioning and etiology; each diagnosis also has defining characteristics such as a cluster of signs and symptoms.

9. Goals are determined from the pattern of functioning and nursing actions from the etiologies.

10. Reasons for standardizing and classifying nursing diagnoses are facilitation of communication, computerization, theory and research, and legal needs.

11. Nursing diagnoses and classification systems are in the process of evolving.

12. Priorities for care can be set on the basis of life-threatening problems, high risk, low risk, and health maintenance.

13. Expected patient outcomes (goals) are written as observable patient behaviors.

14. Independent nursing actions develop during nursing process; collaborative nursing actions are those that facilitate the actions of other health professionals.

15. Action strategies for providing nursing care are monitoring, compensating, teaching, supporting, and motivating.

16. Nursing actions are selected on the basis of the greatest possibility of success with the least risk, discomfort or intrusiveness to the patient.

17. Documentation by the SOAP method includes subjective and objective data, assessment, and plan.

18. Evaluation consists of collecting patient data based on criteria established in the expected patient outcomes.

REFERENCES AND SELECTED READINGS
Contemporary

1. Alfaro, R: Application of nursing process: a step-by-step guide, Philadelphia, 1986, JB Lippincott Co.
2. American Nurses' Association: Nursing and social policy statement, Kansas City, 1980, The Association.
3. Bower, FL: The process of planning nursing care: a theoretical model, ed 3, St. Louis, 1982, The CV Mosby Co.
4. *Calder, M: How we won the team's support for POMR, Nurs 81 11:27-29, 1981.
5. Carlson, JH, Craft, CA, and McGuire, AD: Nursing diagnosis, Philadelphia, 1982, WB Saunders Co.
6. Carnevalli, D: Nursing care planning: diagnosis and management, ed 3, Philadelphia, 1982, JB Lippincott Co.
7. *Carpenito, LJ: Nursing diagnosis: application to clinical practice, ed 2, Philadelphia, 1987, JB Lippincott Co.
8. *Carpenito, LJ: Handbook of nursing diagnosis, Philadelphia, 1985, JB Lippincott Co.
9. *Dickie, GL, and Bass, MJ: Improving problem-oriented medical records through self-audit, Nurs 80 10:487-490, 1980.
10. Duldt, BW, and Giffin, K: Theoretical perspectives for nursing, Boston, 1985, Little, Brown, and Co.
11. Fitzpatrick, J, Whall, A, and Bowie, MD: Conceptual models of nursing: analysis and application, Bowie, Md, 1983, Robert J Brady Co.

---

*References preceded by an asterisk are particularly well suited for student reading.

12. Gettrust, KV, Ryan, S, and Engelman, DS: Applied nursing diagnosis guides for comprehensive care planning, New York, 1985, John Wiley & Sons.

13. *Gordon, M: Manual of nursing diagnosis 1986-1987, New York, 1987, McGraw-Hill Book Co.

14. *Gordon, M: Nursing diagnosis: process and application, ed 2, New York, 1987, McGraw-Hill Book Co.

15. Griffith-Kenney, JW, and Christensen, PJ: Nursing process: application of theories, frameworks and models, ed 2, St. Louis, 1986, The CV Mosby Co.

16. Hurley, M (editor): Classification of nursing diagnoses: proceedings of the sixth national conference, St Louis, 1985, The CV Mosby Co.

17. Johnson, DE: The behavioral system model for nursing. In Riehl, JP, and Roy, C (editors): Conceptual models for nursing practice, ed 2, New York, 1980, Appleton-Century-Crofts.

18. Kelly, MA: Nursing diagnosis source book, Norwalk, Conn, 1985, Appleton-Century-Crofts.

19. *Kim, MJ, McFarland, GK, and McLane, AM: Pocket guide to nursing diagnoses, ed 2, St. Louis, 1987, The CV Mosby Co.

20. Kim, MJ, McFarland, GK, and McLane, AM: Classification of nursing diagnoses: proceedings of the fifth national conference, St. Louis, 1984, The CV Mosby Co.

21. Kim, MJ, and Moritz, DA, editors: Classification of nursing diagnoses: proceedings of the third and fourth national conferences, New York, 1982, McGraw-Hill Book Co.

22. Little, DL, and Carnevali, DC: Nursing care planning, ed 3, Philadelphia, 1983, JB Lippincott Co.

23. *Lunney, M: Nursing diagnosis: refining the system, Am J Nurs 82:456-459, 1982.

24. Marriner, A: The nursing process: a scientific approach to nursing care, ed 3, St. Louis, 1982, The CV Mosby Co.

25. Mayers, M: A systematic approach to the nursing care plan, ed 3, New York, 1983, Appleton-Century-Crofts.

26. McLane, AM (editor): Classification of nursing diagnoses: proceedings of the seventh conference, St. Louis, 1987, The CV Mosby Co.

27. Orem, DE: Nursing: concepts of practice, ed 3, New York, 1985, McGraw-Hill Book Co.

28. Potter, PA, and Perry, AG: Fundamentals of nursing: concepts, process and practice, St. Louis, 1985, The CV Mosby Co.

29. *Price, MR: Nursing diagnosis: making a concept come alive, Am J Nurs 80:668-671, 1980.

30. Rogers, ME: Science of unitary human beings. In Malinsky, V (editor): Explorations in Martha Rogers' science of unitary human beings, New York, 1986, Appleton-Century-Crofts.

31. Roy, C, and Roberts, SL: Theory construction in nursing: an adaptation model, Englewood Cliffs, NJ, 1981, Prentice-Hall.

32. Vaughan-Wrobel, BC, and Henderson, BS: The problem-oriented system in nursing, ed 2, St. Louis, 1981, The CV Mosby Co.

33. Webster, GA: Nomenclature and classification system development. In Kim, MJ, McFarland, GK, and McLane, AM: Classification of nursing diagnoses: proceedings of the fifth national conference, St. Louis, 1984, The CV Mosby Co.

34. Yura, H, and Walsh, M: The nursing process: assessing, planning, implementing and evaluating, ed 4, New York, 1983, Appleton-Century-Crofts.

Classic

35. Fortin, JD, and Rabinow, J: Legal implications of nursing diagnosis, Nurs Clin North Am 14:553-561, 1979.

36. *Maudinger, MO, and Jauron, GD: Developing a nursing diagnosis, Nurs Outlook 23:94-98, 1975.

3

Nursing History and Physical Examination

BARBARA C. LONG

CHAPTER OBJECTIVES

After studying this chapter, the student should be able to:

- Describe ways to enhance a patient interview.
- Describe the purposes of a nursing history.
- Know where to find a sample nursing history and sample head-to-toe physical examination guide.
- Describe the four modalities for physical examination.
- Explain the basis for skin changes.
- Explain the differences between normal and abnormal lung and heart sounds.
- Identify the parameters for describing lung and heart sounds.
- Describe physical changes that may be observed during physical examination of the aged.

The health status of an adult is assessed either separately or conjointly by different health care professionals. The same data may be required by different professionals but for different purposes. For example, both the physician and the nurse require data about the nature of a patient's pain. The physician uses the data for diagnosis and treatment of the conditions causing the pain; the nurse uses the data to help the patient achieve the highest degree of comfort.

Different nurses also collect and analyze different types of data, depending on their knowledge, skill level, and their specific patient population. Thus a clinical nurse specialist who has a private nursing practice will use data and assessment techniques that may be similar or different from the techniques used by the staff nurse working in an acute care hospital.

Subjective data for assessing health status are obtained by asking questions of the patient in either a formal or an informal interview. Data collected in a formal interview for the purpose of planning nursing care is called a *nursing history*. Objective data on health status may be collected by *physical examination* or by general observations.

This chapter will review the assessment methods and specific data useful for providing quality nursing care for adults experiencing pathophysiologic disorders in acute care settings. For information on more comprehensive data collection, the reader is referred to specific health assessment texts.

Guidelines for patient interviews

Modification of environment to facilitate interview

1. Provide privacy by closing door, drawing curtain, etc.
2. Facilitate patient's comfort (comfortable position, water available, etc.).
3. Sit in chair facing patient within a close distance but respecting patient's personal space.
4. Keep environmental noises to a minimum by adjusting TV, radio, etc.
5. Ask visitors to step out of room, if applicable.

Initiation of interview

1. Introduce self.
2. Describe purpose of interview, general content, and approximate length of interview
3. Start with general nonthreatening questions to establish rapport and to demonstrate interest in patient and patient's circumstances.

Progression of interview

1. Keep questions brief and limited to a single topic.
2. Use open or closed questions, depending on the type of data sought. (Open question: "What do you drink with your supper?" Closed question: "Do you drink coffee or milk with your supper?")
3. Avoid leading questions such as "Do you have pain in your chest?" (patient may think this is expected). Instead ask, "Are you having any discomfort? Can you describe it?"
4. Use language that is easily understood by patient. Avoid awkward terms that make you feel uncomfortable (unless no other term is available that patient understands).
5. Allow sufficient time for patient to answer.
6. Use transitional statements when changing topic, for example, "We've been talking about your eating habits, now I'd like to ask you some questions about your bowel movements."
7. Keep the interview focused on data to be obtained. If patient insists on digressing to a particular topic, you can identify this but redirect the interview; for example, "I'd like to hear more about your family but perhaps we can do that later; right now I need to know more about your eating patterns."

Termination of interview

1. Summarize the major ideas offered by the patient.
2. Summarize what you will be doing with the data.
3. Thank the patient for cooperating.
4. State when you will be seeing the patient again.

■ SUBJECTIVE DATA

■ Interviewing

The amount of data collected during an interview depends on the knowledge base and interviewing skills of the nurse and the openness of the patient. Interviewing skills are not intuitive but are developed with experience. A successful interview can be achieved by the following:

1. Modifying the environment to facilitate the interview
2. Listening and showing interest in the patient while simultaneously focusing on the data to be collected
3. Understanding the content base of the interview
4. Using appropriate questions to obtain the data

Guidelines for a successful interview are listed in the box on p. 26. An unsuccessful interview may occur because of factors related to the nurse or the patient situation. Inability to collect data may be the result of the following factors:

1. Lack of time available to the nurse
2. Poor interviewing skills of the nurse
3. Patient condition (for example, pain, decreased consciousness)
4. Patient refusal or inability to answer questions

■ Nursing history

■ PURPOSES

If one of the goals of nursing is to assist people to maintain optimal health, a health history should be obtained by a professional nurse from all persons entering the health care system. The purpose is to obtain data for planning and implementing actions designed to strengthen positive health behaviors and to assist persons to cope with their health problems.

A comprehensive health history can be time-consuming and may not be appropriate in some acute care health centers, particularly if the patient's hospital stay will be short. Data must be collected, however, when a patient is first admitted to the health care center to identify those needs that require nursing interventions.

■ DATA

The nursing history may be a short (10-minute) interview to collect the immediate necessary data with additional data collected subsequently. Whenever possible, however, a more comprehensive nursing history is carried out initially to provide a data base for health teaching.

The nursing history example listed in the box on pp. 28 and 29 takes approximately 30 minutes. The initial questions provide the nurse with the patient's perceptions of his or her health and current problems. Early in the interview data are collected about the presence of pain, since this can affect the course of the interview. A nursing history may begin with general data followed by data pertaining to physiologic functioning (activity, sleep, rest, nutrition, elimination, sensory perception, infection history), relationships with others, and ideas about self (see the box on pp. 28 and 29). Another approach is to collect data for each of Gordon's Functional Health Patterns (see Chapter 2).

■ OBJECTIVE DATA: PHYSICAL EXAMINATION

■ Modalities of physical examination

The four modalities of physical examination are inspection, auscultation, palpation, and percussion (see the box on p. 29).

■ INSPECTION

Inspection can best be described as purposeful looking. It is the simplest modality and yields the most information but is often performed less accurately than other modalities. The key to effective inspection is *knowing what to look for*. A systematic approach to inspection is vital so that valuable data are not lost. Thoroughness is also important; all areas are examined carefully. It is especially important to examine the sacral area and to lift folds of tissue, such as under the breasts or gluteal folds. Embarrassment by the examiner or anticipated embarrassment of the patient may result in inadequate inspection. Most inspection can be carried out without special equipment, but a penlight and tongue blade are helpful aids.

■ AUSCULTATION

Although sounds may be heard by the unaided ear, auscultation is usually carried out with a stethoscope to enhance the examiner's ability to hear sounds coming from within the body cavity. The stethoscope is effective because it eliminates most of the sounds from the environment. Auscultation is used to obtain data about the heart, lungs, and gastrointestinal tract. Turbulent arterial blood flow can also be detected by auscultation.

■ PALPATION

Palpation is often used to confirm data obtained by inspection as well as to provide data concerning temperature, texture, size, consistency, discomfort, and pulsations. The backs of the fingers and hand are most sensitive to temperature; the fingertips are most sensitive to variations in texture.

Light palpation of the abdomen elicits areas of tenderness or distention. Deep palpation of the abdomen is used primarily by physicians or specially prepared nurses seeking data about organ involvement necessary to rule out a pathologic condition.

Sample nursing history

General information

1. Perception of present health status
2. Comparison of present with usual health status (if changed, perception of cause)
3. Medications taken regularly
4. Any allergies: food, medications, contact allergens, inhalants (describe symptoms, measures taken to avoid contact, relief measures)
5. Presence of pain/discomfort (current, past, onset, duration, characteristics, relief measures)
   - Chest pain
   - Joint or muscle problems (pain, stiffness, weakness)
   - Discomfort in extremities (pain, numbness, tingling, swelling, coldness, paleness)
   - Headaches

Physiologic functioning

1. Prescribed activity level
2. Type and frequency of activity (recreation, exercise, work) both usual and current
3. Regular exercise routines and knowledge of benefits of activity
4. Difficulty moving about (describe difficulty and help needed, use of aids)
5. Whether tires easily with activities of daily living (ADL) or desired activity (describe)
6. Any difficulty breathing at rest (describe precipitating factors, duration, position for ease of breathing, type and effectiveness of relief measures)
7. Help needed with ADL
8. Usual hours of sleep per night for past three nights and if this is a change from usual pattern of sleep
9. Naps usually taken (time of day, frequency, length)
10. Feelings about quality of sleep (if poor sleep, perception of cause)
11. Aids taken to promote sleep (dose, frequency, effectiveness, length of time taken)
12. Food and fluid pattern for a typical day (type, amount)
13. Recent changes in amount and type of food and fluids, appetite
14. Weight, usual and current (if overweight or underweight: lifetime pattern, feelings about weight level, reasons for recent changes)
15. Patient's perception of weight level
16. Dentures (fit, comfort)
17. Problems with eating (chewing, swallowing)
18. Frequency of bowel movements (usual, recent changes)
19. Last bowel movement (time, character)
20. Aids usually taken for bowel elimination (type, frequency, effect)
21. Problems with bowel control (onset, perception of cause, effectiveness of measures taken)
22. Problems with urinary control or discomfort (onset, perception of cause)
23. Ability to see, hear, taste, smell, feel sensations (pain, heat, touch) and use of corrective devices
24. Usual condition of skin and mucous membranes (dryness, cracks)
25. Frequency of colds or infections (throat, ear, bladder or kidney, boils)
26. Cough or history of coughs (productivity)
27. History of smoking or exposure to other inhalants
28. Knowledge and ability to summon help if needed (use of call cord)

Sample nursing history—cont'd

Relationships with others

1. Persons or groups most helpful right now
2. Satisfaction with current role (family role, work role)
3. Self as member of a cultural or ethnic group
4. Recent changes in functioning in family, peer group
5. Living arrangements
6. Type and frequency of social activities outside home
7. Satisfaction with leisure time, hobbies, recreational pastimes
8. Anything interfering with role of mother, father, wife, husband
9. Anything (surgery, illness) changing feelings or thoughts about self as man or woman
10. Anything (illness, surgery, medications) affecting sexual function

Ideas about self

1. How do you feel right now? Is this how you usually feel?
2. What kind of person would you say you are?
3. How do you feel about yourself?
4. What do you usually do when things do not go as you plan or when things get tough?
5. Describe your goals or plans for the future.
6. Can you tell me about any spiritual or other beliefs and practices that are helpful to you now?
7. Is there anything else you would like to share with me that would help in your care?

■ PERCUSSION

Percussion is used less frequently in nursing practice than the other modalities. Effective percussion requires skill both in carrying out the technique and in interpreting the resultant sounds, and generally elicits data more pertinent for the medical diagnosis. Percussion can be used to differentiate between abdominal distention caused by gas (tympanic sound) and distention caused by fluid (dull sound).

■ Head-to-toe physical examination

The most common systematic approach used in a physical examination is a head-to-toe approach. This permits examining all areas in a sequential pattern to avoid omitting data. The box on p. 30 lists areas of assessment useful for planning nursing care of adults experiencing pathophysiologic disorders in an acute care center.

■ GENERAL SURVEY

The nurse makes general observations of the patient on entering the patient's room. Items to note are listed below.

☐ State of health

Overall observable indicators should be assessed. Does the person look well, that is, relaxed, in no acute distress, well-nourished, etc? Does the person look ill, that is, cachectic, strained facies, pale and sweating, moving with difficulty, etc?

Modalities of physical examination

Inspection	*Looking* at the skin and mucous membranes, body position and movements, and so on
Auscultation	*Listening* to heart, lung, and bowel sounds, blood pressure sounds
Palpation	*Feeling* or *touching* the skin to determine skin changes, enlargement of underlying structures, or presence of air or fluid
Percussion	*Tapping* an area to establish the presence of air, fluid, or dense tissue

---

☐ State of awareness

Overall awareness should be noted. Is the person able to respond to questions? Is the patient able to remain alert during interview and physical examination? Is the patient oriented to person, place, and time?

☐ State of emotions

Nonverbal cues to the patient's emotional state are identified. Is the person relaxed and smiling? Restlessly pacing the floor or wringing the hands? Tearful? Listless? Have poor grooming? (Unkempt hair and clothing and poor personal hygiene may be observed in a depressed person.)

Head-to-toe physical examination guide

General survey

State of health
State of awareness
State of emotions: mood, distress, grooming
Motor activity, posture, gait
Speech
Odors

General parameters

Height and weight
Vital signs
Skin parameters during inspection of each body
    area: color, elasticity and turgor, moisture, tem-
    perature, lesions

Head

Eyes: symmetry, eyelids, conjunctiva and sclera,
    cornea and lens, pupillary reflex and accom-
    modation, visual acuity, extraocular movement
Ears: external structures, external auditory canal,
    auditory acuity
Hair
Scalp
Face: skin, symmetry of movement, muscle strength
    of jaw, pain sensation
Nose: nares, septum, vestibule
Mouth: lips, teeth, gums, mucous membranes,
    pharynx, tongue

Neck

Swallowing
Position of trachea
Muscle strength
Range of motion
Jugular vein distention
Carotid pulses

Upper back and side

Inspection of skin of back and axilla
Inspection and palpation of spine
Symmetry of respiratory movement
Thoracic diameters
Auscultation of lungs (posterior and lateral)

Anterior chest

Skin turgor over sternum
Respiratory pattern
Slope of ribs
Auscultation of lung sounds
Auscultation of heart sounds
Breast inspection

Abdomen

Inspection
Auscultation of bowel sounds
Palpation of femoral pulses
Testicle inspection

Lower back

Inspection of sacrum and buttocks

Extremities

Inspection of skin
Inspection of nails
Capillary filling
Palpation for pitting edema (legs)
Pulses: radial and brachial on arms, dorsalis pedis
    and posterior tibialis in feet
Sensation
Muscle strength: legs, ankles, arms, hands
Range of motion
Coordination

Whole body coordination

□ **Motor activity, posture, gait**

General posture and activity may provide cues to problems such as fatigue (slumped posture, inactivity), dyspnea (sitting upright and trying to get breath), or pain (refusal to move, clutching a body part). The person's gait when walking may indicate weakness of one side, fear of falling (holding onto furniture), or loss of balance.

□ **Speech**

Slurring of speech, inability to articulate words, or inability to speak the language of the health care professional may create communication problems. Difficulty with speech may be caused by problems of the central nervous system or larynx. If patients cannot speak, can they communicate with sign language or writing materials?

□ **Odors**

Breath or body odors may result from poor personal hygiene, ingestion of certain substances such as food or alcohol, or medical conditions such as diabetes mellitus (acetone), pulmonary infections, uremia, or liver failure.

■ **GENERAL PARAMETERS**

□ **Skin**

The skin provides a considerable amount of information about the person's state of health as well as being subject to lesions and breakdown. Data obtained on the initial physical examination provide information concerning potential for skin breakdown and a baseline of the status of existing lesions for future comparison. In the head-to-toe

Table 3-1   Skin color changes

Color	Physiology	Conditions
Redness	Vasodilation: more rapid blood flow, more oxygenated blood giving a reddish hue (erythema)	Blushing, heat, inflammation, fever, alcohol ingestion, extreme cold (below 15 C), hot flushes
Whiteness (pallor)	Vasoconstriction: slower blood flow, less blood in capillaries	Cold, fear, shock
	Partially obstructed blood flow: less blood in capillaries	Vasospasm, thrombus, narrowed vessels
	Fluid between blood vessels and skin surface	Edema
	Decreased oxygenation of blood from decreased hemoglobin	Anemia
	Loss of melanin	Vitiligo
Bluish	Deoxygenated hemoglobin (cyanosis) seen in earlobes, lips, mucous membranes of mouth, nail beds	Heart or lung disease, inadequate respiration, peripheral blood vessel obstruction
Yellow	Increased bile pigment in blood eventually distributed to skin and mucous membranes and to sclera of eye	Liver disease, obstruction of bile ducts, chronic uremia, rapid hemolysis
Brown	Increased melanin deposits: normal in brown-black races	Aging, sunburn
Dullness	Vasoconstriction in dark skin	Cold, fear, shock

physical examination, the skin is scrutinized throughout the examination whenever a specific body part is assessed. The specific observations include color, elasticity and turgor, moisture, temperature, and lesions or scars.

□ *Color*

The color of the skin depends on the amount of melanin in the cells and the blood supply (Table 3-1). Individuals differ in skin color intraracially as well as interracially. Color also varies on different skin areas of a given individual. Increased skin color is usually seen on exposed areas and in the areola of the nipples.

Lack of melanin in some skin areas may result from a genetic defect or from certain diseases such as hyperthyroidism, pernicious anemia, or adrenal cortical insufficiency. Scar tissue also lacks melanin. Areas of increased melanin often develop normally in aged persons and appear as brown patches on the skin (Fig. 3-1). A normal finding in most persons is pigmented moles. Changes in color of moles, especially to black or greenish black, should be reported to a physician for possible determination of malignancy.

Skin appears lighter with blood vessel constriction and redder with dilation because dilated vessels are closer to the skin surface. Body areas particularly sensitive to vasodilation include a "butterfly" area across the cheeks and nose, neck, upper chest, flexor surfaces of the extremities, and genital areas. Skin and mucous membranes may also appear bluish or darker when there is an excess of deoxygenated blood (cyanosis) or yellow from an excess of serum bile (jaundice).

In dark-skinned individuals pallor is observed by the absence of the underlying red tones that normally give the brown and black skin its "glow" or "living color."[13] Brown skin will therefore appear more yellowish brown, and black

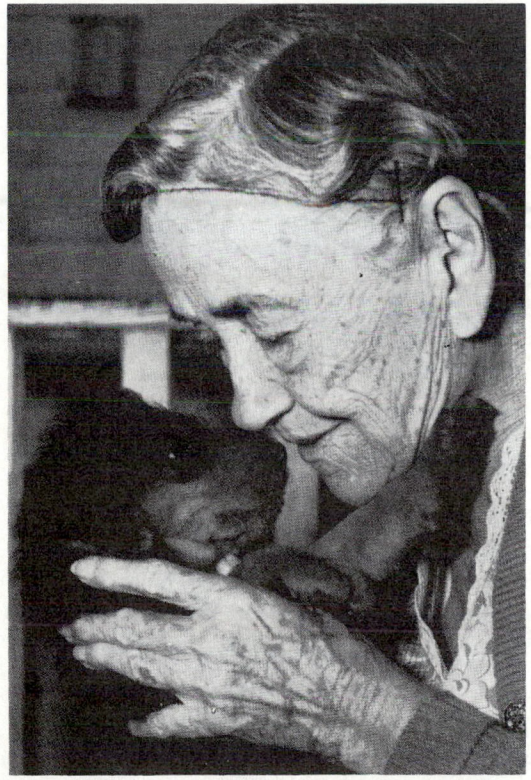

Fig. 3-1   Elderly patients have skin changes. Note discolored spots on skin and tiny raised area on this woman's eyelid. (VanDerMeid from Monkmeyer Press Photo Service.)

skin will appear ashen gray. Generalized pallor and cyanosis may be better observed in the mucous membranes, lips, and nail beds. Erythema in the dark-skinned person is more readily observed as generalized redness of the lips.

☐ *Elasticity and turgor*

Normal skin is elastic and returns to its original position after it has been stretched. It also moves freely over underlying tissue (mobility). Skin may become taut from being stretched over enlarged underlying tissue, such as that caused by fluid (edema). Loose skin over the extremities and neck appears during old age because of loss of underlying subcutaneous tissue.

Turgor is the speed with which skin returns to its normal position after it has been stretched. Decreased turgor results from dehydration and is best assessed over the sternum. A fold of skin is picked up and observed for speed of return to normal; a delay indicates decreased turgor.

☐ *Moisture*

Insensible fluid loss through the skin usually evaporates immediately, and normal skin is usually dry to the touch. Mucous membranes are normally moist and appear dry with dehydration. Increased fluid loss through the skin producing a sensation of moisture occurs when the external temperature is high, when high body temperature (fever) suddenly declines, or whenever the stress response occurs (fear, shock, etc.). The skin of the very young adult may be oily, and that of the elderly person may be very dry.

☐ *Temperature*

Skin temperature increases with vasodilation and decreases with vasoconstriction. Vasodilation results from increased external or internal body temperature or from inflammation. Vasoconstriction results from decreased external or internal body temperature and as a result of sympathetic stimulation, as seen in the stress response. The backs of the fingers are more sensitive than the fingertips and are therefore used in the assessment of skin temperature.

☐ *Lesions*

Different types of lesions may be observed on the skin (Table 3-2). Any lesions other than normal skin changes are described in terms of color, size, shape, texture, effect of pressure, arrangement and distribution over the body, and variety (presence of different types of lesions). Descriptions should be precise, and vague terms such as *small* or *medium* are avoided. Lesions may be discrete or coalesce into each other. They may occur in patches located in certain body areas or occur widely distributed in an even or uneven pattern. The use of correct medical terms when describing skin lesions facilitates communication to others.

Swelling of the skin may result from the presence of fluid in or between tissue cells or from overgrowth of tissue cells (Fig. 3-2). Fluid may appear as fluid-filled sacs on the skin surface or in the tissue. Interstitial fluid results from increased extracellular body fluid (Chapter 8) and is termed *pitting edema* because a finger pressed over the swollen tissue leaves a pit on the skin surface. The amount of

Table 3-2 Skin lesions

Term	Description	Example
Change in color		
Macule	Flat spot less than 1 cm	Freckle
Change in cell growth		
Papule	Raised mass less than 1 cm	Measles spot
Nodule	Raised mass 1 to 2 cm	Mole
Tumor	Raised mass over 2 cm	Epithelioma
Change involving fluid		
Vesicle	Fluid-filled sac less than 1 cm	Small blister
Bulla	Fluid-filled sac more than 1 cm	Large blister
Pustule	Pus-filled sac less than 1 cm	Acne lesion
Wheal	Circumscribed raised skin containing intracellular fluid	Hives
Changes in consistence or integrity		
Plaque	Large raised surface on skin	Psoriasis
Crust	Dry exudate over a lesion	Eczema lesion
Scale	Dry exfoliation of skin cells	Psoriasis
Fissure	Crack in skin surface	Crack in corner of mouth
Ulcer	Erosion of skin surface	Decubitus ulcer
Lichenification	Leatherlike thickening of outer skin layer	Lichen planus

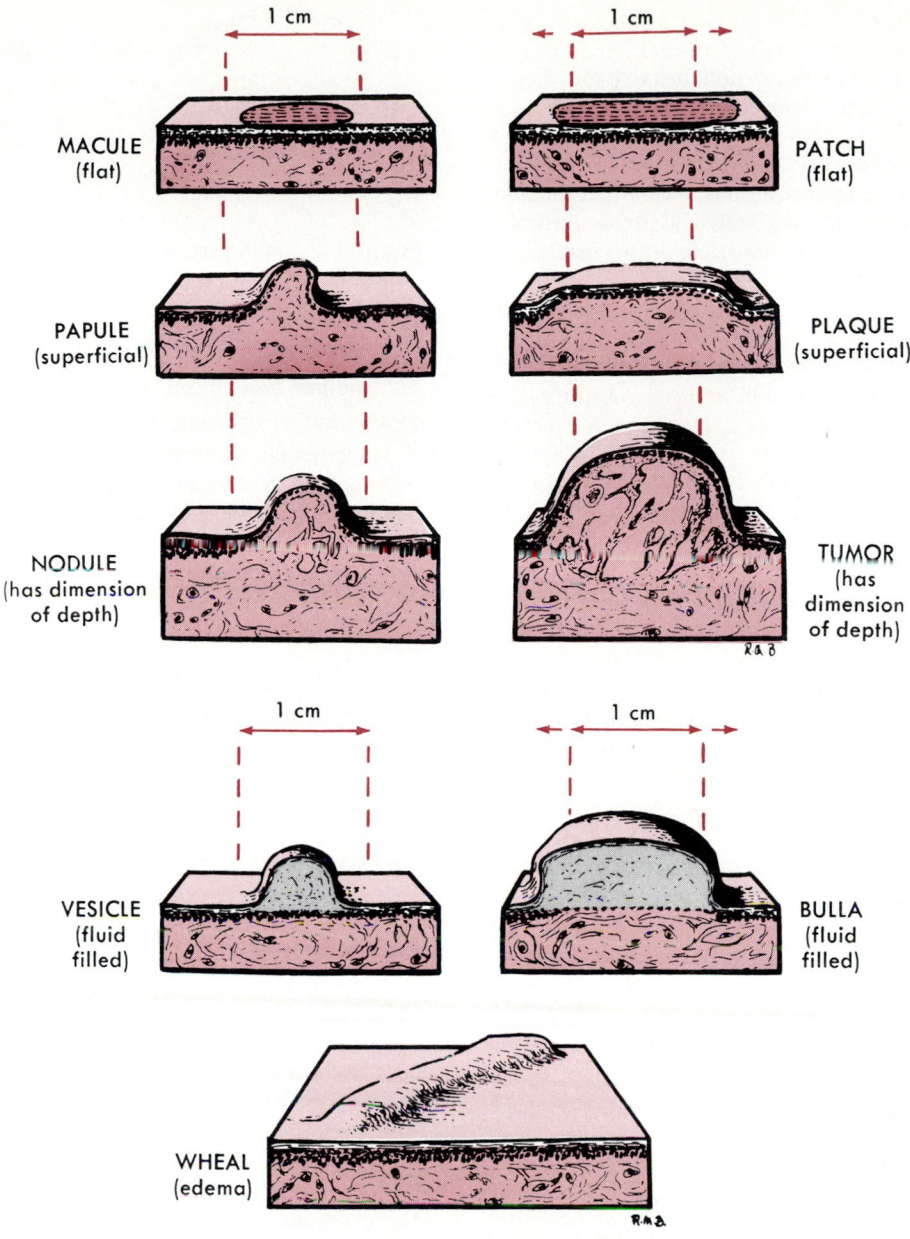

Fig. 3-2 Skin lesions. (From Stewart, WD, Danto, JL, and Madden, S: Dermatology: diagnosis and treatment of cutaneous disorders, ed 4, St. Louis, 1978, The CV Mosby Co.)

pitting is recorded as + to + + + +, depending on the depth of the pit.

Overgrowth of tissue cells has different terms, depending on the size of the growth (Table 3-2). The term *tumor* refers to a growth over 2 cm and is not restricted to malignancy, since tumors can also be benign.

■ HEAD EXAMINATION

Examination of the head includes external structures, visual and auditory acuity, and facial movement.

□ Eyes

The eyes are examined first after the examiner's hands have been washed. The patient is questioned about contact lenses so that a lens is not inadvertently lost during the eye examination.

HEAD

Eyes
Symmetry

Look for presence of false eye.

Eyelids

EXAMINATION TECHNIQUES
Note position of lids to eyeballs and inspect for edema, color, lesions, and ability to close.

ABNORMAL FINDINGS
Drooping of lid (ptosis) may result from muscular weakness or nerve damage, edema from allergies, local inflammation, recent crying, or fluid-retaining states. Redness indicates inflammation. Failure to close may dehydrate cornea.

Conjunctiva and sclera

EXAMINATION TECHNIQUES
Examine conjunctiva by depressing the lower lid while asking the person to look up. The normal conjunctiva is clear and the sclera is white.

ABNORMAL FINDINGS
Redness indicates inflammation. The sclera turns yellow with jaundice.

Cornea and lens

EXAMINATION TECHNIQUES
Shine a light obliquely across eye to detect opacities of cornea and lens.

ABNORMAL FINDINGS
Opacities will appear grayish against black pupil. Opacities interfere with vision.

Pupillary reflex and accommodation

EXAMINATION TECHNIQUES
Pupils are normally equally round and reactive to light and accommodation (PERRLA).
Reaction to light
1. Ask person to look at a distance.
2. Shine a light obliquely and quickly twice across each eye.
3. Note *direct reaction* of pupil to light and *consensual reaction* (reaction of opposite pupil).

ABNORMAL FINDINGS
The pupil of a false eye does not respond to light. Small fixed pupils occur with administration of opium derivative or miotic drug for glaucoma. Dilated fixed pupils occur with anticholinergic drugs, severe brain damage, or severe hypoxia.
Reaction to accommodation
1. Hold your finger about 5 to 10 cm from bridge of the person's nose.
2. Ask the person to look first at a distance, then at your finger.
3. Note pupillary constriction and convergence of the eyes when focus is on finger (near object).

Visual acuity

The ability to see is assessed both with and without glasses or contact lenses. The person is asked to read large print at a distance (note approximate number of feet), then small print about 35 cm (14 inches) from the face. Glasses used only for reading are not used to test far vision.

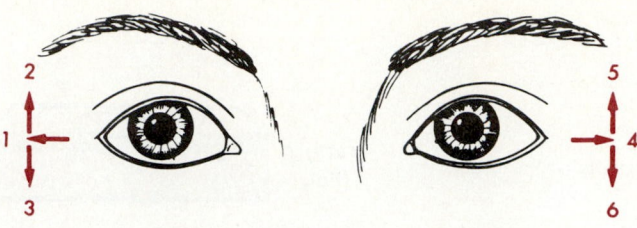

Fig. 3-3 Testing extraocular movement. The numbers indicate the sequence of motion.

Extraocular movement

EXAMINATION TECHNIQUES
Testing ocular movement determines whether eyes are moving in a synchronous fashion.
Method: Have the person follow your finger in an **H** configuration (Fig. 3-3).

ABNORMAL FINDINGS
Asymmetry of movement may cause double vision.

Ears
External structures and external auditory canal

EXAMINATION TECHNIQUES
Inspect auricles and surrounding tissues of external ear for deformities, lumps, or skin lesions. The outer portion of external auditory canal is inspected by pulling auricle up, back, and out and using a penlight for better vision.

ABNORMAL FINDINGS
Ear pain, discharge, and redness are signs of inflammation.

Auditory acuity

To estimate hearing ability, test one ear at a time. Ask the person to occlude one ear with a finger. Stand approximately 1 to 2 feet away and whisper softly two equally accented numbers (such as 14, 25) toward the unoccluded ear. Repeat with the other ear. Be sure person cannot read your lips.

Hair

1. *Appearance:* Lack of shine occurs with age or malnutrition.
2. *Distribution:* Thin sparse hair occurs with age or malnutrition. Alopecia (loss of hair) occurs with chemotherapy or radiation therapy.
3. *Attachment:* Easily plucked hair occurs with malnutrition.
4. *Presence of lice:* Lice may deposit tiny white ovoid nits on hair shafts, especially behind ears.

Scalp

EXAMINATION TECHNIQUES
Part hair in several places and examine for dryness and scaliness of lesions.

ABNORMAL FINDINGS
Scaling may result from dandruff or psoriasis.

Face
Skin

Inspect color, moisture, temperature, texture, and lesions.

Symmetry of movement

EXAMINATION TECHNIQUES
Ask patient to elevate eyebrows and forehead, frown, smile, close eyes quickly and tightly, show teeth, whistle, and blow out cheeks.
ABNORMAL FINDINGS
Asymmetry will be noted with weakness of the facial nerve.

Muscle strength of jaw

EXAMINATION TECHNIQUES
Place both hands against jaws and ask person to
1. Clamp jaws tightly.
2. Move jaw side to side against your hand resistance.
ABNORMAL FINDINGS
Muscle weakness may interfere with mastication.

Pain sensation

EXAMINATION TECHNIQUES
1. Ask person to close eyes.
2. Use two safety pins (to avoid moving across the person's eyes).
3. Ask person to respond to sharp or dull pricks with pin.
ABNORMAL FINDINGS
Pain sensation may be lost with paralysis of the trigeminal nerve.

Nose
Nares

EXAMINATION TECHNIQUES
Inspect nares for flaring or discharge.
ABNORMAL FINDINGS
Flaring occurs with respiratory exertion.

Septum

EXAMINATION TECHNIQUES
Using penlight, inspect nasal septum for marked deviation.
ABNORMAL FINDINGS
Breathing through nose may be impaired by a deviated septum.

Vestibule

EXAMINATION TECHNIQUES
Using penlight, inspect vestibule for color and exudate.
ABNORMAL FINDINGS
Redness and exudate occur with inflammation.

Mouth

EXAMINATION TECHNIQUES
The mouth, like the skin, is an excellent barometer of general health, reflecting general disease and debility as well as good health. A tongue blade and penlight are necessary for inspection.

Lips

EXAMINATION TECHNIQUES
Inspect for dryness or cracks.
Inspect for lesions.
ABNORMAL FINDINGS
These may occur with dehydration or malnutrition.

Teeth, gums, and mucous membranes

EXAMINATION TECHNIQUES
Inspect gums for color, moisture, and lesions
Inspect teeth for caries.
Inspect dentures for comfort and fit.
ABNORMAL FINDINGS
Redness or white "curd" patches on gums occur with inflammation.
Lack of dentures or ill-fitting dentures may interfere with chewing.

Pharynx

EXAMINATION TECHNIQUES
Depress tongue with tongue blade and ask patient to say "Ah."
Touch back of throat with tongue blade to elicit gag reflex.
ABNORMAL FINDINGS
Redness and discharge occur with inflammation; asymmetry with movement of soft palate may interfere with swallowing.
A decreased gag reflex (change from normal) may interfere with swallowing.

Tongue

EXAMINATION TECHNIQUES
Inspect color, coating, and lesions.
Ask person to move tongue up and down, and side to side.
ABNORMAL FINDINGS
A smooth tongue may indicate malnutrition; a thickened white patch may be a premalignant lesion.
Asymmetry of movement may indicate paralysis and interfere with eating.

NECK
Trachea

EXAMINATION TECHNIQUES
Inspect trachea for deviation.
Place a finger on trachea and ask person to swallow.
ABNORMAL FINDINGS
Tracheal deviation may indicate neck mass, pneumothorax, pleural effusion, and atelectasis.
Decreased tracheal movement may indicate decreased ability to swallow.

Muscle strength

EXAMINATION TECHNIQUES
Ask person to shrug shoulders and turn head to each side against your hands.
ABNORMAL FINDINGS
Assess strength of neck muscles.

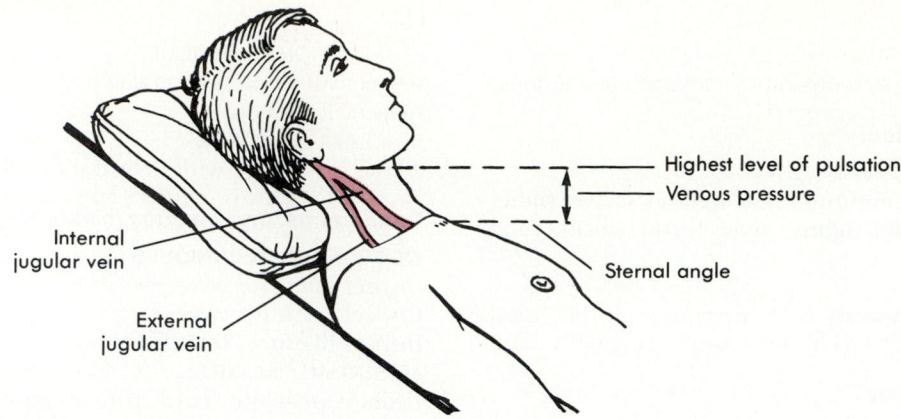

Fig. 3-4 Position of internal and jugular veins used in measuring venous pressure.

Range of motion (ROM)

EXAMINATION TECHNIQUES
Ask person to move head through range of motion.
ABNORMAL FINDINGS
Decreased ROM may interfere with ADL.

Jugular vein distention

EXAMINATION TECHNIQUES
Place person with head elevated 45 degrees. Note uppermost point of visible vein pulsation. Note level of vein pulsation above sternal angle (Fig. 3-4).
ABNORMAL FINDINGS
Distended neck veins (increased pressure) may result from circulatory overload or right-sided heart failure.

UPPER BACK AND SIDE

Spine

EXAMINATION TECHNIQUES
Inspect back for differences in height of shoulders. Palpate length of spine with a finger on each side of spine to detect lateral curvatures.
ABNORMAL FINDINGS
Marked deformities may interfere with respiration or cause fatigue.

Symmetry of respiratory movement

EXAMINATION TECHNIQUES
Place both hands on lateral thorax just below scapula with thumbs at spine and fingers outstretched. Ask person to take a deep breath. Observe and feel equal expansion of thorax.
ABNORMAL FINDINGS
Asymmetry suggests a lung or pleural disorder and interferes with full excursion.

Thoracic diameters

EXAMINATION TECHNIQUES
Usually compare front to back (AP) and side to side (lateral).

ABNORMAL FINDINGS
Barrel chest seen with emphysema or normal with a ratio of 1:1 AP to lateral diameters (normal ratio 1:2).

Auscultation of lungs (posterior/lateral)

EXAMINATION TECHNIQUES
Auscultation of the lungs is described on p. 39.
ABNORMAL FINDINGS
Assess for decreased breath sounds or presence of adventitious (abnormal) sounds.

ANTERIOR CHEST

Respiratory pattern

EXAMINATION TECHNIQUES
Note depth of breathing. Count rate (may also be done when counting heart rate).
Note effort of breathing.
Listen for audible breath sounds (for example, wheezing).
ABNORMAL FINDINGS
Very shallow breathing limits alveolar expansion.
Very deep breathing indicates respiratory effort.
Intercostal retraction and nasal flaring occur with labored breathing.
Audible breath sounds occur with asthma and chronic bronchitis.

Slope of ribs

EXAMINATION TECHNIQUES
Trace one intercostal space anterior to posterior.
ABNORMAL FINDINGS
Rib is more horizontal with emphysema.

Lung sounds

EXAMINATION TECHNIQUES
See p. 39 for auscultation of lungs anteriorly.
ABNORMAL FINDINGS
Assess for decreased breath sounds or presence of adventitious (abnormal) sounds.

Heart

EXAMINATION TECHNIQUES
Count heart rate at apex of heart. Assess rhythm. Listen to heart sounds (see p. 41).

ABNORMAL FINDINGS
Describe abnormal sounds (gallops, murmurs, opening valve snaps and clicks) in terms of timing with S_1 and S_2, anatomic location, pitch, intensity, and character.

Breast inspection

EXAMINATION TECHNIQUES
The female patient is asked if she performs a regular breast self-examination (BSE).

ABNORMAL FINDINGS
Nonperformance of BSE indicates need for patient teaching.

ABDOMEN

Abdominal inspection

EXAMINATION TECHNIQUES
Inspect skin for dryness and lesions.
Check umbilicus for cleanliness and lesions.
Note contour and movements (peristaltic movements and aortic pulsations may be noted in thin persons). Measure distended abdomen with tape measure across umbilicus.

ABNORMAL FINDINGS
Abdominal distention may result from fat, ascites, distended bladder, pregnancy, and tumors. Increased peristaltic waves may be seen with early intestinal obstruction.

Bowel sounds

EXAMINATION TECHNIQUES
Use diaphragm of stethoscope with light pressure to listen for bowel sounds, starting in right lower abdominal quadrant. If not heard in that site, listen in other quadrants.

ABNORMAL FINDINGS
Alterations in bowel sounds occur with diarrhea and ileus.

Palpation of femoral pulses

Palpate presence and strength of femoral pulses.

Testicle inspection

EXAMINATION TECHNIQUES
The male patient is asked if he performs a regular testicular self-examination.

ABNORMAL FINDINGS
Nonperformance of testicular self-examination indicates need for patient teaching.

LOWER BACK

Sacrum and buttocks

EXAMINATION TECHNIQUES
Inspect sacrum and buttocks for redness or lesions.

ABNORMAL FINDINGS
Baseline data on skin of sacrum and buttocks is especially important if patient is malnourished, edematous, or on bed rest.

EXTREMITIES

NOTE: always compare right with left. Assess both legs, then both arms.

Skin

Check size in proportion to body development.
Inspect skin (include all skin areas and skin between toes).
Check skin temperature.

Nails

EXAMINATION TECHNIQUES
Inspect nails for texture and thickness, angle of fingernail to nail base.

ABNORMAL FINDINGS
Nail changes are seen with age and malnutrition.
Clubbing of nails is seen with lung conditions (hypoxia).

Capillary filling

EXAMINATION TECHNIQUES
Check for capillary filling: press your thumbnail against the edge of the person's nail and release quickly.

ABNORMAL FINDINGS
Lack of blanching response or slow return of color may indicate lack of circulation to finger or toe.

Palpation for pitting edema

EXAMINATION TECHNIQUES
Press finger firmly over shin, over dorsum of foot, and behind medial malleolus.

ABNORMAL FINDINGS
Pitting edema is caused by increased fluid in the interstitial spaces.

Pulses

EXAMINATION TECHNIQUES
Assess radial and brachial pulses in arms and dorsalis pedis and posterior tibialis pulses in feet (Table 3-3) for presence, strength, and symmetry.

Table 3-3 Techniques for palpation of peripheral pulses

Pulse	Technique
Radial	Press two fingertips over groove along thumb side of inner wrist
Brachial	Press three fingertips across the medial side of the inner aspect of the elbow, slightly superior
Dorsalis pedis	Press two fingertips gently over the middle dorsum of the foot along the groove between extensor tendons of the big toe and adjoining toe
Posterior tibialis	Press three fingertips gently behind and slightly inferior to medial malleolus of the ankle

ABNORMAL FINDINGS
Decreased pulses may suggest decreased circulation.

Sensation

EXAMINATION TECHNIQUES
Test sensation by means of two safety pins (as with face), starting at fingers or toes and moving toward elbow or knee.
ABNORMAL FINDINGS
Areas that have decreased sensation are at high risk for injury.

Muscle strength
Legs

EXAMINATION TECHNIQUES
For legs, do straight leg raises (one at a time) against hand resistance. Place one of your hands under knee and other hand on top of ankle. Ask person to lift lower leg against your resistance. Then move hand to underneath ankle and ask person to lower leg against resistance (Fig. 3-5).
ABNORMAL FINDINGS
Decreased muscle strength of legs will decrease ability to ambulate and increase risk of fall.

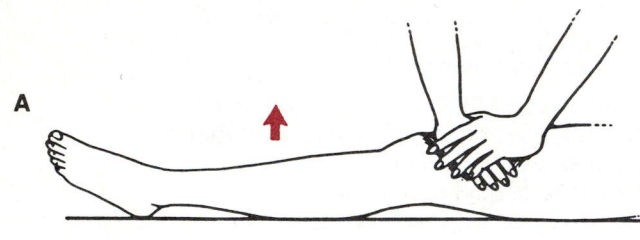

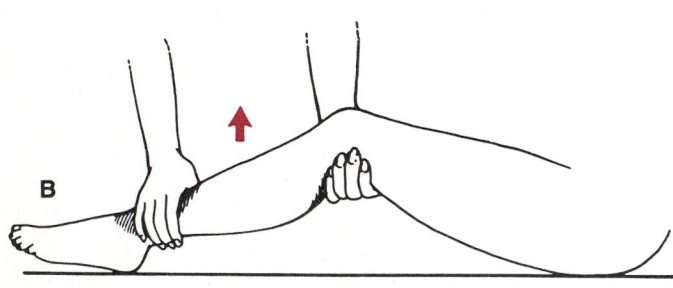

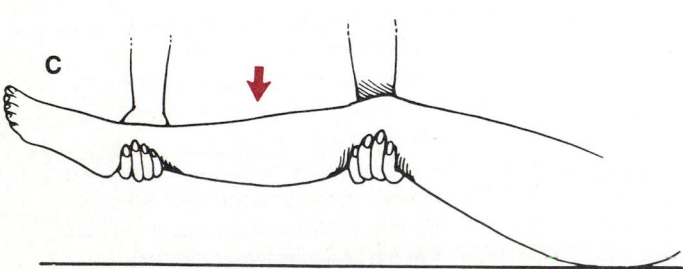

Fig. 3-5 Testing muscle strength in the legs. **A,** Straight leg raises (quadriceps). **B,** Raising lower leg against resistance (quadriceps). **C,** Pulling lower leg against resistance (hamstrings).

Ankles

EXAMINATION TECHNIQUES
Test ankle strength by asking person to push against resistance of your hand placed first on dorsal then plantar aspects of each foot.
ABNORMAL FINDINGS
Decreased ankle strength will increase risk of fall when ambulating.

Arms

EXAMINATION TECHNIQUES
For arms, ask patient to grip your index and middle fingers and to first pull, then push your hands against your resistance.
Test hand strength by asking person to grip two of your fingers tightly.
ABNORMAL FINDINGS
Decreased muscle strength of arms may interfere with ADL.
Hand weakness may interfere with ADL.

Range of motion (ROM)

EXAMINATION TECHNIQUES
Assess ROM of shoulders, elbows, wrists, and fingers. Assess ROM of hips, knees, and ankles.
ABNORMAL FINDINGS
Decreased ROM may interfere with ADL and walking.

Coordination

EXAMINATION TECHNIQUES
1. Finger coordination: Ask person to touch thumb to each finger in rapid succession.
2. Finger-to-nose coordination: Ask person to touch your index finger, then his or her nose several times, first with eyes open and then with eyes closed.
3. Heel-shin coordination: Ask person to place heel on opposite shin and move heel up and down shin.
ABNORMAL FINDINGS
Awkwardness with point to point coordination may suggest motor weakness, loss of position sense, or cerebellar disease. The patient may have some difficulties with ADL and have increased risk of falls.

WHOLE BODY COORDINATION

EXAMINATION TECHNIQUES
1. If person is ambulatory, ask person to walk across room and back to assess gait.
2. Ask person to stand still with arms at side, first with eyes open, then with eyes closed, to assess balance (Romberg sign).
ABNORMAL FINDINGS
Awkward gait and decreased balance may interfere with ambulation and increase risk of falls.

■ Pulmonary auscultation

Auscultation of the lungs enables a nurse to establish baseline data for identifying current and potential lung problems that require nursing interventions, such as de-

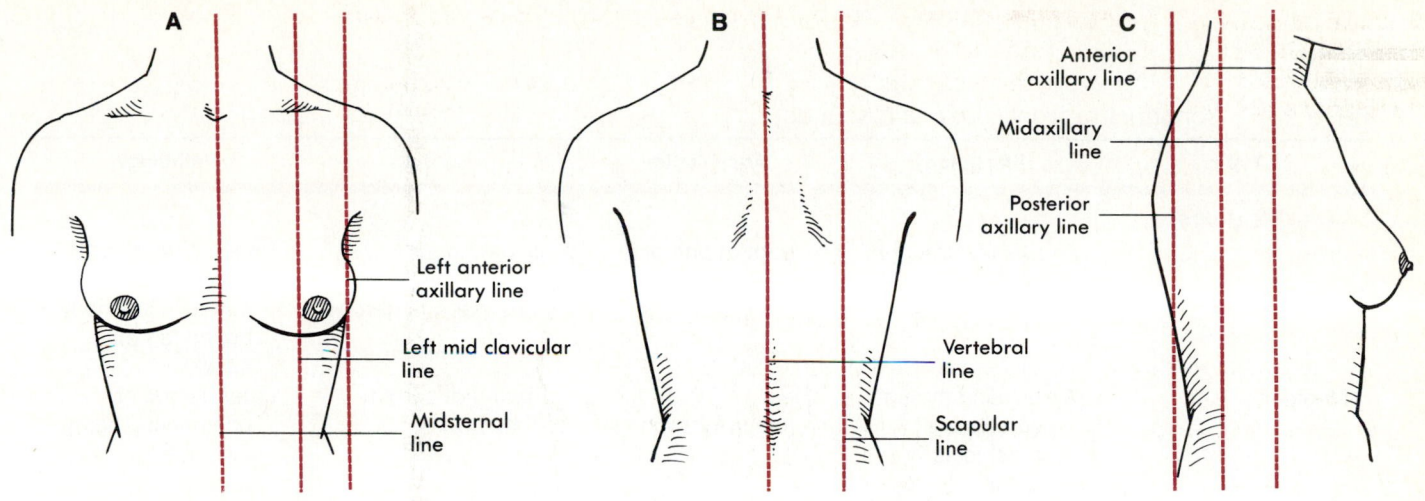

Fig. 3-6   Topographical landmarks. **A,** Anterior thorax. **B,** Posterior thorax. **C,** Lateral thorax.

termining the frequency for breathing exercises or the need for or effectiveness of suctioning. Landmarks for pulmonary auscultation are illustrated in Fig. 3-6.

■ BREATH SOUNDS

Breath sounds result from the movement of air through the lungs and air passages. The sounds are thought to occur as a result of two elements, the vesicular and bronchial elements. The vesicular element occurs when the walls of the alveoli are separated by air entering the alveoli from inspiration. The bronchial element is a hisslike sound resulting from air flowing past the bronchi and across the vocal chords.

The three types of breath sounds that can be heard are vesicular, bronchovesicular, and bronchial (Fig. 3-7). *Vesicular breath sounds* are heard over most of the lungs because of the prominence of the alveoli. The sounds are of a low pitch and have a soft rustling or swishing quality. The sound of the inspiratory phase is longer and higher in pitch than that of the expiratory phase, which is a soft, short, low-pitched, almost inaudible sound. The relative loudness of inspiration may differ among listening sites; the sounds are usually softer at the bases of the lungs.

Bronchovesicular breath sounds are heard as one auscultates toward the main bronchi. Inspiration and expiration are loud and nearly equal in duration and intensity because of auscultating closer to the vocal chords.

Bronchial breath sounds normally are *not* heard over any area of lung tissue, and their presence indicates consolidation or compression of lung tissue or a pleural effusion. These breath sounds are high-pitched and loud; during the expiratory phase they increase in duration, pitch, and intensity.

□ Adventitious (abnormal) lung sounds

Adventitious lung sounds are abnormal sounds superimposed on breath sounds. There are essentially two kinds of abnormal sounds: (1) *crackles* or *rales* (rhymes with pals) caused by air flowing through moisture in the air passages and, (2) *wheezes* or *rhonchi* caused by air flowing through narrowed air passages (Table 3-4). A third type of sound occurs outside the lung; a *pleural friction rub* results from the rubbing of inflamed pleura between the lung and chest wall.

□ General directions for pulmonary auscultation

1. Have person seated if possible for auscultation of posterior lung fields. The female patient may be easier to auscultate anteriorly if she is lying down.
2. Use the diaphragm of the stethoscope. Press firmly to produce a blanched ring when the diaphragm is removed. Hold the diaphragm in such a way as to decrease extraneous sounds (fingers not touching skin and diaphragm, or tubing not touching clothing or other objects).
3. Provide counter support for the person with your free hand.
4. Tell person to (a) turn head away, (b) breathe *slightly* deeper but *not* faster, and (c) breathe through the mouth.
5. Listen in a consistent, systematic manner.
6. At each listening site (Figs. 3-8, 3-9, and 3-10), listen for one full breath and identify:
   • Type of breath sound
   • Intensity of breath sound
   • Presence of adventitious sounds

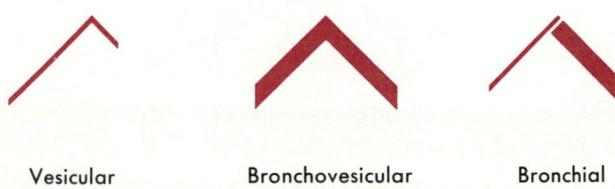

Vesicular   Bronchovesicular   Bronchial

Fig. 3-7   Schematic representation of the three types of breath sounds.

Table 3-4   Abnormal (adventitious) lung sounds

Type	Physiology	Auscultation	Sound	Pathology
Crackles (rales)				
Fine	Air passing through secretions in alveoli	Heard at end of inspiration	Several hairs rubbed together between fingertips	Pneumonia, heart failure (may occur normally in elderly bedridden persons)
Medium	Air passing through secretions in bronchioles or bronchi	Heard midway during inspiration	Fizzing of carbonated drink	Later stages of pneumonia, heart failure, pulmonary edema
Coarse	Air passing through secretions in large airways, especially trachea	Heard at beginning of inspiration	Rough gurgling	Persons with repressed cough reflexes, unable to clear own secretions
Wheezes (rhonchi)	Air passing through narrow passages	Heard mostly during expiration, but may also occur with inspiration	Loud musical gurgling	Obstructive lung disease
Pleural friction rub	Rubbing of inflamed pleura	May occur throughout respiratory cycle, heard best at base of lung at end of expiration	Scratching, grating, rubbing	Inflamed pleura

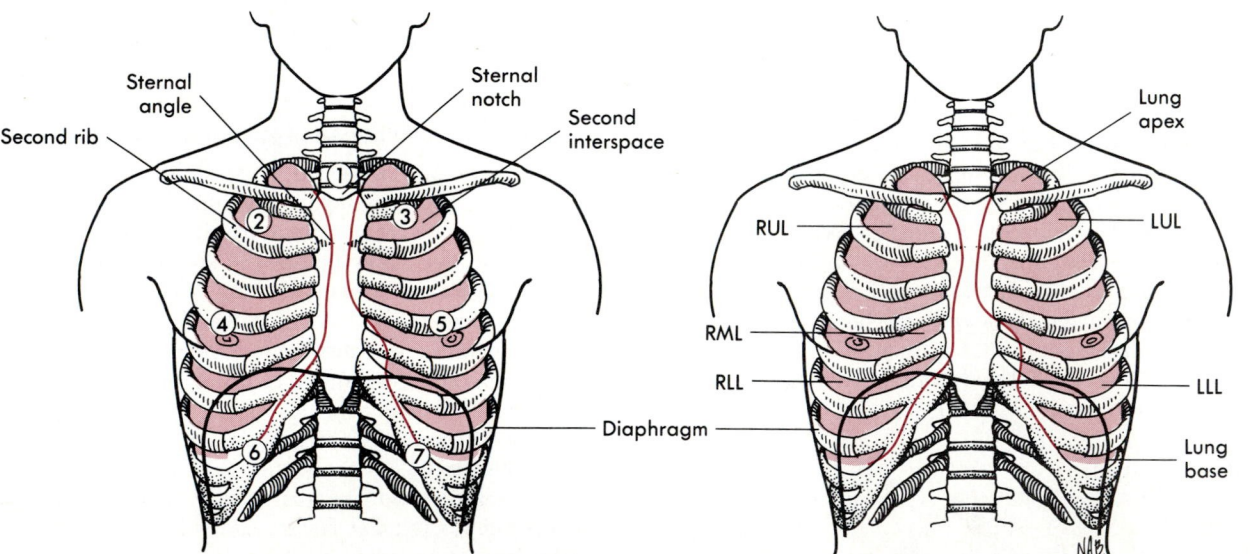

Fig. 3-8   Anterior thorax showing placement of stethoscope when listening to breath sounds and position of lobes of lungs.

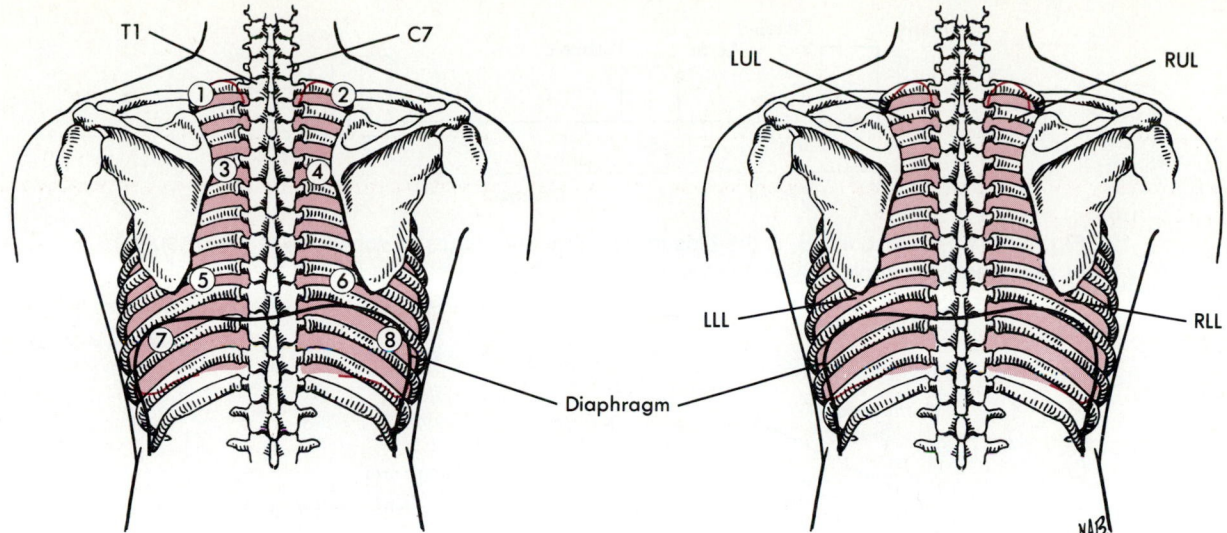

Fig. 3-9   Posterior thorax showing placement of stethoscope when listening to breath sounds and position of lobes of lungs.

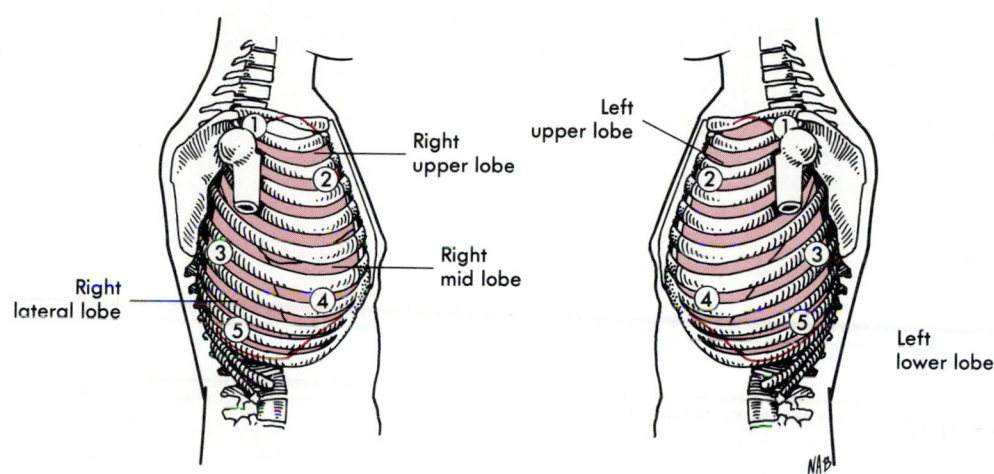

Fig. 3-10   Lateral thorax showing placement of stethoscope when listening to breath sounds and position of lobes of lungs.

■ Cardiac auscultation

Auscultation of heart sounds enables a nurse to establish baseline data for identifying current and potential cardiac problems that require nursing intervention. Cardiac auscultation also assists the nurse in evaluating a patient's progress (for example, effect of activity on heart rate) or in monitoring responses to medications (for example, quinidine or digitalis preparations).

■ HEART SOUNDS

The familiar "lub-dub" heard when taking an apical pulse are the first and second heart sounds (S_1 and S_2) and mark the beginning and end of each ventricular contraction; hence rate, when obtained by auscultation, is determined by counting each set of "lub-dubs" as one beat. Whether these sounds occur regularly or irregularly determines the assessment of cardiac rhythm.

The first heart sound (S_1) is the result of the closure of the *mitral* and *tricuspid* atrioventricular valves (Fig. 3-11). This sound is heard best at the apex of the heart (normally the fifth left intercostal space at the midclavicular line) (Fig. 3-12). The valves do not close at precisely the same time. However, the fact that the time difference between their closure is measured in terms of hundredths of a second and that a greater volume of sound is produced by

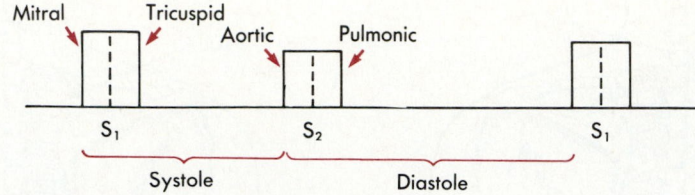

Fig. 3-11 Heart sound S_1 is the closure of mitral and tricuspid valves; S_2 is the closure of aortic and pulmonic valves. Systole is the time interval between S_1 and the start of S_2. Diastole is S_2 to the start of S_1. Diastole is longer than systole.

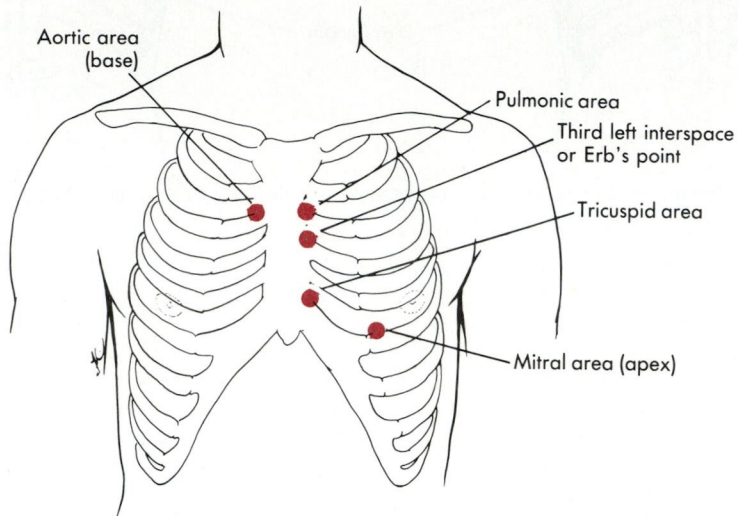

Fig. 3-12 Topographic areas for cardiac auscultation (intercostal spaces).

the mitral valve generally results in only one detectable noise. Occasionally the tricuspid component may be heard along the lower left sternal border.

The second heart sound (S_2) is the result of the closure of the semilunar valves (*aortic* and *pulmonic*). This sound is usually heard best at the base of the heart in the aortic area (second right intercostal space). The aortic valve closes slightly ahead of the pulmonic valve but produces a louder sound, so S_2 is also often detected as only one sound. When auscultating in the pulmonic area (second left intercostal space) one may hear the pulmonic component of S_2 (producing what is then referred to as a *split sound*) in a phasic manner, that is, the splitting is heard for a few beats and then is absent for a few beats. This phasic appearance of a split S_2 is the result of alterations in right ventricular volume (and therefore contraction time) related to the respiratory cycle. Under normal circumstances the split S_2, if heard at all, is detected during inspiration.

□ **Extra heart sounds**

With some exceptions, the occurrence of any additional heart sounds would be considered an abnormal finding. Abnormal cardiac sounds include gallops (S_3 and S_4), murmurs, opening snaps, and clicks.

Ventricular diastolic gallop (S_3) is a faint, low-pitched sound produced by rapid ventricular filling in early diastole

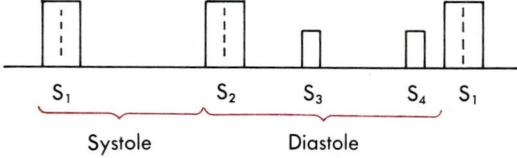

Fig. 3-13 Location of extra heart sound during cardiac cycle.

(Fig. 3-13). Ventricular "gallop" describes the canter of a horse, which is frequently mimicked at heart rates greater than 100 beats per minute. When this sound is present in healthy children and young adults, it is almost always a normal condition and is referred to as a physiologic S_3. An S_3 heard in an older person is usually a pathologic sign and is frequently one of the first signs of serious heart disease or cardiac decompensation as seen in congestive heart failure.

Atrial diastolic gallop (S_4) is a low-pitched sound that occurs late in diastole when atrial contractions eject blood into a noncompliant ventricle. It may be heard in such states as hypertensive cardiovascular disease, coronary artery disease (especially during an attack of angina pectoris), and aortic stenosis.

Murmurs are audible vibrations of the heart and great

vessels that occur because of turbulent blood flow. They may occur either during systole or diastole or through both phases. The intensity may be faint or loud; the pitch may be high (sharp) or low (dull), and the quality is described as harsh, blowing, rumbling, or musical. Murmurs may be organic (structural cardiovascular abnormalities), functional (increased blood flow through normal structures), or physiologic.

Other sounds that may be heard include a high-pitched clicking sound heard during systole (ejection sounds) or a high-pitched snapping sound heard in early diastole (opening snap of stenosed mitral valve).

☐ General directions for cardiac auscultation

1. Locate the landmarks for auscultation: the second and fifth intercostal spaces.
2. Start at either the mitral or aortic areas.
3. Move the stethoscope at very short intervals (inching method) along the fifth interspace to sternum, then along the left sternal border to the second left interspace, then across the sternum to the right second interspace (or vice versa) (see Fig. 3-12).
4. Go through the listening sequence at least two times, first with the diaphragm for high-pitched sounds, then with the bell for low-pitched sounds. It is easier to follow the sequence three times (twice with the diaphragm listening first for normal sounds S_1 and S_2; second, for extra high-pitched sounds; and third, with the bell for extra low-pitched sounds).
5. Press firmly when using the diaphragm, but rest the bell only lightly on the skin.
6. When listening to normal heart sounds, note intensity of sounds and presence of splitting. Splitting of S_1 can be heard best at the tricuspid area and splitting of S_2 at the pulmonic area. The carotid pulse can be used to verify S_1 if needed. If splitting of S_2 is heard, note timing in relation to respiratory cycle.
7. Describe any extra sounds in terms of timing (systolic or diastolic), intensity, pitch character, and location where heard on thorax. For example, a sound might be described as "a high-pitched, blowing, systolic murmur of medium intensity, best heard along the left sternal border."

■ Physical assessment of changes with aging

There is great variation in the degree of change that occurs with aging when comparing one older person with another. Changes caused by aging are irreversible as contrasted with changes caused by illness, which may be reversible. The physical changes seen in older persons are not predictable and may result from the age factor alone or from other factors, such as environment (for example exposure to sun), illness, or genetic traits. Some of the changes that occur with aging are listed in the box at right.

In the physical examination of an older adult some differences may be noted that are normal variations caused by age. These variations may include the following:

Skin. Decreased elasticity; increased wrinkles on sun-exposed areas; increased dryness with flaking and scaling; purple patches, brown spots, cherry angiomas (red); skin tags, seborrheic keratoses (greasy warts)

Hair. Loss of hair, thinner, decreased luster

Face. Increased facial hair in women, coarse hair on men (in ears and nose)

Eyes. Decreased vision, especially for near objects; pupillary response to light may be slower; lens may look gray but have clear vision; may be opaque if cataract developing

Ears. Decreased hearing, especially for high-pitched sounds; sounds may become distorted

Mouth. Teeth worn, darker color; dentures common; decreased salivation

Neck. Decreased range of motion, neck veins more prominent

Thorax. Increased dorsal curve of thoracic spine (kyphosis); increased anterior-posterior diameter; chest expansion may be decreased, decreased size of breasts, pendulous

Abdomen. Increased fat deposits in lower abdomen, weakened abdominal muscles (pot belly)

Extremities. Nails: thickened (especially toenails); ROM: may be decreased; muscle strength: decreased; decreased pain and touch sensation

Whole body coordination. Position sense may be decreased, gait may be unsteady

---

Physical changes with aging

Loss of tissue elasticity

Loss of subcutaneous fat

Altered endocrine function (thyroid, pancreatic, estrogenic, androgenic)

Altered immune response

Alteration in bone and muscle mass

Altered sensory perception (temperature, pressure, pain, touch, taste, vision, hearing)

Respiratory changes (decreased number but increased size of alveoli, rigidity of lung tissue, decreased vital capacity, decreased cough response)

Cardiac changes (decreased cardiac output, decreased contractility, increased time for heart rate to return to normal after activity)

Vascular changes (decreased vessel elasticity, decreased blood flow to coronary arteries, liver, and kidneys, decreased venous muscle tone and decreased efficiency of venous valves, decreased capillary permeability)

Gastrointestinal changes (decreased digestive enzymes, absorption, muscle tone, salivation, gag reflex)

Sleep changes (less time, changes in cycles)

Putting knowledge to practice

- You are planning to do a nursing history and physical examination on a newly admitted patient. What would you say to the patient?
- Examine the sample nursing history guide and physical examination guide. Consider the usefulness of these guides based on your conceptual framework for nursing practice.
- Do a general survey of two or more young adults, middle-aged adults, and older adults. How do the data differ within and among each age group?
- Practice taking a complete nursing history with someone you do not know well. What data were difficult to obtain and for what reason? What transitional sentences were necessary to move from one topic to another?
- Practice doing a head-to-toe physical examination on a family member or friend. Were you systematic? Did it take less than 30 minutes? Write a description of your findings in each category (avoid the use of words such as "normal").

■ SUMMARY

1. A nursing history collects subjective data.
2. A patient interview may be enhanced by modifying the environment, listening carefully while focusing on data to be collected, understanding the content base, and asking appropriate questions.
3. The purpose of a nursing history is to obtain data for planning and implementing nursing actions.
4. Different approaches may be used to collect and analyze patient data but the basic data are the same.
5. Modalities of physical examination include inspection, auscultation, palpation, and percussion. The more commonly used modalities in nursing are inspection and auscultation.
6. The most common systematic approach used in a physical examination is a head-to-toe approach.
7. The skin provides information about a person's state of health in addition to skin lesions themselves. Skin changes may result from changes in blood supply, oxygenation or bile pigments, melanin content, nutrition, or hydration. Skin lesions are noted as changes in color, cell growth, fluid content, or consistence/integrity.
8. Breath sounds can be vesicular, bronchovesicular, or bronchial. Adventitious lung sounds are crackles or rales and wheezes or rhonchi. Abnormal sounds result from air flowing through moisture or narrowed air passages.
9. Lung sounds are auscultated starting at the top and moving downward, always comparing one side with the other. The anterior, posterior, and lateral chests are auscultated.
10. S_1 and S_2 are normal heart sounds. S_1 results from closure of the mitral and tricuspid valves. S_2 results from closure of the aortic and pulmonic valves.
11. Extra heart sounds are S_3 (ventricular diastolic gallop) heard in early diastole, and S_4 (atrial diastolic gallop) heard late in diastole.
12. Murmurs are audible heart vibrations occurring from turbulent blood flow; they may be physiologic, functional, or organic.
13. Physical changes with aging may be noted on all the parameters of physical examination (see p. 43).

REFERENCES AND SELECTED READINGS
Contemporary

1. Bates, B: A guide to physical examination, ed 4, Philadelphia, 1987, JB Lippincott Co.
2. *Boyd-Monk, H: Examining the external eye, Part 1, Nurs 80 10(5):58-63, 1980.
3. *Boyd-Monk, H: Examining the external eye, Part 2, Nurs 80 10(6):58-63, 1980.
4. *Cohen, S, and Viellion, G: Patient assessment: examining joints of the upper and lower extremities, Am J Nurs 81:763-786, 1981.
5. Ebersole, P, and Hess, P: Toward healthy aging: human needs and nursing response, ed 2, St. Louis, 1985, The CV Mosby Co.
6. Gordon, M: Nursing diagnosis: process and application, ed 2, New York, 1987, McGraw-Hill Book Co.
7. Malasanos, L, and others: Health assessment, ed 3, St. Louis, 1986, The CV Mosby Co.
8. Murray, R, and Zentner, J: Nursing assessment and health promotion through the life span, ed 3, Englewood Cliffs, NJ, 1985, Prentice-Hall, Inc.
9. Murray, R, Huelskoetter, MW, and O'Driscoll, DL: Nursing process in later maturity, Englewood Cliffs, NJ, 1980, Prentice-Hall, Inc.
10. Patient assessment series, 21 programmed units, New York, 1980, American Journal of Nursing Co.
11. Seidel, H, and others: Mosby's guide to physical examination, St. Louis, 1987, The CV Mosby Co.
12. *Visich, M: Knowing what you hear: a guide to assessing breath and heart sounds, Nurs 81 11(11): 64-76, 1981.

Classic

13. *Roach, L: Color changes in dark skin, Nurs 77 7(1):48-51, 1977.

---

* References preceded by an asterisk are particularly well suited for student reading.

4

Quality Assurance in Nursing

WILMA J. PHIPPS and MARY LOU MONAHAN

CHAPTER OBJECTIVES

After reading this chapter, the student will be able to:

- Define quality assurance.
- Identify three reasons why quality assurance is an important aspect of the practice of nursing.
- Describe the steps of the American Nurses' Association (ANA) model of quality assurance.
- State the difference between standards and criteria.
- Name five mechanisms involved in implementing quality assurance programs.
- Describe the use of quality indicators as one means for monitoring quality of care.

■ IMPETUS FOR QUALITY ASSURANCE

Nursing is committed to professional excellence in providing the highest quality of care possible. Implicit in this commitment is the responsibility to evaluate the quality and appropriateness of that care. However, it has only been in the last 15 years that attempts have been made to develop an extrinsic, systematic approach to monitor and improve care. The impetus for this change has come from a variety of sources: (1) legislation; (2) changes in third-party reimbursement; (3) economic factors; and (4) the nursing profession itself.

■ Legislation

Since the passage of Medicare/Medicaid legislation in 1965, the federal government has become the largest source of third-party health care payment. Because of this increasing financial commitment, Congress and government officials at all levels are under pressure to ensure: (1) that the services rendered are necessary; (2) that they meet professionally recognized standards of care; and (3) that they contain costs.

■ Third-party reimbursement

To establish some system of accountability for these expenditures, Congress created a system for reviewing these expenses as part of Public Law 92-603, the Social Security Amendments of 1972. This legislation established a nationwide network of professional standards review organizations (PSROs) for review of patient care financed by the federal government. Private insurance carriers such as Blue Cross also established standards for review of the care for which they have been asked to make payment.

These efforts were essentially ineffectual and by 1981 more stringent fiscal measures were passed by Congress in the Omnibus Reconciliation Act, which imposed cost-sharing requirements on Medicare beneficiaries and made substantial reductions in federal contributions to Medicaid. Changes in the Social Security Act in 1982 mandated prospective Medicare payments using the 467 Diagnosis Related Group (DRG) categories. Both of these later legislative changes have resulted in cost-containment strategies that have raised increasing questions of whether the quality of health care has diminished because of the increased emphasis on reducing costs.

■ Economic factors

Because health care costs have assumed an increasing share of the gross national product (GNP) in the past decade, consumers and legislators have increased scrutiny of the components of this cost. Reviewing the cost of illness raises vital questions about the relation of quality of care to cost. For example, the principle of "high cost/low benefit" is defined by poor quality of health care in terms of overdiagnosis or overtreatment, which can lead to excessive health care expenditures even in the absence of any *iatrogenic* or untoward consequences. Poor quality in the form of misdiagnosis, mistreatment, or inadequate nursing care can increase mortality or morbidity, length of hospital stay, and loss of earnings, and, therefore, this poor quality can increase the costs of health care to individuals and to society.

The current economic situation that exists with health care costs growing at an unacceptable rate, budgetary cutbacks, and the implementation of the DRG reimbursement scheme has implications for nursing. More than ever before, the nursing profession must demonstrate the value and benefits of its service if it wishes to retain government and consumer support.

■ Professional standards

Last but certainly not least, the nursing profession itself places as its highest goal the delivery of quality health care. The American Nurses' Association (ANA) published *Standards of Nursing Practice*[23] in 1973 for the purpose of ensuring quality health care to the public (see the box on p. 47). However, primary responsibility for implementing these standards rests with the individual nurse in the practice setting. Individual nurses must be familiar with both general and specific standards pertinent to the patient population for whom they are responsible (for example, the standards of care for the orthopedic patient). These standards identify elements of nursing care that must be met to ensure quality care and to provide a baseline for measuring that quality.

Other professional standards that apply to the nurse in the practice setting are nurse practice acts, medical practice acts, and standards set by the Joint Commission on Accreditation of Hospitals (JCAH).[13] Almost every state has a nurse practice act and a medical practice act. Both of these are external sources of standards for nursing practice. Together they define and delineate, from a legal standpoint, the content and practice of nursing.

Nurse practice acts define nursing practice and identify those activities that fall within the province of nursing. *Medical practice acts* further delineate nursing practice by defining those areas that are the exclusive province of the physician. Such exclusions limit the activities in which nurses may engage. Neither act sets actual standards for practice; rather, they define general areas of activity for both professions and establish the legal relationship of the nurse to society and to related professions.

The JCAH is a voluntary, nongovernmental organization that, since its incorporation in 1951, has established standards for operation of hospitals and other health facilities. It conducts surveys and accreditation programs to promote high-quality care and to ensure that patients receive the optimum benefits that medical science has to offer. It emphasizes organization and administration of functions for efficient patient care. Compliance with JCAH standards is recognized by issuance of certificates of accreditation.

The governing body of the JCAH, the Board of Commissioners, consists of 20 persons appointed by its four

---

American Nurses' Association standards of nursing practice

Standard I: The collection of data about the health status of the client/patient is systematic and continuous. The data are accessible, communicated, and recorded.

Standard II: Nursing diagnoses are derived from health status data.

Standard III: The plan of nursing care includes goals derived from the nursing diagnoses.

Standard IV: The plan of nursing care includes priorities and the prescribed nursing approaches or measures to achieve the goals derived from the nursing diagnoses.

Standard V: Nursing actions provide for client/patient participation in health promotion, maintenance, and restoration.

Standard VI: Nursing actions assist the client/patient to maximize health capabilities.

Standard VII: The client's/patient's progress or lack of progress toward goal achievement is determined by the client/patient and the nurse.

Standard VIII: The client's/patient's progress or lack of progress toward goal achievement directs reassessment, reordering of priorities, new goal setting, and revision of the plan of nursing care.

From American Nurses' Association Standards of Nursing Practice, Kansas City, Mo., 1973, The Association Reprinted by permission of the American Nurses Association

---

member organizations: The American College of Physicians, the American College of Surgeons, the American Hospital Association, and the American Medical Association. Currently, nursing is represented on the commission by the American Hospital Association.

JCAH accreditation is voluntary and is not the same as licensure or certification by state or local authorities. However, accreditation has come to be recognized as a benchmark of quality and is used by some regulatory agencies as one criterion for licensure or certification and by some insurance agencies as a condition for honoring reimbursement claims. In addition to its standards for organization of the nursing service department, a standard on quality of professional services was added in 1976, and delineates the characteristics of a patient care evaluation program. In 1985, this standard required the following:

1. A planned and systematic process for monitoring and evaluating patient care
2. Regular data collection to accomplish monitoring and periodic assessment to evaluate it
3. Action plans and evaluation of action plans to assess whether the plans have improved care
4. Documented reports of findings
5. Documented reports of actions
6. Annual appraisal of the nursing quality assurance program

■ DEFINITION OF QUALITY ASSURANCE

Quality assurance can be described on two levels. In its strictest sense, it is a set of techniques for assuring the maintenance and improvement of standards and the efficiency and effectiveness of nursing care; more broadly, it is an effort to control nursing practice. As such, it involves relationships between nurses and consumers and between nurses and governmental bodies.

Quality assurance can be defined as a process that involves evaluating the degree of excellence of the observable and measurable characteristics of delivered nursing care. The purpose of quality assurance is always twofold. First, it determines that extent to which predetermined standards are being met by a particular nursing program. Second, these findings are used to make decisions about changes that are to be implemented by persons carrying out the program of care. Both must be in place if nursing is to ensure its accountability to the consumer. Although the specific target of each evaluation may differ depending on the information about quality that is desired, the purpose of the evaluation is always the same.

Nurses who are engaged in the delivery of health services cannot escape inclusion of quality assurance reviews in their practice responsibilities. Indeed, some proficiency in evaluation must be part of the modern nurse's basic repertoire.

The quality assurance process is not mysterious. Most nurses are well on their way to expertise in this area by virtue of their basic education and experience. Nurses who are expert in the care of specific patient populations, for example, patients with cardiac disease, possess the knowledge necessary to determine desired health processes and outcomes for that population. These nurses are well acquainted with the direct care processes to be used in assisting clients toward health and wellness. They are also aware of the observable changes that will occur at certain intervals in the course of healing.

Most nurses are not expert, however, in the methods used to conduct these evaluations. The following section describes the steps in the quality assurance review process.

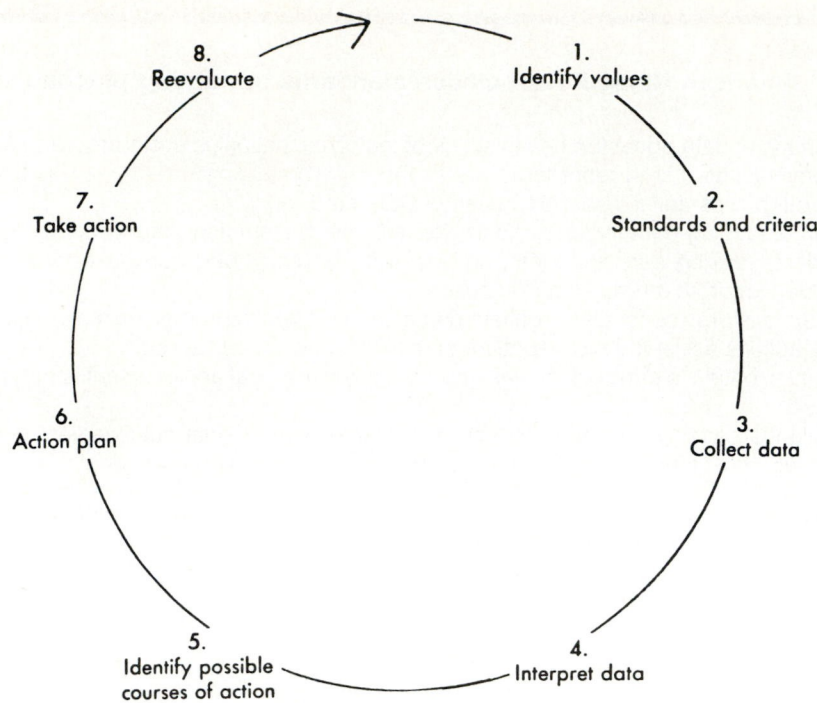

Fig. 4-1 American Nurses' Association model for quality assurance review. (From American Nurses' Association: Quality assurance for nursing care, Kansas City, Mo., 1976, The Association. Reprinted by permission of the American Nurses' Association.)

■ THE QUALITY ASSURANCE PROCESS

A variety of techniques have been proposed to perform the quality assurance review. Presented here is the problem-solving model used by the ANA. Its eight steps include the following:

1. Identify values
2. Identify standards and criteria
3. Measure degree of attainment of standards and criteria
4. Interpret strengths and weaknesses
5. Identify possible courses of action
6. Select a course of action
7. Take action
8. Reevaluate

Each of these steps is discussed and illustrated with a clinical example (Fig. 4-1).

Topics for quality assurance reviews are generally placed in some order of priority based on their frequency and their real or potential impact on patient care. Impact is usually gauged by whether efficiency or effectiveness of patient care is affected. *Efficiency* is generally defined in terms of accomplishing a task with a minimum of resources (time, money, personnel); *effectiveness* is defined in terms of accomplishment of predetermined goals. The focus for the evaluation may be the nurse, the unit or institution, the nursing care, or a combination of the three.

If the focus of the evaluation is the nurse, it can include the actions of a single nurse or of all the nurses in a department, and any area of nursing activity can be examined. For example, is the nursing staff satisfied with the primary nursing program instituted 3 months ago? What criteria do the nursing staff use to determine the frequency of vital sign monitoring in the immediate postoperative period? Are the nursing standards for administration of intravenous therapy being adhered to?

If the nursing unit or institution is the focus of the quality assurance review, it might examine the administrative structure, the physical plant and equipment, or staffing. For example, a review could be implemented to determine whether required educational records for nurses in the critical care units are up to date. Or a review could be done in conjunction with the environmental services department to determine if there is an appropriate number of wheelchairs and IV poles and whether they are all functional.

When nursing care or a nursing care problem is the focus of the review, it is generally best to limit the scope to a certain population (for example, patients with certain diagnoses, surgical procedures, nursing care problems, or degree of illness) so that the project is manageable in terms of all the variables to be considered.

It is critical to remember that the perspective of the consumer must be considered in any evaluation. In selected instances, such as using patient outcomes or in attempting to validate patient care plans with patients themselves, consumer input is essential.

■ Steps in a quality assurance review
■ STEP 1: IDENTIFY VALUES

Before the implementation of the quality assurance model there must be an examination of the *societal, professional,* and *individual values* that guide the health care in the respective agency. The very word *quality* implies that someone somewhere has determined that certain outcomes have more value than others. As applied to nursing care, the individual nurse, nursing unit, hospital, and community will interact to influence the development of criteria to be used in the review process.

To cite some obvious examples, in most Catholic hospitals a high value is placed on human life from the moment of conception; therefore, in a Catholic institution abortions will not be performed. A prevailing societal or cultural value may influence another hospital to favor a youth orientation. The emphasis in health care at that institution may, therefore, be oriented toward teen and young adult programs as opposed to geriatric programs. Whatever setting the nurse happens to be in operates under a set of values that must be identified and understood if the quality assurance review is to be fair and accurate.

■ STEP 2: IDENTIFY STRUCTURE, PROCESS, OUTCOME, STANDARDS, AND CRITERIA

A *standard* is the desirable or achievable level or range of performance of a certain criterion, or a framework against which performance is compared. An example of a standard is, "Every patient will have an admission assessment by a registered nurse." A *criterion measure* is that variable believed to be the indicator of the quality of care, for example, "The assessment form will be completed by the admitting nurse within 8 hours of admission."

The standards for nursing practice are generally developed by clinical nursing leaders in the institution, using their professional expertise as well as professional research and literature. The standards are made operational by construction of the criterion elements. These criteria, which are the actual evaluation criteria, are generally developed by a quality assurance committee, the nursing practice committee, or some similar group.

The actual criteria that are developed can be of three types: structure, process, and outcome (see the box above, right). *Structure criteria* describe the environmental elements, setting, and conditions within which the nurse-patient relationship occurs. It includes the philosophy and objectives of the institution; its fiscal resources, equipment, physical facilities, management structure, accreditation, and licensure; and the quality and characteristics of the professional and technical employees. Examples of structure criteria include, "Hospital beds must be 3 feet apart." "All patients must sign the required consent form before any invasive or surgical procedure." "The current license number of each registered nurse must be on file in the main nursing office."

Process criteria describe the nature and sequence of nursing care activities. For example, process criteria might describe the nursing plan for a patient who demands pain

---

Example of standards and outcomes

Patient goal Adequate pain medication to enable mobilization and pulmonary hygiene.

Structure	Pain medication is available and ordered by physician.
Process	Nursing staff assess patient at least every 4 hours for discomfort.
Outcome	Patient has adequate pain control, and is able to ambulate, cough, and deep breathe.

---

medication every 1½ hours, although he has made a contract with his primary nurse that he will not do so. A teaching plan for a diabetic patient is another example.

Outcome criteria focus on the results of the processes of health care. Many experts consider them to be the ultimate indicators of the quality of patient care. For the patient the outcome should be measurable in terms of change in health, knowledge, or functional status. Examples of outcome criteria for the person with an ostomy are listed in the box on p. 50.

After the criteria have been written, they must be validated, generally by "consensus among peers." The rationale for this validation step is to ensure that all criteria are correct and relevant and reflect nursing practice at the particular institution. Usually, nurses most expert in the selected clinical area are chosen to do the review.

The final step in the criteria writing process is the establishment, by the quality assurance committee and the "nurse experts," of a specific and observable level of performance for each criterion measure. For example, for the outcome criterion "Patient or significant other is able to demonstrate proper technique in insulin administration," at least 90% compliance might be expected. However, for the outcome criterion "Patient is able to apply own stoma appliance," the committee may decide that 80% compliance is appropriate, because many of the patients are elderly, are not completely independent in activities of daily living by the time of discharge, and are frequently discharged to nursing homes.

■ STEP 3: MEASURE DEGREE OF ATTAINMENT OF STANDARDS AND CRITERIA

Multiple methods are available to collect data to assess the attainment of the standards and criteria. The degree to which the actual practice exceeds, meets, or falls below the validated criteria provides the data necessary to evaluate the strengths and weaknesses of the nursing care program. Data collection methods might include *questionnaires, staff interviews, patient interviews, self-assessment questionnaires, performance evaluations, utilization reviews,*

Outcome criteria for the person with a colostomy or ileostomy

The patient or significant other can do the following:
1. Demonstrate how to measure the stoma for an appliance. (The stoma shrinks as healing occurs. Measure the stoma before purchasing more appliances.)
2. Demonstrate proper application of the appliance. (Application includes appliance removal, skin care, and reapplying an appliance.)
3. State plans for follow-up care.
4. State community resources available for obtaining permanent appliances and financial assistance, and list support groups. (Include the name of one surgical supply house, and the telephone number of the Ostomy Association, the Visiting Nurses Association, or some other home care support group.)
5. State need to observe stoma and skin around it for redness, bleeding, or excoriation.
6. Patient or significant other has information packet, which has been reviewed with the nurse.

---

audits, patient or staff complaints, and *direct observation.* Whatever the method selected, the data should be easily accessible, and questions of efficiency and accuracy should be considered.

Specific questions that the quality assurance review committee needs to answer at this point include:
1. Who will collect the data?
2. What will be the source of the data?
3. Where will the data be collected?
4. When will the data be collected?
5. How will the data be collected?

The answers to these questions will assist the committee in deciding whether the review can be accomplished as planned given the inherent requirements for efficiency and accuracy. As a final check, the committee should be certain that each criterion measure is written so that a decision can be easily made as to whether or not the standard has been met.

Once the data has been collected, the results are tabulated, and it is determined whether the percentage of yes and no answers corresponds to the previously established level of performance (that is, percentage of compliance) for each criterion. If the level of performance does not achieve the expectations, the criterion for this evaluation item has not been met.

Table 4-1 illustrates one method for keeping track of a multicriterion evaluation process.

Table 4-1 Criteria tracking form

Outcome criteria for person with colostomy	Level of performance (percentage of compliance)*	Identified problems, strengths, and weaknesses
Patient or significant others can do the following:		
Demonstrate how to measure the stoma for an appliance.	85%	One patient was blind; no documentation on two patients.
Demonstrate proper application of the appliance.	85%	Two patients stated it would have been helpful to have a mirror provided; one patient was blind.
State plans for follow-up care.	60%	Forty percent of patients were being transferred to an extended care facility
State community resources available for purchase of permanent appliances, for financial assistance, and support groups.	80%	Twenty percent of charts audited had one of these components missing.
State need to observe stoma and skin around it for redness and excoriation.	75%	No documentation of this being done on 25% of charts.
Patient or significant other has ostomy informational booklet, which has been reviewed with nurse.	100%	

*Expected compliance in these areas is 100%.

STEP 4: INTERPRET STRENGTHS AND WEAKNESSES

The degree to which the levels of performance have been met serves as the basis for describing the strengths and weaknesses of the nursing care program. However, it is essential that certain subtle factors not be overlooked before final judgments are made. Consider the following: One of the outcome criteria for a patient with a pacemaker is, "The patient or significant other is able to take a pulse." A retrospective nursing audit was done on patients with pacemakers to determine whether the outcome was being met. On nursing unit A, 95% of the patients could take their pulse, whereas on nursing unit C, only 65% of the patients could. Careful inspection of the patient data revealed that, in general, patients on unit C were older, had fewer significant others, and were frequently discharged to extended care facilities. Comparing the two units on these factors provided insights into reasons for their differences that may have been missed if the evaluator had not questioned these differences.

STEP 5: IDENTIFY POSSIBLE COURSES OF ACTION

After identifying the strengths and weaknesses, possible courses of action to correct the weaknesses are developed. The goal of the action plan is elimination of the weaknesses and reinforcement of the strengths of the existing program. Consideration should be given to how best to motivate the nursing staff to implement the desired changes. Generally the best results will be obtained when those staff most affected by the quality assurance review are involved in the planning of subsequent courses of action.

Solutions to the identified problems can be numerous and can include administrative changes, further clinical research into the problem, continuing education, changes in practice, environmental changes, a reward system for improved compliance, or even the organization of peer pressure. Each of the possible solutions has advantages and disadvantages, and the peer group will have to weigh each one.

STEP 6: SELECT A COURSE OF ACTION

After examining the alternatives, the peer group selects the course of action, based on such considerations as the identified problem, available resources, and organizational structure. How the decision is implemented will vary among institutions. After a decision is made, different institutions will make varying decisions about how the plan for change is presented to the administration and how the change is to be implemented. In the case of a nursing practice change, at one institution the director of nursing may wish to make the final decision and at another institution the director of nursing may only wish to be informed of the findings, and the committee may be charged with making appropriate changes.

STEP 7: TAKE ACTION

Improving the quality of nursing care implies change, and sooner or later some *action must be taken*. Implementation of selected action generally includes time frames, persons responsible for overseeing each step of the plan, and selection of a date for reevaluation. This action step is critical to the success of the quality assurance review.

STEP 8: REEVALUATE THE PROCESS

We have added this step to the original ANA model. The rationale for its addition is to illustrate that once a corrective action or other type of action has been taken, the action must be monitored to ascertain if it has been effective in solving the problem. Therefore, once an action has been taken, the cycle begins over again. See the box on p. 52 for a clinical example of a quality assurance review.

MONITORING ACTIVITIES AND INSTRUMENTS

In addition to the problem-focused quality assurance reviews, a variety of methods have been devised for ongoing assessment of the nursing care program. Some of the more frequently used methods are described here.

Incident reports

Whenever an untoward event occurs involving a patient, nurse, or visitor, an incident report must be completed. Generally these are compiled by the hospital and/or the hospital insurance carrier. Increases in certain types of incidents, such as medication errors or patient falls, would be a signal to the quality assurance committee that a review of either of these two areas may be indicated.

Quality indicators (monitors or screens)

Recently the JCAH has mandated that quality indicators be monitored on an ongoing basis. Each department in an institution determines its own quality indicators.

Quality indicators are those items that a health care agency believes are indicators of quality patient care. For example, quality indicators used by a nursing service would depend on the patient population being served and on *high-risk, high-volume events* that need to be monitored. In medical-surgical nursing, quality indicators might include: (1) number of patient falls, (2) ratio of medication errors to the total doses administered, and (3) the number of pressure sores (decubitus ulcers). For each of the quality indicators a threshold of acceptance is set. In the case of falls it might be not more than one patient fall per nursing unit each month.

Quality assurance review topic: learning needs of the patient with a colostomy or ileostomy

Step 1: Identify values

Patient and family education and patient involvement in care are high priorities at this institution. Nurses on the surgical units were concerned that ostomy patients, in particular, were not receiving adequate discharge information.

Step 2: Identify criteria

The outcome criteria (revised in 1985) for the person with a colostomy or ileostomy were selected as the evaluation criteria (see the box on p. 50).

Step 3: Collect data

Charts of 30 patients with the discharge diagnosis of some type of ostomy were selected at random from patients discharged in the previous 6 months. Review of the patient record using the outcome criteria for the person with a colostomy or ileostomy revealed incomplete teaching plans and no record of the patient having received any type of information booklets. (The rule is, "If it isn't documented, it hasn't been done.")

Step 4: Interpret data

The quality assurance committee was certain that the patients had received more information than was documented in the record. But where was such documentation to be found? It was also apparent to the committee that some of the criterion elements required updating.

Step 5: Identify possible courses of action

It was observed that the documentation system for discharge planning for these patients needed to be more efficient, yet more thorough. The surgical nursing staff suggested that the outcome criteria sheet be printed on a Nurse's Note Sheet. Another suggestion was to use a large stamp containing elements of the teaching plan, which could be checked off as completed. A group of experienced nurses was formed, who, with the assistance of the clinical nurse specialist, rewrote and assisted in the validation process for the outcome criteria.

Step 6: Write the action plan

The quality assurance committee met with the surgical nursing staff and concluded that the best choice was to have the outcome criteria overprinted on the Nurse's Note Sheet. The appropriate administrative approval was obtained.

Step 7: Implement the action plan

One member of the quality assurance committee was assigned to oversee the production of the new forms. After they were obtained, the unit nursing staff took the responsibility for introducing them and explaining their purpose to the other staff members. An evaluation was planned for 4 months later.

Step 8: Reevaluate

Four months after the implementation, the surgical nursing staff conducted a repeat review. There was 100% compliance with each criterion element.

By setting the threshold for acceptance a determination can be made as to how well the quality indicator is being met. It is important to establish in advance how and at what intervals data will be collected for each quality indicator.

The appropriateness of each quality indicator needs to be *assessed* on a *regular basis*. If a particular indicator is no longer high risk or high volume, consideration should be given to deleting it. The important thing to remember is that *quality indicators* should not be stagnant but should change as circumstances change.

■ Nursing audit

The nursing audit compares predetermined criteria with the documentation found in the patient record. There are two types of audit: retrospective and concurrent. A *retrospective audit* is a critical examination of nursing actions, with a view toward improvement in practice. A retrospective review is done after the patient has been discharged. The reviewer has the advantage of using data from the patient's entire stay, from admission to discharge, and of evaluating the results for a large series of comparable patients. One advantage of a retrospective audit is that sometimes practitioners gain impressions from single cases in which they are personally involved. These impressions, however, may not be borne out by later systematic study of a large number of cases.

A *concurrent audit* is a critical examination of the patient's progress toward a desired health status (outcome) and patient care management activities (processes) while the care is in progress. Patient questionnaires, interviews, and observation and review of the patient record are possible sources of data for a concurrent review. Concurrent review has the advantage of providing opportunities for making changes in the ongoing care program. Retrospective and concurrent reviews each have their own advantages, and may be used singly or together in a quality assurance review. The term *nursing audit* is being used less frequently; it is being supplanted by the term *evaluation study*.

■ Peer review

Nursing peer review occurs when nurses establish standards and criteria and evaluate the quality of each other's patient care. The peer review process may be performed within a single unit or by specialty, for example, orthopedic nurses. Clinical nurse specialists also frequently have a peer review group that monitors their practice.

■ Patient satisfaction questionnaire

A patient satisfaction questionnaire is generally used when written data regarding a patient's perceptions of his or her hospitalization are needed, for example, by hospital management or a nurse researcher. Many hospitals routinely distribute these questionnaires to all patients and request that they complete them. Other hospitals have patient ombudsmen who visit patients, question them regarding their hospitalization experience, answer any questions they may have, and intervene in their behalf, if necessary.

■ Staff satisfaction surveys

Staff satisfaction surveys, either questionnaires or interviews, are used by the administration to assess general employee satisfaction or to test responses to certain program changes.

■ Utilization review

The utilization review program was mandated by the JCAH in 1978. Its primary goal is the appropriate allocation of hospital resources. This program does not focus primarily on nursing, but it does provide data that may require nursing involvement in a more thorough evaluation.

■ Infection control reports

Because nurses are involved in the direct care of patients, they may at times be included in infection surveillance and infection control programs. Even when the nursing staff is not involved directly, they should be familiar with the monthly report of nosocomial infections on their respective unit. Questions can be raised about nursing procedures and practices that may affect the infection rate on the unit.

■ ETHICAL ISSUES

Several other issues are being raised as part of the quality assurance process. These issues relate to confidentiality of patient information and ethical problems encountered as part of the quality assurance process. Both of these are discussed below.

■ Confidentiality and the quality assurance process

Confidentiality of data is an issue frequently associated with quality assurance. The availability and use of evaluative data about a patient or groups of patients has always been of concern to health professionals. The increasing use of *computerized data* about patients has generated enormous concern for potential *threats to privacy*. Most quality assurance studies can be conducted without the recording of patients' names and are reported in terms of *aggregate data*. Review of care provided to an individual patient requires constant vigilance to ensure protection of the patient's identity.

■ Ethics and quality assurance

Ethical problems can and do influence the quality assurance concerns of nurses. Certainly there are traditional areas of mutual interest: patient education, informed consent, and unnecessary surgery or procedures. But ethical problems probably occur much more frequently than is apparent through patient care evaluation, particularly because quality assurance has focused largely on technical aspects of care—whether appropriate tests are ordered, whether surgical complications were prevented or managed, and whether patient records list the steps taken in treatment.

For several reasons, quality assurance will need to focus more on *ethical decision making* in the future.

First, the rapidly increasing opportunities in patient care will provide more options for patients and providers. A heart transplant for one patient, for example, may mean that a heart must be sacrificed in a comatose patient who is on a ventilator. *Balancing individual rights* with *social good* will become more frequent and more difficult in the future.

Second, as resources continue to diminish, problems of *distributive justice* will arise. It is quite possible that in the future some type of health care *rationing* could exist. Who should receive this service? How much service should they receive? Who should pay? As public policymakers attempt to reduce all care choices to cost-benefit analyses, nurses must be aware of the limitations of these calculations and

---

Putting knowledge to practice

■ Identify one clinical problem and the steps you would use to assess it using the ANA model.
■ Identify four nursing process standards for a patient with impaired mobility.
■ Investigate the impact of the quality assurance program on the quality of patient care in a hospital in which you have clinical experience.

---

the inability of accounting for human pain and suffering mathematically.

Third, nurses as well as other health professionals must participate in these ethical decisions or risk losing their unique influence entirely. For example, in cases of the comatose, terminally ill patient, peer review would focus not only on the clinical aspects of death but also on the human dimension. Did the health care provider confer with the patient and/or family to keep them totally informed? Were the providers guided by the wishes of the patient and family? Did the provider seek competent, objective, and relevant third-party opinions?

None of the decisions can be made irrespective of federal or state laws? But there are questions of quality that lie within the realm of quality assurance activity. In addition to questions of nontreatment, other *ethical dilemmas* must be recognized, analyzed, and resolved within a quality assurance framework. One approach suggests that decisions themselves are less important than the approach taken by the participants. In analyzing problems did they use accurate and necessary information? Was the reasoning logical? Did the decision-maker account for the values and rights of the individual? Use of the systematic quality assurance process has much to offer in this area in the future.

■ SUMMARY

1. Nursing's commitment to professional excellence includes monitoring the quality of care given.
2. Four factors have influenced quality assurance in nursing. These are (1) legislation, (2) changes in third-party reimbursement, (3) economic factors, and (4) professional standards.
3. The ANA Standards of Nursing Practice include 8 standards to be followed by all nurses in giving care.
4. The Joint Commission on the Accreditation of Hospitals (JCAH) is a voluntary organization that accredits hospitals.
5. The JCAH publishes an Accreditation Manual, which includes a standard for quality of professional services. This standard forms the basis for evaluating patient care.
6. The ANA quality assurance model consists of 8 steps:
   a. Identify values.
   b. Identify structure, process, outcome, standards, and criteria.
   c. Measure the degree of attainment of standards and criteria.
   d. Interpret strength and weaknesses.
   e. Identify possible courses of action.
   f. Select a course of action.
   g. Take action.
   h. Reevaluate.
7. Outcome criteria pertinent to a specific patient population must be developed as part of the quality assurance process and before an evaluation of the quality of nursing care can be made.
8. Outcome criteria should be measurable in terms of change in health, knowledge, or functional status of the patient.
9. Structure criteria describe the setting and conditions in which the nurse-patient relationship occurs.
10. Process criteria describe the nature and sequence of nursing care activities.
11. Quality assurance is an ongoing process in which the results of the evaluation of patient care are interpreted to caregivers so that needed improvements in care can be made.
12. Quality indicators are items that a health care agency believes are indicators of quality of care.

REFERENCES AND SELECTED READINGS
Contemporary

1. Aduddell, P, and Weeks, L: A cost effective approach to quality assurance, Nurs Econ 1:279-82, 1984.
2. Bergman, R: Evaluation of nursing care: could it make a difference? Int J Nurs Stud 19:53-60, 1982.
3. *Blake, B: Quality assurance: an ethical responsibility, Supervisor Nurs 12:32-38, 1981.
4. *Brown, BJ: Quality assurance update, Nurs Adm Q 7(3):1-93, 1983.
5. Bulman, T: Ambulatory care: a practical way to quality assurance, Nurs Manage 16(12):19-24, 1985.
6. *Curtis, B, and Simpson, L: Auditing: a method for evaluating quality of care, J Nurs Adm 15(10):14-21, 1985.
7. Davis, K: Nursing and the health care debates, Image 15:67, 1983.
8. Donabedian, A: Criteria, norms and standards of quality: What do they mean? Am J Public Health 71:409-412, 1981.

---

*References preceded by an asterisk are particularly well suited for student reading.

9. Ferguson, D, and Brunner, N: Balancing priorities to attain quality care, Nurs Manage 13:67-69, 1982.

10. Griffith, N, and Megel, M: Quality assurance: an educational approach, Nurs Outlook 29:670-673, 1981.

11. Howe, M: Developing instruments for measurement of criteria: a clinical nursing perspective, Nurs Res 29:100-103, 1980.

12. Inzinga, M: Legislative issues and health care trends: quality assurance, Nurs Adm Legislative Update 8:80-85, 1984.

13. Joint Commission on Accreditation of Hospitals: Accreditation manual for hospitals, Chicago, 1988, The Commission.

14. *Lane, G, Cronin, K, and Peirce, A: Teaching diploma students how to utilize the ANA quality assurance model, J Nurs Educ 21(9):42-44, 1982.

15. *Maciorowski, L, Larson, E, and Keane, A: Quality assurance evaluate thyself, J Nurs Adm 15:38-42, 1985.

16. Padilla, G, and Grant, M: Quality assurance programme for nursing, J Adv Nurs 7:135-145, 1982.

17. Smeltzer, C, Fettman, B, and Rajki, K: Nursing quality assurance: a process, not a tool, J Nurs Adm 13(1):5-9, 1983.

18. Tucker, S, and others: Patient care standards: nursing process, diagnosis and outcome ed 4, St. Louis, 1988, The CV Mosby Co.

20. Westfall, UE: Nursing diagnosis: its use in quality assurance, Top Clin Nurs 5(4):78-88, 1984.

21. Williamson, J, and others: Teaching quality assurance and cost containment in health care, San Francisco, 1982, Jossey-Bass, Inc., Publishers.

Classic

22. American Nurses' Association: Quality assurance for nursing care, Kansas City, Mo, 1976, The Association.

23. *American Nurses' Association: Standards of nursing practice, Kansas City, Mo, 1973, The Association.

24. Marriner, A: The research process in quality assurance, Am J Nurs 79:2158-2161, 1979.

25. *Moore, K: What nurses learn from nursing audit, Nurs Outlook 27:254-258, 1979.

26. Phaneuf, M: The nursing audit, ed 2, New York, 1976, Appleton-Century-Crofts.

UNIT II
Health Promotion

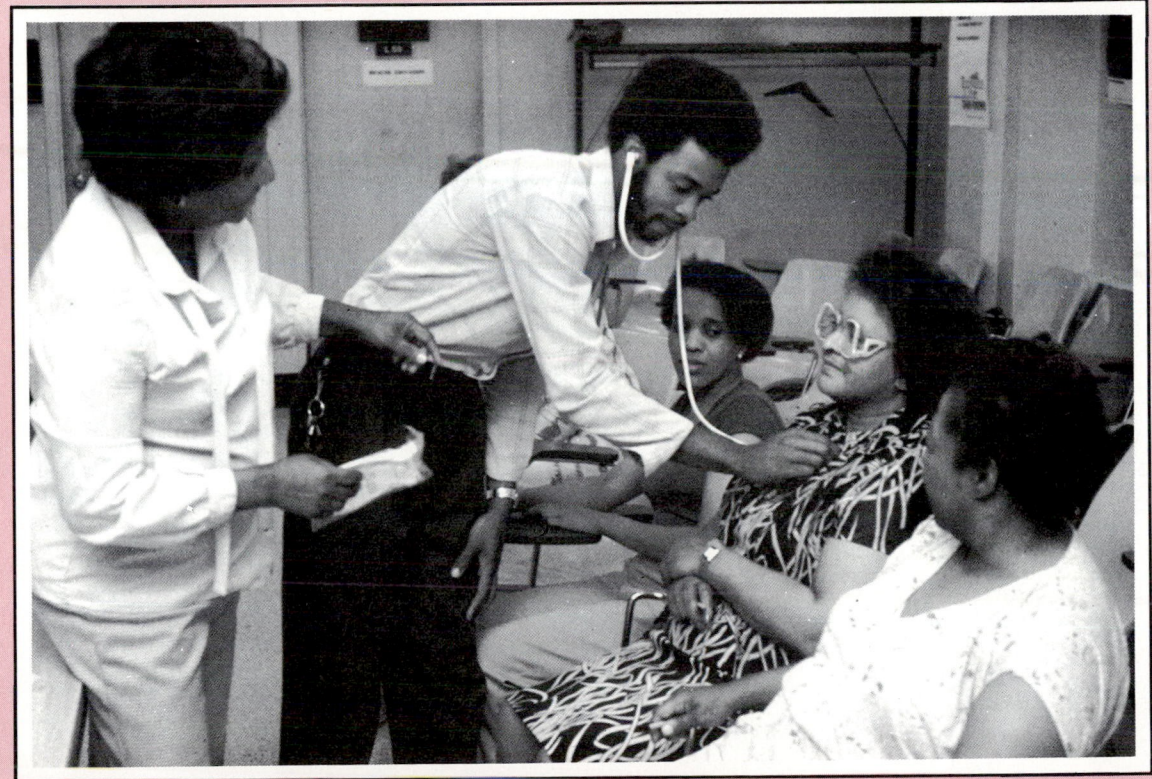

5

Developmental Factors Affecting Health of Adults

RUTH LINCOLN

CHAPTER OBJECTIVES

After reading this chapter, the student should be able to:

- Describe physical development characteristics of each adult age group.

- Describe changes in sexuality characteristics of each adult age group.

- Describe the characteristics of the three adult stages of psychologic development.

- Describe the developmental tasks of young, middle, and late adulthood.

- Identify the health needs of each adult age group.

- Identify the major health concerns of each adult age group.

- Describe general nursing interventions for the elderly patient.

Every person for whom the nurse provides care is engaged in the process of growth and development. Changes in physical and psychosocial development occur in adults as they move from young adulthood to middle adulthood and then to late adulthood.

Growth refers to an increase in size, or change in structure, function, or complexity. *Development* is the patterned lifelong changes in thought or behavior that evolve as the organism matures.[41] It is evident that physical, mental, social, emotional, and spiritual aspects of development are interrelated. However, not all aspects will progress simultaneously.

The most striking difference between adults and children is the lack of orderly progression through the developmental stages in adulthood. Children experience growth and accomplish developmental tasks at approximately the same age. As adults age, they experience increasing complexity and diversity.[17] This is important to recognize when comparing adults to each other.

■ YOUNG ADULTHOOD

Young adulthood, extending from approximately 20 to 45 years of age, is a complex period of life, a time in which the transition from adolescence to adulthood is the primary focus. During the young adult years, energies are directed toward career initiation, social involvement, and establishing a life-style.

■ Physical development

Full growth and development are complete by the early to mid-twenties, and most body systems are functioning at optimal levels (see the box below).

■ Sexuality

Sexuality is an integral part of self-concept. Competence in the area of sexuality is of prime importance during adult years. During young adulthood the body's sexual response is powerful and there is a need to find satisfactory expression. A man reaches peak sexual capacity at about 18 years of age, and a woman generally in her early thirties.

If the expression of sexual feelings is restricted, perhaps because of illness or injury, causing a felt or imagined change in body image, sexual concerns may become paramount. Nurses frequently are asked by young adults for assistance with marital or sexual problems. Unless the nurse is secure in his or her own sexual identity and has had adequate preparation to deal with such matters, he or she will have difficulty assisting others with sexual issues. The nurse must also be aware of appropriate persons to whom referrals can be made (Chapter 33).

■ Psychosocial development

Adulthood is often equated with maturity. It is characterized by a sense of responsibility, maintenance of appropriate impulse control, ability to plan and implement realistic goals, and capacity to enter into intimate relationships.

Everyone does not arrive at young adulthood with the same level of maturity. Emotional maturity varies from person to person, as do intellectual ability and physical characteristics. In addition, an adult who appears reasonably mature under usual circumstances may, under stress, exhibit certain immature behavior, for example, when the stress of illness occurs.

In Erikson's *eight ages of man,* the first adult stage is characterized by *intimacy versus isolation* (Table 5-1). Intimacy involves sharing the self to form a commitment to an intense lasting relationship with another person, a cause, or a creative effort, without fear of loss of identity. Intimacy requires the ability to trust. The inability to develop some form of intimacy leads to increasing feelings of isolation, alienation, and self-absorption.

The successful resolution of this phase of the life cycle is dependent on a positive self-concept. How persons feel about themselves affects relationships and the choices made during this period. A person who feels adequate and competent in setting and achieving goals tends to have positive outcomes. Negative feelings may foster withdrawal and the inability to mobilize resources for positive gains. When caring for the young adult, it is therefore important

---

Physical development in the young adult

1. Posture is erect, and maximum height is achieved.
2. Muscle tone and coordination are optimal.
3. Energy levels are high, and well controlled.
4. Skin is smooth and taut.
5. Tissue repair and healing occur readily.
6. Body rhythms are established.
7. Reproductive capabilities are high.

From Murray, R, and Zentner, J: Nursing assessment and health promotion through the lifespan, ed 2, Englewood Cliffs, NJ, 1979, Prentice-Hall, Inc.

Table 5-1 Psychosocial development in adulthood

Age	Erikson's eight ages of man
Young adulthood: 20 to 45 years	*Intimacy versus isolation* Significant objects, persons, causes
Middle adulthood: 45 to 65 years	*Generativity versus stagnation* Significant persons: spouse, grandchildren, friends
Late adulthood: 65 + years	*Integrity versus disgust, despair* Significant persons: spouse, family members, friends

to assess the individual's self-perception. These data not only provide information about motivation potential, but also form a basis for nursing intervention to help increase the individual's self-esteem.

■ BODY IMAGE

Body image, an important aspect of self-concept, is a mental picture of the body's appearance, as well as the attitudes, emotions, and personality of the individual. At a period of life when acceptance by others is most important, and with society's emphasis on youth, beauty, and physical fitness, any alteration in body function or structure poses a threat to a positive body image. Adaptation to these alterations depends on the nature and meaning of the threat, existing coping mechanisms, and available support systems.

Nursing interventions to help someone deal with a threat to or a change in body image include the following:

1. Careful assessment of the individual's perception of the condition
2. Assistance in helping the person maintain a realistic perception of the threat in relation to total self-image
3. Assistance in identifying useful coping mechanisms (Chapter 7)
4. Identification of support systems

■ Intellectual development

The highest overall performance on intelligence tests is achieved sometime between the late teens and late twenties. Longitudinal evidence has shown, however, that general intelligence remains the same or increases during the adult years.[5]

■ Developmental tasks

The focus of the developmental tasks of early adulthood is the choice of life-style. Although fairly clear boundaries have been established between self and parents by this time, parental attitudes and value systems have been internalized in young adults. Inherent in future life choices

---

Tasks of young adulthood

Leaving the family of origin
Establishing a new home base
Choosing a life-style
Developing sexual bonding
Reexamining commitments
Choosing a vocation

From Levinson, D, and others: The psychosocial development of men in early adulthood and the midlife transition. In Ricks, D, Thomas, A, and Roffields, M (Editors): Life history research in pathology, Minneapolis, 1974, University of Minnesota Press.

is the quest for independence from family socially and economically (see the box below, left).

■ OCCUPATIONAL CHOICE

An occupation is much more than a set of skills and functions. It determines the environment in which the person lives. Occupational choice plays a significant part in shaping the personality by providing a social system, status, roles, and life-style. The choice of an occupation often requires pursuing appropriate education, and thus educational goals and achievements become a very important part of this choice.

The women's liberation movement has exerted a significant influence on women's choices. It is socially acceptable for women to choose a career goal. Among married young adults there is a growing tendency to delay having children until economic and career goals are more solidified.[7] Some women in this age group may choose to have an abortion if they become pregnant at a time that is inconvenient to their career or other pursuits.

■ MARITAL CHOICE

A major decision of early adulthood is whether to marry. Our society continues to support marital status among young adults. While there may be many reasons for entering the marital relationship, marriage is generally recognized as a close and loving partnership between two people where intimacy and affection exist in a free and equal relationship.[41]

The arrival of the first child initiates the roles of parenting. Preparation for parenthood has not been widespread in our society. It is therefore difficult to anticipate many of the stresses of being a parent and the changes required in life-style.

Although the institutions of marriage and family are the most socially acceptable, tolerance for diversity in life-styles is increasing. Communes, living together, single parenthood, childlessness, bisexuality, and homosexuality are among the many choices for young adults.[41] When assessing young adults, nurses should be sensitive to the influence of the person's life-style on health problems.

■ Health needs

The importance of studying growth and development lies in gaining better understanding of those physical and psychosocial variables that determine the health needs of individuals as they progress through life. Physical growth ceases by the time a person reaches young adulthood. Change in life-style is reflected in physical and psychosocial needs of the adult.

■ NUTRITION

The young adult's nutritional needs are not the same as those of adolescents. With cessation of physical maturation there is a reduction in some nutritional requirements, such as calcium and protein, whereas an increase in some nutrients, such as vitamin B₆ and C, is necessary. In addition, young men require additional vitamin E and riboflavin, and young women need additional iron.

Nutritional problems of young adults frequently stem from the increased demands of job, home, children, and economics. The nurse can help the young adult understand the importance of adequate nutrition and of adjusting schedules to allow more time for meals. Young adults should have an understanding of the influence of inadequate nutrition on illness and recovery.

■ EXERCISE, REST, AND SLEEP

Exercise serves several functions in the young adult. It helps to regulate appetite, release tension, aid sleep, tone body muscles, maintain cardiovascular conditioning, and retard aging. Exercise should be regular and appropriate to the person's physical condition (Chapter 6).

As the demands of work, social activities, responsibilities, and educational pursuits increase, the young adult's need for adequate rest and sleep also increases, but in actuality the young adult often goes without proper rest and sleep. Although an individual can adjust to a lack of sleep for a short time, prolonged periods can contribute to altered mental and physical functions.[41]

■ Health concerns

Accidents are the leading cause of death in young adults. Many injuries and illnesses require restriction of activity, which presents social and economic problems.[41] Injury and illness may also necessitate some dependence, creating conflict with developmental tasks.

Acute conditions such as *upper respiratory tract infections* occur more frequently in the young adult than do other acute illnesses. With young adults, the primary responsibility of the nurse is the teaching of preventive measures. Prevention is directed at supporting the body defenses and reducing susceptibility to illness. The nurse should stress avoiding environmental pollutants, keeping alcohol intake at an acceptable level, and observing basic health practices.

Physiologic and psychologic changes resulting in unusual

Major health problems of young adulthood

Accidents (especially motor vehicle)
Acute respiratory tract infections
Periodontal disease
Hypertension
Stress reactions
Suicide
Alcoholism
Drug addiction
Battered women

---

or disturbed adaptive behavior patterns occur when the young adult is unable to cope with newly acquired tasks and responsibilities. Mate selection, marriage, childbearing, college, job demands, social expectations, and independent decision making are all stressors. Stress may be a major factor in the incidence of *gastric* and *duodenal ulcers*. When stressors are perceived as overwhelming, they may result in self-destructive behavior such as *drug abuse and addiction, alcoholism,* or *suicide,* one of the leading causes of death in young adults. Nursing interventions include measures to reduce or cope with stress (Chapter 7).

The major health problems of young adults are listed in the box below, left.

■ MIDDLE ADULTHOOD

The transition from young adulthood to the middle years is developmental rather than a dramatic body change.

As the young adulthood phase begins to taper in the middle to late 30s, perceptions of time, productivity, self, and others begin to change. Individuals approach the middle years with a sharpened sense of awareness as they begin to take stock of life:

Has it been fulfilling?

Am I doing what I really want to be doing?

Am I really going to accomplish my original, probably idealistic goals?

What are my goals in life from now on?

Evaluation of the quality of life already lived and the potential for the future may have a significant influence on adaptation in the succeeding years.

■ Physical development

The adult usually approaches this phase of life functioning at near peak efficiency. As the middle years progress, gradual physiologic changes occur:

1. Hair begins to turn gray.
2. Skin becomes dryer and less elastic.
3. Fatty tissue is redistributed regardless of diet or exercise.
4. Skeletal muscle increases in bulk until about age 50 years; no changes occur in smooth muscle.
5. Sensory changes begin to be noted:
   a. Presbyopia (decrease in near vision) results from decreased elasticity of the eyes.
   b. Auditory acuity gradually decreases.
6. Menopause occurs in women, usually between ages 40 and 55 years (Chapter 34).

■ Sexuality

The physical aspects of aging, together with the many pressures common to this stage of life, affect the attitudes about one's sexuality and sexual functioning.

Some adults view middle age (particularly after menopause) as lessening their physical attractiveness, thus affecting sexual interest and capacity for competent sexual functioning. Others, especially women, feel that the middle years find them at their best sexually. They enjoy the freedom from menstruation and feel an increase in vigor and power. Ambivalence about growing older in a youth-oriented society often breeds feelings of inadequacy relative to one's sexuality. As a result, some adults may become depressed and sexually unresponsive. Others feel a need to retrieve that sense of youthfulness by behaving and dressing in a youthful manner or by having an affair with a younger person.

The middle-aged adult who approaches these years with self-acceptance and appreciation continues into the later years with a satisfying and fulfilling sex life.

Some of the physical changes that accompany menopause may affect the pleasure of sexual intercourse. For example, decrease in the production of vaginal lubrication caused by hormonal changes may result in some discomfort during intercourse. Use of a water-soluble lubricant during intercourse may be helpful.

As men age, certain social and psychologic factors influence their sexual responsiveness. Several recurrent themes relative to waning sexual responsiveness can be noted:

1. Monotony in the sexual relationship or a feeling of being taken for granted
2. Concerns with economic or career pursuits
3. Mental or physical fatigue
4. Physical or mental illness of the individual or spouse
5. Overindulgence in food or drink
6. Fear of failure[22]

Continued sexual activity contributes to the quality of the relationship and to the continuation of sexual activity into the later years.

Because of prevailing cultural attitudes about waning sexual interest in the middle years, sexual concerns are often ignored in the care and rehabilitation of the middle-aged adult. It is very important, therefore, that health care providers become knowledgeable about and sensitive to the sexual needs of patients, particularly those who experience injury or illness that restricts physical activity.

■ Psychosocial development

Erikson has described adaptation to middle age in terms of resolution of the crisis, *generativity* versus *stagnation* (Table 5-1). In a broad sense, generativity includes guiding the next generation, productivity, creativity, and concern for others. When this enrichment and fulfillment are not experienced, stagnation and personal impoverishment occur, to the point of isolation and preoccupation with self.[33]

■ Intellectual development

Mental capacity is unimpaired in the middle years. Active use of mental powers throughout the years will contribute to mental productivity in the later years. The middle-aged adult is encouraged to continue activities that facilitate mental productivity, even during episodes of illness and hospitalization.

Role transitions of middle adulthood

Renewing relationships with partner or significant other
Rediscovering dormant creativity
Taking on civic responsibility
Accepting physical changes of middle age
Developing a wholesome relationship with parents
Learning to parent one's adult children
Preparing for retirement
Acknowledging plateaus in most areas of life
Reevaluating life goals

■ Developmental tasks

The psychologic and social development of the individual in the middle years is best exemplified by role transitions (see the box above). Role transitions involve alteration in self-image, life-style, values, and attitudes. This age group is at the peak of productivity, wields the most power, and demonstrates the greatest social influence.

The ability to change roles and take on new roles smoothly contributes to a creative and productive life during the middle years. Where the focus of life revolved solely around the children, their departure from the home may be felt as loss. What is lost is not only the grown child but also all the attachments associated with the parent role.[42] Furthermore, the health status of one's parents is changing. Illnesses and perhaps impending death often necessitate assuming the role of parent to one's own parent(s). Decisions regarding the care of aging parents may require changes in life-style.

During the middle years, renewal and full development of relationships can occur, and the patterns of child-centered days and of nurturing the intimate relationship of husband and wife change. The individual may enjoy the enrichment of new and renewed relationships and a new sense of freedom. If throughout previous years a couple has not developed mutual support, open communication, and awareness of each other's needs, the development of an enriching relationship may be difficult for the couple to achieve.

For some adults the middle years are a time of peak social influence, prosperity, economic success, and stability. But for others the middle years are approached with a sense of frustration and failure if goals and expectations set earlier have not been reached. The realization that the time has passed for significant achievement of status and success is often crisis producing.

The literature indicates that for many adults a major midlife crisis occurs between the ages of 40 and 50. Both men and women reevaluate their life, relationships, and vocational choices. Divorce, career changes, and life-style changes may be the result of this *stock-taking*.[10] The women's movement has contributed to the motivation of women to seek self-fulfillment and usefulness in a new vocation or avocation.

Productive use of leisure may be a source of contentment for some adults, with the exploration and development of new areas of talent, skill, and hobbies. Involvement in outside activities demonstrates the external orientation characteristic of this period of life. The mobilization of inner resources generates the creativity and productivity that facilitate continued growth throughout the remaining years.

■ Health needs

As individuals change, so do their health needs. Consideration of the needs of proper nutrition, rest, and exercise are most important during the middle years.

■ NUTRITION

Reduced energy requirements together with reduced physical activity dictate a decreased demand for calories. The middle-aged adult needs to lower intake of saturated fats and cholesterol, which may contribute to obesity and atherosclerosis. The diet should contain the basic four food groups (Chapter 6), with an emphasis on protein, minerals, and vitamins. Caloric intake should be based on age, body build, size, and activity.

■ EXERCISE AND REST

Changes in life-style may lead to a lack of exercise, restful sleep, and relaxation. It is important that rest and sleep be balanced with physical activity to keep the body functioning at its optimum (Chapter 6). An assessment of daily activities may give some indication about the kind and amount of exercise necessary. Middle-aged persons should take the following precautions regarding an exercise program[36]:
1. Before starting an exercise program, consult a physician if overweight, have a personal or family history of cardiovascular or respiratory disease, or have a sedentary life-style.
2. Increase exercise gradually.
3. Exercise consistently.
4. Avoid overexertion (10 minutes after exercising, the heart rate should return to baseline status).[36]

■ HEALTH ASSESSMENT

Middle-aged adults should be encouraged to have regular complete medical examinations, including rectal or proctoscopic examination. Women should have regular pelvic examinations, including a Papanicolaou test. Routine dental, vision, and hearing tests will help prevent periodontal disease, glaucoma, and hearing loss. Women should be taught how to do breast self-examination (BSE) once a month following the menstrual period (see Chapter 36).

Major health problems of middle adulthood

Cardiovascular disease
Pulmonary disease
Rheumatoid arthritis
Cancer
Diabetes
Obesity
Alcoholism
Anxiety
Depression

■ Health concerns

Motor vehicle accidents, occupation-related accidents, and falls in the home are leading causes of death in middle age. Fractures and dislocations are the most common injuries. Respiratory conditions are frequent causes of absenteeism from work. Generally, middle-aged women have more disability days from work because of respiratory and other acute disorders, whereas men have more disability days from injury.[41] The major health problems of this age group are listed in the box above.

The close interrelationship between the physical and psychologic makeup of the human body is exemplified in menopause. How a woman reacts depends a great deal on her feelings about herself and her womanhood. If procreation and motherhood have been her major sources of self-esteem and she cannot adapt to physical changes and changing life circumstances, she may become severely depressed and require treatment. Many women adjust to menopause without difficulty (Chapter 34).

Although men do not undergo the same physiologic changes as women do, they often go through a kind of psychologic "change of life." Symptoms may include fatigue, headaches, increased moodiness, impatience, worry, and complaints such as indigestion, heartburn, rapid or irregular heartbeat, and insomnia. These symptoms may be associated with preoccupation with thoughts of aging, anticipation of retirement, loss of career status, and a general feeling of worthlessness.

For the middle-aged person who feels depressed, trapped, frustrated, or isolated, easily accessible escape mechanisms are often alcoholism, drug abuse, or excessive food intake. Hypochondriasis is a symptom of the self-absorbed adult and may be a means of gaining attention. The self-absorbed person is likely to demonstrate regressed, immature behavior resulting in increased dependency. Suicide is a leading cause of death among the middle aged.

Adults may experience numerous highly stressful life events. The use of a stress index, such as Holmes and Rahe's life change units (LCUs), may offer predictive value for predisposition to illness (Table 5-2). The stress index

Table 5-2   Social readjustment rating scale (life change units)

Life event	Mean value	Life event	Mean value
Death of spouse	100	Son or daughter leaving home	29
Divorce	73	Trouble with in-laws	29
Marital separation	65	Outstanding personal achievement	28
Jail term	63	Wife beginning or stopping work	26
Death of close family member	63	Begin or end school	26
Personal injury or illness	53	Change in living conditions	25
Marriage	50	Revision of personal habits	24
Fired at work	47	Trouble with boss	23
Marital reconciliation	45	Change in work hours or conditions	20
Retirement	45	Change in residence	20
Change in health of family member	44	Change in schools	20
Pregnancy	40	Change in recreation	19
Sex difficulties	39	Change in church activities	19
Gain of new family member	39	Change in social activities	18
Business readjustment	39	Mortgage or loan less than $10,000	17
Change in financial state	38	Change in sleeping habits	16
Death of close friend	37	Change in number of family get-togethers	15
Change to different line of work	36	Change in eating habits	15
Change in number of arguments with spouse	35	Vacation	13
Mortgage over $10,000	31	Christmas	12
Foreclosure of mortgage or loan	30	Minor violations of the law	11
Change in responsibilities at work	29		

From Holmes, T, and Rahe, H, J Pyschosom Res 11:213, 1967.

lists 43 events that may cause a crisis for the adult. Some of these are *death of spouse, separation, jail term,* and *change in job.* A high stress level, indicated by a large number of stressful events or several events with high ratings, can identify an individual who is more vulnerable to disease. Nurses should assess hospitalized patients for the number of stressors impinging on them in addition to the current illness. If the adult is at high risk, the nurse may mobilize extra supports for the person and encourage healthy coping mechanisms. The family, as well as the individual, will need encouragement and help.

■ LATE ADULTHOOD

The number of elderly in the United States is increasing dramatically. By the year 2000, the elderly will comprise 12% of the population. The growth rate of those 75 years and older is even greater than that of the elderly as a whole.[37] The reasons for the growth are decrease in infant mortality, control of communicable diseases, improved treatment of acute and chronic diseases, and technological advances in medicine and surgery.

Although 65 years of age is usually considered the beginning of late adulthood, or old age, tremendous individual variation exists. Age is really a sociocultural concept and not wholly physiologic and chronologic. The three main components of the aging process are biologic age, psycho-

logic age, and social age. Some people may be old at 45 years, whereas others are not old at 75 years.

Biologic aging has been explained as programmed senescence (biologic clocks, predetermined sequences) and as random deterioration (mutations, radiation hits, metabolic waste products).[33] No single theory is adequate to explain the multiplicity of changes in the human organism.

■ Physical development

In late adulthood, physiologic function does not correlate with chronologic age. Adult years are not characterized by specific events at particular ages, with the exception of

---

Major components of aging

Biologic age	Position in time relative to potential life span
Psychologic age	Capacity for adapting to the environment
Social age	Role in family, at work, and in the community, as well as interests and activities

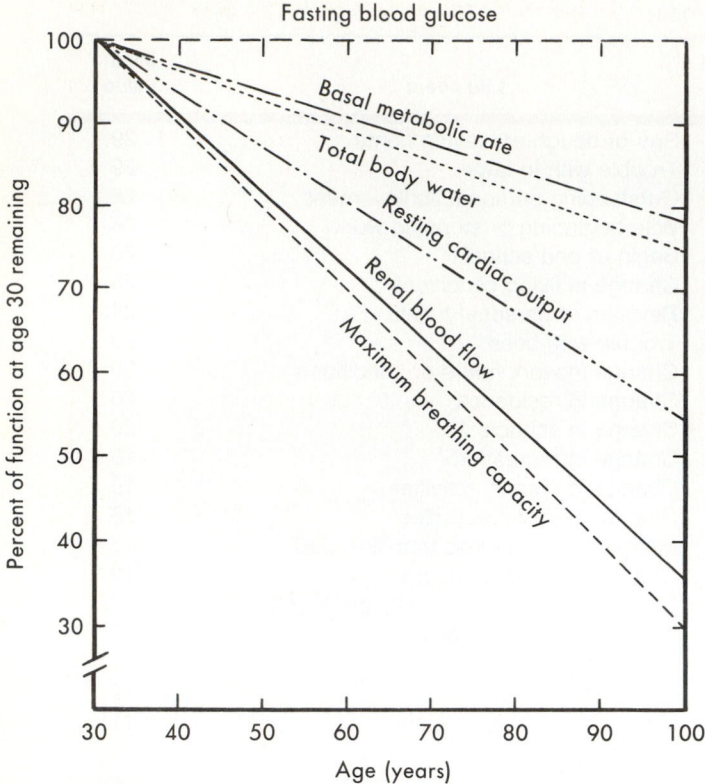

Fig. 5-1 Biologic concepts of aging. (From Shock, NW: Biologic concepts of aging. In Simon, A, and Epstein, LJ (editors): Aging in modern society. Washington, DC, 1968, American Psychiatric Association. Reprinted by permission.)

menopause. Some biologic variables remain constant throughout the lifespan (for example, fasting blood sugar, blood pH, serum electrolytes). Other body functions begin a gradual decline after age 30, continuing into the late decades (Fig. 5-1). Certain generalizations can be made, however.

1. The older the age group, the greater the variability among individuals.
2. The rate of decline varies between body functions.
3. Changes previously thought to be associated with aging have been shown to be a result of a lack of physical conditioning or of disease.

■ PRIMARY AND SECONDARY AGING

Primary aging refers to biologic changes that are universal, gradual, intrinsic, and inevitable. Graying hair and wrinkles are examples of primary aging changes. *Secondary aging* refers to pathophysiologic conditions. These may be more prevalent in the elderly but are not universal. More importantly, secondary changes are treatable and sometimes reversible. In the past, many conditions that were attributed to old age have been proven to be pathologic. Some of these are senility, arthritis, loss of hearing, muscle weakness, and incontinence. The 93-year-old man who complained to his doctor about his gimpy right leg is an

Physiologic changes of aging

Cardiovascular system
  Decreased elasticity of blood vessels
  Decreased cardiac output
  Possible blocking of blood vessels by fatty deposits (atherosclerosis)
  Increased peripheral vascular resistance leading to increased blood pressure
  Slowed circulation
  Decreased efficiency of valves in veins of lower extremities
Respiratory system
  Decreased elasticity of lungs and chest wall
  Decreased recoil of lungs
  Increased residual lung volume
  Decreased forced expiratory volume
  Decreased oxygen pressure (Po_2) (about 4 mm Hg/decade)
Nervous system
  Generalized loss of neurons
  Progressive decrease in weight of brain
  Decreased gag reflex
  Decreased sensory status (vision, hearing, touch, taste, and smell)
Musculoskeletal system
  Decreased lean muscle mass
  Increased body fat
  Decreased muscle strength
  Demineralization of bones (especially vertebrae and femur)
  Decreased joint mobility
Gastrointestinal system
  Decreased intestinal motility
  Decreased control of defecation
Urinary system
  Reduced renal blood flow
  Decreased glomerular filtration rate
  Decreased bladder muscle tone
  Decreased control of voiding

example of primary vs secondary aging. The doctor said, "You're old; you have to put up with aches and pains." The old man retorted, "Tell that to my left leg."

The nurse working with the elderly must know the common aging changes (see the box above). Assessment should include baseline function, prediction of functional changes, and discrimination between primary and secondary aging. Because the elderly themselves often believe the myths regarding what they "must put up with," they need to be encouraged to seek medical treatment for their chronic and acute conditions. Some symptoms, such as weakness and fatigue, are helped by diet and exercise. Often an elderly person can improve aspects of physical functioning.

■ Sexuality

Both men and women maintain interest in sexual activity into the late adulthood years. More women cease having sexual activity after age 65 than do men. The primary reasons for the cessation are lack of acceptable sexual partner for widows or an ailing husband for married women (rather than lack of interest).[15]

Both sexes are influenced by cultural attitudes toward the elderly. Older men and women tend to be thought sexually unattractive and lacking in ability to engage in sex. However, Masters and Johnson[40] have found that although sexual responses are slower, the elderly still have the same phases of excitement, plateau, orgasm, and resolution as younger persons. Men, in particular, can expect adequate sexual performance up to and beyond the eighth decade (see Chapter 34).

Sexual problems occur more frequently for the elderly. Women may have dyspareunia as a result of vaginal thinning and decreased lubrication.[41] These factors are caused by postmenopausal steroid starvation. Men tend to be affected by secondary impotence caused by performance anxiety and low self-esteem. Diabetes, alcohol, and medications for hypertension are other prominent causes of impotence.[41]

Masters and Johnson report a condition known as "widower's syndrome."[40] Following an extended period of sexual inactivity, a man cannot achieve or maintain an erection. An equivalent condition occurs in women in which the vagina constricts and undergoes atrophic changes. The conclusion to be drawn is that those who do not engage in sexual activity lose the ability.

Sexuality is more than the physical act of intercourse. Elderly persons continue to need human companionship and the sharing of love and affection. Nurses need to be aware of the components of sexuality and how the elderly may be affected by chronic illness, loss of a partner, and need for touch. Being sensitive to family dynamics is just as important for a newly married couple in their seventies as for a young couple.[18] Through counseling the nurse can explain aging changes, suggesting vaginal lubrication for women and extra physical stimulation for men. Changes in sexual position and styles of lovemaking are appropriate for those with disabling diseases. Nurses have a vital role in enabling elderly persons to express their needs for love and affection.

■ Psychosocial development

Aging has long been associated with deterioration in function rather than an expansion of abilities. Early theories of aging, such as *disengagement theory* (withdrawal from society)[27] and *activity theory* (finding substitutes for lost function),[34] are inadequate. New evidence is accumulating to support multifactor systems theories to account for the richness and variety encountered in individuals in late adulthood.

Reed proposes the view that adult development is a progressive, not a decremental, phenomenon.[17] She emphasizes the role of person-environment interactions in successful aging and views aging behavior not as decremental, but as "trade-offs." Important concepts are that adults:

1. Have a clearer perception of themselves and others not clouded by the context of the situation
2. Are better equipped to engage in complex and meaningful interactions with others
3. Conceptualize problems better and delegate less complex details to others
4. Are better able to predict future consequences
5. Develop more realistic solutions to problems
6. Are increasingly capable of transforming conflicts into meaningful experiences

The "trade-offs" for the older adult are a decreased intellectual dexterity, decreased flexibility in thinking, and loss of ability to remember details. These may appear as deficiencies to young adults but actually help the elderly provide a stabilizing force for society.

A positive outlook on aging is crucial to the nurse's capacity to evaluate the abilities of the elderly in any setting. An 84-year-old woman admitted to the hospital from a nursing home is not the equivalent of a regressed child. She should be regarded as an experienced adult, integrally related to the environment, no matter what her functional level.

Nurses are challenged to facilitate well-being among adults who have developed useful modes of functioning as they age. Strategies are not appropriate if they are based on physical strength, deftness of function, and speed of recall. The tasks of late adulthood are summarized in the box above.

■ Intellectual development

Intellectual function curves stay relatively stable throughout the life span (Fig. 5-2). Research has shown that many components of cognitive function remain intact in the elderly. Problem solving, verbal ability, recognition, and memory span are examples of areas in which normal elderly persons scored well.[23] Only when the tests were timed and speed was important did results decline.

The implications for the nurse are clear when devising teaching strategies for the elderly. Older adults should be

---

Tasks of late adulthood

Adjusting to declining physical strength and health
Adjusting to retirement and change in financial status
Accepting reorganized family patterns
Adjusting to a new pattern of social and civic responsibilities
Adjusting to death of significant others
Establishing affiliation with one's age group
Maintaining satisfactory living arrangements
Developing point of view about death

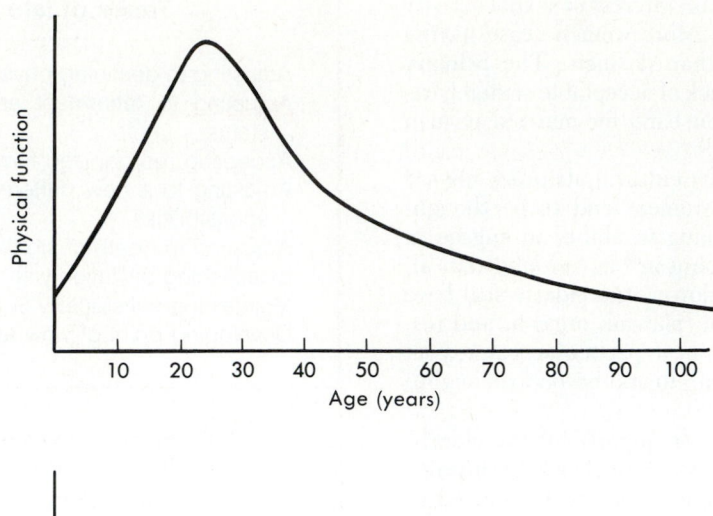

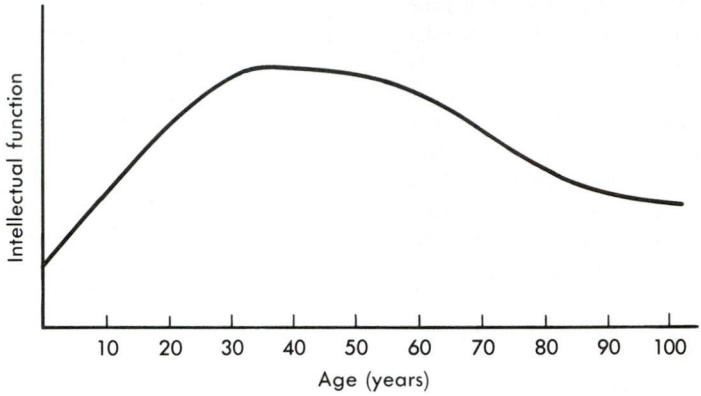

Fig. 5-2   Comparison of physical and intellectual function over life span.

Major health problems of late adulthood

Heart disease
Hypertension
Cancer
Renal disease
Chronic obstructive pulmonary disease
Acute pulmonary disease (pneumonia, pulmonary edema)
Vascular disease (cerebrovascular accident, peripheral vascular disease)
Arthritis
Skin disorders
Accidents
Alcoholism

Stressful life changes for the elderly

Loss of driver's license
Multiple relocations
Hemiplegia
Sensory deficits
Hospitalization
Institutionalization
Mechanical speech difficulties
Loss of children and friends
Dispersal of significant belongings
Incompetency proceedings
Inheritance conflicts
Birth of grandchildren
Moving to a nursing home
Inadequate health insurance coverage

assumed to be able to learn. The content will be retained best if it is related to something familiar, it is sequenced, and there is plenty of time to learn each facet.

■ Health concerns

Nearly all of the body systems are affected by the secondary aging process. Chronic diseases are a major health problem and are much more common among the elderly population (see the box on p. 68, left). Estimates show that 85% of the elderly have one or more chronic diseases. Heart disease and hypertension are the most prevalent, with 50% of persons over the age of 65 years having observable signs of heart disease. Gastrointestinal disorders, rheumatism, and arthritis affect large numbers of the elderly. Visual problems, atherosclerosis, lung disease, and hypertension appear to be associated with lower socioeconomic status.

The figures on prevalence of health problems may be misleading. The important issues are: (1) what is normal functioning and (2) how disabling are the chronic conditions?

Despite chronic disease, 83% of persons over the age of 65 have little difficulty carrying out activities of daily living. Only 5% live in nursing homes, although 35% will be in a nursing home at one time or another. Another 5% are homebound.[24]

The following factors are important to remember when evaluating the physical capacities of the elderly:

1. Organ systems have a great compensatory ability, in spite of loss of cells and tissue through aging (such as in the brain, kidney, heart, and liver).
2. Compensatory mechanisms may fail when the organism is stressed through illness and disease (for example, renal failure can occur with urinary tract infection).
3. The body takes a longer time to return to normal following a stressful event.
4. Once a stressful event has occurred, the individual may not return to baseline function.
5. The immune system is decreasingly effective as the individual ages, causing increased susceptibility to infection. The elderly are much more prone to pneumonia, skin infections, urinary tract infection, and sepsis.
6. The symptomatology of a particular disease is often atypical in the elderly (for example, a myocardial infarction without severe crushing chest pain, an infection without a fever, a gastrointestinal hemorrhage without severe stomach pain).
7. The most typical sign that an individual has had a change in physical well-being is sudden onset of confusion.[26]

Stress situations may produce more pronounced reactions in the elderly and require a longer period of readjustment. The Holmes-Rahe Stress Scale has been criticized for lack of applicability to the elderly. Stressful events peculiar to older adults are found in the box on p. 68.

Variables associated with altered thought processes

Physologic
Pulmonary disease
Cardiovascular disease
Anemia
Infections
Trauma
Dehydration
Electrolyte imbalance
Hypoglycemia/hyper-
  glycemia

Medications
Sedatives/hypnotics
Narcotic analgesics
Antihypertensives
Antiarrhythmics
Anticonvulsants
Diuretics
Digitalis
Tagamet

Environmental
Strange equipment
Unfamiliar surroundings
Restraints
Tubings (IV, Foley)
Strange people

Sensory limitation
Decreased vision
Decreased hearing
Sensory overload
Sensory deprivation

Emotional stressors
Loss of health
Loss of loved ones
Loss of home
Loss of cherished pos-
  sessions
Loss of pets
Expectations of sick role

Adapted from Roberts, B, and Lincoln, R: Cognitive disturbances in hospitalized and institutionalized elders (abstract), Nurs Res 35(2):126-127, 1986.

■ Altered thought processes

The nursing diagnosis "altered thought processes" is a common occurrence among hospitalized elderly adults. Although 75% of the elderly have normal intellectual function, many factors can cause temporary reversible confusion (see the box above). The most significant diagnostic factor is that the disorientation occurred suddenly and recently.

Imagine a relatively independent 72-year-old woman who comes to the hospital with pneumonia. She is stripped of her belongings, taken to a strange room, jabbed with needles, and barraged by questions from strangers. A needle is placed in a vein for antibiotics; her hands are restrained to keep her from pulling it out. Her glasses and hearing aid are in the drawer. She compensates adequately until nightfall. Then she cannot distinguish shapes or outlines. She becomes quite agitated, thrashing about. A sedative does nothing to help her. Suddenly she cries out, loosens her wrists, gets out of bed and falls. The many stressors have overtaxed her hypoxic brain and she has become confused and delirious.

The nurse can prevent or at least minimize these common effects by a few simple measures. Patients should be given detailed, repeated explanations of where they are and what is being done to them. Glasses and hearing aid should be placed on the patient while he or she is awake. Maintaining adequate hydration and pain control is often sufficient to clear confusional status. A friend or relative staying through the night could eliminate the need for restraints, and an antihistamine is preferable to a sedative for sleep.[21]

The nurse should anticipate that any elderly patient is at risk for confusion. When gathering assessment data, the nurse is alert to any previous history of confusional episodes, chronic and acute medical conditions leading to hypoxia or hypoxemia, sensory deficits, and medications that may trigger confusion.

Although temporary confusion is the more common form of altered thought processes, the nurse should be aware that *chronic dementia* may be superimposed. The most common dementia is *Alzheimer's disease,* which afflicts 50% to 60% of those who have organic brain disease (Chapter 19). This devastating condition progressively affects the memory until the patient no longer remembers how to eat, dress, or toilet nor even remembers loved ones' faces.[5] The patient and family need great support and encouragement when the patient with Alzheimer's is hospitalized for an acute illness.

Depression is often confused with dementia and can occur with true dementia; therefore, in many elderly persons, treatable depression is not recognized. If there is any possibility that depression exists, the older person should receive treatment.

■ Health needs and nursing interventions

The goal of medical and nursing care is to keep people functioning at the highest possible level for their age. This includes helping them adjust to living with chronic ailments and continuing degenerative changes.

Similarities between childhood and old age should not be assumed, because they are not valid. Even in the matter of helplessness there is no similarity. Children are in ascendance; they are developing new power daily and marking up achievements over their environment. The aged person's helplessness is infinitely more frustrating because it is increasing rather than decreasing.

Nursing care depends on the physiologic and anatomic changes, the diseases that are present, and the person's emotional makeup and apparent adjustment to the particular situation. Older persons frequently talk at length about their families and the past; their conversations may give clues to interests that should be encouraged and to problems confronting them. Plans should be made to help them maintain as much independence as possible despite their limitations. Community resources are available to assist older persons to maintain independence and meet their social needs (see the box above right).

Community support services for older persons

Senior citizen centers	Social, nutritional, educational, and counseling services
Geriatric day care centers	Assistive daytime nursing care, and social, nutritional, and rehabilitative services may be available
Adult foster home care	Care in private home for the older person who is unable to live alone
Meals on Wheels	Meals delivered to the person's home
Homemaking service	Household chores, shopping, and so on
Transportation service	Arranged pickup by public transportation system
Home health service	Skilled home nursing care
Legal services	Will, settlement of estate

■ PROMOTING SELF-WORTH

When giving nursing care to elderly patients, it is necessary to take special care to build and protect their sense of worth and feelings of adequacy:
1. Call patients by name; avoid using terms such as *grandma* or *grandpa.*
2. Face patients when speaking, and enunciate clearly to prevent embarrassment from not hearing; do not shout.
3. Give explanations clearly and slowly to prevent misunderstanding.
4. Provide written instructions for activities the patient must follow independently.
5. Give as much control as possible over procedures and routines.
6. Involve the patient in all decisions regarding treatment, no matter what cognitive impairments are present.

■ SELF-CARE DEFICIT

All persons prefer to maintain their independence and perform their own activities of daily living. For the elderly, who may see a loss of independence as a real possibility, self-care provides a sense of control of their lives.

1. Place equipment and personal supplies within easy reach.
2. Provide self-help devices such as handrails in halls and bathrooms, sturdy chairs with arms, and assistive devices such as tongs for reaching and special utensils for eating.
3. Clear room of clutter to facilitate use of walkers and wheelchairs.
4. Provide *time* and equipment for personal physical care.
5. Adjust hospital routines whenever possible to correspond to patient's usual daily routines.

■ IMPAIRED SKIN INTEGRITY

The most striking change in the skin of the elderly is dryness. Dryness occurs as *seborrhea* and sweat glands decrease their production of sweat and oils necessary for supple, healthy skin. Testing for skin turgor is difficult in the elderly using the normal measurements; checking skin over the sternum gives more accurate results. Other normal (primary) skin changes are wrinkles (loss of subcutaneous fat), "liver spots" (hyperpigmented areas), senile purpura, and seborrheic keratoses (see Chapter 39). The elderly are also more susceptible to contact dermatitis from jewelry, scented cosmetics, and soap.

Because the skin is likely to be very dry, daily bathing is often contraindicated. Because of dryness, poor circulation, and low resistance, the skin readily becomes infected. A podiatrist should care for very hard nails and other conditions such as calluses and corns.

1. One or two baths a week are sufficient.
2. Mild glycerine soaps are preferred.
3. Bath oils may be used.
4. Apply lotion to dry skin areas immediately after the bath to retain moisture.
5. Soak feet and dry carefully, especially between toes.
6. Use preventive measures to protect skin of elderly patients confined to bed (for example, alternating pressure or egg crate mattress, flotation pad, sheepskin pads, frequent position changes).
7. Brush hair daily with soft-bristled brush.
8. Avoid frequent shampooing; encourage use of conditioner.

■ ALTERED SENSORY PERCEPTION

Elderly who are bed bound for all or part of the day are especially susceptible to pressure sores and shearing lesions. Pressure sores are ischemic areas of breakdown that occur when fragile tissue is compressed between a bony prominence (sacrum, heels, scapulae) and a firm surface such as a mattress or a chair. Shearing lesions arise from loss of outer layers of skin resulting from friction when a person is moved or turned in bed. Treatment of deep pressure sores can cost thousands of dollars. Nurses are in the best position to prevent this serious complication.

Prevention requires meticulous attention to relief of pressure through turning schedules and pressure-reducing devices. Maintaining clean, dry skin, adequate hydration (up to 2400 ml per day), and supplemental nutrition for the malnourished are equally critical to prevention of lesions.

The eyes of older people accommodate more slowly to changes in light. Bright lights or sunlight may be almost unbearable; therefore, blinds may need to be partially drawn. Many elderly persons see poorly in the dark; night lights are used to reduce confusion and to prevent those who get up during the night from having accidents. Cataracts, failing vision, and blindness are common in the aged (Chapter 20). Many older persons require glasses or contact lenses. These visual aids must be protected from damage or loss and need to be kept clean for best use.

The major changes that affect the hearing of elderly adults are difficulties with speech discrimination, loss of ability to hear high pitched tones, and problems with background noises. Nurses should make certain that any hearing aids are functioning correctly and are being used whenever the patient is awake.

■ ALTERED ORAL MUCOUS MEMBRANE

The gums of elderly persons become less elastic and less vascular. They made recede from the remaining teeth, exposing sensitive areas of a tooth not covered with enamel. Progressive diseases of the gum may have caused loss of teeth. Many elderly persons have decayed, broken, or missing teeth. This leads them to avoid foods that are difficult to eat, affecting nutrition.

By 70 years of age, tooth loss is common and may necessitate dentures. Care of dentures and prevention of their loss are part of the general nursing care of elderly patients. Many individuals older than 65 years have oral lesions of which they are unaware. The mouth is assessed for presence of white patches (leukoplakia), irritations, and growths.

■ IMPAIRED MOBILITY

One of the more common problems of secondary aging is joint and muscle disease. Osteoarthritis, rheumatism, and osteoporosis are prevalent among the elderly. As joints stiffen and muscle tone decreases, the individual may develop an awkward, halting gait. It becomes difficult to rise from a chair or to get in and out of cars or buses. Impaired gait, cardiovascular changes, sensory deficits, and osteoporosis, make the elderly susceptible to falls. The factors contributing to falls are listed in the box on p. 72. Falls account for 23% of deaths and injuries in people over the age of 65.

Nurses in the acute care setting must maintain a balance between preventing injury from falls and promoting independence in self-care. Restraints should be kept to a minimum and used only as a last resort. Providing assistive aids for walking (canes, walkers) and keeping self-care items conveniently located will help prevent falls.

Factors associated with falls

Intrinsic

Limited mobility
Decreased vision
Confused mental state
Orthostatic hypotension
Decreased ability to
   maintain equilibrium

Extrinsic

Poor lighting
Unfamiliar environment
Loose slippers
Cluttered equipment
   and furniture

Causes of malnutrition in the elderly

Acute and chronic illness
Limited financial resources
Psychologic factors such as boredom and lack of
   companionship while eating
Loss of teeth
Faulty eating patterns
Fads and notions regarding certain foods
Lack of energy to prepare foods
Lack of knowledge of appropriate nutrition
Decreased digestive enzymes

Suggestions for the older person to keep the musculo-skeletal system healthy while hospitalized include the following:

1. Use a firm mattress for good body alignment.
2. Use light, warm bedcovers, tucked loosely to permit active movement in bed.
3. Place pillow under shoulders, as well as head, to permit good chest expansion.
4. Teach patient exercises to be done daily:
   a. Legs: flexion, extension, abduction, adduction
   b. Arms: cross over chest, extend over head
   c. Neck: raise head from flat position

■ SLEEP PATTERN DISTURBANCE

Elderly people have less stage 4 (deep) sleep and more periods of awakening; REM sleep is often interrupted.[2]

At home the person may get out of bed, read, wander about the house, and even prepare something to eat at odd hours. Some wakefulness can be expected in the elderly patient who is hospitalized. A low bed, night lights, and adequate supervision help prevent accidents. The nurse monitors the extent of wakefulness to ascertain that the patient does have periods of sleep. Elderly patients, like all others, may be unable to sleep. Many sedatives may interfere with REM sleep and cause confusion in the elderly. An antihistamine is the sleeping medication of choice. Altered sleep patterns that are normal in aging need to be differentiated from depression and dementia.

■ PAIN AND DISCOMFORT

Protective adipose tissue under the skin disappears with age, and the volume of circulating blood, particularly to the small outer arteries, may be diminished. This affects the ability to withstand chilling without discomfort. Many elderly persons suffer from mild arthritis and fibrositis, which produce vague muscle and joint pains. Several layers of lightweight clothing are warmer than fewer heavy layers if the person is cold. Many elderly persons wish to wear socks and additional clothing in bed. Provision must be made to prevent drafts in the room while maintaining good air circulation.

■ ALTERED NUTRITION

Many elderly people are undernourished. Some causes of malnutrition are listed in the box above. It is not unusual for the older person's diet to be high in carbohydrates and low in vitamins, minerals, and protein, especially if the person lives alone. Qualitative nutritional needs of the elderly are essentially the same as for other adults except that caloric needs diminish. Increased fiber is beneficial to the gastrointestinal system. Fluid intake is important.

Some elderly persons are obese, even though undernourished. Weight reduction in the aged person should be gradual and supervised by a physician. Sudden loss of weight is poorly tolerated by many elderly persons whose vascular system has become adjusted to the excess weight.

■ ALTERED ELIMINATION

Activity of the intestinal musculature may be decreased with age, and supportive structures in the intestinal walls become weakened. Sensory perception is less acute, so the signal for bowel elimination may be missed. Constipation occurs, and in turn leads to fecal impaction. The very elderly and the somewhat confused patient may need to be reminded to go to the bathroom after meals. Measures to prevent constipation (Chapter 31) take high priority in the care of elderly persons. Any marked change in bowel habits is reported to the physician because cancer of the large bowel and diverticulosis are fairly common among this age group.

Urinary incontinence affects 11% to 30% of hospitalized elderly. Chronic loss of urine is categorized as (1) stress incontinence (dysfunctional internal sphincter), (2) urge incontinence (detrusor instability), (3) reflex incontinence (nerve innervation dysfunction), (4) total incontinence (mixed neurologic and mechanical problems), and (5) functional incontinence (urine loss without organic cause).[19] Women are most affected by urge and stress incontinence, whereas men have more problems with dribbling and retention associated with obstructive disease.

Nurses can best assist those with this socially and psychologically distressing problem through accurate differential diagnosis and strategies based on the diagnosis. Strategies most commonly involve timing of fluids and habit retraining such as bowel or bladder training (see Chapters 31 and 32).

Some patients develop temporary urinary incontinence as a result of a urinary tract infection, inability to get to the bathroom, and altered fluid intake caused by illness and diagnostic testing. The nurse should be alert to early symptoms of incontinence. Reassurance that the loss of urine can be treated will help alleviate the embarrassment and feelings of shame the elderly often have.

Nosocomial infections are a frequent sequela to use of indwelling urinary catheters (Chapter 11). Patients who are catheterized longer than 3 days, are immunosuppressed, or are bed bound are more at risk. The nurse should take great care to cleanse the perineum and use meticulous handwashing practices.

MEETING PSYCHOSOCIAL NEEDS

Elderly patients are often lonely and appreciate just talking with others. Volunteers may provide a service by visiting with the elderly. Many patients appreciate visits with a member of the clergy. When visiting with elderly persons, it should be remembered that, although they commonly talk about events and activities in their own past, they usually are interested in the activities of young persons and of the world about them.

The need to be useful is important to all persons. There are many tasks in which even the elderly person who is ill may be able to participate. At home, the elderly may be able to help with the dishes or with meal preparation. They may be interested in crafts or making useful items. The older person may be quite slow, and great care must be taken not to show impatience, which may discourage further participation.

Elderly persons are usually aware of death as an imminent possibility and sometimes see it as a welcome event. The issue should not be avoided. If the patient shows genuine concern about death, the nurse can encourage discussion of feelings (Chapter 15). The family may also need opportunities to discuss their feelings about death.

■ Special precautions related to diagnosis and treatment

■ MEDICATIONS

Elderly persons consume disproportionately more prescription and over-the-counter drugs than do middle-aged adults because of increased frequency of illness, especially chronic illness. These drugs may not be well tolerated and may produce adverse reactions and interactions or unpredictable responses in the elderly. Age-related physiologic changes contribute to altered responses to drugs in the elderly. The effects of the medications may be altered in various ways (see the box above, right).

Factors affecting drug response in the elderly

Effect	Cause
Decreased drug absorption	Decreased hydrochloric acid
	Altered gastrointestinal motility
Altered drug distribution	Storing of fat-soluble drug in fatty tissue
	Decreased serum albumin for binding of drugs
Altered drug metabolism	Decreased enzyme activity in liver
Decreased drug excretion	Decreased renal blood flow
	Decreased glomerular filtration rate
	Decreased number of functional renal tubules

Drugs have a definite place in the therapeutic regimen in the elderly, but their use must be monitored carefully. In general, *drug levels should be increased or reduced gradually,* and *the fewest possible number of drugs should be used.* If the patient is emaciated or very elderly, the use of full adult doses of drugs should be questioned.

In planning self-administration of drugs with the elderly, it is helpful to determine when it is easiest for the person to remember to take medication. This time is usually tied to some incident of daily living, such as arising or taking meals. The use of a medication checklist may be helpful. Some persons have found it helpful to use something with compartments, such as an egg carton, with the days marked off. One dose is placed in each compartment, and it is easy to see whether the medication has been taken.

■ DIAGNOSTIC TESTS

Diagnostic tests should be judiciously spaced to prevent overtaxing the elderly individual. Routine preparations for tests may need modification to prevent exhaustion or dehydration. Elderly persons may become weak or dizzy from pretest preparations such as multiple enemas or withholding of food. Weak patients should not be left unattended on a treatment table. Persons who are dizzy are advised to sit up slowly and to remain sitting on the table for a few moments before standing. The dizziness is caused by the slow compensation of inelastic blood vessels.

Because of the rapidity with which they develop pressure sores, pads should be placed under the normal curves of the back and under bony prominences in elderly patients who must lie on treatment or operating room tables for lengthy periods. If the patient is placed in the lithotomy position, both legs are placed in (and removed from) the stirrups at the same time to prevent pull on unresilient muscles.

Putting knowledge to practice

- List some of the stresses most common to persons in your own age group. How do these compare with stresses in your parents' age group?
- Talk with and observe persons in age groups other than your own. How do you and they differ in terms of physical development and major concerns in your lives?
- Review the eating patterns of an elderly person of your acquaintance; compare his or her food intake with your understanding of an adequate diet. If there are inadequacies, what are some possible reasons?
- From what you have read in newspapers and heard discussed, what would you select as major problems of elderly people in your community?
- What services are available for the elderly in your community?

■ STANDARDS FOR GERIATRIC NURSING PRACTICE

The American Nurse's Association has developed standards for geriatric nursing practice that embody those interventions considered to be based on knowledge derived from nursing, the natural, behavioral, and applied sciences, and the humanities. The standards address themselves to the following nursing actions:

1. Observing and interpreting signs and symptoms of normal aging, as well as pathologic changes, and intervening appropriately.
2. Differentiating between pathologic social behavior and the usual life-style of the aged person.
3. Demonstrating an appreciation for the heritage, values, and wisdom of older persons.
4. Supporting and promoting physiologic functioning in the aged.
5. Providing protective and safety measures and supporting the aged during stressful situations.
6. Using methods to promote effective communication and socialization of aged persons with individuals, family, and others, thus increasing sensory stimulation.
7. Helping the older person adapt to the physical and psychosocial limitations of his environment, yet fulfill his needs.
8. Assisting with the obtaining and use of helpful mechanical devices for improving function.
9. Resolving personal attitudes about aging, dependence, and death to provide assistance in meeting these crises with dignity and comfort.

■ SUMMARY

1. Growth and development continues throughout the life span.
2. Nurses must be aware of the developmental tasks of each phase of life to understand the impact of illness and disease on the individual.
3. Young adults' main task is to choose a life-style, whereas middle-aged adults are reevaluating their life goals and readjusting expectations.
4. Persons in late adulthood are focusing on their life accomplishments and looking toward life's end, while maintaining their autonomy and dignity.
5. Health concerns differ from young adulthood to late adulthood.
6. Accidents and traumatic injuries are more common in young adults; middle-aged adults contract more cardiovascular disease, cancer, and diabetes.
7. Elderly adults often have more than one chronic illness, with the incidence increasing with age.
8. Nursing care must be tailored according to the specific physical, psychologic, sexual, and social effects of any disease or illness on the individual.
9. Nurses need to be cognizant of the differences between primary and secondary aging changes in elderly.
10. Nursing care should be predicated on the belief that late adulthood is a time of diversity, richness, and increasing complexity.

REFERENCES AND SELECTED READINGS
Contemporary

1. Allen, M: Drug therapy in the elderly, Am J Nurs 80:1474-1475, 1980.
2. Bahr, RT, Sr: Sleep-wake patterns in the aged, J Gerontol Nurs 9:534-537, 1983.
3. Burnside, I: Nursing and the aged, ed 2, New York, 1981, McGraw-Hill Book Co.
4. Burnside, I: Psychosocial nursing care of the aged, ed 2, New York, 1980, McGraw-Hill Book Co.
5. Busse, E, and Blazer, D: Handbook of geriatric psychiatry, New York, 1980, Van Nostrand Reinhold Co, Inc.
6. *Change through environmental interaction makes aging exciting, J Gerontol Nurs 11:35-36, 1985.
7. DeVore, N: Parenthood postponed, Am J Nurs 83:1160-1163, 1983.

---

*References preceded by an asterisk are particularly well suited for student reading.

8. Ebersole, P, and Hess, P: Toward healthy aging, St. Louis, 1981, The CV Mosby Co.
9. Forman, M: Acute confusional states in elderly: an algorithm, Dimen Crit Care 3(4):209-215, 1984.
10. *Grant, R: Women and mid-life crisis, Ladies Home Journal, p. 87+, August 1987.
11. Haug, M, Ford, A, and Sheafor, M: The physical and mental health of aged women, New York, 1985, Springer Publishing Co.
12. Hazard, MP, and Kemp, RE: Keeping the well elderly well, Am J Nurs 83:567-569, 1983.
13. Kaluger, G, and Kaluger, MF: Human development: the span of life, ed 3, St. Louis, 1984, The CV Mosby Co.
14. *Katch, MP: A negentropic view of aging, J Gerontol Nurs 9(12):557, 1983.
15. Palmore, E, and others: Normal aging III, Durham, NC, 1985, Duke University Press.
16. Ramos, LY: Oral hygiene of the elderly, Am J Nurs 81:1468-1469, 1981.
17. Reed, P: Implications of the life-span developmental framework for wellbeing in adulthood and aging, Adv Nurs Sci 6:1, 18-25, October 1983.
18. Travis, S: Older adults' sexuality and remarriage, J Gerontol Nurs 13:9, 1987.
19. Voith, AM: A conceptual framework for nursing diagnoses regarding alterations in urinary elimination, Rehab Nurs 11(1):18-21, 1985.
20. Wells, T: Aging and health promotion, Rockville, Md, 1982, Aspen Systems Co.
21. *Wolanin, MO, and Phillips, LF: Confusion: prevention and care, St. Louis, 1981, The CV Mosby Co.
22. *Woods, NF: Human sexuality in health and illness, ed 3, St. Louis, 1984, The CV Mosby Co.

Classic

23. Birren, J, and Schaie, K: Handbook of the psychology of aging, New York, 1977, Van Nostrand Reinhold Co, Inc.
24. Butler, R: Why survive? Being old in America, New York, 1975, Harper & Row, Publishers.
25. *Butler, R, and Lewis, M: Love and sex after sixty, New York, 1976, Harper & Row, Publishers.
26. Cape, R: Aging: its complex management, Hagerstown, Md, 1978, Harper & Row, Publishers.
27. Cummings, E, and Henry, W: Growing old, New York, 1955, Basic Books, Inc, Publishers.
28. Diekelman, NL: The middle years: a time of change, Am J Nurs 75:997-1001, 1975.
29. Diekelman, NL: The young adult: the choice is health or illness, Am J Nurs 75:1272-1277, 1975.
30. Dresden, SE: The middle years: the sexually active middle adult, Am J Nurs 75:1001-1005, 1975.
31. Ebersole, P, and Hess, P: Toward healthy aging, St. Louis, 1981, The CV Mosby Co.
32. Eliopoulos, C: Gerontological nursing, New York, 1979, Harper & Row, Publishers.
33. Erikson, EH: Childhood and society, ed 2, New York, 1963, WW Norton Co, Inc.
34. Havinghurst, R: Psychology of aging, Bethesda Conference, Public Health Rep 70:836-856, 1955.
35. Holmes, T, and Rahe, H: Social readjustment rating scale, J Psychosom Res 11:213, 1967.
36. Johnson, L: The middle years: living sensibly, Am J Nurs 75:1002-1016, 1975.
37. Lawton, MP: Community planning for an aging society, Strousburg, Pa, 1976, Dowden, Hutchinson, & Ross, Inc.
38. Levinson, D, and others: The psychosocial development of men in early adulthood and the midlife transition. In Ricks, D, Thomas, A, and Roffiede, M (editors): Life history research in pathology, Minneapolis, 1974, University of Minnesota Press.
39. Lidz, T: The person, rev ed, New York, 1976, Basic Books, Inc, Publishers.
40. Masters, W, and Johnson, V: Human sexual response, Boston, 1966, Little, Brown and Co.
41. *Murray, R, and Zentner, J: Nursing assessment and health promotion through the lifespan, ed 2, Englewood Cliffs, NJ, 1979, Prentice-Hall, Inc.
42. *Peplau, H: Life in the middle years: mid-life crisis, Am J Nurs 75:1761-1765, 1975.
43. Reichel, W (editor): Clinical aspects of aging, Baltimore, Md, 1978, Williams & Wilkins Co.
44. Rossman, I (editor): Clinical geriatrics, Philadelphia, 1977, JB Lippincott Co.
45. *Sheehy, G: Passages, New York, 1976, EP Dalton & Co, Inc.

AUDIOVISUAL RESOURCES

Aging, Del Mar, Calif, CRM Educational Films. (Film)

Gramp: a man ages and dies, Baltimore, Mass Media Ministries. (Filmstrip)

Grow old along with me, New York, Focus International. (Film)

Miles to go before I sleep, New York, Learning Corporation of America. (Film)

Patient mental health, psychological growth and adjustment, Oaklawn, Ill, Westinghouse Learning Corp. (Filmstrip and audiotape)

Peege, Princeton, NJ, Phoenix Films. (Film)

Perspectives on aging, Costa Mesa, Calif, Concept Media.

The shopping bag lady, Baltimore, Mass Media Associates. (Film)

6

Health Promotion: Nutrition and Exercise

BARBARA C. LONG

CHAPTER OBJECTIVES

After studying this chapter, the student should be able to:

- Describe factors affecting health-promoting behaviors.
- Identify the major nutrients required for body needs.
- Describe the interrelationships between food and drugs.
- Use the daily food guide to evaluate adequacy of nutrient intake.
- Define obesity and identify medical and nursing interventions to facilitate weight loss.
- Define underweight and identify interventions to facilitate weight gain.
- Discuss difficulties that may occur with tube feedings or total parenteral nutrition.
- Describe the effects and benefits of exercise.
- Describe recommendations for physical fitness programs.
- Differentiate between isometric and isotonic exercises.

■ HEALTH PROMOTION IN MEDICAL-SURGICAL NURSING PRACTICE

Health promotion can be defined as activities directed toward helping persons maintain or achieve a high level of functioning and well-being. Health promotion is an integral part of nursing care for all types of patients and clients in all types of environments of care. In ambulatory care centers, health promotion assumes a major focus. In acute care centers the major focus is assisting patients to regain their health (illness care). However, health care must also be considered, that is, that which is healthy must be maintained.

Health promotion strengthens the person's capacity to withstand physical and emotional stress. Thus the person who is in an excellent nutritional state, has good physical endurance, and copes well with stress is at less risk of developing a pathophysiologic disorder and has resources to use in regaining optimal functioning more quickly if illness or disease does occur.

■ Factors affecting health-promoting behaviors

Why do some persons take actions that promote a high level of functioning, whereas others do not? Pender[43] has identified factors that (1) affect the individual's perceptions, (2) modify behaviors, and (3) influence the likelihood of health-promoting actions.

■ INDIVIDUAL PERCEPTIONS

Motivation to participate in health-promoting behaviors is influenced by the person's perceptions about health and perceptions about self:
1. Perceptions about health
   a. Value placed on health by the person
   b. Desire for the highest achievable health level versus that for maintaining status quo
   c. Evaluation of present health status
   d. Perceived benefits of the health-promoting behaviors
2. Perceptions about self
   a. Perceived control over own behavior (internal versus external control)
   b. Desire for mastery of the environment
   c. Self-concept
   d. Self-esteem

Thus persons who do not value health or see a need to improve their health status, who are not self-motivated, or who have a poor self-concept are less likely to engage in health-promoting behaviors. Nursing approaches in these situations include helping these persons identify their values and explore feelings about themselves with emphasis placed on identifying strengths. Helping these persons set their own goals (thus exerting internal control) will greatly enhance the likelihood of achieving desired behaviors.

■ MODIFYING FACTORS

Pender[43] has identified three categories of modifying factors: demographic (age, sex, ethnicity, education, income), interpersonal, and situational variables. The specific effect of demographic variables on health-promoting behaviors is not clearly established and requires further research.

The major interpersonal factors influencing health-promoting behaviors are the influence of family or friends and the family patterns of health care. Persons more likely to participate are those who have support for the health-promoting behaviors from family or friends and who have been raised in a family in which health-promoting behaviors are valued. Health teaching is enhanced when the patient's support persons are included in the teaching.

Situational factors include the availability of opportunities to engage in health-promoting behaviors. For example, facilitation of a nutritionally balanced weight control program is enhanced by the availability of fruits and vegetables rather than vending machines with candy and potato chips. Nurses can assist patients in exploring alternative ways of achieving their goals.

■ LIKELIHOOD OF HEALTH-PROMOTING ACTIONS

The probability that a person will engage in health-promoting actions is influenced by actual or perceived barriers to action, such as cost, time, or ability, and the presence of cues to action.[43] Nursing approaches include assisting the person in differentiating between perceived and actual barriers and promoting behaviors directed toward overcoming actual barriers.

Cues to action include hearing about activities that promote health either in interactions with others or through the mass media. Nurses can participate in health teaching of patients or encourage patients to read, to listen to radio, or to watch television programs that emphasize health promotion. Nurses also need to be instrumental in the development of these health-teaching tools.

Since health promotion is an integral part of the care of persons with pathophysiologic disorders, promotion of nutrition and exercise will be discussed further in this chapter. Stress management is discussed in Chapter 7.

■ NUTRITION

■ Relationship of nutrition to health

Good nutritional status exists when the necessary nutrients (protein, fat, carbohydrate, minerals, vitamins, and water) are consumed in sufficient amounts and are used appropriately by the body to meet needs regardless of age, sex, life-style, or state of health. All persons need the same nutrients throughout life (see the box on p. 79).

All nutrients are equally important, although they are not required in equal amounts (see Appendix C). The nutrients providing energy (protein, fats, carbohydrates) and water are required in much larger quantities than vitamins that regulate body processes. The differences in

---

Essential nutrients required for health

Water
Protein (essential amino acids)

Isoleucine	Phenylalanine
Leucine	(tyrosine)
Lysine	Threonine
Methionine	Tryptophan
(cystine)	Valine

Carbohydrate: starches, sugars, fiber
Fat: linoleic acid and arachidonic acid (polyunsaturated)
Minerals

Calcium	Manganese
Chloride	Molybdenum
Chromium	Phosphorus
Copper	Potassium
Fluorine	Selenium
Iodine	Sodium
Iron	Zinc
Magnesium	

Vitamins

Vitamin A	Biotin
Vitamin B₆	Folacin
Vitamin B₁₂	Niacin
Vitamin C	Pantothenic acid
Vitamin D	Riboflavin
Vitamin E	Thiamin
Vitamin K	

---

the quantities of various nutrients required by an individual are much greater than the change in amounts of any one nutrient over the life cycle. The amounts of required nutrients vary in predictable patterns. Growth, basal metabolic needs, and physical activity are the major factors responsible for changing nutrient needs. Disease, trauma, variations in metabolism (normal or abnormal), medications, and treatments can also affect needs. The effects of good nutrition are summarized as follows:

Growth and development of tissues/organs
Source of energy for metabolic processes and physical activity
Tissue healing and repair
Resistance to infection

■ NUTRITIONAL DEFICITS

When nutritional supplies are limited, growth, function, or reproduction may be impaired. Since the body exists in a state of dynamic equilibrium, anabolism (tissue building) and catabolism (tissue breakdown) are continuous. Muscles, organs, bones, fat, and blood participate in the constant exchange of materials, with some tissues more active than others. There is some loss of nutrients; therefore,

replacement from food is necessary throughout life. Periods of growth increase requirements for nutrients and energy.

Homeostatic mechanisms tend to protect the body against minor or temporary changes in nutrient status as nutrient reserves are mobilized to meet needs. With nutrient deficits, adaptations occur to conserve body resources. For example, when energy supplies are limited, physical activity and then basal metabolism are reduced. Over time, however, there is gradual nutrient loss in the tissues when a deficit is present. If this process is permitted to continue long enough, classic deficiency diseases, such as scurvy, beriberi, and pellagra, will result from depletions of vitamin C, thiamin, B complex vitamins, and niacin. If untreated, progressive depletion results in death.

Protein-calorie malnutrition is the most common form of nutritional deficiency in the United States.[20] An insufficient intake of calories and proteins containing the essential amino acids may result from inadequate diet (seen in low-income populations) or be associated with some pathologic disorders, such as diseases of the gastrointestinal tract that interfere with intake or absorption of nutrients, or with malignancies that interfere with appetite or increase the use of nutrients. Protein may be lost through body fluids, such as fluid loss from diarrhea or removal of ascitic fluid from the abdominal cavity. Persons with severe protein-calorie malnutrition heal slowly, because there are no resources available for use in tissue building. In addition to protein and calories, vitamins B, C, and K are necessary for tissue healing and clot formation.

Malnutrition increases susceptibility to infection by decreasing the availability of nitrogen and amino acids necessary for production of white blood cells and fibroblasts, which are necessary to counteract an invasion of microorganisms. Infection, in turn, increases the body's need for nutrients that are already depleted. A severely malnourished person may die from a severe infection that would not be fatal to a well-nourished person. The immune response is also impaired by nutritional deficits. Protein-calorie malnutrition is related to a decrease in thymic activity with a reduction in T cell activity (Chapter 37) and with changes in metabolic activity that interfere with phagocytosis of bacteria by white blood cells. Lack of vitamin B₆ and pantothenic acid depresses antibody formation.

■ NUTRITIONAL EXCESS

Nutritional excesses can also produce malnutrition. Mechanisms tend to protect the body by accumulating reserves or, for some nutrients, by increasing the rate of excretion from the body or decreasing efficiency of absorption. When excesses are large or prolonged, increased concentrations of nutrients and alterations in enzyme activities and levels of metabolites develop.

Over time, clinical signs and symptoms develop. The most common example of this type of malnutrition in the U.S. population is *obesity*. Consumption of energy-yielding compounds (for example, protein, fat, carbohydrate, and alcohol) in amounts greater than needed for energy expenditure results in storage of energy as body fat. Eventually these stores of body fat become large enough to affect body functions, mobility, and health. Obese persons have a greater risk of osteoarthritis, diabetes mellitus, cardiovascular disease, hypertension, gallbladder disease, cardiorespiratory dysfunction, and thromboembolic disease.

Excesses of cholesterol and triglycerides in the circulating blood are associated with atherosclerosis and coronary artery disease. These excesses may result from an increased intake of saturated fatty acids associated with increased production by the liver. A high intake of dietary cholesterol will increase the blood cholesterol level; however, the liver normally compensates for the high intake level by synthesizing less cholesterol and converting more cholesterol into bile acids. This compensatory mechanism is altered in some persons, perhaps as a result of genetic factors, and it is these persons specifically who are at a higher risk for atherosclerosis. Most persons in the United States ingest more fat than is needed; therefore, health education should include teaching the substitution of complex carbohydrates for some fats and use of unsaturated rather than saturated fats.

Some persons have an unsupported intuitive feeling that nutrient supplements are essential.[54] Response to these supplements occurs only when persons have been relatively nutrition deficient, have been eating foods marginal in nutrient value, and when the supplement provides the specific nutrient or nutrients that are deficient. There is a point beyond which supplementation does not help the person and may actually cause harm. Continued intake of vitamins and minerals at levels from 10 to 100 times the recommended daily allowance (RDA) is associated with chronic toxicity.

⊞ Assessment

To assess nutritional status, it is necessary to determine the supply of available nutrients, the sources available for metabolic processes, body size, and physical signs. Data are obtained primarily by patient interview, by observing the patient's general appearance, and by physical examination.

■ SUBJECTIVE DATA

Interviewing for the purpose of collecting data is discussed in Chapter 3. Data to be collected to determine nutritional status include the following:

Food intake
    Typical day food/fluid pattern (type, amount)
    Recent changes in amount and type of intake
    Recent changes in appetite
Eating ability
    Dentures (fit, comfort)
    Problems with chewing or swallowing
Weight
    Usual and current weight
    Patient's perception of weight level
      If overweight/underweight: lifetime patterns, feelings about weight, reasons for recent change
Food supplements, medications, drugs (types, duration)

□ Food intake

When collecting data about nutrition, it is especially important to phrase the questions so that patients describe what they typically do eat rather than what they think they should. For example, the question, "Do you usually drink orange juice for breakfast?" implies (1) that breakfast is a desirable or expected behavior and (2) that orange juice is essential. Thus the patient may answer, "Yes," believing that is the expected answer, when in fact neither orange juice nor breakfast is usually eaten. A better approach is to say, "Tell me what you typically eat and drink in a day. What do you usually eat or drink first?" Questioning should elicit a picture of total food consumption for a day including all snacks. Designation by meals or snacks is not really necessary and may bias answers by implying value judgments.[42]

Identification of amount consumed is as important as the type of food. Often people find this difficult to estimate. Persons familiar with cooking may be able to estimate in terms of tablespoons or cups. For the hospitalized patient the equipment or portions on the tray can be used as a basis for comparison.

Changes in appetite or in the amount or type of food or fluids ingested may be the result of illness (for example, anorexia, nausea, vomiting, or pain), self-imposed dietary regimens, or emotional or physical stress.

□ Medications

Some medications may affect nutritional status if taken over a period of time (see box, p. 81, top). Conversely, food can interfere with absorption of oral medications.

Drugs are absorbed more readily if the gastrointestinal tract is free of food. Drugs taken with water when the stomach is empty move rapidly into the small intestines, where much drug absorption takes place. Fatty foods delay gastric emptying for as long as 2 hours; therefore, drugs that are absorbed in the small intestine have delayed absorption if taken with a meal high in fats. Food particularly delays the absorption of antimicrobial drugs, specifically the tetracyclines, the penicillins, and the sulfonamides. However, medications that have a gastric irritant effect may be enhanced if taken with food (see the box on p. 81).

Drugs that are normally slightly acidic, such as aspirin or barbiturates, usually ionize and are absorbed in the stomach. If the stomach pH is increased, such as by milk or antacids, the rate and extent of absorption of these drugs will be decreased. Alteration in stomach acidity may also break down the protective coating of spansules or enteric-coated tablets, resulting in premature release of contents. Acidic liquids, such as lemon, pineapple, or cranberry juices or dry ginger ale may inactivate acid-unstable drugs, such as ampicillin, potassium, penicillin G, cloxacillin, and erythromycin.

Food components can interact with oral medication by the chemical or physical binding of one substance on another, thus interfering with absorption of either the food component or the drug. Tetracycline becomes bound with calcium, aluminum, or magnesium ions when taken with milk or antacids. This decreases absorption of tetracycline.

Effect of some drugs on nutritional status

Aspirin	Malabsorption of folate
	Excretion of vitamin C
Barbiturates	Malabsorption of thiamin, vitamin B₁₂
	Excretion of vitamin C
Corticosteroids	Malabsorption of calcium, zinc, phosphorus
Hydralazine	Excretion of pyridoxine
Methotrexate	Malabsorption of vitamin B₁₂, folate, fat
Mineral oil	Malabsorption of fat-soluble vitamins, calcium, phosphorus
Neomycin	Malabsorption of major nutrients
Oral contraceptives	Possible decreased absorption of vitamin C, B complex vitamins, magnesium, zinc
Penicillin	Loss of potassium
Tetracycline	Malabsorption of calcium, iron, magnesium, pyridoxine
	Excretion of vitamin C, riboflavin, niacin, folic acid
Thiazides	Excretion of potassium, magnesium, zinc, riboflavin

Medications to be taken with food

Aminophylline	Nitrofurantoin
Chlorothiazide	(Macrodantin)
(Diuril)	Phenylbutazone
Ferrous sulfate	(Butazolidin)
Indomethacin	Phenytoin (Dilantin)
(Indocin)	Prednisolone
Metronidazole	Reserpine (Serpasil)
(Flagyl)	Triamterene (Dyrenium)

Foods containing tyramine (cheeses, wines) may interact with monoamine oxidase (MAO) inhibitors, such as phenelzine (Nardil) or tranylcypromine (Parnate), which are depressants, causing hypertensive reactions.

☐ Additional data

If nutritional intake is identified as inadequate, additional data will facilitate analysis and planning:
1. Food and fluid likes and dislikes
2. Financial resources
3. Facilities and ability for purchasing, storing, and preparing food
4. Problems with prescribed diets

■ OBJECTIVE DATA

☐ Height and weight

Height and weight are easily measured and are important data to obtain and use. The most reliable weight measurement is in the morning after voiding and before eating or drinking fluids. The patient's weight and height are compared with a table of recommended values (Table 6-1). One quick estimate for body frame size is to measure the person's wrist. An example is shown below.

Wrist sizes for estimating body frame: medium size

Less than 5 feet 2 inches	5½ to 5¾ inches
5 feet 2 inches to 5 feet 5 inches	6 to 6¼ inches
More than 5 feet 5 inches	6¼ to 6½ inches

☐ Physical examination data

The time elapsing between the lack of nutrient supply and the actual appearance of clinical signs that are obvious on physical examination can be as little as a week or as long as several years. Data from the head-to-toe physical examination (Chapter 3) that may suggest malnutrition include the following:

Hair	Lack of shine, easily plucked
Eyes	Pale conjunctiva, fissures at corner of eyelids
Lips	Redness, edema, fissures at corners of lips
Tongue	Swollen, smooth, raw, enlarged papillae
Teeth	Cavities, loose or missing teeth
Gums	Bleeding gums
Skin	Lack of subcutaneous fat, dryness, petechiae
Nails	Brittle, ridged
Muscles	Decreased muscle tone

➡ Data analysis: nursing diagnoses

■ ANALYSIS OF FOOD INTAKE

Food guides developed to help people choose the kinds and amounts of food to eat for health can be used for rapid evaluation of adequacy of the diet eaten at home or food intake in the hospital. There are many different food guides, since to be effective they must be devised for a specific country or culture and feature the foods readily available and acceptable to the people being evaluated.

A daily food guide used in the United States is shown in Table 6-2. The guide groups staple food items rich in protein, vitamins, and minerals into four major classes according to their major nutrient contributions. Recommendations are made for the number and size of servings to be selected from each food group. To evaluate a diet quickly, one checks to see if the recommended types of food and servings are included in the usual dietary pattern.

Since foods are mixtures of nutrients, the protein, vitamin, and mineral requirements are substantially met when the daily intake includes the recommended servings from each group. The calorie level of the basic diet is low,

Table 6-1 Height and weight tables for adults with desirable weights for persons age 25 and over

Men					Women				
Height		Small frame (lb)	Medium frame (lb)	Large frame (lb)	Height		Small frame (lb)	Medium frame (lb)	Large frame (lb)
Feet	Inches				Feet	Inches			
5	2	128-134	131-141	138-150	4	10	102-111	109-121	118-131
5	3	130-136	133-143	140-153	4	11	103-113	111-123	120-134
5	4	132-138	135-145	142-156	5	0	104-115	113-126	122-137
5	5	134-140	137-148	144-160	5	1	106-118	115-129	125-140
5	6	136-142	139-151	146-164	5	2	108-121	118-132	128-143
5	7	138-145	142-154	149-168	5	3	111-124	121-135	131-147
5	8	140-148	145-157	152-172	5	4	114-127	124-138	134-151
5	9	142-151	148-160	155-176	5	5	117-130	127-141	137-155
5	10	144-154	151-163	158-180	5	6	120-133	130-144	140-159
5	11	146-157	154-166	161-184	5	7	123-136	133-147	143-163
6	0	149-160	157-170	164-188	5	8	126-139	136-150	146-167
6	1	152-164	160-174	168-192	5	9	129-142	139-153	149-170
6	2	155-168	164-178	172-197	5	10	132-145	142-156	152-173
6	3	158-172	167-182	176-202	5	11	135-148	145-159	155-176
6	4	162-176	171-187	181-207	6	0	138-151	148-162	158-179

Metropolitan Life Insurance Co., New York, 1983.
Weights at ages 25-59 based on lowest mortality. Weight in pounds according to frame (in indoor clothing weighing 5 pounds, shoes with 1-inch heels).

Table 6-2 Daily food guide

Food group (servings/day)	Amount/serving	Nutrients supplied
Milk		
2	1 c milk 40 g (1½ oz) cheese 1¾ c ice cream 1 c yogurt	Protein, calcium, phosphorus, riboflavin, other vitamins and minerals (except iron and vitamin C)
Meat protein		
2	60 to 75 g (2 to 3 oz) lean meat, poultry, fish 1 egg ½ c beans, peas, lentils 4 Tbsp peanut butter	Protein, fat, B complex vitamins, (plant products lack vitamin B_{12})
Vegetables/fruits		
4 or more total 1 dark green or deep yellow at least every other day	½ c broccoli, kale, carrots, squash, spinach, sweet potatoes, turnip or mustard greens, apricots, cantaloupe, pumpkin	Vitamin A
1/day (vitamin C sources)	½ c citrus fruits/juices, cabbage, broccoli, brussels sprouts, peppers, strawberries, tomatoes	Vitamin C
2 to 3/day (other)	½ c medium potato or apple, other vegetables or fruits	All fruits/vegetables: vitamins, minerals (low sodium), fiber
Bread/cereal		
4 (whole grain or enriched)	1 slice bread 30 g (1 oz) dry cereal ½ to ¾ c cooked cereal, rice, pasta	Complex carbohydrates, protein, iron, thiamin, riboflavin, niacin

but it is approximately sufficient for adult basal metabolism. Adequacy of energy intake is best judged by evaluation of body weight. In this method of evaluation, fats, oils, and sweets are not tabulated, since they provide primarily energy.

Each food group contributes particular nutrients to the total diet. The absence of any one food group from the diet or particular types of food should alert the nurse that the person has a potential nutrition problem. The box below is an example of an analysis of food intake using the daily food guide.

The daily food guide can also be used for evaluating vegetarian diets. Many people are vegetarians and their reasons vary (for example, religion, food cost, philosophy).

Assessment of a diet history

45-year-old woman with obesity and hypertension; meals eaten at home

7:00 AM

1 c cooked oatmeal
2 tsp sugar
1 c skim milk (fortified)
0 c coffee, plain

10:15 AM

2 c coffee, plain

1:00 PM

Sandwich
   2 slices white bread, enriched
   ½ tsp margarine
   ½ tsp mayonnaise
   60 g (2 oz) meatloaf or luncheon meat
4 cookies (fig bars, gingersnaps)
3 c coffee, plain

4:00 PM

7 cookies
½ c unsweetened fruit (canned, frozen, or fresh)
2 c tea, plain

10:00 PM

8 soda crackers
60 g (2 oz) American cheese
360 ml (12 oz) cola (sweet)
½ c homemade bread-and-butter pickles

Midnight

2 aspirin
1 c tea, plain

Assessment

Food group	Servings
Milk	
Skim milk	1
Cheese	1
Meat-protein	
Meatloaf	1
Fruits, vegetables	
Fruit	1
Vegetable	1
Bread, cereal	
Oatmeal	2
Bread, enriched	2
Crackers	2
Sweets	
Cookies	11
Cola (360 ml [12 oz])	
Pickles, cucumber	
Fats	
Margarine	
Mayonnaise	

Evaluation

Choice from milk group adequate. Meat intake low. Fruit and vegetable intake low; choice of items rich in vitamin C or A happenstance. Bread intake is 6 servings. Intake of sweets, particularly cookies, high. Use of pickles and soda crackers questionable, since patient reports that low-sodium diet was prescribed for her several years ago.

Dietitian was asked to check caloric value. Intake is 1500 to 1600 calories/day, which includes 800 calories from basic food items; remainder from sweets and fat. Protein levels adequate, although source of protein could be improved.

To the reader: Identify nutritional risks for this person; identify appropriate interventions and behavioral goals for her.

From Neville, J: Assessment of nutritional status and dietary counseling. In Phipps, WJ, Long, BL, and Woods, NF: Medical-surgical nursing: concepts and clinical practice, ed 3, St Louis, 1987, The CV Mosby Co.

The diets vary as well. Generally the lactoovovegetarian (includes milk products and eggs) diet is nutritionally sound when a variety of foods is included. Persons on more restricted vegetarian (vegan) diets should be considered at nutritional risk and candidates for more detailed study (refer to dietitian). One potential problem with the vegan diet is vitamin B_{12} insufficiency unless fortified cereal or a dietary supplement is taken. The young adult who has changed to a vegan diet may use body stores of B_{12} for a time (a 5-year store is possible), but is at potential risk, especially if intake of folacin in vegetables is high, masking the signs of megaloblastic anemia.

■ NURSING DIAGNOSES

Possible nursing diagnoses based on collected data include the following:

Knowledge deficit

Altered nutrition: potential for more than body requirements

Altered nutrition: more than body requirements

Altered nutrition: less than body requirements

⊡ Planning: expected patient outcomes

Expected patient outcomes to promote a good nutritional status may include the following:

1. Patient can describe modifications in dietary intake to correct existing or potential nutritional deficits or excesses.

2. Patient can describe desired servings for each food group to meet basic nutritive needs.

3. Patient maintains weight within desired weight ranges.

⊡ Implementation
■ TEACHING

Good nutrition can be promoted by giving positive reinforcement for selection of balanced meals from hospital menus. Teaching patients with specific knowledge deficits includes identification of the patient's motivation to learn. Patients with extensive lack of knowledge about food preparation, particularly with ways of preparing nutritionally balanced meals at low cost, may require the services of a dietitian.

The daily food guide (Table 6-2) is a useful tool for teaching persons a method of evaluating their own food intake. The dietitian may be helpful in developing a specific food guide for persons whose cultural patterns or personal preferences (for example, vegetarians) do not fit the standard food guides.

Persons who have been prescribed a dietary modification may need interpretation of the rationale for the diet and assistance in planning acceptable meals using the prescribed dietary plan (see the box below). The dietitian usually initiates the discussion of a new home-going diet, but the nurse serves as interpreter to the patient by providing explanations about the diet and feedback on how to make changes in current dietary patterns to meet the di-

---

Types of diet modifications

Protein	Increased with losses from tissue catabolism, bleeding, exudates
	Decreased for chronic renal failure or hepatic coma
	Elimination of specific proteins (for example, allergies or malabsorption of gluten)
Fats	Increased to provide essential calories in concentrated form
	Decreased for pain with gallbladder disease
	Modified for disorders of digestion or absorption, lipid metabolism, or to alter serum lipid levels
Carbohydrates	Increased for weight gain
	Decreased for weight loss or diabetes mellitus
	Changed from simple to complex carbohydrates in diabetes mellitus
	Elimination of specific carbohydrates with disorders of carbohydrate intolerance (for example, lactase deficiency)
Vitamins	Increased for vitamin deficiency
	Provided in an alternate form to enhance absorption or use
Minerals	Sodium restriction with hypertension, fluid retention, kidney disease
	Potassium and calcium increased or decreased for lack or excess
	Provided by prescription for deficiency
Liquid, soft, pureed	Postoperative, diseases of gastrointestinal tract, difficulty with chewing or swallowing
Elimination diets	Food allergies

etary prescription. Since the patients are the ones who must implement the dietary changes, they need to internalize the need for a behavior change. This takes active participation in all phases of the learning process. The person who does the cooking (if not the patient) also needs to be involved in the learning process. Dietary changes are more likely to be implemented if the changes can be easily adjusted to the family's usual meal plans.

■ FACILITATING WEIGHT LOSS

□ Etiology of obesity

Obesity is a major health problem in the United States. The incidence of cardiovascular disease, hypertension, diabetes mellitus, and gallbladder disease is high among obese persons.

Obesity is defined as 20% or greater over the established height and weight standards (Table 6-1). *Morbid obesity* is generally defined as 45 kg (100 lb) above the standard. Persons in an overweight category (up to 20% above the standard) who are gaining weight have a potential for malnutrition. The fat cells of obese people contain more fat than do those of lean persons and the number of fat cells may increase in adulthood. In general, obesity results from an increased caloric intake and a decreased energy output.

There are many genetic, psychologic, and social factors that influence the development of obesity (see the box below). Although "fatness" seems to occur in some families, much of this may be a result of learned eating behaviors of high caloric foods rather than genetically influenced.

□ Weight reduction

Obesity exists in two forms: adult onset (hypertrophic) and lifelong (hyperplastic-hypertrophic). Persons with adult-onset obesity (middle-aged spread) have a fixed number of fat cells, but each cell contains excessive fat. These persons respond well to weight-reduction regimens. Persons with lifelong obesity not only have excessive fat in each cell, but also have more fat cells and generally respond poorly to weight reduction regimens. Persons who become massively obese are usually of the lifelong type.

□ Diet

Diet is the most important method of weight reduction. Weight loss for some persons may be achieved by eating three regular, balanced meals a day that include the four basic food groups and avoiding fried foods, sweets, and between-meal snacks. Other persons achieve better results with planned, frequent small meals. Some obese persons omit breakfast but then snack frequently and thus ingest more calories and fewer required nutrients. Therefore, changes in eating patterns are usually required for permanent weight loss.

Persons consuming high levels of calories before weight-reduction diets are likely to be successful in achieving rapid weight loss, because the calorie deficit between need and the recommended diet is large. There is a difference in weight loss patterns between men and women. If both a man and a woman are instructed to adhere to a 1000-calorie intake, the man should lose at a faster rate, not because he is more cooperative but because his calorie deficit is greater.[42]

Rapid weight loss is usually the result of loss of fluid rather than fat. Thus after an initial successful loss of weight on a weight-control diet, a plateau is reached when weight appears to remain constant or decrease only slightly. This can be discouraging to the person who is following the prescribed approach. Reinforcement to continue the regimen is usually needed at this point.

Diets are planned on an individual basis, with the caloric intake planned at a level below the person's caloric need for maintaining weight. The calorie intake should come from complex carbohydrates and proteins. A protein intake of about 1 g/kg of ideal body weight should be maintained. Fats must be decreased. Salt-free diets are of no long-term value for weight reduction, because the weight loss relates to water loss, and the weight will return when salt is added to the diet.

Fasting diets are controversial. Rapid weight loss may be necessary in some instances; however, weight gain following the fasting period is a common occurrence. Most fasting programs use a high-protein liquid; some commercial products use hydrolyzed collagen that is low in nutritional value. Close medical supervision is imperative for fasting diets because risks are high (such as ketosis, metabolic acidosis, hypokalemia, hepatic impairment, renal insufficiency, and death).

Fad diets should generally be avoided, although they usually induce rapid weight loss in a relatively easy way. However, nutrients will be lost (marked protein catabolism with losses of nitrogen, phosphorus, calcium, potassium, sodium, and water). Weight then returns to the original level

---

Factors influencing obesity

Genetic	Heavy bone structure, large muscle mass
Psychologic	Pleasure associated with eating
	Emotional problems (for example, grief, stress, or boredom)
	Interpersonal problems with family, friends, or coworkers
Sociologic	Learned behaviors of overeating or eating high caloric foods
	Reinforcement from others to eat large amounts of high caloric foods
Environmental	Easy availability of high caloric "junk" foods
	Availability of money to spend on high caloric foods

after termination of the diet, because the person's general pattern of eating has not been changed.

□ Exercise

Exercise is an essential component of any weight control program. It promotes expenditure of energy and makes body appearance more pleasing to the person and thus desirable to maintain. Although the actual number of calories used will be few, the combination of diet and exercise promotes loss of fat rather than lean tissue. It is important that the exercise program be agreeable to the person so that it becomes a pattern of behavior to be continued throughout life (see p. 91 for further discussion of exercise).

□ Behavior modification

Behavior modification consists of changing the pattern of eating and exercising. *Without behavior modification, over 90% of obese persons who successfully lose weight either through dietary or medical therapy return to or surpass their original weight within 5 years.*[32]

Behavior modification is accomplished by self-action over a period of time by the following:
1. Setting own goals
2. Self-monitoring
3. Developing a personal reward system
4. Obtaining positive feedback
5. Developing a new self-concept of "thinness"
6. Developing and implementing an activity program

Self-control is important in learning to change eating habits to facilitate weight loss and to maintain desirable body weight. Setting one's own goals and developing a personal reward system can facilitate motivation to participate in the desirable behaviors. Self-monitoring by means of planning the menus and keeping food diaries increases the person's awareness of the foods consumed. (Many persons are unaware of the number of calories consumed, especially by "nibbling.")

Reinforcement from others is a major factor in the success of a weight control program. The effectiveness of weight control groups, such as Weight Watchers, is based on this concept.

□ Surgery

When the person is morbidly obese and when other methods have been diligently tried and have failed, the physician may consider bypass surgery. Criteria for surgery are as follows:

Age 17 to 50[25]

At least two times ideal body weight (100+ pounds over ideal weight)

Morbid obesity for at least 5 years[6]

Have made serious dieting efforts

Highly motivated

No major illnesses

Obese persons are a high surgical risk, however, and the surgeries themselves add additional risks. The surgical procedures are of two types: those that reduce food intake, such as gastric partitioning or gastric bypass (the preferred methods), and those that cause malabsorption (intestinal bypass).

□ *Gastric partitioning*

In this procedure, the stomach is made smaller by placement of sutures either horizontally or vertically through the stomach walls (Fig. 6-1). A small pouch is thus formed that limits the amount of food the person can take without experiencing pain and vomiting. This type of surgery has fewer consequences than bypass surgery because the gastrointestinal tract is not opened and remains intact.

Postoperatively, if irrigation through the nasogastric tube is necessary, only a small amount of fluid (30 ml) is used. Clear fluids are introduced on about the third day and, if they are tolerated, the patient is advanced to a diet of pureed foods. A blenderized diet is followed for 8 weeks, at which time small amounts of soft bland foods and vitamin supplements are introduced gradually. Solid foods are then introduced slowly. Foods to be avoided initially are meat and skin of poultry or fish,[6] foods high in cellulose that are not easily digested, and foods that provide high calories (such as milkshakes and alcohol).[25] Upper abdominal pain radiating to the left shoulder following surgery may indicate perforation of the stomach by the staples. Occasional vomiting is commonly encountered.

□ *Gastric bypass*

A Roux-en-Y gastric bypass is illustrated in Fig. 6-2; the resected jejunum is attached to a closed-off pouch of the upper stomach created by complete horizontal stapling. This procedure involves intrusion of the gastrointestinal

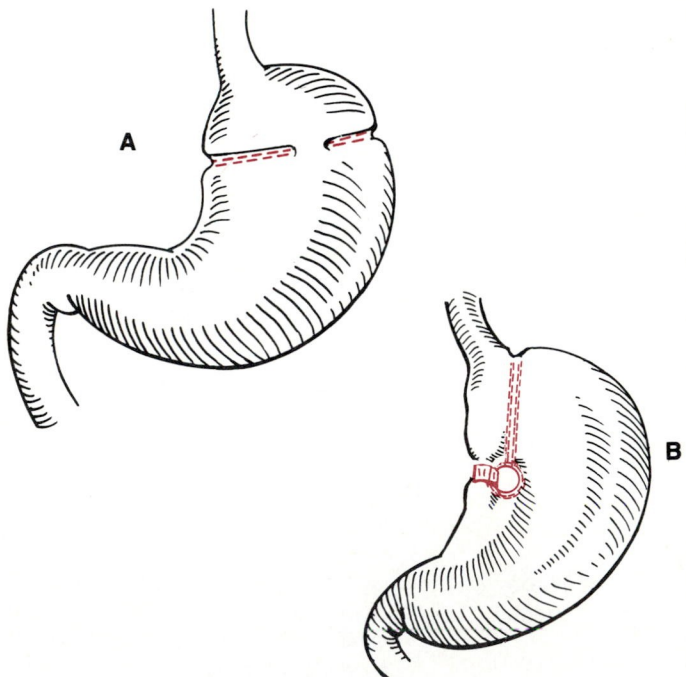

Fig. 6-1 Gastric partitioning. **A,** Horizontal stapling; **B,** vertical stapling.

tract, and the care of the patient is similar to that for other gastric surgeries (see Chapter 31). Complications include dumping syndrome, uncontrolled vomiting, leaks in the suture lines, and pulmonary infections.

□ Intestinal bypass

This least preferred and now seldom used method includes bypassing the ileum and connecting the jejunum to the transverse colon (Fig. 6-3). Diarrhea is usually a problem in the early postoperative period because of the in-

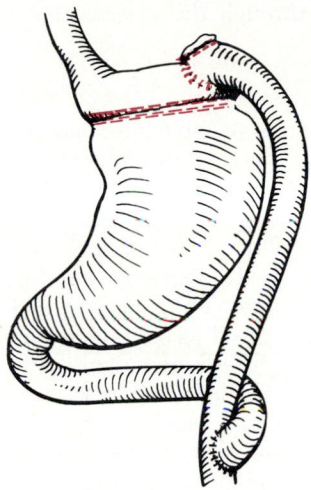

Fig. 6-2   Roux-en-Y retrocolic gastric bypass. Stomach is stapled completely horizontally; jejunum is resected from duodenum and connected to stomach entrance; distal duodenal stump is connected to jejunum to permit drainage of intestinal secretions.

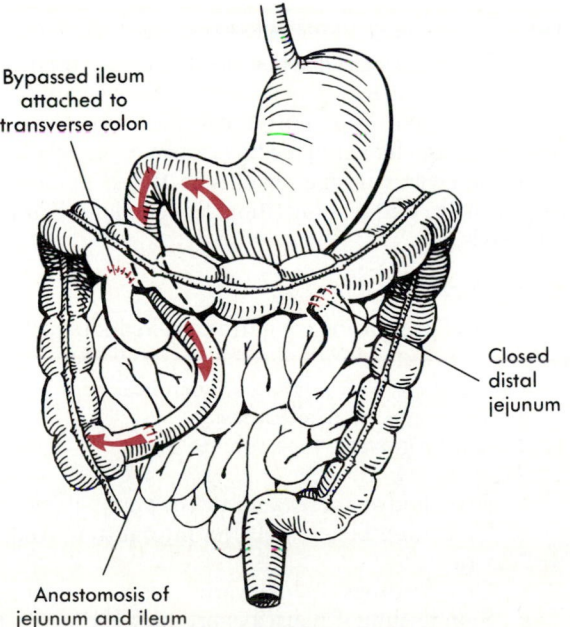

Bypassed ileum
attached to
transverse colon

Closed
distal
jejunum

Anastomosis of
jejunum and ileum

Fig. 6-3   Intestinal bypass.

creased transit time, but eventually most persons stabilize at about five semiformed stools per day. Malabsorption of fat and fat-soluble vitamins usually occurs, and dietary supplements are usually necessary. Protein malnutrition may also occur and leads to hepatic dysfunction. Other complications include prolonged severe diarrhea, polyarthritis, intestinal inflammation, osteomalacia, and oxylate renal stones.

□ Gastric balloon

A newer method to facilitate weight loss is the gastric balloon (Garren-Edward gastric bubble). This is a *temporary* method used in conjunction with dietary control and behavior modification. Indications for the procedure are persons more than 20% above ideal body weight who have failed to achieve weight loss by serious dietary and behavior modification plans alone. Contraindications include a history of peptic ulcer, hiatal hernia, or gastrointestinal surgery, or concurrent use of antiinflammatory agents, anticoagulants, or drugs that cause gastric irritation.[22,44]

The gastric balloon is a polyurethane balloon with a hollow central channel that is inserted by endoscopy into the stomach. The balloon is then inflated with 200 to 220 ml of air through a catheter attached to a self-sealing valve. The balloon occupies about 25% of the stomach capacity and thus produces early satiety. It is also thought to suppress appetite by stimulating the fundus, thus sending inhibitory stimuli to the appetite center in the hypothalamus.[44] The gastric balloon is removed endoscopically after 4 months. If necessary, another balloon may be inserted.

Postprocedure instructions include the following:
1. Drink a 500-calorie liquid diet for 1 week.
2. Progress to 800- to 1000-calorie regular diet.
3. Avoid gastric stimulants (coffee, alcohol, tobacco) and aspirin.
4. Take multivitamin and mineral supplements.
5. Take antacid four times daily (between meals and at bedtime).
6. Attend weekly diet and behavior modification sessions.
7. Participate in an exercise program.

Although the gastric balloon procedure has low risks, about 5% of initial patients developed gastric ulcers that responded to removal of the gastric balloon and ulcer therapy. The balloon may cause nausea, vomiting, crampy pain, and heartburn, especially during the first week.[22]

● ● ●

In summary, maintenance of weight loss is not usually achieved by participation in fad diets or medical therapies, but by a change in eating behaviors and increase in energy expenditure. This requires a long period of time and considerable involvement by the person with support from others. The nurse in an acute care setting cannot achieve this goal; however, the nurse can identify those persons who are obese, explore with them their perceptions and desires about their weight level, and provide support and guidance about ways to begin a weight control program.

Factors influencing anorexia

Offensive sights or smells
Past experiences with foods
Pattern of behavior when coping with stress
Poor oral hygiene
Inflammatory disorders
Nausea or vomiting
Edema or decreased muscle tone of gastrointestinal tract
Liver failure
Abdominal distention
Increased blood temperature (heat, fever)
Drugs (amphetamines)

■ FACILITATING WEIGHT GAIN

□ Etiology of underweight

Underweight is defined as more than 20% below the accepted weight standards. Weight loss is often the first sign of ill health. Loss may be mild or severe, insignificant or serious. It may be caused by
1. Inadequate calorie intake
2. Problems in digestion or absorption
3. Abnormalities in metabolism
4. Excretion of nutrients before they can be used
5. Failure to increase calorie intake when physical activity is increased

Anorexia (lack of appetite) is a mental state, a desire not to eat whether hunger is present or not. A number of factors may contribute to anorexia (see the box above).

□ Encouraging food intake

Persons with inadequate nutrition stores need encouragement to eat, although forced feeding may lead to frustration or nausea and vomiting. Motivating a person with anorexia to eat can be a challenge. Interventions that can correct the cause will lead to improved appetite. Determining the person's likes and dislikes, providing an environment conducive to eating, and providing several small meals rather than three large meals a day may facilitate an adequate nutrition intake.

A high-calorie, high-protein diet is indicated if the patient can eat. The diet is essentially a normal one with added protein and supplementary high-caloric feedings. High-protein diets are contraindicated if there is liver disease because protein catabolism takes place in the liver.

If the person cannot ingest nutrients by the oral route or cannot absorb the nutrients through the intestinal tract, other methods must be used:
1. Enteral feeding via nasoenteral tubes (gastric, duodenal or jejunal) or via ostomy (cervical esophagostomy, gastrostomy, or jejunostomy; see Chapter 31)
2. Parenteral feeding

□ Tube feedings

Nasoenteral tubes are used to provide nutrients when a person with normal intestinal function is unable to ingest sufficient nutrients by oral ingestion, has difficulty swallowing, or has mild to moderate malabsorption (short bowel syndrome). The tube is inserted through the nose and terminates in the stomach, duodenum, or jejunum.

Feeding tubes are soft polyurethane or silicone tubes with a narrow lumen (usually #5 to #10 F), although in some instances a larger bore tube may be necessary. Some tubes have a monofilament or stainless steel stylet for easy passage. A tube with a weighted end may be used to help pass the tube through the pylorus into the intestine, if desired.

□ *Technique*

Administration of tube feedings may be by bolus, gravity drip, or infusion pump. *Bolus* delivery consists of infusing 300 to 400 ml of formula over several minutes four to six times daily.[28] It is appropriate only for persons who can eat and are receiving supplemental tube feedings. The sudden influx of the feeding may cause nausea, cramping, diarrhea, or aspiration. The *gravity* method consists of placing the feeding in a feeding bag attached to the nasoenteral tube and allowing the fluid to run in by gravity. Disadvantages of this method include erratic fluid flow and greater potential of tube blockage. The gravity method may be used for intermittent or continuous administration. Most persons can tolerate 250 to 400 ml per feeding given over 20 to 30 minutes. The *infusion pump* is the preferred method for more constant administration rate and less probability of tube blockage or of diarrhea; however, it is more expensive. Pump accuracy must be checked routinely by comparing the actual drop count with the preestablished rate.

□ *Solutions*

Different types of fluids may be given by tube feedings (Table 6-3). Blenderized whole foods may be used; these are nutritious and less expensive, but they require large-bore tubes and are good culture media for bacteria. Elemental and semielemental feedings are more easily digested and can be given through small-bore tubes, but they are more expensive and less nutritionally complete than liquid whole foods.

□ *Complications*

Methods of preventing complications include the following:
1. *Regurgitation with aspiration:* keep head elevated to at least 30 degrees at all times.
2. *Tube dislodgement:* tape tube to nose.
3. *Tube clogging*
   a. Give fluid at a constant rate (by pump, if possible).
   b. Give water before and after intermittent feedings.
4. *Nausea*
   a. Give feedings at lukewarm (room) temperature.
   b. Stop feeding if nausea is present, and notify physician.

Table 6-3 Tube feedings

	Elemental	Supplemental	Liquid whole foods
Examples	Vivonex Flexical Pregestimil	Precision Vital	Ensure Sustacal Isocal
Content	Simple carbohydrates, amino acids	Complex carbohydrates, peptides	Complex carbohydrates, proteins
Osmolality	500-800 mOsm	450-600 mOsm	300-600 mOsm
Advantages	Given through small-bore tube Well tolerated for prolonged use	Can be given through small-bore tube More effective protein content than elemental	Lower osmolality Moderate price Acceptable flavor More nutritionally complete
Disadvantages	Unpalatable High osmolality Not well tolerated by bolus feeding Excellent culture media for bacteria Expensive Require monitoring of blood glucose and electrolytes	More expensive than liquid whole foods Tend to coagulate in tube Require monitoring of blood glucose and electrolytes	High fat content Tend to coagulate in tube May require a large-bore tube

c. When restarting feeding, administer it more slowly until tolerated.

5. *Bacterial contamination*
   a. Do not let feeding hang for more than 6 hours.
   b. Change equipment every 24 hours.

6. *Dehydration* (thirst, low urinary output, decreased skin turgor)
   a. Give water as necessary; total fluid intake should equal urinary output.
   b. Isoosmolality is 300 mOsm; the greater the osmolality of the feeding, the more water is needed.
   c. Give extra water if the need is increased, such as with fever.
   d. Monitor for decreased skin turgor, thirst, and dry mucous membranes.

7. *Diarrhea*
   a. Initiate feedings slowly at half strength.
   b. Increase concentration and rate gradually (do not change both concentration and rate at the same time).
   c. If diarrhea occurs:
      (1) Decrease rate of fluid flow.
      (2) Administer prescribed antidiarrheal medication through tube.

8. *Hyperglycemia*
   a. Monitor urine for glucose and acetone.
   b. If urine tests positively, decrease rate of feeding flow and notify physician.

□ Home tube feedings

Home tube feedings can be maintained by persons after receiving instruction in insertion and care of the tube, in formula care and insertion, and in monitoring for complications. An enteral infusion pump may be rented or purchased. The person needs to know where in the community to purchase materials (tubes, administration sets, and formula bags).

□ Total parenteral nutrition

Total parenteral nutrition (TPN), also known as parenteral hyperalimentation, is a method of giving concentrated solutions intravenously to maintain protein synthesis. Indications for this therapy are (1) major gastrointestinal diseases, fistulas, or inflammatory diseases; (2) extensive negative nitrogen balance, such as occurs with major body burns, extensive wounds, or cachexia; and (3) gastrointestinal side effects from radiation therapy.

□ *Technique*

Under strict aseptic conditions, an intracatheter is inserted either into the subclavian vein through the chest wall (Fig. 6-4) or into the basilic vein in the antecubital fossa and then threaded through to the superior vena cava. The large amount of blood in the superior vena cava helps to dilute the highly concentrated solution rapidly and thus prevent phlebitis or vein occlusion.

A Hickman catheter is commonly used in place of a standard intracatheter. This catheter is designed so that the end of the catheter can be capped between infusions. At completion of an infusion, the catheter is filled with heparinized saline solution to prevent clotting and is capped until the next infusion.

The catheter is secured with one suture and covered by an air-occlusive dressing. The dressing may be transparent

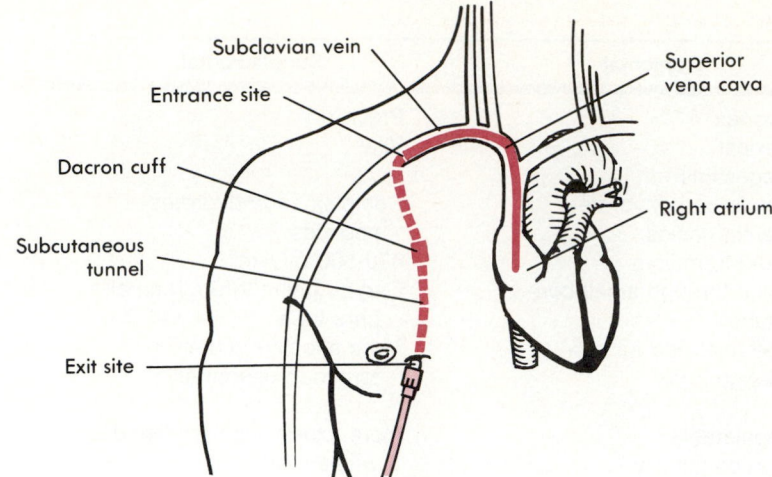

Fig. 6-4 Placement of Hickman catheter for administration of TPN solutions.

(OpSite) or a gauze dressing covered entirely with adhesive tape. The infusion is started with a standard intravenous fluid (5% dextrose) until a radiograph confirms the location of the catheter tip in the superior vena cava.

□ Solutions

Solutions for TPN are good culture media and are prepared under strict aseptic conditions in the pharmacy under a laminar airflow hood. The physician orders the solution contents based on the person's nutritional needs. The solutions are kept refrigerated until ready for use and are then warmed to room temperature before infusion. Prepared formulas should be used within 48 hours to prevent contamination.

TPN solutions usually consist of 500 ml 50% dextrose, 500 ml of 5% to 10% amino acids, electrolytes, minerals, and vitamins.[20] Ten percent to twenty percent fat emulsions may also be added. Dextrose and fat are given for caloric value to spare the proteins for anabolism. Fat provides twice the caloric value of glucose, exerts minimal osmotic pressure, and prevents fatty acid deficiency.[30] Filters are not used with fat emulsions because of filter clogging by large fat particles.[3] Regular insulin may be added to the TPN solution or may be given by injection for glucose utilization.

□ Nursing interventions

Nursing care centers on prevention of infection and air embolism, maintenance of fluid and electrolyte balance, and promotion of activity and comfort (see the box on p. 91). Dressing changes are carried out under aseptic technique. A transparent dressing is usually changed once a week or as necessary. A gauze dressing is changed three times a week or if it becomes wet, soiled, or the tape loosens.[3,53] Some medical centers have a TPN team, and one nurse changes the dressings for all patients to ensure consistency of technique and to reduce the chance of infection. Patients who experience itching under the dressing are cautioned not to scratch or disturb the dressing.

The possibility of air embolism is greater with use of the superior vena cava than with a peripheral vein because the decreased venous pressure as the blood approaches the heart can cause air to be sucked into the tubing. Filters are useful for trapping air as well as bacteria.

In addition to care related to the TPN per se, persons receiving TPN require good mouth care to prevent infection, dryness, and discomfort.

Patients may have many fears and concerns about being fed by intravenous fluids over a long period of time. They should have an understanding of what is occurring and the reason for the frequent dressing changes. They are encouraged to sit at the dinner table to participate in the social interaction. If food is not permitted orally, persons may need aid in coping with stress incurred by the smell of food or watching others eat. If receiving TPN over a long period of time, they may be concerned about regaining taste or normal eating patterns. Being fed only by tube, even though temporary, may create stress from a change in body image. Patients are encouraged to express their feelings and are supported in developing coping patterns to deal with these stresses (see Chapter 7).

□ Complications

Complications of TPN may be mechanical, infectious, or metabolic. *Mechanical* problems may include pneumothorax, hemothorax, air embolism, catheter misplacement, brachial plexus injury, and thromboembolism. These complications are rare with correct catheter insertion and maintenance. *Infection* is a serious complication but can be prevented by using conscientious aseptic technique during catheter insertion and subsequent care.

The major *metabolic* alterations are hyperglycemia or, more rarely, hypoglycemia. Other possible alterations include fluid imbalances; electrolyte imbalances in sodium, potassium, calcium, magnesium, and phosphates; and acid-base imbalances (primarily acidosis). Vitamin D deficiency and vitamin A excess may also occur. Serum levels are monitored several times a week, and urine is tested for sugar and acetone. The patient is weighed daily for the first 2 weeks and three times a week thereafter.

Nursing care of the patient receiving total parenteral nutrition

1. Prevent infection
   a. Maintain strict aseptic technique
   b. Keep solutions cold until ready for use; use within 48 hours
   c. Change dressings 3 times/week for gauze dressings, once a week for polyurethane dressings
2. Prevent air embolism
   a. Tape all connections of the system
   b. Clamp catheter when opening system
   c. Cover insertion site with an air-occlusive dressing (covered with adhesive tape) or transparent polyurethane (Op-Site) dressing
3. Maintain fluid and electrolyte balance
   a. Maintain a continuous uniform infusion rate
   b. If rate is too *slow:*
      (1) Return rate to prescribed rate
      (2) If prescribed rate does not resume, ask person to change position
      (3) Monitor and report to physician signs of *hypoglycemia* (pallor, diaphoresis, tachycardia, hunger, trembling, behavioral changes)
   c. If rate is too *fast:*
      (1) Slow infusion to prescribed rate
      (2) Monitor for signs of *overhydration* (neck vein distention, cough, weight gain)
      (3) Monitor for signs of *hyperglycemia* (sugar in urine, nausea, weakness, thirst, headache)
   d. Monitor daily weights and intake and output
   e. Monitor serum electrolyte, glucose, and blood urea nitrogen (BUN) levels
4. Encourage ambulation, activities of daily living
5. Promote comfort
   a. Provide for good oral hygiene
   b. Provide emotional support to enhance coping

☐ *Home total parenteral nutrition*

Since the advent of home total parenteral nutrition (HTPN) many persons have been able to lead more nearly normal lives, going to work or school, and participating in selected activities, including sexual. These persons infuse the solutions over a 12-hour period overnight and then participate in normal daily activities. Their lives are somewhat limited by being connected to the infusing equipment for the 12 hours, although there are vest systems that support the HTPN solution, tubing, and pump to provide increased mobility. There are also 24-hour battery packs to provide more freedom for the person who is connected to a pump that requires an electrical outlet.[5]

One patient described HTPN as taking energy, concern, and consideration from the whole family.[5] Certainly many family plans must revolve around the patient's need for TPN. Learning to mix, infuse, and disconnect the infusion and care for the equipment may be overwhelming at first for both patient and family. Teaching is started in the hospital by the hospital nurse well before the patient is discharged and is continued at home by the home health nurse. Teaching includes the following:

1. Principles of aseptic technique
2. Opening and setting up bags
3. Starting pump, stopping infusion, flushing tubing, clamping tube
4. Maintaining and troubleshooting equipment
5. Catheter care
6. Monitoring for signs of complications
7. Where to obtain supplies and need for storage space for supplies in the home

Companies that supply HTPN equipment and supplies often have a nutrition support nurse who can provide information as necessary and may have an instruction manual for patient use.[12]

HTPN teams are available to assist the person or family member to carry out TPN care at home. Before the patient is discharged, the home health nurse should meet with other team members and the patient to facilitate the move home. The home health nurse then assists the person with HTPN at home until the person becomes self-sufficient and can manage independently. Contact is maintained with the health team for assistance with changes that are needed and with problems that may arise. The person often requires changes in solution content depending on response to therapy.

Complications of HTPN are similar to those of TPN. However, risk of infection is increased, mostly from *Staphylococcus aureus.*[20] Catheter damage may occur from repeated cross-clamping; however, the catheter may be repaired with a catheter repair kit.[20] An occluded catheter may be opened by instillation of urokinase or streptokinase into the catheter. Unusual metabolic deficiencies may occur with long-term therapy, such as deficiencies in chromium, selenium, molybdenum, and vitamins A and E.[20]

HTPN is expensive but the cost is considerably less than the similar care provided in a health care center. In addition, the person can remain at home and have continuity in activities of daily living.

■ EXERCISE

Many American adults live a sedentary life-style, although there has been a positive trend toward increased exercise in recent years. Most people are aware that activity or mobility is necessary for carrying out tasks of daily living. The need for exercise (activity that requires physical exertion) as a part of one's life-style is less commonly understood or accepted. The topic of exercise is value laden. Persons who do not value exercise as a means of maintaining optimal health often find excuses for not participating in a planned exercise program on an on-going basis.

Exercise does imply effort; if exercise is not valued, the effort will not be taken.

Why is it important for the nurse caring for patients in an acute care center to consider the concept for exercise? Understanding the effects of exercise will assist the nurse in promoting exercise for the hospitalized patient and encouraging all persons to be as active as possible within their limitations and capabilities.

■ Benefits of exercise

A program of regular exercise can have both psychologic and physiologic benefits (see the box below). A physically fit person also generally has greater endurance and faster recovery time (return to resting rate), which contribute to more rapid recovery from illness.

Exercise is important regardless of age. Some elderly persons believe they are too old to begin an active fitness program, but these programs are possible even for persons with chronic illness. The fitness program is individually planned and based on the person's interests, capabilities, and limitations.

Physically, exercise enhances cardiovascular fitness, endurance, muscle strength, flexibility, and weight control. It has positive effects on the musculoskeletal, neurosensory, circulatory, respiratory, gastrointestinal, and urinary systems (see the box at right).

■ Exercise programs
■ CLASSIFICATION OF EXERCISE

Exercises may be classified as aerobic or anaerobic. *Aerobic* exercises are those activities that are supported by aerobic metabolism (the breakdown of carbohydrates and fats to carbon dioxide and water in the presence of oxygen, that is, the Krebs cycle). Aerobic exercises are characterized by activities that involve large muscle groups and that are performed in a rhythmic and continuous nature for more than 15 minutes. Examples of aerobic exercises include brisk walking, jogging, bicycling, swimming, skating, cross-country skiing, and aerobic dancing.

Anaerobic exercises involve anaerobic metabolism (the breakdown of glucose to lactic acid in the absence of oxygen). This occurs with high-intensity activities in which the available oxygen is used up and the anaerobic pathways are then used to provide the necessary additional energy. Anaerobic types of exercises include weight lifting and competitive sports, such as football, soccer, basketball, baseball, volleyball, and hockey. Greater benefits to overall physical fitness and well-being are achieved with aerobic rather than with anaerobic exercises.

■ RECOMMENDATIONS FOR PHYSICAL FITNESS PROGRAMS

Persons with a personal or family history of cardiovascular disease or who are over 35 years of age should have a physical examination before beginning an exercise program. A program is then planned on the basis of the person's tolerance and interests (it should be enjoyable).

Tolerance is evaluated by assessing pulse rate (Table 6-4). For example, a healthy, active 50-year-old person should

---

Benefits of aerobic exercise

Sense of well-being
Enhanced coping with stress
Decreased anxiety or depression
More restful sleep
Maintenance of physiologic functioning at optimum level
Enhanced weight control
Decreased risk factors for coronary artery disease
Better control of hypertension and diabetes mellitus
Assistance with reduction of addictive behavior (for example, smoking, overeating, or drinking)

Physiologic effects of exercise

1. Musculoskeletal system
   a. Maintains muscle strength
   b. Maintains joint flexibility
   c. Maintains endurance (tolerance to continue an activity)
2. Neurosensory system
   a. Maintains coordination
   b. Maintains orientation to environment
3. Circulatory system
   a. Maintains a more constant average work load on heart
   b. Maintains normal blood pressure regulatory adjustment to transient position changes
   c. Promotes venous return through contraction of muscles
4. Respiratory system
   a. Contributes to ease of breathing
   b. Provides stimulus to deep breathing and aeration of alveoli
   c. Provides movement of secretions
5. Gastrointestinal system
   a. Maintains elimination through muscle activity and visceral reflex patterns
   b. Encourages the person to heed defecation reflex
6. Urinary system
   a. Promotes urine formation
   b. Promotes complete emptying of bladder

Table 6-4 Target pulse rates with exercise

Category	Pulse target zone	Pulse return after exercise
Healthy active adults	70% to 85% of maximum heart rate (220 minus age)	Less than 120 in 5 min Less than 100 in 10 min
Obese, low physical conditioning	50% to 60% of maximum heart rate	Baseline level in 10 min
Cardiac disease, following bed rest	No more than 20 beats above baseline	Baseline level in 5 min

aim at maintaining a pulse rate during exercise of 70% to 85% of 170 beats per minute (220 minus 50), that is, within a range of 119 to 145. The pulse is then assessed for the time it takes to return to normal. Tolerance to activity of hospitalized patients who are starting to ambulate (aerobic exercise) after inactivity is assessed in the same manner; that is, the pulse rate should not increase greater than 20 beats per minute over the patient's baseline pulse rate and should return to baseline level within 5 minutes after ambulating.

Exercising should be done on a regular basis; one of the federal government's stated national health goals for 1990 is 20 minutes of exercise three times a week by all persons.[13] All persons should start each exercise period with deep diaphragmatic breathing and stretching exercises. Duration of the exercise period, which depends on the person's conditioning, is usually about 15 to 60 minutes per period. The exercises should be performed at just under the anaerobic threshold (identified by a tightness or "burning" sensation in the muscles and shortness of breath). It is best to start out slowly and gradually extend the program as conditioning improves. If the pulse target zone is exceeded or if the recovery period is extended, the exercise is too strenuous. With inactivity there is a loss of 20% conditioning within 2 to 3 weeks and up to 50% loss by 1 month.[10]

■ TYPES OF EXERCISES

□ Isometric exercises

With isometric exercises, opposing muscles are contracted, thus increasing the tone of the muscle fibers but not changing muscle length or moving the joints. The purpose of these exercises is to maintain muscle strength and tone. There is very little effect on cardiovascular or respiratory conditioning, although isometric exercises may not be easily tolerated by persons with coronary artery disease. Examples of isometric exercises for hospitalized patients are quadriceps-setting exercises and gluteal sets (Chapter 16) to maintain muscle strength in the thighs and buttocks for walking.

Persons doing isometric exercises should be taught to *exhale while exerting effort.* Many persons tend to hold their breath while bearing down (Valsalva maneuver). This increases intrathoracic pressure, causing a decrease in venous return to the heart. When the breath is then released, the intrathoracic pressure decreases, causing a large surge of blood return to the heart and increasing the cardiac work load. Exhaling while exerting effort can prevent the Valsalva effect.

□ Isotonic exercises

With isotonic exercises, muscle length changes and joint movements occur. There is less muscle tension than with isometric exercises. Isotonic exercises maintain and increase muscle strength. Aerobic exercises are one form of isotonic exercises. Some types of isotonic exercises for the hospitalized patient include moving and turning in bed, ambulating, and moving arms and legs against light resistance.

■ Immobility

Immobility may be accompanied by a number of complications that can involve any or all of the major systems of the body (Table 6-5). It is important that those caring for the patient whose mobility is impaired be aware of these potential complications and be skilled in interventions designed to help prevent them. The patient is encouraged to be as active as possible within the activity limitations by moving and turning in bed and by carrying out active range of motion, isometric, and isotonic exercises.

■ SUMMARY

1. Factors influencing health-promoting behaviors include perceptions about health and self, demographic factors, influence of family or friends, family patterns of health care, availability of opportunities to engage in health-promoting behaviors, and actual or perceived barriers to health-promoting actions.
2. All persons need the same nutrients throughout life but not in equally important amounts. Protein, fats, carbohydrates, and water are required in much larger quantities than vitamins and minerals.
3. Nutrient needs are affected by growth, basal metabolic needs, physical activity, disease, trauma, medications, and treatments.
4. The most common nutritional alterations are obesity and protein-calorie malnutrition.
5. Obese persons are at risk for osteoarthritis, DM, cardiovascular disease, cardiorespiratory dysfunction, and thromboembolic disease.

Table 6-5 Complications of immobility

System	Physiologic effect	Dysfunction/pathology	Nursing intervention (preventive)
Cardiovascular	Pooling of venous blood in legs Decreased venous return to heart Decreased cardiac output	Thrombophlebitis Pulmonary embolus Postural hypotension Decreased tolerance for activity when initiated	Range of motion: active and passive Isometric exercises of legs Turn frequently Avoid pressure on major blood vessels Slow mobilization
Respiratory	Pooling of secretions from decreased movement Decreased stimulation to cough Decreased depth of ventilation	Hypostatic pneumonia Atelectasis	Turn and move frequently Active range of motion Deep breathing and coughing
Gastrointestinal	Decreased peristalsis Change in eating/drinking habits Change in position to eliminate (bedpan)	Constipation	Increase fluid intake Good dietary intake of fiber foods Active movement in bed Use of stool softener or suppositories
Urinary	Increased calcium from bone destruction Alkaline urine Urinary stasis	Urinary calculi Urinary retention Urinary tract infection	Increase fluid intake Decrease calcium intake Use commode rather than bedpan if possible
Musculoskeletal	Muscle atrophy and shortening Fibrosis or bony ankylosis of joints Loss of bone matrix with release of calcium	Muscle weakness Contractures Osteoporosis	Active range of motion Isometric and isotonic exercises Positioning of joints to facilitate use
Neurologic	Decreased stimuli	Decreased orientation	Social contacts Diversionary materials
Skin	Friction, pressure, or shearing forces Decreased circulation from pressure Break in skin integrity Maceration from perspiration or urinary incontinence	Abrasions Decubitus ulcers	Frequent assessment Protection of vulnerable areas (foam or alternating pressure mattresses, sheepskin, flotation pads, elbow or heel pads) Turn frequently

---

Putting knowledge to practice

- Make a list of foods you like best. Compare your list with a classmate's list. What are some of the reasons for the differences? Would you eliminate many of these foods if a health professional told you these would place you at high risk for X disease? What factors would influence your decision about complying or not complying?
- Write a list of your food intake over a typical day (be honest!). Compare your food intake with the daily food guide described in this chapter. Does your intake meet the recommendations? What changes, if any, would you make?
- A friend tells you that she had discovered a great discount store for buying vitamin pills so she takes 35 different vitamins a day. What problems could result?
- Compare your weight to the standard tables (do not forget to allow for the shoe heels in height). If you are 20% or more above or below the 100% level (midpoint of the range) for your height and frame, what difficulties might you experience?
- Why would it be ineffective to tell an obese person he/she should lose weight?
- Develop a teaching plan for a patient who will be giving herself total parenteral nutrition feedings at home.
- How often do you engage in 15 minutes or more of aerobic activities each week? What change, if any, would you make to meet recommendations for health promotion?

6. Medications may affect nutritional status; food can, in turn, affect absorption of oral medications.
7. The daily food guide is useful for a quick dietary assessment.
8. Obesity is defined as more than 20% over established height/weight standards; morbid obesity is 45 kg (100 lbs) above the standard.
9. Persons who generally respond well to weight-reduction programs are those with adult onset obesity rather than lifelong obesity.
10. Methods of weight reduction include diet, exercise, behavior modification, surgery, and gastric balloon.
11. Rapid weight loss is usually the result of loss of fluid rather than fat.
12. Without behavior modification, most persons who lose weight by weight control programs return to or surpass their original weight within 5 years.
13. The most effective method of administration of tube feedings is by the infusion pump
14. Tube feeding solutions differ in terms of CHO or protein content, osmolality, consistency, palatability, flavor, and expense.
15. Complications of tube feedings include aspiration, tube dislodgement, tube clogging, nausea, bacterial contamination, dehydration, diarrhea, and hyperglycemia.
16. TPN solutions are deposited into the superior vena cava to provide greater dilution of the highly concentrated solutions.
17. TPN solutions must be prepared and given under strict aseptic conditions to prevent bacterial contamination.
18. Complications of TPN include infection, air embolism, lung injury from tube dislodgement, thromboembolism, electrolyte imbalances, overhydration, hyperglycemia, hypoglycemia, vitamin D deficiency, and vitamin A excess.
19. Home TPN permits persons to lead more normal lives; teaching for HTPN begins in the hospital and is continued in the home until the person can function independently.
20. Exercise enhances cardiovascular fitness, endurance, muscle strength, flexibility, weight control, sense of well-being, sleep, and ability to cope with stress. Exercise also has a positive effect on the body systems, decreases risk factors of coronary artery disease, provides better control of hypertension, and assists in reducing addictive behaviors.
21. Aerobic exercises are those that involve large muscle movements in a continuous and rhythmic manner for more than 15 minutes. Anerobic exercises are high intensity activities that use up available oxygen and are supported by anaerobic pathways.
22. Activity tolerance of healthy active adults is assessed by a pulse rate 70% to 85% of maximum heart rate (220 minus age) that returns to normal within 5 minutes.

23. Isometric exercises are those that include muscle contraction without joint movement. Isotonic exercises include muscle contraction with joint movement.
24. Persons doing isometric exercises should exhale while exerting effort to prevent Valsalva maneuver.

REFERENCES AND SELECTED READINGS
Contemporary

1. *Ackerman, S: The management of obesity, Hosp Pract 18(3):117-121, 125-129, 134-135, 1983.
2. *Anderson, BJ: Tube feeding: is diarrhea inevitable? Am J Nurs 86:705-706, 1986.
3. *Atkins, JM, and Oakley, CW: A nurse's guide to TPN, RN 49:20-24, 1986.
4. *Baj, PA: Liposuction, AORNJ 43:1127-1135, 1986.
5. *Baker, DJ: Ten years of TPN at home, Am J Nurs 84:1248-1249, 1984.
6. Bass, J, and Freeman, JB: Complications of gastric partitioning for morbid obesity, Adv Surg 18:223-255, 1984.
7. *Birdsall, C: When is TPN safe? Am J Nurs 85:73, 1985.
8. Briggs, GM, and Calloway, DH: Bogert's nutrition and physical fitness, ed 11, Philadelphia, 1984, WB Saunders Co.
9. Brozenac, SA: Surgical implants: medication and alimentation devices, AORN J 37:1353-1368, 1983.
10. Cantu, RC: Toward fitness: guided exercise for those with health problems, New York, 1980, Human Sciences Press, Inc.
11. Cantu, RC: Health maintenance through physical conditioning, Littleton, Mass, 1981, PSG Publishing Co, Inc.
12. *Carr, P: When the patient needs TPN at home, RN 49:25-30, 1986.
13. Centers for Disease Control: Status of the 1990 Physical fitness and exercise objectives, MMMR 34(34):521-531, 1985.
14. Clark, JB, Sherry, FQ, and Karb, VB: Pharmacologic basis of nursing practice, ed 2, St Louis, 1986, The CV Mosby Co.
15. *Clark, SR: Compliance and health behavior, Top Clin Nurs 7(4):39-46, 1986.
16. Cornacchia, HJ, and Barrett, S: Consumer health: a guide to intelligent decisions, ed 3, St Louis, 1985, The CV Mosby Co.
17. Dychtwald, K, and MacLean, J: Wellness and health promotion for the elderly, Rockville, Md, 1986, Aspen Systems.
18. Ebersole, P, and Hess, P: Toward healthy aging: human needs and nursing response, ed 2, St Louis, 1985, The CV Mosby Co.
19. Fitzgerald, PL: Exercise for the elderly, Med Clin North Am 69:189-195, 1985.
20. Fleming, CR, and McGill, DB: Total parenteral nutrition. In Beck, JE (editor): Bockus' gastroenterology, ed 4, Philadelphia, 1985, WB Saunders Co.

*References preceded by an asterisk are particularly well suited for student reading.

21. Freeman, JB, and Fairfull-Smith, RJ: Current concepts of enteral feeding, Adv Surg 16:75-112, 1983.

22. Gastric balloon for treatment of obesity, Med Lett 28:77-78, 1986.

23. Getchell, B: Fit: a personal guide, ed 2, Indianapolis, 1986, Benchmark Press.

24. Guiness, R: How to use the new small-bore feeding tubes, Nurs 86 16(4):51-56, 1986.

25. Halpern, NB: Surgery for obesity, Ala J Med Sci 22:53-57, 1985.

26. Haskell, WL, Montoye, HJ, and Orenstein, D: Physical activity and exercise to achieve health-related physical fitness components, Pub Health Rep 100(2):202-210, 1985.

27. Herbert, V: Nutrition cultism: facts and fiction, Philadelphia, 1980, George F Stickley Co.

28. Heymsfield, SB, and Andrews, JS: Enteral nutritional support. In Beck, JE (editor): Bockus' gastroenterology, ed 4, Philadelphia, 1985, WB Saunders Co.

29. *Holm, K, and Kirchhoff, KT: Perspectives on exercise and aging, Heart Lung 13:519-523, 1984.

30. Homsy, RN, and Blackburn, GL: Modern parenteral and enteral nutrition in critical care, J Am Coll Nutr 2:75-95, 1983.

31. *Hutchison, MM: Administration of fat emulsions, Am J Nurs 82:275-277, 1982.

32. Kaye, D, and Rose, L: Fundamentals of internal medicine, St Louis, 1983, The CV Mosby Co.

33. *Kornguth, ML: When your client has a weight problem: nursing management, Am J Nurs 81:553-554, 1981.

34. Krause, MV, and Mahan, LK: Food, nutrition, and diet therapy, ed 7, Philadelphia, 1984, WB Saunders Co.

35. McCain, GH: Sources of health information for consumers and health practitioners, Fam Comm Health 9(2):46-50, 1986.

36. Meguid, MM, Eldar, S, and Wahba, A: The delivery of nutritional support, Cancer 55(Suppl 1):279-289, 1985.

37. *Metheny, NM: Twenty ways to prevent tube-feeding complications, Nurs 85 15(1):47-50, 1985.

38. Miller, BL: Jejunoileal bypass: a drastic weight control measure, Am J Nurs 81:564-568, 1981.

39. *Mojzisik, CM, and Martin, EW Jr: Gastric partitioning, the latest surgical means to control morbid obesity, Am J Nurs 81:569-572, 1981.

40. *Mogan, J: Behavioral treatment of obesity, Occup Health Nurs 32:312-314, 1984.

41. Moore, MC: Do you still believe these myths about tube feedings, RN 50(5):51-55, 1987.

42. Neville, J: Assessment of nutritional status and dietary counseling. In Phipps, WJ, Long, BL, and Woods, NF: Medical-surgical nursing: concepts and clinical practice, ed 3, St Louis, 1987, The CV Mosby Co.

43. *Pender, NJ: Health promotion in nursing practice, ed 2 Norwalk, Conn, 1987, Appleton-Century-Crofts.

44. Schreiber, H, and Guyton, DP: Gastric bubble: therapy of obesity, Ohio State Med J 82:476-479, 1986.

45. Shepard, RJ: Physical activity and growth, Chicago, 1982, Year Book Medical Publishers, Inc.

46. Shannon, BM, and Parks, SC: Fast foods, a perspective on their nutritional impact, J Am Diet Assoc 76:242-247, 1980.

47. Stefee, P: Malnutrition in hospitalized patients, JAMA 244:2630-2635, 1980.

48. Steinhard, AJ, Foster, GD, and Grossman, RF: Surgical treatment of obesity, Adv Psychosom Med 15:140-166, 1986.

49. Van Italie, TB, and Kral, JG: The dilemma of morbid obesity, JAMA 246:999-1003, 1981.

50. *White, JH: Behavioral intervention for the obese client, Nurs Pract 11:27-34, 1986.

51. *White, JH, and Schroeder, MA: When your client has a weight problem: nursing assessment, Am J Nurs 81:550-563, 1981.

52. White, PL, and Mondeika, T: Diet and exercise—synergistic in health and maintenance, Chicago, 1981, American Medical Association.

53. *Wihelm, L: Helping your patient "settle in" with TPN, Nurs 85 15(4):60-64, 1985.

54. *Willett, W, and others: Vitamin supplement use among registered nurses, Am J Clin Nutr 34:1121-1125, 1981.

55. Williams, RM, McMahon, LC, and Macgregor, AM: Gastric bypass with Roux en Y: surgical treatment for morbid obesity, AORN J 43:1094-1105, 1985.

56. Williams, SR: Nutrition and diet therapy, ed 5, St Louis, 1984, The CV Mosby Co.

Classic

57. Cooper, KH: Aerobics, New York, 1972, Bantam Books, Inc.

58. Cooper, KH: The aerobics way, New York, 1977, M Evans & Co, Inc.

59. *Friedman, BJ, and Knight, K: Running for life, health, and pleasure, Am J Nurs 78:602-607, 1978.

UNIT III
Common Problems Encountered in Medical-Surgical Nursing

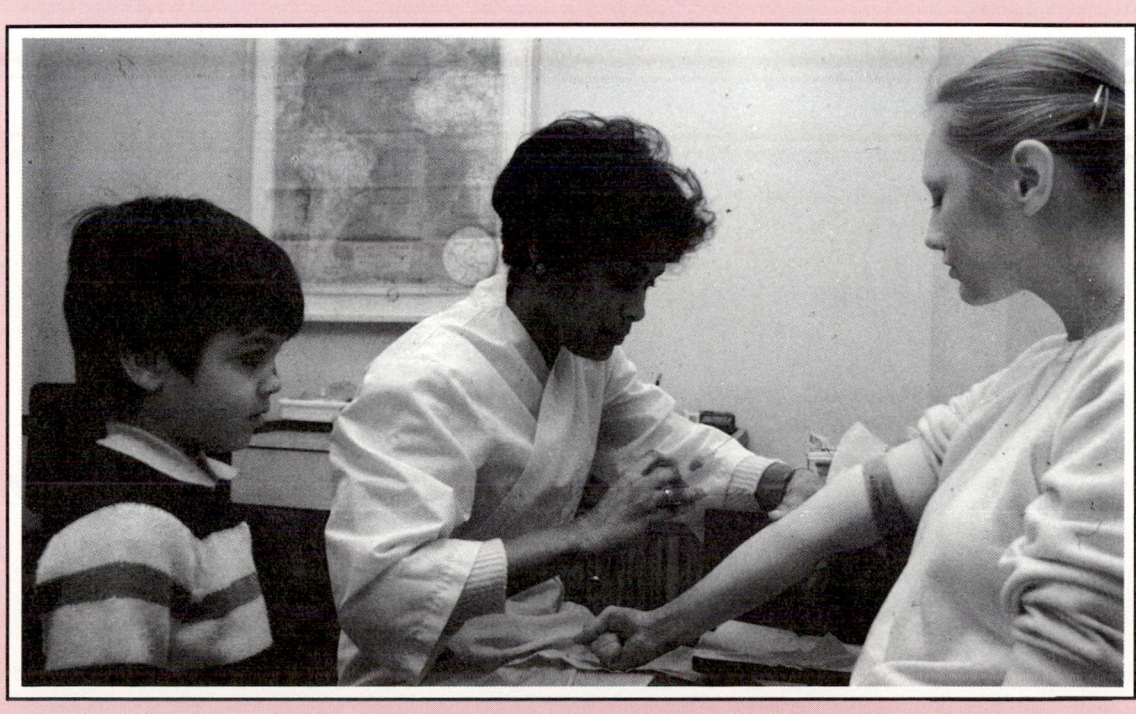

7

Stress and Stress Management

BARBARA C. LONG and MAY WYKLE

CHAPTER OBJECTIVES

After studying this chapter, the student should be able to:

- Differentiate between stress and stressor, and explain the relationship of stress to optimal functioning and growth.

- Identify factors influencing stress response.

- Describe physiologic and behavioral responses to stress.

- Define coping and describe types of coping strategies.

- Identify assessment parameters of and interventions for anxiety.

- Describe the nature of crisis and approach to crisis intervention.

- Describe methods of stress management.

Promotion of health involves activities that facilitate a sense of well-being. This implies a feeling of "ease," which is accomplished in part by coping effectively with internal or external stressors.

Many pathophysiologic disorders that are stress-related can be exacerbated by inadequate techniques for coping with stress.

Selected stress-related disorders

Hypertension	Peptic ulcer
Angina pectoris	Ulcerative colitis
Myocardial infarction	Headaches
Hyperthyroidism	Insomnia
Bronchial asthma	Alcoholism
Allergies	

Nurses can help patients learn how to cope with stress in a positive manner and thus prevent or diminish the effects of stress. This chapter will discuss concepts of adaptation and stress, responses to stress, and stress management.

■ ADAPTATION

Humans can be conceptualized as open systems that respond to stimuli from the internal and external environments. This process of interaction can be termed *adaptation*. In this context, adaptation has neither positive nor negative values. However, many prefer to use the term in a positive sense, to mean the process of interaction with the environment that promotes dynamic equilibrium (homeostasis) and growth. The process that leads to inadequate functioning is then termed *maladaptation*.

Human beings adapt biologically, psychologically, and socially. The goal of biologic adaptation is survival or stability of internal processes. The body has numerous physiologic feedback loops and compensatory mechanisms that help to maintain body processes within the ranges of normal, which facilitate optimal functioning. When the ability to maintain this equilibrium is lost, pathophysiologic disorders result (Fig. 7-1).

Psychologic adaptation is directed toward preservation of self-identity and self-esteem. The person adapting in this mode is mentally healthy, whereas maladaptation leads to mental illness. Social adaptation depends on the socio-cultural expectations of the society of which the person is a member. A maladaptive or socially deviant behavior in one society may be acceptable in another.

■ RESPONSES TO STRESS

■ Stress as a concept

The term *stress* has been used for many years to denote mental strain, for example, the comment "He's under stress." Selye was the first to use the term in a biologic context, that is, the nonspecific response of the body to a variety of noxious stimuli.[24] He termed the stimulus a *stressor*. The stressor may be a stimulus from the internal or external environment, and it places a demand on the system, disrupting the dynamic equilibrium. The stressor may produce a biologic or a behavioral response.

The stress or tension that results from the stressor may have either negative or positive results or both. For example, a person may experience pain (a stressor). The pain may cause anorexia, which may lead to nutrient imbalance and inactivity, which may lead to the side effects of immobility. These are negative results. On the other hand, the presence of pain may guide the person to seek medical intervention. This may lead to removal of the underlying condition causing the pain, a positive result.

Stress is not necessarily something to be avoided, and in fact a certain amount of normal stress (*eustress*) is considered necessary for adaptation. For example, microorganisms can upset cellular function, leading to disequilibrium and death. However, exposure to microorganisms in limited numbers or of decreased strength can help the body develop mechanisms to defend against subsequent exposures. Similarly, exposure to psychologic stressors in everyday living helps develop useful coping methods that facilitate dealing with new stressors. Coping with biologic or psychosocial stressors in an adaptive manner aids optimal functioning and growth. Maladaptation leads to dysfunction and pathophysiologic or psychopathologic disorders.

■ Factors influencing stress responses

A given stressor may cause one person to respond adaptively, a second person to respond maladaptively, and a third person to respond neutrally (that is, little response).

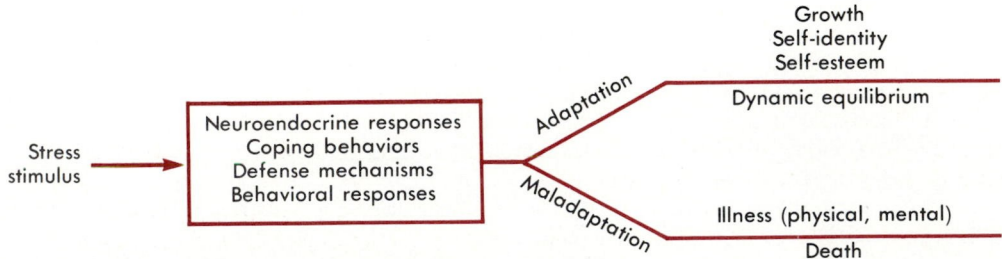

Fig. 7-1   Responses to stressful stimuli may lead to adaptation or maladaptation.

The following factors can influence the type of stress response:

1. Stimulus characteristics
   a. Intensity
   b. Duration
   c. Number
2. Personal characteristics
   a. Meaning of stressor to person
   b. Availability of resources and coping responses
   c. Health status

■ STIMULUS CHARACTERISTICS

A stimulus of low intensity may not be a stressor if the body can deal with it automatically, without disturbing the equilibrium. In general, the greater the intensity of the stimulus, the greater the probability that a stress response will occur.

A sudden, intense stimulus will generally produce a more marked response than a stimulus that develops gradually. The insidious onset often gives the person time to develop coping responses that may not be present with the acute onset. On the other hand, a persistent stressor may deplete the person's energy and eventually exhaust the resources available for coping.

The number of stimuli present at a given time will also affect response. The common phrase "the straw that broke the camel's back" describes the concept by which a specific stimulus may have no effect by itself, but may precipitate a stress response when combined with numerous other stressors.

■ PERSONAL CHARACTERISTICS

The meaning of the stressor for the individual is one of the major factors influencing the stress response. Stressors creating a change that is viewed negatively have a high probability of an increased response. For example, a woman who places great value on her body as a means of personal and sexual gratification will likely experience a greater response to removal of a breast than a woman who places little significance on her bodily appearance.

The individual's *perception* of the stressor (and hence the meaning that is interpreted) is influenced by cognitive ability, verbal skills, past experiences, interpersonal relationships, support person's responses, and feelings of control. A sense of control over the stressor helps to decrease the response. For example, patients who know in advance some measures to decrease postoperative pain (that is, have control over the pain) will usually adapt more effectively in the postoperative period. Persons who have developed a repertoire of coping skills can select one that will facilitate adaptation to a new stressor. Thus persons who have had to cope with numerous intense stressors in the past are often able to cope effectively when crises occur.

When health status is poor, less energy is available to deal with environmental stimuli, and responses to stressors may be affected. Nutritional deficits especially place the person at higher risk of maladaptive responses (see Chapter 6).

■ Integrated psychobiologic response

People respond to stress as a *unified whole*, that is, compensatory or defense mechanisms are initiated to help the individual cope with the stress biologically and psychologically. Some of the evoked responses will be biologic, others will be behavioral, and both frequently occur simultaneously. For example, anxiety can cause sweaty palms, pale skin, and frequent voiding, as well as decreased attention span, decreased ability to follow directions, or immobility. For the purpose of study, however, it is easier to separate physiologic responses from behavioral responses.

■ General adaptation syndrome

A small locally applied stimulus may result in a *local adaptation syndrome* (LAS). The inflammatory process is an example of LAS. Moderate to severe stressors will cause a *general adaptation syndrome* (GAS). The GAS proposed by Selye as a response of individuals to stress consists of 3 stages: alarm reaction, resistance, and exhaustion. The first two stages are repeated continuously throughout life as persons encounter stressors. The exhaustion stage occurs when resistance cannot be sustained, and altered functioning then results.

■ ALARM REACTION STAGE

During the initial alarm stage (shock), the "fight or flight" response is initiated. The individual prepares to counteract the stressor or remove himself or herself from the stressor. If the shock is too severe, a "freeze" response occurs; the person is overwhelmed by the stressor and cannot fight or flee. During the alarm reaction stage, the neuroendocrine mechanisms are activated. If the compensatory mechanisms are sufficient to deal with stressor, the individual returns to the prestressed level (Fig. 7-2, A).

■ RESISTANCE STAGE

Continual and prolonged application of the stressor leads to the resistance stage. During this stage, there is continued adrenocortical activity to facilitate adaptation. Energy is required to maintain a high level of resistance. If the stressor is maintained a sufficient time, stress-related pathophysiologic disorders (p. 100) may result. If adaptation is successful and the stressor removed, the person may return to the prestressed level (Fig. 7-2, B).

■ EXHAUSTION STAGE

If the original stressor is so damaging that it is impossible for the defense mechanisms to be effective or if the stressor is not removed and energy to maintain resistance is depleted, the exhaustion stage occurs (Fig. 7-2, C). Examples of extreme stress situations are arterial bleeding, pressure on the hypothalamus, overwhelming infection, blockage of a major branch of the coronary artery, or sudden death of a spouse. Presenting symptoms may include those seen in the initial shock phase. Unless the primary biologic condition can be controlled promptly, death may ensue.

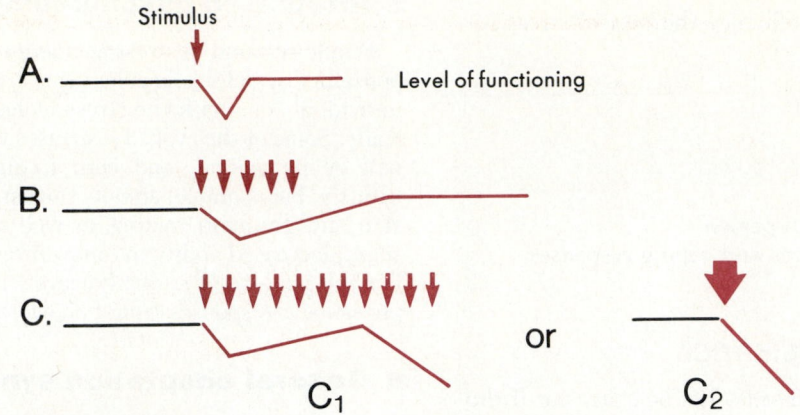

Fig. 7-2 General adaptation syndrome. **A,** Alarm reaction with return to prestressed level. **B,** Continued application of stimulus leads to resistance stage; return to prestressed level may occur when stimulus is removed. **C,** Depletion of resources with continued stimuli or strong damaging stimulus leads to exhaustion.

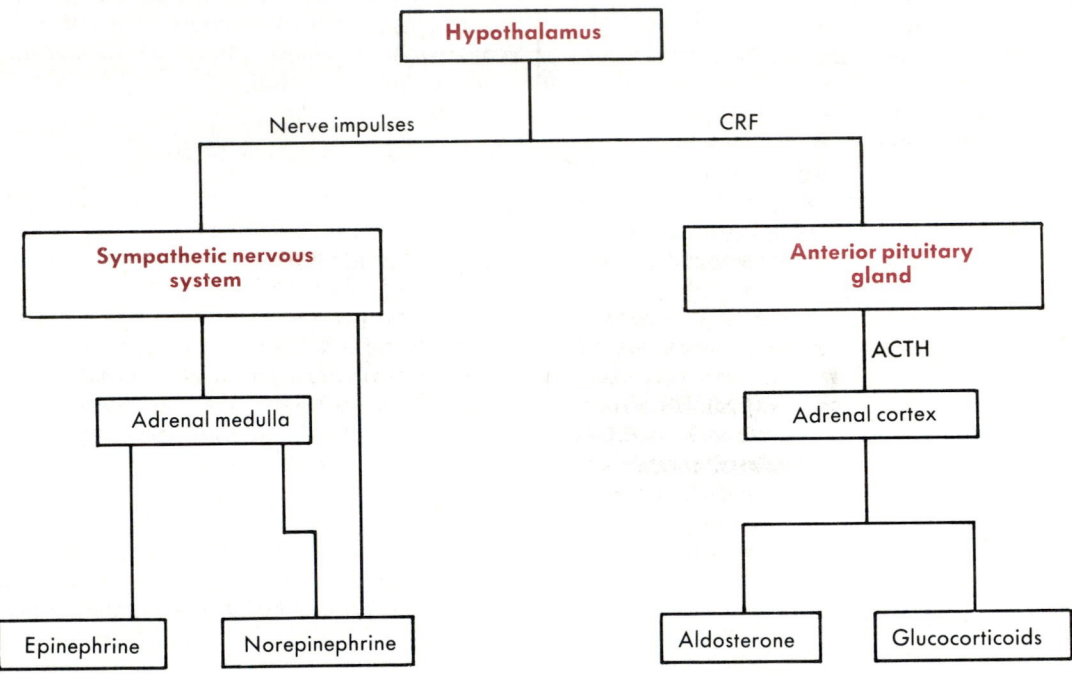

Fig. 7-3 Physiologic response to stress.

Overwhelming psychologic stressors may also lead to mental dysfunction or death.

■ Neuroendocrine response to stress

The hypothalamus responds to stimuli from the peripheral receptors or cerebral cortex by activating two different mechanisms, the sympathetic-adrenal medullary mechanism and the anterior pituitary-adrenocortical mechanism (Fig. 7-3).

The first mechanism, the *sympathetic-adrenal medullary*

mechanism, suppresses functions that are nonessential for life and augments those that facilitate overcoming or escaping the stressful situation. Impulses are conducted from the hypothalamus to the sympathetic centers in the thoracolumbar segments of the autonomic nervous effectors to prepare the body for "fight or flight." An adequate blood supply to the brain and heart is maintained, and the blood supply to the skeletal muscles is increased. Provision is made to maintain the body's water, electrolyte, and temperature balances and to supply extra energy. To achieve these responses, the adrenergic fibers (sympathetic) of the

Effects of sympathetic-adrenal medullary mechanisms

Eye	Pupillary dilation
Heart	Increased rate, contractility and cardiac output
Blood vessels	
Coronary, brain, lungs	Dilated
Skin, mucosa, renal, abdominal viscera	Constricted
Lungs	Relaxation of bronchial muscles, decreased secretions
Gastrointestinal tract	Decreased motility and secretions
Pancreas	Decreased secretion
Liver	Glycogenolysis, gluconeogenesis
Urinary bladder	Relaxed
Glands; salivary, sweat	Increased secretion
Skin	Piloerection (goose bumps)

Effects of adrenal cortical hormones

Aldosterone

Maintenance of fluid and electrolyte balance
  Reabsorption of sodium and water
  Excretion of potassium, ammonium, and magnesium

Glucocorticoids

Provision of emergency fuel and repair materials
  Protein catabolism
  Release of glucose from liver and muscle glycogen
  Gluconeogenesis
  Glycogen synthesis
Stabilization of internal environment
  Reabsorption of sodium and excretion of potassium
  Increased ability of skeletal muscle to contract and delay fatigue
  Stabilization of lysosome membranes in cells
  Increased oxygen transport
  Decreased lactic acidosis
  Increased microcirculatory flow

Table 7-1   Types of coping strategies

Category	Examples
Action	Taking walks, washing floors, gardening
Cognitive	Problem solving
Intrapsychic	Religion, activities to search for meaning of stress
Interpersonal	Use of support persons, talking it over with someone
Emotional	Use of defense mechanisms, such as denial

and released in the pituitary portal veins. CRF stimulates the pituitary gland to increase the amount of adrenocorticotropic hormone (ACTH) released, which in turn causes an outpouring of adrenocorticosteroid hormones. The effects of the adrenal cortical hormones, aldosterone, and the glucocorticoids are to maintain fluid and electrolyte balance, provide for emergency energy and materials for repair, and stabilize the internal environment (see the box at left).

■ Coping

Coping refers to processes or skills that individuals use to deal with events, circumstances, or situations that are out of the ordinary. Coping strategies are overall plans of action for overcoming stressors.[1] Thus coping is a general behavioral response to stress.

People cope with stressors in one or more ways (see Table 7-1). Actions to cope with stress may be adaptive or maladaptive, depending on the achieved level of functioning. Some persons respond to most stressors in one characteristic mode; however, this limits their ability for adaptation when new stressors occur. For example, persons who generally respond to stressors by physical activity are severely hampered when an illness (stressor) that decreases physical

autonomic nervous system are stimulated to produce a chemical called norepinephrine, and the adrenal *medulla* secretes norepinephrine and epinephrine. The effects of the sympathetic-adrenal medullary mechanism are listed in the box at the top of this page.

The second mechanism, the *anterior pituitary-adrenocortical mechanism*, is not activated by nerve impulses but by a neurosecretion called corticotropin-releasing factor (CRF). This chemical is produced in the hypothalamus

mobility occurs. Persons who have developed several coping strategies are better able to cope effectively with new stressors.

■ Defense mechanisms

Defense mechanisms are unconscious processes used by individuals in adjustment to life stresses. They evolve during personality development and serve to protect the personality, satisfy emotional needs, maintain harmony between conflicting tendencies, and reduce the tension of anxiety by modifying reality to make it more acceptable. Defense mechanisms are compromise solutions.

There are two levels of defense mechanisms: those that are considered more primitive and those that are of a higher level (see the box below). Defense mechanisms are used by mentally healthy people as well as by those who are neurotic or psychotic. In the mentally healthy the mechanisms are used less frequently and those mechanisms of a more primitive kind are avoided. Defense mechanisms become pathologic when they are overused.

A defense mechanism is effective when it succeeds in easing intrapsychic tensions. When lower level defense mechanisms fail, a more pathologic process evolves, and the person exhibits psychiatric symptoms. All defense mechanisms are unconscious with the exception of suppression. Two defense mechanisms, denial and repres-

sion, that are frequently manifested by the hospitalized patient are discussed in more detail.

■ DENIAL

One of the defense mechanisms used frequently in dealing with the stress of illness is denial. This mechanism occurs during the early stages of crisis after the initial stressful impact. Denial of the illness helps the person deal with increased tension by protecting the ego (self) from reality. The pattern used by the person is similar to games played by children when they close their eyes and believe no one can see them. "It's not there because I don't see it." That which cannot be perceived is therefore not painful.

During denial intolerable thoughts are disowned. The ego gets rid of unwelcome facts (such as an illness) while still retaining its faculty for reality testing. The person manifests denial by disowning any body changes. For example, patients with coronary disease may deny they have had heart attacks and will blame their discomfort on indigestion. Patients may even deny the severity of the pain and act as though the pain were not present.

Denial works well for the person who has been independent and has a self-image of a strong, self-made individual or who views sickness as a sign of weakness. Denial can be complete or partial and includes a "splitting" of

---

Defense mechanisms

Higher level: less primitive mechanisms

Repression	Ideas painful to consciousness are forced into the unconscious
Suppression	Thoughts or desires are consciously inhibited
Sublimation	Energy of repressed tendencies is transformed and directed to socially acceptable goals
Identification	Person assumes the personal qualities or elements of the personality of another
Compensation	Person makes up, covers up, or disguises real or fancied inadequacies in another area
Displacement	An emotion is transferred or displaced from its original object to a more acceptable substitute that is less threatening
Rationalization	Plausible explanations are given to account for a belief or behavior motivated from unconscious sources

Lower level: more primitive mechanisms

Denial	The disavowal of intolerable thoughts, feelings, or wishes; person refutes external elements of reality that are unpleasant or painful
Regression	Person reverts to a pattern of behavior belonging to an earlier stage of development
Conversion	Painful emotional experience is repressed and later is expressed in the form of a physical symptom
Projection	That which is emotionally unacceptable within the self is rejected and attributed to others
Introjection	Person absorbs the emotional attitudes, wishes, ideals, or personality of others into oneself; the aspirations and self-restraints of others are incorporated into the personality
Reaction formation	Person adopts attitudes and behavior that are opposites of the impulses to which the individual is reacting

thoughts, feelings, and actions; for example, the patient may own the thoughts but deny the feelings.

Approaches that may be useful when working with the person exhibiting denial include the following:

1. Explore fears and anxieties underlying the denial.
2. Avoid direct confrontation of denial.
3. Assist person in controlling selected aspects of care.
4. Provide reassurance of the person's worth as a human being despite being in a dependent state.
5. Reinforce behaviors indicating reality acceptance.
6. Set limits kindly but firmly when denial behavior interferes with treatment.

■ REGRESSION

Regression is a defense mechanism often seen in persons who are ill, because regression facilitates acceptance of the patient role. The ego is acted on rather than acting. Regression makes a dependency relationship possible because of the individual's reversion to behavior patterns of an earlier level of development. Illness necessitates patients placing themselves in the hands of competent others. They often become self-centered and concerned only with their own needs and interests. These interests focus on what is happening to the person and on their acceptance or rejection by care givers. Often regression is a help to patients in that it promotes conservation of energy.

■ Specific behavioral responses

Stress leads to behaviors that are either adaptive or maladaptive. Persons who display adaptive behavior are those who make appropriate use of their coping mechanisms and do not exhibit symptoms of psychologic disturbance. Those with maladaptive behavior are at the end of the spectrum (Fig. 7-4); their psychiatric symptoms are a way of dealing with the increased stress. (For further information on maladaptive behavior consult a psychiatric–mental health text.) Anxiety and common behaviors resulting from the stress of illness are discussed here.

■ ANXIETY

Anxiety is a psychologic response to stress with both physiologic and psychologic components. It is a feeling of dread or uneasiness from an unrecognized source. Anxiety results when a person perceives a threat to the self either physically or psychologically (such as to self-esteem, body image, or identity).

Anxiety is manifested in different levels ranging from mild to severe.[44] In the box below, note the changes in the way the person relates to the environment. Awareness, which is heightened with mild anxiety, begins to decrease until the panic stage, in which perceptions of the environment become distorted. Persons can vacillate among the several levels of anxiety. The level of anxiety engendered and its manifestations depend on the person's maturity, understanding of need tension, level of self-esteem, and coping mechanisms.

Anxiety is an energy that cannot be seen; it is only implied by the individual's actions. This state of *anxiousness* manifested by behavioral changes is communicated interpersonally. Highly anxious persons can transmit the sense of anxiousness to others; for example, a very anxious patient can heighten a family member's anxiety, and vice versa.

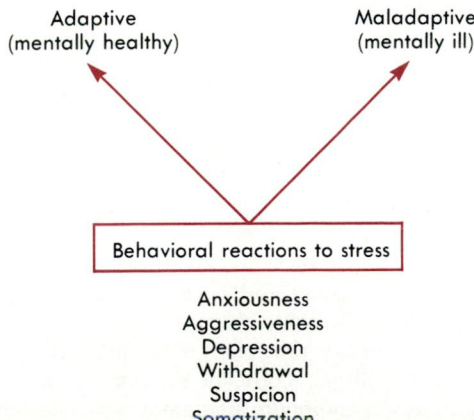

Fig. 7-4 Behavioral responses of persons experiencing anxiety from stress such as illness range from adaptive to maladaptive behavior.

Level	Behavior patterns
Levels of anxiety	
Mild anxiety	Alertness
	Quick eye movements
	Increased hearing ability
	Increased awareness
Moderate anxiety	Decreased awareness of environmental details
	Focus on selected aspects of self (or illness)
Severe anxiety	Disturbances in thought patterns
	Incongruency of thoughts, feelings, and actions
	Perceptual field greatly decreased
Panic	Distorted perceptions of environment
	Inability to see or understand situation
	Unpredictable responses
	Random motor activity

Although the ego attempts to deal with anxiety through the use of defense mechanisms, certain degrees of anxiety are reflected in behaviors resulting from a discharge of energy necessary to restore equilibrium of the individual. These responses range from behavior that is adaptive to behavior that is considered, by our social standards, to be maladaptive (Fig. 7-4). The types of behavioral reactions that occur are influenced by psychosociocultural factors, basic personality development, past experiences, values, and economic status.

■ AGGRESSIVE BEHAVIOR

Whenever self-concept is threatened, individuals may respond by aggression, a way that makes them feel less helpless and more powerful. Aggression is one way of handling anxiety. People are often angry at the loss of health status and question what is happening. They become irritable and uncooperative and may project their anger on others and become demanding. Expression of anger in socially acceptable ways prevents anger from being turned inward, causing depression.

Approaches that prove to be useful when working with a person exhibiting aggressive behavior include the following:
1. Provide opportunities for the person to express feelings and the reasons for the feelings.
2. Accept expressions of hostility without retaliation or making the person feel guilty.
3. Set limits and then anticipate the demands of the patient.

■ DEPRESSED BEHAVIOR

Depression is a normal response to illness, once the illness has been accepted. The person may describe feelings of sadness or unhappiness. Some common signs of depressed behavior include the following:
1. Decreased interaction with others
2. Lack of interest in activities or environment
3. Voiced concern about illness and amount of care required
4. Expressed wish for or concerns about dying
5. Dependent behavior
6. Decreased activity
7. Complaints of fatigue or inability to sleep
8. Crying spells

Any expressions about suicide should be taken seriously and the person referred for counseling.

Approaches useful when working with a person exhibiting depressed behavior include the following:
1. Approach the patient in a serious mood.
2. Convey by action and communication an understanding of what the person must be feeling.
3. Help the person express feelings.
4. Convey acceptance of the right to feel sad.
5. Listen to the person so that the anger can be turned outward.

■ WITHDRAWN BEHAVIOR

Withdrawal is commonly noted during illness. It permits the person to conserve mental and physical energy needed to deal with the stress and to promote repair and restoration. Withdrawn patients usually do not pose as many problems and are apt to be labeled "good" patients. They demand little from others and thus may be overlooked. Withdrawn patients regress more easily to earlier levels of behavior at which they can accept the patient role. They may have feelings of low self-worth.

Approaches that may be useful when working with the withdrawn person may include the following:
1. Spend time with the person, even if you are both silent, to increase the person's self-worth.
2. Provide gentle encouragement to talk, express feelings, and relate to others.

■ SUSPICIOUS BEHAVIOR

A sense of powerlessness or lack of control as a result of stress and anxiety may lead to suspicious behavior. Suspicious patients have difficulty with trust and may have had previous experiences in which they learned to distrust care givers. They are often suspicious of staff, the routines, the medicine, and the procedures. Whispered conversations by others within the person's hearing may reinforce feelings of suspiciousness that others are talking about the person.

Approaches that may be useful when working with persons exhibiting suspicious behavior may include the following:
1. Let the person talk about concerns but do not insist.
2. Keep promises made to the person to promote trust.
3. Avoid an overzealous approach, which may make the person more suspicious.
4. Provide explanations of procedures and routines so the person knows what to expect.
5. Avoid whispering or talking about the person within his or her hearing.

■ SOMATIC BEHAVIOR

A familiar reaction to illness is one that can be called *flight into illness*. Patients somaticize their concerns; that is, they have learned to express anxiety through complaints about a variety of physical symptoms. They may be preoccupied with body functions and feelings of pain. Vague complaints of backache, headache, or fatigue are expressed to legitimize the *attention needed*. Staff often become angry at patients who use somatic behavior because of the vague symptomatic complaints and because staff members feel "caught" if they minimize the symptoms, since there is always the possibility that the complaints are truly connected with an illness. Guilt on the part of staff prevails for some time if a complaining patient who was ignored is diagnosed as having a physical illness.

Approaches that may be useful for the person exhibiting somatic behavior may include the following:

1. Accept all symptoms and report them.
2. Spend time with the person and listen to physical complaints with some limit setting.
3. Use a saturation technique to provide needed attention.

ASSESSMENT

The conclusion that a person is demonstrating anxious behavior can be made when several signs of anxiety are present. With mild anxiety the signs are fewer and less prominent. Signs of anxiety are more overt in persons who are experiencing severe anxiety or panic.

Subjective data may include the following[14,22]:

1. States feeling apprehensive, uncertain, fearful, helpless, or anxious
2. States fears of unspecific consequences
3. States feeling overexcited, rattled, distressed, or jittery
4. States feeling tired and having difficulty sleeping

Data from the initial nursing history and the situation (such as proposed surgery, diagnostic tests) may provide clues to possible etiologies.

Objective data are listed in Table 7-2; observations are made about the person's behavior and interaction in addition to the physiologic signs. Restlessness and an increased awareness of the environment are early signs of anxiety. The person focuses more on the self as anxiety increases. Physiologic signs usually begin with moderate anxiety and are more prevalent and intense during severe anxiety and panic.

→ DATA ANALYSIS: NURSING DIAGNOSES

The nursing diagnosis of *anxiety* is best qualified whenever possible by citing the anxiety level (mild, moderate, severe, or panic, as noted in the box on p. 105). Possible *etiologies* include the following[22]:

Threat to self-concept
Threat of death
Threat to or change in health status, socioeconomic status, role functioning, environment, or interaction patterns
Situational and maturational crises
Interpersonal transmission and contagion
Unmet needs

PLANNING: EXPECTED PATIENT OUTCOMES

The expected patient outcomes will depend on the behaviors demonstrated by the anxious person; the outcomes will indicate a decrease in the exhibited behaviors. Expected patient outcomes for the anxious person may include, but are not limited to, the following:

1. The person states feeling more relaxed and less anxious.
2. The person states sleep is improved.
3. Vital signs return to usual norms.
4. Elimination is regular.
5. Diaphoresis is decreased.
6. Muscles are relaxed and the person rests quietly.
7. The person demonstrates increased ability to follow directions.
8. The person demonstrates effective coping skills.

IMPLEMENTATION

Interventions for the person experiencing stress may include general interventions to reduce the effects of stress, crises intervention for panic, specific support approaches, and stress management therapies.

■ General interventions

Nursing actions support the body's mechanisms for handling stressors and provide an environment that permits the person to mobilize natural defenses.

■ SUPPORTING PROTECTIVE MECHANISMS

Rest is absolutely essential with severe stress to maintain energy supply for metabolic functions essential for life. The person is kept comfortably warm but never overly

Table 7-2 Signs of anxiety

Type	Observations
Physiologic	
Skin	Pale or ashen, moist
Pupils	Dilated
Respirations	Deeper; may or may not be faster
Pulse	Increased rate and strength
Body temperature	Slightly increased
GI tract	Anorexia, nausea, constipation
Urinary tract	Frequency of urination with moderate stress, oliguria with severe stress
Motor system	Restlessness, frequent hand movements with moderate stress; immobility with severe stress
Behavior	Decreased attention span
	Decreased ability to follow directions
	Increased acting out
	Increased somatization
Interaction	Increased number of questions
	Constant seeking of reassurance
	Frequent shifting of topics of conversation
	Avoidance of focusing on feelings
	Focus on equipment or procedures

warm, because overheating causes vasodilation and counteracts the arteriolar constriction necessary to ensure an adequate blood supply to vital organs.

Even minor stress reactions cause annoying discomforts such as backache, generalized muscle tension, and headache. These discomforts can act as additional stressors, and comfort measures such as back rubs, position changes, and back support to relax the muscles are indicated. Pain should be alleviated as much as possible and noise and disturbance should be kept to a minimum. During severe stress, oral food and fluids may need to be withheld until nausea subsides and gastrointestinal tract activity returns to normal.

■ PROVIDING EXPLANATIONS

Structure decreases anxiety and is helpful for the person experiencing mild or moderate anxiety. Explanations are one method of providing structure. Each new experience should be explained to patients and, if possible, related to familiar experiences. The higher the level of anxiety, the more simple should be the explanations.

If patients are to have treatments or tests, they need to be given some idea of what will be done, the preparation involved, and the reasons why the procedure is necessary. To remove the water pitcher and inform patients that they cannot have any more water until after the x-ray examination can generate many anxious thoughts: "What x-ray examination?" "I wonder when it is?" "What will it be like?" "It must be something special if I can't have any water." Lack of knowledge as a cause of anxiety reflects the nurse's lack of consideration for the patient's rights as an individual.

Explanations should be given in the patient's own terms at appropriate times and repeated as necessary. If the patient is very anxious, repeated explanation may be necessary, since extreme anxiety reduces intellectual function. It is useless to give explanations to patients who are severely anxious or sedated or to those who have high temperatures or severe pain. Repetition is often required for older persons and children because they may have short memory spans.

Time spent in giving explanations to relatives is not wasted. Not only does it relieve their anxieties, which may be transmitted to the patient, but it also saves having to untangle misinformation. Often the family is helpful in interpreting necessary instructions to the patient in a manner that the patient understands and accepts.

■ PROMOTING EXPLORATION OF FEELINGS

In most instances a large part of the nurse's work is to encourage patients to express anxieties, to help patients see the universality of fear in their situation, to help them seek outlets for their fears and tensions, and to allay these negative feelings whenever possible. Nurses provide opportunities for the patient to talk, but they should not probe. There is a difference between prying into a patient's thoughts and beliefs and eliciting information that will aid in the understanding of behavior and in planning for care. Without seeming unduly curious, one can usually find some topic of personal interest to the patient that will provide an opening. A picture on the bedside table may create such an example. Nurses who listen with sincere interest and without making judgments about the patient may begin to gain insight into the patient as a person. And more important, the patient may begin to speak about personal fears.

As soon as the patient begins to talk about feelings, the nurse should proceed with conversation, taking cues from what the patient offers. The nurse who feels inadequate or anxious may cut off the conversation. For instance, if a patient says, "You know, I don't think I'll ever get to see my little boy again," a common response is "Oh, don't say that, certainly you will; you're going to be all right," The patient may very well not be all right. Would it not be better to respond, "What makes you feel this way?" Such a response helps the patient explore the subject and leaves opportunity for the patient to examine this concern. The nurse who is willing to listen to patients, to be guided by their reactions, and to work with them rather than to make decisions for them will give them needed emotional support. Solving patient's problems for them, even if it were possible, is not the aim of nursing. Indeed, it would tend to make patients less healthy psychologically.

The art of meaningful communication involves more than just listening; it includes moving the conversation so that the patient's attempts to communicate are assisted. Observing the patient for facial changes and general body movements provides opportunites for the nurse to discover from the individual the full meaning of the situation. For example, consider the patient who sucks in air while talking. The mouth becomes drier and drier as the tongue seems to stick in the mouth. These patients are not at ease and show anxiety even though their words may be quite innocuous. A simple statement such as "Your mouth seems very dry. Would a glass of water help?" allows the nurse the clarify observations. Such an approach gives the patient a chance to tell what is being felt, and to gain understanding by talking about it.

The nurse helps patients examine those problems that they are able to bring into awareness. Underlying problems should be handled by people trained in psychotherapy. A nurse needs to be able to recognize normal anxiety reactions and to report exaggerated reactions that may indicate the need for psychiatric referral.

When any patient's anxiety increases to a high level, the nurse may need to sit with the patient. The nurse's very presence is often reassuring. If possible, the patient is helped to recognize the anxiety by the nurse asking, "Are you uncomfortable?" or "What are you feeling?" In severe anxiety and panic, being there is most important, and touch may be used as a means of reassurance. Some severely anxious persons, however, view touching as an intrusion of their personal boundary, and the nurse needs to keep this in mind. When the patient is able to talk, the nurse helps the patient to describe what is happening, what has happened, and what is expected to happen.

■ SUPPORTING COPING MECHANISMS

There is no one specific or best way to cope with any given situation. What is useful to one individual may be inappropriate for another. The nature of the stressor, the developmental level of the individual, the social and cultural environment, and the physical and interpersonal resources available all influence the style and effectiveness of coping strategies.

It is most useful to help a person to cope in ways that are congruent with previously established styles. Data must therefore be collected to identify the person's usual coping strategies. One method is by asking the question, "What do you usually do when things get tough?" Weisman suggests seven simple questions that may obtain a great deal of information about coping strategies[37]:

1. What problems, if any, do you see this illness creating?
2. How do you plan to deal with them?
3. When faced with a problem you must do something about, what do you do?
4. How does it usually work out?
5. To whom do you turn when you need help?
6. What has happened in the past when you have asked for help?
7. What kinds of problems usually tend to get you upset or down?

These questions establish perception of the current problem, present and usual ways of dealing with problems, sources and responses to help, and recurrent problems that affect coping.

Stress management includes reinforcing appropriate coping mechanisms and helping the person explore alternative strategies if existing coping mechanisms are inappropriate.

■ FACILITATING PROBLEM SOLVING

Some persons solve problems in a haphazard manner. Problem solving can be a means for coping with stress and is more effective if the problem-solving steps are consciously followed. The steps include the following:

1. Gathering data
2. Identifying the problem (or effect of stressor)
3. Identifying factors affecting the problem or stressor
4. Determining goals
5. Exploring alternative ways and consequences of the actions to achieve the goals
6. Implementing action
7. Evaluating effectiveness of actions

If the stressor has been identified, the nurse first assists the patient in exploring feelings and reactions associated with the stressor. Often persons are not consciously aware of what they are feeling and therefore may select inappropriate actions. Persons vary in their ability to identify problems and in their desire to discuss personal feelings, although it is widely accepted that talking does help. If the patient is pushed indiscriminately to talk about problems, the relationship will become superficial and mechanical. The identification of the consequences of actions is often omitted but is an important component if problem solving is to be effective.

Problem solving reduces ambiguity and feelings of loss of control. Persons who do not generally employ conscious problem solving as a means of coping with stressors may benefit from learning about problem solving as a strategy for coping with stress.

■ TEACHING RELAXATION TECHNIQUES

Relaxation exercises are developed from the concept that stress with anxiety does not and cannot exist when the muscles of the body are relaxed. Relaxation exercises do not "cure" stress but do help to minimize effects of stress and give the person a sense of control. A daily program of relaxation exercises has been shown to have an effect on physiologic responses to stress (for example, lowering of elevated blood pressure or elevated blood sugars) and in psychologic responses to stress (for example, decreased level of anxiety). They are also helpful on a short-term basis when anxiety is present.

There are four basic components of relaxation techniques:

1. *Quiet environment:* deleting all possible noise and distractions
2. *Comfortable position:* sitting with no undue muscle tension
3. *Passive attitude:* emptying all thoughts from the conscious mind
4. *Mental device:* focusing on a sound, word, phrase, mental image, object, or breathing pattern to shift the mind from logical, externally oriented thoughts

The important factor is that the person empties the mind of all thoughts and concentrates on the mental device. It is natural for the mind to wander. When this occurs, the person simply redirects the mind back to the mental device. Each relaxation session should take approximately 20 minutes.

There are several approaches to performing relaxation exercises. Two approaches that can be carried out by nursing instructions to patients, without use of special equipment and without physician's orders, are *progressive relaxation* and *Benson's relaxation response.*

Progressive relaxation consists of tensing and relaxing muscle groups and focusing on the feelings of relaxation (see the box on p. 110). The systematic application of progressive relaxation has three major effects, which are as follows[42]:

1. Muscle groups are relaxed more and more with each practice.
2. Each of the major muscle groups is relaxed one after the other. As a new muscle group is added, the previously relaxed portions also relax.
3. More total body relaxation is experienced as the person moves into the relaxation phase. The relaxed state is maintained beyond the relaxation period.

Benson's relaxation response omits the muscle tensing. It is particularly helpful for muscle relaxation in patients

---

Progressive relaxation

1. Assume a comfortable position in a quiet room
2. Begin by focusing on easy breathing
3. Tense specific muscle groups (see step 5) for 5 to 7 seconds, then relax quickly
4. Concentrate for 10 seconds on the sensations of the relaxed muscles
5. Follow a sequence, repeating each muscle group, tensing two or three times:
   a. Hand and arm: clench fist, pull elbow tightly, wrinkle nose, purse lips, smile with teeth tightly clenched
   b. Face: wrinkle forehead, close eyes tightly, wrinkle nose, purse lips, smile with teeth tightly clenched
   c. Neck: pull chin to chest
   d. Trunk: pull shoulder blades together, tighten stomach and buttocks
   e. Leg and foot: push down with leg, point toes upward (dorsiflexion) dominant leg first
6. Repeat process in any areas in which increased tension has been identified

---

who are experiencing pain or discomfort. It is important to remain with the patient to coach and encourage the relaxation.[40]

Benson's relaxation response

1. Assume a comfortable sitting position in a quiet room.
2. Close eyes.
3. Relax body muscles (that is, "let go").
4. Concentrate on breathing. Repeat a word or sound such as "one" or "um-m" after each exhalation.
5. Continue for about 20 minutes.
6. Open eyes.
7. Take time to adjust to surroundings before moving.

■ PROVIDING ANTIANXIETY MEDICATIONS

In some instances, the patient may be prescribed an antianxiety medication to reduce the anxiety symptoms. The antianxiety agents may be divided into two groups, the benzodiazepines and the nonbenzodiazepines (Table 7-3). Note that the dosage of benzodiazepines is less for elderly persons who metabolize the drugs slowly, resulting in a prolonged depressant effect. Dosage should also be reduced for persons with impaired liver or kidney function.

The benzodiazepines are the most frequently prescribed antianxiety agents. These drugs act by inhibiting transmission of stimuli from the limbic system of the brain (septum, amygdala, and hippocampus). Side effects include drowsiness, dizziness, and weakness.

Antianxiety agents produce muscle relaxation and a sense of well-being. The drugs are prescribed for short-term relief of anxiety but not for anxiety from daily stressors. Long-term therapy leads to increased tolerance and dependence; larger doses are then needed to produce the desired effects and drug abuse may ensue.

Persons taking antianxiety agents are cautioned not to take alcohol or other CNS depressants during therapy because of serious complications, even death, as a result of synergistic effects. People also need to be cautious when driving or working around heavy machinery because of possible dizziness.

■ Crisis intervention

Awareness of what occurs during a crisis helps the nurse understand the accompanying behavior. When the ego is met with overwhelming anxiety created by biologic, physiologic, or social threats to the self, a crisis ensues. The ego is not able to cope successfully with the sudden disequilibrium, and the person needs assistance to use the situation as a growth experience.

A crisis occurs when a person is unable to use customary methods of coping when faced for a time with what seems to be an unsurmountable obstacle to an important life goal. A period of disorganization ensues, a period of upset during which many abortive attempts at solutions are made.

■ PHASES OF CRISIS

Shontz describes several phases or stages that occur during crisis.[49] These stages are similar to the stages of death and dying as described by Kübler-Ross.

1. *Initial impact.* During this phase the client experiences shock and depersonalization as reality is clearly perceived. Functioning is organized and automatic with individual centering and docility.

2. *Realization.* In the second phase the existing self-structure collapses. Reality seems overwhelming, and the person experiences high anxiety, panic, and helplessness. There is inability to plan, reason, or understand the situation.

3. *Defensive retreat.* The third phase is one of regression in which there is an attempt to establish previous identity, to return to better times. Reality is avoided, and denial and wishful thinking may ensue to relieve the anxiety. When challenged, the ego reacts with anger and the person may experience rage and disorientation. Thinking is situation-bound, and there is a resistance to change.

Table 7-3 Antianxiety agents

Generic name	Trade name	Usual adult dosage	Elderly dosage
Benzodiazepines			
Alprazolam	Xanax	0.25-0.5 mg tid	0.25 mg bid/tid
Chlordiazepoxide	Librium Libritabs	5-25 mg qid	5 mg bid/qid
Clorazepate	Tranxene	7.5-15 mg bid/qid	7.5-15 mg qd
Diazepam	Valium	2-10 mg bid/qid	2-2.5 mg qd or bid
Halazepam	Paxipam	20-40 mg tid/qid	20 mg qd or bid
Lorazepam	Ativan	1-3 mg bid/tid	0.5-1 mg bid
Oxazepam	Serax	10-30 mg tid/qid	10-15 mg tid
Prazepam	Centrax	10 mg tid or 20-40 mg at bedtime	5 mg bid/tid or 15 mg at bedtime
Nonbenzodiazepines			
Hydroxyzine HCl	Atarax	25-100 mg tid/qid	Same as adult dosage
Meprobamate	Equanil Meprospan Miltown	400 mg bid/tid or 600 mg bid	Same as adult dosage

4. *Acknowledgment*. This is the "yes" stage: "It has happened to me." The individual experiences depression and self-depreciation. Reality imposes itself again and looms large in relating the event to one's life. Without intervention the client may become more disorganized, depressed, and suicidal.

5. *Adaptation*. This is the stage when change occurs if help is adequate. New identity appears along with hope and renewed sense of personal worth. Anxiety is subsequently decreased and satisfaction is increased as a result of the stabilization and reorganization. Functional improvement is noted without actual change in disability status.

The model just offered is a useful approach for explaining what a person experiences during an illness crisis, even though reactions to crisis are individual. People are not equally vulnerable to all categories of stress, but there is thought to be some commonality in the reactions. Knowledge about the commonalities can facilitate plans for nursing intervention.

■ INTERVENTION

The essential element of crisis intervention is the intensive nature of support required to help the ego maintain its integrity and its ability to use coping mechanisms. Crisis, according to Caplan,[41] is self-limiting. Early intervention can prevent maladaptive behavior, and the individual can emerge a stronger person. Acute illness or catastrophic illness often precipitates a crisis reaction. The outcome of a crisis is governed by the kind of interaction that takes place between the individual and key figures in the environment during the time of crisis.

Often because of changes in society, previous guidelines for behavior in stressful situations render the individual helpless. In crisis the individual is helped to find ways to facilitate efforts to enlarge on the experience. A state of disequilibrium produces a felt need to reduce anxiety. The following balancing factors have been identified as being necessary to resolve the problem and to avert crisis:

1. A realistic perception of the event
2. Adequate situational support (staff and family)
3. Adequate coping mechanisms[1]

When one or more of these balancing factors are absent, the result is an increase in anxiety, with immobilization and an inability to avert the crisis (Fig. 7-5)

In crisis, help should be immediate. Staying with the person, talking through the situation, and encouraging catharsis facilitate recognition and expression of feelings and subsequent relief of guilt. Strengthening of coping mechanisms is crucial in preventing the formation of symptoms. Personal growth is facilitated by using problem-solving skills and a hierarchy of needs framework to help the person set priorities.

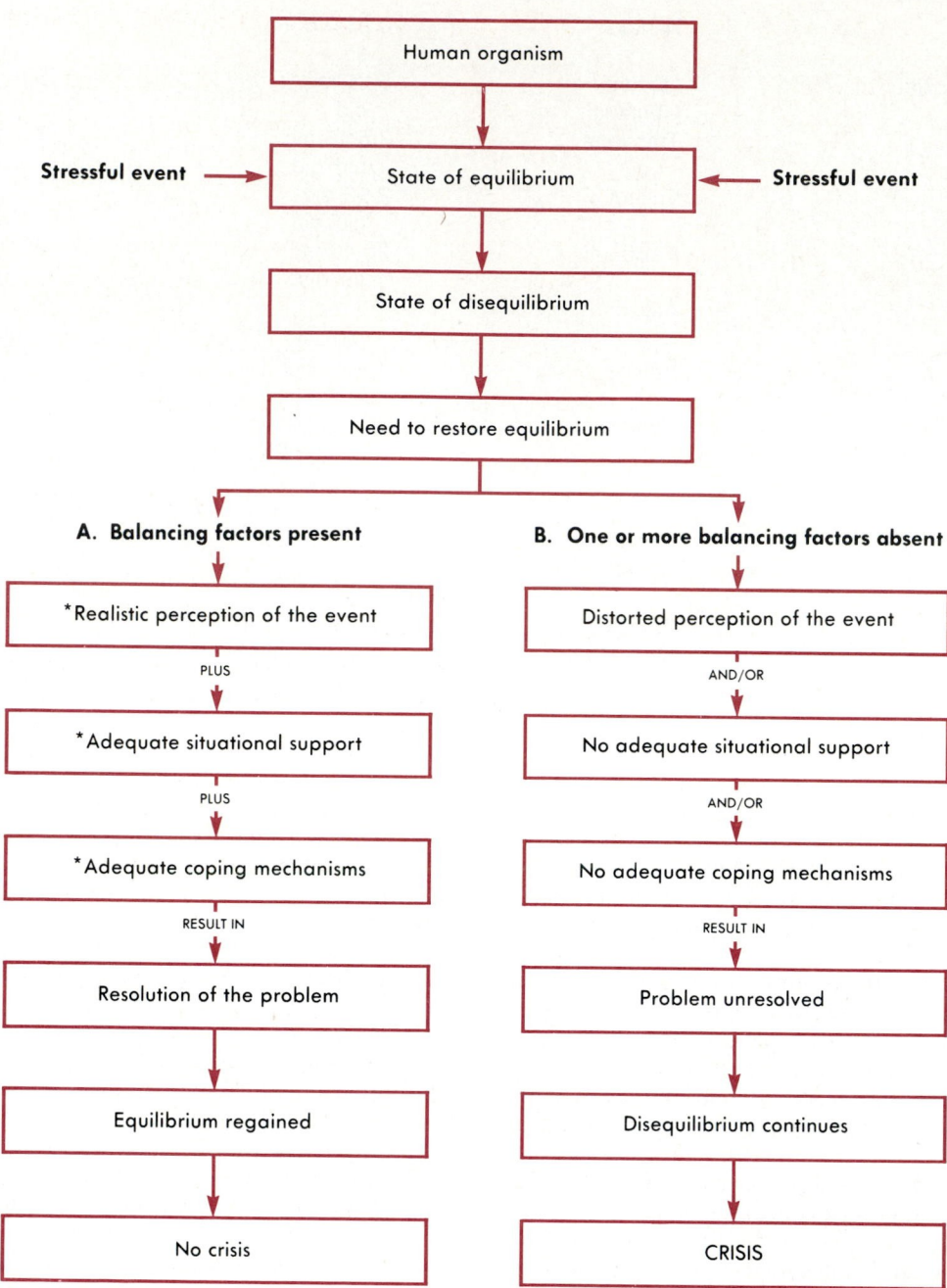

Human organism

→ State of equilibrium ←

Stressful event → State of equilibrium ← **Stressful event**

State of disequilibrium

Need to restore equilibrium

A. Balancing factors present | **B. One or more balancing factors absent**

*Realistic perception of the event	Distorted perception of the event
PLUS	AND/OR
*Adequate situational support	No adequate situational support
PLUS	AND/OR
*Adequate coping mechanisms	No adequate coping mechanisms
RESULT IN	RESULT IN
Resolution of the problem	Problem unresolved
Equilibrium regained	Disequilibrium continues
No crisis	CRISIS

*Balancing factors.

Fig. 7-5 Paradigm: effect of balancing factors in stressful event. (From Aguilera, DC, and Messick, JM: Crisis intervention: theory and methodology, ed 5, St. Louis, 1986, The CV Mosby Co.)

■ Specific support approaches

Persons who are having difficulty coping because of severe or multiple stressors may be referred for individual or group counseling. A person may need assistance and support from the nurse in seeking out and initiating counseling.

Therapeutic groups consist of persons who are experiencing common stressors. Peer support is given because the participants share the common experience. Persons often are able to express their feelings more easily when they know that the group members understand what they are experiencing. Approaches found helpful in solving the common problems are also shared. Therapeutic groups may be self-help groups or be directed by health professionals. Examples of therapeutic groups are Al-Anon (for family member of alcoholics), Parents Without Partners, Reach to Recovery (postmastectomy), "ostomy" groups, and the American Cancer Society's "I Can Cope" program.

■ Stress management therapies

Some approaches to stress management require special training or equipment. Stress management therapists help people design and implement a structured program of change to enable the individual to control and deal more effectively with stress. Some of the therapies include biofeedback, autogenic training, behavioral change programs, and systematic desensitization.

■ BIOFEEDBACK

Biofeedback is a system of learning voluntary control over autonomically regulated body functions so that an individual is able to monitor physiologic response to stress and to replace it with a nonstressful response. For example, if after a stressful day you notice soreness and muscle tension in your shoulders, you can sit quietly and concentrate on relaxing the shoulder muscles to feel the tension slip away.

With biofeedback, machinery is used to "train" the person to monitor certain parameters. For example, muscle activity can be monitored with an electromyograph (EMG) and the stimuli converted into a visual or auditory signal. Using this biofeedback, the person can learn how to replace muscle tension with muscle relaxation. Machines can also be used to measure skin temperature or sweat activity, and a similar feedback approach is used. The person is then weaned from the machine to produce the desired effects without machinery. A comprehensive biofeedback program includes feedback from multiple systems and sites.

■ AUTOGENIC TRAINING

Autogenic training teaches cognitive behavioral change together with physiologic behavioral change through passive concentration to decrease sympathetic nervous system activity. The person repeats a statement verbally with the physiologic state that is being practiced. The physiologic states are heaviness and warmth of extremities, calm and regular heartbeat and breathing, abdominal warmth, and cooling of forehead.[8] The methods are similar to that of transcendental meditation.

■ BEHAVIORAL CHANGE PROGRAMS

Some specific stress-related behaviors, such as smoking or overeating, may be eliminated by behavioral conditioning. The programs consist of the following:

1. Self-monitoring to identify characteristics and situations associated with the behaviors
2. Identifying outcome criteria in precise behavioral terms
3. Developing a formal contract with the therapist stating short-term goals with rewards and frequency of evaluation

The overall goal is a change in the person's behavior. Behavioral change programs are most effective with highly motivated persons; they must sincerely *want* to change the behavior.

■ SYSTEMATIC DESENSITIZATION

Systematic desensitization provides specific stressful stimuli (such as those related to phobias) in increasing doses while the individual practices relaxation skills. The person is first taught effective relaxation skills. Stimuli eliciting the anxiety are then presented in increasing intensity, starting at a minimal level while the person uses the relaxation techniques. Then the person is instructed to relax while imagining the situation in more threatening circumstances. The principle of systematic desensitization is to train the person to behave (relax) in a manner opposite to anxiety behavior (tension). A low initial stimulus that increases in intensity gives the person a sense of control over and of coping with the undesirable stimulus, thus decreasing the anxiety.

■ SUMMARY

1. Adaptation is a process of interaction with the environment that promotes dynamic equilibrium and growth. Maladaptation leads to inadequate functioning.
2. Responses to stress include neuroendocrine response, coping behaviors, defense mechanisms, and specific behavioral responses.
3. Response to stress is influenced by the stimulus (intensity, duration, number) and personal characteristics (perception, meaning, availability of resources and coping responses, and health status).
4. The general adaptation syndrome consists of three stages: alarm reaction, resistance, and exhaustion. The first two stages occur frequently throughout life; death may ensue from exhaustion.
5. The sympathetic-adrenal medullary response prepares the person for "fight or flight" through release of epinephrine and norepinephrine. The hormonal response

---

Putting knowledge to practice

- Should you try to lead a life that is free from stress? Explain.
- Think back over several situations when you were experiencing stress. What type of physical symptoms did you experience? What is the physiologic reason for each symptom that you experienced? Were the symptoms always the same? If not, state why.
- In what way(s) do you cope with stress? What other coping strategies might be useful for you?
- Try one or both of the relaxation techniques described in this chapter. Describe the sensations experienced during relaxation. How did you feel after completing the exercise? What types of difficulties did you have in carrying out the relaxation exercises? Identify a patient situation from your experience where you think relaxation exercises might have been a useful nursing intervention.

---

maintains homeostasis and provides energy and materials for repair through release of aldosterone and glucocorticoids.

6. Types of coping strategies include action, cognitive, intrapsychic, interpersonal, or emotional strategies.

7. Defense mechanisms are unconscious mechanisms used by individuals in adjustment to life stresses. Mentally healthy persons use defense mechanisms occasionally, avoiding more primitive mechanisms.

8. Some specific behavioral responses to stress include anxiety, aggressive behavior, depressed behavior, withdrawn behavior, suspicious behavior, and somatic behavior.

9. Anxiety results when a person perceives a threat to the self, either physically or psychologically.

10. Anxiety may be mild, moderate, severe, or a state of panic. Awareness of the environment decreases and physiologic signs increase as anxiety increases.

11. Rest and relief of discomfort conserve energy for coping with stress; providing explanations provides structure, which helps to decrease anxiety. Exploration of feelings helps to relieve tension associated with stress, and problem solving reduces feelings of loss of control associated with stress.

12. Relaxation is the opposite of tension produced by stress; it also gives the person a sense of control. Basic components of relaxation techniques are quiet environment, comfortable position, passive attitude, and a mental device to remove externally oriented thoughts.

13. The most frequently prescribed antianxiety agents are the benzodiazepines. Alcohol or other CNS depressants should be avoided when taking antianxiety agents.

14. Crisis occurs when anxiety overwhelms the self and the person is unable to use coping mechanisms. Crisis is self-limiting. Balancing factors necessary to resolve crises include a realistic perception of the event, adequate situational support, and adequate coping mechanisms.

15. Stress management therapies include biofeedback, autogenic training, behavioral change programs, and systematic desensitization.

REFERENCES AND SELECTED READINGS
Contemporary

1. *Aguilera, DC, and Messick, JM: Crisis intervention: theory and methodology, ed 5, St. Louis, 1986, The CV Mosby Co.
2. *Agras, S: Panic: facing fears, phobias, and anxiety, New York, 1985, WH Freeman & Co.
3. Beck, C, Rawlins, R, and Williams, S: Mental health–psychiatric nursing: a holistic life-cycle, ed 2, St. Louis, 1987, The CV Mosby Co.
4. *Billings, CV: Come here, nurse! Am J Nurs 86:915-916, 1986.
5. Clark, JB, Queener, SF, and Karb, VB: Pharmacologic basis of nursing practice, ed 2, St. Louis, 1986, The CV Mosby Co.
6. *Crockett, MS: How a disabled, depressed patient learned to break an unhappy cycle, Am J Nurs 86:294-297, 1986.
7. Curtis, J, and Detert, R: How to relax, Palo Alto, Calif, 1981, Mayfield Publishing Co.
8. Danskin, D, and Crow, M: Biofeedback: an introduction and guide, Palo Alto, Calif, 1981, Mayfield Publishing Co.
9. *DeGennaro, M, and others: Antidepressant drug therapy, Am J Nurs 81:1304-1308, 1981.
10. Donovan, M: Relaxation with guided imagery: a useful technique, Cancer Nurs 1:27-32, 1980.
11. Ebersole, R, and Hess, R: Toward healthy aging: human needs and nursing response, ed 2, St. Louis, 1985, The CV Mosby Co.
12. Garland LI, and Bush, CT: Coping behaviors and nursing, Englewood Cliffs, NJ, 1982, Reston Publishing Co.
13. *Gilliss, C: Reducing family stress during and after coronary artery bypass surgery, Nurs Clin North Am 19(1):103-111, 1984.

References preceded by an asterisk are particularly well suited for student reading.

14. Gordon, M: Manual of nursing diagnosis 1986-1987, New York, 1987, McGraw-Hill Book Co.
15. Hahn, AB, Oestrich, JK, and Barkin, RL: Mosby's pharmacology in nursing, ed 16, St. Louis, 1986, The CV Mosby Co.
16. *Harris, B: Drugs and depression, Am J Nurs 86:292-293, 1986.
17. *Harris, E: Antipsychotic medications, Am J Nurs 81:1316-1328, 1981.
18. Hoff, LA: People in crisis: understanding and helping, Menlo Park, Calif, 1984, Addison-Wesley Publishing Co, Inc.
19. Hyman, RB, and Woog, P: Stressful life events and illness onset: a review of crucial variables, Res Nurs Health 5:155-163, 1982.
20. *Jasmin, SA, Hill, L, and Smith, N: Keeping your delicate balance: the art of managing stress, Nurs 81 11(6):52-57, 1981.
21. *Jupp, H, and others: Group cognitive/anxiety management, J Adv Nurs 9:573-580, 1984.
22. Kim, MJ, McFarland, GK, and McLane, AM: Pocket guide to nursing diagnosis, ed 2, St. Louis, 1987, The CV Mosby Co.
23. Kogan, HN, and Betrus, P: Self-management: a nursing mode of therapeutic influence, Adv Nurs Sci 6:55-73, 1984.
24. *Lambert, VA, and Lambert, CE: Psychosocial care of the physically ill, ed 2, Englewood Cliffs, NJ, 1985, Prentice-Hall, Inc.
25. Lazarus, RS, and Folkman, S: Stress, appraisal and coping, New York, 1984, Springer Publishing Co.
26. Mellion, MB: Exercise therapy for anxiety and depression: what are the specific considerations for clinical application? Postgrad Med 77(3):91-95, 1985.
27. *Minot, SR: Depression: what does it mean? Am J Nurs 86:283-287, 1986.
28. Moos, R: Coping with physical illness, ed 2, New York, 1985, Plenum Publishing Corp.
29. *Owen, PL: A dozen tasks vie for your attention at the same time, with no respite in sight—what can you do to keep stress at bay? Am J Nurs 86:52-53, 1986.
30. *Pender, NJ: Health promotion in nursing practice, Norwalk, Conn, 1982, Appleton-Century-Crofts.
31. Pender, NJ: Effects of progressive muscle relaxation training on anxiety and health locus of control among hypertensive adults, Res Nurs Health, 8(1):67-72, 1985.
32. *Robinson, L: Psychological aspects of the care of hospitalized patients, ed 4, Philadelphia, 1984, FA Davis Co.
33. *Ryan J: The neglected crisis, Am J Nurs 84-1257-1258, 1984.
34. *Smith, FB: Patient power, Am J Nurs 85:1260-1262, 1985.
35. Stuart, GW, and Sundeen, SJ: Principles and practice of psychiatric nursing, ed 3, St. Louis, 1986, The CV Mosby Co.
36. Symposium on anxiety disorders, Psychiatr Clin North Am 8(1):1-179, 1985.
37. *Weisman, A: Coping with cancer, New York, 1979, McGraw-Hill Book Co.
38. Wilson, H, and Kneisl, C: Psychiatric nursing, Menlo Park, Calif, 1982, Addison-Wesley Co.

Classic

39. Antonovsky, A: Health, stress, and coping, San Francisco, 1979, Jossey-Bass Publishers.
40. Benson, H: The relaxation response, New York, 1975, William Morrow & Co, Inc.
41. Caplan, G: Principles of preventative psychiatry, New York, 1964, Basic Books, Inc, Publishers.
42. Carlson, CE (editor): Behavioral concepts and nursing interventions, ed 2, Philadelphia, 1978, WB Saunders Co.
43. *Morris, CL: Relaxation therapy in a clinic, Am J Nurs 79:1958-1959, 1979.
44. Peplau, H: A working definition of anxiety. In Burd, S, and Marshall, M (editors): Some clinical approaches to psychiatric nursing, New York, 1963, Macmillan Publishing Co, Inc.
45. Rappaport, L: The state of crisis: some theoretical considerations, Chicago, 1972, University of Chicago Press.
46. *Richter, JM, and Sloan, R: A relaxation technique, Am J Nurs 79:1960-1964, 1979.
47. Selye, H: Stress without distress, New York, 1975, New American Library.
48. Selye, H: The stress of life, rev ed, New York, 1976, McGraw-Hill Book Co.
49. Shontz, F: The psychological aspects of physical illness and disability, New York, 1975, Macmillan Publishing Co, Inc.
50. *Smith, MJT, and Selye, H: Reducing the negative effects of stress, Am J Nurs 79:1953-1955, 1979.
51. Sutterly, DC, and Donnelly, GS: Stress management, Top Clin Nurs 1(1):1-104, 1979.

8

Fluid and Electrolyte Imbalances

BARBARA SOLTIS and MARY KAY LEHMAN

CHAPTER OBJECTIVES

After studying this chapter, the student should be able to:

- Describe the mechanisms for maintaining fluid and electrolyte balance.
- Describe the mechanisms and effects of fluid deficit and excess.
- Describe the mechanisms and effects of deficits and excesses of sodium, potassium, calcium, and magnesium.
- Describe the mechanisms that maintain acid-base balance.
- Differentiate among metabolic and respiratory acidosis and alkalosis, and describe the causes and effects of each type.
- Identify data indicating fluid or electrolyte imbalances.
- Describe the management of patients with fluid and electrolyte imbalances.

The *internal environment* is a term used to describe body water and the constituent electrolytes and other dissolved substances that sustain all the physiologic processes that maintain life. The amount and distribution of water in the various body compartments, as well as the type and amount of electrolytes and nonelectrolytes dissolved in the water, are kept in an extremely delicate balance by a number of control mechanisms. These mechanisms are so effective that normal values have been established for all constituents of the internal environment in healthy individuals. Knowledge of these normal values is used for detection and correction of imbalances that occur during illness.

The assessment and maintenance of a patient's fluid and electrolyte balance is a major nursing responsibility. This chapter describes some basic information about water and electrolytes in the body and the causes and effects of common fluid and electrolyte imbalances. The last part of the chapter discusses nursing measures employed to prevent, identify, and alleviate these imbalances and to relieve discomfort.

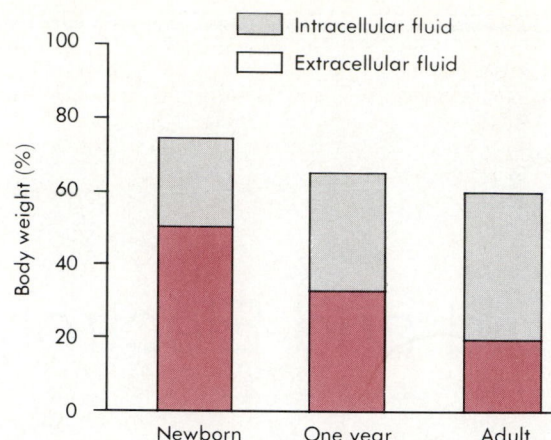

Fig. 8-1 In the newborn more than half of total body fluid is extracellular. As the child grows, proportions gradually approximate adult levels.

■ BASIC MECHANISMS OF FLUID AND ELECTROLYTE BALANCE

■ Body water

A large percentage of body weight is composed of water containing dissolved particles of organic and inorganic substances vital to life. A newborn infant's weight is approximately 75% water, whereas a young adult male's is about 60% and a female's 50% (Fig. 8-1). The percentage of body weight that is water gradually declines with age. Because fat contains little water, the more obese an individual is, the smaller the percentage of weight that is water. Both obese and aged persons have increased risk of morbidity and mortality in situations involving fluid loss because they have less fluid reserve on which to draw.

■ FLUID DISTRIBUTION

Water is distributed throughout the body but is described as being contained in the following three compartments: *intracellular, interstitial,* and *intravascular.* Functionally the fluids in the three compartments are considererd as two fluids, intracellular and extracellular (which includes both the interstitial and intravascular) (Table 8-1). The largest percentage of body water is located in the billions of individual body cells (Fig. 8-2). Gastrointestinal (GI) secretions, urine, sweat, and exudates are considered extracellular water because when they are lost in large amounts, extracellular volume decreases severely.

■ FLUID BALANCE

Body fluid is constantly being lost and must be replaced for normal processes to continue. With an average daily intake of food and liquids, the healthy body easily maintains compartmental balance. The body receives water from in-

gested food and fluids and through metabolism of both foodstuffs and body tissues. Solid foods, such as meat and vegetables, contain 60% to 90% water. Table 8-2 shows the approximate daily intake for an average adult. Note that the normal daily replacement of water equals the normal daily loss. Easily measurable intake (liquid) and easily measurable output (urine) are also approximately equal. These figures therefore serve as guides for determining normal fluid balance and emphasize the great need for recording patient fluid intake and output accurately.

Two vital processes demand continual expenditure of water: the removal of body heat by vaporization of water through the skin and lungs, and the excretion of urea and other metabolic wastes by the kidneys. The volume of water used in these processes varies greatly with external influences such as temperature and humidity.

■ Body electrolyte component

■ TYPES OF BODY ELECTROLYTES

All body fluids contain chemical compounds. Chemical compounds in solution may be classified as electrolytes or nonelectrolytes on the basis of their ability to conduct an electric current in solution. Electrolytes in solution break up into charged particles called *ions.* Sodium chloride in solution exists as positively charged sodium ions, NA^+, and negatively charged chloride ions, Cl^-. Positively charged ions are called *cations.* Negatively charged ions are called *anions.* Proteins are special types of charged molecules. They have a charge that is dependent on the pH of the body fluids. At normal plasma pH (7.4) the proteins exist with a net negative charge. Nonelectrolytes such as urea, dextrose, and creatine remain molecularly intact and are essentially uncharged.

Electrolytes account for most of the osmotic pressure of the body fluids, are important in the maintenance of acid-base balance, and help to control body water volume.

Table 8-1 Body fluid distribution

Compartment	Description	Fluid
Intracellular	Fluid within cells	Intracellular fluid (ICF)
Extracellular	Fluid outside cells	Extracellular fluid (ECF)
Intravascular	Fluid within blood vessels	Plasma
Interstitial	Fluid in tissues (between cells or in body spaces)	Examples: interstitial fluid, lymph, cerebrospinal fluid, intraocular fluid, GI secretions, urine, sweat, exudates

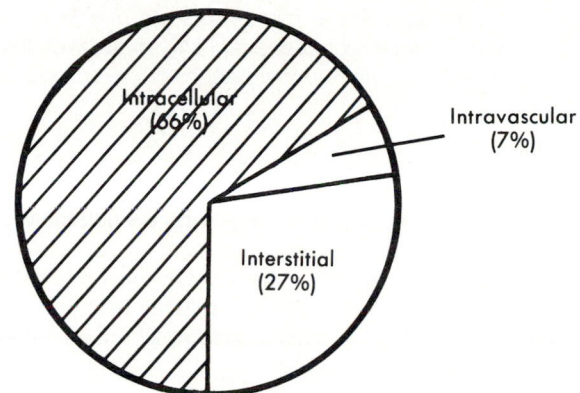

Fig. 8-2 Volumes of body fluids in each fluid compartment.

Table 8-2 Normal fluid intake and loss in an adult eating 2500 calories per day (approximate figures)

Intake		Output	
Route	Amount of gain (ml)	Route	Amount of loss (ml)
Water in food	1000	Skin	500
Water from oxidation	300	Lungs	350
Water as liquid	1200	Feces	150
		Kidney	1500
TOTAL	2500	TOTAL	2500

Table 8-3 Normal electrolyte content of body fluids*

Electrolytes (anions and cations)	Extracellular		Intracellular (mEq/L)
	Intravascular (mEq/L)	Interstitial (mEq/L)	
Sodium (Na^+)	142	146	15
Potassium (K^+)	5	5	150
Calcium (Ca^{++})	5	3	2
Magnesium (Mg^{++})	2	1	27
Chloride (Cl^-)	102	114	1
Bicarbonate (HCO_3^-)	27	30	10
Protein ($Prot^-$)	16	1	63
Phosphate (HPO_4^-)	2	2	100
Sulfate (SO_4^-)	1	1	20
Organic acids	5	8	0

*Note that the electrolyte level of the intravascular and interstitial fluids (extracellular) is approximately the same and that sodium and chloride contents are markedly higher in these fluids, whereas potassium, phosphate, and protein contents are markedly higher in intracellular fluid.

■ DISTRIBUTION OF BODY ELECTROLYTES

The three fluid compartments contain similar electrolytes, but the concentration of the electrolytes in each compartment varies greatly (Table 8-3). Electrolytes move between compartments, but most of the exchange occurs between *interstitial* and *intravascular* fluids.

Differences in individual ion concentrations occur in various *extracellular* fluids. For instance, gastric secretion is acid; hence the concentration of hydrogen ions is high. Pancreatic secretion, on the other hand, is more alkaline than plasma and contains a high concentration of bicarbonate. Gastric and pancreatic secretions and bile all contain high concentrations of sodium ions. Knowing the common electrolytes found in various body fluids is helpful in preventing depletion of necessary substances and in noting early signs of imbalance.

■ ELECTROLYTE BALANCE

In health the ratio of cations to anions in each of the body fluids and the concentration of the various ions in these fluids are relatively constant. Dietary intake and, in some instances intravenous infusions, are the routes by which an individual obtains a supply of electrolytes to replace daily losses and to keep the body in electrolyte balance. Electrolyte loss is mainly through the kidneys, with smaller losses through the skin and lungs and relatively minimal losses through the bowel. The kidneys selectively excrete certain electrolytes, retaining those needed for normal body fluid composition. Hormonal influences affect the kidneys' selective function. For example, the adrenocortical hormone aldosterone favors sodium reabsorption and the excretion of potassium.

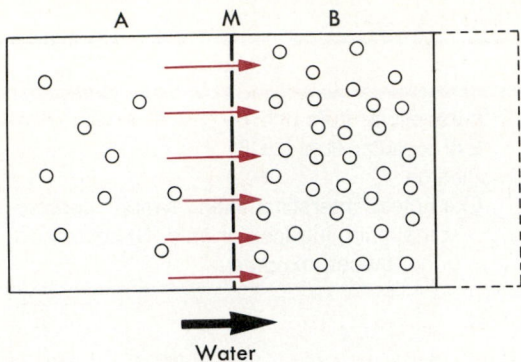

Water

Fig. 8-3 Osmosis: water moves from area of lesser solute concentration (A) through a membrane (M) to area of greater solute concentrations (B) until concentration of solute on both sides of the membrane is equal. Compartment B will have to expand (as shown by dotted lines) to accept the additional water.

■ Mechanisms for fluid and electrolyte movement

Fluids, electrolytes, gases, and small molecules move freely through the semipermeable membranes that separate compartments. This movement occurs constantly as oxygen and nutrients are carried to cells and wastes are removed from cells by the blood. In spite of the constant movement of water and dissolved particles (*solutes*) back and forth, the actual amount of water and concentration of solutes in each compartment remain relatively unchanged when the body is functioning normally. The mechanisms by which water and solutes move are *osmosis, diffusion,* and *filtration.*

■ OSMOSIS

Osmosis is the movement of a *solvent* (water) through a membrane from an area of lower concentration of solute to an area of higher concentration (Fig. 8-3). The water moves to dilute the more highly concentrated solution until an equilibrium is reached on both sides of the membrane. The concentration of solute in any one compartment is called *osmotic pressure* or *osmolality* and is determined by the total number of dissolved particles per unit of solvent.

Because of their large size, protein molecules normally have little movement between compartments. Their presence, especially in the intravascular fluid, creates a pressure called *colloid osmotic* or *oncotic* pressure, which functions to hold water within the compartment.

■ DIFFUSION

Diffusion is the movement of a *solute* from an area of greater concentration to an area of lesser concentration (Fig. 8-4). This is known as *movement along a concentration gradient.* Diffusion includes dispersion of solute throughout the fluid within a compartment, as well as movement of the solute through a membrane that separates two compartments until its concentration is equal on both sides of

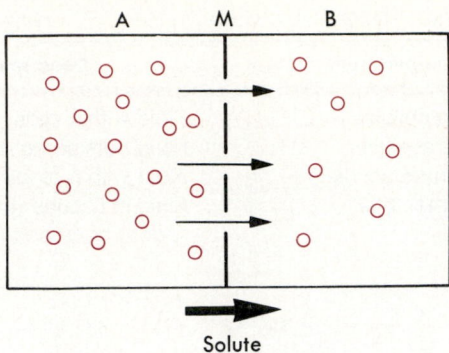

Solute

Fig. 8-4 Diffusion: Solute moves through membrane (M) from area of greater concentration (A) to area of lesser concentration (B) until concentration on both sides is equal.

the membrane. The semipermeable walls of blood vessels and cells contain tiny pores through which small molecules and electrolytes diffuse freely.

Large molecules such as glucose are too large to pass through membrane pores and are assisted in crossing the membrane by *carrier substances;* this process is known as *facilitated diffusion.*

■ FILTRATION

Filtration pressure is another means by which water and diffusible particles are moved through a membrane. Movement occurs because the weight or pressure of the fluid is greater on one side of the membrane than on the other. Filtration pressure is discussed later in this chapter in relation to normal exchange of water and solutes across capillary membranes (p. 124).

■ Hormonal control

Three hormones play a particularly vital role in maintaining fluid and electrolyte balance as follows:
1. Antidiuretic hormone (ADH)
   a. Is produced in the hypothalamus and stored and released from the posterior pituitary gland
   b. Acts on the renal tubules to retain water and to decrease urinary output
2. Aldosterone
   a. Is secreted by the adrenal cortex
   b. Acts on the renal tubules to reabsorb sodium and to excrete potassium
   c. Increases circulatory volume by reabsorbing water along with sodium
3. Parathormone
   a. Produced by the parathyroid glands
   b. Promotes absorption of calcium from the intestine
   c. Promotes release of calcium from bone
   d. Increases the excretion of phosphate ions by the kidneys

Table 8-4 lists the factors that stimulate or inhibit release of these hormones.

Table 8-4 Factors influencing hormone release and effects on fluid and electrolyte balance

Hormone	Factors promoting or inhibiting hormone release	Effect
Aldosterone	***Promotes hormone release***	
	Increased serum potassium	Reabsorption of sodium and water: increased blood volume, hypertension
	Decreased serum sodium	
	Decreased blood volume	Excretion of potassium: hypokalemia
		Excretion of hydrogen ions: alkalosis
	Inhibits hormone release	
	Increased serum sodium	Excretion of sodium and water: decreased blood volume, hypotension
	Decreased serum potassium	
	Increased blood volume	Potassium retention; hyperkalemia
	Spironolactone (diuretic)	Retention of hydrogen ions: acidosis
Antidiuretic hormone (ADH)	***Promotes hormone release***	
	Hypertonic plasma	Reabsorption of water in renal tubules
	Low blood volume	
	Pain, stress	
	Drugs: narcotics, anesthetics	
	Inhibits hormone release	
	Hypotonic plasma	Blocking of water reabsorption: loss of water via kidneys
	Increased blood volume	
	Alcohol ingestion	
Parathormone	***Promotes hormone release***	
	Decreased serum calcium	Loss of calcium from bone
		Increased absorption of calcium from GI tract
		Decreased renal excretion of calcium, increased excretion of phosphate
	Inhibits hormone release	
	Increased serum calcium	Decreased absorption of calcium from GI tract
	Increased calcium and vitamin D in diet	Increased renal excretion of calcium, decreased loss of phosphate

■ FLUID AND ELECTROLYTE IMBALANCE

Almost all medical-surgical conditions threaten fluid and electrolyte balance. There may be deficits or excesses of water or of any electrolyte. Actually several imbalances occur simultaneously because of the interrelationship of body fluids and their electrolytes. For clarity, imbalances of body fluid and of each ion are considered separately.

■ Fluid imbalances

Tonicity is a term used to compare the osmolality of a solution to the normal osmolality of body fluids. As previously mentioned, osmolality is determined by the total number of particles dissolved in a unit of solvent. The osmolality of body fluid is measured in milliosmols or thousandths of an osmol because the number of particles in a

solution is relatively small. Normal osmolality of body fluids is approximately 300 mOsm/L. Solutions relate to normal osmolality in the following ways:

1. *Isotonic:* same osmolality as body fluids
2. *Hypotonic:* less osmolality than body fluids
3. *Hypertonic:* greater osmolality than body fluids

When the body gains or loses fluid in excess of normal fluid balance, the intercompartmental fluid movement that occurs depends on whether the extracellular fluid becomes hypertonic or hypotonic or remains isotonic. The effects of different types of fluid imbalances are illustrated in Table 8-5.

■ FLUID LOSS

There are a number of ways in which body fluids and electrolytes contained therein are lost or made unavailable for normal fluid and electrolyte balance, as summarized in the list on p. 122.

Table 8-5 Fluid imbalances

Fluid imbalance	Pathophysiology	Signs and symptoms	Therapy
Isotonic fluid deficit	Decreased body water and electrolytes; extracellular fluid remains isotonic but volume decreases	Hypotension, increased pulse and respirations, cool skin, delayed vein filling, shock, decreased urinary output	Replacement of water and sodium: oral intake of salty fluids; IV of normal saline
Hypertonic fluid deficit	Decreased body water more than decreased electrolytes; water moves out of cells to dilute extracellular fluid (cellular dehydration)	Thirst; skin flushed, dry, poor turgor; dry coated tongue; increased body temperature; increased hemoglobin and hematocrit levels; apprehension, restlessness	Water taken orally, if possible; IV of 5% dextrose in water; additional water given with tube feedings
Hypotonic fluid excess (water intoxication)	Excess body water without excess electrolytes; water moves into cells causing cells to swell	Behavior changes, confusion, incoordination; sudden weight gain; warm moist skin; lethargy, convulsions	Water restriction; for severe signs, 3% to 5% sodium chloride IV
Isotonic fluid excess (edema)	Excess body water and sodium; excess fluid moves into extracellular spaces	Edema of dependent body parts: pitting over bony prominences; swollen, tight, shiny skin Pulmonary edema: dyspnea; wheezing cough with frothy sputum; cyanosis	Elevation of dependent part; treatment of underlying condition; diuretics, reduced salt intake; treatment of pulmonary edema

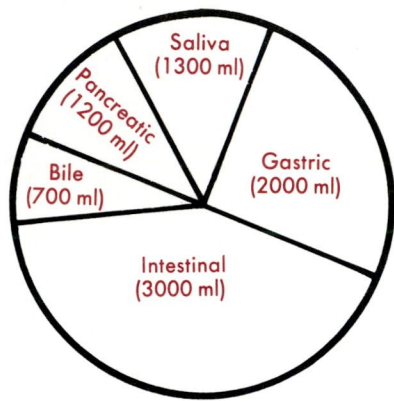

Fig. 8-5 Fluid volume of gastrointestinal secretions.

Losses of fluid and electrolytes

Skin: diaphoresis, oozing from severe wounds or burns
GI tract: profuse salivation, vomiting, diarrhea, GI drainage, enemas
Kidneys: diuretics, polyuria
Hemorrhage
Trapping of fluids: wound swelling, edema, ascites, intestinal obstruction

The GI tract secretes approximately 8 L of fluid daily (Fig. 8-5); therefore, large amounts of fluid may be lost through the GI tract. Loss of both water and solutes leads to *isotonic* fluid deficit with resulting circulatory collapse. Loss of water in excess of solutes leads to a *hypertonic* fluid deficit with resulting dehydration.

☐ Isotonic fluid deficit

Sodium ions constitute most of the osmolality of *extracellular* fluid. If both water and sodium are lost, the result is isotonic fluid loss; the extracellular fluid becomes depleted, and circulating blood volume is decreased (Table 8-5). The body attempts to maintain circulation vital to tissue perfusion by initiating several compensatory mechanisms (see the box on p. 123). If adequate blood volume cannot be maintained by these mechanisms, cardiac output is decreased and blood pressure drops. If volume depletion occurs rapidly, shock may ensue.

Isotonic loss can result from hemorrhage, profuse diaphoresis, and large losses of GI fluids. Treatment is directed toward replacing both fluids and electrolytes.

If plasma proteins are lost from the body, as occurs in hemorrhage, or if they are shifted from the blood to the interstitial fluid, as occurs in burns, the blood volume drops rapidly because fluid from interstitial spaces cannot be mobilized to maintain it, and shock follows (see Chapter 9). Whole blood, plasma, or plasma expanders usually must be given to these patients to replace the protein loss before extensive fluid therapy is effective.

☐ Hypertonic fluid deficit

When water is lost from the body in excess of sodium and other electrolytes or when water intake is inadequate to replace normal losses, the extracellular fluid becomes hypertonic (Table 8-5). Water moves out of the cells by osmosis to dilute the extracellular compartment and *cellular dehydration* results. As both extracellular and intracellular fluids decrease, cell function is impaired because food, oxygen, and waste products are inadequately diffused.

Compensatory mechanisms to maintain circulation

Mechanism 1
1. Decreased intravascular fluid increases the plasma colloid osmotic pressure.
2. Interstitial fluid is pulled back into the blood vessel to equalize pressure (Starling's law of the capillaries, p. 124).
3. Blood volume is increased.

Mechanism 2
1. Blood flow through kidneys is decreased because of the decreased blood volume.
2. Aldosterone is released from adrenal cortex resulting in sodium retention and potassium excretion.
3. Sodium retention increases the reabsorption of water because of osmolality.
4. Urinary excretion is decreased and extracellular fluid is increased.
5. Blood volume is increased.

When solutes are taken in without sufficient water, such as occurs when high-protein tube feedings are given, the extracellular fluid becomes *hypertonic*. The kidneys attempt to remove excess solute by excreting large amounts of urine; this is known as *osmotic diuresis*.

Dehydration may be encountered in patients who have dysphagia (difficulty swallowing), are unaware that they are thirsty (confused, disoriented), hyperventilate excessively, or have severe diarrhea or diabetes insipidus. Treatment consists of water replacement. Intravenous infusion of 5% dextrose in water is given to the patient who cannot take oral fluids. Water is given along with or between tube feedings.

■ FLUID EXCESS

Fluid that is retained in the body in excess of normal is termed overhydration. There may be an excess of water without an increase in electrolytes (hypotonic fluid excess) or an increase in both water and electrolytes (isotonic fluid excess).

□ Hypotonic fluid excess (water intoxication)

If an excess of water is present without an increase in sodium or protein, water enters the cells through osmosis, causing them to swell. This is referred to as *water intoxication* (dilution syndrome) (Table 8-5). This form of overhydration can occur when the water intake is greater than the kidney's ability to excrete it.

Water excess can occur in the following situations:
1. Excess secretion of ADH as seen in acute stress such as trauma, surgery, pain, fear, acute infections, anesthetics, analgesics (morphine, meperidine), and cerebral lesions
2. Low renal blood flow, as seen in congestive heart failure, cirrhosis of the liver, acute renal insufficiency, and Addison's disease
3. Large amount of water given rectally as occurs with repeated enemas

4. Frequent and continuous amounts of water taken orally, especially in the seriously ill patient who drinks sodium-free liquids rather than eating solid foods
5. Absorption of irrigating fluids during transurethral resection of the prostate

The signs and symptoms of acute water intoxication result from the swelling of cells, especially in the brain, and may develop rapidly and dramatically. The patient usually recovers with careful water restriction. If convulsions or coma occur or if serum sodium is below 110 mEq/L, rapid treatment is necessary and may be accomplished by infusion of a small amount of 3% or 5% sodium chloride solution intravenously.

□ Isotonic fluid excess (edema)

If an excess of body water is present with a concomitant increase in sodium (isotonic fluid), the excess fluid is retained in the *extracellular* compartment and leads to the formation of edema (Table 8-5). *Edema* is the accumulation of fluid in the interstitial spaces. A negative interstitial fluid pressure occurs in normal tissue, and cells are held in close approximation to facilitate the exchange of gases, nutrients, and waste products between the cells and capillaries. If fluid accumulates in the interstitial space and is not removed, either by direct return to the blood vessel or through the lymph system, a positive interstitial fluid pressure develops, and cells are pushed farther apart. If a finger is pressed over an edematous area, the indentation made by the finger may remain briefly as the fluid is pushed to another area; this is called *pitting edema*. The fluid refills the interstitial space in the "pit" area within a few seconds.

In the healthy individual, edema does not develop immediately with the initial inflow of fluid into the interstitial spaces because of the body's compensatory mechanisms, that is, the existing negative interstitial fluid pressure and the removal by the lymph system of excess fluids and proteins that accumulate in the interstitial spaces.

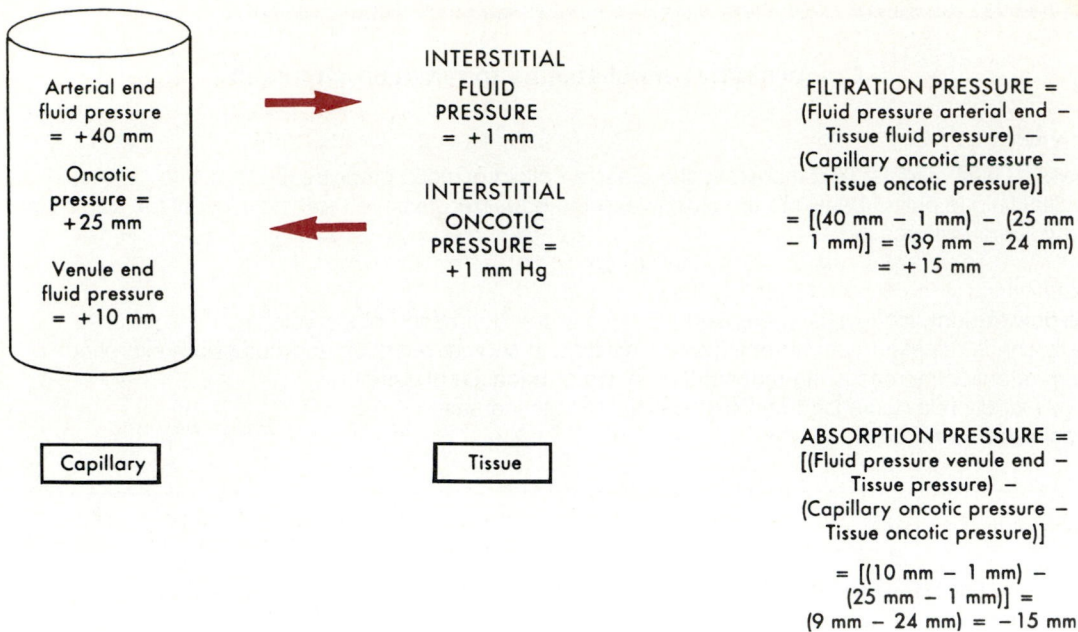

Fig. 8-6 Starling's law of capillaries. An equilibrium exists between forces filtering fluid out of capillary and forces absorbing fluid back into capillary. Note that fluid pressure within capillary is greater than fluid pressure in tissue. This differential (fluid pressure gradient) serves as a filtering force. Note also that oncotic pressure (colloid osmotic pressure) is greater within capillary. This serves as an absorbing force.

□ *Capillary dynamics*

A review of normal capillary dynamics aids in understanding the various factors that can cause edema to develop. Two types of pressures influence the flow of fluid across a capillary membrane: *fluid pressure* (resulting from the hydrostatic force of fluid) and *colloid osmotic pressure* or *oncotic* pressure (pressure resulting from the presence of proteins that do not diffuse across the membrane wall). Fluid pressure within the capillary is much greater than fluid pressure in the interstitial space; this force *filters* fluid out of the capillary. Because a larger number of protein molecules is found in plasma than in interstitial fluid, the oncotic pressure within the capillary serves as a force to *absorb* fluid back into the capillary.

According to Starling's "law of the capillaries," pressures that promote movement of fluid *out* of the capillary are greatest at the *arteriole* end, whereas pressures promoting fluid movement back *into* the capillary are greatest at the *venule* end. An exchange of fluid occurs across the capillary membrane with an overall equilibrium between the forces filtering fluid out of the capillary and the forces absorbing fluid back into the capillary (Fig. 8-6).

□ *Pathophysiology of edema*

Edema was defined as an accumulation of fluid in the interstitial spaces creating a positive fluid pressure. Thus edema can be produced by the following:
1. Increase in capillary fluid pressure
2. Decrease in capillary oncotic pressure
3. Increase in interstitial oncotic pressure (Table 8-6)

The same mechanisms that create edema in the interstitial spaces can create fluid collection in *potential fluid spaces*. These are spaces between two membranes that normally contain only traces of fluid. The main potential fluid spaces are intrapleural (lung and chest wall), pericardial (heart and pericardial sac), peritoneal (intestines and abdominal wall), and joint spaces. Large amounts of fluid also collect in areas of trauma, burn, and surgical wounds. When fluid is abnormally accumulated in any of these places, the condition is referred to as *third-spacing* of fluids. The symptoms of fluid collection in these spaces are usually caused by the pressure of the collected fluid against adjoining organs or structures. Large amounts of fluid may collect in the peritoneal space (*ascites*). This fluid is high in protein and electrolytes. Accumulation of large amounts of fluid in all body tissue is called *anasarca*.

□ *Overloading of vascular system*

A major cause of increased capillary fluid pressure is overloading of the vascular system. This overloading results in an increase in the hydrostatic pressure of the blood, in turn resulting in generalized tissue edema. More important, if the increase in hydrostatic pressure is great enough to push large amounts of fluid into the alveoli of the lungs, it rapidly leads to death from "drowning" in one's own fluids (*pulmonary edema*). The hydrostatic pressure in the pulmonary vessels normally is much lower than that in the general circulation, and therefore any increase is reflected rapidly in the lungs.

Overloading of the vascular system may be caused by

Table 8-6 Causes of edema according to underlying physiologic mechanism

Fluid pressure	Oncotic pressure

Increased capillary fluid pressure
Increased venous pressure
 	
Vein obstruction
   Varicose veins
   Thrombophlebitis
   Pressure on veins from casts, tight bandages, or garters
Increased total volume with decreased cardiac output
   Congestive heart failure
   Fluid overloading
 	
Sodium and water retention: increased aldosterone from:
 	
Decreased renal blood flow
   Congestive heart failure
   Renal failure
Increased production of aldosterone
   Cushing's syndrome
Aldosterone added to system
   Corticosteroid therapy
Inability to destroy aldosterone
   Cirrhosis of liver
	Decreased capillary oncotic pressure
	Loss of serum protein
	
	Burns, draining wounds, fistulas
	Hemorrhage
	Nephrotic syndrome
	Chronic diarrhea
	
	Decreased intake of protein
	
	Malnutrition
	Kwashiorkor
	
	Decreased production of albumin
	
	Liver disease
	
	Increased interstitial oncotic pressure
	Increased capillary permeability to protein
	
	Burns
	Inflammatory reactions
	   Trauma
	   Infections
	Allergic reactions (hives)
	
	Blocked lymphatics: decreased removal of tissue fluid and protein
	
	Malignant diseases
	Surgical removal of lymph nodes
	Elephantiasis

giving too much fluid within a short period of time to a person who cannot dispose of the surplus because of circulatory or renal disease. *Elderly* people tolerate increases in blood volume poorly, because, with inelastic vessels, only relatively small increases in volume are needed to markedly increase hydrostatic pressure. Monitoring the central venous pressure is one method used to determine if overloading is occurring.

Overloading the vascular system also may be caused by increasing the oncotic (pull) pressure of the intravascular fluid by giving proteins so rapidly that the body cannot dispose of those that are in excess of its need. This overloading causes fluids to be pulled into the intravascular compartment from other body fluid compartments. The blood volume increases rapidly, neutralizing the oncotic pressure but increasing the hydrostatic pressure of the vascular system and the oncotic pressure of the interstitial fluid compartment. Fluid is then pushed into the tissues. Overloading is a danger when fluids such as plasma, plasma expanders, albumin, or blood are given to any patient regardless of age or state of health.

☐ *Treatment of edema*

Edema is often treated with diuretics. Some diuretics, such as the thiazides, block sodium reabsorption and consequently water reabsorption by the renal tubules. Other diuretic agents are partially or completely unabsorbable by the renal tubules and tend to carry sodium and water with them into the urine. When diuretics are given, a large amount of fluid is lost from the vascular compartment, increasing its oncotic pressure and causing fluid to be pulled back into it from the tissues. Potassium is usually lost along with sodium and water.

Reducing the salt intake also may reduce edema because the remaining supply of sodium seems to be needed to maintain the isotonicity of the blood and thus is not available for holding water. If edema is caused by venous stasis, elevating dependent body parts and applying supportive stockings helps promote venous return.

■ **Electrolyte imbalances**

Serum electrolytes are measured in milliequivalents per liter (mEq/L), indicating the chemical combining activity of an electrolyte. For example, 1 mEq of the cation sodium is available to combine with 1 mEq of an anion such as chloride or bicarbonate. The concentration of cations in blood serum or plasma is the same as the concentration of anions when expressed in terms of milliequivalents. This is more useful than measuring electrolytes in milligrams per 100 ml, which is only an indication of the amount of an electrolyte by weight and thus gives no information about the relationship between cations and anions. *No single electrolyte can be out of balance without causing some others to be out of balance.*

Sodium, potassium, and calcium are all essential for the *passage of nerve impulses.* Whenever the concentrations of any of these cations are increased or decreased in body fluids, the increase or decrease is reflected in the stimulation of muscles by nerves. The muscles may become weak and atonic because of inadequate stimulation, or they may become somewhat spastic because of excess stimulation. For example, a decrease in calcium concentration in body fluids causes the stimulus to be increased and results in muscle spasms. GI and cardiac symptoms, so often produced by electrolyte imbalances, result in part from changes in neural stimulation on the muscles of these systems.

With cation imbalances, the *distribution of body fluids* is frequently upset. Abnormal collections of fluid probably cause some of the GI symptoms such as nausea, vomiting, and diarrhea. Decreased amounts may cause anorexia, dyspepsia, and constipation. It is thought that edema of cerebral tissues may be responsible for headache, convulsions, and coma.

■ SODIUM

□ Sodium deficit (hyponatremia)

The normal concentration of sodium in the blood is 138 to 145 mEq/L. A low sodium level in the blood (*hyponatremia*) can indicate either a deficit of sodium or an excess of water. Whenever sodium is lost from the body fluids, the fluids become hypotonic. Sodium loss from the intravascular compartment, therefore, causes fluid from the blood to diffuse into the interstitial spaces. As a result,

sodium in the interstitial fluid is diluted. In response to this reduction of the sodium concentration in the extracellular fluid, potassium moves out of the intracellular fluid. Therefore, the patient with sodium imbalance is also likely to have a potassium imbalance.

Sodium depletion results most often from the loss of GI secretions. It can also occur from losses through the skin and in the shifting of body fluids so that the sodium is not accessible for use.

Anyone who is perspiring profusely because of environmental conditions, exercise, or fever is losing large amounts of both sodium and water. If salt is not replaced with water, such as by drinking salty fluids, water intoxication occurs. The causes and symptoms of sodium deficit are summarized in the box below, left.

□ Sodium excess (hypernatremia)

A serum sodium level greater than 145 mEq/L is known as *hypernatremia*. There are actually two kinds of sodium excess, edema and hypernatremia. When there is a sodium and water excess, edema exists; when there is an excess of sodium in relation of water in the extracellular compartment, hypernatremia exists. The causes and symptoms of sodium excess are listed in the box below.

As seen in Table 8-7, hypernatremia does not necessarily indicate an excess of total body sodium.

If fluids are greatly limited or if excess salt is taken into the body and retained because of poor renal function, sodium may be concentrated in body fluids. Excess intravascular sodium causes fluid to be withdrawn from interstitial spaces. Extracellular fluids become hypertonic and draw water from the cells, causing cellular dehydration. If fluids are not given to dilute the sodium and if excretion of sodium is not increased, severe fluid and electrolyte disturbances occur, causing manic excitement, tachycardia, and eventual death.

Causes and symptoms of sodium deficit

Causes	Symptoms
Loss of GI fluids	Headache
Vomiting	Muscle weakness
Diarrhea	Fatigue
GI or biliary drain-	Apathy
age	Postural hypotension
Fistulas	Nausea/vomiting
Loss through skin	Abdominal cramps
Diaphoresis	*Severe prolonged deficit*
Large open lesions	Shock
(burns)	Mental confusion
Shifting of body	Coma
fluids	
Massive edema	
Ascites	
Burns	
Small bowel ob-	
struction	

Causes and symptoms of sodium excess

Causes

More water than sodium is lost from the body
An abnormally large intake of sodium
  Taking too many salt tablets
  IV saline infused too rapidly

Symptoms

Dry, sticky mucous membranes
Low urinary output
Firm, rubbery tissue turgor
Severe prolonged excess
Manic excitement
Tachycardia
Death

Table 8-7 Comparison of serum sodium levels with total body sodium*

Condition	Serum sodium	Total body sodium
Prolonged sweating	Low (hyponatremia)	Low
Diuretics and low sodium diets	Low	Low
Addison's disease	Low	Low
Edema (cardiac, renal, hepatic disease)	Low or normal	High
Excretion of dilute urine, early stages of gastrointestinal sodium loss	Normal	Low
Excess oral or IV sodium intake	High (hypernatremia)	High
Water and sodium loss with water loss > sodium loss	High	Low

*Note that a low or high serum level does not necessarily correspond with total body sodium.

■ POTASSIUM

Potassium is the major cation of the cells. During the formation of new tissue (*anabolism*) or when glucose is converted to glycogen, potassium enters the cell. With tissue breakdown (*catabolism*), potassium leaves the cell. This occurs with trauma, dehydration, or starvation. The normal serum level of potassium is 3.5 to 5.0 mEq/L.

□ Potassium deficit (hypokalemia)

A serum potassium level below 3.5 mEq/L is know as *hypokalemia*. The body's mechanism for conserving potassium is not as effective as that for conserving sodium, and the kidneys may excrete potassium even when the body needs it. Whenever sodium is being retained in the body through reabsorption by the kidney tubules, potassium is excreted. Thus whenever aldosterone secretion is increased, such as in stress, potassium is excreted. Potassium depletion, therefore, is common in many diseases and injuries and during therapy such as surgery. Potassium may also be lost through the urine as a result of certain diuretics such as the thiazides and furosemide (Lasix).

The patient who has a balanced diet withheld for several days, is dehydrated, or is given large amounts of parenteral fluids with no replacement of potassium develops potassium depletion. Dilution of extracellular potassium by the administration of 5% dextrose without potassium supplements and potassium loss caused by catabolism of body proteins account for many electrolyte imbalances in the postoperative patient.

The practice of giving multiple enemas is becoming less common because it is now known that some of the enema fluid is absorbed and dilutes the potassium in the interstitial compartment, upsetting the balance between compartments. Solutions for hypertonic enemas may damage cells in the bowel mucosa, causing potassium loss.

Potassium has a direct effect on cardiac and skeletal muscle function. The patient with potassium deficit shows characteristic electrocardiographic changes of flattened or inverted T waves with a prolonged Q-T interval (see Chapter 25). The most striking symptom of hypokalemia is muscle weakness. Digitalis toxicity can occur in patients taking digitalis if they develop hypokalemia. With severe hypo-

---

Causes and symptoms of hypokalemia

Causes

Decreased potassium intake
Increased potassium loss
    Increased aldosterone activity
    GI losses
    Potassium-losing diuretics
    Loss from cells as in trauma, burns
Conditions causing very large urine output
Potassium shift into cells
    Treatment of acidosis
    Metabolic alkalosis

Symptoms

Muscle weakness
Anorexia, nausea/vomiting
Diminished deep tendon reflexes, lethargy
Cardiac arrhythmias
ECG changes
Severe or prolonged deficit
    Flaccid paralysis
    Kidney damage
    Paralytic ileus
    Cardiac/respiratory arrest

Foods rich in potassium

Fruits
(including juices)

Apricots
Bananas
Grapefruit
Melon
   Canteloupe
   Honeydew
Dried fruits
   Figs, dates, raisins
Oranges

Protein foods

Beef
Chicken
Liver
Pork
Veal
Turkey
Milk
Nuts, peanut
   butter

Vegetables

Asparagus
Dried beans
Broccoli
Cabbage
Carrots
Celery
Mushrooms
Dried peas
Potatoes
   White, sweet
Spinach
Squash

Beverages

Cocoa
Cola drinks
Dry, instant tea
   and coffee

*Most raw vegetables contain potassium, much of which is lost in cooking.

Causes and symptoms of hyperkalemia

Causes

Potassium intake (parenteral or oral) in excess of
   kidney's ability to excrete
Renal failure
Adrenal insufficiency
Potassium enters bloodstream, from injured cells
   with extensive trauma
Metabolic acidosis

Symptoms

Nausea, vomiting
Diarrhea, colic
Cardiac arrhythmias
ECG changes
Numbness, tingling
*Severe or prolonged excess**
   Flaccid paralysis
   Cardiac arrest
    Anuria

*Prolonged potassium excess results in symptoms similar to those of hypokalemia.

---

kalemia, the patient may die unless potassium is administered promptly. The causes and symptoms of hypokalemia are summarized in the box on p. 127.

The safest way to administer potassium is orally. Fresh fruits (especially oranges and bananas) or foods high in protein are good sources of potassium (see the box above). A potassium salt may be prescribed orally; if given in liquid form, it should be given in fruit or vegetable juice or chilled to increase palatability. When potassium is given intravenously, the rate of flow must be monitored closely to prevent hyperkalemia and atrial arrest. The usual rate of infusion should not exceed 20 mEq of potassium per hour.

☐ Potassium excess (hyperkalemia)

A serum potassium level greater than 5.0 mEq/L is termed *hyperkalemia*. This condition does not occur as frequently as hypokalemia, especially if renal function is normal.

As previously stated, whenever there is severe tissue damage, potassium is released from the cells into the extracellular fluids. Because shock usually accompanies this damage, renal function is reduced, and a high blood potassium level results. There is great danger in giving extra potassium to any patient with poor renal function. If the patient is dehydrated or has lost vascular fluid, glucose and water or plasma expanders usually are given until renal function returns. Untreated adrenal insufficiency also is a contraindication for giving potassium.

The patient with hyperkalemia develops spasticity of muscles because of their overstimulation by nerve impulses. The patient complains of nausea, colic, diarrhea, and skeletal muscle spasms. The muscles later become weak because the overstimulation produces an accumulation of lactic acid and because potassium is lost from the muscle cells.

If the condition is not controlled, overstimulation of the cardiac muscle causes the heartbeat to become irregular and eventually stop. ECG evidence of potassium elevation includes tall, peaked, symmetric, or tented T waves with a short Q-T interval. As the blood potassium level increases further, the QRS spreads and atrial arrest occurs. See the box above.

If the patient who has hyperkalemia needs a blood transfusion, *fresh* blood must be used. Cells in blood that has been stored for several days tends to release potassium during storage. A transfusion of stored blood may further increase the patient's serum potassium level.

When hyperkalemia occurs, the patient is allowed nothing orally, and infusion of 10% glucose with 50 units of insulin is often given to induce transfer of potassium from the serum to the intracellular fluid. If the patient is in a state of acidosis (p. 132), correction of the situation results in movement of potassium back to the cell.

Kayexalate, a cation exchange resin, can be given orally

or rectally. It results in the release of sodium and binding of potassium, with the potassium then excreted in the stool. If the patient is in renal failure or if the serum potassium is dangerously high, hemodialysis is necessary. The patient is placed on absolute bed rest until the potassium blood level is returned to normal.

■ CALCIUM

There is a considerable amount of calcium in the human body, most of it located in the bony skeleton and a small amount dissolved in body fluids. Serum calcium level must be maintained at a level of 4.5 to 5.8 mEq/L to maintain vital functions of neuromuscular irritability and blood clotting. Calcium is present in the blood in two forms, free ionized calcium and calcium bound to protein. Only ionized calcium is physiologically active. Both *parathyroid hormone* and *vitamin D* are necessary for normal absorption of calcium from the GI tract, for reabsorption of calcium from bone to maintain the normal serum calcium level, and for prevention of excess calcium loss in urine.

☐ Calcium deficit (hypocalcemia)

A decrease in serum calcium level below 4.5 mEq/L is termed *hypocalcemia*. Some conditions lead to excessive calcium binding, such as the infusion of large amounts of blood containing citrate (citrate binds calcium) and alkalosis (more calcium is bound in an alkaline medium). When these conditions are present, the patient begins to show signs of calcium deficit, because, although the total amount of blood calcium is not changed, there is less physiologically active (unbound, ionized) calcium available.

Patients with pancreatic disease or disease of the small intestine may fail to absorb calcium from the GI tract, and they may excrete abnormally large amounts of calcium in the feces, thus reducing the blood level of calcium. *Hypocalcemia* may also occur during the diuretic phase of acute renal failure as calcium is excreted.

The patient with a calcium deficiency usually first complains of numbness and tingling of the nose, ears, fingers, and toes. If calcium is not given at this time, painful muscular spasms, especially of the feet and hands (carpopedal spasm), muscle twitching, and convulsions may follow (*tetany*). The causes and symptoms of hypocalcemia are summarized in the box above, right. The two tests used to elicit signs of calcium deficiency are as follows:

1. Trousseau's sign
   a. Constrict the circulation of the arm by grasping the wrist or inflating a blood pressure cuff
   b. Positive sign of serious calcium deficit—hand goes into a position of palmar flexion
2. Chvostek's sign
   a. Tap the face lightly over the facial nerve (just below the temple)
   b. Positive sign of calcium deficit—facial muscle twitching

The specific treatment for a low blood level of calcium is the administration of calcium gluconate or calcium chloride orally or intravenously.

Causes and symptoms of hypocalcemia

Causes

Excess binding of calcium ions
    Large amount of citrated blood
    Alkalosis
Dietary deficiency of calcium
Chronic renal failure
Pancreatic disease
Disease of small bowel
Draining intestinal fistulas
Deficiency of parathyroid hormone or vitamin D
Increased magnesium

Symptoms

Osteoporosis, pathologic fractures
Tingling around nose, mouth, ears, fingers, toes
Muscle spasm of feet and hands
Tetany
Nausea, vomiting
Diarrhea
Cardiac arrhythmias, cardiac arrest
Calcium deposits in body tissues

☐ Calcium excess (hypercalcemia)

A serum calcium level above 5.8 mEq/L is called *hypercalcemia*. It may be caused by calcium leaving the bone and concentrating in the ECF (as seen in bone diseases or with prolonged immobilization) or by increased intake and absorption of calcium.

Normal retention of calcium in the bones is believed to be caused by the pressure exerted on bones by active movement or exercise. When a large amount of calcium accumulates in the extracellular fluid and passes through the kidneys, calcium can precipitate and form stones (calculi), a not infrequent complication of immobilization. Calcium precipitates more readily in alkaline solution. This can be a problem in a urinary tract infection, which increases the alkalinity of the urine. See the box on p. 130 for a summary of causes and symptoms of hypercalcemia.

Treatment for hypercalcemia is removal of the cause. Intravenous saline and a diuretic (furosemide) may be given to promote renal excretion of the calcium. Oral or intravenous phosphate may also be given because calcium is excreted when phosphorus serum levels are increased.

Nursing responsibilities for the person with hypercalcemia include the following:

1. Active exercises for immobilized persons
2. Increased fluid intake (3000-4000 ml/day) for both high-risk persons and those with hypercalcemia
3. Prevention of urinary tract infection
4. Gentle handling to prevent pathologic fractures

Causes and symptoms of hypercalcemia

Causes

Loss from bone
Immobilization
Metastatic bone cancer
Multiple myeloma

Excess intake
Dietary
Antacids containing calcium

Increased absorption
Increased parathyroid hormone
Increased vitamin D

Symptoms

Thirst, polyuria
Renal stones
Decreased deep tendon reflexes
Lethargy, coma
Cardiac arrhythmias, cardiac arrest
Decreased muscle tone
Decreased GI motility

Causes and symptoms of hypomagnesemia

Causes

Decreased intake
Prolonged malnutrition
Starvation
Impaired absorption from GI tract
Alcoholism
Hypercalcemia
Diarrhea
Draining intestinal fistulas
Conditions causing large losses of urine

Symptoms

Mental changes
Agitation, depression, confusion
Paresthesias
Tremors
Ataxia
Cramps, spasticity, tetany
Tachycardia
Hypertension
Arrythmias

■ MAGNESIUM

The normal serum magnesium level is within the range of 1.5 to 2.5 mEq/L. About 50% of magnesium is located in bones, 5% in ECF, and the remaining 45% within the cells. It functions in the activation of enzymatic reactions, especially in carbohydrate metabolism. Magnesium has a sedative effect on the CNS similar to that of calcium. High serum levels result in vasodilation and lowering of blood pressure; this is a rare occurrence except with kidney failure.

Metabolically, magnesium is closely interrelated with both calcium and potassium. In the presence of a large amount of calcium in the GI tract, calcium is absorbed in preference to magnesium, and the magnesium is excreted. Conversely, low calcium levels increase magnesium absorption. The kidneys effectively conserve magnesium when intake is low.

□ Magnesium deficit (hypomagnesemia)

Hypomagnesemia is a serum magnesium level below 1.5 mEq/L. It may be caused by impaired absorption from the GI tract, excess loss through the kidneys, or prolonged malnutrition.

A low serum magnesium level leads to increased neuromuscular irritability. Hypomagnesemia is usually manifested by behavioral and neurologic symptoms such as confusion, hallucination, convulsions, increased reflexes, muscle spasms, and paresthesias (see box above).

Nursing responsibilities for the person with hypomagnesemia include the following:
1. Encouraging foods high in magnesium (fruits, green vegetables, whole grain cereals, milk, meats, and nuts)
2. Careful observation and supervision of the patient who is confused or hallucinating
3. Providing for patient safety if convulsions occur

□ Magnesium excess (hypermagnesemia)

Hypermagnesemia is a serum magnesium level greater than 2.5 mEq/L. The action of magnesium is on the myoneural junction where a high magnesium level blocks acetylcholine release, decreasing the excitability of the muscle cells. Hypermagnesemia rarely develops unless there is renal failure, although it has been identified in diabetic ketoacidosis where there is severe water loss. In persons with renal failure, frequent use of magnesium-containing antacids or cathartics can cause toxicity. The vasodilating effect of magnesium is accentuated in hypermagnesemia and can lead to hypotension. There may be loss of deep tendon reflexes, respiratory depression, and cardiac arrest (see the box on p. 131).

Correction of the underlying cause corrects magnesium excess. If renal failure is present, dialysis is necessary. Intravenous calcium gluconate may be a useful temporary treatment, because calcium has an antagonistic effect on magnesium.

Causes and symptoms of hypermagnesemia

Causes

Renal failure
Diabetic ketoacidosis with severe water loss

Symptoms

Hypotension
Vasodilation
    Heat
    Thirst
    Nausea/Vomiting
Loss of deep tendon reflexes
Respiratory depression
Prolonged severe excess
    Coma
    Cardiac arrest

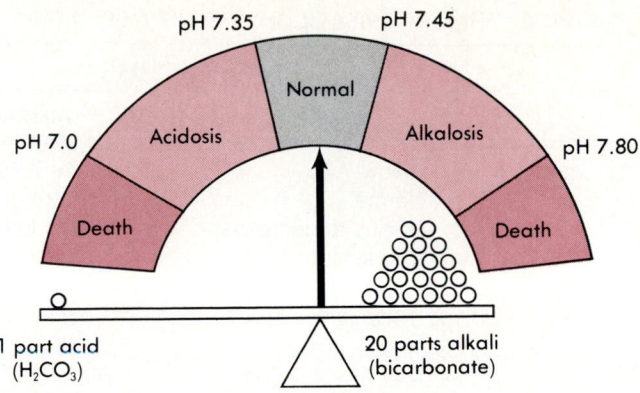

Carbonic acid-base bicarbonate balance

Fig. 8-7   Note that the relationship of 1 part carbonic acid to 20 parts bicarbonate will maintain hydrogen ion concentration (pH) within normal limits. Increase in H_2CO_3 or decrease in HCO_3^- will cause acidosis; similarly, decrease in H_2CO_3 or increase in HCO_3^- will cause alkalosis. (Redrawn from Abbott Laboratories: Fluid and electrolytes, North Chicago, 1970, Abbott Laboratories.)

■ ACID-BASE BALANCE AND IMBALANCE

■ Acid-base balance

■ BUFFER SYSTEM

Cells are sensitive to changes in the pH (hydrogen ion concentration) of body fluids. The maintenance of a stable pH of body fluids is essential to life. Normal body fluid is slightly alkaline (pH 7.35 to 7.45) and is maintained in a relatively stable condition by buffer systems located in the body.

A *buffer* is a substance that can act as a chemical sponge, either soaking up or releasing hydrogen ions so that the pH remains relatively stable. The main buffer systems of the ECF are hemoglobin, protein, and the carbonic acid-bicarbonate system. The latter is the most important clinically. Two types of carbonate are present in body fluids—carbonic acid (H_2CO_3) and bicarbonate (HCO_3^-). The ability of the body to keep the pH of body fluids within normal limits relies essentially on maintenance of the normal ratio of *one part of carbonic acid to 20 parts of bicarbonate* (Fig. 8-7).

Carbonic acid concentration is controlled by the lungs, because if carbon dioxide is retained in large amounts, more is available to combine with water to form carbonic acid in the following chemical reaction:

$$CO_2 + H_2O \rightarrow H_2CO_3$$

The amount of carbon dioxide expelled is varied by the rate and depth of respiration.

Bicarbonate concentration is controlled by the *kidneys,* which selectively retain or excrete bicarbonate, depending on body needs.

■ LABORATORY TESTS

Information about a patient's acid-base status is obtained by testing a sample of arterial blood (arterial blood gas) for the following values:

1. pH (normal 7.35-7.45): measure of hydrogen ion concentration.
2. P_{CO_2} (normal 40 mm Hg): partial pressure of carbon dioxide.
3. Bicarbonate (normal 27 mEq/L): sometimes reported as carbon dioxide content, which is a measure of all carbon dioxide dissolved in the blood as carbonic acid and bicarbonate. The approximate bicarbonate can be determined by subtracting 1 mEq/L from the carbon dioxide content.

The P_{O_2}, partial pressure of oxygen, is also measured and indicates how well the patient is obtaining oxygen, but does not indicate the acid-base status.

■ Acid-base imbalance

When the buffer systems are unable to maintain the hydrogen ion concentration (pH) of the blood within the normal range, the blood becomes more acid (*acidosis*) or more basic (*alkalosis*). If the pH of the blood drops below 6.8 or rises above 8.0, death usually ensues (Fig. 8-7). Carbonic acid (H_2CO_3) excess or deficit is referred to as *respiratory* acidosis or alkalosis, whereas base bicarbonate change is called *metabolic* acidosis or alkalosis. Changes in laboratory values are illustrated in Table 8-8.

Maintenance of the 20:1 ratio of bicarbonate to carbonic acid is crucial to keeping serum pH within the normal range. Actual amounts of both bicarbonate and carbonic

Table 8-8   Serum levels of pH, P_{CO_2}, HCO_3^- seen in acidosis and alkalosis

	Metabolic levels		Respiratory levels	
	Acidosis	**Alkalosis**	**Acidosis**	**Alkalosis**
Serum pH	Below 7.35	Above 7.45	Below 7.35	Above 7.45
P_{CO_2}	Normal	Normal	Increases above 40 mm Hg (because of excessive retention of carbon dioxide)	Decreases below 40 mm Hg (result of excessive loss of carbon dioxide)
	Begins to decrease to less than 40 mm Hg to compensate	Begins to increase to more than 40 mm Hg to compensate		
HCO_3^-	Decreases below 27 mEq/L	Increases above 27 mEq/L	Normal	Normal
			Increases to more than 27 mEq/L to compensate	Decreases to less than 27 mEq/L to compensate
Urine pH	Less than 6.0	More than 7.0	Less than 6.0	More than 7.0

Table 8-9   Types of acid-base disturbances and compensatory mechanisms

Disturbance	Physiologic causes	Method of compensation
Respiratory acidosis	Carbonic acid excess: lungs not removing sufficient CO_2 (hypoventilation)	Bicarbonate production by kidneys increased; bicarbonate retained and chloride excreted instead by kidneys; secretion and excretion of hydrogen ions in urine increased
Respiratory alkalosis	Carbonic acid deficit: lungs removing too much CO_2 (hyperventilation)	Kidneys increase excretion of bicarbonate ions
Metabolic acidosis	Bicarbonate deficit: retention of acid metabolites, diabetic ketoacidosis, excess acid intake (salicylate poisoning), or loss of bicarbonate	Increased rate and depth of respiration cause increased excretion of CO_2 by lungs; formation of bicarbonate ions in the kidneys increased
Metabolic alkalosis	Bicarbonate excess: excess intake (sodium bicarbonate, carbonated drinks) or retention of bicarbonate Potassium depletion Loss of acid	Rate and depth of respiration decreased; lungs retain more CO_2; kidneys excrete bicarbonate

acid may vary, but the pH remains normal as long as the 20:1 ratio exists. For example, if the P_{CO_2} indicator of carbonic acid rises, the bicarbonate rises to keep the normal ratio between these two substances intact. This effort of the body to maintain normal pH when acidosis or alkalosis occurs is known as *compensation.*

There are two other compensatory mechanisms besides the buffer systems. The first is the action of hydrogen ions on the respiratory center in the medulla to *increase or decrease rate and depth of breathing.* As a result, carbon dioxide is removed rapidly or retained to a greater extent in the blood. This decreases or increases carbonic acid content.

The second mechanism is the *excretion of an acid or alkaline urine by the kidneys.* In acidosis the kidney reabsorbs bicarbonate and excretes hydrogen ions with nonbicarbonate ions or as ammonia (NH_4). The reverse occurs with alkalosis (Table 8-9). When conditions leading to acid-base

imbalances occur, the compensatory mechanisms are not completely effective and normal pH can only be attained by correction of the underlying cause.

The major effect of acidosis is depression of the CNS as evidenced by disorientation followed by coma. *Alkalosis* is characterized by overexcitability of the nervous system, and the muscles may go into a state of tetany and convulsions. Acid-base imbalances always produce an imbalance of the body's electrolytes as well; therefore, symptoms of these imbalances also occur.

■ BICARBONATE DEFICIT (METABOLIC ACIDOSIS)

When acid production or addition of acid by ingestion exceeds acid loss, bicarbonates attempt to buffer the acid load; but the bicarbonate supply soon becomes depleted

Causes and effects of metabolic acidosis

Causes

Increased acid production
  Ketoacidosis (uncontrolled diabetes mellitus, starvation)
  Uremic acidosis (kidney failure)
  Lactic acidosis (shock, respiratory or cardiac arrest)
Increased acid ingestion
  Salicylates, ethanol, ethylene glycol
Loss of bicarbonate
  Severe diarrhea
  Intestinal fistulas

Effects

Hyperventilation
  Weakness
  Hyperkalemia
  Disorientation
  Coma

Causes and effects of metabolic alkalosis

Causes

Loss of stomach acid
  Gastric suctioning
  Persistent vomiting
Excess alkali intake
Loss of potassium
Biliary drainage
Intestinal fistulas
Diarrhea

Effects

Numbness, tingling of extremities
Hypertonic muscles, tetany
Bradycardia
Depressed respirations

and a bicarbonate deficit, metabolic acidosis, results (Table 8-9). Bicarbonate may also become depleted by losses of large amounts of alkaline secretions, such as intestinal secretions.

Increased acid production occurs during the development of ketoacidosis, uremic acidosis, or lactic acidosis. In *ketoacidosis,* glucose either cannot be used or is not available for oxidation. The body compensates for this by using body fat for energy, thus producing abnormal amounts of ketone bodies, which are fatty acids. Ketoacidosis also develops whenever a person does not eat sufficient food to meet daily needs and body fat must be burned for energy. It is the reason why extremely low-carbohydrate or high-protein–zero-carbohydrate reduction diets are criticized by nutrition experts.

Lactic acidosis results when lactic acid is produced in large quantities by anaerobic oxygenation, such as occurs with shock. *Uremic acidosis* results from the inability of the failing kidney to excrete the acid end products of metabolism.

Hyperkalemia may result during metabolic acidosis; as the hydrogen ion concentration of the extracellular fluid increases, hydrogen moves into the cell and potassium moves out into the bloodstream.

The patient in acidosis becomes hyperpneic and has deep, periodic breathing. Hyperventilation represents an attempt to blow off carbon dioxide and to lower the P_{CO_2}, thus compensating for the acidosis. If the condition is untreated, disorientation, stupor, coma, and death occur. The box above shows the causes and effects of metabolic acidosis.

Metabolic acidosis is controlled by giving an intravenous solution of sodium bicarbonate or sodium lactate. Sodium bicarbonate sometimes is given orally if it can be retained. Treatment of the condition precipitating the acidosis is then instituted.

■ BICARBONATE EXCESS (METABOLIC ALKALOSIS)

When acid loss is greater than acid production, hydrogen ions are lost from body fluids and bicarbonate excess (metabolic alkalosis) exists. An excess may also occur with an excessive intake of sodium bicarbonate or other alkaline salt, especially if renal function is impaired.

Loss of potassium can also lead to metabolic alkalosis. When potassium is lost from the body, hydrogen ions move into the cells to replace the lost potassium, leaving a decreased hydrogen ion concentration in the extracellular fluid, that is, metabolic alkalosis (Table 8-9).

In metabolic alkalosis, breathing becomes depressed in an effort to conserve carbon dioxide for combination with hydrogen ions in the blood to raise the blood level of carbonic acid (Table 8-9). See the box above for causes and effects of metabolic alkalosis.

Treatment consists of administration of sodium chloride or ammonium chloride. If the condition is associated with a loss of sodium chloride, potassium must be restored because it is lost with the sodium.

■ CARBONIC ACID EXCESS (RESPIRATORY ACIDOSIS)

Any condition that decreases the rate of pulmonary ventilation increases the concentration of dissolved carbon dioxide and hydrogen ions and results in a build-up of carbonic acid known as respiratory acidosis. The excess or carbon dioxide (hypercapnia) can cause *carbon dioxide nar-*

Causes and effects of respiratory acidosis

Causes

Damage to respiratory center in medulla
Depression of respiratory center by drugs (narcotics)
Obstruction of respiratory passages: pneumonia, chronic bronchitis
Loss of lung surface for ventilation
   Atelectasis
   Pneumothorax
   Emphysema
Weakness of respiratory muscles

Effects

Rapid breathing
Visual disturbances
Behavioral changes
Confusion
Drowsiness
Headache
Coma

Causes and effects of respiratory alkalosis

Causes

Hyperventilation syndrome (caused by anxiety, hysteria)
Hyperventilation caused by:
   Fever
   Hypoxia
Pulmonary disorders
CNS lesions
Excess assisted ventilation

Effects

Paresthesias: numbness and tingling around mouth and in extremities
Inability to concentrate
Blurred vision
Dry mouth
Coma

---

cosis. In this condition carbon dioxide levels are so high that they no longer stimulate respirations but depress them. Associated with the decreased respiratory rate are lack of oxygen and hypoxia. During respiratory acidosis, potassium moves out of the cells, producing *hyperkalemia*. Ventricular fibrillation may occur if the blood potassium levels are greatly increased. The box above contains a summary of the causes and effects of respiratory acidosis.

Treatment is aimed at increasing the excursion of the lungs to improve the exchange of carbon dioxide and oxygen. This objective is accomplished by using positive pressure breathing and bronchodilators to assist the patient in exhaling carbon dioxide. Because the respiratory center is narcotized by increased amounts of carbon dioxide, the lowered oxygen tension of the blood maintains respiration. For this reason, oxygen is never given to patients with carbon dioxide narcosis, and low flow oxygen is used when a patient has an impaired ability to exhale carbon dioxide normally.

■ CARBONIC ACID DEFICIT (RESPIRATORY ALKALOSIS)

Excessive pulmonary ventilation decreases hydrogen ion concentration and the formation of carbonic acid, leading to respiratory alkalosis. A common cause of respiratory alkalosis is *hyperventilation*. A person who hyperventilates blows off large amounts of carbon dioxide.

Respiratory alkalosis can be prevented in a person who is hyperventilating by administering a few whiffs of carbon dioxide or by having the person breathe into a paper bag and then rebreathe the exhaled carbon dioxide. Care should be taken in adjusting mechanical respirators so the patient does not breathe too deeply or too rapidly.

The patient may complain of lightheadedness and numbness or tingling of the fingers and toes. If the alkalosis becomes more severe, tetany and convulsions may be present. Serum potassium levels will decrease because potassium moves into the cells as hydrogen ions move out in an attempt to correct the alkalosis. The causes and effects of respiratory alkalosis are shown in the box above.

Treating the underlying condition usually effectively resolves respiratory alkalosis. Respiratory alkalosis becomes especially dangerous when it leads to cardiac arrhythmias caused partly by a decreased serum potassium level. If tetany is present, calcium gluconate is given intravenously. Renal function must be maintained to promote renal compensation of the alkalosis.

■ ASSESSMENT OF FLUID AND ELECTROLYTE BALANCE

■ Patient data

The nurse should be familiar with signs and symptoms of fluid and electrolyte disturbances. Because these symptoms are frequently subtle, it is necessary to have a high degree of sensitivity to the possibility of occurrence in certain persons, as in the following:

1. Has an illness of a type that usually disrupts fluid and electrolyte balance
2. Has medical or surgical treatments that result in imbalances

Table 8-10   Data supporting fluid and electrolyte imbalances

	Signs and symptoms	Imbalance
Change in mental status	Irritable, restless	Sodium or potassium excess
	Confusion, lethargy	Sodium or calcium excess or deficit
		Hypotonic fluid excess
		Isotonic fluid deficit
Head/neck	Dry, sticky mucous membranes	Sodium excess
	Facial puffiness (edema)	Isotonic fluid excess
	Distended neck veins	Isotonic fluid excess
	Thirst, dry mucous membranes, longitudinal furrows on tongue	Isotonic fluid deficit
	Flat neck veins in supine position	Isotonic fluid deficit
Temperature	Increase	Water loss, sodium excess
	Decrease	Fluid excess
GI	Absent bowel sounds (ileus)	Potassium deficit
	Anorexia, nausea, vomiting	Fluid excess or deficit
		Potassium excess or deficit
		Calcium excess
Circulation	Increased blood pressure	Increased circulatory volume
		Magnesium deficit
	Decreased blood pressure	Decreased circulatory volume
		Magnesium excess
	Increased pulse, slow vein filling	Potassium excess or deficit
		Isotonic fluid deficit
	Bounding pulse	Increased circulating volume
		Potassium excess or deficit
	Weak, irregular pulse	Potassium excess or deficit
	Cardiac arrhythmias	Potassium excess or deficit
Respiration	Dyspnea, orthopnea, moist breath sounds	Isotonic fluid excess
	Decreased rate	Magnesium excess
Skin	Pale, cool extremities (without edema)	Decreased circulating volume
	Pitting edema	Isotonic fluid excess
	Poor turgor (test over sternum)	Fluid deficit, sodium excess
	Dryness in groin, axillae	Isotonic fluid deficit
	Flushed dry skin	Sodium excess
Neuromuscular	Numbness, tingling around mouth, fingers, toes	Calcium deficit
	Increased irritability, muscle spasms	Calcium deficit
	Muscle weakness, paralysis	Potassium deficit
	Decreased muscle tone, decreased deep tendon reflexes	Magnesium deficit
	Abdominal cramps	Potassium excess

3. Has considerable limitation of food and fluid intake
4. Sustains significant loss of body fluids

By knowing of conditions that put an individual at risk and making careful ongoing assessments, the nurse can prevent or detect imbalances before they become severe.

Subjective data include thirst, headache, pain, nausea, dyspnea, and orthopnea. The time of origin and a description of symptoms are noted. Objective data, as noted in Table 8-10, can be compared to the baseline assessment obtained at the time of the patient's initial contact with health care providers.

■ Laboratory values

Laboratory determinations of serum levels of the specific electrolytes help in making decisions concerning electrolyte excesses or deficits. When electrolyte disturbances develop slowly, symptoms may not be pronounced, and the problem may be detected only by a determination of the electrolyte concentration in the patient's blood. Serum pH and Pco_2 levels help in identifying acid-base balances (Table 8-8). When there is excess water, hemodilution occurs and the

Table 8-11 GI output

Type of fluid	Consistency	Color	Odor
Gastric	Watery	Pale yellow-green	Sour
			Fruity odor with metabolic acidosis
Biliary	Thicker than gastric	Bright yellow to dark green	Acrid odor and bitter taste
Intestinal	Thick	Dark green to brown	Fecal

hemogolobin and hematocrit levels decrease. With excessive fluid loss, there is hemoconcentration and the hematocrit and BUN levels increase.

■ Additional data

Important data to be considered in assessing fluid balances are comparison of fluid intake to output and changes in patient weight. Acutely ill medical patients and patients undergoing major surgery need to have their fluid intake and output and daily weight closely monitored. The practice of totaling the fluid intake and output every shift or every 24 hours provides additional data for determining whether or not the patient has a fluid imbalance.

■ FLUID INTAKE

The intake record should show the type and amount of all fluids the patient has received and the route by which these were administered. This includes fluids given orally, parenterally, rectally, or fluids administered by tubes and retained by the patient. Foods that are eaten in a semisolid state but are basically liquid, such as gelatin or ice cream are recorded as fluids. To record the fluid intake of ice chips, the amount of ice chips is divided by one half (60 ml of ice chips equals 30 ml water). Patients may receive considerable amounts of fluid through the frequent sucking of ice chips.

■ FLUID OUTPUT

□ Urinary output

Urinary output is recorded as to time and amount of each voiding to help evaluate renal function. If renal function is a major concern, such as in the patient with shock, an indwelling catheter is used so the amount of urine can be recorded every hour and fluid intake regulated accordingly.

□ Wound drainage

Any drainage from a catheter draining a wound is measured and the amount and character of the drainage is recorded. If there is excessive drainage on dressings, it may be necessary to weigh the dressings. Fluid loss equals the difference between the wet weight and dry weight of the dressing.

□ GI drainage

Electrolytes are lost in large amounts with vomiting, diarrhea, and gastric and intestinal drainage. The amount and kind vary according to the type of GI fluid lost. For determination of the amount and type of fluid replacement, vomitus, GI drainage, and liquid stools are measured as accurately as possible and are described as to consistency, color, and odor (Table 8-11). Fluid used to irrigate nasogastric tubes is subtracted from total drainage before the amount of drainage is recorded.

□ Other output

Fluid aspirated from any body cavity, such as the abdomen or pleural spaces, must be measured. This fluid contains not only electrolytes but also proteins.

Diaphoresis is difficult to measure. If the clothing and linen become saturated, there may be as much as 1000 ml of fluid lost in perspiration. Dry and wet weights may be taken to get a more accurate measure of the amount of fluid loss.

■ DAILY WEIGHT

The daily weight record is often the best way to determine the onset of dehydration or the accumulation of fluid either as generalized edema or as "hidden" fluid in body cavities. *An increase of 1 kg in weight is equal to the retention of 1 L of fluid.* If the weight record is to be useful, the patient must be weighed on the same scale and at the same hour each day and must be wearing the same amount of clothing. Usually weights are taken in the early morning before the patient has eaten or defecated but after voiding.

■ URINE SPECIFIC GRAVITY

The specific gravity of urine is a measure of the density (amount of solutes) in a sample of urine compared with the density of pure water (which is 1.000). Normal range for urine specific gravity is approximately 1.003 to 1.030. A person with renal impairment excretes a small amount of dilute urine (low specific gravity) because of the inability of the kidneys to concentrate solutes in the urine. The relationship between specific gravity and fluid deficit or excess is summarized as follows:

Fluid deficit: small urine volume with high specific gravity

Fluid excess: large urine volume with low specific gravity

■ INTERVENTIONS FOR PATIENTS WITH FLUID AND ELECTROLYTE IMBALANCE

Important nursing functions include prevention of fluid and electrolyte imbalance, assessment of patients to recognize and report early signs of imbalance, planning and carrying out actions related to therapy to correct the condition, and relief of symptoms.

■ Prevention of fluid and electrolyte imbalance

Unless preventive measures are employed, many medical-surgical conditions and therapies may lead to fluid and electrolyte imbalance. In some frequently encountered situations, attention to preventive aspects may lessen the possibility of the development of serious fluid and electrolyte imbalance.

■ PREVENTION OF INADEQUATE FLUID INTAKE

Any patient who is unable to ask for fluids, to identify a need for fluid, or to swallow easily may develop a fluid deficit. The fluid intake of these patients is monitored, and specific plans are made to offer fluids at regular intervals. Some conditions placing persons at risk for fluid deficit are as follows: aphasia, catatonia, confusion, disorientation, dysphagia, weakness, and tube feedings.

■ PREVENTION OF IMBALANCES FROM GI FLUID LOSS

☐ Vomiting and diarrhea

Vomiting and diarrhea are common symptoms of many illnesses. Sodium and some potassium are lost in vomiting and diarrhea, whereas chloride is lost only from vomitus. As soon as fluids are tolerated, the patient may be served salty broth and tea or another fluid high in potassium to replace the losses. Dry salty crackers often are tolerated when fluids are not and can be used to replace sodium. These measures often keep the patient from feeling weak and exhausted.

☐ Draining fistulas

A patient with a draining fistula from any portion of the GI tract loses *sodium, calcium,* and some *potassium,* and dietary supplements are needed. Extra milk can replace all the losses if tolerated by the patient. The vitamin D in the milk enables the body to use the calcium in the milk. A person with a permanent fistulous opening, such as an ileostomy, needs to be especially careful to supplement their sodium and potassium intake when vomiting, diarrhea, or fever adds to the already unusually large loss of electrolytes.

☐ Nasogastric drainage

Routine intravenous replacement usually is adequate to compensate for losses through nasogastric drainage, unless the patient has been sucking many ice chips or has had the tube irrigated frequently with water. Both of these practices, although they seem to be harmless because the fluid is removed immediately through the aspiration apparatus, stimulate the secretion of gastric juices. Aspiration of gastric juices of the stomach at rest may lead to loss of electrolytes and fluid. If irrigation of the tube is necessary, normal saline is used.

☐ Enemas

Repeated enemas may result in water intoxication and potassium loss. If there is an order for enemas until the returns are clear, it is best not to give more than three enemas at one time without consulting the physician. If an elderly person living at home complains of pronounced weakness without apparent cause, the person is asked whether cathartics or enemas are being taken. If so, stopping this practice, eating foods with high potassium content, and increasing fluid intake may relieve the symptoms. Methods to combat constipation without taking laxatives or frequent enemas are than taught.

■ PREVENTION OF EXCESSIVE FLUID LOSS FROM SKIN, LUNGS, KIDNEYS

☐ Diaphoresis

Diaphoresis may result from heat, strenuous exercise, or fever. Even the healthy person who is perspiring profusely needs extra salt in the diet and should drink extra fluids. Some salty fluids are needed by the patient with a fever. Patients on salt-restricted diets and those with draining fistulas are especially likely to suffer from sodium depletion and should increase their salt intake slightly when perspiring profusely.

☐ Diuretics

Diuretics are administered to encourage excretion of sodium and water in excess of body needs. However, potassium, which may not be in excess, is also lost with the increased urinary output. The patient receiving diuretics is encouraged to eat foods that are *high in potassium but low in sodium.* Good sources are bananas and other fresh fruits (see the box on p. 128).

Diuretics such as the thiazides may eventually cause sodium depletion; therefore, the person receiving extensive diuretic treatment is taught to observe for symptoms indicating sodium depletion (p. 126) and to report these symptoms to the physician. Table 8-12 lists some commonly used diuretics.

☐ Renal or circulatory impairments

Any patient with renal or circulatory impairment, as may occur in *shock, cardiac failure, renal insufficiency,* or *constriction of blood vessels* because of disease, may develop

---

Usages of common intravenous solutions

Solution	Use
Dextrose	
5% in water	Maintenance therapy when sodium not desirable
5% in saline (0.9%, 0.45%, 0.2%)	Maintenance therapy depending on desired amount of sodium
Sodium chloride (0.9%)	For large losses of sodium, as in loss of GI fluids, burns
One-sixth molar lactate	Replacement of sodium but not chloride
Ringer's lactate	Balanced solution containing Na^+, K^+, Ca^{++}, Cl^-

---

Table 8-12 Common diuretics and their possible effects on fluid and electrolytes

Generic name	Trade name	Possible effect
Thiazides		
Chlorothiazide	Diuril	Hyponatremia, hypochloremia, hypokalemia, decreased extracellular volume, hyper-
Hydrochlorothiazide	HydroDiuril	glycemia, hyperuricemia, decreased calcium excretion
Potent diuretics		
Furosemide	Lasix	Hyponatremia, hypokalemia, decreased ECF, hyperuricemia, hypocalcemia, hypo-
Ethacrynic acid	Edecrin	magnesemia, hypochloremia, alkalosis
Potassium saving		
Spironolactone	Aldactone	Hyperkalemia, hyponatremia, decreased ECF, acidosis
Triamterene	Dyrenium	
Osmotic agent		
Mannitol	Osmitrol	Hyponatremia, hypochloremia, increased ECF, water intoxication if renal excretion is not adequate

---

a fluid and electrolyte imbalance. Common imbalances include the following:

1. Edema from sodium and water retention
2. Hyperkalemia
3. Hyponatremia
4. Acidosis from inadequate tissue oxygenation
5. Overhydration

Patients with the above conditions are instructed to avoid taking too much food containing sodium, potassium, or bicarbonate. They should not drink carbonated beverages. The nurse must be expecially aware of overhydration whenever intravenous fluids are being given to persons with renal or circulatory impairment.

□ Respiratory impairments

Patients with diseases such as emphysema that limit lung excursion and therefore limit gaseous exchange should not take carbonated beverages or bicarbonate of soda. These substances tend to make the blood more alkaline than normal, and respiration is depressed in an effort to correct this imbalance. Depression of respiration is highly unde-

sirable for patients with obstructive lung diseases. Early recognition and treatment of these lung diseases may help prevent acid-base imbalances.

■ Replacement therapy

Fluids may be replaced by various routes as follows: orally (preferred route), by intravenous infusion, or by tube feedings (see Chapter 6).

■ SPACING OF FLUIDS

Fluids given by any route should be spaced throughout a 24-hour period. Not only does this practice help to maintain normal body fluid levels, but it also provides for better regulation of the electrolyte balance by the kidneys and prevents the end products of metabolism and toxic materials from being excreted in concentrated form. In this way the danger of renal damage, formation of calculi, and irritation of the lower urinary tract are reduced. In addition, fluid spacing prevents overloading of the circulation.

Table 8-13   Solutions for intravenous use

Type of solution	Cations (mEq/L)					Anions (mEq/L)			Glucose (g/L)
	Na$^+$	K$^+$	Ca^{++}	Mg^{++}	NH$_4^+$	Cl$^-$	HCO$_3^-$ lactate	PO$_4^-$	
5% Dextrose in water									50
10% Dextrose in water									100
Normal saline (0.9%)	154					154			
3% Saline	513					513			
Ringer's solution	147	4	4			155			
5% Dextrose in Ringer's lactate	130	4	3			109	28		50
Ringer's lactate	130	4	3			109	28		
Ammonium chloride (0.9%)					170	170			
Sodium lactate 1/6 molar	167						167		
5% Dextrose in 0.2% saline	34					34			50
5% Dextrose in 0.45% saline	77					77			50

■ CONCENTRATION OF FLUIDS

Infusing *concentrated solutions* rapidly and in large amounts into the alimentary tract causes the blood volume to drop because large amounts of fluid are needed to dilute the substance. If the circulating volume becomes considerably depleted, irreversible shock can result. The "dumping syndrome," which sometimes occurs after gastric resection, is caused by this abnormal shift of fluid. Concentrated solutions sometimes are given intentionally to reduce cerebral edema.

Concentrated intravenous solutions of sugar or protein should also be given slowly in small amounts because they require fluid for dilution. Hypertonic saline solution may cause fluid to diffuse from the tissues to equalize the concentration of salt in the intravascular compartment. The superior vena cava is the preferred site for infusions of hypertonic solutions, such as parenteral hyperalimentation, because of the rapid dilution by the larger amount of blood at this site. If any of these concentrated solutions flows too rapidly into the vascular system, pulmonary edema can develop.

■ ORAL INTAKE

Adults who have no circulatory or renal malfunction usually need between 1500 and 3000 ml/day of fluid, depending on the amount of food consumed. Patients who have anorexia and are not eating well require more fluid to maintain a fluid balance. Medical prescriptions for fluid restriction are usually given for patients who have fluid excess (edema or water intoxication) or whose kidneys are not functioning well.

A medical prescription may be given to the patient to "force fluids" or the nurse may make the decision that a large intake of fluids is desirable, such as for prevention of urinary stasis with its subsequent complications. No standard amount can be stated because the amount required depends on the following:

1. Size of the patient
2. Patient's circulatory and renal status
3. Amount of food intake
4. Amount of fluid loss (if appropriate)

It must be remembered that people with small or inelastic vascular systems become overhydrated easily. If the person has had a large portion of the body such as a limb removed either by surgery or trauma, the person's size is thereby decreased. If there is a question concerning the amount of fluids a patient should be encouraged to drink, the physician is consulted.

■ PARENTERAL FLUIDS

▫ Type of fluid

The nurse needs to know the common solutions used parenterally (Table 8-13). Some of the reasons for giving the more common intravenous solutions are listed in the box on p. 138. Potassium chloride may be added to maintain normal intake of potassium and to replace losses. Ascorbic acid and vitamin B (Solu-B) may be added for nutritional purposes.

Whole blood, plasma, concentrated albumin, or plasma volume expanders can be given to substitute for blood protein loss and are used to establish normal blood volume and prevent shock. *Dextran* is the most generally accepted plasma volume expander. It increases the oncotic pressure of the blood, thus increasing the reabsorption of fluid from interstitial spaces. This creates an increase in plasma volume. *Low-molecular dextran* decreases the viscosity of the blood, allowing greater blood flow through the capillaries; thus it is useful in treating cardiogenic, hemorrhagic, or septic shock. It may cause prolonged bleeding time and should not be used if renal disease with severe oliguria or anuria is present. The patient is monitored for signs of anaphylactic reaction (apprehension, dyspnea, wheezing, respirations, tightness of chest, itching, hypotension) when dextran is being given.

Intravenous fluids containing electrolytes should be run slowly to allow the body to regulate their use. The patient is monitored for signs of intoxication (excess of fluids or electrolytes) and satisfactory urinary output. Increased serum potassium (hyperkalemia) can be particularly dangerous, because it may cause cardiac arrest. Renal failure and untreated adrenal insufficiency are contraindications for the use of potassium. Many physicians do not start intravenous therapy until chemical analyses of the blood have been reported for the day.

☐ Amount and rate of administration

The administration rate of fluids usually is ordered by the physician and depends on the patient's illness, the kind of fluid given, and the patient's size and age. Approximately 30 ml/kg body weight is needed to meet daily fluid requirements. Fever increases water needs by about 15% for each 1 degree Centigrade rise in a patient's body temperature.[8] If there has been an acute illness resulting in a significant fluid deficit, fluid is replaced at the rate of 1000 ml/kg loss in weight. The physician calculates water needs based on the amount needed to replace losses and the amount required to meet daily needs.

The usual rate for replacement of fluid loss is 3 ml/min; it is rarely run at a rate faster than 4 ml/min. If fluids are given continuously or if they are given when there is impaired renal or cardiac function, they are rarely run faster than 2 ml/min. Intravenous infusions that are run at too rapid a rate (sometimes seen when an infusion is "speeded up" to complete the treatment at a specified time)

may result in overloading of the circulatory system and pulmonary edema. At the first signs of increased blood volume (p. 124) in any patient receiving an intravenous infusion, the rate of flow is reduced and the physician notified.

■ Relief of thirst

Thirst, the first and most insistent sign of dehydration, sometimes causes the patient more misery than surgery or the symptoms of a disease. It may develop even when fluids have been withheld only for a number of hours. If fluid is being withheld intentionally, thirst often is made more bearable by explaining to patients why fluid is withheld and when they can expect to receive some.

Thirst usually is relieved rather readily by taking fluids. If fluids cannot be taken orally, the administration of fluids parenterally usually gives relief. It is often helpful to explain to the patient who is receiving an infusion that the procedure will soon provide some relief from thirst.

Mouth care allays some of the discomfort from thirst and may need to be repeated every hour. If patients can be trusted not to swallow, they may be given ice chips, which are held in the mouth and then spit out. Hard candies often give relief, even though they also must be expelled. The chewing of gum helps some patients.

Pronounced and continued thirst, despite the administration of fluids, is not normal and is reported. In the patient recently returned from surgery, this kind of thirst may indicate internal hemorrhage, elevation of temperature, or some other untoward development. Thirst may also be an indication of hypercalcemia or the onset of diabetes mellitus.

■ SUMMARY

1. Losses of fluid and electrolytes occur through the skin by diaphoresis and oozing form severe wounds or burns; from GI drainage and enemas; from the kidneys because

---

Putting knowledge to practice

- Review the sources and actions of the hormones aldosterone, antidiuretic hormone, and parathormone.
- Review methods of giving fluids intravenously (in your fundamentals text or procedure manual).
- What happens when a 5% salt solution is placed in a container in which it is separated by a semipermeable membrane from a 1% salt solution?
- What happens if a solution containing a protein such as gelatin is separated by a semipermeable membrane from water?
- What happens to the extra salt and water you consume when eating a ham dinner?
- If you (or a close friend) have recently had severe vomiting, diarrhea, or high fever, what symptoms did you observe that might indicate a fluid or electrolyte imbalance?
- Examine the laboratory values on the chart of an acutely ill patient. What values are suggestive of a fluid or electrolyte imbalance? What symptoms did the patient demonstrate?

of diuretic use and polyuria; from hemorrhage; and through the trapping of fluids by wound swelling, edema, ascites, and intestinal obstruction.

2. A low sodium level in the blood can indicate either a deficit of sodium or an excess of water.

3. Muscle weakness, anorexia, nausea or vomiting, diminished deep tendon reflexes, lethargy, cardiac arrhythmias, and ECG changes are symptoms of hypokalemia.

4. Nursing responsibilities for the person with hypercalcemia include active exercises for immobilized persons, increased fluid intake, prevention of urinary tract infections, and gentle handling to prevent pathologic fractures.

5. Carbonic acid concentration is controlled by the lungs; bicarbonate concentration is controlled by the kidneys.

6. Monitoring fluid and electrolyte balance is particularly important in persons with an illness of the type that disrupts fluid and electrolyte balance, with medical-surgical treatments that result in imbalances, with considerable limitation of food and fluid intake, and in persons who have sustained significant loss of body fluids.

7. Assessment of fluid and electrolyte balance includes the monitoring of laboratory values, fluid intake, fluid output (urinary output, wound drainage, GI drainage, fluid from any body cavity, diaphoresis), daily weight, and urine specific gravity.

REFERENCES AND SELECTED READINGS

Contemporary

1. *Barta, MA: Correcting electrolyte imbalances, RN 50(2):30-34, 1987.

2. Cardin, S: Acid-base balance in the patient with respiratory disease, Nurs Clin North Am 15(3):593-601, 1980.

3. Daly, BJ: Intensive care nursing, ed 2, Garden City, NJ, 1986, Medical Examination Co, Inc.

4. *Felver, L: Understanding the electrolyte maze, Am J Nurs 80:1591-1599, 1980.

5. Friedman, FB: Clinical controversies: can we really trust those I & Os? RN 45(4):52-53, 118-120, 1982.

6. Goldberg, PB: Medications that contain sodium, Geriatric Nurs 1:204-205, 1980.

7. *Goldberger, E: A primer of water, electrolytes and acid-base syndromes, ed 7, Philadelphia, 1986, Lea & Febiger.

8. Guyton, AC: Textbook of medical physiology, ed 7, Philadelphia, 1986, WB Saunders Co.

9. Kee, JL: Fluid and electrolytes with clinical applications (programmed approach), ed 4, New York, 1986, John Wiley & Sons, Inc.

10. Keithley, JK, and Fraulini, KE: What's behind that I.V. line? Nurs 82 12(3):33-45.

11. Lane, G, and Peirce, AG: When persistence pays off: resolving the mystery of an unexplained electrolyte imbalance, Nurs 82 12(1):44-47, 1982.

12. Managing special patients' fluids and electrolytes, Nurs 82 12(11):111-113, 1982.

13. McFadden, EA, Zaloga, GP, and Chernow, B: Hypocalcemia: a medical emergency, Am J Nurs 83:226-231, 1983.

14. Methany, N: Preoperative fluid balance assessment, AORN J 33:51-56, 1981.

15. *Methany, N, and Snively, WD: Nurses' handbook of fluid balance, ed 4, Philadelphia, 1983, JB Lippincott Co.

16. Menezel, LK: Clinical problems of electrolyte balance, Nurs Clin North Am 15(3):559-576, 1980.

17. Menezel, LK: Clinical problems of fluid balance, Nurs Clin North Am 15(3):549-558, 1980.

18. Plumer, AL: Principles and practice of intravenous therapy, ed 3, Boston, 1982, Little, Brown & Co.

19. Quinlan, M: Beyond electrolytes: solving the mysteries of calcium imbalance: an action guide, RN 45(11):50-54, 1982.

20. Rando, JT: Fluid and electrolyte management of the adult surgical patient, AANA J 50:49-54, 1982.

21. Sabiston, DC (editor): Textbook of surgery, ed 13, Philadelphia, 1986, WB Saunders Co.

22. Todd, B: Drugs and the elderly: when the patient has a potassium deficiency, Geriatr Nurs 2:373-376, 1981.

23. Weldy, NJ: Body fluids and electrolytes (programmed instruction), ed 4, St Louis, 1983, The CV Mosby Co.

24. Williams, SR: Essentials of nutrition and diet therapy, ed 4, St Louis, 1986, The CV Mosby Co.

25. Woodward, WE, and Woodward, TE: Management of dehydrating diarrhea, Hosp Pract 21(3):60, 63, 67-68, 1986.

26. Wright, TR, and Murray, M: Potassium problems: which patient's in danger? RN 45(6):56-62, 1982.

27. Wyngaarden, JB, and Smith, LH: Textbook of medicine, vol I and II, Philadelphia, 1985, WB Saunders Co.

28. Zerwekh, JV: The dehydration question, Nurs 83 13(1):47-51, 1983.

Classic

29. Haughney, E, and Sica, F: Diuretics: how safe can you make them? Nurs 77 7(2):34-39, 1977.

30. *Kubo, W, and others: Fluid and electrolyte problems of tube-fed patients, Am J Nurs 76:912-916, 1976.

31. *Metabolic acid-base disorders: chemistry and physiology (programmed instruction), I, Am J Nurs 77:1619-1650, 1977.

32. *Metabolic acid-base disorders: physiology abnormalities and nursing actions (programmed instruction), II, Am J Nurs 78:87-108, 1978.

33. *Metabolic acid-base disorders: clinical and laboratory findings (programmed instruction), III, Am J Nurs 78:443-460, 1978.

34. *Tripp, A: Hyper and hypocalcemia, Am J Nurs 76:1142-1145, 1976.

---

*References preceded by an asterisk are particularly well suited for student reading.

9

Shock

GAIL OSTERFIELD

CHAPTER OBJECTIVES

After studying this chapter, the student should be able to:

- Contrast three major types of shock.
- Describe early and late pathophysiologic changes that occur with shock.
- Describe organ damage that may occur with shock.
- Describe different methods of monitoring for shock.
- Describe methods of fluid replacement during shock.
- Identify effects of pharmacologic agents used to treat shock and nursing measures for patients receiving drug therapy.
- Describe therapeutic measures for shock other than fluids and drug therapy.

Shock is a syndrome characterized by hypoperfusion of body tissues. Any condition that prevents cells from receiving an adequate blood supply can interfere with their metabolism and produce shock.

Blood flow is dependent on pressure changes within the vascular compartment. Blood flows from areas of greater pressure to areas of lesser pressure. In the systemic circulation, the mean pressure is highest in the aorta, where the blood leaves the left ventricle, and lowest in the right atrium. In order for the necessary pressure gradients to exist so that blood can flow, the following three factors are necessary:

1. An adequate amount of blood for the heart to pump around the body
2. Ability of the heart to pump blood
3. Blood vessels with good tone, able to constrict and dilate to maintain normal pressure.

Shock results from the disruption of one or more of these factors.

■ ETIOLOGY OF SHOCK

Shock may be classified as hypovolemic, cardiogenic, or vasogenic (see the box below).

■ Hypovolemic shock

Hypovolemic shock is the most common type of shock. Any condition that reduces the *volume* within the vascular compartment by 15% to 25% can result in hypovolemic shock.[30] Common causes include the following:

1. Excessive blood loss: trauma (most common cause), gastrointestinal bleeding, coagulation disorders, surgery
2. Loss of body fluids other than blood: excessive diuresis (diabetic ketoacidosis or other hyperosmolar states), plasma loss from burns, fluid loss from excessive vomiting or diarrhea
3. Movement of fluid into another body space (third space), for example, bowel obstruction (up to 5 or 10 L may collect in bowel) or peritonitis (4 to 6 L may collect in peritoneal cavity within 24 hours)

Types of shock

Hypovolemic   From loss of fluid from vascular system (through blood loss or fluid loss)

Cardiogenic   From inability of heart to pump blood to tissues (decreased cardiac output)

Vasogenic   From massive vasodilation (from interference with sympathetic nervous system or effects of histamine or toxins)

■ Cardiogenic shock

Cardiogenic shock results from the inability of the heart to pump blood sufficiently to perfuse the cells of the body. When stroke volume falls initially, cardiac output may be maintained by an increase in heart rate (Chapter 25); however, an increase in the heart rate may further damage the heart. As the heart rate increases, the period of diastole shortens and the period of systole remains relatively constant. Because the coronary arteries fill during diastole, their filling time is reduced. The heart works for longer periods and requires more oxygen and nutrients. Thus tachycardia can both increase the oxygen need of the heart and decrease its oxygen supply.

Although cardiogenic shock may be caused by various cardiac conditions including cardiac tamponade, restrictive pericarditis, pulmonary embolism, severe valvular disease, or arrhythmias, the most common cause by far is myocardial infarction. Studies have shown that in most patients who die from cardiogenic shock, at least 40% of the left ventricle was damaged by a recent infarction or by a recent infarction plus a previous scar.[34] In spite of improvements in managing cardiogenic shock, the mortality still remains above 80%. (Additional information on cardiogenic shock is given in Chapter 25.)

■ Vasogenic shock

Vasogenic shock is caused by massive dilation of the blood vessels, resulting in disproportion between the size of the vascular space and the amount of blood contained. As arterial blood pressure falls, the difference between arterial and venous pressures decreases. Because blood flow is dependent on pressure differences, blood flow decreases. Blood pools in the blood vessels, resulting in decreased venous return to the heart. Cardiac output falls, and blood pressure decreases even further.

Initially in vasogenic shock, the extremities are warm because of vasodilation. However, as cardiac output decreases and tissue perfusion is reduced, compensatory vasoconstriction occurs.

Loss of vascular tone may result from a number of conditions. *Neurogenic shock* results from interference with the sympathetic nervous system, which helps maintain vasomotor tone. Spinal cord injury, spinal anesthesia, and rarely, brain damage are among the causes. *Anaphylactic shock* occurs when there is massive dilation of the blood vessels from the direct effect on the vessels of a substance such as histamine. Histamine, released by mast cells and basophils, has a powerful dilating effect on blood vessels, particularly capillaries. The endothelial cells that line the capillaries separate and expose the basement membrane, which is permeable to fluid and plasma proteins, resulting in hypovolemia.[28]

Septic shock, another form of vasogenic shock, may result from various infections, including those caused by both gram-positive and gram-negative bacteria, viruses, and fungi, although it most commonly results from gram-negative bacterial infections. The primary sites of infection are usually the urinary tract, respiratory tract, or blood. Organisms that ordinarily dwell in the gastrointestinal tract may cause sepsis and shock if they enter the bloodstream.

Conditions that predispose to septic shock include the following:

1. Age, both very young and very old
2. Immunosuppressive and steroid therapy
3. Chronic disease of the immune system
4. Urologic or gastrointestinal tract surgery

Elderly men are particularly susceptible to septic shock because of the high incidence of prostatic hypertrophy in this group. They are more likely to develop urinary tract infections and to have urologic surgical procedures.

The mechanism by which septic shock occurs is not completely understood. Some believe that early in sepsis, fluid leaks out of the vascular system, and the resultant shock is simply a form of hypovolemic shock.[4] Others see the primary cause as faulty cellular metabolism from the direct effect of the toxin.[14] Although the early pathophysiology of septic shock is not completely understood, it is known that when some organisms enter the bloodstream, they are destroyed by the immune system and a toxin is released. This toxin, in some way, causes the characteristic symptoms of early septic shock (increased cardiac output,

peripheral vasodilation, skin flushing, hyperthermia, increased renal output, and respiratory alkalosis).[32] As septic shock progresses and cardiac output decreases, it resembles other types of shock, with low urinary output, vasoconstriction, and cool moist skin.

■ PATHOPHYSIOLOGY OF SHOCK

■ Early stage

In the early stage of shock the body responds to hypoperfusion as it would to any other stressor. Many of the changes that occur are mediated through the sympathetic nervous system. Stimulation of the sympathetic nervous system results in secretion of epinephrine and norepinephrine by the adrenal medulla. Both alpha- and beta-adrenergic receptors are stimulated throughout the body. Alpha receptors respond by causing vasoconstriction and beta receptors respond by causing vasodilation (beta 1) and increased rate and strength of contraction of the heart (beta 2). The skin and the abdominal organs, which are rich in alpha receptors, receive a decreased blood supply because

Major pathophysiologic changes in shock

Change	Effect
Early stage (compensatory stage)	
Increased epinephrine and norepinephrine Alpha and beta receptors stimulated	Increased cardiac output to send more blood to tissues
Alpha effects Skin	Vasoconstriction and decreased blood supply
Beta effects Heart and skeletal muscles	Vasodilitation and increased blood supply and heart rate
Renin-angiotensin response	Vasoconstriction and secretion of aldosterone; sodium and water retention and potassium loss
Increased glucocorticoids and mineralocorticoids	Sodium and fluid retention to increase intravascular volume
	Potassium loss
Hypoxemia	Hyperventilation; provides more oxygen to tissues; may cause respiratory alkalosis
Decreased hydrostatic fluid pressure	Fluid shifts from interstitial space to capillaries to increase vascular volume
Late stage (noncompensatory stage)	
Decreased blood flow to heart	Impaired cardiac pumping ability (decreased cardiac output); blood pressure decreases
Anaerobic metabolism	Acidosis; decreased ATP; failure of cellular N^+-K^+ pump (K^+ leaves cell, Na^+ and water enter cell); cellular damage
Arteriolar dilation and venule constriction	Fluid shift from intravascular to interstitial space
Decreased blood flow to kidney	Decreased kidney function (oliguria or anuria, retention of nitrogenous waste products)
Decreased blood flow to pancreas	Production of myocardial depressant factor (MDF)

of vasoconstriction. The heart and skeletal muscles, which are rich in beta receptors, receive an increased blood supply because of vasodilation. The heart beats faster and harder and the respiratory rate increases in response to beta stimulation, thereby increasing oxygen delivery to the tissues. All of the compensatory responses mediated through the sympathetic nervous system occur rapidly.

Another compensatory response, mediated through the renin-angiotensin system, occurs more slowly. As cardiac output falls, the blood supply to the kidneys decreases. The juxtaglomerular cells respond by secreting renin, which acts upon a plasma protein, converting it to angiotensin I. This is converted to angiotensin II, which has two major effects: it causes vasoconstriction and it causes the adrenal cortex to secrete aldosterone. Aldosterone causes the kidneys to retain sodium and water and secrete potassium, resulting in an increased blood volume. The secretion of potassium may result in *hypokalemia* during this stage of shock. Decreased cardiac output results in decreased hydrostatic pressure in the capillaries, causing fluid to shift from the interstitial space into the capillaries. This also improves blood volume.

For a short period of time the compensatory mechanisms have a beneficial effect. The most vital organs, the heart and the brain, receive an adequate blood supply at the expense of the less vital organs, such as the kidneys, and other abdominal organs. This allows time for the underlying cause of shock to be corrected. However, if the underlying problem is not or cannot be corrected, the compensatory mechanisms will not be able to continue to perfuse vital organs sufficiently and the mechanisms themselves will have a deleterious effect on the body. Shock will then progress to a later stage. The box on p. 145 summarizes the pathophysiologic changes in early and late shock.

■ Late stage

As shock progresses, blood flow to all body tissues becomes impaired. Cells in vasoconstricted organs receive insufficient oxygen, and aerobic metabolism is replaced by anaerobic metabolism. Energy, in the form of adenosine triphosphate (ATP), is produced very inefficiently. Lactic acid cannot be metabolized in the absence of oxygen, so it

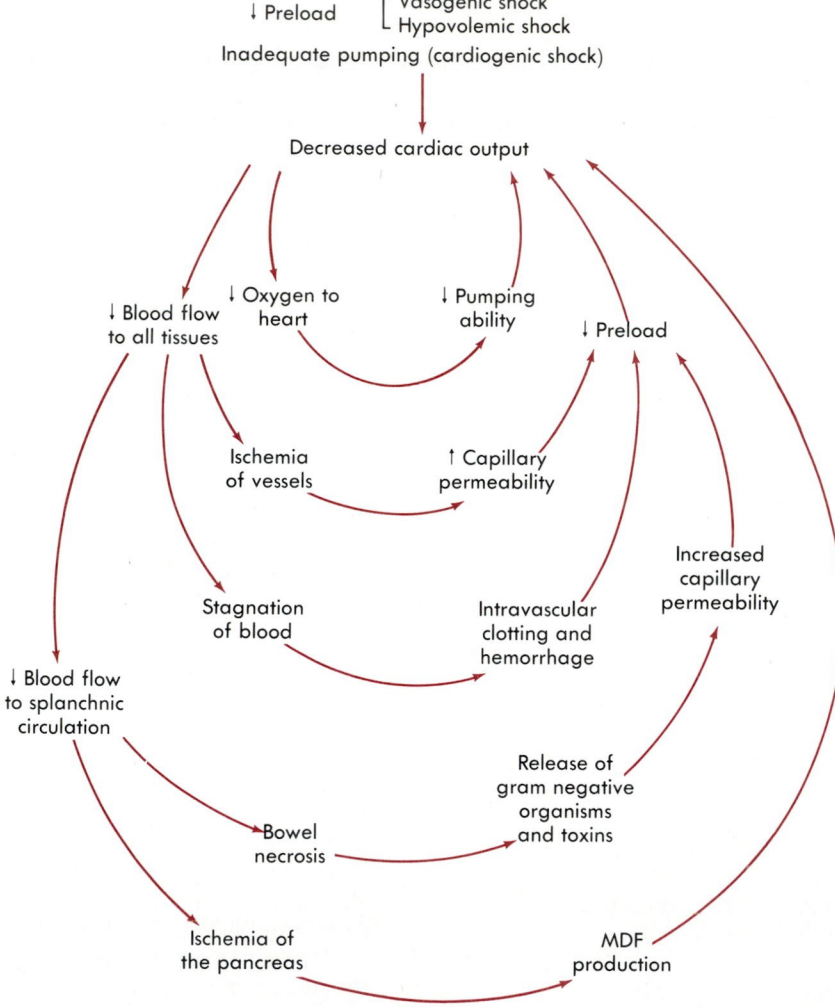

Fig. 9-1 Shock causes shock.

accumulates in the body, resulting in metabolic acidosis. With insufficient ATP, the sodium-potassium pump fails; potassium leaves the cells and sodium and water enter. Organelles within the cells are damaged. Rupture of the cell wall of the lysosomes is particularly dangerous. They normally have an important role in phagocytosis and contain digestive enzymes. When their cell walls are destroyed, the digestive enzymes are released into the cell and autodigestion of the cell occurs.[44] This process can spread from cell to cell, resulting in organ death.

Acid metabolites cause dilation at the arteriole end of the capillaries (precapillary sphincter) and constriction at the venule end of the capillary (postcapillary sphincter), increasing *intracapillary hydrostatic pressure*. This results in a fluid shift out of the capillary, further decreasing blood volume. Increased capillary permeability may occur, particularly in septic shock, as large amounts of *histamine* and *serotonin* are released in response to gram-negative toxins. As proteins leak out of the capillaries, fluid follows and the blood volume is even further reduced. As the blood supply to the kidneys is decreased, *oliguria* or *anuria* occurs. The blood urea nitrogen (BUN) and serum creatinine levels rise. Cellular damage releases potassium into the blood, and the impaired kidneys are unable to excrete it. *Hyperkalemia,* which results, depresses the contractility and conduction in the heart.

Vasoconstriction of the splanchnic vessels in response to sympathetic stimulation causes ischemia of the abdominal organs. Of particular importance is the pancreas. In response to hypoxemia the pancreas produces and secretes a substance called myocardial depressant factor (MDF), which depresses contractility of the heart. As compensatory mechanisms fail, blood supply to the heart decreases and electrical and mechanical activity are impaired.

Shock is a dynamic process with shock itself causing shock[20] (Fig. 9-1). At some point a cycle begins that cannot be interrupted, and an *irreversible stage of shock* ensues. Even if the primary problem that caused the shock is corrected and good supportive care is given, the patient will die. However, the exact point at which shock becomes irreversible cannot be determined. Regardless of the patient's symptoms, all efforts should be made to reverse the progression of shock.

■ ORGAN DAMAGE IN SHOCK

■ Kidneys

The kidneys contain about 2,400,000 nephrons, each of which is capable of forming urine. Each nephron is composed of a glomerulus, made up of capillaries and the collecting tubules (Chapter 32). Under normal conditions the pressure within the glomerulus is sufficiently high to force fluid out of the capillaries into the collecting chamber. When the systolic pressure falls below 70 mm Hg, glomerular filtration ceases and the body is unable to rid itself of fluid and nitrogenous wastes.

The tubules, which are perfused by the peritubular capillaries, suffer from the lack of oxygen and nutrients.

Acute tubular necrosis develops. The tubular epithelial cells slough and block the tubules, causing loss of function of the nephron.

The kidneys often are affected in the early stage of shock, even before systolic blood pressure falls, because the renal vessels respond to sympathetic stimulation and constrict. A decrease in urinary output is often an early sign of shock.

■ Brain

The brain is not affected early in shock. Because it does not contain alpha-adrenergic receptors, its vessels do not constrict in response to the increased levels of epinephrine and norepinephrine, and blood is shunted to the brain (and heart) at the expense of the other organs. As shock progresses and compensatory mechanisms fail, the brain does suffer inadequate perfusion. As *cerebral hypoxia* occurs, restlessness and anxiety, followed by lethargy and coma may be seen. Cerebral function may also be altered by the increasing acidosis and the accumulation of toxic substances.

■ Heart

Although deterioration of cardiac function is a primary problem only in cardiogenic shock, the heart eventually is affected in all types of shock. As cited earlier, in the early stage of shock the heart is spared. As shock increases, the pumping ability of the heart is affected and cardiac output decreases (p. 146). As the heart muscle becomes increasingly hypoxic, it begins to show disturbances of electrical activity. Most *dysrhythmias* have a detrimental affect on cardiac output, and some may be fatal. In the later stages of shock, deterioration of myocardial function is probably the most important factor in the further progression of shock.[20]

■ Lungs

The effect of shock on the lungs has only been more recently determined. During the Vietnam War, many victims of traumatic shock survived the early complications because of the use of massive blood transfusions and renal dialysis. The effect of shock on the lungs surfaced as a later complication. The pulmonary condition that results from hypoperfusion of the lungs has been known by a number of names, including shock-lung, white lung, and Da Nang lung. It is now known as adult respiratory distress syndrome (ARDS) (Chapter 24).

ARDS can result from any condition that causes hypoperfusion of the lungs, but is seen most commonly with traumatic or septic shock.[29] It is characterized by increased permeability of the pulmonary capillaries to proteins and water, resulting in noncardiac pulmonary edema. Type 2 pneumocytes are destroyed, impairing the production of surfactant that normally prevents collapse of the alveoli. Alveoli either become filled with fluid or collapse, and lungs become stiff.

In the early stages, *hypoxemia* results from impaired gas

exchange and *hyperventilation* occurs, resulting in *hypocapnea* and *respiratory alkalosis*. Platelet aggregation in the pulmonary capillaries further damages the lungs. Hypoxemia persists despite administration of increasing amounts of oxygen. As shock progresses, ventilation is impaired and carbon dioxide is retained. *Respiratory acidosis* results. As hypoxemia increases, platelet aggregation increases, and a destructive cycle is initiated.

Gastrointestinal tract

Sympathetic stimulation, which occurs early in shock, causes vasoconstriction and thus decreased blood supply to the organs of the gastrointestinal tract. Bowel function decreases, and *paralytic ileus* may result. If the blood supply is severely impaired for a length of time, necrosis of the intestinal mucosa may occur. Microorganisms normally found in the bowel lyse and release *endotoxins* when they are attacked by the leukocytes in the blood. Shock, from whatever cause, will now also have a septic component. The gastric mucosa commonly ulcerates when it becomes ischemic, which may result in occult bleeding or massive hemorrhage.

Liver

Sympathetic stimulation causes vasoconstriction in the liver. In the early stages of shock this can be beneficial. Normally the liver is capable of storing large amounts of blood in its veins. With vasoconstriction it can release up to 350 ml blood into the general circulation, resulting in improved cardiac output. With continued sympathetic stimulation and decreased blood flow, liver tissue is affected. In *septic shock* there is an increase in oxygen uptake and a decrease in energy production in the liver. All types of shock affect the metabolic functions of the liver including the excretion of bile and cholesterol, gluconeogenesis, detoxification, and protein synthesis.[26]

Table 9-1 Comparison of signs and symptoms in early and late shock by body system

Body system	Early shock	Late shock
Respiratory system	Hyperventilation; ↑ minute volume; ↓ Pco_2; normal Po_2	Respirations shallow; breath sounds may suggest congestion; ↑ Pco_2; ↓ Po_2
Cardiovascular system	Blood pressure normal to slightly lowered; ↑ diastolic pressure; ↓ pulse pressure; cardiac output normal; tachycardia; mild vasonconstriction in hypovolemic and cardiogenic shock	↓ Blood pressure; ↓ cardiac output; tachycardia continues; vasoconstriction worsens in hypovolemic, cardiogenic, and septic shock
Renal system	Normal to slightly depressed urine output; ↑ urine osmolality; ↓ urine sodium concentration	Oliguria or complete renal shutdown; buildup of waste products
	Hypokalemia	Hyperglycemia
Acid-base balance	Respiratory alkalosis	Metabolic acidosis; respiratory acidosis
Vascular compartment	Fluids shift from interstitial space to vascular compartment; thirst	Fluids shift from vascular space to interstitial and intracellular space, causing edema
Skin	Minimal to no changes in hypovolemic and cardiogenic shock; warm, flushed skin in vasogenic shock	Cool, clammy skin in hypovolemic, cardiogenic, and septic shock; cool and mottled skin in other types of shock
Hematologic system	Release of red blood cells from bone marrow to increase vascular volume; platelet aggretation	Disseminated intravascular coagulation
Mental-neurologic system	Restless; alert; confused	Lethargic; unconsciousness
Gastrointestinal-hepatic system	No obvious changes	Perfusion decreases and bowel sounds may be diminished
		MDF production by hypoxic pancreas
		Liver dysfunction
		Possible bowel necrosis

The sinusoids of the liver are lined with Kupffer cells, which are part of the reticuloendothelial system (RES). These cells are very powerful phagocytes and destroy the many bacteria from the colon that reach the liver by way of the portal system. Normally, very few bacteria get past the RES. With the destruction of the RES, bacteria enter the general circulation and produce toxins, which under normal circumstances would be detoxified by the liver. The liver can no longer perform this function, and overwhelming infection and toxicity result.

■ Blood

Disseminated intravascular coagulation (DIC) (Chapter 27) can be a cause or a result of shock. It is characterized by intravascular clotting, resulting in the formation of microthrombi in the capillaries. Some of the factors that activate clotting factors in the blood are acidosis, stagnation, and procoagulant substances such as bacterial toxins [23] Acidosis and stagnation of blood are present in all types of shock, and bacterial toxins are found in septic shock. As clotting occurs in the capillaries, clotting factors in the rest of the body become depleted. Hemorrhage may then occur from incisions, punctures, the gastrointestinal tract, and other sites. A vicious cycle ensues. Intravascular clotting results in even further decrease in tissue perfusion and acidosis. The hemorrhage caused by DIC decreases the cardiac output even further and worsens tissue perfusion. The mortality in patients with DIC in association with infection and shock is 50% to 60%.[18]

▦ ASSESSMENT

The signs and symptoms of shock are summarized in Table 9-1. There are few observable signs in the early stage; the patient may be restless and the pulse and respiratory rates may be increased. Cool, clammy skin, decreased blood pressure, and lethargy or unconsciousness are signs of the later stage. The status of patients in shock is monitored by various methods. The parameters used in assessing shock appear in the box below.

■ Hemodynamic monitoring

Hemodynamic alterations are often the first sign of the onset of shock. The patient's hemodynamic status can be assessed at various levels (Fig. 9-2).

■ VITAL SIGNS

Vital signs are assessed frequently. In the early stages of shock the pulse is usually increased. As shock progresses, the pulse becomes quite rapid and difficult to palpate. Irregularities in the pulse may develop as cardiac dysrhythmias occur.

Early in shock the blood pressure may be normal or even elevated because of compensatory vasoconstriction. Blood pressure can be heard without difficulty at this stage. As shock progresses, the blood pressure may be difficult to auscultate, but it may be possible to obtain the systolic pressure by palpation. If intraarterial pressure monitoring

---

Parameters for assessing status of patient in shock

Hemodynamic monitoring

Blood pressure (cuff and/or intraarterial)
Pulse
Central venous pressure
Pulmonary artery pressure
Pulmonary wedge pressure
Cardiac output
Electrocardiogram

Respiratory monitoring

Respiratory rate, depth
Breath sounds
Blood gases
 pH
 P_{O_2}
 P_{CO_2}
Percent O_2 saturation

Fluid and electrolyte monitoring

Serum electrolytes
Blood lactate and pyruvate levels
Intake
 By mouth
 Intravenous
 Nasogastric
 Irrigation solutions
 Solution in medications
Output
 Urinary
 Gastrointestinal tract
 Sweating
 Dressings
Weight
Serum creatinine level
Blood urea nitrogen level
Serum and urinary osmolality
Urinary specific gravity

Neurologic monitoring

Alertness
Orientation
Confusion

Hematologic monitoring

Erythrocytes
Hematocrit and hemoglobin levels
Leukocytes
Platelets
Prothrombin and partial thromboplastin times
Clotting time
Fibrin degradation products

Other monitoring

Bowel sounds
Skin temperature

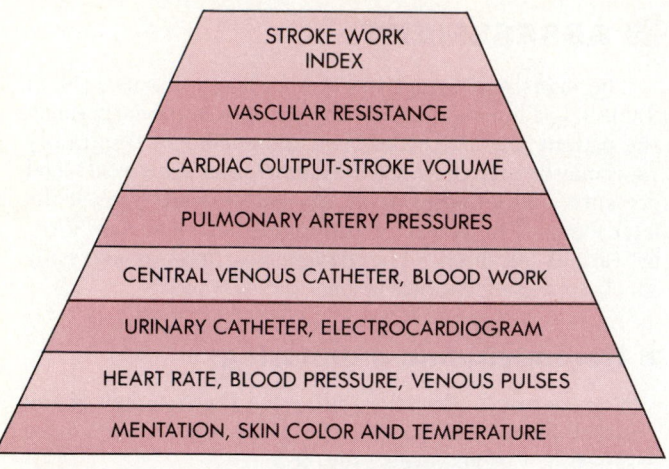

Fig. 9-2 Levels of hemodynamic monitoring. (From Ellerbe, S: Fluid and blood component therapy in the critically ill and injured, New York, 1981, Churchill Livingstone, p. 35)

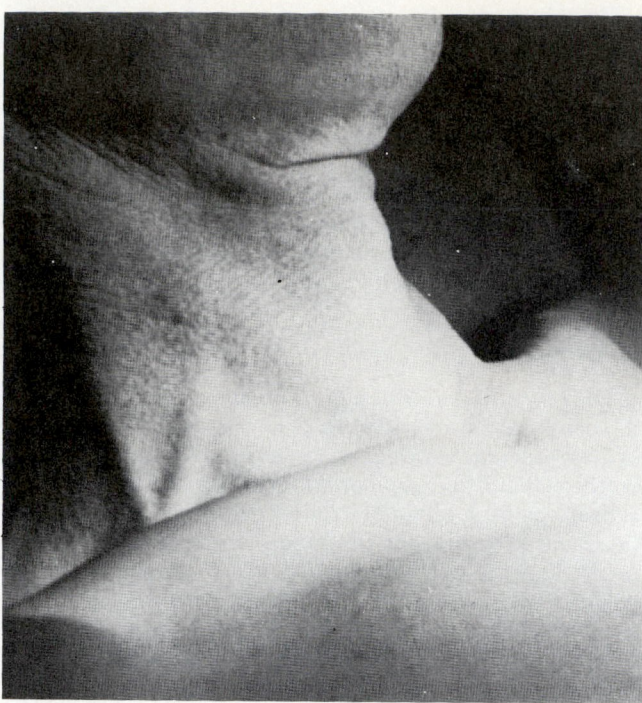

Fig. 9-3 Distended external jugular neck vein of a patient with right-sided heart failure. (From Daily, EK, and Schroeder, J: Techniques in bedside hemodynamic monitoring, ed 2, St Louis, 1981, The CV Mosby Co)

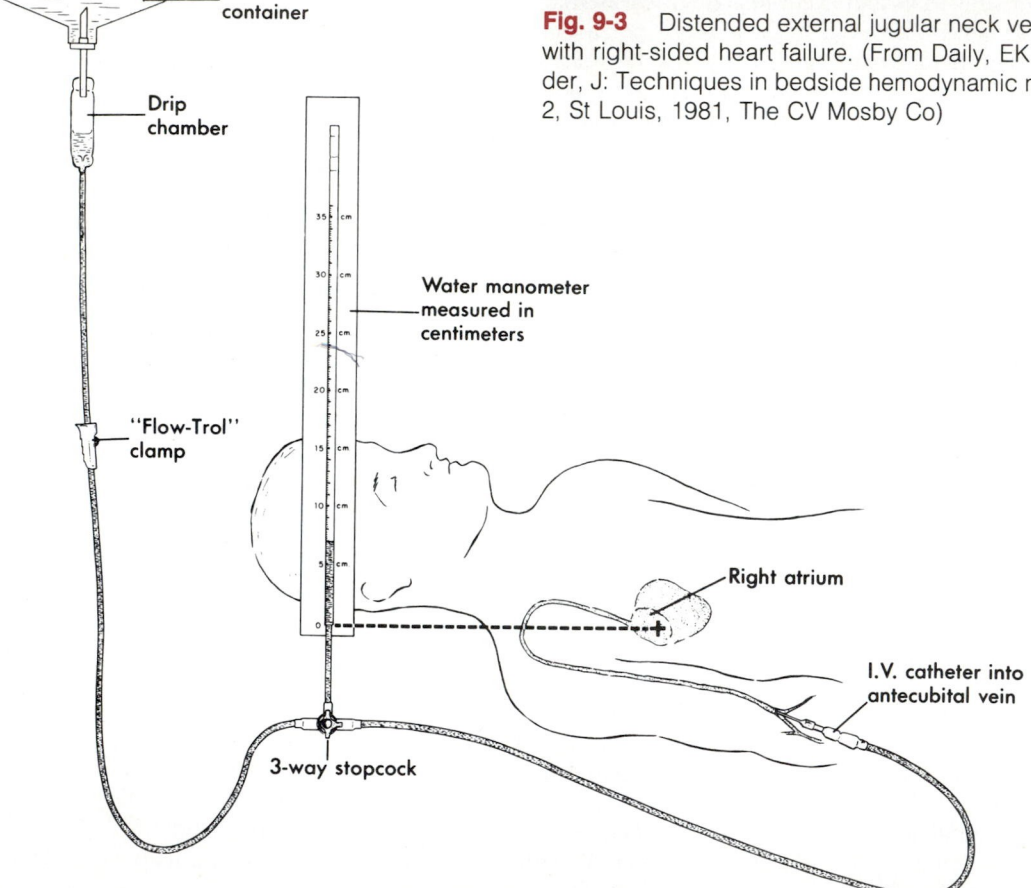

Fig. 9-4 Measurement of central venous pressure (CVP) using water manometer. Zero point on manometer is at level of midright atrium, and CVP reading is 7 cm of water.

is not instituted, Doppler ultrasound (Chapter 26) may be helpful in obtaining the blood pressure.

Venous pulsation in the neck is noted. Both the external and internal jugular veins should be examined. Generally, the external jugular vein is easier to see, but in some patients with heart disease the external jugular veins are occluded by fibrosis or are absent.[43] Normally, *venous pulsations* are visible when the patient is lying flat but not when the head is elevated to 45 degrees (Fig. 9-3). Flat neck veins, when the patient is in a horizontal position, often indicate *hypovolemia,* common in most types of shock.

■ CENTRAL VENOUS PRESSURE

Central venous pressure (CVP) is a more accurate means of determining the fluid status of a patient in shock. CVP measures right ventricular filling pressure, which reflects venous return to the heart. CVP monitoring is most valuable in assessing status in patients with absolute or relative hypovolemia, including those with vasogenic, neurogenic, and hypovolemic shock. It is less valuable in assessment in patients with cardiogenic shock, who may have intravascular fluid excess.

To obtain an accurate CVP reading, a catheter is inserted into a major vein and threaded through the superior vena cava into the right atrium. The catheter is attached by a three-way stopcock to an intravenous infusion and a water manometer (Fig. 9-4). The intravenous solution (usually 5% glucose in water) is allowed to drip slowly into the vein to keep the vein open. When a reading is to be taken, the stopcock is opened to the manometer and the manometer is filled with the intravenous solution. The stopcock is then turned to the venous opening (the patient). The fluid level in the manometer should fluctuate with each respiration. The fluid is allowed to stabilize before a reading is taken, and the highest level of the fluid fluctuating in the column is used for the CVP reading. As soon as the reading is taken, the stopcock is turned to the solution position, and the infusion is continued.

For the CVP reading to be accurate, the patient must be relaxed, and the zero point of the manometer must always be at the level of the right atrium, which in most people is level with the midaxillary line. If the patient cannot be flat in bed, the zero point on the manometer is adjusted to the level of the right atrium in a sitting position. Any change in the patient's position requires that the zero point be reset. The initial CVP reading and the position that the patient was in when it was taken should be recorded, because these will serve as a baseline for comparison with subsequent readings. The patient should be placed in the same position for each reading, since even a slight change in position alters the CVP.

The normal values for CVP will vary with the use of different equipment; however, a range of 5 cm to 15 cm water is acceptable. It is important to note that a change or a trend in the CVP is more important than the actual numeric value.

Central venous catheters can also be used to obtain blood

samples, to assess venous oxygen saturation determinations, and to administer fluids. The catheter insertion site should be kept scrupulously clean to minimize the possibility of phlebitis. Patient movement is not restricted as long as the catheter and tubing are secured adequately and intravenous flow is maintained.

■ PULMONARY ARTERY PRESSURES

The status of the left side of the heart can best be evaluated by the measurement of *pulmonary artery pressure* (PAP) and *pulmonary capillary wedge resection* (PCWP). A mean PAP of less than 10 mm Hg may indicate decreased blood volume resulting in decrease preload in the left ventricle. A mean PAP of more than 20 mm Hg may indicate poor myocardial contractility and left ventricular overload. These pressures are measured with a special triple-lumen balloon tipped (Swan-Ganz) catheter (Fig. 9-5). The catheter is inserted into a vein, usually the *subclavian,* and advanced to the *right atrium.* The balloon is inflated and carried to the right ventricle and then to the pulmonary artery by the blood flow. The balloon is then deflated and the tip of the catheter is left in the *pulmonary artery.* The opening at the tip of the catheter communicates with the distal port. The lumen from the proximal port opens into the right atrium. The distal port is connected to a transducer, which converts the pressure it senses through the catheter to an electrical signal, which is then displayed on a monitor. Thus the pressure in the pulmonary artery can be measured continuously. A continuous flush system is used to maintain patency of the distal lumen. Intravenous fluid is infused through the proximal port. The proximal port can also be used for the administration of medications.

In individuals without lung or pulmonary vascular disease, PAP is a good indicator of how well the left side of the heart is functioning. Pressure changes in the left ventricle are reflected in the left atrium and back to the pul-

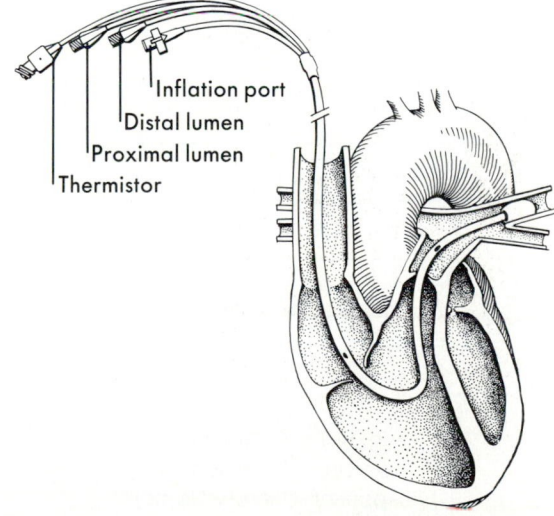

Fig. 9-5 Placement of Swan-Ganz catheter.

Table 9-2 Complications of pulmonary artery pressure monitoring

Complication	Indications	Interventions
Infection	Chills Headache Malaise Generalized aching Flushed face Warm skin Elevated temperature	1. Notify physician immediately. 2. Prepare for removal of catheter. 3. Administer antibiotics as ordered. 4. Provide symptomatic relief.
Ventricular arrhythmias: premature ventricular contractions, or short runs of ventricular tachycardia	"Skipped heart beats" Irregular pulse PVC's noted on cardiac monitor	1. Notify physician immediately. 2. Prepare for repositioning of catheter. 3. Administer antiarrhythmic drugs if problem persists after repositioning.
Sustained ventricular tachycardia, or ventricular fibrillation	Lightheadedness, progressing to loss of consciousness Loss of consciousness Pulselessness Arrhythmia noted on cardiac monitor Respiratory arrest	1. Notify physician immediately. 2. Prepare for repositioning of catheter. 3. Defibrillate.
Pulmonary infarction	Chest pain Hemoptysis Fever Friction rub Elevated LDH Area of opacity on chest x-ray film Decreased paO_2	1. Notify physician immediately. 2. Administer oxygen. 3. Prepare for repositioning or removal of catheter. 4. Provide symptomatic relief.
Valvular damage	Depends on extent of damage Patient may be asymptomatic, or may develop symptoms of congestive heart failure or new murmur	1. Notify physician of development of new murmur or new symptoms.

Modified from Asheervath, J, and Belvins, D: Handbook of clinical nursing practice, Norwalk, Conn, 1986, Appleton-Century-Crofts.

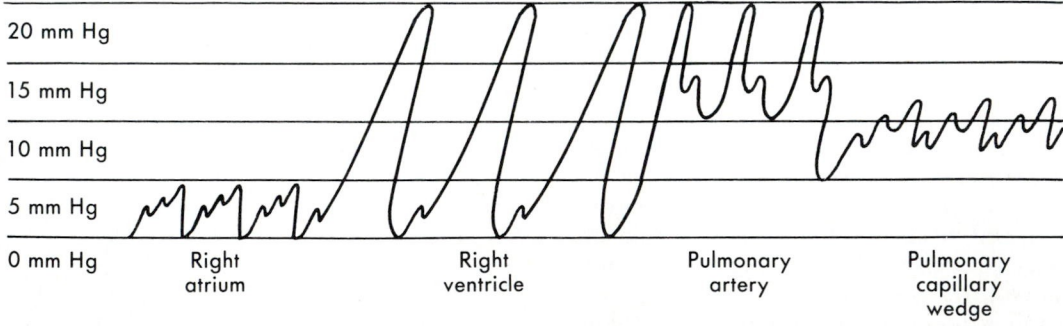

Fig. 9-6 Characteristic waveforms of pulmonary artery pressure monitoring. (From Asheervath, J, and Blevins, D: Handbook of clinical nursing practice, 1986, Norwalk, CT, Appleton-Century-Crofts)

monary artery. If there is any disease in the lungs, however, as frequently occurs in shock, the PAP does not accurately reflect left ventricular pressure. In this case, the PCWP should be obtained. By inflating the balloon, which is near the tip of the catheter, the pulmonary artery can be occluded. This blocks communication between the pressure in the pulmonary artery and the lumen of the catheter, allowing for pressure that is ahead of the occluded artery to be transmitted through the catheter. The PCWP is identical to the left atrial pressure.

The nurse caring for the patient with pulmonary artery pressure monitoring must be aware of the common complications that can occur with this type of invasive monitoring (Table 9-2). The appearance of either a *right ventricular* or *PCWP waveform* on the monitor can have serious consequences for the patient. Dislodgement of the tip of the catheter from the pulmonary artery into the right ventricle can result in the occurrence of *premature ventricular beats* or even *ventricular tachycardia*. Progression of the catheter into a small vessel in the pulmonary vasculature can occlude the vessel and result in *pulmonary infarction*. Prolonged inflation of the balloon can have the same effect. The nurse must be able to distinguish the normal PAP waveform from both right ventricular and PCWP waveforms (Fig. 9-6). It is essential that sterile technique be maintained during the insertion of the PAP catheter and during dressing changes.

■ INTRAARTERIAL MONITORING

Intraarterial monitoring is usually instituted along with pulmonary artery pressure monitoring. A catheter is inserted into a radial, brachial, or femoral artery and attached to a transducer in much the same way as the pulmonary artery catheter (Fig. 9-7). Because this is a high-pressure system, hemorrhage is a possible complication, and the insertion and connections in the system must be monitored frequently. The extremity distal to the insertion site must be monitored for signs of arterial occlusion (color, temperature, movement, presence or absence of pulses, and pain) (Table 9-3). It is essential that sterile technique be maintained during insertion of the catheter and during dressing changes. A patient who is ill enough to require hemodynamic monitoring has little reserve to fight infection.

■ CARDIAC OUTPUT AND CARDIAC INDEX MONITORING

Some pulmonary artery catheters allow for cardiac output and cardiac index to be monitored at the bedside. Such catheters have a port through which fluid can be injected into the right atrium. A *thermistor* is located at the tip of the catheter and attached to a wire that runs through the catheter and is attached to a *cardiac output computer*. Iced saline solution is injected into the right atrium. The solution travels with the blood into the pulmonary artery. The thermistor senses the extent of temperature change, and from this data the computer is able to calculate cardiac output. The normal cardiac index is 2.5 to 3.5 L/min/m².

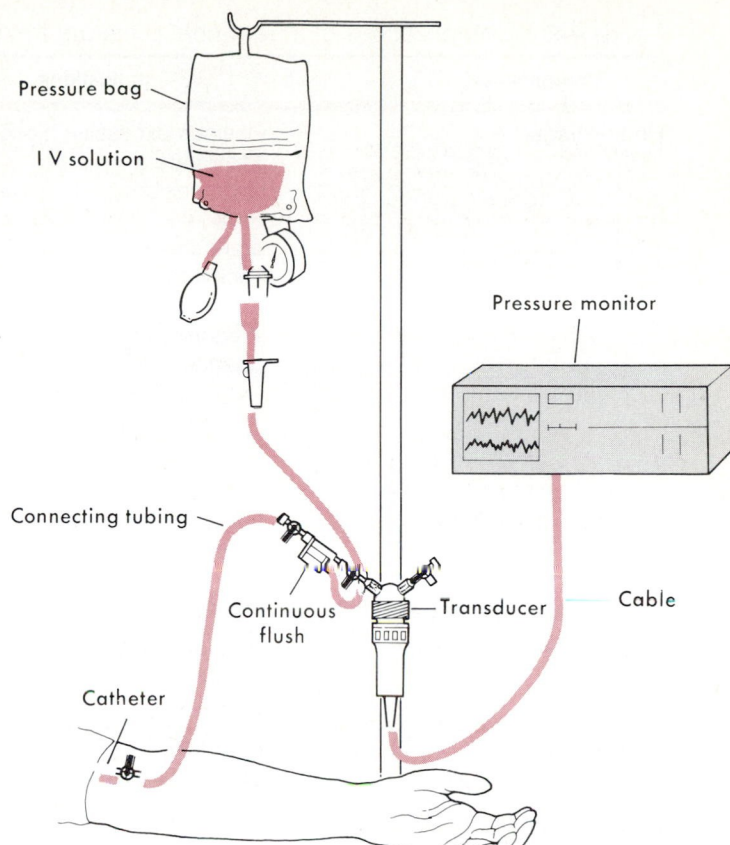

Fig. 9-7 Connections between intraarterial catheter, transducer, monitor, and fluid. (From Daily, EK, and Schroeder, J: Techniques in bedside hemodynamic monitoring, ed 3, St Louis, 1985, The CV Mosby Co)

■ Respiratory monitoring

As cited earlier (p. 147), hypoperfusion of the lungs, common in shock, may result in adult respiratory distress syndrome (ARDS). This may be suspected very early in the course of the disease from changes in the patient's mentation. There may be minor changes in orientation, unusual interpersonal exchanges, and mood changes.[7] The patient is observed for *cough* and *dyspnea*, which develop as ARDS progresses. Changes in respiratory rate and in the color of the mucous membranes and skin are important indicators of pulmonary status. Breath sounds are auscultated. Early in the course of the disease the lungs may be clear, but as ARDS progresses, rales and rhonchi may be heard.

If the patient is receiving *mechanical ventilation*, the amount of pressure required to deliver a specific tidal volume is noted. As the lungs become increasingly stiff, the pressure required to deliver the volume increases. With ARDS, the pulmonary artery pressure may rise, although the pulmonary capillary wedge pressure remains normal.[21]

Arterial blood gases may provide valuable information and are monitored as indicated depending on the patient's condition. Characteristically with ARDS, the PaO_2 falls,

Table 9-3 Complications of intraarterial pressure monitoring

Complication	Indications	Intervention

Hemorrhage	Obvious excessive bleeding
	Tachycardia
	Hypotension
	Pallor
	Diaphoresis
	Tachypnea
	Restlessness
	Dizziness
	Headache
		1. Control bleeding
		  a. If bleeding is occurring at the puncture site, apply pressure.
		  b. If part of the system has become disconnected, turn the stopcocks to stop bleeding immediately.
		2. Attach a syringe containing sterile saline until contaminated parts of the system are replaced with sterile parts.
		3. Notify the physician if a large amount of blood has been lost.
		4. Prepare the patient for blood replacement if loss has been large.

Thrombus or embolus	Pallor, loss of pulse, and coolness distal to the site of the thrombus Pain	1. Notify the physician immediately. 2. Instruct patient to lie quietly.
Infection of catheter site	Redness and warmth at the site Possible fever	1. Notify the physician. 2. Prepare for removal of the catheter. 3. Send the catheter tip for culture.
Bacteremia	High fever Chills	1. Notify the physician. 2. Prepare for removal of the catheter.

Modified from Asheervath, J, and Blevins, D: Handbook of clinical nursing practice, Norwalk, Conn, 1986, Appleton-Century-Crofts.

in spite of ventilation with increasing amounts of oxygen, because of *physiologic shunting* of blood through the lungs to the left side of the heart. Shunting occurs because many alveoli are either collapsed or filled with fluid, and diffusion cannot occur. In the earlier stages of ARDS, when a sufficient number of alveoli are functioning, the $PaCO_2$ is usually normal or more likely low because of the rapid diffusion of CO_2 and of hyperventilation that results from hypoxia. However, as the number of functioning alveoli decreases, the $PaCO_2$ increases.

Arterial blood gas determinations are also used to assess the *acid-base balance* of the patient in shock. In the early stages of shock, mild *respiratory alkalosis* is common from *hyperventilation* that is part of the stress response. As shock progresses and tissues become progressively hypoxemic, anaerobic metabolism takes place and metabolic acidosis occurs. In the advanced stages of shock, when respirations decrease and ARDS becomes progressively worse, respiratory acidosis may also develop.

■ Fluid and electrolyte monitoring

The urinary output and the CVP most accurately reflect fluid status. An indwelling urinary catheter is usually inserted, and the urine output is measured hourly. Other output, such as gastrointestinal drainage, wound drainage, or perspiration, is measured or estimated as accurately as possible. *Body weight* often gives a more accurate assessment of fluid changes than the measurement of intake and output; however, this can be an inaccurate determinant of intravascular volume when "third spacing" of fluid occurs. Noting the presence of *edema*, auscultating the chest for the presence of fluid, and measuring the abdominal girth for the development of *ascites* are means of assessing fluid collection in the third spaces.

In the early stages of shock, the serum potassium concentration may be abnormally low as a result of increased levels of aldosterone in response to stress. However, as shock progresses, the serum K^+ level may become abnormally high as damaged cells release K^+. As urinary output falls, the body is unable to eliminate the excess amounts of K^+ that are accumulating in the serum. If K^+ is administered in the early stage of shock, it is extremely important that the urinary output and serum electrolytes be monitored frequently.

The concentration of other serum electrolytes may be abnormal as a result of acid-base abnormalities, altered renal function, or fluid therapy. Serum enzymes may be elevated because of ischemia and damage to the heart, liver, and pancreas.

■ Neurologic monitoring

In shock, the brain may be adversely affected by *hypoxia, acid-base imbalance,* or *toxins.* Often, subtle changes in mentation are the earliest signs of cerebral hypoxia. The patient is observed for *increasing restlessness*. Sedation should not be given until the patient's status has been assessed further and it has been determined that the restlessness does not have an organic cause. In the late stages, when perfusion of the brain is severely impaired, *loss of consciousness* occurs. Vital signs and arterial blood gas determinations can aid in assessing the cause of subtle neurologic changes.

■ Hematologic monitoring

The *hemoglobin* and *hematocrit* levels are valuable tools for assessing blood loss in hypovolemic shock secondary to hemorrhage. It must be remembered, however, that the hemoglobin and hematocrit levels do not drop immediately with loss of an excessive amount of blood, because plasma is lost along with the blood cells. The blood that remains in the intravascular compartment initially will have a normal concentration of RBCs. Because the kidneys retain water in response to blood loss, the blood becomes more dilute and there is a decrease in the hemoglobin and hematocrit concentrations.

Patients in shock are assessed for the development of DIC. The nurse may be the first to observe that the patient is bleeding for an excessively long time after a venipuncture or that blood is oozing from an incision. If DIC is suspected, laboratory studies are initiated; then clotting factors (including fibrinogen and platelet counts) are decreased, prothrombin time and partial thromboplastin time (aPTT) are prolonged, and fibrin degradation products are increased.

■ Other monitoring

Abdominal assessment is important in the patient in shock. Decreased blood flow to the intestines may result in decreased peristalsis or paralytic ileus (Chapter 31). Decreased or absent bowel sounds are noted. Gastric drainage and stools are assessed for occult blood because of the high incidence of gastrointestinal tract bleeding with shock.

➡ DATA ANALYSIS: NURSING DIAGNOSES

Although there will be some variation according to the individual patient's symptoms and stage of shock, the following nursing diagnoses are appropriate in most patients in shock:

Diagnostic title	Possible etiologies
Activity intolerance	Imbalance between oxygen supply and demand
Ineffective airway clearance	Decreased energy and endotracheal intubation
Anxiety	Threat of death
Ineffective breathing pattern	Inadequate perfusion of respiratory muscles

Diagnostic title	Possible etiologies
Decreased cardiac output	Myocardial hypoxia and myocardial depressant factor
Impaired verbal communication	Endotracheal intubation
Fluid volume deficit (1)	Blood loss, increased capillary permeability, or vasodilation
Impaired gas exchange	Decreased lung compliance, interstitial edema
Potential for infection	Invasive monitoring, Foley catheter, decreased immune response
Altered oral mucous membrane	Endotracheal intubation
Sleep pattern disturbance	Intensity of nursing care
Alterd cardiopulmonary tissue perfusion	Hypovolemia, decreased cardiac output, and redistribution of blood

◱ PLANNING: EXPECTED PATIENT OUTCOMES

Expected patient outcomes for the person with shock may include, but are not limited to, the following:

1. Patient will be able to tolerate activity involved in care without significant decrease in pulse rate.
2. Patient's airway will remain free from secretions.
3. Patient and significant others will remain free of avoidable anxiety.
4. Respiratory rate and tidal volume will be within normal limits.
5. Cardiac output will be within normal limits.
6. Patient will make needs understood by verbal or alternate means of communication.
7. Intravascular volume will return to normal.
8. Blood gasses will be within normal limits.
9. Patient will be free from infection.
10. Oral mucous membrane will remain moist and intact.
11. Patient will have undisturbed periods of sleep.
12. Patient will have normal tissue perfusion.
13. Patient will remain free of injury.

▦ IMPLEMENTATION

■ Assisting with achievement of therapeutic goals

Treatment of shock will vary to some extent, depending on the cause. The cause of the shock must be treated first. Blood must be given if the patient has hemorrhage; antibiotics are given if an infection is present; and epinephrine is given if anaphylaxis has occurred. All types of shock have enough in common, however, that there are some common forms of treatment. In most types of shock, fluid replacement is the first therapeutic measure to be instituted, followed by administration of vasoactive drugs.

■ Assisting with fluid replacement

The need to administer fluids to the patient with hypovolemic shock is obvious. At times, fluid replacement is the only therapy needed in this type of shock. Vasogenic and septic shock are accompanied by hypovolemia because fluid is leaking out of the capillaries. Fluids are always part of the treatment. What is less obvious is that patients with cardiogenic shock *may* also require fluid therapy, although many may require fluid *restriction* or removal of fluid. Before fluid therapy is instituted for cardiogenic shock, a pulmonary artery catheter is inserted and the pulmonary end diastolic pressure measured. If the pressure is less than 20 mm Hg, fluid therapy may be beneficial.[3]

Various fluids may be given to the patient in shock. It is generally agreed that the patient who has sustained a large blood loss will require blood replacement. There is a great deal of disagreement concerning what other types of fluids should be used to treat shock. There are both advantages and disadvantages to all types of resuscitative fluids, including blood.

■ ADMINISTRATION OF WHOLE BLOOD

The administration of whole blood has the obvious advantage of increasing the oxygen-carrying capacity of the blood. It also has many disadvantages (transmission of dis-

Table 9-4 Fluids used for replacement therapy in shock

Type	Uses/indications	Advantages	Disadvantages	Special considerations
Blood and blood products				
Whole blood	Replace blood volume and maintain hemoglobin (Hgb) at 12-14 g/100 ml	Provides intravascular volume Increases oxygen-carrying capacity of the blood	Potential associated risks of hepatitis and allergic reactions Delayed administration because of necessary typing and cross-matching Possibility of type and crossmatch errors	Whole blood should be stored at 0°-10° C (32°-50° F), but warmed at least 20-30 min before administration (never infuse cold blood) Use *fresh* whole blood whenever possible to avoid adverse metabolic changes related to stored blood
RBCs (packed, concentrate) Fresh, frozen (also called leukocyte-poor)	Increase hematocrit to a minimum level of 30% Correct RBC deficiency and improve the oxygen-carrying capacity of the blood	Concentrated form helps to prevent excess fluid administration in patients with cardiogenic shock (increases oxygen-carrying capacity with less volume loading) Associated with fewer risks of metabolic complications when compared to stored whole blood (decreased amount of transfused antibodies, electrolytes, etc.) Provides economic use of blood as a resource; frees other blood components such as platelets and clotting factors to be concentrated and stored	Slow infusion rate because of increased viscosity Decreased content of plasma proteins and coagulation factors when compared to whole blood Inadequate (alone) for volume replacement and correction of hypovolemia Altered blood clotting with administration of more than 20 units; for every 4 units of RBCs over 20, 1 unit of fresh frozen plasma should be administered to replenish clotting factors High cost of frozen (thawed) RBCs	Administer via Y-connector tubing with normal saline to increase infusion flow rate Washed RBCs (resuspended in saline) can be given in shock to decrease red cell adhesiveness (washing decreases the cell's fibrinogen coating)

Table 9-4 Fluids used for replacement therapy in shock—cont'd

Type	Uses/indications	Advantages	Disadvantages	Special considerations
Blood and blood products—cont'd				
Human plasma (fresh, frozen, or dried)	Restore plasma volume in hypovolemic shock without increasing the hematocrit Restore clotting factors (except platelets)	Effective for rapid volume replacement Contains clotting factors	Expensive Deficient in RBCs	Human plasma carries the risk of viral hepatitis and allergic reactions Administer fresh frozen plasma promptly after thawing to prevent deterioration of clotting factors V and VIII
Colloid solutions				
Plasma protein fraction (e.g., plasmanate, plasmaplex)	Expand plasma volume in hypovolemic shock (while cross-matching is being completed) Increase the serum colloid osmotic pressure	Can be used interchangeably with 5% human serum albumin Osmotically equivalent to plasma Associated with low risk of hepatitis	Expensive Deficient in clotting factors Associated with larger number of side effects such as hypotension, and hypersensitivity than those reported with 5% albumin (because of presence of globulins) Hypotension induced by rapid intravenous administration (greater than 10 ml/min)	Plasma protein fraction is prepared from pooled plasma heated to 60° C (140° F) for 10 hr This procedure reduces the risk of transmission of hepatitis viruses Rapid administration of large dosages can alter blood coagulation This solution should be used cautiously in patients with congestive heart failure (caused by added fluid and rapid plasma volume expansion) and in patients with renal failure (caused by added proteins)
Albumin 5% 25% (salt-poor)	Increase the plasma colloid osmotic pressure Rapidly expand the plasma volume	Rare allergic reactions (less than 0.01% in all albumin solutions combined) Rare transmission of hepatitis virus	Potential leakage from capillaries in shock states associated with increased capillary permeability Possible precipitation of congestive heart failure following rapid infusion in patients with circulatory overload and compromised cardiovascular function	Albumin does not contain preservatives; therefore each opened bottle should be used at once Rate of administration of 5% albumin should not exceed 2-4 ml/min 25% albumin is reserved for use in patients with pulmonary or peripheral edema and hypoproteinemia Administer with a diuretic to ensure diuresis

Continued.

Table 9-4 Fluids used for replacement therapy in shock—cont'd

Type	Uses/indications	Advantages	Disadvantages	Special considerations
Plasma expanders				
Dextran Low-molecular-weight dextran (LMWD) (Dextran 40) (Reomacrodex) (Gentran 40) High-molecular-weight dextran (HMWD) (Dextran 70) (Gentran 70-75) (Macrodex)	Rapidly expand plasma volume	All dextrans: associated with low incidence of anaphylactic reactions; less expensive than protein solutions LMWD: associated with fewer allergic reactions than HMWD; facilitates blood flow by decreasing RBC adhesiveness HMWD: leaks from the capillaries less readily than LMWD; can effectively increase plasma volume for up to 24 hr	LMWD: 70% excreted unchanged in urine, so urine osmolality and specific gravity are altered; potential osmotic-nephorisis and renal tubular shutdown; possible bleeding from raw surfaces caused by decreased platelet adhesiveness; side effects include decreased hemoglobin, hematocrit, fibrinogen, and clotting factors V, VIII, and IX HMWD: 50% excreted unchanged in the urine, so the urine osmolality and specific gravity are altered; higher incidence of allergic reactions when compared to LMWD; increases blood viscosity and platelet adhesiveness	Avoid use of dextran in patients with active hemorrhage, hemorrhagic shock, coagulation disorders, and thrombocytopenia Bleeding times can be prolonged when the correct dose of dextran 70 (1.2 g/kg/day) or dextran 40 (2 g/kg/day) are exceeded Administer dextran in dextrose solutions to patients with sodium restriction
Hetastarch (Hespan) (Volex)	Expand plasma volume	Same volume expansion characteristics of albumin but with a longer duration of action (up to 36 hr) Associated with low risk of allergic and anaphylactic reactions (0.085%) Cost of hetastarch is about one half that of plasma protein fraction and albumin Nonantigenic No danger of transmission of hepatitis virus	Potential dilution of plasma proteins and decreased plasma colloid osmotic pressure Potential dilution of clotting factors with resultant coagulation changes Potential circulatory overload in patients with severe congestive heart failure and compromised renal function Increased serum amylase level (>200 mg/100 ml), peaking within 1 hour of intravenous administration of hetastarch and persisting for 3 to 4 days (caused by action of amylase in hetastarch degradation)	Do not use if the solution is cloudy or deep brown or if it contains crystals Monitor clotting studies and platelet counts, observing for prolonged prothrombin and partial thromboplastin times and thrombocytopenia Safety and compatibility of additives with hetastarch have not been established; the manufacturer recommends infusing hetastarch through a separate line, when possible, or piggybacking the second drug Maximum infusion rate in acute hemorrhagic shock is 20 ml/kg/hr Monitor serum albumin; if it falls below 2 g/100 ml, consider substituting albumin for hetastarch

Table 9-4 Fluids used for replacement therapy in shock—cont'd

Type	Uses/indications	Advantages	Disadvantages	Special considerations
Plasma expanders—cont'd				
Mannitol (Osmitrol)	Raise intravascular volume Reduce interstitial and intracellular edema Promote osmotic diuresis	Reduces intracellular swelling Increases urinary output	Potential circulatory overload in patients with congestive heart failure, pulmonary congestion, and renal dysfunction	
Crystalloid solutions (isotonic)				
Normal saline	Raise plasma volume when RBC mass is adequate Replace body fluid	Considered by some to be the single most important salt for maintaining and replacing ECF Increases plasma volume without altering normal sodium concentration or serum osmolality	Potential fluid retention and circulatory overload caused by sodium content	
Lactated Ringer's solution (Hartman's solution)	Replace body fluid Buffer acidosis	Lactate is converted to bicarbonate (in the liver), which buffers acidosis Lactate replaces bicarbonate, preventing precipitation of calcium bicarbonate and calcium carbonate Lactate is more stable than bicarbonate and more compatible with ions present in the solution	Increased lactic acidosis in shock caused by lactate Fluid retention and circulatory overload caused by sodium content	Lactate conversion requires aerobic metabolism; therefore, it should be used cautiously in shock and other hypoperfusion states
Ringer's solution	Replace body fluid Provide additional potassium and calcium	Does not contain lactate, so can be given to patients with hypoperfusion	Potential hyperchloremic metabolic acidosis caused by high chloride concentration Potential fluid retention and circulatory overload caused by sodium content	
Crystalloid solutions (hypotonic)				
½ Normal saline	Raise total fluid volume		Potential interstitial and intracellular edema caused by rapid movement of this fluid from the vascular space Dilution of plasma proteins and electrolytes	
5% dextrose in water (D₅W)	Raise total fluid volume Provide calories for energy (200 cal/1000 ml)	Distributed evenly in every body compartment (acts like free water) Reverse dehydration Prevents hyperosmolar state Maintains adequate renal tubular flow (facilities water excretion)	Dilution of plasma proteins and electrolytes caused by rapid metabolism of glucose and resultant free water	

eases, transfusion reactions, cost) (Chapter 38). If massive transfusions are given, additional problems may result. Because blood for transfusion contains an anticoagulant to prevent it from clotting while it is being stored, the patient who receives large amounts of blood may develop clotting defects. Stored blood is also deficient in platelets and other clotting factors. Massive transfusions of cold blood can result in hypothermia, which can cause cardiac arrhythmias.

Stored blood also contains some debris resulting from the aggregation of platelets, leukocytes, and fibrin. It is believed that some of this debris is able to pass through standard blood filters and is eventually filtered out of the blood by the pulmonary capillaries. This probably causes little difficulty in the patient who receives only a few units of blood, but it is likely to cause a problem for the patient who receives massive transfusions. It is recommended by some that microfilters be used when large quantities of blood are transfused.[16]

The pH in stored blood is lower than in normal blood. The added anticoagulant makes the blood more acid. Also, because blood is stored in an airtight bag, the metabolism that continues is anaerobic, and the end products are *lactic* and *pyruvic acid*. With all of its disadvantages, until a blood substitute is available for general use, blood must be given to maintain relatively normal hemoglobin and hematocrit levels.[11]

Some patients who are losing large amounts of blood may be given transfusions with their own blood, collected from the bleeding site with special equipment. Autotransfusion has been used in patients bleeding massively from an uncontaminated wound as well as in patients who bleed excessively during surgery. While it does eliminate transfusion reactions and hepatitis associated with blood transfusions, it is not without risks. The most common complications of autotransfusion are *hemolysis* resulting in renal failure, coagulopathy, embolization of debris, and sepsis.[39] Its main use is in patients who are bleeding so rapidly that the supply of stored blood is becoming depleted.

■ OTHER TYPES OF FLUID THERAPY

Other fluids given are classified either as crystalloid or colloid solutions (see Table 9-4). Controversy exists concerning which should be used. Those who favor the use of crystalloid solutions believe these are better able to re-

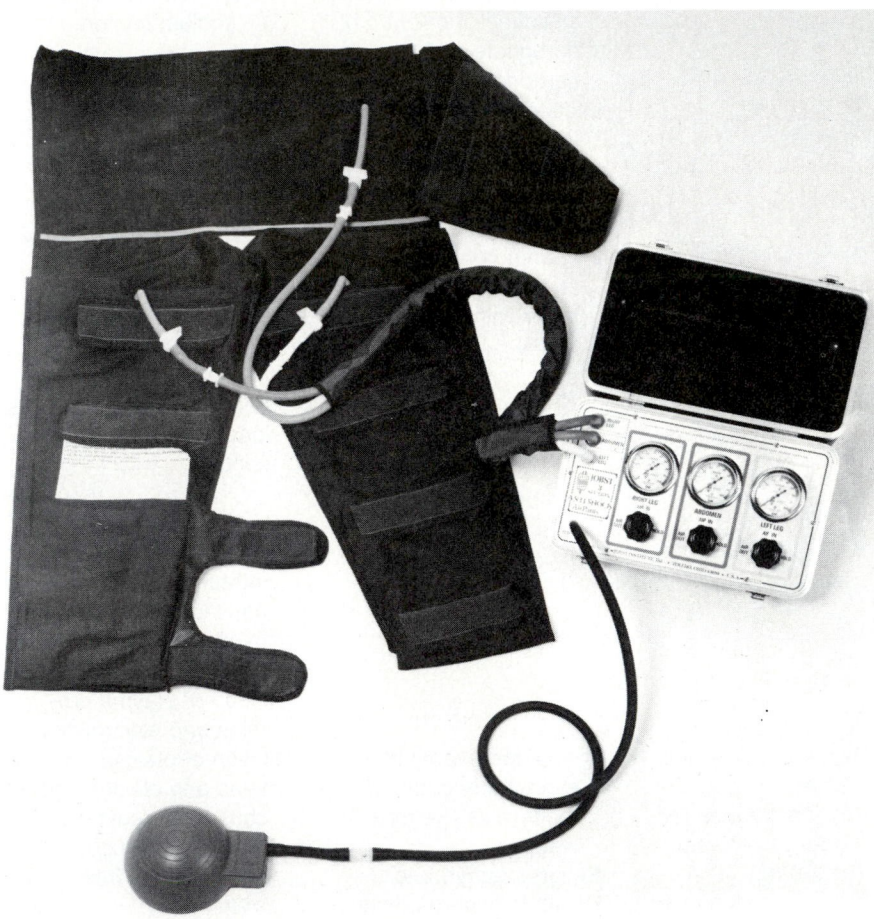

Fig. 9-8   Military antishock trousers (MAST) with inflation device and manometers. (Courtesy The Jobst Institute, Inc, Toledo, OH; from Burrell, LO, and Burrell, AL: Critical care, St Louis, 1982, The CV Mosby Co)

store and maintain urinary output.[14] Some believe that colloid solutions should be given because they remain in the intravascular compartment where the fluid is needed.[33] Still others believe that a proper mixture of the two types of solution should be given.

Regardless of the type of fluid that the patient receives, the nurse must carefully monitor the rate at which it is administered. The patient is assessed frequently for signs of hypovolemia or fluid overload (Chapter 8). Neck veins are observed for distention, and lungs are auscultated for signs of fluid (rales, rhonchi).

■ FLUID REDISTRIBUTION

Another way in which fluid resuscitation may be accomplished is by the use of the MAST suit (Military Anti-Shock Trousers). The suit consists of three inflatable parts, one for each leg and one for the abdomen (Fig. 9-8). When inflated, the trousers "autotransfuse" the upper circulation with up to 2 L blood from the lower extremities, increasing blood to the heart, lungs, and brain.[39] The trousers also increase peripheral resistance, which helps compensate for decreased blood volume. If there is

bleeding in the lower extremities, the MAST suit helps to control bleeding by tamponade (counterpressure). The suit is used as a temporary measure until adequate fluid can be administered. When the suit is to be removed, it must be deflated gradually to prevent a sudden fall in peripheral resistance and a return of shock.

■ Assisting with drug therapy

If fluid therapy alone is not sufficient to reverse the shock state, vasoactive drugs may be given (Table 9-5). Most vasoactive drugs are *catecholamines*, which stimulate *alpha* or *beta receptors* in the body. Generally, stimulation of alpha receptors causes vasoconstriction, and stimulation of beta receptors causes vasodilation. Stimulation of beta receptors also causes the heart to increase its rate (*chronotropic* effect) and strength of contraction (*inotropic* effect). The abdominal viscera, skin, and muscles respond primarily to the alpha effects of the catecholamines.

Mixed alpha- and beta-adrenergic drugs are used most commonly. In the past, drugs that caused vasoconstriction were used primarily because they enhanced the body's normal compensatory mechanisms. One problem was that the

Table 9-5 Vasoactive drugs commonly used to treat shock

	Effect	Advantages	Disadvantages
Mixed α- and β-adrenergic drugs			
Norepinephrine (levarterenol)	β-1: pronounced effect in low doses Positive inotropic and chronotropic effects	May improve cardiac output by increasing rate and stroke volume.	Increase O_2 need of heart
	β-2: weak effect dilation of coronary arteries	May improve blood flow to heart	
	α: pronounced effect especially in higher doses Vasoconstriction	May improve oxygenation of heart by increasing coronary artery perfusion pressure (especially in presence of hypotension)	May decrease cardiac output by increasing afterload Increases O_2 need of heart
Metaraminol (Aramine)	Same as norepinephrine Acts by releasing catacholamine stores in the body	Same as norepinephrine	Same as norepinephrine
Epinephrine	β-1: pronounced effect Positive inotropic and chronotropic effect	May improve cardiac output by increasing stroke volume and rate	Increases O_2 need of heart
	β-2: pronounced, especially in lower doses Dilates coronary arteries and vessels in skeletal muscles	May increase blood supply to heart	May shunt blood away from vital organs because of dilation of vessels in skeletal muscles
	α: pronounced effect in higher doses	May improve oxygenation of heart by increasing coronary perfusion pressure	May decrease cardiac output by increasing afterload Increases O_2 need of heart

Continued.

Table 9-5 Vasoactive drugs commonly used to treat shock—cont'd

	Effect	Advantages	Disadvantages
Mixed α- and β-adrenergic drugs—cont'd			
Dopamine	Dopaminergic receptors: pronounced effect in low (2-5 μg/kg/min) and moderate doses (5-10 μg/kg/min); α effect in high doses (greater than 10 μg/kg/min)	Improves perfusion of kidneys and abdominal viscera	
	β-1: pronounced effect in moderate dose range—positive inotropic and chronotropic effect	Improves cardiac output	Increases O_2 need of heart
	β-2: moderate effect Dilates coronary arteries	Increased blood supply to heart	
	α: pronounced in high doses Offsets dopaminergic and beta effects	May improve oxygenation of heart by increasing coronary perfusion pressure	May decrease cardiac output by increasing afterload Increases O_2 need of heart
Dobutamine	β-1: pronounced effect Positive inotropic effect	Improves the cardiac output by increasing stroke volume	Increases O_2 need of heart
	Minimal chronotropic effect	Lack of rate increase allows more coronary filling time than other inotropic drugs	
	β-2: weak effect Some dilation of coronary arteries α: minimal effect	May improve coronary artery blood flow	
β-Adrenergic drugs			
Isoproterenol	β-1: very pronounced strong positive inotropic and chronotropic effects	Increases cardiac output by increasing stroke volume and rate	Pronounced increase in O_2 need of heart Cardiac arrhythmias
	β-2: very pronounced Dilates coronary arteries and vessels in skeletal muscles Lowers peripheral resistance	May increase blood supply to heart May improve cardiac output by decreasing afterload	Decreased blood pressure may decrease coronary artery perfusion pressure
Vasodilators			
Nitroprusside	Acts directly on smooth muscle, dilating both veins and arterioles	Decreases O_2 need of heart by decreasing both preload and afterload Decreases pulmonary congestion by decreasing preload Increases cardiac output by decreasing afterload	Decreases in peripheral resistance can decrease coronary artery perfusion pressure
Nitroglycerine	Acts directly on smooth muscle Effect on veins: pronounced Effect on arterioles: weak	Decreases O_2 need of heart by decreasing preload and, to a lesser extent, afterload	Decrease in preload can decrease cardiac output and coronary artery perfusion pressure

---

Nursing care of patients receiving vasoactive drugs

1. Monitor blood pressure every 5 to 15 minutes at the beginning of the infusion and every 15 minutes thereafter to maintain a *mean* blood pressure at prescribed level (usually 80 mm Hg).
2. Drug must be diluted in a compatible solution and administered slowly by intravenous pump (for control).
3. Observe peripheral site of infusion (if used) frequently for signs of infiltration (necrosis and sloughing of tissues may occur with infiltration).
4. If infiltration occurs, infiltrate area around site with norepinephrine blocker (Regitine) as prescribed.
5. Monitor urinary output.
6. When discontinuing drug infusion, taper infusion slowly while continuing to monitor blood pressure every 15 minutes.

---

compensatory mechanisms themselves can have an adverse effect on the body. As blood is shunted away from the kidneys to perfuse the heart and brain, renal perfusion decreases and renal failure may result. In addition, bowel necrosis may develop, and the ischemic pancreas may begin to produce myocardial depressant factor. The ischemic liver can no longer perform its important functions.

Vasodilator drugs have been used to counteract the adverse effects of the body's compensatory mechanisms. They decrease the amount of pressure against which the heart has to pump, and thereby have the effect of increasing cardiac output without increasing the work load and oxygen need of the heart. *Fluid therapy must be given along with vasodilator drugs,* or the decrease in peripheral resistance can cause a decrease in venous return, thereby decreasing cardiac output. *Cardiac output* must be maintained when vasodilators are given, or the heart and brain may be poorly perfused. The drug selected will depend to some extent on the cause of shock and how far shock has progressed.

Combinations of drugs may be given. Dopamine and nitroprusside may be given together to increase cardiac output by combining the inotropic effect of dopamine with the decreased peripheral resistance effected by nitroprusside. For these two drugs to work together effectively, adequate fluid must be administered.[46] Low-dose dopamine may be given for its effect on renal and mesenteric perfusion along with dobutamine for its inotropic effect.

Patients receiving *vasoactive drugs* require very careful monitoring (see the box above). Ideally, intraarterial and pulmonary pressure monitoring should be instituted. If the blood pressure is being measured by both cuff and intra-arterial line, the two readings may vary. It is imperative that everyone working with the patient use the same measurements in adjusting the rate of drug infusion.

Steroids are often administered to patients in shock; however, their use is controversial. Many benefits from their use have been suggested, the most important of which is stabilization of lysosomal membranes, thereby preventing the leak of destructive enzymes.[26] The clinical success related to their use has been variable, as has the incidence of complications.[37] Other drugs are being used experimentally at present and may become accepted therapeutic agents in the future; these include calcium channel blockers,[22] Naloxone (a beta endorphin antagonist),[26] and energy substrates.[24]

■ Assisting with cardiac support

When the left ventricle becomes severely impaired, as in cardiogenic shock or in the late stages of any type of shock, its function may be augmented by the use of the *intraaortic balloon pump* (Chapter 25). A balloon-tipped catheter is inserted into the aorta by way of the femoral artery. The catheter is attached to a machine that inflates and deflates the balloon in synchrony with the patient's cardiac cycle. During systole the balloon is deflated as the heart pumps blood into the aorta. During diastole the balloon inflates, enhancing blood flow to the heart, which is perfused during diastole, and to the rest of the body. During the next period of systole, the balloon deflates again, leaving a space in the aorta that must be filled. This causes a reduction in resistance, which allows the heart to eject a large quantity of blood with less effort than would normally be required.

Complications are not uncommon with use of the balloon pump. The most common complication is vascular insufficiency of the extremity distal to the insertion site. Frequent assessments are made of the pulses, color, temperature, movement, and sensation of the extremity, and any abnormality is reported immediately. Infection may occur with this procedure, as with any invasive procedure; therefore, the patient's temperature is also monitored.

The use of the intraaortic balloon is a temporary measure used to enhance cardiac output only until the heart is able to function adequately on its own.

■ Assisting with respiratory support

Most patients in shock have some degree of *hypoxemia*. Oxygen is usually administered because tissues are already suffering from oxygen deprivation from poor blood flow. Because the energy system of the body is impaired, the muscles used in ventilation may not function adequately and breathing may have to be assisted. If symptoms of

ARDS develop, positive end expiratory pressure (PEEP) may have to be used. Positive pressure at the end of expiration prevents surfactant-deficient alveoli from collapsing, resulting in atelectasis (see Chapter 24). Coughing and deep breathing are important, if the patient is able. If the patient is too weak to cough or if an endotracheal tube is in place, suctioning is necessary to keep the airway free of excessive secretions. Meticulous mouth care is necessary while the endotracheal tube is in place, because the mouth remains open and swallowing may be difficult. Turning the patient at least every 2 hours is important to aid in the mobilization of secretions.

■ Preventing injuries

In the early stages of shock, the patient may exhibit *restlessness,* which may then progress to *confusion.* During this time, injury is likely to occur if preventive measures are not taken. If the patient attempts to remove or disconnect lifesaving equipment, soft restraints may have to be applied.

Infections are very common in patients who are in shock, because of the many invasive procedures that are performed. Some potential sources of infection are indwelling catheters, arterial lines, pulmonary artery catheters, intravenous lines, endotracheal tubes, surgical incisions, and traumatic wounds. Meticulous sterile technique must be used with endotracheal suctioning, dressing changes, tubing changes, and urinary catheter care. Patients who are receiving steroids or who have experienced excessive blood loss are at increased risk for developing infection.

Complications of immobility must be prevented. It is not uncommon for the patient in shock to remain in one position for an extended period because of the constant activity that is occurring at the patient's bedside. This immobility can predispose the patient to thrombi, pneumonia, and decubitus ulcers. Frequent turning and maintaining cleanliness of the skin will aid in the prevention of *decubitus ulcers.* If immobility is prolonged, the use of special mattresses may be considered.

■ MAINTAINING COMFORT AND REST

The patient should be kept as comfortable as possible. In the past, patients in shock were kept in the Trendelenberg position (head down), but this is no longer recommended. It is usually suggested that the patient remain flat, with the legs elevated if necessary. If a patient in shock has difficulty breathing, a small pillow may be used to elevate the head slightly.

Rest is important. All nonessential activities should be eliminated because activity increases the body's need for oxygen and nutrients, substances already deficient in the cells of the patient in shock.

Ambient temperature should be kept at a comfortable level. Excessive warmth increases the metabolic rate of the tissues, thereby increasing their oxygen need. Excessive coolness may cause the blood to flow even more sluggishly through the microcirculation, enhancing the formation of microthrombi. Patients with an endotracheal tube in place or who are very lethargic may not be able to express how they feel. Covers should be used according to the room temperature.

Both the conscious patient and the family will probably experience considerable anxiety. The nurse should remain calm and explain all interventions whenever possible. It may be necessary to repeat explanations frequently to both patient and family, because anxiety can interfere with their ability to comprehend and to remember.

⊞ EVALUATION

Evaluation is based on expected patient outcomes and may include the following:

1. Patient will be able to tolerate activity involved in care. Did pulse increase no more than 10 beats per minute? Did skin remain warm and dry? Did respiratory rate remain the same?
2. Patient's airway will remain free from secretions. Are lung sounds clear? Can suction catheter be inserted into airway easily?
3. Patient and significant others will remain free of avoidable anxiety. Are they able to verbalize fears? Are they free of signs of anxiety?
4. Patient will have a respiratory rate and tidal volume within normal limits. Are respirations regular? Is the respiratory rate between 16 and 22 per minute? Is the tidal volume normal for the patient's size?
5. Cardiac output will be within normal limits. Is the mean arterial blood pressure greater than 80 mm Hg? Is the pulse rate between 60 and 100 beats per minute? Is the cardiac index 2.5 to 3.5 L/min/m²? Is the PCWP between 10 and 20 mm Hg?
6. Patient will make his or her needs understood by verbal or alternate means of communication. Is the patient able to make his or her needs known? Is the patient free from anxiety when trying to communicate?
7. Intravascular volume will return to normal. Is the CVP between 6 and 15 cm water? Is the pulse volume normal? Is the pulse rate between 60 and 100 per minute?
8. Blood gases will be within normal limits. Are the blood gases within the following range? PO_2 80 to 100 mm Hg; PCO_2 35 to 45 mm Hg; HCO_3 22 to 26 mEq/L; pH 7.35 to 7.45.
9. Patient will be free from infection. Is the patient's temperature within normal range? Is the leukocyte count between 4500 and 11,000/mm? Are the catheter insertion sites free from redness, swelling, and drainage?
10. Oral mucous membrane will remain moist and intact. Is mucous membrane pink and moist? Are lips free from cracks? Is mouth free of excess mucus?
11. Patient will have adequate rest. Does patient appear rested? Has care been planned to allow for periods of undisturbed sleep?

Putting knowledge to practice

- Review the effects of the sympathetic nervous system on blood vessels of the heart, brain, and peripheral vessels.
- Review the physiologic requirements for the maintenance of adequate blood pressure.
- Explain physiologically why a person who has suffered injuries should not be covered by blankets on a warm day at the scene of an accident.
- Review in your physiology text the difference between alpha receptors and beta receptors.
- Review in your pharmacology text the actions and effects of adrenergic drugs.

---

12. Patient will have normal tissue perfusion. Is the urinary output greater than 30 ml/hr? Is the BUN between 8 and 25 mg/dl? Is the serum creatinine between 0.6 and 1.2 mg/dl? Is the lactic acid level less than 1.9 mEq/L? Is the serum potassium level between 3.8 and 5.0 mEq/L? Is the serum sodium level between 136 and 142 mEq/L? Is the patient's skin warm, dry, and pink? Is capillary refill less than 3 seconds? Is the patient's mental status the same as before the onset of shock?
13. Patient will remain free of injury. Is the patient free from nosocomial infections? Is the patient free of abrasions? Is the patient free of complications of immobility?

■ SUMMARY

1. Shock is a syndrome characterized by hypoperfusion of body tissues.
2. The major classifications of shock are hypovolemic, cardiogenic, and vasogenic shock.
3. Shock results in a derangement of cellular metabolism, and if not treated in the early stages, it can affect all body systems.
4. The early stage of shock is characterized by a stress response.
5. At some point in the progress of untreated shock, the process becomes irreversible and no treatment can save the patient.
6. The management of shock includes the following:
   a. Fluid therapy
      Colloids
      Crystaloids
   b. Drug therapy
      Vasodilators
      Vasoconstrictors
      Inotropes
   c. Supportive care
      Cardiac support
      Respiratory support
      Prevention of injuries

REFERENCES AND SELECTED READINGS
Contemporary

1. Armstrong, P, and Baigrie, R: Hemodynamic monitoring in critically ill patients, Heart Lung 9:1060-1062, 1980.
2. *Asheervath, J, and Blevins, D. Handbook of clinical nursing practice, Norwalk, Conn, 1986, Appleton-Century-Crofts.
3. *Barrow, JJ: Shock demands drugs—but which one's best for your patient? Nurs 82 12(2):34-41, 1982.
4. Blaisdell, FW: Controversy in shock research, Con: the role of steroids in septic shock, Circ Shock 8(6):673-682, 1981.
5. Brinkmeyer, SD: Fluid resuscitation: an overview, J Am Osteopath Assoc 82:326-330, 1983.
6. Chaudry, IH, and Baue, AE: The use of substrates and energy in the treatment of shock, Adv Shock Res 3:27-46, 1980.
7. *Cline, BA, and Fischer, ML: ARDS means emergency, Nurs 82 12(2):63-67, 1982.
8. Clough, DH, and Higgins, P: Discrepancies in estimating blood loss, Am J Nurs 81:331-333, 1981.
9. Corpening, JT: Colloid vs crystalloid fluid resuscitation in shock and injury. In Ellerbe, S: Fluid and blood component therapy in critically ill injured, New York, 1981, Churchill Livingstone.
10. Daily E, and Schroeder, J: Techniques in bedside hemodynamic monitoring, ed 2, St. Louis, 1981, The CV Mosby Co.
11. Dislet, L, and others: Cardiogenic shock in evolving myocardial infarction, Heart Lung 16:649-651, 1987.
12. Demling, RH, and Nerlich, M: Hypovolemic shock resuscitation: an update. In Collins, JA, and others: Massive transfusion in surgery and trauma, Prog Clin Biol Res 108:30-35, 1982.
13. DeSantis, D, and others: Delayed appearance of a circulating myocardial depressant factor in burn patients, Ann Emerg Med 10:22-24, 1981.
14. Elenbass, R: Anaphylactic shock, Crit Care Q 2:85-90, 1980.
15. Ellenbogen, C: Treatment priorities for septic shock, Am Fam Physician 25:163-167, 1982.
16. *Ellerbe, S: Fluid and blood component therapy in the critically ill and injured, New York, 1981, Churchill-Livingstone.
17. Eskridge, R: Septic shock, Crit Care Q 2:55-76, 1980.

---

*References preceded by an asterisk are particularly well suited for student reading.

18. Feinstein, DI: Diagnosis and management of disseminated intravascular coagulation: the role of heparin therapy, Blood 60:284-287, 1982.
19. Glover, JL, and Broadie, TA: Intraoperative autotransfusion. In Collins, JA, and others: Massive transfusion in surgery and trauma, Prog Clin Biol Res 108:160-165, 1982.
20. Guyton, AC: Textbook of medical physiology, ed 6, Philadelphia, 1981, WB Saunders Co.
21. Hardaway, RM: Pulmonary artery pressure vs pulmonary capillary wedge pressure and central venous pressure in shock, Resuscitation 10:47-56, 1982.
22. Hess, ML, and others: Improved myocardial hemodynamic and cellular function with calcium channel blockade (Verapamil) during canine hemorrhagic shock, Circ Shock 10:119-130, 1983.
23. Hudak, CM, Lohr, T, and Gallo, BM: Critical care nursing, Philadelphia, 1982, JB Lippincott Co.
24. Isoyama, T, and others: Effects of naloxone and morphine in hemorrhagic shock, Circ Shock 10:119-130, 1982.
25. Karliner, JS, and Gregorates, G: Coronary care, New York, 1981, Churchill Livingstone.
26. Lefer, AM, and Schumer, W: Molecular and cellular aspects of shock and trauma, Prog Clin Biol Res 111:144-145, 1983.
27. Metheny, N: The interstitial (third space) phenomenon, NITA 6:251-254, 1983.
28. *Myers, JL: Introduction to complications of shock. In Perry, AG, and Potter, PA: Shock: comprehensive nursing management, St. Louis, 1983, The CV Mosby Co.
29. Nicholson, DP: Corticosteroids in the treatment of septic shock and the adult respiratory distress syndrome, Med Clin North Am 67:717-723, 1983.
30. *Niedringhaus, L: Hypovolemic shock. In Perry, AG, and Potter, PA: Shock: comprehensive nursing management, St. Louis, 1983, The CV Mosby Co.
31. *Park, G: Cardiogenic shock, Crit Care Q 2:43-54, 1980.
32. *Perry, AG, and Potter, PA: Shock: comprehensive nursing management, St. Louis, 1983, The CV Mosby Co.
33. Pinsky, MR: Cause-specific management of shock, Postgrad Med 73:127-149, 1983.
34. Rackley, CE: Critical care cardiology, Philadelphia, 1981, FA Davis Co.
35. *Rice, V: Shock: shock, a clinical syndrome—the clinical continuum of septic shock, Critical Care Nurse 4(5):86-109, 1984.
36. Riede, U, Sandritter, W, and Mittermayer, C: Circulatory shock: a review, Pathology 13:299-311, 1981.
37. Schumer, W: Controversy in shock research: the role of steroids in septic shock, Circ Shock 8:667-682, 1981.
38. Schuster, H, and others: The influence of disseminated intravascular coagulation on renal function after experimental hemorrhagic shock, Resuscitation 8:3-28, 1980.
39. Shine, KI, and others: Aspects of the management of shock, Am Coll Phys 93:723-734, 1980.
40. Tilkian, SM, Conover, MB, and Tilkian, AG: Clinical implications of laboratory tests, St. Louis, 1979, The CV Mosby Co.
41. *Visalli, F, and Evans, P: The Swan-Ganz catheter: a program for teaching safe, effective care, Nurs 81 11(1):42-47, 1981.

Classic

42. Denny, M: Septic shock, JEN 3:19-23, 1977.
43. Fowler, NO: Examination of the heart: inspection and palpation of venous and arterial pulses, New York, 1978, American Heart Association.
44. Goldstein, IM: Lysosomes and their relation to the cell in shock, Kalamazoo, Mich, 1975, Upjohn Co.
45. *Hathaway, R: Hemodynamic monitoring in shock, JEN 3:37-43, 1977.
46. Shearer, JK, and Caldwell, M: Use of sodium nitroprusside and dopamine hydrochloride in the postoperative cardiac patient, Heart and Lung 8:302-307, 1979.

10

Pain

BARBARA C. LONG

CHAPTER OBJECTIVES

After studying this chapter, the student should be able to:

- Describe the physiology of pain and the gate control theory of pain transmission.
- Compare factors that influence perception and reaction to pain.
- Identify analgesics effective for mild to moderate and moderate to severe pain, and factors to consider when giving narcotics.
- Describe medical approaches for pain control in addition to medications.
- Describe specific psychologic approaches for pain control.
- Identify guidelines for nursing interventions for pain control.
- Describe nursing measures to modify the pain stimulus and pain response.
- Explain the purpose and methods of the team approach for chronic pain control.

Pain is experienced to one degree or another by all persons. It is, however, a very individualized experience. It has never been satisfactorily defined or understood. It is an unpleasant feeling, entirely subjective, that only the person experiencing it can describe or evaluate. It can be evoked by a multiplicity of stimuli, but the reaction to it cannot be measured objectively. Pain is a learned experience that is influenced by the entire life situation of each person.

Pain accompanies many pathophysiologic disorders, as well as some therapies. It is a sensation that is frequently feared by persons undergoing surgery. Although many persons with cancer do *not* experience it, pain is one of the major concerns people have about cancer.

Relief of pain and discomfort is a major nursing intervention and one that requires skill in both the art and science of nursing. It requires knowledge about concepts related to pain, data collection, and useful therapies. It also requires sensitivity and empathy—an effort on the part of the nurse to try to understand what the patient is experiencing and to communicate understanding and caring. It requires that the nurse use a systematic approach (nursing process) with the patient in pain. Too often when a patient states that he or she has pain, medication is given without valid assessment and evaluation, resulting in undermedication, overmedication, or medication when other interventions would be more effective.

■ PHYSIOLOGY OF PAIN

■ Pain receptors and stimuli

Pain receptors, called *nociceptors,* are free nerve endings on unmyelinated or lightly myelinated afferent neurons. Nociceptors are located extensively in the skin and mucosa and less frequently in selected deeper structures such as viscera, joints, arterial walls, liver, and bile ducts. Nociceptors respond preferentially to harmful stimuli that may be chemical, thermal, electrical, or mechanical. Chemical stimuli for pain include histamines, bradykinin, prostaglandins, and acids, some of which are released by damaged tissues. Anoxia leads to pain by chemicals released by the damaged anoxic tissue. Muscle spasms induce pain by compressing blood vessels, thus leading to anoxia. Stretching of muscle fibers may also lead to anoxia. Tissue swelling may cause pain by creating pressure (mechanical stimulation) on nociceptors of adjoining tissue.

Pain receptors do not adapt to repeated stimulation and, in some instances, may become more sensitive over time. In pathologic conditions, pain sensitivity may be increased (hyperalgesia). For example, sunburned skin may be highly pain sensitized to even the slightest touch (mechanical stimulus).

■ Pain transmission

Pain impulses are transmitted to the spinal cord by two types of fibers: fast myelinated A-delta fibers and slow unmyelinated C fibers. Pain that may be described as "sharp" or "pricking" and that can be easily localized results from impulses transmitted by the A-*delta fibers.* An example of this type of pain is that felt by a needle prick. Pain that may be described as "burning," "dull," or "aching" and that is more diffuse results from impulses transmitted by the C *fibers.* Impulses transmitted over A-delta fibers have an inhibitory effect on those transmitted over C fibers.

The afferent nerve fibers enter the spinal cord through the dorsal root and synapse in the *dorsal horn* (Fig. 10-1). The dorsal horn consists of several layers (laminae) with interconnections. Lamina II and III comprise an area called *substantia gelatinosa* (SG). Substance P is released at synapses in the SG and is thought to be a major neurotransmitter of the pain impulses.

The pain impulses cross the spinal cord over interneurons and connect with *ascending spinal pathways.* There are at least six ascending pathways for nociceptive impulses located in the ventral half of the spinal cord; the most important are the spinothalamic tract (STT) and the spinoreticular tract (SRT). The STT is a discriminative system and conveys information about the nature and location of the stimulus to the thalamus and thence to the cortex for interpretation. Impulses transmitted over the SRT (which goes to the brainstem and part of the thalamus) activate the autonomic and limbic (motivational-affective) responses.

■ Modulating pain mechanisms

■ OPIATE PATHWAYS

Discovery of receptors in the brain to which opiate compounds bind led to the discovery of two naturally occurring endogenous morphinelike pentapeptides (5-amino acid compounds), met-enkephalin and leu-enkephalin. These enkephalins are classified as *endorphins* (from the terms endogenous and morphine). Other endorphins, such as beta-endorphin, have also been identified. The endorphins are thought to suppress pain by (1) acting presynaptically to *inhibit release* of the neurotransmitter substance P or (2) acting postsynaptically to *inhibit conduction* of pain impulses.[44] The endorphins are found in high concentration in the basal ganglia of the brain, thalamus, midbrain, and dorsal horn of the spinal cord.

Descending spinal pathways, from the thalamus through the midbrain and medulla to the dorsal horns of the spinal cord, conduct nociceptive *suppressive* impulses. Serotonin is a neurotransmitter that supports these suppressive impulses.

The endogenous pain suppressive system is more effectively activated by nociceptive stimuli transmitted by A-delta fibers. Electrical stimulation by means of TENS (p. 179) using low frequency and high intensity activates opiate anesthesia. Acupuncture is also thought to use the opiate pathways.[24,58]

■ NONOPIATE PATHWAYS

Descending spinal pathways that do not respond to naloxone (and therefore are nonopiate) are known to exist, but less is known about them. The mechanism is thought

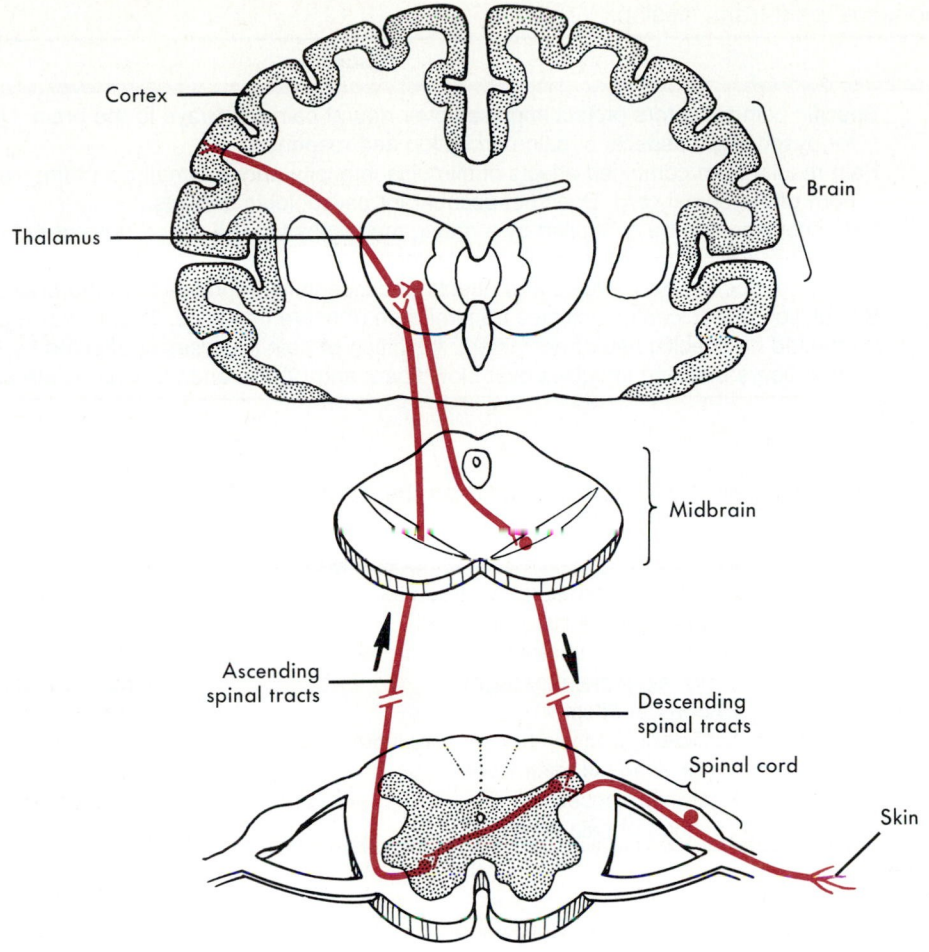

Fig. 10-1 Pathways of pain transmission to and from cortex.

■ Physiologic responses to pain

As stated earlier, impulses transmitted over the SRT ascending pathway activate, in part, the autonomic nervous system, specifically with pain that is severe and of sudden and unexpected onset. This response is similar to the alarm reaction to threat (see Chapter 7), and may include tachycardia, increased blood pressure, pupillary dilatation, diaphoresis, and stimulation of adrenal medullary secretion. In some situations, however, such as with severe visceral pain of sudden onset, there may be vasodilation with subsequent fall in blood pressure and shock.[44]

Noxious stimuli may also produce a reflex contraction of flexor muscles, a withdrawal response to pain. For example, touching a hot object will result in immediate contraction of hand and arm muscles with withdrawal of the hand from the object. Continuous noxious stimulation usually produces a steadily maintained reflex contraction of

to be neural or hormonal.[58] Electrical stimulation by means of TENS using high frequency and low intensity activates the nonopiate system. Biofeedback (p. 182) also effects nonopiate mechanisms.

adjacent or distant muscles.[44] An example of this phenomenon is the abdominal rigidity noted in persons with intraabdominal pain.

■ Theories of pain transmission

Various theories of pain transmission have been proposed (Table 10-1). The specificity and pattern theories were early theories that led to the development of the gate control theory. Although the *gate control theory* does not fully explain pain transmission, it serves as a basis for understanding pain transmission. The concepts of the transmission-inhibition theory are described in the preceding section on physiology of pain.

The gate control theory was proposed by Melzack and Wall in 1965. The theory proposes that the substantia gelatinosa (SG) in the spinal cord acts as a gating mechanism to permit or inhibit passage of pain impulses. The "gate" can be "closed" (so that contact is not made, thus interrupting the pain impulse) by nerve impulses from the A-delta fibers or from the descending pathways. Impulses conducted over large fibers not only close the gate but also are sent immediately to the cortex for rapid identification,

Table 10-1 Theories of pain transmission

Theory	Description
Specificity theory	Specific pain receptors project impulses over neural pain pathways to the brain. Does not account for pyschologic aspects of pain perception and response.
Pattern theory	Pain results from combined effects of stimulus intensity and summations of impulses in the dorsal horn of the spinal cord. Does not account for psychologic aspects.
Gate control theory	Pain impulses can be controlled by a gating mechanism in the dorsal horn of the spinal cord to permit or inhibit transmission. Gating factors include effect of impulses transmitted over fast or slow conducting nerve fibers and effects of descending impulses from the brainstem and cortex.
Transmission-inhibition theory	Stimulation of nociceptors initiates transmission of nerve impulses. Transmission of pain impulses is effected by specific neurotransmitters. Inhibition of pain impulses is effected by (1) impulses over large fibers blocking impulses over slow fibers and (2) the endogenous-opiate suppressive system.

Table 10-2 Factors affecting pain transmission based on the gate control theory

Site	Close gate (block transmission)	Open gate (permit transmission)
Fibers	Impulses transmitted by large fast myelinated A-delta fibers	Impulses transmitted by slow unmyelinated C fibers
	Stimulation of unaffected skin areas (for example, massage)	Stimulation of affected skin areas (for example, sunburned skin)
Brainstem (descending pathway)	Endorphin effect	No endorphin effect
	Sufficient or maximum sensory input (for example, distraction)	Insufficient sensory input (for example, monotony)
Cortex	Past experiences	Past experiences
	Feelings of pain control	Anxiety

evaluation and modification of the sensory inputs.[41] Impulses sent to the brainstem, the center for motivational-affective and sensory-discriminative actions, can influence cognition or evaluation in the cortex. Cortical-spinal nerves then send impulses from the cortex back to the SG to inhibit or permit passage of pain impulses. Note in Table 10-2 the various factors that can open or close the gate.

PAIN EXPERIENCE

The pain experience is influenced by the meaning of the pain for the person, the perception of pain, pain tolerance, and the person's reaction to the pain.

Meaning of pain

Pain has different meanings for each person, which may differ for the same person at different times. In general, most persons view pain as a negative experience, although it may also have some positive aspects. Some examples of the meanings of pain include the following:

Harm or damage
Complication, such as infection
New illness
Recurrence of illness
Fatal disease
Increasing disability
Loss of mobility
Aging
Healing
Necessary for cure
Punishment for sins
Challenge
Appreciation for suffering of others
Something to be tolerated
Release from unwanted responsibilities

Numerous factors influence the meaning of pain for an individual, including age, sex, sociocultural background, environment, and past or present experiences. For example, two women may be experiencing pain from a fractured leg. The 75-year-old woman who lives alone and has few social contacts might interpret the pain on the basis of fear of aging and long-term loss of mobility that could interfere with activities of daily living. The 25-year-old secretary might interpret the pain as an expected nuisance, with the realization that healing will occur and she can get back to work soon.

Pain perception

Perception of pain takes place in the cortex (cognitive-evaluative function) as a result of the stimuli transmitted up the spinothalamic and thalamic-cortical tracts. Pain perception is subjective, highly complex, and individual; it is influenced by factors affecting stimulation of the nociceptors and transmission of the nociceptive impulse, as well as by cortical receptivity and interpretation:

1. Stimulation of nociceptors
   a. Increased number of stimuli
   b. Increased duration of the stimulus
2. Alteration of transmission
   a. Damage to nerve endings
   b. Inflammation, tumors, or injuries to spinal cord
3. Receptivity of cortex
   a. Inflammation, degenerative changes of brain
   b. Depression of brain function
   c. Anesthesia
4. Interpretation in cerebral cortex
   a. Childhood training
   b. Past experience with pain
   c. Cultural values
   d. Religious beliefs
   e. Physical and mental health
   f. Knowledge and understanding
   g. Attention and distraction
   h. Fear, anxiety, tension
   i. Fatigue
   j. State of consciousness

Pain *threshold* refers to the *intensity of the stimulus necessary for the person to perceive pain.* As with other pain characteristics, the pain threshold varies among and within individuals. The pain threshold is not affected by age, sex, fatigue, or minor mood alterations. It may be altered, however, by local skin conditions and by stimuli characteristics (number, intensity, time interval).[44] Pain perception may be decreased or absent during periods of intense stress or emotion.

Damage to nerve endings can block the pain sensation at its origin. For example, persons with third-degree burns may have no sensation of pain despite the severity of the injury because of destruction of nerve endings.

Elderly persons may fail to perceive tissue damage that normally would cause pain and thus alert a younger person. Atrophy of nerve endings, degenerative changes in the pain-bearing pathways, and decreased alertness may reduce the perception of pain in the elderly, and more stimulation may be required to evoke a response.

■ Pain tolerance

Pain tolerance refers to the *intensity of the pain that a person is willing to endure before seeking relief.* A high tolerance means that considerable pain is endured before relief is sought. Pain tolerance varies among individuals. Some persons maintain a relatively stable pattern of pain tolerance; others have different levels of tolerance depending on the situation.[65] Numerous factors can increase or decrease pain tolerance (see the box above).

American society tends to reward high tolerance to pain, as evidenced by phrases such as "Grin and bear it" and "Bite the bullet." Persons with high tolerance may, however, refuse measures to relieve pain, even when continued

---

Factors that influence pain tolerance

Increase tolerance	Decrease tolerance
Alcohol	Fatigue
Drugs	Anger
Hypnosis	Boredom
Warmth	Anxiety
Rubbing	Persistent pain
Distraction	Illness
Faith	
Strong beliefs	

---

pain may delay recovery. Other persons may demand pain medication for what the nurse perceives as only minor pain. Both of these situations may create problems for the nursing staff. It is important that health practitioners *not* make value judgments about how much pain a patient "should" or "should not" endure. It is often expected that men should tolerate pain more than women. Each person is different, and each person's tolerance to pain is part of that person's total pain experience. Each person is also entitled to refuse or receive relief measures without censure.

■ Reaction to pain

People respond to pain in different ways. Some may be fearful, apprehensive, and anxious, whereas others are tolerant and optimistic. Some weep, moan, scream, beg for relief or help, threaten to destroy themselves, thrash about in bed, or move about aimlessly when in severe pain; others lie quietly in bed and may only close their eyes, grit their teeth, bite their lips, clench their hands, or perspire profusely when experiencing pain.

Some people, by training and example, are taught to

Factors that influence reaction to pain

Meaning of pain to individual
Degree of pain perception
Past experience
Cultural values
Social expectations
Physical and mental health
Parental attitudes toward pain
Setting in which pain occurs
Fear, anxiety
Usual way of responding to stressors
Age

Table 10-3 Comparison of acute and chronic pain

Characteristic	Acute pain	Chronic pain
Experience	An event	A situation, state of existence
Source	External agent or internal disease	Unknown or cannot be changed or treatment is prolonged or ineffective
Onset	Usually sudden	May be sudden or develop insidiously
Duration	Transient (up to 6 months)	Prolonged (months to years)
Pain identification	Pain vs. nonpain areas generally well identified	Pain vs. nonpain areas less easily differentiated; intensity becomes more difficult to evaluate (change in sensations)
Clinical signs	Typical response pattern with more visible signs	Response patterns vary; fewer overt signs (adaptation)
Meaning	Meaningful (informs person something is wrong)	Meaningless; person looks for meanings
Pattern	Self-limiting or readily corrected	Continuous or intermittent; intensity may vary or remain constant
Course	Suffering usually decreases over time	Suffering usually increases over time
Actions	Leads to actions to relieve pain	Leads to actions to modify pain experience
Prognosis	Likelihood of eventual complete relief	Complete relief usually not possible

endure severe pain without reacting outwardly. Persons from cultures in which health teaching and disease prevention are emphasized tend to accept pain as a warning to seek help, and expect that the cause of pain will be found and cured.

Numerous factors influence reaction to pain (see the box on p. 169). One cannot predict how any given person will respond, and value judgments should not be made concerning how a patient responds. It is very important to some persons to respond to pain in ways that are part of their sociocultural values.

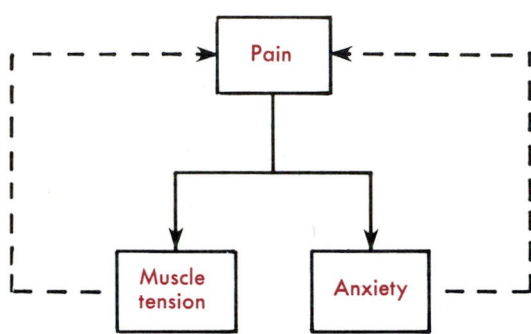

Fig. 10-2 Acute pain.

■ TYPES OF PAIN

■ General types of pain

There are two types of pain syndromes: acute and chronic. Unfortunately, a number of health care professionals provide care for the person experiencing chronic pain as though it were acute pain. There are many differences between acute and chronic pain (Table 10-3), and the approaches to pain relief are usually different, although some of the same techniques may be used.

■ ACUTE PAIN

Acute pain lasts no longer than 6 months. It is essentially a transient episode and informs the person that something is wrong. There is usually sudden onset from a perceived cause, and the painful areas can generally be well identified.

Acute pain is characterized by increased muscle tension

and anxiety, both of which may contribute to increased perception of pain (Fig. 10-2). If the pain is moderate or severe, overt physiologic and behavioral signs facilitate assessment of the pain. The person usually seeks pain relief.

■ CHRONIC PAIN

Pain that persists longer than 6 months is usually classified as chronic pain. Either the source of pain is unknown or the pain cannot be eliminated. The pain sensation often becomes more diffuse, so that it is difficult for the person to identify a specific pain site. The pain may have originally been acute pain but persisted (for example, third-degree burns), or the onset may be so insidious that the person cannot state specifically when it was first experienced.

There are different types of chronic pain. *Intermittent* chronic pain occurs only at specific periods; at other times the person is pain free (migraine headaches). *Persistent* pain

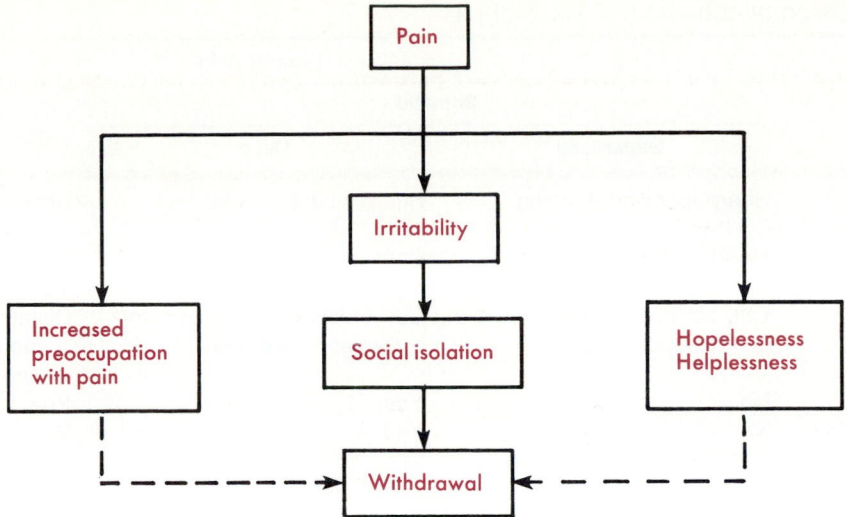

Fig. 10-3 Chronic pain.

is always present, although there may be periods when pain is more or less intense (as seen with low back pain). One form of persistent pain may increase in frequency because of the pathologic condition (pain from incurable cancer). (Cancer pain is discussed in Chapter 12.)

Chronic pain is characterized by irritability (often compounded by insomnia), which leads to decreasing interests and isolation from friends and family. Added to that is the centering of the person's life on the pain experience, with increasing feelings of helplessness and hopelessness as the pain persists. Ultimately the person withdraws from social interactions (Fig. 10-3).

The patient's world centers on ways to modify the pain experience. Some patients go from one physician to another seeking pain relief, which takes time, effort, and money. Even as they seek relief, they often lose faith in the ability of anyone to help them. The lack of continuity of care augments the problems. Physicians themselves may feel helpless when the patient continues to complain of pain. Tender loving care (TLC), which is appropriate for acute pain is *destructive* for chronic pain, because it reinforces the patient role. Acceptance without emphasis on the chronic pain is more effective. The development of pain clinics and inpatient teams has led to successful control of chronic pain for some (but not all) persons with chronic pain.

As a means of differentiating the acute and chronic types of pain, Crue has developed a taxonomy of pain, beginning with acute pain of short duration and ending with continuous intractable pain (unrelieved by therapeutic measures)[10]:

1. *Acute:* lasts a few days, is caused by tissue injury, and can be expected to end when source is removed
2. *Subacute:* similar to acute but persists days to weeks
3. *Recurrent acute pain:* exacerbations of chronic pain
4. *Ongoing cancer pain:* caused by progressive pathology

5. *Intractable benign pain* (adequate coping): pain is continuous but persons are able to live productive lives
6. *Intractable benign pain* (inadequate coping): person is completely disabled by the continuous pain

■ Specific types of pain

■ SOMATIC VERSUS VISCERAL PAIN

Pain may originate in the skin and subcutaneous tissue, (superficial), in the muscles and bones (deep somatic pain), or in the body organs (visceral pain). Somatic and visceral pain differ in their characteristics, particularly in the quality of pain, localization, causes, and accompanying symptoms (Table 10-4).

■ REFERRED PAIN

Referred pain is felt in areas other than those stimulated. It may occur when stimulation is not perceived in the primary areas. For example, the person having a heart attack may complain only of pain radiating down the left arm when in fact the tissue damage is occurring in the myocardium.

Referred pain occurs most often with damage or injury to visceral organs, and the pain is referred to cutaneous surfaces (Fig. 10-4). The origin of referred pain is complex and not clearly understood and may relate to one or more of the following[17]:

1. Referred pain usually occurs in structures that developed from the same embryonic dermatome.
2. Visceral and somatic nerves enter the nervous system at the same spinal level and share the same spinothalamic tracts.
3. Somatic pain is more common and the person has "learned" to interpret signals conducted on certain pathways as being somatic in origin.

Table 10-4 Comparison of somatic and visceral pain

| | Type of pain | | |
| | Somatic | | |
Characteristic	Superficial	Deep	Visceral
Quality	Sharp, pricking, burning	Sharp or dull and aching	Sharp, dull and aching, cramping
Localization	Good	Poor	Poor
Referred pain	No	No	Yes
Provoking stimuli	Cut, abrasion, excessive heat or cold, chemicals	Cut, pressure, heat, ischemia, displacement (bone)	Distention, ischemia, spasms, chemical irritants (no cutting)
Autonomic reactions	No	Yes	Yes
Reflex muscle contractions	No	Yes	Yes

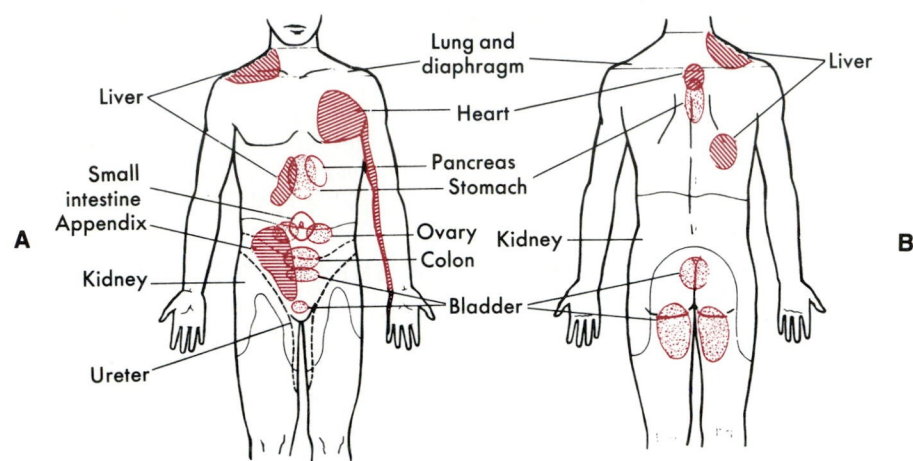

Fig. 10-4 Referred pain. **A,** Front. **B,** Back.

The cutaneous pattern of various referred pains is fairly constant and frequently seen in practice. The nurse should be able to recognize the possibility of visceral organ disease in patients who have appropriate complaints of cutaneous pain.

■ PSYCHOGENIC PAIN

Psychogenic pain is pain for which no physical findings exist; that is, it appears to originate in the person's mind. A sensation is perceived by the person as "pain," and it can be just as intense as pain originating from physical stimuli. Pure psychogenic pain, that is, pain with absolutely no physiologic basis, is rare. More often what is called psychogenic pain is pain that appears to have a greater psychologic basis than apparent physical basis.[65] In some instances pain that has been labeled as psychogenic pain is discovered later to have a strong physical basis not previously identified.

■ PHANTOM LIMB PAIN

Phantom limb pain is pain or discomfort perceived by the individual to be occurring in an extremity that has been amputated. It is more likely to develop in persons who had pain before amputation and may persist long after healing has occurred. The phenomenon of phantom limb pain is poorly understood, and therefore, treatment is not very effective.

■ NEUROLOGIC PAIN

Pain in the neurologic system occurs in different forms. *Neuralgia* is sharp, spasmlike pain along the course of one or more nerves. Two common areas of neuralgia are the trigeminal nerve in the face and the sciatic nerve in the lower trunk. *Causalgia,* a form of neuralgia, is severe burning pain associated with injury to a peripheral nerve in the extremities. The patient may go to great lengths to protect against irritating stimuli (which may be something as simple as the noise of a plane overhead).

▚ ASSESSMENT

▪ Acute pain

When a patient states having pain or asks for pain medication, it is important to make a rapid assessment, collecting both subjective and objective data before taking any actions. Omission of assessment may lead to inadequate pain relief. Consider the example of a young woman who, after pelvic surgery, was crying loudly and demanding pain medication, which was given to her without assessment of the pain. No relief was obtained from the medication. When an assessment was finally made, it was discovered that she had a full bladder of which she was unaware. After she voided, the pain disappeared.

▪ SUBJECTIVE DATA

Data that are useful to obtain *before* pain is anticipated are the patient's expectations for pain relief from health care providers. Many persons are unaware of their expected role in speaking out when they have pain or discomfort. Some patients think they will be considered "complainers" or "bad patients" if they state that they are experiencing discomfort. In this situation, an explanation is given of the subjective nature of pain and the need for patient input to facilitate selection of effective pain relief measures.

The best assessment of pain is the patient's own evaluation. Data need to be gathered about the nature of the acute pain, that is, the location, intensity, quality, timing (onset, duration, frequency, cause), and provoking and palliative factors. One approach for evaluating these characteristics is the use of the mnemonic PQRST[50]:

P Provoking factors: what makes the pain worse or relieves it
Q Quality: dull, sharp, crushing
R Region or radiation: site and radiation to other areas
S Severity or intensity
T Time: onset, duration, frequency, cause

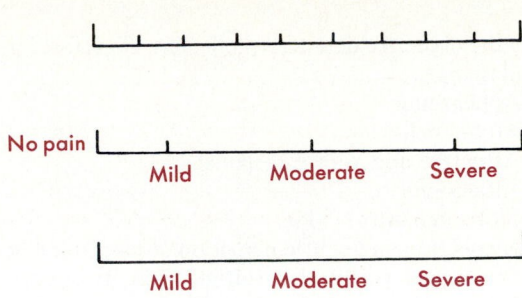

Fig. 10-5 Visual analog pain scales. Person marks line describing intensity of pain.

Pain *intensity* can be determined by various means. One way is to ask the patient to describe the pain or discomfort. Another method is to ask the patient to describe the severity of the pain or discomfort using a pain scale (see the box below, left). The pain scale score can be recorded on a flow chart to provide ongoing assessment of progression of the pain. A third approach is to ask the patient to mark an **X** on a visual analog scale (Fig. 10-5).

When acute pain has subsided, further data can be collected about the *meaning* of pain for the person.

▪ OBJECTIVE DATA

Objective data assist the nurse in identifying possible pain or discomfort in a person who has not reported pain and in helping to clarify the subjective response.

Objective signs of pain are of two types: physiologic and behavioral. *Physiologic* signs of pain result from activation of the sympathetic nervous system (see the box below). With very severe acute pain, neurogenic shock may result from the stressful insult to the system. The *behavioral* signs are not specific to pain; therefore, if the observable data suggest that pain may be present, subjective data must be elicited to validate the assumption.

Pain scales

0—No pain*	0—No pain	0—No pain
1—Mild pain	1—Mild pain	1—Slight pain
2—Discomfort	2—Moderate	2—Moderate
3—Distressing	pain	pain
4—Horrible	3—Severe pain	3—Severe
5—Excruciating	4—As bad as it	pain
	could be	

*NOTE: The first scale is the McGill Pain Scale.

Objective signs of pain

Physiologic signs	Behavioral signs
Pulse: increased rate	Rigid body position
Respirations: increased depth and frequency	Restlessness
	Frowning
Blood pressure: increased systolic and diastolic	Clenched teeth
	Clenched fists
Diaphoresis, pallor	Crying
Dilated pupils	Moaning
Muscle tension (face, body)	
Nausea and vomiting (if pain is severe)	

Specific objective data to be collected, therefore, include the following:

1. Appearance
2. Motor behavior
3. Affective and verbal responses
4. Vital signs
5. Skin: moisture, color
6. Inspection and gentle palpation of painful area; identify trigger points that initiate pain, if present

Sometimes the patient's subjective response differs from the objective signs. For example, the patient may request an analgesic, a back rub, or other measure to relieve pain, but when the nurse arrives to carry out the request, the patient is found to be asleep. It is possible that the patient is exhausted from the pain and thus falls asleep, but the sleeping may be totally unrelated to the continuing presence of pain. It is important to reiterate that pain is what the patient says it is, and although objective data may assist in confirming the existence of pain, the diagnosis cannot be made solely on the basis of the objective data.

■ Chronic pain

■ SUBJECTIVE DATA

Long-term pain requires a much more in-depth assessment of the pain syndrome. Hospitals or pain clinics that use a team approach in providing care to the person with chronic pain often develop their own pain history form or questionnaire (see references 6, 39, 40, and 65 for examples). This history may be collected by one or more health team members, and the data are used by one or more health team members. Types of data collected may include the following:

1. Demographic data
2. Sociocultural data
3. History of the pain pattern from time of onset
4. Factors perceived to increase or decrease the pain
5. Effects of the pain on the person's life-style
6. Meaning of the pain for the person
7. Effects of the patient's pain on other family members or friends
8. Measures used in the past and present for relief of pain

■ OBJECTIVE DATA

Physiologic signs of pain may be absent in the person with chronic pain because of the body's compensatory mechanisms. Although there is adaptation to the pain stimuli, the pain persists. The absence of physiologic signs, therefore, does not indicate absence of pain. Prolonged pain, however, may create changes in the person's appearance over time, perhaps as a result of decreased appetite or lack of interest in appearance because of fatigue or depression.

Behavioral responses to chronic pain are varied and unique to the individual. Here, also, there may be few overt signs to indicate the presence of pain. If the person

is extremely depressed because of the ongoing pain, withdrawal behaviors may be noted.

▶ DATA ANALYSIS: NURSING DIAGNOSES

If pain is present for which specific nursing interventions may be effective, a nursing diagnosis is made of *Pain* (specify location). Possible etiologies may include but are not limited to: physiologic (specify), trauma, diagnostic tests, immobility, improper positioning, overactivity, or pressure points.

Pain may also be an etiologic factor for other nursing diagnoses, such as the following:

Anxiety related to increasing or threatened pain
Ineffective breathing pattern: related to pain in chest or abdomen
Impaired physical mobility: related to pain
Self-care deficit (describe) related to pain
Sexual dysfunction related to pain
Sleep pattern disturbance related to pain

▣ PLANNING: EXPECTED PATIENT OUTCOMES

Expected patient outcomes for the person experiencing pain may include, but are not limited to, the following:

1. Patient states comfort is improved.
2. Pain-related behaviors or signs (specify) are decreased or absent.
3. If pain is present when patient is discharged, patient or significant other can
   a. Describe general measures for pain relief (such as exercises)
   b. Explain prescribed medications (actions, dosages, frequency, side effects)
   c. Describe when to seek medical assistance if pain is not relieved as expected
4. Person with chronic pain can
   a. State plans to participate in ongoing therapies
   b. State plans for increasing independence in activities of daily living

The need to assess the person with pain is ongoing, yet the nurse must begin to plan an approach to the person and the pain, particularly acute pain. The nurse is able to function independently with many interventions, but careful planning with other members of the health care team should ensure that all have the same patient outcomes or goals in mind.

One aspect of the treatment plan that is often forgotten or omitted is the incorporation of measures the patient thinks may help relieve the pain, even if these measures are different from those usually carried out in that institution. Without encouragement, the patient may hesitate to mention these possible remedies, for example, nonprescription liniments, special applications of heat and cold, unusual positioning, or favorite homemade foods or drinks.

If there are no contraindications to the remedy the patient wishes to try, the health care team may consider using it before trying other relief measures.

In some situations it may be appropriate for the patient to help plan the use of pain relief measures. For example, the patient may wish to receive parenteral analgesics at bedtime to improve sleep and to receive a less potent medication that causes less drowsiness before family members visit.

Planning for the same health care team members to care for the patient regularly should result in a more consistent approach and plan of care. Between the small group of health care team members and the patient, a plan of care can be developed in which the patient's decisions are honored, and a daily routine can be devised that will reduce anxiety and frustration about constant changes. This plan should include, if appropriate, such items as specified hours for analgesic administration before uncomfortable procedures, specified blocks of time for rest or napping, and coordination between various departments, such as physical therapy and occupational therapy. For some patients fatigue is a great problem, so regular visits to off-unit departments should be interspersed with rest periods; for other patients the most beneficial plan includes ensuring that they go directly from one department to the next so that time is not wasted getting in and out of bed or performing other painful maneuvers.

■ MEDICAL APPROACHES TO PAIN CONTROL

■ Medications

Medications can relieve pain in various ways. Any medication given to treat the cause of pain will decrease the pain. Pain can also be relieved by interfering with the transmission of the stimulus to alter perception and by decreasing cortical response to the pain. Some drugs, such as narcotics, will affect both perception and response.

■ NARCOTIC ANALGESICS

The opiates are most widely recognized and used for control of moderate to severe pain (Table 10-5). The effects of narcotics vary with the physiologic state of the patient. The very young and the very old are sensitive to the effects of narcotics and require smaller doses to obtain relief from pain. A person of any age may be more depressed physically and emotionally by narcotics during the early morning hours (1:00 to 6:00 AM) than at any other time of the day and should be watched carefully for untoward effects.

Narcotics can cause lowering of the blood pressure and general depression of vital functions, including respiratory depression, bradycardia, and drowsiness. Some of these reactions can be advantageous; for example, with hemorrhage some lowering of blood pressure may be desireable. Hypotension may be a disadvantage in the debilitated patient, who may go into shock from an excessive dosage of a drug. The narcotics are less likely to cause shock if the patient is up and moving about and taking food and fluids, because these activities tend to maintain the blood pressure at a safe level.

□ Concern for addiction

Narcotics are frequently underprescribed by physicians and underadministered by nurses because of concern for addiction. It is important to differentiate tolerance, dependence, and addiction, as summarized below:

Tolerance   Larger doses are needed to produce desired effects
Dependence   Need to continue use of drug to prevent symptoms
Addiction   Behavioral pattern of compulsive drug use, obtaining drug at any cost

Drug tolerance creates a problem in terms of pain relief over time when the stimulus persists or increases. This is

Table 10-5   Commonly used narcotics

Generic name	Trade name	Usual dosage*	Route	Onset	Peak	Duration
Morphine sulfate	—	5-20 mg q 3-4 hr	SC, IM	5-10 min	60 min	4-6 hr
Codeine sulfate	—	15-60 mg q 3-4 hr	SC, PO	5-30 min	30-60 min	3-4 hr
Hydromorphone hydrochloride	Dilaudid	2-4 mg q 4-6 hr	IV, IM, SC, PO	5-15 min	1 hr	4-6 hr
Meperidine hydrochloride	Demerol	50-150 mg q 3-4 hr	IV, IM, SC, PO	10-15 min	30-60 min	2-4 hr
Methadone	Dolophine	2.5-10 mg q 3-4 hr	IM, SC, PO	10 min	1-2 hr	4-6 hr
Pentazocine	Talwin	15-30 mg q 3-4 hr	IM, SC	10-30 min	1 hr	2-3 hr
		50-100 mg q 3-4 hr	PO			

*Must be individualized.

a physiologic response. Physical dependency, appearance of physiologic withdrawal symptoms, may occur if a narcotic is *suddenly* discontinued when a person has been receiving it for a week or more. This *rarely happens*, because as pain decreases the dosage is gradually tapered, and no symptoms are experienced. Physical dependency and drug tolerance are involuntary behaviors.

Persons receiving narcotics for relief of severe pain rarely develop addiction, which is a voluntary behavior. Fewer than 1% of all narcotic addicts in the United States become addicted during hospitalization.[65] Persons more likely to become addicted are those who seek the narcotic for the feeling of well-being it provides rather than for relief of pain.

Persons with moderate to severe acute pain should not be denied full pain control with narcotics. Control of *acute pain* is best achieved by giving smaller doses more frequently (such as 6 to 10 mg morphine sulfate every 3 to 4 hours). Relief of *cancer pain* is best achieved by giving larger doses less frequently (such as 10 to 25 mg morphine sulfate every 6 hours). The use of narcotics for relief of *persistent chronic pain* (other than for cancer) is controversial. In general, efforts are made to reduce narcotic intake and to substitute other analgesics.

Patient-controlled analgesia

One method of providing more adequate pain control with narcotics is the system of patient-controlled analgesia (PCA). The system consists of a syringe-type infusion pump that is filled with the prescribed narcotic and is piggybacked into an intravenous injection port.[56] PCA is activated when the patient pushes a button to release a set amount of narcotic by bolus. A refractory time prevents delivery of another bolus before a preset time interval. The device also records the patient's attempts to receive the narcotic in a given time period. The physician determines the narcotic dosage and the refractory time interval. The usual morphine dosage is 0.5 mg to 1.5 mg per bolus, and the usual refractory time is 5 to 10 minutes.[56]

Experience has demonstrated that persons using PCA tend to take less narcotic than those receiving the standard method of intramuscular injections.[21,51,56] PCA has been used for postoperative pain, for other types of acute pain such as sickle cell crisis, and for cancer pain. Nursing activities related to PCA include maintaining the system, recording the number of times the patient activates the system, and monitoring the patient's pain. The patient should be the only person who activates the PCA (presses the button); this serves as a safeguard to prevent oversedation.

■ NONNARCOTIC ANALGESICS

Mild to moderate pain can generally be controlled by nonnarcotic analgesics, most commonly aspirin, acetaminophen, and the nonsteroidal antiinflammatory agents (NSAIDs).

□ Aspirin

Acetylsalicylic acid (aspirin) is the most widely used analgesic for mild to moderate pain. Salicylates produce analgesia by blocking pain impulses peripherally or centrally, possibly in the hypothalamus, and by inhibiting synthesis of prostaglandins. Aspirin is therefore also an antiinflammatory agent. Aspirin has an onset of 15 to 20 minutes, peak of 1 to 2 hours, and duration of 3 to 4 hours.

Aspirin is a platelet aggregation inhibitor and a weak vitamin K antagonist. It produces an increased bleeding time and prolonged prothrombin time when given in large doses. Therefore, it is contraindicated for persons receiving anticoagulant drugs.

Irritation of the gastric mucosa is a common side effect of aspirin; therefore, it should not be taken on an empty stomach. Aspirin is best taken after meals or with a snack such as a glass of milk. Persons with a history of peptic ulcer should avoid taking aspirin. Aspirin should also be avoided by persons taking phenylbutazone and spironolactone because of drug interaction.

□ Acetaminophen

Acetaminophen (Tylenol, Datril) is comparable to aspirin for analgesic effects but is not antiinflammatory. It causes less alteration in prothrombin level and has fewer side effects but can cause severe liver damage. It is useful for persons who are allergic to aspirin and for whom aspirin is contraindicated.

■ NONSTEROIDAL ANTIINFLAMMATORY DRUGS

The nonsteroidal antiinflammatory drugs (NSAIDs) act primarily by inhibition of prostaglandin synthesis. In lower doses, these drugs have analgesic properties; in higher doses there is antiinflammatory action in addition to an-

---

Table 10-6 NSAIDs commonly used for mild to moderate pain

Generic name	Trade name	Dosage range
Fenoprofen	Nalfon	200 mg q 4-6 hr prn
Ibuprofen	Advil, Motrin	400 mg q 4-6 hr prn
Mefenamic acid	Ponstel	500 mg initially then 250 mg q 6 hr prn (not to exceed 7 days)
Naproxen	Anaprox, Naprosyn	550 mg initially, then 275 mg q 6-8 hr prn
Zomepirac	Zomax	50 to 100 mg q 4-6 hr prn

algesia. The principal uses of NSAIDs are control of moderate pain of dysmenorrhea, arthritis and other musculoskeletal disorders, postoperative pain, and migraine. NSAIDs commonly used for relief of mild to moderate pain are listed in Table 10-6.

NSAIDs, like aspirin, inhibit platelet aggregation with resulting increased bleeding time. Common side effects include gastrointestinal disturbances, dizziness, tinnitus, and headache. Persons who are hypersensitive to aspirin may also be hypersensitive to NSAIDs. Concurrent use of an NSAID with aspirin may lead to increased side effects.

Phenylbutazone (Butazolidin) is an NSAID with potent antiinflammatory properties given for short-term therapy for moderately severe arthritis, gout, or bursitis. Although the drug has analgesic activity, it is not used as a general analgesic for moderate pain because it is poorly tolerated by many persons and has numerous side effects, including hematologic changes, gastric irritation, and fluid and electrolyte disturbances.

OTHER DRUGS FOR PAIN RELIEF

Smooth muscle relaxants may be given for pain from muscle spasms and include propantheline bromide (Pro-Banthine) and drugs of the belladonna group, such as atropine. For example, belladonna and opium (B&O) suppositories are effective in relieving bladder spasms after prostatectomy.

Sedatives and antianxiety agents are sometimes prescribed for persons with pain. These drugs do *not* have analgesic effect but may permit relaxation and decrease anxiety and thus prevent potentiation of pain. The drugs may permit the person to sleep and thus be better able to cope with the pain. In some persons sedatives and antianxiety agents may lead to disorientation and agitation, which can increase the pain and decrease the person's ability to cope. Treating pain with analgesics is the more effective and preferred method.

Counterirritants are over-the-counter (OTC) drugs that relieve local pain by producing counterirritation (stimulation of the large A-delta fibers). Examples of counterirritants include ointments containing methyl salicylate (oil of wintergreen) or ethyl aminobenzoate and oil of cloves (for toothaches).

■ Electrical stimulators

The purpose of electrical stimulators is to modify the pain stimulus by blocking or changing the painful stimulus with stimulation perceived as less painful. The success of this approach is thought to be explained by the gate control theory of pain transmission, that is, blockage of pain stimulus by stimulation of the large sensory fibers. Selected forms of electrical stimulation may activate the opiate or nonopiate descending pathways (see the box below).

TRANSCUTANEOUS ELECTRICAL NERVE STIMULATOR

The transcutaneous electrical nerve stimulator (TENS) is a battery-powered stimulator worn externally. It is a convenient, nonintrusive, nonaddictive type of pain therapy that can be learned easily by the patient. Success is variable.

A number of TENS devices are on the market; all consist of a battery-powered portable pulse generator about the size of a pocket paging device. Control knobs on the generator permit adjustment of the impulse. The generator is connected by a pair of cables to electrically conductive tape electrodes placed at appropriate sites on the skin. The TENS delivers a balanced biphasic potential in a waveform. The more commonly used TENS settings follow[49]:

Pulse width	50 to 100 msec
Frequency	0 to 60
Current flows	20 to 30 ma
(voltage)	50 to 60 ma

TENS appears to be more useful for postoperative pain, posttraumatic pain, phantom limb pain, peripheral neuralgias, low back pain, and muscle and bone pain. It is less effective with cancer pain, inflammatory arthritis, trigeminal neuralgia, or with anxious or depressed persons.[54,57]

TENS electrodes should not be placed over hair, irritated skin, sutures, carotid sinus (may produce bradycar-

---

Methods of electrical stimulation for pain control

Transcutaneous electrical nerve stimulator (TENS)	Manually controlled stimulation of specific pain areas through externally placed electrodes
Percutaneous implanted spinal cord epidural stimulator (PISCES)	Stimulation by an external transistorized receiver of leads inserted percutaneously in epidural space of spinal column
Dorsal column stimulator	Stimulation by a transistorized receiver, implanted surgically in an infraclavicular or abdominal skin pouch, of electrodes surgically implanted on dorsum of spinal cord

dia), laryngeal or pharyngeal muscles (may trigger spasms), or a pregnant uterus.[52] A cardiac pacemaker may interfere with TENS effects. Suggested electrode placement may include (1) directly over the painful area, (2) at trigger points along the nerve pathways, or (3) at trigger points in the same dermatome as the pain.[43]

Routine skin care at the electrode sites includes the following:

1. Remove and clean electrodes at least once a day.
2. Wash skin with soap and water.
3. Allow skin to air dry.
4. Wipe skin with a prep pad before reapplying conductor pad.

If the skin becomes irritated, it may be cleaned with milk of magnesia, rinsed well, then air dried.[43]

■ SPINAL CORD STIMULATORS

Spinal cord stimulators are similar to the TENS except that they are intrusive procedures. Instead of electrode placement on the skin, the electrodes are placed on or near the spinal cord. This is done either surgically over the ventral surface of the spinal cord or percutaneously through the back into the epidural space. Because percutaneous placement of electrodes (PISCES) can be performed under local anesthesia, it is preferred over surgical placement of the dorsal column stimulator electrodes. Postoperative care after dorsal column stimulator implantation includes the same care that follows laminectomy, with monitoring for infection and leakage of cerebrospinal fluid (Chapter 22).

■ Neurosurgical procedures

Constant relentless chronic pain that cannot be controlled by analgesics (*intractable pain*) may be reduced or eliminated by one of various neurosurgical procedures (see Table 10-7 and Fig. 10-6). Other forms of pain control are usually attempted before neurosurgical procedures.

The neurosurgical procedures generally have not been successful. Major limitations include short duration of relief, occurrence of dysesthesia (pain induced by gentle touch of the skin), central pain syndrome (burning sensations in skin areas lacking sensation from surgical afferent interruptions), and possible further neurologic dysfunction.[49]

Neurectomy has limitations in that peripheral nerves may regenerate. Both rhizotomy and anterolateral cordotomy require laminectomy. A more commonly used procedure is percutaneous cordotomy, a closed stereotactic procedure in which the lesion is first located by using three-dimensional coordinates. The anterospinothalamic tracts are destroyed by electrodes inserted percutaneously. The patient is awake to provide feedback, thus providing more accurate site location and better pain relief. The effect usually lasts 18 to 24 months.[49]

Rhizotomy interferes with the ability to perceive heat and cold; therefore, protection from extremes in temperature is important for prevention of injury. The advantages of cordotomy include a wide sense of analgesia below the surgical site while preserving other sensory and motor functions. After surgery there may be temporary leg weakness and loss of bowel and bladder control from edema of the spinal cord; these usually disappear within 2 weeks. If quadriceps setting exercises are begun in the early postoperative period, walking will be less difficult.

Pain pathways in the brain may also be interrupted by stereotactic techniques (tractotomy, thalamotomy, lobotomy). These surgical procedures are usually reserved as a final solution for patients with intractable pain, usually from malignant invasion of cranial or facial structures. Lobotomy usually results in a change in personality.

■ Nerve block

A nerve block involves the injection of substances such as local anesthetics or neurolytic agents (for example, alcohol or phenol) close to nerves to block the conduction of impulses over the nerves. Nerve blocks are frequently used for the symptomatic relief of pain. They are used to treat chronic pain associated with peripheral vascular disease, trigeminal neuralgia, causalgia, and cancer.

A nerve block may be unsuccessful because of difficulty in locating the correct nerve fiber or because of the com-

Table 10-7 Neurosurgical procedures for pain control

Procedure	Method	Use
Neurectomy	Severing of nerve fibers from the cell body	Trigeminal neuralgia (fifth nerve resection); incapacitating dysmenorrhea (presacral neurectomy)
Rhizotomy	Resection of posterior nerve root before it enters spinal cord	Severe pain in upper trunk (for example, lung cancer)
Cordotomy	Severing of ascending anterolateral pain-conducting pathways of spinal cord	Severe pain of lower body (for example, pelvic cancer)
Sympathectomy	Excision or destruction of one or more sympathetic ganglia or nerves	Pain secondary to vascular insufficiency of extremities (for example, Raynaud's disease)

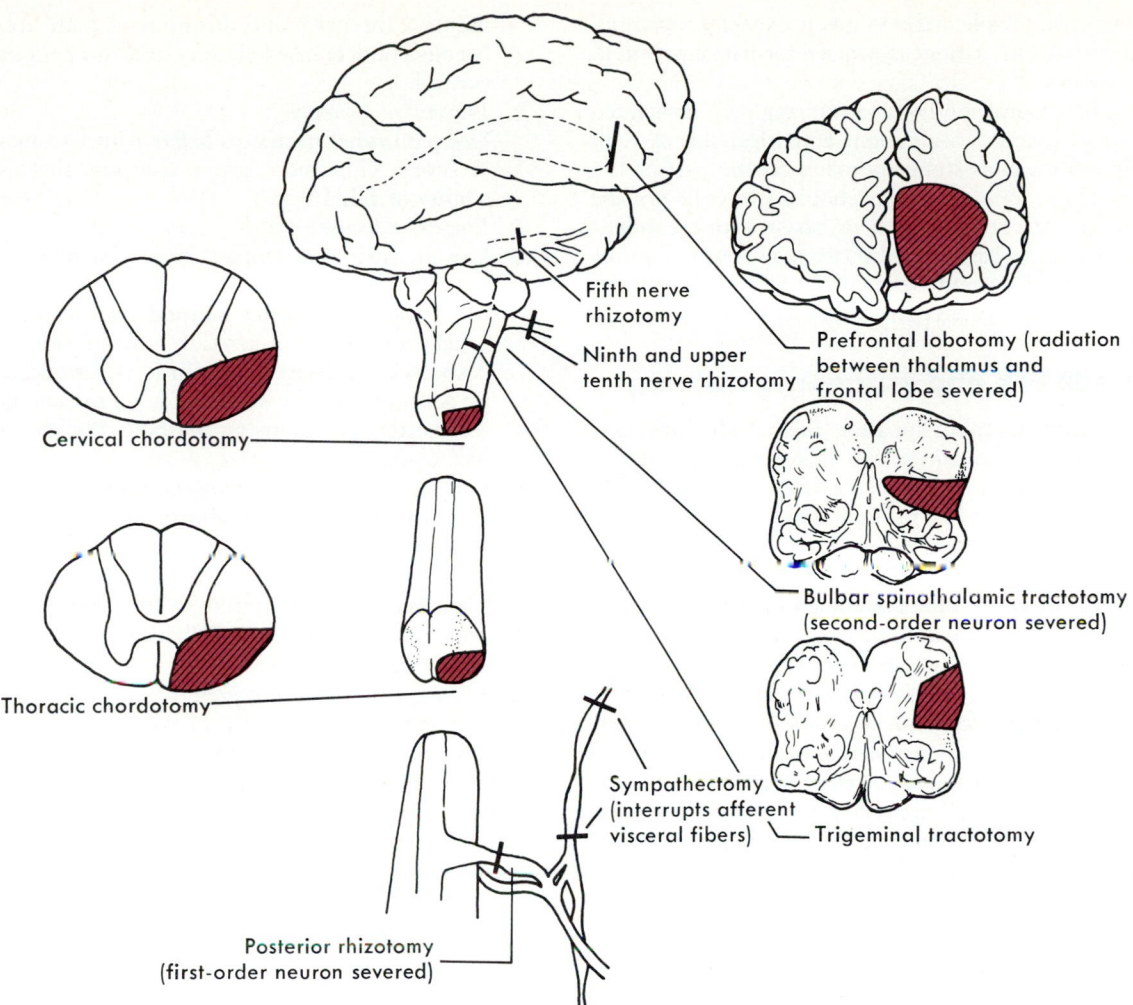

Fifth nerve
rhizotomy

Ninth and upper
tenth nerve rhizotomy

Prefrontal lobotomy (radiation
between thalamus and
frontal lobe severed)

Cervical chordotomy

Thoracic chordotomy

Bulbar spinothalamic tractotomy
(second-order neuron severed)

Sympathectomy
(interrupts afferent
visceral fibers)

Trigeminal tractotomy

Posterior rhizotomy
(first-order neuron severed)

Fig. 10-6 Neurosurgical procedures for pain relief. (From Conway-Rutkowski, BL: Carini and Owens' neurological and neurosurgical nursing, ed 8, St. Louis, 1984, The CV Mosby Co.)

plexity of the pain. Because the nerve fibers, ganglia, and roots contain fibers other than those for pain, and because some of the injected agents may leak out of the injection site and affect other nerves, the nerve block usually produces some other type of neurologic deficit.

■ Acupuncture

Acupuncture is an ancient form of disease treatment that can be used for pain relief. Only recently has the method been used in Western countries. Small needles are skillfully inserted and manipulated at specific body points, depending on the type and location of pain. The gate control theory provides the best explanation for the success of acupuncture: the local stimulation of large-diameter fibers by the needles "closes the gate" to pain. It is not known to what extent the psyche and the power of suggestion contribute to the effectiveness of this therapy. Nursing intervention includes careful client assessment and teaching.

■ PSYCHOLOGIC APPROACHES FOR PAIN CONTROL

■ Behavior modification

Behavior modification consists of a planned change in the way a person behaves by means of rewarding desired behavior and ignoring undesirable behavior. Forms of behavior modification are used unconsciously all the time: a young boy "throwing a tantrum" may be ignored, but as his behavior becomes more appropriate his mother may reward him with her time and attention.

Behavior modification may be useful for persons with chronic pain. For example, one protocol for patients with chronic low back pain is to set a limit of 10 minutes daily for discussion of their pain experiences (with the exception of data-gathering interviews). Pain medications are given on a regular schedule to dissociate the feelings of pain with inappropriate use (reward) of analgesics or other unhealthy behaviors. The medication can be refused, but no additional or stronger medication is given except acetaminophen or aspirin. The patient is praised for participating in desired activities.

In using behavioral methods in altering pain-associated behavior or in encouraging patient activities, success will occur only with a consistent approach on the part of the health care team. While patients should always be praised for their efforts to comply with or assist with treatment regimens, a true behavior modification program requires careful analysis of patient behavior and the development of a specific and comprehensive treatment plan.[12]

■ Biofeedback and autogenic training

Some persons are able to alter their body functions through mental concentration. In biofeedback training a machine that monitors brain wave activity (electroencephalograph [EEG]) is used. The individual concentrates on slowing his or her brain wave activity to rates at which pain and distress are unlikely to cause discomfort (that is, complete relaxation). It may take many months of regular practice to achieve the desired level of control. The nurse should encourage and praise the person's efforts.

In autogenic training the same type of self-regulation is used to alter various autonomic nervous system functions, such as pulse, blood pressure, and muscle tension. Practiced use of transcendental meditation and other methods of concentration and self-control may achieve the same degree of autoregulation without the use of sophisticated physiologic monitoring equipment.

■ Hypnosis

Hypnosis may be used in the treatment of various conditions, particularly when these conditions are aggravated by tension and stress. Individuals are helped to alter their perception of pain through the acceptance of positive suggestions made to the subconscious. Many persons are able to learn self-hypnosis. Individuals vary in their suggestibility and readiness to try this approach. The nurse's most helpful role may be to support the patient's desire to make hypnotism work.

■ NURSING APPROACHES FOR PAIN CONTROL

Specific nursing interventions for pain relief include those related to preventing pain, modifying the stimulus, and modifying the response to pain. General guidelines for pain relief are listed here.

■ Guidelines for pain relief measures

1. *Preparation for painful experiences*
   Prepare patients for what to expect in terms of discomfort and measures of pain control *before* pain occurs, whenever possible (such as before painful tests or treat-

ments). Intensity and duration of pain are decreased because of decreased anxiety and the patient's sense of control.

2. *Preventive approach*
   Use pain relief measures *before* pain becomes moderate or severe. The more severe the pain the less the possibility of relief.

3. *Placebo response*
   Use methods that employ a placebo response, that is, some relief from discomfort not related specifically to the applied pain relief method. If the person expects relief from the pain, anxiety and muscle tension will decrease, and decreased pain is experienced. This can be accomplished by suggestion ("This should help you feel better") or by using methods the patient believes will work.

4. *Patient's ability or will to participate*
   Consider the patient's ability or will to be active or passive in using pain relief measures.[65] Decreased ability results from severe pain, fatigue, sedation, or unconsciousness. Decreased will occurs with some persons with chronic pain who have experienced numerous failures in pain relief.

5. *Varying pain relief measures*
   Use more than one type of pain relief measure when appropriate. For example, give an analgesic, rub the patient's back, and then offer some distraction, or combine an analgesic with relaxation response.

6. *Introducing new pain relief measures*
   Introduce a new method in combination with known effective methods. Some measures, such as distraction or relaxation, require practice; do not discard the new method until after several tries.

7. *Giving analgesics*
   a. Give analgesics before pain becomes severe.
   b. Determine which patients are at high risk for developing pain and assess them frequently for presence of increasing pain.
   c. Consider giving narcotics for a limited time (for example, 24 to 48 hours) on a regular basis rather than as needed when acute severe pain is anticipated, such as after some general surgical procedures.
   d. If the medication will be given "as needed," instruct the patient to report the presence of developing or recurrent pain.
   e. Use the parenteral route in acute intermittent pain to provide immediate, short-term relief.
   f. Use the oral route, when possible, in chronic unfluctuating pain to provide more sustained relief.[15]
   g. Report signs of undermedication to the physician (patient who watches the clock, waiting for the next dose, or patient who states having pain before next dose is due).
   h. When a variable analgesic dose and time schedule is prescribed, avoid the roller coaster effect (using wide variations in dose and timing), providing inconsistent pain relief.
   i. Assess and record the effectiveness of analgesics given.

■ Preventing pain

Although in many instances pain cannot be prevented, it is often possible to avoid additional pain when pain is already present. For example, when moving the body or an extremity, supporting the trunk or extremity will prevent increasing the pain by unilateral pulling on muscles, joints, and ligaments. Interventions include the following list:

1. Using a turning sheet for patients with severe neck, back, or general trunk pain
2. Placing a pillow under a painful joint when helping a patient change position
3. Supporting limbs at the joints rather than the muscle bellies when handling an extremity
4. Using special beds (Stryker frame, Foster bed, CircOlectric bed) for patients with severe general or trunk pain
5. Avoiding bumping or moving the bed suddenly

■ Modifying the pain stimulus

■ CUTANEOUS STIMULATION

Cutaneous stimulation innervates the large A-delta fibers to block the pain stimuli across the small C fibers. Methods of cutaneous stimulation include the following:

1. Lightly rubbing the affected area
2. Back rub
3. Application of heat or cold
4. Whirlpool massage

■ REDUCTION OF NOISE AND VISUAL STIMULI

The patient may experience sensory overload with subsequent potentiation of pain stimuli. If nurses could stand still for 5 minutes in the patient's environment and watch and listen, they might understand that some patients are simply bombarded with noise and visual stimulation. If these are problems, it may be possible to change the environment. Changes include the following:

1. Move the patient to a quieter room away from the center of activity.
2. Dim any bright lights; pull shades if sunlight is intense.
3. Keep verbal interactions at a minimum when pain is severe.
4. Keep television or radio at a reasonable level but not loud.
5. Control the number of persons entering the patient's room according to patient's wishes.

■ REDUCTION OF SOCIAL ISOLATION

When external stimuli are decreased too much, the patient may lack distraction from the pain stimuli; thus pain perception is increased. Social isolation may occur for a variety of reasons: the serious nature of a patient's disease may necessitate being in a private room for an extended period; hospitalization far away from home may mean few family members and friends can visit; extended periods of hospitalization may result in friends losing interest in visiting; or the patient may complain so much that no one cares to visit to hear the monologue repeated.

Each of these causes of isolation may have a different solution. In any event, careful assessment may indicate that social isolation is a problem for the patient. Before determining the plan for addressing this problem, the patient should be consulted about the desire and need to alter the present situation. Possible nursing interventions include the following:

1. Placing the patient with a compatible roommate
2. Planning for frequent contacts with health team members
3. Facilitating visits by family and friends
4. Helping patient to be as comfortable as possible during visits by family or friends

■ THERAPEUTIC TOUCH

A less traditional therapy, that of therapeutic touch, may be helpful to patients in pain. The rationale for the success of therapeutic touch is not clearly understood. The nurse undergoes a brief period of meditation before coming in contact with the patient. During this period the nurse quiets his or her internal energy levels and then touches the patient and transmits the healing energies. Few nurses are trained in the use of therapeutic touch as described. It does seem to be helpful for some patients and some kinds of pain.

■ DISTRACTION AND RELAXATION EXERCISES

Patients can be taught to modify their sensory input to control pain by activities that promote distraction or relaxation.

□ Distraction

Distraction interferes with the pain stimulus, thereby modifying the awareness of the pain. Mild or moderate pain can be modified by focusing on activity in the environment. A very quiet environment providing little or no sensory input can actually intensify the pain experience because the individual has nothing to focus on but the painful stimulus.

Severe pain requires more active participation by the individual in an effort to block out the painful stimulus. This can be enhanced by involving two or more sensory modalities, such as vision, hearing, touch, or movement. The distractors must be powerful enough to involve the individual's total interest without resulting in fatigue. Pain of long duration requires a variety of meaningful distracters. Methods of distraction include the following:

1. Playing games, watching television
2. Talking with someone
3. Listening to favorite music
4. Rhythmic breathing
5. Focusing on an object

□ Waking-imagined analgesia

Waking-imagined analgesia is defined as imagining a pleasant situation when a noxious stimulus is applied.[65] This intervention is similar to distraction except that the person concentrates on trying to relive the sensations that occurred during a previous pleasant experience rather than on enumerating the events that took place. Only a small percentage of the population in pain can use this method of analgesia; more can derive benefit from distraction alone.

□ Relaxation

Full relaxation decreases muscle tension and fatigue that usually accompanies pain. It also helps to decrease anxiety, thereby preventing augmentation of the pain stimulus. Carrying out relaxation techniques also serves as a form of distraction.

Not all persons with severe pain are able to achieve sufficient relaxation to have an effect on decreasing the pain sensation. Relaxation exercises may be especially beneficial for persons with chronic pain to help reduce stress that exacerbates the pain and to help the person achieve a sense of control, of being better able to cope with the pain.

There are numerous forms of relaxation techniques. Two techniques, Progressive Relaxation and Benson's Relaxation Response, are described in Chapter 7. Success with a relaxation technique requires practice and encouragement.

■ Modifying the pain response

■ EXPLANATION OF THE PROBLEM

As a result of nursing assessment, it may become clear that the patient's response to pain is really the manifestation of a lack of knowledge about the cause of the pain. Sometimes a simple explanation about what is causing the pain and how long it will last is all that is necessary. Understanding that pain or discomfort is to be expected may relieve anxiety or help the patient to alter expectations and be better prepared for what will happen. In all cases, an explanation that includes information about pain is given before each diagnostic test.

■ DECREASING ANXIETY

Because anxiety increases pain, measures taken to decrease anxiety may help to decrease pain (see Chapter 7 for a discussion of anxiety). Interventions for the patient with pain include the following:
1. Maintain a calm, quiet manner.
2. Help the patient explore concerns related to the pain (meaning of pain for the patient).
3. Respect the patient's response to pain, even if it differs considerably from what the nurse expects.
4. Hold the patient's hand, if appropriate.
5. Arrange for someone to be with the patient if the patient fears being alone.
6. Talk with family or close friends and help them to allay their anxieties so these are not transmitted to the patient.
7. Teach the family and close friends ways in which they can help the patient, such as massage, encouraging the patient to use distraction or relaxation techniques, or supporting painful parts when moving. People often feel helpless when observing a loved one in pain.

■ TEAM APPROACH FOR CHRONIC PAIN CONTROL

In recent years knowledge of the nature of chronic pain and the need for coordinated efforts of different health care professionals have resulted in the establishment of pain clinics and inpatient pain teams for control of chronic pain.

■ Pain clinics

Most pain clinics use a team approach that includes physicians (internists, dolorologists [pain specialists], surgeons, psychiatrists), nurses, physical and occupational therapists, social workers, psychologists, vocational rehabilitation counselors, and appropriate others. Each pain clinic is organized differently and places greater emphasis on different aspects of pain relief. Usual approaches to pain relief include the following:
1. Behavior modification (with patient's approval)
2. Medications: pain cocktail given at a scheduled time (not pain related) with decreasing amounts of medication
3. Exercise and activity prescriptions
4. Family training to support planned goals/activities.

The responsibility of the nurse varies depending on the available team members and may include patient assessment, documentation of observations, creating and maintaining a therapeutic milieu, providing emotional support for patient and family, and patient teaching. Nurses who work in pain clinics must be skilled in nurse-client interactions, be knowledgeable about the mechanisms of pain and the effectiveness of various treatment modalities, and possess patience and understanding as they assist patients in reaching their goals.

■ Inpatient chronic pain teams

Persons with chronic persistent pain are sometimes admitted to a hospital for evaluation or initiation of treatment by a multidisciplinary health team similar to that in a pain clinic. One example is a team for evaluation and treatment of chronic back pain. Each team member participates in the evaluation individually and collectively and in team conferences to develop a specific treatment plan. The culmination of the hospitalization is a discharge conference with the patient and family members in which future treatment plans and recommendations are presented and discussed.

Protocols are developed for the approach to be used in control of the chronic pain; all persons providing patient care during the hospitalization need to become familiar with the protocols so that a consistent approach is used for pain control. For example, protocols for control of chronic back pain in one large medical center include an initial immobilization phase in which patients are placed in pelvic traction and instructed to move as little as possible (for example, eat in side-lying position). This phase is followed by a mobilization phase in which the patients are encouraged to be active (for example, walk to physical therapy and to the cafeteria for meals and make their own beds). The type of nursing care is therefore different depending on which phase is being implemented.

Nursing responsibilities include patient assessment, documenting observations, carrying out phase-related activities, carrying out designated behavior modification modalities, and patient teaching.

✚ EVALUATION

Evaluation is an important component that is often forgotten in the care of the patient with pain. It is vital that the effectiveness of the interventions should be continued, modified, replaced with another intervention, or discontinued. The essential questions in *acute* pain are as follows.

Does the patient still have pain?

If so, how does it compare with the pain experienced before the intervention?

If it is better but still present, should the same intervention(s) be continued unchanged or modified?

Should new interventions be added?

If it is not better, were sufficient data obtained in the initial assessment to determine the cause of pain?

Are there new data to indicate a different diagnosis?

What are the patient's thoughts about the continuing pain and the modes of intervention?

One method of assessing the extent of *pain relief* is to ask the patient to rate the pain relief on a scale of 0 to 4 (0, no relief; 1, slight relief; 2, moderate relief, 3, considerable relief; 4, complete relief, no pain). The answers can be documented on a flow chart to provide an ongoing assessment of effectiveness of pain relief. The essential questions for *chronic* pain are as follows:

To what extent is the patient participating in the planned therapeutic program?

What is the patient's assessment of present pain?

Pain teams often have special evaluation guidelines specific to their patient population and treatment goals.

■ SUMMARY

1. Pain is a complex universal, yet individualized, experience.
2. Nociceptors are pain receptors that respond to chemical, thermal, electrical, or mechanical stimuli. Chemical stimuli released by damaged tissues include histamines, bradykinins, prostaglandins, and acids.
3. Pain impulses are transmitted over fast A-delta and slow C fibers to the substantia gelatinosa (SG) of the dorsal horn of the spinal cord. Ascending spinal pathways in the ventral spinal cord carry impulses to the thalamus and cortex.
4. Some descending spinal pathways carry pain suppressive (opiate and nonopiate) impulses back to the SG. Pain impulses transmitted over A-delta fibers also have a suppressive effect on impulses over the C fibers.
5. Substance P is a neurotransmitter of pain impulses. Endorphins and serotonin are neurotransmitters of pain-suppressive impulses.
6. The gate control theory proposes that the SG is a gating mechanism that may modify the pain experience by "opening" or "closing" the gate to pain impulse transmission. The gating mechanism is influenced by impulses from A-delta and C fibers and from descending pathways from the brainstem and cortex.
7. The pain experience is influenced by the meaning of the pain for the person, pain perception, pain tolerance, and reaction to pain.
8. Pain perception is subjective, highly complex, and individual. It is influenced by characteristics of the pain stimuli and transmission and by receptivity and interpretation in the cerebral cortex.
9. Pain threshold is the intensity of the stimulus necessary for the person to perceive pain.
10. Pain tolerance is the intensity of the pain the person is willing to endure before seeking relief. Pain tolerance may be increased by drugs, warmth, counterirritation, distraction, and strong beliefs; it may be decreased by fatigue, anxiety, boredom, continuous pain, or illness.
11. Reaction to pain is influenced by the degree of pain perception, past experiences, sociocultural values, health status, anxiety, and age.
12. Acute pain is a sudden short-term event, usually with a known source and self-limiting or readily corrected. The typical clinical signs are usually present and pain areas generally well identified. It leads to action to relieve pain with likelihood of eventual relief. Acute pain is characterized by anxiety and muscle tension.
13. Chronic pain is a prolonged situation, often with an unknown source. Pain areas are less easily defined. Pain may be continuous or intermittent and with few typical clinical signs. It leads to actions to modify the pain experience. Chronic pain is characterized by increased preoccupation with pain, hopelessness, and irritability, all leading to withdrawal.
14. Superficial somatic pain is sharp and pricking, well localized, and usually not accompanied by autonomic reactions. Deep somatic and visceral pain are sharp or dull and aching, poorly localized, and usually accompanied by autonomic reactions.
15. Referred pain is felt in areas other than those stimulated; it is usually visceral in origin.
16. Phantom limb pain is perceived to be occurring in a limb that has been amputated.
17. Pain intensity can be determined by the use of pain scales or visual analog scales in addition to asking the person to describe the pain.

Putting knowledge to practice

■ Why is it important to differentiate acute and chronic pain? Think about two patients for whom you have provided care, one with acute pain and one with chronic pain. In what ways did and should care have differed?

■ Which type of data, subjective or objective, are more valid in diagnosing pain? Explain.

■ Collect subjective and objective data on two of your patients who are experiencing pain, using the assessment parameters described in this chapter. What are the similarities and differences in their experiences with pain? What specific factors are involved? How would your nursing interventions differ?

■ If a patient has moderate or severe acute pain, should the prescribed narcotic be delayed because of concern for addiction? Explain.

■ How do the following terms differ: Pain tolerance and pain threshold? Pain tolerance and drug tolerance? Drug dependence and drug addiction?

■ Interview three or four patients using TENS. Compare and contrast the form of therapy (electrical stimulation frequency and intensity), frequency of use, and effectiveness of therapy.

■ Examine the chart of a patient receiving PCA. How does the narcotic dosage received compare with that of standard prescriptions?

18. Subjective data for pain include the location, intensity, quality, timing (onset, duration, frequency, cause), and provoking or palliative factors.

19. Objective data include appearance, motor behavior, affective and verbal response, vital signs, skin color and moisture, and inspection and palpation of painful areas.

20. Narcotics provide relief of moderate to severe pain. Persons with severe pain rarely develop narcotic addiction. Smaller, more frequent dosages of narcotics are more effective for severe acute pain, whereas larger, less frequent dosages are more effective for severe cancer pain.

21. Patient-controlled analgesia is a system of self-administration by an intravenous setup whereby a prescribed preset bolus of narcotic may be taken but not repeated until a prescribed refractory time has occurred.

22. Aspirin, acetaminophen, and NSAIDs provide relief of mild to moderate pain.

23. Electrical stimulators include TENS and spinal cord stimulators. TENS is a nonintrusive system, easily learned by the patient and useful for postoperative, posttraumatic, peripheral neuralgia, and muscle and bone pain.

24. Psychologic approaches for pain control include behavior modification, biofeedback and autogenic training, and hypnosis.

25. General nursing interventions for pain relief include preparing patients for painful experiences, using pain relief measures before pain becomes severe, using the placebo response, varying pain relief measures, trying new approaches, and giving analgesics as effectively as possible.

26. Specific nursing interventions for pain relief include preventing pain when possible; modifying the pain stimulus by cutaneous stimulation, reduction of noise and visual stimuli, decreasing social isolation, therapeutic touch, distraction, and relaxation exercises; and modifying the pain response by careful explanations and measures to decrease anxiety.

REFERENCES AND SELECTED READINGS
Contemporary

1. *Alberico, JB: Breaking the chronic pain cycle, Am J Nurs 84:1222-1225, 1984.
2. Aronoff, GM (editor): Evaluation and treatment of chronic pain, Baltimore, 1985, Urban & Schwarzenberg.
3. *Bast, C, and Hayes, P: PCA: a new way to spell pain relief: patient controlled analgesia, RN 49(8):18-20, 1986.
4. *Beyerman, K: Flawed perceptions about pain, Am J Nurs 82:302-304, 1982.
5. *Boguslawski, M: Therapeutic touch: a facilitator of pain relief, Top Clin Nurs 2:27-37, 1980.
6. Bond, MR: Pain: its nature, analysis and treatment, ed 2, New York, 1984, Churchill Livingstone.
7. *Booker, JE: Pain: it's all in your head (or is it?) Nurs 82 12(3):46-51, 1982.
8. Casey, KL: Neural mechanisms of pain, an overview, Acta Anesth Scand 74(Suppl):13-20, 1982.
9. *Copp, LA (editor): Recent advances in nursing. Perspectives and pain, New York, 1985, Churchill Livingstone.
10. Crue, BL: The neurophysiology and taxonomy of pain. In Brena, SF, and Chapman, SL (editors): Management of patients with chronic pain, New York, 1983, SP Medical and Scientific Books.
11. *Cummings, D: Stopping chronic pain before it starts, Nurs 81 11(1):60-63, 1981.
12. Dernham, P: Phantom limb pain, Geriatric Nurs 7:34-37, 1986.

*References preceded by an asterisk are particularly well suited for student reading.

13. *Donovan, MI: Relaxation with guided imagery: a useful technique, Cancer Nurs 3:27-32, 1980.
14. *Fordham, M: Neurophysiological pain theories, Nursing (London) 3:365-372, 1986.
15. *Fordham, M: Psychophysiologic pain theories, Nursing (London) 3:360-364, 1986.
16. *Friedman, FB: PRN analgesics: controlling the pain or controlling the patient? RN 46(3):67, 1983.
17. Ganong, WF: Review of medical physiology, ed 12, Norwalk, Conn, 1985, Appleton & Lange.
18. *Goldfrank, L, Bresnitz, E, and Weisman, R: Opiods and opiates, Heart Lung 12:114-116, 1983.
19. Gorman, ES, and Warfield, CA: The use of opioids in the management of pain, Hosp Pract 21(6):48A-48H, 1986.
20. *Grainger, S: No cause, no cure—but he's still in pain, RN 50(2):43-45, 1987.
21. Graves, DA, and others: Patient-controlled analgesia, Ann Int Med 99:360-365, 1983.
22. *Heidrich, G, and Perry, S: Helping the patient in pain, Am J Nurs 82:1828-1833, 1982.
23. *Holderby, RA: Conscious suggestion: using talk to manage pain, Nurs 81 11(5):44-46, 1981.
24. Huhman, M: Endogenous opiates and pain, ANS 4(4):62-71, 1982.
25. Krupp, MA, Schroeder, SA, and Tierney, LM: Current medical diagnosis and treatment 1987, Norwalk, Conn, 1987, Appleton & Lange.
26. Lasagna, L: Pain and its management, Hosp Pract 21(10):92C-92Y, 1986.
27. Levine, J: Pain and analgesia: the outlook for more rational treatment, Ann Intern Med 100:269-276, 1984.
28. *McCaffery, M: How to relieve your patient's pain: fast and effectively . . . with oral analgesics, Nurs 80 10(11):58-63, 1980.
29. *McCaffery, M: Patients shouldn't have to suffer: how to relieve pain with injectable narcotics, Nurs 80 10(10):34-39, 1980.
30. *McCaffery, M: Relieving pain with noninvasive techniques, Nurs 80 10(9):26-31, 1980.
31. *McCaffery, M: When your patient's still in pain, don't just do something, sit there, Nurs 81 11(6):58-61, 1981.
32. *McCaffery, M: Would you administer placebos for pain? Nurs 82 12(2):80-85, 1982.
33. *McCaffery, M: Problems with meperidine, Am J Nurs 84:525, 1984.
34. *McCaffery, M: Giving meperidine for pain: should it be so mechanical? Nurs 87 17(4):61-64, 1987.
35. McDonnell, DE: TENS in treating chronic pain, AORN J 32:401-410, 1980.
36. McGuire, DB (editor): Cancer pain seminar, Sem Oncol Nurs 1:81-150, 1987.
37. *McGuire, L, Dizard, S, and Panayotoff, K: Managing pain: in the young patient . . . in the elderly patient, Nurs 82 12(8):52-57, 1982.
38. *McGuire, L, and Wright, A: Continuous narcotic infusion, Nurs 84 14(12):50-55, 1984.
39. Meinhart, NT, and McCaffrey, M: Pain: a nursing approach to assessment and analysis, Norwalk, Conn, 1983, Appleton-Century-Crofts.
40. *Meissner, JE: McGill-Melzak pain questionnaire, Nurs 80 10(1):50-51, 1980.
41. Melzack, R, and Wall, PD: The challenge of pain, New York, 1983, Basic Books, Inc.
42. *Meyer, TM: TENS: relieving pain through electricity, Nurs 82 12(9):57-59, 1982.
43. *Moore, DE, and Blacker, HM: How effective is TENS for chronic pain? Am J Nurs 83:1175-1177, 1983.
44. Mountcastle, VB (editor): Medical physiology, ed 14, St. Louis, 1980, The CV Mosby Co.
45. *Olsson, G, and Parker, G: A model approach to pain assessment, Nurs 87 17(5):52-57, 1987.
46. *Panayotoff, K: Managing pain in the elderly patient, Nurs 82 12(8):53-55, 1982.
47. Pearson, BD: Pain control: an experiment in imagery, Geriatric Nurs 8:28-30, 1987.
48. *Rogers, AG: What to expect from the most common analgesics, RN 46(5):44-46, 1983.
49. Rudy, EB: Advanced neurological and neurosurgical nursing, St. Louis, 1984, The CV Mosby Co.
50. Sheehy, SB, and Barber, J: Emergency nursing: principles and practice, ed 2, St. Louis, 1985, The CV Mosby Co.
51. Tamsen A, and others: Patient-controlled analgesic therapy: clinical experience, Acta Anaesth Scand 74(Suppl):157-160, 1982.
52. *Taylor, AG, and others: How effective is TENS for acute pain? Am J Nurs 83:1171-1174, 1983.
53. Todd, B: Narcotic analgesia for chronic pain: drugs and the elderly, Geriatric Nurs 7:53-55, 1986.
54. Tyler, ET, Caldwell, C, and Ghia, JN: Transcutaneous electrical nerve stimulation, Anesth Analg 81:449-455, 1982.
55. Wall, PD, and Melzack, R (editors): Textbook of pain, New York, 1984, Churchill Livingstone.
56. Warfield, CA: Patient-controlled analgesia, Hosp Pract 20:32L-32P, 1985.
57. Warfield, CA, and Stein, JM: Pain relief by electrical stimulation, Hosp Pract 18:207-218, 1983.
58. Watkins, LR, and Mayer, DJ: Organization of endogenous opiate and nonopiate pain control systems, Science 216:1185-1192, 1982.
59. *West, BA: Understanding endorphins: our natural pain relief system, Nurs 81 11(2):50-53, 1984.
60. Whitman, HH: Sublingual morphine, a novel route of narcotic administration, Am J Nurs 84:939, 1984.
61. *Wilson, RW, and Elmassian, BJ: Endorphins, Am J Nurs 81:722-725, 1981.
62. Wolf, ZR: Pain theories: an overview, Top Clin Nurs 2:9-18, 1980.
63. Wright, Z: From I.V. to P.O.: titrating your patient's pain medication, Nurs 81 11(7):38-43, 1981.

Classic

64. *Davitz, LJ, Sameshima, Y, and Davitz, J: Suffering as viewed in six different cultures, Am J Nurs 76:1296-1297, 1978.
65. McCaffery, M: Nursing management of the patient with pain, ed 2, Philadelphia, 1979, JB Lippincott Co.
66. Sternback, RA (editor): The psychology of pain, New York, 1978, Raven Press.

11

Infection Control

GRACE A. ROTTER, DORA RICE, and ELIZABETH CAMERON ECKSTEIN

CHAPTER OBJECTIVES

After studying this chapter, the student should be able to:

- Describe the chain of infection.

- Identify high-risk factors for infection.

- Describe white blood cell response to infection.

- Identify community approaches to infection control and describe immunization programs.

- Define nosocomial infections and measures of prevention and control (bacteremia, urinary, wound, and respiratory infections).

- Identify two systems of isolation precautions and describe general approaches for each.

■ HISTORICAL PERSPECTIVE

Infection control has become a recognized discipline only in the last decade, although the principles governing it have been in existence for some time. In the middle of the nineteenth century Semmelweiss, an obstetrician in Vienna, demonstrated the significance of hand washing in combating the transmission of infection. He showed that when the students and physicians were required to wash their hands and rinse them in a chlorinated lime solution before a delivery, the incidence of puerperal fever decreased markedly. The idea that hand washing alone could prevent the spread of disease met with much opposition by his colleagues. Better acceptance came after Pasteur, Lister, and Koch developed the germ theory of disease and related asepsis to the prevention of the spread of disease. At about the same time, Nightingale made significant contributions to sanitation and isolation practices. From this evolved an era in which medical asepsis was practiced more by ritual than with the true understanding of the scientific principles on which it was based.

A turning point came during World War II when the sulfonamides and penicillin were first used successfully to treat infections. As new antibiotics were developed, a false sense of security developed about infection control. It soon became apparent, however, that antibiotics were not the sole answer to infection control. Organisms, once well controlled by antibiotics, demonstrated the ability to develop resistant strains. In the late 1950s and the 1960s outbreaks of penicillin-resistant *Staphylococcus aureus* infections were common, and gram-negative organisms such as *Pseudomonas,* which were previously considered nonpathogenic (incapable of producing disease), were suddenly implicated as the cause of infections acquired in the hospital. Along with drug resistance and the emergence of newly recognized pathogens came an increase in the number of persons at risk for secondary infections. An increase in life expectancy, the use of immunosuppressive agents, and an increase in the use of invasive procedures to diagnose and treat disease all increased the risk of infection in certain persons.

The rise in the number of hospital infections made apparent the need to examine preventive and control measures, including a reemphasis on aseptic techniques. In 1970 an international conference to address the problem of hospital-acquired infections was held in Atlanta. As a result, the Centers for Disease Control (CDC) in Atlanta set forth guidelines for prevention and control of infections in hospitals. The CDC is constantly updating and revising its recommendations based on epidemiologic studies and research findings. The American Hospital Association (AHA) and the Joint Commission on Accreditation of Hospitals (JCAH), a major private accrediting agency, looked at the ethical and economic issues concerning hospital-acquired (nosocomial) infections and established standards for programs in infection control. The purpose of these programs was to decrease morbidity and mortality of infections, as well as to reduce the cost of infections that could have been prevented. Consumer awareness of the problem also contributed to the attention given the issue of infection control. In the early 1970s only 10% of U.S. hospitals had infection surveillance and control programs; by the end of the decade nearly all had them.

The field of infection control is a challenging one, with the identification of new pathogens (for example, human immunodeficiency virus or HIV) and advances in research uncovering new information that may change current thinking and practices. Infection control practitioners (ICPs) serve as a valuable resource, since they interact with virtually every department in a hospital as they survey for infections and teach staff how to prevent and control infection. The ICP is an important link between personnel from various hospital departments. When there is a question or problem regarding infection control, the ICP should be called on without hesitation.

The current epidemic of acquired immunodeficiency syndrome (AIDS), caused by the HIV, has presented infection control practitioners with the challenge to develop a system of isolation that would prevent transmission of this and other frequently undiagnosed infections in health care settings and the community. Body substance isolation (BSI) is a new system developed by ICPs Jackson and Lynch. This system emphasizes universal precautions when in contact with the body fluids of all patients.

This chapter presents an overview of the role of the nurse in the prevention and control of infection. For further information regarding a specific infectious disease, the reader should consult the chapter in which the site of the disease is discussed, for example, Chapter 31 for hepatitis, Chapter 25 for tuberculosis, and so on.

■ THE INFECTIOUS DISEASE PROCESS

■ Definitions

A number of definitions are useful when describing certain conditions related to the infectious disease process. These are presented in Table 11-1.

The question of whether a person has an infection or colonization can be difficult to answer. What is important to realize is that persons who are colonized, as well as infected persons, can easily serve as a source of infection to themselves and to others who are at risk.

■ Chain of infection

Essential to appropriate intervention in the prevention and control of infection is an understanding of the infectious disease process. All infectious diseases occur as a result of a sequence of events (Fig. 11-1). These events involve (1) a causative agent, (2) a reservoir, (3) a portal of exit, (4) a mode of transmission, (5) a portal of entry, and (6) a susceptible host.

First there must be a *causative agent,* or pathogen. This can be a bacterium, virus, fungus, rickettsia, protozoan, or helminth (worm). The causative agent exists in a *res-*

Table 11-1   Selected definitions related to the infectious disease process

Term	Definition
Pathogen	Microorganism or substance capable of producing disease
Pathogenicity	Capability of a pathogen to infect and produce disease; determined by ability to survive and multiply outside host, virulence, dose, host specificity, and resistance of host
Invasiveness	Injury to host as a result of presence and spread of pathogen through body tissues
Toxigenicity	Injury to host as a result of effects to host of toxins produced by pathogen
Incubation period	Period of time after pathogen enters host and before clinical symptoms of infection appear
Infection	Presence in the body of a pathogen that multiplies and produces effects injurious to the host
Apparent (symptomatic, clinical)	Clinical signs and symptoms present
Inapparent (asymptomatic, subclinical)	No perceivable signs or symptoms present
Acute	Rapid onset, immediate host response, severe symptoms, and usually short course
Chronic	Insidious onset, delayed host response, mild symptoms, and long course
Latent	Pathogen ever-present in host, symptoms present only intermittently, often in response to a stimulus; pathogen dormant at other times
Localized	Focal point of symptoms or injury
Generalized	Systemic, whole body involvement
Superinfection	New infection by a pathogen different from one that caused initial infection
Colonization	Presence of pathogenic microorganisms in or on a host that do not produce injury or incite an injurious body response
Normal flora	Presence of nonpathogenic microorganisms that normally reside in various body locations without invasion or harm (May become pathogenic if introduced into an area in which they do not normally reside)
Contamination	Presence of pathogenic micoorganisms on inanimate objects or in substances

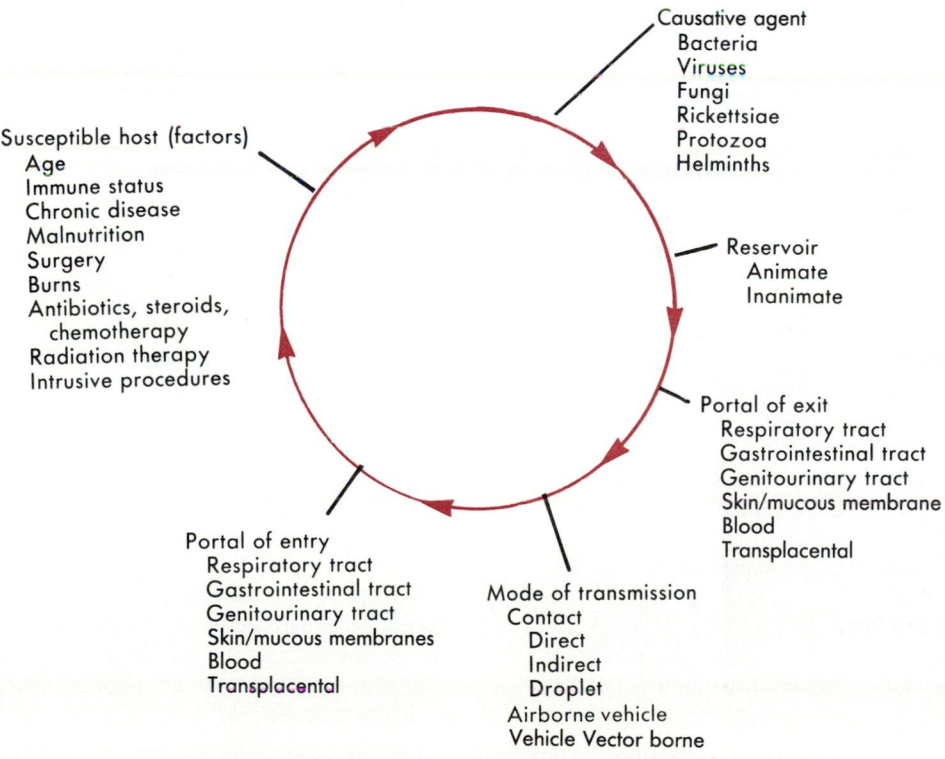

Fig. 11-1   The infectious disease process.

ervoir. The reservoir can be animate (human or animal) or inanimate (soil, water, intravenous solutions, or equipment). Human reservoirs can be either persons with an acute clinical infection or persons who are asymptomatic *carriers,* who harbor the infectious agent but do not develop the infection. Carriers can (1) *be incubating* the agent before the onset of signs and symptoms, (2) have an *inapparent infection (subclinical),* (3) be in the *convalescent stage* of an infection, or (4) be *chronic carriers* of the agent. Hepatitis B virus and HIV are examples of infectious agents that can be transmitted by human carriers in all of these stages. Often the reservoir for an agent responsible for an outbreak of an infection is not readily apparent and, in fact, may never be identified. If the process of infection is well understood, however, appropriate and effective control measures can be instituted even though the original source of the causative agent is not known.

The agent must have a *portal of exit* from the reservoir. If the reservoir is human, the exit can be (1) the respiratory tract, (2) the gastrointestinal tract, (3) the genitourinary tract, (4) the skin or mucous membranes, (5) the blood, or (6) across the placenta.

Once the agent has left the reservoir, it needs a *mode of transmission* to a host. There are four modes of transmission: contact, airborne, vehicle, and vector. These modes and examples of how infection is spread by each mode are explained in the box below.

After the infectious agent has been transmitted to a host, it must gain entry into the host. The *portals of entry* are similar to the modes of exit from the human reservoir and include the respiratory tract, the gastrointestinal tract, the genitourinary tract, the skin or mucous membranes, the blood, and across the placenta.

The final step in the process after the inoculation of the host is the maturation and multiplication of the infectious agent. Entry of an infectious agent into a host does not mean that the agent will proliferate and cause infection. Infection depends on the dose and virulence of the agent and the *susceptibility of the host.* The healthy human body is extremely resistant to infection; however, when the basic biologic defense mechanisms of the body are compromised, an infectious organism has a much greater chance of causing an infection. Chapter 38 deals with many of the factors of biologic defense exhibited by the host to prevent infection and injury. Some of the factors that affect host susceptibility to infection are included in the box on p. 193.

From the preceding it is evident that no one factor alone is responsible for an infection. Rather, there are a number of variables—the *agent,* the *environment,* and the *host*—that determine the outcome and to which prevention and control measures are directed. To intervene effectively in the infectious disease process it is important that all of these concepts be understood.

■ Assessment

The incubation period for an infection is variable, depending on the condition of the host. However, it is often predictable and diagnostically significant. The establishment of an infection within the human body leads to a number of specific and generalized manifestations. The

---

Examples of modes of transmission of infection

Mode	Example
I. Contact	
A. Direct: (source to host)	HIV infection, gonorrhea, syphilis
B. Indirect: by way of intermediate object	
1. Hands	*Staphylococcus aureus* wound infection
2. Fomites (e.g., hypodermic needle)	Hepatitic B, HIV infection
3. Surgical instruments	*Staphylococcus aureus* wound infection
C. Droplet (large particles)	Meningococcal meningitis, influenza
Host inhales droplets expelled from reservoir	
II. Airborne: host inhales droplet nuclei (1 to 5 micrometers) in air	Chickenpox (varicella), pulmonary tuberculosis
III. Vehicle: ingested or administered substance	
A. Food, water	Hepatitis A, salmonellosis
B. Blood products	Hepatitis B, HIV infection
C. IV fluids	Enterobacter bacteremia, fungemia
IV. Vector: animate intermediary (usually insect)	Malaria, Rocky Mountain spotted fever, yellow fever, Lyme disease

---

Factors affecting host susceptibility to infection

Age	Young and old—most susceptible
Impaired immune status	HIV infection, leukemia, immunosuppressive drugs, radiation therapy, steroids
Chronic diseases	Diabetes, cancer, COPD, end-stage renal disease
Poor nutritional status	
Invasive devices	Intravenous catheters, chest tubes, urinary catheters, artificial airways
Surgery	
Impaired skin integrity	Burns, decubitus
Altered body flora	Antibiotics, antacid therapy

---

exact signs and symptoms elicited in the host depend on the agent responsible for the infection and the site of the infection. (For details on host response to specific infectious disease, see the particular chapter that discusses the disease site.) Early recognition of infection is a crucial step to initiating prompt treatment. There are some general subjective, objective, and diagnostic findings that can alert the nurse to suspect an infection, even if the causative agent is not known. These are summarized here.

The normal WBC count in blood is 5000 to 10,000 WBC/mm³. With the presence of a serious infection the number of WBCs rises above 10,000/mm³ in response to the infectious inflammation. Leukocyte values between 10,000 and 20,000 are considered slightly elevated; 20,000 to 40,000 moderately elevated; and greater than 40,000 greatly elevated. In a few infectious diseases the number of WBCs in circulation actually drops, which is also a significant piece of diagnostic data.

Five types of mature WBCs are found in circulation:

neutrophils, eosinophils, basophils, lymphocytes, and monocytes. Each type of WBC plays a more or less specific role in body defense (Chapter 38); therefore, different diseases produce different reactions among the white cell populations in the blood. These changes in patterns of distribution are detected not just by counting the total number of WBCs in a stained blood smear but also by classifying them according to morphology and calculating the relative percentage of each cell type present. This type of account is known as a differential count. The differential count may provide information that can be correlated with other clinical data to help diagnose a situation. Table 11-2 provides some general correlations between leukocyte response and infectious diseases.

None of the signs and symptoms present in localized or generalized infections are diagnostic in themselves. Many can be demonstrated by other disease processes. They can, however, serve as helpful clues in the diagnosis of a suspected infectious process (see the box on p. 194).

Table 11-2 White blood cell response to infections

Leukocyte response	Associated infectious process
Increase in neutrophils (neutrophilia)	Acute local and systemic infections caused by bacteria (especially pyogenic bacteria), rickettsia, some viruses, and a few protozoa
Decrease in neutrophils (neutropenia)	Salmonellosis, brucellosis, whooping cough, overwhelming bacterial infections, influenza, infectious mononucleosis, infectious hepatitis, mumps, rubella, rubeola, and some rickettsial and protozoan diseases
Increase in eosinophils (eosinophilia)	Allergic reactions, chronic skin disease, helminthic infections, and scarlet fever
Increase in lymphocytes (lymphocytosis)	Chickenpox, mumps, measles, infectious mononucleosis, influenza, whooping cough, syphilis, tuberculosis, salmonellosis, viral hepatitis, and viral pneumonia; sometimes in convalescence from acute bacterial infection
Decrease in lymphocytes (lymphopenia)	AIDS/AIDS related complex (ARC)
Increase in monocytes (monocytosis)	Tuberculosis, chickenpox, brucellosis, mumps, syphilis, and certain rickettsial diseases; may occur in certain viral and protozoan diseases and in convalescent phase of acute bacterial infections

Signs and symptoms of infection

Localized infections

Subjective complaints	Objective findings
1. Pain	1. Edema, redness, warmth of area
2. Tenderness	
3. Warmth	2. Exudate or drainage that is bloody, serous, cloudy, clear, creamy or purulent
4. Redness	
5. Swelling	
6. Itching	

Respiratory infections

1. Sore throat	1. Fever
2. Rhinitis	2. Increased pulse rate
3. Congestion	3. Elevated white blood cell count
4. Cough	
5. Sputum	4. Positive throat culture
6. Chest pain	5. Positive x-ray findings
7. Shortness of breath	6. Positive sputum culture
	7. Abnormal breath sounds

Gastrointestinal infections

1. Nausea	1. Fever
2. Vomiting	2. Increased pulse rate
3. Diarrhea	3. Elevated white blood cell count
4. Anorexia	
5. Abdominal cramps	4. Positive guaiac test
	5. Abnormal bowel sounds
6. Distention	

Genitourinary infections

1. Dysuria	1. Fever
2. Frequency	2. Elevated white blood cell count
3. Urgency	
4. Hematuria	3. Positive urine culture
5. Purulent or foul discharge	
6. Flank or pelvic pain	

Generalized infections

Subjective complaints	Objective findings
1. Fatigue	1. Fever
2. Malaise	2. Increased pulse rate
3. Weakness	3. Hypotension
4. Headache	4. Altered mental status
5. Light-headedness	5. Shock
6. Congestion	6. Confusion
7. Muscle aches	7. Convulsions
8. Joint pain	8. Jaundice (in some infections)
9. Decreased appetite	9. WBC may be elevated

■ Diagnostic tests

Diagnostic tests are important in the diagnosis of an infection. Some of the diagnostic tests used to obtain data are the following:

Bacterial, viral, and fungal cultures, gram stain
Antibody detection
Blood counts
Skin tests
Radiologic tests
Gallium scans
Ultrasound examinations
CT scan

Specimens for microbiologic testing are perhaps the most frequently ordered when an infection is suspected.

Proper collection and handling of laboratory specimens are essential to ensure accurate laboratory results. Inappropriate collection or handling of specimens may lead to unnecessary delays in test results or to inaccurate results, thus affecting the therapy given to the patient. When an infection is suspected, cultures are taken of the suspected site. If the patient has a fever and the site of infection is unknown, cultures are commonly taken of the blood, urine, sputum, and any other possible sites of infection. This may include spinal fluid cultures, aspirates of body fluid, or intravenous catheter tips. *It is imperative that these cultures be obtained before the initiation of antibiotic therapy whenever possible, since antibiotics can suppress any bacteria that are present and give inaccurate or false-negative culture results.* Cultures should be obtained in a manner that avoids contamination. Aseptic preparation of the site to be cultured, observance of aseptic technique, and placing specimens in an appropriate container are crucial factors to be observed in ensuring the best example. Once obtained, the specimen must be properly stored and transported promptly to the laboratory. Each institution should have guidelines for the proper method for collecting and handling specimens for the laboratory (see the box on p. 195).

Interpretation of laboratory results is sometimes difficult. Certain body sites have bacteria known as normal flora, which reside there in a commensalistic (intimate) relationship with the host. These bacteria do not cause infection in the normal host. The skin, upper respiratory tract, vagina, urethra, and bowel are examples of body sites in which normal bacterial flora can be found. The bacteria found vary from site to site, and knowing the normal flora is helpful in discerning the significance of laboratory culture results. A *Clinician's Dictionary Guide to Bacteria and Fungi*[20] is an excellent publication that lists in detail the normal flora of various sites. It must be emphasized that laboratory results alone cannot be used to make diagnostic and therapeutic decisions. Rather, they are used in conjunction with the clinical status of the patient to make appropriate diagnostic and therapeutic decisions.

Knowledge about the infectious disease process and about how to recognize or suspect an infectious process is vital to the prevention and control of infectious diseases in both community and hospital settings. Each component

---

General guidelines for specimen collection

Objective

To obtain specimen containing infecting pathogen that is free of contamination

Method

1. Wash hands.
2. Prepare site aseptically.
3. Collect specimen using aseptic technique; wear gloves if appropriate; avoid coughing, sneezing or talking.
4. Obtain adequate amount of specimen.
5. Collect and transport in sterile container appropriate for type of specimen.
6. Label requisition with patient's name, location, date and time of collection, type of specimen, how obtained (clean void or catheter urine), test requested, and current antibiotic therapy.
7. Store properly and transport promptly to laboratory.
8. Keep record of test.

---

of the process must be understood for appropriate assessment of real or potential infection risks. The nurse can then intervene to minimize or eliminate that risk. Prevention and control of disease are addressed in the remainder of this chapter.

INFECTION CONTROL IN THE COMMUNITY

An infectious disease is termed a communicable disease when it is highly transmissable to other persons. Smallpox is an example of a communicable disease that, through cooperative efforts worldwide, has been successfully eradicated. The methods used to eradicate smallpox throughout the world can serve as a model of how to eliminate other communicable diseases. The eradication of smallpox also demonstrates the importance of accurate reporting of communicable diseases to the proper authorities so that prevention and control measures can be instituted.

The community health nurse plays a vital role in the collection of data, surveillance activities, immunization programs, education, and other control measures. Physicians and health care facilities have a responsibility to report communicable diseases promptly to the health department. Health agencies in the community can use the reported data to determine potential or real problems, to identify the causative agent and its source (if possible), and to identify the population at risk. A method to control the problem, care for the exposed, and protect the population at risk can then be devised and implemented.

The AIDS epidemic has posed the greatest communicable disease threat in recent years. Since first identified as a communicable disease in 1981, much has been learned through epidemiologic research. AIDS was first described in homosexual males and then in intravenous drug users and hemophiliacs. This discovery helped to identify the

routes of transmission as sexual contact, contaminated needles, and blood transfusion. Later, the perinatal route was identified as a means of transmission. In 1983 the virus was first isolated in the United States and named human T lymphotrophic virus III (HTLV III). The French named this same virus lymphadenopathy virus (LAV). Later, the virus was renamed human immunodeficiency virus (HIV). Since first recognized as a communicable disease, no new routes of transmission have been identified.

In April 1985 the screening of all blood and blood products for HIV antibody was begun. This has almost eliminated blood transfusions as a source of HIV infection. Today, those most at risk for HIV infection are persons who engage in high-risk behaviors: having multiple sexual partners, sharing intravenous needles, and being a sexual partner of a person who engages in high-risk behaviors. In addition, HIV infection may be transmitted from an infected mother to fetus in utero from maternal circulation or during labor and delivery from the ingestion of blood and blood products. Casual contact *has not* been identified as a means of transmission. Nonsexual cohabitants of HIV-infected persons have not become infected.

Until a cure or vaccine is available, the only effective control measure is education. Educational programs emphasize the routes of transmission, identify high-risk behaviors, and instruct in safer sexual practices. Nurses participate in AIDS education programs in schools, in the media, community centers, and churches. Nurses are also engaged in HIV counseling. It is essential that the nurse be well informed and provide accurate information in a sensitive and and nonjudgmental manner.

AIDS is discussed in more detail in Chapter 38.

Prevention and control measures

One method of prevention and control of disease in the community involves environmental control measures such as sanitation techniques that ensure a pure water supply and proper disposal of sewage and other potentially infectious materials. These measures have been legislated into building codes, state laws, and federal regulations. Similarly, there are regulations regarding health practices in institutions that handle, package, and prepare foods. Another example of an environmental control measure is the spraying of a designated area to kill mosquitos, which are implicated in the spread of viral encephalitis. Spraying usually is done only after an outbreak has been identified.

Depending on the communicable disease, care of exposed persons and protection of the population at risk for contracting the disease may entail prophylaxis, immunization, or only careful monitoring of new cases. Often, simple adherence to basic principles of hygiene is sufficient. Determination of additional required measures should be made by the local or state health department. Attempts are made to reach those at risk and inform them of the preventive measures. Education of the public is a key component of these efforts.

In the United States there has been a significant reduction in recent years in the incidence of infectious diseases, such as measles, whooping cough, and poliomyelitis, which can be prevented by immunization. Concern is being expressed, however, about the decrease in the number of children presently being immunized, despite the fact that these immunizations can often be obtained free of cost. Additionally, concern is being expressed that federal monies used to support local immunization efforts may be reduced to such a level that free immunizations will no longer be equally available in all 50 states. Infections formerly seen only in children are now being seen more frequently in adults because of the failure of the population to develop acquired immunity during early childhood.

A more recent concern because of air travel is the elimination of the barriers of time and distance and the possibility of a person with an infectious disease being brought from a remote area of the world to a major population center where the disease can be readily spread to a susceptible public.

The dramatic control of several infectious diseases has been caused by the development and use of a variety of *inactivated vaccines* and *live attenuated antigens*. The potential for eradication of common infectious diseases brings with it major responsibilities for public health agencies, physicians, and nurses. Ways must be found not only to carry out planned programs of immunization, but also to educate the public to the hazards of apathy and failure to maintain proper levels of immunization. Continued progress in control and eradication requires that there be commitment to continue to add to knowledge about immunization patterns, to evaluate effectiveness and risks of antigens used, and to monitor the levels of protection present in a population.

■ Immunization programs

Immunization programs have played and continue to play a primary role in the control of infectious disease throughout the world. The body can be stimulated to produce

---

Artificial immunization

Active

Produce own antibodies after being inoculated with vaccine made from attenuated, killed organisms, or modified toxins (toxoids).
Examples: Smallpox, diphtheria, tetanus, pertussis, rubella, mumps, rubeola, polio (OPV), pneumococcal, hepatitis B, influenza, typhoid, Haemophilus B polysaccharide vaccine.

Passive

Injected with antibodies produced by other persons or animals. This protection is temporary, lasting a few weeks without stimulating antibody production in the recipient.
Examples: immune human serum globulin, hepatitis B immune globulin (HBIG), mumps hyperimmune gamma globulin, rabies human immune globulin, tetanus immune globulin, varicella zoster–immune globulin.

---

antibodies against some specific diseases without actually having the disease (*active artificial immunity*). Temporary protection sometimes can be provided by injecting antibodies produced by other persons or animals into the bloodstream of a human being (*passive artificial immunity*).

Recommendations concerning current immunization schedules are found in the *Red Book* published by the Committee on Infectious Diseases of The American Academy of Pediatrics and in *Morbidity and Mortality Weekly Reports,* which present recommendations of the United States Public Health Service's Advisory Committee on Immunization Practices (ACIP). The reader should refer to these resources when there are questions about proper immunization practices, prophylaxis, interruption in immunization schedules, or adverse reactions and side effects. A summary of active and passive immunization appears in the box above.

■ ACTIVE IMMUNIZATION

If 90% of the population is protected against organisms that required continued passage through human beings to reproduce and live, the disease caused by the organism can be virtually eliminated because there are too few susceptible hosts for organism spread. Smallpox has been eliminated from the world in this way. This type of protection of a group is called *herd immunity*. It is ineffectual, however, against organisms such as tetanus bacilli that can exist indefinitely (in the soil), and in this instance each person must be immunized to be protected. If the disease is one not prevalent in the environment, such as diphtheria in the United States, or is not spread from person to person

Table 11-3 Recommended schedule for active immunization of normal infants and children (See individual ACIP recommendations for details)

Recommended age	Vaccine(s)	Comments
2 months	DTP-1, OPV-1	Can be given earlier in endemic areas
4 months	DTP-2, OPV-2	6-week to 2-month interval desired between OPV doses to avoid interference
6 months	DTP-3	An additional dose of OPV at this time is optional in areas with a high risk of polio exposure
15 months	MMR, DTP-4, OPV-3	Completion of primary series
24 months	HbPV	Can be given at 18-23 months for children in day care centers
4-6 years	DTP-5, OPV-4	Preferably at or before school entry
14-16 years	Td*	Repeat every 10 years throughout life

From Morbid Mortal Week Rep 35(37):578, 1986.

*Adult tetanus toxoid and diphtheria toxoid in combination; contains same dose of tetanus toxoid as DTP or DT and a reduced dose of diphtheria toxoid. Pertussis is not given after age 7.

DTP = Diphtheria, tetanus, pertussis; OPV = Oral polio vaccine; MMR = Measles, mumps, rubella; HbPV = Haemophilus b polysaccharide vaccine.

by direct contact, such as tetanus, the inoculation must be repeated at regular intervals to maintain protection. This inoculation is called a *booster dose,* and usually one tenth of the original inoculating dose is sufficient.

An inoculation often causes a local tissue response. Symptoms of inflammation (redness, tenderness, swelling, sometimes ulcerations) appear at the site of the injection, and symptoms of widespread tissue involvement (slight febrile reactions, general malaise, muscle aching) for 1 or 2 days are not uncommon. The initial inoculation produces delayed symptoms because the immune response system must become sensitized to the antigen. There usually is an accelerated and less severe systemic reaction to subsequent inoculations because the immune response is stimulated at once. The local reaction also is less severe than that which occurs following the initial inoculation because the organisms have less opportunity to produce inflammation.

Active artificial immunization against many bacilli and viruses is now available. All persons should be encouraged to avail themselves of the protection advised by health officials in their local area. They also should be advised to keep a permanent record of the date of each immunization.

■ PRIMARY IMMUNIZATION SCHEDULES

In the United States, the ACIP recommends that all children be immunized against diphtheria, pertussis, (whooping cough), tetanus (DPT); measles, mumps, and rubella (MMR); and poliomyelitis (OPV). Haemophilus b polysaccharide vaccine (HbPV) is also recommended for children attending day care centers (Table 11-3). Children who have not been immunized as infants can be immunized at any age. All susceptible children, adolescents, and adults should be immunized unless contraindicated.

Routine vaccination against smallpox is no longer recommended by the CDC because the side effects and complications of the vaccine are greater than the danger of

acquiring the disease. The vaccine is indicated only for laboratory workers who are directly involved with smallpox or closely related orthopox viruses. However, the U.S. armed forces require smallpox vaccination for recruits.

At the present time, immunization against typhoid fever is recommended only when there is exposure to a typhoid carrier in the household, when there is an outbreak of typhoid in a community, or for travelers to countries where typhoid is endemic (always present).

Immunization to protect against other diseases is given on a selective basis; that is, groups at a high risk are immunized. Hepatitis B vaccine is an excellent example of a vaccine that is only recommended for persons at high risk of acquiring the virus (see the box below).

Because of the prevalence of *influenza* and its potential for causing death, the ACIP recommends immunization against influenza for all individuals at increased risk of

---

Persons for whom hepatitis B vaccine is recommended

Nonimmunized health care workers having blood or needle-stick exposures
Clients and staff of institutions for the developmentally disabled
Hemodialysis patients
Homosexually active men
Users of illicit injectable drugs
Recipients of certain blood products
Household and sexual contacts of hepatitis B carriers
Infants born to hepatitis B positive mothers

Morbid Mortal Week Rep 36(23):357, 1987.

adverse consequences from infection of the lower respiratory tract. This includes persons over 60 years of age and persons over 2 years of age who have chronic cardiac, respiratory, metabolic, or renal disease or diseases that impair the person's immune system.

The use of pneumococcal vaccine against *Streptococcus pneumoniae* is under investigation. There is not yet enough data for the ACIP to formulate formal recommendations about the routine use of the vaccine for immunization in the general population. It is currently being administered to adults and children over 2 years of age with chronic illnesses who are at increased risk of complications associated with pneumonoccal infections. A single dose is given only once. The duration of protection is unknown. Further investigation of the use of vaccines for protection against other bacterial infections is under way and could offer promise in improving immune defenses in immunocompromised patients.

■ PASSIVE IMMUNIZATION

Passive immunization usually is reserved for situations in which the disease would be detrimental to the person. For example, it is rarely given to prevent a disease such as chickenpox or mumps in children because they are at an optimal age for the body to respond immunologically with minimal inflammatory response. On the other hand, an adult exposed to the same diseases often would be given antibodies because adults may have a severe pathologic response. Immunization is given to all age groups exposed to pathogens that cause serious diseases such as hepatitis, poliomyelitis, diphtheria, tetanus, or rabies. Antivenins, which are given to people bitten by poisonous snakes or black widow spiders, or other examples of passive immunologic products.

Products used for passive immunization may be specific to the disease. Antitoxins and immune animal and human sera are examples. These materials contain elevated levels of immune globulins, which can specifically detoxify the toxin, neutralize the virus, or inactivate the bacterium. The whole blood of a patient who has recently recovered from a disease against which antibodies are produced also may be used. Antitoxins are available for diphtheria, tetanus, botulism, gas gangrene, and the venom of snakes. *Immune animal serum* is available against rabies; *human immune serum* is available for mumps, measles, pertussis, poliomyelitis, and tetanus.

Immune serum globulin (ISG), or gamma globulin (γ-globulin), is an antibody-rich fraction of pooled plasma from normal donors. The rationale for pooling plasma is that someone among the donors will have had the diseases and will have developed antibodies against them. The *globulin fraction* of the plasma carries the antibodies, and because it is known not to transmit the virus of hepatitis, it is considered safe to use. Because of occasional side effects, it is now recommended that the use of immune serum globulin be limited to those disorders in which its efficacy has been definitely established. These are measles prophylaxis or modification, viral hepatitis type A prophylaxis or modification, viral hepatitis type A prophylaxis or modification, and immune deficiency diseases. Immune serum globulin is considered to be of *questionable value* in the following situations: (1) prevention of rubella in the first trimester of pregnancy, (2) prevention or modification of varicella in certain high-risk patients, (3) prevention or modification of viral hepatitis type B after accidental inoculation, and (4) life-threatening bacterial infections.

Special human immune serum globulins are derived from the sera of persons previously immunized or convalescing from specific diseases. Tetanus immune globulin (human) is of value in prophylaxis and treatment of tetanus in persons who have not received prior immunization. Pertussis immune globulin (human) and mumps immune globulin (human) are of uncertain or unproved value in the prevention and treatment of pertussis and mumps, respectively. Hepatitis B immune globulin (human) is available for prophylaxis after exposure to hepatitis B. Zoster immune globulin (human) is available for restricted use for prophylaxis against chickenpox.

■ NURSING RESPONSIBILITIES IN IMMUNIZATION

The greatest responsibility of the nurse in immunization programs is to teach the public the advantages of immunization and encourage widespread participation in programs recommended by the local public health officer.

□ Teaching

In teaching it is advisable to provide the public with the following information: against what disease protection is being given, why immunization is desirable, and when booster doses should be obtained. The relative safety of the immunization and the advantages of immunization early in life should be stressed.

The nurse is responsible for assessing persons before immunization because there are some contraindications to receiving certain immunizing substances. Those that are prepared in chicken or duck embryos may cause an allergic reaction in persons who are allergic to eggs. Many people are allergic to horse serum, and substances containing horse serum, such as tetanus antitoxin, should never be given unless a small amount of the substance has been injected intradermally (a sensitivity test) and after 20 minutes produces no "hive" reaction about the injection site. *Active immunologic products* should not be given while a person has a cold or other infection because the inflammatory reaction from the immunization will be greater than usual.

Live attenuated virus vaccines should not be given to persons with alterations in their immune status, since virus replication after administration may be unchecked in these individuals. OPV viruses are excreted by the recipient of the vaccine and are communicable to other persons, so individuals who live with an immunocompromised person should not receive OPV. If a person has a febrile illness, it is usually best to wait until recovery before vaccination is given. Pregnant women should not receive live *attenuated virus* vaccines because of the theoretical risk to the fetus. Live attenuated virus vaccines should not be given at the same time as passive immunization, since passively acquired antibodies can interfere with the response to live attenuated virus vaccines.

Before leaving the clinic, the person or family members should be instructed about the expected effects of an inoculation and told to contact the physician or to report to a hospital emergency room if any other symptoms develop. The person is cautioned not to scratch any lesion produced by an inoculation. If a severe local reaction with redness, swelling, and tenderness occurs, the physician may order the application of hot, wet dressings. If the lesion is open, these dressings should be sterile.

When antitoxins, antisera, or antivenins are given, the patient is kept under observation for 20 to 30 minutes. Symptoms of severe allergic response usually will appear within that period of time.

Persons employed in health care facilities should maintain their immune status against poliomyelitis, diphtheria, and tetanus. Persons with negative tuberculin tests should be retested every 6 months.

Yearly chest x-ray examinations are no longer recommended for the routine management of persons with positive tuberculin skin tests. After the initial chest x-ray examination following a skin test conversion, yearly chest x-ray examinations have not been shown to be of significant clinical value and are not cost effective in monitoring persons for early disease. Persons with frequent exposure to blood or blood products should maintain their immune status against hepatitis B. Immunity against measles, rubella, and chickenpox should be assessed upon employment in a health care facility. Influenza vaccine is recommended for persons with frequent contact with high-risk individuals. High-risk individuals include adults and children with chronic disorders of the cardiovascular and pulmonary systems and residents of long-term care facilities.

☐ Home care

Persons with communicable diseases are frequently cared for at home. The community health nurse is often asked to teach family members how to care for the patient and how to protect family members, friends, and neighbors. The same principles apply in the home as in the hospital.

Regardless of the disease, good hand washing technique should be practiced and gloves should be worn for contact with any body substance. A smock or apron can be worn to protect the clothes from soiling. A mask, if indicated, can be improvised from any closely woven absorbable material, or disposable ones can be purchased at a pharmacy. All liquid wastes can be flushed down a toilet. Garbage and other wastes containing body substances can be wrapped in newspaper and placed in a plastic bag before discarding in a rubbish container. Dishes should be washed in hot, soapy water. Separate dishes are not required. Laundry should be washed in a washing machine with a detergent. Chlorine bleach or a disinfectant should be added if linen is soiled with body substances. The local health department should be consulted for full information regarding specific communicable diseases.

The special problems the nurse encounters in controlling *hospital-acquired infections* will be the focus of the remainder of this chapter.

■ INFECTION CONTROL IN THE HOSPITAL

■ Scope of the problem

A *nosocomial* infection is one that is not present or incubating at the time a person is admitted to the hospital but develops after admission. A *community-acquired infection* is one that is present or incubating at the time of admission to the hospital. The nurse should be aware of the problem of nosocomial infections, their effects on patient morbidity, mortality, and increased hospital costs, as well as the legal aspects concerning them. The nurse also should be knowledgeable about the types of infections seen most often, the common pathogens and how they are transmitted, factors that predispose a patient to a nosocomial infection, how to recognize persons at risk of infection, and the prevention and control measures necessary to decrease the incidence of nosocomial infections.

At least 2 million persons, or about 5% of all patients admitted to U.S. hospitals each year, develop nosocomial infections. In addition to the considerable morbidity and mortality caused by these infections, their diagnoses and treatment (including additional days of hospitalization) cost more than $1 billion per year.[21] The JCAH requires that those institutions seeking accreditation have a program of infection control centered around monitoring (1) patients with infections, (2) patient care practices, (3) antibiotic usage, (4) health of personnel, and (5) the environment of the institution. The AHA and the CDC have developed guidelines for the prevention and control of infectious diseases for use in patient care centers. Because of these external forces, as well as providing the best possible care for their patients, hospitals are recognizing the need to increase infection surveillance and to upgrade programs to prevent nosocomial infections.

As seen in Table 11-4, the incidence of nosocomial infections varies with the type of hospital, and this can be attributed to differences in the size of hospitals, the severity of illness in the patient population, the susceptibility of the patient population, and the number of personnel who have hands-on contact with the patients. The patient with the greatest risk of developing a nosocomial infection is one with a chronic illness, a prolonged hospital stay, and the most direct contact with various hospital personnel (that is, physicians, students, nurses, or therapists). These factors hold true not only for variations of infection rates from institution to institution, but also for variations in infection rates within an institution. Certain patient care areas are considered to be *high-risk areas* for developing nosocomial infections. These areas understandably are those that care for patients who have decreased host de-

Table 11-4 Infection rates per 1000 discharges by site and hospital category, 1984

	UTI	SWI	LRI	BACT	CUT	OTH	All sites
Nonteaching hospital	9.9	3.6	4.2	1.3	1.1	2.0	22.2
Small teaching hospital	13.9	6.0	5.4	1.9	1.8	4.7	33.8
Large teaching hospital	14.2	6.6	7.7	3.9	2.6	6.4	41.4

From Centers for Disease Control: CDC Surveillance Summaries, 1986; 35 (No. 1SS).
UTI = Urinary tract infection; SWI = Surgical wound infection; LRI = Lower respiratory tract infection; Bact = Primary bacteremia; CUT = Cutaneous infection; OTH = Other.

fenses or in whom invasive procedures and devices are common. Areas generally considered to be high risk are (1) intensive care units (including neonatal units), (2) burn units, (3) dialysis units, and (4) oncology units. The infection rate in these areas may be well over 20%.

■ Persons at risk

The nurse needs to be able to recognize those patients who are at the greatest risk of a nosocomial infection. Some of the factors that predispose a person to infection are mentioned on p. 193. Probably the single most important factor predisposing a patient to acquiring a nosocomial infection is the severity of the patient's underlying disease.

A patient admitted to the hospital with an infection may develop during the hospitalization a *superinfection* with another organism. Often this superinfection is with a more virulent or drug-resistant organism. For example, a patient admitted with a leg ulcer infected with *Staphylococcus aureus* may develop further infection (not colonization) with *Pseudomonas aeruginosa*. Furthermore, if this infection progresses to involve the bloodstream, then a *secondary bacteremia* has occurred. Infection can occur secondary to (1) an existing infection, (2) an underlying disease process, or (3) an anatomic defect that may be causing obstruction. An example of this is the man who has benign prostate hypertrophy (BPH) and who develops a urinary tract infection secondary to the obstruction caused by the BPH.

The most common site for a nosocomial infection is the urinary tract; 75% of these infections are related to instrumentation, including indwelling urinary catheters, catheterizations, and urologic procedures. Infected surgical wounds, followed by lower respiratory tract infections, and then bloodstream infections (some associated with the use of intravascular lines) are the next most frequently encountered types of nosocomial infections. Together these sites account for about 80% of all nosocomial infections.

■ Pathogens causing nosocomial infections

The different types of pathogens commonly responsible for nosocomial infections and their most common reservoirs are listed in Table 11-5. In the past 2 decades there has been a decline in the number of nosocomial infections caused by gram-positive bacteria, especially staphylococci and streptococci; however, *S. aureus* is still the single most common organism causing nosocomial surgical wound infections. At the same time, there has been an increase in the incidence of nosocomial infection caused by gram-negative bacteria, particularly members of the family Enterobacteriaceae and the genus *Pseudomonas*, which now cause 60% to 65% of all nosocomial infections. These gram-negative organisms collectively are responsible for nearly all nosocomial urinary tract infections, 70% of the bacteremias, and the majority of respiratory tract and surgical wound infections. *P. aeruginosa* is present throughout the hospital environment, especially where there is a persistent presence of water (in sinks, irrigating solutions, or nebulizers). Patients who are receiving antibiotic therapy, who are immunodeficient, or who are subject to invasive procedures are particularly susceptible to infections by these organisms. Antibiotic drug resistance can present a serious problem when treating these patients.

Serratia marcescens and *Serratia liquefaciens* are gram-negative organisms that are being seen with increased frequency in nosocomial infections. The reservoirs for these organisms are soil and water, and they are found in the hospital in similar reservoirs as *Pseudomonas*. The colonized body fluids of patients have also been identified as a reservoir for *Serratia* organisms. Previously thought to be nonpathogenic, *S. marcescens* was used because of its red pigmentation to mark air flow and settling patterns of bacteria. It is now recognized as a pathogen that can cause severe infection in a susceptible host. One problem with *Serratia* organisms has been their ability to rapidly develop resistance to antibiotics. This can have devastating consequences in an intensive care or burn unit when an outbreak occurs. Because its mode of transmission is through direct or indirect contact on the hands of personnel or on contaminated articles, good hand-washing and aseptic techniques are the most effective measures to prevent outbreaks of infection.

Candida albicans is a yeastlike fungus that can cause infection, especially in immunocompromised patients or in patients receiving antibiotics. These patients have a decrease in their normal flora, which provides a niche for *Candida* organisms to settle in and proliferate. *Candida* vaginitis and oral thrush are common complications of antibiotic therapy. Antibiotics suppress bacterial growth but do not affect fungal growth; special antifungal agents are

Table 11-5   Common reservoirs of some pathogens

Pathogen	Common reservoir
Gram-positive cocci	
Staphylococcus aureus	Anterior nares, skin (especially hands) of human carriers, contaminated objects
Group A Streptococcus	Nose and throat of human carriers, GI tract of humans
Enterococcus	
Gram-negative rods	
Escherichia, Klebsiella, Enterobacter, Proteus, Salmonella, Serratia, Pseudomonas, Providencia	GI tract, food, water, soil, contaminated solutions and objections, other infected patients
Anaerobes	
Clostridium	Soil, contaminated environment
Bacteroides	Oropharynx, bowel
Fungi	
Candida albicans	Normal flora in some people, contaminated environment
Viruses	
Varicella	Human carriers
Herpes	Human carriers
Rubella	Human carriers
Hepatitis B	Human carriers, contaminated objects
Poliomyelitis	Human carriers, contaminated food, water, and environment
Human immunodeficiency virus	Human carriers

necessary to control these infections unless the normal flora returns following discontinuance of the antibiotics.

Methicillin-resistant *Staphylococcus aureus* (MRSA) is a pathogen causing increasing concern among health care givers. Methicillin is one of the penicillins specifically developed to treat *S. aureus* infections. Since *S. aureus* is a common surgical wound pathogen, the concern is that MRSA infections will be more difficult and expensive to treat. Currently the antibiotic of choice for treating MRSA infection is vancomycin. This antibiotic is only available for intravenous administration and may be ototoxic and nephrotoxic. It is considerably more expensive than the methicillin-group antibiotics. Once introduced into an institution, MRSA becomes endemic, and eradication measures have been largely unsuccessful. The hands of health care givers have been associated with cross-infections. Transfer of MRSA-colonized patients between health care institutions has been refused because institutions are afraid of the spread of this pathogen.

■ Prevention and control measures

In the hospital there are many potential sources of infection, including patients, personnel, visitors, equipment, and linen. The patient may become infected with organisms from either the external environment (*exogenous*) or, as is often seen in the severely immunocompromised host, from their own internal organisms (*endogenous*). Virtually any microorganism can be a potential pathogen to the immunocompromised patient. Most of the causative organisms are present in the external environment of the patient

and are introduced into the body through direct contact or contaminated materials. In many instances nosocomial infections could be prevented by strict aseptic technique when giving care to the patient and by using greater restraint in the use of invasive procedures and antibiotics. A summary of some of the prevention and control measures is presented in the box on p. 202. The reader is referred to the CDC manual of *Guidelines for the Prevention and Control of Nosocomial Infections*[28] for greater detail.

■ PREVENTION OF URINARY TRACT INFECTIONS

As mentioned previously, *urinary tract infections* (UTIs) are the most common nosocomial infections seen in the hospital. The majority of these infections are associated with catheterization and instrumentation of the urinary tract. Urinary catheters should be used only when absolutely necessary. If a catheter must be used, it should be discontinued as soon as medically feasible, since the longer the catheter is in place, the greater the risk of developing an infection. As small a catheter as possible should be used to minimize urethral trauma.

Intermittent catheterization should be considered for patients requiring long-term urinary catheterization because this technique has been shown to reduce the infection risk. External urinary drainage devices such as condom catheters, however, have not been shown to significantly reduce the risk of urinary tract infection.

Strict aseptic technique is necessary when inserting the catheter to prevent transmission of bacteria into the blad-

---

Prevention of and control measures for nosocomial infections

Control of external environment (exogenous sources of infection)

Health care providers

1. In good health—do not care for patients when ill
2. Keep immunizations current
3. Practice effective hand washing between each patient
    a. If skin dry, rough, broken, seek appropriate attention
    b. If active herpes simplex infection of hand (herpetic whitlow), do not give direct patient care until lesion healed
4. Wear gloves when contact with any body substance is anticipated

Housekeeping and sanitation

1. Bed linens not shaken in air or thrown on floor
2. Proper disposal of wastes—solid and liquid
3. Proper cleaning and sterilization of contaminated articles
4. Proper ventilation for adequate air exchanges
    a. Modern hospitals—patients' rooms under negative pressure
    b. Negative pressure keeps air from patients' rooms from moving into hallways
5. Proper mopping and damp dusting to remove dust and other environmental reservoirs of infection

Control of internal environment (endogenous sources of infection)

1. Preventive measures aimed at increasing patient's defense mechanisms and thus reducing risk of infection
    a. Teach patient about good nutrition
    b. Teach patient about personal hygiene, especially hand washing
2. Be aware that normal flora of patient can be disrupted when patient is receiving antibiotics or chemotherapy and colonization may occur
    a. Give antibiotics on time as scheduled
    b. Teach patient about appropriate use of antibiotics and dangers of taking them when not prescribed by physician

---

der. Bacteria that are present around the catheter meatal junction can also be transmitted on the tip of the catheter into the bladder along the thin layer of mucus that surrounds the catheter in the urethra. For this reason, the catheter should be securely anchored to prevent it from moving in and out of the urethra. Movement of the catheter can track bacteria into the urethra and up into the bladder along the mucous sheath. Furthermore, the catheter-meatal junction should be kept clean; the patient incontinent of stool can pose a problem in this regard. In some institutions antiseptic agents are used to cleanse the meatus and antimicrobial agents are applied around the catheter-meatal junction. *Both of these practices are considered controversial.* Good hand-washing techniques by personnel, cleansing of the patient's meatal area with soap and water, and proper anchoring of the catheter are considered to be effective ways to reduce the incidence of UTIs in patients with indwelling catheters.

Another portal of entry for bacteria is through the distal catheter–proximal drainage tube junction. Every time the system is disconnected there is an increased risk of introducing bacteria into the system. For this reason a sterile closed drainage system should be maintained. The tubing should be kept from kinking and obstruction. Bladder irrigations should not be a routine practice. If irrigation is

necessary, a sterile disposable syringe and sterile solution should be used, and the catheter-tubing junction should be disinfected before disconnection. If frequent irrigations are necessary, as in patients who have had a transurethral prostatectomy (TURP) in which blood clots are common, a three-way catheter drainage system with continuous bladder irrigation is recommended. In this way a closed system is maintained. Urine specimens should be obtained from the rubber portal on the drainage tubing. The portal should be cleansed with an antiseptic before insertion of the sterile needle into the portal.

Another portal of entry of bacteria into the system is through the collection bag. The bag should be kept below the bladder level at all times to prevent reflux of urine into the bladder. It also should be kept off the floor and the emptying spout should be cleansed with an antiseptic before and after the urine is emptied from the bag. The container used to collect the urine from the bag must be used for only one patient; it should not be shared between patients. Catheters should not be changed on a routine basis. Rather, they should be replaced only when they become obstructed, requiring frequent irrigations, or when concretions are detected in the tubing, which can lead to obstructed flow. A final control measure in preventing nosocomial UTIs is to place patients with urinary catheters in separate rooms. This is helpful in preventing cross-infection between patients.

PREVENTION OF SURGICAL WOUND INFECTION

Surgical wound infection is primarily related to the degree of contamination, endogenous or exogenous, during the surgical procedure and to specific host factors (underlying illnesses and the presence of a remote untreated infection at the time of surgery). The degree of contamination is related to the anatomic wound site, the wound classification, and the duration of surgery. Operations involving the abdominal cavity, as well as wounds classified as contaminated or dirty, increase the patient's risk of surgical wound infection. Surgical procedures lasting longer than 2 hours also increase the risk of postoperative infection. The duration of the surgical procedure is often considered a function of the surgeon's skill and experience. The surgical wound infection rate is rarely affected by the postoperative nursing care, since the closed wound serves as a barrier to further contamination from exogenous organisms. However, aseptic technique during dressing changes and when emptying closed wound drainage systems is important for all personnel having contact with the surgical wound. Studies have shown that the most effective approach to reducing surgical wound infection in both high- and low-risk patients involves two components. The first consists of an ongoing surgical wound infection surveillance program with routine reporting of surgical wound infection rates back to the surgeons. The second component is the use of a hospital epidemiologist with specific training in hospital infection control who is an active member of the Hospital Infection Control Committee. Findings from the Project Study on the Efficacy of Nosocomial Infection Control demonstrated that hospitals in which programs featured both components had a 35% reduction in high-risk and 41% reduction in low-risk surgical wound infection rates.[31] Keeping the surgeons and operating room nurses informed about specific infection rates results in a heightened awareness of the importance of aseptic technique and efficiency during surgery. Other measures that minimize the risk of infection include the appropriate use of prophylactic antibiotics, limiting the period of preoperative hospital stay, preoperative bathing with antiseptics, hair removal (preferably by depilatory or clipping) in the period immediately before the surgery, and traffic control in the operating room.

The box below has a summary of the ways in which surgical wounds are classified.

PREVENTION OF RESPIRATORY TRACT INFECTIONS

Nosocomial pneumonia is associated with the highest mortality rate of all nosocomial infections. Respiratory intubation is a major risk factor because endotracheal, nasotracheal, and tracheostomy tubes bypass the patient's defense mechanisms of the upper respiratory tract. The importance of proper maintenance and decontamination of respiratory therapy equipment in preventing nosocomial pneumonias is well established. Hand washing is essential before and after contact with patients and respiratory assistive devices because these devices contain moisture, making them ideal reservoirs for gram-negative organisms such as *Pseudomonas* and *Serratia* species. In addition, gloves should be worn for handling all respiratory secretions and devices. Suctioning is a sterile procedure necessitating the use of sterile equipment and irrigants (Chapter 23). Surgical procedures that lead to impaired coughing are also a risk factor. Preoperative teaching stressing the importance and proper technique of coughing and deep breathing is essential to the success of postoperative pulmonary toilet. Inappropriate use of antibiotics should be avoided to minimize oropharyngeal colonization with gram-negative organisms, which, if aspirated, may lead to a more serious pneumonia. Debilitated patients should be protected from the hazards of aspiration when eating or being fed.

Surgical wound classification

Wound classification	Description and example
Clean	Wounds in which the GI or respiratory tract is not entered; no inflammation or break in aseptic technique. Cholecystectomy, hysterectomy
Clean contaminated	Clean operation in which the GI or respiratory tract is entered. Colon resection
Contaminated	Nonpurulent inflammation, gross spillage from GI tract, fresh traumatic wounds, or major breaks in sterile technique. Gunshot wound
Dirty or infected	Old traumatic with dead tissue, pus encountered, or perforated viscus found. Ruptured abscess

■ PREVENTION OF BACTEREMIAS

Many blood infections (bacteremias) occur secondary to infections at another site; thus prevention may depend a great deal on control of the underlying infection. Some bacteremias are the result of the use of intravascular devices and systems. The sources of infection in these instances are the hands of personnel, the patient's skin, or infusions that are contaminated either from mishandling by hospital personnel or, less commonly, at the time of manufacture. Intravenous and intraarterial catheters should be inserted under aseptic conditions, and catheter insertion sites should be cared for aseptically. A sterile dressing should cover the insertion site. The insertion site is inspected frequently for any sign of infection, such as redness, swelling, exudate, purulence, or warmth. The patient may also complain of pain at the site. Peripheral catheters should be changed every 48 to 72 hours or more often if there is a complication such as infiltration or phlebitis. The catheter is secured to prevent in-and-out movement and tracking of bacteria into the cannula site. Aseptic technique should be followed when mixing and adding drugs, changing the infusion, or manipulating connections or stopcocks. It is recommended that the tubing be changed every 48 to 72 hours (24 to 48 hours for hyperalimentation). Before hanging a solution, the nurse should check it for turbidity and particulate matter and for leaks in the system. Solutions should be discarded after 24 hours. Hyperalimentation solutions require special adherence to these practices, since they are composed of nutrients that are an excellent culture media for organisms. *Candida* infections are commonly seen in patients who are receiving hyperalimentation, particularly among those who are immunocompromised.

Category-specific isolation precautions

Strict isolation

Strict isolation is designed to prevent transmission of highly contagious or virulent infections that may be spread by both air and contact.

Specifications for strict isolation

1. Private room is indicated; door should be kept closed. In general, patients infected with the same organism may share a room.
2. Masks are indicated for all persons entering the room.
3. Gowns are indicated for all persons entering the room.
4. Gloves are indicated for all persons entering the room.
5. Hands must be washed after touching the patient or potentially contaminated articles and before taking care of another patient.
6. Articles contaminated with infective material should be discarded or bagged and labeled before being sent for decontamination and reprocessing.

Diseases requiring strict isolation

Diphtheria, pharyngeal
Lassa fever and other viral hemorrhagic fevers, such as Marburg virus disease*
Plague, pneumonic
Smallpox*
Varicella (chickenpox)
Zoster, localized in immunocompromised patient or disseminated

Contact isolation

Contact isolation is designed to prevent transmission of highly transmissible or epidemiologically important infections (or colonization) that do not warrant Strict isolation. All diseases or conditions included in this category are spread primarily by close or direct contact. Thus masks, gowns, and gloves are recommended for anyone in close or direct contact with any patient who has an infection (or colonization) included in this category. For individual diseases or conditions, however, one or more of these three barriers may not be indicated. For example, masks and gloves are not generally indicated for care of infants and young children with acute viral respiratory infections, gowns are not generally indicated for gonococcal conjunctivitis in newborns, and masks are not generally indicated for care of patients infected with multiply resistant microorganisms, except those with pneumonia. Therefore, some degree of "overisolation" may occur in this category.

From Garner, JS, and Simmons, BT: CDC guidelines: nosocomial infections, Infect Control 4:261-283, 1983.
*A private room with special ventilation is indicated.

■ PROTECTION BY ISOLATION

The purpose of isolation is to protect both the health care giver from exposure to infectious agents and the patient from cross-infection. In 1983 the Centers for Disease Control (CDC) published revised guidelines for isolation precautions in hospitals. Two systems were offered for use. One was based on categories of isolation, and the other listed disease-specific isolation precautions. Hospitals were advised to choose the system most appropriate for their needs. There were seven major categories of isolation: strict, contact, respiratory, tuberculosis (AFB), enteric, drainage/secretion, and blood/body fluid. Protective isolation was eliminated as a category because it has not been shown to reduce the risk of infection in the immunocompromised patient.

The current AIDS epidemic has emphasized the need for health care givers to consider the blood and body fluids of all patients as potentially infectious. Although it has been shown that the risk of HIV transmisson to health care givers is low, other pathogens such as hepatitis A virus, hepatitis B virus, non-A and non-B hepatitis virus, cytomegalovirus, herpes simplex virus, Epstein-Barr virus, and *Staphylococcus aureus* are more easily transmitted in health care settings. Infections with these agents are frequently undiagnosed before initial contact with the patient. Therefore, taking precautions with the body fluids of all patients will both protect the health care giver and reduce nosocomial transmission of pathogens. In August 1987 the CDC published new recommendations for the prevention of HIV transmission in health care settings. These guidelines recommend the elimination of a separate blood/body fluid category, because these precautions are to be taken with all patients. Some hospitals have eliminated all the old isolation categories and implemented a system called *body substance isolation* (BSI). BSI protects both the health care worker and patients because it is not dependent on a diagnosis to initiate precautions. Following are explanations of (1) category-specific isolation and universal blood/body fluid precautions (see the box on pp. 204-208) and (2) BSI (see the box on p. 209).

Category-specific isolation precautions—cont'd

Specifications for contact isolation

1. Private room is indicated. In general, patients infected with the same organism may share a room. During outbreaks, infants and young children with the same respiratory clinical syndrome may share a room.
2. Masks are indicated for those who come close to the patient.
3. Gowns are indicated if soiling is likely.
4. Gloves are indicated for touching infective material.
5. Hands must be washed after touching the patient or potentially contaminated articles and before taking care of another patient.
6. Articles contaminated with infective material should be discarded or bagged and labeled before being sent for decontamination and reprocessing.

Diseases or conditions requiring contact isolation

Acute respiratory infections in infants and young children, including croup, colds, bronchitis, and bronchiolitis caused by respiratory syncytial virus, adenovirus, coronavirus, influenza viruses, parainfluenza viruses, and rhinovirus
Conjunctivitis, gonococcal, in newborns
Diphtheria, cutaneous
Endometritis, group A *Streptococcus*
Furunculosis, staphylococcal, in newborns
Herpes simplex, disseminated, severe primary or neonatal
Impetigo
Influenza, in infants and young children
Multiply resistant bacteria, infection of colonization (any site) with any of the following:
1. Gram-negative bacilli resistant to all aminoglycosides that are tested (in general, such organisms should be resistant to gentamicin, tobramycin, and amikacin for these special precautions to be indicated)
2. *Staphylococcus aureus* resistant to methicillin (or nafcillin or oxacillin if they are used instead of methicillin for testing)
3. *Pneumococcus* resistant to penicillin
4. *Haemophilus influenzae* resistant to ampicillin (beta lactamase positive) and chloramphenicol
5. Other resistant bacteria may be included if they are judged by the infection control team to be of special clinical and epidemiologic significance.

Continued.

Pediculosis
Pharyngitis, infectious, in infants and young children
Pneumonia, viral in infants and young children
Pneumonia, *Staphylococcus aureus* or group A *Streptococcus*
Rabies
Rubella, congenital and other
Scabies
Scalded skin syndrome, staphylococcal (Ritter's disease)
Skin, wound, or burn infection, major (draining and not covered by dressing or dressing does not adequately contain the purulent material) including those infected with *Staphylococcus aureus* or group A *Streptococcus*
Vaccinia (generalized and progressive eczema vaccinatum)

Respiratory isolation

Respiratory isolation is designed to prevent transmission of infectious diseases primarily over short distances through the air (droplet transmission). Direct and indirect contact transmission occurs with some infections in this isolation category but is infrequent.

Specifications for respiratory isolation

1. Private room is indicated. In general, patients infected with the same organism may share a room.
2. Masks are indicated for those who come close to the patient.
3. Gowns are not indicated.
4. Gloves are not indicated.
5. Hands must be washed after touching the patient or potentially contaminated articles and before taking care of another patient.
6. Articles contaminated with infective material should be discarded or bagged and labeled before being sent for decontamination and reprocessing.

Diseases requiring respiratory isolation

Epiglottitis, *Haemophilus influenzae*
Erythema infectiosum
Measles
Meningitis
    Haemophilus influenzae, known or suspected
    Meningococcal, known or suspected
Meningococcal pneumonia
Meningococcemia
Mumps
Pertussis (whooping cough)
Pneumonia, *Haemophilus influenzae,* in children (any age)

Tuberculosis isolation (AFB isolation)

Tuberculosis isolation (AFB isolation) is an isolation category for patients with pulmonary tuberculosis who have a positive sputum smear or a chest x-ray film that strongly suggests current (active) tuberculosis. Laryngeal tuberculosis is also included in this isolation category. In general, infants and young children with pulmonary tuberculosis do not require isolation precautions because they rarely cough, and their bronchial secretions contain few AFB, compared with adults with pulmonary tuberculosis. On the instruction card, this category is called AFB isolation to protect the patient's privacy.

Specifications for tuberculosis isolation (AFB isolation)

1. Private room with special ventilation is indicated; door should be kept closed. In general, patients infected with the same organism may share a room.
2. Masks are indicated only if the patient is coughing and does not reliably cover mouth.
3. Gowns are indicated only if needed to prevent gross contamination of clothing.
4. Gloves are not indicated.
5. Hands must be washed after touching the patient or potentially contaminated articles and before taking care of another patient.
6. Articles are rarely involved in transmission of tuberculosis. However, articles should be thoroughly cleaned and disinfected, or discarded.

Category-specific isolation precautions—cont'd

Enteric precautions

Enteric precautions are designed to prevent infections that are transmitted by direct or indirect contact with feces. Hepatitis A is included in this category because it is spread through feces, although the disease is much less likely to be transmitted after the onset of jaundice. Most infections in this category primarily cause gastrointestinal symptoms, but some do not. For example, feces from patients infected with "poliovirus" and coxsackieviruses are infective, but these infections do not usually cause prominent gastrointestinal symptoms.

Specifications for enteric precautions

1. Private room is indicated if patient hygiene is poor. A patient with poor hygiene does not wash hands after touching infective material, contaminates the environment with infective material, or shares contaminated articles with other patients. In general, patients infected with the same organism may share a room.
2. Masks are not indicated.
3. Gowns are indicated if soiling is likely.
4. Gloves are indicated when touching infective material.
5. Hands must be washed after touching the patient or potentially contaminated articles and before taking care of another patient.
6. Articles contaminated with infective material should be discarded or bagged and labeled before being sent for decontamination and reprocessing.

Diseases requiring enteric precautions

Amebic dysentery
Cholera
Coxsackievirus disease
Diarrhea, acute illness with suspected infectious etiology
Echovirus disease
Encephalitis (unless known not to be caused by enteroviruses)
Enterocolitis caused by *Clostridium difficile* or *Straphylococcus aureus*
Enteroviral infection
Gastroenteritis caused by
    Campylobacter species
    Cryptosporidium species
    Dientamoeba fragilis
    Escherichia coli (enterotoxic, enteropathogenic, or enteroinvasive)
    Giardia lamblia
    Salmonella species
    Shigella species
    Vibrio parahaemolyticus
    Viruses—including Norwalk agent and rotavirus
    Yersinia enterocolitica
    Unknown etiology but presumed to be an infectious agent
Hand, foot, and mouth disease
Hepatitis, viral, type A
Herpangina
Meningitis, viral (unless known not to be caused by enteroviruses)
Necrotizing enterocolitis
Pleurodynia
Poliomyelitis
Typhoid fever *(Salmonella typhi)*
Viral pericarditis, myocarditis, or meningitis (unless known not to be caused by enteroviruses)

Drainage/secretion precautions

Drainage/secretion precautions are designed to prevent infections that are transmitted by direct or indirect contact with purulent material or drainage from an infected body site. This newly created isolation category includes many infections formerly included in wound and skin precautions and discharge (lesion), and secretion (oral) precautions, which have been discontinued. Infectious diseases included in this category are those which result in the production of infective purulent material, drainage, or secretions, unless the disease is included in another isolation category that requires more rigorous precautions. For example, minor or limited skin, wound, or burn infections are included in this category, but major skin, wound, or burn infections are included in contact isolation.

Continued.

Category-specific isolation precautions—cont'd

Specifications for drainage/secretion precautions

1. Private room is not indicated.
2. Masks are not indicated.
3. Gowns are indicated if soiling is likely.
4. Gloves are indicated for touching infective material.
5. Hands must be washed after touching the patient or potentially contaminated articles and before taking care of another patient.
6. Articles contaminated with infective material should be discarded or bagged and labeled before being sent for decontamination and reprocessing.

Diseases requiring drainage/secretion precautions

Abscess, minor or limited
Burn infection, minor or limited
Conjunctivitis
Decubitus ulcer, infected, minor or limited
Skin infection, minor or limited
Wound infection, minor or limited
These infections are included in this category provided they are *not* (1) caused by miltiple resistant microorganisms, (2) major (draining and not covered by a dressing or dressing does not adequately contain the drainage) skin, wound, or burn infections, including those caused by *Staphylococcus aureus* or group A *Streptococcus,* or (3) gonococcal eye infections in newborns. See contact isolation if the infection is one of these three.

Universal blood/body fluid precautions

Since medical history and examination cannot reliably identify all patients infected with HIV or other blood-borne pathogens, blood and body fluid precautions should be consistently used for all patients.

Specifications for universal blood/body fluid precautions

1. Gloves are worn for touching blood and body fluids, mucous membranes, or nonintact skin of all patients, for handling items or surfaces soiled with blood or body fluids, and for performing venipuncture and other vascular access procedures. Gloves should be changed after contact with each patient.
2. Masks and protective eyewear or face shields should be worn during procedures that are likely to generate droplets of blood or other body fluids to prevent exposure of mucous membranes of the mouth, nose, and eyes.
3. Gowns or aprons should be worn during procedures that are likely to generate splashes of blood or other body fluids.
4. Hands and other skin surfaces should be washed immediately and thoroughly if contaminated with blood or other body fluids. Hands should be washed immediately after gloves are removed.
5. Disposable articles contaminated with body substances should be bagged and discarded according to local and state regulations.
6. Care should be taken to avoid needle stick injuries. Used needles should not be recapped or bent; they should be placed in a designated puncture resistant container as close to point of use as possible.
7. Blood spills should be cleaned up promptly with a solution of 5.25% sodium hypochlorite diluted 1:10 with water or an approved "hospital disinfectant" that is also tuberculocidal.

Universal blood and body fluid precautions protect the caregiver from blood-borne communicable diseases. Diseases recognized as being transmitted by blood include:
Acquired immunodeficiency syndrome (AIDS)
Arthropod-borne viral fevers (for example, denque, yellow fever, and Colorado tick fever)
Babesiosis
Creutzfeldt-Jakob disease
Hepatitis B (including HBsAg carrier)
Hepatitis, non-A, non-B
Leptospirosis
Malaria
Rat-bite fever
Relapsing fever
Syphilis, primary and secondary (skin and mucous membrane lesions)

Body substance isolation

All body substances are potentially infectious. Feces, sputum, and wound drainage always contain infectious organisms, whereas blood, urine, and other body fluids sometimes contain infectious organisms. The colonized, subclinical, and diagnosed infections are all communicable. However, category-specific or disease-specific isolation only protect against the diagnosed communicable infection. Therefore, protection against communicable disease transmission (health care worker and patient) can be achieved only by taking precautions with the body substances of all patients. Precautions should be determined by the anticipated interaction with a patient's body substances. Under this system, labeling patients with diagnosed infections would serve as a hindrance and support a double standard of practice. For example, a double standard exists when caregivers wear gloves when handling the urine of a patient with diagnosed *Serratia* urinary tract infection but not when handling the urine of other patients. Under BSI, the caregiver would be instructed to wear gloves for handling the urine of all patients.

Specifications for body substance isolation

1. Gloves for contact with mucous membranes, nonintact skin, and moist body substances. Gloves are changed after each patient contact.
2. Gown or plastic apron if soiling of clothing is likely.
3. Mask and eye protection if splashing of moist body substances is likely.
4. A private room is indicated if personal hygiene is poor or if body substances contaminate the environment.
5. Trash and linen bagged securely to prevent leakage.
6. Needles are disposed of uncapped and unbent at the point of use in a puncture-resistant container.
7. Blood spills of all persons should be cleaned by a gloved person using a solution of 5.25% sodium hypochlorite (household bleach) diluted 1:10 in water or a hospital disinfectant that is tuberculocidal.
8. A sign explaining BSI technique is placed in each patient's room.
9. Patients with airborne transmitted diseases require a private room with a sign to alert persons to check with the nurse before entering the room. Special ventilation is indicated. A mask is required to enter the room of a patient with pulmonary tuberculosis or meningococcal disease. Only immune persons should enter the room of a patient with chickenpox.

From Lynch, P, and Jackson, M: Isolation practices: How much is too much or not enough? Asepsis: The Infection Control Forum 8(4):2-5, 1986.

☐ General principles of isolation

Some general principles apply regardless of the type of isolation. Gowns, gloves, and masks should be used only once and then discarded in an appropriate receptacle before leaving the patient's room. Supplies should be available convenient to each patient's room. Hands must be washed before and after patient contact, even when gloves are a required part of the isolation procedure. Masks become ineffective when they are moist and therefore should never be reused. They should be worn over the nose and mouth and should not hang around the neck and then be reused. Disposable used articles and other waste should be placed in an impervious bag and the bag should be securely closed before it is discarded. Mattresses and pillows should be covered with impervious plastic.

The reader can see the similarity between the CDC's universal blood/body fluid precautions and BSI. The difference is that BSI does not require the other categories except for airborne transmitted diseases because the BSI technique prevents the transmission of the diseases in the other categories. There is redundancy in the CDC's category-specific and universal blood/body fluid precaution system.

■ SUMMARY

1. Infection control programs originated to decrease morbidity, mortality, and cost of nosocomial infections.
2. The sequence of events in the chain of infection involve (1) a causative agent, (2) a reservoir, (3) a portal of exit, (4) a mode of transmission, (5) a portal of entry, and (6) a susceptible host.
3. Modes of transmission are (1) contact (direct, indirect, and droplet), (2) airborne, (3) vehicle, and (4) vector.
4. In a serious infection, the WBC count usually rises above $10,000/mm^3$.
5. Whenever possible, appropriate cultures should be obtained before the initiation of antibiotic therapy.
6. In the United States, the ACIP recommends that children be immunized against diphtheria, pertussis, and tetanus (DPT); measles, mumps, and rubella (MMR); and poliomyelitis (OPV).
7. Health care givers who have frequent contact with blood and blood products should be immunized against hepatitis B virus.
8. Passive immunity is temporary, lasting a few weeks without stimulating antibody production in the recipient.

Putting knowledge to practice

- List six factors that put a hospitalized patient at risk of developing an infection.
- Define the following terms: (1) active immunity, (2) active acquired immunity, (3) passive immunity, and (4) herd immunity.
- What is the danger of giving antibodies in horse serum? What is the procedure that should be followed before injecting this type of solution?
- Plan a teaching program to encourage susceptible persons to obtain influenza immunization.
- What is the most common nosocomial infection? What measures could nurses take to reduce the incidence of this nosocomial infection?
- What measures can nurses take to prevent occupationally acquired diseases?

---

9. A nosocomial infection is one that is not present or incubating at the time a person is admitted to the hospital but develops after admission.
10. A community-acquired infection is one that is present or is incubating at the time of admission to the hospital.
11. Hand washing is the single most important measure in preventing cross-infections.
12. Urinary catheterization is associated with increased risk for nosocomial urinary tract infection.
13. Aseptic technique is an important factor in preventing nosocomial infection.
14. Two systems of isolation are (1) CDC category-specific isolation with universal blood/body fluid precautions and (2) body substance isolation (BSI).
15. Adherence to currently recommended isolation practices is the best protection that health care workers have from occupationally acquired infection.
16. Health care workers should direct problems concerning any aspect of infection control to the infection control nurse, the hospital epidemiologist, or the infection control committee in their institution.

REFERENCES AND SELECTED READINGS
Comtemporary

1. Albert, RK, and Condie, F: Handwashing patterns in medical intensive care units, N Engl J Med 304:1465-1466, 1981.
2. American Academy of Pediatrics: Report of the Committee on the Control of Infectious Diseases, ed 19, Evanston, Ill, 1982, The Academy.
3. American Hospital Association: AIDS/HIV infection policy: ensuring a safe hospital environment, AHA Report, pp. 1-27, 1987.
4. Gerherding, JL, and Henderson, DK: Design of rational infection control policies for human immunodeficiency viral infection, J Infect Dis 156(6):861-864, 1987.
5. Valenti, WM: Universal precautions: the data base emerges, Am J Inf Control, 16(2):39-40, 1988.

*References preceded by an asterisk are particularly well suited for student reading.

6. American Public Health Association: Control of communicable disease in man, ed 14, New York, 1985, The Association.
7. Bennett, JV, and Brachmann, PS (editors): Hospital infections, Boston, 1986, Little, Brown & Co.
8. *Bond, GB: Infection control: Serratia—an endemic hospital resident, Am J Nurs 81:2183-2186, 1981.
9. Castle, M: Hospital infection control, New York, 1980, John Wiley & Sons, Inc.
10. *Centers for Disease Control: Recommendations for prevention of HIV transmission in health-care settings, Morbid Mortal Week Rep 36(2S):3-17, 1987.
11. Centers for Disease Control: Perspectives in disease prevention and health promotion: Public Health Services Guidelines for counseling and antibody testing to prevent HIV infection and AIDS, Morbid Mortal Week Rep 36(31):509-515, 1987.
12. Centers for Disease Control: Human immunodeficiency virus infection in the United States: A review of current knowledge, Morbid Mortal Week Rep 36(49):1-14, 1988.
13. Centers for Disease Control: Guidelines for effective school health education to prevent the spread of AIDS, Morbid Mortal Week Rep 37(2S):1-14, 1988.
14. Centers for Disease Control: Recommendation of the Immunization Practices Advisory Committee (ACIP): Update on Hepatitis B prevention, Morbid Mortal Week Rep 36(23):353-366, 1987.
15. Centers for Disease Control: Recommendations of the Immunization Practices Advisory Committee (ACIP): Prevention and control of influenza, Morbid Mortal Week Rep 36(24):373-387, 1987.
16. Centers for Disease Control: Recommendations of the Immunization Practices Advisory Committee (ACIP): New recommended schedule for active immunization of normal infants and children, Morbid Mortal Week Rep 35(37):577-579, 1986.
17. Centers for Diease Control: Recommendations of the immunization practice advisory committee (ACIP): Immunization of children infected with human immunodeficiency virus, Morbid Mortal Week Rep 37(12):181-183, 1988.
18. Centers for Disease Control: Nosocomial infection surveillance, 1984, Morbid Mortal Week Rep 35(1SS):17-29, 1986.

19. Centers for Disease Control: Recommendations of the Immunization Practices Advisory Committee (ACIP): Update: pneumococcal polysaccharide vaccine usage, Morbid Mortal Week Rep 33(20):273-281, 1984.

20. A clinican's dictionary guide to bacteria and fungi, ed 4, Indianapolis, 1981, Eli Lilly Co.

21. Dixon, RE (editor): Nosocomial infections, New York, 1981, Yorke Medical Books.

22. Dixon, RE: Nosocomial respiratory infections, Infect Control 4:376-381, 1983.

23. Farke, BF, Kaiser, DL, and Wenzel, RP: Relationship between surgical volume and incidence of postoperative wound infection, N Engl J Med 305:200-204, 1981.

24. *Fernsebner, B: Antibicrobial therapy for surgical patients, AORN J 36:479-486, 1982.

25. *Fernsebner, B: Patients at risk for nosocomial infections, AORN J 38:613-620, 1983.

26. Friedland, GH, and Klein, RS: Transmission of the human immunodeficiency virus, N Engl J Med 317(18):1125-1135, 1987.

27. Garibaldi, RA, and others: Meatal colonization and catheter-associated bacteremia, N Engl J Med 303:316-318, 1980.

28. Garner, JS, and Simmons, BP: Guideline for isolation precautions in hospitals, Infection Control 4(4):245-325, 1983.

29. Gerberding, JL, Bryant-LeBlanc, CE, and others: Risk of transmitting the human immunodeficiency virus, cytomegalovirus, and hepatitis B virus to health care workers exposed to patients with AIDS and AIDS-related conditions, J Infectious Diseases 156(1):1-8, 1987.

30. Haley, RW: Managing hospital infection control for cost effectiveness, 1986, AHPI.

31. Haley, RW, and others: The efficacy of infection surveillance and control programs in preventing nosocomial infections in US hospitals, Am J of Epid 121(2):206-215, 1985.

32. Haley, RW, and others: Identifying patients at high risk of surgical wound infection, Am J Epidem 121(2):206-215, 1985.

33. Hawley, GB: Bacterial infection from intravascular monitoring devices, Infect Control 4:399-401, 1983.

34. *Jackson, MM, and others: Why not treat all body substances as infectious? Am J Nurs 87(9):1137-1139, 1987.

35. *Jenner, EA: Catheterization and urinary tract infection: preventing catheter associated urinary tract infections, Nurs 83 2(suppl.):1-3, 1983.

36. *Jenner, EA: Infection control in hospital and community. Identification of the infected patient, Nurs 83, 19(suppl.):1-3, 1983.

37. *Kaye, W: Catheter and infusion-related sepsis: the nature of the problem and its prevention, Heart Lung 11:221-228, 1982.

38. Kunin, C: Detection, prevention, and management of urinary tract infections, ed 4, Philadelphia, 1987, Lea & Febiger.

39. Larson, E: Clinical microbiology and infection control, St Louis, 1984, Blackwell Scientific Publications.

40. Labet, C, and Roderick, M: Infection control in the use of intravascular devices, Crit Care Q 3:67-80, 1981.

41. Lynch, P, Jackson, MM and others: Rethinking the role of isolation practices in the prevention of nosocomial infections, Ann Intern Med 107(2):243-246, 1987.

42. *Mooney, BR, and Armington, LC: Infection control—how to prevent nosocomial infections, RN 50(9):21-23, 1987.

43. *Moore, M, and Abbott, NK: Can handwashing practices be changed, Am J Nurs 80:80, 1980.

44. *O'Donnell, J: Antibiotic prophylaxis in surgical infection, Heart Lung 12:20-22, 1983.

45. *Seal, DV, and Ward, K: Catheterization and urinary tract infection: basic techniques for aseptic catheterization of the urinary tract, Nurs 83 2:5-6, 1983.

46. Symposium on infection control, Nurs Clin North Am 15(4):entire issue, 1980.

47. *Taylor, LJ: Infection control in the hospital and the community: prevention of the spread of infection, Nurs 83 2(suppl):3-4, 1983.

48. Youmans, GP: The biological and clinical basis of infectious diseases, ed 2, Philadelphia, 1980, WB Saunders Co.

Classic

49. American Hospital Association: Infection control in the hospital, ed 4, Chicago, 1979, The Association.

50. Band, JD, and Maki, DG: Safety of changing intravenous delivery systems at intervals longer than 24 hours, Ann Intern Med 91:173, 1979.

51. Barrett-Conner, E, and others: Epidemiology for the infection control nurse, St Louis, 1978, The CV Mosby Co.

52. Buxton, J, and others: Contamination of intravenous infusion fluids: effects of changing administration sets, Ann Inter Med 90:764, 1979.

53. Infection control: topics in clinical nursing, vol 1, no 2, Germantown, Md, 1979, Aspen Systems Corp.

54. *Knittle, MA, Eitzman, DV, and Baer, H: Role of hand contamination of personnel in epidemiology of gram negative nosocomial infections, J Pediatr 86:433-437, 1976.

12

Cancer

SUSAN MOELLER SCHNEIDER, MARGARET VETTESE ZACK,
and ROSEMARIE M. HOGAN

CHAPTER OBJECTIVES

After studying this chapter, the student should be able to:

- Discuss the epidemiologic variables related to cancer and the nurse's role in cancer epidemiology.
- Outline the pathophysiology of malignant tumors, focusing on the concepts of tumor growth and metastasis.
- List several factors that contribute to carcinogenesis.
- Describe the nurse's role in cancer prevention and health education.
- Conduct a holistic assessment of the oncology patient and identify appropriate nursing diagnoses.
- Explain the rationale for four categories of cancer therapy and discuss nursing interventions for patients receiving those therapies.
- Formulate a plan of care for the patient with advanced cancer.

Cancer was recognized in ancient times by skilled observers who gave it its name (from the Latin *Cancri*, crab) because it stretched out in many directions like the legs of a crab. It would be preferable if the image of the crab, suggested by Hippocrates for superficial cancer in the advanced stages, could be dropped, because it maintains a legend of incurability. Forms of cancer are found in plants and in humans and other animals. The term is somewhat general and is used interchangeably with *malignant tumor* and *malignant neoplasm.*[47]

One of the least understood facts about cancer is that the name designates more than 200 diseases that have in common the production of abnormal cells that do not obey the laws of normal tissue growth.[39] Therefore, cancer should never be looked on as a disease entity but only as a traditional term that describes a neoplastic process.

■ DEFINITION OF TERMS

The term *neoplasm* comes from the Greek word meaning "new growth" or "new formation." Normally, cell division is an orderly process with a distinct purpose of organism development or replacement of destroyed or injured cells. When cells divide without such a distinct purpose, they form neoplasms, sometimes referred to as *tumors.* Strictly speaking, a tumor is a swelling caused by any number of conditions, for example, inflammation or trauma. However, the terms *neoplasm* and *tumor* often are used interchangeably.

Oncology, a term used in association with the treatment and study of cancer is the study of tumors (from the Greek *onkos,* mass). Neoplasms are classified broadly by distinguishing between those which are "benign" and those which are "malignant." A *malignant* neoplasm (that is, a cancer) will cause death if it is not controlled. A *benign* neoplasm usually will not cause death unless by its location it interferes with vital functions.[36]

■ ATTITUDES TOWARD CANCER

Cancer has become one of the more curable chronic diseases.[4] Progress is evidenced by people's knowledge about the disease and the means to prevent it, more sophisticated diagnostic techniques revealing more cancers in the early curable stages, and improved methods of treating cancer, particularly with radiotherapy and chemotherapy.

More effective management of the side effects of therapy has improved survival rates. Advances in antimicrobial treatments and transfusion technology have helped to combat the life-threatening complications of sepsis and hemorrhage.

Despite this progress, few diseases cause greater feelings of anxiety and apprehension. A diagnosis of cancer still may carry with it a social stigma. In many ways, cancer has replaced tuberculosis as a metaphor for contemporary social ills—dirty, deadly, setting the "victim" apart.[67] The myths surrounding malignant disease, often focusing on incurability, help foster feelings of hopelessness and dread.

Nurses may also have the same negative attitudes that exist in society. For this reason it is extremely important that all nurses examine their own feelings about cancer and try to work them through, both by increasing their knowledge of the diseases and treatments and by discussing feelings openly with members of the health team. Nurses who have worked through their feelings are more able to be of assistance to patients and their families than nurses who have not done so.

The nurse's role in helping cancer patients is broad in scope and area of influence. The nurse must have correct knowledge of prevention, control, and treatment of cancer and be able to apply this information in a variety of settings. Teaching about cancer is not limited to the hospital or clinic setting but takes place in industry, at PTA meetings, and at other public forums. In addition to teaching about prevention, the nurse has an active role in treatment and control programs in all settings in which clients are found. Clients and their families look to the nurse for assistance and guidance in all phases of illness from detection to terminal care.

To be effective as a helping person, the nurse must be aware of the emotional impact that the diagnosis of cancer has on the patient and family, because this emotional response affects every aspect of nursing care. Cancer nursing is a challenge to the creativity, skill, and commitment of the nurse.

■ EPIDEMIOLOGY

Cancer is a disease that is universal in scope. It has existed since the beginning of history and affects humans wherever they live and whatever their race, color, level of culture, and material progress.[44]

Cancer ranks second to heart disease as the cause of death in the United States, but significant progress has been made in prevention and treatment. In the early 1900s few cancer patients had any hope of long-term survival. By the 1960s, 1 in 3 was alive at least 5 years after treatment. Today about 527,000 Americans, or 1 out of 2 cancer patients, will be saved.[1] This success can be attributed to the following:

1. Diagnosis of more cancers in the early, localized stage
2. Treatment of more patients within 4 months of diagnosis
3. Development of new diagnostic and treatment modalities, especially chemotherapy

Despite these advances, it was estimated that about 483,000 persons would probably die in 1987 who might have been saved by earlier diagnosis and prompt treatment. There has been a steady rise in the age-adjusted national death rate for cancer, from 143:100,000 population in 1930 to 176:100,000 in 1981. ("Age-adjusted" denotes a method used to make valid statistical comparisons by assuming the same age distribution among different groups being compared.) The major cause of the increased death rate has been cancer of the lung. Death rates for other major sites are leveling off or declining (for example, stomach and breast cancers).

■ Epidemiologic variables for cancer

Although, in general, cancer shows no respect for economic or social status, there are some variations with regard to sex, site, age, race, and geographic location.

■ SEX AND SITE

The average incidence of cancer is similar in both sexes. Overall survival rates (proportion of people alive 5 years after diagnosis) for some cancers have increased, such as those for cervical cancer. Rates for most other cancers have leveled off in the past 25 years. The average cancer mortality in developed countries is higher for men than for women.

Trends in age-adjusted cancer death rates per 100,000 population (1930 to 1985) indicated the following:

1. For both sexes
   a. Steady decrease in cancer of the liver and stomach
   b. Steady increase in cancer of the lung caused by cigarette smoking
   c. Steady increase, then leveling off, in cancer of the pancreas
2. For males
   a. Slight increase, then leveling off in prostate and colorectal cancer

3. For females
   a. Steady decrease in cancer of the uterus and breast
   b. Noticeable decrease in colorectal cancer[1]

Fig. 12-1 compares cancer incidence and deaths by site and sex.

■ AGE

Although more than three quarters of the deaths from cancer occur in persons over 55 years of age, cancer is the leading cause of death in women between 30 and 54 years of age, and more children aged 3 to 14 years die of cancer than of any other disease. However, mortality among children with cancer has declined.[1]

■ RACE

Cancer incidence and mortality are higher for blacks than for whites. Statistics indicate that blacks have significantly lower survival rates for cancer of the breast, colorectum, prostate, and testis.[1] Esophageal cancer has declined in whites but has risen rapidly in blacks of both sexes. Although incidence of invasive cervical cancer has declined in women of both races, the survival rate for white women is significantly higher than for black women. Endometrial cancer is the one cancer for which the incidence rate in white women is double that in black women.[1]

Most differences in the cancer rates of black and white populations are attributed to environmental and social factors rather than to inherent biologic characteristics. One American Cancer Society survey showed that urban blacks

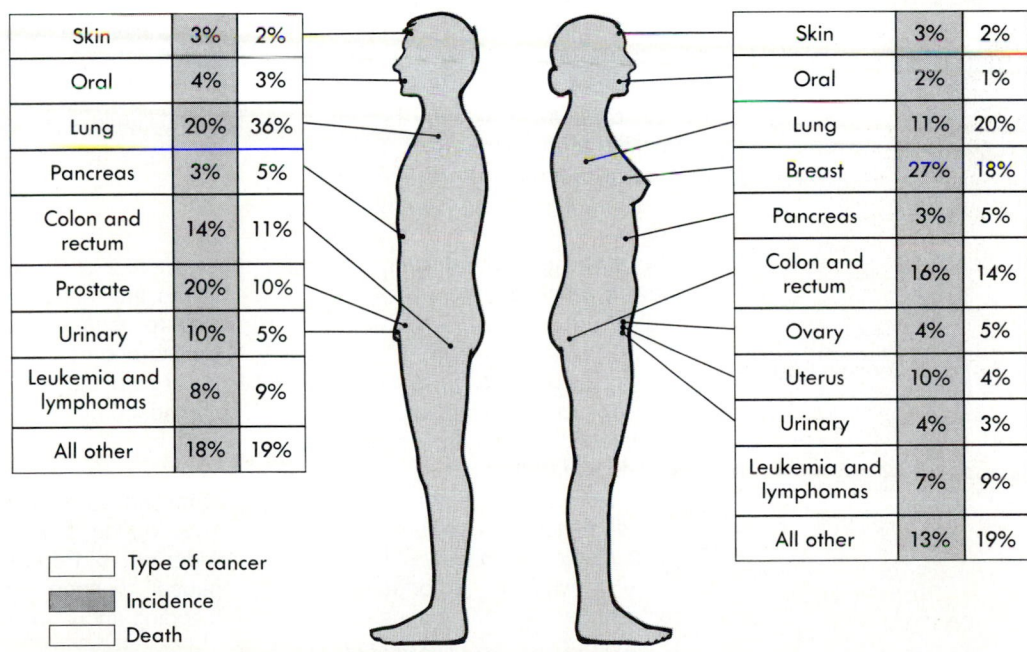

Fig. 12-1 Comparison of cancer incidence and deaths by site and sex (1987 estimates). (From American Cancer Society, 1987 Cancer Facts and Figures, New York, 1987, The Society.)

tend to be less knowledgeable about warning signals and less apt to seek medical care if symptoms do occur. These blacks also tended to underestimate the prevalence of cancer and the choices of cure. Increased risk of exposure to industrial carcinogens and limited educational opportunities among those in the lower socioeconomic group may also be contributing factors, because a higher percentage of blacks are in the lower socioeconomic group.[1]

■ GEOGRAPHIC FACTORS

No place or country on earth is free of cancer, although differences in the geographic distribution of cancer occur.[39,64]

1. The cancer mortality in the Syrian Arab Republic is less than 100:100,000 population. The U.S. rate is 176:100,000 population, and Scotland has the highest rate with more than 200:100,000 population.[1]
2. Cancer of the stomach is common in Japan, Singapore, and Hong Kong, whereas it is somewhat rare in the United States and Brazil.[1]

3. Cancer of the breast is more common in the United States and Western Europe than it is in Japan.
4. Ugandans, Nigerians, and South African blacks are at lower risk for cancer of the lung, stomach, large intestine, uterus, and kidney.

Genetic differences between populations may contribute to international variations. However, observations of what happens to cancer incidence when people migrate from one country to another show that environmental (for example, air pollution) and cultural (for example, diet) factors play a more important role than genetic differences in the rate changes that occur.[14]

■ Nurse's role in cancer epidemiology

Cancer is not only a threat to life, but its cost in loss of income and disruption of the lives of families cannot be estimated. Nurses must be in the forefront of the thousands of health professionals who are working to eradicate the disease. Cancer epidemiologic research has contributed to cancer prevention and control by identifying epidemi-

---

Table 12-1 Risk and epidemiology for six major cancer sites

Site	Estimated new cases 1987*	Estimated deaths 1987*	Risk factors	Comments
Breast	130,900	41,300	Over age 50, personal or family history of breast cancer, never had children, first child after age 30	Leading cause of death from cancer in women
Colorectum	145,000	60,000	Personal or family history of colon and rectum cancer, personal or family history of polyps in colon or rectum, ulcerative colitis, diet high in beef and/or deficient in fiber content	Considered a highly curable disease when digital and proctoscopic examinations are included in routine check-ups
Lung	150,000	136,000	Heavy cigarette smoking, history of smoking 20 or more years, exposure to certain industrial substances such as asbestos, particularly for those who smoke	Leading cause of cancer among men, and rising mortality among women
Mouth	29,800	9,400	Heavy smoking and drinking, use of chewing tobacco	Many more lives could be saved, because the mouth is easily accessible to visual examination by physicians and dentists
Skin	25,800†	7,800	Excessive exposure to the sun, fair complexion, occupational exposure to coal tar, pitch, creosote, arsenic compounds and radium	Readily detected by observation and diagnosed by simple biopsy
Uterus	47,800‡	9,700	Cervical cancer: early age at first intercourse, multiple sex partners. Endometrial cancer: history of infertility, failure of ovulation, prolonged estrogen therapy, late menopause, combination of diabetes, high blood pressure, and obesity	Uterine cancer mortality has declined 70% during past 40 years with wider use of Pap test; post-menopausal women with abnormal bleeding should be checked

*American Cancer Society, 1987 Cancer facts and figures, New York, 1987, The Society.
†Estimated new cases of nonmelanoma skin cancer about 500,000.
‡If carcinoma in situ is included, cases total 88,000.

ologic trends that can be used to determine individuals and groups at high risk for cancer. Nurses can play a vital role in cancer prevention by assessing people's cancer risks and teaching them about environmental and personal carcinogenic risk factors, including recommendations for prevention and early detection. Table 12-1 summarizes important epidemiologic aspects and risk factors for the six major cancer sites.

■ PATHOPHYSIOLOGY

■ Characteristics of malignant cells

Normal tissue contains large numbers of mature cells of uniform size and shape. Each cell contains a nucleus of uniform size. Within each nucleus are the chromosomes, a specific number for the species, and within each chromosome is deoxyribonucleic acid (DNA). DNA is a giant molecule whose chemical composition controls the characteristics of ribonucleic acid (RNA), which is found both in the nucleoli of cells and in the cytoplasm of the cell itself and which regulates cell growth and function. When ovum and sperm unite, the DNA and RNA within the chromosomes of each will govern the differentiation and future course of the trillions of cells that finally develop to form the adult organism. In the development of various organs and parts of the body, cells undergo differentiation in size, appearance, and arrangement; thus the histologist or the pathologist can look at a piece of prepared tissue through a microscope and know the portion of the body from which it came.

Some abnormal changes in cell growth are malignant growths. Other types of cellular growths are benign (nonmalignant). Benign neoplasms involve cellular proliferation of adult or mature cells growing slowly in an orderly manner in a capsule. These tumors do not invade surrounding tissue but may cause harm through pressure on vital structures within an enclosed structure such as the skull. Benign tumors remain localized, do not metastasize (spread), and do not recur after they are completely removed (see Table 12-2).

A malignant cell is one in which the basic structure and activity have become deranged in a manner that is unknown and from a cause or causes that are still poorly understood. It is believed, however, that the basic process involves a disturbance in the regulatory functions of DNA. It is known that the DNA molecule is affected by radiation in certain instances, and it is speculated that it may be affected by other factors as well.

In the neoplastic cell, normal restraints on growth are defective. It is believed that malignant neoplasms occur as the result of faulty mechanisms inside the cell nucleus.[9]

DNA, the permanent genetic material in nuclear chromosomes, contains information necessary for cell replication, the chemical code for cell growth and development. To convey this information, RNA serves as a messenger. Any small change in DNA (mutation) causes a distortion of biologic information, which may result in the affected cells running wild. Malignant neoplasm is the result.[8] The

Table 12-2 Characteristics of benign and malignant neoplasms

Characteristics	Benign	Malignant
Cell characteristics	Cells resemble normal cells of the tissue from which the tumor originated	Cells often bear little resemblance to the normal cells of the tissue from which they arose; there is both anaplasia and pleomorphism (assumption of two or more different forms)
Mode of growth	Tumor grows by expansion and does not infiltrate the surrounding tissues; encapsulated	Grows at the periphery and sends out processes that infiltrate and destroy the surrounding tissues
Rate of growth	Rate of growth is usually slow	Rate of growth is usually relatively rapid and is dependent upon level of differentiation; the more anaplastic the tumor the more rapid the rate of growth
Metastasis	Does not spread by metastasis	Gains access to the blood and lymph channels and metastasizes to other areas of the body
Recurrence	Does not recur when removed	Tends to recur when removed
General effects	Is usually a localized phenomenon that does not cause generalized effects unless by location it interferes with vital functions	Often causes generalized effects such as anemia, weakness, and weight loss
Destruction of tissue	Does not usually cause tissue damage unless location interferes with blood flow	Often causes extensive tissue damage as the tumor outgrows its blood supply or encroaches on blood flow to the area; may also produce substances that cause cell damage
Ability to cause death	Does not usually cause death unless its location interferes with vital functions	Will usually cause death unless growth can be controlled

From Porth, C: Pathophysiology: concepts of altered health states, Philadelphia, 1982, JB Lippincott Co.

Characteristics of malignant cells

1. Nuclei are larger and irregular in shape.
2. DNA is coarsely distributed and tends to appear near nuclear membrane.
3. Nucleoli are large, usually increased in number, and contain more chromatin than usual.
4. Mitosis is increased and atypical in appearance.
5. Abnormal multipolar mitoses and multinucleated cells may appear.
6. Cytoplasm is comparatively scanty and stains more deeply than normal cytoplasm (greater RNA concentration).
7. Cells vary in size from normal cells.
8. Surface characteristics of cells related to the cell membrane are altered: loss of contact inhibition, failure to form intracellular junctions, and impaired cell-to-cell communication.

---

malignant cells lose the normal specialized function of the normal cell or may take on new characteristics and functions.

A characteristic of malignant cells that can be observed through a microscope is *loss of differentiation,* or loss of likeness to the original cell (parent tissue) from which the tumor growth originated. This loss of differentiation is called *anaplasia,* and its extent is a determining factor in the degree of malignancy of the tumor.

Anaplasia is characterized by alterations in intracellular macromolecular synthesis and intercellular relationships and associations. Two types of anaplasia have been identified. In positional or organizational anaplasia, the usual distinct histologic patterns in tissues are altered. In cytologic anaplasia, there is increased or altered nucleic acid synthesis in growing tissues.[14] Anaplasia is one of the most reliable indicators of malignancy. It is seen only in cancers and does not appear in benign neoplasms.

Other characteristics of malignant cells that can be seen through a microscope are the presence of nuclei of various sizes, many of which contain unusually large amounts of chromatin, and the presence of mitotic figures (cells in the process of division), which denotes rapid and disorderly division of cells. The proportion of cells actively proliferating in malignant tumors is generally greater than that of normal cells.

Malignant tumors have no enclosing capsule; thus they invade adjacent or surrounding tissue, including lymph and blood vessels, through which they may spread to distant parts of the body to set up new tumors (*metastases*). Unless completely removed or destroyed, they tend to recur after treatment, and their continued presence causes death by replacing normal cells and by other means not fully understood. Characteristics of malignant cells are summarized in the box above.

■ GROWTH OF MALIGNANT NEOPLASMS

The term *neoplasm* has been defined as a relatively autonomous growth of tissues, the term *autonomy* meaning that a malignant tumor is not subject to the "rules and regulations" that govern cells and cell interaction of the

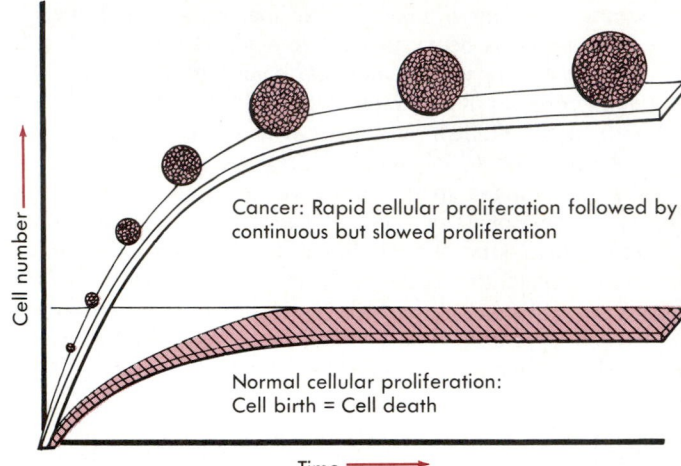

Fig. 12-2 Gompertzian function. (From Cancer: chemotherapy and care, Pt. 1, Bristol Laboratories, Division of Bristol-Myers Co.)

healthy individual. This autonomy is relative in that the tumor is not completely independent of the tissue from which it arose.

There are considerable differences in the rate of growth of malignant tumors. The growth rate is often referred to in terms of tumor *doubling time.* Different types of tumors often have varying doubling times. For example, lymphomas generally have a faster doubling time than cancers of the bone. It is also possible for tumors of the same tissue type to have different doubling times. A breast cancer may spread rapidly in one individual, whereas the growth in another individual could be extremely slow for a period of time and then could later accelerate. In general, it is has been calculated that a tumor mass will double in size 30 times before it is 1 cm in size, when there is a chance for it to be clinically detected[3] (Fig. 12-2). Occasionally, a tumor grows so slowly that it can be removed completely after a long period of time. This characteristic probably accounts for the good results obtained in a few circumstances even when treatment has been delayed. No phy-

CANCER SPREADS IN MANY WAYS:

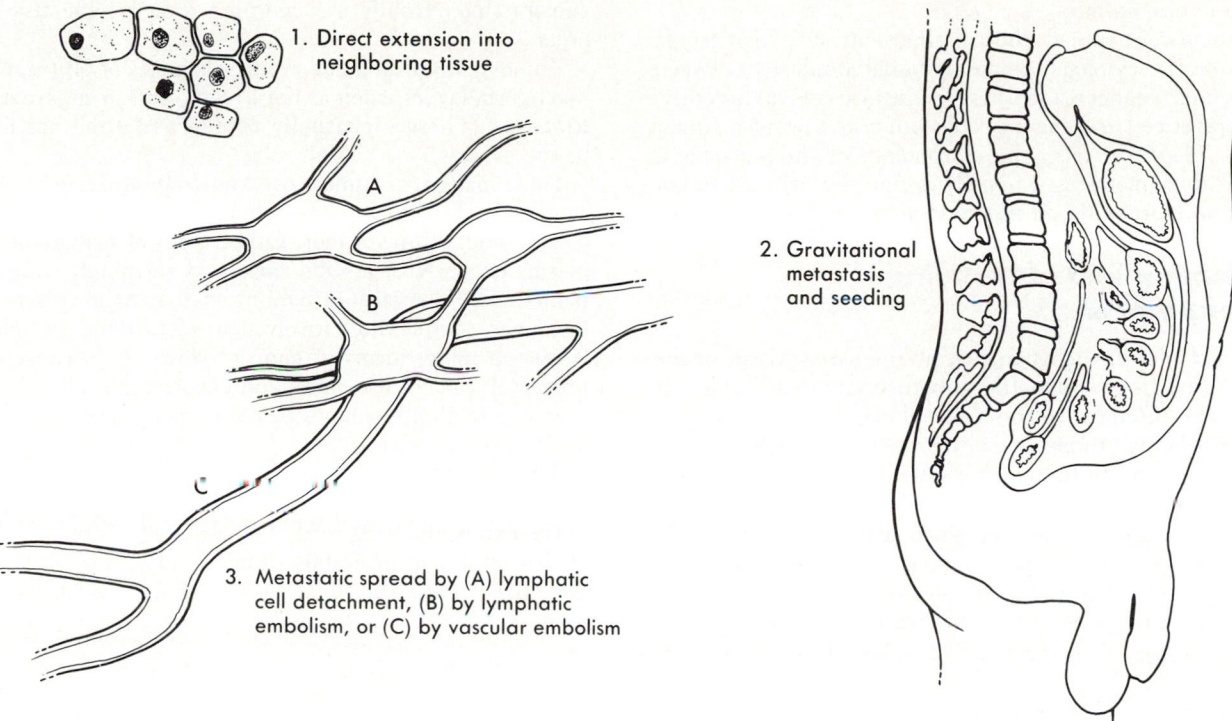

1. Direct extension into neighboring tissue

2. Gravitational metastasis and seeding

3. Metastatic spread by (A) lymphatic cell detachment, (B) by lymphatic embolism, or (C) by vascular embolism

Fig. 12-3   Modes of dissemination of cancer.

sician, however, ever relies on this possibility to justify delay in treatment. Occasionally, a malignant tumor grows slowly for a long time and then undergoes change, and the rate of growth increases enormously.

■ SPREAD OF CANCER

The rate of growth of a malignant neoplasm determines its capacity to spread. Cancer may spread by direct extension, by gravitational metastasis, or by metastatic spread (Fig. 12-3).

□ Direct extension or invasion

Direct extension or invasion of neighboring tissue produces the typical local effects of ulcerating, bulky, hemorrhagic masses or indurative, fibrosing lesions with tissue fixation, distortion of the structure, and the pitting of the skin seen in some breast cancer. Infection may accompany this local infiltration. Because of local spread, any cancer excision must include a margin of surrounding tissues to ensure removal of all malignant cells.

□ Gravitational metastasis and seeding

Gravitational metastasis involves the erosion of cancer cells into body cavities and their dropping onto the serous membrane lining the cavity. The pathway is determined by gravity or movements of the body. A tumor may penetrate the wall of the stomach and its cells implant on the surface of the peritoneal cavity. In the peritoneal cavity, cells tend to gravitate to the pelvis. Cells from neoplasm of the pleura of the thoracic cavity may "drop" to the diaphragm. Cancer cells can also be implanted by the surgeon into the operative area, causing metastatic lesions (mechanical transplantation).

□ Metastatic spread

Metastatic spread ocurs when cancer cells invade vascular or lymphatic channels and travel to distant parts of the body where implantation occurs. In *lymph vessels,* cells may detach and become emboli, which lodge in the regional lymph nodes that receive their drainage from the tumor site. Spread continues to the next group of nodes and into the other organs. Cells also may gain access to the bloodstream by way of the thoracic duct.

Vascular embolism of malignant cells may occur through the veins or arteries to various parts of the body depending on the vascular drainage of the organs involved. The liver is a common metastatic site for cancers originating in the gastrointestinal tract, pancreas, and spleen because of routing through the portal vein before entering the general circulation. Because venous blood travels through the lungs, this is another common site for secondary growth via the venous system. Cancer cells in the arterial system frequently form secondary neoplasms in the bone and the brain, especially if the primary site is in the lungs, where cancer cells can gain direct access to the left heart and systemic circulation.

In metastatic spread, there is almost always a high degree of histologic, cytologic, and functional similarity between the primary cancer and these metastases. Consequently, the type of cell and the probable site of the primary tumor can be identified from the morphology of the metastasis. In addition, metastases usually mimic the primary tumor in the formation of cell products and secretions.

■ Naming and classifying neoplasms

Tumors derive their names from the parent tissue or the tissue type from which the growth originated (Table 12-3). This is often called the tissue of origin. In general, the names of benign tumors carry the suffix *-oma* following the name of the parent tissue, for example, *neuroma* or *fibroma*. Malignant tumors generally are of two types, those of epithelial and those of mesenchymal (connective tissue) origin. The term *carcinoma* denotes a malignant tumor of epithelial cells, and the term *sarcoma* denotes a malignant tumor of connective tissue cells. Hematopoietic or blood-

forming tissues are involved in malignant processes that are disseminated from the beginning, in contrast to solid tumors that initially are confined to a specific tissue or organ.

Tumors containing embryonic elements of all three primary germ layers, such as hair, teeth, and so on; are called *teratomas*. These are usually benign and often are found in the ovaries.

Some malignant tumors are known by the names of the scientists who first described them, for example, Hodgkin's disease and Wilm's tumor. Other types of malignant neoplasms occur with a wide variety of seemingly unrelated names. The diversity in naming malignant neoplasms reflects the complexities involved in identifying and classifying the many forms of cancer. However, a consistent, universal system of naming and classifying tumors is necessary to facilitate communication among researchers and health professionals.

There are two major methods for classifying cancers: *grading* according to histologic criteria and *staging* according to the extent of the spread of the disease. Tumors may be graded by roman or arabic numerals into four grades; the higher the grade, the worse the prognosis,[47] as summarized on p. 221.

Table 12-3 Names of neoplasms

Tissue type	Benign	Malignant
Epithelium		
Skin and mucous membrane	Papilloma	Squamous cell carcinoma
Glands	Adenoma	Adenocarcinoma
Connective tissue		
Fibrous	Fibroma	Fibrosarcoma
Adipose	Lipoma	Liposarcoma
Cartilage	Chondroma	Chondrosarcoma
Bone	Osteoma	Osteosarcoma
Blood vessels	Hemangioma	Hemangiosarcoma
Lymph vessels	Lymphangioma	Lymphangiosarcoma
Muscle tissue		
Smooth muscle	Leiomyoma	Leiomyosarcoma
Striated muscle	Rhabdomyoma	Rhabdomyosarcoma
Nerve tissue		
Nerve fiber end sheath	Neuroma	Neurogenic sarcoma
Ganglion cells	Ganglioneuroma	Neuroblastoma
Glia cells	Astrocytoma	Glioblastoma multiforme
Hematopoietic tissue		
Plasma cells		Multiple myeloma
Lymphoid		Lymphatic leukemia
Miscellaneous		
Placenta	Hydatiform mole	Chorioepithelioma (choriocarcinoma)

Histologic grading

G1	Well-differentiated
G2	Moderately well-differentiated
G3, G4	Poorly to very poorly differentiated

A grade 1 tumor is the most differentiated (more like the parent tissue) and, therefore, the least malignant; grade 4 is the least differentiated (more unlike the parent tissue) and has a high degree of malignancy. These classifications are useful to the physician in knowing whether the tumor may be expected to respond to radiation treatment as well as in planning all other aspects of the patient's treatment. Usually, malignant tissue is slightly more sensitive to irradiation than normal tissue.

Determination of the extent of the spread of cancer (staging) and the site of the original tumor is vital for planning therapy. The International Union Against Cancer has devised the TNM system of classification: *T*, tumor; *N*, regional lymph nodes; *M*, distant metastases. Adding a number to the letters (for example T1, T2, N1, N2) indicates the extent of the malignancy. This system provides a type of shorthand notation to describe the particular tumor (see box below). The purpose of the TNM system is to define categories for all cases and also allow subsequent and more detailed information to be added. A TNM classification has been identified for major cancer sites,

and the choice of treatment depends on the clinical TNM stage, both for the primary tumor and the lymph nodes.

Different staging systems exist for some specific types of cancer. An example of this is the Dukes classification system for adenocarcinoma of the colon (Chapter 31). However, the American Joint Committee for Cancer Staging and End-Result Reporting advocates uses of the TNM system because it can be easily understood and applied to all tumor types. The consistent terminology of the TNM system facilitates communication among health care providers.

■ Physiologic changes with aging

The incidence of cancer is higher in the elderly population than in any other age group, and the chances of developing cancer increase with each decade after an individual reaches the age of 60. While a variety of physiologic changes occur with the aging process that makes the host more vulnerable to malignant growth (see later chapters for specific changes), perhaps the most significant change is the exhaustion of the immune system. Antibody functioning becomes impaired and normal cells are subject to attack when the immune system falsely identifies them as foreign substances. The compromised immune system leaves the host more vulnerable to the development of malignancies and less capable of combating those malignancies when they do occur.[32]

Another theory regarding the increase of cancer incidence in the elderly is that a lifetime of exposure to carcinogens eventually leads to the development of cancer. The physiologic changes of aging do not naturally result in tumor formation, but it is the result of prolonged exposure to cancer-causing agents. Regardless of the cause of cancer in the elderly population, nurses need to remember to assess the patient thoroughly for the signs and symptoms of cancer.

Because many older adults have chronic illnesses, early warning symptoms of malignancy are often attributed to other health conditions or are overlooked as part of the aging process.[32] As a result, many elderly patients are seen initially with advanced malignancies that are less amenable to treatment.

■ ETIOLOGY: CARCINOGENESIS

The factors that contribute to the development of cancer are many and at present are not fully understood; however, certain health practices are known to decrease the possibility that cancer may occur. Since cancer is not a single disease entity, it is not likely that there is a single cause. Cancer probably occurs as the result of the interaction of many risk factors or because of long-term exposure to a single carcinogenic agent. Factors involved in carcinogenesis include host susceptibility, environmental carcinogens, habits and customs, and viruses (see the box on p. 222).

TNM staging classification system

Tumor

T0	No evidence of primary tumor
TIS	Carcinoma in situ
T1, T2, T3, T4	Ascending degrees of tumor size and involvement

Nodes

N0	No regional nodes demonstrably abnormal
N1a, N2a	Demonstrate regional lymph nodes, metastasis not suspected
N1b, N2b, N3	Demonstrable regional lymph nodes; metastasis suspected
Nx	Regional nodes cannot be assessed clinically

Metastasis

M0	No evidence of distant metastasis
M1, M2, M3	Ascending degrees of metastatic involvement of the host including distant nodes

---

Some carcinogenic factors

Host susceptibility

Genetic factors
  Cancer family syndrome (CFS)
  Familial polyposis of colon
  Multiple endocrine adenomatosis (MEA)
  Retinoblastoma
Hormonal factors
  Estrogens
Precancerous lesions
  Polyps of colon and rectum
  Pigmented moles
  Cervical dysplasia
  Paget's bone disease
  Senile keratosis
  Xeroderma pigmentosum
Chronic irritation
  Coal tars and products in industry
  Sunlight overexposure
  Restrictive clothing
  Chronic use of laxatives
Immunologic factors
  Early childhood and old age
  Immunodeficiency disease
  Immunosuppressive therapy

Viruses

Herpesvirus hominis (HSV-2)—cervical cancer
Epstein-Barr virus—Burkitt's lymphoma

Psychosocial factors

Stressful life changes
Depression
Low social support and high need

Environmental factors

Ionizing radiation
  Radiographs
  Radioisotopes
Chemical pollutants
  Polycyclic hydrocarbons (soot, tar, pitch, mineral oils)
  Arsenic compounds
  Asbestos
  Aromatic amines
  Chromium compounds
  Benzol
  Nitrosamines (meat preservatives)
  Nitrates (food additives)
  Aflatoxin 13 (mold on nuts and grains)
  Vinyl chloride
  Diethylstilbestrol (DES)
  Red dyes (food coloring)
  Sweeteners (cyclamates and saccharin)

Health practices

Smoking
Nutrition
  Diets high in refined foods and low in roughage (colon cancer)
  Smoked foods ingestion
  High caloric intake
  Vitamin A, B (riboflavin), and C deficient diets
Alcohol
Sexual practices
  First coitus at an early age
  Multiple sex partners
  Uncircumcised sex partners

■ Host susceptibility

■ GENETIC FACTORS

Studies of genetic factors have focused on specific cancer sites and the disease in general. Chromosomes have been studied to find evidence of the genetic origin of cancer. Chromosomal abnormalities associated with neoplasia may consist of extra or missing chromosomes or the presence of abnormal chromosomes. The question is whether these changes are the cause or the effect of cancer.

A second indication of genetic origin is that cancer cells are a population of cells descendant from a single cell of origin (clones). Future generations of cancer cells are always malignant; they inherit and pass on the trait.

Finally, there is a possibility that cancer arises from an innate genetic inability, possibly a defect in mitotic regulation. Theoretically, in normal cells mitosis is either in-hibited or induced by diffusible substances. The repressor substances are called chalones. Cancer cells may fail to be regulated by the chalones either because the chalones may not be secreted, or if they are, they fail to respond.[50]

Familial polyposis of the colon, a precursor of cancer, is indisputably hereditary. There is also a high incidence of breast cancer in a vertical line of descent, such as from mother to daughter. Risk of breast cancer in the first-degree relatives of a patient is five times that of the general population. Heredity in some way seems to be connected with bronchogenic cancer. It seems to interact with cigarette smoking to cause a synergistic effect.[56]

In general, inherited cancers are a direct expression of an inherited defect, but these syndromes are rare and account for only a small percentage of familial cancer.[60] Studies have shown that the pattern of inheritance is not usually that of single mendelian gene, and it is still not known whether the incidences of many specific cancers are a result of a combination of genetic and environmental factors.

■ HORMONAL FACTORS

Hormones do not appear to be primary carcinogens, but rather they seem to influence carcinogenesis in the following three ways:

1. By a preparative action on the target tissues, making them susceptible to the carcinogenic agent
2. By a "permissive" influence of carcinogenesis allowing the process to progress
3. By a conditioning effect on the tumor

Hormones are capable of restraining or enhancing growth of tumors that have developed. Hormone therapy (p. 246) and some surgical therapies (hypophysectomy and oophorectomy) are based on this fact.

Evidence exists that tissues that are endocrine responsive (for example, breasts, endometrium, and prostate) do not develop cancer unless they are stimulated by their growth-promoting hormones. Estrogens have been associated with cancers such as adenocarcinoma of the vagina, hepatic tumors, breast tumors, and uterine cancer.[58]

In addition to tissue stimulation by the hormone, carcinogenesis may be determined by the length of time of the hormonal effect. The longer the preparative influence of the hormone, the greater the chance of cancer development.

■ PRECANCEROUS LESIONS

Certain benign lesions and tumors have a tendency toward malignant change. These cancers are preventable if minor precursor conditions are treated carefully. Precancerous lesions are a large and heterogenous group. In some cancer is inevitable, whereas in others the risk is so low that medical management disregards the cancer risk. For example, the risk of cancer is high in xeroderma pigmentosa, a rare skin disease, but low in leukoplakia (white patches) of the mucous membranes, especially of the oral cavity, larynx, and vulva.[63]

■ CHRONIC IRRITATION

It is also known that cancer may follow chronic irritation of any part of the body. There are many ways to prevent irritation that may lead to cancer. Effort is being made in industry to protect workers from coal-tar products known to contain carcinogens. Masks and gloves are recommended in some instances, and workers are urged to wash their hands and arms thoroughly to remove all irritating substances at the end of the day's work. Occupational health nurses participate in intensive educational programs to help workers understand the need for carrying out company rules that may help prevent cancer.

Prolonged exposure to wind, dirt, and sun may also lead to skin cancer. Skin cancer of the face and hands is particularly common among outdoor workers who have fair complexions and who do not protect themselves from exposure. The incidence of skin cancer and melanoma is much higher in the "Sun Belt" region of the United States.

Any kind of chronic irritation to the skin should be avoided, and moles that are in locations where they may be irritated by clothing should be removed. Shoelaces, shoetops, girdles, brassieres, and shirt collars are examples of clothing that may be a source of chronic irritation. Glasses, earrings, dental plates, and pipes that are in repeated contact with skin and mucous membrane may contribute to cancer. Cancer of the mouth is sometimes associated with rough jagged teeth and the constant irritation of tobacco smoke or alcohol. Indiscriminate use of laxatives is believed to have possible carcinogenic effects on the large bowel.

■ IMMUNOLOGIC FACTORS

It may be possible that failure of the normal immune mechanism may predispose to certain cancers. The change from normal to malignant cells is relatively common. These new cells are antigenically different and are recognized as such by the body's immune system. If the immune response is initiated, the malignant cell will be destroyed. That a kind of immune surveillance system may exist is suggested by the following evidence:

1. The two peaks of high incidence of tumors in humans are in early childhood and old age.
2. Individuals with rare immunodeficiency diseases in which there is a defect in cellular immunity have increased evidence of tumor development.
3. Individuals receiving immunosuppressive drugs to prevent organ transplant rejection have an increased evidence of neoplasia.[53]

Cancer itself appears to suppress the immune response early in the disease, as well as late in its progression. It has not been definitely established that cancer develops because of failure in immune surveillance, and at present there is not enough data to make a strong case.[33] (The role of the immune system and cancer therapy is discussed later in this chapter and in Chapter 37.)

■ Environmental factors

It has been estimated that 70% to 90% of human cancers result from environmental factors and that we have the knowledge to prevent 30% to 40% of cancers in the United States. Occupational exposure causes 1% to 5% of human cancer, and the Environmental Protection Agency indicates that as many as 50,000 chemical substances, *excluding* pharmaceutical and food additives in common use, are carcinogenic.[64]

There are several types of chemical and physical carcinogens (cancer-producing substances). Various carcinogens may have an additive or enhancing effect on one another, and even small amounts of these substances may constitute a hazard. Carcinogens act on different organs depending on the portal of entry and the distribution in the body.

IONIZING RADIATION

Radiographs and radium may cure cancer, but in other cases they cause it. Ionizing radiation consists of electromagnetic waves or material particles that have sufficient energy to ionize atoms or molecules (that is, remove electrons from them) and thereby alter their chemical behavior. In adequate amounts, it destroys the cells.

Every living thing from the beginning of time has been exposed to small amounts of radiation from the sun and from certain natural elements in the earth, such as uranium, that emit gamma rays (γ-rays) in the process of their decay. This is called natural background radiation. No problem regarding radiation existed until after 1895, when the Roentgen ray (x-ray) machine was developed and became widely used in diagnosis of disease. The development of this machine was followed by the discovery of radium and the use of both radium and radiographs for treatment of disease such as cancer. With developments in the field of nuclear energy, it has been possible to produce radioactive isotopes of a number of the elements, although only a few of them, such as gold, iodine, cobalt, and phosophorus, have medical application at the present time. The problem of overexposure and possible harm to patients and to personnel caring for them has increased greatly with the increased use of radiographs in diagnosis and treatment and the more recent use of radioisotopes in diagnosis and treatment. Also, radiation-producing substances are being used to greater extents in the work and home environments.

No one really knows how much exposure to radiation is safe for persons working with patients and for patients having repeated radiographs taken for various purposes. Relatively small amounts of exposure have produced serious damage in experimental animals, but humans have not lived through enough generations of relatively high exposure for conclusive evidence of safe levels to be obtained. It is reasonable to assume that the less exposure one has the better. This does not mean that a patient receiving radiation treatment should not receive adequate nursing care. There are ways to protect persons from exposure, and hospitals are required to have protective procedures and guidelines for persons who care for patients receiving radiation therapy. Nurses should be familiar with the procedures used in the institution in which they are employed.

The ionizing effect of radiation on the body cells remains, so that exposure is cumulative throughout life. Exposure of the entire body enormously increases the amount of radiation received. For this reason all of the body except the part being treated is protected from exposure when relatively high doses are given for therapeutic purposes.

The amount of exposure the patient receives from a series of radiographs taken for diagnostic purposes depends on the machine used and the technical skill involved. Usually, the fluoroscopic examination entails more exposure than radiography. To prevent excessive exposure with fluoroscopy, physicians allow time for their eyes to accommodate to the darkened room so that the patient can be observed with a lower intensity of the machine. The exposure of the average nurse working in a hospital and occasionally assisting a patient while a radiograph is taken is almost negligible.

Badges are worn by persons whose daily work exposes them to radiation. The badge, which contains photographic film capable of absorbing radiation, is developed each month. A darkening or blackening of the film indicates excessive exposure. Personnel who are becoming overexposed are removed, at least temporarily, from direct contact with radiation.

Because of the possible danger to the fetus, particularly between the second and sixth weeks of life, radiographs are seldom taken of pregnant women. Also, pregnant women usually are not employed in radiology departments or in caring for patients who are receiving radioactive materials internally.

CHEMICAL POLLUTANTS

Air pollution has been blamed for the rising cancer incidence in the twentieth century. Ten polycyclic aromatic hydrocarbons have been recognized as carcinogenic.[47] Tar and pitch and their derivatives and mineral oils containing aromatic hydrocarbons were discovered to be carcinogenic many years ago. Bladder cancer from aromatic amines is an occupational disease of workers in the rubber industry. The risk of contacting lung cancer is 15 to 30 times greater among those exposed to chromium compounds. Other common occupational cancers are respiratory cancers from asbestos and leukemia resulting from long-term inhalation of benzol.

A liver carcinogen, aflatoxin 13, has been isolated from a common mold that grows on peanuts, soybeans, fruit, some meats, and mild and cheddar cheese. A rare form of vaginal cancer in young women has been linked to the ingestion by their mothers of diethylstilbestrol (DES) prescribed to prevent spontaneous abortion.

In 1969 cyclamates, which were widely used as sugar substitutes, were banned when experimental studies revealed that in high doses they could produce cancer of the bladder in mice. Saccharin has also been identified as being carcinogenic in a study of rats, and the Food and Drug Administration has recommended that it not be used as an artificial sweetener. The use of some hair dyes has also been implicated in cancer.

Chemotherapeutic agents used to treat cancer are also considered carcinogens. Because these agents alter the ability of cells to replicate, they are capable of affecting healthy cells as well as tumor cells. Although data are inconclusive regarding how much risk is involved with handling antineoplastic agents, many groups recommend using protective gowns, gloves, and masks. These medications should be prepared under a vertical laminar air flow hood. Nurses should be familiar with the policies and procedures that exist within the institution where they are employed.[23]

Health practices

TOBACCO USE

There is now no question that the rise in lung cancer during the past 70 years can be attributed to the increased use of cigarettes. The American Cancer Society estimates that cigarette smoking is responsible for 83% of lung cancer cases among men and 43% among women—more than 75% overall. Those who smoke two or more packs of cigarettes a day have lung cancer mortality 15 to 25 times greater than nonsmokers, according to the 1982 Surgeon General's Report.[2] In the past, more men than women smoked, and men smoked more heavily; however, the gap has been narrowing. The rise in the number of women smokers has captured the attention of cigarette manufacturers, who have increased their advertising efforts in this direction, to the point of designing cigarettes expressly for women.

Tobacco use accounts for about 30% of all deaths from cancers (some examples are mouth, pharynx, larynx, esophagus, pancreas, and bladder) and is also linked to heart disease, gastric ulcers, chronic bronchitis, and emphysema.[2] If smoking is discontinued, even after a habit of 30 years, there is a decrease in the evidence of lung cancer. Not smoking for 10 to 15 years reduces the risk of cancer to equal that of a person who has never smoked.[39]

The American Cancer Society recently reported a steady decline in the proportion of adult smokers in the United States. Overall, by 1980 the percentage of men and women smokers in the population had dropped to 32%. There are more than 33 million ex-smokers now living in the U.S. Of these, 95% quit on their own, without the aid of any organized program. However, for smokers who need more intensive assistance and group support, smoking cessation clinics are available in most communities.[1]

After the release of the Surgeon General's Report on Smoking and Health in 1964, the National Interagency Council on Smoking and Health was formed. This group, composed of 27 public and private health, educational, and youth organizations, has as its major objective combating smoking as a health hazard. Several of these participating organizations have produced films and other educational materials that are available to schools, organizations, and individuals. Assistance in securing films and other materials can be obtained from the Library, National Clearinghouse for Smoking and Health, Public Health Service.* One of the main concerns of the Interagency Council is how to convince young people not to start smoking.

Smokeless tobacco has also been identified as a carcinogen and has been shown to cause cancer of the oral cavity. The trend among adolescents of using smokeless tobacco as snuff or chew has been linked to the rise in cancer of the mouth. The cancer occurs in the mucous membranes

*5401 Westbord Ave., Bethesda, MD 20016

along areas where the tobacco is placed.[2] In recent years the scope of antismoking campaigns in the schools has broadened to include education regarding the hazards of smokeless tobacco. Antitobacco education in schools is conducted through school courses, assemblies, and exhibits.

Many smokers have switched to brands of cigarettes with filters that reduce the tar and nicotine (T/N) exposure. Although low T/N smokers may find it easier to quit smoking and the lung cancer mortality is reduced somewhat, many people only smoke *more* of filtered cigarettes, resulting in no reduced lung cancer risk. In addition, certain filtered brands have been found to deliver more carbon monoxide than those without filters.[1,69]

Switching from a cigarette to a pipe or cigar also may reduce the risk of lung cancer but not the risk of cancer of the lips, pharynx, and esophagus. The smoke from pipes and cigars contains the same amount of tar and nicotine as cigarettes. It simply is not inhaled.[69]

The question of hazards for nonsmokers who breathe the smoke of others' cigarettes is not resolved, but recent studies have aroused concern. Two studies have shown increased risk of lung cancer among wives of cigarette smokers; however, another study found little, if any, risk for "passive smokers." The American Cancer Society's new Cancer Prevention Study II is including an assessment of the cancer risk among passive smokers.[1]

Nurses have a responsibility, both as well-informed citizens and as professional persons, to be aware of the most recent antismoking programs and to interpret them to the public. One of the best ways for nurses to do this would be to stop smoking themselves. According to the American Cancer Society, approximately 24% of female nurses smoke and 41% of male nurses smoke.[17]

NUTRITION

Nutritional habits are increasingly being investigated and implicated in the etiology of cancer. A high incidence of cancer of the colon occurs in populations whose diet is high in refined food and low in nonabsorbable cellulose "roughage" or fiber. Evidence indicates that the incidence of colonic carcinoma is low among persons who eat a largely vegetarian diet that has relatively few animal products[54] and is especially low in fats. Breast cancer appears to be associated with a diet high in animal fat, but the precise relationship has not been identified.[48]

Other factors in the daily diet may be responsible for cancer. These are not only specific carcinogenic agents but also certain nutritional deficiencies. Breast and colon cancers have also been correlated with nutritional deficits, especially with vitamins A, B (riboflavin), and C, although these may play an indirect role.[49] Ingestion of smoked foods, which contain benzopyrene, has been correlated with an increased incidence of stomach cancer. Some epidemiologic and experimental evidence suggests that high caloric intake may lead to cancer and caloric deprivation may prevent it. Obesity may increase the risk of endometrial cancer.[30]

Some foods may protect against cancer. The food additive

butylated hydroxyanisole (BHA) and butylated hydroxytoluene (BHT) seem to inhibit cancer. Although reports are conflicting, some investigators believe vitamins A, B, and C actually have anticancer effects. The *Lactobacillus bulgaris* and *Streptococcus thermophilus* microorganism found in yogurt have been found to inhibit tumor cell proliferation.[49]

Many food substances contain additives, contaminants, and naturally appearing substances such as aflatoxin, which may be carcinogenic. Food additives being studied include food dyes, flavoring agents, and antimicrobial preservatives such as sodium and potassium nitrite and nitrate. Although some potential carcinogens are present in the diet, the time trends do not indicate that additives now in use are significant in the etiology of cancer. The present government policy is to keep the levels of potential carcinogenic agents in food as low as feasible, recognizing that it is almost impossible to state with absolute certainty that any ingested chemical is safe.[54]

The Delaney clause to the food additive amendment to the Federal Food, Drug and Cosmetic Act requires that no substance producing tumors in experimental animals should be permitted in food for human beings. The problem is that effects from ingesting carcinogenic agents may not be seen for decades because of the long latency periods. Childhood exposure, particularly, may provide the time for cancer to appear.[49]

ALCOHOL

There is a significant association between alcohol intake and cancer of the mouth, pharynx, larynx, and esophagus. However, alcoholism is often associated with smoking and with vitamin and dietary deficiencies, whose roles in the etiology of cancer are not known. It is speculated that alcohol and nutritional deficiencies enhance carcinogenesis by increasing the metabolic activities of specific tobacco carcinogens.[49] Tumors of the involved sites occur with greater frequency in men, blacks, lower socioeconomic groups, increasingly urbanized societies, and the elderly.[14]

SEXUAL PRACTICES

Carcinoma of the uterine cervix is less common in virgins than in married women. It is higher in those who have first coitus at an early age, who have an early first marriage, and who have had multiple sex partners. Cervical cancer is more frequent in women who have had multiple pregnancies, but this factor decreases in importance when the groups of women compared started their sex life at the same age. The development of cancer seems to be connected with coitus rather than pregnancy.

Carcinoma of the penis is virtually unknown among circumcised men. The means by which circumcision provides protection is not clear, but it is probably related to better hygiene. There is also a lower incidence of cancer of the uterine cervix in women whose sexual partner has been circumcised and in cultures in which the men, even though not circumcised, have a high standard of genital hygiene.[51]

The correlation with sexual experience and breast cancer is the reverse of that for the uterine cervix. Breast cancer patients have usually been married and become pregnant later in life. Lactation may provide some protection against breast cancer, since women who have breast-fed their infants show a lower incidence of breast malignancy. Cancer of the breast is reported to be unknown among Eskimo women and to be relatively rare among Japanese women; both cultures practice breast-feeding.

Viruses

There is strong evidence from animal studies that viruses play an important role in carcinogenesis, but evidence for viral etiology of human cancers is much less convincing. The strongest evidence of a causal relationship to cancer in humans is from studies of the DNA Epstein-Barr virus (EBV), a human virus known to be the etiologic agent of infectious mononucleosis and suspected in Burkitt's lymphoma and nasopharyngeal cancer. However, a positive serum test for EBV antibody (indicating past exposure) has been found in healthy adults, suggesting that other factors need to be involved for cancer to develop.[39,42]

Cervical cancer may result from a virus introduced into the cervix during sexual intercourse. This virus may be a member of the herpes group, *herpesvirus hominis* (HSV-2). Carriers of HSV-2 in the population are generally uncircumcised males with poor personal hygiene.[68]

Even if the evidence of viral etiology were more conclusive, consideration needs to be given to the question of whether the virus is transmitted horizontally, from host to host, or vertically, from generation to generation via the viral chromosome. In addition, successful immunization against a virus would require the following:

1. Suppression of the genetic expression of the virus
2. Sufficiently high incidence of the type of cancer to justify the cost of immunization
3. Consideration of previous natural exposure to the virus
4. Consideration of the effects of the immunization on any other etiologic factors that may be linked to the occurrence of the cancer[42]

The viruses found in animal tumors indicate that viruses may act individually or as co-carcinogens in causing malignancy in humans.[68] The question is no longer, however, whether viruses have a role in the cause of cancer but when they will be definitely implicated and whether one or many will be involved.

Psychosocial factors

Stressors such as life changes, loss of a significant other, and personality variables have been suggested as etiologic factors in the development of cancer. Some researchers believe that stress alters the body's immune system, making a person more susceptible to cancer. Depression has also been linked to cancer deaths by causing changes in immune mechanisms.

Social support in the form of institutions, family and

friends also may be an important variable. The individual with low social support and high need may be at a higher risk for developing cancer. In addition, lack of social support may adversely affect coping responses to therapy and to the illness. At the present time, however, how one defines the nature of social support and the degree to which it is present or lacking is unclear.

Conclusions

Carcinogenesis is a dynamic process that is influenced by many independent and poorly defined variables. The initial molecular changes are irreversible, but they may not be expressed when cooperative conditions are absent. Changes in these conditions may alter the carcinogenic process, resulting in either acceleration, inhibition, or even reversal of the process. Etiologic agents may be co-carcinogens. A genetic predisposition for a "weak" immune system along with a viral infection may lead to cancer, or oncogenic viruses may act as suppressants of the immune system. Chemical carcinogens may activate latent viral genes or inhibit the immune system's effectiveness in destroying cancer cells.

Nurses have a vital role to play in communicating to the public the factors involved in carcinogenesis. They can clarify misconceptions, as well as do health teaching, so that known carcinogenic practices may be eliminated. They can also set an example of good health practices for the general public, perhaps a more difficult role. As knowledgeable and concerned citizens, nurses must be initiators and supporters of efforts to have carcinogens removed from the environment.

PREVENTION AND HEALTH EDUCATION

Health teaching

The American public is more widely read and informed about health problems than ever before. Health-seeking behavior and a desire to be more knowledgeable about health problems are indicated by the frequency of articles about topics such as cancer in the lay press. The topic of cancer is also discussed more openly than ever before. Nurses have a major responsibility in the prevention of cancer. Because of their knowledge about the disease and their opportunity for contact with the public in the inpatient and outpatient setting, nurses have the opportunity to teach about cancer and to help motivate patients to seek treatment.

Case finding is a responsibility of all nurses. The nurse must be able to (1) counsel and direct patients to the proper sources of help, (2) have information about those conditions that are known to predispose individuals to the development of the disease, and (3) educate the public about these factors. In addition, the nurse must be sensitive to the needs of patients who may be afraid and embarrassed when confronted with the possibility of cancer.

Since prevention of cancer is a primary goal of health professionals, the nurse must be aware of and able to communicate to others the importance of good health habits and the importance of avoiding conditions that predispose to cancer.

Early detection and treatment

The approach to early detection of cancer is worldwide. General criteria for cancer screening and testing programs have been drawn up by the epidemiology section of the American Public Health Association, and these criteria have been adapted by the World Health Organization. Multiphasic screening and a periodic health examination are being accepted by the public. In some cases diagnosis can be made months before the development of symptoms causes the person to seek care.

Cancer detection is expensive. Education of the public often includes convincing them that a periodic health examination is a sound investment. Some cities have cancer detection centers where a complete physical examination including chest radiograph, Papanicolaou smear, breast examination, proctoscopy, urinalysis, and blood count are performed for a moderate fee. Nurses should be aware of clinics in their area where persons needing such resources may be referred.

The American Cancer Society has revised its guidelines for cancer-related checkups to provide essentially the same benefits with greatly reduced cost, risk, and inconvenience. Protocols for the early detection of cancer in asymptomatic persons are listed in Table 12-4. In general, persons over 20 years of age should have a cancer-related checkup every 3 years, and those over 40 should have one every year. These checkups should also involve health counseling including information about personal cancer risk factors.[19] Women should request that the Pap test (Papanicolaou stain) be done if it was inadvertently overlooked by the health care provider. The Pap test still is one of the best means of preventing death from cervical cancer.

Early detection of cancer can decrease mortality. The guidelines of the American Cancer Society have been developed for people *without* symptoms; however, those who have any signs or symptoms suggestive of cancer should report them immediately to a physician. The nurse must know and be able to explain the significance of the American Cancer Society's seven warning signals and seven safeguards (see boxes on p. 228). Any of these signs should be investigated medically, but their occurrence does not necessarily mean that the person has cancer.

All persons should know the most common sites of cancer. In women these are the breast, uterus (cervix), lung, and colorectum (Fig. 12-1). Women should be taught to examine their breasts each month immediately after the menstrual period or, for postmenopausal women, on a designated day each month. Such self-examination is a much better method of detecting early breast cancer than an annual physical examination (see Chapter 36). Women of all ages should know the importance of reporting an ab-

Table 12-4 Guidelines for cancer related checkups*

Test or examination	Sex	Age (yr)	Recommendation
Papanicolaou test	Female	Over 20; under 20 if sexually active	Every 3 years after two initial negative tests 1 year apart
Pelvic examination	Female	20-40	Every 3 years
		Over 40 or at menopause	Yearly
Endometrial tissue sample	Female	At menopause if high risk	High risk: history of infertility, obesity, failure of ovulation, abnormal uterine bleeding, estrogen therapy
Breast self-examination	Female	Over 20	Monthly
Breast physical examination	Female	20-40	Every 3 years
		Over 40	Yearly
Mammogram	Female	35-40	One baseline mammogram
		40-50	Every 1-2 years
		Over 50	Yearly
Stool guaiac slide test	Male and female	Over 50	Yearly
Digital rectal examination	Male and female	Over 40	Yearly
Sigmoidoscopic examination	Male and female	Over 50	Every 3-5 years after two initial negative examinations 1 year apart

*American Cancer Society recommendations, 1987.

Cancer's seven warning signals

Change in bowel or bladder habits
A sore that does not heal
Unusual bleeding or discharge
Thickening or lump in breast or elsewhere
Indigestion or difficulty in swallowing
Obvious change in wart or mole
Nagging cough or hoarseness

Cancer's seven safeguards

Lung: Don't smoke cigarettes.
Colorectum: Have a proctoscopic exam as part of a regular checkup after age 40.
Breast: Practice monthly breast self-examination.
Uterus: Have a Pap test as part of a regular checkup.
Skin: Avoid overexposure to the sun.
Oral: Have a regular mouth examination by physician or dentist.
Complete body: Have an overall physical checkup annually or at 3-year intervals, depending on age.

---

normal vaginal bleeding or other discharge occurring between menstrual periods or after menopause. (Further information about cancer of specific organs can be found in appropriate chapters of this text.)

Testicular cancer accounts for only 1% of all male cancer, but it is the commonest carcinoma in the 15- to 35-year-old age group.[15] Men, especially those in this young population, should be taught testicular self-examination (see Chapter 34). Testicular cancer, if diagnosed early, has an excellent chance for cure if treated with surgery and/or radiation therapy.

Two common misconceptions that lead the person to ignore symptoms should be corrected. The first is a belief that a disease as serious as cancer must be accompanied by weight loss. Weight loss is usually a late symptom of cancer, yet the person often remarks, "I wasn't losing weight so I thought nothing serious could be wrong." Another reason for neglect of cancer is that it may not cause pain, and again the person believes the absence of pain means that the indisposition is minor. It must be repeatedly

emphasized to the public that pain is not an early sign of cancer and that cancer often is far advanced before pain occurs.

Nurses also have a role in prevention and early detection of genetic cancer. They systematically obtain family cancer histories, teach about health maintenance, and do genetic counseling.[60] They may be involved in centralized familial cancer registries analogous to the monitoring of communicable diseases by health departments. Familial cancer registries would be helpful in pooling data on suspected cancer-prone families, as well as in disseminating current methods of surveillance and management of the conditions.[59]

In addition to being knowledgeable about measures for prevention and early detection of cancer, nurses must be aware of current therapeutic modalities and their rationales. Because of lack of information, misinformation, or fear of the effects of treatment, persons may put off seeking help. Clearly presented information about therapy will help to allay anxiety and confusion.

■ Factors that interfere with health-seeking behaviors

Even though there is more widespread knowledge of cancer, a more positive attitude toward the disease is essential if individuals are to follow good health practices and seek help when warning signs of cancer are noted. The public underestimates the incidence of cancer although they are aware of and concerned about it. This suggests that defense mechanisms are at work. The public does not view the conventional types of therapy as optimal, although they have a high level of awareness of cancer's warning signals. Less-educated people and men in general are less likely to have physical examinations.[37] These are all factors that may interfere with health-seeking behaviors.

Unfortunately, anxiety and fear may immobilize the individual. Despite all the public announcements that have been made in the last few decades, there are still people who think of cancer as a disgraceful disease that must be hidden from others. Cancer is talked about in whispers by some people who look on it as a punishment for past sins, a shameful disease, or a disgrace to the family. This attitude stems partly from the fact that cancer in its terminal stages may be a painful and demoralizing disease that is sometimes accompanied by body odor and other signs of physical debility that are deeply etched on the consciousness of friends and relatives. Actually, there is no characteristic odor of cancer, although diseased tissue that breaks down and becomes infected with odor-producing organisms will be as unpleasant as any other infected wound. The essential point—so often missed by the public—is that this tragic situation is an unusual one.

Some people fear cancer and shun persons who have the disease because they believe it is contagious. Scientific speculation on the possibility that a virus may be the cause has added to this fear. At this time, there is no conclusive evidence that cancer can be spread among humans in a way similar to the spread of infectious diseases, and absolute proof of the specific role of viruses in human malignancy is still not available.

The positive aspects of cancer care should be emphasized. It is estimated that approximately one half of the persons for whom a diagnosis is made are cured by medical treatment. Many more could perhaps be cured by medical treatment if the cancer is diagnosed early enough. Only a third have cancer occurring in locations in which the disease advanced beyond permanent medical aid before sufficient signs appear to warn the patient of trouble. In spite of these facts, some persons think it is useless to report symptoms early, since they believe that if they do have cancer they cannot be cured. It can only be hoped that the recent publicity given to well-known persons who have been treated for cancer will help overcome some of these beliefs. If nothing else, the open discussion of the diagnosis and treatment in all types of media should result in a better informed public than ever before.

■ Cancer quackery

Fatal delay in seeking medical care may occur because of the patient's reliance on a "quick, painless cure." Despite public education and efforts of the medical profession to control extravagant claims of a few unethical practitioners, cancer quackery still exists, feeding on the ignorance and fear of the cancer patient and family.[44,73]

Quacks rely on testimonials of people they have "cured." Books and testimonials in magazines may be so appealingly written that the reader gets the impression that the content is factual and accurate. Electronic gadgets, dietary regimens, and various drugs and enzymes have all been purported to cure cancer.

Two drugs still available mostly outside the United States are krebiozen and Laetrile, a substance derived from apricot kernels. Use of Laetrile for cancer therapy has been outlawed by the FDA, whose regulations prohibit the transportation of Laetrile across state lines. In response to active lobbying by various groups, however, 11 states in 1977 passed legislation legalizing use of Laetrile within their borders. The American Cancer Society and The American Medical Association do not recommend use of Laetrile or krebiozen, since neither drug has been scientifically demonstrated to result in objective benefit to the person or show evidence that metastatic growth has been controlled.

In 1979 the National Cancer Institute (NCI) announced that it would sponsor human testing of Laetrile. In 1981 investigators reported that the drug was a failure as a cancer treatment based on a study of 156 patients at four medical centers. These patients had advanced cancer, usually of the lung, breast, colon, and rectum, that could not be treated by standard methods. In additon to intravenous and oral administration of the drug, the patients received the metabolic program prescribed: vitamins, pancreatic enzymes, and a diet containing fresh fruits, vegetables, and whole grains. Within 1 month cancer had progressed in 50% of the patients and cancer had progressed in 3 months in 90%. Only one fifth were alive after 8 months, findings comparable to no therapy at all.

Laetrile advocates state the the drug was not pure Laetrile and charge that the study was designed to discredit Laetrile. However, NCI stated that the drug was structurally the same as that used in Mexico's Laetrile clinics. The tragedy in the use of these drugs is the false security the treatment gives to patients. The security results in delay in seeking medical care until it is too late.

Federal legislation is aimed at controlling quackery, and the FDA has published a booklet, *The Big Quack Attack: Medical Devices,* that describes various methods of quackery and directs consumers where to report complaints regarding practitioners of these methods.*

*FDA Office of Public Affairs, Rockville, MD 20857.

Organizations and programs offering services to the cancer patient and the family

Organization	General description
National organizations and affiliates	
American Cancer Society* 90 Park Ave. New York, N.Y. 10016	Voluntary organization offering programs of cancer research, education, and patient service and rehabilitation
CanSurmount	Composed of patient, family member, trained volunteer (also a cancer patient), health professional. Volunteers visit hospitals and homes.
I Can Cope	Addresses the education and psychological needs of people with cancer.
International Association of Laryngectomees	Voluntary umbrella organization of 225 local clubs (varying names) that promote and support total rehabilitation program. Volunteers visit hospitals.
Reach to Recovery (Breast Cancer)	Provides rehabilitation support for women who have had mastectomies. Volunteers visit hospitals.
Cancer Information Service	Telephone information and referral service supplemented by printed materials.
The Concern for Dying 250 W. 57th St. New York, N.Y. 10019	Nonprofit educational organization distributes the living will, a document that records patient wishes concerning treatment.
Leukemia Society of America 211 E. 43rd St. New York, N.Y. 10017	Offers financial assistance and consultation services for referrals to other means of local support to cancer patients with leukemia and allied disorders.
Make Today Count P.O. Box 222 Osage Beach, Mo. 65065	More than 200 chapters comprising patients and family members, with the general goal of living each day as fully and completely as possible.
The National Hospice Organization 1901 N. Ft. Meyer Dr. Suite 307 Arlington, Va. 22209	Membership organization consisting of groups providing or preparing to provide hospice care; institutions concerned with care of the terminally ill and their families.
United Cancer Council, Inc. 650 E. Carmel Dr. Suite 340 Carmel, Ind. 46032	Federation of voluntary cancer agencies that seeks the control of cancer through a three-point program of service, education, and research. Agencies are funded by the United Way of Giving.
United Ostomy Association 36 Executive Park Irvine, Calif. 92714	Nonprofit organization with more than 500 chapters in United States and Canada. General goal is to provide ostomy patients with mutual aid, moral support, and education. Members visit hospitals.

From Rosenbaum, E: Living with cancer, St. Louis, 1982, The CV Mosby Co.
*For information on the following programs, contact the American Cancer Society.
†Direct services in tristate metropolitan areas of New York, New Jersey, and Connecticut.

Organizations and programs offering services to the cancer patient and the family—cont'd

Organization	General description
Regional organizations and programs	
Cancer Call PAC (People Against Cancer) American Cancer Society 37 S. Wabash Ave. Chicago, Ill. 60603	Emotional support telephone service; volunteers are recovered cancer patients and family members.
Cancer Care, Inc., of the National Cancer Foundation 1180 Ave. of the Americas New York, N.Y. 10036	Voluntary social service agency providing professional counseling and planning to patients with advanced cancer and their families.
TOUCH, Coordinator, Cancer Control Program University of Alabama in Birmingham 104 Old Hillman Bldg. Birmingham, Ala. 35294	General goal is to provide assistance to cancer patients and their families in forming realistic, positive attitudes toward cancer and its treatment.
Psychosocial Counseling Service UCLA-Jonsson Comprehensive Cancer Center 10833 LeConte Ave. Los Angeles, Calif. 90024	Telephone counseling service directed to psychosocial needs of patients and care givers.

■ Organizations involved in cancer education, detection, and rehabilitation

■ FEDERAL ORGANIZATIONS

Federal recognition of the need to give intensive assistance to educational programs in cancer began in 1926 when Congress proclaimed April of each year as National Cancer Control Month. In 1937 the National Cancer Institute was created within the National Institutes of Health. This institute, with generous support from the federal government, conducts an extensive program of research in the field of cancer.

Cancer patients may also obtain help from both Medicare and Medicaid. The Community Services Administration provides services through state agencies such as Welfare and Aging or direct grants. The Rehabilitation Services Administration will arrange and pay for services that help the cancer patient return to productive living.[2] With the passage of the National Cancer Act of 1971, impetus was given for the development of Cancer Clinical Research Centers. The goal was to translate research results into medical practice so that no one will be denied professional advice and care because of lack of facilities and knowledge. These centers combine research capability, demonstration of recent techniques and therapy, and community outreach programs.

Nurses can be articulate speakers for the cause of cancer care and cure, since they are intimately aware of the effects of cancer in threat to life and cost in dollars, disrupted lives, and human suffering. Nurses must assertively express to their representatives in government the importance of a combined effort to eradicate cancer.

■ NATIONAL AND REGIONAL ORGANIZATIONS

The nurse should know of other sources of information and help for persons who have cancer. Organizations and programs offering services to the cancer patient and the family are listed in the box on p. 230 and above.

▨ ASSESSMENT

■ Subjective data

The physician obtains a careful medical history inquiring into family history to determine those with a familial tendency for cancer, social history, marital and sex history, habits, occupation, and past medical history, since all may provide valuable clues to the presence of cancer.

It is especially important that the nurse obtain baseline data in relation to the cancer patient's health and health habits, since the treatment of cancer often involves complex changes in the patient's ability to meet psychologic, physiologic, and sociologic health needs. By careful collection of data the nurse can plan and carry out the complex nursing care that may be needed by the patient with cancer.

■ KNOWLEDGE OF DIAGNOSIS

Some initial data are needed to plan care. The first important question to be answered is whether the patient knows the diagnosis. This information should be recorded on the nursing care plan and discussed with other health team members. This will ensure that the person does not receive different answers to the same questions from the health care providers. Some hospitals have partially overcome this problem by having regular meetings of all the members of the professional staff at which the information given to each patient is reviewed. If meetings of this type are not being held, nurses should take the initiative in planning such a meeting.

The nurse should also elicit from both the patient and the physician what the patient has been told. Because of anxiety and the need for denial to protect the ego, the patient may have only heard part of the information given by the physician or have misinterpreted the information. The nurse can identify any discrepancies to plan care on the basis of the patient's perceptions of the illness.

Members of the medical profession differ in their opinions regarding whether the patient with cancer should be told the diagnosis. The decision is usually made by the physician after consultation with the patient's family. The present trend is toward telling patients they have cancer. When patients are not informed, the reasons seem to be related much more to the physician's own attitudes and emotional reactions than to concern about patient's reactions. The nurse may help by discussing with the physician the reactions of the patient and the feelings expressed. It is the nurse's responsibility and sometimes a challenge to work effectively for the ultimate benefit of the patient within the seeming limitation it may impose.

Many spiritual advisers recommend telling the truth. Some persons, however, may not want to know the diagnosis and may ask and then answer their own questions negatively. Some do not ask for the diagnosis because they do not wish to have confirmed what they already suspect. Some insist on knowing the diagnosis and are preoccupied with every detail of their progress and treatment in a detached but completely abnormal fashion. Finally, there are some who wish to know the facts and who can accept them in a realistic way when given an opportunity to discuss their feelings with others. Some physicians prepare the patient over a period of time and tell the complete truth when they feel the patient is ready to accept it.

It is also important to determine how long the patient has known the diagnosis. The patient who has just been told may be going through the initial grief reactions. The person who has known for many years may have made a realistic adaptation and may see cancer as a chronic disease and not as a death sentence. The nurse should ascertain from the physician whether the cancer has already metastasized and, if so, whether the patient is aware of this fact. Responses of the patient with metastatic cancer will be different from those of the patient who can be more hopeful of a cure.

■ COPING SKILLS

Coping skills should be identified, because the diagnosis of cancer is an enormous test of the person's inner resources, as well as those of friends and family. Some persons cope by directly verbalizing fears and seeking support from others, whereas other persons are less direct. Some deal with problems with a problem-solving approach; other try to avoid dealing with the problem.

The patient's and family's interpersonal, physical, and financial resources must be determined. What kind of support can be expected from the family? The financial burden the patient anticipates because of the therapy may affect the reaction to the disease.

■ PSYCHOLOGIC RESPONSE TO CANCER

Once the diagnosis of cancer has been made, the patient and family may be overwhelmed and immobilized. As one patient stated, "I cried all day Saturday, Sunday, and Monday. My daughter and my husband wanted to help but they didn't know what to do or say. I know my daughter was scared that she'd get cancer, too." Not all patients can openly express their feelings. Consequently, the nurse may have difficulty gathering data in order to assess and plan intervention. Some individuals are stoic, feeling it is a sign of weakness to display their psychologic devastation in public. The nurse must be alert for subtle cues that may indicate that intervention is needed.

□ Grief

The general psychologic responses to a diagnosis of cancer are those accompanying the grieving process (see Chapter 15). The patient and family may go through a period of denial, during which there may be a delay in beginning therapy. Anxiety, depression, regressive behavior, and anger may all be manifested (see Chapter 7).

To many the diagnosis of cancer signifies the end of life itself, the ultimate loss. Nurses must be careful that they do not communicate any negative reactions to cancer. Beginning practitioners must look at their own attitudes toward the disease.

□ Guilt

Guilt is also a frequent psychologic response. Cancer patients may feel that the disease is punishment for actions of their past life. They may also feel guilty if they have delayed seeking treatment.

□ Sense of isolation

Perhaps one of the most prevalent reactions described by patients with cancer is a sense of isolation, of being cut off from those persons and things that are important to them. Patients with cancer may report that there is a gradual break in relationships. In some cases the isolation is patient initiated, in others it may result from actions of significant others because of their negative attitude toward the disease. Perhaps the most profound isolation is psychologic isolation, an inability to relate to and derive comfort from others, the feeling of being alone in a crowd.

□ Sexual disequilibrium

Nurses must be comfortable with their own sexuality and sensitive to the patients' responses, which may indicate that sexual tension is present.

Cancer is particularly destructive to the sexual relationship. It may so occupy the patient's life that all energy is directed to the illness. Sexual roles change. There may be fear that sexual activity may either cause the cancer to spread or that the well partner may "catch" it. Treatment modalities that affect the genital organs may cause sexual dysfunction, and the psychologic responses of anxiety, anger, depression, and body image disturbance may do violence to the sexual relationship[21] (see Chapter 35).

□ Fantasies of death and dying

Some patients report that they are overwhelmed with fantasies of death and dying. Most patients are more concerned about the process of dying, fearing pain, mutilation, and deterioration in both their physiologic and psychologic status, than with death itself. Patients may be open about their fantasizing, but they are more apt to communicate this in less obvious ways. Patients may focus their attention and discussion on the suffering and pain of others. They may express concern about the future of their families and may speculate what will happen to their loved ones. The nurse must be alert to these signs that patients need to talk about their view of their future.

■ Objective data

■ LOCAL EFFECTS

Benign tumors cause serious problems if they obstruct the lumen of tubular structures such as the ureter, trachea, or intestinal tract. Intraspinal and intracranial tumors cause problems because of the pressure they exert in a closed space. Tumors may also degenerate or by the pressure they exert cause atrophy and ulceration of overlying epithelium.

Malignant tumors may produce the same problems as benign tumors. In addition, because of their size and ability to infiltrate and destroy surrounding tissue, there is danger of obstruction, hemorrhage, ulceration, and secondary infection.

■ SYSTEMIC EFFECTS

The term *paraneoplastic syndrome* is used to describe the systemic effects of cancer. These can be divided into the following categories: (1) hematologic, immunologic, and vascular abnormalities; (2) hormonal and endocrine effects; (3) neuromyopathies; (4) skin and connective tissue disorders; (5) gastrointestinal disorders; and (6) general and metabolic disorders.[62]

Anemia, leukopenia, and platelet deficiency may result from replacement of bone marrow by cancer cells. Patients with cancer of the gastrointestinal tract often develop anemia secondary to chronic blood loss and malabsorption. Tumors of the endocrine glands usually cause an increase in secretion from the glands, resulting in various syndromes such as Cushing's disease or hyperthyroidism. In addition, some malignant tumors of the lung secrete trophic hormones, which can result in conditions resembling Cushing's syndrome.[14]

When there is a metastatic implant in the peritoneal or pleural cavity, this causes an increased production of serous fluid, and the patient develops either pleural effusion or ascites (peritoneal).

Degenerative changes can occur in the central nervous system of patients with advanced cancer, even in the absence of metastases to the area. The patient may show signs of cerebellar disease and peripheral neuritis. There may be severe muscle weakness or dermatomyositis, and hemorrhage may occur if blood vessels are eroded by the growing tumor.

There is destruction of muscle protein, impaired cellular respiration (often a complication of anemia), and neuromyopathies followed by failure of important muscle masses, such as intercostal and abdominal muscle. This results in poor pulmonary ventilation, stasis of secretions, and pneumonia. Smooth muscle failure in the urinary bladder wall and the intestinal tract results in urinary tract infection or constipation.

Cachexia is almost universal in malignant disease at some point in its development and is usually a sign of advanced cancer. It is characterized by anorexia, hypermetabolism, excess of energy consumption over nutritional supply, and wasting as a result of negative protein and fat balance in the body. Weight loss may be gradual or rapid.

The following four factors are involved in the etiology of cachexia[62]:

1. It is possibly caused by inhibition of the hypothalamic appetite center. Appetite may fail to increase in the face of the increased nutrient needs of the tumor.
2. There is altered gastrointestinal function, malabsorption of nutrients, especially in the small intestine, and exudation of protein and electrolytes.
3. There is increased use of nutrients by some tumors that require more amino acids and vitamins than do normal tissues. There may also be insufficient use of available nutrients.
4. There is increased excretion of nutrients such as urinary excretion of electrolytes and metabolic products.

In addition, other factors that may be implicated include immobilization, drugs, and reactive depression that may accompany metastatic cancer. Along with this may be insomnia and a feeling of hopelessness, which also may contribute to anorexia and cachexia. There is an increased susceptibility to infection.

Therapy for the cachectic state is rarely successful unless the underlying cancer is treated. Glucose plus insulin, or androgens for males, may stimulate anabolism.[37]

Pain does not always occur with cancer; when it does occur, it is usually a late sign. Cancer pain is described later in the chapter (p. 254).

The paraneoplastic syndrome often results in devastating effects on the individual host; many of these effects are similar to the side effects of antineoplastic therapy. A common myth held by some general health care consumers is that the treatment for cancer is worse than the disease itself. It is important to remember that cancer, if left untreated, will eventually result in death. All health care professionals have an obligation to inform the public about the importance of early detection and treatment.

Table 12-5 Cancer diagnostic tests

Diagnostic test	Description
Physical examination	External and internal physical assessment to evaluate clinical signs and symptoms related to local or distant effects of cancer growth and development; internal assessment done through pelvic exam and/or rectal examination
Biopsy	Histologic testing (frozen or permanent section) to confirm malignancy and to determine type of cancerous cell and degree of cellular aplasia/differentiation (that is, grading)
Incisional biopsy	Surgical removal of section of neoplasm
Excisional biopsy	Removal of entire growth if tumor is small
Aspiration needle biopsy	Removal of small plug of tumor by use of needle and syringe
Cytology	Collection and slide preparation of exfoliated cells without the tissue framework provided in a biopsy; the Pap smear to determine abnormal or cancerous cells in the cervix is the most familiar example
Clinical laboratory tests	Include routine blood and urine studies as well as other biochemical and chromosomal analyses (for example, measurement of the enzyme acid phosphatase for cancer of the prostate)
Body imaging	
X-ray examinations	Provide good visualization of chest and bone (contrast to surrounding tissue); mammography (to detect breast cancer) differs from ordinary chest x-ray examination in that it uses very slow, nonpenetrating radiation and very sensitive film
Xerography	Uses a specially charged plate of selenium-coated metal, resulting in a detailed picture of soft tissue
Computed tomography (CT scan)	Uses an x-ray beam in conjunction with a computer permitting detailed study of small parts deep in the body without the necessity of invasive procedures
Nuclear magnetic resonance (NMR) scanner	Uses a very strong magnet combined with radio frequency waves and a computer to produce x-ray-like images of body chemistry in heart, brain, and other organs; no radiation is present
Contrast examination	Addition of contrast material for x-ray examination via swallowing of a liquid (for example, barium for gastrointestinal visualization) or injection of a dye into blood or lymph vessels (for example, lymphangiography)
Nuclear scans (radioactive isotopes)	Introduction of radioactive substance into body to detect primary or metastatic cancer; the isotopes concentrate in the tumor (hot spot) or in the normal tissue surrounding the tumor (cold spot) and create an image on a scintillation detector or on photographic film
Ultrasound (echography)	An electronic instrument detects and records echoes of sound when they are reflected at junction of tissues with different densities; not useful, at present, for lungs or stomach
Endoscopy	Uses a telescope-like optical instrument to look at the internal organs; x-ray examination or biopsy may be done simultaneously; instruments are named for the organs they visualize: • Bronchoscope: lungs • Laparoscope: abdomen • Cystoscope: bladder • Gastroscope: stomach • Sigmoidoscope: lower colon • Proctoscope: rectum

■ Diagnostic studies

The nurse needs to be able to give a simple description of various diagnostic procedures to patients and families. The tests may involve the use of complex equipment as well as the injection or ingestion of various substances. The patient's anxiety may be high, and the nurse's ability to give factual information often will help decrease anxiety. Specific procedures before, during, and after diagnostic testing may vary slightly from institution to institution, requiring that the nurse be knowledgeable about the common as well as the possible unique characteristics of a diagnostic test. Table 12-5 lists and describes briefly the most common diagnostic procedures when the patient presents with signs and symptoms suggestive of malignancy.

■ Nursing intervention during assessment phase

The emotional climate produced during the period of diagnostic examination and initial treatment is very important in determining whether patients will continue diagnostic examination, treatment, or repeated follow-up care after discharge. The care they receive in the hospital may shape their attitudes toward the disease and may determine whether they can return home and either care for themselves or be cared for by the family. An important nursing function in the care of patients with cancer is building up faith in the physician and in the clinic or the medical center where care is received. The patient needs to feel certain that everything possible is being done and that new measures will be tried if there is any promise whatsoever of their being helpful.

Many patients must undergo extensive diagnostic examinations and surgery in large medical centers a long distance from their homes. Some patients have reported that, although they were confident that they were in "good medical hands," such confidence did not make up for the feelings that they were not always known as individuals. They needed desperately to feel that at least one person knew and understood them. Some patients experience near panic at the thought of their loved ones coming to visit and being unable to locate them. In most instances it is best for the patient to be accompanied by a relative or a close friend. It should also be recognized that even a patient in familiar surroundings may feel very much alone when awaiting diagnostic tests or surgical treatment for known or suspected cancer.

Both patient and family need something to help pass the time during the period of diagnostic tests and treatment and between steps of treatment such as surgery or x-ray therapy. Psychologic relief may sometimes come from keeping occupied with usual daily activities. Anxious relatives also receive satisfaction from doing things that the patient would do, if possible, thus preserving parts of cherished routines.

Members of the family often need direction in their activity when they have just learned that a loved one has cancer. They may need to talk over immediate and long-term plans with someone not close to the family situation. The nurse can sometimes be this listening person. At other times the family can best be served by a social caseworker, who will help them talk through and think through a course of action.

▶ DATA ANALYSIS AND PLANNING

A sound personal philosophy and an objective, positive attitude toward the disease based on knowledge will help the nurse who is caring for the patient with cancer. The nurse should be able to give support and hope to the patient and family or friends.

Following an assessment that includes subjective and objective data, the nurse analyzes the information and formulates nursing diagnoses. Because cancer is a chronic illness that often involves numerous body systems, the list of pertinent nursing diagnoses can be extensive. It is often a challenge for the nurse to identify all of the pertinent diagnoses that will require nursing interventions for a specific person.

The following four principles should be considered by the nurse when planning nursing interventions that are patient centered:

1. Persons have a right to be part of the treatment team.
2. Persons have the right to choose the desired degree of privacy or communication.
3. The nurse must respect the coping mechanisms of patients who are trying to maintain themselves through a difficult illness.
4. The nurse must remember not to give the appearance of hurrying, thus blocking communications.

The plan of care that a nurse develops for a patient with cancer needs to be individualized to reflect problems unique to a particular disease, treatment regimen, or the personality and life situation of the patient. Table 12-6 provides guidelines for data analysis and planning by listing common problem areas, nursing diagnoses, and expected outcomes for the patient and family. The section that follows will detail the nursing interventions for the patient experiencing one or more of the four treatment modalities and for the patient with chronic pain and cancer that is terminal.

▦ IMPLEMENTATION

Often several physicians are involved in determining the appropriate treatment for cancer. The medical team decides on the choice of treatment on the basis of the biologic characteristic of the tumor, its clinical stage (p. 221), and the condition of the patient. The histologic type of the tumor is particularly important in determining the treatment to be used.

Therapy may be curative (removal of all traces of the disease from the body) or palliative (directed only toward relieving symptoms). At the present time there are four major forms of treatment: surgery, radiotherapy, chemotherapy, and immunotherapy. The latter is the newest form

Table 12-6 Guidelines for data analysis and planning for patients with cancer

Problem area and possible nursing diagnoses*	Possible etiologies†	Expected patient outcomes*

Coping
  Anxiety
  Ineffective individual coping
  Ineffective family coping: compromised
  Altered family processes
  Fear (specify)
  Grieving (specify)
    Anticipatory
    Dysfunctional
  Powerlessness
  Body image disturbance
  Altered role performance
  Self-esteem disturbance
  Personal identity disturbance
  Social isolation
  Spiritual distress
	Threat to self-concept, threat of death, personal vulnerability, maladaptive coping styles, ambivalent family relationships, potential for loss of physiologic functioning, lack of ability to perform role, inadequate or impaired support systems, perceived helplessness, change in lifestyle, separation from religious/cultural ties, long-term illness	Within a level consistent with physical, psychosocial, and spiritual capacities and their value system, the person and family:
		1. Use appropriate resources for support in coping
		2. Communicate feelings about living with cancer
		3. Participate in care and ongoing decision making
		4. Identify alternative resources when present coping strategies do not provide support
		5. State accomplishable goals

Comfort
  Pain
  Sleep pattern disturbance
	Chronic physical disability, tumor necrosis, metastatic lesions, obstruction, pressure, ischemia, distention, environmental changes, anxiety	The person and family:
		1. Report alterations in comfort level
		2. Identify measures to modify psychosocial, environmental, and physical factors that influence comfort and enhance the continuance of valued activities and relationships
		3. State the source of pain, the treatment, and the expected outcome of proposed intervention
		4. Describe appropriate interventions for potential or predictable problems of pain and sleep management program

Nutrition Altered nutrition: less than body requirements	Chewing or swallowing difficulties, anorexia, nausea, emesis, impaired taste sensations, fatigue	1. Identify foods that are tolerated and those that cause discomfort or aversion 2. State measures that enhance food intake and retention 3. Select appropriate dietary alternative to provide sufficient nutrients when usual foods are not tolerated 4. State methods of modifying consistency, flavor, or amounts of nutrients to ensure adequate nutrient intake 5. State dietary modifications compatible with cultural, social, and ethnic practices 6. State foods and fluids that provide optimal comfort during the terminal stage of illness

*From Oncology Nursing Society and American Nurses Association Division on Medical-Surgical Nursing Practice: Outcome standards for cancer nursing practice, Kansas City, Mo, 1979, American Nurses Association.
†Based on suggested etiologies for nursing diagnoses from the North American Nursing Diagnosis Association, 1986.

Table 12-6   Guidelines for data analysis and planning for patients with cancer—cont'd

Problem area and possible nursing diagnoses	Possible etiologies†	Expected patient outcomes
Protective mechanisms (immune, hematopoietic, integumentary, and sensorimotor systems) Fluid volume deficit Potential for injury (specify) Knowledge deficit Altered oral mucous membrane Impaired skin integrity	Neutropenia, thrombocytopenia, radiation, dehydration, ineffective oral hygiene, malnutrition, immobility, chemotherapy, cognitive limitation, lack of interest in learning, unfamiliarity with information resources	1. List measures to prevent skin breakdown, mucosal trauma, infection, and bleeding 2. Identify signs and symptoms of infection, bleeding, and sensorimotor dysfunction 3. Contact an appropriate health team member when initial signs and symptoms of infection, bleeding, or sensorimotor dysfunction occur 4. State measures to manage infection, bleeding, or sensorimotor dysfunction
Mobility Impaired physical mobility	Intolerance to activity, decreased strength and endurance, pain/discomfort, musculoskeletal impairment, depression	1. State the cause of the immobility, the treatment, and the outcome of treatment 2. Describe an appropriate management plan to optimally integrate the alteration in mobility into life-style 3. Describe optimal levels of activities of daily living in keeping with disease state and treatment 4. Identify health services and community resources available for managing changes in mobility 5. Use measures to aid or improve mobility 6. Demonstrate measures to prevent complications of decreased mobility
Elimination Constipation Diarrhea Altered patterns of urinary elimination	Immobility, inadequate nutrition, inadequate fluid intake, chemotherapy, medications, radiation, alterations in peristalsis	1. State appropriate actions if changes in elimination patterns occur 2. Describe the relationship between adequate elimination and physiologic integrity 3. Identify and manage factors that may affect elimination, such as diet, stress, physical activity, and neurogenic conditions 4. Develop a plan for managing an altered elimination route within personal life-style
Sexuality Sexual dysfunction	Change in body image, altered body structure, lack of knowledge, lack of privacy, psychologic stress, chemotherapy, radiation, fatigue	1. Client and partner identify potential or actual alterations in perception of sexuality or sexual function 2. Client and partner identify alternate methods of expressing sexuality

Continued.

Table 12-6 Guidelines for data analysis and planning for patients with cancer—cont'd

Problem area and possible nursing diagnoses	Possible etiologies†	Expected patient outcomes

Ventilation
  Respiratory function, altered
    Ineffective airway clearance
    Ineffective breathing patterns
    Impaired gas exchange
	Infection, tumor, obstruction of airways, chemotherapy, radiation, fatigue, pain, anxiety, anemia	1. State plans for daily activity that demonstrate maximum conservation of energy
		2. List measures to reduce or modify pulmonary irritants from the environment, such as smoke, dry air, powders, and aerosols
		3. Describe the effect of environmental extremes on ventilatory function and oxygen use
		4. State effective measures to maintain a patent airway
		5. Identify reasons for altered ventilation, such as decreased hemoglobin, infection, anxiety, effusion, and obstructed airway
		6. Identify an appropriate plan of action should altered ventilation occur
		7. Develop a plan for managing an altered airway

of treatment for cancer. Combinations of the four treatment modalities are often employed to achieve the best result for each patient.

■ Surgery

Surgery, the oldest method of treating cancer, may be either curative or palliative. The best treatment for cancer at present is complete surgical removal of all malignant tissues before metastasis occurs. Surgery must often be extensive and may require adjustments beyond those needed in many other conditions. There may not be time to accustom oneself gradually to the idea of surgery and the effect it can have on one's body and life-style. The individual often faces the prospect of mutilating surgery with only the hope that it will cure the cancer and be lifesaving. Concern about what will happen to the family may be utmost in the patient's mind. Obviously, the patient and family need empathy and understanding as they attempt to accept the recommendation for immediate surgery.

The operative procedures used to treat various types of cancer are discussed in the appropriate chapters of this book.

■ RADIOTHERAPY

Radiotherapy, or the use of radiation in the treatment of disease, has been used in the treatment of cancer for about 80 years. The principal radiation agents are: (1) x-ray, which consists of electromagnetic radiation produced by waves of electrical energy traveling at a very high speed; (2) radium, which is a radioactive isotope occurring freely in nature; and (3) the artificially induced radioactive isotopes produced by bombarding the isotopes of elements with highly energized particles in a cyclotron. The most common sources of radiation for external beam therapy are the linear accelerator, the cobalt-60 teletherapy machines, and the betatron. These machines produce radiation of varying types of energy, which control the depth of penetration of the x-rays into tissues.

Radiotherapy is effective in curing cancer in some instances; in other instances it controls the growth of cancer cells for a time. Because it may deter the growth of cancer cells, it may relieve pain even when extension of the disease is such that cure is impossible.

□ Principle underlying radiotherapy

Radiotherapy is based on the fact that rapidly reproducing malignant cells are more sensitive to radiation than are normal cells. Therapeutic doses of radiotherapy are calculated to destroy or delay the growth of malignant cells without destroying normal tissue. Rotation of either the target site in the patient or the radiation beam makes it possible to deliver a high total dose to the tumor while at the same time only part of the dose reaches the noncancerous tissue surrounding it.

The radiation used medically consists of alpha- (α-), beta- (β-), and gamma- (γ-) rays (Fig. 12-4). α- and β-rays cannot pass through the skin. γ-Rays, however, have been found to penetrate several inches of lead, although lead shielding offers a considerable degree of protection.

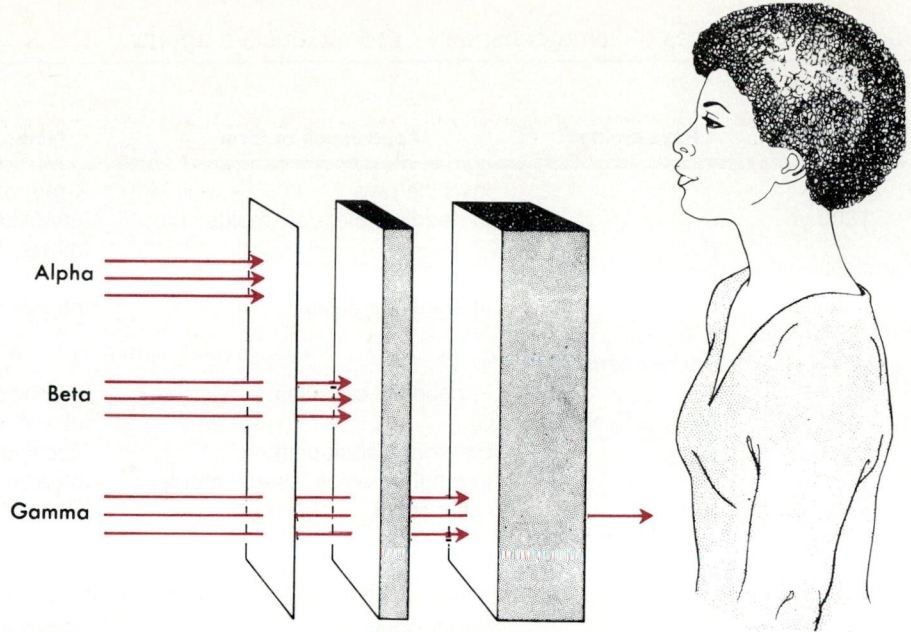

Fig. 12-4 Relative penetrating power of three types of radiation. (From Bouchard-Kurtz, R, and Speese-Owens, N: Nursing care of the cancer patient, ed, 4, St. Louis, 1981, The CV Mosby Co.)

X-rays, which are similar to γ-rays, require lead protection.

Radiation can be delivered to the patient *externally* by exposure to rays, such as from an x-ray machine or from cobalt 60, or *internally,* either by placing radioactive material such as radium within the tissues or body cavity (sealed internal radiation) or by administering the materials intravenously or orally so that they are distributed throughout the body (unsealed internal radiation).

☐ Protection of health workers from radiation hazards

Radiation delivered externally (including x-rays) can do harm to persons working with the patient *only during* the time that the patient is being treated. This is true also of the radiation from some radioactive substances used for other methods of treatment. Patients with internal radiation who emit γ-rays, however, may expose other persons to radiation for varying periods of time, and the time one can be exposed safely to the patient is important in planning care. The time interval required for the radioactive substance to be half dissipated is called its *half-life* (Table 12-7). This period varies extremely widely, but as the end of the half-life is reached, danger from exposure decreases.

Exposure to radiation can be controlled three ways: *time, distance,* and *shielding.* All emanations are subject to the physical law of inverse-square. For example, a person who stands 2 meters away from the source of radiation receives only one fourth as much exposure as when standing only 1 meter away. At 4 meters, only one sixteenth of the exposure will be received. Therefore, increasing the distance from the emanations decreases the exposure (Fig. 12-5).

When a patient such as an infant must be held for x-ray treatment, the nurse or person who holds the patient must be careful to keep at arm's length or as far away as possible and to avoid having any body part in the direct path of the rays. *Leadlined golves and a lead apron, which act as a shield to reduce exposure, should be worn by anyone who attends patients during x-ray treatment or during examination by fluoroscopy.*

When the nurse knows the kind of substance used, the kind and amount of rays it emits, its half-life, and its exact location in the patient and considers these facts in relation to control of exposure, safe and adequate care for the patient can be planned.

Nurses wishing to know about radioactive substances can obtain information from the Division of Radiological Health of the Public Health Service or from their state health department. Several drug companies also publish pamphlets that contain helpful information. In cities with large medical facilities a radiation physicist may be consulted.

■ EXTERNAL RADIOTHERAPY

☐ Preparation of the patient

Teaching the patient and family is an important aspect of care. Orientation programs, information booklets, and weekly group sessions for patients and families are useful methods of communicating information. In group meetings, topics such as scheduling, whom to see for assistance with special problems, or care of the skin are discussed. There is an opportunity to discuss fears and misconceptions

Table 12-7 Characteristics and uses of some commonly used radioactive agents

Radiation source	Half-life (where applicable)	Rays emitted	Appearance or form	Method of administration
X-ray	—	γ	Invisible rays	X-ray machine
Radium	1600 yr	α β γ	In needles, plaques, molds	Interstitial (needles) Intracavitary (plaques, mold)
Radon	4 days	α β γ (low intensity)	In seeds, needles	Interstitial (seeds, needles)
Cesium (^{137}Cs)	33 yrs	β γ	In needles, capsules	Interstitial (needles) Intracavitary (capsules)
Cobalt (^{60}Co)	5 yr	β γ	External (cobalt unit) Internal (needles, seeds, molds)	Machine (teletherapy) Interstitial (needles, seeds)
Iodine (^{131}I)	8 days	β γ (low intensity)	Clear liquid	By mouth
Phosphorus (^{32}P)	14 days	β	Clear liquid	By mouth, intracavitary, intravenous
Gold (^{198}Au)	3 days	β γ	Purple liquid	Intracavitary
Iridium (^{192}Ir)	74 days	β γ (low intensity)	In needles, wires, seeds	Interstitial
Yttrium (^{90}Y)	3 days	β	Beads, needles	Interstitial

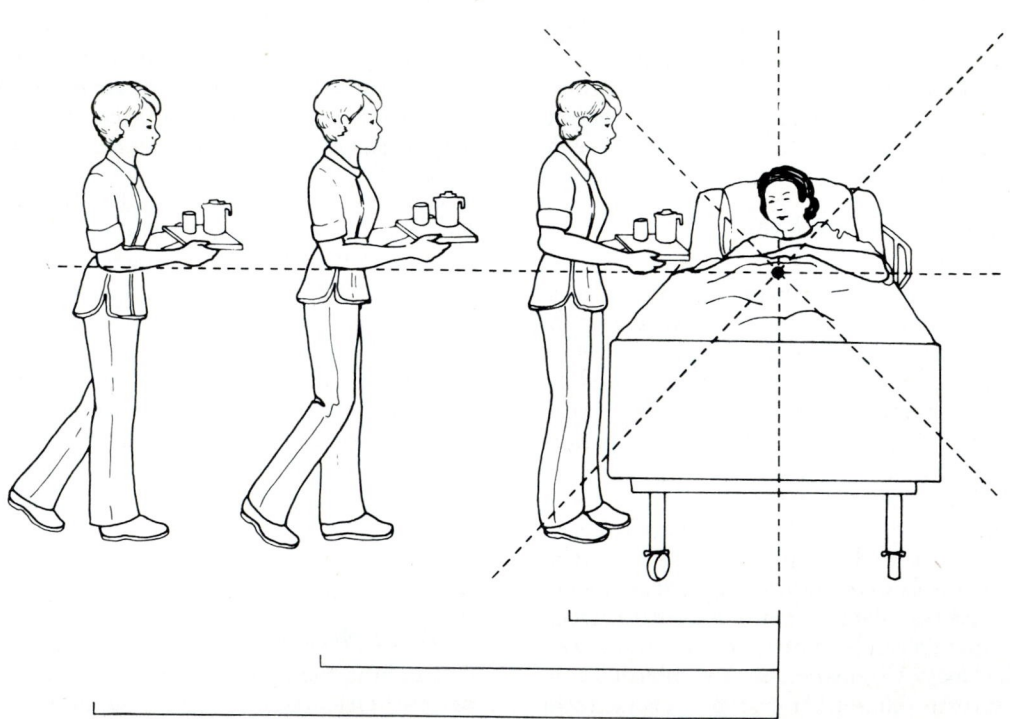

Fig. 12-5 Nurse nearest source of radioactivity (patient) is exposed to more radioactivity. (Adapted from Bouchard-Kurtz, R, and Speese-Owens, N: Nursing care of the cancer patient, ed 4, St. Louis, 1981, The CV Mosby Co.)

about radiation and cancer. Both inpatients and outpatients can attend.

Patients who are to receive radiation therapy should know that they will be attended by radiotherapists who will be stationed outside the treatment room and who will observe the treatment and be in communication at all times. The patient must often lie absolutely still for a period of time, a very tiring experience. There is no pain associated with radiation therapy.

□ Procedure

In giving treatment, rays can be directed at the tumor from several different angles so that normal tissue receives a minimum of exposure. The areas through which rays pass are known as *ports*. Different ports may be used on different days, or the position may be changed at intervals during a daily treatment so that only a certain amount is given through each of several ports. The patient may be placed on a rotating device such as a rotating chair so that although the tumor mass receives the full dose of radiation, skin areas receive less exposure.

In medical centers where hyperbaric oxygen chambers are available, patients may receive radiation therapy while receiving hyperbaric oxygen. The rationale for this combined therapy is that malignant cells, in which the oxygen tension is increased, are more susceptible to the effects of radiation. At the same time, the sensitivity of normal cells to the radiation effects is not increased.[55]

□ Early reaction

When radiation therapy is used, some degree of radiation reaction may occur. Early reactions include blanching or erythema of the skin and mucous membranes, possibly progressing to dry or moist desquamation. If the mucosa of the mouth, pharynx, bladder, or rectum is affected, there may be pain, inhibition of the normal secretions, and impairment of functions.

When treatment is directed toward abdominal organs or any deep tissues there is almost always some skin reaction. There may be itching, tingling, burning, oozing, or sloughing of the skin. The term *burn* should never be used in referring to this reaction, since it implies incorrect dosage. Reddening may occur on or about the tenth day, and the skin may turn a dark plum color after about 3 weeks. The skin may also become dry and inelastic and may crack easily.

Gastrointestinal reactions to radiation therapy are more common when treatment includes some part of the gastrointestinal tract or when the ports lie over this system. The patient may have nausea, vomiting, anorexia, malaise, and diarrhea. This difficulty is usually not discussed with the patient before treatment is started because it is thought that the power of suggestion may contribute to symptoms. Almost all patients who receive moderate or large doses of radiation, however, have these symptoms in varying degrees.

Radiation therapy also causes depression of the hematopoietic system and in turn a low white blood cell count, predisposing the patient to infection. Sloughing of tissue

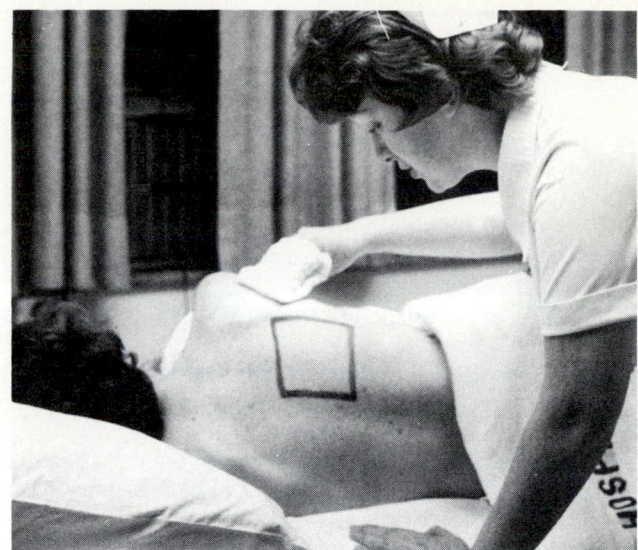

Fig. 12-6 When bath is given, care must be taken not to remove skin markings used to guide radiologist in giving x-ray treatments.

and subsequent hemorrhages are complications that must be considered when radiation is used in any form. Ambulatory patients are told that they should call the physician at once should any sloughing of tissue occur.

□ Late reaction

Effects of radiation may be apparent months or years after therapy. Genital tissue, muscles, and kidneys may be affected, resulting in painful radionecrosis.[51] Radiation causes destruction of fine vasculature, and the skin may show signs of atrophy (thinning and blanching), pigmentation, and telangiectasis. If there is severe vascular damage or if there are other complications that require further surgery, the irradiated tissues may fail to heal.

□ Nursing care of patients receiving external radiation

Nursing care is directed toward preventing skin breakdown, decreasing gastrointestinal upset, and preventing infection (see the box on p. 242). The area to be treated is usually outlined by the radiologist at the time of the first treatment. Occasionally, a small tattoo mark is used instead of the conspicuous skin markings when treatment is given to exposed parts of the body. Marks must not be washed off until the treatment is completed, because they are important guides to the radiologist (Fig. 12-6). Medicated substances that may contain heavy metals such as zinc are not permitted on the skin until the series of treatments is completed, because they may increase the radiation dosage.

If the radiation dosage has been high and blanching or discoloration of the skin has resulted, the patient may be advised to avoid exposure to temperature changes for several years. The patient may have to take much cooler baths

---

Nursing care of patients receiving external radiation

1. *Preventing skin breakdown*
   a. Skin preparation: cleansing.
   b. Care must be taken *not* to remove skin markings used to guide radiologist.
   c. Vegetable fat or oil may be ordered to protect the affected skin.
   d. Medicated solutions, ointments, or powders that may contain heavy metals such as zinc are *not* permitted on the skin.
   e. Consult radiologist about skin care for local radiation reactions; do not remove crusts.
   f. Keep dressings loose; use nonirritating tape and avoid pulling on affected skin.
   g. Teach patient to avoid constricting clothing or friction of any kind on exposed skin.
   h. Teach patient to avoid excesses of heat and cold to affected skin surfaces.
2. *Decreasing gastrointestinal upset*
   a. Advise resting before and after meals to control nausea and vomiting.
   b. Breakfast is usually the best tolerated meal of the day.
   c. Suggest frequent small meals during the day.
   d. Sour beverages and effervescent liquids may relieve nausea.
   e. Suggest high-protein, high-carbohydrate, fat-free, low-residue diet to prevent nausea and vomiting; low-roughage diet for diarrhea.
   f. Administer palliative medications, as ordered.
3. *Preventing infection*
   a. Teach patient to avoid persons with upper respiratory infections.
   b. Use protective isolation if white blood count is low.
   c. Administer antibiotic drugs, as ordered.

---

or showers than formerly and may have to avoid sunbathing or any other extreme of temperature. If x-ray treatments have been given to a woman's face, she must be cautioned regarding the use of cosmetics to cover discolored skin. They may contain heavy, irritating oils and should not be used until consultation with the physician.

When treatment must be given to any part of the head, patients may ask about the possiblity of loss of hair. Whether hair will return after falling out depends on the amount of radiation received. Attractive scarves and wigs are useful for patients with alopecia or when returning hair is too thin.

■ INTERNAL RADIOTHERAPY

Internal radiation may be delivered by sealed or unsealed methods. In either type special precautions may be necessary, depending on the amount of radioactive material used, its location, and the kind of rays being emitted (Table 12-7). Special precautions may be taken if more than a tracer diagnostic dose has been given. Hospitals in which therapeutic doses of radioactive isotopes are administered are required to have a radiation safety officer. Quite often this person is a physicist. The radiation safety officer determines the precautions to be observed in each situation. Most hospitals have printed instruction sheets stating the precautions to be followed for each substance used. Personnel should be fully acquainted with all precautions and should be supervised in carrying them out. Generally, the patient will be placed in a single room or in a double room with another patient who is also receiving radiation therapy. A radiation precaution sign should be placed on the door to the patient's room, and visitors should be restricted.

□ Sealed internal radiotherapy

Brachytherapy is used to deliver a concentrated dose of radiation directly to the malignant lesion or tumor area. Usually this involves insertion of radioactive substances within hollow cavities or within tissues. The radioactive isotopes commonly used are cobalt 60, iridium 192, iodine 125, phosphorus 32, cesium 137, gold 198, and radium 226.[41] These radioactive substances may be used in the form of molds, plaques, needles, wires, special applicators, or ribbons that are carefully placed and left in position for a specified length of time (Fig. 12-7). Emanations from the radioactive substances may also be sealed in tiny gold tubes (seeds) and left indefinitely within the tissues into which they are inserted (Fig. 12-8). The half-life of the seeds is much less than that of the substances from which their emanations come.

A fairly common site for the implantation of seeds is the mouth. Plaques and molds also are used for lesions in the mouth. Sealed internal radiation also is used widely in treatment of cancer of the cervix.

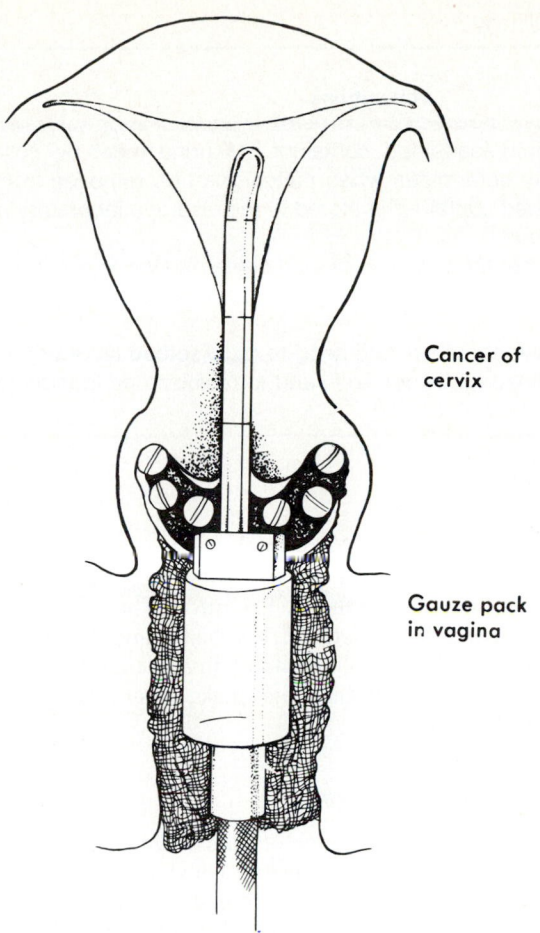

Fig. 12-7   Ernst applicator in place for treatment of cancer of cervix. Note gauze packing in vagina to help maintain applicator in position.

□ *Prevention of radiation hazards*

Safe practice for the nurse caring for a patient receiving sealed internal radiotherapy depends on the principles of time, distance, and shielding (p. 239). Radioactive materials for sealed internal therapy usually are kept in a lead-lined container in the radiology department and are inserted into the patient in the operating room. They should never be touched with bare hands. A pair of forceps should be kept in the patient's room for handling in case the radioactive implant becomes dislodged.

Sealed radioactive material is often reused. On removal from a patient the radioactive material should be cleansed using the precautions just described and returned to the radiology department in a lead-lined container at once so that it may be safe from accidental handling or loss. Even if it is not to be reused, it is returned in a lead-lined container. To prevent accidental loss in cleansing, radioactive material is cleansed in a basin of water instead of in an open sink. If a brush must be used, it must be grasped with forceps so that close contact with the material is avoided.

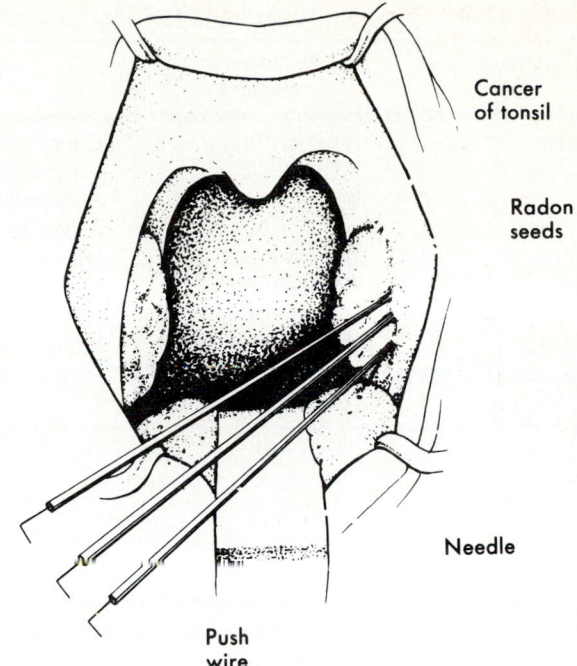

Fig. 12-8   Radium emanations may be sealed in tiny gold tubes (radon seeds) and left indefinitely within tissue into which they are inserted. Schema shows insertion into tonsil.

Exposure is sometimes termed *external* in that it can occur only by direct exposure to the encased radioactive substance. It cannot result from contact with linen, vomitus, or urine or from touching the patient. Knowing where the radioactive material is implanted helps the nurse to plan activities of care. If, for example, the substance is in the patient's mouth, there is less exposure if one stands toward the foot of the bed. If it is in the uterus or bladder, standing at the head of the bed is safer.

□ Unsealed internal radiotherapy

Unsealed internal radiation is delivered to the patient by mouth as an "atomic cocktail" or as a liquid instilled into a body cavity. Exposure for persons caring for the patient can result from direct contact with emanations from the substance in the patient (external exposure) or from contact with the patient's discharges that contain the radioactive substances (internal exposure). It may be inhaled, ingested, or absorbed through the skin. The exposure varies with each of the substances used, and safety for the nurse and others caring for the patient depends on a thorough knowledge of the substance used and its action within the body. If only tracer doses (very small amounts) of radioactive substances are used, as for diagnostic purposes, no precautions are necessary.

□ *Prevention of radiation hazards*

Special precautions that need to be taken when using radioactive iodine, phosphorus, or gold are listed in Table

Table 12-8 Special precautions for unsealed internal radiotherapy

Substance or object	Radioactive element	Precautions
Urine	Iodine (^{131}I)	Urine emptied directly into lead-lined container. *All* urine must be collected (amount of radioactivity determines when patient may be removed from isolation). Urine in lead-lined container is stored in radioisotope laboratory until it can be safely disposed of.
Linen	Iodine (^{131}I)	Monitor with Geiger counter for contamination; if contaminated, place in special
Equipment	Phosphorus (^{32}P) Gold (^{198}Au)	container marked "Radioactive" and send to radioisotope laboratory.
Vomitus	Phosphorus (^{32}P)	Place vomitus in lead-lined container and send to radioisotope laboratory.
Wound drainage	Phosphorus (^{32}P) Gold (^{198}Au)	Place dressings in lead-lined container and send to radioisotope laboratory.

12-8. With radioactive iodine, small amounts will be present in sputum, vomitus, perspiration, or feces, but special precautions are needed *only for urine.* The nurse should know the approved hospital procedure to safely dispose of any urine spilled on the floor.

No linen or equipment is removed from the room until it is monitored with a Geiger-Muller counter for contamination. Paper dishes are usually used and then burned. If the nurse's skin should become contaminated, it should be washed thoroughly with soap and water and then monitored. If contamination remains, washing should be continued until monitoring shows that additional cleansing is not necessary.

When the patient is removed from isolation, all equipment is monitored and carefully scrubbed by attendants who have been instructed in safe methods by persons who are in charge of the administration of the radioactive substances. It is then remonitored. The room is aired until monitoring shows that radioactivity is negligible and that the room is safe for any other patient. Airing takes at least 24 hours.

☐ **Nursing care of patients receiving internal radiotherapy**

Nursing interventions consist of the following:
1. Teach routine and reasons for precautions
2. Decrease isolation by providing radio or television for outside contact and encouraging permissible interaction with nursing staff
3. Plan trips into room to include several tasks
4. Promote comfort: complete bath before treatment, clean bed linens, turn sheet, pillow positioning

The patient should know that isolation is temporary, that the restrictions will be removed on a certain day, and that members of the nursing staff will be available but that they will work quickly and will remain in the room only long enough to carry out essential activities. The patient can assist in notifying family and friends about the restriction on visitors and how long it will last. The patient should also know how the radioactive substance is eliminated to lessen worry about being a danger to others, particularly after therapy is concluded.

Trips made in haste into the patient's room are disturbing psychologically, because they imply that the patient is not acceptable to others. The nurse who plans thoughtfully might deliver a letter, fresh water, and the newspaper and make pertinent observations in less time than the one who plans less well and must make several trips into the patient's room.

■ Chemotherapy

Advances in knowledge of cancer growth and chemotherapeutic agents have led to concomitant advances in cancer treatment. Improvement in overall survival and longer disease-free intervals can be directly ascribed to the use of chemotherapeutic agents, particularly in combination chemotherapy regimens and as adjuvant therapy.

■ BENEFITS OF CHEMOTHERAPY

Chemotherapy is potentially curative in gestational choriocarcinoma, acute lymphocytic leukemia (ALL), Ewing's sarcoma, advanced Hodgkin's disease, diffuse histiocytic lymphoma, Burkitt's lymphoma, testicular cancer, and ovarian cancer. Prolonged disease-free or controlled intervals may be achieved by chemotherapy in the treatment of several non-Hodgkin's lymphomas, multiple myeloma, breast cancer, and oat cell carcinoma of the lung. In other advanced malignancies, such as colorectal carcinoma, chemotherapy rarely produces a complete response and only a few such patients experience an increased survival time. In the treatment of chronic myelogenous leukemia (CML) and chronic lymphocytic leukemia (CLL), although the duration of life may not be prolonged, the quality of life may be enhanced by chemotherapy because of control of symptoms. Patients and families may be told that incurable does not mean untreatable or uncontrollable.

In the care of an individual patient with cancer, the expected benefit of chemotherapy (cure, control, or palliation) should be known by the physician, nurse, and patient. This allows for realistic goal setting by the care givers, patients, and family. Such background also provides a perspective from which to view side effects. The potential for cure, prolonged disease-free survival, or reduction of symptoms is a benefit that most often outweighs the risk and discomfort of short-term toxicity and side effects. Conditions in which risk may outweigh benefits include overt or occult infections, bleeding dyscrasias, bone marrow depression, severe metabolic disturbances, renal or liver dysfunction, and pregnancy.

Adjuvant chemotherapy refers to chemotherapy administered after surgical removal of all known cancer present in the body. It is aimed at the destruction of micrometastases thought likely to be present but too small to be detected by current diagnostic techniques. Left untreated, the micrometastases have a high potential for tumor growth and cancer recurrence. With the use of chemotherapy at a time when the malignant cell population is small and likely to be susceptible, complete tumor cell eradication is possible. The goal is cure.

Adjuvant chemotherapy is now generally considered to be indicated after mastectomy in all women with involved axillary lymph nodes at the time of surgery and it has demonstrated a significant decrease in recurrence rates and prolonged disease-free intervals. Adjuvant chemotherapy also appears to be beneficial in osteogenic sarcoma and Wilms' tumor. Evidence is currently equivocal regarding its benefit in other malignancies, such as colon cancer and malignant melanoma. The precise role of adjuvant chemotherapy will be more clearly delineated during the next decade, but it is already established as one of the major developments in health care.

A feeling of well-being and knowledge that all diagnostic tests are negative for cancer understandably may cause the patient to question the need for adjuvant therapy. This is emphasized when side effects are experienced. A sensitivity to these feelings, coupled with the knowledge of the expected benefit of therapy, is the basis for both patient teaching and the supportive encouragement often needed for continued therapy.

Despite an intellectual understanding of the benefits of chemotherapy, it is sometimes difficult for a nurse to maintain an appropriately optimistic and realistic outlook if all one sees are those patients who did not respond to or are no longer responsive to therapy, manifest severe toxicity, or are dying. The practitioner must take into account the setting in which patients are seen. Hospital-based nurses tend to see patients at the time of diagnosis, when they are critically ill, or during the final days of life. The public health nurse may see the patient at comparable points of illness while providing nursing care in the home. Discussion between the nurse and primary physician, contact with the outpatient clinic, and readmission to the same nursing unit are useful ways of acquiring a more complete picture of an individual's response to treatment. Such positive experiences are a means of nurturing one's own beliefs in therapy so that a realistic and at times very optimistic approach to caring for, supporting, and teaching the chemotherapy patient exists.

■ PATHOPHYSIOLOGIC PRINCIPLES OF CHEMOTHERAPY

Normal and malignant cells progress through various phases in the cell cycle as they replicate. Cancer chemotherapy is based on the action of certain drugs that create changes in the cell cycle phases and interrupt cell growth

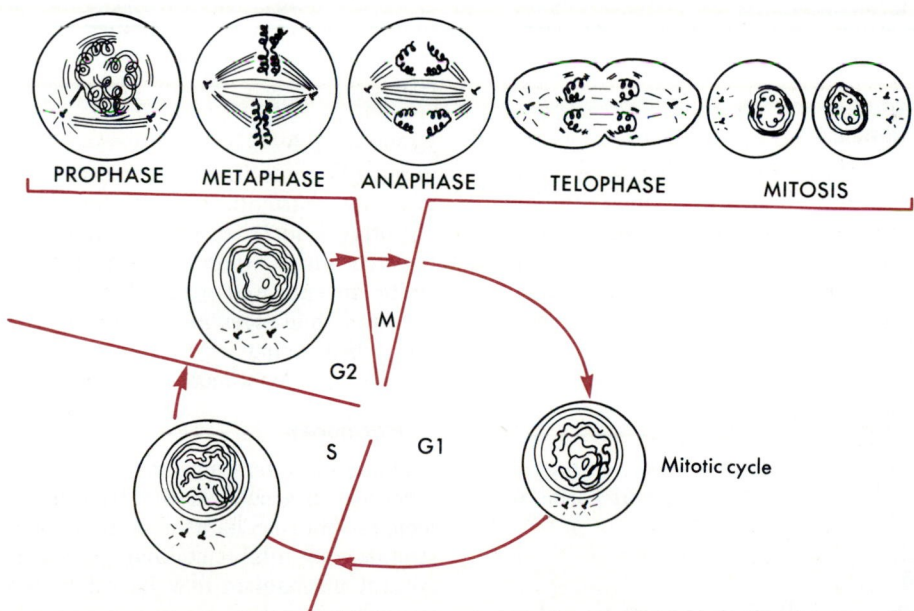

Fig. 12-9 Cell cycle. *G1*, RNA/protein synthesis; *S*, DNA synthesis; *G2*, RNA/protein synthesis and interphase; and *M*, mitosis (Adapted from Krakoff, I: Cancer chemotherapeutic agents: American Cancer Society professional education publication, New York, 1977, American Cancer Society.)

and replication. They specifically do this by disrupting production of essential enzymes, damaging structural proteins, and inhibiting DNA, RNA, and protein synthesis or direct interaction with DNA.

Some drugs are termed *cell cycle specific* because they are effective during a particular point of the cell cycle (Fig. 12-9). Antimetabolites interfere with DNA synthesis and affect the S phase of the cell cycle, whereas Vinca alkaloids, often called mitotic inhibitors, interfere with cell replication during the M phase. Drugs that are active throughout the cell cycle (*cell cycle nonspecific*) include the alkylating agents, antibiotics, and steroid hormones. Combinations of cycle-specific and cycle-nonspecific drugs have proved useful in planning treatment regimens. The goal is to use a combination of drugs that will destroy cancer cells at various stages of the replication process.

One major factor that influences the response of a cancer to chemotherapy is the fraction of tumor cells in replication at a given time, a percentage that varies among different tumors, individual patients, and at different times in the same patient. Malignancies with high growth fractions (proportion of cells in active cycle) and short cell cycle time (for example, leukemia) are most vulnerable to chemotherapy.[24]

☐ Cell population growth

The concept of cell population growth recognizes the fact that the population of both normal cells and cancer cells contains more dividing cells when the overall cell population is small and fewer dividing cells when the overall cell population is large.[20] This relates to chemotherapy in that the choice of drug differs for large, slow-growing tumors as opposed to small tumors whose cell population is likely to be more rapidly proliferating. The latter, because of their sensitivity to interference with DNA, are susceptible to phase-specific drugs, whereas the large, slow-growing tumor is more likely to respond to phase-nonspecific drugs.

☐ Log cell kill hypothesis

The log cell kill hypothesis states that any dose of a chemotherapy drug will destroy only a fraction of the malignant cells.[20] Treatment must be repeated multiple times to eradicate the cancer. Moreover, clinical symptoms disappear before all malignant cells are destroyed, so treatment must often be continued even when all apparent evidence of disease has disappeared.

■ CHEMOTHERAPEUTIC AGENTS

Drugs may be classified as alkylating agents, antimetabolites, plant (*Vinca*) alkaloids, antibiotics, and hormones (Table 12-9).

☐ Alkylating agents

The alkylating agents are cell cycle nonspecific and act against already formed nucleic acids by cross-linking DNA strands, thereby preventing DNA replication and the transcription of RNA.

☐ Antimetabolites

The antimetabolites act by interfering with the synthesis of chromosomal nucleic acid. Antimetabolites are analogues of normal metabolites and block the enzyme necessary for synthesis of essential factors or are incorporated into the DNA or RNA and thus prevent replication. Most antimetabolites are pyrimidine analogues, purine analogues, or folic acid antagonists and are, in general, cycle specific.

☐ Vinca alkaloids

Vincristine sulfate and vinblastine sulfate are plant alkaloids that act as mitotic inhibitors. These agents exert their cytotoxic effect by binding to proteins within the cells. The *Vinca* alkaloids are cell cycle specific. Although these two agents are similar in composition, mechanism of action, and metabolism, their antitumor spectrum, dose, and clinical toxicity differ.

☐ Antibiotics

Those antibiotics that demonstrate antitumor activity appear to affect either the function or synthesis of the nucleic acids. In addition, antimitotic and cell surface effects may be caused by these agents. The cytotoxic antibiotics are cell cycle nonspecific agents.

☐ Steroids

The corticosteroids are produced by the adrenal cortex and include mineralocorticoids and glucocorticoids. It is the glucocorticoids that, in addition to their use in numerous nonmalignant diseases, are effective in the treatment of many neoplastic disorders. In some malignancies (for example, lymphomas, breast cancer, multiple myeloma, acute lymphocytic leukemia, and chronic lymphocytic leukemia) steroids exert a direct antitumor effect. Steroids are also able to reduce edema and inflammation around a tumor and, therefore, are useful for symptom relief. Many side effects are associated with long-term steroid use, most notably a compromised immunologic response to infection, osteoporosis, and a cushingoid syndrome. Steroids in cancer treatment regimens are often given intermittently and for short periods of time and are not often associated with the debilitating side effects associated with chronic, long-term use. Patients often describe an improved sense of well-being and an increased appetite while receiving prednisone. With completion of a prescribed course of therapy, a brief period of fatigue, malaise, and emotional lability may be experienced.

☐ Hormones

Hormonal alteration may be a desired therapeutic goal when tumor growth is directly influenced by certain hormones. The mechanism whereby the steroid hormones stimulate or inhibit cellular growth is not clear; an important mechanism may be interference or alteration at the cell membrane.

Estrogen receptor assays are now routinely done at the time of mastectomy for breast cancer. This technique has made it possible to evaluate the ability of a breast tumor

Table 12-9 Agents used in cancer chemotherapy

Agent	Mechanism of action	Major toxic manifestations
Alkylating agents		
Chlorambucil (Leukeran) Melphalan (Alkeran) Cyclophosphamide (Cytoxan) Busulfan (Myleran)	Interfere with DNA replication by attacking DNA synthesis throughout cell cycle (cell cycle nonspecific)	Bone marrow depression with leukopenia, thrombocytopenia, and bleeding; cyclophosphamide may cause alopecia and hemorrhagic cystitis
Antimetabolites		
Methotrexate (MTX) 6-Mercaptopurine (6-MP) 5-Fluorouracil (5-FU) Cytarabine (Cytosar)	Structural analogs of essential metabolites and therefore interfere with synthesis of these metabolites (cell cycle specific)	Bone marrow depression, oral and gastrointestinal ulceration
Antibiotics		
Doxorubicin (Adriamycin) Bleomycin (Blenoxane) Dactinomycin (Cosmegan) Daunomycin (Daunorubicin) Mithramycin (Mithracin) Mitomycin (Mutamycin)	Interfere with DNA or RNA synthesis, varying with the drug (cell cycle nonspecific)	Stomatitis, gastrointestinal disturbances, and bone marrow depression Doxorubicin causes cardiac toxicity at cumulative doses over 500 mg/m² Bleomycin can cause alopecia and pulmonary fibrosis, but only minimal bone marrow depression
Plant alkaloids		
Vinblastine (Velban)	Interfere with mitosis (cell cycle specific)	Alopecia, areflexia, bone marrow depression
Vincristine (Oncovin)		Neurotoxicity with ataxia and impaired fine motor skills, constipation and paralytic ileus
Steroid hormones		
Androgens (Neo-Hombreol) Estrogens (DES) Progestins (Depoprovera) Adrenocorticosteroids (Prednisone)	Alter the host environment for cell growth (cell cycle nonspecific)	Specific for the actions of the hormone

Adapted from Porth, C: Pathophysiology: concepts of altered health states, ed. 2 Philadelphia, 1987, JB Lippincott Co.

to bind estrogen and thus project the probable sensitivity of the tumor to hormonal therapy.

■ COMBINATION CHEMOTHERAPY

Increased knowledge of how specific cytotoxic drugs exert their effect and of the potential for the emergence of tumor cells resistant to a specific therapy, similar to antibiotic resistance, has led to the use of combination chemotherapy. Combination chemotherapy demonstrates a therapeutic effect superior to a single agent therapy for many cancers. Drugs considered for combination chemotherapy are those that (1) are active when used alone, (2) have different mechanisms of action, (3) have a biochemical basis for possible synergism, (4) do not produce toxicity in the same organs, and (5) produce toxicity at different times after administration.[57] Repeated brief courses of drug therapy are given to reduce immunosuppressive effects.

■ DOSE CALCULATIONS

The dosage range for a particular drug is determined at the time of clinical trial and regimen development. Given these guidelines, the dosage for a specific individual must be calculated before starting therapy. Although some regimens may still prescribe milligrams per kilogram, drug doses are usually stated in terms of body surface area, and therefore, the doses are given in milligrams per square meter (m²).[56] An individual's height and weight are used to determine body surface; therefore, it is very important that height and weight be measured *accurately*.

■ METHODS OF ADMINISTRATION OF CHEMOTHERAPEUTIC AGENTS

The route of administration is based on the metabolism and absorption of a given drug. The route of choice is that which will deliver the optimal amount of drug to the tumor. Chemotherapeutic agents are given orally, intravenously, intramuscularly, intraarterially, and by local instillation (that is; intrapleurally or intrathecally). If tumor cells are in an area that drugs cannot reach, cancer cells will survive with a consequent increase in disease recurrence. An example is the sanctuary effect afforded leukemic cells by the meninges in patients with acute lymphocytic leukemia. For this reason, local instillation of chemotherapy via an Ommaya cerebrospinal reservoir or intrathecally (directly into the spinal fluid by lumbar puncture) is used to treat tumor cells present in the CNS.

Before administering a cytotoxic drug, the clinician consults a reference for usual dosage, acceptable routes of administration, and any precautions that should be taken

Table 12-10 Treatment recommendations for vesicant extravasation

Antineoplastic agent	Local antidote	Application of heat or cold
Nitrogen mustard	Isotonic sodium thiosulfate	Cold
Doxorubicin	Hydrocortisone or dexamethasone and/or sodium bicarbonate	Cold
Vinblastine	Hyaluronidase	Warm

From Oncology Nursing Society: Cancer chemotherapy guidelines for nursing education and practice, Pittsburgh, 1984, The Society.

for that particular drug. Since protocols may deviate from drug manufacturers' guidelines, discussion with the prescribing physician may also be indicated.

□ Oral administration

Many cytotoxic drugs are given in pill form. Since these may be prescribed on a daily basis to be taken at home, careful instructions need to be given to patients. Areas to be discussed include the importance of taking the drug as prescribed, the relationship to meals, fluid intake, and the use of an antiemetic.

□ Intravenous administration

The clinician must know specific properties for each drug to be administered. Of particular importance is the identification of those drugs that are vesicant (produce blisters). If infiltration and extravasation of a vesicant occur, extensive tissue damage and necrosis may result. Nitrogen mustard, doxorubicin (Adriamycin), vincristine, and vinblastine are the principal vesicant drugs. The intravenous site is evaluated before the administration of these drugs. If *any* suspicion of an infiltration or leak exists, the site is changed. Most often, vesicant drugs are given via the side arm of a running IV. If extravasation occurs, immediate action is taken to minimize damage. Guidelines for treating extravasation vary and nurses should be aware of the policies that exist for the agency in which they are employed. Refer to Table 12-10 for suggestions.

For patients with poor venous access, either an indwelling Hickman catheter (Fig. 12-10) or an implantable infusion port (Fig. 12-11) may be used for chemotherapy administration. Nursing care considerations for these two types of venous access devices are described in the boxes

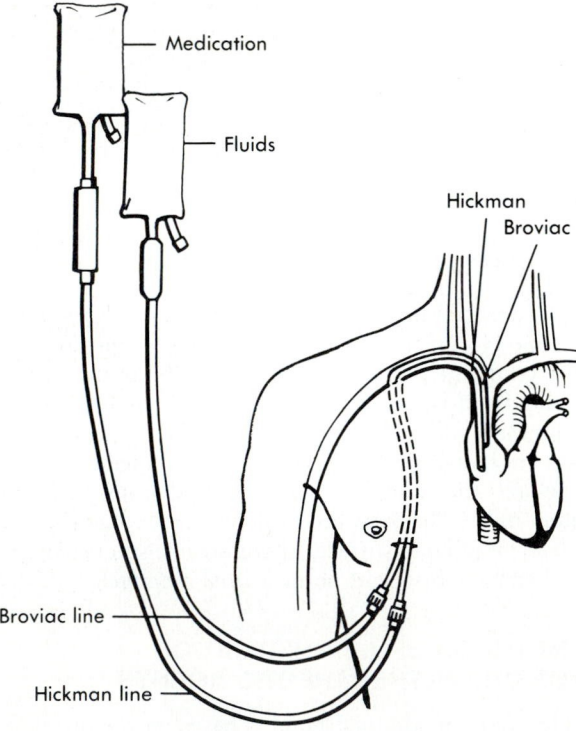

Fig. 12-10 Double lumen Hickman/Broviac catheter.

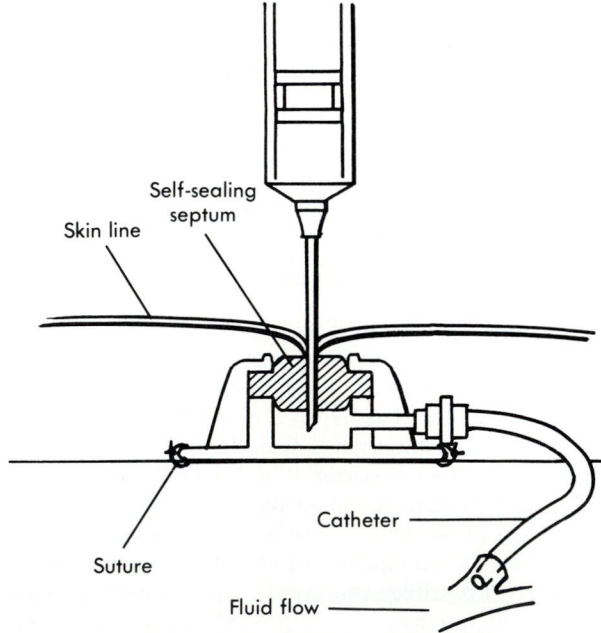

Fig. 12-11 Implantable infusion port. Drugs are administered through self-sealing infusion port.

below. The skin around the catheter insertion site or implanted infusion port is inspected for redness, swelling, or drainage. Showering and bathing are permitted.[17]

☐ Perfusion

Regional and isolation perfusion is a means of delivering a high dosage of a drug directly to a tumor. This is accomplished by the placement of a catheter into an artery that provides the blood supply to the area being treated. By this method, a high percentage of the drug is delivered because it is not diluted in the general circulation.

Intraarterial perfusion is used occasionally for cancers of the head and neck and of the liver and as adjuvant chemotherapy with radiotherapy for advanced cancer of the cervix. Because infusions may be continuous for long periods of time (several hours to days), the patient may be restricted in activity. However, intra-arterial perfusion can be accomplished in ambulatory patients by means of a portable infusion pump (Fig. 12-12). Aspects of nursing care include assessment of the catheter insertion site, care of the line to maintain placement and prevent infection, and observation for bleeding. Outpatients need careful and detailed instruction so that these same criteria can be maintained in the home. Hospital nurses involved in the discharge planning of such patients need to ensure that the community-based nurse also be informed of these detailed instructions.

■ SIDE EFFECTS AND NURSING INTERVENTION

Some degree of injury to normal cells often occurs with treatment by chemotherapeutic agents. The basis for normal cells being affected is their rate of proliferation. Many normal tissues have a high proliferation capacity, in some instances exceeding that of malignant disease. It is these rapidly proliferating tissues (the bone marrow, gastrointestinal epithelium, and hair follicles) that bear the brunt of the toxic effects of many of the cytotoxic drugs.

Routine care of Hickman/Broviac catheters

1. Irrigate catheter daily with 3 ml heparin-saline solution (10 U heparin/ml) to prevent clotting.
2. Irrigate briskly—may help prevent outflow obstruction.
3. Clamping is *not* recommended; clamp over protective covering if necessary.
4. Change dressing every other day for 2 to 3 weeks after insertion using meticulous aseptic technique, then apply bandage to exit site.
5. Prevent undue tension on catheter; tape to patient at all times.
6. Change cap(s) every 7 days.
7. Obtain repair kit for catheter from manufacturer.

From Goodman, SG, and Wickham, R: Venous access devices: an overview, Oncol Nurs Forum 11(5):16-23, 1984.

Maintenance of implantable infusion port

1. Puncture with Huber point needle only.
2. Irrigate every 4 weeks with 3 to 5 ml heparin-saline solution (100 U heparin/ml).
3. Use 20 ml normal saline flush after blood drawing.
4. Irrigate arterial ports once a week with 3 to 5 ml heparin/saline solution (100 U heparin/ml).
5. Flush catheter after each use.
6. No restriction on patient because port is implanted.

From Goodman, SG, and Wickham, R: Venous access devices: an overview, Oncol Nurs Forum 11(5):16-23, 1984.

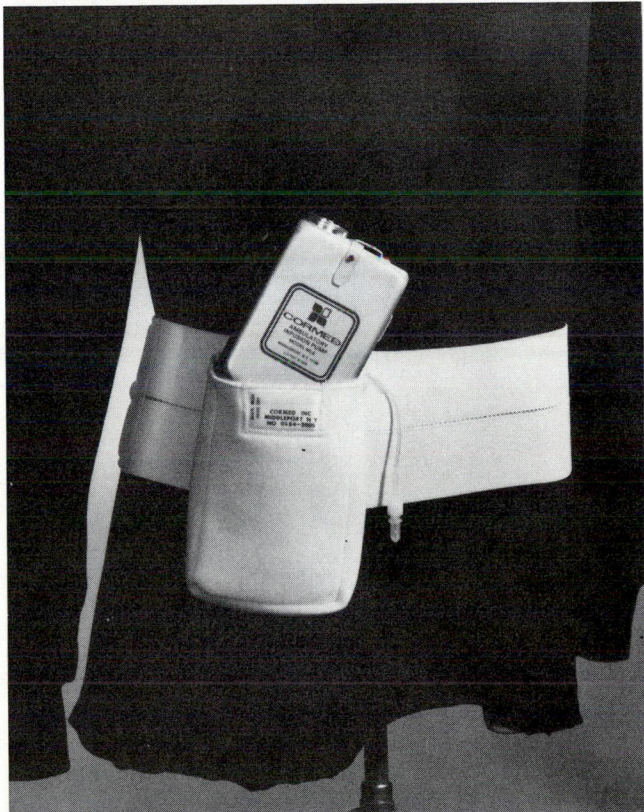

Fig. 12-12 Lightweight, battery-operated infusion pump for ambulatory patient. Flow rate is adjustable. Power pack operates for 7 days before needing recharging. (Courtesy CORMED, Inc, Middleport, NY.)

□ Bone marrow suppression

Recognition of the bone marrow suppressive (myelosuppressive) potential of the chemotherapeutic agents is critical to the care of patients receiving chemotherapy. It is the major life-threatening toxicity associated with chemoterapy. Frequent blood counts are done to monitor this toxicity, and astute attention must be given to the results of the white blood count, platelet count, and hemoglobin, with appropriate modification of drug dosage. Patients who have received previous chemotherapy or radiation therapy, particularly to areas of bone marrow reserve (sternum, hips, or pelvis) may have an increased sensitivity to myelosuppression. Blood counts are done before the administration of chemotherapy and at regular intervals to assess the predictable lowest point, which varies with the drugs used. Nursing care of patients with neutropenia, thrombocytopenia, and anemia are discussed in Chapter 27.

□ Infection

The prevention of infection is of utmost importance in the care and teaching of the cancer patient. Body areas with high potential for infection should be inspected daily. The *skin and mucous membranes*, especially the mouth, axillae, and perineal areas, are infection prone. Assessment of the *respiratory tract* is also important to identify early signs of respiratory infection. Patients are susceptible to middle-ear infections, sinusitis, and pharyngitis. Pneumonia is especially prevalent in patients with leukemia and in elderly persons. Families of patients are instructed not to visit if they have colds.

Injections are usually avoided. Aseptic technique must be scrupulously maintained during intravenous infusions and dressing changes. In preventing all types of infection, good medical asepsis and especially careful handwashing by the medical and nursing staff are important.

□ *Use of patient isolation*

If the white blood count is low, reverse isolation may be ordered to prevent infection. Reverse isolation is not usually effective unless life islands or laminar airflow units are used. The *life island* consists of a special large plastic canopy placed around and over the patient's bed. All equipment is sterilized and the air is filtered to remove airborne bacteria. Objects are passed in and out through locks irradiated by ultraviolet light. Patient contact is through arm-length gloves built into the side of the canopy.

Laminar airflow units are rooms that have a constant flow of purified air flowing across the width and breadth of the room (Fig. 12-13). Anyone in the room remains downstream from the patient. If the patient must be touched, a mask, cap, and gown are worn. The advantage of the laminar airflow room is that it is large and allows more freedom of movement than the life island.

One problem with any type of isolation is that the patient

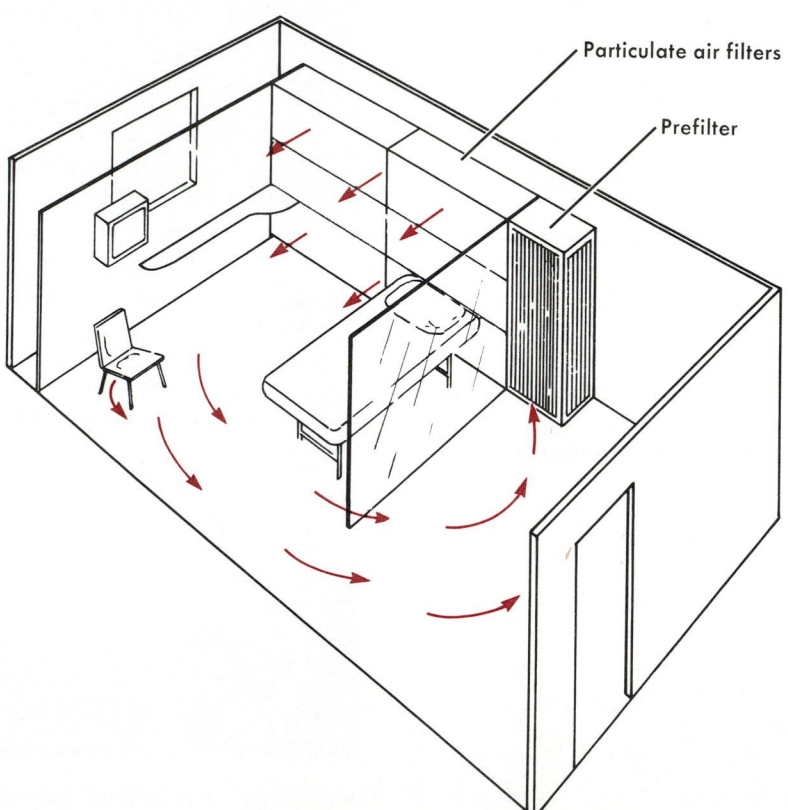

Fig. 12-13 In laminar airflow units constant flow of purified air flows across width and breadth of room. (From American Cancer Society: Proceedings of the National Conference on Cancer Nursing, New York, 1973, The Society.)

may experience sensory deprivation and social isolation. In addition, when reverse isolation is terminated, the patient may feel unsafe, vulnerable, and angry because of removal from the protected environment.

□ Gastrointestinal effects

Changes in bowel habits commonly occur but usually do not require intervention. If diarrhea becomes marked or persists, an antidiarrheal medication such as diphenoxylate with atropine (Lomotil) may be prescribed. Metamucil is also recommended to increase bulk. Persons receiving vincristine are assessed for signs of paralytic ileus and are instructed to report constipation.

Stomatitis, an inflammation of the mucous membranes of the oral cavity, may range from an erythema of the oral mucosa to mild or severe ulceration. Methotrexate, 5-fluorouracil, doxorubicin, dactinomycin, and bleomycin are the chemotherapeutic drugs most frequently used with stomatitis. Patients may also develop a superimposed *Candida* infection of the mouth and esophagus, and oral nystatin is usually prescribed. Good mouth care is encouraged.

Nausea and vomiting

Nausea and vomiting are among the most uncomfortable and distressing side effects of chemotherapy. For the ambulatory patient, nausea may interfere with the ability to continue daily work. Persistent vomiting may result in fluid and electrolyte imbalance, general weakness, and weight loss. Decline of nutritional status renders the patient more susceptible to infection and perhaps less able to tolerate therapy. Such physiologic symptoms can accompany or precipitate psychologic responses that might include depression and withdrawal. Every effort must be made to minimize chemotherapy-induced nausea and vomiting. The onset and duration vary greatly among patients and with the drug given.

Antiemetics vary in success. Tetrahydrocannabinol (THC) taken in pill form produces an antiemetic effect in some patients who have not benefited from the commonly prescribed prochlorperazine (Compazine). Metoclopramide hydrochloride (Reglan) may be helpful for persons receiving cisplatin, and lorazepam (Ativan) is often effective in producing a relaxed state during which an individual is less sensitive to stimuli that can induce feelings of nausea. Timing of food and fluid intake in relation to treatment is often ascertained by the patient, as are the types of foods that are best tolerated. Relaxation techniques are useful for some patients.

□ Alopecia

Alopecia (loss of hair) may occur by two mechanisms. If the hair roots are atrophied, alopecia occurs readily. The hair either falls out spontaneously or by hair combing, often in large clumps. If the hair shaft is constricted because of atrophy or necrosis, the hair will break off very near the scalp. The root remains in the scalp and a patchy, thinning pattern of hair loss occurs.[56] Hair loss may occur on other parts of the body in addition to the scalp. Loss of leg, arm, pubic, axillary, and facial hair is seen less often, although loss of eyebrows and eyelashes may occur.

The pattern and extent of hair loss cannot be accurately predicted for a given patient. When the treatment is given with a drug known to cause alopecia, the patient needs to be told that severe hair loss can begin within a few days or weeks of treatment and that partial or complete baldness can quickly ensue. *Drug-induced alopecia is never permanent.* Occasionally, hair growth may return while chemotherapy treatment continues. Given this perspective, coupled with the goal of disease control or cure, most patients tolerate the hair loss with minimal distress, although it is common and normal that some feelings are expressed about the hair loss.

□ Effects on skin

Vesicant drugs may cause severe tissue necrosis if infiltration should occur. Other skin reactions that might occur are hyperpigmentation, nail changes, and an increased sensitivity to the sun (photosensitivity).

□ Organ toxicities

Liver toxicity is uncommon but may occur. There may be a transient increase in liver enzymes. Alteration in liver function has been associated with Ara-C, methotrexate, and 6-mercaptopurine. *Cardiac* status is carefully moni-

---

Drugs commonly causing alopecia

Bleomycin	ICRF-159
Cyclophosphamide	Hydroxyurea
Dactinomycin	Methotrexate
Daunomycin hydrochloride	Mitomycin
Doxorubicin hydrochloride	VP-16-213
5-Fluorouracil	Vincristine

From Knopf, M, and others: Cancer chemotherapy treatment and care, New Haven, Conn, 1979, Yale Comprehensive Cancer Center.

Drugs not causing alopecia

5-Azacytidine	Melphalan
Busulfan	Mercaptopurine
Carmustine	Mithramycin
Chlorambucil	Nitrogen mustard
Cisplatin	Procarbazine
Cytarabine	Semustine
Dacarbazine	Streptozotocin
Ftorafur	Triazinate
Hexamethylmelamine	Zinostatin
Lomustine	

From Knopf, M, and others: Cancer chemotherapy treatment and care, New Haven, Conn, 1979, Yale Comprehensive Cancer Center.

Nursing care of patients receiving chemotherapy

Bone marrow suppression or infection

1. Check blood counts
2. Assess infection-prone areas daily to identify early signs of infection
3. Maintain medical asepsis through careful handwashing
4. Maintain intact skin and mucous membranes
   a. Teach avoidance of bumping and breaking skin
   b. Maintain aseptic technique during IV infusion and dressing changes
   c. Keep fingernails short
   d. Teach good perineal hygiene
   e. Teach avoidance of excessive friction and importance of vaginal lubrication
   f. Teach avoidance of anal intercourse
   g. No enemas, rectal medications, or rectal thermometers
   h. Encourage fastidious oral hygiene with a soft toothbrush
   i Inspect mouth daily for ulcers and white patches
   j. Use lubricants to prevent drying and cracking of lips
5. Maintain optimal respiratory function
   a. Assess for early signs of respiratory infection
   b. Auscultate lung sounds
   c. Instruct family/friends not to visit if they have colds
6. Maintain reverse isolation if ordered

Gastrointestinal effects: stomatitis, nausea, vomiting

1. Administer oral nystatin, as ordered
2. Use a rinse and lidocaine before meals to lubricate and provide an analgesic effect
3. Use a cleansing rinse of plain water or dilute hydrogen peroxide after meals
4. Administer antiemetic as ordered
5. Determine from patient best time for food and fluid intake in relation to treatment
6. Teach relaxation techniques and imagery, if appropriate

Alopecia

1. Explain that drug-induced alopecia is not permanent
2. Allow expression of feelings about hair loss
3. Scalp tourniquets or scalp hypothermia via ice pack may be ordered for patients with solid tumors to minimize hair loss with some agents (for example, vincristine, adriamycin)
4. Encourage use of wigs, hats, and scarves

Effects on skin

Inspect administration site for signs of infiltration or extravasation

Organ toxicities

1. Assess signs and symptoms of liver dysfunction (see Chapter 30)
2. Monitor cardiac status (arrhythmias, congestive heart failure) (see Chapter 25)
3. Assess signs and symptoms of pulmonary toxicity (see Chapter 24)

Urinary effects: hemorrhagic cystitis, renal toxicity

1. Maintain hydration by encouraging drinking of large amounts of fluid (if receiving cyclophosphamide)
2. Monitor renal function: check serum creatinine or creatinine clearance (with cisplatin or streptozotocin)

Sterility

1. Assess knowledge of known and possible effects on fertility
2. Provide birth control and reproductive counseling, as appropriate

tored in patients receiving doxorubicin. A baseline echo-cardiogram is usually done before beginning treatment and at regular intervals while therapy continues. Two forms of cardiac damage may occur: arrhythmias, most commonly associated with a preexisting cardiac disease, and a delayed moderate to severe congestive heart failure.[57] Other drugs associated with some potential for cardiac toxicity are daunorubicin (Daunomycin) and high-dose cyclophosphamide (Cytoxan). *Pulmonary* toxicity may occur with methotrexate and some of the alkylating agents. The most common cause of chemotherapy-induced pulmonary toxicity is bleomycin. Pulmonary fibrosis can occur and may be irreversible. Each time bleomycin is administered, the pulmonary status of the patient is assessed by auscultation and questioning regarding the presence of cough or shortness of breath.

□ Urinary effects

Hemorrhagic cystitis occurs in about 10% of patients being treated with cyclophosphamide but rarely occur with other agents.[24] Patients receiving cyclophosphamide are encouraged to drink a large amount of fluid to minimize this effect. Taking the cyclophosphamide early in the day may also be of some benefit. Renal toxicity is associated with several drugs, but most notably with cisplatin and streptozotocin. Before the administration of each dose of these drugs renal function is evaluated by either a serum creatinine or a 24-hour urine collection for creatinine clearance.

□ Sterility

Cancer chemotherapy reaches the reproductive organs at dose levels similar to those achieved at the site of the target tumor. The potential exists for a disruptive effect on genetic and fetal development.[61] It is recognized that chemotherapy, particularly some of the alkylating agents, may cause transient or permanent sterility. Patients on chemotherapy need to be informed of the known and possible effects on fertility. Birth control and reproductive counseling need to be factors included in patient teaching. If a nurse does not feel comfortable or qualified to discuss the topic, resources useful to the patient and spouse should be identified. Sperm banking before the initiation of therapy offers male patients the option of future conception. Following completion of chemotherapy, conception and the birth of normal, healthy children are possibilities for couples. It is customary to recommend that procreation be avoided until at least 18 months after completion of treatment.

■ Biologic response modifier therapy (immunotherapy)

■ PATHOPHYSIOLOGY

The role of biologic response modifier (BRM) therapy in the prevention and treatment of cancer is being studied. The term *BRM* actually applies to the broad category of biologic agents that have the potential to control the growth and metastasis of neoplasms. Immunotherapy is a subcategory of BRM therapies.[40]

Many scientists believe cancer occurs in the body more frequently than once in a lifetime; however, in most cases clinical evidence of the disease is not apparent. It is postulated that there is a natural immunity against the development of the disease and that cancer cells are destroyed almost as quickly as they develop.[66] Studies of cancer show that when the normal cell becomes malignant, it often undergoes biochemical changes resulting in formation of new cellular antigens that cause an immune response. Clinical malignancy may occur as a result of failure in the immunologic surveillance system of the body.

The immune response has two major components. The first, or *cellular immune response* (see Chapter 38), produces lymphocytes capable of destroying tumor cells on contact. These lymphocytes (T cells) undergo division and are released into the bloodstream when stimulated by an antigen. In addition to destroying cancer cells on contact, T cells may release cytotoxins, which cause holes in the cell membrane, eventually resulting in lysis or death of the malignant cell.

The second component of the immune response is *antibody production* resulting from activation of lymphocytes (B cells). When stimulated by antigens, B cells proliferate and differentiate into plasma cells, which are the major source of antibody production.

At the present time, the immune response can handle only a limited number of tumor cells, up to 10 million. After a growth to 100 million cells, the immune response is not capable of preventing further growth. Once the cancer is large, it cannot be totally controlled by the immune system, so immunotherapy cannot be the primary mode of cancer therapy at the present time. It is used after surgery, radiotherapy, and chemotherapy have removed the bulk of the tumor.

Much is yet to be learned about the immunology of cancers. The number of cancers once thought to be immunogenic and responsive to immunotherapy is less than originally supposed. If cancer vaccines are developed, they will be effective in tumors caused by viruses, and these are probably limited in number. Even if a cancer-carrying virus is isolated, it must be attenuated so it can be given safely.

■ APPROACHES USED IN BIOLOGIC RESPONSE MODIFIER THERAPY

Biologic response modifiers can be described as therapeutic agents that alter the interaction between tumor and host by influencing the host's biologic response to cancer cells. There the two major categories of BRM therapies are distinguished by their mode of action. The first group consists of agents that *stimulate the general immune capacity* of the host. This group consists primarily of immunomodulators, including chemicals and synthetic compounds, that promote host resistance. The second group consists of effector cells, antibodies, and cytokines that have the ability to directly *destroy the tumor cells* or to indirectly *suppress the growth and metastasis of tumor cells.*[40] A discussion of several specific BRM therapies follows.

■ CYTOKINES AND LYMPHOKINES

The term *cytokine* is a general term referring to the soluble products of cells, whereas *lymphokine,* a more specific term, can be defined as soluble cell products from lymphocytes. Interferon is a cytokine; interleukin-2 is classified as a lymphokine.

□ Interferons

Interferons are a family of secretory glycoproteins produced by leukocytes in response to viral infections or to other stimuli. Interferons induce cellular resistance to a broad spectrum of viruses and are a first line of defense against viral infections (see Fig. 38-4). In addition, they may protect against intracellular parasites, neoplastic changes in cells, and the tumor growth itself. They appear to have an inhibitory effect on DNA synthesis and cell growth and may suppress the tumor directly.[33] Interferon's antitumor effect develops from its ability to augment natural killer (NK) cells (Chapter 37) and to stimulate the expression of antigens on the surface of lymphocytes and macrophages.[40]

When exposed to a virus, all nucleated cells are capable of interferon production. Three cell types produce interferon: leukocytes produce alpha interferon, fibroblasts produce beta interferon, and lymphocytes produce gamma interferon. Each type of interferon is distinctive in its ability to alter immunologic and biologic responses. Synthetic interferon has been manufactured by gene-cloning techniques.

Although interferon is not the cure for cancer that had been hoped initially, current research reports that interferon has antitumor activity against several cancers, including leukemia, lymphoma, and selected solid tumors. The FDA has approved interferon for use in treatment of hairy cell leukemia.[40]

Nursing intervention for persons receiving interferon therapy includes monitoring for side effects: fever, local discomfort at the injection site, and minimal nausea and vomiting. Acetaminophen (Tylenol) is given for discomfort and antiemetics for nausea and vomiting. At some centers nurses teach patients to give their own intravenous or intramuscular injections.[31] Nurses must be careful not to raise false hopes in patients who may view interferon as a last-resort therapy.

□ Interleukin-2

Interleukin-2 (IL-2) stimulates formation of T cells and natural killer cells. Preliminary indications from clinical trials suggest that IL-2 may be useful as a curative agent for some malignancies and be beneficial in combination with other treatment modalities. It is administered by intravenous bolus or continuous infusion, by subcutaneous injection, and by peritoneal infusion. Identified side effects include confusion, psychosis, pulmonary edema, impaired renal functioning, arrhythmias, and hypotension.[22] IL-2 is one of the more promising BRM therapies.

■ MONOCLONAL ANTIBODIES

Monoclonal antibodies are produced by first injecting a mouse with a specific tumor antigen. The mouse's spleen cells are then removed and fused with myeloma cells. This fusion promotes the survival of the cells in cultures where they are cloned. The clones are then injected into a mouse. The result is a monoclonal hybridoma that secretes monoclonal antibodies that can be harvested from mouse and administered to humans.

Numerous clinical trials with monoclonal antibodies are currently being conducted, against both hematopoetic malignancies and solid tumors. Some studies are investigating the use of monoclonal antibodies conjugated with toxic substances.[40] Radioactive isotopes and cytotoxic agents are attached to antibodies to deliver these substances directly to the neoplasm. Monoclonal antibodies are administered by slow intravenous infusion. Side effects include but are not limited to fever, chills, and localized tumor pain.

■ THYMIC FACTORS

The two most common factors produced by the thymus gland are thymosin fraction 5 (TF-5) and thymosin alpha 1 (Tα-1). TF-5 is an extract of calf thymus and appears capable of restoring immunologic functioning when the thymus gland is absent or repressed. Tα-1 is a derivative of TF-5 and can be synthetically produced. Phase I research has demonstrated that thymic factors have immunostimulating capacities in immunosuppressed cancer patients. Some immunorestorative capacity has also been suggested using Tα-1 in clinical trials.[40]

■ NURSING INTERVENTIONS FOR BRM THERAPY

Clinical trials of biologic response modifiers are currently being conducted in many health care centers, and nurses must be familiar with the research protocols being tested in their particular setting. Consent forms need to be obtained. Medications are often administered in rigid schedules and nurses are particularly involved in monitoring for side effects. In general, BRM therapies can cause fever, malaise, arthralgias and myalgias, as well as anaphylactic types of reactions. These treatments are relatively new, and the incidence and severity of side effects are still being established. Thorough documentation of adverse reactions and their response to symptom management is essential. Patient teaching should emphasize the need to report all side effects, regardless of how subtle they may be.

■ Cancer pain

Pain is one of the most feared effects of cancer, although, contrary to popular belief, it is frequently the last symptom to appear. Even in terminal stages, 60% of persons with cancer will experience mild or no pain. The etiology of cancer pain is complex since it has physical, psychologic, social and spiritual aspects.

STAGES OF CANCER PAIN

Three stages of cancer pain have been described: early, intermediate, and late. Early pain usually occurs after initial surgery for diagnosis or treatment and usually subsides after the third day; thus this pain is an acute episode, that is, short term and temporary.

Intermediate-stage pain results from postoperative contraction of scars and nerve entrapment or from cancer recurrence or metastasis. This pain may subside or may be controlled by palliative therapy such as radiation, chemotherapy, neurosurgery, and analgesics. Therapy itself may initiate the pain.[38]

Late-stage pain occurs in terminal cancer when therapy no longer controls the disease. This pain is chronic, may slowly increase in intensity, and at times may be intractable. Severe chronic pain occurs in only about 20% of patients who die from cancer.[28]

PATHOPHYSIOLOGY

Malignant neoplasms cause pain by five physiologic changes: bone destruction, obstruction of lumens (viscera or vessels), peripheral nerve involvement, pressure of growing tumors causing ischemia or distention, and inflammation, infection, or necrosis of the tissue.

Bone destruction with infraction (fractures without displacement) is the most frequent cause of pain, usually resulting from metastatic lesions. Bone destruction may cause increased sensitivity over the area or sharp, continuous pain.

Obstruction of a viscus, such as in the gastrointestinal or genitourinary tract, causes severe, colicky, crampy-type pain. Visceral pain is dull, diffuse, and poorly localized. Obstruction of an artery, vein, or lymphatic vessel may initiate arterial ischemia, venous engorgement, or edema. This pain is dull, diffuse, and aching.

Infiltration or compression of peripheral nerves or nerve plexuses causes continuous, sharp or stabbing pain sometimes accompanied by hyperesthesia or paresthesia.

Infiltration or distention of the integument, fascia, or tissue initiates a severe localized pain that is dull and aching, increasing in intensity as tumor size increases. An example of this is the pain resulting from distention of the abdomen by ascites or the stretching of the skin by carcinoma of the neck.

Finally, inflammation, infection, and necrosis of the tissue itself may cause pain by producing either pressure or ischemia. Chemical mediators of pain are present during inflammation and necrosis.

PSYCHOSOCIAL ASPECTS

The psychologic component of cancer pain is associated with the patient's perception of the threat and stress of cancer and varies from individual to individual. Three categories of stressors have been identified: injury or threat of injury as a result of the cancer, loss or threat of loss (body part or death), and frustration of drives as a result of disabilities from the cancer per se or from the effect of

therapies. Patients may respond with depression, decreased self-esteem, hostility, and irritability.

The sociologic effects include decreased interaction and participation in activities of daily living. There is decreased productivity characterized by absenteeism from work, economic problems, and deterioration in family relationships. The spiritual effects of pain are evidenced by loss of hope and trust and an overwhelming feeling of despair, rejection, and sense of isolation.

Side effects of cancer pain include fatigue, sleeplessness, anorexia, and decreased movement followed by the complications of immobility, namely, muscle weakness, decubiti, contractures, and respiratory dysfunction.

INTERVENTION

Medical therapy in early-stage pain focuses on therapy directed at the cancer per se. Late-stage pain is treated symptomatically by analgesia, neurosurgery, and nerve blocks. Surgical procedures to relieve the pain include simple intercostal nerve block where feasible, surgical section of posterior sensory roots adjacent to the spinal cord, and spinothalamic tractotomy (interruption of pain- and temperature-conducting tracts). Dorsal column stimulators and transcutaneous electrical stimulators (see Chapter 10) may be helpful in selected cases.

Cancer pain, as other types of severe pain, may occupy the patient's entire attention and, unless treated vigorously, may demoralize the patient and interfere with eating, resting, or sleeping. Interventions are directed toward helping the patient live as normal a life as possible and cope with the pain. Pain tolerance is increased when the patient's energy is preserved for enjoyable activities. General comfort measures to promote rest and sleep, good body positioning, and nutrition may do much to increase the patient's pain tolerance. Teaching patients conscious muscle relaxation during which they systematically contract and relax muscle groups throughout the body may decrease pain resulting from muscle tenseness as well as anxiety associated with the pain (see Chapter 10).

Diversionary activities help decrease the patient's perception of the pain by distraction. These activities may be physical (work, walking, rocking, swimming), social, or mental (watching television, reading, crafts). Some patients find imagery (waking-imagined analgesia) helpful. Others may try to separate the pain from their bodies thereby "quieting the mind by letting the body drop away."[38]

☐ Medications

Drugs may be the one significant method that alleviates the pain of cancer. Aspirin is the most effective single analgesic for mild to moderate pain.[28] There is an additive and perhaps synergistic effect between aspirin and codeine; therefore, combinations of these drugs are useful in moderate acute pain and in chronic aching pain.

In severe chronic cancer pain the narcotics, with the exception of codeine and oxycodone, are the most effective. Although there are no significant differences among the various drugs in potency or side effects, there are significant differences in the duration of action. Those with long duration of action are preferred for relief of chronic cancer pain. Tolerance and dependence related to these drugs is less common with cancer pain than when the narcotics are used for acute pain.[28]

There are three important principles in the administration of narcotics. The first is that the optimal dose must be determined, and initial pain control may require seemingly large doses of the narcotics. The second principle is to start with a dose that is too high rather than one that is too low since the person may become anxious if there is no analgesia despite analgesic administration. This anxiety may exacerbate the pain. The third and most important principle is that the narcotic must be *administered regularly*, not prn. Each dose must be given before the previous dose loses effect. Prevention of pain recurrence usually requires less analgesia than treatment of pain after it has recurred.

Oral administration is preferred. Parenteral therapy produces higher initial serum and tissue levels of the narcotic, but the oral doses are as effective as parenteral doses in maintaining drug levels in the body. Intramuscular and subcutaneous injections are more difficult to administer and are painful to patients with marked muscle wasting. In addition, parenteral administration may make the patient dependent on others for drug administration.[62]

Phenothiazines are the principal adjunct drug given to control severe chronic cancer pain. They are effective as antiemetics and also have an antianxiety effect.

Nurses provide the psychologic and social support necessary to help the cancer patient cope with severe pain. Administration of analgesics over the 24-hour period and explanations of the physiologic and pharmacologic effects of the drugs can be very helpful to patients and their families (see Chapter 10).

■ Psychologic support of patient and family

Cancer nursing demands not only caring *for* the patient but also caring *about* the patient, who may be angry, depressed, and perhaps physically unattractive because of the effects of the disease or its treatment. Communication is vital in meeting the needs of the cancer patient and the family. Validating assumptions and assisting patients in describing, clarifying, and identifying reasons for feelings are important to promote communications. In addition, the nurse must try to make explanations clear and uncomplicated. Getting feedback from the patient is one way to ensure that the message has been received.

■ NURSING INTERVENTIONS TO HELP THE PATIENT COPE

Since the threat to life and the potential for other losses are great for patients with cancer, they need especially to have their existing coping mechanisms supported or to receive support if coping mechanisms are inadequate to meet their needs.

Each patient's reaction to cancer is unique, so there can be no easy formula for care. The nurse must be able to work with and accept patients' behavior and coping style. Avoidance of false reassurance and pat answers that block communication will contribute to patient comfort. Openness, honesty, and creativity of the nurse are essential. The nurse reinforces patients' hope but is careful to avoid giving false hope, which can be more devastating than none at all. At times patients may need to deny their illness, while at other times they may want to talk about it.

Trusting patients' resilience and their will to try and helping them live as fully as possible are all appropriate interventions. When patients complain, perhaps the best response is, "Tell me how you feel. Perhaps we can do something about it." Self-esteem is maintained by fostering patients' independence, even if this only involves taking part in decision making about the care to be given.

Persons working with these patients must have confidence in themselves and the ability to suspend their own concerns, needs, and desires to concentrate on patients' problems. To do this one must be able to tolerate a high level of anxiety and to look at problems on both a feeling (affective) and a thinking (cognitive) level.

Listening carefully and attentively to concerns of patients helps to calm fears. In addition, nurses who are knowledgeable about cancer, who can answer questions and clear up misconceptions, help promote the patient's psychologic well-being.

■ NURSING INTERVENTIONS TO HELP THE FAMILY COPE

The interventions that help the patient cope are also important in helping the family cope. The nurse must get to know them and their reactions. They may feel guilty, helpless, and angry, just as the patient does. Letting them know that their feelings are normal may increase their comfort. Families should not be pushed into responsibilities that they cannot handle. Some want to participate in care, others are overwhelmed by the disease and are afraid to or may not want to help. Their feelings need to be respected.

Teaching the family is a major responsibility. They should be reminded not to cut the patient off from family activities and concerns. If possible, the patient should be included in family decision making and planning. In their desire to help their loved ones, families may unintentionally contribute to the patient's sense of isolation by shielding him or her from family concerns.

■ INTERDISCIPLINARY APPROACH TO CARE

The skills of many members of the health team may be required to meet the needs of the cancer patient. Clear, concise communication of ideas about care and the planned interventions is essential for coordination, continuity, and integration of care. Team conferences help establish goals and promote the sharing of expertise. The social worker, occupational therapist, minister, and psychologist may all be needed to contribute to the patient's well-being. The nurse, who spends the most time with the patient, may be the first person to recognize that the patient and family could benefit from the services of health team members.

Rehabilitation of the cancer patient to an optimal level of functioning through the efforts of many health team members results in a more satisfying life for the patient and the family. Often the community health nurse is called on to give care, teach, counsel, and support the patient and family after discharge.

■ Supportive care of the patient with cancer that is terminal

■ PLANNING CARE

When all possible therapies have failed to control the spread of cancer, the patient and family have many special problems. They need encouragement and help in living as normally as possible, in planning for the late stages of the patient's illness, and in adjusting to death and its implications for the family.

Before nurses can help the patient and family, they must have developed a mature philosophy that allows acceptance of death as an eventual reality for everyone. This philosophy is not acquired overnight. The nurse needs the opportunity to discuss feelings about caring for the patient whose death is imminent, since the nurse's attitude toward death and suffering will affect the ability to plan and give care to the patient with advanced cancer. (See Chapter 15 for a discussion of death and dying.)

No one can say with certainty when death will come. The patient may ask about the length of time remaining, but no absolute answer can be given. Physicians may have made a statement to the patient about life expectancy. The nursing staff should know what the patient has been told, since the patient's willingness to participate in self-care and attitude toward the illness may be influenced by perception of life expectancy.

Nursing diagnoses for the patient with cancer that is terminal

Ineffective airway clearance
Constipation
Altered family processes
Fatigue
Fear (specify)
Grieving (specify)
 Anticipatory
 Dysfunctional
Altered nutrition: less than body requirements
Pain
Powerlessness
Bathing/hygiene self-care deficit
Impaired skin integrity
Social isolation
Altered oral mucous membrane

Planning, doing, and achieving are the best way to prevent the hopelessness and despair that may overwhelm the patient. Every effort must be put forth to meet the patient's physiologic needs so that higher order psychologic needs may be expressed. The patient who is in pain or feels "dirty" will probably have difficulty expressing concerns and fears.

Other factors to consider in planning care are the personality of the patient, feelings about death and illness, and the reactions of those significant others whose opinion the patient values. The goal of nursing care should be to relieve physical, mental, and spiritual distress. The most common nursing diagnoses for the patient with cancer that is terminal are listed in the box below.

■ PLANNING FOR HOME CARE

At least half of all deaths from cancer occur in the patients' homes. Planning for home care of the patient without completely disrupting the rest of the family takes the concerted efforts of many people. Patients must always be consulted, and their wishes should be respected in the early stages of the disease. In the final stages they may be too ill to be bothered or concerned with making decisions. The physician, the social worker, and the nurse must work together with the local community agencies, such as the American Cancer Society, to ensure continuity of care from the hospital to the home. The principles governing suitability for home care are similar to those for any patient receiving home care, although the patient with cancer may not live as long as many others with chronic long-term illnesses. Medical and nursing supervision must be available; it must be possible for required care to be given; both patient and family must want the patient home; and home facilities must be suitable. Rehabilitaton teams may also be sent into the home to help the patient and family.

The growth of the *hospice* concept, a place where patients may come for short or long periods for nursing care and then return to their homes as their condition warrants, is exciting. The hospice tries to maintain a homelike setting while relieving the family of the emotional and physical burden of constant care. Hospice programs provide medical, social, and psychologic support for patients and their families so that dying can be truly dignified.

The hospice concept may also be implemented by home care for the patient with the inpatient facility as a backup for home care. If a family wishes to go away on a trip, for example, the patient may request to stay in the hospice. The ultimate goal of the hospice is for the family to develop its ability to give care; thus the relationship of the hospice to the family becomes primarily one of consultation and referral. The family is aided in remaining the patient's primary support system.

Hospice staff are multidisciplinary and are employed and evaluated based on their interests and abilities to care for the terminally ill person. The focus of activities is care rather than cure, with an emphasis on symptom control. Actions are identified to help the patient and family deal with their chief concerns.

■ NURSING INTERVENTION TO MEET PSYCHOLOGIC NEEDS OF PATIENTS WITH ADVANCED STAGES OF CANCER

□ Avoiding false hope

Occasionally, there is a mistake in diagnosis or the disease is in some way arrested for a long time. If the patient assumes that one of these occurrences may take place, the nurse should not suggest facing probable reality. The nurse must, however, avoid encouraging false hopes. Many patients accept their prognosis philosophically, with the hope that a cure for cancer will be found before their disease is far advanced. Some patients are better able to accept the situation if their religious faith can be strengthened. Some patients and their families find it helpful to live each day as fully as possible without looking too far ahead. Sometimes patients with cancer have few symptoms and are able to carry on quite well until shortly before death.

Nurses also must be careful that they do not experience false hope. The inability to fulfill the hope to sustain life may make it more difficult for nurses to accept the patient's death and they may see themselves as having failed.[46]

□ Encouraging social and vocational activities

Patients with advanced cancer should resume their regular work if they can possibly do so, for work makes them feel as though they are still an active part of their group and worthy of the approval of others. It was said many centuries ago that employment is a person's best physician, and this concept applies particularly to persons whose existence is seriously threatened by cancer. Social activities and all experiences associated with normal family life should be continued whenever possible. There is probably no greater service the nurse can give to patients with uncontrollable cancer than to help them continue their everyday lives in any way possible. Family members often need guidance in seeing the patient's need to live as normally as possible. Sometimes the patient appears almost unduly concerned with the details of some aspect of the immediate treatment and almost oblivious to the entire problem. Such a patient senses that success with the immediate treatment is the only way to remain up and about or to carry on at that time.

□ Decreasing fear of helplessness

Patients may be haunted by fear of brain involvement, loss of mental faculties, and the possibility that they may become completely helpless and dependent on others. By these fears they express a basic human wish: the wish to leave the world with as much dignity as possible. The nurse should urge the patient and family to discuss such fears with the physician. The patient may feel that the physician is too busy and that questions are too trivial to justify the use of the physician's time. Some questions, however, are not trivial at all, and a satisfactory answer to them adds tremendously to the patient's peace of mind. Metastasis to the brain in persons who have other metastases is somewhat rare, and some patients suffer more from fear of damage to the brain than is justified. The patient should know that good general hygiene, good nutrition, being up and about for part of each day, and doing deep-breathing exercises with attention to posture all help to prevent helplessness. A positive approach to all problems certainly shortens the time of helplessness and makes the patient more content.

■ NURSING INTERVENTIONS TO MEET PHYSIOLOGIC NEEDS OF PATIENTS WITH ADVANCED STAGES OF CANCER

□ Increasing comfort

Giving good nursing care to the patient with an advanced stage of cancer is challenging. Promoting the patient's comfort should be high on the list of goals. Nursing measures that increase rest and sleep and reduce pain will help maintain the patient's physical and psychologic well-being.

□ Maintaining nutrition

Cachexia is a frequent problem. Anorexia may accompany therapy, and the increased protein needs of the body resulting from tumor growth may be difficult to meet. Mealtimes should be incorporated with family visiting, or patients can eat together if possible. A high-protein diet enhances the response from therapy, and an adequate intake of calories spares protein for cell building. Because chewing may be difficult, food should be cut in small pieces and creamed or combined with cooked vegetables, rice, or noodles. Meat may also be ground or used as a base for soups or stews. Fish, cottage cheese, and eggs are also good sources of protein.

Intravenous hyperalimentation (total parenteral nutrition [TPN]) may be used as an adjunct to therapy. TPN has not been found to stimulate tumor growth and it may result in a return of immune system competence, a decrease in sepsis, wound healing, and an increase in response to chemotherapy.

□ Maintaining elimination

Diarrhea may be a problem, but constipation is more likely. If the patient is receiving narcotics, especially opium derivatives, peristalsis is decreased. Patients receiving the plant alkaloid vincristine (Oncovin) may develop neurotoxicity, causing a high fecal impaction. Increasing the intake of roughage and fluids in the diet, maintaining activity, and using stool softeners may be helpful. Enemas and laxatives may be necessary.

□ Maintaining personal hygiene

Careful and meticulous hygiene is essential. Careful bathing and attention to skin, hair, and clothing will all promote self-esteem in the patient. Odors from body exudates, draining wounds, and incontinence may occur. Soiled dressings and bed linen are changed immediately. Judicious use of deodorizers is helpful, but deodorizers do not take the place of good hygiene.

□ Preventing the effects of immobility

Pressure sores may be a severe problem. The combination of inactivity, poor nutrition, and incontinence seen in patients with advanced cancer predisposes them to skin breakdown. Maintaining the patient's activity by getting him or her out of bed as much as possible will prevent pressure and also promote the patient's joint mobility and muscle strength.

□ Teaching the patient and family

The nurse is involved in teaching during most interactions with the patient and family. Careful explanations about care and sensitivity to what the patient thinks and feels about the disease contribute to the nurse's effectiveness in promoting change in the patient's behavior. When possible, self-care activities should be emphasized. Maintaining the patient's independence whenever possible should be the goal while recognizing that the time may come when dependence is necessary.

⌗ EVALUATION

Because of the diversity and complexity of cancer, evaluation of care is especially dependent on the expected patient outcomes that have been identified. Care is based on the person's level of physical and psychosocial capacities and value systems. General questions that can be asked include the following:

1. Have identified learning needs been met with patient teaching?
2. Have the person and significant others had opportunities to express feelings and concerns?
3. Has the person participated in decision-making as desired?
4. Has hope been maintained, without giving false hope?
5. Is the person as comfortable as possible?
6. Are good ventilation, nutrition, and elimination being maintained?
7. Are usual activities of daily living being carried out, with assistance given as needed?
8. Is the person active within existing limits?

■ SUMMARY

1. The term cancer ... have in common ... more than 200 diseases that do not obey the law ... tion of abnormal cells that
2. Early diagnosis and ne ... al tissue growth. creased the survival rate ... ent advances have increased two persons with cancer ca... day one out of every
3. Malignant cells are characteri... nuclei, increased rates of mitosis, larger irregular appearance, loss of contact inhibition, and increa... ncentration of RNA.
4. Cancer spread occurs by three routes: dire... or invasion, gravitational metastasis or se... tension metastasis via blood or lymph vessels. ..., and
5. The chances of developing cancer increases with each decade after an individual reaches age 60. This may result from an exhaustion of the immune system or from a life-long exposure to environmental carcinogens.
6. Environmental factors, host susceptibility, health practices, and psychosocial factors are all factors that contribute to carcinogenesis.
7. The most common sites of cancer in women are the breast, uterus (cervix), lung, and colorectum.
8. The most common sites of cancer in males are the prostate, lung, and colorectum.
9. Psychologic responses to cancer can range from stoicism to extreme anger. Loneliness, depression, denial, anxiety, and guilt are common reactions.
10. The term paraneoplastic syndrome is used to describe the systemic effects of cancer.
11. Surgery is the oldest treatment for cancer and involves removal of the tumor for cure or palliation.
12. Radiotherapy uses radiation to destroy or delay the growth of the rapidly reproducing malignant cells.
13. Chemotherapeutic drugs bring about changes in the cell cycle phases and interrupt cell growth and replication.
14. Biologic response modifier therapies are therapeutic agents that alter the interaction between the tumor and the host by influencing the host's biologic response to cancer cells.

Putting knowledge to practice

- If you have a family member who has had cancer, did the person know the diagnosis? What were the person's reactions to the illness? What was the family reaction?
- What might be some possible reasons why the person with cancer might hesitate to share the diagnosis with other persons? What effects might withholding this information incur?
- Review the chart of a patient with a diagnosis of cancer. What has been the patient's psychologic response to the illness? What have been the psychologic and physiologic responses to therapy? What measures could be taken to help the patient to cope?
- What resources are available in your community to provide assistance for the person with cancer?

...n by five physiologic
15. Malignant neoplasm: ...struction of lumens, pe-
changes: bone dest...fection and necrosis of tis-
ripheral nerve in... pressure of growing tumors, and infla...ges, 60% of persons with cancer
sue.
16. Even in term... d or no pain.
will experi...

...AND SELECTED READINGS*

Contem...an Cancer Society, 1987, Cancer facts and figures,
1. A...York, 1987, The Society.
2. ...merican Cancer Society: Cancer manual, ed 7, Boston, 1986, The Society.
3. American Cancer Society: Clinical oncology: a multidisciplinary approach, ed 6, New York, 1983, The Society.
4. Baird, SB: Economic realities in the treatment and care of the cancer patient, Top Clin Nurs 2:67-80, 1981.
5. *Bersani, G, and Carl, W: Oral care for cancer patients, Am J Nurs 83:533-536, 1983.
6. *Bjeletich, J, and Hickman, R: The Hickman indwelling catheter, Am J Nurs 80:62-65, 1980.
7. Blumberg, F, Flaherty, M, and Lewis, J: Cancer in the adult. In Coping with cancer, Bethesda, Md, 1980, National Cancer Institute.
8. Bouchard-Kurtz, RE, and Speese-Owens, NF: Nursing care of the cancer patient, ed 4, St. Louis, 1981, The CV Mosby Co.
8a. Bruera, E, and MacDonald, RN: Overwhelming fatigue in advanced cancer, Am J Nurs 88:99-100, 1988.
9. *Bullough, B: Nurses are teachers and support persons for breast cancer patients, Cancer Nurs 4:221-225, 1982.
10. *Carpenito, LJ: Nursing diagnosis: application to clinical practice, ed 2, Philadelphia, 1987, JB Lippincott Co.
10a. Coyle, N: A model of continuity of care for cancer patients with chronic pain, Med Clin North Am 71:259-270, 1987.
11. *Creeland, CS: The impact of pain on the patient with cancer, Cancer 54:2635-2641, 1984.
12. Crowley, M, and Baker, M: Preparing nurses for Hickman catheter care: a self-learning module, Oncol Nurs Forum 7(4):17-19, 1980.
13. *Daeffler, R: Oral hygiene measures for patients with cancer, Cancer Nurs 3:347-355, 1980.
14. DeVita, V Jr, Hellman, S, and Rosenberg, SA: Cancer principles and practice of oncology, ed 2, Philadelphia, 1985, JB Lippincott Co.
15. Drasga, RE, Einhorn, LH, and Williams, SD: The chemotherapy of testicular cancer, CA 32:66-77, 1982.
16. Garfinkel, MA, and Stellman, SD: Cigarette smoking among physicians, dentists, and nurses, CA 36(1):2-8, 1986.
17. *Goodman, SG, and Wickham, R: Venous access devices: an overview, Oncol Nurs Forum 11(5):16-23, 1984.
17a. Groenwald, SL: Cancer nursing: principles and practice, Boston, 1987, Jones & Bartlett, Publishers.
18. *Groer, M, and Pierce, M: Guarding against cancer's hidden killer: anorexia-cachexia, Nurs 81 11(6):39-43, 1981.
19. Guidelines for the cancer-related check-up, CA 30:195-196, 1980.
20. Haskell, C: Cancer treatment, Philadelphia, 1980, WB Saunders Co.
21. *Hogan, R: Human sexuality: a nursing perspective, ed 2, New York, 1985, Appleton-Century-Crofts.
22. Jassak, PF, and Stricklin, LA: Interleukin-2: an overview, Oncol Nurs Forum 13(6):17-22, 1986.
23. Jones, RB, Frank, R, and Mass, T: Safe handling of chemotherapeutic agents, CA 33(5):258-263, 1983.
24. Kaempfle, S: The effects of cancer chemotherapy on reproduction: a review of the literature, Oncol Nurs Forum 8:11-18, 1981.
25. *Kelly, PP, and Tinsley, C: Planning care for the patient receiving external radiation, Am J Nurs 81:338-342, 1981.
26. Kennedy, M, and others: Chemotherapy related nausea and vomiting: a survey to identify problems and interventions, Oncol Nurs Forum 8:19-22, 1981.
27. *Koren, MD: Cancer immunotherapy: what, why, when, how? Nurs 81 11(1):34-41, 1981.
28. Krim, M: Toward tumor therapy with interferons: interferon's production and properties, Blood 55:711-721, 1980.
29. *Kripman, AG: Drug therapy and cancer pain, Cancer Nurs 3:39-46, 1980.
30. LaFortune, S, and Gloriant, FS: Nursing diagnoses in cancer chemotherapy, in theory and practice, A J Nurs 81:2013-2022, 1981.
31. McAdams, CW: Interferon: the penicillin of the future, Am J Nurs, 80:714-718, 1980.
31a. *McGuire, DB: Advances in control of cancer pain, Nurs Clin North Am 22:677-690, 1987.
32. *McIntire, SM, and Cioppa, AL: Cancer nursing: a developmental approach, New York, 1984, John Wiley & Sons.
33. McKhann, C: Cancer immunotherapy: a realistic appraisal, CA 30:286-293, 1980.
33a. *Nieweg, R., and others: A patient education program for a continuous infusion regimen on an outpatient basis, Cancer Nurs 10:177-182, 1987.
34. *Northouse, LL: Living with cancer, Am J Nurs 81:960-962, 1981.
35. Oncology Nursing Society: Cancer chemotherapy guidelines for nursing education and practice, Pittsburgh, 1984, The Society.
36. Porth, C: Pathophysiology: concepts of altered health states, ed. 2, Philadelphia, 1987, JB Lippincott Co.
37. Public attitudes toward cancer and cancer tests, New York, 1980, American Cancer Society.
38. *Rankin, M: The progressive pain of cancer, Top Clin Nurs 2:59-73, 1980.
39. Rosenbaum, EH: Living with cancer, St. Louis, 1982, The CV Mosby Co.
40. Suppers, VJ, and McClamrock, EA: Biologicals in cancer treatment: future effects on nursing practice, Oncol Nurs Forum 12(3):27-32, 1985.
41. *Varricchio, CG: The patient on radiation therapy, Am J Nurs 81:334-337, 1981.
42. Varricchio, CG: Cultural and ethnic dimensions of cancer

---

* References preceded by an asterisk are particularly well suited for student reading.

nursing care: introduction, Oncol Nurs Forum 14(3):57-58, 1987.

43. *Welch, DA: Assessment of nausea and vomiting in cancer patients undergoing external beam radiotherapy, Cancer Nurs 3:365-371, 1980.

Classic

44. American Cancer Society: A cancer source book for nurses, New York, 1975, The Society.
45. Boeker, EH (editor): Symposium on radiation uses and hazards, Nurs Clin North Am 2:1-113, 1967.
46. *Buehler, JA: What contributes to hope in the cancer patient, Am J Nurs 75:1353-1356, 1975.
47. Committee on Professional Education of International Union Against Cancer (editors): Clinical oncology: a manual for students and doctors, New York, 1973, Springer-Verlag.
48. *Donovan, MI, and Pierce, SG: Cancer care nursing, New York, 1976, Appleton-Century-Crofts.
49. Fagin, C, and Dubin, L: Causes of cancer, Cancer Nurs 2:435-441, 1979.
50. Fisher, B, and others: Ten year follow-up of patients with carcinoma of the breast, Surg Gynecol Obstet 140:528-534, 1975.
51. George, MM: Long-term care of the patient with cancer, Nurs Clin North Am 8:623-631, 1973.
52. Golden, S, and others: Chemotherapy and you: a guide to self-help during treatment, NIH pub. no. 80-1136, Washington, DC, 1978, National Institute of Health.
53. Herman, CS: Immunology: the method to our madness, Cancer Nurs 2:359-363, 1979.
54. Higginson, J, Terracini, B, and Agthe, C: Nutrition and cancer: ingestion of foodborne carcinogens. In Schottenfeld, D (editor): Cancer epidemiology and prevention, Springfield, Ill, 1975, Charles C Thomas, Publisher.
55. Horton, J, and Hill, GJ: Clinical oncology, Philadelphia, 1977, WB Saunders Co.
56. Knopf, M, and others: Cancer chemotherapy treatment and care, New Haven, Conn, 1979, Yale Comprehensive Cancer Center.
57. Krakoff, T: Cancer chemotherapeutic agents, New York, 1977, American Cancer Society.
58. Lippsett, MB: Interaction of drugs, hormones, and nutrition in the causes of cancer. In Proceedings of the American Cancer Society and National Cancer Institute's National Conference on Nutrition in Cancer, New York, 1979, American Cancer Society.
59. Lynch, HT, and others: Hereditary cancer: ascertainment and management, CA 29:2116-229, 1979.
60. *McGuire, DB: Familial cancer and the role of the nurse, Cancer Nurs 2:443-451, 1979.
61. McKhann, C, and Yarlott, MA: Tumor immunology, CA 25:187-197, 1975.
62. Pitot, HJC: Fundamentals of oncology, New York, 1978, Marcel Dekker, Inc.
63. Rosai, J, and Ackerman, LV: The pathology of tumors: precancerous and pseudomalignant lesions, CA 28:331-342, 1978.
64. Schottenfeld, D, and Haas, JF: Carcinogens in the workplace, CA 29:173-183, 1977.
65. *Schreier, AM, and Lavenia, J: The nurse's role in nutritional management of radiotherapy patients, Nurs Clin North Am 12:173-183, 1977.
66. Silverstein, MJ, and Morton, DL: Cancer immunotherapy, Am J Nurs 73:1178-1181, 1973.
67. Sontag, S: Illness as a metaphor, New York, 1977, Farrar, Straus and Giroux, Inc.
68. Winters, WD, and Morton, DL: Immunobiology. In Schottenfeld, D (editor): Cancer epidemiology and prevention, Springfield, Ill, 1975, Charles C Thomas, Publisher.

13

Substance Abuse

ELIZABETH SCHENK

CHAPTER OBJECTIVES

After studying this chapter, the student should be able to:

- Name four negative compulsions that are considered addictions.
- Define the difference between tolerance (behavioral, pharmacologic, and cross tolerance) and dependence (physical, psychologic, and cross dependence).
- Name one legal effort and one educational effort to prevent alcoholism and chemical dependency.
- Define the term *enabling* and term *intervention*.
- State two theories of the development of alcoholism.
- Name five disorders directly associated with alcoholism.
- Discuss alcohol withdrawal, including delirium tremens, and actions taken to prevent or reduce withdrawal.
- Define drug addiction and drug habituation.
- Name the six basic types of drugs, citing examples, how they are used, street names, effects and side effects, pathophysiology, and symptoms of overdose.
- Discuss why nurses are at increased risk for chemical dependency.

Terms used to describe responses to drugs/alcohol

Tolerance	Decreased susceptibility to effects because of long-term ingestion of drugs/alcohol
Behavioral tolerance	Few changes in social behavior or activities despite ingestion of large amounts of drugs alcohol
Pharmacologic tolerance	Adaptive metabolic changes that occur despite ingestion of large amounts of drugs/alcohol
Cross tolerance	Decreased sensitivity to other drugs as a result of tolerance to drugs/alcohol
Dependence	Need to continue use of drugs/alcohol to prevent symptoms
Physical dependence	Withdrawal symptoms occur when the drugs/alcohol are withheld
Psychologic dependence	Need to take the drugs/alcohol to prevent occurrence of symptoms
Cross dependence	Suppression of abstinence symptoms by withdrawal of another drug

---

The area of *substance abuse* is gaining increased attention as more and more nurses are working in this specialty. It is commonly accepted that substance abuse includes a complex set of behaviors that are covered under the term *addiction*. These addictions include *alcoholism, drug addiction, overeating, compulsive gambling,* and other negative compulsions. It is possible and likely that persons will have one or more of these addictions at the same time. An example is the alcoholic who is also a drug addict and a compulsive overeater. Only alcoholism and drug addiction will be discussed in this chapter.

Alcoholism and drug addiction are commonly referred to as *chemical dependency.* This is in recognition of the fact that alcohol is a drug and that the person addicted to alcohol is also at great risk for drug addiction.

Dependency includes both *physical* and *psychologic dependency.* Terms used to describe responses to drugs and alcohol are listed in the box above.

■ PREVENTION AND HEALTH EDUCATION

Problems that occur as a result of substance abuse can have devastating results. These results have an impact on almost every body system and produce changes that are *chronic* and *debilitating.*

■ Primary prevention: prevention of disease

Although the cause of substance abuse is not clearly defined, efforts to prevent its occurrence have been made on several fronts. These include the following:
1. Legal
   a. Efforts to restrict sale of alcohol to minors
   b. Stringent legal consequences for use of drugs
   c. Strict DWI laws and serious consequences for driving while intoxicated

2. Education
   a. Teaching young children about the dangers of alcohol use and abuse
   b. Working to increase self-esteem of children so that they can better withstand peer pressure
   c. Educating family members and employers to assist the alcoholic or drug addict into treatment and to stop enabling behavior

Alcoholics are usually surrounded by persons who *enable* them to use and abuse. An example of this is the spouse who calls in to work for the sick mate and tells the employer that the mate is sick with the flu, when in reality the person has a hangover. Without this *enabling behavior,* the alcoholic is often forced to seek help sooner.

■ Secondary prevention: early detection

Early diagnosis and treatment of substance abuse can be important in assisting abusers to once again become a productive member of society and save themselves and others from expense and heartache.

Some still believe that it is only when the alcoholic desires and seeks help with his or her alcohol problem that treatment can be effective. Unfortunately, often by the time an alcoholic seeks help, many things have been lost. Recently the emphasis has been on the use of a process called *intervention* to assist the alcoholic in receiving help. This is sometimes called *raising the bottom.*

Interventions are *planned confrontations* by individuals who care about the person. Rules for intervention include the following[26]:
1. Meaningful persons present facts or data. The employer of the person can often be a very meaningful participant.
2. The data presented are specific and descriptive of events that have happened or conditions that exist.
3. The tone of the confrontation is nonjudgmental.
4. The chief evidence should be tied into alcohol or drug use.

5. The evidence of behaviors is presented in detail and should be explicit.
6. The goal of the intervention is to have the alcoholic see and accept reality so that the need for help is accepted.
7. The choices available for treatment should be offered. If possible, immediate help should be available.

It is often difficult to make the diagnosis of alcoholism or drug abuse without objective evidence. Some indications of problems include the following:

1. Frequent illnesses and related illnesses
2. Undue preoccupation with the intake of drugs or alcohol
3. Mood swings
4. Violent or acting-out behavior
5. Denial about the use of substances
6. Financial difficulties
7. Loss of control over use
8. Use of alcohol or drugs in such a way as to endanger physical health, interpersonal relationships, and/or economic functioning
9. Use of substance as universal answer to all problems
10. Loss of ability to express feelings
11. Use of defense mechanisms, including a strong denial of the problem that drugs or alcohol is causing

■ Tertiary prevention: prevention of complications

It is important to consider tertiary prevention for the patient with substance abuse. These complications occur not only because of the effects of the substance itself, but also because of the nutritional deficits that usually accompany the problem. These problems include *infections, neuropathy,* and *myopathies.* Complications for persons with drug addictions often occur as a result of acquired disease from dirty needles or equipment. These complications will be discussed later in this chapter.

Many patients with substance abuse will have to deal with these complications long after they have stopped the use of the substance.

■ ALCOHOLISM

Alcoholism is very common and may complicate the problems of persons with other health problems. It is recognized today as a treatable disease.

Alcoholism is the third major health problem in the United States.[21] Conservative estimates are that at least 90 million persons use alcohol and that at least 10% of them are alcoholics or *"problem drinkers."* In addition, alcohol negatively affects the health or functioning of another 30 million persons. It has been estimated that 70% of alcoholics are male, but the number of females who are alcoholic is increasing.[34] Women are more likely to hide their problem and are not as likely to be detected. Also, drinking has increased at an alarming rate among adolescents.

Of all deaths in the United States, 10% are alcohol related, as are 80% of all suicides. From 25% to 35% of all patients in the medical-surgical units of general hospitals are suffering from alcohol-related problems. Industries are estimated to lose at least $10 billion yearly because of alcoholism. This figure includes the cost of time lost from work, misjudgments, spoiled materials, and broken machines.

The use of alcohol predates recorded history. It has been used in rites of passage, to celebrate significant events, and to mourn the dead. Alcohol has also been used as magic, as a medicine, and as a part of worship services.

There have been many changes in attitudes and laws about the use of alcoholic beverages in the United States. In 1642 Maryland made drunkenness punishable by a fine. In 1790 the U.S. government passed a law that gave every soldier a daily portion of hard liquor. In 1919 a law was passed that prohibited the production and sale of alcoholic beverages in the United States. This period of *Prohibition* was repealed in 1933.[34]

Numerous theories have been suggested to explain the cause of alcoholism.[34] These theories have been divided into three main categories that include the following:

1. Physiologic theories
   a. Genetotropic-etiologic: related to genetically determined biochemical defect
   b. Endocrine-etiologic: caused by dysfunction of endocrine system
   c. Genetic: alcoholism in part genetically determined (risk of sons of alcoholic men developing alcoholism over their lifetime is 30% to 50%). Identical twins of an alcoholic parent will be alcoholic in 60% of cases)[52]
2. Psychologic theories
   a. Oral fixation: resulting from lack of a warm, loving relationship with a mother figure as a child
   b. Behavioral learning theory: association of alcohol ingestion with positive experience leads to alcoholism
3. Sociocultural or cultural-etiologic theories
   a. Cultural: relationship between various groups in society and incidence of alcoholism (Jews, Mormons, and Moslems have low rate, whereas Frenchmen have high rate)
   b. Moral etiologic: alcoholism a moral fault or sin of alcoholic

Research is on-going to determine the causes of alcoholism. Thus far, no one theory can completely explain the syndrome. It is apparent, however, that alcoholics share common personality characteristics that usually include dependency, denial, and delusion. Also, alcoholism does tend to occur in families. It is likely that the root of alcoholism is multicausal.

■ Pathophysiology

Alcohol abuse can become a problem over a variable period of time. Some persons can drink large amounts for years without becoming alcoholic, whereas other persons

---

Disorders associated with alcoholism

Hepatic	Alcoholic hepatitis, Laennec's cirrhosis, fatty liver
Gastrointestinal	Gastritis, pancreatitis, duodenal ulcers, malabsorption syndromes, cancer of mouth and esophagus
Neurologic	Peripheral neuropathy, Wernicke-Korsakoff's syndrome, organic brain disease
Cardiovascular, hematologic	Cardiomyopathy, hypertension, familial type-IV hyperlipidemia, hypoglycemia, anemia, hyperuricemia, coronary artery disease, congestive heart failure
Musculoskeletal	Skeletal myopathies
Immunologic	Increased susceptibility to infections

---

become alcoholic after just a short period of heavy drinking. The alcoholic begins to develop an increasing physical dependence on and tolerance for alcohol. The drinking becomes uncontrollable and secretive. *Blackouts* (loss of memory from episodes of drinking) may start to occur. Feelings of guilt, shame, and remorse may occur, and the alcoholic drinks more to relieve these feelings. The person *drinks to live and lives to drink.*

Alcohol is a central nervous system (CNS) *depressant.* It affects the brain by suppressing the activity of the neurotransmitter gamma aminobutyric acid (GABA), an inhibitory neurotransmitter. The so-called stimulating effects of alcohol occur because the first areas affected by the suppression of GABA are the higher centers of the brain governing self-control and judgment, which are inhibitory functions. Slowing the release of GABA to those areas results in a seemingly "stimulating" effect. As alcohol continues to accumulate in the brain, areas of the limbic system and brainstem become inhibited. Unconsciousness may set in and the brain can become so overwhelmed by alcohol that it can stop functioning. Other organ systems are also affected. (See the box above.)

The active ingredient in alcoholic beverages is *ethyl alcohol* or *ethanol.* Most American beers contain 3% to 6% alcohol, wine 2% to 21% alcohol, and hard liquors 40% to 50% alcohol. A 12-ounce bottle of beer, a 4-ounce glass of wine, and 1½ ounces of hard liquor contain similar amounts of alcohol.

Alcohol is absorbed in both the stomach and intestine. It does not require digestion. Absorption is hastened by increased alcohol concentrations and an empty stomach. After absorption, alcohol is distributed equally throughout the body, passing across cell membranes. Between 2% and 10% of the alcohol will be lost through the lungs through breathing. Some is also lost in the urine. About 90%,

however, is broken down by a metabolic process that occurs primarily in the liver. This accounts for the high level of liver damage in persons who are alcoholic.

Alcohol has a diuretic effect, caused partly by the increased amounts of fluid ingested. Increased amounts of electrolytes, especially potassium, magnesium, and zinc, may be excreted in the urine of a heavy drinker. Also, continued use of alcohol has a toxic effect on the intestinal mucosa; this results in decreased absorption of thiamine, folic acid, and vitamin B_{12}.

Because alcohol is not converted to glycogen, it cannot be stored and provides 200 kcal per ounce but no minerals or vitamins. These *empty calories* can add weight to a person who, at the same time, is suffering from malnutrition. See Fig. 13-1.

The amount of alcohol in the blood at any one time is called the *blood alcohol level.* This level depends on the amount ingested and the size of the individual. Most laws designate blood alcohol levels of 100 mg/100 ml (0.10%) as the legal limit for intoxication. Increasing blood alcohol levels have increasingly more serious side effects (Table 13-1).

■ FETAL ALCOHOL PROBLEMS

Fetal alcohol problems occur in newborns whose mothers drank during pregnancy. These women have a higher incidence of infants with birth defects and an increase in spontaneous abortions, stillbirths, and infant deaths. Even moderate drinking can result in the birth of children with significant lags in mental and motor development.[22]

The actual *fetal alcohol syndrome* occurs in children whose mothers drank several times daily. The syndrome can include the following:

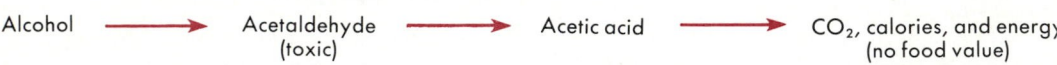

Alcohol ⟶ Acetaldehyde (toxic) ⟶ Acetic acid ⟶ CO_2, calories, and energy (no food value)

Fig. 13-1   Metabolism of alcohol.

Table 13-1 Effects of blood alcohol levels on average-sized nontolerant adult

Blood alcohol levels (per 100 ml of blood)	Effects
50-75 mg	Pleasant, relaxed state, mild sedation, loosening of inhibitions
100-200 mg	Overt signs of intoxication: loosening of tongue, clumsiness, beginning emotional changes
200-400 mg	Severe intoxication: difficulty speaking, stumbling, emotional lability
400-500 mg	Stupor, coma
Over 500 mg	Usually fatal

Symptoms of delirium tremens (DTs)

Increased phsychomotor activity and tremulousness

Confusion and disorientation

Fearfulness

Signs of vasomotor lability

Tachycardia

Temperature elevations (100° to 105° F)

Delusions and hallucinations (visual and tactile, including terrifying animal images and crawling skin sensations)

---

1. Mental retardation
2. Microcephaly
3. Growth deficiencies
4. Malformations of skeletal and urogenital systems

■ ALCOHOL WITHDRAWAL

With sustained drinking, a physiologic dependence on alcohol and increasing tolerance occurs. When the alcohol is unavailable, the person suffers *withdrawal*. Symptoms range from *mild tremors* to *severe agitation* and *hallucinations*. The type and severity of symptoms depends on several factors. Alcoholics at high risk include the following:
1. Older persons
2. Persons who have had previous delirium tremens (DTs) or seizures
3. Persons with coexisting acute illnesses
4. Persons with nutritional deficiencies

See the box below for symptoms of the alcohol withdrawal syndrome.[22]

□ Tremors

The tremors associated with alcohol withdrawal usually are observed 6 to 48 hours after withdrawal from alcohol.

Symptoms of alcohol withdrawal syndrome

Diaphoresis, tachycardia, and elevated blood pressure

Tremors

Nausea or vomiting

Anorexia

Restlessness

Hallucinations

Convulsions

Delirium tremens

They may persist from 3 to 5 days. The hands are involved first, but the temors may become generalized with involvement of the extremities, tongue, and trunk.

□ Seizure disorders

Seizures usually occur from 12 to 24 hours after the last drink. Usually these are *grand mal* seizures and are not preceded by an aura. They are followed by a postictal period, however.

□ Delirium tremens

Delirium tremens, or DTs, is an *acute complication* of alcohol withdrawal that is a serious medical concern. It is a pathologic state of consciousness that results from interference with brain metabolism. DTs that are treated have a 5% mortality rate, whereas untreated ones have a 15% mortality rate. Signs of impending alcohol withdrawal include *restlessness and irritability, headache, nausea, insomnia,* and *nightmares*. Before the onset of full-blown DTs, withdrawal signs may include *visual and tactile hallucinations* that are followed by *seizures*.

The onset of DTs is often sudden and dramatic. It usually occurs 3 to 4 days after the last drink. The condition lasts from 2 to 3 days to a week, but at times it can last 4 to 5 weeks. It may follow injury, infectious disease, anesthesia, or surgery and may develop in patients who have not revealed their alcoholic status to the physician.[22] See the box above for symptoms of DTs.

■ WERNICKE-KORSAKOFF'S SYNDROME

At one time Wernicke-Korsakoff's syndrome was felt to be the result of the neurotoxic results of long-term alcohol use. It is now known, however, that nutritional deficiency is the causative factor. The specific nutritional deficiency in most of the cases is thiamine.

Symptoms present with this syndrome include ocular disturbances, which may include nystagmus and a paralysis of the lateral rectus muscle of the eye. Ataxia may be present, along with symptoms of disturbed mental functioning. The latter can include symptoms of delirium tremens as well as apathy, listnessness, psychosis, and severe confusion. Other problems associated with Korsakoff's psychosis are often seen; these include a problem with memory and confusion.

With this syndrome, the patient may recover from the initial illness, but amnestic psychosis continues. The patient may very well be left with a serious residual mental illness that will require close supervision and intensive care.

Assessment

■ SUBJECTIVE DATA

1. Normal using or drinking patterns
2. Date and time of last drink or use
3. Substances used
4. Quantity used
5. Past history of blackouts, tremors, hallucinations, or DTs
6. Past periods of abstinence
7. Normal dietary patterns
8. Any legal problems
9. Any family problems
10. Any occupational problems
11. Family history of alcoholism
12. Other medications used

It is important to realize that the two cardinal symptoms of untreated alcoholism are *denial and delusion*. As a result, the information gathered from the patient may not always be accurate, and it is helpful to validate it with a family member of significant other.[52]

■ OBJECTIVE DATA

1. Abnormal response to preoperative medication, anesthetics, or sedatives
2. Presence of tremor (usually worse in the morning)
3. Morning nausea
4. Abnormal laboratory studies
5. Presence of pellagra—redness, dryness, scaling, and edema of skin
6. Body weight in relation to height
7. Mental functioning
8. Memory loss
9. General behavior
10. Vital signs (especially tachycardia or hypertension)
11. Presence of ascites
12. Positive blood alcohol or urine alcohol level
13. Petechiae
14. Presence of polyneuropathy

■ CRITERIA SYSTEM

The National Council on Alcoholism divides alcoholism into a *major and minor criteria system* and outlines the development of alcoholism on two tracks as follows.[49]

□ Major criteria

Track I
Physiologic
1. Withdrawal syndrome
2. Tolerance
3. Blackout periods
Clinical
1. Alcoholic hepatitis
2. Laennec's cirrhosis
3. Wernicke-Korsakoff syndrome
Track II
Behavioral, psychologic, attitudinal
1. Drinking despite medical contraindications
2. Drinking despite social contraindications
3. Subjective complaint of loss of control

□ Minor criteria

Track I
Physiologic and clinical
1. Odor of alcohol on breath
2. Alcohol facies
3. Abnormal liver function test
4. Blood-alcohol level over 300 mg/100 ml at any time
Track II
Behavioral
1. Gulping drinks
2. Morning drinking
3. Missing work
4. Frequent automobile accidents
Psychologic and attitudinal
1. Frequent talk about drinking
2. Drinking to release stress
3. Spouse complains about drinking
4. Family disruption

■ DIAGNOSTIC TESTS

Routine blood tests will often reveal abnormalities that are directly related to alcoholism. These include elevated liver enzymes (serum glutamic-oxaloacetic transaminase [SGOT], serum glutamic pyruvic transaminase [SGPT], alkaline phosphatase, and bilirubin). Hypoglycemia may also be present if glycogen stores have been depleted. In addition, hypoalbuminemia and hyperglobulinemia are present in patients with cirrhosis of the liver. Magnesium is often decreased in persons who are alcoholic, usually because of poor dietary intake. It is not uncommon to find anemia and other indications of poor nutrition in alcoholic patients. Patients may have an increased mean corpuscle volume (MCV) when the complete blood count is done. This and an elevated gamma glutamyl transferase (GGT) are strong indicators of a possible diagnosis of alcoholism.

Other diagnostic tests will demonstrate the concomitant diseases that usually accompany alcoholism.

Data analysis: nursing diagnoses

Nursing diagnoses are determined from assessment of patient data. Possible nursing diagnoses for the person

Text continued on p. 272.

NURSING CARE PLAN

Person with substance abuse

DATA: Jane Thomas is a 50-year-old secretary who was admitted to the emergency room after having been found lying in the snow. She was disoriented and had the smell of alcohol on her breath. Her blood alcohol level was 0.23. Her temperature was 97.4° and the respiratory rate was 10. Blood pressure was 90/56 and her pulse was 50. Physical examination showed an enlarged liver, as well as petechiae over parts of her body. She had dry skin in general. Laboratory studies showed low hemoglobin and hematocrit levels, a low RBC count, and elevated liver function test results. X-ray films showed two broken ribs. The urine screen was positive for Valium. The patient was started on Librium 25 to 50 mg q4h. She was admitted for observation and detoxification.

Because of her intoxicated state, it was difficult to obtain a nursing history. Her husband stated that she drank at least a pint of gin per day. In addition she was taking Valium that had been prescribed by her family doctor. Her husband stated that she hadn't been eating well for several months. He wasn't sure when the drinking started, but knew it had been going on for several years.

Collaborative nursing actions include those to prevent further complications caused by possible aspiration or alcohol withdrawal. Immediate reporting of signs and symptoms may prevent serious effects. Nursing actions include monitoring for the following:

1. Signs of respiratory difficulty caused by secretions or alcohol effects: slower, shallower breathing; inability to rouse; aspiration of vomitus.
2. Signs of alcohol withdrawal: diaphoresis, tachycardia, hypertension, tremors, nausea or vomiting, restlessness, or hallucinations
3. Seizures: presence of abnormal muscle movement without aura
4. Signs of delirium tremens: visual and tactile hallucinations, nightmares, insomnia, extreme restlessness or irritability

Nursing diagnosis: Ineffective airway clearance: related to tracheobronchial secretions and cognitive impairment

Expected patient outcomes	Nursing interventions	Rationale
Patient will maintain adequate airway	Observe patient careully for aspiration	Aspiration may occur because of nausea and impaired mental status
	Have suction machine at bedside	Suction may be needed to clear airway
	Keep head of bed at 30 degrees	Position will help respiratory effort

Nursing diagnosis: Ineffective breathing pattern: related to cognitive impairment from effects of alcohol

Expected patient outcomes	Nursing interventions	Rationale
Patient will maintain adequate breathing pattern	Assess respiratory rate at regular intervals	Effects of alcohol can cause respiratory depression
	Give no medications that would further compromise respirations (such as morphine)	Some medications potentiate the effects of alcohol

Nursing diagnosis: Potential fluid volume deficit: due to decreased access to fluids and diuretic effect of alcohol

Expected patient outcomes	Nursing interventions	Rationale
Patient's fluid volume will be maintained at optimal level	Keep accurate intake and output records	Comparing of intake vs output will give indication of fluid volume
	When patient more alert, offer fluids, including juices	Extra fluid will help correct fluid deficit
	Use intravenous fluids as ordered	IVs may be necessary in the presence of nausea or vomiting

Continued.

Person with substance abuse—cont'd

Nursing diagnosis: Hypothermia: related to malnutrition and alcohol ingestion, as well as time spent in snow

Expected patient outcomes	Nursing interventions	Rationale
Patient's temperature will be within normal limits	Monitor patient's temperature frequently	Temperature should increase gradually
	Check extremities for signs of frostbite	Decreased body temperature and time in snow may have caused decreased blood supply to the area
	Use extra blankets on bed to help patient warm to normal temperature	Use of blankets should be adequate to assist in warming patient

Nursing diagnosis: Potential for infection: due to decreased nutrition and fractured ribs

Expected patient outcomes	Nursing interventions	Rationale
Patient will not develop atelectasis	Encourage coughing and deep breathing q4h	Patient may be reluctant to breathe deeply because of fractured ribs
	Assist patient in changing position q2-3h	Changing position will assist with lung expansion

Nursing diagnosis: Potential for injury: trauma, related to lack of awareness of environmental hazards

Expected patient outcomes	Nursing interventions	Rationale
Patient will be free of injury from withdrawal from alcohol	Give Librium as ordered to prevent withdrawal symptoms	Most alcoholic patients require use of medication
	Orient patient frequently to place and time	Patient may be confused
	Keep bed side rails up	Used to prevent falling from bed
	Observe for signs of delirium tremens or seizures	Patient may need more aggressive medical treatment
	Give multivitamins, including B vitamins and thiamine as ordered	B vitamins and thiamine needed to prevent or decrease complications such as Wernicke-Korsakoff syndrome

Nursing diagnosis: Altered nutrition: less than body requirements, due to anorexia and disinterest in eating

Expected patient outcomes	Nursing interventions	Rationale
Patient's nutritional status is improved	Encourage snacks	Patient may not be able to tolerate large meals because of nausea or gastritis
	Encourage well-balanced meals	Good nutrition is important in preventing long term complicaitons from alcoholism
	Consult with dietician about need for special diet	Abnormal liver function studies may necessitate protein restriction

Mrs. Thomas is successfully detoxified from alcohol using Librium over the next 3 days. She is persuaded to accept treatment and is transferred to a nearby treatment facility. At this time additional nursing diagnoses are evident. These include the following (pp. 271-272).

NURSING CARE PLAN

Person with substance abuse—cont'd

Nursing diagnosis: Impaired adjustment: related to disability requiring change in life-style and altered locus of control

Expected patient outcomes	Nursing interventions	Rationale
Patient will make positive adjustment to disease concept	Educate patient about disease concept of alcoholism	Education will help with adjustment
	Encourage patient to share experiences with other patients in group and informally	Peer support will assist with adjustment
	Encourage patient to complete assignments directed at breaking down denial	Self-knowledge will assist in adjustment
	Have patient attend AA meetings	Necessary for long-term adjustment

Nursing diagnosis: Anxiety: related to situational crisis

Expected patient outcomes	Nursing interventions	Rationale
Patient will demonstrate minimal anxiety	Encourage patient to share feelings and concerns	Sharing feelings will ease anxiety
	Educate patient about importance of not taking medications to ease anxiety	Patient will not be able to medicate feelings
	Teach patient relaxation exercises	Will ease anxiety
	Have patient keep feelings log	Will help patient identify sources of anxiety
	Educate patient on 12 steps of AA	Turning life and will over to higher power will lessen anxiety

Nursing diagnosis: Altered family processes: related to situational crisis

Expected patient outcomes	Nursing interventions	Rationale
Patient's family will demonstrate positive family processes	Encourage patient's family to attend family program	Knowledge of disease will assist family to recover
	Encourage patient to keep in contact with family	Their support of patient is important to her recovery

Nursing diagnosis: Knowledge deficit (alcoholism) related to lack of exposure and lack of interest in learning

Expected patient outcomes	Nursing interventions	Rationale
Patient will verbalize understanding of alcoholism	Teach patient about disease concept of alcoholism	Well-informed patient will be better able to stay sober
Patient will verbalize understanding of need to abstain from alcohol and mood-altering drugs	Teach patient about drugs to avoid	See above
Patient will verbalize knowledge of complications of substance abuse	Teach patient about complications	See above
Patient will verbalize knowledge of importance of good nutrition	Teach patient about optimal nutrition	Good nutrition is important to prevent complications of alcoholism
Patient will verbalize knowledge of relaxation techniques	Teach patient about ways to reduce stress	Patient will no longer be able to medicate stress
Patient will verbalize knowledge of importance of aftercare, including AA	Teach patient about importance of aftercare	Aftercare has been found to be essential for continued sobriety

Continued.

NURSING CARE PLAN

Person with substance abuse—cont'd

Nursing diagnosis: Powerlessness: due to alcoholism

Expected patient outcomes	Nursing interventions	Rationale
Patient will verbalize knowledge of powerlessness	Assist patient in learning about and taking first step in AA	First step of AA involves admitting powerlessness Recognition of powerlessness is important for continued recovery

Nursing diagnosis: Self-esteem disturbance: related to change in life-style

Expected patient outcomes	Nursing interventions	Rationale
Patient will verbalize positive self-concept	Give patient positive reinforcement of work and breakthroughs	Will assist in building self-esteem
	Demonstrate to patient that she is not unique	Alcoholics tend to think they are unique
	Encourage patient to share with other alcoholics	They will be support to her

Nursing diagnosis: Spiritual distress: related to separation from religious/cultural ties

Expected patient outcomes	Nursing interventions	Rationale
Patient will verbalize less spiritual distress	Encourage patient to learn about 12 steps of AA	12 steps of AA will assist patient in regaining sense of spirituality
	Ask chaplain to see patient if she wishes	Source of support
	Encourage patient to talk about prayers at AA meetings	This may surprise patients at first
	Encourage patient to talk about difference between spirituality and religion	Many patients may be turned off by formal religion

with alcoholism may include but are not limited to the following:

Diagnostic title	Possible etiologies
Activity intolerance	Generalized weakness
Ineffective airway clearance	Fatigue, tracheobronchial obstruction
Anxiety	Change in health status/role functioning
Body image disturbance	Loss of body functions, change in life-style
Ineffective family coping: disabling	Maladaptive coping styles
Ineffective individual coping	Maturational crises
Altered family process	Situational crisis
Bowel incontinence	Neuromuscular impairment

Diagnostic title	Possible etiologies
Fluid volume deficit (1)	Decreased fluid intake, abnormal fluid loss
Altered health maintenance	Lack of ability to make deliberate judgments
Ineffective home maintenance management	Individual disease, insufficient family resources
Hypothermia	Malnutrition
Total incontinence	Neurologic dysfunction
Potential for infection	Decreased nutrition, decreased immune response
Potential for injury	Sensory deficits, lack of awareness of environmental hazards
Knowledge deficit	Lack of exposure/recall, cognitive limitation

Diagnostic title	Possible etiologies
Impaired physical mobility	Decreased strength and endurance, perceptual/cognitive impairment
Noncompliance (specify)	Alcoholic life patterns
Altered nutrition: less than body requirements	Anorexia, inability to obtain food
Pain	Alcohol withdrawal
Powerlessness	Alcoholism, drug addiction
Feeding, bathing/hygiene, dressing/grooming, toileting self-care deficit	Intolerance to activity/fatigue, perceptual/cognitive impairment
Self-esteem disturbance	Inability to hold job, do necessary tasks, altered thought processes
Sensory/perceptual alterations: visual, auditory, tactile	Altered sensory reception/transmission, integration
Impaired skin integrity	Hypothermia, mechanical forces, immobility
Sleep pattern disturbance	Pain/discomfort
Impaired social interaction	Self-concept disturbance, altered thought processes
Social isolation	Unacceptable social behaviors
Spiritual distress	Separation from religious/cultural ties
Altered thought processes	Neurologic disorders
Altered cerebral tissue perfusion	Decreased cerebral blood flow
Altered patterns of urinary elimination	Sensorimotor impairment, urinary infection
Potential for violence: self-directed or directed at others	Inability to control behavior, toxic reactions to medications

Planning: expected patient outcomes

Expected patient outcomes for the patient with alcoholism may include, but are not limited to, the following:
1. Patient maintains optimal levels of anxiety.
2. Patient demonstrates minimal anxiety.
3. Patient maintains a normal body temperature.
4. Patient is continent of bowel and bladder.
5. Patient has minimal complications from incontinence.
6. Patient has minimal discomfort.
7. Patient maintains a patent airway.
8. Patient maintains adequate hydration.
9. Patient states plans to stop drinking or using drugs.
10. Patient demonstrates the ability to maintain abstinence at home.
11. Patient remains free of infection.
12. Patient does not experience injury.
13. Patient has optimal mobility.
14. Patient maintains optimal nutrition.
15. Patient has minimal deficits in ADL.
16. Patient verbalizes an improved self-concept.
17. Patient does not have sensory-perceptual alterations.
18. Patient demonstrates minimal complications as a result of sensory-perceptual alterations.
19. Patient maintains intactness of skin.
20. Patient maintains normal sleep pattern.
21. Patient demonstrates improved social interactions.
22. Patient maintains a support system.
23. Patient has decreased spiritual distress.
24. Patient maintains cerebral perfusion.
25. Patient does not demonstrate violent behavior.
26. Patient verbalizes powerlessness over drugs or alcohol.
27. Patient and family demonstrate improved and effective coping mechanisms.
28. Patient and family verbalize knowledge of disease and treatment.

Implementation

ASSISTING WITH THE ACHIEVEMENT OF THERAPEUTIC GOALS

Management of acute withdrawal

Care for the alcoholic patient in the acute phase usually involves *detoxification efforts* to prevent acute *withdrawal*. Detoxification is undertaken in a controlled environment where the patient can be monitored and complications prevented, as possible.

Medications

Medication used in the initial period of detoxification includes chlordiazepoxide (Librium) or a similar drug. The drug is used in decreasing doses for its sedating and anticonvulsant effect during detoxification. The dosage can be as great as 50 mg every 3 hours in the first 24 hours. Anticonvulsant therapy that includes phenytoin (Dilantin), as well as magnesium sulfate (2 ml of a 50% solution every 8 to 12 hours for several doses) are also used. Dilantin is likely to be continued past the initial period of detoxification if the patient has a history of seizures.

Because of the nutritional problems common with the disease of alcoholism, multivitamin supplements are usually prescribed. These include thiamine combined with other B-complex vitamins.

Specific medications may differ from setting to setting. In some settings alcohol will still be used to accomplish detoxification. Whatever the medication used, it is wise to remember that many alcoholics need to receive medication, sometimes in large doses, to safely withdraw from alcohol.[40] There is no reason for the alcoholic to suffer because health professionals believe that they deserve to feel some pain. Unfortunately, these beliefs sometimes still exist.

Delirium tremens

Treatment of delirium tremens (DTs) consists of the use of tranquilizing drugs such as chlordiazepoxide (Librium) or diazepam (Valium) and sedatives such as paraldehyde given rectally, intramuscularly, or orally. High-calorie and high-vitamin diets may have to be given by nasogastric tube. The patient needs to be protected from physical injury and observed carefully for signs of cardiac failure. Restraints, including leather restraints, may have to be used, but, if at all possible, they should be avoided because they increase agitation.

□ Wernicke-Korsakoff syndrome

Treatment of Wernicke-Korsakoff syndrome includes strict abstinence from alcohol and the administration of large dosages of B-complex and C vitamins. A danger in treating patients with Wernicke-Korsakoff syndrome is the use of intravenous glucose solution. This solution may exhaust the patient's last reserve of B vitamins and cause rapid worsening of the disease. Because of this, B vitamins must be added when parenteral glucose is given.

When severe brain damage has occurred, long-term custodial care may be required. Family members who assume the care of the patient require much support and education.

□ Rehabilitation

The object of all treatment for alcoholism is to assist patients in completely stopping drinking alcohol. When they do stop drinking, they are taught that they can never take one drink without the danger of relapse. Studies have tried to demonstrate that alcoholics may be taught to become so-called social drinkers, but this has not been substantiated. Alcoholics who are not currently drinking are never considered cured, only recovering. Various methods of long-term care are used. These include some of the methods described in the following paragraphs.

□ *Behavior modification*

Behavior modification may be used to discourage drinking behaviors. The best known aversive agent is *disulfiram* (Antabuse), which blocks the enzymatic action necessary to metabolize alcohol. If the person drinks, the drug will cause symptoms of nausea, vomiting, palpitations, and general ill feelings with even a small sip of alcohol. The person is then conditioned to avoid alcohol. Disulfiram is usually used with other therapy and may help the alcoholic attain a period of sobriety so that other therapy may be effective.

□ *Group therapy*

Much of the goal of group therapy with the alcoholic is to enable the person to see the relationship between the use of alcohol and the negative consequences that have been suffered. In one sense, this is a form of behavior modification. When the alcoholic becomes sober, many of the problems that have occurred can be seen clearly for the first time.

An important part of the treatment of the alcoholic is *positive reinforcement.* This usually occurs in the context of interpersonal relationships with the nurses and other staff, as well as with other patients. Caring, emotional support, and encouragement are very important. This is demonstrated within the context of honesty and also by pointing out negative behaviors, defense mechanisms, and problems.

□ *Rehabilitation groups*

Alcoholics Anonymous (AA) is a group of self-acknowledged alcoholics whose aim is to stay sober and to help other alcoholics gain sobriety. There are AA groups who meet regularly in most communities. Meetings are of various types and include the following:

1. Open meetings—may be attended by anyone
2. Closed meetings—limited to persons who are alcoholic
3. Lead meetings—a recovering alcoholic tells the personal story of alcoholism
4. Discussion meetings—topic is discussed

There are meetings in most communities for women only, men only, young people, gay persons, and in larger communities, the deaf. There is no charge for attendance at the meetings, but a free-will offering is usually taken.

Local AA groups are sometimes listed in the telephone

Twelve steps of Alcoholics Anonymous

1. We admitted we were powerless over alcohol—that our lives had become unmanageable.
2. Came to believe that a power greater than ourselves could restore us to sanity.
3. Made a decision to turn our will and our lives over to the care of God as we understood him.
4. Made a searching and fearless moral inventory of ourselves.
5. Admitted to God, to ourselves, and to another human being the exact nature of our wrongs.
6. Were entirely ready to have God remove all these defects of character.
7. Humbly asked him to remove our shortcomings.
8. Made a list of all persons we had harmed, and became willing to make amends to them all.
9. Made direct amends to such people whenever possible, except when to do so would injure them or others.
10. Continued to take personal inventory and when we were wrong promptly admitted it.
11. Sought through prayer and meditation to improve our conscious contact with God as we understood Him, praying only for knowledge of His will for us and the power to carry that out.
12. Having had a spiritual awakening as a result of these steps, we tried to carry this message to alcoholics, and to practice these principles in all our affairs.

directory, and larger communities will publish and distribute directories of meetings. A phone call to AA (often called the central office) will bring help in the form of telephone conversation, or an AA member may visit the alcoholic desiring help.

In some communities some AA members are reluctant to have persons with other addictions attend AA meetings. This is partly owing to a lack of information about the disease of chemical dependency; it is also based partly on fear. With improved methods of diagnosing drug abuse and alcoholism, especially among younger persons, many AA groups are faced with the addition of younger people who have not suffered the same number or kind of consequences that the older members may have.

The AA philosophy focuses on the opportunity for the alcoholic to share *personal experiences* of alcohol abuse and control. Participation in AA may or may not be accompanied by the participation of the patient in other types of treatment. The success of AA has led to the formation of other groups that share the same twelve-step spiritual approach (see the box on p. 274). These groups include Al-Anon, Families Anonymous, Narcotics Anonymous, Overeaters Anonymous, Emotions Anonymous, Cocaine Anonymous, and Gamblers Anonymous.

The twelve steps assist the alcoholic in admitting his or her powerlessness over alcohol and other drugs. This is seen as essential for continued sobriety. Some persons may have a difficult time at first with the concept of a higher power or God. They are often encouraged to use the power of the group as a higher power, until they are able to recognize and accept a sense of *spirituality*. This sense of spirituality is not the same as religion or church.[48]

■ ASSISTING WITH COMFORT AND ADL

□ Promotion of nutrition

Many alcoholics enter treatment with a history of poor nutritional habits. They may have received as much as a third of their daily intake of calories from alcohol. They may often have been too intoxicated to eat or have had no appetite for normal food. Also, alcohol is the most common cause of acute gastritis, which can result in severe vomiting, contributing to poor nutrition. Often they have consumed many "empty calories" but are malnourished. In the initial detoxification period, diet is as tolerated, including liberal fluids. Intravenous fluids are usually not necessary. As the condition of the alcoholic improves, appetite usually improves also. The emphasis is on three well-balanced meals a day, with free access to snacks. Many patients find that they crave sugar during this initial period. Usually this is not discouraged because withdrawal from alcohol is the first priority.

Patients usually benefit from an assessment by a nutritionist or dietician. Education about the importance of improved nutrition is essential. If the alcoholic patient has developed liver involvement with cirrhosis, dietary modifications may become necessary. The reader is referred to the section in Chapter 30 on cirrhosis for further information.

Teaching for the patient with alcoholism

Disease concept of alcoholism
Medical aspects of the disease, including complications
Need for continued abstinence
Importance of expressing feelings to stay sober
Defense mechanisms
Drugs to avoid
Products that contain alcohol (for example, mouthwash)
Importance of being honest with physician and dentist
Signs and symptoms of impending relapse
Importance of aftercare, including AA

□ Counseling and teaching

Education about the disease of alcoholism is extremely important for the alcoholic. See the box above for important topics that need to be covered.

Any education of the alcoholic should also include the family or significant other. These persons also became sick in the midst of the alcoholic becoming sicker and need understanding and education to help themselves and the alcoholic to recover.

Many over-the-counter drugs contain alcohol. One example of this is many of the different brands of mouthwash. The alcoholic also needs to know that the use of any mood-altering chemical may lead to relapse.

✚ Evaluation

Evaluation of the patient with chemical dependency involves input from the patient, as well as the family members or significant other. Questions to ask include the following:

1. Is the patient sober?
2. Is the patient able to function with minimal anxiety?
3. Is the patient able to hold a job?
4. Is the patient's medical problem under good control?
5. Is the patient demonstrating positive coping mechanisms?
6. Is the patient attending aftercare, including AA?
7. Is the patient free of infection?
8. Is the patient able to carry on home maintenance activities?
9. Is the patient able to carry on ADL with minimal difficulty?
10. Does the patient verbalize a more positive self-concept?
11. Is the patient sleeping normally?
12. Is the patient's nutritional status improved?
13. Is the patient free of traumatic injury?
14. Is the patient's skin intact?
15. Is the patient having less spiritual distress?

16. Is the patient free of violent behavior?
17. Is the patient interacting with others in a more socially acceptable way?
18. Does the patient have a stable support system?
19. Is the patient able to verbalize knowledge of the disease concept of alcoholism?
20. Is the patient able to verbalize knowledge of any prescribed medications?
21. Can the patient explain the importance of notifying his or her doctor or dentist about the history of alcoholism?
22. Is the patient able to state what medications and other products to avoid?
23. Is the patient verbalizing powerlessness over alcohol and/or drugs?

■ DRUG ABUSE

Since alcohol is in itself a drug, alcoholism and drug abuse are considered part of the disease of chemical dependency. There is an increasing tendency for persons who abuse substances to mix a variety of drugs and alcohol. Much of the information already covered in the section on alcoholism also pertains to drugs.

The history of nonmedical drug use is thousands of years old. As early as 5000 BC, the Sumèrians referred to a "joy plant." This is believed to be a reference to the opium poppy plant.[35] Since then drugs have played a significant role in almost every culture. Different drugs have assumed importance in different periods of history. For instance, today cocaine is more problematic than ever before, especially in the form of "crack." Another recent problem is the class of designer drugs, which were unheard of several years ago.

In recent years drug abuse has risen sharply. There are no reliable statistics on drug abusers, and experts disagree about what actually constitutes drug abuse. The use of drugs has risen sharply among young adults and adolescents. Drugs are often readily available in most elementary and secondary schools and on college campuses.

The terms habituation and addiction have been used to define the nature and extent of drug use. *Drug habituation* includes repeated use of a drug to a point where there is *psychologic dependence*. *Drug addiction* involves *craving, psychologic dependence,* and *physical dependence.* The latter includes development of tolerance for increasing dosages of the drug and the appearance of withdrawal symptoms on cessation of the drug. *Drug dependence* is another term that may be used. This refers to a psychologic or physical dependence on a drug that is taken regularly.[35] (See Table 13-2.)

According to the Controlled Substance Act of 1971, there are five basic kinds of drugs:
1. Stimulants
2. Depressants
3. Hallucinogens
4. Narcotics
5. Cannabis

To this list could be added deliriants such as glue and paint thinner.

■ Stimulants

Stimulants are *natural and synthetic drugs* that have a strong *stimulating effect* on the central nervous system.

Table 13-2 Effects of mind-altering drugs

Drug	Tolerance	Physical dependence	Psychologic dependence
Narcotics	High	High	High
Barbiturates	Moderate	High	High
Glutethimide (Doriden)	Moderate	High	High
Methaqualone (Quaalude, Sopor)	Moderate	High	High
Tranquilizers	Moderate	Moderate	High
Amphetamine	High	Low to moderate	High
Cocaine	Low	Low to moderate	High
LSD	Moderate	None	Moderate
Mescaline	Low	None	Moderate
Phencyclidine (PCP, angel dust)	Low	None	Low
Marijuana	Low	None	Moderate

Street names for stimulants

Pep pills	Speed
Dexies	Crystal
Bennies	Meth
Ups	Whites

They are accompanied by a feeling of alertness and self-confidence.

Drugs included in this category are amphetamines, cocaine, caffeine, and nicotine.

■ AMPHETAMINES

Amphetamines and amphetaminelike drugs are *synthetic psychoactive drugs* that are available legally by prescription. They are available in both capsule and tablet forms. A powdered or crystalline form of amphetamine is *methamphetamine*, which must be injected. It is no longer legally produced in injectable form.

Medical uses of amphetamines include the treatment of *narcolepsy, obesity, fatigue,* and *depression.* Ritalin, an amphetamine-like drug, is used to treat children who are hyperactive. Common brand names of amphetamines include dextroamphetamine (Dexedrine), metamphetamine (Methedrine), and amphetamine (Benzedrine). See the box above for common street names for amphetamines.[30]

□ Pathophysiology

Amphetamines are *CNS stimulants.* When swallowed or injected, they speed up the activity of the heart and brain. Other results include the following:
1. Dilation of the pupil of eye
2. Increase in pulse and blood pressure
3. Reduction of fatigue
4. Reduction of appetite
5. Increase in concentration
6. Sense of confidence and well-being

However, when the feeling of alertness wears off, the person experiences *fatigue* and *depression.*

Amphetamines have the potential to produce *tolerance* but usually not physical withdrawal. However, psychologic dependence is common.

Side effects of amphetamine usage include *restlessness, dizziness, insomnia, headaches, diarrhea, constipation,* and *lack of appetite.* Persons who ingest a large amount of amphetamines over a period of time may experience extreme agitation and anxiety. They may become paranoid and suffer from a temporary *paranoid psychosis* that is a psychiatric emergency. Death by overdose does not usually occur, but death may occur from *cerebral hemorrhage* or *heart attack.* Persons can also collapse from exhaustion because the use of amphetamines hides a sense of fatigue. Withdrawal from the drug can lead to profound depression and may lead to suicide.[35]

■ COCAINE

Cocaine is a psychoactive drug that comes from the leaves of the South American cocoa bush. It was first used by the members of early South American tribes. When the Spanish conquistadors discovered the Inca empire, they also found cocaine. They encouraged its use when they found that the natives worked longer and harder and needed less food when they used cocaine.

The active ingredient in cocaine was isolated in its pure form in the nineteenth century. During that time the drug was also used as an ingredient in many products, including *syrups, nasal sprays, cigarettes,* and *liquors.* At one time it was an ingredient in Coca-Cola and was also recommended as a treatment for alcoholism. In 1914 the nonmedical use of cocaine was prohibited by the Harrison Narcotic Act. During the past 15 years, cocaine has become increasingly popular as a recreational drug.[23,31]

Medical uses for cocaine include use as an *anesthetic* of choice for certain procedures and surgery involving the nose, throat, larynx, and lower respiratory passages. It may also be used as an ingredient in Brompton's mixture, which is used for terminal cancer patients.

Cocaine is used by *sniffing, smoking,* or *injecting.* When it is sniffed or snorted, the effect of the drug is realized when the cocaine is absorbed into the nose. Cocaine may also be *free-based.* This is a process of heating the drug to separate it from whatever adulterants it may contain. When free-base cocaine is injected, it produces a high that is more intense and more short-lived than when cocaine is smoked.

A newer form of cocaine that is available is called "crack." Crack is less expensive than other forms of cocaine and is available in crystal form. Crack is considered to be even more addicting than other forms of cocaine.

See the box below for common street names for cocaine.[31]

□ Pathophysiology

Cocaine acts as a *CNS stimulant.* Results of the use of cocaine include the following:
1. Stimulation of respiration and heart rate
2. Raising of blood pressure and blood sugar levels
3. Suppression of appetite
4. Dilation of the eyes

Street names for cocaine

Blow	Snow
Coke	Superblow
Dust	Toot
Flake	White
Nose candy	White girl
Rock	Crack

---

5. Constriction of certain blood vessels
6. Increase in levels of physical activity
7. Insomnia
8. Trembling
9. Sensations of extreme euphoria
10. Feelings of energy, power, confidence, and talkativeness

There is a letdown effect of *cocaine crash* that occurs when the effect of the drug wears off.[31]

Chronic sniffing of cocaine can destroy the nasal tissues. Smoking it can cause lesions in the lungs. Tolerance and psychologic dependence can develop, and an overdose can cause *convulsions, respiratory paralysis,* and *death.* A cocaine psychosis has been reported that is characterized by a loss of pleasure, loss of orientation, hallucinations, insomnia, concern with minor details, stereotyped behavior, and an increased potential for violence. Abrupt withdrawal from cocaine does not lead to physical symptoms of withdrawal.

■ CAFFEINE

Caffeine is the most accepted and used psychoactive substance in the United States. Many beverages and other products contain caffeine. Because of its availability and widespread use, most persons do not view caffeine as a drug.

The use of tea leaves in China dates back at least 4000 years. In the 1200s the Arabians used coffee. Caffeine was first isolated from coffee in 1820. In its pure state, caffeine is a white powder or white needle-shaped crystals. It has been used as an additive in carbonated beverages since the early 1900s.

Medically, caffeine is present in many headache remedies, cold medications, diuretics, diet aids, and other prescriptions. See the box below, left for the amount of caffeine in commonly used beverages.

□ Pathophysiology

Caffeine *stimulates* the CNS and the digestive system and the kidneys. Body metabolism is increased, and the blood pressure is raised. Urination is also increased, and the secretion of gastric acid is stimulated. Large doses of caffeine cause *tachycardia, headaches* and *nervousness, insomnia,* and *stomach distress.* Physical dependence occurs with a regular intake of 350 mg for an adult. The withdrawal symptoms include *severe headaches, irritability,* and *tiredness.*[4]

Caffeine makes most people feel energetic and alert. Too much caffeine can precipitate an *anxiety attack.* Long-term involvement can lead to depression, persistent anxiety, low-grade fever, nausea, ringing in the ears, and chronic insomnia. A fatal dose of caffeine is considered to be about 10 g or 10,000 mg. Some research has indicated that excessive use of caffeine may contribute to the development of heart disease and bladder cancer.[4]

■ NICOTINE

Over 50 million Americans smoke more than 600 billion cigarettes yearly. It is one of the most physically damaging and addictive habits that a large number of people engage in. Smoking has been linked to heart and blood vessel disease, chronic bronchitis and emphysema, and cancer of the lungs, larynx, mouth, esophagus, bladder, pancreas, and kidneys. It is far easier to become addicted to cigarettes than to alcohol or other drugs.[3] Tobacco is used by *smoking, chewing,* or *inhaling.* Snuff is usually placed between the gums and the cheek.

The tobacco plant belongs to the genus *Nicotina,* a member of the *nightshade* family. Evidence has been found that cigarette use occurred as far back as 200 AD. When Columbus reached the New World, the sailors saw the natives smoking and soon picked up the habit. The cigarette-rolling machine was invented in the 1880s. This added greatly to the number of people who abused tobacco. In 1964 the surgeon general of the United States issued a report that linked smoking with several diseases. Cigarette packages are now so labeled. *Cigarette smoking is the chief preventable cause of death in present day society.*[3]

□ Pathophysiology

The nicotine in tobacco acts as a *stimulant* to the CNS. Nicotine is present in the brain within a few seconds of the beginning of smoking. Smokers claim that smoking produces relaxation; however, smoking releases epinephrine, which may cause psychologic stress. Nicotine acts as an *appetite suppressant.* In large doses it produces *tremors, decreased urine output,* and a *rapid respiratory rate.*

Withdrawal symptoms occur with the stoppage of cig-

Caffeine content of products	
Coffee (per cup)	
Brewed	75 to 155 mg
Instant	60 to 90 mg
Decaffeinated	2 to 4 mg
Carbonated sodas	
(All colas, Dr Pepper, Mountain Dew, Sunkist Orange)	30 to 70 mg
Chocolate	
Hot cocoa	30 to 70 mg
Candy (1 ounce)	6 mg
Over-the-counter drugs	
Anacin, Excedrin, Vanquish, Doan's Pills	16 to 65 mg
No-Doz, Vivarin	100 to 200 mg
APC tablets	30 to 100 mg
Diet aids	
AYDS, Dexatrim, Prolamine	140 to 200 mg
Tea	25 to 75 mg

arette smoking. See the box above for symptoms of withdrawal. The craving for a cigarette often continues for an extended period of time.[3]

Depressants

Depressants are *synthetic* drugs that have a *depressant* action on the CNS. Drugs included in this category are the following:

1. Sedatives or methaqualone
2. Barbiturates
3. Tranquilizers

SEDATIVES OR METHAQUALONE

Methaqualone is a *nonbarbiturate sedative-hypnotic.* It is the active ingredient in the drugs *Quaalude* and *Mequin.* It is no longer available as a prescription drug but has become a street drug. It is taken orally. It cannot be injected because it is nonsoluble.

Methaqualone was first made in the early 1950s as a treatment for malaria in India. It was used as a sedative in Europe in the 1960s and was first manufactured in the United States in 1965. It became available as a street drug in the 1960s and 1970s. When it first became available, it was thought not to be addicting.[37]

See the box below for street names for methaqualone.

Pathophysiology

Methaqualone is a *CNS depressant* that is unrelated to other sedatives or barbiturates. It slows the CNS and *impairs coordination, walking,* and *talking.* It also possesses *anticonvulsant, anesthetic,* and *cough-suppressant effects.* Its

primary effect is drowsiness. If the user resists the sleep-inducing effects of the drug, he or she experiences a mellow sense of well-being.

The repeated use of methaqualone produces tolerance, as well as physical and psychologic dependency. Withdrawal from the drug produces *headache, fatigue, dizziness, nausea, anxiety, skin problems, abdominal cramps, seizures,* and *vomiting* if the withdrawal is not accomplished under medical supervision. Withdrawal requires the use of a medication such as diazepam or phenobarbital.

Overdoses of methaqualone occur when the CNS-depressing effects of the drug slow the person's rate of breathing to the extent that unconsciousness occurs. Most overdoses occur when the drug is combined with other drugs such as alcohol that *potentiate* its action. Symptoms of overdose include *delirium, coma, restlessness, convulsions,* and *vomiting.*[37]

BARBITURATES

Barbiturates are *synthetic* drugs that are classified as *"sedative hypnotics."* They arise from barbituric acid. They are used medically to treat high blood pressure, epilepsy, and insomnia, and to sedate patients before and during surgery. Barbiturates are often available on the street.

Barbiturates are swallowed (capsule or elixir), used as a suppository, or injected. The drug was first synthesized in the early 1900s by two German scientists. Currently, about ten derivatives of barbituric acid are in use.

There are many common street names for barbiturates. They refer to the drug type, the drug effect, the drug name, or the color of the particular capsule. See the box below for common street names.[35]

Pathophysiology

Barbiturates cause *depression* of the CNS, including *slowing of physical and mental reflexes.* The continued use of these drugs can cause physical and psychological dependence, as well as tolerance. Barbiturates produce a feeling of well-being, euphoria, and relief from anxiety. Some side effects of barbiturates include *difficulty in breathing, lethargy, allergic reactions, nausea,* and *dizziness.*

Alcohol and other CNS depressants tend to potentiate the effects of barbiturates. Accidental overdoses are common. A person who is physically dependent on barbiturates will experience various withdrawal symptoms on the stopping of the drug. Mild withdrawal includes *irritability, rest-*

lessness, anxiety, and *sleep disturbances.* An extreme form of barbiturate withdrawal can be life threatening and includes symptoms of *convulsions* and *delirium.* Detoxification includes appropriate medication, which may include a long-acting barbiturate given in diminishing dosages.[35]

■ TRANQUILIZERS

Minor tranquilizers are *psychoactive drugs* that are taken to reduce anxiety. They may also be used as a *muscle relaxant.* They are the most commonly prescribed drugs in the world today. Tranquilizers are available in prescription form in capsule, tablet, and liquid forms. Illicitly, they are sometimes injected. Common types of tranquilizers are those found in the benzodiazepine family and include the following:

1. Chlordiazepoxide (Librium)
2. Diazepam (Valium)
3. Prazepam (Antrax or Vestram)
4. Oxazepam (Serax)
5. Lorazepam (Ativan)
6. Clorazepate (Tranzene)

The presence of these drugs is relatively new; the first tranquilizer was developed in 1950. Diazepam was first marketed in 1963.[35]

☐ Pathophysiology

Minor tranquilizers *slow* the activities of the CNS. They also have *anticonvulsant* and *muscle-relaxant properties* and produce a *sense of well-being.* When the effects of the drug wear off, users frequently experience an *increased level of anxiety.* Tranquilizers cause physical and psychologic dependence, and tolerance to them can develop.

Side effects reported for these drugs include *skin rash, headache, nausea, impairment of sexual function, dizziness,* and *light-headedness.* Other CNS-depressing drugs potentiate the action of the tranquilizers. Signs of an overdose include *sleepiness, confusion, loss of consciousness,* and *diminished reflexes.*

Withdrawal symptoms of minor tranquilizer use may not appear for a week after cessation of the drug. These symptoms include *anxiety, sweating, insomnia, vomiting, tremors, delirium,* and *seizures.* The patient must be detoxified with medications in a controlled environment.

■ HALLUCINOGENS

Hallucinogens are natural and synthetic drugs that affect the mind and produce *changes in perception* and *thinking.* One drug included in this category is phencyclidine (PCP), which will be discussed separately from the hallucinogens.

Hallucinogens include *lysergic acid diethylamide (LSD), mescaline, psilocybin,* and *3,4-methylenedioxyamphetamine (MDA).* They are found on the streets in a wide range of forms, including powder, peyote buttons, mushrooms, capsules, and tablets. LSD may be found as tablets, pellets, blotter paper, chips, and sheets of paper containing tattoos or stamplike pictures of cartoon figures. Hallucinogens are

---

Common street names of hallucinogens	
LSD	Acid, barrels, blotter, domes, microdots, purple haze, windowpane
Mescaline	Buttons, cactus, mesc, mescal buttons
MDA	Love drug, mellow drug of America
Psilocybin	Magic mushroom, shroom

---

taken orally, although MDA can be sniffed and injected. They may be put on sugar cubes or mixed in other food. See the box above for common street names of hallucinogens.[33]

Psilocybin and mescaline have been used in religious rites by cultures in the Western hemisphere for centuries. MDA was first synthesized in the 1930s and used as an appetite suppressant. LSD was first synthesized in 1938, and the first "trip" that was documented occurred in 1943 when the drug was accidentally ingested.

The use of LSD was prohibited in 1965. Before that time it had been used as a therapeutic treatment for neurotic and psychotic patients. Some experiments have also been conducted in the use of this drug with alcoholics and terminal cancer patients.[33]

☐ Pathophysiology

Most of the effects of hallucinogens are *psychologic,* although *nausea* and *vomiting* are not uncommon reactions. These drugs act as stimulants at first and produce *anxiety, depressed appetite, dilated pupils,* and *increases in body temperature, heart rate,* and *respirations.* With psilocybin, dizziness, numbness of the face, and shivering may also occur. Tolerance to these drugs occurs rather quickly (usually after 3 days of use), and there is cross tolerance among the four drugs.[33]

Hallucinogens also may have a profound psychologic effect on most people. The effect has been described as a process of *amplification,* with the drug acting as a *catalyst.* Hallucinogens amplify the users' experience of the environment and put them in touch with thoughts and feelings. In low doses, MDA produces a peaceful euphoria. With higher doses, it mimics LSD experiences minus the hallucinations.

All four drugs produce *altered sensory awareness.* The senses become more acute, and it is thought that colors can be heard and sounds seen. Fantasies and illusions occur, along with hallucination-like happenings, although the user is aware that they are not real. With LSD the mood changes can be rapid. Past and present experiences meld together, and some have described a feeling of "oneness, compassion, and love for all things."

The feelings brought on by MDA, mescaline, and psilocybin last from 6 to 8 hours, whereas those of LSD usually last from 8 to 12 hours. Toward the end of the "trip," the person will gradually reenter reality. A person's attempts to resist the effects of the drug seem to increase the chances of a negative experience, or a *bad trip*.

Flashbacks may occur with the use of hallucinogens. In these the user reexperiences the effects of the drug without having taken it. Bad trips are described as being characterized by *tremendous confusion, unpleasant sensory images*, and *extreme panic*. Care during these situations includes getting the person into a nonstimulating environment and staying with the person until the effects of the trip wear off. Reassurance of the fact that the person is experiencing a drug trip is helpful. Some sources cite the giving of niacin (500 mg) as a way to bring the person down from a bad trip.[33]

Although there have been no reports of deaths from LSD, there have been documented instances in which the person died as a result of trying to do something impossible while on a "trip." An example of this is trying to fly; that is, the person actually believes he or she will be able to fly.

■ PHENCYCLIDINE

Phencyclidine (PCP) is a synthetic drug that is generally described as an *anesthetic-hallucinogen*. However, it is chemically unrelated to hallucinogens such as LSD or mescaline.

PCP was first synthesized in 1957 and tested as a general anesthetic for humans. Testing stopped in the mid-1960s because of side effects of *agitation* and *delirium*. It presently is available as an anesthetic agent for use by veterinarians. In the 1960s and 1970s the drug became available as a street drug. It was banned from legal manufacture in 1978 but is still produced illegally.

PCP, produced as a white or yellowish white powder, has a variety of forms, including tablets and capsules. As angel dust it is sprinkled on tobacco or marijuana and smoked. When it is combined with marijuana it is called *sheba*. PCP may also be injected or snorted. See the box below for common street names for PCP.[38]

□ Pathophysiology

Different doses of PCP provide different physical effects. These can be found in the box at top, right.

Psychologic effects of PCP ingestion last from 1 to 6 hours, with 24 hours needed to return to baseline. Research seems to indicate that the bad trip rate of PCP is

---

Common street names for PCP

Angel dust	Embalming fluid
Animal tranquilizer	KJ killer
Crystal	Peace pill
Dust	Synthetic marijuana
Hog	

Physical effects of PCP

Dose	Effects
5 mg	Physical sedation
	Numbness of extremities
	Loss of muscle coordination
	Dizziness
	Constricted pupils, blurred or double vision, and involuntary eye movement
	Flushing and profuse sweating
	Nausea and vomiting
	Increase in blood pressure, heart rate, and respiratory rate (breathing is shallow)
5 to 10 mg	Marked drop in blood pressure, breathing, and heart rates
	Shivering, increased salivation, and watering of the eyes
	Loss of balance, dizziness, and rigidity of muscles
	In some cases, repetitive movements, such as rocking
	Analgesic and anesthetic properties apparent
Over 10 mg	Extreme agitation followed by seizures or coma
	Symptoms similar to mental confusion and delusion similar to schizophrenia

From Scott, L: PCP (pamphlet), Charlotte, NC, 1981, The Drug Center, Inc.

---

five times that of other drugs. Chronic users may have flashbacks. The dose of PCP may indicate the nature of the effects. These are found in the box on p. 282.

Although there is disagreement about whether PCP is physically addicting, there is wide agreement that it is psychologically habit-forming.

PCP overdoses are dangerous because the person may die as a result of *respiratory or cardiac arrest*. Symptoms of PCP intoxication include variable responses such as the following[38]:

1. Violence or combativeness to near unconsciousness
2. Little or no response to pain
3. Inability to speak
4. Elevated blood pressure and pulse rate with slight fever

The person intoxicated by PCP becomes more agitated by noise, bright lights, and talking.

PCP may result in psychosis that lasts from several days to 2 weeks. It is often mistaken for acute schizophrenia. Individuals may be actively suicidal and become depressed when the acute psychosis has passed.

Psychologic effects of PCP

Low dose	Euphoria and sense of alcohol-like intoxication
	Changes in body image
	Mood swings from ecstasy to panic
	Hallucinations and confusion about time and space
	In final stage in some cases, a sense of despair and emotional isolation
	Feeling of paranoia
	Sense of impending death
Moderate dose	Increase in effects felt at low dose
	Loss of sense of contact with environment
High dose	Symptoms of mental and emotional confusion similar to schizophrenia

From Scott, L: PCP (pamphlet), Charlotte, NC, 1981, The Drug Center, Inc.

Table 13-3 Narcotics

Name	Medical use	Route of administration
Heroin	None in the United States	By injection or sniffing
Morphine	Ease pain	By injection, smoking, or by mouth
Opium	Ease pain, treat diarrhea, and suppress cough	By mouth or smoking
Codeine	Suppress cough and reduce pain	By mouth or injection
Meperidine	Relieve pain	By mouth or injection
Methadone	Ease pain and help those dependent on her-	By mouth or injection

From O'Brien, R, and Cohen, S: The encyclopedia of drug abuse, New York, 1984, Facts on File, Inc.

■ NARCOTICS

Narcotics are drugs that are derived from the opium poppy or produced synthetically. The use of narcotics has been recorded far back in history. Synthetic production of narcotics has occurred in the past 30 to 50 years. In general, narcotics lower the perception of pain.

Heroin is one narcotic that is abused to a great extent. The shift has been toward younger addicts of heroin. On the streets, heroin is known as *H, horse, junk, hard stuff, smack,* or *scag.* The use of heroin is an expensive habit; addicts may resort to crime to support it.

There are several different forms of narcotics. See Table 13-3 for a listing of these drugs, their medical use, and route of administration.

□ Pathophysiology

Effects of the use of narcotics include *shallow breathing; reduced hunger, thirst,* and *sexual drive;* and *drowsiness.* The person may also experience *euphoria, lethargy, heaviness of limbs,* and *apathy.* The ability to concentrate is lost, along with judgment and self-control. Overdoses of narcotics can cause coma, convulsions, respiratory arrest, and death. As in the case of heroin, when the drug is injected, there are associated risks of hepatitis, acquired immune deficiency syndrome (AIDS), and other infections such as septicemia. Narcotic addicts develop both *tolerance* and *physical and psychological addiction.* Withdrawal may be painful and should be done under medical supervision. Clonidine (catepres) is often used for purposes of detoxification from

narcotics. The heavier the usage, the longer detoxification may take. Symptoms of withdrawal may include nausea, cramps, chills, sweating, watery eyes, running nose, and restlessness.[35]

■ CANNABIS

Cannabis, or *marijuana,* comes from the Indian hemp plant. It can grow wild or is fairly easily cultivated. Marijuana is usually smoked as a cigarette (joint, reefer) or in a pipe. Other paraphernalia may be used, including "bongs." There are many slang terms for marijuana, including *dope, grass, herb, joint, pot, reefer, roach, smoke, snuff,* and *weed.*

Marijuana has been used as both a medical and nonmedical drug for more than 3000 years. It has been used since the 1850s in the United States. Its popularity as a street drug began to occur in the twentieth century. It is still one of the most popular and commonly abused drugs, especially among young people.[35]

Hashish, or *hash,* is a resinous extract of the leaves and flowering part of the marijuana plant. It is more concentrated than marijuana and has more intense effects.

Marijuana's role in reducing eye pressure in glaucoma patients and controlling side effects of cancer chemotherapy, especially nausea, is being evaluated in research studies.

□ Pathophysiology

Physical effects of marijuana include drying of the eyes and mouth, increase in appetite, reddening of the eyes, and impairment of short-term memory. It also impacts the way stress affects the heart and circulation, and it raises the heart rate and blood pressure. Lowered body temperature, loss of coordination, and possible confusion and distortion of reality may occur. In addition, research indicates that marijuana may affect chromosome segregation during cell division. Because marijuana is a fat-soluble molecule, parts of it may be stored in the body for up to 30 days or more.[35]

Psychologic effects of marijuana include an *altering of perception* of sight, sound, touch, sense of time, and taste. The user usually has a feeling of well-being and intoxication, although depression and panic may occur. Psychologic addiction develops in users. Crisis situations may occur in the form of an anxiety reaction to the marijuana high. A calming and reassuring approach has been found to be helpful.

■ DELIRIANTS

Deliriants are any chemicals that give off fumes or vapors that, when inhaled, produce symptoms similar to intoxication. They may also be called *inhalants*. Vasodilators such as amyl and butyl nitrite are also considered inhalants.

The fumes or vapors from inhalants are sniffed through the nose, or the vapors are put into a bag or captured in a balloon to increase the concentration of the inhaled fumes.

The history of the use of inhalants is traced back to ancient Greece. Sniffing commercial products and solvents was first documented in the 1950s. There is no medical use for commercially prepared inhalants. Of course, the vasodilators and anesthetic agents have a legitimate medical purpose.

The deliriants or inhalants have a *psychoactive* or *mood-altering effect* when the vapors are inhaled or sniffed. Most fall into one of the three following categories[35]:

1. Solvents
2. Aerosol sprays
3. Anesthetics

Solvents include commercial products that are *not* commonly thought of as drugs. These include glue, gasoline, kerosene, lighter fluid, pain products, lacquer thinner, spot remover, and nail polish remover. Products such as hair spray, deodorant, insecticides, and cookware sprays are examples of *aerosols*. *Anesthetics* that are used recreationally include ether, chloroform, and nitrous oxide.

☐ Pathophysiology

Almost all inhalants are *CNS depressants* that *slow the* user's *heart rate, brain activity,* and *breathing.* Other effects include slurred speech, blurred vision, inflamed mucous membranes, light-headedness, ringing in the ears, watering eyes, loss of coordination, and excessive nasal secretions. With high doses, the user may lose consciousness or have seizures. The effects are immediate and usually last 20 to 45 minutes.

Symptoms of inhalant use include *bloodshot eyes, nosebleed,* and *halitosis.* The prolonged use of inhalants may lead to liver, kidney, blood, and bone marrow damage. The sniffing of *toluene,* found in gasoline and commercial cleaners, has been linked to *irreversible brain damage.* This may be demonstrated as forgetfulness, inability to think clearly, depression, irritability, hostility, and paranoia.

Some inhalants cause tolerance. Physical dependence is a possibility. Symptoms of withdrawal have included chills, hallucinations, headaches, stomach pains, cramps, and delirium tremens.

The psychologic effects of deliriants include a feeling of stimulation and energy. At higher doses, the user may feel intoxicated. The development of psychologic dependency is likely.

Use of large amounts of aerosols or solvents can cause death as a result of *cardiac arrest* following arrythmias. Death from inhalants is usually caused by *suffocation* because of the displacement of oxygen in the lungs. Sniffing inhalants from a bag or balloon increases the risk of suffocation. Misuse of commercial aerosol products used to chill food have been reported to cause death by freezing of the lungs of the user.

The CNS effect of inhalants are *potentiated* by other CNS depressants. This increases the chances of overdose.[35]

Assessment

■ SUBJECTIVE DATA

Subjective data of drug use include the same factors listed in the assessment section for alcoholism found on p. 268. One of the obstacles to early detection and treatment of addiction is the reluctance of parents to admit that their son or daughter is a drug user. Even members of the health professions "overlook" the often obvious symptoms of drug addiction, or having confronted the user, fail to report their findings to the parents or authorities.

■ OBJECTIVE DATA

Objective data for drug abuse include the factors listed in this section under alcoholism. In addition, the individual may show the following symptoms:

1. Abrupt changes in behavior; mood swings
2. Loss of interest in school, work, sports, and social or other activities
3. Frequent talking and reading about drugs
4. Loss of appetite
5. Presence of "track marks"

Breaks in the skin are an objective sign that must be noted when assessing for drug addiction. If the person has been *mainlining* (that is, injecting the drug directly into the vein), needle marks, scars, or small scabs can be seen on the hands and forearms or the instep. However, many other veins are used as points of entry to conceal addiction, including the dorsal vein of the penis or the conjunctival artery of the eyelid.

Because of the expense involved, users often sell their belongings, steal, or become prostitutes to get money to supply their drug habit. Each day abuse of drugs costs the American economy millions of dollars.

Occasionally, patients must be given narcotics to control pain over a long period of time and nurses may worry about them becoming addicted. It is rare, however, for addiction

Table 13-4 Acute intoxication and withdrawal of mind-altering drugs

| Drug group | Acute intoxication | | Withdrawal symptoms |
	Symptoms	Treatment	
Narcotics	Respiratory depression, bradycardia, hypotension, cold clammy skin, decreased body temperature; deep sleep, stupor, or coma; pinpoint pupils	Maintain ventilation, provide oxygen Give narcotic antagonist: naloxone (Narcan) 0.4 mg IV Monitor vital signs every 15 to 30 min until patient is conscious Treat for shock	*Not life threatening* Early; restlessness, irritability, drug craving, yawning, lacrimation, diaphoresis, rhinorrhea; followed by "yen" sleep (intense desire to sleep; sleeps restlessly) Later: awakens with more severe symptoms, nausea, vomiting, anorexia, abdominal cramps, bone and muscle pain, tremors, piloerection ("gooseflesh")
Other CNS depressants	Same as narcotics (above)	Lavage if recent oral ingestion Maintain ventilation, provide oxygen Monitor vital signs every 15 to 30 min until patient is conscious Position patient side-lying or prone, not supine Treat for shock Hemodialysis for renal shutdown	*May be life threatening* Insomnia, restlessness, tremors, anorexia, followed by convulsions, and symptoms similar to delirium tremens (confusion, visual and auditory hallucinations), fever, dehydration
CNS stimulants	Labile cardiovascular symptoms (flushing or pallor, pulse and blood pressure changes, arrhythmias), hyperpyrexia, mental disturbances (agitation, paranoia, hallucinations), convulsions, circulatory collapse	Give chlorpromazine, 25 to 50 mg IM Provide a quiet environment Orient patient to reality Monitor vital signs until stable	*Withdrawal is not severe* Somnolence, apathy, irritability, depression, fatigue
Hallucinogens	Physiologic toxicity low at doses that produce strong psychologic effects Acute panic reaction ("bad trip") may lead to suicide "Flashback" episodes Prolonged psychotic disorders (paranoia, depression) Phencyclidine: CNS depression or stimulation may lead to death	Provide quiet, supportive environment and constant attention Give diazepam (Valium), 2 to 10 mg IM for severe anxiety	No evidence of withdrawal symptoms
Cannabis	Adverse reactions infrequent Simple depression, paranoid ideation, confusion, disorientation, hallucinations	Provide support and reassurance Give tranquilizer for agitation	*Withdrawal symptoms rare* Insomnia, anorexia

to develop in those patients given narcotics for real pain, and nurses should not let the fear of the development of addiction keep them from administering prescribed narcotics to patients hospitalized and in severe pain.

■ DIAGNOSTIC TESTS

One diagnostic test used to test for drug abuse is urine or blood drug testing. Some employers are now beginning to demand "clean urines" as a condition of employment. Members of sports teams are asked to give samples at regular intervals. Jobs may be lost as a result of drugs in the urine.

The amount of time after use that drugs can be detected in the urine varies from a very short time for alcohol and cocaine to a long time for benzodiazepines and cannabis. In fact, cannabis may be found in the urine for as long as a *month* after the last use. It is possible to have a minimally positive drug test for cannibis because of a long period of "passive inhalation" from close contact with someone smoking and exhaling marijuana fumes. Also, some persons have claimed that positive results for narcotics may be possible with the use of large amounts of some nonnarcotic analgesics.

Urine testing is usually not used to detect alcohol because it is metabolized very rapidly. Alcohol blood levels are much more accurate. The breathalyzer is used by law enforcement agencies to determine alcohol levels in the blood.

Although some persons are concerned that routine testing violates civil liberties, efforts will continue to develop an accurate objective method for determining whether a person is under the influence of drugs or alcohol.

Other diagnostic tests that may be used include testing for hepatitis. Blood cultures may show the presence of septicemia.

➡ Data analysis: nursing diagnoses

See this section in the discussion of alcoholism in this chapter (p. 268).

▟ Planning: expected patient outcomes

The reader is referred to this section in the part of this chapter dealing with alcoholism (p. 273). The nursing diagnoses and patient outcomes are the same whether the person is abusing alcohol or another drug.

▟ Implementation

The treatment of withdrawal from drug abuse has been discussed in each section under the specific drugs. Table 13-4 lists the symptoms and treatment for acute intoxication and withdrawal. Rehabilitation follows the same guidelines discussed for the treatment of the alcoholic (p. 274). Today, most treatment centers treat alcoholics and drug addicts together because the majority of persons receiving treatment for chemical dependency have a history of abuse of both alcohol and drugs.

One difference between drug and alcohol abuse is that in most cases the possession and use of drugs is *illegal*. In the United States the addiction to narcotics has been considered a crime since the passage of the Harrison Narcotic Act in 1914.[35]

■ ASSISTING WITH THE ACHIEVEMENT OF THERAPEUTIC GOALS

☐ Methadone maintenance

One approach to the treatment of narcotic addiction is the *methadone maintenance program*. Methadone is a synthetic drug, and the average narcotic user's daily dose is much less expensive than that for heroin or morphine. The drug is given legally as a part of a rehabilitation program that should include group or individual therapy or both. Methadone reduces the severity of heroin withdrawal, and the user can maintain employment while undergoing treatment. Methadone itself is addictive and the use of it must be tapered off or the person may continue the habit the rest of his or her life. Because methadone is easily available through legal channels and permits the person to work, some experts believe that using it is essentially the same as taking maintenance doses of other drugs such as insulin, steroids, or digoxin. There are other experts, however, who believe that methadone treatment should be abolished because it promotes substance abuse.

☐ Residential communities

Another form of treatment that has occurred is the use of residential communities such as Synanon, which was founded in California and has chapters across the country. Other centers include the Phoenix and Horizon Houses (New York), Marathon House (Rhode Island-Massachusetts area) and Gateway House (Chicago). Such centers are usually listed in local telephone directories.

The treatment in such communities consists of helping individuals through the withdrawal state and then attempting to help them *increase self-understanding* and to *change their life-style*. Therapy is provided by the group. Rules of these community are strict, and breaking them results in severe consequences. The programs range in length from 18 to 36 months. Many addicts stay in the community after they no longer use drugs and they help to rehabilitate other addicts.

Halfway houses are shorter term residential settings that admit persons after they have completed residential treatment and assist them in reentry to the community. The usual length of stay in a halfway house is 3 to 6 months.

■ ASSISTING WITH COMFORT AND ADL

☐ Cocaine withdrawal

Many persons have described the addiction to cocaine as especially difficult to treat. Although the drug does not produce physical tolerance, the psychologic tolerance is especially strong. Research has also indicated that long-term cocaine use has yielded symptoms similar to those of Parkinson's disease. Cocaine is believed to affect the same areas of the brain as Parkinson's disease. Because of this, bromocriptine (Parlodel) has been used to assist in controlling the symptoms occurring with withdrawal from cocaine and to prevent relapse.

□ Risk of disease

Because many addicts inject drugs they are at risk for diseases such as hepatitis and AIDS. Often addicts share needles and equipment or reuse them without sterilizing them between periods of use. Addicts may also demonstrate resistance to more responsible use because of the character traits that accompany their disease.

Estimates of intravenous drug users who test positive for the AIDS virus are from 50% to 75% in some metropolitan areas such as New York City. Efforts to assist them in using clean equipment or using new equipment have not been very successful up to this point. Some have advocated supplying the addict with clean needles for no charge. This is not suggested to condone drug use, but as a means to prevent the spread of disease. The risk of AIDS for drug users is especially critical because they spread the disease to both men and women and to infants born to these women. Because of their mental condition while under the influence of drugs they may not remember the persons with whom they had sexual contact or shared drug equipment.

□ Counseling and teaching

The teaching for the patient with substance abuse is the same as that for the alcoholic patient (p. 275). It is especially important to teach about over-the-counter drugs that may be a hazard to the recovering person. These include benadryl, which is included in some over-the-counter cold medications, and diet pills.

⌗ Evaluation

The evaluation of care of the patient who is a drug abuser is the same as that for the alcoholic patient (see p. 275).

■ IMPAIRED NURSES

Over the last several years many states have developed programs to assist nurses who are impaired by either alcohol or drugs. This has occurred for a number of reasons, one of the main ones being that the rate of chemical dependency among nurses and other health providers is *greater* than that of the general public. Part of the reason for this is that health care workers have greater access to mood-altering substances. For instance, nurses may handle narcotics every day and may succumb to the temptation to use them. Before the inception of *Peer Assistance Programs,* through either state boards of nursing or state nursing associations, the nurse would often be fired and would be free to migrate to another facility, where the cycle of drug abuse would continue.

In March 1978 nurses from several states attended a meeting held in Manhattan to discuss the problems of the alcoholic nurse. By 1980 two organizations of nurses interested in alcoholism were active in encouraging help for impaired nurses. These were the Drug and Alcohol Nursing Association (DANA) and the National Nurses Society on Addiction (NNSA). In 1981 the American Nurses Association (ANA) created a Task Force on Addiction and Psychological Disturbance to formulate guidelines for state nursing associations to develop programs to help the impaired nurse. At the 1982 ANA convention, the American Nurses Association adopted a resolution that recognized its responsibility to assist the nurse who is impaired.

In 1980 two states, Maryland and Ohio, had peer assistance programs in place. By April 1982 four state programs were in place; and as of fall 1983, 25 states either had programs in place or were planning to start one. As of 1987, only a few states do not have such a program.[1,7]

Peer Assistance Programs have several goals: (1) to assist the nurse who is impaired to receive treatment; (2) to protect the public from the untreated nurse; (3) to help the recovering nurse reenter nursing in a systematic, planned, and safe way; and (4) to assist in monitoring the continued recovery of the nurse for a period of time, usually 2 years. The reentry of the nurse may include the restriction from handling narcotics for a period of time.

The basis of these programs is one nurse helping another nurse. Most volunteers in these programs are nurses who are recovering themselves or are working in the field of chemical dependency or psychiatric nursing. The program can work very effectively in states where the Peer Assistance Program, the state board, hospital administration, and law enforcement agencies all work together to assist the impaired nurse and safeguard the public.

■ SUMMARY

1. Substance abuse includes a complex set of behaviors known as addictions.
2. Examples of addictions include alcoholism, drug addiction, compulsive overeating, and compulsive gambling.
3. Alcoholism and drug addiction are commonly referred to as chemical dependency.
4. Dependency includes both physical and psychologic dependency and is defined as the need to continue use of drugs/alcohol to prevent withdrawal symptoms.
5. With increased use of alcohol and drugs, the person develops tolerance, which is defined as a decreased susceptibility to the effects of the substance.
6. Efforts to prevent substance abuse have included legal and educational efforts.
7. Enabling behavior by spouses and employers allows a person to continue the use of drugs and alcohol.
8. Interventions are planned confrontations by individ-

uals who care about the person and present meaningful data in a nonjudgmental way.

9. The goal of an intervention is to have the substance abuser recognize and accept reality so that the need for help is accepted.

10. Alcoholism is the third major health problem in the United States, affecting at least 9 million persons.

11. Theories concerning the cause of alcoholism include physiologic, psychologic, and sociocultural or cultural-etiologic theories.

12. Alcohol is a central nervous system depressant that affects the brain by suppressing the activity of the neurotransmitter gamma aminobutyric acid (GABA).

13. The so-called stimulating effects of alcohol occur because the first areas of the brain affected are the higher centers affecting self-control and judgment.

14. The active ingredient in alcoholic beverages is ethyl alcohol or ethanol.

15. Ninety percent of alcohol is metabolized in the liver.

16. Because alcohol is not converted to glycogen, it cannot be stored and provides 200 kcal but no minerals or vitamins.

17. The amount of alcohol in the blood at any one time is called the blood alcohol level.

18. The fetal alcohol syndrome occurs in children whose mothers drank several times daily; it includes mental retardation, microcephaly, growth deficiencies, and malformations of skeletal and urogenital systems.

19. Alcohol withdrawal includes symptoms ranging from mild tremors to severe agitation and hallucinations.

20. Delirium tremens (DTs) is an acute complication of alcohol withdrawal. It is a serious medical concern that has a 5% to 15% mortality rate and requires aggressive treatment.

21. Medication used in the initial period of detoxification inlcudes chlordiazepoxide (Librium), phenytoin (Dilantin), magnesium sulfate, and multivitamins.

22. Wernicke-Korsakoff's syndrome is a complication of alcoholism that includes symptoms of psychosis, amnesia, and apathy.

23. Alcoholics Anonymous (AA) is a group of self-acknowledged alcoholics whose aim is to stay sober and to help other alcoholics to gain sobriety

24. Using the twelve steps of AA will assist the alcoholic to accept his or her powerlessness over alcohol.

25. Alcohol is considered a drug.

26. Drug habituation is repeated use of a drug to a point where there is psychologic dependence.

Putting knowledge to practice

- Define substance abuse.
- What are addictions? List several addictions that are common today.
- Define chemical dependency.
- Differentiate between dependence and tolerance.
- What is enabling behavior?
- What legal and educational efforts have been made to help prevent substance abuse?
- What efforts do you think would be helpful in decreasing alcoholism and drug addiction?
- Is alcohol a drug? Why?
- What is the goal of an intervention?
- What are three important points to consider with an intervention?
- What are three common theories used to explain the cause of alcoholism?
- How does alcohol affect the brain?
- What is the active ingredient of alcohol?
- What is meant when it is said that alcohol produces "empty calories"?
- What is the blood alcohol level? what is the level that indicates intoxication?
- What are the possible complications suffered from withdrawal from alcohol? How are they prevented?
- What is Wernicke-Korsakoff's syndrome?
- What medications are commonly used in the treatment of alcohol withdrawal?
- What are the common classes of addictive drugs?
- Define drug habituation and drug addiction.
- What is the most accepted and used psychoactive substance in the United States today?
- What are flashbacks?
- What are bad trips?
- What is Alcoholics Anonymous? What are their twelve steps?
- Why is a nurse more at risk for substance abuse?
- What measures are in place in your state to assist nurses with addictions?

27. Drug addiction includes craving, psychologic dependence, and physical dependence.
28. The basic categories of drugs include stimulants, depressants, hallucinogens, narcotics, cannabis, and deliriants.
29. Caffeine is the most accepted and used psychoactive substance in the United States and is found in many beverages and health products.
30. Flashbacks may occur with the use of hallucinogens and include reexperiencing the effects of the drug without retaking the drug.
31. Drug addicts who inject drugs are at increased risk for the development of AIDS and hepatitis.
32. Nurses are at increased risk for the development of chemical dependency.

REFERENCES AND SELECTED READINGS
Contemporary

1. *American Nurses Association: States start assistance programs for impaired nurses, Am Nurse 15:6, 1983.
2. Arundell, R: Barbiturates (pamphlet). Charlotte, NC, 1981, Charlotte Drug Educational Center, Inc.
3. Arundell, R: Tobacco (pamphlet), Charlotte, NC, 1982, Charlotte Drug Educational Center, Inc.
4. Arundell, R: Caffeine (pamphlet), Charlotte, NC, 1981, Charlotte Drug Educational Center, Inc.
5. Barr, M, and Learner, W: The impaired nurse: a management issue, Nurs Economics 2:190-193, 1984.
6. Bean, M: Alcohol and adolescents, Minneapolis, 1982, Johnson Institute.
7. Bissell, L, and Haberman, P: Alcoholism in the professions, New York, 1984, Oxford University Press, Inc.
8. *Bissell, L, and Jones, R: The alcoholic nurse, Nurs Outlook 29:96-101, 1981.
9. Blume, S: Alcoholism and depression, Minneapolis, 1984, Johnson Institute.
10. Brisbane, F, and Womble, M, editors: Treatment of black Americans, New York, 1985, The Haworth Press.
11. *Brodsley, L: The hospitalized alcoholic: avoiding a crisis, Am J Nurs 82:1865-1873, 1982.
12. Caroselli-Karinja, M: Drug abuse and the elderly, J Psychosocial Nurs 23:25-30, 1985.
13. *Cohn, L: The hospitalized alcoholic: the hidden diagnosis, Am J Nurs 82:1861-1864, 1982.
14. Davis, J: Endorphins: new waves in brain chemistry, Garden City, NY, 1984, The Dial Press.
15. Deutsch, C: Broken bottles and broken dreams: understanding and helping the children of alcoholics, New York, 1982, Teachers College Press.
16. Didlday, RC: What the SNAs are doing in Georgia, Am J Nurs 82:581-582, 1982.
17. Effinger, J: Women and alcoholism, Top Clin Nurs 4:10-19, 1983.
18. Finley, B: Primary and secondary prevention of substance abuse in nurses, Occup Health Nurs 11:8-14, 1982.
19. Geller, A: Alcohol and sexual performance, Minneapolis, 1984, Johnson Institute.
20. Geller, A: Alcohol and anxiety, Minneapolis, 1983, Johnson Institute.
21. Goby, M, editor: Alcoholism, treatment, and recovery, St. Louis, 1984, The Catholic Health Association of the United States.
22. Haber, J, and others: Comprehensive psychiatric nursing, ed 2, New York, 1983, McGraw-Hill Book Co.
23. Hankes, L: Cocaine: today's drug, J Florida Med Assoc 71:234-239, 1984.
24. Harakel, BM: What the SNAs are doing in Ohio, Am J Nurs 82:582-583, 1982.
25. Harris, E: Sedative and hypnotic drugs, Am J Nurs 81:1329-1334, 1981.
26. Johnson, V: Intervention, Minneapolis, 1987, Johnson Institute.
27. Kimball, B: The alcoholic woman's mad, mad world of denial and mind games, Center City, Minn, 1987, Hazelden Foundation.
28. Mann, M: Marty Mann's new primer on alcoholism, New York, 1981, Holt, Rinehart & Winston.
29. Milkman, H, and Shaffer, H (editors): The addictions: multidisciplinary perspectives and treatments, Lexington, 1985, DC Heath & Co.
30. Newman, S: Amphetamines (pamphlet), Charlotte, NC, 1981, Charlotte Drug Educational Center, Inc.
31. Newman, S: Cocaine (pamphlet), Charlotte, NC, 1981, Charlotte Drug Educational Center, Inc.
32. Newman, S: Valium (pamphlet), Charlotte, NC, 1981, Charlotte Drug Educational Center, Inc.
33. Newman, S: Hallucinogens (pamphlet), Charlotte, NC, 1982, Charlotte Drug Educational Center, Inc.
34. O'Brien, R, and Chafetz, M: The encyclopedia of alcoholism, New York, 1982, Facts on File, Inc.
35. O'Brien, R and Cohen, S: The encyclopedia of drug abuse, New York, 1984, Facts on File, Inc.
36. *Reed, M: The dependent nurse—drugs or alcohol, Nurs Times 79:19-25, 1983.
37. Scott, L: Quaaludes (pamphlet), Charlotte, NC, 1982, Charlotte Drug Educational Center, Inc.
38. Scott, L: PCP (pamphlet), Charlotte, NC, 1981, Charlotte Drug Educational Center, Inc.
39. *Schwertz, P: The hospitalized alcoholic: an alcohol treatment team, Am J Nurs 82:1878-1879, 1982.
40. *Strasen, L: Acute alcohol withdrawal in the critical care unit, Crit Care Nurs 2:24-26, 30-31, 1982.
41. *Sullivan, E: A descriptive study of nurses recovering from chemical dependency, Arch Psych Nurs 1(3):194-200, 1987.
42. Symposium on alcoholism and drug addiction, Nurs Clin of North Am 19:77-87, Spring 1984.
43. Talbot, G: Substance abuse and the professional provider: the need for new attitudes about addiction, Alabama J Med Sciences 21:150-155, 1984.
44. Twerski, A: It happens to doctors too, Center City, Minn, 1982, Hazelden Publications.
45. Valiant, G: Natural history of alcoholism: causes, patterns, and paths to recovery, Cambridge, Mass, 1983, Harvard University Press.

---

* References preceded by an asterisk are particularly well suited for student reading.

46. *Weist, J: The hospitalized alcoholic: hospital dialogue . . . verbal intervention . . . what to say, Am J Nurs 82:1874-1877, 1982.

47. Zimberg, S: The clinical management of alcoholism, New York, 1982, Brunner Mazel, Inc.

Classic

48. Alcoholics Anonymous, ed 3, New York, 1976, Alcoholics Anonymous World Services Inc.

49. Criteria Committee, National Council of Alcoholism, criteria for the diagnosis of alcoholism, Am J Psych 129:127-135, 1972.

50. Gerrein, JR, and Rosenberg, CM: Disulfiram maintenance in outpatient treatment of alcoholism, Arch Psych 28:798-801, 1973.

51. Gitlow, S, and Peyser, H, editors: Alcoholism: a practical treatment guide, New York, 1980, Grune & Stratton, Inc.

52. *Heinemann, E, and Estes, N: Assessing alcoholic patients, Am J Nurs 76:785-789, 1976.

53. *Johnson, V: I'll quit tomorrow, San Francisco, 1980, Harper & Row.

54. *Lewis, LW: The hidden alcoholic: a nursing dilemma, Nurs 75 5(7):20-30, 1975.

55. Nelson, K: The nurse in a methadone maintenance program, Am J Nurs 73:870-874, 1973.

56. Wilner, D, and Kassebaum, G: Narcotics, New York, 1965, McGraw-Hill Book Co.

14

Chronic Illness

WILMA J. PHIPPS and PATRICIA BUERGIN

CHAPTER OBJECTIVES

After studying this chapter, the student should be able to:

- Differentiate between acute and chronic illness.
- Describe factors that influence chronic illness.
- Identify areas of assessment of the chronically ill person.
- Describe physical and psychosocial interventions for chronic illness.
- Define rehabilitation and the roles of team members (especially the nurse) and of the patient.
- Describe different patterns and facilities for continuing care.
- Identify major health goals related to chronic health problems to be achieved by 1990.

Prevention and control of chronic disease constitute one of the major health problems in the United States today. In the past the impact of chronic diseases on individuals, families, and communities has been overlooked. Recently, there has been an increasing awareness in the United States of great pockets of unmet needs among people with long-term health problems. These individuals have needs that extend beyond the strictly medical. Their problems demand the use of multiple sources of help and care. In many cases the coping capacities of chronically ill individuals are reduced because of advancing age, serious functional impairment and disability, and limited personal, social, and financial resources.

Chronic disease is not an entity in itself but an umbrella term that encompasses long-lasting diseases, which are often associated with some degree of disability. Each chronic illness is unique and has a different impact on the individual, family, and community. Nevertheless, common problems and complications that accompany the various chronic health problems can be studied in general to help the nurse understand and care for individuals with specific long-term illnesses.

The incidence and prevalence of chronic diseases have increased since the beginning of the twentieth century. This increase has been brought about by a number of developments including decreased mortality from infectious diseases, improved sanitation, and the development of effective vaccines and mass immunizations. Today only 1% of people who die before age 75 in the United States die from infectious diseases. Although the mortality from infectious diseases declined between 1900 and 1980, the proportions of deaths from major chronic diseases such as heart disease, cancer, and stroke increased more than 250%.[32]

Recent figures from the Bureau of Census, indicate that approximately 110 million people in the United States have one or more chronic illnesses.[18] This means that about 50% of the U.S. population have one or more chronic health problems. As a consequence, nearly 32.4 million persons have some limitations in their ability to carry out activities of daily living (ADL). The age groups of those with limitations are (1) 11 million are under age 45, (2) 11 million are between 45 and 64 years of age, and (3) 10.3 million are 65 years of age or older.[18]

Since the late 1960s, there has been a decline in the mortality from heart disease (particularly ischemic heart disease) and cerebrovascular diseases. These decreases have contributed to increased longevity in the United States. This gain in longevity is believed to be the result of an increased emphasis on health and physical fitness.

At the same time, the National Health Survey of 1982 identified major disparities in the health of black Americans and other minorities in the United States when compared with the white population.[13] As a result of these findings, the Secretary of the U.S. Department of Health and Human Services (DHHS) established a Task Force on Black and Minority Health. The findings of the task force are discussed on p. 294.

According to the surgeon general's report, 80% of the over-65 population has one or more chronic illnesses.[28] As mentioned above, there has been a decline in mortality from heart disease (particularly ischemic heart disease) since the late 1960s. In fact, 1977 was the first year in which cardiovascular causes were responsible for less than 50% of all deaths in the United States.[27] Longevity of the total U.S. population has increased by 3.1 years since 1970, compared with a gain of 0.8 year in the sixties. This gain in longevity is undoubtedly the result of improved health measures (such as a diet lower in staturated fat) taken by individuals.

■ DEFINITION OF ACUTE AND CHRONIC ILLNESS

An *acute illness* is one caused by a disease that produces symptoms and signs soon after exposure to the cause, that runs a short course, and from which there is usually a full recovery or an abrupt termination in death. Acute illness may become chronic. For example, a common cold may develop into chronic sinusitis. A *chronic illness* is one caused by disease that produces symptoms and signs within a variable period of time, that runs a long course, and from which there is only partial recovery. The National Health Survey defines chronic conditions as follows: (1) the conditions were first noticed 3 months or more before the date of the interview, or (2) they belong to a group of conditions (including heart disease, diabetes and others) that are considered chronic regardless of when they began.[13] This follows the pattern of the Commission on Chronic Illness which in 1949 defined chronic illness as any impairment or deviation from normal that has one or more of the following characteristics.

1. The illness or impairment is permanent.
2. The illness or impairment leaves residual disability.
3. The illness or impairment is caused by nonreversible pathologic alteration.
4. The illness or impairment requires a long period of supervision, observation, or care.

The symptoms and general reactions caused by chronic disease may subside with proper treatment and care. The period during which the disease is controlled and symptoms are not obvious is known as a *remission*. However, at a future time the disease may become active again with recurrence of pronounced symptoms. This is known as an *exacerbation* of the disease.

Exacerbations of chronic disease often cause the patient to seek medical attention and may lead to hospitalization. The needs of a patient who has an acute illness may be very different from those of the patient with an acute exacerbation of a chronic disease. For example, a young person may enter the hospital with complaints of fever, chest pain, shortness of breath, fatigue, and a productive cough. If the diagnosis is pneumonia, the patient usually can be assured of recovery after a period of rest and a course of antibiotic treatment. However, if the diagnosis is rheumatic heart disease and if the patient is being admitted to the hospital for the third, fourth, or fifth time, the reassurance needed will not be so definite, clear-cut, or easy to give. In such a case it is necessary to begin planning care that will extend beyond the period of hospitalization, taking into consideration many aspects of the patient's total life situation. The concerns of the patient who has repeated attacks of illness will be very different from the concerns of the one who has a short-term illness.

Further, the needs of patients who are admitted to the hospital with an acute illness but who also have an underlying chronic condition must not be overlooked. For example, elderly patients who enter the hospital with pneumonia may receive treatment for the pneumonia and recover from their illness. However, they may still be hampered by the arteriosclerotic heart disease and arthritis that they have had for years. Also these two chronic conditions may have been aggravated by the acute infection, or the return to former activity may be hindered by joint stiffness resulting from bed rest and inactivity. Consideration of a patient's several diagnoses can help in preventing new problems associated with the chronic illness.

Strauss[2] has described the following problems experienced by persons with chronic illness:

1. Preventing and managing medical crises
2. Controlling symptoms
3. Following prescribed regimen
4. Maintaining normal interactions with others
5. Adjusting to recurrent patterns in the course of the disease
6. Arranging payment for treatment

IMPACT OF CHRONIC ILLNESS ON SOCIETY

According to the National Health Survey, 80 million people have one or more chronic conditions. The survey classified chronic conditions in the following categories: (1) selected skin and musculoskeletal conditions, (2) impairments (visual, hearing, speech, paralysis, deformity, or orthopedic impairment), (3) selected digestive conditions, (4) selected conditions of the genitourinary, nervous, endocrine, metabolic, and blood and blood-forming systems, (5) selected circulatory conditions, and (6) selected respiratory conditions.[14]

Many of these conditions cause a limitation of activity, which affects the life-style of the chronically ill. One of the trends that has been documented is that the impact of acute illness has seemed to diminish, whereas the burden of chronic health problems and related disability has increased. Limitation of activity is a measure of long-term disability resulting from chronic health problems or impairment and is defined as the inability to carry on the major activity for one's age group, such as cooking, keeping house, going to school, or going to work.[17] Approximately 15% of the population experience some limitations in their activities, whereas almost half of the persons over 65 years of age are limited in their activities by one or more chronic conditions. Some activity limitations are associated with mental disabilities, but most are the result of physical handicaps caused by heart conditions and arthritis. Since chronic disability increases in direct proportion to age, persons over 65 years of age are most prone to severe chronic disability.[6]

The inability to work or to move about influences greatly the kind of medical treatment and health supervision needed by persons who have a chronic illness. Some persons only need periodic medical examination and perhaps continuing treatment with medications; others may require complete physical care. Some have a disease that progresses very slowly without remissions, while others may have episodes of acute illness and then seem comparatively well for a time. Each person requires a thorough assessment to determine the stage of the illness, the course the illness is likely to take, the type of care needed, and the method by which that care will be delivered if the individual is to be helped appropriately.

Factors that influence chronic illness

AGE

Different age groups have different kinds of experience with acute and chronic diseases. The young are more likely to experience short, intense, acute conditions that are quickly over. The elderly are more likely to have long, drawn-out chronic diseases; nevertheless, it is true that anyone can have either an acute or a chronic disease at any age. Chronic illness and disability may date from birth (e.g., spina bifida with neurologic damage), or it may originate in childhood, adolescence, or early adult life (e.g., multiple sclerosis, rheumatoid arthritis). The major chronic illnesses among those 65 years and over identified in the National Health Survey were: *arthritis, diabetes, heart disease,* and *hypertension.*

Because of strides made in pediatric medicine, children who 30 years ago would have died from diseases such as cystic fibrosis are living longer. The reduction in death rates among the younger age groups has allowed a higher percentage of the population to reach the age of greatest risk from chronic diseases. Cancer develops far more frequently in older people. Because the average age of our population continues to rise, one out of four people now alive will eventually contract cancer.[1]

Much remains to be learned about interactions of the normal, pathologic, and physiologic changes of aging with various diseases. A common question that is asked is "When does aging end and illness begin?" Differences found in age groups or changes found in individuals as they age represent normal aging; that is, a universal, intrinsic process of growth and development that is inevitable, irreversible, unpreventable, but ultimately detrimental. Even though aging, a normal process, is distinct from chronic disease, a pathologic process, chronic illness is often concomitant with aging. The problems of aging and chronic disease are influenced in major ways by each other; for example, the social problems confronting the aged are strongly influenced by the presence and severity of chronic disabilities. Remissions and exacerbations are possibilities with chronic illness; they are not with aging.

■ CULTURAL VALUES

Western culture tends to be cure oriented, therefore, health care for acute conditions is often more valued than is health care for the chronically ill. In contrast to the exciting aspects of sophisticated and mechanical technology, caring for chronically ill persons is often considered boring. The continual struggle to cope with day-to-day living soon becomes tedious for ill persons, their families, and health professionals. The rewards of treating chronic illness cannot be measured by a cure but by the prevention of complications and by helping individuals function at their optimal level.

The cultural context has many symbolic meanings, beliefs, and values that health professionals need to understand to meet individual's health needs. Some individuals may view their chronic disease as a form of punishment from God. Thus they may experience a sense of guilt. Individuals who view their chronic disease as a "leper phenomenon" may experience a sense of social rejection. Others may see their chronic illness as a destructive force without meaning or simply as a physical response of their body. Appreciation of the person's beliefs and behavior in the context of his or her cultural heritage rather than denial of the cultural influence increases understanding between the health professional and the chronically ill person. Differences need not imply deviance. It is possible to introduce health practices in a manner congruent with the individual's cultural values.

■ RACE AND ETHNICITY

Race or ethnic group membership is a factor that influences chronic health problems. Race-specific rates measure the association between disease occurrence and race. Data on specific conditions indicate not only that some problems are more prevalent among nonwhites (blacks, American Indians, and Asiatics) but also that many nonwhites fail to receive necessary care. For example, nonwhites are more than three times more likely to die of hypertension than whites of the same age group.[13] The findings of the Task Force on Black and Minority Health, which were released late in 1985, found that 60,000 excess deaths occur each year in minority populations. Six causes of death were identified that together account for more than 80% of the excess mortality. The health problems related to excess deaths are listed below in alphabetical order:

Cancer: 16% of excess mortality among black males under age 70 and 10% among black females.

Cardiovascular disease and stroke: 24% of excess mortality among black males and 41% among black females.

Chemical dependency (measured by deaths resulting from cirrhosis of the liver, associated with excessive use of alcohol): 13% of excess mortality among Native American males and 22% among Native American females under age 70 years of age.

Table 14-1 Number of selected reported chronic conditions per 1000 persons by race and age: United Stages, 1982

Type of chronic conditions	White		Black	
	65-74	75 years and over	65-74	75 years and over
Arthritis	499.8	482.9	595.3	395.0
Diabetes	86.3	75.3	203.1	96.5
Heart disease	235.7	323.4	142.3	198.2
Hypertension	369.7	394.9	533.7	468.1

From National Center for Health Statistics, Division of Interview Health Statistics, data from National Health Interview Survey, 1982.

Diabetes: 38% of excess deaths among Mexican-born Hispanic females.

Homicides and accidents (unintentional injuries): 60% of excess mortality among Hispanics under age 65 years of age.

Unintentional injuries cause 44% of excess death among male and 30% among female Native Americans. Homicides and unintentional injuries account for 19% of excess mortality among black males under age 70 and 38% among those under age 45. The figures for black females are 6% and 14%, respectively. A substantial portion of excess deaths in this category may be associated with excessive use of alcohol and other drugs.

Infant mortality: of excess deaths among black females up to age 45 years, death in the first year of life accounts for 35%.[11]

Table 14-1 compares the rates of four major chronic illnesses for white and black Americans.

■ Cost of disability

Each chronically ill person and family are subjected to great personal and emotional losses that must be dealt with—loss of self-esteem, loss of status within the family, loss of independence, feelings of rejection, and feelings of helplessness are only a few. These can be more devastating than economic deprivation, which is a constant problem.

The economic cost to the patient and family is considerable. The cost of hospitalization rises yearly. Frequent or extended hospitalization and medical expenses can be ruinous if the patient is inadequately insured or if he or she is unable to qualify for insurance programs. Many are forced to seek public assistance merely to survive. Placement in quality nursing homes is frequently financially impossible for patients or their families to manage. The cost of medications to control or maintain a patient's health status may require a major portion of the family budget. Additional expenses may include special diets and equipment, home modifications (e.g., ramps or widening of doors for wheelchairs), transportation, and support services provided by homemakers, day or live-in attendants, or nurses.

The ability of the individual family to pay its own way is determined in part by which member of the family becomes disabled. Studies show that if the wife is disabled, the family suffers less economic deprivation than if the husband is disabled. However, three fourths of the chronically ill persons unable to carry on their major activity are men.[29]

Some financial assistance is provided by Medicare. This federally administrated program provides hospital and medical insurance protection for individuals 65 years of age and over as well as for people under 65 who are disabled and eligible for Social Security benefits. Persons under age 65 who are medically indigent because of health problems may be eligible for assistance through the Medicaid program.

However, recent changes in federal funding have altered Medicare and Medicaid programs. Persons over age 65 receiving Social Security have a higher fee deducted from their monthly payments to pay for their Medicare premiums. In addition, most persons covered by Medicare purchase supplemental health insurance to cover expenses not covered by Medicare.

There have been severe cutbacks in Medicaid, which is administered at the state level, and eligibility requirements have been made more stringent.

Thus persons with chronic illnesses may have considerable difficulty in paying for prescribed therapy. For example, antiinflammatory agents used to treat arthritis are very expensive. Many of these medications cost between $0.75 and $1.00 each and the usual dose is three times daily.

In considering the cost of disability to the community, it must be realized that most individuals who are unable to work must be supported by others, either from private or from public funds. There are 3 million adults between the ages of 18 and 64 years who are unable to work because of chronic disabilities. There are an additional 9.4 million who are partially limited in their ability to work.[28]

■ CHRONICALLY ILL PERSONS AND THEIR FAMILIES

The effects of chronic illness on individuals and their families are numerous and varied. The first impact of the disability may nearly immobilize them. Time must be provided them to talk through their concerns and fears before they can be expected to begin coping with their new situation.

Marked changes often take place, and are often required to take place, in family living as a result of chronic illness. Some families may find themselves drawn closer together. Other families may drift apart, the individual members being incapable of helping one another. At times, chronic illness may threaten an individual's basic emotional stability, and the whole situation may be unbearable to others. Sometimes the individual's emotional needs may not have been apparent to the family early in the illness, but when such needs grow obvious, relatives feel inadequate to cope with the situation. The length of illness, periodic hospitalizations, and increased financial, emotional, and social burdens are stressors that threaten the family's integrity.

Many persons struggle on their own to assume the full financial burden of the illness and consequently expose other members of the family to lower standards of nutrition, housing, and care. Many times relatives move in with one another, arguments develop, and family ties are strained or broken. Public assistance may be acceptable to some families, whereas others find it impossible to accept.

Chronic illness imposes additional problems of learning how to cope with restrictions on activities of daily living, how to prevent or identify medical crises that occur, and how to carry out treatment regimens as delineated by the health care provider. Family members also need to learn about the restrictions, not only to be of assistance to the chronically ill person, but also because their own activity patterns may be disrupted by the person's activities.

Because chronic illness may have periods of exacerbation when symptoms become more acute and medical crises may occur, patients and family members need to know which symptoms must be reported to the health care provider as well as the time interval for reporting these symptoms. They also need to know how to contact the provider and what measures to take if a medical crisis occurs. For example, the person who has a history of myocardial infarction and that person's family members must know what to do if the person experiences severe chest pain. Should the person be taken immediately to a hospital emergency room or should the physician be contacted first? Patient and family should plan in advance the sequence of actions to take during a medical crisis, depending on the nature and extent of the presenting symptoms.

■ Compliance and noncompliance

Persons with chronic illness are often labeled as "compliant" or "noncompliant" in carrying out regimens prescribed for them. There are many factors that influence the person's ability or motivation to carry out the prescribed regimen. If the person does not carry out the regimen (noncompliant), it does not necessarily mean that the individual is refusing to do so deliberately, although this may sometimes occur.

Before the nursing diagnosis of noncompliance is made, the nurse needs to assess the situation to determine the reasons that the patient is not complying with therapeutic recommendations. The etiology of noncompliance includes the patient's value system (health beliefs, cultural influence, spiritual values).[8] The following are some possible reasons for nonadherence to a prescribed therapy:

1. Failure to understand or internalize the reason for the recommendations
2. Procedures that are difficult to learn and carry out
3. Time required to carry out therapy
4. Inability to pay for prescribed therapy
5. Side effects of therapy (medications, exercises, etc.)
6. Being embarrassed when carrying out regimen in front of others
7. Social isolation and lack of support and positive reinforcement

Conflicts occur within the family structure when one family member recognizes the importance of carrying out the prescribed regimen but another does not. For example, a wife may see the need for continuing checkups and medication for her husband's hypertension, whereas he may perceive this as a needless expense since he feels well and has no symptoms. Persons vary from time to time in the extent of compliance. Individuals who are not hospitalized are their own health care agents and they (or their significant others) determine the actions that are taken.

Coping mechanisms that have been developed should not be tampered with unless, based on a thorough understanding of the situation, viable and more appropriate alternatives can be proposed. If the goal of maintaining the chronically ill person in the optimal state of health is being interfered with by the individual's or the family's attitudes or capacities, a change in those attitudes or capacities is necessary, but it must be a change that is mutually acceptable.

■ Prevention of chronic illness

Because chronic disease evolves over time and pathologic changes may become irreversible, the goal is to detect risk factors as early as possible.

Generally, prevention means inhibiting the development of a disease before it occurs. The term includes several levels of prevention to interrupt or slow the progression of disease (see the box below).

Chronically ill persons and their families require long-term care. The nursing profession has been concerned with chronic health problems and the challenge involved in providing long-term nursing care to chronically ill individuals and their families.

The American Academy of Nursing has made the following statement regarding long-term care:

Long-term care is the provision of that range of services— physical, psychological, spiritual, and social, including socio-economic—needed to help people attain, maintain, or regain their optimal level of functioning. It includes health maintenance

---

throughout the life span as well as care during acute and protracted illness and disability. Such care is the legitimate province of nurses who now are making social contributions through health teaching and promotion, prevention of illness, and rehabilitation.[20]

In the past nursing has followed the general pattern of providing health services by placing the emphasis on acute and episodic care rather than on health promotion and health maintenance. However, there is an emerging consensus among the health community that the health strategy must be changed dramatically to emphasize the prevention of disease. In the same vein, the American Academy of Nursing has proposed that "nursing assume major responsibility for health promotion, maintenance, and teaching within the context of its definition of long-term care."[20]

⊞ Assessment

Before a plan of care can be devised for the chronically ill person, a thorough assessment of needs and capabilities must be carried out. Included in such an assessment are the individual's physical, psychologic, social, and financial status.

■ PHYSICAL STATUS

Because medical diagnoses do not accurately reflect the physical status and functioning of the chronically ill person, the use of a profile system or assessment tool may be instituted as a guide for those working with the patient. One such tool[26] provides a guide for grading the patient in six different categories: (1) physical condition including cardiovascular, pulmonary, gastrointestinal (GI), genitourinary, endocrine, or cerebrovascular disorders; (2) upper extremities, structure and function, including the shoulder girdle and cervical and upper dorsal spine; (3) lower extremities, structure and function, including the pelvis and lower dorsal and lumbar sacral spine; (4) sensory components relating to speech, vision, and hearing; (5) excretory function, including the bowels and bladder; and (6) mental and emotional status. The ability of the person to carry out activities of daily living (for example, dressing, feeding, bathing, brushing teeth, combing hair, toileting, and moving from place to place) specifically need to be assessed. The completed assessment should indicate in what areas the patient has difficulty and the extent of that difficulty. Such a guide can be used in planning goals for care, both immediate and long term, and will be useful in assisting the individual and the family to make realistic plans for care. Because a chronic condition is not static, reassessment should be carried out at regular intervals whether there is improvement or regression.

The impact of chronic illness on the person's desire for or ability to participate in sexual activities should be assessed. Changes in body appearance, shortness of breath, and musculoskeletal or neurologic impairments may make it seem to the person that they can no longer be sexually active. In addition, the side-effects of certain medications tend to decrease sexual desire or cause impotence.[7]

┌───┐

Levels of prevention

Primary

Health promotion
Specific protection against diseases

Secondary

Early detection of disease
Prompt intervention to halt progression of disease

Tertiary

Rehabilitation (appropriate to the stage of disability)
Prevention of further complications
Restoration of optimal functioning to highest possible level

└───┘

The nurse should determine if concern about sexual ability is a problem for the person, and if it is, appropriate action including referral can be taken. (See Chapter 33 for more information about sexuality in health and illness.)

■ PSYCHOLOGIC STATUS

Assessment of the individual's psychologic needs and capabilities includes determining attitudes and stage of adaptation to the illness, feelings concerning how illness affects the family or significant others, and the person's own goals in regard to living with an illness.[30] For example, individuals who are almost totally helpless as a result of an accidental spinal cord injury may seem to have no interest in learning ways to help themselves. Their families may react in the same manner and be of little help to them. Both the individuals and their families need interest and support from professional persons as they learn to cope with the change in their life situations.

Feelings of anxiety, frustration, irritability, bitterness, and guilt may be expressed by some chronically ill persons who face unending pain and loss of economic and social security. Some persons become obsessed with their health problems, and spend much of each day thinking about what will happen and what to do. Guilt may result from being unable to work and support oneself or from the belief, as a result of a search for some purpose or reason for the affliction, that one must deserve the suffering. *Depression* is common among chronically ill persons, especially those who feel powerless. Powerlessness can be the result of feeling unable to control or overcome what has happened to one.[7]

■ SOCIAL AND FINANCIAL STATUS

Social and financial status must be considered, as they relate specifically to the kind of support and resources available to the individuals in meeting their goals. It would be unrealistic, for example, to plan for a hydraulic bathtub chair if the patient could not afford it, family members were unavailable to help operate it, or the patient's apartment manager would not permit it to be installed. Alternative methods of helping the patient to take a tub bath would have to be explored.

The social assessment includes living arrangements, family roles, support of significant others, cultural and social group memberships, education, and vocational and avocational activities. The data collected through the performance of this kind of thorough assessment should make it possible to devise a plan of care directed toward the accomplishment of attainable goals that are mutually acceptable to the patient, the family, and the caregivers.

➡ Data analysis: nursing diagnoses

Nursing diagnoses are determined from assessment of patient data. Possible nursing diagnoses for the person with a chronic illness may include, but are not limited to, the following:

Diagnostic title	Possible etiologies
Activity intolerance	Bed rest, immobility, generalized weakness, sedentary life-style
Impaired adjustment	Disability requiring change in life-style, inadequate support systems, impaired cognition, sensory overload, altered locus of control, incomplete grieving
Anxiety	Threat to self-concept, threat of death, threat of change in health status and/or socioeconomic status, role functioning
Constipation	Change in life-style, immobility, inadequate nutrition, inadequate fluid intake
Ineffective breathing pattern	Neuromuscular impairment, pain, musculoskeletal impairment
Impaired verbal communication	Aphasia, physical impairment
Ineffective family coping: compromised	Inadequate or incorrect information, temporary family disorganization and role changes, prolonged disability of significant person
Diversional activity deficit	Long-term hospitalization
Fear	Loss of body part, long-term illness, pain, life-style changes
Altered health maintenance	Altered communication skills, decreased motor skills
Impaired home maintenance management	Individual/family member disease/injury, insufficient family resources, lack of knowledge/role modeling, inadequate support systems
Hopelessness	Prolonged activity restriction, failing physical condition, long-term stress
Functional incontinence	Altered environment, sensory, cognitive, or mobility deficits
Reflex incontinence	Neurologic impairment
Potential for injury: trauma	Sensorimotor deficits, lack of awareness of environmental hazards
Knowledge deficit	Lack of exposure/recall, cognitive limitation
Impaired physical mobility	Intolerance to activity, decreased strength/endurance, pain/discomfort, cognitive impairment, neuromuscular impairment, musculoskeletal impairment
Altered nutrition: less than body requirements	Chewing or swallowing difficulties, inability to obtain food

Diagnostic title	Possible etiologies
Pain	Immobility, improper positioning, pressure points
Powerlessness	Health care environment, illness-related regimen, lifestyle of helplessness
Feeding, bathing/hygiene, dressing/grooming, toileting self-care deficit	Intolerance to activity/fatigue, pain/discomfort, perceptual/cognitive impairment, musculoskeletal impairment, depression
Body image disturbance	Loss of body parts/functions, severe trauma, change in body appearance, immobility, change in life-style, change in social environment
Self-esteem disturbance	
Personal identity disturbance	
Altered role performance	
Sexual dysfunction	Altered body structure, physiologic limitations
Impaired skin integrity	Mechanical forces (pressure, shearing), immobility
Impaired social interaction	Self-concept disturbance, absence of supporting others, therapeutic isolation

⊞ Planning: expected patient outcomes

Outcomes for specific chronic disease are discussed in the chapters dealing with those diseases. However, it may be stated on a general basis that on discharge from the hospital patients with chronic disease or their family members should be able to do the following:

1. Demonstrate or explain measures that must be taken to avoid further preventable disability.
2. Demonstrate or explain self-care activities of which they are capable.
3. Identify activities for which help is needed.
4. Explain who will be available to help them with those activities and on what basis that help will be available.
5. Explain what community resources are available to them for help and how they may obtain that help.
6. Discuss in reasonable detail their plans for follow-up care and reevaluation.

■ Intervention

■ PHYSICAL CONSIDERATIONS LIMITING DISABILITY

The first focus in intervention for the chronically ill person is on prevention and reduction of disability and on enabling the person to remain a socially functioning individual in every respect. Some of the disability seen among the chronically ill might have been prevented if prompt, aggressive, suitable medical and nursing care had been available at the onset of the illness. Many of the difficulties that limit the chronically ill may not have been caused by the disease itself but may have developed because of immobility during the acute phase of the illness.

Keeping the person's body in good alignment, maintaining joint range and strength, and preventing decubitus ulcers are physical measures that must constantly be borne in mind. (For further information see Chapter 22.) A careful plan of rest and activity helps preserve physical resources and makes the day purposeful. If assistance is needed, it should be given until the persons can manage the activity by themselves or until an alternative method of management can be taught.

☐ Promoting self-care

Recognizing what is meaningful to the individual is a primary step toward helping develop self-care. Physical needs become of paramount importance to chronically ill persons. Meeting these physical needs provides a way to convey to such individuals an interest in their progress and welfare. It is important to be allowed to perform as much of their own care as possible. Persons who have been independent in self-care before hospitalization, should not be allowed to regress in these abilities if at all possible. Helping them to take their own baths, to attend to toilet needs, and to groom themselves can give some sense of accomplishment and help them maintain their self-respect. Helping them to be dressed appropriately promotes a sense of wellness. Success in performing portions of their own self-care may be stimulating enough to strengthen the persons' motivation so that they and their families may make amazing strides in thinking through and working out future problems themselves. For their planning to be realistic and ultimately functional, all health care personnel must teach chronically ill persons the total physiologic ramifications of their disability as well as methods of coping with those ramifications.

Persons who are in their homes or in substitute homes should be encouraged to dress in regular, comfortable street clothing rather than in pajamas or gowns. Visitors coming into the home and members of the family who constantly see such individuals dressed in bedclothes think of them as sick and are reminded of their illness. Seeing them dressed as they ordinarily would be helps to maintain normal attitudes, relationships, and expectations.

■ PSYCHOSOCIAL CONSIDERATIONS

The care of chronically ill persons requires alertness of feeling, seeing, and hearing. Continued warmth and interest are necessary to the well-being of any chronically ill person. Very often it is a relationship based on an understanding of these requirements that helps the individual to become highly motivated. It may be taxing to listen to the same questions and to say the same things day after day, but the nature of chronic illness may require this attention, and the manner in which responses are given will convey warmth and interest. The world of chronically ill persons, whether they are in the hospital or elsewhere, becomes narrowed and circumscribed. They treasure and are interested in those things and those people who are

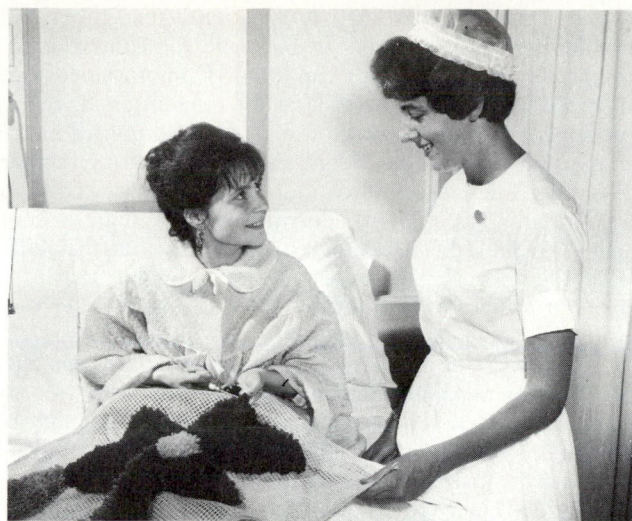

Fig. 14-1 Occupational therapy provides patient with purposeful activity. Interest shown by the nurse encourages patient to complete project.

close to them. Their conversations may be largely about themselves, their immediate environment, a few close objects, and the persons who are close to them. Although they may be confined to bed and to their room, others can keep them up-to-date on outside news. Depending on their level of adaptation to their illness, they may welcome hearing about outside events, or they may not be able to think beyond themselves. When they reach the stage of being able to look beyond themselves, newspapers, magazines, radio, television, or creating something with their own hands (Fig. 14-1) may help to keep up their interest in others and in outside events.

□ Supporting coping skills

Coping skills may be challenged by persistent, ongoing problems such as chronic pain, recurring medical expenses, or continuing difficulties in carrying out activities of daily living. Usual coping methods may become impossible; for example, a person who usually copes by expending energy in physical activity may become unable to do so. The person who usually copes by discussing problems with family members will need to find an alternative method if family communication patterns break down. The person can be helped to identify usual coping methods and to explore alternative approaches when necessary.

It is important to recognize that chronically ill persons or their families may suffer from unresolved sadness known as chronic grief. Chronic grief may be defined as accumulated or prolonged grief. Chronic grief extends over long periods of time with permanent characteristics in a large number of sufferers. It carries with it a potential for decreased functioning. The causes are varied, and new waves of grief are constantly triggered. One example is that of the mother of the retarded child who has accepted her

situation and is coping well, but over and over is faced with unattainable goals, repeated frustrations, and an uncertain future. Another example is grief caused by the losses associated with aging: youth, dreams, jobs, hair, friends, family, health, visual acuity, social role, money, body parts, and mobility. Each loss is accompanied by grief, which builds on previous grief like bricks placed by the mason creating a wall. In chronic grief the patient may be faced with repeated acute episodes. These episodes may coincide with exacerbation of the condition, facing a new limitation, or meeting new indignities. Each new episode requires a renewed struggle back and forth through the various stages of grief.[31]

The nurse can assist by listening and helping the person explore feelings and the content related to these feelings. Because the grief is ongoing, family members can also be helped to identify their feelings and to strengthen the communication patterns within the family structure for mutual support of its members.

□ Clarifying nurse-patient values

Nurses who work with chronically ill persons need to be able to distinguish between their own values, standards, and goals and those of the patient. In day-to-day contact with individuals who are making little or no progress, it is tempting to make plans for their future because of a sincere interest in helping them. This is particularly true when the patient's age is similar to one's own. There may be a feeling that something must be done to speed progress. One may become frustrated by the feeling of wanting to do something or wanting to see some marked change. However, it must be recognized that management of chronically ill persons requires a slow-moving, persistent pace with possibly little or no change for a long time. The person's physical and mental condition must be maintained at its present level or improved, and effort must be made to further progress and to encourage the family's adaptation to the patient's condition. Eagerness and readiness to progress will be determining factors for the future. The "doing" in the care of the chronically ill person is not always an active, physical "doing" with the hands. Many times the maintenance of a positive approach and attitude and a demonstration of real interest are the greatest help to the patient. Teaching patients to perform activities related to their own care independently rather than performing those activities for them may also lead to progress.

□ Assisting the person to adjust to a disability

Success in learning to adjust to living with a disability depends on the person's premorbid personality, total life experience, and premorbid family relationships, as well as the current behavior and motivation the person presents. Certainly, some rehabilitation can occur in any health agency; nevertheless, the greater the number of rehabilitation disciplines that can be made available as needed to individuals, the greater is their chance of achieving their highest potential. The rehabilitative process, as with any form of education, is involved as deeply in the motives and purposes of the teacher as in those of the learner.

□ Supporting the person with a progressive disability

Health care personnel must also be prepared to provide care for patients whose disease will follow a course of progressive disability, for example, multiple sclerosis or rheumatoid arthritis. In these instances, goals of care must be modified to retard the downhill progression of disability rather than to achieve maintenance or improvement of physical status. Helping the patient and family cope with progressive deterioration and, in some cases, eventual death is a demanding task. Those who wish additional information relating to this aspect of care are referred to the literature treating this subject.[31,23]

Persons with a disability, whether it is obvious to others or unrecognizable, should not be viewed from the standpoint of their disability alone. Usually the greatest need is for comprehensive health services and continuing care. Comprehensive care is that which is provided to patients according to their needs in an appropriate, continuous, and dynamic pattern. Accommodating the plan of care to the needs and goals of individual patients rather than to those of the providers of care is the essence of comprehensive care.

■ REHABILITATION

Rehabilitation is the process of assisting the individual with a handicap to realize his or her particular goals, physically, mentally, socially, and economically. As such, "rehabilitation" is an active concept and must be clearly differentiated from the concept of "maintenance" care. Fol-

lowing a thorough assessment of patient's disabilities and capabilities, assumptions can be made regarding the potential for improving their condition. If improvement can be made, patients are candidates for rehabilitation. If improvement cannot be made, care is directed toward maintaining the current condition, that is, preventing further disability. The process of rehabilitation can be viewed more appropriately as patient education rather than patient "care." It must be remembered, however, that the rehabilitation of every patient reaches an end point; that is, a point at which no further progress is possible. At that point, the focus of care reverts to that of maintenance.

The purpose or extent of rehabilitation ranges from employment or reemployment for the handicapped person to the more limited achievement of developing the ability to provide his or her own daily care. This latter accomplishment can be just as important to the individual as earning money and may represent that person's greatest life achievement. This might be true, for example, for a person who was born with a severe physical handicap such as cerebral palsy.

■ Multidisciplinary approach

The number of professional people required to assist the patient and family with rehabilitation varies. Most often the patient, the family, the physician, and the nurse can work out a practical plan. If a patient's problems are complex, other members may be added to the team. Typically, such a team consists of a physician, nurse, social worker, vocational counselor, psychologist, speech pathologist, occupational and physical therapists, and a caseworker from

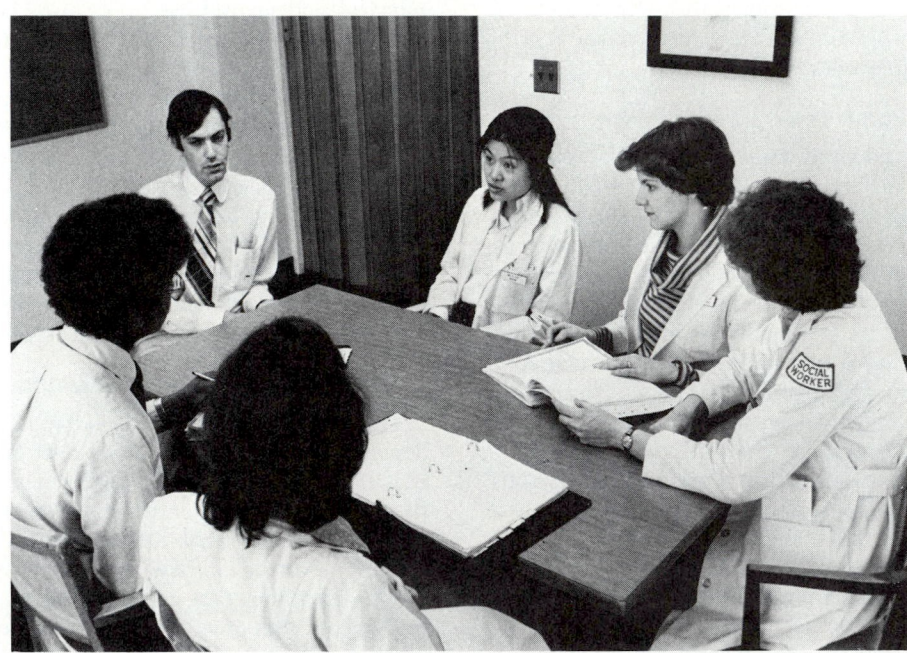

Fig. 14-2 The team approach to rehabilitation is essential. Here, physicians, nurse, physical therapist, and social worker review a patient's program and progress.

the patient's social agency. Teamwork requires that members of the team be able to use their special knowledge and skill and understand the value of their contribution to the patient's care. In addition, team members need some understanding of each other's professional functions and contributions. One of the cooperative efforts of the involved team members is to meet regularly to thoroughly evaluate patients and their abilities. Based on this assessment, each patient and the team devise a plan to foster readjustment, compensation, and the learning of new ways of managing self-care and living. In Fig. 14-2 some of the members of a team review a patient's rehabilitation program.

■ Rehabilitation centers

Persons with complex problems of rehabilitation may need to receive care at specialized centers for rehabilitation or they may receive care at home combined with visits to day rehabilitation centers. The variety of specialized centers includes teaching and research centers (centers located in and operated by hospitals and medical schools), community centers with facilities for inpatients, community out-patient centers, insurance centers, and vocational rehabilitation centers. In addition to centers that provide multiple services for the physically disabled, there are specialized centers for rehabilitation of the blind, deaf, mentally ill, and mentally retarded. Most centers offer a wide range of services that usually fall into the following three areas:

Physical
  Physical, nursing, and medical evaluation
  Physical therapy
  Occupational therapy
  Speech therapy
  Medical and nursing supervision of appropriate activities
Psychosocial
  Evaluation
  Personal counseling
  Social service
  Psychometrics
  Psychiatric service
  Recreational therapy
Vocational
  Work evaluation
  Vocational counseling
  Prevocational experience
  Appropriateness of vocational program to job opportunities
  Trial employment in sheltered workshops
  Vocational training
  Terminal employment in sheltered workshops
  Placement

There are several advantages for patients participating in organized programs for rehabilitation. They have an opportunity to see and be with others who have similar or more extensive disabilities. Often they progress more rapidly when they realize that others have similar difficulties and are overcoming them. Group therapy often arouses a competitive spirit, and a formerly reluctant person may become willing and diligent. On the other hand, all personnel need to be alert to patients who have had the opposite reaction. Patients who see others advance in activity while they either do not improve or progress very slowly may become so discouraged that they give up trying.

On a rehabilitation unit, activities are scaled so that individuals can see their own progress in comparison with their beginning abilities. Patients may take an active interest in keeping their own scores. After a program of therapy has been planned and is scheduled as to time of day, patients can help to keep themselves on the schedule by having a copy of it at the bedside. Individuals can then be helped to gradually assume more and more responsibility for getting themselves ready for scheduled activities. In addition, a master plan of activities for all patients on the unit can be a useful device for nurses, physicians, and therapists. The plan can be kept in a central place on the unit and should list name, activity, and time of activity for each patient. This type of plan is helpful, too, when a patient's progress is to be reevaluated.

A public program for vocational rehabilitation has been serving the nation since 1920. The program involves a partnership between the state and the federal governments. Services for disabled persons are provided by state divisions of vocational rehabilitation. The federal government, through the Social and Rehabilitation Service (SRS), administers grants-in-aid and provides technical assistance and national leadership for the program. Opportunities and services are available in each of the 50 states, the District of Columbia, and Puerto Rico. All persons of working age with a substantial job handicap resulting from either physical or mental impairment are eligible for help or assistance. The purpose of this service is to preserve, develop, or restore the ability of disabled persons to earn a living. The individual services offered are medical care, counseling and guidance, training, and job finding. All 50 states have separate rehabilitation programs for the blind. Application for such services can be made to the SRS or to the agency in the state for serving the blind.

■ Role of the nurse in rehabilitation

The concepts of comprehensive nursing care and rehabilitation can be considered synonymous. Helping the patient and the family to help themselves is an integral part of nursing care. Nurses who work with patients who have disabilities have two major responsibilities: (1) to see that disability from disease is limited as much as possible and (2) to see that a rehabilitation program is planned and implemented. Details of the nurse's role and responsibilities are listed in the box on p. 302.

One of the most important aspects of giving continuing care to a patient with a disability is the nurse's own attitude, perseverance, and expectations. Improvement may be slow, and patients may reach a "plateau" in their progress. Such a time can be critical for patients because they may become discouraged and not wish to continue with their program of care. Realistic encouragement can often

The nurse's role and responsibilities

I. Limit disability from disease as much as possible.
  A. Prevent complications.
    1. Early recognition of symptoms of patient's condition worsening.
      a. Review signs and symptoms and pathology of the chronic illness so as to recognize changes.
      b. Review signs and symptoms of complications frequently associated with the chronic illness, that is, infection.
    2. Prevent deformities.
      a. Maintain proper body alignment.
      b. Position limbs to prevent contractures.
      c. Turn frequently, keep skin clean and dry to prevent skin breakdown.
      d. Provide adequate nutrition.
      e. Provide adequate fluid intake to maintain bladder and bowel program.
      f. Take precautions to prevent infection.
II. Plan and implement a rehabilitation program appropriate to the patient.
  A. Determine patient's own goals for rehabilitation.
  B. Plan appropriate nursing interventions based on mutually agreed on goals.
    Early in rehabilitation nurse may have to assume total responsibility for assisting with activities of daily living (ADL), bathing, intake of food and fluids, bowel and bladder programs, maintaining skin integrity, turning patient, and so on.
  C. Plan nursing interventions that encourage patient to assume responsibility for own ADL as soon as possible.
    1. Set short-term goals with patient.
    2. Goals should be realistic and attainable.
    3. Reinforce patient's progress (no matter how small) with positive feedback.
    4. Work with other members of the rehabilitation team in providing a consistent, coordinated rehabilitation plan.
    5. Keep patient's significant others informed of patient's progress so they can give positive feedback to patient.
    6. Reassess goals periodically and set new goals as possible.
    7. Teach patient, family, and, if necessary, the employer about patient's limitations and rehabilitative expectations.

sustain patients so that they will not regress until some improvement is noted.

Patients in a rehabilitation program must often learn and practice special physical techniques to strengthen muscles and to improve mobility. Such measures as physical exercise to improve walking, activities to improve self-care abilities, and the use of prostheses require the special knowledge and skills of physical and occupational therapists. To be effective in the rehabilitation process, nurses must have an understanding of the techniques used by the various therapists so that they can plan and work cooperatively with them in caring for the patient. This knowledge is also used to help the patient employ appropriate techniques in carrying out activities of daily living (ADL).

■ Role of the patient in rehabilitation

The most important contributions to patients' rehabilitation are made by the patients themselves. The patient, the nurse, the physician, the social worker, the occupational therapist (Fig. 14-3), and sometimes others planning together can arrive at the best plans for the future, but the patient's attitudes, acceptance, and motivation are the most important considerations. If the patient cannot adjust to the disability, whatever it may be and however extensive it may be, attempts at rehabilitation usually are hindered. Patients are the individuals who really make the decisions, and they change at their own pace. If they are agreeable to suggestions but make little or no effort to try them, one should question whether they really have accepted them.

Self-care is encouraged within existing limitations. The patient's behavior from day to day can be the first indication of the direction of positive motivation. For example, if the patient makes every effort to resume normal daily activities such as feeding, bathing, and dressing, one can be quite certain that this is a person with a sincere desire to be independent. As patients become ready for more advanced activities such as ambulation and work in the occupational therapy shop, they need continuing genuine interest and support (Figs. 14-3 and 14-4). As obstacles present themselves, patients may be able to accept them and eventually overcome them. Patients who are truly motivated toward

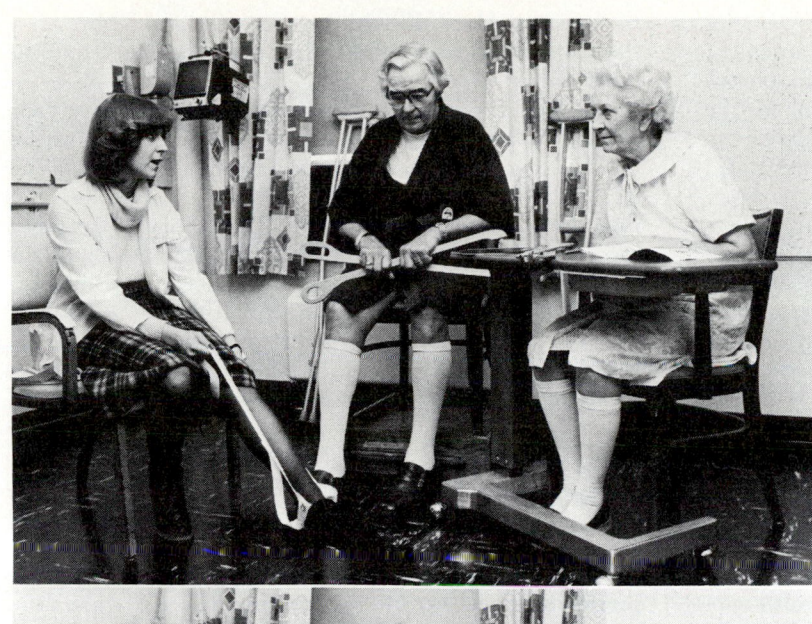

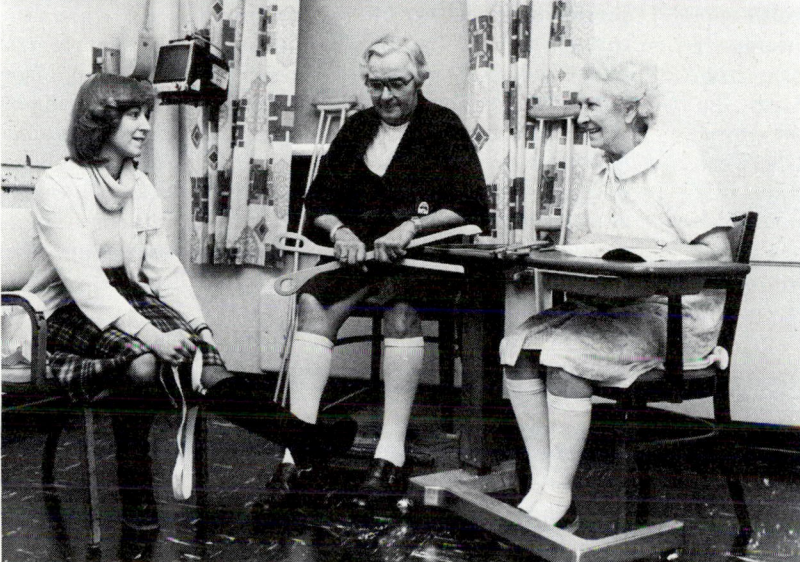

Fig. 14-3 The occupational therapist is concerned with helping patients make necessary adaptations in activities of daily living to permit independent functioning. Here the occupational therapist demonstrates the use of a stocking aid that to the delight of the patients really works.

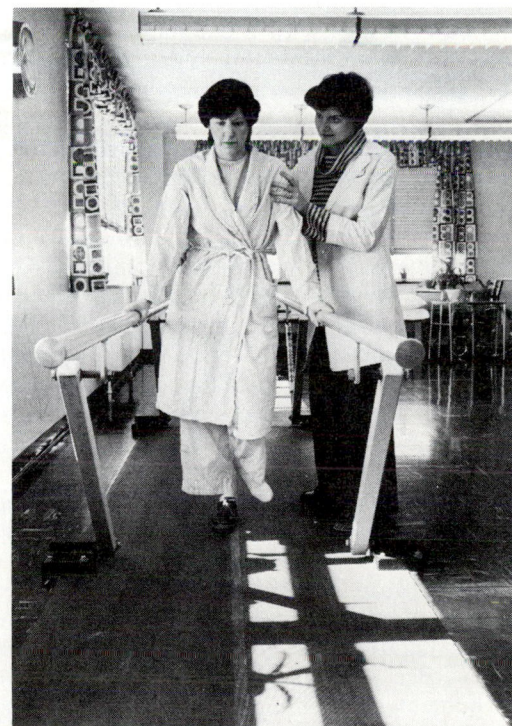

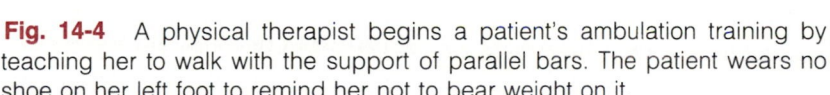

Fig. 14-4 A physical therapist begins a patient's ambulation training by teaching her to walk with the support of parallel bars. The patient wears no shoe on her left foot to remind her not to bear weight on it.

helping themselves never seem to give up, finding ways of accomplishing activities that professional personnel might believe impossible. Each person working with the chronically ill has seen that many times life has meaning for the individual even though it may not be readily apparent to others. However, there are some patients who, when faced with an added burden, cannot accept it and give up trying. Guidance and support for the families of such patients become tremendously important. Health care personnel who understand these attitudes and behaviors can help make life more satisfying for the chronically ill person and can positively influence the behaviors of the family, professional coworkers, and the public.

CONTINUING CARE

Traditionally, health care professionals have assumed responsibility for the patient's well-being within the hospital and little to no responsibility for the person and family in the home setting. This dichotomy between health care in the home and hospital facility in the case of chronically ill individuals interferes with a smooth transition from hospital to home. The major portion of health care for persons with chronic illnesses takes place in the home; thus there needs to be ongoing communications between the client and health professionals. Strauss[31] advocates that sick people participate more in their care within health facilities and that health care professionals play a larger role in aiding chronically sick people and their families to cope with their problems at home.

Home health care

Most persons with a chronic or long-term illness can care for themselves or be cared for at home, and most actually prefer to be at home, where family and friends are close by and where they can still participate in family life. Many chronically ill persons require health care supervision at home. The arrangements that can be made vary greatly and depend on the needs of the individual and the facilities available. Many persons are ambulatory and, during remissions, are able to visit their local clinic. Others manage with visits from their personal physicians and with periodic workups in the physician's office. The assistance of a home health nurse or aide who goes into the home may also be necessary. Many chronically ill persons with disabilities also visit special rehabilitation units of hospitals or outpatient centers for daily or periodic instruction and practice in physical skills and job training.

Nurses from voluntary and official health agencies help the chronically ill in their homes. Nurses who visit the home to assist the individual or family members to accomplish daily care need to understand the patient. Chronically ill persons are often misjudged by even the closest members of the family because of blinding emotional ties or lack of knowledge and understanding. Families need to be helped to understand the limitations and necessary restrictions on

the patients. Hopefully this process will have begun while the patient was hospitalized, but it will need to continue in the home setting.

The benefits and the necessity of self-care as a valid part of the health care system are receiving new recognition. Although the main impetus for this recognition has come from consumers, health care providers are increasingly incorporating self-care into the delivery of primary care. One definition of self-care is "an action taken by the consumer or patient to reduce to the degree possible, incremental debilitation resulting from chronic disease."[31] The increasing prevalence and importance of chronic illness as a principal cause of disability and death place greater demands on the person and family for involvement in self-care.

Self-help groups

Self-help groups are associated with self-care. These groups may or may not include the guidance of health care providers. They provide social support to their members through the creation of a caring community, and they increase members' coping skills through the sharing of information, experiences, and problem solutions. Examples of self-help groups include those for women who have had mastectomies and those for individuals who have colostomies, diabetes, or obesity. There are now self-help groups or clubs for patients with a variety of conditions. Nurses should learn what groups are available to patients in their community. A telephone call to a health agency such as the American Cancer Society, American Heart Association, or American Lung Association can elicit information about clubs available to patients who have the specific condition served by the agency.

In some hospitals nurses have been instrumental in setting up support groups for families of patients with chronic health problems.

It can be expected that more support groups, both those for patients and those for families, will be developing in the near future. Some of the impetus for these groups can be traced to changes in health care reimbursement. With the move to prospective reimbursement and the use of diagnosis related groups (DRGs) as a basis for reimbursement for patients whose care is being paid for with federal dollars (Medicare and Medicaid), the need for such groups will increase. Prospective reimbursement has resulted in shorter hospital stays for both acute and chronic illnesses. As a result, patients and their families need to be better prepared to care for the patient in the home since patients are sent home sooner than in the past and their needs for continuing care are greater.

Facilities for continuing care

It is impossible to include here all of the many facilities that provide continuing care. Each of the programs that will be mentioned has its own criteria for acceptance of patients for the services it renders. Before application for service is made, a determination of the individual patient's eligibility for that service must be carried out.

■ AMBULATORY CARE

The term *ambulatory care* is used interchangeably with *outpatient care* and refers to first contact health care services as well as to continuing contact services in settings that do not require overnight stays. There has been a marked increase in the use of ambulatory care facilities because of the increase in chronic illness and the increase in cost of inpatient services. A good ambulatory care service constitutes one of the most important elements of the hospital's contribution to community health. There is a trend toward development of ambulatory care facilities in neighborhood health centers to assist the disabled, the aged, or the disadvantaged person obtain needed health care. An ambulatory care center usually provides long-term follow-up care needed by the person with a chronic illness, in addition to preventive health care, diagnostic workups, and treatment of acute illnesses for which hospitalization is unnecessary.

■ HOME CARE

Before World War II the home was the place where medical treatment was given. Well-to-do persons rarely thought of going into a hospital, and they received the services of a private physician in their own home. The family was responsible for the day-to-day care. Poor families were among the first persons to use hospitals. The philosophy of home care can be traced as far back as 1796, when the Boston Dispensary provided medical care to the sick poor in their homes. One of the first institutions to study and demonstrate the advantages of continuous medical care for patients at home was University Hospital in Syracuse, New York, in 1940. By 1950, 16 New York City hospitals were offering this service. In 1959 the Commission on Chronic Illness defined care of the aged and disabled as one of the foremost national health problems and recommended the development of home nursing care as an alternative to institutionalization.

One of the most obvious reasons for the development of home care programs was to provide care to patients with long-term illnesses who did not need the around-the-clock services of an institution and yet who were too ill to go to an outpatient center. Caring for patients at home is what the individual and the family often want, and it also releases hospital beds for use by acutely ill patients.

Recently home care has begun to be used for care of acutely ill patients who are discharged from the hospital earlier in their recovery than they were in the past. The introduction of prospective reimbursement for hospitals under DRGs has meant that many patients are being discharged while they still need skilled nursing care. As a result many hospitals have set up home care programs to supply nursing care and other services to their patients after discharge. Hospitals that have not set up their own programs are contracting with the visiting nurse associa-

tion and other community agencies to supply nursing care for their patients after discharge.

Frequently the issue arises as to who should pay for home health services and who should be reimbursed for health care provided. The American Nurses Association's (ANA's) position is that reimbursement systems should foster care of individuals in their homes based on the following premises[21]:

1. Home care is humane and respectful of the dignity and integrity of the individual.
2. Home care or care within the community can be less costly than institutional care.
3. Nursing care is the primary element in home care.
4. Payment systems for home care should recognize nurses as the major providers of home care, and as such their services should be reimbursed on their own authority.

Home care is not the solution for all patients. For those living in smaller dwellings, adequate space for the patient and other members of the family may be at a premium. The choice of home care, independent living center, or institutional care will depend largely on the desires of the patient and the family. Despite many inconveniences some families wish to have the patient with them. The family's understanding of the patient and their ability to assist one another will make a great difference in choosing between home care or other living arrangements. Not only may space be inadequate, but many times it is impossible to have a member of the family in attendance with the patient during the day. Members of the family who work cannot afford to sacrifice jobs to stay with the patient. However, many families find it easier financially to have the patient at home and are able to make satisfactory arrangements even though the facilities are limited.

Many communities now provide portable meals (Meals-on-Wheels) for homebound persons. Most programs provide one hot meal daily and unheated food for at least one other meal. The cost differs widely and depends on the services offered, such as special diets, and on the sponsorship of the plan. Volunteer groups frequently act as delivery messengers. The local public health nursing service usually participates actively in the plan by selecting suitable patients and by being a resource for the workers who encounter health problems on their "rounds." This service alone often makes it possible for a chronically ill or aged person to remain at home.

□ Home health aide services

Home health aide services have developed with the increased use of home care plans, particularly since Medicare plans came into existence. The greater number of persons eligible for home health aide services under Medicare has spurred the growth of such services, not because the services were not needed before, but because the cost of such services would have been prohibitive for most of the persons who needed them. Home health aides, who provide actual physical care to the patient, are trained and assigned to home care through a central office that coordinates plans of care, often in collaboration with community health nursing agencies. The community health nurse assists by evaluating the home situation and the patient's need for physical personal care. Consequently, the community health nurse supervises the home health aide in the provision of continuing care.

With the emphasis on shorter hospital stays, a number of proprietary agencies have entered the home health care field. These agencies provide a variety of health care services for a fee. Increasingly, insurance companies are reimbursing for these services since it is cheaper to provide care to the patient in his or her own home than in the hospital. Changes in home health care are occurring very rapidly and nurses will need to keep abreast of changes in their own communities.

□ Homemaker services

Homemaker services also have developed with the increased use of home care plans. These services are increasingly in demand in many communities and may be sponsored by a public or voluntary health or welfare agency. Homemakers provide service to families with children and to the person who is convalescing, aged, or acutely or chronically ill. Homemakers are trained to assist in homes where the responsible family manager is temporarily unable to perform his or her usual responsibilities because of illness or absence.

■ DAY CARE CENTERS

In a number of communities some nursing homes are expanding their facilities and services to include day care centers. There are a great number of chronically ill persons who are able to live with their families, but who require 24-hour attendance. Often the caretaker in the family has to work 8 hours a day. Homemaker or home health aide services are generally not available 8 hours a day, 5 days a week. Day care centers fill this gap in care by providing a place where the chronically ill person can be looked after on a daily basis. Nursing services, physical and occupational therapy, recreational facilities, meals, and in some instances, transportation to and from the center are provided. This kind of service may allow a person to remain at home with the family rather than having to resort to full-time institutional care.

■ RESPITE CARE CENTERS

Some nursing homes maintain a specified number of beds for respite care. As the name implies, these beds are available on a short-term basis to provide respite for families who have a chronically ill person at home. The day-to-day care of the patient, often on a 24-hour-per-day basis, is a very trying experience for any family. To provide the family or primary caretaker with a period free of this responsibility, respite care may be the answer. Usually the cost of respite care is not reimbursable, however, it may be the only alternative if the primary caregiver cannot continue to care for the family member without a respite.

Community health agencies, such as the Visiting Nurse Association, are also providing respite services in some cities. They will supply respite care in the patient's own home for part of a day, for 24 hours, or for extended periods of time depending on need. As mentioned above, the cost of this service is usually not reimbursable.

■ INDEPENDENT LIVING CENTERS

Some persons with chronic illnesses may be unable to cope with the demands of maintaining a home but wish to live as independently as possible. There are a variety of options available in some communities that range from living units where persons cook their own meals but are provided with maintenance of the living unit to assisted living units where persons can have their own physical living area but are assisted with activities of daily living, as necessary. Living units in such centers are designed with such features as hand rails for support in ambulation and wide doors to facilitate passage of wheelchairs.

■ FOSTER HOMES

Care in foster homes is a service that is now being widely used in many communities. Carefully selected families volunteer to take chronically ill persons into their own homes and provide the nonprofessional care that is needed. The family is paid either by the patient or the patient's family, from public funds, or by some social agency. The plan is primarily for those patients who have no family and cannot live alone, but who neither desire nor need institutional care.

■ INSTITUTIONAL SETTINGS

Many patients and families have to resort to institutional care for the patient because their own facilities are not suitable, no member of the family can be in attendance during the day, community alternatives are not available, or the kind of care needed by the person requires close professional supervision. A large or a limited selection of outside facilities may be available, depending on the community. These include chronic disease hospitals, skilled care facilities, convalescent homes, rest homes, homes for the aged, and nursing homes. The patient's potential for rehabilitation, need for maintenance care, or the level of physical disability are factors that will determine eligibility for placement in any of these facilities.

■ COMMUNITY RESOURCES

Nurses must know the community resources available to patients to interpret to them and their families what resources they may be able to obtain, the types of service from which they may benefit, and what kinds of referrals they need for obtaining those services (see list of community resources). When care is to be continued beyond the hospital setting, the hospital nurse should clearly com-

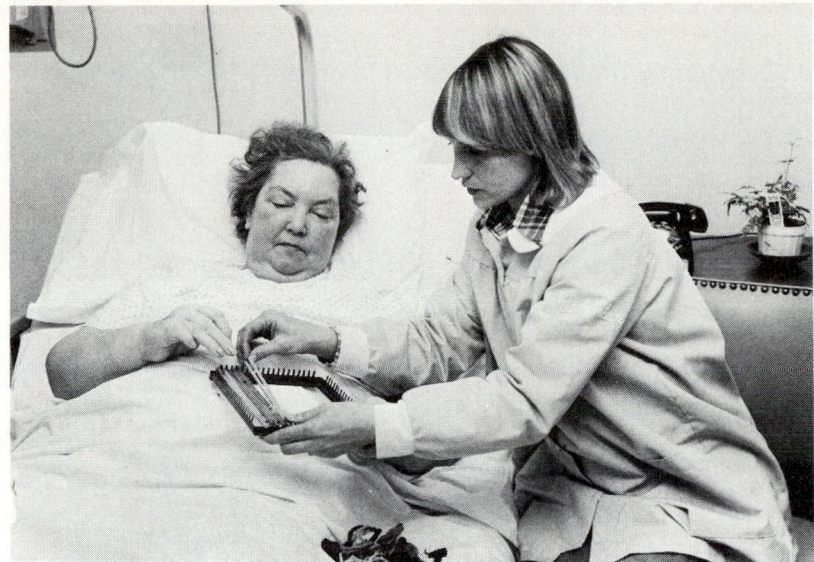

Fig. 14-5 Volunteers can actively involve patients in activities that provide diversion as well as a sense of accomplishment. Nurses often provide assistance or encouragement for completion of projects.

municate to the continuing care agency data pertinent to the care of the patient to provide continuity in the transfer of services. Teamwork and continuity are the keys to successful rehabilitation and management services for patients, and they must be practiced in all stages of care if patients are to realize their fullest potential.

There has been an increasing interest in providing programs for the chronically ill and in assisting chronically ill or disabled persons to assume a more active role in their communities. Volunteer workers may assist patients, both in hospitals and in homes (Fig. 14-5). Institutions receiving federal funds are required to make aids such as ramps available to individuals who are unable to climb stairs or who are in wheelchairs. With the development of structural changes that facilitate mobility, some persons with physical limitations are becoming more actively involved in local activities and associations. Nurses can assist by supporting the further development of these structural changes in all community buildings and by encouraging the participation of chronically ill persons in community activities of interest. Various kinds of information may be obtained from national organizations involved with chronic illness and disability. Many of these agencies have services available in the community. Programs, facilities, and legislation of this nature reflect an increasing awareness on the part of the public of the difficulties that are faced by the chronically ill or disabled (see the box on p. 308).

■ FOCUS ON THE FUTURE

In 1979, the Surgeon General's Report established five goals concerned with major health problems in the United States. The time frame for the achievement of these goals was to be 1990.[32] Recent changes in priorities at the federal level make it doubtful that many of the goals will be achieved by that date. However, it is important that nurses be aware of these goals and their relationship to chronic health problems. The goals are listed below:

1. *To continue to improve infant health and, by 1990, to reduce infant mortality by at least 35%, to fewer than 9 deaths per 1000 live births.* The two principal threats to infant survival and good health are low birth weight and congenital disorders, including birth defects. Low birth weight may be associated with long-term health problems such as mental retardation, cerebral palsy, and other conditions that impede growth and development. Many birth defects, including congenital disorders, mental retardation, and genetic diseases are immediate serious hazards to infants. Many others, if not diagnosed and treated immediately after birth or during the first year of life, can affect health and well-being in the later years.

2. *To improve child health, foster optimal childhood development, and, by 1990, to reduce deaths among people aged 1 to 14 years by at least 20%, to fewer than 34 per 100,000.* The major cause of death among children is accidents, followed by cancer, birth defects, influenza and pneumonia, and homicide. But not all health problems are reflected in mortality figures. Habits and attitudes developed during childhood can lead to adult disease and disability. As many as 40% of school children ages 11 to 14 are estimated to already have one or more of the risk factors associated with heart disease: overweight, high blood pressure, high blood cholesterol, cigarette smoking, poor physical fitness, or diabetes.

3. *To improve the health and health habits of adolescents and young adults and, by 1990, to reduce deaths among people aged 15 to 24 by at least 20%, to fewer than 9.3 per 100,000.*

Community resources involved in chronic health problems

Various kinds of information may be obtained by writing these national organizations. In addition, services of the various agencies are usually available at the local level.

General

American Association of Diabetes Education
3553 W. Peterson Ave.
Chicago, IL 60659

American Association of Retired Persons
1909 K St., N.W.
Washington, DC 20006

American Cancer Society
777 3rd Ave.
New York, NY 10017

American Diabetes Association
1 W. 48th St.
New York, NY 10020

American Heart Association 44 E. 23rd St.
New York, NY 10010

American Lung Association
1740 Broadway
New York, NY 10019

American Parkinson Disease Association
147 E. 50th St.
New York, NY 10022

Arthritis Foundation
221 Park Ave. S.
New York, NY 10003

Leukemia Society of America, Inc.
211 E. 43rd St. New York, NY 10017

Mental Health Materials Center
419 Park Ave. S.
New York, NY 10016

Muscular Dystrophy Association, Inc.
810 7th Ave.
New York, NY 10019

National Aid to Retarded Citizens (formerly N.A.R.
Children)
2709 E. St.
Arlington, TX 76011

National Association for Visually Handicapped
305 E. 24th St.
New York, NY 10010

National Asthma Center
875 Avenue of the Americas
New York, NY 10001

National Council on the Aging
1828 L. St. NW
Washington, DC 20036

National Kidney Foundation
116 E. 27th St.
New York, NY 10016

National Multiple Sclerosis Society
205 E. 42nd St.
New York, NY 10017

Nutrition Foundation, Inc.
489 5th Ave.
New York, NY 10017

Stroke Clubs of America
805 12th St.
Galveston, TX 77550

United Ostomy Association
1111 Wilshire Blvd.
Los Angeles, CA 90017

Rehabilitation

American Coalition of Citizens with Disabilities
1346 Connecticut Ave. N.W., Rm. 817
Washington, DC 20036

Architectural and Transportation Barriers Compliance
Board
330 C St. W.W., Rm. 1010
Washington, DC 20201

Closer Look, National Information Center for the
Handicapped
Box 1492
Washington, DC 20013

Mainstream, Inc.
1200 15th St., N.W., Rm. 403
Washington, DC 20005

National Center for a Barrier-free Environment
8401 Connecticut Ave.
Washington, DC 20015

National Center for Law and the Handicapped
1235 N. Eddy St.
South Bend, IN 46617

National Congress of Organizations of the Physically
   Handicapped
7611 Oakland Ave.
Minneapolis, MN 55432

National Paraplegia Foundation
333 N. Michigan Ave.
Chicago, IL 60601

Paralyzed Veterans of America
7315 Wisconsin Ave. N.W.
Washington, DC 20014

President's Committee on Employment of the
   Handicapped
111 20th St. N.W., Rm. 636
Washington, DC 20210

Prevention/wellness

American Association of Fitness Directors in Business
   and Industry
President's Council on Physical Fitness and Sports
Room 3030
400 Sixth Ave. S.W.
Washington, DC 20201

Bureau of Health Education
Centers for Disease Control
Atlanta, GA 30333

Center for Health Promotion
American Hospital Association
840 N. Lake Shore Dr.
Chicago, IL 60611

Know Your Body Project
American Health Foundation
320 East 43rd St.
New York, NY 10017

Society of Prospective Medicine
Department of Family Medicine
University of South Florida
12901 North 30th St.
Tampa, FL 33612

Well Aware About Health
University of Arizona Health Sciences Center
P.O. Box 43338
Tucson, AZ 85733

Wellness Associates
42 Miller Ave.
Mill Valley, CA 94941

Wholistic Health Center
137 S. Garfield Ave.
Hinsdale, IL 60521

Despite improvements in health over the past 75 years, death rates for adolescents and young adults are increasing. The principal health problems of this age group include violent death and injury, sexually transmitted diseases, alcohol and drug abuse, and emotional problems. Young men are at particular risk, since their death rate is almost three times that of young women. Although chronic diseases are not among the major causes of death at this period of life, the life-styles and behavioral patterns that are shaped during these years may determine later susceptibility to chronic diseases.

4. *To improve the health of adults, and, by 1990, to reduce deaths among people aged 25 to 64 by at least 25%, to fewer than 400 per 100,000.* The leading causes of death in this age group are heart disease, cancer, stroke, and cirrhosis of the liver. Accidents are a prominent problem for the younger members of this group, but overall the chronic diseases predominate. In addition to causes of death, disability from mental illness presents a major health problem. More than one third of all deaths in this group are caused by cardiovascular diseases, principally coronary artery dis-

ease and stroke. However, such deaths have declined in recent years and account for most of the recent decreases in mortality.

5. *To improve the health and quality of life for older adults and, by 1990, to reduce the average annual number of days of restricted activity resulting from acute and chronic conditions by 20%, to fewer than 30 days per year for people aged 65 and over.* Today there are 24 million people aged 65 years and over in the United States, accounting for 11% of the population. This group is the fastest growing segment of the population. By the year 2030 there will be more than 50 million Americans in the over-65 group, and they will represent nearly 17% of the population. The leading causes of death for this age group are heart disease, cancer, stroke, influenza, and pneumonia. The long-term goal of a health-promotion and disease-prevention strategy for older people must be not only to achieve further increases in longevity but also to allow such individuals to seek independent and rewarding lives in their older age—lives that are unlimited by the many health problems that are within their capacity to control.

Even though it is possible to identify health goals for a nation, it is far more difficult to carry them out so that the effect is noticeable to the individual seeking health care.

The challenge of providing health care to all people includes the challenge to promote the full participation of individuals and physical and mental disabilities. The United Nations proclaimed 1981 as the International Year of Disabled Persons (IYDP). The United States Council for the IYDP worked to strengthen public understanding of the needs and contributions of 35 million people. The council defined the following long-term national goals of and for the disabled:

1. Expanded educational opportunities
2. Improved access to housing, buildings, and transportation
3. Greater opportunity for employment
4. Broader recreational, social, and cultural activities
5. Expanded and strengthened rehabilitation programs and facilities
6. Increased biomedical research aimed at conquering major disabling conditions
7. Reduced incidence of disability through accident and disease prevention
8. Increased application of technology on behalf of persons with disabilities
9. Expanded international exchange of information and experience to benefit the disabled everywhere

The commitment of health care providers must be not only to find ways to help the disabled and other chronically ill individuals cope with chronic health problems but also to educate individuals in the prevention of disease and the promotion of health.

■ SUMMARY

1. Chronic health problems is one of the major health problems in the United States.
2. The incidence and prevalence of chronic diseases have increased in this century and can be expected to increase even more as the population ages.
3. The Bureau of the Census estimates that approximately 110 million persons in the United States have one or more chronic illnesses.
4. There are major disparities in the health of black Americans and other minorities in the United States when compared with the white population.
5. The characteristics of chronic illnesses include one or more of the following: (1) illness or impairment that is permanent, (2) residual disability, and (3) nonreversible pathologic alteration, which requires a long period of care.
6. Chronic illnesses may be present from birth or develop during childhood, adolescence, early adult life, or old age.
7. Today some children with chronic illnesses such as cystic fibrosis live into early adulthood because of more effective treatment.
8. Major chronic illnesses of adults include arthritis, diabetes, heart disease, and hypertension. The rates for arthritis and hypertension are higher in blacks than in whites.
9. Cultural values determine how both nurses and patients view chronic illness.
10. The economic costs of chronic illness are considerable and many persons will require some type of financial assistance.
11. Failure to understand or internalize the reason for therapeutic recommendations, procedures that are difficult to learn and carry out, time necessary to carry out therapy, side effects of therapy, inability to pay for prescribed therapy and social isolation and lack of support and positive reinforcement are possible reasons why a person may be noncompliant with therapeutic recommendations.
12. It is important that nurses be involved in prevention of chronic illness.
13. There are 3 levels of prevention: primary, secondary, and tertiary, and the nurse has an important role to play at each level.
14. Primary prevention involves health promotion and specific protection against disease (such as immunization against poliomyelitis).

Putting knowledge to practice

■ What types of patients do you think are most in need of rehabilitation? Outline the rehabilitation needs of a patient you are now caring for or have cared for in the past.

■ What proportion of the patients on the hospital unit to which you are assigned have a chronic illness as either their primary or secondary diagnosis? What proportion has more than one chronic health problem? What age group is affected most by more than one chronic health problem?

■ What resources are available in your community for the care of the chronically ill? Are the facilities adequate for the number of persons needing care? How are these facilities supported financially?

■ From what you have learned in anatomy, outline in detail the physical movements necessary to rise from a sitting position in a chair to a standing position. Describe how you would assist a patient to stand while allowing him or her to be as independent as possible.

15. Secondary prevention includes early detection of disease and prompt intervention to halt progression of disease.
16. Tertiary prevention includes rehabilitation appropriate to the stage of disability, prevention of further complications, and restoring optimal functioning to the highest possible level.
17. Depression is common among the chronically ill, especially those who feel powerless about controlling or overcoming what has happened to them.
18. Rehabilitation is best carried out in a setting where a multidisciplinary team of nurses, physicians, physical and occupational therapists, social workers and, when necessary, speech therapists are available to work together in planning the therapeutic regimen for the patient and in assisting and supporting the patient with the prescribed therapy.
19. The two major roles of the nurse working with persons with disabilities are (1) to limit disability from disease as much as possible and (2) to see that the rehabilitation program is planned and implemented.
20. The nurse should be familiar with the facilities for continuing care in his or her community and the eligibility requirements for each facility.

REFERENCES AND SELECTED READINGS

Contemporary

1. American Cancer Society: 1987 Cancer facts and figures, New York, 1987, The Society.
2. *Anderson, SV, and Bauwens, EE: Chronic health problems: concepts and application, St. Louis, 1981, The CV Mosby Co.
3. Centers for Disease Control: Morbidity and mortality report, Feb. 28, 1986, Vol. 35, No. 8, Massachusetts Medical Society.
4. Expectation of life in the United States at a new high, Stat Bull 61(4):13-15, 1980.
5. *Johnson, JH, editor: Rehabilitation Nursing, Nurs Clin North Am 15:2, June, 1980.
6. Kottke, F, Stilwell, GK, and Lehman, J: Krusen's handbook of physical medicine and rehabilitation, ed 3, Philadelphia, 1982, WB Saunders Co.
7. *Lambert, VA, and Lambert, CE, editors: Adaptation to chronic illness, Nurs Clin North Am 22:527-644, 1987.
8. *Leslie, FM: Nursing diagnosis: use in long-term care, Am J Nurs 81:1012-1014, 1981.
9. *Martin, N, Holt, NB, Hicks, D: Comprehensive rehabilitation nursing, New York, 1981, McGraw-Hill Book Co.
10. Morris, R, editor: Allocating health resources for the aged and disabled, Lexington, Mass., 1981, Lexington Books.
11. National Center for Health Statistics: Vital statistics of the United States, 1980, Vol 11, Mortality, Part B, DHHS, Pub No. (PHS) 85-1102, Washington, DC, 1985, US Government Printing Office.
12. Pollock, SE: Human responses to chronic illness: physiologic and psychosocial adaptation, Nurs Res 35:90-95, March-April 1986.
13. Public Health Service: Vital and health statistics: current estimates from the Health Interview Survey (1981) U.S. Department of Health, Education and Welfare, series 10, No. 141, Rockville, Md, Oct 1982.
14. Public Health Service: Vital and health statistics: health characteristics of persons with chronic activity limitations (1979), US Department of Health and Human Services, series 10, No. 137, Rockville, Md, Dec 1981.
15. *Ryan, S, and Wassenberg, C, editors: Community health and home care nursing, Nurs Clin North Am 15:2, June, 1980.
16. Strauss, AL, and others: Chronic illness and the quality of life, ed 2, St. Louis, 1984, The CV Mosby Co.
17. Thom, A: Home health care agencies in the 1980s, Home Health Care Serv Q 3:5-24, 1982.
18. US Department of Commerce, Bureau of the Census, Statistical abstract of the US, 1986, US Government Printing Office.
19. *Wright, BA: Value-laden beliefs and principles for rehabilitation, Rehabil Lit 42:266-269, 1981.

Classic

20. *American Academy of Nursing: Long-term care: some issues for nursing, Kansas City, Mo, 1976, American Nurses Association.
21. *American Nurses Association: A national policy for health care: principles and positions, Kansas City, Mo, 1977, The Association.
22. Crate, M: Nursing functions in adaptation to chronic illness, Am J Nurs 65:72-76, 1965.
23. Garrett, JF, and Levine, ES: Psychological practices with the physically disabled, New York, 1962, Columbia University Press.
24. Lefkowitz, B: Health differentials between white and non-white Americans, Washington, DC, 1977, US Government Printing Office.
25. *Martin, N, King, R, and Suchinski, J: The nurse therapist in the rehabilitation setting, Am J Nurs 70:1694-1697, 1970.
26. Moskowitz, E, and McCann, CB: Classification of disability in the chronically ill and aging, J Chronic Dis 5:342-346, 1957.
27. *Olson, EV, editor: The hazards of immobility, Am J Nurs 67:780-797, 1967.
28. Rettig, RA: End-stage renal disease and the cost of medical technology. In Altman, SH, and Blendon, RJ, editors: Medical technology: the culprit behind health care costs? DHEW Pub No. PHS-79-3216, Washington, DC, 1979, US Government Printing Office.
29. Rush, H: Rehabilitation medicine, ed 4, St. Louis, 1977, The CV Mosby, Co.
30. *Sorensen, K, and Armis, DB: Understanding the world of the chronically ill, Am J Nurs 67:811-817, 1967.
31. Strauss, AL: Chronic illness and the quality of life, St. Louis, 1975, The CV Mosby Co.
32. US Department of Health, Education and Welfare: Healthy people. Surgeon General's report on health promotion and disease prevention, Washington, DC 1979, US Government Printing Office.

*References preceded by an asterisk are particularly well suited for student reading.

15

Dying, Death, and Loss

BENITA C. MARTOCCHIO

CHAPTER OBJECTIVES

After studying this chapter, the student should be able to:

- Differentiate among dying, death, and loss; define clinical death.
- Identify some rights of dying persons and describe a "living will."
- How do autonomy, informed consent, and paternalism relate to quality of life for the dying person?
- Describe four attitudinal dimensions of death: denial, defiance, desire, and acceptance.
- Describe the stages/phases of dying proposed by Kubler-Ross, Pattison, and Martocchio.
- Describe effects on the family when a family member dies.
- Differentiate among grief, bereavement, and mourning, and describe the grief syndrome.
- Identify assessment parameters for the dying person.
- Describe general nursing interventions for grievers and the dying person.

Despite the amazing advances of science, nursing, and medical knowledge, dying is and will continue to be a part of living. The fact is that at some future time we will cease "to be." In a sense we are dying even as we are living. To conceptualize living and dying as the opposite ends of a continuum creates a false dichotomy. Living and dying are not opposite ends of a continuum; they are the continuum.

When we interact with persons who are known to have a life-threatening disease, we are more directly confronted with their dying and our own finiteness. This confrontation evokes anxiety, and thus we become more aware of the dying component of living. Although we may identify with the suffering and sorrow of persons as they live their dying, we interact with living persons. To appreciate our own and others' responses to loss, dying, and death, we need an understanding of the context in which they occur and our own views and reactions within varying contexts.

Even though dying and grief are personal and vary from one person to another, it is the purpose of this chapter to share understandings and to offer general guidelines that assist in caring for persons who are dying and in helping family members who are sharing the experience. Loss is the underlying theme. Perhaps the most beneficial way to learn to care effectively for dying persons and their families is to understand our own perspectives and those of others on loss, dying, and death.

■ SOCIETAL AND SOCIAL DIMENSIONS

■ Dying and death are different

Dying is different than death. *Dying,* a part of living, is a *process*—the process of coming to an end. *Death,* the permanent cessation of all vital functions, the end of human life, is an *event* and a *state*. The event is the moment of death; the state is that of being dead.[11]

Both dying and death have unique aspects that evoke fears, anxieties, and uncertainties. Some aspects of dying, such as physical and emotional pain, the loss of others, the inability to function in familiar ways, may occur under other circumstances (for example, illness, retirement relocation) and therefore are not unique to dying. The unique aspect of dying is that it ends in death. People have no prior experiences to help them to understand what it means to be dead. Questions surface: Can dead persons think? Can they have feelings? What is it like to be dead? Is there another life? Where will they go?

■ My death: your death

The knowledge that death is imminent or probably within a predicted period of time adds reality to feelings of fear, anxiety, and uncertainty.[13,26] As a result, persons facing imminent death experience these emotions differently than do healthy persons who are speculating about what it is like to be dying. Healthy persons speak of death in the abstract: they talk about the death of another or

project it into the distant future. People cannot imagine the actual end of their own lives on earth. Casual comments such as, "We all have to die some day," "We are all dying from the time we are born," or "Everyone has to die of something," reflect what Freud called "unconscious immortality." The fact that people can continue to think about others who have died causes them to believe unconsciously in their own immortality. But hearing of someone else's dying or death forces them to face their own finiteness.

Neither the casual comments nor the unconscious belief in one's own immortality are good or bad in and of themselves. However, they offer little in the way of understanding or support when made to a dying person or to the family. The statements are usually in response to the discomfort felt when someone says that death is imminent. A more understanding response might be, "I'm sorry to hear that."

Views toward dying and death vary considerably depending on whether the discussion is about *my* death or *your* death or if the discussion is about a member of my family or your family.

Even when we are discussing hypothetic situations, our closeness to dying or to a dying person can influence our views and our responses. The same data are seen differently from different perspectives. We can use age as a common factor and consider how our responses may change. For example, *my* father is 75 years old, and *your* father is 75 years old. When death appears imminent, our thoughts may vary depending on the referent of *my* or *your* father. For example, *my* father is still young; *your* father has lived a long and a good life.

It is important to identify the referrant under discussion whether we are talking in theoretic terms or about practical situations. In other words, from whose perspective are we evaluating the situation, my perspective, your perspective, the patient's perspective, or a family member's perspective?

Lack of recognition of different perspectives leads to poor communication, faulty nursing judgments, and inappropriate nursing interventions.

■ Age and premature death

There was a time when people did not make a connection between aging, loss of bodily functioning, or general progressive debilitation and dying. For example, primitive people believed that if there were no accidents or magically induced illnesses, no one would die.

The expectations of living have changed as life expectancies have changed. During the Roman period, life expectancy was 20 years and increased to about 35 during the Middle Ages. By the late 1800s Americans could anticipate living 50 years; few persons lived into their 60s or 70s. In contemporary American life, people not only anticipate living more than 70 years, they expect to do so as active functioning individuals.

Many people believe that any age is too young to die. In contemporary society, death is perceived as unnecessary, premature, and clinically unnecessary. The concept of clinical death is well entrenched.[21] People do not die of natural causes or of old age. They die while receiving treatment for a recognized diagnosed clinical problem, for example, heart disease, stroke, disseminated intravascular coagulation (DIC), or total body failure. As a consequence, many deaths can be interpreted as avoidable, unnecessary, and premature.

If death is always interpreted as avoidable, unnecessary, or premature, it follows that someone must be blamed. Who can we blame—the physician, the hospital, society? Perhaps we blame the person who died for not getting help sooner, for surely if they had sought help sooner they would not have died. It is this interpretation of death as always being avoidable that contributes to conflict and guilt. People die; death is a part of living. We can give the best care we know and people will die. In fact sometimes the very mechanisms that saves lives creates dilemmas by prolonging life or dying.

Rights of dying persons

Some health care consumers are demanding that dying and death no longer be hidden behind closed doors. As a consequence, there is a movement to recognize that dying persons have rights.[6]

One right of dying persons is the right to know they are seriously ill and that they may die. The assumption is that such information will ensure that they will have more control over what happens to them. As a result, they can participate in decisions about their care and can complete unfinished business.

Another right is to die in an atmosphere of hopefulness. Persons have a right to die in peace and dignity unencumbered by tubes and machines and surrounded by loved ones. They have a right to privacy. Dying persons are entitled to be cared for by sensitive, caring, knowledgeable people who attempt to understand them and their loved ones. They are entitled to die as free from pain or other dicomforts as is possible. Comfort contributes to dying with a sense of self-esteem and gives meaning to life.

■ THE LIVING WILL

The concern that patients be allowed to die with dignity has led to the development of the living will. The living will is a document that is directed toward any individual who may become responsible for the person's health, welfare, or affairs. It may be directed toward the person's family, lawyer, clergyperson, or physician or representatives of any medical facility in which the person may be.

Living wills generally request that under conditions when (1) the individual can no longer take part in decisions about his or her own future and (2) there is no reasonable expectation for recovery, the individual be allowed to die and not be kept alive through use of artificial or extraordinary means. Most wills also request that the person be kept free of suffering and pain although the medications may hasten the moment of death.

At the present time, living wills are not legally enforceable in all states. In addition, there are many questions

---

Example of a living will

To my family, my physician, my lawyer, my clergyman
To any medical facility in whose care I happen to be
To any individual who may become responsible for my health, welfare, or affairs

Death is as much a reality as birth, growth, maturity, and old age; it is the one certainty of life. If the time comes when I, (Name), can no longer take part in decisions for my own future, let this statement stand as an expression of my wishes, while I am still of sound mind.

If the situation should arise in which there is no reasonable expectation of my recovery from physical or mental disability, I request that I be allowed to die and not be kept alive by artificial means or "heroic measures." I do not fear death itself as much as the indignities of deterioration, dependence, mental incapacity, and hopeless pain. I, therefore, ask that medication be mercifully administered to me to alleviate suffering even though this may hasten the moment of death.

This request is made after careful consideration. I hope you who care for me will feel morally bound to follow its mandate. I recognize that this appears to place a heavy responsibility on you, but it is with the intention of relieving you of such responsibility and of placing it on myself in accordance with my strong convictions, that this statement is made.

_____
(Signature)

Witnessed
Copies to: (names of persons)

related to the conditions under which a living will can or should be honored. What is important for purposes of this chapter is that a living will can help caregivers and family members to know what the dying person's wishes were, at least at the time of the writing.

Copies of living wills are usually given to family members, physicians, the person's attorney, and a member of the clergy. People are advised to sign and date them, at least yearly. The wills are more likely to be honored if they are written or signed immediately before the person's becoming unable to express his or her own wishes about dying care. The box on p. 315 is an example of a living will.

A sharing of philosophy of life and desires related to the process of dying with loved ones and primary health care providers is perhaps a more effective way of assuring death with dignity or what has been referred to as a "good death."

◼ Good death/bad death

Many nurses, and in fact people in general, express concern over dying with dignity or dying a "good" death. Is there such a thing as a "good death?" There is no one "good" death but many. There is no one right way to die, just as there is no one right way to live.

There are many views about what constitutes a good death. To die as one lived, to die without pain, to die in the company of loved ones are all answers.

There are many ways to die well. A good death involves individual perceptions of the living-dying process, as well as shared observations of the death event. A death is more likely to be labeled as good when dying is viewed as a part of living and not as a separate phenomenon. A good death also is associated with the way all persons involved interact with each other preceding and during the event. The death is more likely to be seen as good if there is harmony than if there is conflict.

Sometimes nurses refer to deaths as normal or abnormal. Deaths are perceived as normal or good when most or all persons involved perceive that all was done that could be done, that the actions were appropriate and accepted by most persons involved. In these instances there is a sense of loss, but the loss is accompanied by a sense of fulfillment and closure. Nurses label deaths as bad or abnormal when there is conflict over the type of treatment, the length of treatment, and when there are bad feelings about a lack of honesty, especially with family members.

Thus, whether a death is seen as good or bad does not always have to do entirely with the way the person died. Sometimes it has to do with who is present and how they interpret what is happening in the situation. People's attitudes toward dying influence how they interpret the situation and how they act and interact with others.

◼ ETHICAL DIMENSIONS

With the advent of modern therapeutics, the capacity to prolong life has improved to a great extent, but the improvement has been accompanied by some difficult consequences. More and more often death is caused by some-

one's decision rather than the failure of the heart to pump blood or the lungs to breathe.

Death becomes impersonal when the body and the tubes and machines become one and when there is only a deteriorating organ system present. The situation becomes so confusing that those involved have conferences to determine whether life or death is being prolonged.

When a dying person has been termed nonperson and seems neither dead nor alive, all involved persons search for resolution of a situation where neither grief nor hope is appropriate. Family members long to return to normal living. They search for help in making life and death decisions for loved ones who are no longer able to contribute to decision making. Staff members search for relief from a situation fraught with dilemmas.

Discussions of such issues as "quality of life," "right to die," "death with dignity," "living wills," and "informed consent" in lay literature and professional literature demonstrate the extent and awareness of the conflicts associated with modern therapies that may extend life but at a great cost. Concern over decisions regarding life and death issues has led to the development of organizations that represent differing views. The Hemlock Society,[9] the Society for the Right to Die,[20] and the Americans United for Life are examples of a few of these organizations.

Many ethical issues evolve around indications for medical and nursing interventions. These issues arise from such questions as the following: When should medical therapies be started or stopped? When should life supports be discontinued? What constitutes death? Who should decide?

◼ Terminating or withholding treatment

In principle, the most obvious ethical justification for terminating or withholding treatment is that it is ineffective. There is no moral obligation to perform useless or futile interventions. In fact, in some instances it can be argued that some therapies do more harm than good. This justification seems clear but is not particularly useful in clinical practice, because it is difficult to distinguish between long-term and short-term efficacy and to judge how long to wait before identifying a therapy as not effective. In addition, it is difficult to evaluate when or if withdrawing treatment constitutes euthanasia.

◼ Euthanasia

Euthanasia comes from the Greek words meaning good or pleasant death. It implies that under some circumstances death may be preferable to life for an individual. Euthanasia or "mercy killing" is a topic surrounded by controversy. At the present time, there is no agreement on whether death is ever preferable to life for an individual or on what constitutes euthanasia.

Several distinctions are made when discussing euthanasia, the more common being active/passive and voluntary/involuntary. *Active euthanasia* refers to an act that directly and intentionally shortens a person's life. It is an act of *commission*. *Passive euthanasia*, an act of *omission*, usually refers to letting die by either withholding or withdrawing a treatment that might prolong a person's life.

Voluntary euthanasia refers to the involvement of the dying person in the manner and procedures leading to the person's death. The involvement may be through active participation during the dying period or by making wishes known through a living will or other means before the period of imminent death. Sometimes it is necessary to presume the intent of voluntary euthanasia by considering what the patient would have wanted if able to participate in the decisions regarding the circumstances of the death. The latter is especially true in unexpected events such as accidents, strokes, and cardiac disease, in which the person may have lost consciousness and may not have had the opportunity to express wishes regarding the circumstances of dying. In this situation, a clearly written living will that is carried out in good faith serves as a safeguard of the dying person's rights.

A look at questions related to euthanasia reveals a continuum ranging from a strict belief in the sanctity of life (antieuthanasia, treating at all costs) to passive euthanasia (letting die) to active euthanasia (ending life).

A persistent moral issue is the question of whether letting die is morally equivalent to killing, or omission equivalent to commission. Active and passive euthanasia are intentional choices. The distinction seems to be that of the intent of the action. Letting die in the sense of not instituting extraordinary efforts or by discontinuing extraordinary treatments is morally permissible and is not considered "killing." In fact, most physicians accept that killing a patient is morally wrong and thus not permissible, but in some circumstances it may become morally required to let a patient die.[23] Nurses generally accept the same view.

In some circumstances, "to let die" instead of "to kill" implies that there is some possibility that the patient may recover, go into remission, or survive long enough for some new therapy to be discovered. It is an attempt to "buy time" for the patient. The difficult question is: Is the bought time quality time; that is, is it a meaningful enriching experience, or is it a hard time filled with meaningless suffering?

■ Quality of life

What constitutes quality of life? Who can predict what quality of life is or will be during the dying process? Can one person judge the quality of life of another, especially if the other is dying?

Dying persons may perceive quality of life differently from those who are living with an acute or chronic illness or who are well. What constitutes quality of life differs from person to person and for any one person during the various stages of life. What contributes to the *meaningfulness of life* may be a more cogent question than what constitutes quality of life when considering the dying person. For example, depression can be expected but how much and for how long? A person can live with pain, anxiety, and fear but how much and for how long? How much control does the person have over the situation? Can we increase the control they can have in the situation, al-

though they have lost control over dying? Do the symptoms detract from the meaning of life from the perspective of the dying person? Many ethical principles are called into play when considering meaningfulness of life. Patient preferences are important because they make explicit the values of autonomy and self-determination.

■ AUTONOMY

Dying persons must have freedom to choose a style of dying and then be assisted in that choice. Autonomy addresses the individual's right to control his or her own fate. Respect for the patient's autonomy is the moral stance that deters a person from interfering with another person's beliefs and actions. The legal counterpart of autonomy is *self-determination* or the legal right of every human being of adult years and of sound mind to determine what shall be done with his or her body.[10]

■ INFORMED CONSENT

Determining what shall be done implies making *informed* choices. Meaningful information presented in an understandable fashion is necessary to make informed choices or to give what is referred to as *informed consent*.

Informed consent, then, becomes an important factor in supporting meaningfulness of life. It includes giving dying people sufficient information about their diagnoses, prognoses, and possible therapies so they make informed choices about how they will live or die and about who will help them and in what ways. Informed consent is a person's agreement to allow something to happen on the basis of a full disclosure of facts needed to make an intelligent decision. Informed consent reinforces the value of personal autonomy.

Informed consent assumes that the person has the emotional and mental ability to understand, to process data, and to make decisions. This ability is sometimes referred to as competence or mental capacity. *Mental capacity* refers to the ability to understand the situation and make decisions about it. The mentally capable dying person has the

---

Assessment of mental capacity

Orientation to time, place, person, and situation
Ability to recall recurrent and past events and to sequence events logically
Ability to understand abstract ideas
Ability to make reasoned judgments
Psychological state, mood, and affect that may affect ability to make choices (for example, anxiety, fear, depression, suicidal ideation, hallucinations, delusions, illusions)
History of psychiatric disorders that could impact on present judgments

right to refuse or to request treatment. As in other situations, it is not a simple matter. What makes a person mentally capable or incapable? The box on p. 317 suggests some of the components of a systematic assessment of mental capacity and factors that could influence judgments.

■ PATERNALISM

A significant ethical and legal problem associated with the principle of autonomy is the problem of paternalism. Paternalism is a refusal to accept or acquiesce to another person's wishes, choices, or actions for that person's own benefit.[3] Traditionally medical practice and, by association, nursing practice has been paternalistic. Physicians have concealed diagnoses and prognoses from patients "for their own good." Nurses, although often not in agreement with concealing information, act in a paternalistic way by participating in the subterfuge to "protect the patient from conflict." The ethical questions are: Is paternalism ever justified? If so, under what circumstances? More specifically, should all dying persons be told they are dying? When, by whom, and in what manner should they be told? Does lack of total disclosure constitute paternalism?

■ Definitions of death

Much controversy surrounds the question, What is death? Is death the irreversible cessation of respiration and circulation, or is death the irreversible cessation of all functions of the entire brain, including the brainstem?

The term *brain dead,* introduced in recent years, causes much confusion. Originally it referred to a person whose heart and lungs were activated by a respirator but whose centers in the brain stem were destroyed. Removal from the support system would end in death caused by the inability of the person to resume spontaneous breathing. In addition, brain dead means that the person is dead in the sense that a functioning brain is the seat of identity. However, what decisions can be made about persons in a "persistent vegetative state"? They show no evidence of cortical functioning but continue to have sustained capacity for spontaneous breathing and heart beat.

Use of different definitions are appealed to as a rationale for different actions. Each appeal or action has its own consequences. For example, the use of brain dead definitions provides more latitude for organ transplants and experimentation. The rationale for this latitude is that "harvesting organs" is done to aid the living. A worthy endeavor, but does harvesting organs lead to violation of the dead? What are the constraints? Are the bodies being used with the consent of the donor, or is consent unnecessary once a person is dead?

No clear rules dictate decisions in these matters. Decisions depend upon discretion and reflection on basic values. They are accompanied by conflict, insecurity, and discomfort. The conflict and emotions that accompany decisions about the life or death of another are entirely appropriate because they are irreversible.

The important thing in any ethical dilemma, regardless of whether it is dealing with euthanasia, quality of life, or treatment decisions, is to be aware of the values or forces that lead us to make decisions. An understanding or our own values and perspectives does not give explicit answers to dilemmas but does help us to be consistent and to communicate with others in a way that is understandable. This does not ensure agreement, but it does facilitate discussion and attention to multiple perspectives and to the consequences of actions.

■ ATTITUDINAL DIMENSIONS

Death, denial, death defiance, death desire, and death acceptance are four prevailing societal attitudes toward death. As these general attitudes are discussed, it is important to remember that they may vary in different situations, depending on whose death is involved.

Recognition of the prevailing attitudes and their differences helps health care professionals to understand the process of dying, serves as a guide when interacting with others, helps them to avoid conflicts among themselves, and most importantly, enhances communication and thus patient care.

No attitude is good or bad; attitudes are different. Our behavior reflects our attitudes. If we recognize our own attitudes toward dying and death in a particular situation, as well as those of the others involved, we may understand better why all of us feel the way we do and why we are acting the way we are. This recognition and understanding may not always lead to agreement, but it can contribute to modifications of behavior and to decreased conflict in decision making. These attitudes are explored briefly in the following sections.

■ Death denial

Western society has been described as a death-denying society.[22] Many people avoid the subject of dying and death. Health professionals, particularly physicians, have been described as being unwilling to talk to patients about their dying.[24] Both health professionals and family members often justify their stance by expressing the belief that they are "protecting" the dying person.

The question is, whom are they protecting? In most situations they are protecting themselves; that is, consciously or unconsciously, they weigh the impact on themselves and decide or choose not to act because of fear of the reaction or response. The following questions often arise: What will happen to me? Will I lose emotional control? Will the other person shout, cry, or become angry? Will the family become angry? Will the physician become angry? Will I know what to do or say?

In nursing a death-denying attitude has taken on a negative connotation. But *no attitude in and of itself is good or bad*—it just is. The actions and consequences of an attitude can be evaluated as good or bad. For example, a death-denying attitude may contribute to a lack of open communication about dying, but it may also contribute to continuing care in bleak situations. A behavior or action such as continuation of care may reflect more than one attitude, such as both death denial and death defiance.

■ Death defiance

Defiance of death is a part of the Judeo-Christian heritage. Throughout the ages people have fought for causes or ideologies, despite knowing that they might die in the attempt. The attitude is reflected in hospitals, especially in critical care units or during emergency situations. The cause is to save a life; the battle is with death.

Although it is not the staff who die in the battle, they are open to loss. If the patient dies, the staff lives with the sense of a battle lost. Moreover, they face once again the finiteness of their own lives and the inevitability of death, despite modern technology.

Death defiance is helpful as we fight for life; it is not helpful when we do not also attend to the realities of the situation.

■ Death acceptance

Death acceptance is viewing death as a normal, natural, and integral part of living. Becker,[22] a prominent philosopher, defined the resignation to and acceptance of our limited existence as the central task for achieving maturity. With this acceptance, death becomes the conclusion of life's plan. It sounds so simple. It calms the fears and pains of dying, of facing our own immortality. But like the other attitudes toward death, this attitude is not a panacea. In fact, Schneidman[19] helps us to regain our perspective when he points out how romantic this attitude can be.

Death acceptance is for some the ultimate achievement of maturation, a form of self-actualization. The maturation is achieved by the dying person, it is not an attitude to be forced on them by others.

■ Desire for death

The fourth attitude, the desire for death, is more common in our society than people generally know or like to admit. People may desire their own death or the death of others.

Many circumstances give rise to the desire to die or for someone else to die. One major reason is the search for relief from misery. Misery takes many forms; pain, loneliness, disability, fear, uncertainty, and economic and emotional crises are but a few.

Other reasons contributing to the desire to die are associated with a relief from misery but are expressed in a different way. Some persons search for reunion with loved ones. Still others look forward to death as a last phase in the fulfillment of life.

Recognition of how people express their desire to die is important. In many instances the expression of the desire to die is the dying person's or family member's way of confirming recognition that death is inevitable within a predictable period of time in the near future.

■ DIMENSIONS OF DYING PERSONS

The discussion of dying and death has been in somewhat global terms. Now let us turn more directly to discussing dying persons and their characteristics.

■ Chronicity of dying

The nature of dying has changed. Because of modern therapies and technology, patterns of illness have shifted from acute infectious diseases to chronic conditions; as a result, dying has become a chronic process. With the exception of some acute problems such as myocardial infarction, severe infections, and fatal accidents, most dying persons experience chronic problems with multiple pathophysiologic alterations. These alterations are usually permanent and result in disability with a need to adjust to loss and to accommodate to change. Multiple series of losses can affect a person's behavioral responses and ability to cope.

Dying takes on the characteristics of chronic illness. Dying persons, just as other chronically ill persons, express feelings of being socially displaced or isolated. They grieve over the loss of former activities and abilities. They express sorrow over the continued loss of friends, business associates, and acquaintances. They talk of being alive and yet not able to live. They are expected to be present rather than future oriented.

Whenever the anticipated life span is *perceived as shortened,* a person may be viewed as chronically ill or dying and treated accordingly. For example some elderly persons are perceived and perceive themselves as not having enough time left to make future-oriented plans or decisions. The same perception is associated with some persons with diagnoses associated with dying and disability, such as cancer, stroke, and multiple sclerosis. Some people with shortened life spans may perceive themselves or be perceived by others as not deserving services or not being worthy of the efforts of others, since they will not live long enough.

Thus dying persons may be displaced, isolated individuals, not allowed to live their living. Furthermore, the chronicity of their dying may force them into experiencing a social death while they are functionally and biologically very much alive. Many factors contribute in promoting social dying long before the event of death; these factors will be discussed.

■ Stages and phases of dying

One factor that may hasten social dying is indiscriminately applying to an individual some theoretical findings based on groups. Kubler-Ross[27] described a series of stages through which people pass in response to their dying (see the box on p. 320). Physicians and nurse scientists, family members, and dying persons have challenged the usefulness of the stages of dying for guiding care. Weisman[29] identified no well-defined behavioral responses typical of individual persons facing death and suggested changing the

Kübler-Ross's stages of dying

Shock and disbelief
Denial
Anger
Bargaining
Depression
Acceptance

concept of stages to that of phases of dying. Pattison[28] proposed three phases of dying—acute, chronic living-dying, and terminal—as clinically useful for understanding the behaviors accompanying dying. These ideas suggest that stages or phases should be used as *guidelines* of how some people may respond but not as rigid categories into which *all* people can or should be placed.

The stages and phases of dying are sensitizing schemes to help us in being open to assessing what is "going on" in a situation so that we may understand it better. Our ultimate goal is quality care for dying persons and their families. Understanding, observation, and assessment assist in determining appropriate intervention to better achieve that goal.

■ Patterns of living-dying

Another tool to help understand the nature of dying is the patterns of living-dying described by Martocchio[11] and confirmed by Dufault.[13]

The four major patterns (Fig. 15-1) and their various combinations are based on the clinical courses of dying patients. They describe what has occurred, not what will occur. In other words, they are descriptive, *not* predictive. They are useful for understanding the variations of behavior among dying persons. They also demonstrate the futility of expecting persons to pass through a series of stages of behavior in any fixed sequence.

■ PEAKS AND VALLEYS PATTERN

The pattern of peaks and valleys is characterized by a period of greater health (peaks) and periods of crises (valleys). Dying persons refer to the peaks as "hopeful highs" and the valleys as "terrible or depressing lows." Although there are times of greater health, the overall course is downward to the event of death. Many hospitalizations and many moments of increased expectation and dashed hopes are associated with the experience of dying in this pattern. The uncertainties are great; fluctuations in behavior and difficulties in planning and in adjustment are to be expected as goals and plans change.

■ DESCENDING PLATEAUS PATTERN

The pattern of descending plateaus is characterized by an unpredictable number of progressive degenerative steps with plateaus (periods of stable health), lasting an indeterminate period of time. Again, the overall general course is downward. People do not return to their former level of health or functioning after each crisis. Like the peaks and valleys pattern, the course is fraught with the uncertainty of whether another crisis will occur and cause more debilitation.

This pattern is associated with expressions of futility and anger. Dying persons and family grieve the loss of functional ability despite concerted rehabilitative efforts to maintain or regain it.

■ DOWNWARD SLOPES PATTERN

The downward slopes pattern, the third pattern, is characterized by a consistent, persistent, easily discernible downward course. Unlike the other patterns, death is expected within a predictable period of time measured in hours or days. In most instances, the dying person loses consciousness, and there is little time to prepare family members for the death of their loved one. These deaths usually occur in critical care units.

■ GRADUAL SLANTS PATTERN

The fourth pattern of living-dying, gradual slants, is characterized by an ebb of life, gradually and almost imperceptibly culminating in death. Generally these persons experience a debilitating bodily insult from which there is little recovery. In many instances the person is no longer conscious and life is maintained by life support systems, such as respirators.

This pattern is associated with many of the following questions:

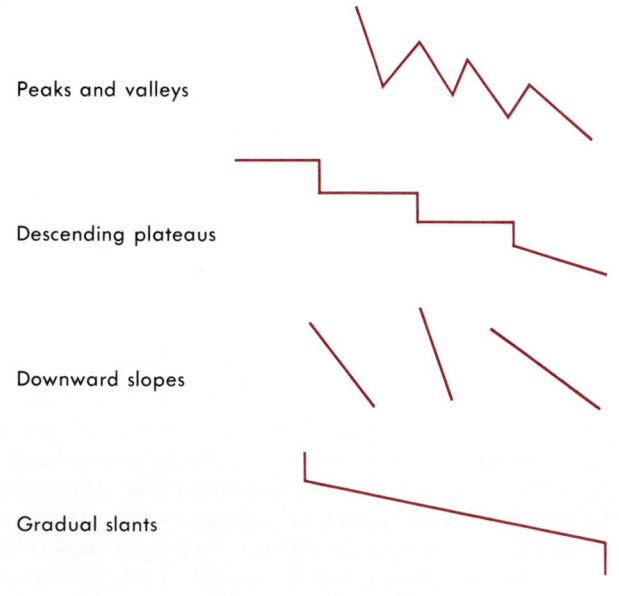

Peaks and valleys

Descending plateaus

Downward slopes

Gradual slants

Fig. 15-1   Martocchio's patterns of living-dying.

When should life support systems be discontinued?

Where should these persons be cared for?

Who should be responsible for their care?

In reality, many combinations of the four patterns may occur in one person's experience of living-dying. For example, a person's pattern may change from peaks and valleys to a downward slope, or from a downward slope to a gradual slant.

■ Choice: a right

All dying persons eventually learn of their fate. They should be free to choose what role, if any, they will play in the circumstances.

Dying persons describe a system of filtering out or listening to that which they wish to know or to realize. They tell us of how they listen to or look at the facts initially but do not hear them or see them until later. People allow the facts to permeate their minds at their own pace. Dying people, or any person facing an extreme crisis, can describe reaching an emotional readiness when they suddenly hear or see the facts and wonder how long they have been there. Sometimes facts have to be introduced more than once by various people and in various ways. Sometimes patients look for confirmation of what they heard or what they saw, that is, of what they think they know.

The person who recognizes that death is imminent but is not allowed to talk about it or is locked behind an impermeable wall of silence with no way to escape to the comfort of loving arms or to the closeness of a relationship with a loved one is condemned to total isolation. No rationalization or self-protection exists to support such punishment of dying persons or their loved ones.

How does this happen? Fear is probably the greatest cause. Families and health care providers blunder into subterfuge and into tragedy. No one anticipates all the lies that will be needed to support the first lie. No one anticipates the energy that will be spent futilely guarding the secret that all know.

There is tremendous hurt and anger when the truth becomes recognized. Would the person have chosen to live differently during the time that can never be returned? What happens to the confidence the person may have had in the nurses, physicians, and health system?

On the other hand, there are patients who sincerely choose not to see or to hear, who choose not to know. If that is their *informed choice*, then it is not appropriate to push them to know that which they do not wish to see or to hear. To force them to see or hear that which they wish to deny is as cruel and as inhumane as the conspiracy of silence. The refusal of the patient to know or to discuss the facts creates its own set of problems.

The foremost problems, both with lying to patients and with refusal by patients to acknowledge or discuss the facts of dying, are the creation of barriers to comforting and supporting care and communication among interactors and the inability to share feelings and concerns on the basis of the reality of the situation.

■ Role of confidant

Nurses can introduce the element of choice by fulfilling the need for a confidant who will initiate and allow honest talk. The role of confidant is a necessary but not an easy role. Talking of dying is not easy and periods of awkwardness and expressions of fear are inevitable.

Dying persons look to the confidant for honesty and acceptance as they search for understanding of their state. They are not searching for pity, consolation, or sympathy. They are uncomfortable with the pity and helplessness that they see in the eyes of others.

They look to the confidant to voice their deepest fears. They do not voice such fears to business associates; they cannot expect casual friends to understand. They do not reveal their most terrible anxieties to those they love; they protect loved ones from their panic.

The role of confidant is primarily to listen and to reassure as the dying person grapples with the experience of dying. The confidant can help to make the period of shifting from living to dying a time of deepening feelings of closeness or reinforcing family relationships, a time to say what needs to be said and done.

Dying persons do not confide in every nurse. Nor will the person they select as confidant necessarily be a nurse. Dying persons, just as any other persons, will be selective. Nurses are obligated to offer opportunities to be selected; to demand to serve in the role of confidant is inappropriate and, in fact, impossible.

■ Dying: an achievement or a failure

Although most dying people express resentment, fear, or sorrow over the major changes in their lives forced on them by their progressive debilitation, some view dying as an achievement. Some persons, especially those with a prolonged course of living with dying, focus on living their dying so as to die well. They speak about their dying to selected people and at selected times.

People who see dying well as an achievement are sometimes described by health professionals as denying or defying death. These people recognize their dying but choose therapy or choose to go home and participate in their customary activities. If you listen carefully to what they tell you, you will see that they intend to live their dying the way they wish, and thus from their own perspective they die well. These persons seem to do more than adjust and accommodate. They rise to an unseen challenge and in so doing expand their living rather than extend their dying.

A minority of persons may perceive dying as a personal failure or attribute it to external forces. Some dwell on all they could have accomplished were it not for their illness. They usually exude a sense of powerlessness and futility and express overt anger. Others with the same perception appear depressed, helpless, and resigned to their situation.

Remember that how people perceive their dying may change throughout the course of their dying. Attitudes, like physical capabilities, do not remain static. Dying encompasses the whole person; it is an emotional, behavioral, and physical process.

■ FAMILY DIMENSIONS

Thus far we have focused on the dying person, but the impact of the knowledge that death is imminent extends beyond the dying person to their families, social groups, and the society in which they live.

■ Cohesive or disruptive force

The experience of dying may serve as a cohesive force in some families and a disruptive force in others. In general, families who have responded to stresses or crises as a unified force in the past will offer each other strength and support. For families who have strained relationships, the dying experience may promote further strain.

Family members generally express remorse over the fact that a family member had to come face-to-face with death before they realized how much they needed each other or cared for each other. The recognition, without assistance in learning how to make the relationships grow, will not necessarily lead to greater social and emotional solidarity.[13]

■ Family control

Dying persons, at times, use their dying to control the behaviors of family members. When dying persons use dying as a means of control for self-gain or as a weapon, the result is anger, resentment, and perhaps retaliation by family members. Retaliation usually takes the form of not visiting, not phoning, or visiting for only short periods. The family members are attempting to protect themselves from the tyranny of the dying person even while they wish to be close and loving.

The problem becomes more grave for family members and dying person alike if the dying person is being cared

---

┌───┐

Factors to consider in home care of the dying

Who will be the caretakers?
Who will relieve the caretakers?
How is the home arranged?
Are the doors large enough to accommodate wheelchairs?
Can rooms be arranged to accommodate commodes or other necessary equipment?
Would a hospital bed or other hospital equipment be helpful?
Are the people in the home prepared for the changes they must make in their own life-styles?
Was the decision made as a family?

└───┘

---

for at home. Dying persons usually recognize the antagonism of family members but may interpret it as inappropriate, since, after all, they are dying. More frequently, the dying person may feel rejected and unloved and may not understand that the family loves the person but not the behaviors.

Family members may recognize their own behavior as a response to the dying person's manipulation, but at the same time they feel guilty about their responses because the other person is dying and they do care. The problem is best addressed openly and honestly, but it is usually difficult to resolve. It is difficult to deal with expressions of anger, resentment, and of long-term depression under the best of circumstances. They are almost impossible to deal with when one person is dying. The focus must be on love for the dying person but displeasure with the offensive behavior.

■ Dying at home

Biomedical technologic advances continue to shift the locus of dying to the institution, while the hospice movement has begun to deinstitutionalize dying. Consequently, more and more persons are encouraged to die in the privacy of their homes surrounded by family.

To have those we love die at home, cared for by family, may fulfill the romantic ideas we have surrounding dying, but it takes proper, careful, and advanced planning. Two major factors to be considered are the economic situation and the dying person's wishes. Other important factors pertain to the environment and available caregivers (see the box at right). Unless all factors are discussed in advance, family members may be ill-prepared to deal with the most simple tasks. They may not know how to change an occupied bed, change dressings, irrigate wounds, and administer medications. They may be concerned about how, what, or even whether to feed the dying person. Nurses choose and have been educated to become nurses, but family members are expected suddenly to assume nursing responsibilities that they may not desire or feel prepared to do. These expectations may lead to feelings of entrapment, anger, frustration, fear, and despair.

Support can usually be provided family members of dying persons by social care agencies such as hospices. The family members need help in learning to provide the required care and support for their concerns and feelings. They also need planned times for their own social activities, as well as for grocery shopping and other necessities.

■ GRIEF

People experience many losses throughout their lifetimes. Not all losses are attributable to deaths, but the most disruptive losses are associated with the deaths of loved ones because of the many life changes imposed on the survivors. The most profound loss is the death of a spouse or life-mate or of a child because of the closeness and intertwining nature of the relationship.

■ Grief, bereavement, and mourning

Grief and bereavement are frequent companions of adulthood. Loss occurs with increasing frequency as people age. *Bereavement* is the response to loss caused by *death*. It is a subjective state that occurs as a result of having suffered the loss of a person with whom there had been a significant loving relationship. *Grief*, or perhaps more accurately stated, the *process of grieving* is the total response (thoughts, feelings, and behaviors) to the emotional suffering caused by loss.[11] Grieving has somatic and psychologic dimensions. *Mourning* is behavior that is shaped by cultural values, norms, and mores.

An uncomplicated grief syndrome more or less follows a predictable course and distinctive symptoms. In general, the symptoms include a period of shock and somatic distress, feelings of hostility, guilt, and abandonment, interruption of life's usual activities, preoccupation with thoughts of the deceased, and finally a recovery period, or a working through to the state of healthy integration. Bereavement often takes months to years. Manifestations of grieving are likely to vary greatly among individuals.

Understanding the process of grieving and recognizing the behavioral manifestations that usually occur can assist nurses in preparing survivors for what they can expect or in helping them understand their feelings or somatic symptoms. Timing of the sharing of information and the type and amount of information given at any one session are important. Grieving persons are helped by sharing their experiences. Recognizing the "normal" nature of their experiences, even those that seem somewhat bizarre, opens the way for sharing.

■ SHOCK AND DISBELIEF

The initial response begins at the time of death and usually lasts for several weeks beyond the funeral. Regardless of whether the death was anticipated or not, the immediate response is shock, numbness, and disbelief. The survivors may feel a sense of unreality, and, as a consequence, they may appear to be "taking the death well." After the funeral this feeling of unreality or numbness changes to feelings of pain and separation. Survivors may experience some somatic symptoms (see the box below).

Bereaved persons exhibit *extremes of behavior*. They may become sedentary and do little of nothing except nap. They may be so hyperactive that they are unable to sit quietly or to sleep. They may experience extremes of mood such as profound sadness, anger, depression, or guilt, or find themselves laughing without an explanation. They may have difficulty concentrating. Coupled with these extremes in mood and behavior may be a continuance of disbelief, although the death is comprehended intellectually. *Searching behaviors* are common and include dreams in which the deceased is alive and experiences of "seeing" the person or "feeling" the deceased person's touch. During this phase, offers of comfort are often rejected because the bereaved person is focusing on the deceased.

■ YEARNING AND PROTEST

For several weeks the bereaved have feelings of yearning and protest. They may feel anger toward the deceased for leaving them, toward God for allowing the death to occur, toward the caregivers for not returning the deceased to health. They may be jealous of others who still have their loved ones. They may wish they had been the one to die. During this period, they may find it difficult to share their feelings or thoughts with others because they question their own sanity. Knowing that others have had similar thoughts and feelings sometimes is beneficial.

■ ANGER, DISORGANIZATION, AND DESPAIR

As the bereaved begin to focus more on themselves and as the numbness and rage begin to fade, the reality and permanence of loss begins to be recognized. Survivors may experience a sense of confusion, aimlessness, an inability to make decisions, a loss of motivation or interest, and a loss of confidence. During this period, they feel lonely and depressed and experience a general loss of meaning to their lives.

All those experiences that the bereaved person formerly shared with the deceased now seem irrelevant. They experience extremes of mood. The intensity of their feelings often is frightening to them. Memory lapses and difficulty in concentrating, although common and temporary, increase their feelings of anguish. They fear loss of emotional control and become centered on themselves as a defense. Friends or other family members may interpret this behavior as selfish and either reprimand the persons or withdraw. Neither behavior is helpful to the bereaved. At the same time, the bereaved may smoke or excessively use chemicals such as drugs or alcohol.

The wish and need to cry fulfills an important function in acknowledging the loss and in receiving support from others. Memories and mental images of the deceased are void of negative characteristics. Feelings of guilt, remorse, fear, and regret may surface. Opportunities to reminisce and to share feelings with others are helpful.

■ IDENTIFICATION

The bereaved may adopt the behavior, admired qualities, and mannerisms of lost loved ones. Some persons may take on the symptoms of the last illness and care must be taken

---

Physical symptoms associated with grief

Muscular weakness, tremors, fatigue
Tightness of the throat, deep sighs
Diaphoresis, cold and clammy sensations
Anorexia

to distinguish symptoms associated with physical illness from those associated with loss. Symptoms associated with loss will abate as the loss is resolved.

■ REORGANIZATION AND RESTITUTION

The feelings and symptoms of grieving gradually subside; they do not suddenly disappear. Bereaved persons tell us they have periods of depression and periods of well-being as life begins to make sense once again. Reorganization and restitution generally begin approximately 6 months after the loss and last for a few years. The process may be considerably longer or shorter and still be within normal range. Contrary to old popular beliefs, although life stabilizes, the pain of loss may remain for a lifetime. Reactions to loss recur around circumstances that are poignant reminders of the deceased, such as birthdays, anniversaries, and holidays.

■ Factors affecting the response of survivors

Many factors combine to affect the degree of stress and the particular response of survivors to a death. The major factors relate to the following:
1. The type of relationship lost (the closer the relationship, the greater the impact of loss)
2. The nature of the death (whether it is perceived as a "good" or "bad" death [p. 316])
3. The characteristics of the survivor (such as physical and mental health and number and nature of grief and crises)
4. The social and cultural milieu
5. The nature of the support network

Persons who are at higher risk for incomplete or delayed grieving are those who experience a loss of socioeconomic status, have poor health before the loss, lack social support, are unable to express grief, or had a pattern of high dependence on the deceased. A sudden death or short illness may also delay grieving because the person did not have an opportunity to begin the process of grieving before the death.

■ NURSING PRACTICE CONSIDERATIONS

Nursing care of the dying consists of providing care for family and friends in addition to the dying person. These persons may not experience the grieving process in the same way. Dying people may grieve over the loss of physical function, the loss of past abilities, the ultimate loss of life, and separation from all they know and love. At the same time, significant others may grieve over the potential loss of the loved one, the hurt they feel, and the emptiness they anticipate.

Although each person's experience of dying and grieving is unique and personal, there are similarities. Knowledge of the uniqueness of the perceived experience and knowl-

---

> **Nursing assessment: input from dying person and significant others**
>
> **General perception of each individual**
>
> Awareness of clinical diagnosis and prognosis
> Philosophy of living while dying
> Expected physiologic and behavioral changes
> Past experiences with major illness or crises
> Shared experiences with major illnesses or crises
>
> **Perceived strengths, desires, and hopes**
>
> Personal abilities and coping techniques
> Personal support systems
> Availability of resources
> Beliefs, religious convictions, cultural views of dying, death, and bereavement
> Past experiences with death
> Expectations about care, dying, use of life supports (present and future)

---

edge of some expected common responses assist nurses in assessing each situation, planning care, intervening, and evaluating both the plan of care and the interventions for dying people and their significant others.

▣ Assessment

Nursing assessment is an ongoing process throughout the term of the dying person-family-nurse relationship. It will continue and become the family-nurse relationship at the death of the patient. A thorough initial assessment with direct input from the dying person and significant others provides the basis for relationships. Assessment parameters are listed in the box above.

Another important aspect of nursing assessment is that of the nurse's own personal responses, beliefs, and attitudes in each individual situation involving dying persons and their families. In addition, the nurse needs to assess his or her own personal and professional support systems.

➡ Data analysis: nursing diagnoses

Nursing diagnoses are determined from assessment of patient data. Most nursing diagnoses will reflect the underlying pathophysiologic disorders. In addition, a major nursing diagnosis for both the dying person and the significant others will reflect the grieving process and may include one of the following:

Diagnostic title	Possible etiologies
Anticipatory grieving	Potential death of self or loved one
Dysfunctional grieving	Actual or perceived loss of loved one

Timing planned nursing interventions

Times for physical care
Social interaction times
Times for privacy for family members and patient
Quiet times alone for reflection, grieving, or rest
Times for reassessment
Times for group planning and evaluation

Planning: expected patient outcomes

As with assessment, planning is a joint venture. Successful planning incorporates the goals of the family and the dying person, as well as goals of nurses and other health care providers. Time is an important factor in planning care for the dying person (see the box above); time is set aside for special activities to enhance meaningfulness for the dying person and significant others, as well as the quality of care provided for the remaining days of life.

Expected patient outcomes may include but are not limited to the following:
1. The dying person
   a. Is as comfortable as possible
   b. Makes decisions regarding care, as possible
   c. Expresses feelings and thoughts with a significant person (nurse or other professional, family, friend), as desired
2. Significant others
   a. Express their grief
   b. Provide effective care to the dying person, as desired and necessary
   c. Identify community resources for support

Nurses also need to plan for their own health maintenance. They need to consider (1) their own time commitments, (2) availability of support from other health professionals, and (3) consideration of actual or potential value conflicts and means of dealing with the conflicts. The planning is done in relation to each individual situation involving a dying person or the significant others of the dying person.

Implementation

INTERVENTIONS WITH GRIEVERS

Some principles of care for grievers apply to both the dying persons and the survivors, whereas other guidelines relate specifically to survivors. The survivor category includes the following guidelines:
1. Make contact; establish a relationship.
2. Do not allow grievers to remain isolated.
   a. Be present and have others present.
   b. Suggest self-help groups and assist grievers in attending.

3. Maintain a family perspective.
   a. Remember that the family is changed.
   b. Include family members in care of the dying person.
4. Give people "permission" to grieve.
   a. Display nonjudgmental attitudes and behaviors; be neutral.
   b. Communicate compassionate support through verbal and nonverbal behavior; for example, if the person starts to cry and turns toward the caregiver, lean forward, relax, do not turn away; allow the griever to cry.
5. Reach out
   a. Take the initiative; reach out in a concrete way. Don't say, "Call me if you need me." Be specific in how you can assist or get others to assist (for example, "How about if I call your sister to accompany you to select the casket?" "Suppose I arrange for you to attend a widow-to-widow meeting?").
   b. Do not take refusals personally or give up.
   c. Repeat offers of assistance; grievers initially may not be able to respond to and appreciate offers of help initially but may do so with time.
6. Be physically and emotionally present to offer security and support.
   a. Use physical contact (hugging, touching, hand-holding); these actions are important early in the process to convey that the griever is not alone. There may be some exceptions, as some people do not like to be touched (watch nonverbal responses).
   b. Encourage family members to be present after the attention of the funeral is over; social supports generally are decreased weeks or months after a death.
   c. Encourage regular expression of feelings to help minimize the tendency to become overwhelmed and unable to function.
   d. Encourage others to take charge of routine functions and responsibilities of the bereaved; for example, run errands, prepare meals.
   e. Help family members to focus on one problem at a time.
   f. Address problems to which practical solutions can be found before addressing more complicated problems.
7. Teach alternative methods for relaxation and coping, as necessary.

INTERVENTIONS FOR THE DYING PERSON

The nursing needs of dying persons are the nursing needs of living persons. The range of activities are as broad as for any diverse population. Nursing intervention may occur in a variety of settings, either at home or in various institutional settings.

Direct physical care is one major part of caring for dying persons. Maintenance of comfort, both physical and emotional, is of the essence. Teaching others involved in direct care the maintenance of comfort allows their participation and promotes their feelings of competence and well-being. Teaching how dying persons may use medication for comfort and at the same time dispelling expressed fears of patient addiction may help the dying person and family alike. The nurse recognizes and respects cultural differences and fears about addiction. Addiction in dying persons is improbable and, in the last days of living, inconsequential.

Another nursing responsibility is to be well informed about organized support systems, agencies, and independent resources within the community and to be prepared to assist patients and their families in contacting and using these resources. Inquiries related to the many alternative modes of care for dying persons, such as hospice care, other forms of home care, nursing home care, other forms of institutional care, should be answered openly and honestly. If the nurse cannot answer the patient or family's questions, they should be referred to those who can supply the answers.

Nursing intervention may include participation in resuscitative efforts and the maintenance of dying patients on life-support systems. Along with direct patient care in these circumstances, nurses are responsible for communicating with and supporting family members or for assuring that someone is providing this service.

In essence, nurses assist patients and families in maintaining control over their individual lives as much as is possible to ensure dignity and self-esteem. This control is accomplished through the actions discussed above.

SUPPORT FOR NURSE

If nurses are to care effectively for patients and families, they need to maintain their own well-being. Planned sessions, within the confines of confidentiality, to discuss thoughts and feelings about a particular situation may be helpful. Recognition that others, health professionals, volunteers, and family members, have much to contribute and are as committed and concerned about the patient's welfare is of importance.

Withdrawal from a situation may be necessary in some rare situations but should occur only when other nursing personnel are available to maintain the care of the patient and significant others.

Peer support is most beneficial to nurses caring for dying persons. Peer support may be accomplished through formal and informal groups. In addition to groups, one-to-one interactions with a trusted peer or personal significant other may alleviate some of the stress related to working with dying persons. More importantly, such relationships serve as an appropriate avenue for recognizing and reinforcing the inherent rewards of providing nursing care for people who are living their dying and those who are sharing the experience.

Evaluation

Each nurse is responsible for evaluating his or her own practice as it relates to each situation. Comfort and satisfaction of the patient may be used as criteria. Nursing intervention may be evaluated through a preestablished evaluation system (see the box on p. 000). Use of these systems contribute to the development and feelings of well-being of nurses by affording support in the decision process.

At the conclusion of a nurse-patient relationship that includes the death of the patient, a nurse will feel a loss. Evaluation of his or her contribution to the relationship gains importance, especially for each nurse's well-being. Recognition of specific successful interventions and contributions leads to feelings of achievement and success.

SUMMARY

1. Living and dying are not opposite ends of a continuum; we are living until the point of death.
2. Dying is a process of coming to the end of life; death is an event or state of cessation of life. Loss is the underlying theme of death; it is what is felt when something of value is gone.

Evaluation methods in the care of dying persons

Care of patient and significant others

Observation of responses to interventions
Discussion of goals and how they have been achieved
Discussion of alternative methods to achieve goals more effectively
Mutual evaluation of continued appropriateness of goals
Mutual identification of new or revised goals and means to achieve these goals

Preestablished nursing evaluation systems

Formal and informal peer review of goals and interventions
- Open discussion of problems
- Venting of feelings
- Sharing of positive responses

Specific criteria developed by groups of nurses involved in caring for dying persons

---

Putting knowledge to practice

- Examine current literature for discussion of ethical issues related to dying and death.
- Write a list of your family practices related to death; in what ways do these practices provide support for survivors?
- How would you respond to a patient who asks you, "Am I going to die?" What would be your response or feelings if a nurse responded in a similar way to you if you were the patient?
- Arrange to provide care for a patient whose condition is terminal. What cues does the patient give you of wanting to talk about dying or death? How do the concepts presented by Kubler-Ross, Pattison, or Martocchio help you understand the patient's experience?
- What support services are available to dying persons and their families in your community?
- If possible, visit a hospice agency in your community. What is their philosophy of care? What services do they provide?

---

3. Views of death vary considerably depending in part on the person's perspective of the personal relationship.
4. Rights of dying persons include the right to know they may die, to die in an atmosphere of hopefulness and caring, to privacy, to be free of pain when dying, and to die with a sense of self-esteem.
5. Living wills, although not yet legally enforceable in all states, provide moral direction of the dying person's wishes regarding the conditions of death.
6. Euthanasia may be active (acts that shorten a person's life) or passive (letting die by withholding or withdrawing treatment). The opposite of euthanasia is antieuthanasia or treating the dying person at all costs.
7. The concept of quality of life (or meaningfulness of life) includes autonomy (the right to determine one own's fate) and informed consent (making choices based on necessary information). Paternalism is a refusal to accept patient autonomy when providing health care.
8. The controversy surrounding the legal definition of death centers on whether death is the cessation of respiration and circulation or the cessation of all functions including the entire brain.
9. Death denial is the avoidance of the subject of dying and death; it may have negative or positive results.
10. Death defiance is acting in ways that may contribute to death even when knowing the possible consequences.
11. Death acceptance is viewing death as a normal, natural, and integral part of living.
12. Death desire is wishing for the death of self or of others and is often related to relief from misery. The desire to die may be an expression of the inevitability of imminent death.
13. The stages of dying according to Kubler-Ross are shock and disbelief, denial, anger, bargaining, depression, and acceptance.
14. The three phases of dying according to Pattison are acute, chronic living-dying, and terminal.
15. The patterns of living-dying according to Martocchio are peaks and valleys (periods of greater health and

crises), descending plateaus (progressive degenerative steps), downward slopes (consistent discernable downward course), and gradual slants (gradual, almost imperceptible, ebbing of life).
16. Dying may serve as a cohesive force in families who have responded well in the past to crises or as a disruptive force for families who have strained relationships.
17. Choosing to die at home must take into consideration the desires of the dying person and the resources (economic, psychologic, physical) of the family members; careful planning, instruction, and support are often required and may be provided by hospice programs.
18. Grief is the emotional suffering caused by loss; bereavement is the response to loss caused by death; mourning is death-related behavior influenced by sociocultural factors. The phases of the grief syndrome include shock and disbelief; yearning and protest; anger, disorganization and despair; identification; and reorganization and restitution.
19. Interventions for grievers include establishing a relationship, preventing isolation of grievers, encouraging family support, giving people permission to grieve, reaching out in concrete ways, and teaching alternative methods of relaxation and coping.
20. Interventions for dying persons include promoting comfort and providing information on care to family members and on availability of community resources.

REFERENCES AND SELECTED READINGS
Contemporary

1. *Anderson, GC, and others: Living wills: do nurses and physicians have them: Am J Nurs 86:271-275, 1986.
2. *Bandman, B, and Bandman, E: Nursing ethics in the life span, Norwalk, Conn, 1985, Appleton-Century-Crofts.
3. Childress, JF: Who should decide: paternalism in health care, Oxford, 1982, Oxford University Press, Inc.

---

*References preceded by an asterisk are particularly well suited for student reading.

4. Curtin, L: Nursing ethics: theories and pragmatics, Bowie, Md, 1982, Robert J Brady Co.

5. Davis, AJ, and Aroskar, MA: Ethical dilemmas and nursing practice, ed 2, New York, 1983, Appleton-Century-Crofts.

6. Donovan, ML, and Girton, SE: Cancer care nursing, ed 2, New York, 1984, Appleton-Century-Crofts.

7. *Gass, KA: Coping strategies for widows, J Gerontol Nurs 13(8):29-33, 1987.

8. *Graham, J: In the company of others, New York, 1982, Harcourt Brace Jovanovich, Inc.

9. Hemlock Society: Supporting the option of active voluntary euthanasia for the terminally ill, Los Angeles, 1985, The Society.

10. Jonsen, AR, Siegler, M, and Winslade, WJ: Clinical ethics, New York, 1982, Macmillan Publishing Co.

11. *Martocchio, BC: Living while dying, Bowie, Md, 1982, Robert J Brady Co.

12. *Martocchio, BC: Grief and bereavement: healing through hurt, Nurs Clin North Am 20(2):327-341, 1985.

13. *Martocchio, BC, and Dufault, Sr K: Dying, a part of living. In Diamond, M (editor): Advances in geriatrics, long-term nursing, vol 1, New York, 1983, Pro Scientia, Inc.

14. Mitchell, C: Dilemmas in practice: steadying the hand that feeds, Am J Nurs 87:293-296, 1987.

15. Mitchell, C and Rutherford, PA: Dilemmas in practice: the fragile survivor, Am J Nurs 87:603-606, 1987.

16. Oerlemans-Bunn, M: On being gay, single, and bereaved, Am J Nurs 88:472-476, 1988.

17. Rando, TA: Grief, dying and death, Champaign, Ill, 1983, Research Press Co.

18. Raphael, B: The anatomy of bereavement, New York, 1983, Basic Books, Inc.

19. Schneidman, ES: Voices of death, New York, 1980, Harper & Row, Publishers.

20. Society for the Right to Die: Support of dying with dignity, New York, 1985, The Society.

Classic

21. *American Nurses Association: Code for nurses, Kansas City, 1976, The association.

22. *Becker, E: The denial of death, Riverside, NJ, 1973, Free Press.

23. Branson, R, and Casebeer, K: The Quinlan decision: observing the role of the physician, Hastings Cent Rep 6(I, Feb 6):8-11, 1976.

24. *Feifel, H: The functions and attitudes toward death: death and dying, attitudes of patient and doctor, New York, 1965, Group for Advancement of Psychiatry.

25. Illich, I: Medical nemesis: the expropriation of health, New York, 1976, Pantheon Books.

26. *Kalish, RA: Death and dying in a social context. In Binstock, RH, and Shanes, D (editors): Handbook of aging, New York, 1976, Van Nostrand Reinhold Co.

27. Kubler-Ross, E: On death and dying, New York, 1969, Macmillan Co.

28. Pattison, EM: The experience of dying, Englewood Cliffs, NJ, 1977, Prentice-Hall, Inc.

29. *Weisman, AD: The realization of death: a guide for psychological autopsy, New York, 1974, J Aronson.

UNIT IV
Perioperative Nursing

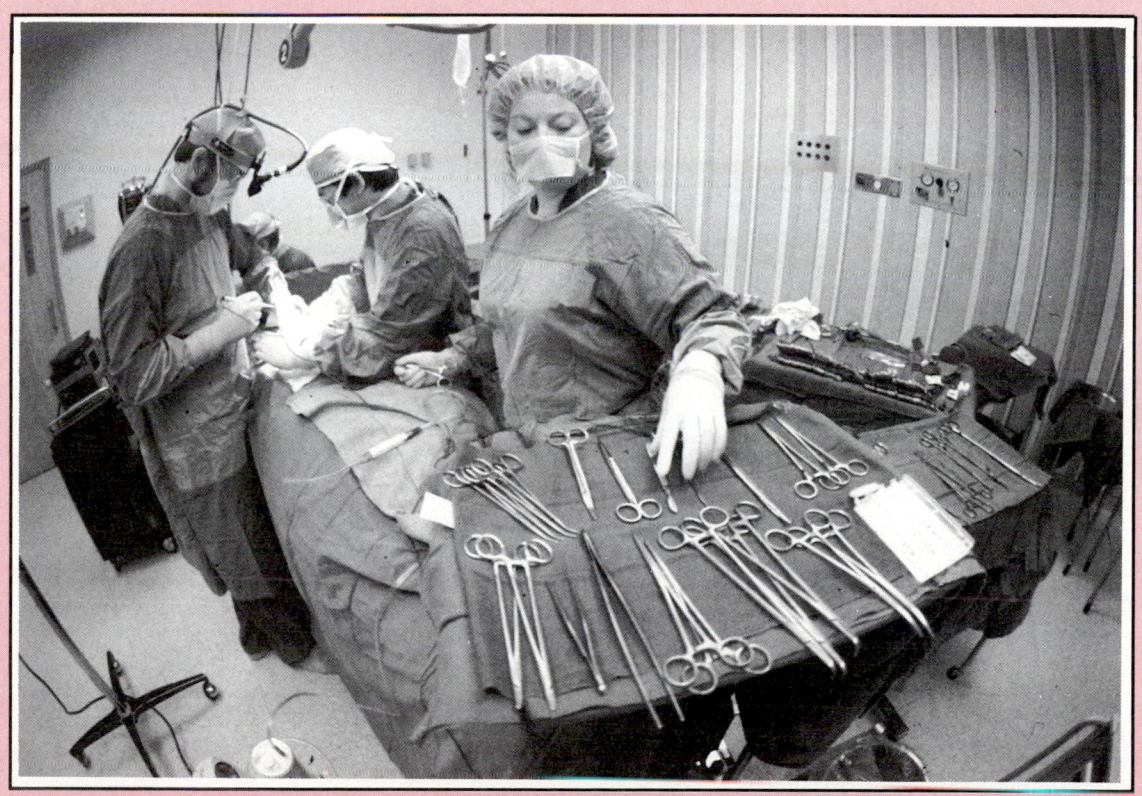

16

Preoperative Intervention

BARBARA C. LONG

Surgery is one of the major modes of medical therapy. It is a stressful experience as it involves a threat to body integrity and sometimes a threat to life itself. Pain frequently occurs. The nurse is in a position of assisting the person in coping with the stressors, in seeking relief from the pain, and in returning to optimal functioning.

The surgical (perioperative) experience can be divided into three stages: preoperative, intraoperative, and postoperative. The next three chapters discuss knowledge basic to the care of the patient during each of the three stages.

TYPES OF SURGERY

Classification

Surgeries may be classified in several ways, such as by location, extent, or purpose of the surgery.

LOCATION

Surgery may be performed externally or internally. In *external surgery* the skin or underlying tissues are readily accessible to the surgeon. External surgery has disadvantages; it may result in scarring or disfiguration that may be readily visible, leading to great concern and distress for some patients. *Plastic surgery* (Chapter 39) is an example of external surgery; it is directed toward reconstruction and repair of deformed tissues. *Internal surgery* involves penetration of the body. The scars of internal surgery may not be visible but may lead to complications such as adhesions. Surgery of major internal organs may lead to decreased function if sufficient tissue is removed.

Surgery may also be classified by location of body parts or systems, such as cardiovascular surgery, chest surgery, neurologic surgery, and so on. Information specific to these types of surgery can be found elsewhere in the text.

EXTENT

Surgery may be classified as minor or major. *Minor surgery* is simple surgery that presents little risk to life. It may be performed in a surgeon's office, a clinic, or an outpatient or inpatient surgical suite. Many minor surgeries are performed with the patient under local anesthesia, but general anesthesia may also be used. Although the operation is termed "minor," it is frequently not viewed as a minor episode by the patient and may evoke some fears and concerns.

Major surgery is usually performed under general anesthesia in an inpatient surgical suite. It is more serious than minor surgery and may involve risk of life. There is a trend toward an increased number of surgical procedures being performed in hospital ambulatory centers in which persons are admitted to the center on the morning of surgery, remain there for their immediate postoperative care, and are then discharged to their homes before the end of the day. Some major surgical procedures, such as herniorrhaphy, are now being performed in this manner.

PURPOSE

There are several purposes for performing surgery (Table 16-1). The surgeon explains the method and purpose for the proposed surgery to the patient and family. Because the preoperative period is often a time of increased anxiety for the patient or family, they may not perceive or understand the reason for the surgery and may require further clarification, which the nurse can provide.

Surgical procedures

Most surgical procedures are given names that describe the site of the surgery and the type of surgery performed. For example, a hysterectomy is the removal of (-ectomy) the uterus (hyster-).

Common surgical suffixes

-ectomy	Removal of an organ or gland
-rrhapy	Suturing or stitching
-ostomy	Providing an opening (stoma)
-otomy	Cutting into
-plasty	Plastic repair
-scopy	Looking into

Some surgeries, however, carry the name of the surgeon who developed the technique, such as the Heineke-Mikulicz procedure (widening of the pyloric opening of the stomach).

Table 16-1 Purposes of surgery

Type of surgery	Reason performed	Examples
Diagnostic	Determine cause of symptoms	Biopsy, exploratory laparotomy
Curative	Removal of diseased part	Appendectomy
Restorative	Strengthen weakened areas	Herniorrhaphy
	Correct deformities	Mitral valve replacement
	Rejoin a separated area	Bone pinning
Palliative	Relieve symptoms without curing disease	Sympathectomy
Cosmetic	Improve appearance	Rhinoplasty

■ EFFECTS OF SURGERY ON THE PATIENT

Surgery is a potential or actual threat to a person's integrity and thus may produce both physiologic and psychologic stress reactions. The physiologic stress reaction is directly related to the extent of the surgery, that is, the more extensive the surgery, the greater the physiologic response. The psychologic response, however, is not directly related. A relatively minor surgical procedure, such as removal of a cyst from the face, may evoke a greater psychologic response than removal of an organ such as the spleen because of the former's potential for scarring. Removal of the uterus, however, may evoke a greater response than would removal of the spleen. This is because of the implications and values attached to the uterus.

■ Physiologic responses

Major surgery is a stressor to the body and evokes a neuroendocrine response. The response, which consists of sympathetic nervous system and hormonal responses (Table 16-2), serves to protect the body from the threat of injury (Fig. 16-1). (Review Chapter 7 for the neuroendocrine response to stress.) When the stress to the system is severe or if blood loss is excessive, the body's compensatory mechanisms are overwhelmed, and shock is the result. Certain types of anesthesia used may also contribute to shock formation.

Metabolic responses also occur. Carbohydrates and fats are metabolized to produce energy. Body proteins are broken down to provide a supply of the amino acids used to build new tissues. Those amino acids that are not used are broken down to nitrogen end products, such as urea, and excreted. This leads to a *negative nitrogen balance*, that is, nitrogen loss exceeds nitrogen intake. All of these factors lead to weight loss after major surgery. A high protein intake is necessary for restoration of needed proteins for healing and for restoration of optimal functioning.

■ Psychologic responses

Persons differ in the way they perceive the meaning of surgery, and thus they respond in different ways. There are, however, some common fears and concerns. Some of the fears underlying preoperative anxiety are elusive, and the person may not be able to identify the cause. Others are more specific. Following is a list of these fears.

General	Specific
Fear of unknown	Diagnosis of malignancy
Loss of control	Anesthesia
Loss of love from significant others	Dying
	Pain
Threat to sexuality	Disfigurement
	Permanent limitation

Fear of the unknown is most common. If the diagnosis is uncertain, fear of malignancy is frequent, regardless of the probability of occurrence. Fears concerning anesthesia are usually related to dying, "going to sleep and never waking up." Some persons are concerned about what they will say when they are awakening from anesthesia; if they do speak, their words often make little sense. Fears concerning pain, disfigurement, or permanent disability may be realistic or may be influenced by myths, lack of information, or lurid stories told by friends. The patient may also have other concerns related to hospitalization, such as job security, loss of income, and care of family.

Persons with anxiety so high that they cannot talk about and begin to cope with their anxiety before surgery frequently experience difficulty in the postoperative period. They are more apt to be angry, resentful, confused, or depressed. They are also more vulnerable to psychotic reactions than are persons with lower levels of anxiety.

Lack of any emotional response to surgery may indicate denial; this precludes dealing with and coping with the anxiety before surgery. Some anxiety enables the individual to identify and begin to cope with feelings. These persons usually have a smoother postoperative course.

Table 16-2 Effects of physiologic responses to surgery

Response	Positive effect	Negative effect
Sympathetic nervous system		
Vasoconstriction	Maintain blood pressure, adequate blood flow to heart and brain	
Increased cardiac output	Maintain blood pressure	
Decreased GI activity		Anorexia, gas pains, constipation
Hormonal		
Increased glucocorticoid secretion (adrenal cortex)		
Sodium retention	Increased blood volume	Potassium loss
Protein and fat catabolism	Increased energy, amino acids available for healing	Weight loss
Increased platelet production	Prevent bleeding through clotting	Possible thrombus formation
Increased ADH secretion (posterior pituitary)	Increased blood volume	Possible fluid overload

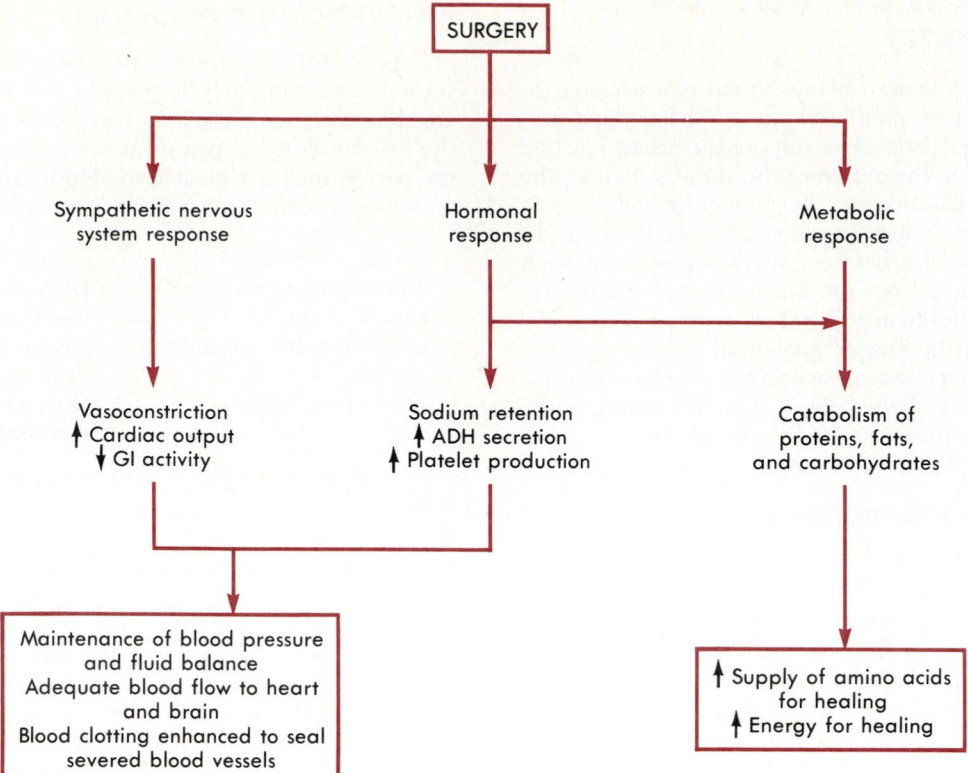

Fig. 16-1 Positive effects of the pathophysiologic responses to surgery.

■ Elderly persons' response to surgery

The ability of the elderly patient to tolerate surgery depends on the extent of physiologic changes that have occurred with the aging process, the duration of the surgical procedure, and the presence of one or more chronic diseases. Elderly persons vary greatly in the extent to which physiologic changes occur. The changes that affect responses to surgery are cardiovascular, renal, pulmonary, and musculoskeletal (Table 16-3).

The greater the number of changes present, the greater the potential for the development of a postoperative complication. Heart rate changes in the elderly occur more slowly than in younger persons; therefore, the pulse rate *may not* be a good index in assessment of shock, and a longer period of time may be necessary to wait for pulse stabilization after activity.

The duration of the surgical experience can affect the response of elderly persons to surgery. Surgery of short duration is more easily tolerated. Presence of chronic diseases such as pulmonary, cardiac, or CNS disease limits the elderly person by prolonging recovery or by increasing the risk of mortality. Certain types of surgery present low or high risks for elderly persons:

Lower risk	Higher risk
Elective	Thoracic
Away from diaphragm	Radical head and neck
Not involving infections	Closure of wound dehiscence
Permitting early mobility	Perforated ulcer
Requiring minimal narcotics	Colostomy following obstruction

Table 16-3 Potential postoperative complications in elderly persons

Dysfunction	Possible effects
Decreased circulation	Shock, wound infection, thrombophlebitis
Decreased kidney function	Prolonged response to anesthesia, fluid and electrolyte imbalances (especially overhydration)
Decreased respiratory function	Atelectasis, pneumonia
Decreased mobility	Atelectasis, pneumonia, thrombophlebitis, constipation or fecal impaction

■ RISK FACTORS FOR SURGERY

A number of variables influence physiologic and psychologic responses throughout the surgical experience.

■ Age

Surgery can be performed on persons of any age, from newborns (and even on the fetus) to the very aged. Persons at extremes of age are less able to tolerate stress such as tissue trauma (surgery) or infection. The specific factors influencing the surgery of the elderly are noted in the previous section.

■ Nutrition

Malnourished persons (nutritional deficits or excess) are poorer surgical risks than the well nourished and are more likely to develop postoperative complications. *Undernourished* persons already have diminished reserves of carbohydrates and fats. Body proteins will be used to provide the necessary energy requirement to maintain metabolic functioning of cells; thus nitrogen imbalances will be greater than normal and less protein will be available for healing. Wound healing becomes considerably delayed in undernourished persons, and wound separation and infection may occur. If surgery is not an emergency, it is delayed until the patient's nutritional status is improved.

The *obese* person presents numerous risks during the surgical experience:

Respiratory complications
Vital signs fluctuations
Wound separation and infection
Incisional hernias
Thrombophlebitis

The organs are enlarged and excessive demands are placed on the cardiovascular sysem. Fatty tissue lacks circulation so wounds heal more slowly. Obese persons have greater difficulty expanding their chests, moving in bed, and walking.

Conditions predisposing the person to preoperative malnutrition include chronic inflammatory disorders, liver and renal disease, gastrointestinal cancer, and congestive heart failure.

■ Neuroendocrine response ineffectiveness

The neuroendocrine response assists the person in coping with the stress of surgery. If this response is ineffective, postoperative complications such as shock and delayed wound healing may occur. In addition, anesthesia may be tolerated poorly, and fluid and electrolyte imbalances are more likely to occur because of insufficient adrenocortical activity. Persons with diseases of the adrenal gland or the sympathetic nervous system or those who are under a great deal of stress before surgery may do less well postoperatively. Infants and the elderly also have diminished neuroendocrine responses.

■ Chronic disease

The existence of one or more chronic diseases does not necessarily increase surgical risk. The nature and extent of the diseases and the degree to which they are under control are the important variables.

Pulmonary disease, such as chronic obstructive pulmonary disease (COPD), may affect the person's response to the anesthetic and ability to cope with respiratory problems after surgery (see Chapter 18). In persons with a history of recent respiratory infection, surgery will be delayed until they are in optimal condition.

Cardiovascular disease can affect the individual's response to surgery because a heart that pumps effectively and blood vessels that constrict effectively are necessary for the prevention of shock and of fluid imbalances. Body responses to hemorrhage and inflammation also depend on an adequate supply of red and white blood cells. Surgery is usually postponed if possible when the cardiovascular status of the patient is not at the optimal level of functioning.

Renal insufficiency can increase the risk of surgery because of difficulty in the removal of increased amounts of electrolytes, especially potassium, and waste products from catabolism. Persons with renal disease are prone to develop fluid overload from parenteral fluids if urine production is not adequate.

The patient with *diabetes mellitus* should have the disease well controlled before surgery and monitored closely during and after surgery. Glucocorticoid activity and potassium changes following surgery can influence insulin utilization (see Chapter 28).

■ Smoking

Smoke irritates the tracheobronchial tree, resulting in increased secretions that impinge on the airway and decrease ventilation. Therefore, heavy smokers are at higher risk for developing postoperative pulmonary complications. Most surgeons prefer that persons who are heavy smokers decrease their smoking for a period of time before surgery.

■ INFORMED CONSENT

Written permission must be obtained from the patient for each operation performed and is usually obtained for major diagnostic procedures, such as a thoracentesis, cystoscopy, or bronchoscopy, that involves entering the body cavity. The consent implies that the patient has been provided with the knowledge necessary to understand (1) the nature of the procedure to be performed, (2) the available options, and (3) the risks associated with each option. Signed permission protects the patient from undergoing unauthorized surgery and protects the surgeon and hospital against claims of unauthorized surgery or that the patient was unaware of the risks involved.

Legal responsibility for obtaining informed consent from the patient resides with the physician. Oral consent is as binding as written consent.[8] Physicians will document that

Preoperative nursing assessment

Subjective data

1. Knowledge and past experiences
   a. Understanding of proposed surgery
      (1) Site
      (2) Type of surgery to be done
      (3) Information from surgeon regarding extent of hospitalization, postoperative limitations
      (4) Preoperative routines
      (5) Postoperative routines
      (6) Preoperative tests
   b. Previous surgical experiences
      (1) Type, nature, response
      (2) Time interval
2. Psychologic readiness for surgery
   a. Concerns or fears about proposed surgery
   b. Usual coping methods
   c. Religion and its meanings for patient
   d. Cultural beliefs or practices related to surgery
   e. Family and close friends
      (1) Accessibility (distance)
      (2) Perception of family and friends as source of support
   f. Changes in sleep patterns
   g. Increased urinary frequency
3. Physiologic status
   a. Medications that may interfere with anesthesia or contribute to postoperative complications (Table 16-4)
   b. Allergies: medications, soaps, adhesive tape
   c. Sensory: difficulties with vision or hearing
   d. Nutrition: adequacy of dietary intake (food, fluids), nausea, anorexia
   e. Elimination: problems with constipation, last bowel movement, problems with urination
   f. Motor: difficulties with ambulation, movement of arms and legs, arthritis, previous orthopedic surgery (joint replacement, spinal fusion)
   g. Prosthetic devices: dentures, artificial eye or limb
   h. Comfort: ability to sleep, presence of pain or discomfort, expectations regarding relief of postoperative pain

Objective data

1. Speech patterns: repetition of themes, change of topic, avoidance of topics related to feelings (anxiety); ability to understand English
2. Degree of interaction with others (anxiety)
3. Behavior: excessive hand movements, restlessness, withdrawal or excessive activity (anxiety)
4. Height and weight
5. Vital signs
6. Sensory: ability to see and hear
7. Skin: turgor, presence of lesions, rashes or bruising
8. Mouth: dentures, condition of teeth and mucous membranes
9. Chest: breath sounds (presence, character), chest expansion, ability to do diaphragmatic breathing, heart sounds (baseline for postoperative comparison)
10. Extremities: muscle strength (especially legs), character of peripheral pulses before vascular or limb surgery
11. Motor ability: any limitation to walking, sitting, or moving in bed, coordination with ambulation

the necessary information has been provided the patient. Signing of the official consent form is primarily evidence that the *consent process* has occurred—that the patient is aware of the concept of informed consent. The signatures of the health care personnel (as required by specific states or hospitals) merely provide witness to the signature of the patient or family member. Thus the nurse's signature does not reflect the substance of the informed consent process.

What then is the role of the nurse in the decision-making process? In the role of patient advocate, the nurse identifies that the patient has discussed with the physician the risks and benefits of the procedure and the alternatives. If this has not been done, the nurse consults with the physician. The professional nurse then uses skills of teaching and counseling to clarify any patient misconceptions and to facilitate the decision-making process by the patient. This process should occur before the patient receives any sedation. Patients may decide to refuse surgery, and it is their right to do so. Nurses have the responsibility to see that the decision is an *informed* decision.

If an adult is incapable of giving informed consent, consent must be obtained from the next of kin. The order of kin relationship for an adult, as determined from legal intestate succession, is usually spouse, adult child, parent, sibling.[28] A parent or legal guardian usually provides consent for a minor child. "Emancipated minors," that is, persons who are married or earning their own livelihood and retaining the earnings, can sign their own permit. The signature of the husband or wife of a married minor is also acceptable.

In an emergency situation, the surgeon may operate without written permission of the patient or family, although every effort is made to contact a family member or guardian if time permits. Consent in the form of a telephone call is permissible in this situation.

ASSESSMENT

Data are collected by the nurse in the preoperative period to identify the patient's (1) knowledge of events that will occur, (2) psychologic readiness for surgery, and (3) physiologic status before surgery. Specific data to be collected are listed in the box on p. 336.

■ Patient knowledge

A major nursing strategy in the preoperative period is teaching the patient about forthcoming events and exercises that can be used in the postoperative period to decrease the potential for complications. Before teaching can take place, it must be determined what the patient knows about the proposed surgery and the preoperative and postoperative routines.

■ Psychologic readiness for surgery

The degree of anxiety felt by the patient needs to be assessed. Patients may not be able to identify specific concerns, and further exploration may be necessary. If the

Table 16-4 Medications that can adversely affect anesthesia or surgery

Medication	Effect
Antibiotics	Potentiate muscle relaxants
Anticoagulants	Increase bleeding and hemorrhage
Antihypertensives	Affect anesthesia and compensatory ability (hypotension may occur)
Aspirin	↓ Platelet aggregation
	Potentiates effect of anticoagulants
Diuretics (thiazides)	Possible potassium imbalance
Steroids	↓ Neuroendocrine response
	Antiinflammatory effect, may delay wound healing
Tranquilizers	Potentiate effect of narcotics and barbiturates
	Hypotension

nurse has identified clues from the patient's behavior that moderate to severe anxiety is present, these complications need to be validated with the patient. (Review Chapter 7 for further information about anxiety, if necessary.) If the collected data indicate that the patient is severely anxious or if the patient describes fear of dying while in surgery, report this information to the physician for further evaluation. Surgery may need to be postponed in these situations.

Knowledge of the meaning of religion for the patient can help the nurse identify a possible source of support. The effect of family members or significant others on the patient's level of anxiety needs to be determined. Some family members or friends increase the patient's anxiety by transmitting their own anxiety—hovering over the patient, displaying anxious behaviors, or offering false reassurances. Others are calm, and it is observed that the patient's anxiety is reduced when they are present.

Changes in sleep patterns or frequent urination also provide clues about increased anxiety. Major causes of insomnia are worry, fear, and concerns about the future.

Signs of anxiety in the preoperative patient are no different from those in other persons. Physical signs include an increased pulse rate and respiratory rate, moist palms, constant hand movements or motor-verbal activity, and restlessness.

■ Physiologic status

Data are collected in the preoperative period concerning the patient's physiologic status to obtain baseline data for comparison in the intraoperative and postoperative phases and to identify potential postoperative problems requiring preoperative intervention. Admission histories and physical examinations by the physician and nurse are good sources of pertinent data. The physician may order special tests (Table 16-5) to detect the presence of diseases that may affect the perioperative course. Patients often need explanations concerning the necessity for the sometimes numerous tests.

Table 16-5 Preoperative tests to establish baselines and detect presence of diseases that can affect patient responses in intraoperative or postoperative phases

System	Test	Disease or condition
Respiratory	Chest radiograph	Tuberculosis or other pulmonary disease
	Vital capacity	Tuberculosis, chronic obstructive lung disease, bronchitis, asthma
	Pulmonary function	
	Blood gas studies	
Circulatory	Electrocardiogram	Cardiac arrhythmias, myocardial damage
	Blood studies	
	WBC and differential	Chronic infection
	RBC, hemoglobin, hematocrit	Anemia
	Electrolytes	Electrolyte imbalances
	Platelet count, bleeding and clotting times, prothrombin	Liver disease, blood dyscrasias
	Typing and crossmatching	Compatibility for transfusion
	Blood volume	Heart disease
Renal	Urine studies	
	Bacteria	Urinary tract infection
	Albumin, specific gravity	Kidney disease
	Blood studies	
	Creatine, BUN, NPN, electrolytes	Kidney disease
Metabolic	Blood sugar, urine sugar, acetone	Diabetes mellitus
		Starvation

■ ABILITY TO COMMUNICATE

Data relating to the senses and language indicate the patient's ability to understand directions and to receive support during the perioperative experience. Deficits need to be communicated with the operating room staff.

■ OXYGENATION

Respiratory data are especially important for determining the person's ability to expand the lungs, the risk for postoperative atelectasis or pneumonia, and the ability to carry out deep breathing exercises. Circulatory data are particularly important when the patient is elderly or is undergoing vascular or heart surgery. Persons with chronic lung, heart, or peripheral vascular disease may have more difficulties with tissue oxygenation in the postoperative period.

■ NUTRITION

The height-to-weight ratio indicates whether the patient is overweight or underweight (see Chapter 6). Persons who are at risk for postoperative nutritional deficiency should be identified early. Inadequate dietary intake, nausea, anorexia, and poor conditions of the mouth and teeth will influence preoperative nutritional intake and may be factors to consider in the postoperative period.

■ ELIMINATION

Decreased activity after surgery predisposes a patient to constipation. Persons with a history of chronic constipation have a higher probability for developing constipation or fecal impaction postoperatively.

■ ACTIVITY

Mobility and ambulation are important activities in the postoperative period for preventing postoperative complications. The patient's ability to move and walk preoperatively will determine actions that must be taken to enhance maximum mobility.

■ COMFORT

Many persons are not aware of the hospital's routines or the nursing staff's expectations regarding the giving of medications for postoperative pain. The routines need to be clarified with the patient to prevent misunderstandings.

➡ DATA ANALYSIS: NURSING DIAGNOSES

Nursing diagnoses are determined from assessment of patient data. Possible preoperative nursing diagnoses may include, but are not limited to, the following:

Diagnostic title	Possible etiologies
Anxiety	Threat of death, threat to role functioning, threat of unmet needs, fear of the unknown
Fear	Anesthesia, surgery (type), loss of body part, anticipated pain, possible lifestyle changes

Diagnostic title	Possible etiologies
Potential for infection	Lack of knowledge, decreased nutrition
Potential for injury: trauma	Sensory/motor deficits, lack of awareness of environmental hazards
Knowledge deficit (events pertaining to surgery)	Lack of exposure/recall, information misinterpretation, cognitive impairment, severe anxiety

PLANNING: EXPECTED PATIENT OUTCOMES

Expected patient outcomes for the preoperative patient may include, but are not limited to, the following:

1. Patient demonstrates no more than moderate anxiety.
2. Patient describes (if conscious) the surgery to be performed and has signed the operative consent form.
3. Patient describes the sequence of events and physical activities expected in the early postoperative period (turning, deep breathing and coughing).
4. Patient wears a legible identification band that has been checked.
5. Patient does not wear nail polish, hairpins or wigs, dentures, or jewelry to the O.R. (articles have been stored for safekeeping).
6. Patient voids before going to the O.R.
7. Patient receives preanesthetic medication as ordered.

IMPLEMENTATION

Assisting with achievement of therapeutic goals

MEDICAL INTERVENTIONS: CORRECTION OF EXISTING DEFICIENCIES

Postoperative complications can be minimized if existing medical conditions are treated or are under good control before surgery. Measures to treat wound infections are carried out before secondary closure or skin grafting. Dehydration from vomiting and diarrhea is treated with parenteral fluids to reestablish fluid and electrolyte balance.

Patients with chronic diseases should be at their optimal health level before surgery. The undernourished patient is placed on a high-protein, high-carbohydrate diet rich in vitamins B_1, C, and K. Supplementary vitamins may be ordered. If an oral diet is poorly tolerated or poorly absorbed, total parenteral nutrition (TPN) will be initiated. The obese patient is placed on a weight-reducing diet. Both the undernourished and the obese patient should understand the rationale for the diets. They may need a considerable amount of support and encouragement to maintain the diets.

Patients with chronic obstructive pulmonary disease are frequently placed on vigorous respiratory therapy to ensure maximal ventilation and to decrease postoperative respiratory complications. This therapy usually includes postural drainage, aerosol inhalations, and antibiotics. Smoking is discouraged for all patients preoperatively and especially for patients with lung disease. Diabetes mellitus should be under good control.

PREOPERATIVE PREPARATION

Diet

Except in bowel surgery for which patients may be placed on a low residue diet, a regular diet is permitted the day before surgery, but no food is allowed 8 hours before surgery. The diet should be in accordance with the pre-existing conditions. Fluids are usually withheld at least 4 hours before surgery. Presence of food or fluids in the stomach increases the possibility of aspiration of gastric contents should the patient vomit while under anesthesia. This can lead to aspiration pneumonia. If it should be discovered that the patient has consumed food or fluids when ordered "nothing by mouth" (NPO), the surgeon should be notified, since this may necessitate rescheduling the surgical procedure. If a local or spinal anesthetic is planned, a light meal may be permitted.

Patients who are dehydrated will usually have parenteral fluids initiated before surgery. If it is anticipated that the patient may have decreased peristalsis after surgery (as a result of anesthesia or manipulation of the abdominal viscera), a nasogastric tube may be inserted before surgery.

Bowel preparation

Enemas are usually given preoperatively only for surgery of the GI tract or of the pelvic, perineal, or perianal areas. If a preoperative enema is ineffectual, it may be repeated. The purpose of the preoperative enema is to prevent injury to the colon, to provide better visualization of the surgical area, and to prevent constipation or fecal impaction postoperatively.

If enemas are to be given until the returns are clear, it is important to remember that fluid excess and potassium deficits can occur with repeated enemas. It is common practice to check with the physician if returns are not clear after the third enema. One method is to give up to three enemas the evening before surgery, and then if the returns are still not clear to repeat the enemas the following morning. Repeated enemas are very tiring for the patient and may irritate rectal and bowel mucosa. If antibiotic enemas are ordered for the purpose of decreasing intestinal bacteria before intestinal surgery, synthesis of vitamin K by the intestinal bacteria may be inhibited. Supplementary vitamin K may be given to prevent bleeding after surgery.

Skin preparation

The purpose of preoperative skin preparation is to free the operative site of as many microorganisms as possible. In many instances showering well with hexachlorophene soap will suffice. In certain types of surgery, such as orthopedic implants where infections can lead to dysfunction, a special cleansing routine is prescribed. No soap, alcohol, or alcohol-based solutions should be used in conjunction with hexachlorophene solutions as these substances decrease the antiseptic properties of hexachlorophene.

Hair is removed from the surgical site because microorganisms cling to the hair. A depilatory may be used if the skin is not sensitive to the depilatory. Shaving of the hair may be ordered either the night before or immediately before surgery. A sharp disposable razor is used with good lighting. Shaving must be *against the grain* of the hair shaft for a closer shave. The skin should not be scratched or nicked since microorganisms can harbor in broken skin surfaces.

Shaving of hair on certain areas of the body may have a special meaning for some persons. These areas include face, head, and pubic area. If the entire head is to be shaved, it is frequently carried out after the patient has been anesthetized. The eyebrows are not shaved. Pubic hair is shaved only when necessary; the regrowth of this hair is uncomfortable to many patients.

Some hospitals have specified procedures delineating the size of the area to be shaved. The surgeon usually specifies which of the areas is to be shaved. An area larger than the anticipated incision is shaved to permit flexibility in location and size of incision.

■ Counseling and teaching

■ PSYCHOLOGIC PREPARATION FOR SURGERY

Both patient and family need opportunities to discuss their concerns and fears about the forthcoming surgery. The assessment of the patient's psychologic readiness for surgery provides the nurse with data about the patient's specific fears and concerns.

Having opportunities to talk with a supportive, knowledgeable individual helps persons begin to identify the reasons for their anxiety and to marshal coping responses. It

---

┌───┐

Helpful information for preoperative patients and families

Preoperative tests—reason, preparation
Preoperative routines
Special equipment needed
Transfer to operating room (time, checking procedures)
Recovery room
  Place where patient will awaken
  Frequent monitoring of vital signs
  Return to room when vital signs stable
Probable postoperative therapies
  Need for increased mobility as soon as possible
  Need to keep respiratory passages clear
  Anticipated treatments (for example, I.V.)
  Pain medication routines (timing sequence, "as needed" [p.r.n.] status)

└───┘

---

is helpful for the nurse to plan for a quiet unhurried time to sit down with the person or family and give an opportunity to ask questions and to talk about concerns. Touch is often a helpful form of communication, sending the message, "I care," and some persons will talk more readily while receiving a back rub. Knowing that a nurse is interested and cares helps to reduce anxiety. If the person knows also that anxiety is a normal reaction to the threat of surgery, it may help to remove the often self-imposed expectation, "I shouldn't be nervous."

Loss of control is one of the fears associated with surgery. Allowing persons to participate in decision making in regard to their own care, when feasible, helps them partially meet the need for control. Identifying and carrying out measures to help the patient meet physical needs in the preoperative phase may help provide a feeling of security about having postoperative needs met and thus allay some anxiety.

Teaching is an important function of the nurse in the preoperative phase and helps to allay anxiety when the patient knows what to expect. Also, if persons are to move toward self-care and independence, they need to know early the what, why, and how of activities that will help them regain an optimal level of functioning after surgery. Waiting until the patient has sufficiently recovered from the insult of surgery before teaching is started means a considerable loss of time, and learning may be less effective. In addition, the patient may be discharged before teaching is completed.

■ EXPLANATION OF EVENTS

Fear of the unknown can be decreased by an understanding of the events that will occur. The amount of information to give preoperatively depends on the background, interest, and stress level of the patient and the family. A good rule to follow is to ask patients what they would like to know about forthcoming surgery and to base responses on the types of questions asked. Simple explanations are indicated for persons under considerable stress or those with severe pain. A highly anxious person may not take in and remember information given. Information helpful for preoperative patients is listed in the box on the left.

■ DEEP BREATHING AND COUGHING EXERCISES

Some persons are at high risk for developing postoperative pulmonary complications such as atelectasis or pneumonia (see the box on p. 341, left). These persons need to carry out deep breathing and coughing exercises in the early postoperative period.

Coughing is *contraindicated*, however, in intracranial surgery and surgery of the eye, ear, nose, and throat, because it either increases pressure, causing tissue damage and dislodging of sutures, or dislodges a clot (Table 16-6). Waiting until after surgery to teach persons how to carry out the exercises decreases the effectiveness of the outcome, since anesthesia and pain will decrease the ability to retain information.

The person needs to know how to perform diaphragmatic breathing, as this increases lung expansion by permitting the diaphragm to descend fully. Many males normally breathe diaphragmatically, whereas few females do. With diaphragmatic breathing, the abdomen *rises with inspiration and falls with expiration*. The nurse assesses the person's normal breathing pattern by placing a hand lightly on the person's abdomen and asking the person to take a deep breath. If diaphragmatic breathing does not occur naturally, the person can be taught to inspire deeply while pushing the abdomen up against the hand.

The method for deep breathing and coughing exercises is listed as follows:

1. Lie in semi-Fowler's or high Fowler's position with knees flexed to relax abdomen and allow full chest expansion.
2. Place a hand lightly on the abdomen.
3. Breathe in slowly through nose, letting chest expand and feeling abdomen rise against hand.

4. Hold breath for 3 seconds.
5. Exhale slowly through pursed lips (abdomen contracts).
6. Inhale and exhale 3 more times. *Following last inspiration cough forcefully* to expel any secretions.
7. Rest.
8. Repeat steps 3 through 7 two more times.

If thoracic or high abdominal incisions are present, the person can "splint" the incision with a pillow during coughing to relieve stress or pull on the incision.

■ LEG EXERCISES

Venous stasis in the postoperative period may lead to thrombophlebitis (blood clot). Persons at high risk include those who (1) will have decreased mobility after surgery, (2) have a history of decreased peripheral circulation, or (3) undergo cardiovascular or pelvic surgery. These patients will need to carry out exercises postoperatively to prevent venous stasis in the legs. Tightening and relaxing leg muscles (see the box below) help to "pump" the blood along the veins. Valves in the veins prevent back flow of blood.

Persons who will be restricted to bed rest for several days after surgery will need to exercise the legs to maintain muscle tone to facilitate ambulation at a later date. These persons need to learn to carry out quadriceps drills and gluteal tightening exercises.

■ MOBILITY

Moving and turning in bed helps to prevent pulmonary and circulatory complications, prevent decubiti, stimulate

---

High-risk factors: pulmonary complications

Inhalant anesthesia	Tight abdominal
Thoracic surgery	binders
Upper abdominal surgery	Body casts
Smoking	Obesity
Chronic lung disease	Elderly

Table 16-6 Surgeries for which coughing is contraindicated or modified

Surgery site	Effect of coughing
Intracranial	Coughing increases intracranial pressure (ICP), leading to cerebral trauma
Eye	Coughing increases ICP, which then increases intraocular pressure, causing pressure on suture line
Ear	Mouth must be kept open if coughing occurs to prevent pressure backup through eustachian tube to middle ear, causing pressure on suture line
Nose	Mouth must be kept open if coughing occurs to prevent dislodgement of clot with subsequent bleeding
Throat	Vigorous coughing may dislodge a clot with subsequent bleeding

---

Postoperative leg exercises

Muscle pump exercises
1. Contract calf and thigh muscles
2. Relax leg muscles
3. Rest
4. Repeat at least 10 times

Quadriceps drill
1. Bend knees with foot flat on bed
2. Straighten leg on bed
3. Lift heel, pressing back of knee against bed
4. Repeat at least 5 times

Gluteal tightening exercises
1. Pinch buttocks together
2. Attempt to move leg to side of bed
3. Relax
4. Repeat at least 5 times

peristalsis, and decrease pain. During the preoperative period, persons can be taught how to use the side rails effectively for turning. They can also be taught how to sit up on the side of the bed with the least amount of pull on the incision:

1. Move to edge of bed
2. Raise head of bed to high Fowler's position
3. Drop feet over side of bed
4. Push up to sitting position with hand closest to edge of bed

■ Assisting with comfort

Anxiety often causes sleeplessness and restlessness. If the patient is extremely restless, an antianxiety agent may be given for 1 to 2 days before surgery. Ambulation is encouraged before surgery to give the patient a feeling of well-being, to stimulate circulation and ventilation, and to maintain muscle tone. Fatigue is to be avoided, and patients with chronic illnesses may need planned periods of rest.

The person should be permitted to sleep on the morning of surgery for as long as possible and to rest undisturbed until shortly before administration of preanesthetic medication. Many persons prefer to take their bath or shower the evening before surgery rather than in the morning. The person who has bathed the night before is given an opportunity to wash hands and face and to perform mouth care. The person is reminded that he or she should not swallow water if fluids by mouth are not permitted.

Comfort also implies readiness for surgery and that the patient is able to marshal effective coping mechanisms. Family are advised to arrive at least 1 hour before the scheduled time for surgery. The patient should have an opportunity to have last-minute questions answered. Explanations for last-minute routines are given if this was not done previously. If the surgery is to be delayed even for a short time, both the patient and family should be informed.

■ Carrying out final preparation for surgery

■ PREVENTION OF INJURY

Measures taken to protect the patient from errors of identification or injury include the following:

1. Check identification band for secureness and legibility.
2. Remove hair pins and wigs; protect hair with a cap.
3. Remove jewelry; wedding ring may be taped to patient's finger.
4. Remove nail polish (for assessment of circulation during surgery).
5. Remove contact lenses and store in proper container.
6. Remove any prostheses (dentures, false eyes, and so on); store prostheses in a safe place.
7. Leave hearing aid in place if patient is unable to hear without the aid (inform operating room nurse).

8. Apply antiembolic stockings if patient is at high risk for thromboembolism or shock (elderly, marked varicosities, pelvic surgery, time-consuming surgery).
9. Have patient empty bladder immediately before receiving preanesthetic medication.

■ PREANESTHETIC MEDICATION

A sedative is usually ordered the night before surgery to ensure a full night's sleep. If additional sedation or medication for pain is given during the night, it must be given at least 4 hours before the preanesthetic medication to prevent oversedation.

Preanesthetic medications, commonly referred to as *premedication,* are given when the patient is "on call" for the operating room (usually about 45 to 90 minutes before surgery is anticipated). Preanesthetic medications are given to decrease anxiety, to provide a smoother induction and maintenance of anesthesia, to diminish undesirable reflexes during emergence from anesthesia, to decrease salivary and respiratory secretions, and to block vagal impulses that produce bradycardia.

The effects of commonly used preanesthetic medications are listed in Table 16-7. Adults frequently receive a combination of drugs. Dosages may be decreased in the elderly.

Any delay in giving the medication is reported to the anesthesiologist. All preoperative routines are completed before the preanesthetic medication is given. The patient should remain in bed following administration of the medication to promote maximum effect and to prevent falls from dizziness. The side rails are raised, the bed is placed in low position, the call signal is placed within reach, and the patient is instructed not to get out of bed.

One major desired effect before surgery is decreased anxiety. It must be reemphasized that psychologic preparation of the patient for surgery is the most effective approach to help allay anxiety. The administration of preanesthetic medication without any attempt at psychologic preparation may render the patient drowsy, but it does not reduce anxiety.

Some drugs other than preanesthetic agents, such as insulin, antihypertensive agents, and cardiac medications, may be prescribed for the day of surgery. Oral medications are given with only a small sip of water. Administration of these medications is recorded on the chart before patient transfer to surgery.

■ RECORDING

A check-off list that includes the final preparations is often used. A final nurse's note is written listing the times the patient voided, when the patient leaves for surgery, and any final pertinent remarks regarding the patient's condition and emotional response. Presence of any handicaps such as blindness or deafness should be noted for use by the surgical staff.

Before the patient leaves for surgery the chart is checked for completeness as to the following:

Table 16-7 Commonly used preanesthetic medications

Drug	Desired effects	Undesired effects
Sedative-hypnotics		
Pentobarbital sodium (Nembutal)	Reduces anxiety, promotes relaxation and sleep	May cause excitement or confusion in elderly persons or in those with severe pain
Secobarbital sodium (Seconal)	Same as above	Same as above
Flurazepam hydrochloride (Dalmane)	Promotes relaxation and sleep	
Chloral hydrate	Same as for flurazepam	
Narcotics		
Morphine sulfate	Reduces anxiety, promotes relaxation, decreases preoperative pain, decreases amount of anesthetic needed	Depresses respiration, circulation, and gastric motility; may cause nausea and vomiting
Meperidine hydrochloride (Demerol)	Same as for morphine sulfate	Same as for morphine sulfate
Antianxiety agents		
Promethazine hydrochloride (Phenergan)	Reduces anxiety, antiemetic	Postoperative hypotension
Chlorpromazine (Thorazine)	Same as for promethazine hydrochloride	Same as for promethazine hydrochloride
Hydroxyzine (Vistaril, Atarax)	Reduces anxiety, produces drowsiness, antiemetic	Geriatric patients are more sensitive to usual adult dose
Neuroleptanalgesic agent		
Fentanyl and droperidol (Innovar)	General quiescence, state of indifference, decreased motor activity, analgesia, antiemetic	Respiratory depression, muscle rigidity, hypotension
Vagolytic agents		
Atropine sulfate	Decreased secretions, prevention of laryngospasms	Excessive dryness of mouth, tachycardia
Scopolamine hydrochloride (Hyoscine)	Decreased secretions, amnesia, state of indifference, sedation	Excessive dryness of mouth
Glycopyrrolate (Robinul)	Same as atropine sulfate	Same as atropine sulfate

1. Skin preparation done and checked by nurse
2. Vital signs (temperature, pulse, respiration, blood pressure) charted
3. Premedications charted
4. Regular medication charted
5. Weight and height recorded (for use by anesthesiologist)
6. Operative permit signed, witnessed, and attached to chart
7. All recent laboratory, radiographic, and ECG reports attached to chart

✠ EVALUATION

Questions to ask may include the following:
1. Is the patient's anxiety level no more than moderate?
2. Does the patient understand the nature of the surgical procedure to be performed, and has the operative permit (consent form) been signed?
3. Has the patient been taught the physical activities to be performed in the early postoperative period, as pertinent (turning, deep breathing and coughing, and leg exercises)?

4. Is the patient wearing a legible identification band that has been checked?
5. Have all removable objects been stored for safekeeping?
6. Has nailpolish been removed?
7. Did the patient void just before receiving premedication?
8. Has the premedication been given and charted?
9. Is the chart complete?

■ TRANSPORTATION TO OPERATING ROOM

Personnel transporting the patient bring the stretcher from the operating room and identify themselves to the nurse. The unit nurse assigned to prepare the patient for surgery checks the patient record, accompanies the transportation attendant to the patient's bedside, checks the patient's identification band, and signs the patient identification form. This form is usually then attached to the stretcher. Patients should be protected from drafts. Since the operating room is kept cool, cotton blankets are used to keep the patient warm.

The patient's family or close friends are provided with the following information:
1. Where to wait until patient returns to the unit
2. Availability of coffee shop, cafeteria, and so on
3. Expected time intervals
   a. Patient is sent to surgery 45 to 60 minutes before surgery actually commences
   b. Surgery may be delayed if the previous surgery took longer than anticipated
   c. Patient will be sent to a postanesthesia room (recovery room) after surgery for varying periods of time
4. Method of receiving information when surgery is completed
5. Visit by surgeon after surgery (if this is the policy)
6. What to expect when patient returns from surgery (condition, special equipment, and so on)

■ AMBULATORY SURGERY

Although certain types of minor surgeries have been performed on an outpatient basis for many years, only in recent years has there been a sharp increase in certain major surgeries being performed on an ambulatory basis. Also, larger numbers of persons are having these surgeries. One major reason for these changes has been the emphasis on cost containment in health care services.

■ Preoperative considerations

Ambulatory surgery is directed toward the healthy person requiring uncomplicated surgery.[7] The surgery itself must not be one that requires expert postoperative care.

Success in ambulatory surgery depends on several factors, including preoperative testing and teaching facilities, physical status of the patient, and home care support persons.

■ PREOPERATIVE TESTING AND TEACHING

Preoperative screening is performed several days before the anticipated surgery. A complete medical and nursing history is as important before ambulatory surgery as it is for inpatient surgery. The kind and number of preoperative laboratory studies varies, ranging from none to a complete workup.[29] On the basis of cost versus benefits to the patient, physicians have recently begun to question the necessity for extensive preoperative testing in the absence of indications from the preoperative history and physical examination. Many physicians, however, still order multiple preoperative screening tests because of fear of malpractice suits.[19]

Patient and family teaching is of the utmost importance to ensure effective postoperative care, including monitoring. Psychologic preparation is the same as for the inpatient (p. 340), and a tour of the facility may help decrease a patient's anxiety (fear of the unknown). The minimum preoperative information is listed in the box below. It is particularly useful to provide *written* instructions whenever possible, especially for activities the patient and family are to carry out.

■ PHYSICAL STATUS

Most ambulatory surgical patients are either healthy or may have a mild systemic disease, such as diet-controlled diabetes mellitus, moderate obesity, chronic bronchitis, old MI, or mild hypertension. In selected instances persons with a severe systemic disease but who are in a stable condition may be considered.[29] Persons who are poor risks for ambulatory surgery include those with brittle diabetes mellitus, with morbid obesity, or with a systemic disease that places them in constant threat, such as cardiac, pul-

---

Preoperative teaching for the ambulatory surgical patient

Knowledge about the proposed surgery
Preoperative routines
  Arrival time
  Clothes to wear
  Restrictions (food, fluids)
  Responsible person to accompany the patient to and from the facility
Expected activity in the surgical center
Postoperative routines (in center and at home)
Home support: type needed

monary, renal, hepatic, or endocrine insufficiency.[29]

Age, per se, is not a limiting factor, and in fact, many elderly persons have increased benefits from ambulatory surgery versus inpatient surgery. Benefits for the elderly include decreased risk of complications such as pneumonia or infection, increased mental and physical functioning because the environment is less foreign, decreased cost, and maintenance of contacts with family and friends.[7] Additional care requirements may be needed for elderly persons, including providing time and attention needed for adjustment.

■ HOME CARE SUPPORT PERSONS

Having a responsible person who is physically and intellectually capable of providing any necessary home care is of utmost importance to the ambulatory surgical patient. This person should accompany the patient on the preoperative visit, if at all possible, and be included in the preoperative teaching session with the nurse.

■ Day of surgery

Presurgical preparations are usually similar to those of inpatient surgeries, such as removal of loose prostheses, wearing of identification band, presurgical voiding, and preanesthetic medication. The physician and anesthesiologist do a final physical checkup before surgery.

In the postoperative period, patients frequently are not routinely given medication for postoperative pain, both because pain is often not severe and because the person must not be sedated or dizzy before leaving for home. Some surgeons administer long-acting local anesthetics to reduce postoperative pain.[7]

Most ambulatory surgical centers have specific criteria that must be met before the patient is discharged. Vital signs must be stable and the patient fully awake. Nausea, vomiting, and dizziness preferably should be absent or at least minimal, and there should be no respiratory distress.

The person must be able to swallow, cough, and ambulate at the preoperative level. Home care instructions are repeated, especially with the home caregiver, and are provided in writing. The patient and caregiver must know specific signs and symptoms to be monitored, what to do if these occur, and the specific person or agency to notify.

■ SUMMARY

1. Surgery may be classified by location (external or internal or body system) or by extent (major or minor).
2. The purpose of surgery may be diagnostic, curative, restorative, palliative, or cosmetic.
3. Surgery is a stressor; therefore, it evokes neuroendocrine and metabolic responses to stress. Neuroendocrine responses include vasoconstriction, increased cardiac output, decreased GI activity, increased glucocorticoid secretion, and increased ADH secretion. Metabolic responses include utilization of carbohydrates and fats for energy and protein catabolism.
4. Anxiety and fear are common responses to anticipated surgery. Persons with severe anxiety are poor candidates for surgery.
5. Risk factors for surgery include extremes of age, malnutrition, neuroendocrine response ineffectiveness, selected chronic diseases, and smoking.
6. Patients must know about the nature and risks of the proposed surgery and available options for care before signing a consent form (informed consent). The physician is responsible for obtaining informed consent; the nurse facilitates the process and ensures that the consent form has been signed before surgery.
7. Data are collected by the nurse in the preoperative period to identify the patient's knowledge about surgery and psychologic response (for planning of preoperative care); physiologic data are collected to establish a baseline for future comparison and to identify potential postoperative problems.

Putting knowledge to practice

■ What general reactions do you believe you would have if told you must have immediate major surgery? What questions would you want answered? Compare and contrast your reaction and questions with those of a classmate.

■ Examine the charts of several patients on your clinical unit who have had surgery for the following: Do the preoperative notes provide data concerning the patient's readiness for or concerns about surgery? Was the preoperative teaching carried out? What were some of the preanesthetic medications given?

■ Examine the informed consent form of your agency. What is your responsibility in this situation?

■ Talk with several surgical patients about their concerns before surgery. In what ways were the nursing staff helpful? What do the patients think would have been more helpful?

■ Role play with fellow students preparing the patient on the day of surgery. Use any preoperative checklist forms used by your agency.

8. Preoperative medical care includes treatment of existing medical conditions, including nutritional status, to facilitate optimal health status (except in emergency surgery).
9. Dietary restrictions for adults having major surgery usually include no food for 8 hours and no fluids for 4 hours before surgery.
10. The skin is usually prepared by careful cleansing. Shaving is best done in the operating room immediately before surgery to prevent infection.
11. Psychologic preparation of the patient for surgery includes helping the person explore concerns or fear about surgery and providing desired information about the perioperative experience.
12. Teaching of necessary postoperative patient activities, such as deep breathing and coughing exercises, leg exercises, and turning in bed, are best taught in the preoperative period.
13. Final preparations before the patient is transported to surgery include removing nonattached objects and nail polish, ensuring proper patient identification, providing a hair cap, and asking the patient to void.
13. Preanesthetic medications are given to decrease anxiety; facilitate induction, maintenance, and emergence from anesthesia; decrease secretions; and prevent bradycardia. The patient must remain in bed after premedication has been given to facilitate drug effects and to prevent falls from dizziness.

REFERENCES AND SELECTED READINGS
Contemporary

1. Alexander, J, and others: The influence of hair removal methods on wound infections, Arch Surg 118:347-352, 1983.
2. American College of Surgeons' Committee on Pre- and Postoperative Care: Manual of preoperative and postoperative care, ed 3, Philadelphia, 1983, WB Saunders Co.
3. Association of Operating Room Nurses, Inc: Standards of nursing practice, Denver, 1980, The Association.
4. *Blackwood, S: Back to basics: the preop exam, Am J Nurs 86:39-44, 1986.
5. *Breslin, EF: Prevention and treatment of pulmonary complications in patients after surgery of the upper abdomen, Heart Lung 10:511-514, 1981.
6. *Connaway, CA, and Blackledge, D: Preoperative testing center: central location to evaluate and educate patients, AORN J 43:666-670, 1986.
7. *Crawford, FJ: Ambulatory surgery: the elderly patient, AORN J 41:356-369, 1985.
8. *Cushing, M: Informed consent: an MD responsibility? Am J Nurs 84:437-440, 1984.
9. *Does preop medication promote stress? Am J Nurs 84:1202, 1984.
10. Evaluating the usefulness of routine preoperative tests, AORN J 45:696, 1987.
11. *Fraulini, KE: Coping mechanisms and recovery from surgery, AORN J 37:1198-1208, 1983.
12. *Fuchs, P: Before and after surgery, stay right on respiratory care, Nurs 83 13(5):47-50, 1983.
13. *Greenwood, BS: Check out your patient's presurgery fears, Nurs 82 12(7):34-35, 1982.
14. Gruendemann, BJ, and Meeker, MH: Alexander's care of the patient in surgery, ed 8, St. Louis, 1987, The CV Mosby Co.
15. Hathaway, D: Effect of preoperative instruction on postoperative outcomes: a meta-analysis, Nurs Res 35:269-275, 1986.
16. *Hogue, E: What you should know about informed consent, Nurs 86 16(6):47-48, 1986.
17. *Horsley, J, and Crane, J: Structured preoperative teaching, New York, 1981, Grune & Stratton, Inc.
18. Johnston, M: Preoperative emotional states and postoperative recovery, Adv Psychosom Med 15:1-22, 1986.
19. Kaplan, EB, and others: The usefulness of preoperative laboratory screening, JAMA 253:3576-3581, 1985.
20. *Kathol, DK: Anxiety in surgical patient's families, AORN J 40:131-137, 1984.
21. Kneedler, J, and Dodge, G: Perioperative patient care, Boston, 1983, Blackwell Scientific Publications, Inc.
22. Luce, JM: Clinical risk factors for postoperative pulmonary complications, Resp Care 29:484-495, 1984.
23. *Mackie, RM, and Peddie, RP: Perioperative care plan guides, AORN J 40:192-201, 1984.
24. Mason, JH: General surgery. In Steinberg, FU (editor): Cowdry's The care of the geriatric patient, ed 6, St. Louis, 1983, The CV Mosby Co.
25. *McHugh, NG, Christman, NH, and Johnson, JE: Preparatory information: what helps and why, Am J Nurs 83:780-782, 1982.
26. Mortensen, M, and McMullin, C: Discharge score for surgical outpatients, Am J Nurs 86:1347-1349, 1986.
27. Rogers, M, and Reich, P: Psychological intervention with surgical patients: evaluation outcomes, Adv Psychsom Med 15:23-50, 1986.
28. Way, LW: Current surgical diagnosis and treatment, ed 7, Los Altos, Calif, 1987, Lange Medical Publications.
29. *Wetchler, BV: Patient selection criteria for 1987: ambulatory surgery, AORN J 44:30-36, 1987.
30. Wetchler, BV: Postanesthesia scoring system: discharging ambulatory surgery patients, AORN J 41:382-384, 1985.
31. *Williams, D: Preoperative patient education: in the home or in the hospital? Orthop Nurs 5(1):37-41, 1986.
32. Wong, J, and others: A randomized trial of a new approach to preoperative teaching and patient compliance, Int J Nurs Stud 22(2):105-115, 1985.
33. Worley, B: Preadmission testing and teaching: more satisfaction at less cost . . . surgical admissions, Nurs Manage 17(12):32-33, 1986.

*References preceded by an asterisk are particularly well suited for student reading.

17

Intraoperative Intervention

JUDITH L. GREIG

CHAPTER OBJECTIVES

After studying this chapter, the student should be able to:

- Explain the concept of perioperative nursing care.
- Identify the members of the surgical team and describe their individual responsibilities.
- Identify the basic rules of surgical asepsis.
- Explain the rationale for operating room attire and personnel health habits.
- Identify factors that promote patient safety in the operating room.
- Describe five common positions for patients undergoing surgery and specify the nursing care planning involved.
- Describe the various methods of administering anesthestics and identify the common agents used for each.
- Identify the various methods available for monitoring patients during surgical procedures.
- Describe nursing interventions to ensure safe patient care when the surgical procedure has been completed and before transfer to the recovery area.

Each surgical patient is unique, and, therefore, surgery on each is a unique experience. Patients bring with them to the operating suite an individual set of feelings and values that must be considered in planning nursing care during the intraoperative period.

The operating room nurse functions as the patient's advocate during surgery. This role has been viewed in the past as being entirely technical in nature. One cannot deny that an operating room nurse must possess knowledge of skills, procedures, instruments, and supplies to function as an effective team member. Not all of operating room nursing is technical, however, and the integration of nursing process into this arena of care has become the accepted standard for operating room nurses. These nurses are responsible for providing a safe, caring, and efficient environment in which the surgical team can function to provide the best outcome for each patient.

■ CONCEPTS BASIC TO OPERATING ROOM NURSING

■ Perioperative nursing

The perioperative role of the professional operating room (O.R.) nurse consists of nursing activities performed during the preoperative, intraoperative, and postoperative phases of the patient's surgical experience (Fig. 17-1). The extent of activities depends on the nurse's knowledge and skill, varying from a basic competency level to a level of excellence.

Each phase of this role begins and ends at an appointed time in the chain of events involved in surgical intervention; each includes a variety of nursing activities that can be performed using nursing process. The *preoperative phase*

begins when the decision for surgical intervention is made and ends when the patient is transferred to the operating room table. The scope of nursing activities involved can be as broad as beginning assessment of the patient in the clinic or at home through a preoperative interview, or it can be as limited as doing a preoperative assessment in the holding area of the surgical suite.

The *intraoperative phase* begins when the patient is transferred to the operating table and ends with transfer to the recovery area. Again, the activities performed by the nurse can be as broad as recognizing the patient's potential for skin breakdown in certain areas and taking special precautions or as limited as simply positioning the patient on the table according to the basic principles of good body alignment.

The *postoperative phase* begins with admission of the patient to the recovery area and ends with a follow-up evaluation. The scope of care can be as broad as seeing the patient in a home or clinic setting or as limited as the nurse communicating to personnel in the recovery area pertinent information relative to the patient's surgery. Table 17-1 illustrates a sample list of nursing activities in the three phases of perioperative nursing.

Perioperative nursing is seen as a goal for care practiced by operating room nurses. This role has been developed through the efforts of the Association of Operating Room Nurses (AORN), a volunteer organization of registered nurses concerned with the care of patients before, during, and after surgery. By practicing the perioperative role, the O.R. nurse brings together traditional and extended nursing activities during the intraoperative period. Thus the more recently developed preoperative and postoperative assessment, teaching, and evaluation functions are integrated from both a technical and professional aspect.

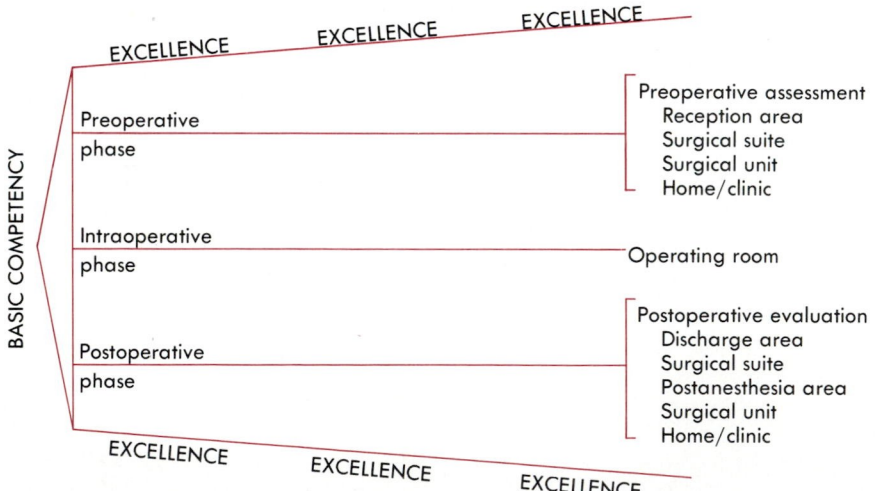

Fig. 17-1 Perioperative nursing practice: a continuum. (From A model for perioperative nursing practice, AORN J 41:192-193, 1985. Reprinted with permission from AORN, Inc, 10710 E Mississippi Avenue, Denver, CO, 80231. All rights reserved.)

Table 17-1   Examples of activities in the perioperative role

Preoperative phase	Intraoperative phase	Postoperative phase

Preoperative assessment
Home/clinic
1. Initiates initial preoperative assessment
2. Plans teaching methods appropriate to patient's needs
3. Involves family in interview
Surgical unit
1. Completes preoperative assessment
2. Coordinates patient teaching with other nursing staff
3. Explains phases in perioperative period and expectations
4. Develops a plan of care
Surgical suite
1. Assesses patient's level consciousness
2. Reviews chart
3. Identifies patient
4. Verifies surgical site
 	
Planning
1. Determines a plan of care
 	
Psychological support
1. Tells patient what is happening
2. Determines psychological status
3. Gives prior warning of noxious stimuli
4. Stands near/touches patient during procedures/induction
5. Communicates patient's emotional status to other appropriate members of the health care team
	Maintenance of safety
	1. Assures that the sponge, needle, and instrument counts are correct
	2. Positions the patient
	  a. Functional alignment
	  b. Exposure of surgical site
	  c. Maintenance of position throughout procedure
	3. Applies grounding device to patient
	4. Provides physical support
	
	Physiological monitoring
	1. Calculates effects on patient of excessive fluid loss
	2. Distinguishes normal from abnormal cardiopulmonary data
	3. Reports changes in patient's pulse, respirations, temperature, and blood pressure
	
	Psychological monitoring (prior to induction and if patient conscious)
	1. Provides emotional support to patient
	2. Continues to assess patient's emotional status
	3. Communicates patient's emotional status to other appropriate members of the health care team
	
	Nursing management
	1. Provides physical safety for the patient
	2. Maintains aseptic, controlled environment
	3. Effectively manages human resources
		Communication of intraoperative information
		1. Gives patient's name
		2. States type of surgery performed
		3. Provides contributing intraoperative factors, e.g., drain, catheters
		4. States physical limitations
		5. States impairments resulting from surgery
		6. Reports patient's preoperative level of consciousness
		7. Communicates necessary equipment needs
		
		Postoperative evaluation
		Recovery area
		1. Determines patient's immediate response to surgical intervention
		Surgical unit
		1. Evaluates effectiveness of nursing care in the OR
		2. Determines patient's level of satisfaction with care given during perioperative period
		3. Evaluates products used on patient in the OR
		4. Determines patient's psychological status
		5. Assists with discharge planning
		Home/clinic
		1. Seeks patient's perception of surgery in terms of the effects of anesthetic agents, impact on body image, distortion, immobilization
		2. Determines family's perceptions of surgery

■ Standards of perioperative nursing practice

Standards have been developed to guide the practice of operating room nursing.[18] These standards are based on nursing process and serve as a model to measure the quality of patient care delivered. The standards include all aspects of nursing process (assessment, planning, implementation, and evaluation) pertinent to the planned surgical intervention.

Standards of care and the use of nursing process during the intraoperative period are viewed as paving the way for nurses in the operating room to expand knowledge, increase sensitivity to individuals' needs, and be accountable to patients as consumers. This also provides continuity of care in an integrated manner using preoperative assessment, intraoperative intervention, and postoperative evaluation.

■ Intraoperative patient care team members

■ OPERATING TEAM

The intraoperative patient care team members are commonly subdivided into two basic categories: scrubbed sterile members and nonsterile members.

The *scrubbed sterile* team members usually include the following:

1. Primary surgeon
2. Assistants to the surgeon (may vary in number and qualifications; however, most medical staff bylaws state, "A qualified physician shall assist during all major operations."[19])
3. Scrub nurse or technician

The *nonsterile* team members may include the following:

1. Anesthesiologist or anesthetist
2. Circulating nurse
3. Others (technicians to operate complicated monitoring devices or equipment such as the heart-lung machine, biomedical engineers, pathologist if a frozen tissue section is necessary, and so on)

■ SCRUB NURSE

Nursing responsibilities in the operating room are commonly divided into the roles of scrub nurse and circulating nurse. The scrub nurse may or may not be a nurse, as this role can be carried out by a registered nurse, practical or vocational nurse, or a trained technician. Scrub nurse activities may include the following:

1. Preparing sterile supplies and equipment needed for the operation
2. Assisting the surgeon and surgical assistants during the procedure
3. Teaching new personnel, if qualified to do so
4. Assisting in accounting for needles, scalpel blades, sponges, and instruments used during the procedure, using the established *count* procedure

To carry out these activities effectively the scrub nurse must possess thorough knowledge of aseptic technique, manual skill and dexterity, physical stamina, the ability to work under pressure, and a sincere concern for accuracy and accountability in performing in a manner consistent with optimal patient care.

■ CIRCULATING NURSE

The circulating nurse plays a role in the overall management of the operating room. This person is vital to the effective flow of patient care before, during, and after the surgical procedure. Although the surgeon is in charge of the operative site, the circulating nurse is relied on to coordinate all activities of the room and to manage the nursing care required for the patient. The circulating nurse is often the one team member who is in a position to have an overall picture of patient care needs and to be the patient's advocate. Consistent with such responsibility,

it is considered vital to the perioperative role that this individual be, at minimum, prepared as a registered professional nurse.

Circulating nurse activities may include the following:

1. Assessing, planning, implementing, and evaluating nursing activities to meet individual patient needs.
2. Creating and maintaining a safe and comfortable environment for the patient. This often involves diligent observation for breaks in aseptic technique and initiation of appropriate measures to correct the situation.
3. Providing assistance to any team member as necessary (directing and anticipating the performance and needs of the scrub nurse and providing extra supplies and equipment as needed to any team member).
4. Maintaining communication between team members in the operating room and any necessary contact with other health care professionals and patient's family.
5. Identifying any potential environmental dangers or traumatic situations involving the patient or team members and taking appropriate action to correct or assist with the problem.

■ ALLIED PERSONNEL

There are a number of other persons who function in an indirect relationship in contributing to the needs of each surgical patient. These persons may include clerical personnel, blood bank employees, laboratory technicians, nursing assistants, pharmacists, central service employees, pathologists, radiologists, and laundry personnel.

■ OPERATING ROOM SUITE DESIGN

The design of an operating room suite offers a challenge to the planning team to optimize efficiency by creating realistic traffic and work flow patterns for patients, personnel, and supplies. Designs also need to allow for flexibility for future needs. Since no one plan meets all hospitals' requirements, each O.R. suite is designed on an individual basis to meet projected and specific community needs.

Operating room zones

Protective	Locker rooms, lounges, offices, patient receiving areas
Clean	Clean storage areas, scrub areas, recovery room
Sterile	Operating rooms, storage of sterile supplies
Dirty	Disposal area for all used materials

Specific traffic patterns are determined dependent on the entrances and exits for both personnel and materials. Traffic control can be aided by designating a 4-zone concept (see the box on page 350).

Infection control practices that are related to design may include but are not limited to the following:

1. Walls that are smooth and easily washable
2. Cabinets that are recessed to facilitate cleaning
3. No windows
4. Sliding doors (as opposed to swinging doors) that decrease air turbulence
5. Presence of adequate air filtration system
6. Ceiling-mounted lighting units on a single post as opposed to lights on tracks. (Ceiling light tracks are not readily accessible for cleaning, and handles are likely to become contaminated.)
7. Disposal systems for contaminated equipment that are uniform for all cases

Temperature and humidity are also important design factors. High relative humidity should be maintained. Moisture provides a relatively conductive medium, allowing static to leak to earth as fast as it is generated. Temperature is purposely cool to deter bacterial growth. The combination of increased humidity and decreased temperature is also desirable for maintaining the patient's exposed tissue.

A *communication system* is a vital link to summon routine or emergency assistance or to relay appropriate information to and from the operating room team. An intercom system is commonly used, but team members must be aware of the type of information that is shared over an intercom if the patient is awake. Call light systems outside the operating room door may be used to summon selected persons such as orderlies or housekeeping personnel.

■ NURSING PRACTICE IN THE OPERATING ROOM

■ Aseptic technique and infection control

Aseptic technique is the foundation on which modern surgery is based. Asepsis means the absence of any infectious agents; therefore, aseptic technique is aimed at eliminating microorganisms present in the surgical environment. This also includes those microorganisms living harmlessly on the body surface or within. They must be prevented from reaching the open wound to allow healing by first intention.

Principles of bacteriology and microbiology are applied in developing infection control programs to be followed by all operating room personnel. Such programs involve specific guidelines for O.R. attire, sterilization and packaging of supplies, scrubbing, gowning and gloving, and methods of housekeeping.

When following infection control principles, self-discipline and a *surgical conscience* are imperative. A surgical conscience may be described as a Surgical Golden Rule;

that is, "Do unto the patient as you would have others do unto you."[19] This implies that the nurse takes appropriate action to rectify any break in technique whether the person is alone or observed by others. Thus the nurse must be as conscientious about monitoring his or her own technique as when observing other team members.

■ BASIC RULES OF SURGICAL ASEPSIS

Definite rules must be followed during surgery to create and maintain a sterile field with a well-defined margin of safety for the patient. Strict adherence to the following rules eliminates or minimizes possible contamination:

1. Only sterile materials may be used within a sterile field. If there is any doubt about the sterility of an item, it is considered unsterile.
2. Gowns of scrubbed team members are considered sterile in the *front from shoulder to waist level and sleeves to 2 inches above the elbow*. Unsterile areas of gowns are shoulders, neckline, axillary region, and back. Scrubbed persons should not allow their hands or any sterile item to fall below waist or tabletop level.
3. Draped tables are considered to be sterile on top surface only. Any item that extends over the table edge is considered contaminated and cannot be brought back up to tabletop level.
4. Sterile surfaces should contact only other sterile areas. Unsterile team members must avoid reaching over a sterile field. Scrubbed persons should stay close to the sterile field, and if they change positions, they should turn back to back or face to face.
5. Edges of any sterile package or container are considered unsterile. Sterile boundaries are not always well defined; therefore, the following rules are accepted guidelines:
   a. Cap edges of a bottle of sterile solution are considered contaminated once the cap is removed. Since the cap cannot be replaced without contaminating the pouring edges, the sterility of the bottle contents is no longer certain and the remainder is discarded.
   b. Package wrappers are usually considered to have a 1-inch safety margin around the edge. The flap ends are secured in the hand of the person opening them to keep the flap ends from dangling loosely (Fig. 17-2).
   c. Peel-back packages should not be torn open but rather pulled back to expose sterile contents. The inner edge of the heat seal is considered to be the boundary between sterile and unsterile.
6. The sterile field should be created as close to the time it is going to be used as possible. The degree of contamination is proportional to the length of time items are left uncovered. Sterile areas are kept in continuous view, and once supplies are opened, someone must remain in the room to ensure sterility.
7. Sterile barriers that have been permeated are considered contaminated. Filtration of airborne microorganisms through materials (as when an item is dropped on the floor), passage of liquids through materials, and undetected holes are modes of contamination.

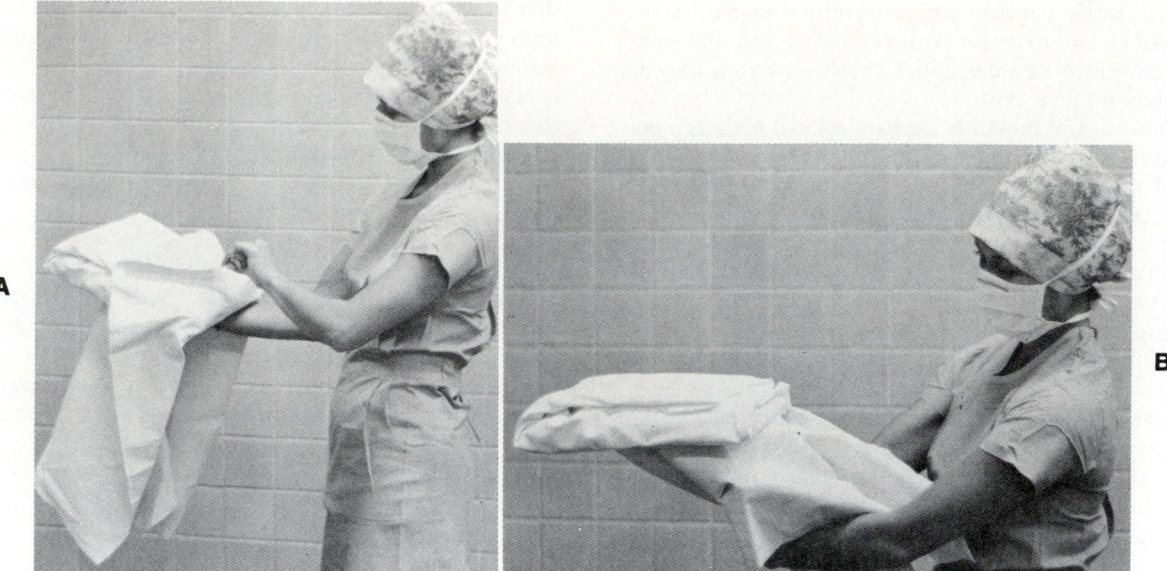

Fig. 17-2 **A,** When opening a sterile package, the circulating nurse opens the corner nearest the body last to avoid potential contamination of the inner pack. **B,** To prevent unsterile corners of outer wrapper from touching the scrub nurse or sterile field, the circulating nurse draws back corners of opened wrapper when presenting the inner package. (From Gruendemann, BJ, and Meeker, MH: Alexander's care of the patient in surgery, St. Louis, 1983, The CV Mosby Co.)

■ O.R. ATTIRE AND PERSONNEL HEALTH HABITS

Adherence to proper practices regarding the attire worn by health care workers within the operating room greatly lessens the risk of their serving as potential sources of infection for the patient. It is known that large quantities of bacteria are present in the nose and mouth, on the skin, and on the wearing apparel of persons who enter the operating room. For this reason, areas must be provided for staff members to remove personal attire, to put on appropriate O.R. attire, and to enter the operating room suite directly without passing through a contaminated area.

Daily body hygiene practices and clean hair also help prevent wound infections. Hair is a fertile source of bacteria, and other body areas may shed bacterial and dead cells into an open wound. Policy should prevent personnel who have active infections of any kind or who are known to be carriers of infection from entering the operating room suite.

□ Uniform

Street clothes should not be worn in restricted areas of the surgical suite. There should be a visible line beyond which no one may go without proper attire (Fig. 17-3). Clean operating room apparel made of fabric that meets the National Fire Protection Association standards should be available to anyone requiring entrance into restricted areas. Scrub pants with close-fitting cuffs are superior to scrub dresses; such cuffs prevent the liberation of bacteria from the perineal and thigh area. Shirts are tucked inside pants to prevent accidental contact with sterile areas and to contain skin shedding. It is also recommended that nonsterile team members wear long-sleeved warm-up jackets to prevent shedding from bare arms. If scrub dresses are worn, they are secured at the waist and panty hose are worn to reduce bacterial shedding. Operating room attire that becomes visibly soiled or wet is changed, and all O.R. apparel is laundered by the hospital laundering facilities.

□ Head coverings

All possible head and facial hair, including sideburns and neckline are completely covered before donning other O.R. attire. This prevents the possibility of hair or dandruff being shed onto the scrub suit. Caps should be flame resistant, provide comfort, and fit snugly. Cleanliness of homemade caps is debatable; if they are used, it is recommended that they be laundered by hospital facilities. Disposable head coverings are discarded in designated containers before the person leaves the operating room suite.

□ Masks

All personnel should wear disposable high filtration masks in specified restricted areas of the surgical suite. The mask must completely cover the mouth and nose and be secured to prevent venting at the sides. This prevents droplets from the oro- or nasopharynx from being expelled

Fig. 17-3   Proper operating room attire. **A,** The scrub top should be tucked into pants, or, **B,** should conform to the waist to reduce dispersal of bacteria. Ankle closures on scrub pants ensure containment of potential contaminants. **C,** The scrub dress should be secured at the waist. Advocates of scrub dresses believe that bacteria can be contained as effectively with panty hose as with pantsuits. **D,** The warm-up jacket worn over the scrub suit provides maximum coverage of skin. (From Gruendemann, BJ, and Meeker, MH: Alexander's care of the patient in surgery, St. Louis, 1983, The CV Mosby Co.)

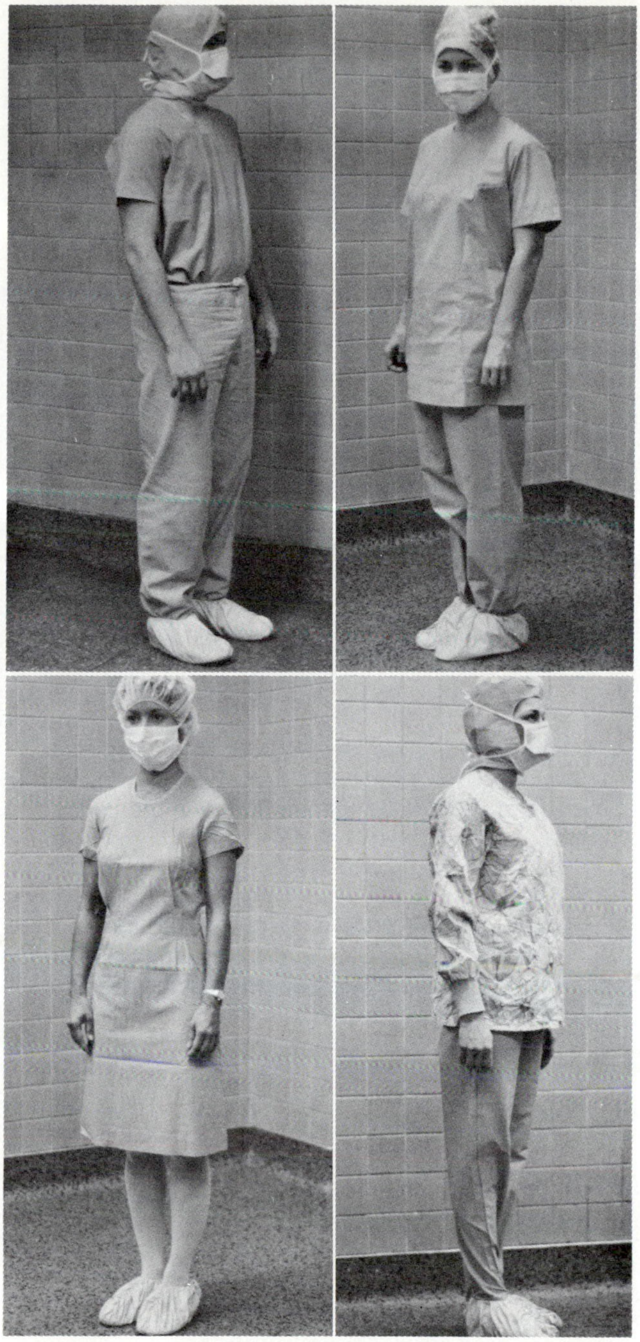

into the surgical environment. Masks must also be handled properly during and after use. They should be either on or off and not dropped loosely around the neck; if allowed to dangle, bacteria that have been filtered onto the mask will become dry and airborne. When masks are removed, only the strings are touched to reduce contamination of the hands from the nasopharyngeal area. Masks are changed between cases and more often if they become moist during a long case.

□ **Shoe coverings**

All persons entering the restricted areas of the surgical suite should wear shoe covers. When the same shoes are worn in the O.R. for successive operations, they will have a very high bacterial count and a potential for cross-infection.

Shoe covers must be conductive in areas where static spark is a hazard, and conductivity is checked when entering the restricted area and at intervals throughout the tour of duty. Care must be taken to make sure that the black carbon strip is placed inside the shoe between the sock or hose in good contact with the inner sole. This provides conductivity, or an electrical gound, for the wearer.

Shoe covers are removed when leaving restricted areas, and clean ones are reapplied on returning. This prevents cross-contamination with other areas of the hosptial. In the interest of safety, clogs, sandals, and tennis shoes should not be worn in the operating room. Clogs can be a hazard when a person tries to move quickly, and if sharp objects are accidentally dropped, sandals and tennis shoes provide little protection.

□ **Other considerations**

Additional considerations in relation to O.R. attire may address the amount and type of jewelry that may be worn. Dangling necklaces and earrings may fall into the sterile field. Excessive rings or rings with sharp stones interfere with good handwashing technique as well as possibly injuring the patient during transfers.

No operating attire, including surgical uniforms, caps, and shoe covers, should be worn outside the surgical suite as this creates a two-way hazard. Any contaminants coming in contact with the operating room team members can become airborne and find susceptible hosts outside the surgical suite. Conversely, bacteria present outside the suite may be carried back on O.R. attire. If this practice is not feasible, head and shoe coverings are removed and the scrub clothes are covered by a clean, buttoned lab coat when a person leaves the suite. On return, the scrub clothes are changed.

■ **SCRUBBING, GOWNING, AND GLOVING**

Only personnel who are free of upper respiratory infections and skin problems should scrub. Abrasions and cuts tend to ooze serum that may serve as a medium for bacterial growth.

The major objective of the surgical scrub is to reduce the microbial skin count as much as possible and to leave an antimicrobial residue on the skin to prevent regrowth. This is achieved by mechanically cleansing the hands and lower arms to remove skin oil, dirt, and microbes.

The exact procedure to be followed and the selection of materials used may differ among hospitals. The most frequently used antimicrobial agents include povidone-iodine, hexachlorophene, and chlorhexidene gluconate. When scrubbing, it is recommended that light friction be applied as opposed to hard scrubbing. This will produce dilation of blood vessels with better circulation, which helps recondition the skin; on the other hand, scrubbing with harsh bristles can cause desquamation of the dermis. The use of synthetic disposable sponges in place of brushes has become popular; however, reusable or disposable nylon brushes have been shown to be equally effective.

The actual scrub procedure may be based on the *time*

Surgical scrub guidelines

Suggested action

1. Remove all hand jewelry. Make last-minute adjustments of head covering, mask, and eyeglasses.

2. Adjust water to a comfortable warm temperature. (Most scrub sinks have automatic or knee controls for water flow.)

3. Wet hands and forearms and apply antimicrobial soap or detergent on palms via foot control. Rub palm surfaces together and add water as needed to make a lather.

4. Using friction, wash the hands and arms thoroughly to a level at least 2 inches above the elbow. The amount of time required may vary with the cleansing agent used and the amount of soil present.

5. Hands and arms should be rinsed thoroughly, being careful to keep the hands higher than elbows. Avoid splashing water onto clothing.

6. A sterile brush or sponge (either prepackaged or from a dispenser) should be obtained. A metal or plastic nail cleaner should be included and used to clean under the fingernails while hands are held under running water.

7. An antimicrobial agent should be applied to the brush or sponge if not already impregnated. Starting at the fingertips, the nails and subungual area should be scrubbed vigorously with the brush held perpendicular to them. All sides of each finger are scrubbed, followed by the back and palm of the hand.

8. The arms are scrubbed on each side with a circular motion to 2 inches above the elbow. (The time spent in steps 7 and 8 may be established by setting a time limit for the scrubbing of one part after another or by counting a particular number of strokes for each side of each part.)

9. The hands and arms are rinsed thoroughly with the brush being discarded into the proper container. Hands and arms are held up in front of the body with elbows slightly flexed as the person enters the operating room.

Rationale

1. Jewelry harbors microorganisms and also serves as a potential source of foreign bodies in the operative wound.

2. Warm water is believed to enhance cleansing action because it has a lower surface tension than cold.

3. Detergents and soaps lower surface tension of water and emulsify oil.

4. Microbes are removed by physical and mechanical separation as well as chemical antisepsis. By washing one handbreadth above contaminated areas, recontamination of hands and forearms during rinsing and drying is more readily avoided.

5. This allows water to run off at the elbow and prevents contaminated water from above the elbow from running down onto scrubbed hands. If the scrub attire becomes wet, the moisture may cause contamination of the sterile gown by wicking action.

6. Special attention should be given to the subungual space where microbes can accumulate. Orangewood sticks should not be used because they cannot be sterilized properly afterward.

7. and 8. Hospital policy should be established, and the procedure posted in the scrub area. The individual's conscientious attention to detail is of utmost importance.

9. Rinse procedure should be followed as in step 5. Same rationale applies.

method or the *anatomic brush-stroke method*. Both methods are effective if properly carried out. The time method involves scrubbing the fingers, hands, and arms for an allotted period of time for each area. The brush-stroke method prescribes a number of brush strokes to be applied lengthwise with the brush or sponge for each surface of the fingers, hands, and arms. There is no difference in microbial reduction whether the scrub lasts 5 or 10 minutes. The same scrub procedure should be used consistently, whether it is the first or last scrub of the day.

Before beginning the surgical scrub, the hands are inspected for cuts or skin problems. Nails should be short to avoid glove puncture, and no polish is preferred to prevent a harbor for microbes. The head covering is adjusted to ensure that all hair is contained, and a fresh mask should be properly applied. (Surgical scrub guidelines are described in the box on p. 354.)

After the scrub, the team member is ready to put on sterile gown and gloves. The procedure for gowning and gloving may vary, depending on the type of materials used (linen or disposable) and gown design, and whether the gloving will be done by self or by another team member. Sterile gloves may be applied using an open or closed method. The closed method is usually preferred, since bare skin on the hands and wrists are not exposed during the process. (For detailed discussion on the procedures, see references 19 and 37.)

■ Safety and protection of the patient

■ ADMITTING PATIENT TO THE OPERATING ROOM AREA

Most hospitals have an established procedure for admission into the holding area of the O.R. suite. The holding area is ideally a quiet, restful area where patients can gain optimal benefit from any premedication they have received. This is also an area where patients may feel terribly alone. They now come face to face with their impending surgery. Separation from family members has become a reality, and any fears the patient might have are likely to resurface.

The professional nurse's first goal is to establish a meaningful relationship with the patient. The nurse greeting the patient can decrease the patient's apprehension by a friendly introduction and by talking to the patient in a positive manner. The patient is told that the circulating nurse will be in constant attendance once the patient is admitted to the surgical room, and an explanation is given of what is being done in preparation for the surgery. If the nurse treats the patient with respect and warmth, answers any questions, and sees to the patient's comfort at the time, much will be accomplished toward instilling security and confidence in the entire O.R. team. Any necessary delays are explained to the patient and also relayed to the waiting family.

The circulating nurse has a number of important things to do when admitting the patient to the operating room such as the following:

1. Ask the patient to state his or her name, the operative procedure to be done, and the site of the operation, if pertinent.
2. Check the patient's name and hospital number on the chart and compare it with the name and number on the patient's identification band.
3. Check for a signature on the operative permit and determine if properly signed, dated, and witnessed. The procedure on the permit must agree with the scheduled procedure.
4. Review the chart, checking for the following:
   a. The medical history and physical examination results, which must be completed before surgery begins
   b. Laboratory reports and x-rays (abnormalities are reported to the surgeon and anesthesiologist)
   c. Availability of blood if the patient was typed and crossmatched
   d. Allergies and any previous reactions to the anesthetic or transfusions
5. Check for jewelry, wigs, contact lenses, prostheses, dentures, and objects in the mouth.
6. Observe the patient for any signs of adverse effects to preoperative medication and ask patient if anything has been taken by mouth if an NPO order was written.

■ TRANSFERRING AND POSITIONING PATIENT FOR SURGERY

Based on the scheduled procedure and the surgeon's preferences, the circulating nurse should be able to anticipate the basic patient position required. The final responsibility for the position of the patient on the O.R. table is shared by the nurse, surgeon, and anesthesiologist. During the preoperative assessment, the patient's height, weight, and individual health problems that may relate to safe transfer and positioning have been determined and recorded.

No matter what position is to be assumed, good positioning is important to the following:

1. To adequately expose the operative area
2. To make the patient accessible for induction of the anesthetic and administration of intravenous solutions or drugs
3. To minimize interference with circulation as a result of pressure on a body part
4. To provide protection from injury to nerves as a result of improper positioning of arms, hands, legs, or feet
5. To provide for the maintenance of respiratory function by avoiding pressure on the chest to allow for adequate ventilation of the lungs and by holding the jaw forward to keep it from dropping on the chest
6. To provide for the patient's privacy by proper draping and avoiding unnecessary exposure

Specific nursing care planning may involve deciding the appropriate method of transfer, determining equipment and positioning aids needed, and deciding if additional personnel will be needed to carry out the plan safely. Imple-

Table 17-2 Commonly used operative patient positions

Position	Description	Comments
Supine	Flat on back with arms at side, palms down, legs straight with feet slightly separated (Fig. 17-4, A)	Most commonly used position, used for hernia repair, exploratory laparotomy, cholecystectomy, gastric and bowel resection, and mastoidectomy
Prone	Patient lies on abdomen with face turned to one side, arms at side with palms pronated, elbows slightly flexed; feet elevated on pillow to prevent plantar flexion (Fig. 17-4, B)	Patient is anesthetized in supine position, then placed prone; used for surgery on back, spine, and rectal area
Trendelenburg	Head and body are lowered into a head-down position and held in place with padded shoulder braces; knees are flexed by "breaking" table (Fig. 17-4, C)	Respiratory excursion is decreased from upward movement of viscera; used for surgery on lower abdomen and pelvis
Reverse Trendelenburg	Head is elevated and feet lowered	Used for biliary surgery
Lithotomy	Patient lies on back with buttocks to edge of table; thighs and legs are placed in stirrups simultaneously to prevent muscle injury; head and arms are secured to prevent injury (Fig. 17-5, A)	Used for perineal, rectal, and vaginal surgery; elastic wraps may be used on legs to prevent thrombus formation
Lateral	Patient lies on side; table may be bent in middle (Fig. 17-5, B)	Used for renal surgery

mentation of the plan includes certain safety measures which may include the following:

1. The O.R. table and transfer cart are securely locked
2. A physician assumes responsibility for movement of an unsplinted fracture
3. All muscles, nerves, and bony prominences are positioned or padded to avoid injury
4. Heavily sedated patients and the elderly are moved slowly and gently to prevent shearing forces on the skin and to allow the circulatory system to adjust
5. Care is taken to see that no tubings (for example, intravenous lines, urinary catheters) are dislodged or obstructed
6. Restraints are placed snugly over a blanket covering the patient, avoiding contact with the skin. Straps should not interfere with circulation or exert pressure on nerves or bony prominences
7. Sterile tables are positioned high enough to prevent any pressure on the patient's body
8. Sterile team members are reminded not to lean on any part of the patient.

The patient may be positioned on the operating room table in a number of different positions (Table 17-2 and Figs. 17-4 and 17-5). Whatever the position, special attention is given to prevent injury to the patient's arms and legs and to prevent pressure on any one given area.

One major problem that may occur is the pooling of blood in dependent areas. Sudden shifting of blood when the supine position is reassumed following surgery may place a strain on the cardiovascular system with a precipitous drop in blood pressure. For this reason, the patient is always returned *slowly* from the operative position to the

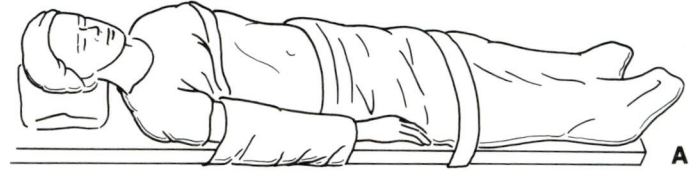

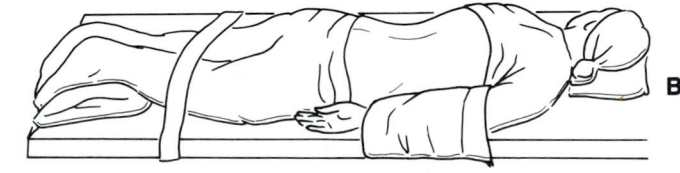

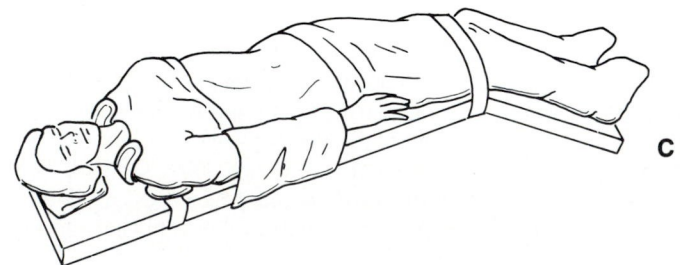

Fig. 17-4 Three commonly used operative positions. **A,** Supine. **B,** Prone. **C,** Trendelenburg.

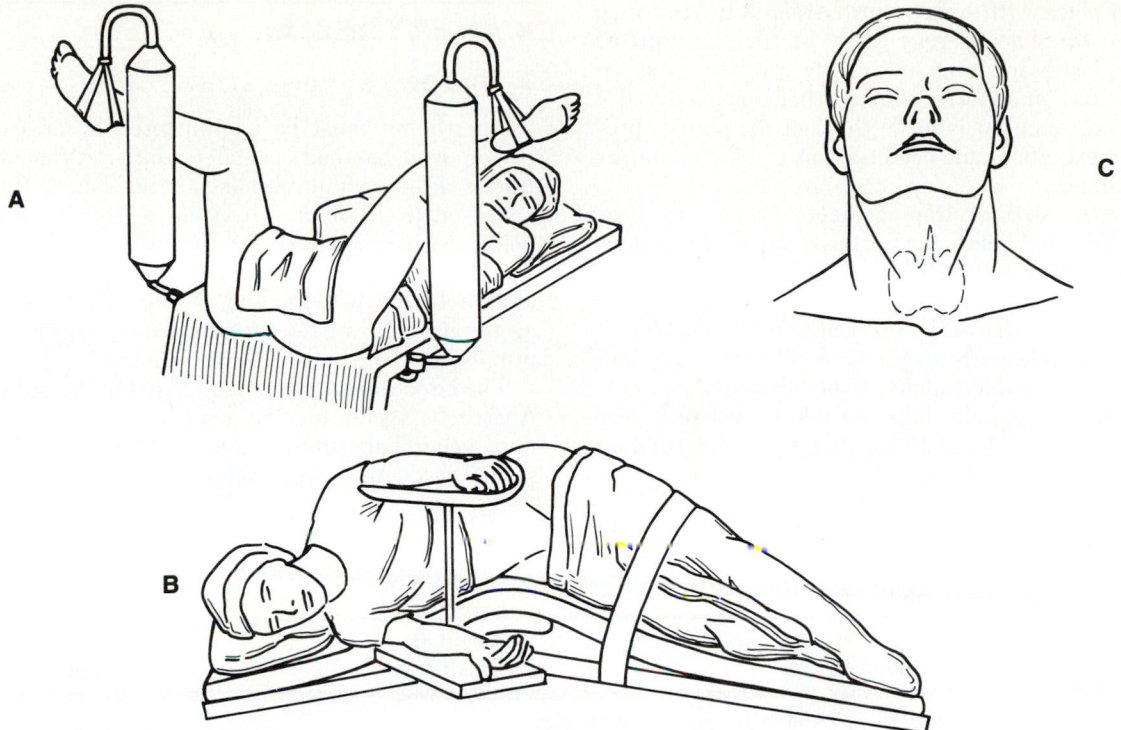

Fig. 17-5 Three operative positions for specialized surgery. **A,** Lithotomy. **B,** Lateral. **C,** Thyroid exposure.

supine position. Elderly persons and persons with preexisting cardiovascular problems are at high risk and are monitored carefully.

■ SKIN CLEANSING AND PREPARATION

The purpose of preoperative skin preparation is to establish an operative site as free as possible from dirt, skin oils, and transient microbes, as well as reducing the resident microbial count to as low as possible. This should be accomplished in the shortest period of time with the least amount of tissue irritation. If the skin *prep* is to be done while the patient is awake, the nurse explains the procedure to the patient, providing for comfort and minimizing exposure.

Removal of hair from the operative site should only be done as necessary and as near the time of surgery as possible. Alternatives for hair removal include a depilatory, electric clippers, and shaving with a razor. Studies have revealed that differences in wound infection rates are higher for patients shaved preoperatively than for patients with no preoperative shave or on whom a depilatory is used.[11] If a shave is ordered, it should be done by a person who has demonstrated skill in the procedure to avoid nicking and cutting the skin. Such skin breaks can allow cutaneous bacteria to proliferate and increase the chances of infection.

After hair is removed, the operative site is prepared with an antimicrobial agent(s). The agent used, the method of

application, and the exposure time of the skin to the agent is determined by institutional policy and the surgeon's preference. Criteria used in selection of the agent include the following:

1. Spectrum of activity (gram-positive or gram-negative organisms, activity in presence of blood or pus)
2. Speed of action
3. Potential for skin irritation and sensitivity
4. Flammability characteristics (especially if electrosurgery will be used)
5. Possible incompatibility or inactivation by alcohol, soap, detergent, or organic matter

Supplies used for the final skin preparation are arranged on a separate sterile table. The scrub begins at the proposed incision line and proceeds to the periphery of the area involved. A soiled sponge is never brought back over a scrubbed area. Open wounds and body orifices are prepared last, even when these areas are the proposed incision line.

■ STERILE DRAPING

The purpose of draping is to create a sterile field around the operative site. An effective barrier eliminates the passage of microorganisms between sterile and nonsterile areas and leaves a minimal area of skin exposed.

Towels or self-adhering plastic sheeting are commonly used to drape the area immediately surrounding the operative site. Towels may be made of cotton muslin or synthetic disposable materials. If muslin is used the towels are held in place with towel clips, while synthetics may have their own self-adherent edge. Sterile, waterproof, antistatic, plastic sheeting, commonly referred to as an *incise drape*, has an adhesive backing that is applied to dry skin. The skin incision is made through the plastic, preventing skin excretions and bacteria from coming in contact with the wound.

Various other sizes of draping sheets are used to cover the areas above and below the operative area. The patient and the operating table are covered with sterile drapes in such a manner as to allow exposure of the surgical site and isolation of the area of the surgical wound. Fenestrated sheets are available with openings of different sizes and shapes. Several reusable and disposable materials are available; they are not equally impermeable to moisture over time, and this is considered during draping for determining the necessary number of layers.

■ ANESTHESIA

■ Usage

Anesthetics must be administered by an experienced person who has had special training. Although surgical nurses do not administer anesthetic agents, they may be called on to assist the physician or nurse anesthetist in doing so. It is essential for the nurse to have an understanding of drug interactions, of the preanesthetic preparation of the patient, and of the effects of anesthetic agents given during the operative phase to provide effective nursing care in the postoperative period.

The effects of anesthesia are listed in the box on p. 359. Anesthetic agents may be given to produce unconsciousness (general anesthesia) or to produce loss of sensation in specific body areas (regional anesthesia). *Local* anesthesia

Table 17-3 Types of anesthetic

Type	Action and effect	Method of administration	Definition
General	Blocks awareness centers in brain; produces unconsciousness, body relaxation, loss of sensation	Inhalation	Vapors from liquids and gases under pressure, administered through a tube and/or mask
		Intravenous	Drug given directly into vein, usually used for induction
Regional	Inhibition of excitatory process in nerve endings or fibers; analgesia over a specific body area with consciousness retained	Nerve block	Injection of drug to anesthetize an isolated nerve
		Intravenous regional block with tourniquet (Bier block)	Injection of drug intravenously into an extremity
		Field block	Series of injections of drug into tissues surrounding the operative site
		Spinal (intrathecal)	Injection of drug into subarachnoid space of spinal cord (Fig. 17-6)
		Epidural	Injection into space surrounding dura mater without breaking dural membrane
Local	Blocks transmission of nerve impulses at site of action; analgesia over limited tissue area with consciousness retained	Topical	Drug applied directly to surface, mucous membrane, or open wound
		Infiltration	Injection of drug into tissue at site of incision
Hypoanesthetic	Artificially induced passive state of consciousness in which there is increased amenability to suggestions and commands, reduced awareness, and restricted attentiveness	Hypnosis	Induction of the anesthetic state by hypnosis; may be combined with use of small dose of IV anesthetic or muscle relaxant
Acupuncture	Blocks painful stimuli by *gate control theory* and by stimulating release of endorphins with consciousness retained	Use of needles or surface electrodes	Needles or electrodes are connected to an electronic machine that creates current flow between these electrodes

can be considered a form of *regional* anesthesia (Table 17-3). Hypoanesthesia (usually hypnosis) is rarely used, and acupuncture, although commonly carried out in Oriental countries, is seldom used.

Choice

The choice of anesthetic is based on many factors: the physical condition and age of the patient; the presence of coexisting diseases; the type, site, and duration of the operation; and the personal preferences of the anesthetist. The anesthesiologist evaluates each patient carefully and selects the anesthetic agents best suited for that individual. An apprehensive patient may not respond well to a regional anesthetic.

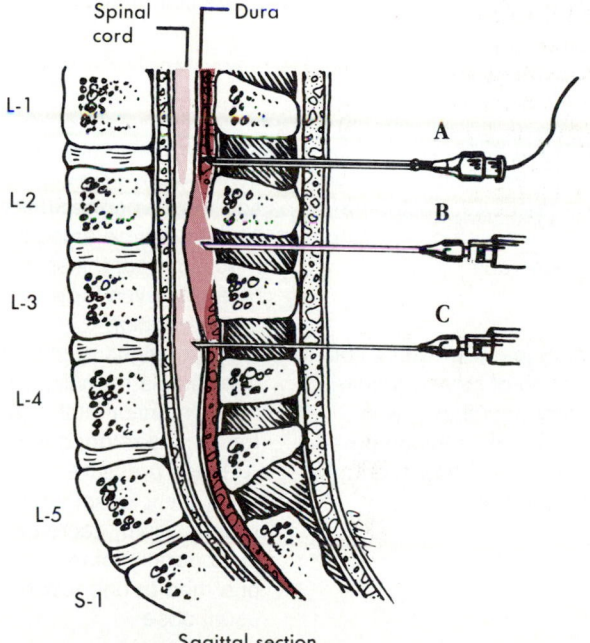

Fig. 17-6   Position of needles and injection sites. **A,** Epidural catheters. **B,** Epidural anesthesia. **C,** Spinal anesthesia. (From Gruendemann, BJ, and Meeker, MH: Alexander's care of the patient in surgery, ed 7, St. Louis, 1983, The CV Mosby Co.)

Preparation of patient for anesthesia

Patients have many anxieties related to anesthesia (see the box above). Most anxieties can be dispelled if the patient and family are well informed about the anesthetic selected for use and the care taken by the physician and nurse in assessing the patient's physical condition. The patient is encouraged to discuss any questions or concerns about the anesthetic with either the anesthesiologist or the surgeon.

The patient can be assured there will be close surveillance during anesthesia and in the immediate postoperative period. Very few patients talk while under anesthesia, and what is said is usually unintelligible so that talking need not be of great concern to the patient. Persistent anxiety on the part of the patient regarding the anesthetic should be discussed with the surgeon and the anesthesiologist.

A premedication is commonly ordered to assist in sedating the patient, and if necessary, in drying secretions that may interfere with safe deliverance of a general anesthetic. This is usually administered before the patient's arrival in the operating room suite but may be given there if there is a holding area for surgical preps within the O.R. suite or in an emergency.

After the patient is transferred to the operating room table, an intravenous infusion is started and any necessary noninvasive monitoring equipment is connected (for example, electrocardiogram leads, blood pressure cuff, stethoscope, and so on.) The desired anesthetic will then be administered.

It is very important that the circulating nurse remain near the patient during induction of the anesthetic. The nurse may be called on to protect the patient physically if an unusual reaction occurs. It is possible for the patient to become excited and move excessively, requiring additional restraint to prevent self-injury. Stimulation of the patient in the form of noise or moving body parts is avoided as this may cause vomiting, retching, or laryngospasm, which in turn may lead to hypoxia. If this occurs, the anesthesiologist may require the nurses' assistance with suctioning equipment and with observing the monitors. Emotional support can be very important, and simply hold-

Table 17-4 Comparison of selected anesthetic agents

Name	Method of administration	Advantages	Disadvantages	Special nursing considerations
Nitrous oxide	Inhalation	Rapid induction and recovery; nonirritating; nonflammable but supports combustion	Possible hypoxia with excessive amounts	Monitor for signs of hypoxia
Halothane (Fluothane)	Inhalation	Rapid induction; low incidence of postoperative nausea or vomiting; nonirritating; nonflammable	Shivering with emergence; circulatory-respiratory depressant	Monitor vital signs closely
Methoxyflurane (Penthrane)	Inhalation	Decreased need for analgesics in immediate postoperative period; nonflammable	Prolonged induction; renal toxicity (dose dependent); postoperative nausea or vomiting	Position to prevent aspiration if vomiting occurs
Enflurane (Ethrane)	Inhalation	Rapid induction and recovery; some muscle relaxation on its own; nonflammable	Circulatory/respiratory depression (dose dependent); expensive; shivering with emergence	Monitor vital signs frequently
Cyclopropane	Inhalation	Rapid induction; adequate muscle relaxation	Highly flammable; possible cardiac irritability and arrhythmias; emergence excitement; postoperative nausea, vomiting, headache	Monitor pulse frequently for irregularities; position to prevent aspiration with vomiting
Isoflurane (Forane)	Inhalation	Smooth and rapid introduction; good muscle relaxant; nonirritating; cardiovascular stability	Expensive	Hypotension may occur
Ether	Inhalation	Inexpensive; good muscle relaxation; decreased need for postoperative analgesia	Irritating to mucous membranes; prolongation of anesthesia; postoperative nausea or vomiting; flammable	Supervise constantly in early postoperative period; position to prevent aspiration; suction if large amounts of mucus present; inspect face and eyes for blistering or irritation
Thiopental sodium (Pentothal Sodium)	IV	Rapid smooth induction and recovery	Laryngospasm with stimulation of larynx; respiratory depression with high doses; blood pressure may drop suddenly	Monitor for signs of stridor, neck tissue retraction, cyanosis; monitor vital signs for ↓ respiratory depth or ↓ blood pressure
Droperidol and fentanyl	IV	Rapid smooth induction and recovery; nontoxic to liver, kidneys, or heart; less analgesia required postoperatively	Hypoventilation	Monitor for ↓ respiratory rate or depth; decrease postoperative narcotics to one third to one fourth usual dose
Ketamine	IV	Profound analgesia with no loss of consciousness; amnesia for surgical event	Unpleasant dreams in early postoperative period and sometimes later; does not block visceral pain	Maintain quiet environment postoperatively

Continued.

Table 17-4   Comparison of selected anesthetic agents—cont'd

Name	Method of administration	Advantages	Disadvantages	Special nursing considerations
Midazolam (Versed)	IV	Induction of anesthesia can be achieved within a narrow dose range and a short period of time; high incidence of partial or complete impairment of recall for several hours	Depresses respiration and causes fluctuation in vital signs	Monitor for respiratory depression and hypotension
Sufentanil (Sufenta)	IV	Rapid, primary anesthetic agent to induce and maintain anesthesia	Hypotension or hypertension, tachycardia, dysrhythmia, bronchospasm	Monitor for blood pressure changes, nausea and vomiting, and respiratory depression
Procaine Cocaine Tetracaine Dibucaine Lidocaine Carbocaine Bupivacaine Chloroprocaine	Tissue injection (local); spray	No loss of consciousness	CNS stimulation or seizures; cardiac depression; absorbed into bloodstream	Monitor for excitability, twitching, pulse, or blood pressure changes, pallor, respiratory difficulty

ing the patient's hand has been reported by many to be a great comfort.

Malignant hyperthermia is a potential life-threatening condition that can occur at induction of anesthesia or at any time postoperatively. It is usually triggered in persons who have an inherited defect in the membrane of the skeletal muscle by certain anesthetic agents (such as potent inhalation anesthetics). The defect is believed to be present in the sarcoplasmic reticulum, where the triggering agent sets off the release of calcium. The high intracellular calcium level of the muscle cells dramatically accelerates their metabolic rate. A number of resulting chemical changes, if not controlled, may lead to high fever, metabolic alterations, and brain damage. The primary treatment modalities include: packing the patient in ice; hyperventilating with 100% oxygen; and administering chilled intravenous fluids, diuretics, steroids, and dantrolene (Dantrium).

■ General anesthesia

General anesthesia is produced by inhalation or by injection into the bloodstream of anesthetic drugs. Certain drugs that produce general anesthesia when administered intravenously, such as thiopental sodium (Pentothal sodium), are used to put the patient to sleep and are almost always supplemented with other agents to produce surgical anesthesia.

Frequently a combination of inhalation anesthetic agents such as nitrous oxide and oxygen may be used with muscle relaxants and narcotics. This form of combined drug administration is referred to as *balanced anesthesia*. The com-

bination of drug effects provides analgesia, hypnosis, and adequate muscular relaxation as well as sleep. The choice of agents (Table 17-4) depends on the anesthesiologist's judgment and the individual patient's needs.

General anesthesia affects all the physiologic systems of the body to some degree. It chiefly affects the central nervous, respiratory, and circulatory systems. The anesthesiologist judges the depth of anesthesia by the changes produced in these systems. These changes are observed by monitoring heart rate (with stethoscope and ECG), blood pressure, respiratory rate, and oxygen saturation (with an oximeter).

■ STAGES OF GENERAL ANESTHESIA

The stages of anesthesia may vary, depending on the drug used, the rapidity of induction, and the skill of the anesthesiologist. Since current practice is to induce anesthesia with a rapid-acting intravenously administered drug before inhalation anesthesia, a rapid transition through the early stages may occur. The classic, distinct stages are best seen when diethyl ether is used. All stages will not be observable with all anesthetics (Table 17-5). Characteristics of each stage are listed in box below.

■ INHALATION ANESTHESIA

Inhalation anesthesia is produced by having the patient inhale the vapors of certain liquids or gases. Oxygen is always given with these anesthetic agents. The gas mixture may be administered by mask or into the lungs through an

Table 17-5 Stages and planes of ether anesthesia and selected central nervous system effects

Central nervous system effects	Stage 1	Stage 2	Stage 3 planes				Stage 4
			1	2	3	4	
Consciousness	Maintained Analgesia Euphoria Some distortion of perceptions Variable amnesia	Lost	Absent	Absent	Absent	Absent	Absent
Respiration	No alteration or increased rate with some irregularity	Rapid, irregular	Regular	Regular but expirations longer than inspirations	Diaphragmatic	Thoracic ceased Diaphragmatic depressed	No respiratory movement Respiratory paralysis
Skeletal muscles	Normal tone	Tone increased	Small muscles relaxed	Large muscles relaxed	Complete relaxation	Complete relaxation	Diaphragm paralyzed
Eyes							
Pupils	Reaction to light	Dilated	Constriction	Middilation		Dilated	Dilated
Movements	Unchanged	Increased	Increased	None	None	None	None
Tear secretion			Decreased	Decreased	Decreased	Absent	
Reflexes							
Lid	Present	Present	Absent	Absent	Absent	Absent	Absent
Corneal	Present	Present	Present	Absent	Absent	Absent	Absent
Pharyngeal or "gag"			Absent				
Laryngeal				Absent			
Cough					Absent in large bronchi	Absent in small bronchi	
Heart rate	Unchanged	Increased	Decreased				
Blood pressure	Unchanged	Increased	Normal	Normal	Decreased	Decreased	Decreased
Venous pressure	Unchanged	Increased	Unchanged				Increased

From Hahn, AB, Barkin, RL, and Oestreich, SJK: Pharmacology in nursing, ed 16, St. Louis, 1986, The CV Mosby Co

---

Stages of anesthesia

Stage 1 Extends from beginning of administration of anesthetic to beginning of loss of consciousness
Stage 2 Extends from loss of consciousness to loss of eyelid reflexes; often called the stage of *excitement or delirium*
Stage 3 Extends from loss of eyelid reflex to cessation of respiratory effort; called stage of *surgical anesthesia* Patient is unconscious; muscles are relaxed; reflexes are abolished
Stage 4 Stage of *overdose* or danger; death will follow if anesthetic is not immediately discontinued

---

endotracheal tube inserted into the trachea. The use of endotracheal intubation ensures an airway can be maintained when the chest wall is open. The endotracheal tube may have a balloon that is inflated after insertion. The balloon fills the tracheal space, lessening the chance of aspiration of gastric contents. Regardless of the skill of the anesthesiologist, an endotracheal tube cannot help causing some irritation to the trachea and subsequent edema. If it is difficult to intubate the patient, which may occur because of anatomic differences, it is not uncommon for the patient to complain of a sore, irritated throat postoperatively.

Some of the more common inhalant anesthetics are described in Table 17-4. The use of *nitrous oxide* is limited because it cannot be administered alone in adequate concentrations to produce deep muscle relaxation. The effect of nitrous oxide is additive with other anesthetics and is used extensively as an adjunct to halothane, enflurane, and methoxyflurane. Its greatest use is an agent for induction and as a component of balanced anesthesia for prolonged or complicated surgery. In low concentrations, nitrous oxide may provide adequate anesthesia for intraabdominal procedures in patients who are in profound shock, debilitated, or who are critically ill and cannot tolerate other anesthetic agents.

Cyclopropane quickly produces unconsciousness and adequate relaxation for most abdominal surgery. Emergence excitement is common. During the administration of this gas, extreme care must be taken to prevent the production of any electric charge that might cause it to be ignited.

Halothane (Fluothane) is easily inhaled and is usually administered through special vaporizers with nitrous oxide and oxygen. It is nonirritating, and laryngospasm is infrequent. Halothane does not provide adequate muscle relaxation, and a separate muscle relaxant must be used. It is contraindicated in patients with hepatic or biliary disease.

Isoflurane (Forane) is a depressant anesthetic similar to halothane. It provides adequate muscle relaxation and induction is smooth and rapid.

Ether is seldom used in the United States today because of its flammability and disagreeable side effects. Because it does have a wider margin of safety with minimal effects on the cardiovascular system, it may be used in areas of the world where sophisticated monitoring equipment is unavailable.

■ INTRAVENOUS ANESTHESIA

Thiopental sodium (Pentothal sodium) is the drug used most frequently for induction of anesthesia. It produces unconsciousness quickly. It may also be given to relieve severe, prolonged convulsive states. If large doses of thiopental have been used, the patient may sleep for a long time and should be observed for signs of respiratory depression. Some patients appear to waken quickly only to return to the anesthetized state when undisturbed. Thiopental is detoxified in the liver and excreted by the kidneys; therefore, in patients with liver or kidney disease, elimination of the drug may occur more slowly. Thiopental may be used for brief surgical procedures such as closed reduction of a fracture or dislocation or incision and drainage of an abscess.

Innovar is a combination of a potent tranquilizer (droperidol) and a powerful narcotic analgesic (fentanyl). Orientation returns quickly without restlessness or emergence delirium. Because of the tranquilizing component (droperidol), the patient requires less analgesia in the postanesthesia period. Innovar has lost some of its original popularity because of the depression of alveolar ventilation and respiratory rate that persists longer than the analgesic effect. When Innovar is used along with nitrous oxide, the resulting state is referred to as *neuroleptanesthesia*. As the nitrous oxide is discontinued, the patient will become conscious but remain in a detached state of awareness.

Ketamine produces an anesthetic state termed *dissociative anesthesia*. The patients are anesthetized as far as recollection or awareness is concerned, but they may appear awake since movement may occur and the eyes remain open. Ketamine is chemically related to the hallucinogens, and unpleasant dreams during awakening and extending into the postoperative period may constitute a drawback. To help overcome these effects, a small dose of diazepam (Valium) may be given, or more importantly the patient is left undisturbed during the emergence phase. Ketamine is useful in diagnostic procedures such as neuroradiology and for superficial procedures of short duration; it is not useful for visceral surgery as it does little to block visceral pain.

■ Muscle relaxants

The use of skeletal muscle relaxants (neuromuscular blocking agents) in combination with anesthetics is frequently employed. These drugs have the following uses:
1. Facilitate endotracheal intubation
2. Prevent laryngospasm
3. Produce adequate muscle relaxation during anesthesia
4. Reduce the amount of general anesthetic needed

Nondepolarizing agents, such as metocurine, pancuronium bromide, gallamine triethiodide, and tubocurarine chloride, may be referred to as stabilizing agents and are preferred in longer procedures. Depolarizing blocking agents, such as succinylcholine and decamethonium bromide, are used in shorter procedures.

Muscle relaxants cause respiratory depression or paralysis; thus the patient must be observed closely for signs of respiratory distress during and after administration of the drug. Patients developing respiratory problems will require intubation and mechanical ventilatory assistance.

Delayed recovery can result in patients who have received nondepolarizing relaxants along with certain other drugs. Drug interactions may occur with the use of antibiotics, causing a synergistic effect in which paralysis will be prolonged. This is more likely to occur if the antibiotics are given intravenously or if the peritoneal cavity is irrigated with antibiotic solution. Synergism also occurs with inhalation anesthetics and nondepolarizing agents.

■ Regional anesthesia

Regional anesthesia is produced by the injection or application of a local anesthetic agent along the course of a nerve or at the site of the stimulus, thus abolishing the conduction of all impulses to and from the area supplied by that nerve. The patient experiences no pain in the operative area and remains awake during the entire procedure because the anesthetic affects a particular region only; it does not affect cortical functions. Regional anesthesia is used for treatments, diagnostic measures, examinations, and surgery.

The drugs used to produce regional anesthesia are usually called local anesthetics (Table 17-4). Care is taken that the drugs are given in a localized area in the smallest dose necessary to produce anesthesia, since absorption in the bloodstream may cause CNS stimulation and depression of the heart. Epinephrine may be added to the solution of local anesthetic drug to produce vasoconstriction in the area of injection. Vasoconstriction tends to reduce the rate of absorption, to extend the length of anesthesia, and to reduce hemorrhage.

At the first sign of toxic reactions (see the box above), an intravenous injection of a short-acting barbiturate such as thiopental sodium is administered. Oxygen may also be necessary, and it is important that a patent airway be maintained. If the reaction is caused by an idiosyncratic reaction to the drug, circulatory failure may occur and emergency

---

Signs of toxicity to local anesthetics

Excitability (laughing, crying, excessive talking)
Twitching
Pulse or blood pressure changes
Pallor of the skin
Respiratory difficulties

---

measures such as CPR must be started. Patients should be questioned regarding any previous sensitivity to these drugs.

Regional anesthesia may be given by infiltration, nerve block, epidural block, spinal injection, or topically (Table 17-3).

Spinal anesthesia is not used for surgery of the upper part of the body because it causes paralysis of the diaphragm and the intercostal muscles used in respiration. With spinal anesthesia the patient may be conscious of pulling sensations throughout the operation but experiences no pain. Occasionally a feeling of faintness and nausea may result from these sensations. Because of the sympathetic blockade, hypotension may occur with both spinal and epidural anesthesia.

One of the limitations of spinal anesthesia is that the patient may be awake during the operation, although the preoperative medication may decrease awareness of the surroundings. A screen restricts the patient's vision from the surgical area and a towel may be placed over the eyes. The conversation and activities of the members of the operating room staff should be carried on with the patient's consciousness in mind.

Following spinal anesthesia the patient should be quiet in bed in a supine position. Safety needs must be considered since sensation may not return to the anesthetized area for 1 to 2 hours. The patient is monitored for signs of respiratory or circulatory depression.

Headache may occur following spinal anesthesia and is thought to result from leakage of spinal fluid at the puncture site. The headache usually occurs 24 hours after the puncture and may last several days or a week, occasionally longer. It may be prevented by keeping the patient flat and quiet after surgery and promoting hydration to replace the lost spinal fluid.

■ Other types of anesthesia

■ INDUCED HYPOTHERMIA

Hypothermia refers to the reduction of body temperature below normal to reduce oxygen and metabolic requirements. Extracorporeal cooling, a method of bloodstream cooling, consists of removing the blood from a major vessel, circulating it through coils immersed in a refrigerant, and returning it to the body through another vessel. Blood-stream cooling is the fastest method for producing hypothermia and is used primarily for patients undergoing surgery, particularly open-heart surgery. The patient is given heparin to prevent the blood from clotting during surgery.

The most widely accepted method of nonintrusive hypothermia today is the use of cooling blankets (Fig. 17-7). The patient is placed on, and may be covered by, body-sized vinyl pads containing many coils. The pads are connected to a reservoir filled with alcohol and water. A pump fills the coils and circulates the solution through the coils. A recording thermometer monitors the patient's temperature and an electric unit heats or cools the solution to a preset temperature. Hypothermia may be used for a variety of illnesses when extremely high temperatures occur. (The care of the patient receiving prolonged hypothermia is described in the box below.)

■ INDUCED HYPOTENSION

Hypotension may be induced for the purpose of decreasing bleeding at the operative site in selected instances such as radical head and neck or pelvic surgery. Hypotension can be induced by deep anesthesia with an inhalant anesthetic such as halothane or by an intravenous anesthetic that affects the autonomic nervous system. Vital signs are monitored closely in the early postoperative period.

■ Monitoring patient during anesthesia
■ MONITORING METHODS

During surgery requiring anesthesia, the patient's body is subjected to a variety of stressors. Potent drugs, required body positions, aggravation of preexisting disease processes,

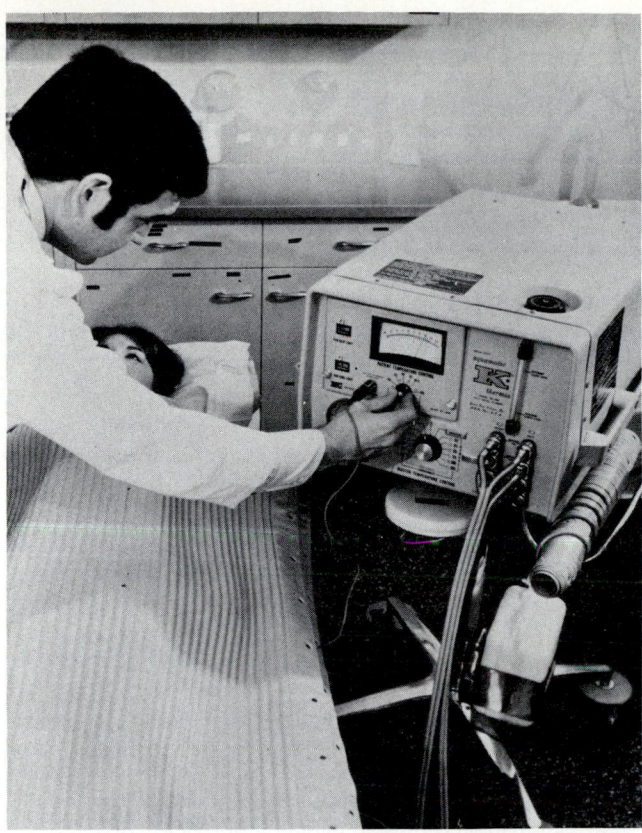

Fig. 17-7 Hypothermia can be produced by means of a cooling blanket. Cold alcohol and water are circulated through the coils by a pressure pump. (Courtesy Hamilton Industries, Two-Rivers, Wis.)

Nursing care of the patient during prolonged hypothermia

1. Prepare patient for procedure
2. Give complete bath before procedure; protect skin with a thin coating of emollient
3. Insert indwelling catheter (if ordered) for monitoring urinary output
4. Monitor patient
   a. Monitor vital signs for sudden increases or decreases or rapid fluctuations
   b. Note shivering and give prescribed medication (usually chlorpromazine hydrochloride)
   c. Observe skin for signs of pressure, edema, discoloration
5. Turn patient every 2 hours and maintain good body alignment
6. Provide fluids and nutrients as ordered (usually by intravenous or tube feedings)
7. Provide good oral hygiene
8. Cleanse and protect eyes if corneal reflexes and eye secretions are decreased
9. When hypothermia is terminated:
   a. Apply blankets to rewarm patient
   b. Monitor return of normal body temperature and remove blankets as necessary

Table 17-6 Monitoring during anesthesia

Parameter	Method	Comments
Arterial blood pressure	Sphygmomanometer (indirect)	Used in all situations Automatic equipment available Arm is protected from injury
	Arterial catheter (direct)	Catheter usually inserted percutaneously in radial artery Used for continuous monitoring in complex procedures and for induced hypotension
Cardiac	Stethoscopy	Stethoscope taped to chest Pressure sensitive units may be placed in esophagus Units attached to anesthesiologist's ear by indwelling ear piece
	ECG	Usually consists of a screen and print-out system Chest and extremity electrodes used Other electrosurgical equipment may affect ECG recordings
Central venous pressure	Water manometer	Used for evaluation of overall circulatory status Serves as a guide during blood and fluid administration Aids in preventing too rapid fluid replacement that could lead to pulmonary edema
Arterial blood gases	Blood samples	Used for evaluation of acid-base status and pulmonary gas exchange
Body temperature	Thermistor	Thermistor inserted in esophagus or rectum Used for events that are preceded by hypopyrexia or hyperpyrexia
Urinary output	Indwelling urinary catheter	Hourly measurements made Used for evaluation of blood volume and fluid administration
Blood loss	Weighing of blood-soaked sponges	Used to estimate blood loss from surgical procedure Dry weight of sponges is subtracted from wet weight
	Measurement of blood in suction systems	Estimate is also made of blood on drapes and team members' gowns

and bleeding may all contribute to situations that interfere with respiration and circulation and contribute to altered physiology.

Many devices are now available to augment the measurement of patient's responses to these stressors. Most of this equipment is expensive, takes up extra space in the operating room, and may constitute an electrical safety hazard. Involved personnel must still use skills of looking, listening, and palpating, even when sophisticated monitoring equipment is in use (Table 17-6).

A variety of other monitoring devices may be used depending on the complexity of the procedure being performed and the physical condition of the patient. Computers are being used more extensively in monitoring and processing patient data and greater use of the computer is envisioned in the future.

■ ELECTRICAL SAFETY HAZARDS

Monitoring of patient safety during anesthesia must also take into consideration electrical safety hazards. The operating room is an area containing many potential life threatening and mechanically injurious situations related

to electrical shock, burns, fire, and explosions. It is imperative that team members have up-to-date knowledge of the equipment and supplies most often involved in such incidents.

Federal regulations govern the marketing and safety standards of electronic devices used in operating rooms, and the Joint Commission on Accreditation of Hospitals (JCAH) has standards that must be met. The most significant hazards, however, are inadequately trained personnel, malfunctioning equipment caused by improper maintenance, inappropriate design of operating room suites, and inappropriate surveillance of equipment by O.R. team members.

■ TERMINATION OF SURGERY

One of the most crucial periods for the surgical patient is the immediate postoperative phase after surgery has been completed and the patient is transferred to the appropriate recovery area. During this period, the operating room nurse may be involved in a variety of activities related to providing effective patient care.

■ Dressings and drains

The circulating nurse will assist in the application of the outer layer of any necessary dressings. Dressings are used to protect the wound from trauma and contamination, to absorb drainage, and to support or immobilize the incisional area. Pressure dressings may be applied to aid in minimizing edema and to assist with hemostasis.

A wide variety of gauzes, pads, and tapes are available for use. The type used will depend on the area of the body involved, the amount of drainage anticipated, and the pressure that is necessary. Montgomery straps may be used if frequent dressing changes or wound inspections are anticipated. In some instances the application of a splint or cast will be required.

Some surgeons prefer that the wound be covered with a transparent spray dressing. This commonly stays on for 3 to 6 days and may either peel off or be removed with solvent. This type of dressing is particularly suitable for areas where gauze dressings could become contaminated with urine or feces.

Other surgeons prefer that the wound be left uncovered and open to the air to allow the incisional area to heal with the aid of air and light. It also allows for easy observation, prevents possible tape reactions, and increases comfort and maneuverability for certain patients.

A variety of drains may also be inserted at the time of surgery (see Chapter 18). Drains are used to expedite the removal of air and fluids such as blood, serum, bile, and pus from the involved site. The type and exact location of the drains are recorded and reported to the recovery room nurses.

■ DOCUMENTATION

Written documentation is important for communicating to other health team members the nursing actions that were performed in the intraoperative period and the patient outcomes. If the perioperative role is to be effectively implemented, operating room nurses must be accountable by documenting what they do.

Some facilities have the operating room nurse document information on the same form used for all nursing notes. Others have found it more expedient to develop a separate form that combines a checklist format along with areas for narrative comments (see reference 11).

■ Transfer of patient to recovery room

After appropriate dressings have been applied, the circulating nurse checks to see that the patient is clean. A clean gown and blanket are applied.

Special care must be taken in moving the patient from the operating room table to the recovery stretcher or bed. At least four people are usually required to transfer the unconscious patient safely while keeping the body in proper alignment. Care must be taken not to allow the patient to slip between the table and the stretcher and that no body tissues have shearing forces applied to them. Arms and legs must be carefully supported and IV sites splinted to prevent dislodging the needle. The anesthesiologist pro-

tects the head and neck from injury during the transfer. A patient lifting frame or roller device is very helpful when moving heavy patients.

The patient is lifted or rolled *slowly* to avoid circulatory depression, and the actions of all involved persons are carefully synchronized. The patient is placed in a comfortable position appropriate for maintaining an unobstructed airway and adequate circulation. It is important that the patient be constantly observed during this time as changes in position can stimulate vomiting, cause respiratory obstruction, hypotension, or cardiac arrest.

Before moving the stretcher or bed, siderails are pulled up and restraint straps fastened. All drainage systems are connected as indicated, and drainage bags are kept below the level of tubing to prevent retrograde flow.

The patient chart and nursing care plan are sent with the patient along with any other supplies that will be needed. In some hospitals the circulating nurse accompanies the patient and anesthesiologist to the recovery room so that a nursing report can be given to the nurse admitting the patient. Various other personnel may go along during the actual transfer, depending on the condition of the patient.

■ EVALUATION

Although desired outcomes will vary, depending on the individual needs that are assessed for each patient and the planned nursing activities that are carried out, the patient outcomes (based on standards of perioperative nursing practice) may be desirable for any surgical patient as follows:

1. The person shows evidence of managing preoperative anxiety.
2. The person is safely transported to the operating room and moved with proper assistance and good body alignment.
3. The person receives optimal emotional support and consideration from health team members from the time of admission to the O.R. suite until anesthetic has taken effect.
4. The person experiences minimal pain and exposure during transfer to the O.R. table.
5. The person experiences no adverse effects as a result of the following:
   a. Improper positioning or restraints
   b. Solutions used to prepare the skin
   c. Improper maintenance, application, or use of electrical equipment
   d. Foreign objects such as sponges, needles, or instruments being left in the surgical wound
   e. Improper application of the surgical dressing
   f. Transfer from the O.R. table to cart
6. Drapes are applied in a manner that provides minimal skin exposure and maximal skin protection from infection.
7. The person receives proper monitoring while receiving anesthetic and until completion of transfer to recovery area.

---

8. Documentation includes presence of drains and actions taken to meet identified needs.

■ SUMMARY

1. Perioperative nursing includes nursing activities performed by the professional nurse during the preoperative, intraoperative, and postoperative periods.
2. Members of the scrubbed sterile surgical team include the primary surgeon, assistant surgeons, and scrub nurse or technician.
3. Members of the nonsterile surgical team include the anesthesiologist (or anesthetist), circulating nurse, and other persons as needed (such as technicians, biomedical engineer, or pathologist).
4. A professional nurse serves as the circulating nurse and plays a vital role in overall O.R. management.
5. Principles of strict aseptic technique must be followed in the O.R. to prevent infection.
6. Rules for wearing correct O.R. attire and following good health habits are essential for lessening the risk of personnel serving as loci of infection.
7. Procedures for scrubbing before surgery differ among health care agencies; persons should be free of upper respiratory infections and skin problems that could serve as a medium for bacterial growth.
8. Factors that promote patient safety in the O.R. include reducing patient anxiety, following correct procedures for patient identification, reviewing the chart for completeness of necessary information and for identification of allergies, checking for possible hazards, and observing the patient for adverse effects of preoperative medication.
9. Some commonly used operative positions include supine, prone, Trendelenburg, reverse Trendelenburg, and lateral. Care must be taken in placing persons in each position to prevent patient injury.
10. Anesthesia may be general, regional, or local; it may be administered by inhalation or intravenously, by regional block, field block, spinal, epidural, topical, or infiltrative means. Hypnosis or acupuncture may also be used.
11. Anesthesia may produce amnesia, analgesia, hypnosis, or muscle relaxation, thus decreasing either awareness of or decreased sensation to pain.
12. Four stages may be noted with some types of anesthetic (especially diethyl ether); the extent to which the stages are seen depends on the drug used, rapidity of induction, and skill of the anesthesiologist or anesthetist.
13. Induced hypothermia consists of reducing body temperature below normal to reduce oxygen and metabolic requirements; it may be effected by extracorporeal cooling during surgery, by the use of cooling blankets, or by submerging the person in ice.
14. Parameters monitored during anesthesia include arterial blood pressure, cardiac arrhythmias, arterial blood gasses, central venous pressure, body temperature, urinary output, blood loss, and patient safety.
15. Nursing care requirements following surgery include application of external dressings (as necessary), connection of drainage tubes to receptacles as indicated, applying clean gown and blanket, moving the patient to the recovery stretcher, monitoring the patient, documenting actions and nursing care plan, transferring the patient to the recovery room, and reporting on the patient's condition and special needs.

REFERENCES AND SELECTED READINGS
Contemporary

1. *Allen, P: Applying standards to practice, AORN J 31:805-813, 1980.
2. American Nurses' Association Division on Medical-Surgical Nursing Practice and Association of Operating Room Nurses: Standards of perioperative nursing practice, Kansas City, Mo., 1981, American Nurses' Association.
3. American College of Surgeons, Subcommittee on Control of Surgical Infections: Manual on control of infection in surgical patients, ed 2, Philadelphia, 1984, WB Saunders Co.
4. AORN Ad Hoc Committee on Basic Competencies: Developing basic competencies for perioperative nursing, AORN J 35:871-884, 1982.

---

*References preceded by an asterisk are particularly well-suited for student reading

5. AORN Committee on Nursing Practices: Using revised standards, AORN J 36:363-377, 1982.
6. AORN, Inc: AORN recommended practices for inhospital sterilization, AORN J 32:222-244, 1980.
7. AORN, Inc: Patient outcome standards for perioperative nursing, AORN J 39:400-402; 40:578-580, 1984.
8. AORN, Inc: Proposed recommended practices: Radiation safety in the operating room (including lasers), AORN J 40:881-886, 1984.
9. AORN, Inc: Recommended practices for aseptic barrier materials for surgical drapes, AORN J 37:249-250, 1983.
10. AORN, Inc: Recommended practices for basic aseptic technique. In AORN Standards and Recommended Practices for Perioperative Nursing, Part III, Sections 2-1-4, Denver, 1985. AORN, Inc.
11. AORN, Inc: Recommended practices for documentation of perioperative nursing care, AORN J 35:744-748, 1982.
12. AORN, Inc: Recommended practices: monitoring the patient receiving local anesthesia, AORN J 39:1080-1083, 1984.
13. AORN, Inc: Recommended practices: OR attire, AORN J 39:710-720, 1984.
14. AORN, Inc.: Recommended practices: OR sanitation, AORN J 39:838-844, 1984.
15. AORN, Inc: Recommended practices for preoperative skin preparation of patients, AORN J 37:244-248, 1983.
16. AORN, Inc: Recommended practices: Surgical scrubs, AORN J 39:1084-1088, 1984.
17. AORN Inc: Recommended practices for traffic patterns in the surgical suite, AORN J 35:750-758, 1982.
18. AORN Standards and recommended practices for perioperative nursing, Denver, 1985, AORN, Inc.
19. Atkinson, LJ, and Kohn, ML: Berry and Kohn's Introduction to operating room techniques, ed 6, New York, 1986, McGraw-Hill Book Co.
20. *Bartley, J, and Chamberlin, DA: The barriers to infection, Today's OR Nurse 5(7):226-29, 1983.
21. *Brennan, PE: Preoperative visits: controlling the stress, Today's OR Nurse 4:9-13, 1982.
22. *Brock, AM: How do the aged cope with surgery? Today's OR Nurse 6:16-25, 1984.
23. Brukhardt, SS: Patient monitoring in the operating room: an introduction and overview, J Oper Room Res Inst 3:10-22, 1983.
24. *Chansky, ER: Reducing patients' anxieties: techniques for dealing with crises, AORN J 40:375-377, 1984.
25. Copp, F., and others: Covergowns and the control of operating room contamination, Nurs Res 35:263-268, 1986.
26. Cordner, JW: Logic of operating room nursing, ed 3, Oradell, NJ, 1984, Medical Economics Books.
27. Crow, S: Minimizing the risk of infection in the compromised patient, Gown Glove 3:4-5, 1981.
28. Danner, D: Patients rights emphasized in informed consent ruling, Malpract Dig. 10:1-2, 1983.
29. Dripps, RD, and others: Introduction to anesthesia, ed 7, Philadelphia, 1988, WB Saunders Co.
30. Fernsebner, B: Patients at risk for nosocomial infections, AORN J 38:613-620, 1983.
31. Fernsebner, B: A protocol for malignant hyperthermia, AORN J 31:814-818, 1980.
32. *French, MM, and Phillips, KF: When seconds count: treating malignant hyperthermia, RN 47(11):26-31, 1984.
33. Greelhoed, GW, and others: A comparative study of surgical skin preparation methods, Surg Gynecol Obstet 157:265-268, 1983.
34. Greene, NM: Neurologic complications associated with regional anesthesia, Curr Rev Clin Anesth 2:202-208, 1982.
35. Groah, LK: Operating Room Nursing: the perioperative role, Reston, VA, 1983, Reston Publishing Co.
36. Groah, L, and Reed, EA: Your responsibility in documenting care, AORN J 37:1174-1188, 1983.
37. Gruendemann, BJ, and Meeker, MH: Alexander's care of the patient in surgery, ed 8, St. Louis, 1987, The CV Mosby Co.
38. Hahn, AB, Barking, RL, and Oesterich, SJK: Pharmacology in nursing, ed 16, St.Louis, 1986, The CV Mosby Co.
39. Kaul, AF, and Jewett, JF: Agents and techniques for disinfection of the skin, Surg Gynecol Obstet 152:677-685, 1981.
40. Kneedler, JA, and Dodge, GH: Perioperative patient care, Boston, 1983, Blackwell Scientific Publishers.
41. LeMaitre, G, and Finnigan, JA: The patient in surgery, ed 5, Philadelphia, 1988, WB Saunders Co.
42. Mackie, R, and others: Perioperative care plan guides, AORN J 40:192-201, 1984.
43. Mathieu, A, and Burke, JF: Infection and the perioperative period, New York, 1982, Grune & Stratton.
44. McCredie, JA, editor: Basic surgery, ed 2, New York, 1986, Macmillan Publishing Co, Inc.
45. McVay, CB: Anson's and McVay's surgical anatomy, ed 6, Philadelphia, 1984, WB Saunders Co.
46. *Metheny, N: Perioperative fluid balance assessment, AORN J 33:51-56, 1981.
47. Nursing Practice Committee: A model for perioperative nursing practice, AORN J 4L:188-194, 1985.
48. Petty, C: Assisting the patient receiving a regional anesthetic, Point View 21:16-17, 1984.
49. Phippin, M: OR nurses' guide to preventing pressure sores, AORN J 36:205-212, 1982.
50. Rogers, AL, and Sturgeon, CL, Jr: Malignant hyperthermia: a perioperative emergency, AORN J 41:369-374, 1985.
51. Sabiston, DC: Davis-Christopher's textbook of surgery, ed 13, Philadelphia, 1986, WB Saunders Co.
52. Schwartz, SI, and others, editors: Principles of surgery, ed 4, New York, 1984, McGraw-Hill Book Co.
53. Weiner, MB, and Pepper, GA: Clinical pharmacology and therapeutics in nursing, ed 2, New York, 1985, McGraw-Hill Book Co.
54. Yoder, ME: Nursing diagnosis: applications in perioperative practice, AORN J 40:183-188, 1984.

Classic

55. *Foster, C, and others: Effects of surgical positioning, AORN J 30:219-221, 1979.
56. Kneedler, J, and others: From standards into practice, AORN J 28:603-642, 1978

18

Postoperative Intervention

BARBARA C. LONG

CHAPTER OBJECTIVES

After studying this chapter, the student should be able to:

- Identify nursing interventions to meet patient needs in the postanesthetic period.
- Discuss the rationale for collection of data necessary to plan nursing care when the patient returns to the clinical unit.
- Describe the types and process of wound healing and interventions that promote wound healing.
- Explain wound dehiscence and evisceration and appropriate nursing interventions.
- Identify postoperative respiratory and circulatory problems, assessment parameters, and preventive measures.
- Describe possible postoperative problems with fluid and electrolyte balance, nutrition, elimination, and inactivity, and the assessment parameters and preventive measures.
- Describe measures to promote patients' physical and psychologic comfort in the postoperative period.

The postoperative period begins as soon as the operation is completed. If a general anesthetic has been given, the patient is usually taken to a recovery (postanesthesia) room for the postanesthetic phase.

POSTANESTHETIC PHASE

The immediate postanesthetic period is critical. The patient must be observed diligently and must receive intensive physical and psychologic support until the major effects of the anesthetic have worn off and the overall condition stabilizes. The nurse is largely responsible for the care of the patient at this time.

The patient is accompanied to the recovery room by the anesthesiologist and another member of the operating room professional staff. The recovery room nurse assesses the patient's status, obtains report, and begins recording the recovery room notes.

Much of the ongoing nursing care provided in the immediate postanesthetic period depends on the surgical procedure performed and is discussed elsewhere in this text (see specific surgical care for each body system). Some outcomes, however, are the same for all patients: pulmonary ventilation, circulation, and fluid and electrolyte balance are maintained, injury is prevented, and comfort is promoted.

Maintaining pulmonary ventilation

In the immediate postanesthetic period, two of the most common causes of inadequate pulmonary exchange are airway obstruction and hypoventilation.

■ AIRWAY PATENCY

Airway obstruction most frequently occurs as a result of the tongue, which is relaxed against the pharynx (Fig. 18-1) or of secretions or other fluids collecting in the pharynx, trachea, or bronchial tree. This can be prevented by proper positioning, use of an artificial airway, or removal of secretions.

□ Positioning

Until protective reflexes have returned, the best position for the majority of patients is a *side-lying* or *semiprone* position with the head tilted back and the jaw supported forward. It is important to remember that aspiration can occur unless the *whole body* is turned. Turning the patient's head while the chest and shoulders remain in the back-lying position is useless.

□ Artificial airway

An oropharyngeal or nasopharyngeal airway is often left in place after administration of a general anesthetic to keep the passage open and the tongue forward until pharyngeal reflexes have returned (Fig. 18-2). These artificial airways are made of rubber, plastic, or metal. They are removed as soon as the patient begins to awaken and has regained coughing and swallowing reflexes. After this time their presence can be irritating and can stimulate vomiting or laryngospasm. The pharyngeal reflex can be tested by touching the posterior pharynx with a tongue blade to produce gagging.

□ Removal of secretions

If the patient cannot cough up and expectorate secretions, they must be removed by suctioning. Pharyngeal

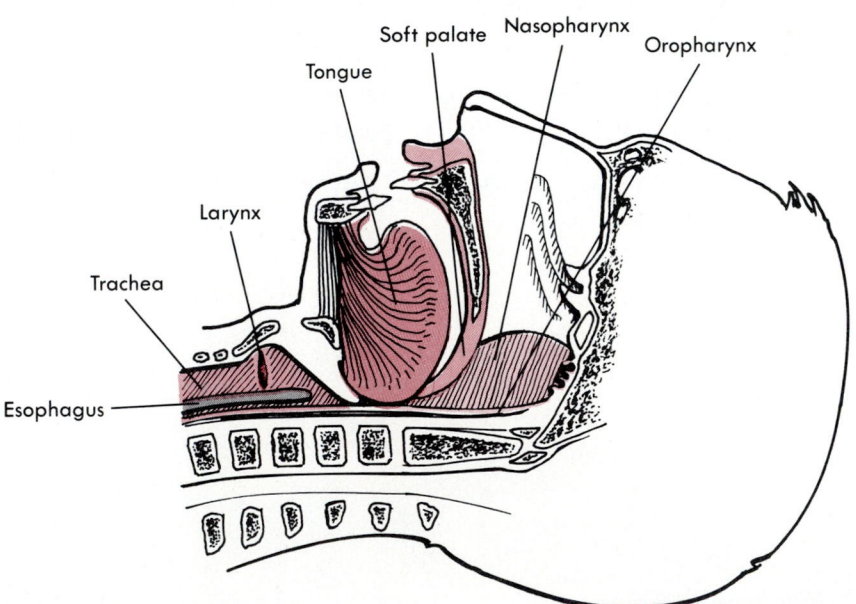

Fig. 18-1 Obstruction of airway by tongue blocking oropharynx in unconscious person lying in supine position.

suctioning is usually all that is necessary, although intra-tracheal suctioning may be indicated.

■ ADEQUATE VENTILATION

Immediate postoperative hypoventilation can result from drugs (anesthetics, narcotics, tranquilizers, sedatives), incisional pain, obesity, chronic lung disease, or pressure on the diaphragm. Oxygenation and ventilation can be enhanced by oxygen therapy and breathing exercises.

□ Oxygen therapy

Oxygen is usually given postoperatively because after anesthesia almost all patients have decreased pulmonary expansion and areas of atelectasis, both of which result in hypoxemia. Oxygen is administered by nasal cannula, disposable face mask or shield, or endotracheal or tracheostomy tube if one is in place. Patients with thoracic or upper abdominal incisions or with preexisting pulmonary disease may be given oxygen for several hours or even into the next day.

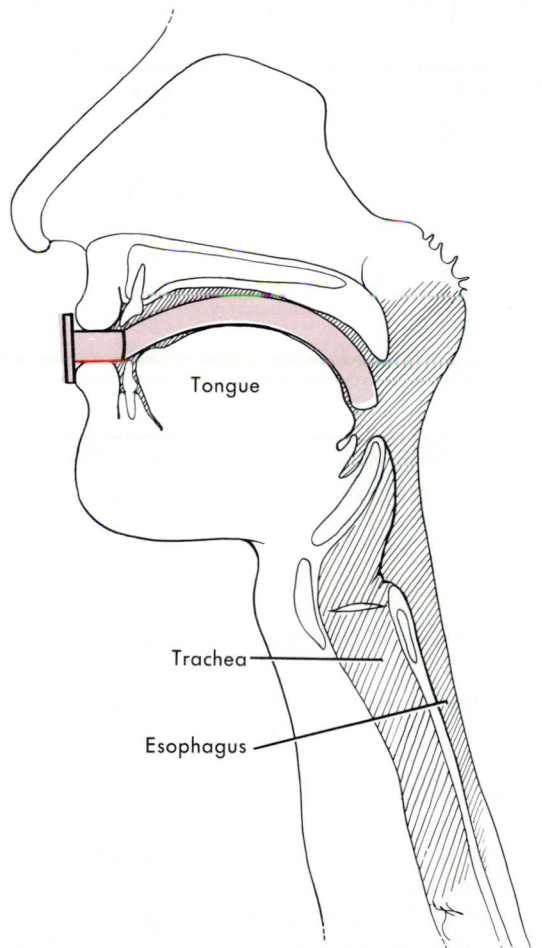

Fig. 18-2 Airway in place to prevent tongue from falling back against pharynx and blocking airway.

□ Breathing exercises

Deep-breathing exercises are started as soon as the patient is conscious and able to follow directions. Considerable encouragement and repetition of directions are needed because of amnesia related to the anesthetic. If the patient is unconscious or will not breathe deeply when stimulated, the nurse can hyperventilate the lungs passively using a breathing bag and mask.

■ Maintaining circulation

Hypotension and cardiac arrhythmias are the most common cardiovascular complications in the immediate postanesthetic period. Early recognition and management of these complications before they become serious enough to diminish cardiac output depend on frequent assessment of the patient's vital signs.

The blood pressure, pulse, and respirations are usually taken every 15 minutes until stable, then every half hour for 2 hours, and then every 4 hours until ordered otherwise. In many hospitals the monitoring of vital signs every 15 minutes extends for as long as the patient is in the recovery room and for at least 1 hour after leaving the recovery room. The rate, volume, and rhythm of the pulse are carefully observed and the character and rate of respiration are noted. Preoperative vital signs are used as a baseline for comparison.

■ HYPOTENSION

Many factors can cause circulatory changes that result in lowering of blood pressure in the postoperative patient (see the box below). A mild decrease in blood pressure from the normal preoperative range is not uncommon during the early postoperative period. It is usually well tolerated in healthy patients and does not require treatment. Shock must be prevented because the brain, heart, kidneys, and other vital organs do not tolerate long periods of hypoxemia. Measures to control shock are immediately instituted when signs of shock occur (Chapter 9).

Possible causes of postoperative shock

Moving patient from operating table to bed
Jarring patient (bed) during transport
Reactions to drugs and anesthesia
Loss of blood and other body fluids
Cardiac arrhythmias
Cardiac failure
Inadequate ventilation
Pain
Residual sympathectomy from conductive anesthesia

■ CARDIAC ARRHYTHMIAS

Hypoxemia and hypercapnia are common causes of postoperative cardiac arrhythmias, especially premature beats and sinus tachycardia. These arrhythmias often can be suppressed by adequate ventilation. Other common causes of postoperative cardiac arrhythmias include pain, hypovolemia, gastric distention, and acidosis. Significant arrhythmias are treated by attention to the underlying cause when possible. Antiarrhythmic drugs may be prescribed (Chapter 25).

■ Maintaining fluid and electrolyte balance

In most patients admitted to the recovery room, administration of intravenous fluids is the immediate postoperative means of maintaining fluid and electrolyte balance. Careful monitoring of the intravenous fluids is essential to ensure adequacy of replacement and prevention of fluid overload (Chapter 8).

■ Maintaining safety and comfort
■ PREVENTING INJURY

After anesthesia, side rails on the stretcher or bed are generally raised and left so until the patient is fully awake. The patient is turned frequently and placed in good body alignment to prevent nerve damage from pressure and muscle and joint strain from lying in one position for a long time.

■ PROMOTING PHYSICAL COMFORT

Incisional pain is a common complaint after surgery, and from the patient's point of view it is probably the most significant postoperative complication. In the immediate postanesthetic period, narcotic analgesics are given for pain when warranted, but this should be done with the realization that pronounced depression of the respiratory, circulatory, or central nervous system may follow. Because the patient generally has not completely recovered from the effects of the anesthetic, the first postoperative dose of a narcotic is usually reduced to about *one half* the dose to be received after full recovery from anesthesia. Pain medication for restlessness is given only after it has been determined that the restlessness is not a result of hypoxia.

■ PROMOTING PSYCHOLOGIC COMFORT

The immediate postanesthetic period is often frightening for the patient. Psychologic support is imperative for physical as well as emotional well-being. While awakening from anesthesia, the patient needs frequent orientation to place and reassurance of not being alone. The patient also needs to know that the operation is over and that recovery from anesthesia is satisfactory. Careful explanations of procedures being carried out are given even when it appears that the patient is not alert. The need for privacy is considered at all times. Patients who receive this type of sup

port frequently recover from anesthesia faster, with fewer complications and less incisional pain.

■ Discharge from recovery room

Patients are discharged from the recovery room when the following criteria have been met:
1. Vital signs are stable and indicate adequate respiratory and circulatory function.
2. Patient is awake or easily aroused and can call for assistance if needed.
3. Postsurgical complications have been thoroughly evaluated and are under control.
4. After regional anesthesia, motor and partial sensory functions have returned to all anesthetized areas.

Acutely ill patients who require further close supervision are transferred to an intensive care unit. Most patients are transferred to a clinical unit. The unit is notified to expect the patient, and all pertinent information concerning the patient's status is communicated to the nurse who will continue to provide postoperative nursing care. The recovery room nurse writes a discharge summary note before the patient leaves the recovery room.

■ ADMISSION OF PATIENT TO CLINICAL UNIT

■ Preparation on clinical unit

The patient's room is prepared to facilitate patient transfer and monitoring (see the box below). The family is notified of the patient's expected return.

Most surgeons discuss the results of the operation with the family immediately after surgery and also visit the patient to describe briefly what was found and to provide reassurance. The family is frequently highly anxious concerning the patient's condition and may not perceive or understand all that the surgeon tells them. Patients frequently experience periods of amnesia during the hours when they first regain consciousness and may not remem-

---

Preparing room for patient's return from surgery

1. Make an open surgical bed to facilitate easy transfer of patient.
2. Provide sufficient covers (patient may feel cold).
3. Clear a passageway to the bed.
4. Provide necessary equipment
   a. Intravenous pole
   b. Sphygmomanometer
   c. Any special equipment as designated by recovery room nurse.

ber what they have been told. The nurse needs to know what information was given to the patient and family to be able to answer their questions. The family also needs to know what to expect when the patient returns to the unit.

■ SAFETY

Bed siderails are kept raised until the patient is fully awake and responding or to prevent the heavily medicated patient from falling. The patient is instructed early regarding permissibility of ambulation and the need to call for assistance for initial attempts. The call cord should be easily accessible to the patient.

■ FAMILY MEMBERS

If family members are present in the room when the patient returns, they may be asked to step outside until the patient has been transferred and assessed. Before leaving the patient, the nurse invites the family to return, explains equipment, and describes the patient's state of awareness and comfort. Family members who understand what is occurring can offer support to the patient. Explanations should be simple but concrete and accurate.

▦ ASSESSMENT

■ Initial assessment

As soon as the patient is positioned on the bed in the clinical unit, the nurse makes a rapid assessment of the patient's condition. Parameters to assess include respiratory, circulatory, and neurologic status, dressing, patient comfort and safety, and functioning of equipment (see the box below).

■ SUBJECTIVE DATA

The patient is asked for symptoms of discomfort after having been transferred to the bed and positioned in supportive body alignment. This gives the nurse a quick indication of the level of alertness and symptoms of discomfort. An indirect question such as, "How do you feel?" will elicit data concerning nausea or pain without focusing on a specific area where there may be no discomfort. Pain perception is frequently increased at this time because of the movement from stretcher to bed. It is important to find out location, onset, and change in pain intensity and not to assume that the pain is incisional.

Nausea occurs less frequently postoperatively with the use of newer anesthetics. There is greater possibility of nausea when the stomach has been manipulated extensively during the surgical procedure or if considerable amounts of narcotics have been administered. The emesis basin should be easily available but not in sight if vomiting is a possibility.

■ OBJECTIVE DATA

☐ Respiratory status

Respirations may be increased or decreased (see Table 18-1). If hypoventilation is present, oxygen may be given if a nasal cannula is in place.

Very noisy respirations may be heard without the aid of a stethoscope. Noisy respirations may be caused by airway obstruction from the tongue falling back against the pharynx or from secretions. The patient with noisy respirations

---

Patient assessment on return from recovery room

Respiratory status	Patency of airway
	Respirations: depth, rate, character
	Breath sounds: presence, character
Circulatory status	Pulse, blood pressure, temperature
	Skin color, temperature
	Capillary filling
Neurologic status	Level of consciousness
Dressing	Presence of drainage
	Presence of tubes to be connected to drainage systems
Comfort	Presence of pain, nausea, vomiting
	Patient positioned for comfort and to facilitate ventilation
Safety	Necessity for side rails
	Call cord within reach
Equipment	Monitors connected and functioning
	Intravenous fluids: rate, amount in bag, patency of tubing
	Drainage systems (for example, nasogastric, chest, urinary): type, patency of tubing, connection of appropriate container, character and amount of drainage

Table 18-1 Some causes of vital sign changes in early postoperative phase

Vital sign	Increase	Decrease
Temperature	Stress reaction (low-grade fever)	Cold operating room and recovery room
Pulse rate	Jarring during transfer	Digitalis overdose
	Shock, hemorrhage	Cardiac arrhythmias
	Hypoventilation	
	Acute gastric dilation	
	Pain	
	Anxiety	
	Cardiac arrhythmias	
Respiratory rate	Hypoventilation: poor positioning, tight chest or upper abdominal dressing, obesity, gastric dilation	Drugs: anesthetics, narcotics, sedatives
Blood pressure	Anxiety ($\uparrow$ systolic)	Jarring during transfer
	Pain	Severe pain
	Distended urinary bladder	Cardiac arrhythmias
		Shock: fluid loss, hemorrhage, acute gastric dilation

is assisted in coughing and then positioned side-lying if possible. Suctioning may be indicated if coughing does not clear the airway.

If respirations are not noisy, the lungs are auscultated to establish a baseline for future comparison and to identify adventitious sounds (Chapter 3). Absent breath sounds indicate hypoventilation of the lobe (Table 18-1). Coarse rales (crackles) indicate secretions in air passages. Presence of adventitious sounds indicates the need for energetic ventilatory exercises. Deep-breathing and coughing measures are instituted immediately in all patients who have had general anesthesia (Chapter 16).

□ **Circulatory status**

The pulse, blood pressure, skin color and temperature, and capillary filling are assessed (Table 18-1). Signs of shock or hemorrhage are reported immediately to the surgeon. Hypotensive changes may be related to shock, although other signs of shock usually occur before changes in blood pressure. The skin often feels cool to the touch after surgery as a result of coolness of the surgical suites, hypovolemia from blood loss, or vasoconstriction from stress. Restlessness is an early sign of shock.

After surgery of the extremities, local circulation is assessed by the presence and strength of peripheral pulses *distal* to the operative site or plaster cast. If the dressing is too tight, it should be loosened, if permissible, or reported at once to the physician.

□ **Level of consciousness**

Level of consciousness can be ascertained by asking the patient to respond to simple questions or commands. Variations in consciousness level from alertness to drowsiness will be observed. If the patient is not easily aroused, these data are compared with the patient's consciousness status at the time of discharge from the recovery room. A decrease in consciousness level may indicate shock (from jarring motions during the transfer) and should be reported to the surgeon at once along with any other pertinent data.

□ **Dressing**

The entire dressing is inspected with the covers pulled back or the patient turned as necessary. A dressing applied to the side, such as after kidney surgery, may appear dry on the top visible area if the patient is supine but may have excess drainage on the lower portion as a result of gravity. Excess drainage is reported immediately.

Whenever it is anticipated that fluid may collect in a body area postoperatively, leading to delay in healing, the surgeon usually inserts a tube or drain (Table 18-2) to permit escape of the fluid. One end of the tube or drain is placed in or near the organ or cavity to be drained, and the other end is passed through the body wall, usually through a separate stab wound.

After most types of surgery, the surgeon usually changes the dressing for the first time. If small amounts of unexpected drainage are observed, especially bright red drainage, the area can be outlined with a pen on the dressing so that the rate of drainage can be easily determined. Dressings that *cannot* be changed by the nurse are reinforced with dry dressings if drainage penetrates the outer layer; this prevents bacterial contamination by capillary action through the wet dressings. If these additional dressings become wet, they are removed and replaced with new dressings, leaving the original dressing intact. Dressings that *can* be changed by the nurse are changed as often as necessary to prevent maceration of the skin and to promote patient comfort.

□ **Body position**

The patient is placed in a position of comfort that aids good ventilation. Except after spinal anesthesia or in certain types of eye surgery or neurosurgery when the bed must remain flat, most patients prefer the head of the bed slightly elevated. The patient who is not very alert needs to be placed in a position of good alignment. There should be no strain on the area surrounding the incision. Pillows should *not* exert pressure on the popliteal area (behind the knee), because this leads to venous obstruction.

Table 18-2   Surgical tubes and drains

Type	Purpose	Examples	Comments
Tubes	Prevent blockage of drainage	T-tube (Fig. 18-3)	Connect to drainage system as ordered
	Drain an area by suction	Abramson all-purpose tube (Fig. 18-4)	
		Saratoga sump tube (Fig. 18-4)	
Drains	Drain an area by gravity	Penrose drain (Fig. 18-5)	Use a safety pin to prevent drain from sliding back into abdomen
		Cigarette drain (Fig. 18-5)	Encase outer end of drain in a dressing

Fig. 18-3   T tube for draining common bile duct.

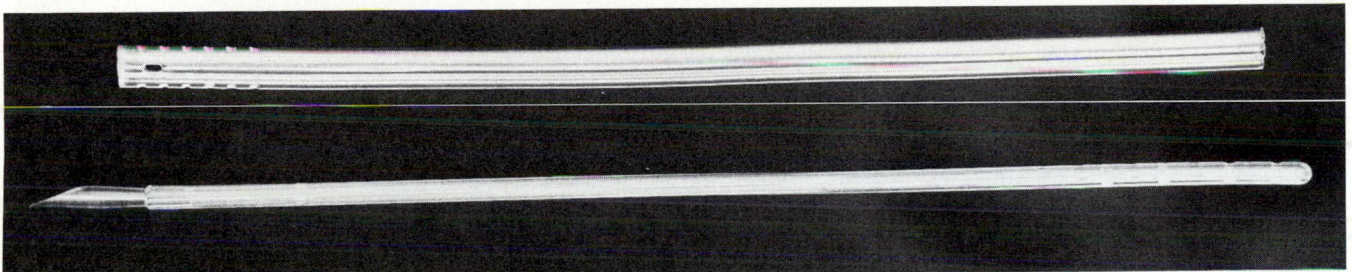

Fig. 18-4   Surgical drain tubes. *Top,* Abramson all-purpose drain has three lumens: for aspiration, irrigation, and instillation. *Bottom,* Saratoga sump drain has a tube within a tube for low-pressure suction.

Fig. 18-5   Wound drains. *Top,* Penrose drain. *Bottom,* Cigarette drain.

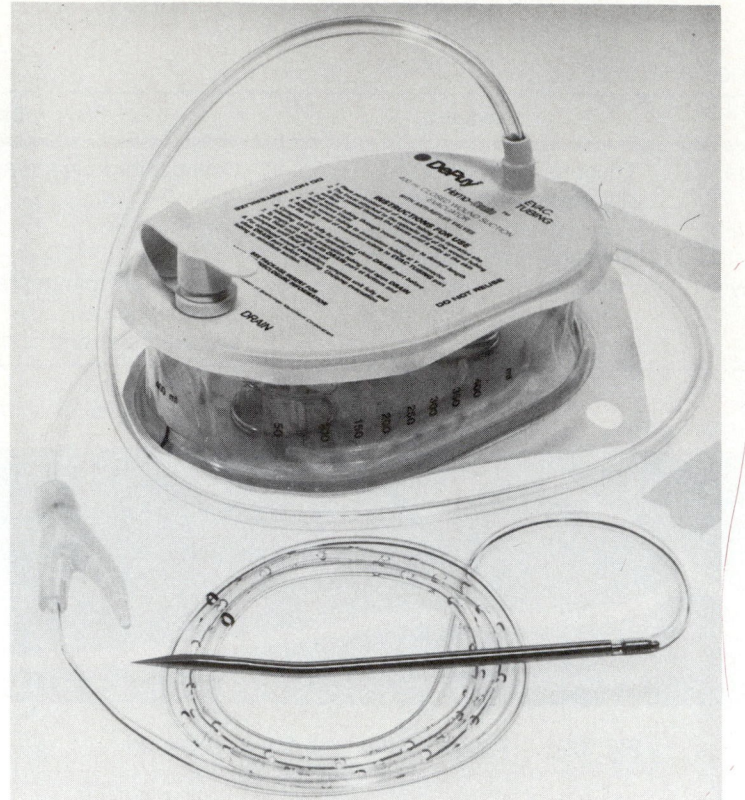

Fig. 18-6 Hemo-drain for low-suction wound drainage. Unit is compressed, then drain cap closed. Inner spring expands slowly, creating suction through tube. (Courtesy De Puy, Warsaw, Ind.)

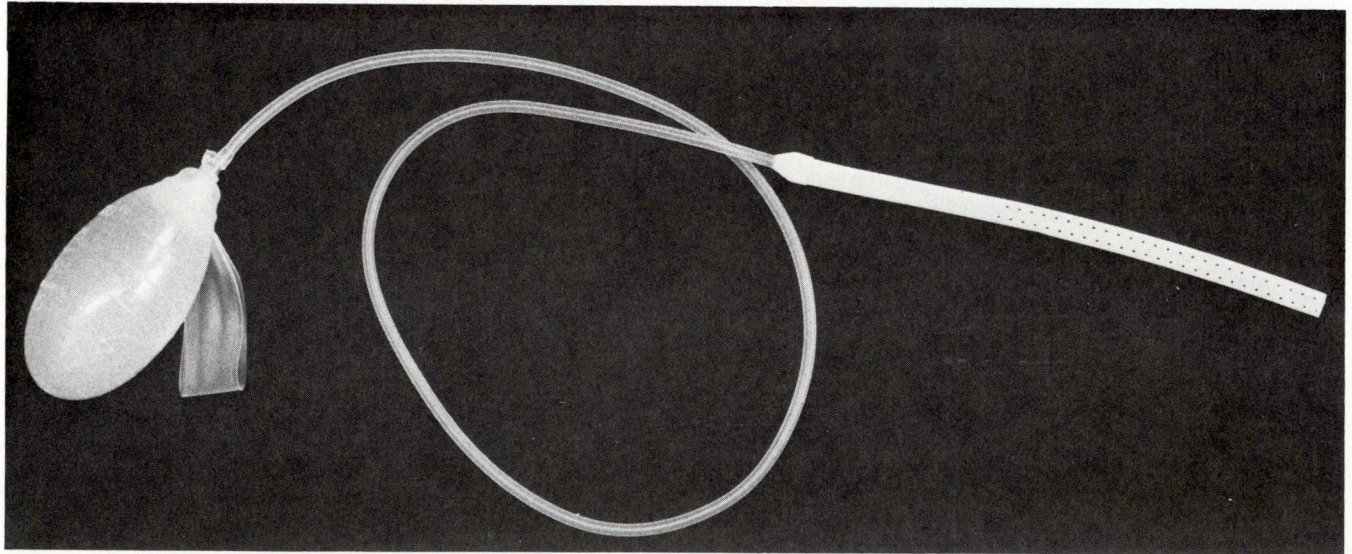

Fig. 18-7 Jackson-Pratt wound suction apparatus. After emptying through spout, reservoir bulb is kept compressed until spout is closed. Slow expansion of bulb creates low-pressure suction.

■ ASSESSMENT OF FLUID LINES

Fluids may be ordered to be given intravenously or instilled in body cavities for irrigation, such as in the bladder (see Chapter 32). The contents of the fluid containers, the patency of the tubing, and the rate of fluid administration are checked. Fluids are usually given intravenously at rates ranging from minimal (to keep the line open, K/O) to 3 ml/min. If the rate is greater than 3 ml/min, and if the physician's order sheet is not available in the patient's room, the rate should be slowed, the order checked immediately, and the rate adjusted appropriately. Rate of administration varies with the amount of fluid lost, size and age of the patient, and the underlying illness (Chapter 8). The patient and family should be instructed early concerning permissibility of fluids taken orally.

Drainage from tubes can be accomplished by either gravity or suction (Table 18-3). All tubing is connected to the drainage receptacle and checked for patency. The amount of fluid in each receptacle is marked on the receptacle and recorded as baseline for future comparison.

■ Data from patient's chart

After the patient has been assessed and positioned comfortably and safely, the nurse gathers additional data from the patient's chart (Table 18-4) before planning and initiating general postoperative care.

➡ DATA ANALYSIS: NURSING DIAGNOSES

The collected data are recorded in the nursing admission notes and used to identify the specific needs of the patient in the postoperative period. The preoperative condition of the patient, type of surgery performed, and strengths and resources of the patient are determining factors in postoperative discomfort or complications. In planning the pa-

Table 18-3 Drainage systems

Tube	System
Nasogastric tube	
Levine tube	Intermittent low electric suction
Sump tube	Constant low electric suction
Urinary catheter	Gravity urinary drainage system
Chest tube	Waterseal drainage system (gravity or suction)
Incisional tubes	Low negative pressure: Hemovac (Fig. 18-6), Jackson-Pratt (Fig. 18-7), or low constant electric suction

Table 18-4 Chart data useful in planning postoperative care

Data	Direction for action/interpretation
Surgeon's orders	
Activity	Extent permissible
Fluids, food	Intravenous: type, amount, rate
	Oral: type
Medications	Type and frequency of medications to be taken as needed
	Medications to be started immediately
Other orders	Special orders to be carried out depending on type of surgery
Surgical notes	
Postoperative diagnosis	Interpretation to patient/family
Type of surgery	Special nursing interventions
	Interpretations to patient/family
Anesthetic	
Inhalant	Need for deep-breathing measures
Muscle relaxants	Assessment of respiratory distress
Spinal	Supine position postoperatively; headache may occur
Estimated blood loss (EBL) and fluid replacement	Potential for fluid and electrolyte imbalance or transfusion reactions
Drains	Possible drainage on dressing
Recovery room notes	
Vital signs before transfer	Identification of changes related to transfer
Patient progress	Identification of persistent problems
Medications given	Times when drugs given and patient response
Urinary output	Status of renal function or urine retention

tient's care the nurse uses previously collected data, present data, knowledge of factors related to specific types of surgery (as illustrated in succeeding chapters of this text), and specific postoperative needs and possible postoperative complications.

Possible nursing diagnoses for the postoperative patient may include, but are not limited to, the following:

Diagnostic title	Possible etiologies
Anxiety	Threat to self-concept; threat or change in health status, socioeconomic status, role functioning; unmet needs
Constipation	Anesthesia, inactivity, inadequate nutrition, stress
Ineffective breathing pattern	Increased respiratory secretions, dry sticky secretions, decreased thorax expansion, pain, tight bandages or casts, abdominal distention, medications
Pain	Incisional pain, decreased circulation from tight dressings or cast, abdominal distention, full bladder, inactivity (gas pains)
Comfort, altered: nausea	Anesthetic, narcotics, electrolyte imbalance
Fluid volume excess	Age (elderly), large fluid volume intake
Potential for injury: wound dehiscence	Excessive coughing, distention, dehydration, obesity
Potential for injury: falls	Weakness, dizziness (medications), prolonged immobility
Knowledge deficit, postoperative routine, preventive measures, specific care requirements	Lack of exposure or recall, information misinterpretation
Impaired physical mobility	Pain, decreased strength and endurance, multiple tubes
Altered nutrition: less than body requirements	Anorexia, weakness, pain, nausea
Potential impaired tissue integrity	Inactivity, shock, obesity, pressure on popliteal area, tight dressing or cast
Urinary retention	Position for voiding, anesthetic, narcotic, pelvic surgery

PLANNING: EXPECTED PATIENT OUTCOMES

Expected patient outcomes for the postoperative patient may include, but are not limited to, the following:
1. No injury occurs during hospitalization.
2. The incision heals normally without infection.
3. No avoidable complications (atelectasis, pneumonia, thrombophlebitis, overhydration) occur.
4. Elimination patterns are reestablished.

5. Weight loss is minimal or stabilized.
6. The patient carries out activities of daily living at an optimal level, although fatigue may still be present.
7. The patient has an opportunity to explore individual concerns.
8. At discharge the patient or significant other can explain
   a. Treatments to be carried out at home, if any
   b. Medications to be taken at home (name, dosage, frequency, side effects)
   c. Any dietary changes required by the surgery
   d. Activity limits incurred by the surgery and any exercise programs to be carried out at home
   e. When and where to go for follow-up care by the surgeon

IMPLEMENTATION

Promoting wound healing

PATHOPHYSIOLOGY OF WOUND HEALING

Understanding the pathophysiology of wound healing and the factors that influence wound healing provides the basis for some of the postoperative nursing care, particularly wound care, dietary requirements, and need for physical activity.

Result of wound healing

Wounds may heal by *regeneration* of the tissue or by *scar* formation. Injured cells that have the capacity to regenerate (Fig. 18-8) will do so if the underlying structure has not been destroyed. Muscle and nerve cells rarely undergo mitotic division and are unable to regenerate. When muscle cells are injured, satisfactory performance may result by hypertrophy of marginal cells. Nerve cells in the central nervous system do not regenerate. In the peripheral nervous system there is no regeneration if the cell body is

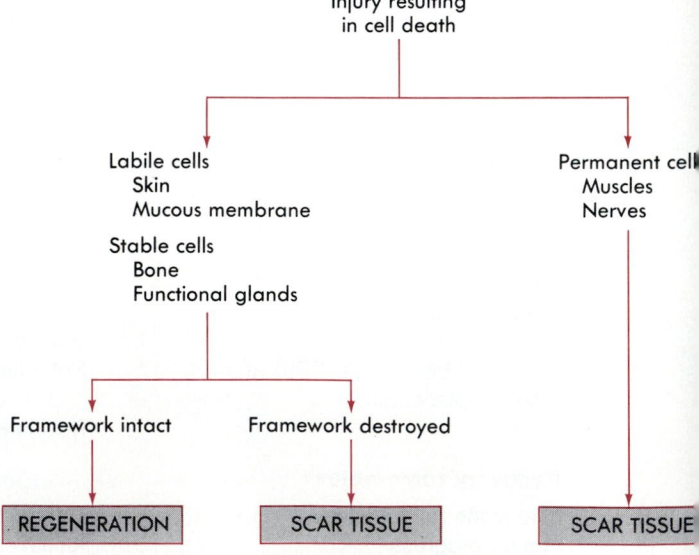

Fig. 18-8 End results of wound healing.

destroyed; however, if the axon is injured, there is partial degeneration of the axon, followed by regeneration.

In a typical surgical incision, muscle tissue is cut into. Although the epithelial cells regenerate over the scar tissue, the epithelial layer is so thin that the scar tissue is visible.

☐ Types of wound healing

Tissue may heal by primary, secondary, or tertiary intention (Fig. 18-9).

☐ Primary intention

All layers of the wound are closely approximated by suturing. If not infected, they heal quickly with minimum scarring.

☐ Secondary intention

Ulcers with edges that cannot be sutured heal by filling the area in from the bottom. The wounds are open, with increased chance of infection, and heal slowly with considerable scarring.

☐ Tertiary intention

The wound is sutured several days after wounding. The wound is more contaminated than with primary intention, so scarring is greater.

☐ Process of wound healing

Regardless of the type of wound healing, the process is the same. The difference is in length of time for each phase of healing and the extent of granulation tissue

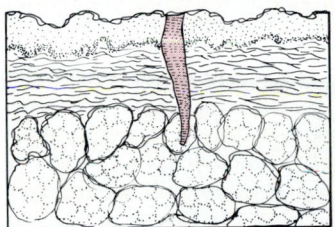 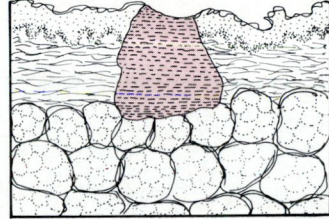 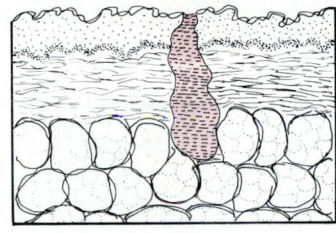

Fig. 18-9 Types of wound healing: primary, secondary, and tertiary intention.

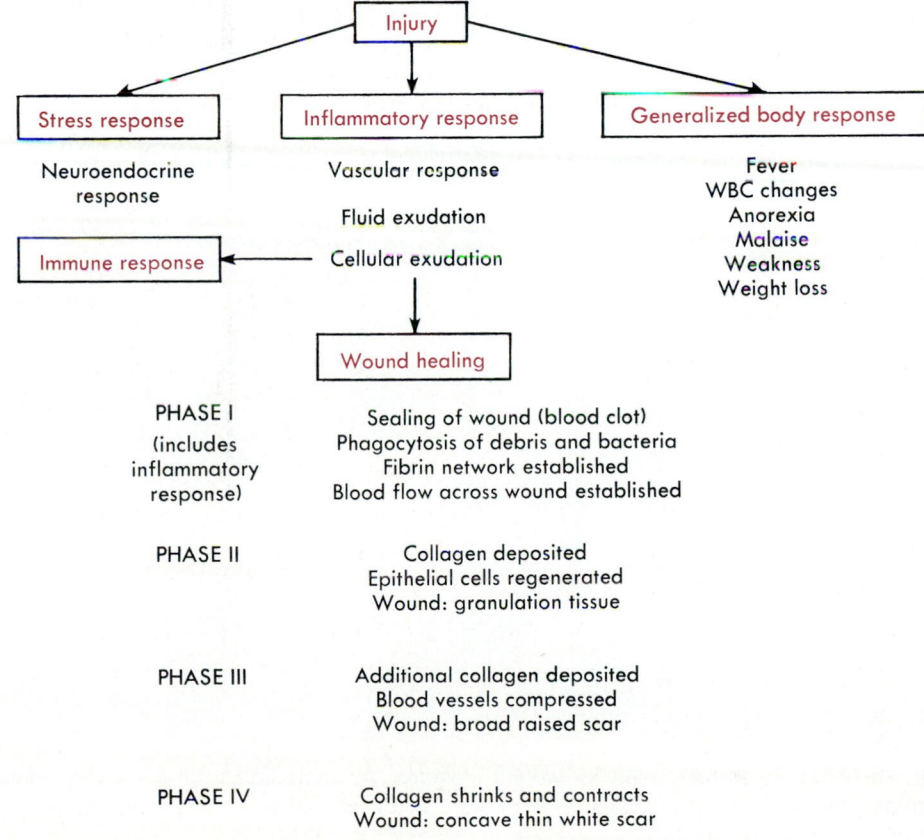

Fig. 18-10 Response of body to injury.

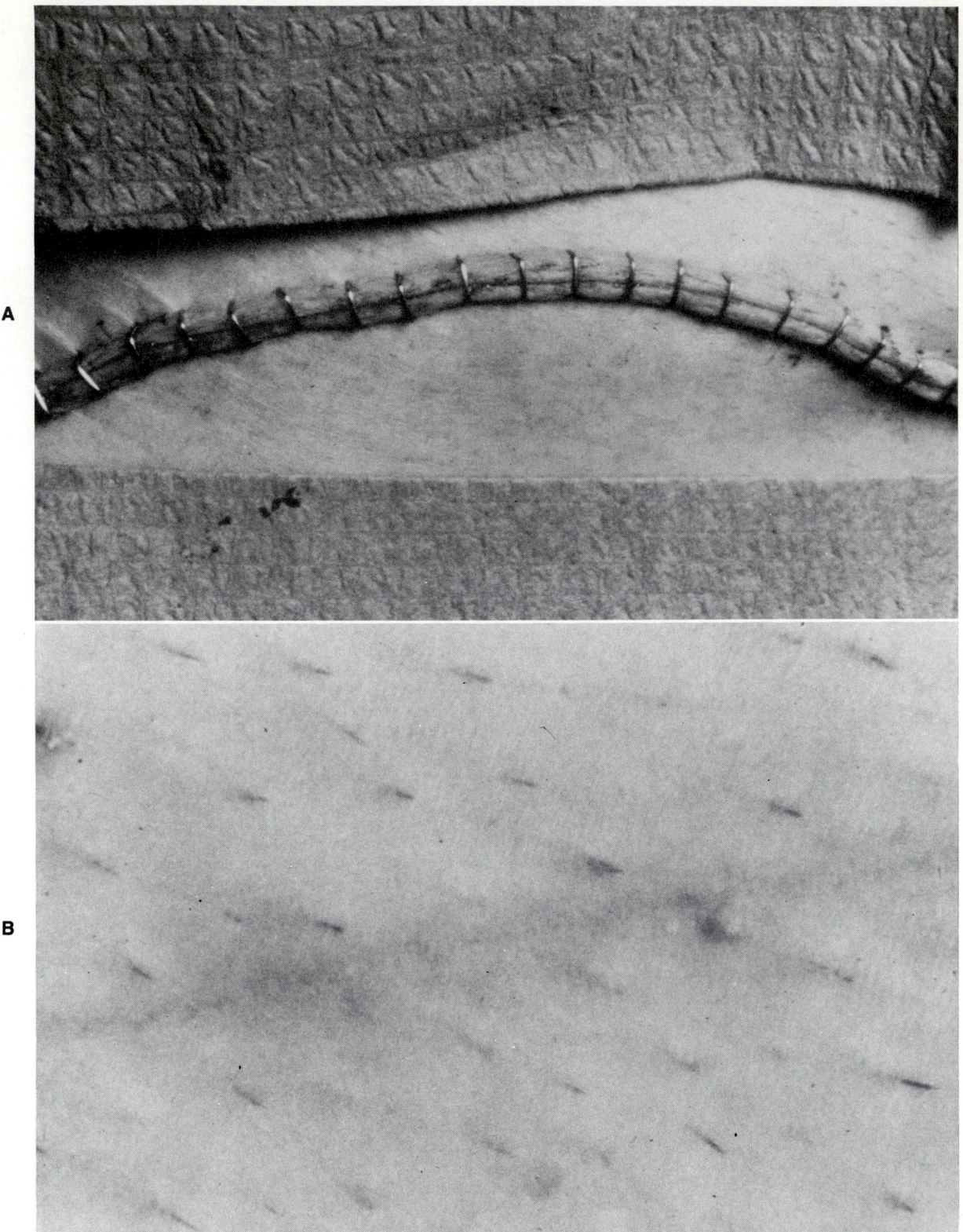

Fig. 18-11   Skin staples used for wound closures. **A,** Immediately after surgery. Note staples grasping only superficial layer of skin. **B,** Same site 6 months later. (Courtesy Ethicon, Inc, Somerville, NJ)

formed. When tissue is injured, two major responses occur: the stress response (Chapter 7) and the inflammatory response (Chapter 37). The inflammatory response serves to prepare the tissue so that wound healing can take place (Fig. 18-10).

In *phase I* of wound healing, leukocytes (white blood cells) ingest bacteria and debris. Fibrin is deposited throughout the clot that fills the wound, and new blood vessels develop across the wound using the fibrin threads as a framework. A thin layer of epithelial cells migrate across the wound and help to seal the wound. The wound strength is low but sutured wounds will hold together if sutured correctly. After major surgery the patient looks and feels ill during this first phase, which lasts 3 days.

Phase II lasts from 3 to 14 days after surgery. The leukocytes start disappearing and the space begins to fill with *collagen*, a white protein fiber. All layers of epithelial cells are completely regenerated in about 1 week. The new tissue is a highly vascular connective tissue, reddish from the numerous blood vessels, and is called *granulation tissue*. If scraped, this tissue will bleed readily. The patient begins to look and feel better.

The collagen that is deposited will provide good support for the wound in 6 to 7 days. Thus sutures are often removed about this time, depending on the site and extent of surgery. Skin sutures that are commonly used include black silk, fine wire, metal skin clips, and metal staples (Fig. 18-11).

During *phase III*, collagen continues to be deposited. This compresses the new blood vessels, and blood flow decreases. The wound now looks like a broad pinkish raised scar. During this phase, which lasts from about the second to the sixth week after surgery, the patient should avoid heavy use of the affected muscles.

The final phase, *phase IV*, lasts for several months after surgery. The patient may complain of itching around the wound. Although collagen continues to be deposited during this time, the wound shrinks and contracts. If the wound is near a joint, contractures may occur. Because of the shrinkage the wound becomes a concave thin white line. Scar tissue is acellular, avascular collagen tissue. It will not tan with sunlight nor sweat nor produce hair.

■ INTERVENTIONS TO PROMOTE HEALING

1. Promote intake of foods high in protein and vitamin C. Protein is needed for the formation of collagen. Vitamin C also facilitates collagen formation and helps maintain the integrity of the capillary walls.
2. Carry out measures to increase circulation (p. 387). Healing requires that the necessary cells to fight infection and nutrients be brought to the wound and that the debris and dead cells be removed.
3. Avoid antiinflammatory drugs (such as steroids) when healing is desired; inflammation is a desired part of the healing process.
4. Prevent infection that delays healing:
   a. Change soiled wet dressings immediately.

   b. Use strict aseptic technique when changing dressings.
   c. Cover moist dressings with a dry sterile cover.
5. Irrigate contaminated wounds well to remove foreign substances that create an excessive inflammatory reaction and infection, which delay healing.
6. Maintain suction of wound catheters. Fluid remaining in a wound space delays healing.

■ CARE OF THE SURGICAL WOUND

Surgical wounds, because they are aseptically created, generally heal well and quickly. For psychologic reasons and to prevent trauma until epithelialization occurs, the wound is usually covered initially by a dressing.

Incisional coverings may be gauze, semiocclusive, or occlusive dressings. Gauze dressings permit air to reach the wound; semiocclusive dressings permit oxygen but not air to pass; occlusive dressings permit neither air nor oxygen to pass. Occlusive and semiocclusive dressings are thought to promote healing by keeping wounds moist (yet sterile) so epithelial cells can slide more easily over the surface of the wound during epithelialization.[33]

A gauze dressing is usually required when drainage is present that may contact and macerate the skin. If an open drainage system is present, the open end of the drain should be encased in an absorbable dressing to protect the skin; this dressing is changed frequently. Fewer open drainage systems are being used, however, in preference for closed drainage systems.

■ WOUND DEHISCENCE AND EVISCERATION

□ Pathophysiology

Wound *dehiscence* (disruption) is partial to complete separation of the wound edges. Wound *evisceration* is protrusion of abdominal viscera through the incision and onto the abdominal wall (Fig. 18-12).

Wound dehiscence is rare in persons under 30 but occurs in 5% of persons over age 60 who are having laparotomy. It occurs in 1% of all persons having abdominal surgery.[48] Thoracic wounds are less apt to dehisce than abdominal wounds.

Wound separation that occurs during the first 3 postoperative days (phase I of wound healing) are usually a result of inadequate surgical closure. During the next 10 days, wound separation is usually associated with postoperative complications, such as excessive coughing or vomiting, distention, dehydration, or infection. Many of these complications can be prevented by careful assessment and continued monitoring and by the institution of vigorous preventive measures (ventilatory exercises, ambulation, adequate fluid intake, aseptic technique) on the part of the nurse. Wound separation during phase III (after 2 weeks) is usually associated with metabolic factors such as cachexia, hypoproteinemia or avitaminosis, increased age, decreased resistance to infection, malignancy, multiple trauma, or hypothermia. These factors can also cause wound separation at an earlier time.

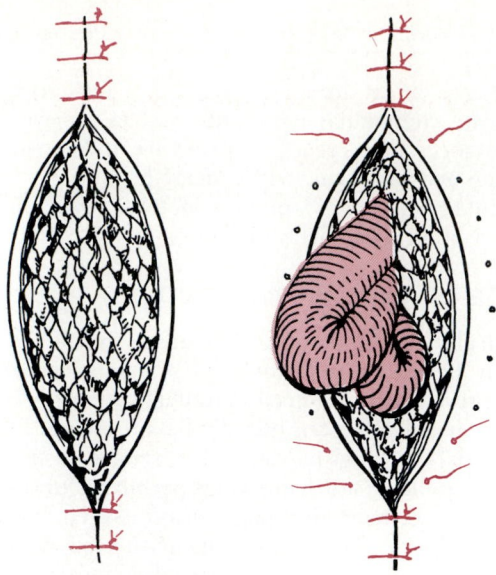

Fig. 18-12 **A,** Wound dehiscence. **B,** Wound evisceration.

□ **Assessment**

The patient may complain of a "giving" sensation at the incision or a feeling of wetness. If evisceration has occurred and a loop of bowel is obstructed, the patient will complain of severe pain at the incision. On inspection the dressing will be found to be saturated with clear pink drainage. The wound edges may be partially or entirely separated, and loops of intestine may be lying on the abdominal wall. Signs of shock may be present.

□ **Intervention**

1. Notify physician.
2. Put patient in bed in low Fowler's position to ease strain on the incision.
3. Tell patient to lie quietly and not cough, eat, or drink until seen by the physician.
4. Cover protruding viscera with a dressing moistened with warm sterile saline solution to prevent tissue dryness and necrosis.
5. Remain with the patient until the physician arrives if evisceration is present; monitor vital signs for shock.

The treatment for wound dehiscence or evisceration is immediate closure of the wound under local or general anesthesia. If the patient is in shock, the preanesthetic medication may be omitted. Convalescence is usually prolonged, although the wound usually heals surprisingly well after secondary closure.

■ Maintaining adequate respiration

■ PATHOPHYSIOLOGY

Postoperative patients are at high risk for developing pulmonary complications (Table 18-5). The pulmonary complications are often preventable by nursing manage-

ment. The most common respiratory complications are atelectasis and hypostatic pneumonia.

In *atelectasis* a bronchiole becomes blocked by secretions and the distal alveoli collapse as the existing air is absorbed, producing hypoventilation (Fig. 18-13). A major bronchus or many small bronchioles may be involved. The latter situation is frequently undetected because there are few symptoms. The extent of atelectasis is determined by the site of the blockage; if the main stem bronchus to one lung is blocked, that *lung* will be atelectatic. If a bronchus to a lobe is blocked, that *lobe* will be atelectatic.

Hypostatic pneumonia is inflammation of the lung from stasis of secretions. Both atelectasis and hypostatic pneumonia decrease oxygenation, prolong recovery, and add to the patient's discomfort.

■ ASSESSMENT

The patient is assessed frequently during the first 24 to 48 hours after an inhalant anesthetic, depending on the number of risk factors present. A person at high risk may need to be assessed as often as every hour. Assessment includes monitoring respirations and chest expansion, auscultating the lungs, evaluating the productiveness of the cough, and observing for signs of atelectasis and pneumonia (see the box on p. 385).

■ INTERVENTION

After general anesthesia most patients will need to ventilate their lungs well *at least* every 1 to 2 hours during the first postoperative day, and then every 3 to 4 hours while awake for several days if not active. The decision for the type and frequency of preventive respiratory measures is based on each patient's risk factors and hour-by-hour and day-by-day response. Measures effective in increasing ventilation in one patient may be less effective in another patient.

□ **Ventilatory measures**

A number of ventilatory measures (Table 18-6) can be used in the postoperative period to prevent atelectasis by inflating the alveoli as fully as possible. Once the alveoli are fully inflated, they will remain open for at least 1 hour. The two most effective ventilatory maneuvers that lead to maximum alveolar inflation are the yawn and the incentive spirometer (Fig. 18-14). Guidelines for using ventilatory measures are described in Table 18-7.

□ **Positioning and turning**

If the patient lies in one position with continuous pressure from body weight against the chest wall, proper ventilation and drainage of secretions on that side of the chest are not possible and atelectasis can develop (Fig. 18-15). Turning and changing of position frequently (at least every 2 to 3 hours) provide for better ventilation of the lungs. The patient should be encouraged to help in the turning. Alternating the height of the bed is useful: high Fowler's position facilitates diaphragm movement; low Fowler's or

Table 18-5   Risk factors in development of postoperative pulmonary complications

Risk factors	Effect
Increased respiratory secretions	
Smoking	Irritation of lining of tracheobronchial passages
Intubation	Decreased ciliary action to remove secretions
Inhalant anesthetics	Secretions will block bronchial passages or alveoli
Chronic lung disease	
Upper respiratory infection	
Dry sticky secretions	
Chronic lung disease	Difficult to cough up secretions
Dehydration	Secretions will block bronchial passages
Decreased thorax expansion	
Pain (chest, upper abdomen)	Lung does not expand fully, resulting in hypoventilation
Obesity	of alveoli
Age	
Tight binders or casts	
Skeletal abnormalities (for example, scoliosis)	
Decreased diaphragm mobility	
Abdominal distention	Decreased lung expansion, leading to hypoventilation
Surgery of chest or upper abdomen	
Muscle relaxants	
Neurologic deficit	
Depression of respiratory center	
Sedatives	Depressed respirations result in hypoventilation
Narcotics	
Acid-base imbalance	
Aspiration of gastric contents	
Vomiting	Causes aspiration pneumonia

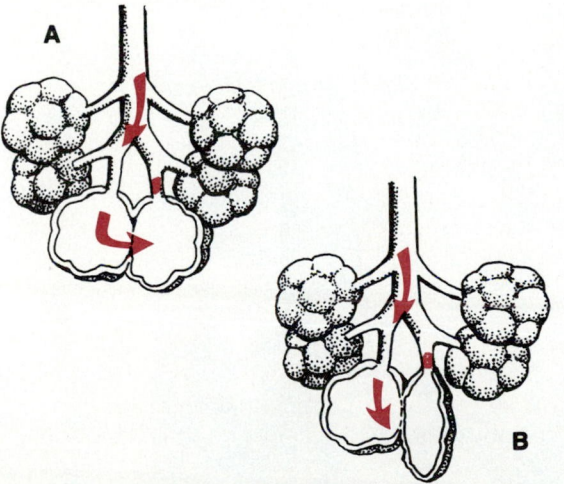

Fig. 18-13   Mucous plug blocking alveolar duct in obstructive atelectasis. **A,** Aeration of blocked alveolus through interalveolar duct with deep inspiration. **B,** Collapse of blocked alveolus with shallow inspiration.

Signs of postoperative pulmonary dysfunction

Hypoventilation	Rapid shallow respirations
	Absent or diminished breath sounds in lower lobes
	Decreased chest expansion
Increased secretions in airways	Rales heard on auscultation
	Nonproductive cough
Atelectasis	Signs may be absent
	Fever, increased pulse and respirations; dyspnea, cyanosis, and shock if a large bronchus is blocked
Hypostatic pneumonia	Fever, dyspnea, chest pain, cough productive of mucopurulent sputum

Table 18-6 Common postoperative ventilatory maneuvers

Manuever	Method	Comments
Yawn	Inhale deeply with mouth open (yawn), hold breath for 3 seconds, exhale	Easy to do; good deep breath when yawn occurs
Incentive spirometer	Breathe in through mouthpiece as deeply as possible, hold breath 3 seconds, exhale; work toward increasing inspiratory effort	Promotes sustained maximal inspiration; requires minimal instruction; avoid using at mealtimes (may cause nausea)
Deep breathing	Inhale deeply through nose using diaphragm (abdomen rises), exhale slowly through pursed lips	Effectiveness depends on depth of respirations; patients with chest or abdominal incisions tend to limit depth; patients need encouragement

Table 18-7 Guidelines for using ventilatory measures in postoperative patients

Nursing interventions	Rationale
Schedule ventilatory measures 30 minutes after narcotic is given, if possible	Facilitates patient cooperation
Place patient in high Fowler's position, if permitted	Facilitates diaphragm and chest expansion
Auscultate lungs	Baseline assessment
Suggest patient take three to five normal breaths between each deep inspiration	Prevents dizziness from hyperventilation
After patient takes three to five deep breaths, ask patient to cough *deeply*	Removes loosened secretions; shallow cough is ineffective and causes fatigue
Splint chest or abdominal incision with towel, small pillow, or hand before cough, if necessary	Prevents additional pain and muscle strain; provides support to incision to encourage deep cough
Auscultate lung	Comparison with baseline for evaluation of effectiveness

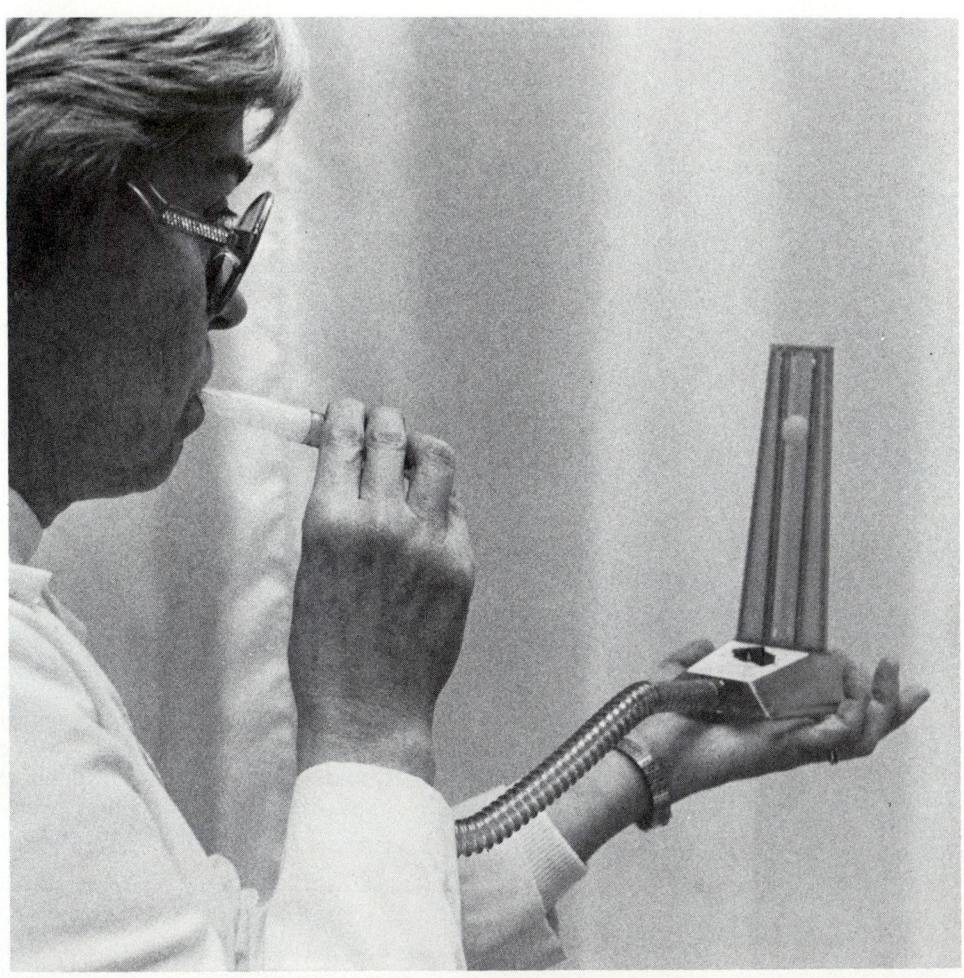

Fig. 18-14 Incentive spirometer. Ball rising with inspiration is a visual cue for patient. Ball remains up as patient holds breath for 3 seconds.

a flat position facilitates drainage and expectoration of respiratory secretions.

■ Maintaining circulation

■ PATHOPHYSIOLOGY

Thrombophlebitis, which results from venous stasis, is a preventable postoperative complication in many situations. Platelets adhere to the venous wall, especially at bifurcation of vessels, with resultant thrombus formation (Fig. 18-16). Venous stasis occurs postoperatively for a number of reasons (see the box at right).

■ ASSESSMENT

If a patient complains of any discomfort in a leg, examine the leg (with gentle palpation) for redness and tenderness along the course of a vein if a superficial vein is involved or for tenderness and edema if a deep vein is involved.

There is usually pain on dorsiflexion of the foot (Homan's sign) and fever.

■ PREVENTION

1. Use elastic stockings, both in and out of bed, on patients at high risk to promote venous return by counter-pressure on leg muscles.
2. Teach patient to avoid sitting for long periods (pressure on popliteal area) and to elevate feet on a stool when sitting to promote venous return.

Risk factors for postoperative thrombophlebitis

Intrinsic factors	Older age, obesity, malnutrition, contraceptive use
Pathologic condition	Malignancy, congestive heart failure, history of previous deep-vein thrombosis, polycythemia
Types of surgery	Pelvic, abdominal, thoracic; fracture of hip or lower extremity
Effects of surgery	Anesthesia, shock, decreased mobility
	Prolonged sitting with legs crossed
	Pressure on popliteal area
	Tight dressings or cast on lower extremities

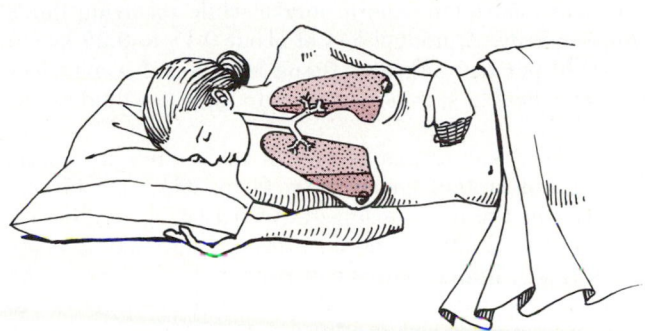

Fig. 18-15 Schematic of lungs illustrating pooling of secretions in dependent alveoli.

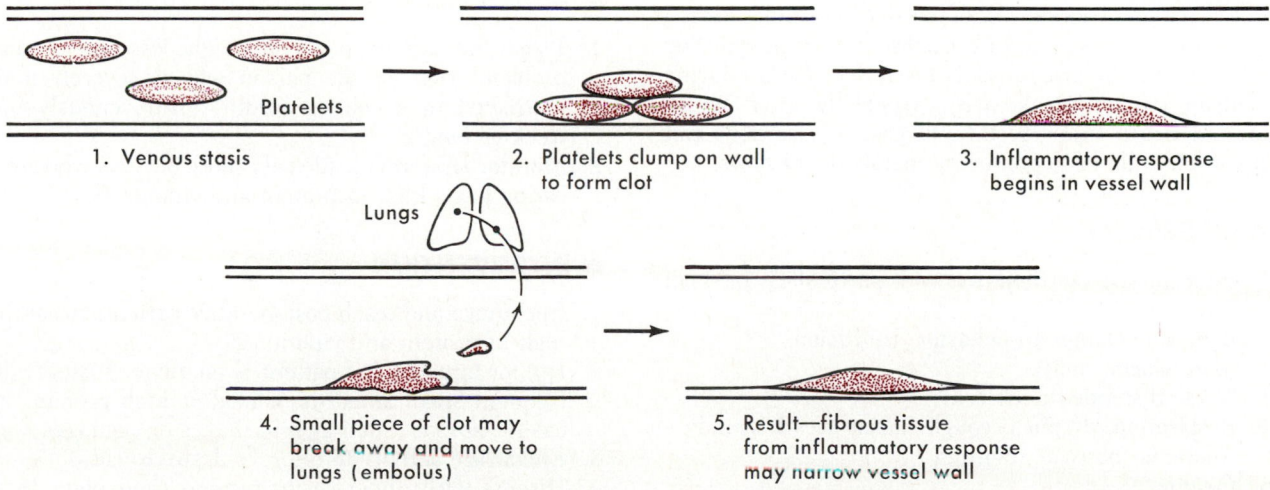

Platelets

1. Venous stasis

2. Platelets clump on wall to form clot

3. Inflammatory response begins in vessel wall

Lungs

4. Small piece of clot may break away and move to lungs (embolus)

5. Result—fibrous tissue from inflammatory response may narrow vessel wall

Fig. 18-16 Diagram illustrating formation of thrombus on wall of vein following venous stasis resulting in narrowing of blood vessel.

3. Avoid any pressure on popliteal area (for example, pillow under knee) that can impede venous return.
4. Avoid leg massage postoperatively; massage may loosen a newly formed clot, causing an embolus.
5. Teach and encourage leg exercises (Chapter 16) for the inactive patient.
6. Encourage early ambulation.

■ INTERVENTION

The care of the patient with thrombophlebitis is discussed in Chapter 26. At the first sign of possible thrombophlebitis, ask the patient to return to bed and notify the physician. Rest, heat, elastic bandages, and anticoagulant therapy are usually prescribed. Monitor the patient for signs of pulmonary embolus (chest pain, dyspnea).

■ Maintaining fluid and electrolyte balance

■ PATHOPHYSIOLOGY

Fluid is lost during surgery through blood loss and increased insensible fluid loss through the lungs and skin. During the surgical procedure the blood loss is estimated and fluids are replaced intravenously.

For at least the first 24 to 48 hours after surgery, fluids are retained by the body because of the stimulation of antidiuretic hormone (ADH), as part of the stress response to trauma and the effect of anesthesia. During surgery there is also renal vasoconstriction and increased aldosterone activity, leading to increased sodium retention and subsequent water retention. *Overhydration* can occur with vigorous fluid replacement, especially in very small or elderly persons. Both water intoxication and pulmonary edema can occur, depending on the type and amount of fluids given. (For further information on fluid overload, see Chapter 8).

Sodium and potassium depletion can occur in the postoperative patient from the loss of blood or body fluids during surgery or the loss of gastrointestinal secretions by vomiting and through nasogastric tubes. Potassium is also lost during catabolism (tissue breakdown), especially after severe trauma or crush injuries. Loss of gastric secretions can result in chloride loss, producing metabolic alkalosis.

■ ASSESSMENT

Monitor for signs of fluid overload, particularly in small or elderly persons:
1. Behavior: change in behavior, confusion
2. Skin: warm, moist
3. Neck: distended neck veins
4. Respiration: dyspnea, cough, moist breath sounds
5. Anorexia, nausea, vomiting
6. Fatigue
7. Weight gain (weigh high-risk patients)

■ INTERVENTION

Intravenous administration of fluids is monitored carefully so that fluids are given evenly over the entire 24 hours. (For further information on intravenous fluids, see Chapter 8.) If signs of fluid overload appear, slow the intravenous fluid to a keep-open rate and notify physician.

Fluids are started orally as soon as peristalsis is present. Sips of water are offered first to see if fluids can be tolerated. Some persons better tolerate sucking on ice chips. Ice chips must be recorded as fluid intake (two parts ice equal one part water). As soon as the patient can tolerate drinking fluids, the physician discontinues the intravenous fluid administrations.

■ Maintaining adequate nutrition

■ PATHOPHYSIOLOGY

Convalescence after surgery can be shortened if protein deficiency does not develop. The best way to supply essential foods is orally. Weight loss usually occurs after surgery as a result of catabolism, nutrients used for healing, and inadequate caloric intake while receiving fluids intravenously. A gradual loss of about 0.15 to 0.25 kg (⅓ to ½ lb) per day indicates tissue loss. Rapid weight loss indicates *fluid* loss: rapid weight gain indicates fluid retention.

Two food substances of special importance in wound healing are protein and vitamin C (p. 383). During catabolism in the early postoperative period, a negative nitrogen balance occurs; more nitrogen is lost than is taken in. Nitrogen is an essential constituent of amino acids, the building blocks of proteins. Protein intake is necessary to restore nitrogen balance and to provide the necesary amino acids for anabolism. Vitamin C is stored only in small amounts in the tissues, so must be supplied daily from an external source.

■ ASSESSMENT

1. *Weigh* the patient in whom weight loss may present a problem, that is, the person who is severely undernourished or receiving feedings intravenously for 1 week or longer.
2. Monitor *meal trays* to identify those persons who are not eating foods high in protein and vitamin C.

■ INTERVENTION

1. Encourage and teach postoperative patients to eat foods high in protein and vitamin C.
2. Do not force food if patient is anorexic. Instead, offer frequent small amounts of food or high protein, high calorie liquids (such as milkshakes or eggnogs).
3. Encourage activity to improve desire to eat.
4. Discuss with underweight persons their plans for obtaining the desired nutrients after discharge.

■ Maintaining elimination

■ URINE ELIMINATION

□ Pathophysiology

A patient who is well hydrated usually voids within 6 to 8 hours after surgery. Although 2000 to 3000 ml solution usually is given intravenously on the day of surgery, the first voiding may be 200 ml or less, and the total urinary output for the day may be less than 1500 ml. The small amount of urinary output results from the loss of body fluid during surgery, increased insensible fluid loss, vomiting, and increased secretion of antidiuretic hormone. As body functions stabilize, fluid and electrolyte balance returns to normal in about 48 hours.

Urinary retention, or the inability to void, may occur in the early postoperative period for several reasons (see the box below). *Urinary tract infections* may occur in patients who must have prolonged bed rest after surgery, have a history of urinary tract infections, have had pelvic surgery, or have indwelling catheters.

□ Assessment

1. Monitor urinary output until output equals fluid intake.
2. If patient does not void sufficiently, especially within 6 to 8 hours after surgery, assess for urinary retention (suprapubic distention, sensation of full bladder, suprapubic discomfort).
3. If patient complains of frequency of urination with burning, check body temperature, send a clean voided urine specimen to laboratory for culture and sensitivity (if protocols permit), and notify physician.

□ Intervention

If urinary retention is present, carry out measures to facilitate voiding (Chapter 32). Catheterization may be delayed longer than the usual 8 hours postoperatively in the hope that the patient will void normally. Bethanechol chloride (Urecholine) may be ordered by the physician for acute postoperative urine retention; it may be given orally or subcutaneously but not by intramuscular injection because this may induce circulatory collapse.

If the bladder must be catheterized repeatedly after surgery, an indwelling catheter may be inserted. Fluids are then encouraged up to 3000 ml, unless contraindicated, to prevent urinary stasis.

■ BOWEL ELIMINATION

□ Pathophysiology

Peristalsis will be decreased for at least 24 hours after abdominal or pelvic surgery and for several days after surgery of the gastrointestinal tract. No bowel movement can occur when peristalsis is absent or significantly decreased. *Constipation* occurs frequently after major surgery for several reasons (see the box below). A bowel movement may be intentionally delayed after burns of the buttocks or extensive rectal surgery (by administration of paregoric orally) to prevent additional trauma.

□ Assessment

1. Monitor daily for bowel movement. If absent, ask if patient is passing flatus.
2. After abdominal surgery, record signs of returning peristalsis (bowel sounds, passing flatus).
3. Examine stool for amount and consistency; small dry, hard stool indicates constipation.
4. Assess for potential constipation:
   a. Narcotics given frequently or in high doses
   b. Inactivity
   c. Fluid intake less than 1200 ml/day
   d. Previous history of constipation

□ Intervention

1. Institute measures to *prevent* constipation for the first 2 or 3 days after major surgery:
   a. Facilitate fluid intake of 2000 to 3000 ml/day
   b. Encourage maximal activity within prescribed limits
   c. Provide bathroom privileges as early as possible
2. If no bowel movement within 3 or 4 days after surgery:
   a. Give prune juice, if permissible and desirable
   b. Consult physician about a laxative order. A hypertonic (Fleet) enema or small soapsuds enema may be necessary if laxative is ineffective
   c. Encourage intake of foods high in fiber, if permissible

---

Causes of postoperative urinary retention

Recumbent position
Nervous tension
Anesthetic; decreased bladder sensation and ability to void
Narcotic: decreased bladder sensation
Pelvic surgery: interference with innervation of bladder muscles, local edema

---

Causes of postoperative constipation

Neuroendocrine response to stress (decreased gastrointestinal motility)
Anesthetic agents
Narcotics
Inactivity
Decreased intake of high-fiber foods

Causes of postoperative vomiting

Anesthetic agent
Narcotic
Abdominal distention (fluid, gas)
Pain
Electrolyte imbalances
Drug idiosyncrasies

■ Promoting comfort

The major discomforts after surgery are nausea and vomiting, abdominal distention and gas pains, and incisional pain.

■ NAUSEA AND VOMITING

Nausea and vomiting, which occur less frequently with the newer anesthetic agents, may be related to a number of factors (see the box above). Persistent postoperative vomiting is usually a symptom of pyloric obstruction, intestinal obstruction, or peritonitis. Vomiting tires the patient, puts strain on the incision, and causes excessive loss of fluids and electrolytes. Choking while vomiting may lead to aspiration pneumonia.

Interventions for the person who is experiencing nausea and vomiting include the following:

1. Side-lying position to prevent aspiration
2. No food or fluids until vomiting subsides
3. Sips of fluid (ice chips, ginger ale, hot tea) or dry solid food (crackers) after vomiting subsides
4. Frequent oral care
5. Prescribed antiemetics given parenterally

■ ABDOMINAL DISTENTION AND GAS PAINS

□ Pathophysiology

Postoperative *distention* results from accumulation of nonabsorbable gas in the intestines caused by a reaction to the handling of the bowel during surgery, by swallowing of air during recovery from anesthesia or attempts to overcome nausea, and by passing of gases from the bloodstream to the atonic portion of the bowel. Distention will persist until the tone of the bowel returns to normal and peristalsis resumes. It is experienced to some degree by most patients after abdominal and renal surgery.

Gas pains are caused by contractions of the unaffected portions of the bowel in an attempt to move the accumulated gas through the intestinal tract.

□ Assessment

If the patient complains of diffuse or cramping abdominal pain, monitor the following:

1. Measurement of abdominal girth with tape measure to determine degree of distention
2. Percussion of distended abdomen for drumlike (tympanic) sounds
3. Presence of signs of shock from acute gastric dilation

□ Intervention

If the stomach is distended, the fluid and gas can be aspirated with a nasogastric tube. General distention or gas pains from sluggish intestinal peristalsis can be relieved by passage of flatus.

There are a number of interventions that may be helpful in moving the gas along the colon and facilitating passage:

1. Ambulation: most effective method to stimulate peristalsis and get the gas moving so it can be expelled
2. Avoidance of very hot or cold liquids that tend to cause gas buildup: sucking ice chips does not have the same effect because the water warms before it reaches the stomach[34]
3. Exercise to stimulate movement of the gas from right to left and prevent buildup[34]:
   a. Lie on back with legs extended and a pillow under knees.
   b. Bend right knee, moving it toward abdomen.
   c. Put hands on knee and pull down toward abdomen.
   d. Hold position for count of 10.
   e. Lower leg slowly.
   f. Take 2 to 3 slow deep breaths.
   g. Repeat action with left leg.
   h. Repeat steps *a* through *g* 3 to 4 times.
4. Pelvic rock to stimulate peristalsis[19]:
   a. Lie on back.
   b. Exhale slowly while contracting abdominal muscles, simultaneously pressing small of back to bed.
   c. Relax and then repeat actions several times.
5. Abdominal massage to help push gas along colon[34]:
   a. Make a fist with both hands.
   b. Place one fist on lower right abdomen, rolling knuckles upward.
   c. Keeping first fist in place, put second fist above it and roll upward.
   d. Work hand over hand up to lower edge of ribs, across abdomen, then down left side (following course of the colon).
6. Rectal tube for 20 minutes every 4 hours as necessary: tube stimulates lower colonic peristalsis and permits easy passage of the gas past the anal sphincters
7. Heat to the abdomen (heating pad or hot water bottle): heat expands the gas, stimulating peristalsis; this method most effective combined with a rectal tube
8. Prescribed enema to stimulate peristalsis

■ PAIN

□ Pathophysiology

Pain is common after nearly all types of surgical procedures in which there has been cutting, pulling, or manipulation of tissues and organs. It may result from stimulation of nerve endings by chemical substances released at the time of surgery or from tissue ischemia caused by interference of blood supply to the part, such as by pressure, muscle spasm, or edema. After surgery other factors can add to the sensation of pain, such as infections, distention, muscle spasms surrounding the incisional area, and tight dressings or casts (see the box above).

Postoperative pain usually lasts 24 to 48 hours but may continue longer depending on the extent of the surgery, the pain threshold of the patient, and response to pain (Chapter 10). The presence of pain can prolong convalescence because it may interfere with return to activity.

☐ Assessment

When the patient complains of pain in the postoperative period, do not assume that the pain is incisional. It is important to try to ascertain the possible cause of the pain. Subjective data include origin, area involved, nature of the pain, and possible cause from the patient's point of view. Objective data include observation of facial expressions, body position, activity, muscle rigidity, and pulse rate. If the patient is having severe pain, the assessment should be made gently and quickly but thoroughly.

☐ Intervention

It is often impossible to prevent postoperative pain, but it can be minimized so that the patient is relatively comfortable. Patients with adequate preoperative instructions and confidence in the surgeon, the nurse, and the outcome of the surgery usually have less postoperative pain than apprehensive patients because they have less tension. Measures to reduce anxiety and apprehension will also help reduce pain. Relief of pain may encourage the patient to move and breathe more deeply, thus preventing postoperative complications, which cause more pain.

If the cause of pain is determined to be other than incisional, measures are taken to relieve the cause. Emptying a full bladder can relieve what was thought to be pain from a lower abdominal incision. Elevation of a part may relieve venous stasis. Loosening of a tight bandage, if permissible, will relieve ischemic pain.

Incisional pain can be relieved by nursing measures and by analgesics.

1. Encourage patient to move in bed or to ambulate, to decrease pain from muscle tension and increase circulation to the part.
2. Move the injured part as a whole; for example, move trunk as one unit.
3. Support an injured limb during a move (a pillow is a useful support).
4. Teach patient to use siderails in moving to decrease incisional pull.
5. Teach relaxation and distraction techniques, if suitable (Chapter 7).
6. Give medications according to the guidelines for acute pain (Chapter 10).
   a. Narcotics are usually required on a regular basis for 12 to 48 hours after major surgery.
   b. Patients receiving meperidine (Demerol) are monitored for signs of orthostatic hypotension (dizziness, fainting, rapid pulse) during ambulation.
   c. Nonnarcotics may provide relief after 48 to 72 hours following major surgery.

Transcutaneous electrical nerve stimulation (TENS) is an additional method for postoperative pain relief (see Chapter 10). The conductive tape electrodes are usually applied to the skin on either side of the incision. The electrodes are then connected by a pair of cables to a battery-powered portable pulse generator about the size of a pocket paging device. The stimulation is patient-controlled.

For relief of postoperative pain, a *high-frequency* (80 to 100 Hz) *low-intensity* (12 to 20 mamp) impulse appears to be the most effective.[44] The intensity is determined preoperatively on a trial-and-error basis by the patient who locates a point just below the threshold of discomfort. A tingling sensation may be experienced. The patient can vary the intensity according to the pain level. The best results are obtained when the TENS is used at periodic intervals, such as for a 60-minute period, rather than continuously. It may be helpful to provide stimulation for about 30 minutes before painful activities, such as coughing exercises or ambulation.

TENS is not for all patients. Effectiveness appears greater for relief of muscle or bone pain, and less for poorly localized visceral pain.[44] Patients using TENS require lower amounts of analgesic medications postoperatively.[43] TENS has been shown to decrease postoperative complications such as atelectasis by alleviating incisional pain.[2,44] It permits earlier ambulation and decreases the side effects of narcotics. TENS should not be used with demand cardiac pacemakers or during the first trimester of pregnancy.

■ Maintaining activity

■ PATHOPHYSIOLOGY

Early ambulation has been a significant factor in hastening postoperative recovery and preventing postoperative complications. Numerous benefits are derived from the

---

Effects of early postoperative ambulation

Increased rate and depth of breathing	Prevention of atelectasis and hypostatic pneumonia
	Increased mental alertness from increased oxygenation to brain
Increased circulation	Nutrients required for healing are more available to wound
	Prevention of thrombophlebitis
	Increased kidney function
	Decreased pain
Increased micturition	Prevention of urinary retention
Increased metabolism	Prevention of loss of muscle tone
	Restoration of nitrogen balance
Increased peristalsis	Promotion of expulsion of flatus
	Prevention of abdominal distention and gas pains
	Prevention of constipation
	Prevention of paralytic ileus

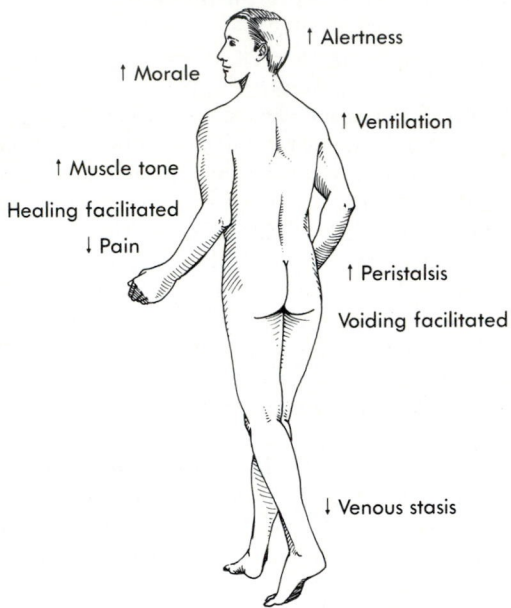

Fig. 18-17 Benefits from early postoperative ambulation.

exercise of getting in and out of bed and walking during the early postoperative period (see the box above and Fig. 18-17). Ambulation is usually contraindicated when there is a severe infection or thrombophlebitis.

■ ASSESSMENT

Before helping the patient to ambulate for the first few times after major surgery, an assessment is made of the patient's level of alertness to follow directions, cardiovascular status, and motor status:

1. Level of alertness: ask patient simple questions or to follow simple commands

2. Cardiovascular status
   a. Assess pulse and respiratory rate and depth while supine, then after sitting
   b. Observe skin color for pallor while sitting
   c. Note complaints of dizziness when sitting
3. Motor status
   a. Assess muscle strength of legs (Chapter 3)
   b. Assess sitting ability:
      (1) Assist patient to sitting position on side of bed
      (2) Ask patient to maintain an erect position while being gently pushed sideways.

It is also important to know of any limitations to ambulation present preoperatively. The patient with arthritis or arteriosclerosis may take longer to move and to adjust to standing and walking. The patient who used a walker preoperatively will need assistance for a longer time before progressing to using the walker again.

■ INTERVENTION

1. Encourage muscle strengthening exercises before ambulation:
   a. Bend knees, lower knees, press back of knees hard against bed.
   b. Alternately contract and relax calf and thigh muscles 10 times using the following cycle: contract, relax, rest.
2. Have patient sit on side of bed (legs dangling) to become accustomed to upright position before ambulating the first time. Be sure *pulse has stabilized* (returned to baseline) before ambulation is attempted:
   a. Clamp off nasogastric tube until patient has ambulated, then reconnect.
   b. Keep urinary tube connected to drainage bag; carry bag or pin bag to inside of robe.
   c. Attach intravenous bag to a movable pole.

4. Use two people to assist a weak patient receiving intravenous fluids to ambulate.
5. Encourage patient to walk farther at each ambulation.

The word *ambulate* means to move from place to place, to walk. Sitting in a chair is not considered ambulation. After ambulating, the patient may sit in a chair if permitted, but should be advised to stand and walk at intervals and to elevate the legs while sitting to prevent venous pooling in the extremities. Sitting in a chair for long periods is to be avoided.

■ Helping meet psychologic needs

■ PSYCHOLOGIC FACTORS

Some of the concerns that were present preoperatively may continue into the postoperative period. These concerns fall into essentially three categories: concerns specific to the surgery performed, concerns over loss of a body part, and concerns about the future. Future concerns include those related to changes in sexuality, economic status, prognosis, or permanent effects. Sexuality may be threatened by enforced absence from home or by a specific surgical procedure. Sexual concerns may center around the effect of the surgery on the spouse or parent relationship or on sexual performance itself.

■ ASSESSMENT

Anxieties will be expressed in many different ways. It must be remembered that expressions such as anger, resentfulness, crying, excessive joking, inappropriate laughter, or withdrawal may all be signs of anxiety and are often seen in the postoperative period. Some of these feelings may be projected against the surgeon, nurse, housekeeping aide, food, and such.

■ INTERVENTION

Sitting down and talking with surgical patients about their concerns is as important a nursing action in many instances as any of the physical activities. Time must be planned for this. If a specific concern is expected, such as sexual functioning after a perineal prostatectomy, the topic may have to be introduced by the nurse who has established rapport with the patient in order to let the patient know that it is permissible to talk about it.

■ Discharge planning

During hospitalization the patient and family should be prepared for any care that must be given at home, and any necessary arrangements for convalescent care should be completed several days before discharge. Patients are helped to become as self-sufficient as possible before being discharged so they do not have to depend any more than necessary on the assistance of relatives and friends.

If dressings are needed, the patient may be given a 48-hour supply to take home unless a family member has already obtained them. The patient and family must know where in the community they can get dressings and other needed materials. A community health nurse is a useful resource person when treatment of almost any kind is to be provided at home.

On discharge the patient is given an appointment for a follow-up examination in the surgeon's office or clinic. This appointment is usually for 1 to 2 weeks after discharge. The patient should understand the importance of returning for the medical examination (which is usually included in the surgeon's operating fee).

With modern surgical techniques the wound is usually healing well by the time of discharge from the hospital. Therefore, the convalescent period usually is relatively short, and most patients may return to their usual activities and occupation within 2 to 4 weeks. Normal activities should be resumed gradually. Driving is usually permitted 2 weeks after major surgery, but the patient should avoid any heavy lifting, pushing, or pulling for at least 6 weeks following surgery.

⊞ EVALUATION

Evaluation is based on the identified patient outcomes, which vary greatly, depending on the type of surgery performed and the patient response to surgery. Some questions to ask may include:

1. Have postoperative complications or injury been avoided?
2. Is the incision healing well?
3. Has weight been stabilized?
4. Have usual elimination patterns been reestablished?
5. Does the person state feeling comfortable?
6. Has the person had an opportunity to explore concerns related to surgery?
7. Does the person know the medication therapy, treatments, dietary restrictions, or activity prescription to be carried out at home and when to report for follow-up care?

■ SUMMARY

1. The most common problems encountered in the postanesthetic phase are airway obstruction, hypoventilation, hypotension, cardiac arrhythmias, and pain.
2. Measures to prevent postanesthesia pulmonary problems include side-lying position, artificial airway until patient begins to awaken, suctioning secretions that patient is unable to cough up, oxygen therapy, and initiation of breathing exercises.
3. The first postoperative dose of a narcotic is usually reduced about one-half the usual dose because of synergistic effects with anesthetics that may produce depression of the CNS and respiratory system.
4. Common causes of vital sign changes in the early postoperative period include shock, pain, anxiety, hypo-

---

Putting knowledge to practice

- Examine the charts of several postoperative patients. What types of preventive respiratory measures were used? What was the effect? How did the patients compare in their response to postoperative ambulation? Did some need more encouragement than others? Did any postoperative complications occur? If so, what risk factors were present? What changes in vital signs occurred during the early postoperative period as compared to the preoperative baseline? What were possible reasons for these changes?
- Arrange for an observational experience in a recovery room, if possible. What patient assessments were made by the nurse? Write down a list of activities carried out by the nurse: identify activities that were preventive in nature and describe the effect of these activities.
- Examine the operating room notes, recovery room notes, and surgeon's postoperative orders of a postoperative patient; discuss in clinical conference how the data are pertinent to planning the patient's care.
- Admit a patient who has just returned from the recovery room, performing an assessment and writing a care plan.

---

ventilation, jarring during transfer, distended urinary bladder, and drugs.

5. Regeneration of tissue or scarring depend on the types of injured cells (skin, mucous membrane, muscles, nerves) and intactness of the underlying structure.

6. Healing by primary or tertiary intention involve suturing of the incision, immediate or delayed; healing by secondary intention consists of filling the area in from the bottom.

7. Responses that occur following tissue injury include stress, inflammatory, immune, and generalized body responses followed by wound healing.

8. Phase I of wound healing includes the inflammatory response, reestablishment of blood flow across the wound, and initiation of epithelialization.

9. Phase II of wound healing consists mainly of filling in the spaces with collagen and completing epithelialization.

10. During the phases III and IV of wound healing, further collagen is deposited, compressing the new blood vessels, then shrinking and contracting.

11. Interventions to promote wound healing include intake of protein and vitamin C, avoidance of antiinflammatory drugs, and prevention of wound infection and of fluid buildup in wound spaces.

12. Wound dehiscence (separation of wound edges) and wound evisceration (protrusion of viscera through incision) may be prevented during phase II of wound healing by early institution of ventilatory exercises, ambulation, adequate fluid intake, and aseptic technique during dressing changes.

13. Persons at high risk for postoperative pulmonary complications are those with increased or dry respiratory secretions, decreased thorax expansion, decreased diaphragm mobility, depression of respiratory center by drugs, or aspirated gastric contents.

14. Measures to prevent postoperative thrombophlebitis include providing elastic stockings for persons at high risk, avoiding pressure on popliteal area or leg massage, and encouraging leg exercises and early ambulation.

15. Water intoxication or pulmonary edema are more likely to occur postoperatively in elderly persons receiving intravenous fluids.

16. The patient is monitored in the early postoperative period for urinary retention; measures are taken to encourage voiding.

17. Constipation may be prevented postoperatively by encouraging maximal fluids and ambulation, as permitted, and by providing bathroom privileges as early as possible.

18. Incisional pain can be relieved or modified by medication in combination with encouraging the person to move in bed and ambulate, teaching relaxation and distraction techniques, and supporting injured parts.

19. Gas pains may be relieved by ambulation, avoidance of very hot or cold liquids, specific exercises or massage, rectal tubes, heat to the abdomen, or enemas.

20. Early ambulation increases alertness, ventilation, muscle tone, and peristalsis; decreases pain and venous stasis; facilitates healing and voiding; and promotes increased morale.

REFERENCES AND SELECTED READINGS

1. *Aldrete, JA: Assessment of recovery from anesthesia, Curr Rev Recov Room Nurs 1:161-168, 1980.
2. Ali, J, Yaffe, CS, and Serrette, C: The effect of transcutaneous electric nerve stimulation on postoperative pain and pulmonary function, Surgery 89:507-512, 1981.
3. American College of Surgeons: Manual of pre- and postoperative care, ed 3, Philadelphia, 1983, WB Saunders Co.
4. *Blackwood, S: Back to basics: the preop exam, Am J Nurs 86:39-44, 1986.
5. *Bray, CA: Postoperative pain: altering the patient's experience through education, AORN J 43:672-683, 1986.

---

* References preceded by an asterisk are particularly well suited for student reading.

6. *Brozenec, S: Caring for the postoperative patient with an abdominal drain, Nurs 85 15(4):55-57, 1985.

7. *Burge, S, and others: How painful are postop incisions? Am J Nurs 86:1263-1265, 1986.

8. *Carroll, PF: Artificial airways: real risks, Nurs 86 16(8):56-59, 1986.

8a. Coleman, DL: Control of postoperative pain: nonnarcotic and narcotic alternatives and their effect on pulmonary functioning, Chest 92:520-528, 1987.

9. *Crocker, CG: Acute postoperative pain: cause and control, Orthop Nurs 5(2):11-15, 1986.

10. *Deters, GE: Managing complications after abdominal surgery, RN 50(3):27-32, 1987.

11. Drain, CB: Comparison of two inspiratory maneuvers on increasing lung volumes in postoperative upper abdominal surgical patients, AANA J 52:379-388, 1984.

11a. Drain, CB, and Christoph, SS: The recovery room: a critical care approach to postanesthesia nursing, ed 2, Philadelphia, 1987, WB Saunders Co.

12. Equipment: wound care, taking a drain check, Am J Nurs 84:1039-1040, 1984.

13. *Faherty, BS, and Grier, MR: Analgesic medication for elderly people post-surgery, Nurs Res 33:369-372, 1984.

14. Flynn, ME: Influencing repair and recovery, Am J Nurs 82:1550-1558, 1982.

15. *Flynn, ME, and Rovee, DT: Promoting wound healing, Am J Nurs 82:1543-1549, 1982.

16. *Fuchs, P: Before and after surgery, stay right on respiratory, Nurs 83 13(5):47-50, 1983.

17. *Greenwood, BS: The before and after of good postoperative pulmonary care, Nurs 82 12(12):68-69, 1982.

18. *Hughes, JM: Postoperative pulmonary care: past, present, future, Crit Care Q 6(2):67-71, 1983.

19. *Kearns, PC: Exercises to ease pain after abdominal surgery, RN 49(7):45-48, 1986.

20. *Keithley, JK: A unified approach to assessment of the surgical patient, Am J Nurs 82:612-614, 1982.

21. *Kleinbeck, SVM: Simplifying postoperative assessment, AORN J 38:344-345, 348, 1983.

24. Kneedler, J, and Dodge, G: Perioperative patient care, Boston, 1983, Blackwell Scientific Publications, Inc.

25. *Leeson, L: Pain and the postoperative patient, Nurs (Oxford) 2:1289-1290, 1985.

26. Marini, JJ: Postoperative atelectasis: pathophysiology, clinical importance, and principles of management, Resp Care 29:516-528, 1984.

27. *McConnell, EA: After surgery: how can you avoid the obvious and not so obvious hazards, Nurs 83 13(2):74-84, 1983.

28. *Miller, KM: Deep breathing relaxation: a pain management technique, AORN J 45:484-488, 1987.

29. *Montanari, J: Action STAT! Wound dehiscence, Nurs 86 16(2):33, 1986.

30. Mortenson, M, and McMullin, C: Discharge score for surgical outpatients, Am J Nurs 86:1347-1348, 1986.

31. *Neary, JM: Transcutaneous electrical nerve stimulation for the relief of post-incisional surgical pain, AANA J 49:151-155, 1981.

32. *Neuberger, GB, and Richling, JB: A new look at wound care, Nurs 85 15(2):34-41, 1985.

33. *Neuberger, GB: Wound care: what's clear, what's not, Nurs 87 17(2):34-37, 1987.

34. *Nichols, RR: Simple remedies for postoperative gas pain, RN 49(2):42-44, 1986.

35. *Pastras, AZ: The operation's over but the danger is not, Nurs 82 12(9):50-56, 1982.

36. *Postoperative complications: how to help the patient when everything goes wrong, Nurs 81 11(3):50-55, 1981.

37. *Predicting postoperative pulmonary problems, Am J Nurs 84:1357, 1984.

38. *Robusto, N: Advising patients on sex surgery, AORN J 32:55-61, 1980.

39. Schomburg, FL, and Carter-Baker, SA: Transcutaneous electrical nerve stimulation for post laparotomy pain, Phys Ther 63:181-193, 1983.

40. *Schumann, D: How to help wound healing in your abdominal surgery patient, Nurs 80 10(4):34-40, 1980.

41. *Shea, M, and McCreary, M: Early postoperative feeding, Am J Nurs 84:1230-1231, 1984.

41a. *Smith, CE: Detecting acute abdominal distention: what to look for, what to do. In The Nursing Institute's CE test handbook, vol 3, Hicksville, NY, 1988, Springhouse Book Co.

42. Stone, HH: Infection in postoperative patients, Am J Med 81(1A):39-44, 1986.

43. *Taylor, AG, and others: How effective is TENS for acute pain? Am J Nurs 83:1171-1174, 1983.

44. Tyler, ET, Caldwell, C, and Ghia, JN: Transcutaneous electrical nerve stimulation: an alternative approach to the management of postoperative pain, Anesth Analg 61:449-455, 1982.

45. Tyler, ML: The respiratory effects of body positioning and immobilization, Resp Care 29:477-480, 1984.

45a. *Wound management: update 88, Nurs 88 18(6):33-37, 1988.

46. Warfield, CA, and Stein, JA: Pain relief by electrical stimulation, Hosp Prac 18:207-218, 1983.

47. Warfield, CA, and Warfield, GR: Postoperative analgesia, Hosp Prac 19:85-92, 1983.

48. Way, LW: Current surgical diagnosis and treatment, ed 6, Los Altos, Calif, 1983, Lange Medical Publications.

49. *Weaver, TE: New life for lungs . . . through incentive spirometers, Nurs 81 11(2):54-58, 1981.

50. Willis, N: The effect of relaxation on postoperative muscle tension and pain, Nurs Res 31:236-238, 1982.

UNIT V
Sensorimotor Problems

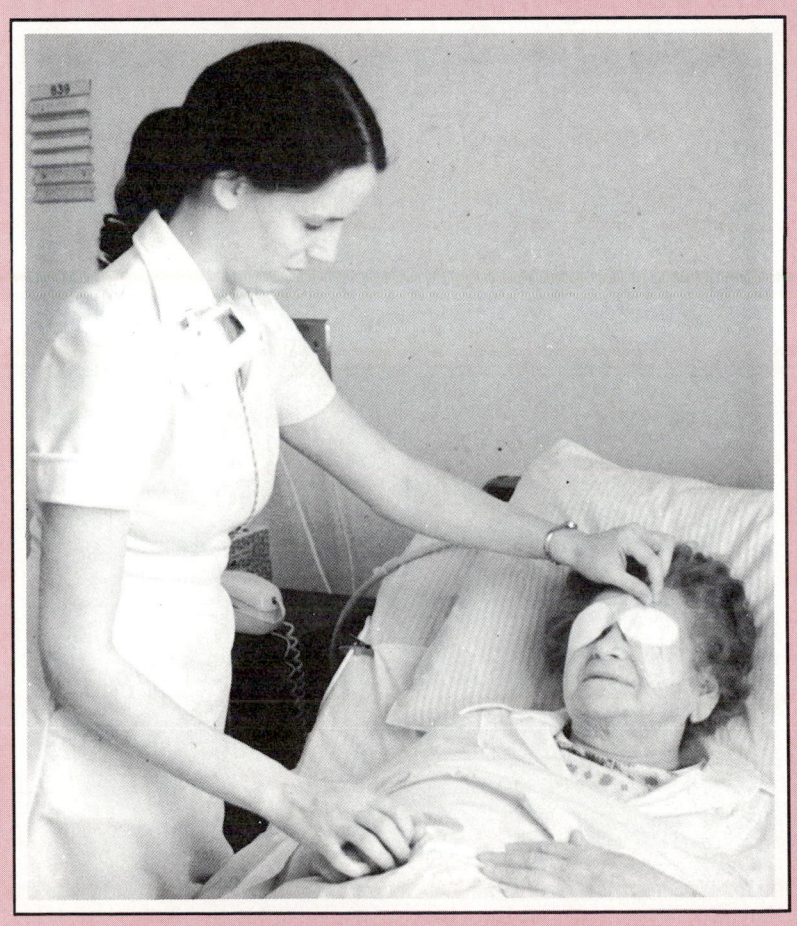

19

The Patient with Neurologic Problems

ELIZABETH SCHENK

CHAPTER OBJECTIVES

After studying this chapter, the student should be able to:

- Explain the difference in types of neurons and how they transmit impulses.
- List the divisions of the central nervous system, peripheral nervous system, and the autonomic nervous system.
- List four physiologic changes in the nervous system that occur with aging.
- Explain three components of the neurologic assessment.
- Explain the importance of primary, secondary, and tertiary prevention in problems of the nervous system.
- State five symptoms of increased intracranial pressure.
- List five nursing actions to decrease intracranial pressure.
- List two degenerative diseases and three infection-related diseases of the nervous system and explain the pathophysiology involved.
- Define cerebrovascular accident, cerebral thrombosis, cerebral embolism, transient ischemic attack, and cerebral hemorrhage.
- State two complications of brain surgery.

■ ANATOMY AND PHYSIOLOGY

The application of the nursing process to patients with neurologic problems requires knowledge of the structure and function of the nervous system. The nervous system works as an electrical conductance system. It coordinates and controls all activities of the body. These activities can be divided into the following four kinds of functions:

1. Receiving information (stimuli) from the internal and external environment over sensory (afferent) pathways
2. Communicating information between distant parts of the body (periphery) and the central nervous system
3. Computing or processing the information received at various reflex (spinal cord) and conscious (higher brain) levels to determine responses appropriate to existing situations
4. Transmitting information rapidly over varied motor (efferent) pathways to organs for body action control or modification

■ Neuroglia cells

While the basic structural and functional unit of the nervous system is the neuron, *neuroglia cells* serve as an adjunct. Neuroglia cells make up almost half of the microscopic structures of the spinal cord and brain. They provide nourishment, support, and protection for the neurons. Four different types of neuroglia cells have been identified. These cells and their functions are listed below:

1. Astrocytes
   a. Maintain chemical environment for conduction and transmission of impulses
   b. Maintain nutritional needs of neurons
   c. Store information
   d. Support structures of neurons
   e. Participate in the blood-brain barrier
2. Ependyma
   a. Produce CSF

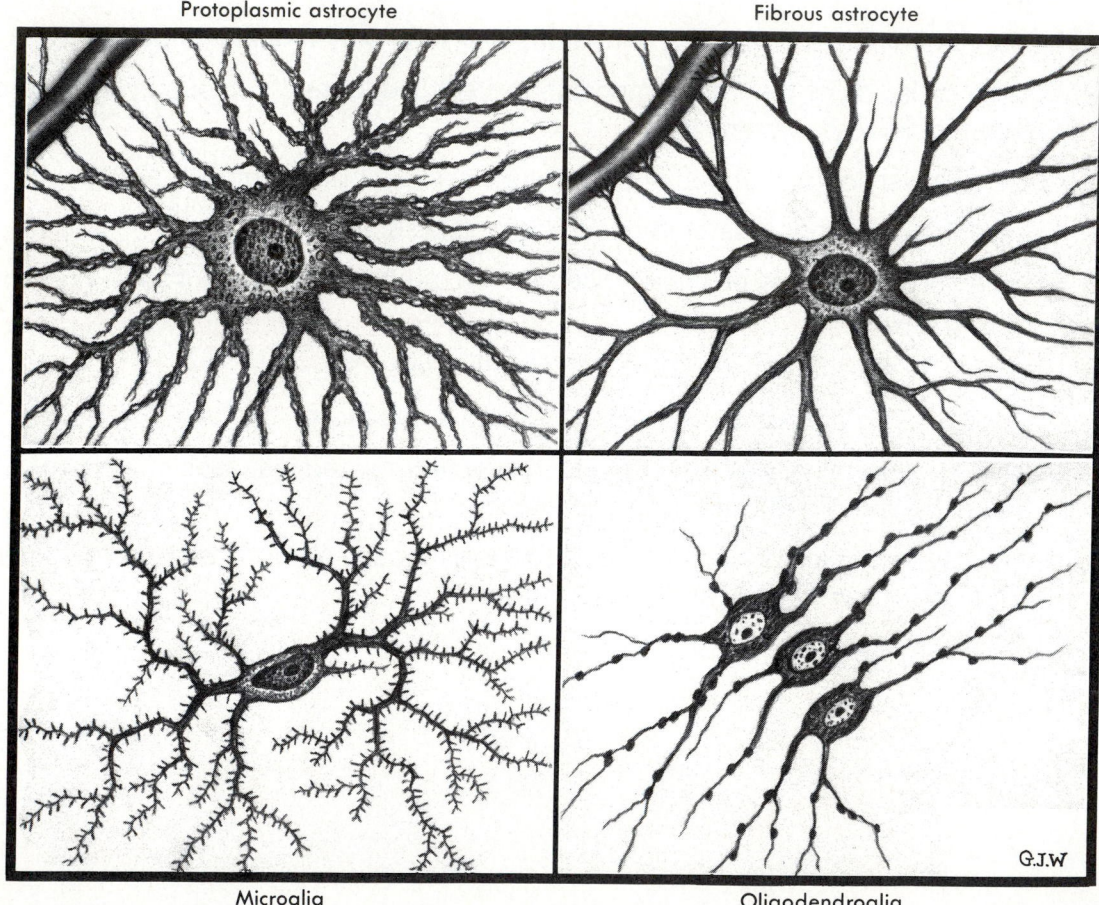

Protoplasmic astrocyte

Fibrous astrocyte

Microglia

Oligodendroglia

Fig. 19-1 Types of neuroglia cells. (From Thompson, JM, and others: Clinical nursing, St. Louis, 1986, The CV Mosby Co.)

3. Microglia
   a. Take part in phagocytosis
4. Oligodendroglia
   a. Produce lipid-protein complex that forms myelin sheaths around axons

All of the cells, except microglia, arise from the embryonic ectoderm. Because they can divide and multiply by mitosis they serve as a source for tumors of the nervous system (Fig. 19-1).

Neuron

The basic structural and functional unit of the nervous system is the *neuron*. It is a highly specialized and differentiated cell, but it has all the basic biologic and biochemical properties of other body cells. The neuron's specialized properties are excitation and electrical-chemical conduction. The neuron consists of a *cell body* (soma, or perikaryon) with two extensions: *dendrites*, which receive infor-

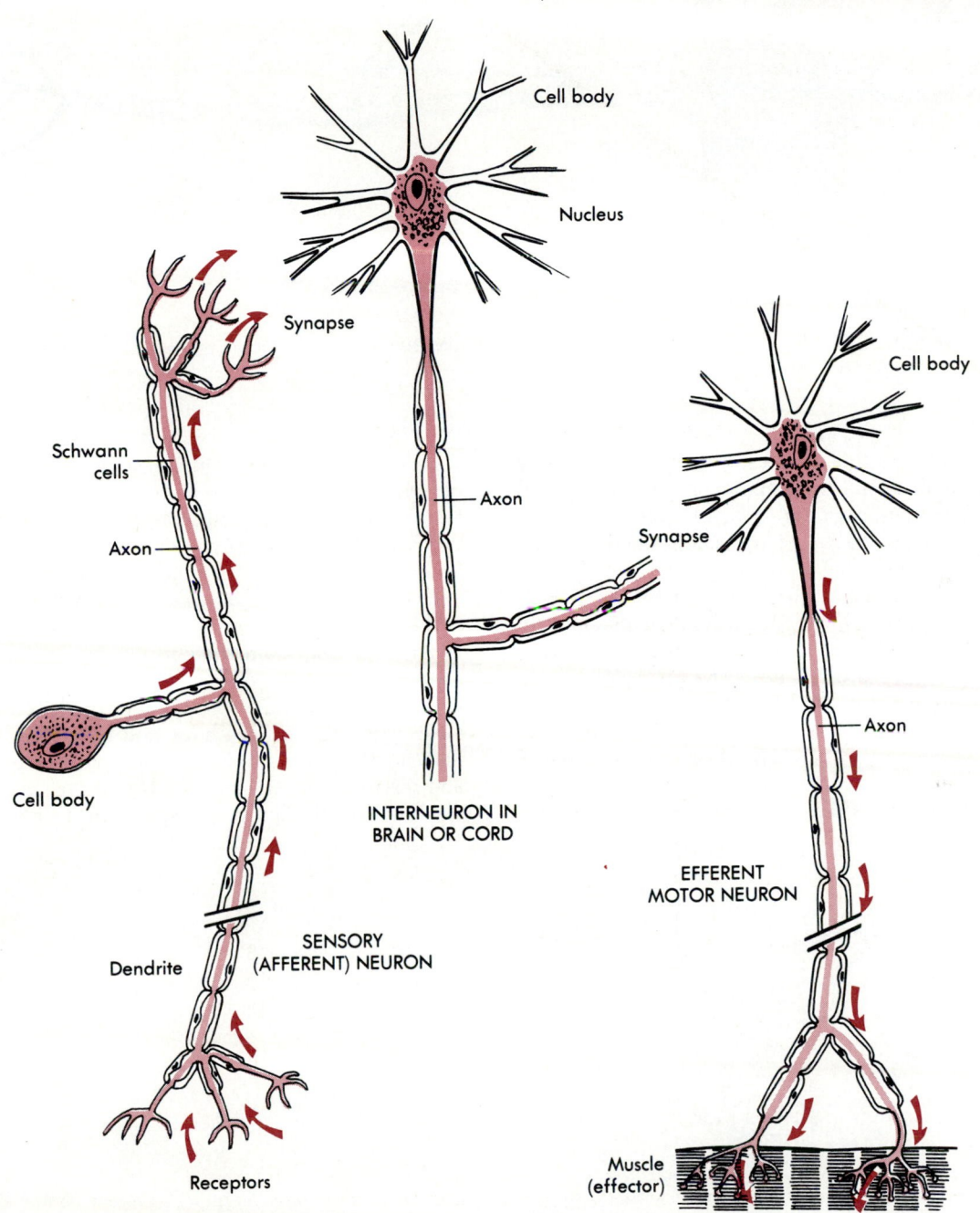

Fig. 19-2 Diagram of neurons showing the cell body (soma), dendrites, and axon. Direction of impulse conduction indicated by arrows.

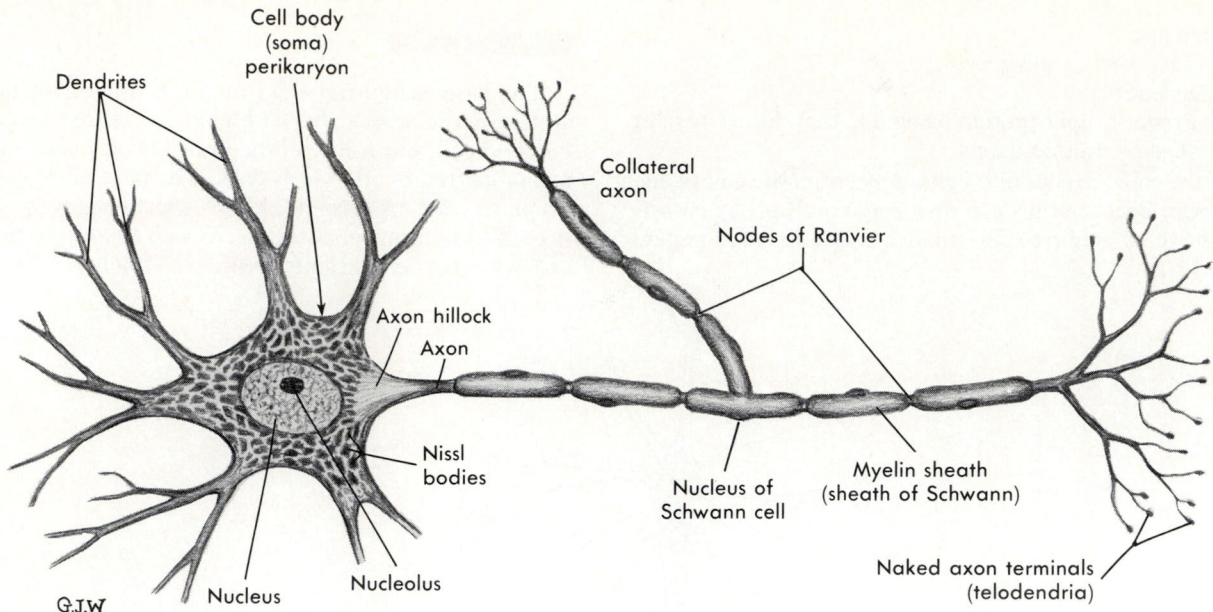

Dendrites

Cell body
(soma)
perikaryon

Collateral
axon

Nodes of Ranvier

Axon hillock

Axon

Nissl
bodies

Nucleus of
Schwann cell

Myelin sheath
(sheath of Schwann)

Naked axon terminals
(telodendria)

G.J.W   Nucleus   Nucleolus

Fig. 19-3 Peripheral nerve. (From Thompson, JM, and others: Clinical nursing, St. Louis, 1986, The CV Mosby Co.)

mation from axon terminals at special sites called synapses, and *axons,* which transmit information away from the cell body to adjacent neurons (Fig. 19-2). A cell membrane encloses the outer boundary of the soma, dendrite, and axon (Figs. 19-2 and 19-3).

One centrally located nucleus is typically found in each neuron. This nucleus is the repository for deoxyribonucleic acid (DNA). Inside the nucleus is a *nucleolus* containing ribonucleic acid (RNA) (Fig. 19-4). *Cytoplasm,* granular in nature, surrounds the nucleus and contains other organelles such as *mitochondria, neurofilaments, microtubules,* the *Golgi complex,* and *Nissl bodies.* Each carries out a specific function related to the neuron.

Neurons can be classified according to structure and

function. Structurally, the divisions include the number of processes. *Unipolar neurons* have only one process or pole; the general sensory neuron is an example of a unipolar neuron. The *bipolar neuron* contains two poles: one dendrite and one axon. These neurons are found in the rods and cones of the retina, the mucous membrane of the nose, and in other special sensory areas. The multipolar neuron consists of one axon and one or more dendrites (Fig. 19-5).

Neurons may also be classified by the length of the axon. *Golgi type I neurons* are large and have long axons. They make up the long fiber tracts of the spinal cord, cerebellum, and cerebral cortex. *Golgi type II cells* are smaller cells that are found in the brain and spinal cord. They have short

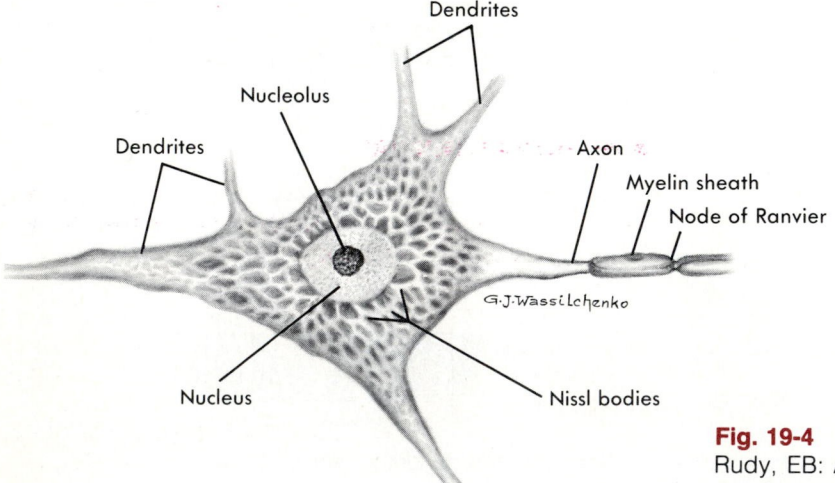

Dendrites

Nucleolus

Dendrites

Axon

Myelin sheath

Node of Ranvier

G.J.Wassilchenko

Nucleus

Nissl bodies

Fig. 19-4 Diagram of neuron with composite parts. (From Rudy, EB: Advanced neurological and neurosurgical nursing, St. Louis, 1984, The CV Mosby Co.)

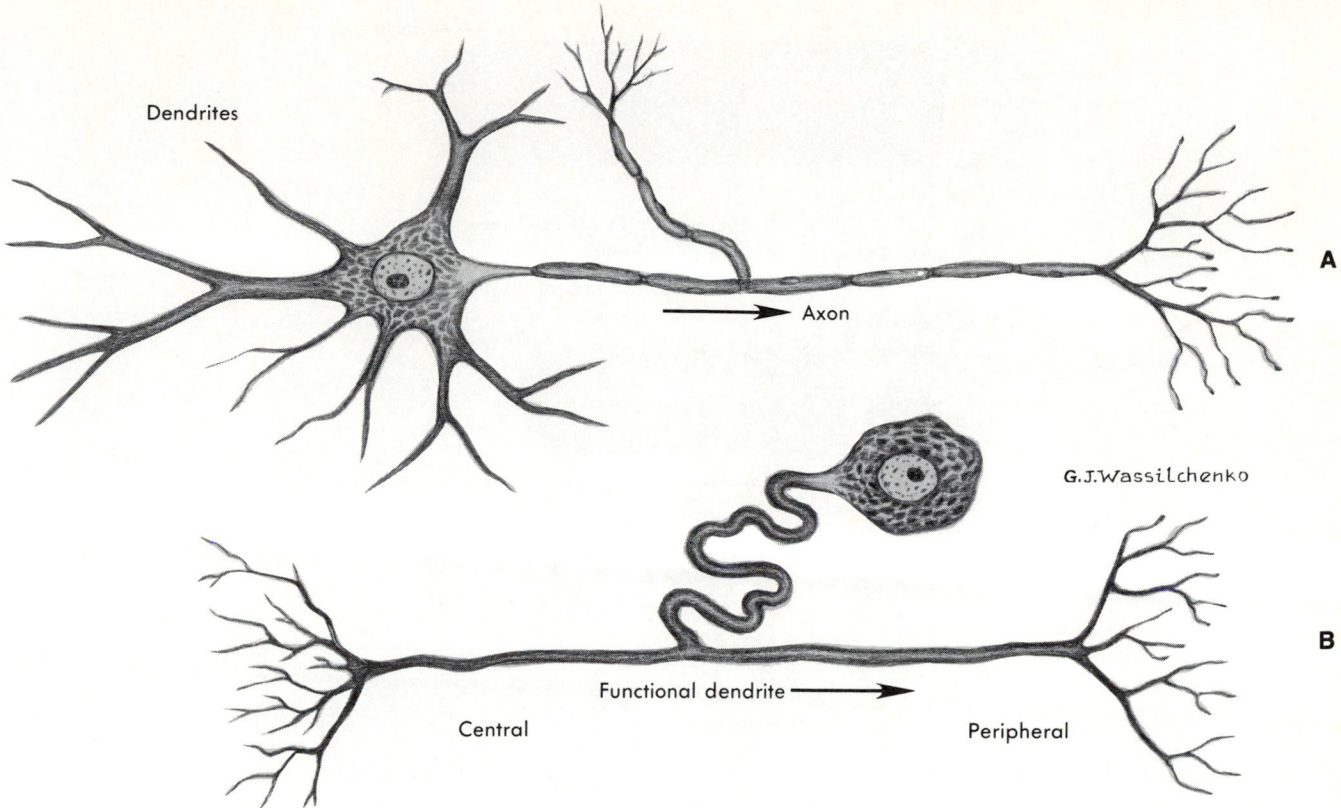

Dendrites

Axon

A

G.J.Wassilchenko

Functional dendrite

Central

Peripheral

B

Fig. 19-5   Types of neurons. **A,** Multipolar. **B,** Unipolar. (From Thompson, JM, and others: Clinical nursing, St. Louis, 1986, The CV Mosby Co.)

axons that branch repeatedly. The purpose of these neurons is to establish complex circuits in the nervous system.[48]

Neurons are functionally known as *afferent, internuncial,* or *efferent.* Afferent neurons are sensory neurons that conduct impulses from the periphery *to* the central nervous system. Internuncial neurons are found in the central nervous system and assist in impulse conduction. Efferent or motor neurons transmit impulses *from* the central nervous system to the periphery.

Neurons are grouped in chains in the peripheral nervous system to form *nerves.* These collections are called *fiber tracts* in the central nervous system.

Collections of neurons are connected in complex ways. The connection determines what each collection of neurons is capable of doing. The neurons are organized into circuits, some of which are simple and made up of relatively few neurons and others that are very complicated. A single neuron may be a part of several different neurologic circuits and thus may have a role in several functions.

Many of the important functional properties of the neuron lie within the *cell membrane.* The membrane is permeable to oxygen, carbon dioxide, and certain inorganic ions, and it is impermeable to organic compounds (proteins) and

other inorganic ions. The characteristic of the membrane is called *differential permeability.*

The neuron also can be characterized by the property of *excitability.* Excitability means that the resting potential of neurons is unstable under certain conditions, as when the membrane of the neuron is stimulated. This unstable condition gives rise to *action potentials.* Action potentials can only arise from excitable cells. All nervous system functions occur from the phenomenon of the action potential (Fig. 19-6).

■ **ACTION POTENTIAL**

Two phases occur within the action potential—*depolarization* (positive state) and *repolarization* (return to the more normal resting potential). When resting, the nerve fiber is charged, with the inside of the cell membrane negatively charged in relation to the outside. A high concentration of sodium exists extracellularly, and a high concentration of potassium exists intracellularly. When the nerve fiber is stimulated, there is an influx of sodium and a loss of intracellular potassium by diffusion. The cell becomes positive, and the action potential (depolarization) occurs. Following depolarization, the ion flow is reversed

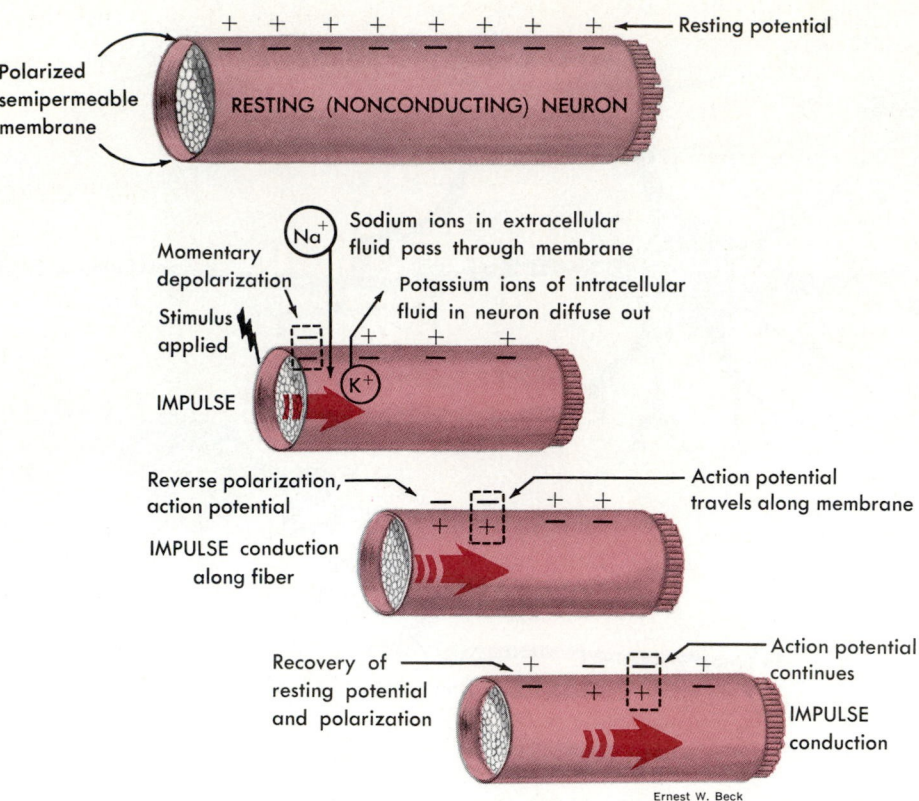

RESTING (NONCONDUCTING) NEURON

Resting potential

Polarized semipermeable membrane

Momentary depolarization

Stimulus applied

IMPULSE

Na⁺

Sodium ions in extracellular fluid pass through membrane

Potassium ions of intracellular fluid in neuron diffuse out

K⁺

Reverse polarization, action potential

IMPULSE conduction along fiber

Action potential travels along membrane

Recovery of resting potential and polarization

Action potential continues

IMPULSE conduction

Ernest W. Beck

Fig. 19-6   Upper diagram represents polarized state of membrane of nerve fiber when it is not conducting impulses. Lower diagrams represent nerve impulse conduction: a self-propagating wave of negativity or action potential travels along membrane. (From Anthony, CP, and Thibodeau, GA: Textbook of anatomy and physiology, ed 12, St. Louis, 1987, The CV Mosby Co.)

and the membrane is returned to its resting state. During depolarization and part of the repolarization process, there is a time interval called the *absolute refractory period*. During this time the nerve cannot be restimulated. This prevents repetitive excitation of the nerve.

When an action potential is generated it proceeds automatically to completion regardless of the type of stimulus that started the depolarization. This means that a strong stimulus does not cause a larger action potential. The action potential also spreads over the entire membrane without a decrease in velocity. The velocity is related to the size of the axon (velocity is higher with a larger diameter) and whether myelin is present.

Myelin is an excellent insulator of axons. The myelin sheath is deposited around the axons by Schwann's cells, and this layer may be as thick as the axon itself. Myelin prevents almost all ion flow across the axon and its membrane. However, at distances of approximately 1 mm, the sheath is interrupted by *nodes of Ranvier*. At these small, uninsulated areas, ions can flow easily between the extracellular fluid and the axon.

The presence of myelin causes such fibers to be called *large fibers;* those without myelin are called *small fibers.*

Large fibers have a greater conduction velocity because (1) the jumping effect allows depolarization to proceed quickly and (2) energy is conserved, since only the nodes depolarize. Large fibers appear white because of the myelin; the *white matter* of the nervous system is made up of myelinated fibers.

Many action potentials of neurons originate in a receptor neuron where internal and external stimuli are normally received. A receptor is like a transducer and can change one form of energy into another form. A receptor, however, responds or depolarizes to *only one* type of stimulus. For example, the retina of the eye responds only to the stimulus of light, which is converted to electrical energy and travels over the optic nerves to the visual cortices for perception.

SYNAPSES

Neurons make contact with one another at sites called *synapses.* Transmission occurring across a synapse is a chemical process that occurs because of the release of neurotransmitters. The synapse consists of the *presynaptic terminal,* the *synaptic cleft,* and the *postsynaptic membrane.* Three types of interneuronal synapses occur. When the axon of one neuron synapses with the cell body of another neuron, it is called *axosomatic*. *Axodendritic* synapses occur between the axon of one neuron and the dendrites of another. Finally, *axoaxonic* synapses occur when one axon connects with another axon.

The end of the axon contains a chemical substance that is released by the action potential. The substance diffuses across the synapse to the adjacent cell membrane. *Synaptic transmission* is both *excitatory* and *inhibitory* in nature. Excitatory neurotransmitters react with receptor sites on the postsynaptic membrane to enhance permeability to sodium, chloride, and potassium ions. Inhibitory neurotransmitters decrease the postsynaptic membrane permeability to sodium, while increasing the permeability to potassium and chloride ions. The membrane becomes *hyperpolarized*. The amount of neurotransmitter released depends on the amount and speed of impulses stimulating the presynaptic terminal. Whether a neuron fires is dependent on the sum of the excitatory and inhibitory inputs.

At least 30 different neurotransmitters can affect transmission of an impulse at the synapse. Chemicals allowing excitatory transmission are *acetylcholine*, *norepinephrine*, *dopamine*, and *serotonin*. Those inhibiting transmissions are *gamma aminobutyric acid (GABA)* in brain tissue and *glycine* in the spinal cord.

■ Divisions of the nervous system

Macroscopically, the nervous system has two major divisions. These are the *central nervous system* and the *peripheral nervous system*.

■ CENTRAL NERVOUS SYSTEM

The central nervous system (CNS) is made up of collections of neurons and their connections into the brain and spinal cord. Areas of the brain and spinal cord are distinguished where cell bodies are concentrated into *nuclei* and groups of axons run in *tracts* that interconnect the parts. The brain and spinal cord are structurally continuous. The brain is housed in the skull and the spinal cord in the vertebral column.

□ Skull

Surrounding the brain is the skull, a bony structure that encloses and protects it (Fig. 19-7). The skull is divided into two primary sections: the *cranium* and the *bones of the face*. Only the former will be discussed here.

The cranium is made up of eight bones that are joined by a series of fixed joints called *sutures*. The bones are

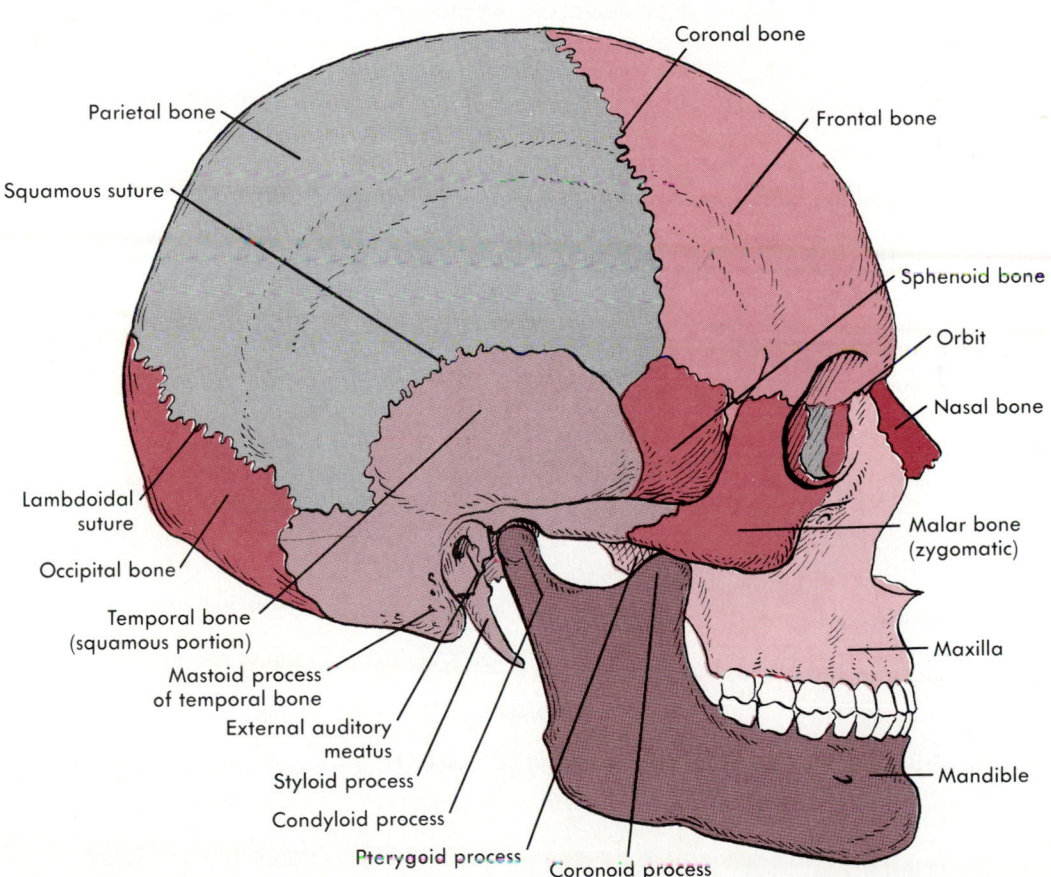

Fig. 19-7 Lateral view of skull. (From Anthony, CP, and Kolthoff, NJ: Textbook of anatomy and physiology, ed 9, St. Louis, 1975, The CV Mosby Co.)

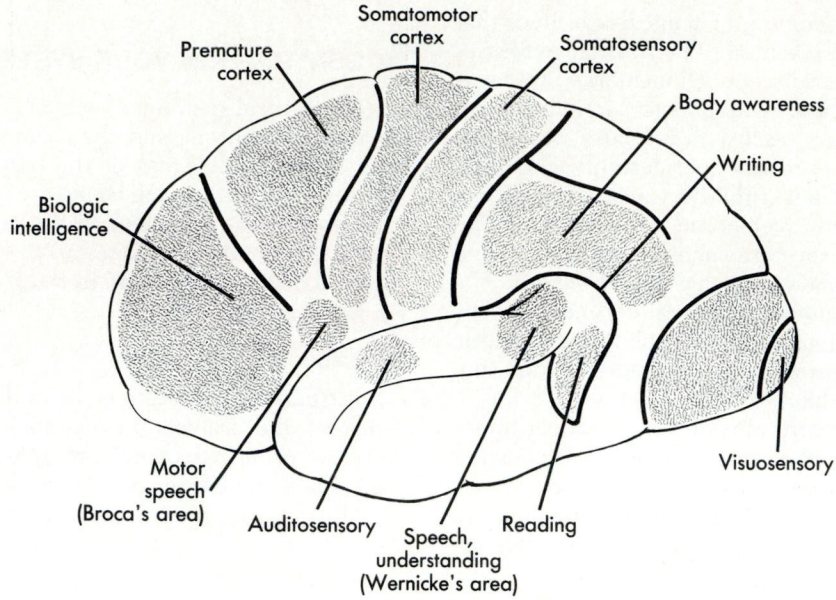

Fig. 19-8 Lateral view of the cerebrum, showing the lobes.

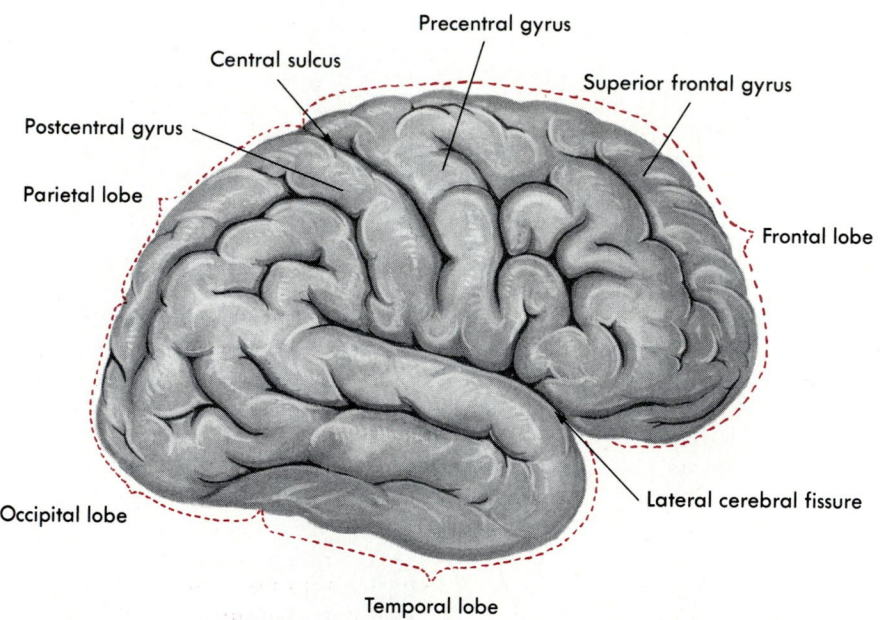

Fig. 19-9 Lateral view of the skull, showing the cranial bones and sutures that separate them.

made up of three layers that are called the *outer table,* the *diploe,* and the *inner table.* The outer and inner table are solid, whereas the diploe is spongy. The inner table forms an inner cavity that is divided as follows:

1. Anterior fossa—contains frontal lobes
2. Middle fossa—contains temporal, parietal, and occipital lobes
3. Posterior fossa—contains brainstem and cerebellum

The *foramen magnum* is a large oval shaped opening at the base of the skull. It is at this level that the spinal cord and brain connect.

□ Brain

The brain weighs about 3 pounds and is divided grossly into the following three main areas: (1) the cerebrum, (2) the brainstem, and (3) the cerebellum.

□ Cerebrum

The cerebrum of each hemisphere (right and left) is composed of the following four major lobes: the *frontal, parietal, temporal,* and *occipital.* The cerebrum is the largest part of the brain and is covered on the outside by the cerebral cortex, which is approximately ¼ inch thick and contains over 14 billion neurons. It receives and analyzes all impulses, controls voluntary movement, and stores knowledge of all impulses received.

The cerebrum is longitudinally divided into right and left hemispheres. The major folds of the cortex divide each hemisphere into four lobes. Each cerebral lobe, named for the overlying cranial bone, carries out specific functions such as general sensation, perception, special senses, perception, and speech (Figs. 19-8 and 19-9).

Deep within the cerebrum are the *basal ganglia.* These are masses of gray matter (cell bodies) and include the caudate nucleus, putamen, and globa pallidus. The basal ganglia function as part of the extrapyramidal system and control postural adjustment and fine voluntary movements, especially those of the hands and lower extremities.

One function of the cerebrum deserves special mention—that of speech. Speech is a function of the dominant hemisphere, which is on the left side of the brain for all right-handed people and most left-handed people. The two identified speech centers are Broca's area and Wernicke's area. *Broca's area* is in the frontal lobe adjacent to the motor cortex and controls verbal, expressive speech. *Wernicke's area* is in the posterior part of the temporal lobe and may extend to adjacent parts of the parietal lobe. It is responsible for reception and understanding of language. An area in the frontal lobe governs ability to write words, and an area in the occipital lobe controls ability to understand written material. The specific functions of the cerebral cortexes are listed in the box above.

□ Brainstem

The *brainstem* lies deep in the center of the hemisphere and connects with the spinal cord at the level of the medulla (Fig. 19-10). It carries all nerve fibers passing between the brain hemisphere and the spinal cord; additionally, all

Specific functions of cerebral cortexes

Frontal cortex	Conceptualization Abstraction Judgment formation Motor ability Ability to write words Higher level centers for autonomic functions
Parietal cortex	Highest integrative and coordinating center for perception and interpretation of sensory information Ability to recognize body parts Left versus right Motor movement
Temporal cortex	Memory storage Auditory integration Hearing
Occipital cortex	Visual center Understanding of written material

cranial nerves except cranial nerve I arise from it. Several structures are contained in the brainstem. These include the diencephalon, the midbrain, the pons, and the medulla oblongata. The specific functions of each of the structures that are located in the brainstem are listed in the box on p. 409.

Of special importance is the core of tissue that extends throughout the entire brainstem called the *reticular formation* (Fig. 19-11). This interconnecting network of cells is the integrating center for respiration, cardiac function, motor systems, and states of consciousness. Stimulating these cells leads to wakefulness, and decreasing stimulation results in sleepiness (as in anoxia caused by increased intracranial pressure).

□ Cerebellum

The cerebellum is located below the posterior cerebrum and is about one fifth the size of the cerebrum. It has two lateral hemispheres and a medial part called the *vermis.* It controls skeletal muscles to produce coordinated movement, equilibrium, and erect posture. It acts with the cerebrum to coordinate muscle activity and produce skilled movement. Voluntary movements can proceed without the cerebellum, but they are clumsy and incoordinated (as in *asynergia* and *cerebellar ataxia*). The cerebellum receives both sensory and motor impulses, and it can detect errors in muscle synergy and adjust muscular control within the body.

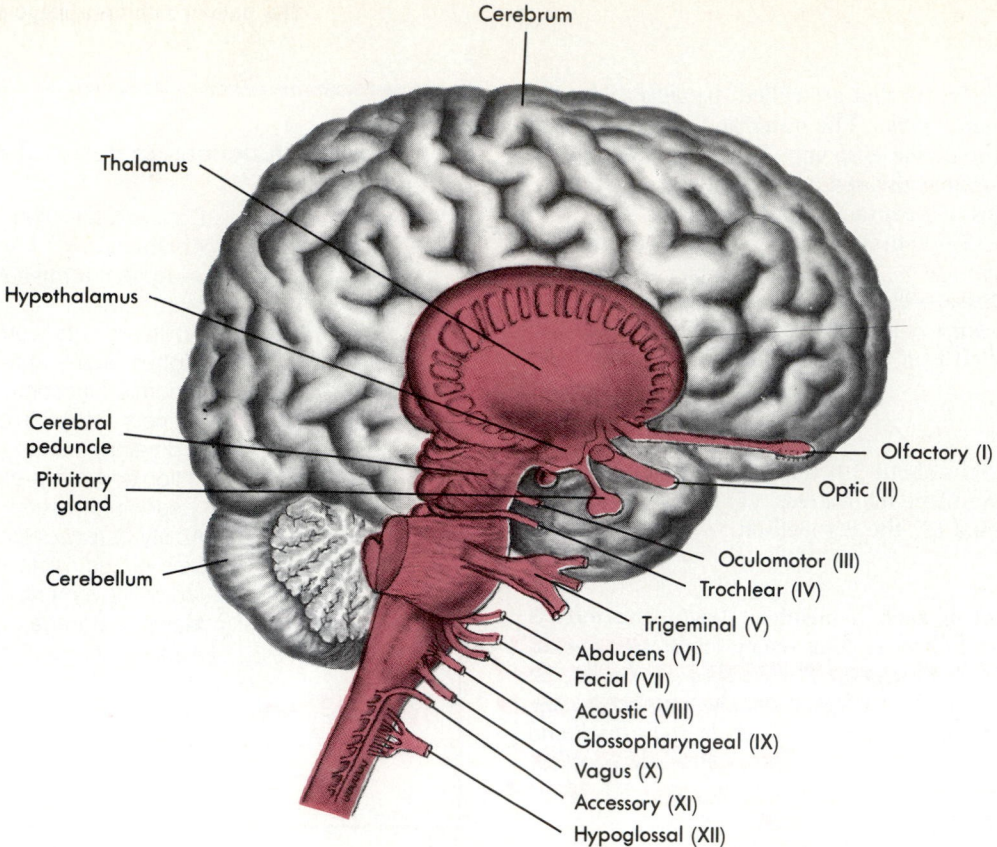

Fig. 19-10   Lateral view of the brain, showing the brainstem. Also shown are the cranial nerves, which arise from it. (From Rudy, EB: Advanced neurological and neurosurgical nursing, St. Louis, 1984, The CV Mosby Co.)

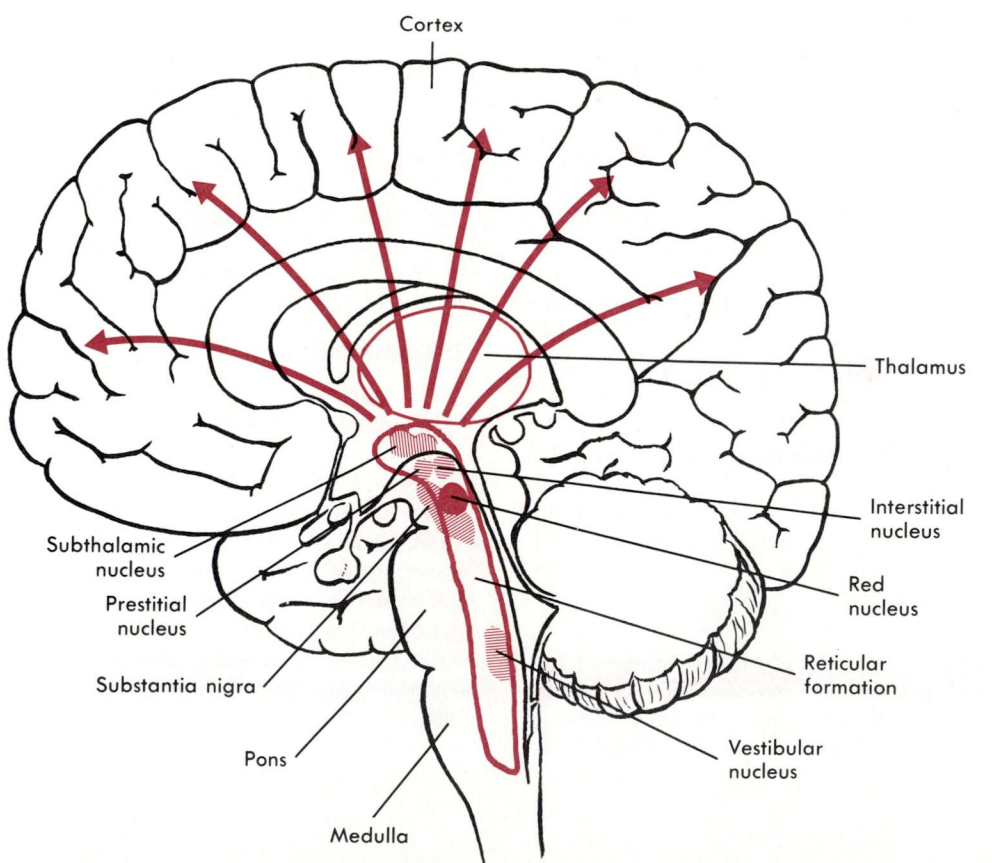

Fig. 19-11   Reticular activating system. (From Thompson, JM, and others: Clinical nursing, St. Louis, 1986, The CV Mosby Co.)

Brainstem functions

Diencephalon (thalamus and hypothalamus)

Receives sensory impulses (pain, temperature, and touch)
Acts as relay station
Controls pain threshold
Acts in synthesis of vasopressor and oxytocin
Helps maintain wakeful state
Controls temperature
Generates emotional response

Pons

Pneumotaxic center (rhythmicity of respirations)
Connection between medulla, midbrain, and cerebellum
Origin of cranial nerves V, VI, VII, and VIII

Midbrain

Motor movement
Relay of impulses
Postural reflex patterns
Auditory reflexes
Righting reflex
Some control of vision
Origin of cranial nerves III and IV

Medulla

Cardiac, vasomotor, and respiratory center
Center for cough, swallowing, and hiccuping
Role in reticular activating system
Origin of cranial nerves IX, X, XI, and XII

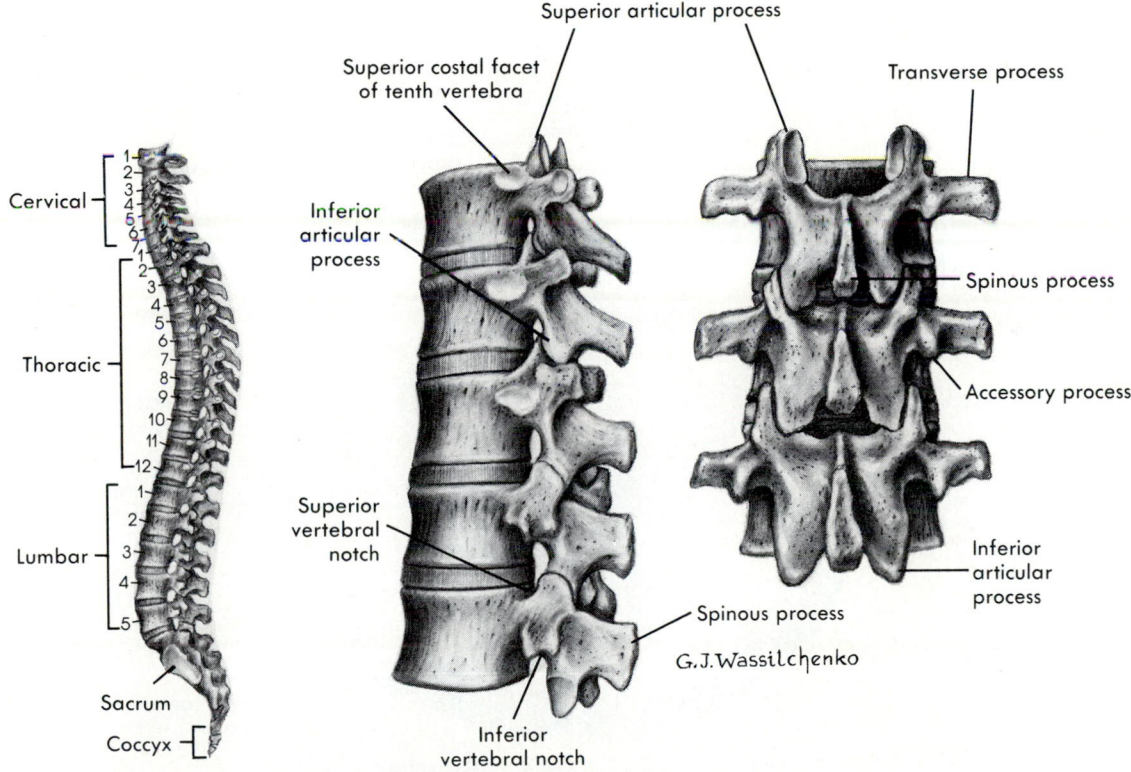

Fig. 19-12 Vertebral column and anatomical structure of vertebrae. (From Rudy, EB: Advanced neurological and neurosurgical nursing, St. Louis, 1984, The CV Mosby Co.)

☐ Spinal vertebrae

The vertebral column is divided into these five regions: *cervical, thoracic, lumbar, sacral,* and *coccygeal.* The total number is 33 and is divided as follows:

1. 7 cervical
2. 12 thoracic
3. 5 lumbar
4. 5 sacral vertebrae fused to form the sacrum
5. 3 to 5 fused bones forming the coccyx

Each vertebrae is separated from those above and below by *cartilage* and *fibrous tissue* called *intervertebral discs.* The *vertebral foramen* is the center of the spinal cord and is part of the vertebral canal containing the spinal cord and spinal meninges. Muscles and ligaments are attached to the vertebrae at the vertebral processes (Fig. 19-12).

☐ Spinal cord

The spinal cord is the downward continuation of the medulla oblongata. It starts at the level of the foramen magnum and ends at L2. The cord tapers in the lower thoracic region into a cone-shaped structure called the *conus medullaris.*

The spinal cord includes H-shaped central gray matter (cell bodies) surrounded by white matter composed of ascending and descending tracts. The gray matter resembles a butterfly (Fig. 19-13). The front or ventral horn consists of multipolar neuronal structures such as cell bodies and dendrites that form the efferent neurons of the ventral roots and the spinal nerves. The dorsal horn contains cell bodies and dendrites of afferent neurons and sensory receptors from the periphery. The gray matter also contains internuncial neurons that send impulses from one level to another, from the dorsal to ventral horns and from one lateral half of the spinal cord to the other. The ascending pathways transmit sensory information from receptors in the periphery to the spinal cord and brain. The descending pathways transmit impulses from the brain to the motor neurons in the spinal cord *(upper motor neurons)* or to the peripheral nervous system *(lower motor neurons).* Some examples of ascending and descending spinal cord tracts are found in Fig. 19-13.

The spinal cord is also the site of reflex pathways. Reflexes do not require relay to the brain level for action—they are an example of the simplest neural circuit. A reflex action consists of a specific stereotyped motor response to an adequate sensory stimulus. The response may involve skeletal muscle movement. A reflex may involve only one spinal cord level, or it may involve more spinal cord levels (segmental reflex). One example of the simple reflex arc is the knee jerk (Fig. 19-14).

☐ Circulation of the brain and spinal cord

The arterial system of the brain includes the larger conducting arteries and the penetrating smaller vessels that enter the brain at right angles after branching off from the conducting vessels. The smaller vessels supply nutrients

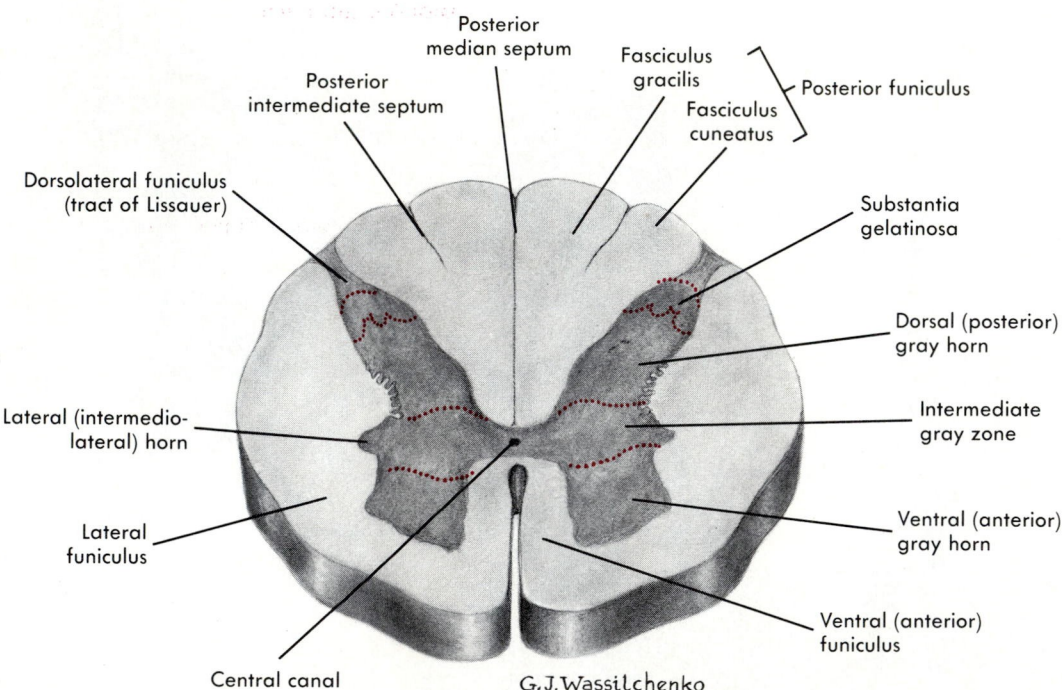

Fig. 19-13 Cross section of spinal cord illustrating subdivisions of white and gray matter. (From Rudy, EB: Advanced neurological and neurosurgical nursing, St. Louis, 1984, The CV Mosby Co.)

to the neurons. The conducting arteries and the areas they supply include the following:

1. Internal carotid arteries—80% of blood supply
   a. Anterior cerebral arteries
      (1) Medial surface of the frontal and parietal lobes
      (2) Basal ganglia
      (3) Portions of the internal capsule and corpus callosum
   b. Middle cerebral arteries
      (1) Lateral surfaces of parietal, frontal, and temporal lobes
      (2) Precentral (motor) gyri
      (3) Postcentral (sensory) gyri
2. Vertebral arteries—20% of blood supply
   a. Basilar artery
      (1) Brainstem
      (2) Cerebellum

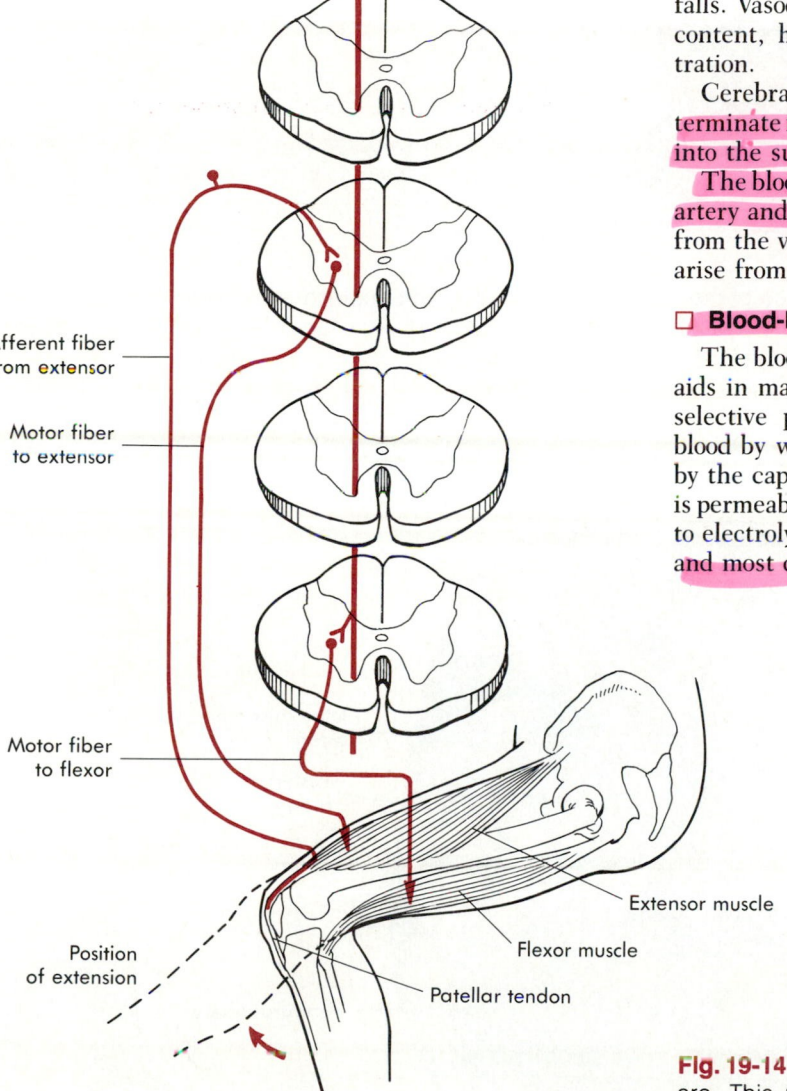

Afferent fiber from extensor

Motor fiber to extensor

Motor fiber to flexor

Position of extension

Extensor muscle

Flexor muscle

Patellar tendon

b. Posterior cerebral arteries
   (1) Portions of temporal and occipital lobes
   (2) Vestibular organs
   (3) Cochlear apparatus

The posterior cerebral artery connects to the middle cerebral artery by the posterior communicating branches. The anterior cerebral arteries connect through the anterior communicating branches. The purpose of this connection in the Circle of Willis is to ensure circulation in case of a problem in any of the four main arteries. Branches of cerebral arteries reach all parts of the brain (Figs. 19-15 and 19-16).

Circulation to the brain has several unique characteristics. Systemic circulation favors the CNS overall, balancing parts to assure a constant supply of nutrients (glucose and oxygen) to the brain. The brain is also able to change its blood flow to respond to changes in blood pressure. In the presence of increasing blood pressure, cerebral vessels constrict, whereas they dilate when blood pressure falls. Vasodilation also occurs with elevated carbon dioxide content, hypoxia, and an elevated hydrogen ion concentration.

Cerebral veins have no valves. All veins of the brain terminate in sinuses created by the dura mater. They empty into the superior vena cava via the jugular vein.

The blood supply to the spinal cord comes from the spinal artery and two radicular arteries. The spinal artery arises from the vertebral arteries, whereas the radicular arteries arise from the aorta.

□ **Blood-brain barrier**

The blood-brain barrier is a physiologic mechanism that aids in maintaining the homeostasis of the brain through selective permeability. Normally, substances enter the blood by way of capillaries into the cerebrospinal fluid or by the capillaries into the extracellular fluid. The barrier is permeable to O_2, CO_2, and water. It is slightly permeable to electrolytes but is impermeable to fixed acids and bases and most drugs.

Fig. 19-14 Deep tendon reflex that demonstrates the reflex arc. This reflex is called the knee jerk or patellar tendon reflex.

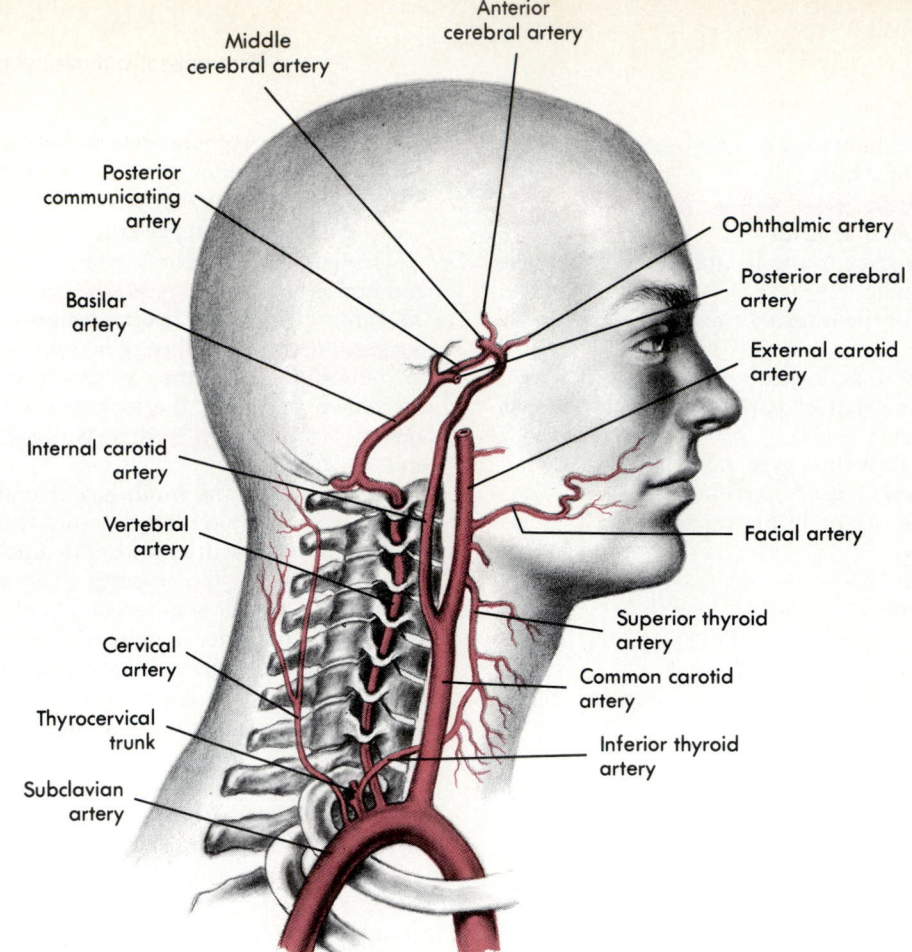

Fig. 19-15 Conducting arteries of the brain, including the internal carotid arteries and the vertebral arteries. (From Rudy, EB: Advanced neurological and neurosurgical nursing, St. Louis, 1984, The CV Mosby Co.)

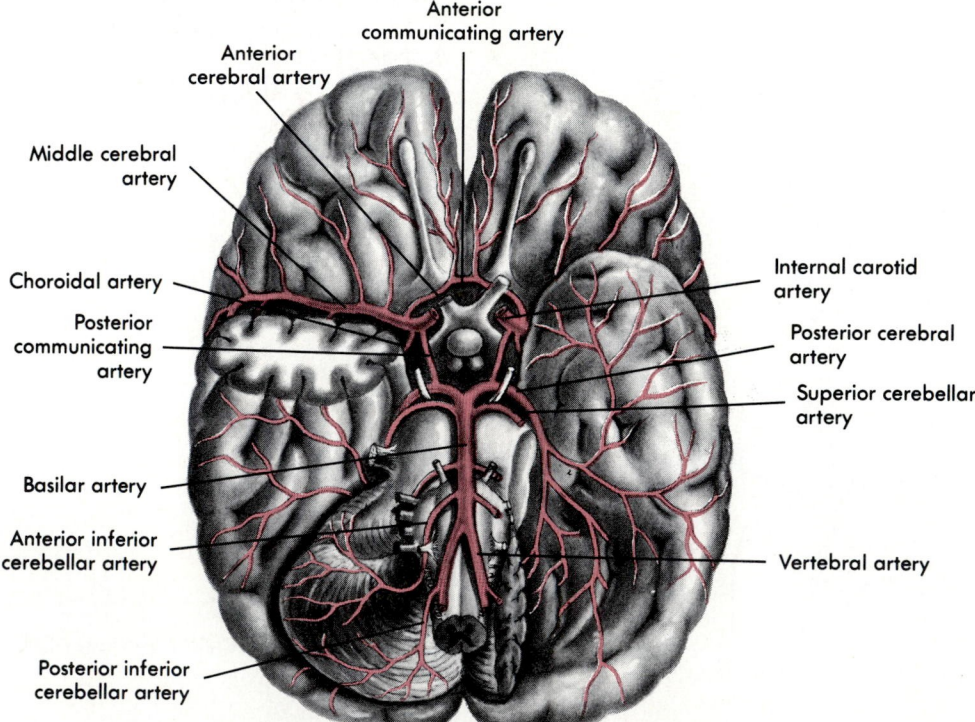

Fig. 19-16 Blood supply of the brain showing the penetrating vessels and the circle of Willis. The internal carotids and the vertebral arteries anastomose at the circle of Willis. (From Rudy, EB: Advanced neurological and neurosurgical nursing, St. Louis, 1984, The CV Mosby Co.)

☐ Cerebrospinal fluid (CSF)

Cerebrospinal fluid (CSF) is found in the ventricles of the brain, in the central canal of the spinal cord, and in the subarachnoid space. It serves as a fluid cushion for the tissue of the nervous system and helps support the weight of the brain. The cerebrospinal fluid is formed in the vessels of the choroid plexus. In a 24-hour period the choroid plexus secretes approximately 500 to 570 ml of CSF. However, only 125 to 150 ml is circulating at any one time. After circulating around the brain and spinal cord, the fluid returns to the brain and is absorbed from the subarachnoid space through the arachnoid villi. The cerebrospinal fluid then enters the venous system and follows the pathway through the jugular vein to the superior vena cava into systemic circulation (Fig. 19-17).

Normally there are up to 8 lymphocytes/ml of spinal fluid. An increase in the number of cells may indicate an infection, such as tuberculosis or a viral infection. Bacterial infections such as tuberculous meningitis often lower the blood sugar level, as well as the chloride levels. Spinal fluid protein is increased in the presence of degenerative disease and/or brain tumor. Blood in the spinal fluid indicates hemorrhage from somewhere in the ventricular system. See the box at right for normal characteristics of CSF.

Normal characteristics of cerebrospinal fluid (CSF)

Specific gravity	1.007
pH	7.35 to 7.45
Chloride	120 to 130 mEq/L
Glucose	50 to 80 /100 ml
Pressure	50 to 200 mm water
Total volume	80 to 200 ml (15 ml in ventricles)
Total protein	15 to 45 mg/100 ml (lumbar)
	10 to 25 mg/100 ml (cisternal)
	5 to 15 mg/100 ml (ventricular)j
Gamma globulin	6% to 13% of total protein
Cell count	
RBC	none
WBC	0-5
	0-10 cells (all lymphocytes and monocytes)

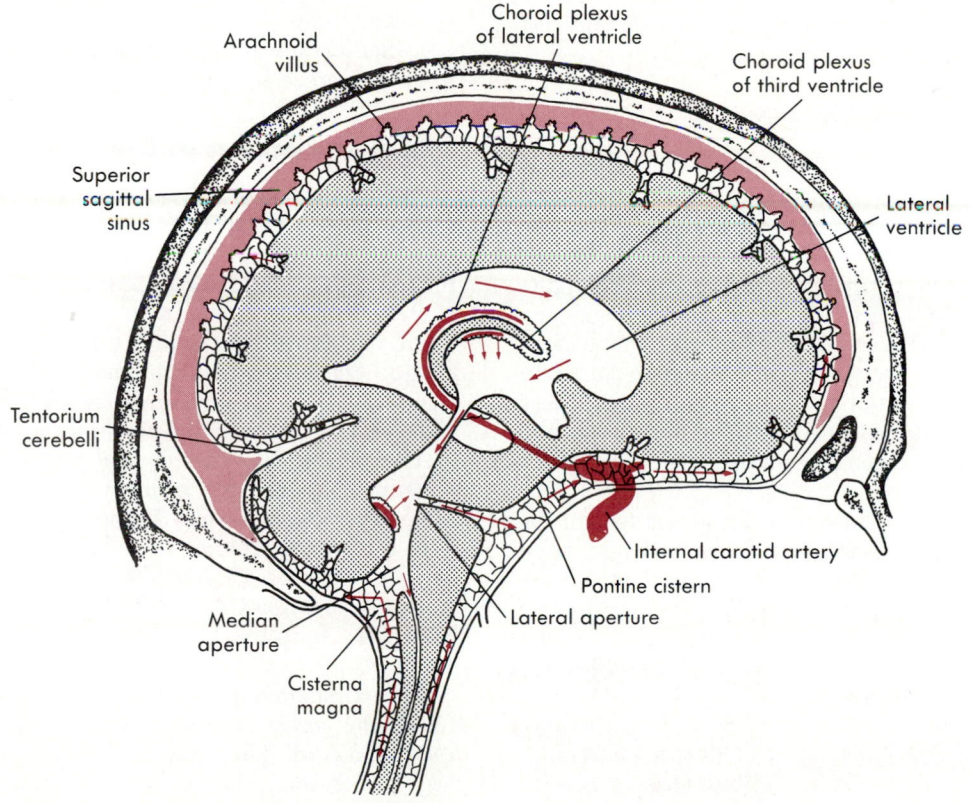

Fig. 19-17 Path of circulation of cerebrospinal fluid from its formation in the ventricles to its absorption into the superior sagittal sinus. (From Nolte, J: The human brain, St. Louis, 1981, The CV Mosby Co.)

☐ Ventricles

The ventricular system is made up of four cavities. The two lateral ventricles are found within each cerebral hemisphere and are the largest cavities. They are separated by a thin layer called the *septum pellucidum*. Each of the lateral ventricles communicates with the central ventricle, which communicates with the fourth ventricle. Parts of the lateral, third, and fourth ventricles are lined with a dense layer of capillaries called the *choroid plexus*.

☐ Meninges

The coverings of the nervous tissue in the brain and spinal cord are called the meninges. These coverings help support, protect, and nourish the vital tissues below. The outermost is the *dura mater*. It is a very tough membrane with two layers. One of these meningeal layers sends four processes deep into the brain. These processes form fibrous compartments for protection of the brain. The *arachnoid* is a delicate membrane that lies beneath the dura and closely covers the brain. Projections called *arachnoid villi* extend into the overlying dura. The innermost of the meninges is the *pia mater*, which is a vascular membrane with many minute plexuses of blood vessels. The same three meninges are also found in the spinal cord.

Three potential spaces are associated with the meninges. These include the following:

1. Extradural (external to the dura)
2. Subdural (between the dura and the arachnoid)
3. Subarachnoid (between the arachnoid and the pia mater)

■ PERIPHERAL NERVOUS SYSTEM

The peripheral nervous system (PNS) is basically a set of common channels located outside the CNS. Peripheral nerves are individual nerves or bundles of nerves that are either motor, sensory, or "mixed" (both sensory and motor fibers) in nature. The peripheral nervous system consists of 12 pairs of cranial nerves, which carry impulses to and from the brain, and 31 pairs of spinal nerves, which carry impulses to and from the spinal cord. Each spinal nerve innervates a specific part of the body for sensation; these parts are called *dermatomes*. Several spinal nerves may also join together to form a complex network of nerve fibers called plexuses.

Peripheral nerves that transmit information toward the CNS are *afferent* or sensory in nature, and peripheral nerves that transmit information away from the CNS are *efferent* or motor in nature. In the peripheral nervous system the motor and sensory nerves usually travel together but separate at the cord level into a *posterior* or *sensory root* and an *anterior* or *motor root*.

The peripheral nervous system is divided into the *somatic* and *autonomic nervous systems*. The somatic nervous system innervates skeletal (striated) muscles. Fibers of axons liberate the neurotransmitter *acetylcholine* at the skeletal muscle cells; this produces an action potential and movement.

■ AUTONOMIC NERVOUS SYSTEM

Body functions regulated by the *autonomic nervous system* include those of the cardiovascular, respiratory, and endocrine systems. Regulatory efforts have the goal of preserving homeostasis. Fibers of the autonomic nervous system synapse once after leaving the CNS at a site called the *ganglion*. The neurotransmitter is *acetylcholine*. The autonomic nervous system can be subdivided into the *sympathetic nervous system* and the *parasympathetic nervous system*. The sympathetic system functions to maintain homeostasis and to provide defense against stressors. During stress, sympathetic responses include an *increase* in blood pressure and heart rate and *vasoconstriction* of peripheral blood vessels. The parasympathetic system conserves and restores regulatory functions.

■ Sensory system pathways

Stimulation of receptor neurons in the body is the first step in sensation. These receptor neurons provide the brain with information about the internal and external environments. The general sensory system includes the following:

1. Receptor neurons, which respond to specific stimuli
2. Posterior roots of the peripheral or afferent sensory nerves, which carry nerve impulses (action potentials) toward the CNS
3. Ascending or sensory tracts within the spinal cord and brain
4. Sensory area of the cerebral cortex, in which stimuli are perceived and interpreted

■ Motor system pathways

Once sensation has been perceived by the brain, corrective action or response is initiated. This action is conveyed by the descending motor pathways, which include the *corticospinal (pyramidal) tracts*, the *extrapyramidal system*, and the *cerebellar system*. The corticospinal system is primarily concerned with skilled, voluntary movement of skeletal muscle. Fibers that combine to form the corticospinal tracts arise from the upper motor neurons, which are located in most areas of the cerebral cortex.

After fibers leave the cerebral cortex they travel to the medulla, in which the majority of fibers *decussate* (cross over) to the opposite side. These fibers eventually synapse with the anterior horn cells, which are in the spinal cord and the motor nuclei in the brainstem. These cells are the *lower motor neurons* and are the final communication pathway with muscles via the myoneural junction (Fig. 19-18).

The extrapyramidal tracts provide separate pathways between the cortex, the basal ganglia, the brainstem, and the spinal cord. These include all descending motor pathways other than the corticospinal tracts, and they are named for their points of origin and termination. Generally, the extrapyramidal tracts help maintain muscle tone and control of gross autonomic skeletal muscle movement.

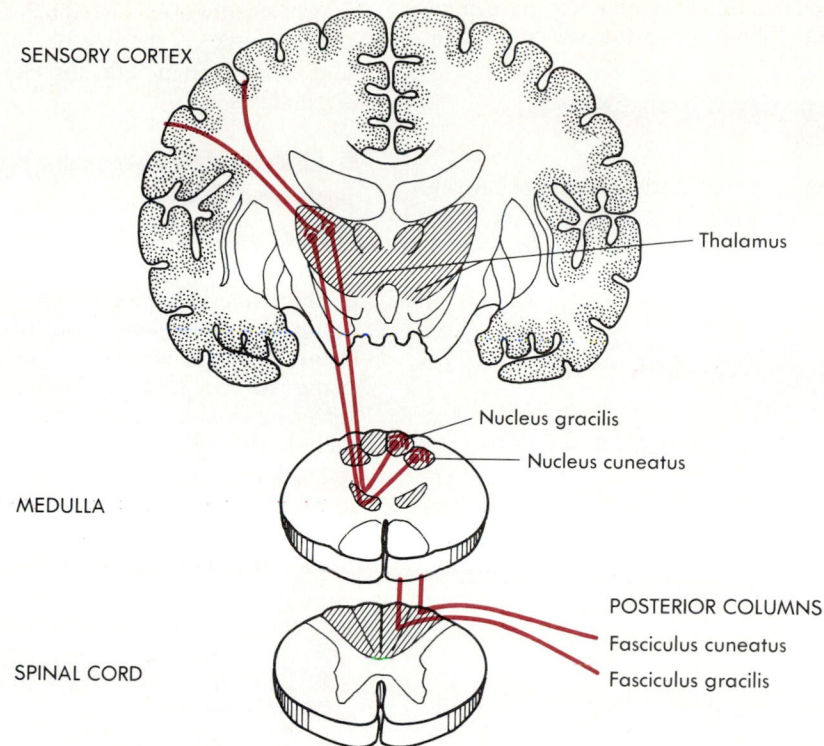

SENSORY CORTEX

Thalamus

Nucleus gracilis
Nucleus cuneatus

MEDULLA

POSTERIOR COLUMNS
Fasciculus cuneatus
Fasciculus gracilis

SPINAL CORD

Fig. 19-18   Pathways for fine touch, deep touch and pressure, vibration, and proprioception. Note how stimuli entering through dorsal route (posterior) travel on same side as posterior columns to medulla where they cross to opposite side, ascend to thalamus, and end in somasthetic area where perception occurs.

Visceral efferent pathways from the spinal cord control the action of involuntary or smooth muscles located within the walls of hollow organs, tubes, the heart, and glands.

■ Physiologic changes with aging

Studies have shown that the nervous system does change with aging. The effect of these changes is variable. The brain itself significantly *decreases in weight* with aging, along with a substantial loss of neurons. Those cells not destroyed undergo structural changes. Brain cells are lost at a rate of 1% a year after 50 years of age.[48] The loss is inconsistent, so that some parts of the brain lose cells at a faster rate. The cortex generally loses cells at a faster rate than the brainstem. There may be a general decline in interconnections of dendrites. Also senile plaques and neurofibrillary plaques, as well as the age pigment lipofuscin, are found in neuronal cells. In addition, there is a significant *reduction of cerebral blood flow, a decrease in brain metabolism, and a decrease in oxygen utilization.*

The aged may also experience an altered *sleep/wakefulness ratio* and a *decreased ability to regulate body temperature.* These suggest changes in the function of the hypothalamus in the aging.

The control of the autonomic nervous system over various functions of the body is unpredictable and labile in the elderly, but some changes do occur. Additionally, sensory and motor conduction *decreases in velocity of nerve impulses* occur with aging, sensory conduction decreasing faster than motor. This occurs especially in peripheral nerves and more often in females. In the spinal cord the blood supply to the white matter has been found to be decreased, leading to diminished reflexes in the lower extremities (distal).

It is important for the nurse to realize that normal changes that occur with aging in the nervous system cannot be equated with senility, Alzheimer's disease, or organic brain disease. These conditions occur in a small number of older persons, and many aged persons reach advanced ages without any deterioration in the ability to think.

■ PREVENTION AND HEALTH EDUCATION

Problems that occur in the nervous system can have devastating results. These results often have impact on almost every body system and produce changes that are chronic and debilitating. Problems in other body systems, if discovered and treated in a timely fashion, can have much more satisfactory results than those in the nervous system.

■ Primary prevention: prevention of disease

Many of the problems of the nervous system have no known cause and thus cannot be prevented. For other problems, however, preventive measures can be emphasized. Neurologic problems can be divided into several main categories as follows.

■ PROBLEMS RESULTING FROM VASCULAR DISEASE

Neurovascular diseases can at times be prevented, or their results can at least be minimized. Many of the cerebrovascular diseases are thought to occur more frequently as a result of the presence of certain risk factors. These same factors also increase the risk of cardiac disease:

1. Cigarette smoking
2. Hypertension
3. Hypercholesteremia
4. Obesity
5. Stress-related occupations and a hectic pace of life

■ PROBLEMS RESULTING FROM METASTASIS

Cigarette smoking has been identified as a major cause of lung cancer. This is significant to the nervous system because neoplasms of the lung often metastasize to the brain. In fact, a significant number of lung malignancies are discovered subsequent to signs and symptoms of brain metastasis.

■ PROBLEMS RESULTING FROM TRAUMA

Some actions can play an important role in preventing head injuries and spinal cord injuries. Factors that can influence the outcome include the following:

1. Use of seat belts in automobiles
2. Use of helmets while riding motorcycles or snowmobiles
3. Practice of firearm safety—keeping guns away from children
4. Minimal use of drugs and alcohol
5. Not driving after drinking or taking drugs
6. Safe use of motor vehicles—no showing off or speeding
7. Use of precautions while swimming and especially not diving into shallow water

■ PROBLEMS RESULTING FROM INFECTIONS

Neurologic diseases resulting from infections can sometimes be prevented. Because ear or sinus infections can be a source of brain abscess or meningitis, it is important that these infections be treated. Also, because several of the neurologic diseases related to infections are spread through sexual contacts, the practice of responsible sex is important. This may include abstinence, monogamy, or the use of condoms.

■ Secondary prevention/early detection

Early detection of neurologic diseases often is difficult. Many initial symptoms are so vague that it is easy to deny or minimize their importance. Also, some changes may occur over such a long period of time that adaption to them occurs. Certain warning symptoms can be found in such vague patterns that patients may be thought at first to be suffering from hysteria. The symptoms that are significant include the following:

1. Headaches that first occur after middle age or change in character, especially ones that are worse in the morning or awaken a person from sleep
2. Clumsiness or loss of function in an extremity
3. Changes in visual acuity
4. Any new or worsened seizure activity
5. Numbness or tingling in one or more extremities
6. Pain that is neurologic in nature
7. Galactorrhea
8. Cessation of menses
9. Personality changes

■ Tertiary prevention/prevention of complications

It is important to mention the issue of tertiary prevention for the patient with neurologic dysfunction. Unfortunately, many of these patients are prone to iatrogenic complications, as well as functional disabilities. These occur secondary to the neurologic problems and include contractures, decubiti, and eye damage, as well as other hazards of immobility.[71] It is extremely important for the nurse working with neurologically impaired patients to be aware of rehabilitative concepts and apply them in the nursing care. Many patients with neurologic dysfunctions may also benefit from formal inpatient rehabilitative care after the acute hospitalization.

■ COMMON NEUROLOGIC MANIFESTATIONS

The practice of neurologic nursing is concerned with problems of the nervous system that have a variety of causes. Whatever the cause, various symptoms occur, at times related to both organic and functional causes. Because of the nature of the anatomy and physiology of the nervous system, *organic lesions or trauma result in clinical manifestations related to the site affected, regardless of the underlying pathologic condition.* Other manifestations result not from the damaged site itself, but from other parts of the nervous system that are affected by the damaged site.

One example of this is a lack of control or regulation. The nurse must realize that patients with neurologic problems may have to make significant changes in life-style and adaptation. The psyche and the body are one in the person; often there is no clear-cut distinction of symptoms. A person is an open system in which many subsystems interplay.

In this section, we will discuss neurologic manifestations resulting from alterations in neurologic function and structure that are common to many pathologic conditions. A brief review of neurologic assessment is helpful in this discussion.

Neurologic assessment

Complete neurologic assessment is usually performed in phases and is dependent on the condition of the patient and the urgency in collecting the data. It includes a history and neurologic examination. The reader is referred to Chapter 3 for a discussion of assessment.

Neurologic examination of the conscious adult includes physical examination of the following:

1. Mental status
   a. Level of consciousness
   b. Orientation
   c. Mood and behavior
   d. Knowledge
   e. Vocabulary
   f. Memory
2. Cranial nerve function (Table 19-1)
3. Language and speech
4. Meningeal signs
5. Sensory status
   a. Touch
   b. Pain
   c. Temperature
   d. Proprioception
6. Motor status
   a. Gait and stance
   b. Muscle strength
   c. Muscle tone
   d. Coordination
   e. Involuntary movements
   f. Muscle stretch reflexes

More detailed descriptions of selected portions of the examination will be covered in specific parts of this chapter. The reader is also referred to a neurologic nursing text for additional information.

In clinical settings, it is not feasible or essential to completely repeat the total neurologic exam during the shift-to-shift assessment of the patient. In many settings, such as intensive care units, the neurologic checks are done every hour. When doing these checks, certain features have been identified as most important. Generally these include the following:

1. Orientation
2. Level of consciousness
3. Ability to speak
4. Muscle strength
5. Involuntary movements
6. Any abnormal posturing

Table 19-1   Assessment of cranial nerve function

Nerve	Function	Assessment
Olfactory (I)	Sensory—smell	Identification of odors
Optic (II)	Sensory—vision	Visual acuity; inspection of fundi; determination of visual fields
Oculomotor (III)	Motor—pupil constriction, elevation of upper eyelid, extraocular movements	Tested together for extraocular movements; also pupil reflex for CNIII
Trochlear (IV)	Motor—downward/inward eye movements	
Trigeminal (V)	Motor—jaw movement Sensory facial sensation	Jaw strength; facial sensation; corneal reflex
Abducens (VI)	Motor—lateral eye movements	
Facial (VII)	Motor—facial muscles Sensory taste on anterior two thirds of tongue	Facial movements; identification of tastes
Acoustic (VIII)	Hearing—cochlear divison	Whisper
	Balance—vestibular division	Caloric stimulation test
Glossopharyngeal (IX)	Sensory—pharynx and posterior tongue, with taste	Identification of tastes
	Motor—pharynx Sensory—pharynx and larynx	Gag reflex; uvula motion; soft palate movement; hoarseness
Vagus (X)	Motor—palate, pharynx and larynx	
Spinal accessory (XI)	Motor—stemocieidomastoid, upper part of trapezius	Shoulder and neck motion
Hypoglossal (XII)	Motor—tongue	Tongue motion

Adapted from Bates, B: A guide to physical examination, ed 2, Philadelphia, 1979, JB Lippincott Co.

Glasgow Coma Scale

	Stimuli	Score
Eyes open	Spontaneously	4
	To speech	3
	To pain	2
	None	1
Best verbal response	Oriented	5
	Confused	4
	Inappropriate words	3
	Incomprehensible	2
	None	1
Best motor response	Obeys commands	5
	Localizes to pain	4
	Flexes to pain	2
	None	1

■ GLASGOW COMA SCALE

One way to standardize observations of patients is the Glasgow Coma Scale. It was developed in 1974 and consists of assessment of three parts of the neurologic assessment. These include the following:

1. Eye opening
2. Best motor response
3. Best verbal response

The stronger the stimulus needed to obtain a response, the lower the score assigned to the part (see the box above). The number value assigned to each parameter is added to

yield an objective score. The score for normal persons who are not neurologically impaired is 14. The lowest possible score is 3. Any score of 7 or less is commonly accepted as a definition of coma[64] (Fig. 19-19).

■ Headache

Headache is a common symptom experienced by many patients. It can result from many pathologic processes, and its significance also is variable. *The source of recurring headache should be determined through careful physical examination with appropriate neurologic assessment.* Persons have been known to self-treat headaches for months, believing them to be nothing to worry about, only to learn later that the pain was caused by a more serious problem such as a brain tumor. Because of the site of some tumors in the brain, headache may be the only symptom for many months.

■ PATHOPHYSIOLOGY

Headache may have many causes. Some of these are as follows:

1. Expanding masses such as neoplasms
2. Intracranial bleeding
3. Inflammation of the meninges as in meningitis
4. Other infections of the brain and spinal cord
5. Head trauma
6. Cerebral hypoxia
7. Dilation of the cerebral blood vessels
8. Psychologic factors such as stress
9. Systemic disease including eye, ear, and sinus problems
10. Allergies

The exact pathophysiology of head pain is not known. Although the skull and brain tissues are not capable of sensory pain, pain arises from the scalp and its blood vessels

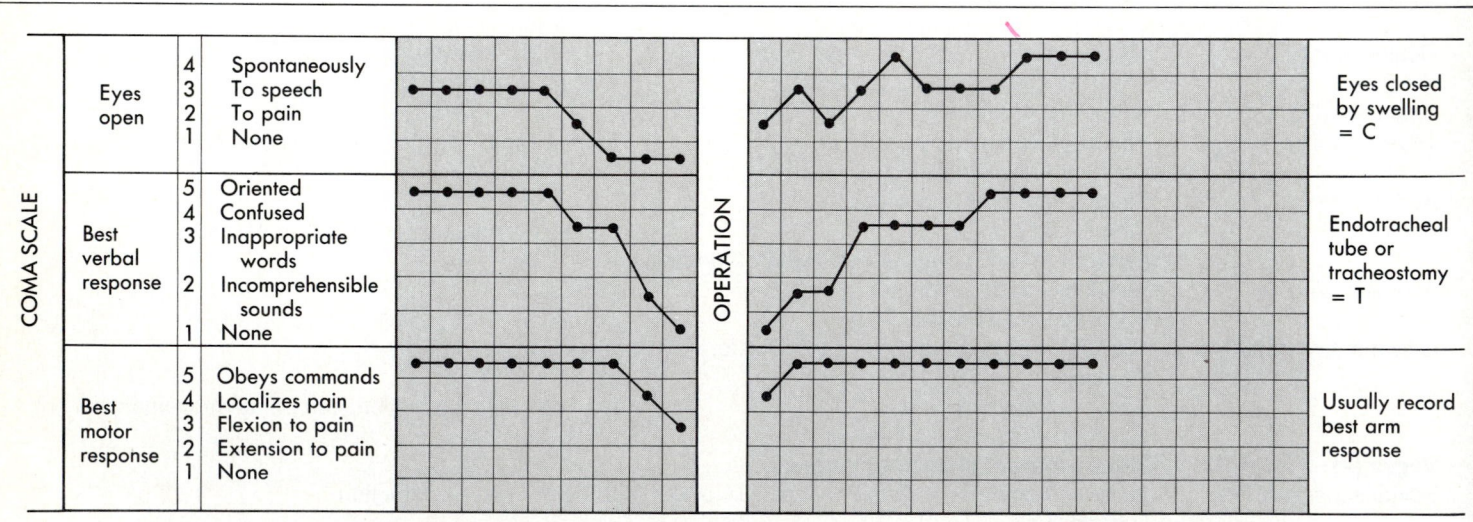

Fig. 19-19 Glasgow Coma Scale, demonstrating measurement of level of consciousness. Notice change in patient's condition just before and after surgery.

Table 19-2 Comparison of migraine, cluster, and tension headaches

Type	Onset	Frequency	Duration	Nature	Prodromal symptoms/ associated symptoms	Treatment
Migraine headaches	Occur at any age Strongly hereditary More common in women than men	Episodic, tend to occur with stress or life crisis May occur with menstruation	Hours to days	Occur slowly; pain becomes severe, with one side of head affected more than other	Prodromal: visual field defects, confusion, paresthesias Associated: nausea, vomiting, chills, fatigue, irritability, sweating, edema	Ergotamine tartrate Methysergide maleate Inderal Nonnarcotic analgesics Relaxation techniques Application of heat or cold
Cluster headaches	Early adulthood; precipitated by alcohol or nitrates More common in men	Episodes clustered together in quick succession for few days or weeks with remissions that last for months	Few minutes to few hours	Pain intense: throbbing, deep, often unilateral; begin in infraorbital region and spread to head and neck	Prodromal: uncommon Associated: flushing, tearing of eyes, nasal stuffiness, sweating swelling of temporal vessels	Avoidance of dietary tyramine, nitrate, and gluconate Narcotic analgesics during acute phase, often intramuscularly
Tension headaches (muscle contraction)	Often in adolescence; related to tension or anxiety No family history	Episodic; vary with stress	Variable, can be constant	Dull, constant, uncommon aggravating pain, vary in intensity; usually bilateral and involve neck and shoulders; pain may be poorly defined	Prodromal: uncommon Associated: sustained contraction of head and neck muscles	Nonnarcotic analgesics Relaxation techniques Amitriptyline (Elavil)

and muscles, from the dura mater and its venous sinuses, from the blood vessels at the base of the brain, and from some cervical cranial nerves. Blood vessels dilate and become congested with blood. Headaches are divided into the following three categories[48]:

1. Vascular
   a. Migraine
   b. Cluster
   c. Hypertensive headaches
2. Tension
   a. Psychogenic problems (tension or stress)
   b. Medical problems (cervical arthritis)
3. Traction-inflammatory
   a. Infection
   b. Intracranial or extracranial
   c. Occlusive vascular structures
   d. Arteritis

See Table 19-2 for details about and comparison of three specific types of headache.

ASSESSMENT

Both subjective and objective data are important in determining more about the cause and nature of the headache.

□ Subjective data

1. Patient's understanding of headache and possible causes.
2. Awareness of any precipitating factors such as stress
3. Measures that relieve symptoms, including medications
4. Location, frequency, pattern, and character of head pain, including site of return, time of day, and intervals between headaches
5. Initial onset of headache
6. Presence of any prodromal symptoms
7. Presence of associated symptoms
8. Family history of headaches (especially important with migraine)
9. Situations that make headache worse
10. Presence of allergies

□ Objective data

1. Behavior: signs indicating stress or anxiety or pain
2. Change in ability to carry on daily activities
3. Abnormalities on physical assessment part of neurologic examination
4. Temperature
5. Sinus drainage

Information about the patient's understanding of the nature and precipitating factors is helpful for planning necessary teaching. It is not unusual for the patient to manifest little objective data in the presence of subjective complaints.

Headache pain may be made worse by stress or tension. Knowledge of the patient's perception of the effect of stress on the symptoms is important in planning for measures that relieve or reduce effects of stress.

Migraine headaches are unusual in that there are prodromal signs and symptoms that occur before the acute attack. These may include the following:

1. Visual field defects
2. Confusion
3. Paresthesias
4. Paralysis in rare cases

During the actual attack, signs and symptoms may include nausea, vomiting, sensitivity to light, chilliness, fatigue, irritability, sweating, edema, and other autonomic signs.

In assessing headache several key points are considered. These include the following:

1. Localized type of head pain is usually associated with migraine headaches or an organic disorder.
2. Generalized headache is usually related to psychologic causes or the presence of increased intracranial pressure.
3. Migraine headaches may change from one side of the head to the other.
4. Headaches that occur with increased intracranial pressure usually are present on awakening and may awaken the person from sleep.
5. Sinus headaches typically occur early in the morning and increase in intensity as the day progresses.
6. Many headaches are related to stress.
7. Pain described as dull, nagging, aggravating, and ever present often occurs with psychogenic headaches.
8. Organically caused pain tends to be constant and progressive in nature.
9. Migraine headaches may be associated with menstruation.
10. Headaches may be precipitated by eating foods containing monosodium glutamate, sodium nitrate, or tyramine, as well as by alcohol.
11. A family history of headache is important, especially with migraine headaches.
12. Sleeping too long, fasting, or inhaling toxic fumes in work situations with inadequate ventilation can cause headaches.
13. Oral contraceptives may make migraine headaches worse.
14. Any secondary gains that patients receive from headaches must be assessed.

□ Diagnostic tests

It is important to evaluate headaches that are not slight and transient. Usual testing includes a neurologic examination, including a CT scan. The CT scan is becoming more available as a way to easily and safely detect abnormalities in the CNS (Fig. 19-20). It has replaced many invasive and painful procedures that neurologic patients previously were subjected to during a diagnostic workup. See the box on p. 421.

The MRI scan may also be done.[43] See the box on p. 422 for information. Another scan that is similar to the CT and the MRI is the PET scan (positron emission tomography). In this scan the patient receives an injection of deoxyglucose with radioactive fluorine. The head is

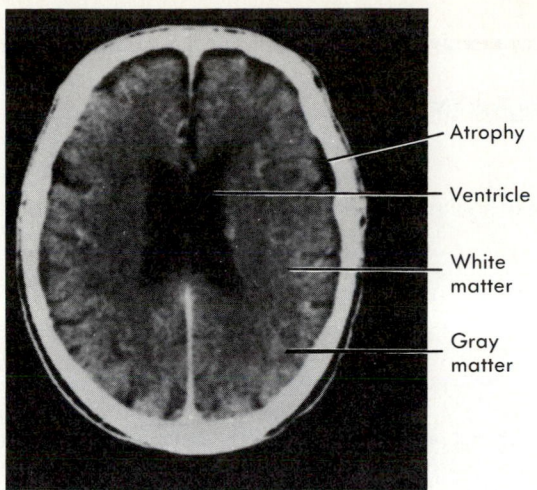

Atrophy

Ventricle

White matter

Gray matter

Fig. 19-20 CT scan printouts. CT brain scan differentiates between gray and white brain matter. (From Ballinger, PW: Merrill's atlas of radiographic positions and radiologic procedures, ed 5, St. Louis, 1982, The CV Mosby Co.)

scanned and a color composite picture is obtained. Various shades of colors indicate levels of glucose metabolism.

A lumbar puncture may also be performed. A lumbar puncture is not done, however, if there is evidence of increased intracranial pressure or if a brain tumor is suspected, since the quick reduction in pressure produced by removal of the spinal fluid may cause brain herniation. In this situation a CT scan must be done first. The box on p. 423 outlines the procedure for lumbar puncture.

At times, because of anatomic abnormalities or other causes, a lumbar puncture may not be possible. At these times a cisternal puncture may be attempted. The cisternal puncture is made between the first cervical vertebra and the base of the skull (Fig. 19-22). See the box on p. 424 for a description of this procedure.

Other tests that may be done include a brain scan (Fig. 19-23) and plain skull films (see the box on p. 424).

The skull x-ray films will demonstrate bony abnormality as well as congenital changes, but will not yield the information that more sophisticated procedures do.

Computed tomography (EMI, CT, or CAT scan)

Purpose

Detection of cerebral and spinal cord pathology using a technique of scanning without radioisotopes.

Preparation of patient

1. No special physical preparation
2. Patient teaching
   a. Explain procedure
   b. Time: Approximately 20 to 30 minutes for CT scan without contrast medium; 60 mintues if scans with and without contrast medium are done.
   c. Sensation: Procedure is painless, except for slight discomfort when IV is started for injection of contrast medium. Also, there is some discomfort in lying still and possible feelings of claustrophobia as a result of head being positioned in head holder.
   d. Patient must maintain motionless position until scan is completed.
3. If contrast medium is used, history of allergy to iodine (seafood) is determined before medium is given.

Procedure

1. Patient lies supine with the head positioned within a rubber head-holder to prevent air gaps between the machine and scalp.
2. Head is scanned in two planes simultaneously and at various angles. Each image is a specific layer of brain tissue.
3. The computer calculates tissue absorption in contiguous layers of brain tissue and diplays a printout. Selected photographs of the printouts are taken.
4. Tumor densities are compared with the normal brain tissue. (Tumors, infarctions, bone displacement, and the ventricles are well visualized.)
5. If a contrast study is desired, the patient receives the contrast medium and the scanning process is repeated.

After procedure

1. No adverse effects except the risk of transient increased intracranial pressure in patients with masses or other brain pathology.
2. Plan period of rest as needed for the patient.

Magnetic resonance imaging (MRI)

Purpose

Detection of cerebral and spinal cord pathology using a technique of scanning using magnetic forces to image body structures

Preparation of patient

1. No special physical preparation
2. Patient teaching
   a. Explain procedure
   b. Time: approximately 45 to 60 minutes
   c. Sensation: Procedure is painless, except for discomfort in lying still and possible feelings of claustrophobia as a result of head being positioned in head holder
   d. Patient must maintain motionless position until scan is completed
   e. Machine makes different noises during procedure that could startle patient
   f. Because scan involves a magnetic force, patient should remove all credit cards, watches, or other metal from clothing before entering scan room
3. Patient should be questioned about presence of metal in body (orthopedic appliances, aneurysm clips, pacemakers)

Procedure

1. Patient lies supine with the head positioned in a head holder.
2. Machine slowly scans parts of the brain or spinal cord. Images appear on a monitoring screen.
3. Magnetic field is used to measure the activity of the tissues.

After procedure

1. No adverse effects

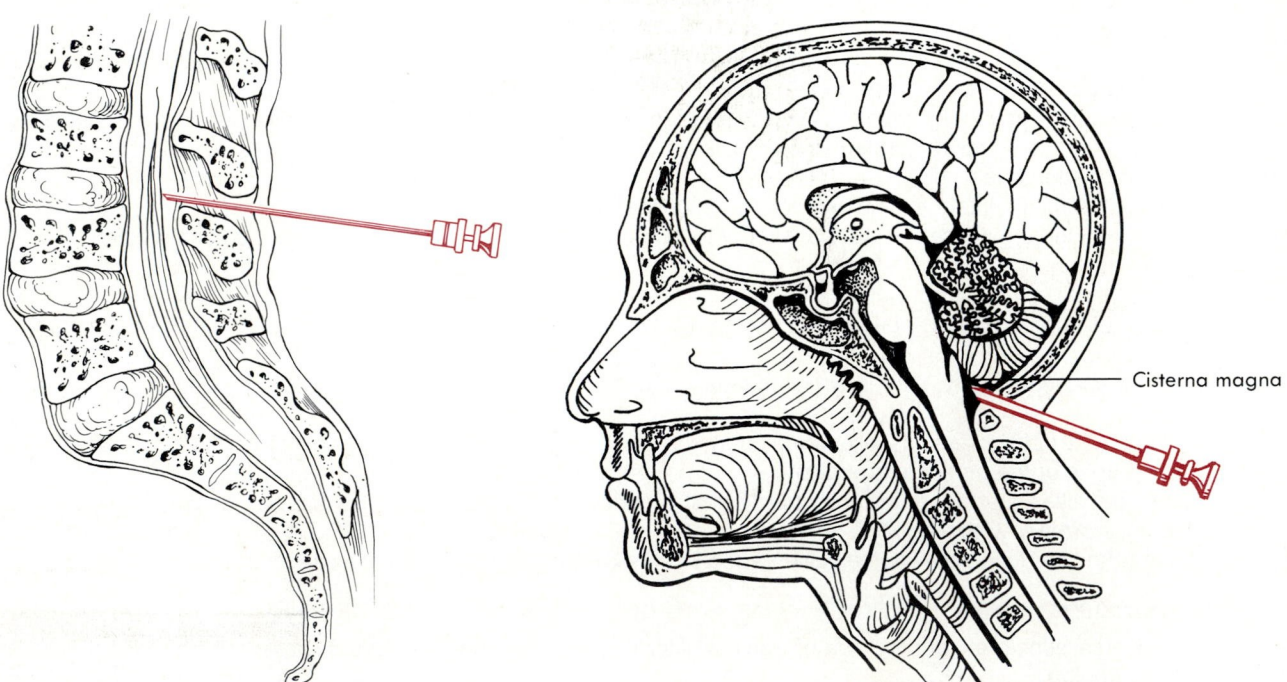

Fig. 19-21 Position and angle of needle when lumbar puncture is performed. Note that needle is in fourth lumbar interspace below level of spinal cord.

Fig. 19-22 Cisternal puncture. Position of needle when cisternal puncture is performed. Note needle length and short bevel.

Cisterna magna

Lumbar puncture

Purpose

To obtain cerebrospinal fluid (CSF) for examination or relief of pressure.

Preparation of patient

1. Usually a permit is signed by patient or family member.
2. Occasionally sedation is given before procedure.
3. Patient teaching
   a. Explain procedure
   b. Time: approximately 10 to 15 minutes.
   c. Sensation: slight pain and pressure may be felt as the dura is entered. A sharp shooting pain down one leg may be felt, caused by the needle coming close to a nerve.
   d. Other: Remind patient to lie still and not to move suddenly.

Procedure

1. Patient is usually positioned on the side with both knees and head flexed at an acute angle to allow maximum lumbar flexion and separation of interspinous spaces. Occasionally patients may be positioned sitting up and leaning over the bedside table.
2. Local anesthetic is usually used to anesthetize the lumbar area.
3. Under strict aseptic technique the needle is inserted below the level of the spinal cord at the L4-L5 or L5-S1 interspace (Fig. 19-21).
4. Inner needle is removed to allow drainage and measurement of spinal fluid.
5. Level of fluid column in manometer used to measure pressure is read.
6. Fluid is collected for various tests or to relieve pressure. Occasionally the first specimen of spinal fluid contains blood from slight bleeding at the site of puncture. This specimen should not be sent for cell count.
7. *Queckenstedt's test* may be performed to test for subarachnoid block. The jugular veins are compressed for 10 seconds, first on one side, then on the other side, and then on both sides at the same time. Any change in spinal fluid pressure during the compression is noted.
8. Needle is withdrawn.

After procedure

1. Patient lies flat in bed for several hours.
2. Site of puncture should be observed for any leakage of CSF.
3. Headache is fairly common and is thought to be caused by the loss of spinal fluid through the dura mater. The sharpness and size of the needle, the skill of the physician, whether the patient lies flat, and the patient's emotional state may determine if a headache occurs.
4. Headaches are usually treated with bed rest, analgesics, and ice applied to the head.

Cisternal puncture

Purpose

To obtain CSF for examination, or for instillation of contrast medium for diagnostic studies

Preparation of patient

1. Usually a permit for surgery is signed.
2. Back of patient's neck may be shaved.
3. Procedure is performed in the patient's bed or in treatment room.
4. Patient is positioned in a side-lying position at the edge of the bed or treatment table with the head bent forward.
5. Patient teaching
   a. Same as for lumbar puncture.
   b. Procedure may be more frightening to the patient because of the close proximity of the procedure to the brain.

Procedure

1. Same as for lumbar puncture except for different site (between C1 and base of skull).
2. Head of patient should be held firmly during procedure so it does not rotate.

After procedure

1. Patient observed immediately for dyspnea, apnea, or cyanosis.
2. Headache occurs less frequently than with lumbar puncture.

Brain scan

Purpose

Detection of cerebral pathology using radioactive isotopes and a scanner.

Preparation of patient

1. No physical preparation of patient.
2. When mercury is used as the isotope indicator, a mercurial diuretic (meralluride [Mercuhydrin]) is administered several hours before the procedure. This allows a greater concentration of radioactive mercury to be circulated to brain tissue, since melluride minimizes the uptake of mercury by the kidneys.
3. Patient teaching
   a. Explain procedure.
   b. Time: approximately 45 minutes for the actual scan.
   c. Sensation: minimal discomfort associated with the IV administration of the radioactive iosotope. Some patients may find it uncomfortable to lie still for the scan.

Procedure

1. Patient is injected with radioisotope (mercury or sodium pertechnetate Tc 99m)
2. While patient lies still, usually in supine position, scanner is passed over head. This picks up concentrated areas of uptake. Several scans are taken.

After procedure

1. No adverse effects.
2. Plan period of rest as needed for the patient.

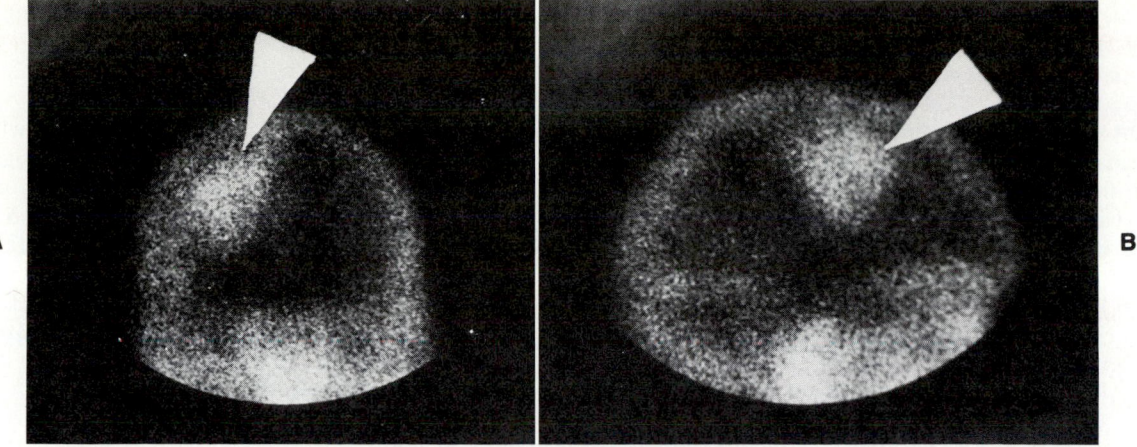

Fig. 19-23 Brain scans. **A,** Anteroposterior view. **B,** Lateral view. White pointers indicate tumor seen in both views. (From Pagana, K: Diagnostic testing and nursing implications: a case study approach, St. Louis, 1982, The CV Mosby Co.)

→ DATA ANALYSIS: NURSING DIAGNOSES

Nursing diagnoses are determined from assessment of patient data. Possible nursing diagnoses for the person with headache may include, but are not limited to, the following:

Diagnostic title	Possible etiologies
Anxiety	Threat/change in health status/ role functioning/situational/ maturational crisis
Pain	Headache
Ineffective individual coping	Situational crises, maturational crises
Knowledge deficit	Lack of exposure, information misinterpretation, cognitive limitation, lack of interest in learning, unfamiliarity with information sources
Self-care deficit	Pain/discomfort, depression, severe anxiety
Sleep pattern disturbance	Pain/discomfort, anxiety

PLANNING: EXPECTED PATIENT OUTCOMES

Expected patient outcomes for the person with headache may include, but are not limited to, the following:
1. Anxiety is decreased.
2. Headache pain is decreased.
3. Patient can explain prescribed medication (dosage, action, side effects, and frequency).
4. Patient demonstrates improved coping mechanisms.
5. Patient can demonstrate prescribed relaxation techniques.
6. Patient can explain the importance of continuing medical supervision for chronic headache.
7. Patient can carry out ADLs with minimal difficulty.

8. Patient can identify any factors that trigger headache.
9. Patient can explain the danger of continued use of over-the-counter drugs for chronic, recurring headache.
10. Patient is able to sleep 6 hours per night.

IMPLEMENTATION

☐ **Assisting with achievement of therapeutic goals**
☐ *Medications*

Treatment for headache often includes the use of selected medications. These will be described in terms of their use for migraine, cluster, and tension headaches.

MIGRAINE HEADACHES. *Acetylsalicylic acid* (aspirin) is seldom effective for classic migraine but may be helpful after the headache has developed. *Ergotamine tartrate* preparations taken early in the attack may prevent the headache from developing. These drugs are the treatments of choice in migraine, and their success in relieving the headache is often considered diagnostic of migraine. Ergotamine tartrate preparations act by constricting cerebral blood vessel walls, thus reducing cerebral blood flow. It may be administered orally, sublingually, or rectally in 2 to 4 mg dosages. It is also available for injection in 0.25 to 0.5 mg dosages. Ergot preparations are also available in combination with other drugs such as *caffeine, phenobarbital,* and *belladonna.* Ergot preparations have the side effects of nausea, vomiting, numbness and tingling, muscle pain, and changes in heart rate. They also stimulate uterine smooth muscle, so they cannot be taken by pregnant women. Other drugs that may be substituted include nonnarcotic analgesics, such as *phenacetin, acetaminophen,* or *propoxyphene (Darvon),* as well as narcotics, such as *codeine. Propranolol hydrochloride (Inderal)* has been used to prevent migraine headaches with limited success. Methysergide maleate (Sansert) has been used in the prophylactic treatment of migraine and other vascular headaches.

CLUSTER HEADACHES. Because the pain associated with cluster headaches is so severe, narcotic analgesics are often prescribed during the acute attack. Often these must be administered intramuscularly for optimal relief.

Patients with cluster headaches usually feel fine between attacks, so no analgesia is needed during these times.

TENSION HEADACHES. The nonnarcotic analgesics are often prescribed for tension headaches. These include acetaminophen, propoxyphene, phenactin, and acetylsalicylic acid. Narcotic analgesics such as codeine may be prescribed along with diazepam (Valium) for relief of tension. It is far better, however, to counsel the patient to develop other ways to relieve the headache.

☐ Promotion of rest and relaxation

Since stress and emotional upsets may precipitate some headaches and make others worse, measures are taken to facilitate relaxation and rest. Relaxation techniques (Chaper 8), planned sleeping hours, and rest periods as needed may prove helpful. Because alcohol has been found to be significant in causing cluster headaches, it should not be used as a way to relieve tension.

Some patient who have tension headaches have found relaxation by regular physical exercise to be helpful.

☐ Dietary counseling

It may be helpful to educate the patient about foods that may cause headaches or make them worse. These include those containing tyramine, nitrates, or glutamate. For example, MSG is often present in Chinese cooking. Other foods that may provoke headache are included in the following list:

1. Vinegar
2. Chocolate
3. Yogurt
4. Alcohol
5. Fermented or marinated foods
6. Ripened cheeses
7. Herring
8. Cured sandwich meats
9. Excessive caffeine
10. Pork

☐ Psychotherapy

Patients with chronic headaches may respond to psychotherapy. It may be used to help the patient develop awareness of stressors, as well as to deal with feelings about being the victim of headache pain.

☐ Assisting with comfort and ADL

Other treatments that have been found to be helpful with headache include cold packs applied to the forehead or base of the brain. Pressure applied to the temporal and carotid arteries may be helpful depending on the cause of the headache. Patients who are having migraine headaches, especially, may be most comfortable lying in a dark room with minimal auditory stimulation.

☐ Identification of triggering factors

Discovery of triggering factors associated with severe recurring headaches will need to be made through ongoing assessment of the person's personality, habits, and ADL. Clues may be obtained from seeking information about the person's goals and aspirations, work habits, family relationships, coping mechanisms, and the relaxation patterns. The person may be asked to keep a diary of activities and the occurrence of headaches, as well as the nature of the headaches and how they were treated. Triggering factors may include the following:

1. Fatigue
2. Alcohol
3. Stress
4. Climatic changes
5. Hunger
6. Menstruation
7. Allergies

■ Teaching

Teaching is an important part of nursing care of the patient with head pain. The box below lists appropriate teaching activities.

⊞ EVALUATION

Evaluation of headaches is based on the nursing outcomes and should be done in conjunction with the patient. Questions to ask include the following:

1. Is the use of medication within medical guidelines?
2. Is the patient keeping follow-up appointments?
3. Is the patient functioning optimally?
4. Is the patient following medical advice?
5. Is the patient able to sleep?
6. Is pain decreased?

Teaching for the patient with headache

1. Avoid factors found to trigger or increase headache.
2. Use relaxation measures (such as biofeedback) when emotional tension is present.
3. Maintain regular sleep patterns.
4. Take medications as ordered—be aware of their side effects and report these to physician.
5. Follow up with medical care as indicated.
6. Allows others to assist with activities during headaches.
7. Structure home and work environment to keep stressors at a reasonable level.

■ Neurologic pain

■ PATHOPHYSIOLOGY

Neurologic pain other than headache is commonly seen in nursing. It it sometimes difficult to distinguish between pain produced by lesions within the nervous system that cause objective sensory abnormalities and peripherally produced, somatic pain in a distant organ (see the box below). Although in practice pain may be viewed from the standpoint of neural transmission, the transmission of pain impulses is not fully understood. Neurologic pain may arise from lesions involving peripheral cutaneous nerves, the sensory nerve roots, the thalamus, and the central pain tract (spinothalamic) at some level (Fig. 19-24). Pain receptors are not adaptable. Pain impulses continue at the same rate as long as the stimulus is present. They are specific for pain only. Pain receptors can be activated by the following:

1. Cellular damage
2. Certain chemicals such as histamine
3. Heat
4. Ischemia
5. Muscle spasms
6. Sensations of heat, cold, and itching that go beyond a specific level of intensity

Pain that is described as unbearable and does not respond to treatment is classified as *intractable*. It is chronic and often disabling.

ASSESSMENT

Both subjective and objective data are important to assess in the patient with neurologic pain. Again, it should be remembered that pain is highly subjective, and there may not be a great deal of objective data to accompany the subjective complaints.

□ Subjective data

1. Patient's understanding of the pain
2. Any precipitating factors
3. Measures that relieve symptoms, including medication
4. Site, frequency, and nature of pain
5. Usual coping patterns when under stress
6. Presence of associated symptoms
7. Measures that make pain worse

□ Objective data

1. Behavior: signs indicating pain or stress
2. Change in ability to carry out ADL
3. Muscle weakness or wasting

Site of problem and resulting neurologic pain

Site of problem	Results	Characteristics of pain
Peripheral cutaneous nerves	Pain usually limited to anatomic area supplied by affected nerve or nerves	Often described as burning sensation, but can be described as sharp or dull and aching Pain may be constant or permanent Often described as severe Also called local pain
Root pain	Limited to dermatomes supplied by affected sensory nerve roots (pain from lesion arising from deep somatic and visceral stimulus may radiate beyond dermatomes) (Fig. 20-8)	Aggravated by anything that causes direct or indirect movement of spinal cord (sneezing, coughing, or straining)
Central lesion within thalamus	Pain confined to contralateral side of body	Pain described as burning, pulling, and swelling Often aggravated by emotional stress and fatigue Influenced by cutaneous stimulation
Central spinothalamic tract	Pain sensation distributed to level of tract involved Hemisection of spinal cord produces loss of pain and temperature sensation on contralateral side at a level one or two segments below injury	May be similar to thalamic pain, but less disturbing

4. <mark>Vasomotor responses (flushing, for example)</mark>
5. <mark>Spinal reflexes and sensory examination</mark>

The quality of pain and its distribution are important factors to assess. Pain may vary from mild to excruciating. Terms with which the nurse should be familiar include those listed in the box on p. 429.

As stated earlier, neurologic pain may arise from lesions involving peripheral cutaneous nerves, the sensory nerve

roots (posterior), the thalamus, and the central pain tract. Each of these sources produces characteristic pain.

□ **Diagnostic tests**

It is extremely difficult to evaluate pain objectively. Electrical stimulation may be attempted to define the pain to a greater extent. The person with intractable pain may undergo psychologic testing as part of the workup. Tests

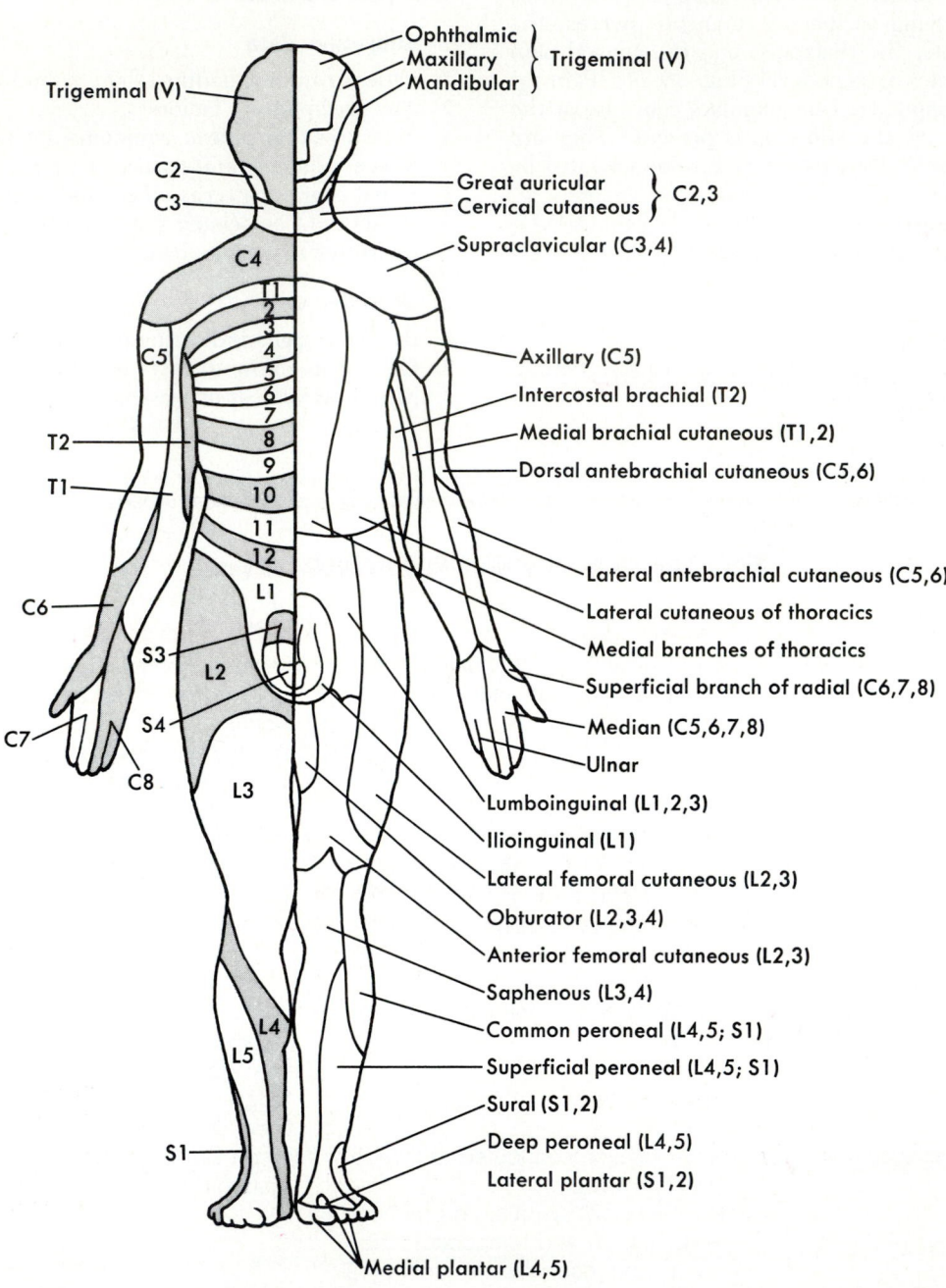

Fig. 19-24 Peripheral distribution of sensory nerve fibers, anterior view. *Right,* distribution of cutaneous nerves. *Left,* dermatomes (shaded) or segmental distribution of cutaneous nerves.

Types of pain sensation

Paresthesia	Abnormal sensation
Hyperalgesia	Increased pain sensation
Hypoalgesia	Decreased pain sensation
Analgesia	Blocked pain sensation
Dysesthesia	Pain sensation caused by stimulus that normally would not be painful
Referred pain	Pain that occurs in a site other than its origin
Causalgia	Intense, continuous, burning pain
Local pain	Occurring as a result of direct stimulation of pain receptors

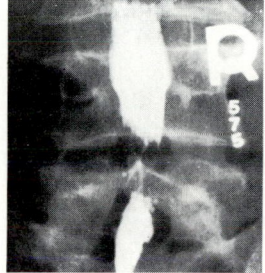

Fig. 19-25   Myelogram showing almost complete block in interspace between fourth and fifth lumbar vertebrae. (From Moseley, HF (editor): Textbook of surgery, ed 3, St. Louis, 1959, The CV Mosby Co.)

to rule out causes of the pain may be indicated, including the myelogram (see the box on p. 430). This is commonly done when back pain is present (Fig. 19-25).

DATA ANALYSIS: NURSING DIAGNOSES

Nursing diagnoses are determined from assessment of patient data. Possible nursing diagnoses for the person with neurologic pain may include, but are not limited to, the following:

Diagnostic title	Possible etiologies
Anxiety	Threat/change in health status
Chronic pain	Chronic physical/psychosocial disability
Ineffective individual coping	Situational crises
Impaired home maintenance management	Individual disease/injury, inadequate support systems

Diagnostic title	Possible etiologies
Knowledge deficit	Lack of exposure/recall
Impaired physical mobility	Intolerance to activity/decreased strength and endurance, pain/discomfort, neuromuscular impairment
Sleep pattern disturbance	Pain/discomfort

PLANNING: EXPECTED PATIENT OUTCOMES

Expected patient outcomes for the person with neurologic pain may include, but are not limited to, the following:
1. Patient's pain is decreased.
2. Patient demonstrates minimal difficulty in carrying out ADL.
3. Patient demonstrates physical methods that can be used for pain control.
4. Patient describes positioning methods and their relationship to pain.
5. Patient explains the relationship between pain and emotional upsets.
6. Patient demonstrates minimal anxiety.
7. Patient states the plan for follow-up care.
8. Patient explains medications to be taken, including dosage, action, side effects, and frequency.
9. Patient demonstrates good management of sleep and rest patterns.
10. Patient demonstrates improved coping mechanisms.
11. Patient has minimal restrictions in physical mobility.
12. Patient demonstrates ability to maintain home.

IMPLEMENTATION

☐ Assisting with achievement of therapeutic goals
☐ *Medications*

Treatment for patients with neurologic pain may include the use of medications. These often include the nonnarcotic analgesics—acetaminophen, propoxyphene (Darvon), phenacetin, and acetylsalicylic acid. Narcotic analgesics such as codeine may be prescribed along with diazepam (Valium) or amitriptyline hydrochloride (Elavil). The emphasis should be on helping the patient learn other measures to control pain.

☐ *Promotion of rest and relaxation*

As with headache, stress and emotional upsets may precipitate neurologic pain or make it worse. Rest and relaxation should be facilitated. Relaxation techniques, planned sleeping hours, and rest periods throughout the day may be helpful. Relaxation techniques used include biofeedback and meditation.

Some patients with pain, especially pain defined as intractable, may respond well to psychotherapy. It can help the patient develop awareness of stressors and how they influence the perception of pain.

Myelogram (metrizamide and Pantopaque)

Purpose

To identify lesions in the intradural or extradural compartments of the spinal canal by observing the flow of radiopaque dye through the subarachnoid space.

Preparation of patient

1. Permit must be signed.
2. If metrizamide dye is to be used the patient should not take the following drugs for 24 to 48 hours before the test:
    a. Phenothiazines
    b. Tricyclic antidepressants
    c. CNS stimulants
    d. Amphetamines
3. With metrizamide dye, fluids are encouraged.
4. Lower extremity strength and sensation should be assessed for baseline.
5. Patient teaching
    a. Explain procedure.
    b. Time: approximately 2 hours.
    c. Sensation: slight pain and pressure may be felt as dura is entered. Some patients find varied positions they must assume during procedure uncomfortable.

Procedure

1. Patient is usually positioned on the side with both knees and head flexed at an acute angle to allow maximum lumbar flexion and separation of interspinous spaces. Cisternal puncture may also be done (Fig. 20-6).
2. Local anesthetic is used to anesthetize the puncture site.
3. Under strict aseptic technique needle is inserted at L4-L5 or L5-S1 or cisternally.
4. Inner needle is removed to allow drainage, measurement of pressure, and collection of specimens.
5. Dye is instilled and needle removed.
6. Patient is turned to varied positions to visualize the spinal cord while fluoroscopic and radiologic films are taken.
7. After the procedure is completed, Pantopaque dye is removed via another lumbar puncture. Leaving it in would cause serious irritation to the meninges.
8. Metrizamide dye is water soluble and does not need to be removed.
9. With metrizamide dye the patient usually undergoes a CT scan of the spinal cord 4 to 6 hours after the myelogram.

After procedure

1. Pantopaque myelogram
    a. Patient lies flat in bed overnight.
    b. Site of puncture should be observed for leakage of CSF.
    c. Headache is fairly common.
    d. Strength and sensation of lower extremities should be assessed.
2. Metrizamide
    a. Patient's head and thorax must remain elevated 30° to 50° for at least 8 hours and then elevated at least 30° for 24 hours.
    b. Fluids are encouraged.
    c. Common side effects include nausea, vomiting, seizures (peak time of risk is 4 to 8 hours after procedure), and some nonspecific behavior changes.
    d. Strength and sensation of lower extremities should be assessed after procedure.
    e. Site of puncture should be assessed for leakage of CSF.
    f. Avoid drugs previously listed—they lower seizure threshold. (When nausea occurs after a metrizamide myelogram, prochlorperazine [Compazine] cannot be used. Drugs that may be used include benzquinamide [Emete-Con].)
    g. The advantages of metrizamide outweigh the risks. It is less viscous than iodine-based dye and therefore permits better visualization of smaller areas.

☐ *Nonsurgical methods of pain relief*

Neurologic pain has been found to respond to other methods of pain control. These include transcutaneous electrical nerve stimulators and spinal cord stimulators. Both use electrodes applied near the site of pain or on or around the spine. The goal is to modify the sensory input by blocking or changing the painful sensation with a stimulus that is perceived to be less painful or nonpainful.

Acupuncture has also been used to treat patients with neurologic pain. See Chapter 10 for a further explanation of these procedures.

☐ *Nerve block*

A nerve block involves the injection of a substance such as a local anesthetic or alcohol or phenol close enough to a nerve to block the conduction of impulses. It is used to treat chronic pain that may result from trigeminal neuralgia, cancer, or peripheral vascular disease.

☐ **Assisting with comfort and ADL**

Patients having neurologic pain may be extremely uncomfortable. The nurse should help the patient attain a position of comfort. For example, the patient with root pain should avoid movements that cause direct or indirect movement of the spinal cord. Significant nursing activities include the following:

1. Patient should not lie in a horizontal plane for long periods, as this causes tension or traction on the thoracic and sacral nerve roots.
2. Sitting may help to relieve tension on the nerve roots.
3. When moving a person with root pain, sharp flexion of the neck and extension of the legs should be avoided as much as possible.
4. Straining during bowel movements can intensify pain—stool softeners are often indicated

The identification of any triggering factors of neurologic pain is important. This can be done by a thorough assessment of personality, habits, and ADL. The person may be asked to keep a diary of ADL and the occurrence of the pain.

☐ *Surgery*

In cases of intractable pain that does not respond to medical and nursing actions, surgery may be necessary to reduce or abolish pain. Neurosurgical procedures that may be done include the following:

1. Neurectomy—interruption of the peripheral or cranial nerve supplying a specific part of the body. The nerve fibers to the affected area are severed from the cord. Fibers controlling movement and position sense are also interrupted. Cannot be used to control pain in the lower extremities.
2. Rhizotomy—resection of a posterior nerve root just before it enters the spinal cord. Cannot be used with pain in the lower extremities because position sense is lost. Involves a laminectomy.
3. Cordotomy—pain pathways in spinothalamic tract (anterior and lateral aspect of the cord) on the side opposite the cord are severed. This results in a wide

sense of analgesia, while other sensory and motor functions are preserved. In a percutaneous cordotomy, a spinal needle is inserted laterally between C1 and C2. A wire electrode is inserted into the lateral cord, and a lesion is made to destroy ascending pain fibers.

These procedures all have potential complications that must be considered before the decision is made to do surgery. For example, with cordotomy, the patient may expect to have problems with postural hypotension, temperature sensation, and possibly bladder and motor function. Also, patients may have a temporary paralysis or leg weakness and loss of bowel and bladder control that results from edema of the cord. Usually this disappears in several weeks.[80]

☐ **Counseling and teaching**

Teaching is an important part of nursing care for the patient with neurologic pain. Appropriate teaching activities are listed in the box above.

⊞ EVALUATION

Evaluation of the patient with peripheral nerve or intractable neurologic pain considers how the person is functioning in spite of the pain. Questions to consider include the following:

1. Is the use of medications within guidelines?
2. Is the patient following up with appointments?
3. Is the patient able to carry on normal functions?
4. Is the patient cooperating with medical advice?
5. Is the patient using physical methods to control the pain in a correct way?
6. Is the patient sleeping at least 6 hours a night?
7. Is the patient able to manage home maintenance activities?
8. Is the patient's mobility improved?
9. Is the patient showing little anxiety and good coping strategies?

Teaching for the patient with neurologic pain

1. Avoid factors that increase pain
2. Use relaxation measures such as biofeedback and meditation when emotional tension is present
3. Maintain regular rest and sleep pattern
4. Take medication as prescribed
5. Be aware of physical methods of controlling pain (such as positioning) and use them
6. Follow up with medical care as indicated
7. Structure home and work environment to keep stressors at a minimum

---

Causes of increased intracranial pressure

Space-occupying lesions that increase tissue volume

Cerebral contusions
Hematomas
Infarctions
Abscesses
Intracranial tumors

Cerebrospinal problems

Increase in production of cerebrospinal fluid
Blockage in ventricular system
Decreased absorption of cerebrospinal fluid

Cerebral edema

Use of contrast dye that changes homeostasis of brain
Overhydration with hypotonic solution
Aftereffects of trauma to brain

■ Increased intracranial pressure

■ PATHOPHYSIOLOGY

Increased intracranial pressure is a complex manifestation that is the consequence of multiple neurologic conditions. It often occurs suddenly and requires surgical intervention.

The contents of the skull, or cranial contents, are brain tissue, vascular tissue, and cerebrospinal fluid. The brain makes up 80% of the intracranial content, blood volume makes up 10%, and the cerebrospinal fluid makes up the remaining 10%.[23] Any increase in the volume of one of the cranial contents results in increased intracranial pressure, because the cranial vault is rigid, closed, and nonexpandable. Specific causes of increased intracranial pressure are listed in the box above.

An increase in any one of the cranial contents is usually accompanied by a reciprocal change in the volume of one of the others. Brain tissue cannot expand without serious effects in the flow and amount of cerebrospinal fluid and cerebral circulation. Space-occupying lesions displace and distort the brain and vacular tissues as pressure increases. The buildup of pressure may occur slowly (days or weeks) or rapidly, depending on the cause. At first, one hemisphere of the brain will be more involved, but eventually both hemispheres will be affected.

As pressure increases within the cranial cavity, it is at first compensated for by venous compression and cerebrospinal displacement. As the pressure continues to rise, the cerebral blood flow decreases and inadequate perfusion occurs. This inadequate perfusion initiates a vicious cycle causing the Pco_2 to increase and the Po_2 and the pH to fall. These changes cause vasodilation and cerebral edema. The edema further increases the intracranial pressure, causing increased compression of neural tissue and an even greater increase in intracranial pressure.

When the pressure exceeds the brain's ability to compensate, pressure is exerted on surrounding structures where the pressure is lower. This movement of pressure is called *supratentorial shift* and can result in two kinds of herniation. *Central* or *transtentorial herniation* is the downward displacement of the cerebral hemispheres through the tentorial notch. This compresses the diencephalon and brainstem. The other type of herniation is called *uncal herniation* and occurs when expanding masses in the middle fossa or temporal lobe shift over the lateral edge of the tentorium, pushing the uncus toward the midline.[11] As a result of herniation, the brainstem is compressed at variable levels, which in turn compresses the vasomotor center, the posterior cerebral artery, the oculomotor nerve, the corticospinal nerve pathway, and the fibers of the ascending reticular activating system (Fig. 19-26). The life-sustaining mechanisms of consciousness, blood pressure, pulse, respiration, and temperature regulation fail.

▦ ASSESSMENT

☐ Subjective data

1. Patient's understanding of condition
2. Presence of visual changes: diplopia or blurred vision
3. Ability to think
4. Presence of pain, especially headache
5. Ability to carry on daily activities
6. Presence of nausea

☐ Objective data

1. Level of consciousness
2. Pupillary signs
3. Vital signs
4. Focal motor or sensory signs
5. Presence of vomiting or hiccuping
6. Eye changes including papilledema
7. Speech patterns

The detection of increased intracranial pressure must occur early when it is still reversible and before the stage of decompensation. The ability to make accurate observations, to interpret observations intelligently, and to record observations carefully is the most important part of nursing care for patients with increased intracranial pressure.

☐ *Level of consciousness*

A decreasing level of consciousness is an early sign of increased intracranial pressure. Any change in the level of consciousness is one of the most important observations for the nurse to make, report, and record. Restlessness, disorientation, and lethargy may be the first signs seen.

The observations are recorded in terms of *behaviors* and

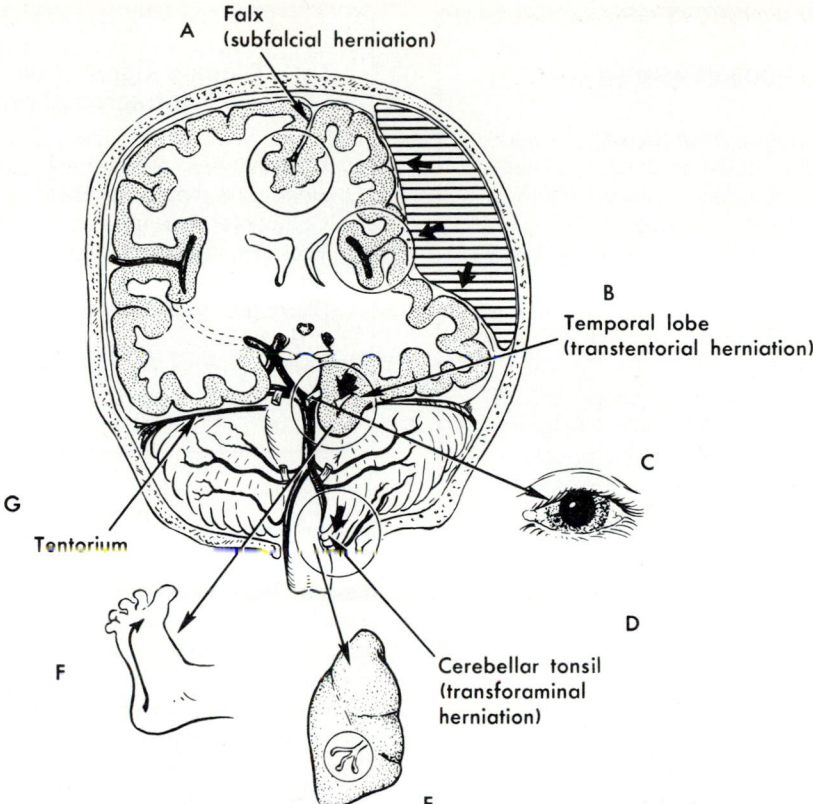

A
Falx
(subfalcial herniation)

B
Temporal lobe
(transtentorial herniation)

C

G

Tentorium

D

F

Cerebellar tonsil
(transforaminal
herniation)

E

Fig. 19-26 Consequences of increased intracranial pressure. Expanding temporoparietal epidural hematoma with medial and downward pressure has produced subfalcial, transtentorial, and transforaminal internal herniations. Note distortion of falx, *A,* bulging of medial temporal lobe at tentorial edge, *B,* and herniation of cerebellar tonsil with descending pressure on brainstem. *D.* Also note how major blood vessels are collapsed in encircled areas. Some consequential effects of continuing and/or expanding pressure on neural structure with alterations in body functions are detailed: *C,* homolateral dilation and fixation of pupil with ptosis of eyelid; *E,* life-threatening respiratory arrest through indirect effects on respiratory centers in brainstem; *F,* contralateral Babinski sign showing extension of great toe and fanning of other toes on plantar stimulation. (Coronal view of head, ventral view of brainstem.) (Modified from an original painting by Frank H Netter, MD; from Clinical symposia. Copyright by Ciba Pharmaceutical Co., Division of Ciba-Geigy Corp., Summit, N.J. All rights reserved.)

symptoms and not in terms of labels. Flow sheets that document neurologic changes in an objective way are helpful, especially when frequent neurologic checks are being done.

The Glasgow Coma Scale is another way to document the neurologic patient's condition. See p. 418 for a description of this tool. A description of levels of consciousness is presented in the box on p. 434.

☐ *Pupillary signs*

Pupil responses are controlled by cranial nerve III (the oculomotor nerve). This nerve carries sensory, motor, and parasympathetic fibers, as well as sympathetic fibers. As the brain herniates, the oculomotor nerve is compressed by the herniating tissue, the pupilloconstrictor fibers in the top part of the nerve being the first affected. The ipsilateral pupil (when the lesion is in one hemisphere) remains dilated and is incapable of constricting. The pupil appears larger than that of the affected side and does not react to light. As cerebral pressure increases and both hemispheres are affected, bilateral pupil dilation and fixation occur—the pupil may respond to light slowly. Dilating pupils are a sign of impending tentorial herniation. When pupils dilate or change in ability to react, the physician should be notified immediately. A pupil that is fixed and dilated is sometimes referred to as a "blown pupil" and is an ominous sign (Fig. 19-27).

Levels of consciousness

Alert	Responds appropriately to auditory, tactile, and visual stimuli
Loss of ability to abstract	Inattentiveness, slowed thinking, difficult to arouse
Confusion	Disorientation, inability to follow simple commands
Stupor	Responds to verbal commands with moaning or groaning, if at all
Semicomatose	Loss of ability to cooperate, responds only to pain—response may range from purposeful to decerebrate or decorticate
Comatose	Loss of ability to respond to any external stimuli and loss of all brain functions[12]

Classic signs of early increased intracranial pressure

Restlessness, disorientation, or lethargy
Headache may be present
Contralateral hemiparesis
Vital signs relatively stable
Pupils dilated ipsilaterally
Blurring of vision, decreased visual acuity, or diplopia
Vomiting usually not present
Normal temperature

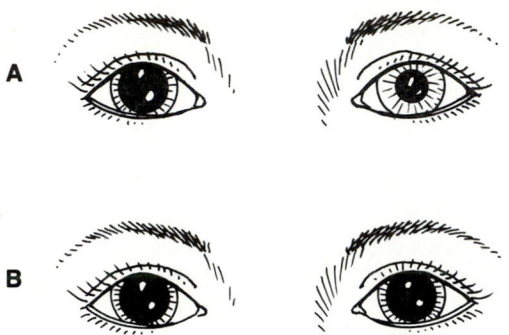

Fig. 19-27 **A,** Unequal pupils, also called anisocoria. **B,** Dilated and fixed pupils, indicative of severe neurological deficit.

□ Visual disturbances

Another sign of increased intracranial pressure that occurs fairly early is some type of visual disturbance. These may include *diplopia* or *blurring* or *decreased visual acuity*. Diplopia usually results from paralysis or weakness of one of the muscles that controls the eye movement.

Vomiting usually occurs in patients who have lesions below the tentorium. This vomiting usually occurs without the presence of nausea.

□ Blood pressure and pulse

The effect of increased intracranial pressure on pulse and blood pressure is variable. Compensatory changes occur in the cerebral vasculature relative to hypoxia. Herniation, however, causes ischemia of the vasomotor center. This excites the vasoconstrictor fibers, causing the systolic

blood pressure to rise. If the intracranial pressure continues to increase, blood pressure may fall, especially the diastolic blood pressure. An increased systolic blood pressure followed by a sharp drop in blood pressure is often seen as the patient's condition deteriorates.

Pressure in the vasomotor center also increases the transmission of parasympathetic impulses through the vagus nerve to the heart; as a result the pulse rate slows. Slowing of the pulse rate in conjunction with a rising systolic blood pressure is a significant observation that should be reported. For consistency, blood pressure and pulse should be taken in the same arm.

A widened pulse pressure, increased systolic blood pressure, and bradycardia are together referred to as *Cushing's response*. It is considered an important diagnostic characteristic of late-stage increased intracranial pressure.[23]

It is important to assess the trend of blood pressure and pulse. Indications of Cushing's response should be reported immediately.

□ Headaches

The patient with increased intracranial pressure (ICP) may complain of a headache. It is thought to result from venous congestion and the tension in the intracranial blood vessels as the cerebral pressure rises. The location and duration of the headache should be elicited from the patient. Headache that occurs with increased intracranial pressure usually increases in intensity with coughing, straining at stool, or stooping. Headache is usually present in the early morning and may awaken the patient from sleep.

It is important to realize that patients do not always complain of headache. Even if they do, the complaints may be vague and uncertain (see the box above for signs of ICP). As the intracranial pressure increases, the headache usually becomes worse.

□ Respiration

Herniation produces respiratory dysrhythmias that are variable and related to the level of the brainstem compression or failure. The breathing pattern may be deep and stertorous or periodic (Cheyne-Stokes) respirations. Another breathing pattern found with increased intracranial pressure is *ataxic breathing*. This is an irregular and unpredictable breathing pattern with random shallow and deep breaths and occasional pauses. This type of breathing is seen in patients with medullary damage.[23] As intracranial pressure increases to fatal levels, respiratory paralysis occurs. The beginning of periods of apnea is significant. It is important to remember that the patient with a decreased level of consciousness will require assistance in keeping the airway clear. Persons with acute increased intracranial pressure require supplemental oxygen to prevent hypoxia, which can further increase intracranial pressure.

□ Temperature

Failure of the thermoregulatory center because of compression occurs later with increased intracranial pressure and gives rise to high, uncontrolled temperatures. Hyperthermia must be controlled because it increases the metabolism of brain tissue.

□ Focal motor and sensory symptoms

Compression of the upper motor neuron pathway (corticospinal tract) interrupts transmission of impulses to the lower motor neuron, and progressive muscle weakness occurs. This often begins with the presence of drift and may progress to hemiparesis and hemiplegia. *Drift* is tested by asking the patient to close the eyes and extend the arms straight out in front for about 30 seconds. If one arm is weakened, it will drift downward without the patient being aware of it. Testing of the lower extremities includes the ability to push and pull against the tester, the ability to dorsiflex and plantar flex the feet, and the ability to do straight leg raises.

The presence of the *Babinski sign, hyperreflexia,* and *rigidity* are additional signs of decreased motor function. Seizures may occur. Herniation of the upper part of the brainstem produces *decerebrate rigidity* (fixed posture with arms, legs, and trunk extended and with flexion of the palms and plantar joints) or *decorticate rigidity* (fixed posture with flexion of the arm, wrist, and fingers, with adduction of the arm and extensors and internal rotation of the legs) (see Fig. 19-28). The worsening of existing motor defects is significant, and such signs should be reported to the physician.

□ Papilledema

The *blind spot* of the retina measures the size and shape of the optic papilla or optic disk. As intracranial pressure increases, the pressure is transmitted to the eyes through the cerebrospinal fluid and to the optic disk. Because the meninges of the brain reflect out around the eyeball, they permit the direct transmission of pressure along the spaces through the cerebrospinal fluid. As the optic disk swells, the retina is also compressed. The damaged retina cannot detect light rays. Visual acuity is lessened as the blind spot enlarges (Fig. 19-29).

Papilledema is also referred to as *choked disk,* which is caused by the engorgement of the retinal veins.

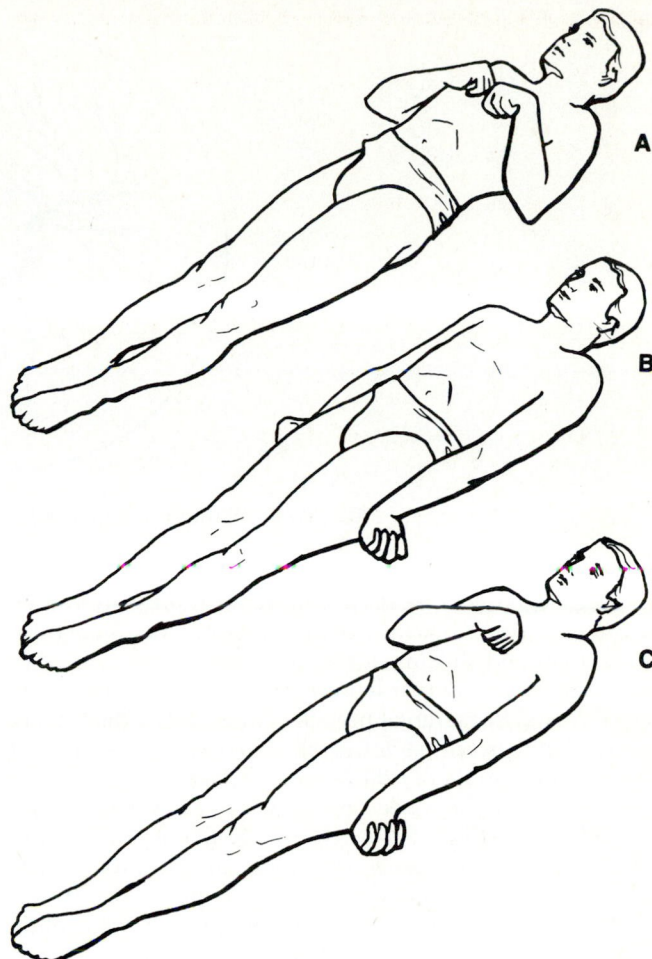

Fig. 19-28 Decorticate and decerebrate responses. **A,** Decorticate response. Flexion of arms, wrists, and fingers with adduction in upper extremities. Extension, internal rotation, and plantar flexion in lower extremities. **B,** Decerebrate response. All four extremities in rigid extension, with hyperpronation of forearms and plantar extension of feet. **C,** Decorticate response on right side of body and decerebrate response on left side of body. (From Zschoche, D: Mosby's comprehensive review of critical care, ed 3, St. Louis, 1985, The CV Mosby Co.)

□ Vomiting

Projectile vomiting may be associated with increased intracranial pressure. The significance of vomiting and its frequency and character must be associated with other clinical signs.

□ Hiccuping

Compression of the vagus nerve (cranial nerve X) causes spasmodic contraction of the diaphragm. This compression occurs as brainstem herniation occurs. Hiccuping in a patient who is at risk for increased intracranial pressure or who has other symptoms should be reported to the physician immediately.

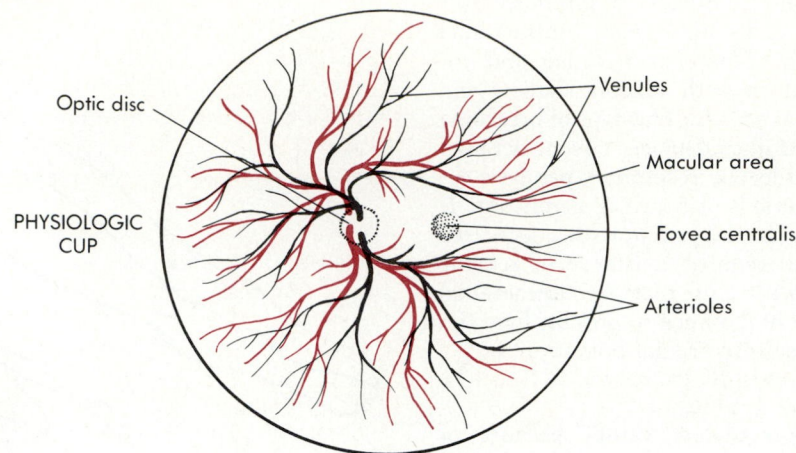

Optic disc

Venules

Macular area

PHYSIOLOGIC CUP

Fovea centralis

Arterioles

Fig. 19-29 Structures of the left eye as visualized through the funduscope.

□ **Diagnostic tests**

The diagnosis of increased intracranial pressure can be made with the CT scan, which can show actual structural herniation and shifting of the brain. The displacement of the brain to the right or left occurs at a relatively late stage of increased intracranial pressure. Most of the time, however, acute increased intracranial pressure is a medical emergency, and there is little time for diagnostic tests. The diagnosis must be made on the basis of observation and neurologic testing. Although the frequency of "neuro checks" is often ordered by the physician, the nurse should use judgment to decide whether more frequent assessments and recordings are indicated. The presence of even subtle changes may be very significant.

In some postoperative or critically ill patients internal measuring devices are used to diagnose increased intracranial pressure. One of the most common requires the placement of a hollow screw through the skull into the subarachnoid space. The screw is attached to a Luer-Lok, which is connected to a transducer and oscilloscope for continuous monitoring. The transducer is fastened level with the screw for accurate readings. A manometer may be attached for intermittent readings, or constant monitoring is available with the monitor.

It has become evident that the traditional clinical signs of increased intracranial pressure do not always correlate with the actual pressure changes as seen on the monitor. Many of the classic signs of increased pressure do not appear until the pressure has reached extremely high levels, and the chance to reverse the rising pressure and prevent permanent brain damage has already passed.

◗ **DATA ANALYSIS: NURSING DIAGNOSES**

Nursing diagnoses are determined from assessment of patient data. Possible nursing diagnoses for the person with increased intracranial pressure may include, but are not limited to, the following:

Diagnostic title	Possible etiologies
Ineffective airway clearance	Perceptual/cognitive impairment, trauma
Ineffective breathing pattern	Neuromuscular impairment
Impaired verbal communication	Physical impairment
Hyperthermia	Illness/trauma
Potential for injury: trauma	Sensorimotor deficits
Impaired physical mobility	Neuromuscular impairment
Pain	Increased intracranial pressure
Sensory/perceptual alterations	Altered sensory reception/transmission/integration
Altered thought processes	Neurologic disorder
Altered cerebral tissue perfusion	Decreased blood flow

◗ **PLANNING: EXPECTED PATIENT OUTCOMES**

Expected patient outcomes for the person with increased intracranial pressure may include, but are not limited to, the following:

1. Patient's airway is patent.
2. Patient has minimal pain.
3. Patient's breathing pattern is effective.
4. Patient's ability to communicate with others is maintained.
5. Patient maintains optimal levels of mobility.
6. Patient does not have an injury resulting from trauma.
7. Patient has minimal problems as a result of sensory-perceptual alterations.
8. Cerebral tissue pressure is adequate.
9. Cerebral edema is reduced.
10. Patient cooperates to a high degree with the therapeutic plan.

IMPLEMENTATION

☐ Assisting with achievement of therapeutic goals

The prevention of increased intracranial pressure may not be possible, but prevention of further rises in pressure and resulting damage to brain tissue is crucial. The detection of early signs is important to prevent irreversible effects.

The medical treatment of patients with increased intracranial pressure depends on the cause of the pressure. For example, if it is caused by an intracranial tumor, the tumor is removed surgically (p. 507). If surgery is not possible (or not indicated), efforts are made to reduce the pressure through the use of drug therapy or direct physical measures.

☐ *Mechanical decompression*

Rapidly rising intracranial pressure is often relieved by mechanical decompression. This may include a craniotomy, in which a bone flap is removed and then replaced or a craniectomy, in which the bone flap is removed and not replaced. This latter procedure is commonly performed to decompress the brain when pressure is high.

Other means of decompression may include continuous ventricular drainage or drainage of any subdural hematoma.

☐ *Medications*

The three types of drugs usually administered to patients with increased intracranial pressure are *osmotic diuretics, corticosteroids,* and *anticonvulsants.* Osmotic diuretics are also referred to as *hyperosmolar drugs.* They draw water from the edematous brain tissue. The traditional osmotic diuretic is mannitol. It starts to reduce increased intracranial pressure within 15 minutes and its effects last for 4 to 6 hours. It is important for the patient receiving this drug to have a Foley catheter in place because of the large amounts of urine that usually are produced. Glycerol is another osmotic diuretic that is sometimes given, but it has the disadvantage of causing rebound swelling of brain tissue and must be given orally.

The corticosteroid most likely to be given is dexamethasone. An antacid may be given with it. Monitoring blood glucose levels is important because steroids can affect carbohydrate metabolism and glucose utilization.

Anticonvulsants are given to prevent seizures. Phenytoin (Dilantin) is the most commonly prescribed drug. It can be given intravenously but is not recommended to be given intramuscularly.

Narcotics and other drugs that cause respiratory depression are avoided.

☐ Conservative measures

Conservative measures to reduce venous volume may be implemented. The head of the bed is elevated to 30 to 45 degrees to promote venous return, and the neck is kept in a neutral position. Positioning to avoid flexion of the hips, waist, and neck is important. Rotation of the head, especially to the right, has been found to increase intracranial pressure. Any patient at risk from increased intracranial pressure is discouraged from doing any isometric exercise. Passive range of motion exercises are appropriate and will not increase systemic blood pressure because they are not resistive. Spacing of nursing activities is important in maintaining lower pressure levels.[31,32,63]

Fluid intake may also be restricted. When osmotic diuretics are administered, urine output must be carefully monitored. An indwelling catheter is often used. The Valsalva maneuver is eliminated to the extent it is possible because it causes increased intrathoracic pressure, which indirectly increases intracranial pressure. This includes not allowing the patient to become constipated or to strain during defecation. Suctioning should be performed only when necessary (and then with the patient well preoxygenated) because it causes coughing and gagging. Suctioning should not be performed at the same time as other procedures that could cause increased intracranial pressure.

Oxygen therapy via mask or cannula is administered to improve brain oxygenation. Endotracheal intubation may be necessary. With the use of controlled ventilation, the PCO_2 can be lowered to below normal, which causes a slightly alkalotic pH. The decrease in the PCO_2 and the increase in the pH will decrease vasodilation and thereby decrease intracranial pressure.

A hypothermia blanket may be necessary to control the patient's body temperature. Increased temperature may lead to accelerated brain damage. Care must be taken when using the blanket not to bring the patient's temperature down too quickly or to leave the blanket on for too long a period of time. The temperature of a neurologically impaired patient will tend to continue to decrease after the blanket is turned off.[23]

☐ Internal monitoring devices

Internal monitoring devices are being used more frequently to diagnose and monitor increased intracranial pressure. Three basic monitoring systems are used. These include the following:

1. Ventricular catheter—consists of cannula that is implanted through burr holes into the anterior horn of the lateral ventricle of the nondominant cerebral hemisphere. The catheter is connected to a transducer and recording device.
2. Subarachnoid bolt or screw—one of earliest methods is inserted through skull into the subdural or subarachnoid space. The screw is attached to a transducer and oscilloscope so that continuous monitoring may be done.
3. Epidural sensory—placement of a fiberoptic sensor in the epidural space through a burr hole in the skull. The sensor cable is connected to the monitor.

Monitoring produces pressure waves that can be evaluated to indicate pathology (Fig. 19-30).[45]

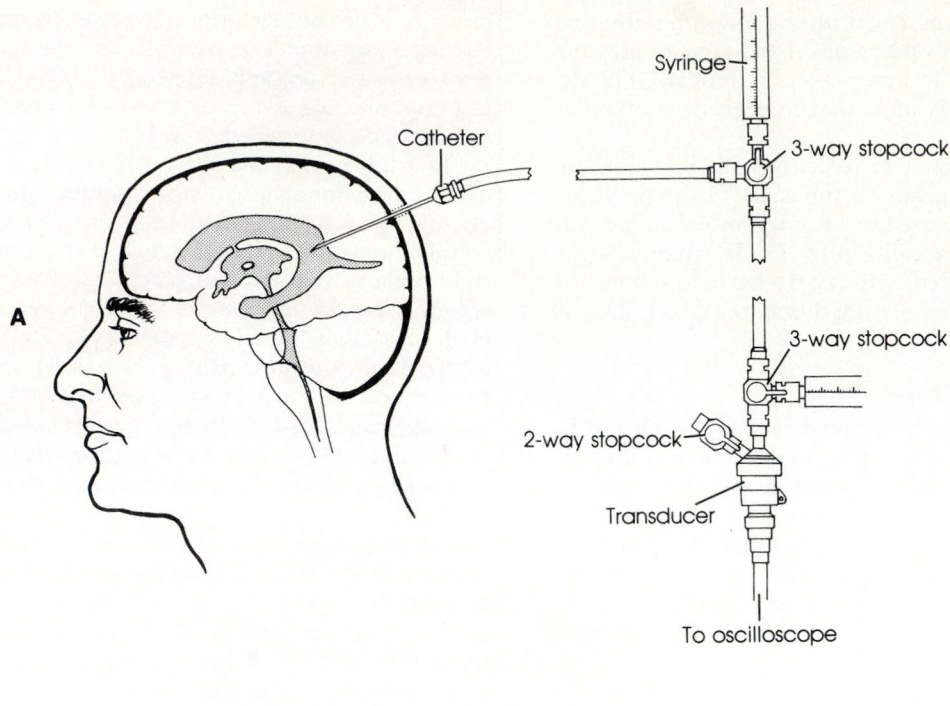

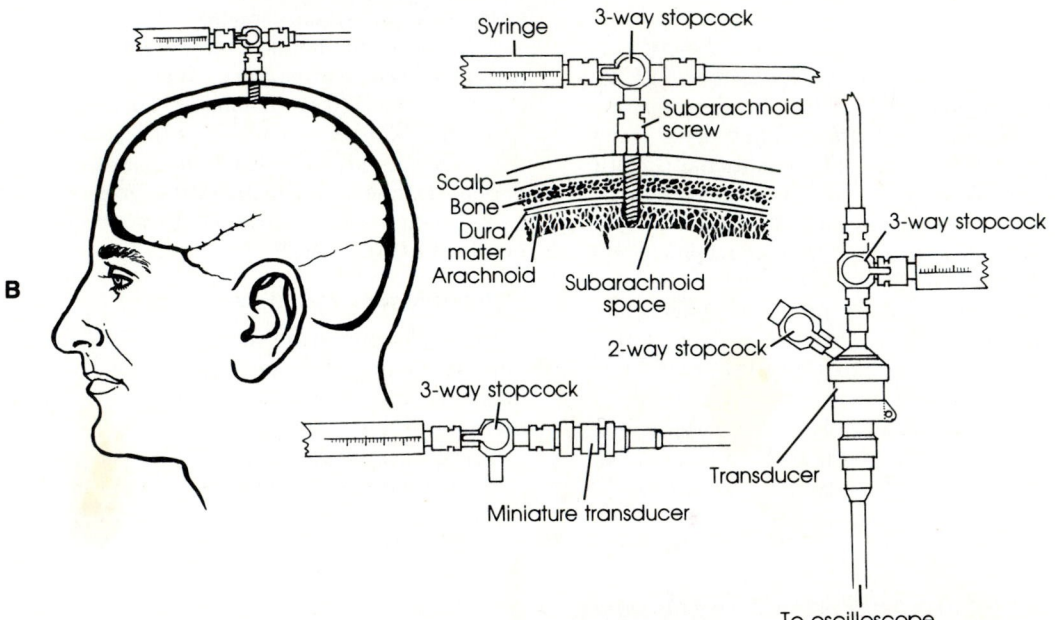

Fig. 19-30 Equipment for pressure monitoring. **A,** Ventricular pressure monitoring. Catheter is inserted through burr hole in skull into lateral ventricle and attached to transducer and oscilloscope to monitor intracranial pressure. **B,** Subarachnoid screw pressure monitoring. The subarachnoid screw is inserted through a burr hole in the skull and attached to a transducer and oscilloscope for continuous monitoring. (From Rudy, EB: Advanced neurological and neurosurgical nursing, St. Louis, 1984, The CV Mosby Co.)

⊞ EVALUATION

Evaluation of the patient with increased intracranial pressure includes frequent checks to evaluate neurologic status. Questions to ask include the following:

1. Is effective respiration occurring?
2. Are signs and symptoms of increased intracranial pressure decreased?
3. Is fluid intake limited and is careful measuring of intake and output occurring?
4. Are the patient and family being supported, and is the patient being kept as comfortable as possible?
5. Is the patient's safety monitored and in good control?
6. Are nursing measures being spaced in a way to avoid further increases in intracranial pressure?
7. Is the patient's temperature maintained?

■ Alterations in muscle tone and motor function

■ PATHOPHYSIOLOGY

Motor function disturbances are the most commonly encountered neurologic symptoms. Because the nervous system is designed primarily for the movement of the body in space and of the various parts in relation to each other, damage to it often causes serious problems in mobility. A loss of function, either motor or sensory, is called *paralysis*. A lesser degree of paralysis is called *paresis*. Damage to sensory pathways that are concerned with motor function may occur at the same time as the loss of motor function.

Injury or disease of motor neurons results in alterations

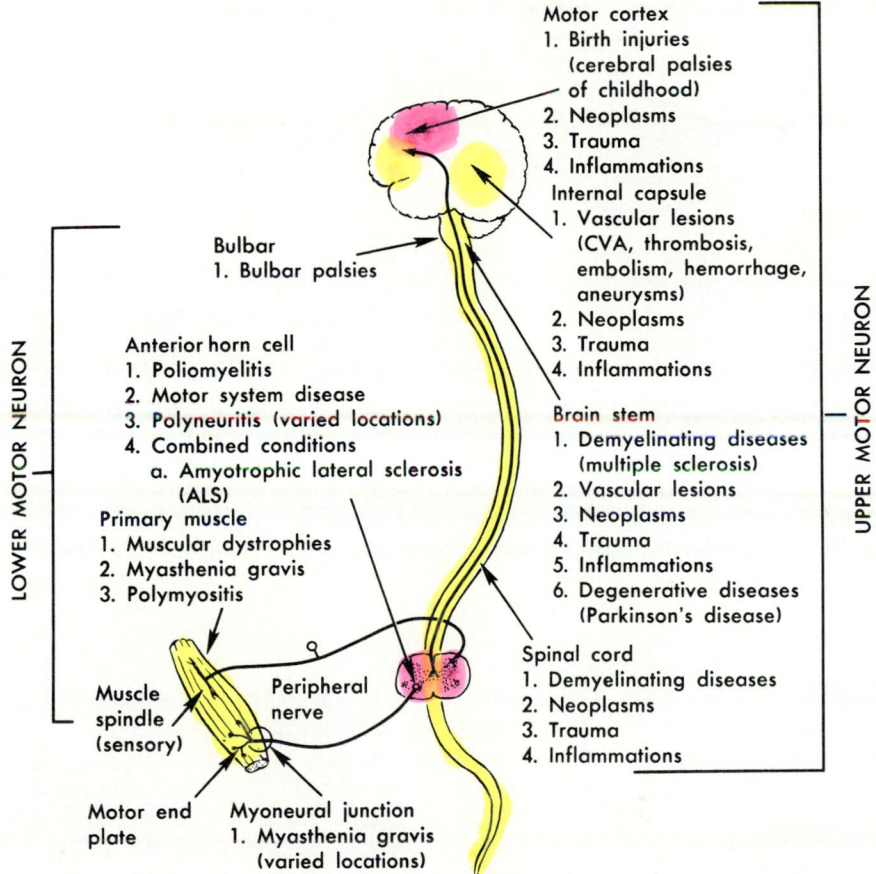

Fig. 19-31 Disturbances in motor function are classified pathologically along upper and lower motor neuron structures. It should be noted that the same pathologic condition occurs on more than one site in upper motor neuron shown on right. A few pathologic conditions involve both upper and lower motor neuron structures, as in amyotrophic lateral sclerosis, for example. Other lesion sites include myoneural junction and primary muscle, making it possible to classify conditions as neuromuscular and muscular, respectively. (Modified from Chusid, JG: Correlative neuroanatomy and functional neurology, ed 15, Los Altos, Calif, 1970, Lance Medical Publications.)

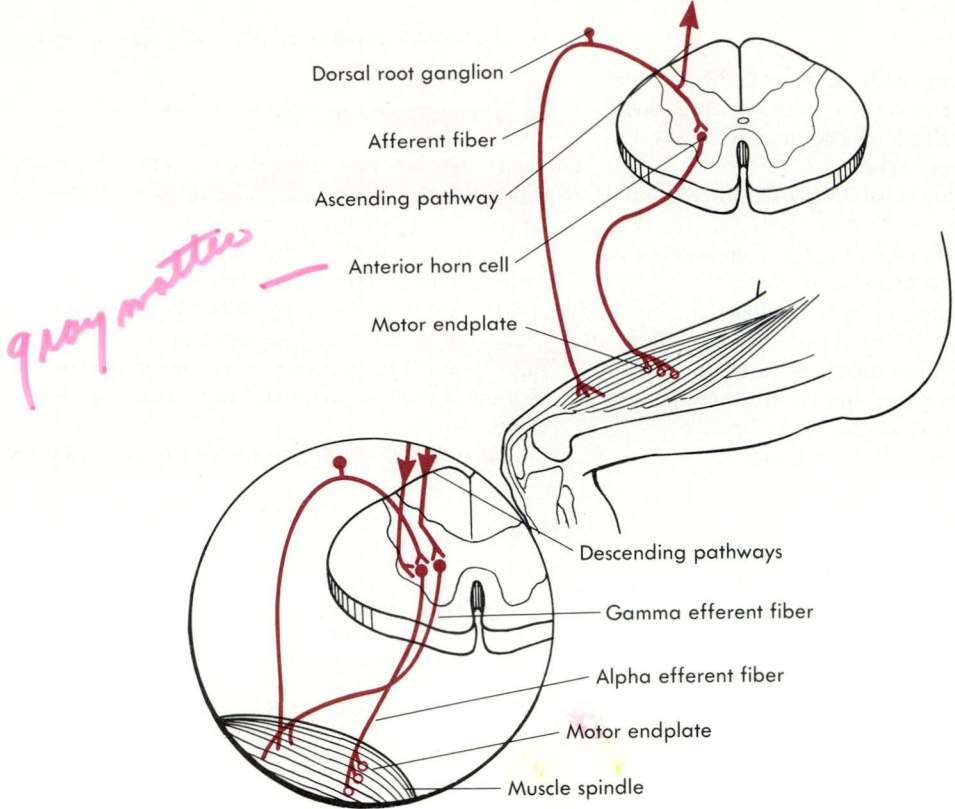

gray matter

Fig. 19-32 Structures making up lower motor neuron including motor (efferent) and sensory (afferent) elements. Shown on left is anterior horn cell in anterior gray column of spinal cord and its axon terminating in motor end-plate as it innervates extrafusal muscle fibers in quadriceps muscle. Detailed in enlargement are sensory and motor elements of γ-loop system. γ-Efferent fiber is shown innervating polar or end region of muscle spindle (sensory receptor of skeletal muscle). Contraction of muscle spindle fibers stretch central portion of spindle and cause afferent spindle fiber to transmit impulse centrally to cord. Muscle spindle afferent fibers in turn synapse on anterior horn cell and are transmitted by way of α-efferent fibers to skeletal (extrafusal) muscle, causing it to contract. Muscle spindle discharge is interrupted by active contraction of extrafusal muscle fibers. (Modified from Truex, RC, and Carpenter, MB: Human neuroanatomy, ed 6, Baltimore, 1969, The Williams & Wilkins Co.)

of muscle strength, tone, and reflex activity. The specific clinical manifestations differ according to whether the lesion involves an upper motor neuron or a lower motor neuron (Fig. 19-31).

□ Lower motor neuron signs

The lower motor neurons (LMNs) consist of a large anterior horn cell located in the gray matter of the spinal cord (Fig. 19-32). They are also found in the motor cranial nuclei of the brainstem. This anterior horn cell, in conjunction with the anterior spinal nerve and the peripheral nerve involved, forms a motor unit that affects skeletal muscle activity (voluntary and reflex). When a lesion selectively involves some part of the lower motor neuron, the results include the following:

1. Flaccid muscle weakness or paralysis
2. Loss of reflex activity
3. Loss of muscle tone
4. Atrophy confined to the involved muscle or muscles

The degree of muscle weakness is directly related to the extent and severity of the lesion.

The involved muscles become *flaccid* because the motor unit has been damaged and normal reflex activity has been interrupted. This flaccidity also is manifested in *hypotonia* and *hyporeflexia* and/or *areflexia* (reduced or absent muscle stretch reflexes). This interruption of the motor unit results in localized muscle atrophy or wasting. This atrophy also increases with nonuse of the muscle. In some LMN lesions, the affected muscle exhibits small localized, spontaneous, and involuntary contractions called *fasciculations*.

☐ Upper motor neuron signs

Upper motor neurons (UMNs) originate in the motor strip of the cerebral cortex and in multiple brainstem nuclei (Fig. 19-33). These axons then pass through the brainstem, deccusate (cross) in the medulla, and descend in the spinal cord via the corticospinal tracts. These fibers synapse with LMNs in the spinal cord. The collective working of both the UMN and LMN is essential for fine, orderly, and smooth muscle movements.

When an UMN lesion is rostral to the medulla, as in a cerebrovascular accident, deficits will occur contralateral to the lesion and will result in *hemiplegia*. The distribution or degree of paralysis is not always equal or the same within hemiplegic distribution. The following are upper motor neuron signs:

1. Paresis or paralysis of voluntary muscle tone and spasticity
2. Hyperreflexia
3. Late atrophy from disuse
4. Increased muscle tone

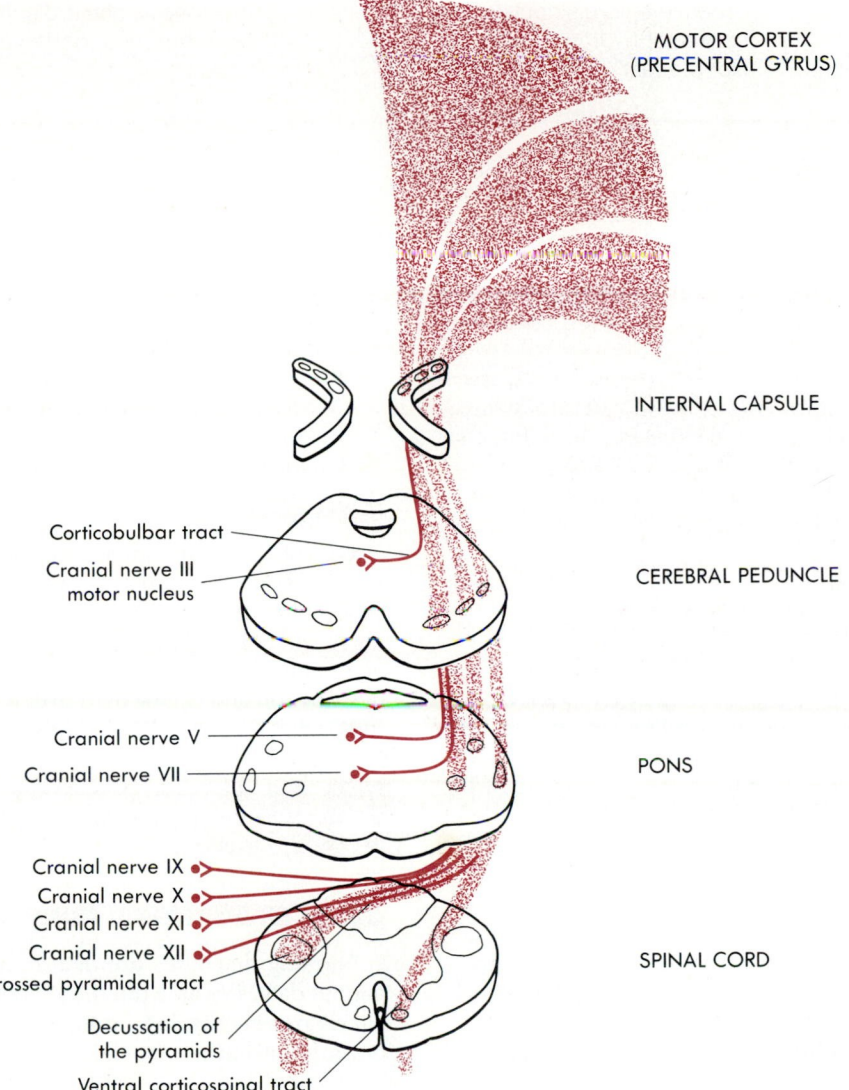

MOTOR CORTEX
(PRECENTRAL GYRUS)

INTERNAL CAPSULE

Corticobulbar tract

Cranial nerve III
motor nucleus

CEREBRAL PEDUNCLE

Cranial nerve V

Cranial nerve VII

PONS

Cranial nerve IX

Cranial nerve X

Cranial nerve XI

Cranial nerve XII

Crossed pyramidal tract

Decussation of
the pyramids

Ventral corticospinal tract

SPINAL CORD

Fig. 19-33 Structures making up upper motor neuron, or pyramidal system. Pyramidal system fibers are shown to originate primarily in cells in precentral gyrus of motor cortex; converge at internal capsule; descend to form central third of cerebral peduncle; descend further through pons, where small fibers are given off to cranial nerve motor nuclei along the way; form pyramids at medulla, where majority of fibers decussate; and then continue to descend in lateral column of white matter of spinal cord, where they synapse with anterior horn cells at all segments of cord. A few fibers descend without crossing at medulla level. (Modified from original painting by Frank H Netter, MD: Reproduced with permission from The Ciba Collection of Medical Illustrations. Copyright 1983 by the Ciba-Geigy Corp. All rights reserved.)

Clinical syndromes of UMN and LMN lesions

Motor component	UMN characteristics	LMN characteristics
Reflex	Hyperreflexia, extensor toe sign (Babinski's sign)	Hyporeflexia or areflexia
Muscle tonus	Hypertonia, clasp-knife spasticity, clonus	Hypotonia, flaccidity
Muscle movement	Paralysis or paresis of movements in hemiplegic distribution, etc.	Paralysis or paresis of individual muscles in peripheral nerve distribution
Muscle wasting	Late atrophy from disuse	Early atrophy or denervation
Muscle fasciculations	Not present	Present

Initially, the muscles affected by an upper motor lesion are *flaccid (hypotonic)* and *hyporeflexic.* Gradually, and with variability, the reflex arcs become increasingly hyperreactive. Then paresis, or paralysis of voluntary muscle movement, occurs with increased tone and spasticity. The spasticity is characterized by *increased resistance to passive movement, hyperreflexia,* and *clonus.* (Clonus can be defined as a forced series of alternating contractions and partial relaxation of a muscle that occurs in some neurologic diseases.) An unilateral Babinski sign is present on the hemiparetic side.

Upper motor neuron lesions caudal to the medulla produce deficits ipsilateral to the lesion. Spinal cord injury is an example of this. If the cord is transected, the lesion extends into both halves of the spinal cord; deficits will be demonstrated as quadriplegia, or paraplegia, with loss of motor function, muscle tone, and reflex activity, as well as somatic and visceral sensations below the level of injury. The box above lists clinical syndromes of UMN and LMN lesions.

ASSESSMENT

Both subjective and objective data are important in determining more about any abnormal muscle movements.

☐ Subjective data

1. Patient's understanding of the problem and possible causes
2. Initial onset of problem
3. Measures that improve symptoms
4. Presence of clumsiness or incoordination
5. Presence of any abnormal sensation

If the lesion occurs suddenly, such as in spinal cord injury from trauma or a cerebrovascular accident, subjective symptoms of the muscle weakness may be minimal. Frequently, subjective symptoms occurring early in an illness involving abnormal muscle movements or sensations are ignored.

☐ Objective data

1. Coordination
2. Muscle strength
3. Muscle tone
4. Any atrophy of muscles
5. Presence of clonus or fasciculations
6. Ability to move muscles, abnormal gait
7. Reflexes
8. Change in ability to carry on daily activities

☐ Diagnostic testing

One of the most common diagnostic procedures to evaluate muscle dysfunction is electromyography (see the box on p. 443). In motor disease, electrical activity of various types and abnormal patterns appear in resting muscle. An electromyogram (EMG) provides direct evidence of motor dysfunction and can be used to detect a dysfunction located in the motor neuron, the neuromuscular junction, or muscle fibers. It is particularly helpful in the diagnosis of lower motor neuron disease, primary muscle disease, and defects in the transmission of electrical impulses at the neuromuscular junction.

➡ DATA ANALYSIS: NURSING DIAGNOSES

Nursing diagnoses are determined from assessment of patient data. Possible nursing diagnoses for the person with alterations in muscle tone and motor function may include, but are not limited to, the following:

Diagnostic title	Possible etiologies
Body image disturbance	Loss of body functions, change in body appearance
Constipation or incontinence	Neuromuscular impairment, immobility, inadequate nutrition/fluid intake
Impaired home maintenance management	Decreased motor skills
Potential for injury	Motor deficits

Electromyogram (EMG)

Purpose

To measure the contraction of a muscle in response to electrical stimulation.

Preparation of patient

1. No special preparation.
2. Patient teaching
   a. Explain procedure.
   b. Time: approximately 45 minutes for one muscle study.
   c. Sensation: some discomfort when electrodes are inserted—persons with sensory neuropathies may have more intense pain. Some discomfort when electrical current is used.
   d. Muscle may ache for a short time after the procedure.

Procedure

1. Electrodes are inserted into selected skeletal muscle.
2. Electrical current is passed through electrodes.
3. Machine graphs the variations of muscle potentials (voltage).

After procedure

1. Observe for signs of bleeding at site of electrode insertion.
2. Plan rest period for patient.
3. Medicate patient as needed for discomfort.

Diagnostic title	Possible etiologies
Knowledge deficit	Lack of exposure/recall, unfamiliarity with information sources
Feeding, bathing/hygiene, dressing/grooming, toileting self-care deficit	Neuromuscular impairment
Sexual dysfunction	Physiologic alterations
Impaired skin integrity: actual or potential	Mechanical forces, immobility
Impaired swallowing	Neuromuscular impairment
Altered patterns of urinary elimination	Sensorimotor impairment, urinary infection

◪ PLANNING: EXPECTED PATIENT OUTCOMES

Expected patient outcomes for the person with alterations in muscle tone and motor function may include, but are not limited to, the following:

1. Patient's skin will remain intact and free of breakdown.
2. Patient's mobility will be at optimal level without contractures.
3. Patient describes dosage, function, side effects, and toxic effects of medications to be taken.
4. Patient demonstrates measures to prevent muscle or joint deformities.
5. Patient describes measures to prevent skin breakdown.
6. Patient describes and demonstrates range of motion.
7. Patient lists signs of skin breakdown that require professional assessment.
8. Patient directs bowel and bladder program.
9. Patient has regular bowel evacuations without diarrhea or constipation.
10. Patient demonstrates activities of daily living that can be done alone and can describe methods of assistance for those functions that are dependent.
11. Patient states plans for follow-up care.
12. Patient remains free of infection.
13. Patient verbalizes positive self-concept.
14. Patient remains free of traumatic injury.
15. Patient demonstrates safe swallowing mechanism.
16. Patient is sexually active if desired.

◪ IMPLEMENTATION

Successful nursing care of the patient with motor dysfunction includes those activities that prevent complications such as decubitus ulcers or joint contractures, as well as those that develop the person's optimal level of functioning.

☐ Assisting with therapeutic goals
☐ *Safety needs*

Patients with paralysis have significant safety needs. Protection of the patient from falling is a major one. When left alone, hemiplegic patients need to have the side rail raised on the side of the bed next to their affected side. A chair restraint may be helpful when the patient is up in a chair.

Also, the eye on the affected side of the body should be protected when the lid remains open and there is no blink reflex. If this is not done, damage to the cornea will occur, leading to corneal ulcers and blindness. Irrigation with a physiologic solution of sodium chloride, followed by artificial tear solution (methylcellulose) is sometimes used. An eye pad may be used to keep the eye closed. If a pad is used, it must be changed daily and the eye cleaned and carefully examined for signs of infection or drying of the cornea. Eye shields are preferable to pads, because there is no danger of lint entering the eye.

☐ *Skin care*

Skin over bony prominences needs to be inspected regularly for signs of pressure. Paralyzed persons are at risk for decubitus formation. The following several factors account for this:

1. Muscles are not being used.
2. Interference with autonomic reflexes that monitor and maintain vasomotor tone may result in altered circulation to the paralyzed areas.
3. Accompanying sensory loss may prevent the individual from perceiving pain and pressure, the warning symptoms of tissue injury.

Persons who are physically capable of activity are taught to turn themselves in bed and to reposition themselves independently. Paraplegics are taught how to shift their weight in bed; for the quadraplegic patient these activities are done by the staff. Weight shifts done in a wheelchair or other chair are also important. These may include controlled leaning from one side to another or push-ups done by the patient to relieve pressure for a short time every hour or so. Most patients are taught to do a weight shift for 5 minutes every hour. If the patient is not able to independently do a weight shift, then the staff must do it. However, patients are taught to take the responsibility to remind the staff when it is time for the weight shift. If the person also has a loss of sensation, no external heat such as hot water bottles or heating pads should be used (the heat may not be felt and a burn could result). Paralyzed or weakened areas should be inspected daily for any signs of skin irritation; a mirror or other devices to assist in this assessment is imperative so that all areas can be visualized.

☐ *Activity needs*

The limbs of a person who has acute hemiplegia, as with the person who has paraplegia or quadriplegia, are often flaccid at first. Spasticity with a tendency to muscle contracture develops gradually. The joints then become flexed and fixed in useless positions with deformity unless preventive measures are taken by the nurse. Joint capsules and ligaments around the immobile joint shorten, and the limb may be drawn into a flexor or an extensor contracture with or without muscle spasm.

Based on assessment of the joints that are vulnerable to contracture and deformity formation, the nurse should carefully place the limbs in a normal anatomic position to prevent deformity. Counterpositioning may be used. In hemiplegia, for example, the affected upper limb is pulled inward at the shoulder joint and the wrist drops; in the lower limb the knee flexes and the foot drops. In *counterpositioning* the nurse positions the patient so that the shoulder and upper arm are in abduction, the elbow is flexed, the wrist is dorsiflexed, the knee is in a neutral position, and the foot is dorsiflexed. If the person is supine, a pillow can be placed between the upper arm and body to hold the arm in abduction. Hand splints are often used to prevent hand deformity. Footboards may be used to prevent footdrop, although some feel that these contribute to increased spasticity and should not be used routinely for patients with UMN lesions. High-topped tennis shoes can be effective to prevent foot deformity if initiated early enough. A sling may be useful for shoulder subluxation.

Physical therapists and occupational therapists can provide splints, braces, and casts that can be an adjunct to positioning.

The prone position is excellent for patients who are able to tolerate it. Not only is the chance of skin breakdown decreased with this position, but the position also causes extension of the hip and knee joints by means of gravity.

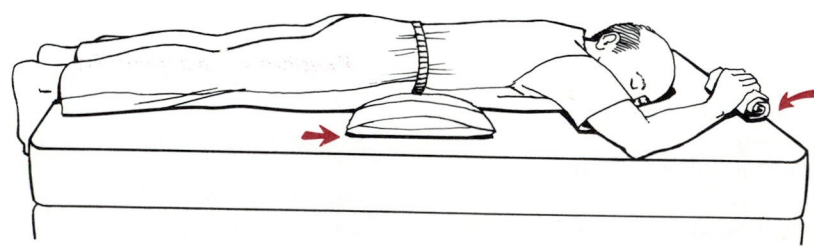

Fig. 19-34   Patient lying prone with feet extending over end of mattress. Note small pillow under midsection and hand is flexed around rolled towel.

Many patients are able to comfortably assume this position. A pillow placed under the chest may make the patient more comfortable and make breathing easier (Fig. 19-34).

Positioning of the paralyzed person is extremely important. Knee flexion and foot-drop are serious complications that must be prevented. The development of a flexion contracture at the knee joint interferes with the person's ability to bear weight in an upright position and to transfer independently. As a result, the level of self-care and independence may be diminished. Subluxation of a shoulder joint in a person with hemiplegia, related to inadequate support of the joint when in an upright position, causes pain and limits therapy. Keeping the paralyzed person upright or semiupright for long periods of time results in hip deformities. Most joint deformities in a paralyzed person are preventable with early and continuing nursing interventions.

In addition to positioning, interventions for the person with paralysis include range of motion (ROM) exercises to all joints. These may be passive (carried out by the nurse) or active (carried out by the patient). Passive ROM is indicated at least three times daily for all joints that the person cannot voluntarily move.

☐ Medications

Patients having ongoing problems with spasticity may be given skeletal muscle relaxants to decrease tone and involuntary movements and to help relieve anxiety and tension. Common side effects include drowsiness and dizziness, which are potentiated when the medications are used in combination with alcohol, barbiturates, sedatives, hypnotics, or tranquilizers. Some commonly prescribed medications are the following:
1. Baclofen (Lioresal)—a derivative of GABA (an inhibitory neurotransmitter). Acts on the spinal cord.
2. Dantrolene sodium (Dantrium)—acts directly on skeletal muscle by impairing Ca^{++} release from the sacroplasmic reticulum. Can cause additional side effects of muscle weakness, slurred speech, drooling, and anuresis.
3. Diazepam (Valium)—centrally acting muscle relaxant and antianxiety agent.

☐ Nutritional needs

Patience and persistence are necessary in giving food and fluids to the person with hemiplegia. So much difficulty may be encountered in swallowing food and fluids because of paralysis that the patient may believe that effort is not worthwhile. Important nursing measures are listed in the box above, right.

Some patients may have severe dysphagia and require prefeeding and feeding exercises. This activity often is shared by nurses, speech therapists, and occupational therapists. In patients at severe risk of aspiration, a *video fluoroscopy* with barium may be used to rule out aspiration. This procedure requires the patient to swallow small amounts of liquid or semisolid barium while fluoroscopy is being done.

Nursing measures to improve nutrition

1. Make patients feel that problem is not overwhelming.
2. Give positive feedback to patient when any improvement is noted.
3. Avoid foods that cause choking, such as mashed potatoes.
4. Check affected side of mouth for accumulation of food and subsequent poor mouth hygiene—it may be helpful to irrigate mouth after eating.
5. Encourage patient to feed self as soon as possible.
6. Dentures should be used if at all possible.
7. Make sure patient is sitting up at 90 degrees.
8. Keep patient's head up and chin slightly tucked. Head should not be extended.
9. Encourage patient to tip head toward unaffected side while swallowing.
10. Do not mix liquids and solid foods.
11. Encourage patient to take small bites.

Self-help devices for feeding are available. These include utensils with universal cuffs (Fig. 19-35), covered plastic cups, plate guards, and the Asepto syringe.

☐ Elimination needs

The person with paralysis from an UMN or LMN lesion may have problems with bowel and bladder control. This is discussed in Chapters 31 and 32.

☐ Assisting with comfort and ADL
☐ Activities of daily living

During the rehabilitative and acute phases, patients with paralysis are taught how to carry out ADL to the extent that they are able. A variety of self-help devices are available that assist with dressing with one hand, for example. The occupational therapist becomes involved in many of these activities, including homemaking. It is important to stress the concept of the rehabilitative team in managing these patients. Volunteers may also be included in helping the patient find meaningful diversional activities.

☐ Psychologic adjustment

The person with paralysis will need assistance in adjusting to the change in the body. The loss of the ability to function independently when paralyzed is traumatic. The person also may have fears of rejection by loved ones, concerns about the future, and loss of self-esteem. A grief reaction similar to that described for the stages of death and dying may occur. At times, persons may relate to the paralyzed portion of the body as though it were not a part

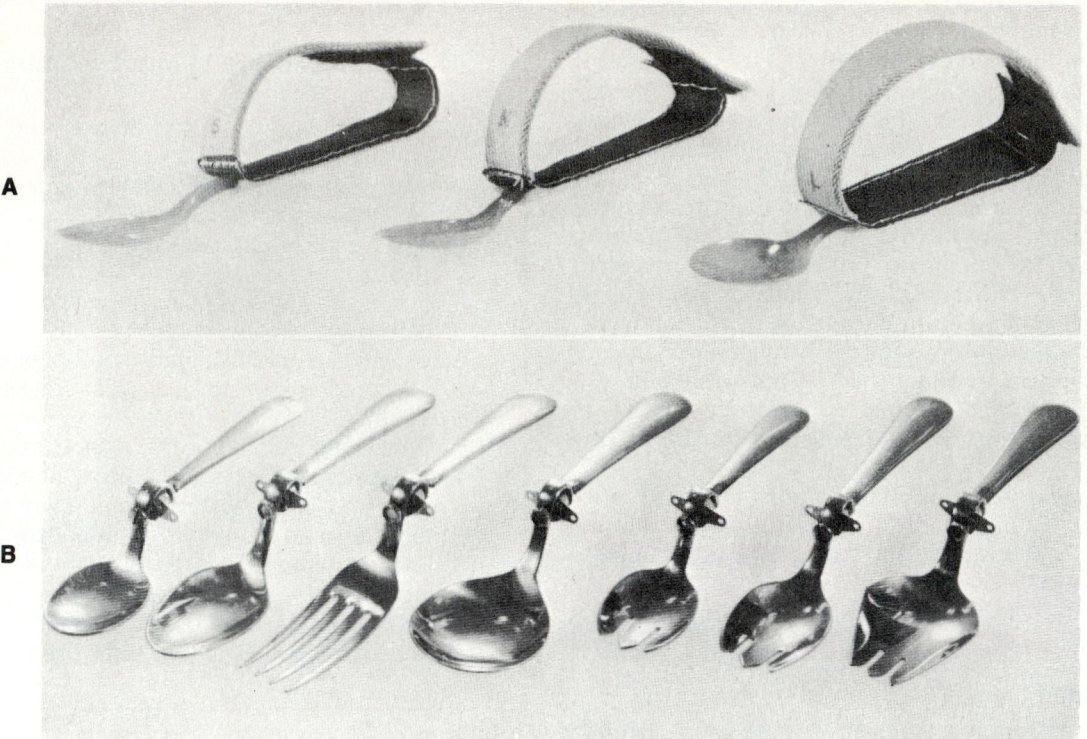

Fig. 19-35 Self-help devices for quadriplegic. **A,** Spoons with small, medium, and large universal cuff attachments that fit over hand. **B,** Swivel spoons, forks, and sporks (combination spoon and fork, last three on right), which are used with universal cuff. (Courtesy Fred Sammons, OTR, Chicago, Ill.)

of them. Nursing interventions to help the patient cope with the loss of function and change in body image are essential.

☐ Counseling and teaching

Teaching is an extremely important part of caring for the person with motor problems. Appropriate teaching activities are outlined in the box on p. 448.

⌗ EVALUATION

Evaluation of the patient with motor dysfunction is made based on the perception of the patient and measurement against the defined patient outcomes. Questions to consider include the following:

1. Is the patient knowledgeable about range of motion?
2. Is the patient receiving adequate nutrition?
3. Is the patient as independent in ADL as possible?
4. Is the patient's fluid intake adequate?
5. Is the patient's skin intact?
6. Is the patient doing skin checks or asking staff to do them?
7. Are the joints freely moveable?
8. Does the patient assume control of bowel and bladder program?

9. Can the patient state plans for follow-up care?
10. Does the patient verbalize knowledge of the medication regime?
11. Does the patient verbalize a positive self-concept?
12. Is the patient free of infection?
13. Does the patient remain free of traumatic injury?
14. Is the patient swallowing without difficulty?
15. Is the patient involved in sexual relationship if desired?

■ Alterations in sensory function

■ PATHOPHYSIOLOGY

The presence of a lesion anywhere within the sensory system pathway, from the receptor to the sensory cortex, alters the transmission or perception of sensory information. The parietal lobe cortex is of major importance in interpretation of sensation with the exception of sight, hearing, smell, taste, and thermoregulation. Loss, decrease, or increase in sensation of pain, temperature, touch, and proprioception, singly or in combination, results in difficulty in daily living. Because these sensations normally help the person to be aware of alterations in the

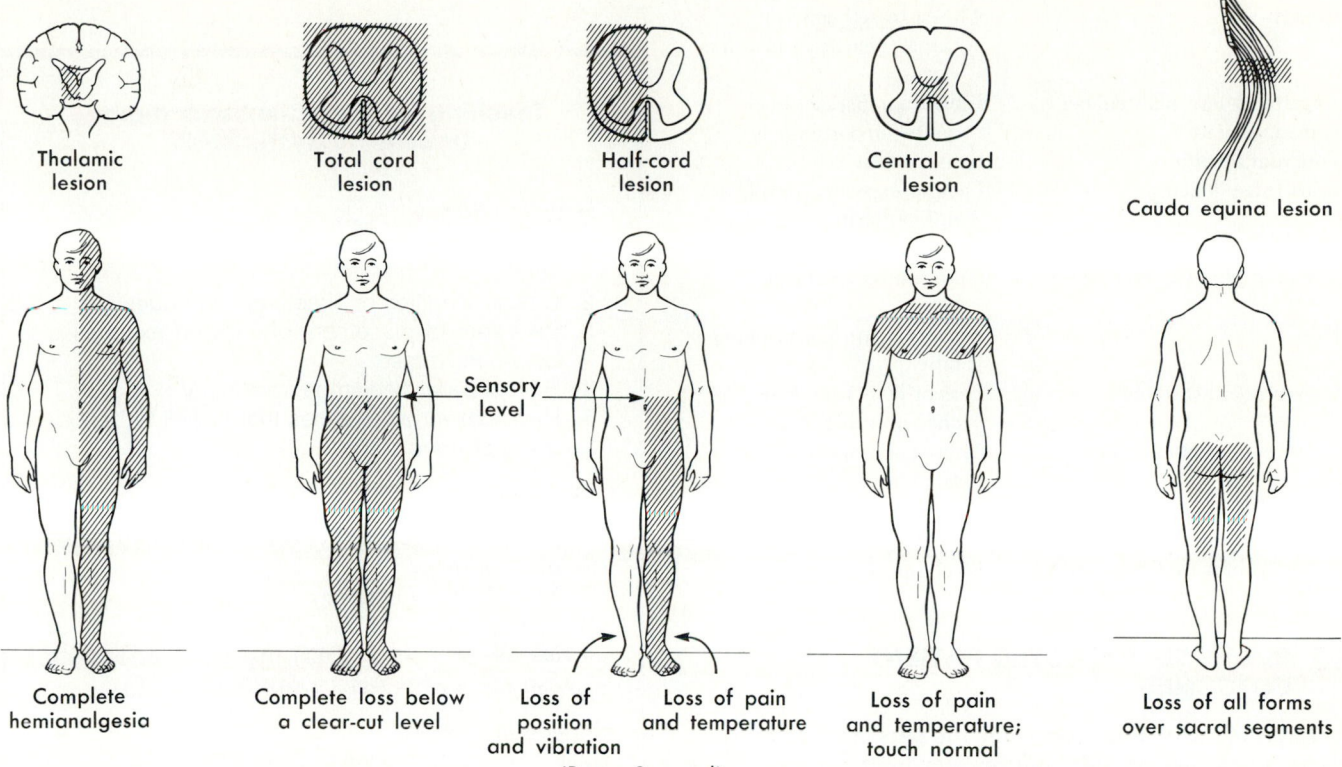

Thalamic lesion   Total cord lesion   Half-cord lesion   Central cord lesion   Cauda equina lesion

Sensory level

Complete hemianalgesia

Complete loss below a clear-cut level

Loss of position and vibration   Loss of pain and temperature

(Brown-Sequard)

Loss of pain and temperature; touch normal

Loss of all forms over sacral segments

Fig. 19-36   Common patterns of sensory abnormality. Upper diagrams show site of lesion; lower diagrams show distribution of corresponding sensory loss. (Adapted from Bickerstaff, ER: Neurology for nurses, ed 2, London, 1971, English Universities Press Ltd, and Hodder & Stoughton, Ltd.)

internal and external environments, any alteration in sensation lessens the ability to be completely and accurately protected.

One specific loss is that of *proprioception,* or the ability to know the position of the body and its parts without looking directly at the part. Lack of control of body temperature, or *hyperthermia,* is another dysfunction and occurs as a result of malfunction in the thermoregulatory center in the brain, such as that which occurs following brain surgery near the hypothalamus or from head injury.

Fig. 19-36 presents common patterns of sensory loss. A cerebral lesion results in various alterations in sensation contralateral to the lesion. This distribution results because all sensory fibers have decussated (crossed) before reaching the sensory cortex of the cerebrum. On the other hand, transection of the spinal cord results in total bilateral sensory loss distal to the lesion, because all pathways have been severed. The characteristic distribution of deficits with Brown-Sequard syndrome is ipsilateral (same side) loss of proprioception and vibratory sense and contralateral (opposite side) loss of pain, temperature, and crude touch sensation.

ASSESSMENT

The sensory examination is the most difficult part of the neurologic examination. Subjective data are collected as follows.

☐ Subjective data

1. Patient's understanding of the sensory disturbance
2. Measures that relieve symptoms, including medications
3. Site of sensory abnormality
4. Onset of sensory problem
5. Presence of associated symptoms
6. Alteration in sensation
   a. Pain   d. Proprioception
   b. Touch   e. Stereognosis
   c. Temperature

➡ DATA ANALYSIS: NURSING DIAGNOSES

Nursing diagnoses are determined from assessment of patient data. Possible nursing diagnoses for the person with sensory dysfunction may include, but are not limited to, the following:

Diagnostic title	Possible etiologies
Anxiety	Threat to self-concept, threat/change in health status
Impaired home maintenance management	Individual disease, inadequate support systems
Potential for injury	Sensory deficits
Knowledge deficit	Lack of exposure/recall, unfamiliarity with information sources
Impaired physical mobility	Neuromuscular impairment
Pain	Sensory disturbance, immobility
Body image disturbance	Loss of body functions, change in life-style
Sensory/perceptual alterations	Altered sensory reception/transmission/integration
Sexual dysfunction	Physiologic limitations
Potential impaired skin integrity	Mechanical forces

PLANNING: EXPECTED PATIENT OUTCOMES

Expected patient outcomes for the person with sensory dysfunction may include, but are not limited to, the following:

1. Patient can demonstrate how to compensate for each sensory deficit or loss.
2. Patient can explain safety factors needed in activities of daily living to protect against injury.
3. Patient can demonstrate how to inspect the affected body parts for injury.
4. Patient can state signs and symptoms that would indicate worsening of the condition and the need to seek medical assistance.
5. Patient demonstrates minimal anxiety.
6. Patient verbalizes a positive self-concept.
7. Patient remains free from traumatic injury.
8. Patient's skin is clear.
9. Patient has minimal dependence in ADL and home maintenance.
10. Patient's discomfort or pain is minimal.
11. Patient compensates for any sexual disability.
12. Patient can state plans for follow-up care.

IMPLEMENTATION
Teaching

The most important nursing intervention for the patient with sensory dysfunction is teaching the person and family protective measures in relation to the sensory deficit or alteration (see the box at right). Teaching the person to use noninvolved senses to an increased extent helps to avoid injuries. For example, teaching the person with hypoesthesia (lessened touch) to visually inspect involved body parts regularly will help to prevent injuries.

Teaching for the patient with motor or sensory dysfunction

Safety needs

1. Always lock wheelchair when transferring patient
2. Check condition of affected eye frequently
3. Be aware of placement of affected extremities before movement
4. Protect paralyzed limbs from injury
5. Have patient wear shoes that fit well for ambulating or transferring

Skin care

1. Regular inspection of skin surfaces, using mirror or other device
2. Need to turn frequently
3. Weight shifts
4. No use of heating pads, hot water bottles, or excessively hot water for bathing

Activity needs

1. Range of motion
2. Proper positioning
3. Frequent changes in position

Medications

1. Use of medication, side effects, dosage, and timing
2. Reporting of side effects to physician
3. Importance of not combining medication with other mood-altering drugs or alcohol

Nutrition-diet

1. Foods that can be easily tolerated
2. Measures to decrease swallowing difficulty
3. Use of special appliances to assist with eating

ADL

1. Teaching techniques of bathing, grooming, dressing
2. Importance of having meaningful recreational activities
3. Bowel and bladder care

Other teaching

1. Importance of good fluid intake
2. Follow-up care—where to procure equipment, supplies
3. Methods for relieving feelings of frustration

⊞ EVALUATION

Evaluation of the patient with sensory dysfunction involves the patient and family. Questions to consider include the following:

1. Is the patient carrying out ADL in a safe manner?
2. Is the patient successfully compensating for sensory deficits?
3. Is the patient inspecting affected body parts for injury?
4. Is the patient following through with the prescribed follow-up care?
5. Can the patient state signs and symptoms that indicate the need to notify the physician?
6. Is the patient sexually active?
7. Is the patient free of pain or discomfort?
8. Is the patient verbalizing a positive self-concept?
9. Is the patient maintaining independence in home maintenance?

Major health problems of the neurologic system

Functioning of the neurologic system can be interrupted for a variety of reasons. These include the following:

1. Interference with impulses because of conduction of impulses
2. Interference because of degenerative changes
3. Interference because of vascular problems
4. Interference because of infection
5. Interference because of trauma
6. Interference because of tumors

Some common neurologic disorders are listed in the box at right.

■ INTERFERENCE WITH FUNCTION BECAUSE OF PROBLEMS WITH CONDUCTION OF IMPULSES

■ Epilepsy or seizures

Epilepsy (convulsive disorder) is one of the oldest diseases known to humans. (For purposes of this text the terms *epilepsy, seizure disorder,* and *convulsive disorder* will be used interchangeably.) Seizures occur in all races, and affect males and females equally. There is no apparent geographic distribution. Epilepsy can begin at any age, but in many the onset is before the age of 20. The incidence is about 1 in every 200 to 300 persons. Between 2 and 4 million persons in the United States are affected by epilepsy. Many of these are children.

There are numerous ways to classify seizures. One common way is the International Classification of Epileptic Seizures. In this classification, seizures are identified as

---

Health problems of the neurologic system

1. *Interference with function because of problems with conduction of impulses*
   a. Epilepsy or seizures
   b. Myasthenia gravis
2. *Interference with function because of degenerative diseases*
   a. Multiple sclerosis
   b. Parkinson's disease
   c. Amyotrophic lateral sclerosis (ALS)
   d. Alzheimer's disease
   e. Neurofibromatosis
3. *Interference with function because of vascular conditions*
   a. Cerebrovascular accident (CVA)
   b. Intracerebral hemorrhage
4. *Interference with function because of infection/inflammation*
   a. Meningitis
   b. Encephalitis
   c. Brain abscess
   d. Poliomyelitis
   e. Guillain-Barré syndrome
   f. Neurosyphilis
   g. AIDS
5. *Interference with function because of trauma*
   a. Craniocerebral
   b. Spinal cord
   c. Peripheral nerve
6. *Interference with function because of tumors*
   a. Intracranial
   b. Intraspinal

---

partial (beginning locally), generalized (bilaterally symmetric and with no local onset), unilateral, or unclassified. Another way to classify seizures is based on the clinical features of the attack. The five groups in this type of classification are the following:

1. Grand mal (major or generalized)
2. Petit mal
3. Psychomotor
4. Jacksonian and focal
5. Miscellaneous (myoclonic, akinetic)

Table 19-3 shows the characteristics of each type of seizure.

■ PATHOPHYSIOLOGY

Epilepsy may be defined as a transitory disturbance in consciousness or in motor, sensory, or autonomic function with or without loss of consciousness. It is associated with

Table 19-3 Characteristics of seizures

Type of seizure	Etiology	Characteristics	Clinical signs	Aura	Postictal period
Grand mal	Most common	Generalized, characterized by loss of consciousness for several minutes	Aura Cry Loss of consciousness The fall Tonic-clonic movements Incontinence	Yes Flashing lights Smells Spots before eyes Dizziness	Yes Need for sleep 1 to 2 hrs Headache common
Petit mal	Usually occur during childhood and adolescence Frequency decreases as child gets older	Sudden impairment in or loss of consciousness with little or no tonic-clonic movement Occurs without warning Has tendency to appear a few hours after arising or when person is quiet	Sudden vacant facial expression with eye focused straight ahead All motor activity ceases except perhaps for slight symmetric twitching about eyelids Possible loss of muscle tone Consciousness returns	No	No
Psychomotor	Occur at any age	Sudden change in awareness associated with complex distortion of feeling and thinking and partially coordinated motor activity Longer than petit mal	Behaves as if partially conscious Often appears intoxicated May do antisocial things such as exposing self or carrying out violent acts Autonomic complaints may occur Chest pain Respiratory distress Tachycardia Gastrointestinal distress Urinary incontinence	Yes Complex hallucinations or illusions	Yes Confusion Amnesia Need for sleep
Jacksonian-focal	Occur almost entirely in patients with structural brain disease	Dependent on site of focus May or may not be progressive	Commonly begin in hand, foot, or face May end in grand mal seizure	Yes Numbness Tingling Crawling feeling	Yes
Myoclonic	May antedate grand mal by months or years	May be very mild or may have rapid, forceful movements	Sudden involuntary contraction of muscle group, usually in extremities or trunk No loss of consciousness	No	No
Akinetic	Not common	Peculiar generalized tonelessness	Person falls in flaccid state Unconscious for minute or two	Rarely	No

sudden, excessive, and disorderly electrical discharges in the neurons of the brain that result in the sudden, violent, involuntary contraction of a group of muscles. The patterns or forms of seizures vary and are dependent on the area of the brain from which the seizure arises. The pattern is stereotyped in the individual, although variations may occur with progression of cerebral lesions.

Seizures can involve essentially all parts of the brain at once, as in the generalized type, or only a minute focal spot. In the first type, the excessive neuronal discharges are thought to originate in the brainstem portion of the reticular activating system; these then spread throughout the CNS including the cortex and the deeper parts of the brain. The process may last from a few seconds to as long as 3 to 5 minutes, or it may stop immediately, as in a *petit mal seizure*. Stoppage of a seizure is thought to result from fatigue of the neurons involved in precipitating the seizure or by inhibition of certain structures within the brain. The excessive neuronal discharges may result in a *tonic convulsion*, with the contraction of all muscles at once, or a *clonic convulsion*, with alternate contraction and relaxation of opposing muscle groups. This gives the characteristic jerking movements of the body. Seizures are followed by inhibition of cerebral function with a variable length. This is called the *postictal period*.

When recurrent generalized seizure activity occurs at such frequency that full consciousness is not regained between seizures, it is called *status epilepticus*. This is a medical emergency and requires intensive medical and nursing care to prevent death from brain damage secondary to prolonged hypoxia and exhaustion.

Seizures occur in many childhood and adult illnesses. Causes include the following:

1. Cerebral anoxia
2. Hypoglycemia
3. Disturbance of calcium balance
4. Electrolyte imbalances
5. Disturbance in hydration
6. Injection of drugs and poisons with convulsive activity
7. Numerous metabolic disturbances and disorders
8. Infections that cause high temperature elevations
9. Generalized inflammatory processes
10. Degenerative tissue disorders
11. Hysteria

In many patients with epilepsy, a localized organic lesion serves as the focus for the abnormal neuronal discharges from the damaged brain tissue. These organic lesions include the following:

1. Neoplasms
2. Inflamed areas or abscesses
3. Sclerosis
4. Vascular formations or hematomas
5. Congenital malformations
6. Trauma
7. Other space-occupying lesions[36]

ASSESSMENT

Assessment of both subjective and objective data is important in the patient who is having a seizure (see the box below).

□ Subjective data

1. Patient's understanding of the seizure disorder and what might be causing it
2. Awareness of precipitating factors
3. Presence of an aura
4. Postictal feelings
5. Presence of amnesia

An *aura* is defined as the set of symptoms that occurs before the seizure. An aura occurs in about 50% of all patients with *grand mal seizures* and usually includes a change in sensation or a change in affect. The exact char-

---

Observations to be made about a person having a seizure

Aura	Presence or absence; nature if present; ability of patient to describe it (somatic, visceral, psychic)
Cry	Presence or absence
Onset	Site of initial body movements; deviation of head and eyes; chewing and salivation; posture of body; sensory changes
Tonic and clonic phases	Movements of body as to progression; skin color and airway; pupillary changes; incontinence; duration of each phase
Relaxation (sleep)	Duration and behavior
Postictal phase	Duration; general behavior; ability to remember anything about the seizure; orientation; pupillary changes; headache; injuries present
Duration of seizure	Length from aura to relaxation phase
Level of consciousness	Length of unconsciousness if present
Presence of injury	Injury to mouth, lips, tongue, or soft tissues from seizure Injury to extremities

Electroencephalogram (EEG)

Purpose

To provide evidence of focal or diffuse disturbances of brain function produced by organic lesions by measuring the electrical activity of the brain (Fig. 19-37).

Preparation of patient

1. No special preparation.
2. Patient is encouraged to be quiet and rest before the procedure.
3. Scalp and hair should be clean.
4. Patient teaching
   a. Explain procedure.
   b. Time: 1 hour or more.
   c. Sensation: not painful—electrodes are applied to scalp with collodion.

Procedure

1. Patient usually sits in a comfortable chair or lies on a cot with eyes closed. Testing is done in a special room where outside electrical acitivity is eliminated.
2. Electrodes are fixed to the scalp, usually with collodion, in a set pattern to cover all scalp areas.
3. The basic resting rhythm is affected by opening the eyes or altering attention.
4. Recordings can be made while the patient is asleep or when sleep deprived.
5. Comparisons are made of different patterns of the recordings.

After prodecure

1. Patient should be allowed to rest if tired.
2. Patient should be assisted if necessary in washing hair and removing collodion from scalp.

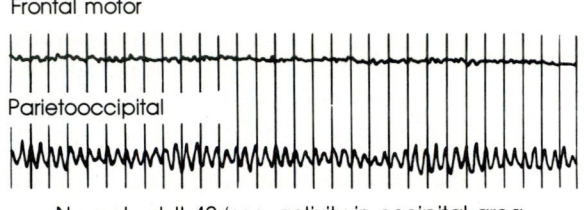

Frontal motor

Parietooccipital

Normal adult, 10/sec. activity in occipital area.

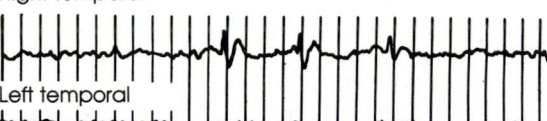

Right temporal

Left temporal

Complex-partial (temporal lobe) epilepsy.
Right temporal spike focus.

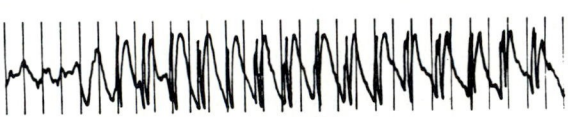

Absent attacks (petit mal seizures).
Synchronous 3/sec. spikes and waves.

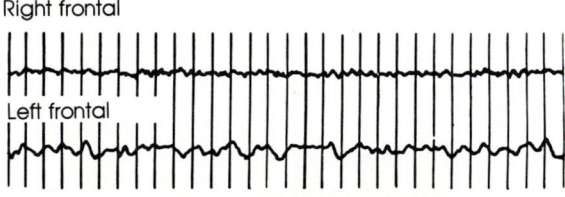

Right frontal

Left frontal

Brain tumor. Left frontal slow wave focus.

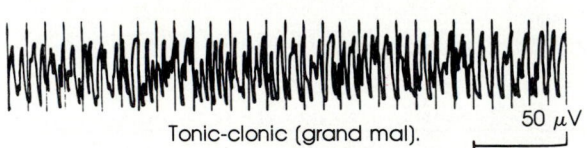

Tonic-clonic (grand mal).

50 µV

1 sec

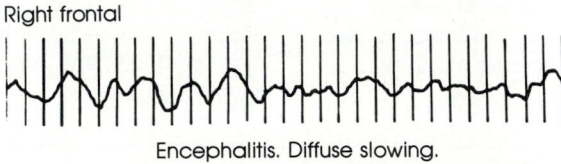

Right frontal

Encephalitis. Diffuse slowing.

Fig. 19-37 Tracings of electroencephalogram. The normal tracing is demonstrated, as are several pathologic states.

acter of the aura varies from person to person but may include numbness, flashing lights, dizziness, tingling of the arm, smells, or spots before the eyes. The patient may not be able to describe the aura precisely, but it gives conclusive evidence of the impending seizure and allows the patient to seek privacy and safety before it occurs.

During the postictal phase the individual is groggy and acts confused. Complaints of headache or muscular pain are common. A deep sleep usually follows. During this phase the pupils may remain dilated and plantar reflexes may be abnormal. After a variable period of time the patient awakens and is frequently unaware of the occurrence of the seizure. A dull headache and depression are common.

□ **Objective data**

1. Number of seizures occurring within a specific time
2. Behavior: signs of stress or fatigue
3. Character of seizure
4. Injuries sustained

□ **Diagnostic tests**

By far the most common test used to evaluate siezure disorders is the electroencephalogram (see the box on p. 452). It is safe and noninvasive and allows for more specific diagnosis.

➡ **DATA ANALYSIS: NURSING DIAGNOSES**

Nursing diagnoses are determined from assessment of patient data. Possible nursing diagnoses for the person with seizures may include, but are not limited to, the following:

Diagnostic title	Possible etiologies
Anxiety	Threat to self-concept, threat/change in health status/role functioning/socio-economic status
Ineffective airway clearance	Tracheobronchial obstruction
Potential for injury	Sensorimotor deficits
Knowledge deficit	Lack of exposure/recall, information misinterpretation, unfamiliarity with information sources
Sensory/perceptual alterations: visual, auditory, kinesthetic, gustatory, tactile, olfactory	Altered sensory reception/transmisison/integration
Social isolation	Alteration in physical appearance, altered state of wellness

■ **PLANNING: EXPECTED PATIENT OUTCOMES**

Expected patient outcomes for the person with seizures may include, but are not limited to, the following:

1. Seizures are reduced or at least do not increase in severity or number.
2. Patient demonstrates a patent airway.
3. Patient remains free of traumatic injury.

4. Patient shows a low level of anxiety.
5. Patient can describe medication to be taken, including action, side effects, toxic effects, and dosage schedule.
6. Patient can explain the importance of taking medication regularly even when the seizures are controlled.
7. Patient can explain the importance of avoiding alcohol while taking anticonvulsant drugs.
8. Patient explains how to use available community resources.
9. Patient and significant other can explain the necessary measures to carry out if a seizure does occur.
10. Patient shows social participation.
11. Patient wears medical alert tag.

■ **IMPLEMENTATION**

□ **Assisting with the achievement of therapeutic goals**
□ *Medications*

Treatment of patients with a seizure disorder almost always includes the use of one or more of the anticonvulsant drugs (see Table 19-4). The choice of medications depends on the type of seizure. Anticonvulsant medications act generally on the cerebral cortex and are not selective in acting on the part of the brain involved in abnormal neuronal discharges.

The dosages of anticonvulsant drugs are difficult to establish and regulate because of the high incidence of side effects and the toxicity of the drugs. The drug of choice is introduced in an average therapeutic dose, and the dose is increased until seizure control is reached. If toxicity is reached before control of the seizures, the dose is decreased to the previous nontoxic or tolerated dose. Additional secondary drugs may be introduced at this time to aid in seizure control.

Failure to take the prescribed medication or to take an adequate dose is often the cause of failure in treatment. Tests to determine the blood level of the anticonvulsant are helpful in providing an accurate check on the therapeutic and toxic levels of the medications taken.

□ **Surgical treatment**

Surgical treatment of seizures is becoming less common, but it may still be used in some cases in which medical therapy is not effective. *Cortical resection* is one surgical approach. It involves removal of the brain tissue in which the focus of electrical discharge is located. The localization of tissue must occur in a part of the brain that is easily accessible to surgery and that can be removed without leaving the person with a serious disability.

Another surgical approach involves *stereotactic* procedures using electrical stimulation. This technique is used to interrupt the pathways of seizure activity, to destroy the foci, or to alter the actions of the cortical nerve cells.

□ **Assisting with comfort and ADL**

Because most persons with seizures do not have symptoms between attacks and because a majority of seizures

Table 19-4 Anticonvulsants used to prevent seizures

Drug	Use related to seizure type	Toxic effects
Phenytoin sodium (Dilantin)	Grand mal, focal, psychomotor	Ataxia, vomiting, nystagmus, drowsiness, rash, fever, gum hypertrophy, lymphadenopathy
Phenobarbital (Luminal)	Grand mal, focal, psychomotor	Drowsiness, rash
Primidone (Mysoline)	Grand mal, focal, psychomotor	Drowsiness, ataxia
Ethosuximide (Zarontin)	Petit mal, psychomotor, myoclonic, akinetic	Drowsiness, nausea, agranulocytosis
Trimethadione (Tridione)	Petit mal	Rash, photophobia, agranulocytosis, nephrosis
Diazepam (Valium)	Status epilepticus, mixed	Drowsiness, ataxia
Carbamazepine (Tegretol)	Grand mal, psychomotor	Rash, drowsiness, ataxia
Valproic acid (Depakene)	Petit mal, absent seizures	Nausea, vomiting, indigestion, sedation, emotional disturbance, weakness, altered blood coagulation
Clonazepam (Clonopin)	Petit mal, akinetic, myoclonic ?Grand mal seizures	Drowsiness, ataxia, hypotension, respiratory depression

can be controlled by medication, the person with seizures should be encouraged to lead as normal a life as possible. Until seizures are controlled, however, the person should avoid dangerous activities such as driving a car, working on or about machinery, or swimming. Once the person has achieved seizure control for a significant period and has learned the importance of taking the medication regularly and avoiding alcoholic beverages, these restrictions can be relaxed. Maintaining adequate rest and nutritional intake is also important.

The issue of driving a car is one that often poses a problem. Epilepsy does impose driver limitations. Usually 1 year without seizures should elapse before the person is eligible to drive and then only if seizures are completely controlled.

The use of alcohol should be avoided. Also, the person should be taught the importance of good mouth care if receiving long-term phenytoin (Dilantin) therapy, because gingival hyperplasia is a common side effect.

□ *Care during a seizure*

The primary goals of the nurse and family caring for a patient having a seizure are protection from injury and observation and recording of the seizure activity. Specific actions are listed in the box below.

□ **Counseling and teaching**

Teaching is an important part of the care of the patient with seizures. This includes the patient, as well as members of the family, who should learn to care for the person during and after a seizure. Involvement of the family or significant other during the hospitalization is essential. One of the more important things for the family to learn is the need to be calm and accept the family member's seizures.

Teaching for the patient with a seizure disorder includes the actions defined in the box on p. 455.

Nursing actions during a seizure

1. Never leave the person alone.
2. If patient is in upright position, lower to floor or bed and move adjacent articles and equipment away to prevent injury.
3. Loosen constricting clothing, especially around the neck.
4. Turn head to one side to aid with airway.
5. No effort should be made to restrain the person manually or with restraints.
6. If the jaws are not already clenched when seizure is first observed, a padded tongue blade may be inserted between the back teeth to prevent injury to the tongue and mouth tissues. The mouth should not be pried open—this may cause injury to the patient or to self.
7. Pad side rails if the patient is confined to bed or has seizures during sleep. Pillows should not be used for padding because of danger of suffocation.
8. Accurate observations should be made and recorded.

Teaching for the patient with a seizure disorder

1. Use of medication, including side effects, dose, timing; reporting side effects to physician
2. Importance of avoiding the use of alcohol with anticonvulsants
3. Safety measures to avoid injury in case of seizures
4. Good oral hygiene if patient is taking phenytoin
5. Importance of adequate rest and diet
6. Importance of taking medication even when free of seizures
7. Community resources
8. Restrictions concerning driving
9. Importance of follow-up care
10. Importance of verbalizing feelings
11. Need to avoid excessive stress
12. Importance of wearing medical alert bracelet
13. Importance of not overprotecting self

⊞ EVALUATION

As with other conditions, evaluation of the patient experiencing seizures is made using the feelings and input of the patient. Questions to consider include the following:
1. Is the number of seizures decreased?
2. Is the patient taking the medication as prescribed?
3. Are blood levels of the prescribed anticonvulsants within normal limits?
4. Is the patient refraining from dangerous activity?
5. Can the patient explain daily routine that includes adequate rest?
6. Is the patient able to identify available community resources?
7. Is follow-up care occurring as prescribed?
8. Is the patient verbalizing feelings?
9. Is the patient wearing a medical alert bracelet?
10. Is the patient socializing with others?

■ Myasthenia gravis

Myasthenia gravis is a neuromuscular disease that affects the lower motor neurons and muscles. Excessive fatigue occurs along with weakness of muscles, especially those involved with the face, eyes, larynx, and pharynx and the process of respiration. The fatigue and weakness worsens with exercise and is improved with rest. It affects about 1 in 20,000 persons.

The cause of myasthenia is unknown, although it is thought to be an autoimmune disease. It characteristically starts between the ages of 20 and 30 or in late middle age. In younger persons, women are affected more than men, but in older persons men are affected to a greater extent. Familial occurrence is rare.[21]

■ PATHOPHYSIOLOGY

No structural change in the muscle or nerve is observed in cases of myasthenia gravis. Nerve impulses fail to pass to muscles at the myoneural junction. It is not known specifically why the motor nerve impulses fail to pass to the muscle and cause it not to contract. This is believed to be caused by a *decrease in the release of acetylcholine* from the presynaptic terminals or a *blockage of or a reduction in the number of postsynaptic membrane receptor sites*. It is known that circulating antibodies to the acetylcholine receptor (AChR) are present and are believed to cause the myasthenic weakness.

About 10% of patients with myasthenia have been found to have a thyoma, and nearly 70% have changes in the cellular structure of the thymus gland (usually hyperplasia). The role of the thymus gland in the pathophysiology of myasthenia gravis is unclear.

In severe cases, the respiratory muscles and bulbar cranial nerves may be involved, leading to severe respiratory infection and possible death. However, sensation is not lost and the involved muscles usually do not atrophy.

▦ ASSESSMENT

☐ **Subjective data**
1. Patient's understanding of disease
2. Fatigue—when it occurs and where it occurs
3. Profound muscle weakness
4. Presence of diplopia
5. Difficulty in keeping eyelids open and mouth closed or chewing and swallowing
6. Effect of stress on the symptoms
7. Patient's perception of muscle weakness

☐ **Objective data**
1. Documented muscle weakness on neurologic testing
2. Presence of ptosis of eyelids
3. Documented weight loss
4. Breath sounds
5. Muscle atrophy

Exacerbation of the disease occurs with upper respiratory infections, emotional tension, and menstruation. Because of the slow and insidious onset of myasthenia gravis and the occurrence of symptoms with stress, patients with this disease are sometimes misdiagnosed as suffering from neurosis or hysteria.

It is important to differentiate between myasthenia gravis and Eaton-Lambert syndrome, a condition associated with cancer that has many of the same symptoms as myasthenia gravis. Because the onset of Eaton-Lambert syndrome may precede the discovery of the cancer by months

---

Comparison of myasthenia gravis and Eaton-Lambert syndrome

	Myasthenia gravis	Eaton-Lambert syndrome
Onset	Slow and insidious	Slow and insidious
Vision	Diplopia common	Diplopia not as common
Muscle involvement	Cranial nerves; arms and hands; trunk and lower limbs affected (difficulty with walking and sitting); distal muscles not as affected as proximal muscles	Muscles of trunk as well as those of pelvis and shoulder girdle are most commonly involved
Weakness	Weakness and generalized fatigue that comes on quickly	Increased weakness with exertion, but there may be temporary increase in muscle power at first

---

or years it is important that the patient be checked thoroughly for malignancy. Cancers associated with Eaton-Lambert syndrome are the following:

1. Oat cell carcinoma of the lung (most common)
2. Rectal carcinoma
3. Cancer of the stomach
4. Cancer of the prostate
5. Cancer of the breast

The clinical differences between myasthenia gravis and Eaton-Lambert syndrome are described in the box above.

☐ Diagnostic tests

Diagnosis of mysthenia gravis is partially made on the basis of EMGs that rule out other muscle disorders. A specific diagnostic test that is used is the endrophonium chloride (Tensilon) test. Edrophonium is a very short-acting anticholinesterase drug. The procedure for the test is as follows:

1. Edrophonium and normal saline are drawn up in separate syringes.
2. Each is injected intravenously separately.
3. It is important that the patient not be aware which solution is being given.
4. Increased strength in a predetermined muscle group with the administration of edrophonium is a positive test.

The results occur in 30 seconds to 1 minute and usually last only a few minutes.

A chest x-ray examination or CT scan of the chest may be done to determine the presence of a thyoma. The curare test may be done if all other tests are normal or questionable. Because curare causes respiratory paralysis, equipment and personnel to intubate the patient should be available. The curare test may be definitive when other tests are not.[48]

➡ DATA ANALYSIS: NURSING DIAGNOSES

Nursing diagnoses are determined from assessment of patient data. Possible nursing diagnoses for the person with myasthenia gravis may include, but are not limited to, the following:

Diagnostic title	Possible etiologies
Activity intolerance	Generalized weakness
Ineffective airway clearance	Tracheobronchial infection/obstruction/secretion
Anxiety	Threat of death, change in health status/role functioning
Ineffective breathing pattern	Neuromuscular impairment
Impaired verbal communication	Physical barriers
Constipation	Immobility, inadequate nutrition
Knowledge deficit	Lack of exposure/recall, unfamiliarity with information sources
Impaired physical mobility	Intolerance to activity/decreased strength, neuromuscular impairment
Altered nutrition: less than body requirements	Chewing or swallowing difficulties
Feeding, bathing/hygiene, dressing/grooming, toileting self-care deficit	Intolerance to activity/fatigue

⊢ PLANNING: EXPECTED PATIENT OUTCOMES

Expected patient outcomes for the person with myasthenia gravis may include but are not limited to the following:

1. Patient and family verbalize adequate knowledge of myasthenia gravis.
2. Patient has a patent airway.
3. Patient demonstrates an effective pattern of breathing.
4. Patient maintains an optimal level of mobility.
5. Patient can explain the action, side effects, and

toxic effects of each anticholinesterase or cholinergic drug.

6. Patient can explain the reason for taking the medication at the exact time.
7. Patient can explain the need to monitor effects of medication on respiration, swallowing, and general muscle strength.
8. Patient can list drugs that act on the neuromuscular junction and are contraindicated.
9. Patient can explain the need to avoid overexertion and emotional tension.
10. Patient demonstrates minimal self-care deficits.
11. Patient has minimal difficulty with impaired verbal communications.
12. Patient has minimal anxiety.
13. Patient evacuates bowel on a regular basis without constipation.
14. Patient maintains optimal nutrition.

IMPLEMENTATION

□ Assisting with the achievement of therapeutic goals
□ *Medications*

Two medications that are used in myasthenia gravis are neostigmine (Prostigmin) and pyridostigmine (Mestinon). These drugs block the action of cholinesterase at the myoneural junction and allow acetylcholine to act. Atropine or other anticholinergic agents that block the effects of acetylcholine can be used to treat the side effects of neostigmine and pyridostigmine. Treatment is planned so that the patient receives the drug in the amount tolerated without side effects and yet is able to carry out activities essential for normal living. Usually, the patient is allowed to adjust the dosage. Ambenonium chloride (Mytelase) may also be given in doses of 10 to 25 mg. orally 3 or 4 times daily. Corticosteroids such as prednisone are sometimes used as an adjunct to other drug therapy.

It is often difficult to distinguish between *myasthenic crisis* (too little drug) and *cholinergic crisis* (too much drug), because both conditions cause severe muscle weakness. Administering edrophonium (Tensilon) intravenously differentiates between the two conditions. A positive test (increase in strength) indicates underdosage of the drug. An increase in weakness is a sign of overdosage.

□ *Respiratory care*

Respiratory complications are common for the patient with myasthenia gravis, and for this reason they are usually advised not to live alone. They are also cautioned to avoid crowds or other circumstances where infections are common. Upper respiratory infections are seen because patients may not have the energy needed to cough effectively and may develop pneumonia or airway obstruction. Aspiration is common. Many patients have airway equipment at home.

During acute episodes of the disease, the following are important:

1. Tracheostomy set at bedside, because respiratory status may change rapidly

2. Serial determinations of vital capacity, minute volumes, and tidal volumes
3. Suction as necessary
4. Nasogastric tube if swallowing is too dangerous (patient will not be able to cough to indicate if tube is in trachea, so careful assessment of the position of tube is important)
5. With severe impairment in respiratory function, the patient will probably require endotracheal intubation and ventilator assistance (see Chapter 24 for further discussion of the patient on mechanical ventilation)

□ Assisting with comfort and ADL

Patients with severe symptoms of myasthenia gravis may be too weak to do anything for themselves. The nurse may have to turn and position the patient in addition to doing most of the other ADL. It is important to remember that the patient with myasthenia gravis will remain alert and will often be very frightened. Psychologic support and reassurance are essential.

□ Counseling and teaching

The patient with myasthenia gravis often has a great deal of control over his/her medication schedule and can do much to prevent respiratory problems. A well-informed patient is more likely to stay healthy. Teaching should include the points listed in the box on p. 458.

EVALUATION

Evaluation of the patient with myasthenia gravis is important. Involving the patient in this process is essential. Questions to consider are the following:

1. Is the patient taking medication as ordered?
2. Can the patient explain the action, time element, and side effects of the medication?
3. Does the patient know what drugs to avoid? (See the box on p. 458.
4. Is the patient free of respiratory infection?
5. Does the patient demonstrate knowledge of any necessary equipment?
6. Is the patient's weight stable?
7. Is mobility maintained at optimal levels?
8. Is the patient able to carry on ADL independently?
9. Are the patient's bowel habits regular without constipation?
10. Is the patient expressing minimal anxiety?
11. Is the patient's verbal communication effective?

INTERFERENCE WITH FUNCTION BECAUSE OF DEGENERATIVE DISEASES

The term *degenerative diseases* is used to refer to neurologic diseases in which there is a premature senescence of nerve cells, there is a known or suspected metabolic disturbance, or the cause of the disease is unknown. In-

---

Teaching for the patient with myasthenia gravis

1. Medications
   a. Importance of taking medication at time prescribed
   b. Dose individually determined and related to the activity of the person
   c. How to adjust dose to maintain muscle strength
   d. Side effects and how to monitor
   e. Medications to avoid
   f. Importance of not taking medications with fruit, tomato juice, coffee, or other medications
   g. Importance of not taking over-the-counter drugs without checking with physician
2. Respiratory care
   a. Avoid crowds during peak times for upper respiratory infections
   b. Eat only when sitting up
   c. Importance of seeking medical treatment at first sign of upper respiratory infection
3. Pattern of acitivity
   a. Acitivities planned around time of day when fatigue is lessened
   b. Importance of frequent rest periods
   c. Plan so that minimum amount of energy is used in activities that are essential to remaining relatively self-sufficient, and conserve energy for other activities the patient wishes to take part in
   d. Activity and exercise to tolerance should continue
   e. Need for diversional activities
   f. Independence and socialization encouraged
4. Nutritional concerns
   a. Importance of maintaining adequate nutrition
   b. Importance of eating only when sitting up
   c. Adequate fluid intake (at least 2,000 ml/day)
5. Other considerations
   a. Importance of expressing fears
   b. Need to wear medical alert tag
   c. How to avoid constipation

Drugs to be avoided by persons with myasthenia gravis

1. Muscle relaxants
2. Barbiturates
3. Morphine sulfate
4. Tranquilizers
5. Neomycin (potentiates muscle weakness because of effect on myoneural junction)

---

cluded in this section are five such diseases. They are the following:

1. Multiple sclerosis
2. Parkinson's disease
3. Amyotrophic lateral sclerosis (ALS)
4. Alzheimer's disease
5. Neurofibromatosis (Von Recklinghausen's disease)

See Table 19-5 for a comparison of these five diseases.

Another degenerative disease is syringomyelia. This is a destruction of the gray and then white matter of the spinal cord that occurs as a result of the development of *syrinxes* (cysts filled with CSF). As a result, nerve pathways in the spinal cord, are destroyed and nerve impulses are interrupted. This disease will not be discussed in further detail but it is one that the nurse should be aware of.

■ Multiple sclerosis

Multiple sclerosis is a common degenerative neurologic disease. At least 50,000 persons suffer from it. The cause remains unknown despite research. Several hypotheses have been advanced as to the cause:

1. Genetic—it has been found that relatives of persons with multiple sclerosis have a much higher incidence of the disease than the general population. A person with an identical twin with the disease has a 20% risk of having the disease.
2. Epidemiologic—persons living in temperate climates have an increased risk of the disease. When they move to another region, they retain the same risk.

Table 19-5 Comparison of degenerative neurologic diseases

Disease	Pathologic signs	Effect	Medical treatment
Multiple sclerosis	Multiple foci (patches) of nerve degeneration throughout the brain and spinal cord	Demyelination causes nerve impulses to be interrupted (blocked) or distorted (slowed)	No specific treatment Symptomatic treatment Judicious use of ACTH or other corticosteroids
Amyotrophic lateral sclerosis	Destruction of myelin sheath of motor neurons of lateral tracts of spinal cord and brain	Demyelination causes nerve impulses to be interrupted (blocked) or distorted (slowed)	No specific treatment Symptomatic and supportive care
Parkinson's disease	Destruction of nerve cells of basal ganglia of brain	Decreased dopamine (neurotransmitter substance with anticholinergic effect)	Anticholinergic alkaloids Synthetic anticholinergic drugs Levodopa Carbidopa-levodopa Surgery in selected cases
Alzheimer's disease	Degeneration of neurofibrils and presence of plaque in brain	Destruction of neurons leading to impairments in intellectual functioning	No specific treatment Symptomatic and supportive care
Neurofibromatosis (Von Recklinghausen's disease)	Numerous fibromas of spinal or cranial nerves and skin, café au lait spots on the skin and developmental anomalies	Tortuous interfacing of tissue cords that result in multiple tumors	No medical treatment except supportive care Tumors removed surgically Genetic counseling

3. Viral—the serum and cerebrospinal fluid of patients with multiple sclerosis has been found to contain antibodies to many viruses, including measles, mumps, herpes simplex, and influenza.
4. Immunologic—most persons with multiple sclerosis have been found to have abnormalities of the spinal fluid indicative of autoimmune disease.

The onset of symptoms usually occurs between the ages of 20 and 40. The course of the disease is estimated to be 12 to 25 years. Several studies have demonstrated an increased incidence of multiple sclerosis among siblings and even distant relatives. The highest number of persons with multiple sclerosis live in the Great Lakes area, the Pacific Northwest, and the north Atlantic states. There has been no evidence to suggest a sexual mode of transmission.

■ PATHOPHYSIOLOGY

Multiple foci of demyelination are distributed randomly in the white matter of the brainstem, spinal cord, optic nerves, and cerebrum. During the demyelination process (primary degeneration), the myelin sheath and the sheath cells are destroyed, but there is early sparing of the axon cylinder. The outer myelin sheath destruction causes interruption or distortion of the impulse so that it is slowed or blocked. There is evidence of partial healing in areas of degeneration, which accounts for the transitory nature of early symptoms. In later stages the degeneration may extend to gray areas of the cord and limit healing. Although the outer surface of the brain appears normal, brain weight may be decreased and the ventricles may be enlarged.

Because of the wide distribution of areas of degeneration,

the variety of signs and symptoms in multiple sclerosis is greater than in other neurologic diseases. It is a chronic, remitting, and relapsing disease. The majority of persons recover from their early episodes, with remissions lasting for a year or more. Exacerbations may be aggravated or precipitated by fatigue, chilling, and emotional disturbances. In rare cases the disease may terminate in death within a few years of onset.

▨ ASSESSMENT

Early symptoms of multiple sclerosis are usually transitory. Many persons may be considered neurotic because of the wide variety and temporary nature of symptoms and the emotional instability produced by the disease. Subjective symptoms are important in making the diagnosis.

□ Subjective data

1. Patient's understanding of disease
2. Presence of eye problems
   a. Diplopia
   b. Scotomas (spots before the eyes)
   c. Blindness
3. Presence of weakness or numbness of part of the body such as hand
4. Presence of unusual fatigue
5. Presence of tremor
6. Presence of emotional instability
7. Presence of bowel and bladder problems
8. Presence of impotence in men
9. Loss of joint sensation and proprioception
10. Presence of vertigo

☐ Objective data

1. Documented abnormalities in neurologic testing
   a. Nystagmus
   b. Scanning speech
   c. Muscle weakness and spasms
   d. Changes in coordination
   e. Spastic ataxic gait
2. Behavior: presence of euphoria, emotional, lability, mild depression
3. Urinary incontinence, frequency, or retention
4. Difficulty in swallowing
5. Intentional tremors of upper extremities

It is suspected that the presence of euphoria is caused by patients' attempts to reassure themselves that their condition is not serious. Motor signs associated with multiple sclerosis have UMN characteristics. Pain is not a common symptom.

☐ Diagnostic tests

Examination of the cerebrospinal fluid usually shows elevated gamma globulin level and an increased white blood cell count. An electroimmunodiffusion determination will be done. A CT scan may demonstrate enlargement of the ventricles. Cerebral atrophy is present in advanced disease.

Even in early stages of multiple sclerosis, abnormal visual and brainstem evoked potentials are present. The visual evoked response will show optic atrophy in the majority of cases. Evoked potentials are electrical measurements of physiologic maturation of the human nervous system. They provide information about the primary sensory areas of the cortex.

➡ DATA ANALYSIS: NURSING DIAGNOSES

Nursing diagnoses are determined from assessment of patient data. Possible nursing diagnoses for the person with multiple sclerosis may include, but are not limited to, the following:

Diagnostic title	Possible etiologies
Ineffective airway clearance	Decreased energy/fatigue, obstruction/secretion
Anxiety	Threat/change in health status/role functioning
Body image disturbance	Change in body appearance, immobility, change in life-style
Constipation or incontinence	Neuromuscular impairment, weakened perineal muscles, immobility
Impaired verbal communication	Physical impairment
Impaired home maintenance management	Individual disease, inadequate support systems
Functional or total incontinence	Neurologic impairment
Potential for infection	Decreased nutrition, lack of knowledge

Diagnostic title	Possible etiologies
Potential for injury: trauma	Sensory/motor deficits, lack of awareness of environmental hazards
Knowledge deficit	Lack of exposure/recall, cognitive limitation, unfamiliarity with information sources
Impaired physical mobility	Perceptual/cognitive impairment, neuromuscular impairment
Altered nutrition: less than body requirements	Chewing or swallowing deficits
Pain	Improper positioning, immobility
Feeding, bathing/hygiene, dressing/grooming, toileting self-care deficit	Neuromuscular impairment
Sensory/perceptual alterations: visual	Altered sensory reception/transmission/integration
Sexual dysfunction	Physiologic limitations
Potential impaired skin integrity	Mechanical forces, immobility
Altered thought processes	Neurologic disorders, anxiety, isolation
Altered patterns of urinary elimination	Sensorimotor impairment, urinary infection

⊞ PLANNING: EXPECTED PATIENT OUTCOMES

Expected patient outcomes for the person with multiple sclerosis may include, but are not limited to, the following:

1. Patient has a patent airway.
2. Patient demonstrates minimal anxiety.
3. Patient's bowel patterns are continent to the degree possible, and complications of any incontinence or constipation are minimal.
4. Patient has minimal discomfort.
5. Patient's verbal communication is maintained.
6. Patient has minimal impairments in home management.
7. Patient has minimal complications because of urinary incontinence.
8. Patient remains free of infection.
9. Patient remains free of traumatic injury.
10. Patient/family can verbalize knowledge of disease.
11. Patient can explain the action, side effects, and toxic effects of prescribed medications.
12. Patient maintains adequate nutrition.
13. Patient can explain the plan for inclusion of hobbies and other diversional activities.
14. Patient maintains optimal mobility.
15. Patient has minimal deficits in self-care activities.
16. Patient verbalizes a positive self-concept.
17. Patient can state plans for follow-up care.
18. Patient can state how to secure community help.
19. Patient's skin is intact.
20. Patient and/or family can compensate for impaired thought processes.
21. Patient continues to function sexually if desired.
22. Patient has minimal problems with sensory-perceptual alterations.

IMPLEMENTATION

□ **Assisting with the achievement of therapeutic goals**
□ **Medications**

At present there is no specific treatment for multiple sclerosis. Favorable results seem to occur with the use of adrenocorticotrophic hormone (ACTH) and the corticosteroids. Their efficacy remains controversial. Some physicians prefer oral prednisone or intramuscular or oral dexamethasone (Decadron). ACTH may be given intramuscularly or intravenously. The effects of ACTH and the steroids on the demyelinating process is unknown. It is known from testing that (1) nothing is gained from long-term treatment, and (2) some gain is possible from taking high doses of steroids at the start of an exacerbation, because the episode then seems to resolve more rapidly.[20]

□ **Elimination**

Urinary frequency and urgency may respond to timed doses of propantheline bromide (Pro-Banthine). Prevention of urinary tract infection remains a problem, and such infections are a major cause of death. Cholinergic drugs such as bethanechol (Urecholine) may be helpful for the patient with atonic bladder. Oxybutynin chloride (Ditropan) is used to treat neurogenic bladder. It acts by exerting a direct antispasmodic effect on smooth muscles. Some patients are given prophylactic doses of medications such as trimethoprim and sulfamethoxazole (Bactrim, Septra) or nitrofurantoin (Macrodantin). Cystometric studies can be helpful in defining the specific bladder problem.[62]

The patient should be encouraged to drink adequate fluids. Several glasses of cranberry juice a day may be helpful in decreasing urinary tract infection.

It may be necessary to have the patient take a stool softener such as docusate sodium (Colace) to prevent constipation.

□ **Nutrition**

A well-balanced diet with plenty of high-vitamin foods is important. Obesity should be avoided because it makes it more difficult for the patient to maneuver and to meet daily needs. High-fiber foods and prune juice may help reduce constipation.

□ **Skin care**

Many persons with multiple sclerosis have motor involvement that prevents them from moving about freely and changing position readily. Also, they may have sensory disturbances that affect how they sense pressure. As a result, decubiti can easily develop. Patients must be taught the importance of turning at least every 2 to 3 hours. Other devices such as air mattresses may also be helpful.

□ **Assisting with comfort and ADL**
□ **Activity and rest**

Persons with multiple sclerosis should have a daily routine for rest and activity. They are usually advised to exercise regularly but never to the point of extreme fatigue. During an acute exacerbation, patients are often kept as quiet as possible, bed rest is maintained, and all activities are limited.

One side of the body is usually affected more than the other. The patient may learn to stabilize the gait by leaning toward the uninvolved side. Having the foot slap forward in taking a step may sometimes be overcome by putting the heel down in a pronounced fashion and rolling the weight forward on the side of the foot.

The judicious use of passive and active exercises, when the person is not in acute exacerbation, can be useful in maintaining function. Drugs such as diazepam (Valium) and dantrolene sodium (Dantrium), as well as baclofen (Lioresal), have been used to prevent spasticity.

Effort is made to maintain activity and work as long as possible. Patients can be helped to plan their activities so that they may continue to function even when the disease is well advanced.

□ **Control of environment**

Hot baths should be avoided because the heat can increase weakness in the person with multiple sclerosis. Traveling in hot weather should be carefully planned to prevent travel during the warmest part of the day.

Persons with multiple sclerosis need a peaceful, relaxed environment. They may have slowness of speech and slowness in the ability to respond. Members of the family may need help in understanding this problem and meeting it calmly. The person may have sudden explosive emotional outbursts of crying or laughing. Reminding the patient of something sad may stop the laughing, and holding the patient's mouth open may stop the crying.

□ **Counseling and teaching**

Teaching is important for both the patient with multiple sclerosis and his/her significant others. In late stages of the disease all functions of care usually have to be assumed by someone other than the patient. Teaching needs are listed in the box on p. 462.

EVALUATION

Evaluation should include the patient and caregivers. Questions to consider include the following:
1. Is the patient taking medication as ordered?
2. Can the patient explain the use of the medication?
3. Is an exercise program being followed?
4. Can daily functions be accomplished?
5. Is the patient infection free?
6. Is elimination occurring without difficulty?
7. Is the skin free of pressure sores?
8. Can the patient explain how community agencies may be of assistance?
9. Is the patient reporting for follow-up care?

■ Parkinson's disease

Parkinson's disease is one of the more common diseases of the nervous system. It is also referred to as idiopathic Parkinson's and paralysis agitans. The disease was first

---

Teaching for the patient with multiple sclerosis

1. Use of medications, including side effects, dose, timing; importance of reporting side effects to physician
2. Importance of good fluid intake
3. Importance of spacing activities so that time is left for relaxation and fun activities
4. Range of motion exercises, as well as other exercises
5. Good, balanced diet
6. Emotional reactions of persons with multiple sclerosis
7. Safety factors to prevent injury
8. Positioning for prevention of decubiti
9. Importance of skin inspection
10. Importance of avoiding temperature extremes
11. Community resources and how to obtain them
12. Disease process
13. Compensatory techniques for visual problems

---

described in 1817 by James Parkinson. It affects both men and women in their middle and late years (50 to 60 years old). The mean age at onset is 60 years of age, and the prevalence of the disease increases with age. The incidence is about 130 per 100,000 population. It affects all races and classes of persons. The course of Parkinson's disease varies from person to person.

■ PATHOPHYSIOLOGY

The pathologic process that occurs with Parkinson's disease is basically a *depigmentation* of the *substantia nigra* of the basal ganglia. The loss of neurons in the substantia is severe. Also, selective depletion of dopamine occurs and can be correlated with the degree of striatal degeneration. Without dopamine inhibitory influence is lost and excitatory mechanisms are unopposed.

The cause of Parkinson's disease includes viral, toxic, vascular, and genetic etiologies, as well as some unknown factors. The characteristic symptoms are also sometimes found in arteriosclerotic patients, leading some to believe that arteriosclerosis may be a causative factor. Drug-induced parkinsonian syndromes occur with drugs that interfere with the synthesis or storage of dopamine or interfere with the striatal dopamine receptors. These drugs include the following:

1. Reserpine (Serpasil)
2. Phenothiazines
3. Butyrophenones (e.g., haloperidol)

▦ ASSESSMENT

Like many of the other neurologic diseases, Parkinson's disease starts with subtle symptoms and progresses slowly. The person may not be able to recall the onset of symptoms.

☐ Subjective data

1. Patient's understanding of disease
2. Complaints of fatigue
3. Presence of incoordination
4. Defects in judgment and emotional instability
5. Heat insensitivity

☐ Objective data

1. Presence of tremor (pill-rolling motion of the fingers or resting tremor)
2. Muscular response to movement (bradykinesia)
3. Postural reflexes
4. Appearance of face (masklike facies)
5. Presence of drooling
6. Shuffling gait
7. Trunk forward extension
8. Sensory testing
9. Inability to carry out daily activities
10. Presence of dementia (in about 30% of cases)
11. Presence of constipation, sometimes severe
12. Abnormal swallowing
13. Presence of scaly erythematous eruptions of skin, particularly near the ears and eyebrows and in scalp and nasolabial folds

The tremor is the outstanding sign of the disease. Two other frequent signs are muscular weakness with rigidity and loss of postural reflexes. It is essentially a problem of motion. Muscle rigidity prevents normal response and results in characteristic changes. These changes include a masklike appearance of the face and slowed, monotonous speech; drooling; shuffling gait that is propulsive and may not be able to be stopped until any obstruction is met; and moist and oily skin.

☐ Diagnostic tests

No test is diagnostic of Parkinson's disease. The clinical examination and history, along with the response of the patient to administration of medication used to treat Parkinson's disease, confirms the diagnosis.

If there is a history of chronic dementia, the CT scan may show cerebral atrophy. The EEG may show minimal slowing, or it may be normal. Upper GI studies may show delayed emptying of the stomach and hypomotility.

DATA ANALYSIS: NURSING DIAGNOSES

Except for "Sensory perceptual alteration: visual" (which is not a diagnosis for Parkinson's disease), the list of nursing diagnoses is the same as for multiple sclerosis (p. 460).

PLANNING: EXPECTED PATIENT OUTCOMES

The expected patient outcomes for Parkinson's disease are the same as for multiple sclerosis (p. 460).

IMPLEMENTATION

☐ **Assisting with the achievement of therapeutic goals**
☐ *Medications*

Treatment for Parkinson's disease is palliative and symptomatic and depends on pharmacologic manipulation of the disease. The severity of symptoms and the presence of associated disease processes determine the drugs to be

Table 19-6   Medications used in Parkinson's disease

Medication	Action/effects	Side effects	Comments

Anticholinergic alkaloids
  Scopolamine hydrochloride
  Hyoscyamine sulfate
	Act against cholinergic excitatory effects
	More effective in lessening muscle rigidity than in controlling tremor
		Central and peripheral cholinergic actions
		  Blurring of vision
		  Dryness of mouth and throat
		  Constipation
		  Urinary retention or urgency
		  Ataxia
		  Dysarthria
		  Mental disturbances
			Optimal results depend on dosage that provides compromise between improvement and development of side effects

Synthetic anticholinergic drugs Trihexyphenidyl hydrochloride (Artane) Benztropine mesyulate (Cogentin) Procyclidine hydrochloride (Kemadrin) Biperiden hydrochloride (Akineton)	Some degree of CNS anticholinergic action, but incapable of restoring striatal balance	Same as above	Same as above
Antihistamine drugs Diphenhydramine hydrochloride (Benadryl)	Exerts mild central anticholinergic properties	Sleepiness Dry mouth	Does not affect underlying process of Parkinson's disease
Levodopa	Assists in restoring striatal dopamine deficiency	Kidney, liver damage Nausea, vomiting Orthostatic hypotension Insomnia Agitation and mental confusion	Side effects common
Amantadine hydrochloride (Symmetrel)	Acts by blocking the reuptake and storage of catecholamines and allowing accumulation of dopamine in extracellular or synaptic sites	Mental confusion Visual disturbances Seizures	May not be effective for longer than 3 months
Carbidopalevodopa (Levodopa with inhibitor of the enzyme dopa decarboxylase)	Inhibitor limits metabolism of levodopa peripherally and provides more levodopa to brain	Same as levodopa	Fewer side effects than levodopa used alone

used. Particular drugs and their characteristics can be found in Table 19-6. These drugs have had a dramatic effect on the course of the disease. With proper medications many of the symptoms never develop.

After prolonged treatment with some of the drugs, there may be an increased appearance of side effects as well as a decrease in the effectiveness of the medication. It has been found helpful to admit some patients into the hospital for a *drug holiday*, during which all medications are withdrawn for a period of time. The medications are then restarted, and often much smaller doses are able to produce favorable results. This type of drug holiday must take place in the hospital. Complications such as aspiration pneumonia can occur because immobility, rigidity, and other symptoms will return when the drugs are withdrawn.[16]

□ Surgery

A surgical procedure has been used with some success in the treatment of selected patients with Parkinson's disease. It includes destroying portions of the globus pallidus (to relieve rigidity) or the thalamus (to relieve tremor) in the brain by stereotactic methods through the use of cautery, removal, or injection of alcohol. Operative techniques involving cooling or freezing with liquid nitrogen have been attempted with good results in selected cases. Medications used to control rigidity and tremor are discontinued several days preoperatively so that symptoms will be at their maximum during the surgery. Preoperative and postoperative care are the same as for the patient undergoing cranial surgery and will be discussed later in this chapter. Many patients cannot be treated surgically. Results seem best in younger patients with unilateral involvement following other diseases and who have marked tremor and rigidity.

□ Assisting with comfort and ADL
□ Activity

Special attention should be paid to posture. Lying on a firm bed without a pillow may help to prevent the spine from bending forward. Lying in the prone position also helps. Holding the hands folded behind the back when walking may help to keep the spine erect and prevent the arms from falling stiffly at the sides. The tremor is often less apparent when persons are sitting in an armchair, since they can grip the arms of the chair and partially control the tremor in their hands and arms.

□ Feeding

Feeding the patient becomes a real problem when the disease is far advanced because of the danger of aspiration; aspiration pneumonia may be fatal. Unless the disease is well controlled by medication, drooling can be a problem and increases with general excitement. A bib can be used to protect the clothing during naps. When patients are dressed, garments with generous pockets for tissues will help them be less conspicuous and more comfortable.

□ Elimination

The patient with Parkinson's disease may feel urgency and hesitancy in voiding. Measures appropriate for the patient with multiple sclerosis also apply to those with Parkinson's disease. Fluids are forced to at least 2000 ml per day. Cranberry juice is encouraged to acidify urine. Medications such as methenamine mandelate may be prescribed.

Chronic constipation may be a real concern. The patient should be on a diet high in residue and roughage. Fluids are encouraged and stool softeners, suppositories, and prune juice are often helpful. Mild cathartics such as milk of magnesia are used if required.

□ Counseling and teaching

Teaching is important for the caregiver and the patient with Parkinson's disease. The teaching is the same as that for the patient with multiple sclerosis (p. 462).

⊞ EVALUATION

The evaluation of the care of the patient with Parkinson's disease is based on the expected patient outcomes and is the same as for the patient with multiple sclerosis (p. 461).

■ Amyotrophic lateral sclerosis

Amyotrophic lateral sclerosis (ALS) is a degenerative motor neuron disease that affects upper or lower motor neurons lying within the brain or spinal cord or a combination of the two. At first, the characteristic disability involves atrophy of the muscles of the hands, forearms, and legs. In later stages of the disease all muscles are involved. It is sometimes called Lou Gehrig's disease because the famous New York Yankee baseball player died of ALS. It affects men more than women and usually first appears in middle age, between the ages of 40 and 70. It also may occur in the younger or older person. There may be a familial element to the disease. Death usually occurs within 2 to 3 years from the time of diagnosis, but some patients may live 5 to 20 years.

The cause of ALS is unknown. Genetic or external agents, metabolic disturbances, inappropriate nutrition, and systemic infection or trauma have been suggested as possible causative agents.

■ PATHOPHYSIOLOGY

In ALS the myelin sheaths are destroyed and replaced with scar tissue. There is direct involvement of the lateral tracts of the spinal cord, with possible involvement of the medulla and the ventral tracts, and loss of large motor neurons. The nerve impulses are distorted or blocked. Symptoms depend on which motor neurons are affected.

⊞ ASSESSMENT

□ Subjective data

1. Patient's understanding of disease
2. Presence of fatigue
3. Dysphagia
4. Difficulty with tasks involving fine finger movements

☐ **Objective data**

1. Inability to carry out ADL
2. Muscle testing on neurologic examination
3. Evidence of involvement of brainstem and medulla
4. Weight loss
5. Serum CPK elevation

In ALS progressive muscle weakness, atrophy, and fasciculations are present. Spasticity of the flexor muscles is common. With involvement of the brainstem and medulla dysphagia, dysarthria, jaw clonus, tongue fasciculations, and respiratory difficulty occur. As the disease progresses, disability relative to both upper and lower limbs occurs, and one side of the body becomes more involved. The person remains alert, and there is no sensory loss. Death usually occurs within 5 years of diagnosis because of respiratory problems or bulbar paralysis.

☐ **Diagnostic tests**

Initial testing may include an EMG (p. 443) to rule out other muscle disease. A muscle biopsy may also be helpful in establishing the diagnosis of ALS.

DATA ANALYSIS: NURSING DIAGNOSES

The nursing diagnoses for the patient with ALS are the same as those for the patient with multiple sclerosis (p. 462) except that the diagnosis of "Sensory perceptual alteration: visual" is not a diagnosis relevant to ALS.

PLANNING: EXPECTED PATIENT OUTCOMES

The expected patient outcomes for ALS are the same as for multiple sclerosis (p. 460).

IMPLEMENTATION

☐ **Assisting with the achievement of therapeutic goals**

Treatment is directed toward relieving the symptoms of the disease. Prostheses are often supplied to support the weakened muscles. As the disease progresses, respirations are affected. At this time constant nursing attention is required. Providing adequate nutrition to the patient is a real challenge, and a nasogastric or gastrostomy tube may be necessary. A cervical esophagostomy also may be done. In some cases, mechanical ventilation may be instituted, although this is an action that needs to be well considered by the patient and the family. Some patients may elect not to be placed on a respirator. Attention to prevention of skin breakdown and contractures is important.

☐ **Assisting with comfort and ADL**

Nursing interventions include assistance with ADL as limb defects occur. Emotional support is extremely important. Patients and their families should be involved in making decisions about the types of interventions that will be used as the disease progresses. Some patients will decide to use ventilators at home as respiratory muscles become involved, whereas other patients will decide not to use any supportive devices. Because the patient remains alert until death, nurses should remember that they are dealing with someone who is probably very afraid.

EVALUATION

Because the outcomes in ALS are similar to those of multiple sclerosis, refer to that part of the chapter for the appropriate questions to ask (p. 461). An additional reference question is whether the patient is maintaining weight.

■ Alzheimer's disease

Alzheimer's disease is a degenerative disorder that affects the cells of the brain and causes impairment of intellectual functioning. It is recognized as the most common cause of dementia in the older adult. It affects men and women equally. Most newly diagnosed persons are in late middle age, but the disease has been documented in some persons as young as 40 years old.

One of the difficulties in making a definitive diagnosis of Alzheimer's disease is that evidence is often obtained only from an autopsy.

■ PATHOPHYSIOLOGY

The changes in the brains of patients with Alzheimer's disease are visible in the cerebral cortex. The first change is the presence of microscopic "plaques" found in brain tissue. These plaques consist of a core surrounded by strands of fiberlike material. In addition, there is degeneration of some of the small fibers (neurofibrils) that run through the body of the nerve cells. These changes were first discovered in 1907 by the German neurologist Alzheimer.[58]

ASSESSMENT

☐ **Subjective data**

1. Patient's understanding of disease
2. Mental status part of neurologic examination
3. Onset of symptoms

☐ **Objective data**

1. Inability to carry on ADL
2. Behavior: evidence of agitation, restlessness
3. Presence of incontinence

The patient with Alzheimer's disease goes through three rather distinct stages. These stages are described in the box on p. 466.

The diagnosis of Alzheimer's disease is made after ruling out conditions in which there is memory loss. These include the follwing diseases:

1. Pernicious anemia
2. Drug reactions
3. Hormonal imbalances
4. Depression
5. Drug or alcohol abuse

Clinical stages of Alzheimer's disease

Stage one

Mild mental impairment
Forgetfulness
Impairment in judgment
Decrease in initiative
Lack of spontaneity

Stage two

Confusion
Agitation
Irritability
Extreme restlessness
Incontinence of urine and stool
Need for constant supervision

Stage three

Total inability to care for self
Inability to communicate
Total incontinence

---

6. Brain tumor
7. Chronic meningitis
8. Head trauma
9. Pick's disease
10. Parkinson's disease with dementia

The signs and symptoms of Alzheimer's disease occur progressively, but the rate at which they occur varies between individuals. In a few cases, the decline may be very rapid, but in most cases deterioration is gradual. Cause of death is often pneumonia or other infections.

□ Diagnostic tests

No diagnostic test is specific for Alzheimer's disease. A CT scan is used to rule out other abnormalities. Often neuropsychologic testing can reveal characteristic changes in the ability to think. A family history of Alzheimer's aids in the diagnosis.

→ DATA ANALYSIS: NURSING DIAGNOSES

The possible nursing diagnoses for the patient with Alzheimer's disease are the same as for the patient with multiple sclerosis (p. 460), with the following additions:
Sleep pattern disturbance
Violence, potential for
The violence that sometimes occurs in the patient with Alzheimer's disease occurs most often when the patient does not understand what is happening or what nursing care is being done. It is not an intentional harmful act, but an effort to avoid that which is not understood.

PLANNING: EXPECTED PATIENT OUTCOMES

The expected outcomes for the patient with Alzheimer's disease are the same as those for the patient with multiple sclerosis. One difference is that in many cases the person with Alzheimer's disease is mentally incompetent, so that the caregiver needs to have major involvement in planning for the outcomes. The patient may not be able to have real input into them.

IMPLEMENTATION

□ Assisting with the achievement of therapeutic goals

No treatment can cure, reverse, or stop the progression of Alzheimer's disease. Nursing care is directed toward maintaining nutrition, continence, hydration, and safety. Emotional support of both the patient and family is important. Appropriate drugs can sometimes be used to lessen anxiety, agitation, and unpredictable behavior.

□ Safety

One large area for intervention concerns safety. Because of forgetfulness, patients with this condition often do dangerous things. This includes walking outside without appropriate clothing, turning on burners, getting lost, and setting things on fire. The family must make plans to protect the patient from these hazards. This includes removing burner controls from the stove at night, double-locking all doors and windows, and keeping the person under supervision at all times. One very frustrating part of the illness is that many of the patients sleep for only short periods of time and are awake most of the night. This must be worked out if the caregiver is to get any rest.

EVALUATION

Evaluation of the patient with Alzheimer's disease focuses on the patient outcomes. Refer to the evaluation section for multiple sclerosis for appropriate questions to ask (p. 461). An additional question is whether the person is safely carrying out daily activities.

■ Neurofibromatosis

Neurofibromatosis is a genetic disorder transmitted as an *autosomal dominant trait* by either parent. It is also called *multiple neuroma* or *neuromatosis*.

The disease affects one of every 3,000 births and can occur with spina bifida, meningocele, or seizures. About half of the patients with neurofibromatosis have no family history of the disease. Malignant degeneration occurs in a small number of cases, and mental retardation occurs in about one tenth of persons affected with the disease. Men are more commonly affected than women. The clinical symptoms usually appear in later childhood or adolescence and continue to develop with advancing age.

Neurofibromatosis is characterized by the following:
1. Numerous fibromas of spinal or cranial nerves and skin.
2. Café au lait spots on the skin
3. Developmental disorders of bone, muscle, and viscera

Neurofibromatosis can be classed as *central* (affecting the intraspinal and intracranial nervous system), *peripheral* (primarily affecting peripheral nerves), or *visceral* (involvement of the viscera and autonomic nervous system).[48]

■ PATHOPHYSIOLOGY

With neurofibromatosis there is proliferation of *fibroblasts,* or *Schwann cells.* This results in interlacing of tissue cords to form tumors in multiple areas. The size of the tumors varies from very small to several centimeters in size. The majority of the tumors occur as nodules along the course of involved nerves. Superficial dermal tumors may also occur, mainly over the trunk; these are asymptomatic. Other tumors such as meningiomas and glioblastomas may also occur.

Café au lait spots are composed of melanin located on the epidermis of the skin. They are pale brown macules, usually uniform in color and round or oval and range in size from 0.5 to 15 cm in diameter. The presence of 5 or more spots that are at least 1.5 cm in diameter is called *Crowe's sign* and is considered sufficient evidence to make the diagnosis of neurofibromatosis. The macules are usually found in the axilla, over the trunk, and over the pelvis.

■ ASSESSMENT

□ Subjective data

1. Complaints of facial numbness or weakness
2. Family history of disease
3. Onset of symptoms
4. Understanding of the disease

□ Objective data

1. Presence of multiple cutaneous neurofibromas
2. Presence of cafe au lait spots
3. Presence of associated problems, including endocrine or skeletal
4. Presence of visual loss or deafness
5. Limitations in ADL

□ Diagnostic tests

Analysis of the cerebrospinal fluid of patients with neurofibromatosis will show elevated protein levels. A myelogram will indicate whether spinal cord tumors are present, and the CT scan will be used to determine whether intracranial tumors are present. Skull films may be done to determine if cerebral tumors have caused bone erosion.

➡ DATA ANALYSIS: NURSING DIAGNOSES

Nursing diagnoses are determined from assessment of patient data. Possible nursing diagnoses for the person with neurofibromatosis may include, but are not limited to the following:

Diagnostic title	Possible etiologies
Anxiety	Threat to self-concept, change in health status
Body image disturbance	Change in body appearance
Knowledge deficit	Lack of knowledge/recall
Impaired physical mobility	Pain/discomfort
Pain	Neurofibromatosis, immobility
Social isolation	Alteration in physical appearance

If the patient suffers the effects of a spinal cord tumor or brain tumor, the nursing diagnoses applicable to those diagnoses will apply. The reader is referred to those areas in the chapter.

▣ PLANNING: EXPECTED PATIENT OUTCOMES

Expected patient outcomes for the person with neurofibromatosis may include, but are not limited to, the following:

1. Patient expresses minimal anxiety.
2. Patient has minimal discomfort.
3. Patient maintains mobility at the highest possible level.
4. Patient can verbalize knowledge of the disease and symptoms to watch for.
5. Patient verbalizes a positive self-concept.
6. Patient maintains social contacts

▦ IMPLEMENTATION

□ Assisting with the achievement of therapeutic goals

The care of the patient with neurofibromatosis consists mainly of excision of the tumors. There is no medical treatment known to be effective. If the patient develops increased intracranial pressure, monitoring may be indicated. A shunt may be done if hydrocephalus is present.

Supportive care includes genetic counseling and psychosocial support.

□ Teaching

Teaching for the patient with neurofibromatosis includes education about the disease, as well as its hereditary nature.

╫ EVALUATION

Evaluation of the patient with neurofibromatosis considers how the patient is able to function within the confines of the disease. Questions to consider include the following:

1. Is the patient free of pain?
2. Is the patient verbalizing a positive self-concept?
3. Is the patient verbalizing minimal anxiety?
4. Is the patient maintaining optimal mobility?
5. Is the patient knowledgable about the disease?
6. Is the patient involved socially with other people?

INTERFERENCE WITH FUNCTION BECAUSE OF VASCULAR CONDITIONS

Interference with function because of vascular conditions is common in neurologic nursing. In this section of the chapter the following two conditions will be discussed:

1. Cerebrovascular accident
   a. Thrombosis
   b. Embolism
   c. Hemorrhage
2. Intracerebral hemorrhage

Cerebrovascular accident

Cerebrovascular accident (CVA) is the most common disease of the nervous system and is ranked as the third leading cause of death in the United States. Approximately 200,000 deaths occur annually, with another 200,000 persons having residual effects. Stroke effects persons in all age groups, but the greatest number occurs in persons between 75 and 85 years of age. In this section, the term *cerebrovascular accident* will be discussed as a general term. Most neurologists and neurosurgeons, however, refer more specifically to the cause of the CVA. These causes are as follows:

1. Thrombosis
2. Embolism
3. Hemorrhage (this is discussed on p. 474)

The medical and nursing care may differ for each, depending on the specific cause (see the box below). *Stroke* is another term used when referring to CVA; clinically, stroke refers to the sudden and dramatic development of focal neurologic deficits.

Cerebrovascular accidents can be precipitated by many underlying factors and are frequently associated with other chronic diseases that cause vascular problems. These include heart disease, hypertension, kidney disease, peripheral vascular disease, and diabetes mellitus. Other risk factors for stroke include obesity, high serum cholesterol, cigarette smoking, stress, and a sedentary life-style. Women who use oral contraceptives are also at increased risk. The presence of more than one risk factor increases the risk of a stroke.

Conditions causing CVA

Thrombosis

Atherosclerosis in intracranial and extracranial arteries
Adjacency to intracerebral hemorrhage
Arteritis caused by collagen (autoimmune) disease or bacterial or arteritis
Hypercoagulability such as in polycythemia
Cerebral venous thromboses

Embolism

Valves damaged by rheumatic heart disease (RHD)
Myocardial infarction
Atrial fibrillation (this arrhythmia causes variable emptying of left ventricle, blood pools and small clots form and then at times the ventricle will be emptied completely with release of small emboli)
Bacterial endocarditis and nonbacterial endocarditis causing clots to form on endocardium

Hemorrhage

Hypertensive intracerebral hemorrhage
Subarachnoid hemorrhage
Rupture of aneurysm
Arteriovenous malformation
Hypocoagulation (as in patients with blood dyscrasias)

Generalized hypoxia

Severe hypotension, cardiopulmonary arrest, or severe depression in cardiac output caused by arrhythmias

Localized hypoxia

Cerebral artery spasms associated with subarachnoid hemorrhage
Cerebral artery vasoconstriction associated with migraine headaches

---

■ PATHOPHYSIOLOGY

The brain is very dependent on oxygen and has no reserve oxygen supply. When anoxia occurs, as in CVA, cerebral metabolism is promptly altered, and cell death and permanent damage can occur within 3 to 10 minutes. Any condition that alters cerebral perfusion will cause hypoxia or anoxia. Hypoxia first leads to cerebral ischemia. Short-term ischemia (less than 10 to 15 minutes) causes temporary deficits but no permanent deficits. Long-term ischemia causes permanent cell death and results in cerebral infarction, with accompanying cerebral edema.

The type of permanent focal deficits will depend on the area of the brain that has been affected. The area of the brain affected depends on which cerebral vessels are involved. The vessel most commonly affected is the middle cerebral artery; the second most commonly affected is the internal carotid artery. Permanent focal deficits may be unknown when the patient is first seen because of generalized cerebral ischemia that may resolve.

□ Cerebral thrombosis

Thrombosis is the most common cause of a CVA, and the most common cause of cerebral thrombosis is atherosclerosis. Additional disease processes commonly found with thrombi are hypotension and other types of vascular injury such as arteritis. CVA secondary to thrombosis is seen most often in the 60- to 90-year-old group. Thrombi usually occur in larger vesels and are associated with damage to the vessel wall at the point where the occlusion occurs. The internal carotids are a common source of thrombi.

The onset of symptoms of CVA secondary to thrombosis tends to occur during sleep or soon after arising. This is thought to be related to the fact that elderly persons have decreased sympathetic activity, and recumbency causes a lowering of blood pressure, which can lead to brain ischemia. These persons often also have postural hypotension and poor reflex response to changes in position. Neurologic signs and symptoms very frequently worsen for the first 48 hours after thrombosis.

□ Cerebral embolism

Embolism is the second most common cause of CVA. Patients who have CVAs secondary to embolism are usually younger, and most commonly the emboli originate from a thrombus in the heart. The myocardial thrombus is most commonly caused by rheumatic heart disease with mitral stenosis and atrial fibrillation.

Emboli usually affect small vessels and are commonly found at points of bifurcation where the vessels narrow. They most frequently occur in the middle cerebral artery. Another type of emboli is called septic and originates from bacterial endocarditis.

□ Transient ischemic attack

The term *transient ischemic attack* (TIA) refers to transient cerebral ischemia with temporary episodes of neurologic dysfunction. The neurologic dysfunction can be profound with complete loss of consciousness and loss of all sensory and motor function, or there may only by focal deficits. The most common deficit is contralateral weakness of lower face, hands, arms, and legs, transient dysphasia, and some sensory impairment. Ischemic attacks may occur over days, weeks, or months—between attacks the neurologic examination is normal. TIAs most commonly precede cerebral thrombotic attacks. They can be caused by any of the causes of CVA.

The major importance of TIAs is that they warn the patient and health care professional of the existence of an underlying pathologic condition. At least one third of patients who have TIAs will have a CVA in 2 to 5 years. A person with a TIA needs to be aggressively assessed to determine if preventive measures can be taken.

▥ ASSESSMENT

□ Subjective data

1. Patient's understanding of disease or symptoms
2. Characteristics of onset of symptoms
3. Presence of headache—nature and location
4. Any sensory deficits
5. Visual ability—presence of diplopia, blurred vision
6. Ability to think clearly
7. Any other concomitant symptom

□ Objective data

1. Motor strength—paresis or plegia is common
2. Change in level of consciousness, including unconsciousness
3. Signs of increased intracranial pressure
4. Respiratory status
5. Ability to verbalize—presence of aphasia

The exact clinical picture varies depending on the area of the brain affected. The most common focal signs and symptoms are caused by disruption of flow through the midcerebral artery. These symptoms include the following:

1. Contralateral paralysis or paresis
2. Contralateral sensory loss
3. Sensory and motor loss most noticeable in face, neck, and upper extremities
4. Dysphasia or aphasia; occurs if dominant hemisphere is affected (left hemisphere in right-handed persons and most left-handed persons)
5. Spatial-perceptual problems, changes in judgment and behavior, neglect of paralyzed side, and inability to recognize paralyzed extremity as own (*anosognosia*) if nondominant hemisphere is affected
6. Contralateral *homonymous hemianopsia*

Aphasia is a disorder of language caused by damage to the speech-controlling areas of the brain. It includes all areas of language, including speech, reading, writing, and understanding.[7,8,66] These abnormalities can occur in a variety of ways as follows:

1. *Sensory aphasia*—inability to comprehend spoken word (also called receptive aphasia)

Comparisons between left and right hemiplegia

(handwritten: R hemisphere) *(handwritten: Left hemisphere)*

	Left hemiplegia	Right hemiplegia
Language	Usually intact	Receptive or expressive aphasia in varying degrees
Speech	Dysarthria	Dysarthria
Sensation	Left sensory loss	Right sensory loss
	Left homonymous hemianopsia	Right homonymous hemianopsia
Perception	Decreased awareness of left side of body	Normal awareness of right side of body
	Other perceptual problems	
Movement	Left-sided paralysis or paresis	Right-sided paralysis or paresis
	Apraxia *(handwritten: movement problem (voluntary))*	Less often apraxic
Behavior	Impaired judgment	Judgment intact
	Increased emotional lability	Increased emotional lability
Memory	Deficit of new spatial information	Deficit of new language information

---

Cerebral arteriogram (angiogram)

Purpose

To visualize the cerebral arterial system by injecting radiopaque material. Allows detection of arterial aneurysms, vessel anomalies, ruptured vessels, and displacement of vessels by mass lesions

Preparation of patient

1. Patient is given clear liquids morning of procedure.
2. Patient must be assessed for allergy to iodine.
3. If femoral approach is to be used, it is helpful to assess and mark the locations of the bilateral pedal pulses.
4. If the carotid artery is used, the neck circumference is measured as part of the baseline data.
5. Sedation may be given the night before and just before the procedure.
6. If the femoral approach is used, the groin site may be shaved the night before.
7. Immediately before the procedure, baseline vital signs, pulses, and neurologic checks should be done and recorded.
8. Patient teaching
   a. Explain procedure.
   b. Time: approximately 2 to 3 hours.
   c. Sensation: some discomfort in lying still for several hours. At the time of dye injection, most patients complain of feeling extremely hot and seeing flashes of light.

Procedure

1. Patient is positioned supine on the x-ray table.
2. Local anesthetic is used to anesthetize the area of puncture site.
3. Catheter is introduced percutaneously.
   a. In a four-vessel study, catheter is inserted into the femoral artery, innominate, carotid, and vertebral arteries.
   b. Each vessel is injected with the contrast dye as serial x-ray films are taken.
   c. Carotid or vertebral vessels may be used directly.
4. Catheter is withdrawn and pressure is applied to puncture site for at least 5 minutes.

After procedure

1. Patient is usually kept in bed overnight.
2. Vital signs are checked frequently (may be as often as every 15 minutes for a period of several hours), as well as neurologic checks with each vital sign check.
3. Site of puncture is assessed frequently for presence of hematoma.
   a. Femoral: check pulses distal to site for evidence of arterial occlusion.
   b. Carotid: check for difficulty breathing or swallowing; measure neck girth frequently.
4. Dye used in angiogram may raise intracranial pressure and cause decreased extremity strengths or change in level of consciousness.

Digital subtraction angiography (DSA)

Purpose

To identify abnormalities of the cerebrovascular system, using a process that removes overlying structures in an image, so that the clinically significant details can be displayed with enhanced visibility.

Preparation of patient

1. Permit must be signed.
2. Food may be restricted before procedure.
3. Patient should be asked about allergy to iodine.
4. Patient teaching
   a. Explain procedure.
   b. Time: approximately 45 to 60 minutes
   c. Sensation: some discomfort associated with the start of the IV. Injection of the dye may be uncomfortable. Some patients may find need to lie still uncomfortable.

Procedure

1. Patient is positioned supine on the x-ray table.
2. Local anesthetic may be used to anesthetize the area of puncture site.
3. Catheter is introduced into vein, usually in the arm for cerebral studies.
4. Dye is injected as films are taken.
5. Catheter is withdrawn.

After procedure

1. Vital signs are checked on return to floor.
2. Circulatory status of arm is assessed.
3. Injection site is checked for presence of hematoma.
4. Usually no activity restrictions—procedure can be done on an outpatient basis.
5. The computer performs the subtraction, a process that removes underlying structures in an image, so that the clinically significant details can be displayed with enhanced visibility.

---

2. *Motor aphasia*—inability to use the symbols of speech (also called expressive aphasia)
3. *Global aphasia*—inability to understand the spoken word, as well as to speak[18]

☐ Diagnostic tests

A lumbar puncture (p. 423) is usually performed and may reveal increased spinal fluid pressure. If the CVA is caused by hemorrhage, blood will be present in the spinal fluid. The CT scan may show an area of decreased density. The MRI scan will visualize this pathology also. A brain scan can demonstrate diminished perfusion.

Following TIAs, a cerebral angiogram may be done to discover blocked or occluded vessels. In some cases a digital substraction angiogram (DSA) is done instead. See the boxes on p. 470 and above for details of the procedure.

▶ DATA ANALYSIS: NURSING DIAGNOSES

Nursing diagnoses are determined from assessment of patient data. Possible nursing diagnoses for the person with a stroke may include, but are not limited to, the following:

Diagnostic title	Possible etiologies
Ineffective airway clearance	Obstruction/secretion, perceptual/cognitive impairment
Anxiety	Change in health status/role functioning
Body image disturbance	Loss of body functions, immobility change in life-style
Ineffective breathing pattern	Neuromuscular impairment
Impaired verbal communication	Aphasia, physical impairment
Constipation or incontinence	Immobility, inadequate nutrition, neuromuscular impairment
Impaired home maintenance management	Individual injury, impaired cognitive functioning, inadequate support systems
Total incontinence	Neurologic dysfunction
Knowledge deficit	Lack of exposure/recall, cognitive limitation, unfamiliarity with information sources

Diagnostic title	Possible etiologies
Impaired physical mobility	Neuromuscular impairment, perceptual/cognitive impairment
Unilateral neglect	Neurologic illness/trauma
Altered nutrition: less than body requirements	Chewing or swallowing difficulties
Pain	Immobility, improper positioning, stroke
Feeding, bathing/hygiene, dressing/grooming, toileting self-care deficit	Perception/cognitive impairment, neuromuscular impairment
Sensory/perceptual alterations: visual, kinesthetic, tactile	Altered sensory reception/transmission/integration
Sexual dysfunction	Physiologic alterations
Potential impaired skin integrity	Mechanical forces, immobility
	Neuromuscular impairment
Altered thought processes	Neurologic disorders
Altered cerebral tissue perfusion	Decreased blood flow
Altered patterns of urinary elimination	Sensorimotor impairment

⊞ PLANNING: EXPECTED PATIENT OUTCOMES

Expected patient outcomes for the person who has had a stroke may include, but are not limited to, the following:

1. Patient demonstrates a patent airway.
2. Patient verbalizes minimal anxiety.
3. Patient has an effective breathing pattern.
4. Patient has minimal discomfort.
5. Patient has minimal problems because of altered verbal communication.
6. Patient develops alternative means of communication.
7. Patient shows optimal ability to manage activities of daily living and home maintenance.
8. Patient has minimal complications as a result of incontinence.
9. Patient's continence is improved.
10. Patient remains free of traumatic injury.
11. Patient or caregiver can demonstrate exercises to maintain function.
12. Patient or caregiver can explain medication regimen—side effects, times, doses, and route.
13. Patient safely compensates for visual field cuts, perceptual, motor, and sensory losses.
14. Patient can maintain an adequate nutritional status.
15. Patient's skin is intact.
16. Patient verbalizes plans to compensate for disability in terms of sexual performance.
17. Patient's swallowing is intact.
18. Patient's cerebral circulation is adequate.
19. Patient can state plans for follow-up care.
20. Patient can explain the importance of frequent position changes and can demonstrate such positioning.

⊞ IMPLEMENTATION

☐ **Assisting with the achievement of therapeutic goals**
☐ *Care in the initial phase*

Goals in the initial phase are directed toward survival needs and preventing further brain damage. Care must take into account that some patients may be unconscious. Neurologic assessment is performed at regular intervals to detect changes in status, as well as any complications. Any indication of rising intracranial pressure should be reported at once. Drugs to reduce intracranial pressure, such as dexamethasone (Decadron) may be given. The patient may have an intracranial monitoring device in place. See p. 437 for a description of these devices.

The use of anticoagulants is controversial. In an attempt to prevent further thrombosis or emboli, heparin may be given if it is certain that the cause of the CVA is cerebral thrombosis or emboli and not cerebral hemorrhage.

☐ *Care in the acute phase*

Goals for the care in the acute phase are directed toward preventing complications from the original CVA, from the immobility and dependency it causes and from the loss of function caused by focal deficits.

MOTOR FUNCTION. Since the CVA frequently results in some paralysis, refer to p. 439 for a discussion of the care of the person with loss of motor function.

NUTRITION. Fluids may be restricted for the first few days after a CVA in an effort to prevent edema of the brain. In patients who are comatose or who have swallowing difficulties, it may be necessary to use intravenous fluids, or a nasogastric tube may be inserted and tube feedings started. When patients are more alert, food and fluids are offered in small amounts. Returning as soon as possible to a regular diet and a normal fluid intake is desirable.

ACTIVITY. Rest and quiet are important even if the CVA has not been serious enough to cause complete loss of consciousness. The length of time the patient remains in bed depends on the type of CVA and the judgment of the physician in regard to early mobilization.

Prevention of joint deformity is initiated during the acute stage. This includes positioning of affected limbs in anatomic position and ROM exercises. There should be a regular schedule for turning the patient to avoid the danger of circulatory stasis, hypostatic pneumonia, and decubitus ulcers.

ELIMINATION. Urinary output should be noted carefully and recorded for several days after a CVA. Retention of urine may occur, but it is more likely that the patient will be incontinent. If urinary incontinence occurs, the patient should be told that control of elimination should improve day by day. Offering a bedpan or urinal immediately after meals and at other regular intervals is a start to bladder training. A retention catheter may be used for the first several days. In the male patient who is not retaining urine, an external catheter may be very helpful.

Fecal incontinence also is a fairly common occurrence following a CVA. Some patients develop constipation, and impaction can develop rapidly. Elimination must be noted carefully, since diarrhea may develop in the presence of an impaction, thus causing it to go unnoticed. Suppositories such as bisacodyl (Dulcolax) may be prescribed, along with stool softeners. Warm oil–retention enemas are sometimes given when impactions occur. The patient must be cautioned not to strain at the stool. The patient also usually needs assistance in getting on and off the bedpan. Side rails that can be held onto while turning or a trapeze that can be reached with the unaffected arm and hand will help the patient move independently.

□ *Care in the rehabilitation phase*

The greatest challenge for the nurse in care of the patient who has had a CVA comes after the patient is past the point of danger, because then the long, slow process of learning to use whatever abilities remain or can be relearned must be faced. Also, adjustments to limitations must be faced and made if meaningful life is to continue.

The nurse is an important member of the rehabilitation team. Three nursing goals include the following:
1. Prevention of further impairment
2. Maintenance of existing abilities
3. Restoration of as much function as possible

Knowledge of the physical arrangements for after-hospital care is important in setting priorites and planning care.

RETURN OF FUNCTION Return of motor impulses and movement in involved extremities occurs in stages. These stages can last from hours to months. Recovery may also halt at a specific stage and progress no further. Brunnstrom has defined these recovery stages in degrees of *synergy*. Synergy has been defined as muscles acting together as a bound unit in stereotyped movement patterns.[57] See the box above, right for these stages.

Return of motor function and impulses is significant for the future use of the affected part but presents new problems. Muscles that draw the limbs toward the midline become very active, and the arm may be held tightly adducted against the body. The affected lower limb may be held inward and adducted to, or even beyond, the midline. Muscles that draw the limbs into flexion are also stimulated, with the result that the heel is lifted off the ground, the heel cord shortens, and the knee becomes bent. In the arm, flexor muscles draw the elbow into the bent position, the wrist is flexed, and fingers are curled in palmar flexion.

Persistent nursing efforts must be directed toward prevention of further impairment. It is important that no part of the body remains in a position of flexion long enough for the occurrence of muscle shortening and joint changes that might interfere with free joint action. Appropriate interventions include the following:
1. Passive exercise—stimulates circulation and may help to reestablish neuromuscular pathways
2. Active exercise started as soon as possible

Recovery stages	
Flaccidity	No voluntary motion, lack of muscle tone
Partial synergy	Muscle tone develops and muscles contract either voluntarily or with spasticity. Patient can move extremities in part of synergy pattern.
Synergy	Spasticity moderate to severe. Patient can move joints through all or most of synergy pattern.
Breaking out of synergy	Spasticity decreased. Patient can perform combinations of movements that are out of synergy.
Partially isolated	Less influence of spasticity. Movement combinations are less like stereotyped patterns.
Isolated	Near normal movement with good control of voluntary movement and little spasticity.

3. Attention to the unaffected limbs to maintain strength—includes keeping unaffected leg in position of slight internal rotation
4. Early ambulation—facilitates vasomotor tone and has positive psychologic effects on the patient and family members

The *Bobath technique* is a treatment approach designed to normalize muscle tone. This is done by providing as many sensations of normal muscle tone, posture, and movement as possible. The goal of the treatment is to redirect short-term memory toward an appreciation of normal movement of the paralyzed side by incorporating techniques of weight bearing, counter-rotation, and protraction of the shoulder girdle and pelvis. The reader is referred Johnson and Olson[23a] and to a rehabilitation nursing text for further description of this technique.

When patients begin to move about and try to help themselves, they may have several problems that can affect ability to proceed. They may have loss of position sense, so that it is awkward for them to handle their bodies normally, even when they have the muscular coordination to do so. They may have dizziness, spatial-perceptual deficits, diplopia, and alteration of skin sensations. They may also have to work harder to receive a normal amount of air on inhalation because the involved side of the chest does not expand easily.

SURGERY. After the patient's condition is stable (with a CVA), or after one or more TIAs, surgery may be used for selected patients. If the symptoms are associated with an atherosclerotic lesion in the extracranial system (internal carotid artery or common carotid artery), a carotid end-arterectomy may be performed.

A carotid endarterectomy involves the reaming out of the diseased vessel under either local or general anesthesia. Postoperative care includes the following:

1. Close attention to neurologic signs (changes in strength, mentation, speech, and level of consciousness)
2. Observation for bleeding in the incisional area
3. Observation for swelling of the neck or complaints of dysphagia
4. Availability of tracheostomy tray in case of severe respiratory distress.[81]

Revascularization procedures are now possible with the use of stereoscopic microscopes. Commonly, the superficial temporal artery is anastomosed to an artery within the brain such as the midcerebral artery. Other vessels can be used. The purpose is to provide for greater blood flow. The surgery usually does not resolve any permanent deficits, but it may prevent further problems. The care of the patient preoperatively and postoperatively is similar to that for any patient with cranial surgery, but it also includes the following:

1. Checking for pulse in anastomosed vessel
   a. Doppler
   b. Gentle palpation
2. Keeping graft areas free of pressure
   a. Eyeglass frames bent out so as not to occlude vessel
   b. No other restricting bands around head

The patient will have a postoperative angiogram to assess the patency of the vessel.[32,35]

☐ Assisting with comfort and ADL
☐ Emotional support

If the patient who has had a CVA survives the first few days, consciousness usually returns, and some of the paralysis may disappear. It is then that great understanding is needed to help the patient accept his or her limitations. Using quiet assurance, a nurse can help the patient feel that progress toward recovery and self-sufficiency has begun and will continue.

The patient who has sustained a CVA may be overly emotional, and this reaction, combined with the fear and frustration on becoming aware of his or her condition, may be upsetting to the family. Crying is common. Family, staff, and sometimes other patients need reassurance that they are not the cause of the reaction.

☐ Perceptual problems

Following a stroke, persons may have difficulty relating to themselves and their environment. After the acute stage, a multibed environment is advocated, since the sensory input from others is helpful. Hemianopsia, or decreased visual field, occurs commonly. Approaching patients from the side of intact vision and teaching them to scan with their eyes will help make them more aware of stimuli and help prevent injury. Diminished awareness or denial of the affected side (anosognosia) can occur and can be a safety hazard. This possibility should be considered when the

patient runs into objects or allows the affected arm or leg to drag behind.

☐ Activities of daily living

The patient is evaluated regarding the ability to carry out the usual ADL and is assisted by the occupational therapist or nurse in becoming independent in each activity to the extent possible. Rehabilitation in this way is essentially a teaching-learning process in which the patient is actively involved.

☐ Counseling and teaching

The teaching for a patient with cerebrovascular accident is the same as that for the patient with a motor problem (p. 448).

⊞ EVALUATION

See p. 446 for a description of evaluation questions for the patient with motor dysfunction and p. 449 for those of a patient with a sensory dysfunction.

■ INTRACRANIAL HEMORRHAGE

Intracerebral or intracranial hemorrhages include bleeding into the subarachnoid space or into the brain tissue itself. These hemorrhages cause damage to the brain by destroying and replacing brain tissue. Nursing and medical treatment of a patient with an aneurysm and intracranial hemorrhage can be significantly different from that of a patient with a CVA.

Intracranial hemorrhages are the third most common cause of CVAs. The peak incidence of aneurysms is in the 35- to 60-year-old age group. Women are affected slighly more often than men. A ruptured cerebral aneurysm is the most common cause of subarachnoid hemorrhage not related to trauma. Bleeding may be from a vessel on the surface of the brain, and the bleeding may be limited to the subarachnoid space. Bleeding from a vessel in the brain substance may form a cerebral hematoma and extend through the brain tissue to the ventricles.

The most common causes of cerebral hemorrhage are as follows:

1. Berry aneurysms—usually congenital defects
2. Fusiform aneurysms—from atherosclerosis
3. Mycotic aneurysms—from necrotic vasculitis and septic emboli
4. Arteriovenous malformations—tangled, interconnected vessels that allow blood to pass directly from the artery to the vein[61]
5. Rupture of cerebral arterioles—from hypertension, which causes thickening and degeneration

■ PATHOPHYSIOLOGY

Any of the causes listed can result in subarachnoid hemorrhage, intracerebral hemorrhage, or a combination of the two. The most common site for berry aneurysms is the anterior portion of the Circle of Willis at the junction between the internal carotid and posterior communicating arteries. Multiple aneurysms are found in many persons.

Aneurysmal rupture occurs when a small hole occurs in a part of the aneurysm. The hemorrhage spreads rapidly, producing localized changes and irritation to the cerebral vessels. The bleeding is usually halted by the formation of a plug consisting of fibrin-platelets and by tissue compression. Within 3 weeks the hemorrhage begins to undergo resorption. Recurrent rupture is a serious risk 7 to 10 days after the initial hemorrhage. The rupture of a vessel causes disruption of the blood flow to a selected area, focal ischemic changes, and infarction of brain tissue. In addition, the sudden release of blood has the effect of a concussion, and unconsciousness occurs. It also causes a rapid rise in cerebrospinal fluid pressure with displacement of the brain. Bleeding into brain tissue itself can cause damage by dissecting the brain along the fiber tracts. In addition, hemorrhage may produce a filling of the ventricular system or produce a hematoma that distorts brain tissue.

Blood itself is a noxious agent, and as it is hemolyzed it irritates the blood vessels, the meninges, and the brain. The blood and the release of vasoactive substances promote arterial spasms, which can further decrease cerebral perfusion. This arterial spasm, or vasospasm, usually occurs from 4 to 10 days after the hemorrhage and causes constriction or narrowing of the cerebral arteries. These vasospasms are serious complications: they can cause focal neurologic decline, ischemia of the brain, and infarction.

About 50% of patients with rupture of an aneurysm recover from the initial episode, but at least 50% of these persons will have recurrences of hemorrhage if untreated. Recurrence may occur within 2 weeks, and the danger of death occurs and increases with each bleeding episode.

ASSESSMENT

The assessment for intracerebral hemorrhage includes the factors identified in the subjective and objective assessment for the patient who has had a CVA. Symptoms of an intracranial hemorrhage include the following:

1. Sudden, explosive headache
2. Photophobia
3. Neck rigidity
4. Nausea and vomiting
5. Loss of consciousness
6. Convulsions
7. Respiratory distress
8. Shock

DATA ANALYSIS: NURSING DIAGNOSES

Possible nursing diagnoses for the patient with an intracerebral hemorrhage are the same as for the patient who has had a CVA (p. 471).

PLANNING: EXPECTED PATIENT OUTCOMES

In addition to those patient outcomes defined for the patient with a CVA (p. 472), these additional outcomes are important:

1. Patient does not develop signs of increased ICP.
2. Patient does not develop complications from the immobility.
3. Patient can explain the need for surgery and relevant factors.
4. Patient can explain any restrictions in activity.

IMPLEMENTATION

☐ Assisting with the achievement of therapeutic goals

The immediate treatment for intracranial hemorrhage is to keep the person absolutely quiet to prevent additional bleeding. An antifibronolytic agent (aminocaproic acid [Amicar]) may be used to seal the clot. Other nursing actions to be used may include those listed in the box below.

☐ Surgery

The only satisfactory treatment for aneurysm is surgery. Surgery is not usually performed to repair arteriovenous anomalies or hypertensive vascular disease. If an intracerebral hematoma has formed, it may be evacuated after the patient's condition is stable. Before surgery can be performed, angiography must be performed to determine location of the aneurysm. The time after the acute rupture until the surgery is performed varies with the person, their age, the intensity and kind of symptoms present, and the judgment of the surgeon to determine when surgery will be recommended (see the box on p. 476).

Surgery consists of a craniotomy and location of the aneurysm. When found, the aneurysm may be obliterated by ligation at its neck with the application of a silver clip. If the base of the aneurysm is too large for ligation to be practical, it may be coated with a liquid, adherent, plastic substance that hardens to form a firm support about the

---

Nursing care of the patient with an intracranial hemorrhage

1. Use gentleness in moving patient.
2. Keep room darkened.
3. Keep patient resting in bed—head of bed is usually elevated 30 degrees. Occasionally bathroom privileges are allowed.
4. Give patient no ice water.
5. Initiate a bowel program to prevent constipation and straining at stool.
6. Allow few visitors.
7. Decrease stimuli in room—no TV or radio in severe cases.
8. Take no rectal temperatures.
9. Encourage patient to seek assistance for change in position.

Postoperative care of the patient with intracranial surgery

1. Monitoring
   a. Assess neurologic status including ability to move, level of orientation, and alertness and pupil checks.
   b. Assess degree and character of drainage.
      (1) Amount of drainage and bleeding should be minimal.
      (2) Initial head dressing can be reinforced as necessary.
      (3) Often incision is left open to air after first several days.
2. Promoting mobility
   a. Turning to either side is permitted except when large brain tumors have been removed. If this is the case, patient is not turned to affected side as gravity may cause displacement of brain structures.
   b. For supratentorial surgery, the head of the bed is elevated at least 30 degrees.
   c. If infratentorial surgery was performed, the bed is flat or elevated only slightly and a small pillow is placed under the nape of the neck. Neck flexion is avoided.
   d. Early ambulation is encouraged to prevent complications of bed rest. Observe carefully for signs of postural hypotension and raise head of bed gradually; patient should always sit before standing.
3. Promoting decreased ICP
   a. Space nursing activities to allow patient to rest between them.
   b. Coughing and vomiting should be avoided.
   c. Suctioning should be done only as necessary, and then gently and cautiously.
4. Protecting safety of patient
   a. Use of soft hand restraints if restraints are necessary.
   b. Use of mittens as alternative to restraints; make sure fingers are separated and fingers are placed around large roll. Change mitt at least daily—give range of motion to hand at this time.
   c. Keep side rails up at all times.
5. Promoting electrolyte balance
   a. Accurate intake and output with measurement of specific gravity. Frequent testing for sugar and acetone if patient is taking steroids.
   b. Resumption of diet as soon as possible; assess for difficulty in swallowing or absence of gag reflex.
   c. Monitor electrolyes for evidence of abnormalities.
6. Promotion of comfort
   a. Medicate for comfort with codeine sulfate or nonnarcotic analgesic.
   b. Ice cap to head for headache may be helpful.

---

weakened vessel wall. If the aneurysm has not ruptured but has produced symptoms, attempts may be made to produce thrombosis by use of an electrical current and other means.

□ Other procedures

Not all aneurysms can be treated surgically at the site of the lesion. If surgery is not feasible, the common carotid artery in the neck may be completely or partially obliterated to lessen the flow of blood to the site of the aneurysm and reduce the chances of hemorrhage. This is contingent on whether sufficient blood can be supplied from collateral vessels to preserve brain function. The procedure usually is performed in stages over several days. A clamp (Silverstone or Salibi) with a detachable screw stem that can be tightened gradually is used. Usually the surgeon adjusts it each day, and the nurse assesses the patient closely and is instructed to release the clamp at once if there is evidence of inadequate blood supply, as shown by decreased neurologic status. Immediate removal of the clamps may prevent irreversible complications such as hemiplegia, aphasia, and loss of consciousness. If complete occlusion can be tolerated, the vessel may be permanently ligated. Serial embolizations of blood vessels that "feed" the aneurysm may also be done via the femoral or axillary route. The procedure is similar to a cerebral angiogram, and the postoperative care is the same. Thrombus formation with resultant cerebral embolism may complicate the patient's postoperative course following any surgery for a cerebral aneurysm.

□ Counseling and teaching

If the patient with an intracranial hemorrhage has neurologic deficits consistent with a CVA, the teaching is the same. Additionally, the points listed in the box on p. 477 are important.

Teaching for the patient with intracranial hemorrhage

1. Importance of following activity restrictions
2. Importance of keeping as free of stress as possible
3. Very specific teaching about what activites are restricted
4. Use of medication and what it does
5. Information about preoperative and postoperative care will be useful

---

✚ EVALUATION

These questions should also be asked in the evaluation of a patient who has had a CVA:

1. Is the patient's neurologic status stable?
2. Is the patient cooperating with the activity restrictions?
3. Is the patient relatively calm?
4. Does the patient verbalize understanding of the restrictions?
5. Does the patient verbalize understanding of surgery planned?

■ INTERFERENCE WITH FUNCTION BECAUSE OF INFECTION/ INFLAMMATION

Interference with function because of infection/inflammation is a fairly common occurrence. Specific conditions to discuss include the following:

1. Meningitis
2. Encephalitis
3. Brain abscess
4. Poliomyelitis
5. Guillain-Barré-Strohl syndrome (polyneuritis)
6. Herpes zoster
7. Neurosyphilis
8. AIDS

Because these conditions contain many common characteristics, they will be discussed together.

The nervous system may be attacked by a variety of organisms and viruses and may suffer from toxins of bacteria and viruses. These toxins reach the nervous system through a variety of routes. Untreated chronic otitis media and mastoiditis, chronic sinusitis, and fracture in any bone adjacent to the meninges may be the source of infection. Some organisms such as the tubercle bacillus reach the nervous system by means of the blood or lymphatic system. Meningitis can occur as a complication of an invasive procedure such as a lumbar puncture. The exact route of some other organisms is not known.

■ Meningitis

■ PATHOPHYSIOLOGY

Meningitis is an acute infection of the meninges. It is usually caused by one of the following organisms:

1. Pneumococci
2. Meningococci
3. Staphylococci
4. Streptococci
5. *Haemophilus influenzae*
6. Aseptic agents (usually viral)

The effect of the bacteria or other organisms in the subarachnoid space is an inflammatory reaction in the pia and arachnoid and in the CSF. Pus accumulates in these areas. The bacteria or its toxin, if not treated in a timely manner, may injure cranial and spinal nerves and other structures. In addition, the purulent material that occurs may obstruct the flow of CSF, resulting in hydrocephalus. The longer the infectious process occurs before it is treated, the more complications and neurologic sequalae that can occur.

Meningitis can be classed as bacterial (leptomeningitis) or aseptic. The term aseptic meningitis was first introduced in 1925 and was first thought to refer to a specific disease. It is now recognized as a complex of symptoms that result from many infective agents, the majority of which are viral. *Herpes simplex* is an example of a virus that can cause aseptic meningitis. Any other pathogenic organism, such as the tubercle bacillus, that gains access to the subarachnoid spaces can also cause meningitis. The incidence of bacterial meningitis is higher in fall and winter when upper respiratory tract infections are common. Children are more often affected than adults because of frequent colds and ear infections.

Pathologic changes that occur include any or all of the following:

1. Hyperemia of the meningeal vessels
2. Edema of brain tissue
3. Increased ICP
4. Generalized inflammatory reaction with exudation of white blood cells into the subarachnoid spaces
5. Associated hydrocephalus caused by exudate blocking the small passage between the ventricles

▦ ASSESSMENT

Subjective and objective assessment are important in any patient with an infection of the nervous system. This assessment includes characteristics that are common to all the infections/inflammations discussed in this section.

☐ Subjective data

1. Patient's understanding of process and possible causes
2. Any history of infection such as upper respiratory infections
3. Measures that relieve symptoms
4. Presence of discomfort, including headache or stiff neck

5. Initial onset of symptoms
6. Presence of difficulty in thinking
7. Presence of muscle weakness, soreness, or incoordination

☐ **Objective data**

1. Behavior: signs indicating discomfort or disorientation
2. Change in ability to carry out daily activities
3. Abnormalities on physical assessment part of neurologic examination
4. Temperature
5. Presence of vomiting
6. Pulse and blood pressure
7. Respirations
8. Abnormal CT results
9. Meningeal irritation
10. Evidence of presence of seizures

The onset of meningitis is usually sudden and characterized by severe headache, stiffness of the neck, irritability, malaise, and restlessness. Nausea, vomiting, delirium, and complete disorientation develop quickly. Temperature, pulse rate, and respirations are increased. Two pathologic signs that occur with meningitis are the following:

1. *Kernig's sign*—the inability of the patient to extend the legs completely without extreme pain
2. *Brudzinski's sign*—flexion of the hip and knee when the neck is flexed

☐ **Diagnostic tests**

Most of the infections affecting the nervous system can be diagnosed by examining the cerebrospinal fluid. A CT scan and an EEG may also be used. These procedures were discussed earlier in this chapter.

➡ DATA ANALYSIS: NURSING DIAGNOSES

Nursing diagnoses are determined from assessment of patient data. Possible nursing diagnoses for the person with meningitis may include, but are not limited to, the following:

Diagnostic title	Possible etiologies
Ineffective airway clearance	Tracheobronchial infection/obstruction/secretion
Anxiety	Threat of change in health status
Bowel incontinence	Neuromuscular impairment
Impaired breathing pattern	Neuromuscular impairment
Impaired verbal communication	Aphasia
Impaired home maintenance management	Individual disease, impaired cognitive functioning
Hyperthermia	Illness/trauma
Total incontinence	Neurologic disease
Potential for injury: trauma	Sensorimotor deficits
Knowledge deficit	Lack of exposure/recall

Diagnostic title	Possible etiologies
Impaired physical mobility	Neuromuscular impairment
Altered nutrition: less than body requirements	Chewing or swallowing difficulties
Pain	Meningeal irritation
Feeding, bathing/hygiene, dressing/grooming, toileting self-care deficit	Neuromuscular impairment
Potential impaired skin integrity	Mechanical forces, immobility
Ineffective swallowing	Neuromuscular impairment
Ineffective thermoregulation	Illness
Altered thought processes	Neurologic disorder
Altered cerebral tissue perfusion	Decreased blood flow
Altered patterns of urinary elimination	Sensorimotor impairment, urinary infection

⊞ PLANNING: EXPECTED PATIENT OUTCOMES

Expected patient outcomes for the person with meningitis may include, but are not limited to, the following:

1. Patient demonstrates a patent airway.
2. Patient demonstrates minimal anxiety.
3. Patient's bowel movements are continent to the extent possible and there are minimal complications of any incontinence or constipation.
4. Patient has minimal discomfort.
5. Patient's verbal communication is maintained.
6. Patient has minimal impairments in home management.
7. Patient has minimal complications because of urinary incontinence.
8. Patient remains free of traumatic injury.
9. Patient (if able) or family can verbalize knowledge of disease.
10. Patient and/or family can explain the action, side effects, and toxic effects of medications to be taken.
11. Patient maintains adequate nutrition.
12. Patient's temperature remains normal.
13. Patient maintains optimal mobility.
14. Patient has minimal deficits in self-care activities.
15. Patient can explain plans for follow-up care.
16. Patient compensates for difficulties in thought processes.
17. Patient's skin is intact.

⊞ IMPLEMENTATION

☐ **Assisting with achievement of therapeutic goals**

Treatment of meningitis consists of massive doses of the antibiotic or antibiotics specific for the causative organism. Treatment with multiple antibiotics is common. Culture and sensitivity studies demonstrate the most effective antibiotic. Usually a course of at least 10 days of parenteral administration is needed. The antibiotic may also be given directly into the spinal canal (intrathecally). The use of hyperosmolar agents or steroids may be necessary to decrease cerebral edema. Anticonvulsants may be given to prevent seizures.

Nursing care for the patient with meningitis includes the following:

1. General care given a critically ill patient
2. Darkened room, with noise kept to a minimum, because sensory stimulation can cause seizures
3. Careful neurologic checks at frequent intervals
4. Padded side rails

Residual damage from meningitis includes deafness, blindness, paralysis, and mental retardation. These complications are usually the result of chronic arachnoiditis. Hydrocephalus may also develop, requiring a shunting procedure.

Isolation of the patient depends on the causative organism. Check the infection control manual of your institution for specific guidelines.

⊞ EVALUATION

Evaluation of the patient with meningitis includes answers to the following questions:

1. Is the patient breathing effectively?
2. Is the patient demonstrating minimal anxiety?
3. Is the patient having minimal complications from incontinence?
4. Is the patient having regular bowel movements without diarrhea or constipation?
5. Is the patient's mobility at the optimal level?
6. Is the patient free of other infections?
7. Is the patient able to compensate for any alterations in thought processes?
8. Is the patient maintaining optimal nutrition?
9. Is the patient having minimal difficulties in ADL?
10. Is the patient free of pain?
11. Is the patient free of injury?
12. Can the patient or family explain the medication regime?
13. Can the patient or family state plans for follow up?
14. Can the patient or family verbalize knowledge of the disease process?
15. Is the patient's skin intact?
16. Can the patient communicate with those around him?
17. Is the patient making progress toward continence?

If the patient has motor dysfunction, appropriate questions can be found on p. 446.

▪ Encephalitis

▪ PATHOPHYSIOLOGY

Encephalitis is an inflammation of the brain tissues and its covering. Occasionally, the meninges of the spinal cord are also involved. It can have a variety of causes, including the following:

1. Syphilis
2. Exogenous poisoning such as that which follows the ingestion of lead or arsenic or inhalation of carbon monoxide
3. Reaction to toxins produced by infections such as typhoid fever, measles, and chickenpox
4. Reaction to vaccination
5. Various viruses, including arbovirus (those transferred by biting arthropod to humans)

Encephalitis caused by a virus and occurring in epidemic form was first described by von Economo in Austria, and the name *von Economo's disease* is still used to identify the widespread epidemic in the United States that followed the influenza epidemic in 1918. von Economo's disease was also called *sleeping sickness,* a term still used by laypersons. The demonstration that viruses can affect the central nervous system after a prolonged incubation period has resulted in considerable search for viral agents in many chronic neurologic diseases.

▦ ASSESSMENT

The subjective and objective data for encephalitis are the same as for meningitis (p. 477). The onset of encephalitis is often abrupt, with a high fever, headache, meningeal signs, nuchal rigidity, and vomiting. Drowsiness or coma and focal or generalized convulsions usually develop within 24 to 48 hours after onset of symptoms. Focal neurologic signs develop, such as hemiplegia and cranial nerve palsies. There are typical findings in the CSF. Mortality may be as high as 60%.[48]

▶ DATA ANALYSIS: NURSING DIAGNOSES

The reader is referred to the nursing diagnoses in the discussion of meningitis (p. 478).

▦ IMPLEMENTATION

Nursing care consists of symptomatic or supportive care and careful observation. Any change in appearance or behavior should be reported becasue the progress of this disease sometimes is extremly rapid. Bed rest is advocated. If disorientation is present, the patient must be attended constantly. During the time when temperature is increased, sponge baths or other hypothermia methods are used. There is no specific medical treatment for this disease. No isolation is necessary because encephalitis is not transmitted from person to person. Prevention of arboviral infections includes destruction of larvae and elimination of breeding places. Control includes avoiding bites of the mosquito or tick vectors.

⊞ EVALUATION

Evaluation includes those questions defined under the evaluation section of meningitis (at left).

■ Brain abscess

The frequency of abscesses in the areas of the brain is site specific, with most found in the cerebrum (75%) and cerebellum (25%). Some abscesses, as many as one fifth, have multiple foci.[48] Of patients with brain abscesses, 30% to 60% may die and those surviving may have different types of residual deficits, including paralysis and seizures.

A brain abscess is almost always secondary to a foci of infection somewhere else in the body, such as extension of chronic middle ear, sinus, or mastoid infections. The bacteria gain access to the cranial vault directly through bone, through the dura matter, across the subarachnoid and subdural spaces, or along venous routes. Common sites of the primary infection include the following:

1. Ear
2. Sinus or mastoid
3. Lung
4. Heart
5. Pelvic organs
6. Teeth
7. Skin

The three most common organisms involved are the streptococci, staphylococci, and pneumococci. Brain abscesses are most common in older children and young adults but may be seen at any age.

Complications from ear infections account for almost one half of all brain abscesses. These abscesses are often found in the frontal lobe. Abscesses originating from infections in the frontal, ethmoid, and sphenoid sinuses are also found in the frontal lobe. The sphenoid sinuses may also seed into the temporal lobe. If the abscess is disseminated through the blood stream, the abscesses are multiplied and found in the white matter. Penetrating head injuries, compound skull fractures, and osteomyelitis of the skull lead to the formation of brain abscesses.

■ PATHOPHYSIOLOGY

The first stage of brain abscess is characterized by local edema, hyperemia, infiltration by leukocytes, and softening of the parenchyma. Septic thromboses of some vessels occur, and the surrounding brain tissue becomes necrotic and edematous. Days to weeks after the beginning stages there is a process of central liquefaction and necrosis of brain tissue with the formation of a cystic wall of pus. This becomes encased by a wall that is thinner on the ventral side with a predisposition to rupture. If rupture occurs, the infection extends through the entire brain, leading to meningitis.

ASSESSMENT

The questions to ask in collecting data from the patient with a brain abscess are the same as for the patient with meningitis (p. 477). With a brain abscess, there may be a history of infection. The most common symptom is a constant or intermittent headache that is not relieved by medication and that is increased by straining (see the box above, right).

Symptoms of brain abscess

1. Constant and severe headache
2. Drowsiness
3. Confusion
4. Mental slowness
5. Focal or generalized seizures
6. Fever with bradycardia
7. Signs and symptoms of increased ICP
8. Nuchal rigidity

The evolution of symptoms is variable. In some patients there may be a rapid progression of symptoms ending in death, whereas in others the course is more benign. Generally, however, the mortality is high with brain abscess, and residual disability often results.

□ Diagnostic tests

The diagnosis of brain abscess is made primarily on the basis of the history and examination of the CSF. EEG changes are present (significant slowing at the site of the abscess), and there will be areas of increased uptake on the CT scan. The brain scan is able to locate abscesses that are over 1 cm in size. Arteriography can be helpful in locating temporal lobe abscesses or cerebellar abscesses. The lumbar puncture is contraindicated if intracranial pressure is increased because of the danger of causing brain herniation.

➡ DATA ANALYSIS: NURSING DIAGNOSES

The nursing diagnoses and the expected patient outcomes are the same for the patient with brain abscess as for the patient with meningitis (p. 478).

⊞ IMPLEMENTATION

□ Assisting with the achievement of therapeutic goals

Treatment consists of administering the appropriate antibiotics, often for extended periods of time. Combined antibiotics along with broad-spectrum antibiotics may be used. Antibiotics that are used include penicillin, chloramphenicol (Chloramycetin), and nafcillen (Unipen). If anaerobic bacteria have been identified, metronidazole (Flagyl) may be used. Agents to reduce ICP may be necessary. Ongoing assessment for signs and symptoms of increased ICP is important. These patients often must undergo long hospitalizations and periods of treatment; as a result, they may need a great deal of psychologic support.

Surgical treatment consists of aspiration or complete excision and evacuation of the abscess. The method of evacuation depends on the site and accessibility.

◼ Poliomyelitis

Poliomyelitis is an acute febrile disease caused by poliomyelitis virus types 1, 2, and 3. Paralysis is more common with type 1. With discovery of the Salk vaccine, its wide use since 1956, and the availability of the Sabin vaccine, this disease has become quite rare. At one time it was a serious crippler of children and young adults.

◼ PATHOPHYSIOLOGY

The incubation period for poliomyelitis is from 7 to 21 days. The virus attacks the anterior horn cells of the spinal cord where the motor pathways are located and may cause motor paralysis. Sensory perception is not affected, because posterior horn cells are not attacked. Poliomyelitis sometimes takes a somewhat different form and attacks primarily the medulla and basal structures of the brain, including the cranial nerves. This is called *bulbar paralysis*. If the medulla is involved, the patient may need respiratory assistance.

◼ Guillain-Barré-Strohl syndrome (polyneuritis)

Guillain-Barré-Strohl syndrome is also known as acute inflammatory polyradiculoneuropathy and postinfectious polyneuritis. It is often serious because of the extent to which the nervous system is involved. It involves an acute type of peripheral nerve syndrome resulting in widespread inflammation and demyelination of the peripheral nervous system. The disease affects persons of all ages and is seen equally in men and women. The cause is unknown, but it is thought to be either a viral agent or a result of an autoimmune reaction.

NURSING CARE PLAN

Person with Guillain-Barré-Strohl syndrome

DATA: Mr. Doe is a 45-year-old married auto mechanic with a history of progressive weakness that began in his feet and legs. For the past day he has not been able to walk. He is also complaining of shortness of breath. He gives a history of an upper respiratory tract infection 2 weeks before admission. On admission he demonstrated weakness of all four extremities. His tidal volume was decreased and his respiratory rate was 32. He complained of discomfort in his lower extremities. The sensory examination was WNL. He was alert and oriented ×3. He was admitted to the neurologic unit for observation. He was started on corticosteroids and his respiratory rate closely monitored. The day after admission the patient demonstrated paralysis of muscles below the waist.

The nursing history identified the following:
1. He is unsure about what has happened to him and the reason for his weakness.
2. He expresses anxiety about what to expect.
3. He seems to have a close relationship with his wife.
4. Leisure activities are mainly sports activities.

Collaborative nursing actions include those to prevent further complications caused by muscle weakness and respiratory weakness. Immediate reporting may prevent serious effects (respiratory arrest, clot formation). Nursing actions include monitoring for the following:
1. Signs of respiratory compromise: decreased tidal volume, increased shortness of breath, tachypnea, cyanosis, restlessness.
2. Signs of pulmonary embolism: chest pain, hemoptysis.
3. Signs of DVT (deep vein thrombosis): difference in leg girth, positive Homan's sign, leg pain, difference in temperature of legs.

Nursing diagnosis: Anxiety related to change in health status

Expected patient outcomes	Nursing interventions	Rationale
Patient verbalizes minimal anxiety	Explain to patient procedures being done	Explanations will help minimize anxiety
	Allow him time to verbalize feelings	Expression of fears will lessen anxiety
	Encourage his wife to spend time with him	Family members are an important source of support

Continued.

NURSING CARE PLAN

Person with Guillain-Barré-Strohl syndrome—cont'd

Nursing diagnosis: Ineffective breathing pattern: to neuromuscular impairment

Expected patient outcomes	Nursing interventions	Rationale
Patient will have adequate breathing pattern	Assess respiratory rate, tidal volume, and color frequently	Ongoing assessment will detect critical changes
	Notify MD of any changes immediately	Changes in respiratory status can occur quickly
	Keep head of bed at 30 degrees	Position helps respiratory effort
	Give supplemental oxygen as ordered	Lowered oxygen levels in blood are common with impaired respiratory efforts

Nursing diagnosis: Comfort, alteration in: leg pain related to Guillain-Barré syndrome

Expected patient outcomes	Nursing interventions	Rationale
Patient states that leg pain is improved	Position for comfort	Positioning may relieve pain
	Administer mild analgesic such as acetominophen	Pain relief
	Teach relaxation measures as appropriate	Promotes rest and eases pain

Nursing diagnosis: Potential for injury: related to possible trauma

Expected patient outcomes	Nursing interventions	Rationale
Contractures do not develop	Position patient with limbs in normal anatomic position	Will prevent flexion contractures
	Change position q 2 hr	
	Perform passive or active ROM to all extremities several times a day	Activity stretches muscles and keeps joints moveable
	Assist out of bed at least daily	Change in position helps prevent complications of immobility
	Apply elastic stockings and keep legs elevated when up in chair	Assists with venous return and helps prevent stasis

Nursing diagnosis: Knowledge deficit: related to lack of exposure

Expected patient outcomes	Nursing interventions	Rationale
Patient can describe nature of disease and possible complications	Review nature of disease with frequent reinforcement	Teaching can raise patient's level of cooperation
		Reinforcement of earlier teaching helps promote retention

Continued.

NURSING CARE PLAN

Person with Guillain-Barré-Strohl syndrome—cont'd

Nursing diagnosis: Impaired physical mobility: related to neuromuscular impairment

Expected patient outcomes	Nursing interventions	Rationale
Patient has minimal impairments in mobility	Allow patient to do as much for self as possible See actions under "Injury, potential for"	Active exercise has positive effect on patient

Nursing diagnosis: Bathing/hygiene, dressing, toileting self-care deficit: related to neuromuscular impairment

Expected patient outcomes	Nursing interventions	Rationale
Patient carries out ADL at highest ability level	Provide basic ADL needs as necessary but encourage patient to do what he can	Self-care will promote positive self-concept
	Provide sufficient time to do ADL	Doing ADL with deficits often takes more time
	Work with therapists to optimize patient's learning needs	Team work can accentuate care

Nursing diagnosis: Body image disturbance, personal identity disturbance: role performance related to loss of body functions and immobility

Expected patient outcomes	Nursing interventions	Rationale
Patient verbalizes positive self-concept	Provide information about disease and expected progress	Understanding of disease will improve self-concept
	Provide privacy	Patient may be embarrassed by need for physical care
	Provide care but encourage patient to do as much for self as possible	Ability to care for self will improve self-concept
	Encourage family to visit	Visitors will cheer patient
	Give family chance to share their concerns	If family concerns are met, they can be more supportive of patient
	Encourage family to maintain previous role relationships, if possible	There is comfort in knowing that role in family is intact
	Identify patient's strengths and weaknesses	Can assist nurse in planning care with patient

Nursing diagnosis: Potential impaired skin integrity related to mechanical forces and pressure

Expected patient outcomes	Nursing interventions	Rationale
Skin remains intact	Monitor pressure areas for signs of skin breakdown	Early detection of pressure can allow time for measures to prevent breakdown
	Use turning sheet when turning patient to prevent shearing effect	Shearing forces lead to skin breakdown
	Turn patient q2h	Turning prevents pressure areas
	Keep skin clean and dry	Moisture leads to skin breakdown
	Use air mattress or water mattress or special bed	Can assist with relief of pressure areas

■ PATHOPHYSIOLOGY

With this disease patchy demyelination occurs in peripheral nerves, nerve roots, root ganglia, and spinal cord. Axons are generally spared so recovery may occur early, although they may be affected in severe cases.

There may be variations in the pattern of onset of weakness, as well as in the rate of progression of symptoms. The progression may stop at any point. If cranial nerves VII, IX, and X are involved, the patient may have difficulty in swallowing, speaking, and breathing. The vital centers in the medulla may be affected.

The pathology also is related to infiltration of the peripheral nervous system with mononuclear cells. It is thought that sensitized lymphocytes have a part in the demyelination, since more than half of the individuals affected have had a nonspecific infection 10 to 14 days before the onset of the disease. Many persons developed symptoms of Guillain-Barré after receiving swine flu vaccine in the early 1980s.

Symmetric muscle weakness and lower motor neuron paralysis (flaccidity) are present with Guillain-Barré syndrome. The paralysis usually starts in the lower extremities and moves upward to include the thorax, upper extremities, and the face. Paresthesias may occur. Respiratory failure is possible if the intercostal muscles are affected; without mechanical ventilation there is a 10% to 20% mortality. Autonomic symptoms, such as fluctuating blood pressure, also occur. The bowel and bladder are rarely affected.

Of the persons suffering from Gullain-Barré syndrome, 85% will regain complete function. The recovery period is variable, ranging from weeks to years. Those not recovering completely will have some degree of permanent neurological deficit. Generally, recovery from the disease occurs in the *reverse* of how paralysis or weakness occurred.

■ ASSESSMENT

☐ Subjective data

1. Patient's understanding of the disease
2. History of infection in recent past
3. Initial onset of symptoms and nature of symptoms
4. Presence of muscle weakness

☐ Objective data

1. Abnormalities found in the physical assessment part of the neurologic examination
2. Presence of increased temperature
3. Presence of muscle weakness
4. Abnormalities found with arterial blood gases
5. Presence of dyspnea
6. Blood pressure abnormalities

➡ DATA ANALYSIS: NURSING DIAGNOSES

See section on the patient with meningitis (p. 478).

■ IMPLEMENTATION

☐ Assisting with achievement of therapeutic goals

A priority goal is the maintenance of respiratory function. Close observation of respiratory function is necessary. This should include serial measurements of the patient's vital capacity, tidal volume, and minute volume. Patients who develop respiratory failure require mechanical ventilation and may require tracheostomy. Arterial blood gas monitoring is common. The patient may also require nutritional maintenance intravenously or through a nasogastric tube. If the patient has severe paralysis and is expected to have a long recovery period, a gastrostomy tube may be inserted. Special eye care is important to prevent corneal damage.

Adrenocortical steroids are used at times to treat symptoms. Convalescence may require many months. Attention to the prevention of iatrogenic complications such as contracture, decubitus ulcers, muscle atrophy, and loss of range of motion is imperative to allow complete recovery.

■ Neurosyphilis

■ PATHOPHYSIOLOGY

In the late or chronic stage of syphilis, infection may involve the brain and spinal cord. The oculomotor nerves may be involved, causing inability of the pupil to react to light (*Argyll Robertson pupil*). *Tabes dorsalis* is the name given to the involvement of the posterior columns of the spinal cord and the posterior nerve roots. Sensory symptoms predominate. The patient may have severe paroxysmal pain anywhere in the body, the most common location being in the stomach (gastric crisis). There may be areas of severe paresthesia. A common finding in tabes dorsalis is loss of position sense in the feet and legs. The patient is unable to sense where the feet are placed resulting in a highly characteristic slapping gait. Walking in the dark is increasingly difficult because the person relies on vision in placing the feet. Visual loss or blindness also can occur. Tabes dorsalis can cause trophic changes in the joints so that stability is lost (*Charcot's joint*).

General paresis is the term used to designate another late manifestation of syphilis in which there are degeneration of the brain and deterioration of mental function, as well as evidence of other neurologic disease.

■ Herpes zoster

Herpes zoster, also known as shingles, is a common disease occurring at higher rates among the old and in patients with lymphomas, cancer, and Hodgkin's disease.

■ PATHOPHYSIOLOGY

The causative organism is the varicella virus, similar to the one that causes herpes simplex. It may occur as a result of a reactivation of the viral infection that lies dormant in the ganglion following a primary case of chickpox. It is not communicable, except to persons who have not had chickenpox. An acute inflammatory reaction takes place in the spinal or cranial sensory ganglions, the posterior gray matter of the cord, and the meninges.

The rash seen in herpes zoster consists of a vescicular, cutaneous eruption within a dermatome. It may be preceded by severe itching, pain in the area, fever, and malaise. Segmental weakness and atrophy may exist in the same area as the sensory changes. A small percentage of patients first seek medical attention for ophthalmic herpes, with the rash and pain occurring along the distribution of the trigeminal nerve.

ASSESSMENT

☐ Subjective data

1. Complaints of pain
2. Any sensory changes
3. Complaints of malaise
4. Complaints of itching

☐ Objective data

1. Fever
2. Presence of rash—vesicular cutaneous eruption within a dermatome
3. Presence of weakness or atrophy in the area of sensory changes

DATA ANALYSIS: NURSING DIAGNOSES

Nursing diagnoses are determined from assessment of patient data. Possible nursing diagnoses for the person with herpes zoster may include, but are not limited to, the following:

Diagnostic title	Possible etiologies
Potential for infection	Decreased immune response
Knowledge deficit	Lack of exposure/recall
Impaired physical mobility	Pain/discomfort
Pain	Herpes
Feeding, bathing/hygiene, dressing/grooming self-care deficit	Pain/discomfort
Impaired skin integrity	Rash
Sleep pattern disturbance	Pain/discomfort, itching
Impaired social interaction	Therapeutic isolation

PLANNING: EXPECTED PATIENT OUTCOMES

Expected patient outcomes for the person with herpes may include but are not limited to the following:

1. Patient has minimal discomfort.
2. Patient remains infection free.
3. Patient can explain prescribed medication (dosage, action, side effects, and frequency).
4. Patient has minimal difficulty with ADL.

5. Patient's skin integrity improves.
6. Patient is able to sleep at least 6 hours per night.
7. Patient has minimal complications from therapeutic isolation.
8. Patient maintains optimal mobility.

IMPLEMENTATION

☐ Assisting with the achievement of therapeutic goals

Treatment for herpes zoster consists mainly of supportive care with medication for control of pain. The pain may persist for some time after the rash disappears. Phenytoin (Dilantin) and carbamazerine (Tegretol) may be helpful for control of persistent pain. Steroid therapy started early in the disease course is believed to shorten the course but is not recommended for patients with suppressed immune responses. Special emphasis should be placed on rest, nutrition, and hydration during the acute period.

☐ Control of environment

Isolation may be necessary for staff who have not had chickenpox. This is especially true for the pregnant employee. Also, patients with malignancies, lymphomas, or Hodgkin's disease who have not had chickenpox should be protected from exposure to the patient.

Because the virus is spread by direct contact and airborne routes, strict isolation is often necessary, at least until drainage from any lesions stop. The protective measures are listed in the box below.

EVALUATION

Evaluation of the patient with herpes zoster includes the following questions:

1. Is the patient having minimal pain?
2. Is the patient free of infection?
3. Is the patient able to state the required medications including dosage, side effects, times, and expected results?

Isolation measures for patient with herpes zoster

1. Private room with private toilet facilities
2. Gown, masks, and gloves required of caregivers
3. Strict hand washing
4. Linen handled as isolation linen
5. Double-bagging of dressings
6. Disposable dishes if possible
7. Transport patients only as necessary
8. Isolation procedure for visitors

4. Is the patient's mobility optimal?
5. Is the patient able to sleep at least 6 hours per night?
6. Is the patient's rash improving?
7. Is the patient compensating for the therapeutic isolation?

■ Acquired immunodeficiency syndrome

Acquired immunodeficiency syndrome (AIDS) is a disease that has serious implications on the nervous system. About 40% of AIDS patients have neurologic symptoms; in fact, with approximately 10% of all AIDS patients the initial presenting problem is neurologic.

As of 1987 over 40,000 cases of AIDS had been reported to the Centers for Disease Control. More than 60% of these patients had died. The average age of males with AIDS was 36.8 years, and the average age of females was 34.9 years.[38]

■ PATHOPHYSIOLOGY

AIDS is believed to be caused by *HIV*, previously known as *HTLV III*, lymphadenopathy-associated virus (LAV), and AIDS-associated retrovirus (ARV). HIV is a *retrovirus that causes persistent cellular infection by destroying T helper lymphocytes, resulting in a compromised immune system*. As a result, the patient with AIDS has an increased susceptibility to many life-threatening infections.

It is possible for patients to be infected without having AIDS. To have the disease in the full sense the patient must have the following:
1. Infection with the virus
2. Impaired immunity
3. Life-threatening infections or neoplasms

Many of these persons do not have AIDS but are infected with the virus have *AIDS-related complex (ARC)*. These persons have symptoms that include *lymphadenopathy, diarrhea,* and *fatigue*. Of the estimated 60,000 to 120,000 persons in the United States with ARC, it is estimated that 6% to 20% of these persons may develop AIDS in the next 2 years.[38]

Patients develop neurologic symptoms either as a result of infection with HIV itself or as a result of associated infections.

Patients with AIDS may have *ADC (AIDS dementia complex)*, which is also known as subacute encephalitis. Patients with ADC may manifest early signs of difficulty in concentrating or recent memory loss. This progresses to a global cognitive dysfunction with confusion, a vacant stare, and little spontaneous or verbal behavior.[38]

Opportunistic infections seen with AIDS include the following:
1. Aseptic meningitis
2. Herpes simplex or herpes zoster
3. Cytomegalovirus
4. Progressive multifocal leukoencephalopathy (PML): a demyelinating disorder
5. Toxoplasmosis
6. Cryptococcal fungal infections: cryptococcal meningitis

Finally, patients with AIDS may develop neoplasms of the CNS; these include primary malignant lymphomas.

▯ ASSESSMENT

The reader is referred to the assessment section for patients with meningitis for assessment factors (p. 478). The neurologic symptoms of AIDS vary because of the various neurologic problems that exist.

□ Diagnostic tests

CT scans are helpful in the diagnosis of neurologic problems related to AIDS. The MRI may also be used and often gives a more diagnostic imaging. Biopsies of brain tissue have also been used to diagnose specific problems.

▱ DATA ANALYSIS: NURSING DIAGNOSES

The reader is referred to the section on meningitis (p. 478).

▯ PLANNING: EXPECTED PATIENT OUTCOMES

The reader is referred to the section on meningitis (p. 478).

▤ IMPLEMENTATION

Treatment of the patient with neurologic problems related to AIDS depends on the nature of the infection. Unfortunately, no treatment is available for many of the problems, such as AIDS dementia complex.

Infections that result from the herpes virus may be treated by acyclovir (Zovirax). Brain abscesses may be treated with pyrimethamine (Daraprim), an antimalarial agent, and sulfadiazine. Cryptococcal infections are usually treated with antifungal agents such as amphotericin-B.[38]

▤ EVALUATION

The reader is referred to the section on meningitis (p. 479).

■ INTERFERENCE WITH FUNCTION BECAUSE OF TRAUMA

Interference with neurologic function can occur as a result of trauma. Parts of the nervous system commonly subjected to trauma include the craniocerebrum, the spinal cord, and the peripheral nerves. Traumatic lesions usually result from direct physical force or from sustained compression.

Craniocerebral trauma

Craniocerebral trauma, or head injury, causes death or serious disability in people of all ages. Head injury is the second most common cause of major neurologic deficits and the major cause of death between ages 1 and 35. About 77,000 persons die each year in the United States from craniocerebral trauma. Another 50,000 persons survive yearly with mild to severe permanent disabilities.

Brain injury causes more deaths than does injury to any other organ. Causes of head injury include motor vehicle accidents, falls, industrial accidents, assaults, and sports-related accidents. In some states the repeal of laws requiring motorcyclists to wear helmets has resulted in an estimated threefold increase in death and injury from damage to the brain sustained in motorcycle accidents.

PATHOPHYSIOLOGY

Craniocerebral trauma may result in injury to the scalp, skull, and brain tissues, either singly or collectively. Some of the variables that may modify the extent of the injury to the head include the following:

1. Location and direction of the impact
2. Rate of the energy transfer
3. Surface area of the energy transfer
4. Status of the head at the time of the impact

Injuries vary from minor scalp wounds to concussions and open fractures of the skull with severe damage to the brain. The amount of obvious damage is not indicative of the seriousness of the trouble. General effects of moderate to severe head injury include *cerebral edema, sensory and motor deficits,* and *increased intracranial pressure.* Later damage can occur as a result of *brain herniation, cerebral ischemia,* and *hypoxemia.*

Injuries to the brain can result from direct or indirect trauma to the head. Indirect trauma is caused by *tension strains* and shearing forces transmitted to the head by stretching of the neck. Direct trauma occurs when the head is directly injured. This results in *acceleration-deceleration* with *cavitation* (release of dissolved gases from the CSF, blood, or brain tissue). The release of gases damages nervous tissue. Direct trauma also results in rotation of the skull and its contents. These forces can occur at the same time or in succession and can damage the brain by compression, shearing, or tension.

Acceleration injuries occur when the head is struck by a moving object and set in motion. As a result of acceleration forces, *bruising* or *contusion* of the occipital and frontal lobes and the brainstem and cerebellum, may occur.

Deceleration injuries occur when the head strikes a solid immovable object with a rapid deceleration of the skull. The brain decelerates more slowly.

Acceleration-deceleration movements that occur with lateral flexion, hyperflexion, hyperextension, and turning cause the cerebrum to rotate about the brainstem, resulting in *shearing, stretching,* and *distortion of neural tissue.* The stretching or tension causes fracture of the axons.

Head injuries can be *open* or *closed.* Open head injuries result from skull fractures or penetrating wounds. The amount of injury with this type of wound is determined by the velocity, mass, shape, and direction of the impact. Usually there is some type of skull fracture. These include:

1. Linear—simple break in bone
2. Comminuted—two or more common breaks that divide the bone into more than two fragments
3. Depressed—bone forced below the line of normal contour
4. Compound—can be linear, comminuted, or depressed

Fractures at the base of the skull are usually serious because of their location. When one is sustained, vital centers, cranial nerves, and nerve pathways may be permanently damaged. Trauma and the resulting edema may obstruct cerebrospinal fluid flow directly or indirectly, with resultant increased intracranial pressure. If the injury has caused a direct communication between the cranial cavity and the middle ear or the sinuses, meningitis or a brain abscess may develop. Bleeding from the nose and ears suggests a basal fracture. Serosanguineous drainage from these orifices may contain cerebrospinal fluid and should be noted.

Damage of brain tissue caused by trauma

	Characteristics	Structural alteration	Effects
Concussion	Characterized by immediate and transitory impairment of neurologic function caused by mechanical force	No	May be loss of consciousness that is instant or delayed—usually reversible
Contusion	Likened to bruising with extravasation of blood cells	Yes	Injury may be at site of impact (coup) or at opposite site (contrecoup) Often damage to cortex
Laceration	Tearing of tissues caused by sharp fragment or shearing force	Yes	Hemorrhage is serious complication

Closed head injuries include concussions, contusions, and lacerations. See the box on p. 487 for a comparison of these injuries.

The effect of a blow on the cranium to the brain tissues within the skull is one of sudden movement. This effect can be likened to what happens as one stops suddenly when moving quickly with an open dish of fluid—some of the fluid spills. The only difference is that instead of spilling in the closed cavity, the brain tissue strikes the bony covering forcibly. A contusion or laceration directly below the site of the cranial impact is called a *coup* lesion. A lesion opposite the impact site is callled *contrecoup*. Damage to the brain tissues may include concussion, contusion, or laceration.

Lacerations of the scalp bleed profusely because of its large blood supply. Hemorrhage resulting from craniocerebral trauma may occur at the following sites:

1. Scalp
2. Epidural
3. Subdural
4. Intracerebral
5. Intraventricular

Two of these, *epidural* and *subdural hematomas*, require careful and continuous observation by the nurse and pose special problems to the patient with a head injury. Epidural hematomas form as blood collects rapidly between the dura and skull. Bleeding in this area is commonly caused by laceration of the middle meningeal artery, which is capable of producing rapid clot formation. Common sites for bleeding include sites of basal and temporal skull fractures. If lethargy or unconsciousness develops after the patient regains consciousness, an epidural hematoma may be suspected. Bleeding needs to be controlled promptly and the blood evacuated.

A subdural hematoma forms as venous blood collects below the dural surface. Because the bleeding is under venous pressure, the hematoma formation is relatively slow. The clot formation will, however, cause pressure on the brain surface and may eventually displace brain tissue. If the expanding clot is not evacuated it can cause increased ICP with compression of vital areas. The focal neurologic signs of clot formation are related to the site of the clot. If a patient who has been conscious for several days to weeks after a head injury becomes unconscious or develops neurologic symptoms, a *subdural hematoma* should be suspected. Subdural hematomas can be classed as follows:

1. Acute—occurs within 24 to 48 hours
2. Subacute—occurs within 48 hours to 2 weeks
3. Chronic—can occur weeks or months after the injury. These occur most commonly in the 60-70 year age range. At times, the cause of the hematoma is uncertain.

Intracerebral hemorrhage usually occurs in the frontal or temporal regions.

Most deaths from head injury are from cerebral edema caused by damage rather than the actual primary destruction of vital centers. Brain edema is a major cause of increased ICP. Along with the swelling, local and systemic disturbances in circulation occur with resulting anoxia.

The brain damage may be severe and not related to the demonstrated structural damage.

ASSESSMENT

Subjective data

1. Patient's understanding of injury and resulting pathology—also patient's ability to understand
2. Information about nature of the injury—how it happened
3. Presence of headache, nausea, or vomiting
4. Presence of diplopia or other visual problems
5. Unusual sensations (paresthesias, ringing in ears)
6. History of bleeding from ear, nose, eye, or mouth
7. History of loss of consciousness
8. Use of alcohol or durgs
9. Time of most recent food intake

Objective data

1. Respiratory status (presence of patent airway, need for suctioning, need for intubation and mechanical ventilation)
2. Arterial blood gases
3. Level of consciousness and alertness
4. Pupils: size, equality, reactivity
5. Orientation
6. Motor status
7. Vital signs
8. Presence of bleeding
9. Presence of vomiting
10. Speech patterns—abnormalities
11. Presence of increased intracranial pressure

Because many persons with head injury, especially from motor vehicle accidents, have sustained other injuries, the intrathoracic and intraabdominal areas are checked carefully and the limbs are examined for fractures and injuries to nerves or arteries.

Diagnostic tests

Diagnostic tests performed for patients with head injury include skull x-ray films, CT scan, MRF, and possibly cerebral angiography. These procedures were described earlier in this chapter. Other diagnostic tests such as skull and chest films rule out other injuries.

DATA ANALYSIS: NURSING DIAGNOSES

Nursing diagnoses are determined from assessment of patient data. Possible nursing diagnoses for the person with craniocerebral trauma may include, but are not limited to the following:

Diagnostic title	Possible etiologies
Ineffective airway clearance	Tracheobronchial infection/obstruction/secretion, perceptual/cognitive impairment, trauma

Diagnostic title	Possible etiologies
Anxiety	Threat of death, change in health status/role functioning
Body image disturbance	Severe trauma, immobility
Impaired communication	Aphasia
Altered growth and development	Effects of physical disability
Altered health maintenance	Perceptual/cognitive impairments
Impaired home maintenance management	Individual disease, impaired cognitive functioning, inadequate support systems
Hyperthermia	Trauma
Bowel incontinence	Neuromuscular impairment
Total incontinence	Neurologic dysfunction
Potential for infection	Decreased nutrition, decreased immune response
Knowledge deficit	Lack of exposure/recall, cognitive limitation
Impaired physical mobility	Perceptual/cognitive impairment, neuromuscular impairment
Noncompliance	Perceptual/cognitive impairment
Altered nutrition: less than body requirements	Chewing or swallowing difficulties
Pain	Head injury, trauma/diagnostic tests, immobility
Feeding, bathing/hygiene, dressing/grooming, toileting self-care deficit	Perceptual/cognitive impairment
Sensory-perceptual alterations: visual, auditory, olfactory, tactile, kinesthetic	Altered sensory reception/transmission/integration
Sexual dysfunction	Physiologic limitations, lack of significant other
Potential impaired skin integrity	Mechanical forces, immobility
Impaired social interaction	Poor communication skills, altered thought processes
Social isolation	Alteration in physical appearance, alteration in mental status, unacceptable social behavior/values
Ineffective thermoregulation	Trauma/illness
Altered thought processes	Neurologic disorders, hypoxia
Altered cerebral tissue perfusion	Decreased blood flow
Altered patterns of urinary elimination	Sensory-motor impairment, urinary infection

PLANNING: EXPECTED PATIENT OUTCOMES

Expected patient outcomes for the patient with craniocerebral trauma may include, but are not limited to, the following:

1. Patient can maintain a patent airway.
2. Patient's anxiety is minimal.
3. Patient can maintain an effective breathing pattern.
4. Patient can maintain communication, whether it be verbal or an alternate means of communication.
5. Patient has minimal complications as a result of incontinence.
6. Patient has regular bowel movements without diarrhea or constipation.
7. Patient has minimal discomfort.
8. Patient maintains optimal growth and development.
9. Patient has few problems with health maintenance.
10. Patient can function at optimal levels in home maintenance.
11. Patient's temperature remains normal.
12. Patient remains free of injury.
13. Patient maintains optimal mobility.
14. Patient remains free of infection.
15. Patient compensates for unilateral neglect.
16. Patient complies with the treatment prescribed.
17. Patient can maintain optimal nutrition.
18. Patient has minimal deficits in ADL.
19. Patient maintains a positive self-concept.
20. Patient learns to compensate for sensory-perceptual alterations so that problems are minimized.
21. Patient can maintain a sexual relationship, if desired.
22. Patient's skin remains intact.
23. Patient maintains optimal social interaction.
24. Patient has minimal antisocial behaviors.
25. Patient has intact swallowing.
26. Patient maintains cerebral perfusion.
27. Patient regains bowel and bladder continence if able.
28. Patient can explain and demonstrate prescribed therapy to follow at home.
29. Patient can explain homegoing medication regimen (side effects, desired effects, time, dose, and route) to be followed at home.

IMPLEMENTATION

Assisting with the achievement of therapeutic goals

Immediate care is directed toward lifesaving measures and the maintenance of normal body function until the time when recovery is assured. The major aims of medical and nursing management are as follows:

1. To be constantly alert for changes in the patient's condition, especially changes that indicate any increase in ICP
2. To sustain the patient's vital functions until recovery allows the functions to resume
3. To manage complications that will be life threatening and interfere with full recovery

Respiratory care

It is extremely important to maintain a patent airway and ensure adequate oxygenation. Anoxia with a buildup of carbon dioxide can produce cerebral hypoxia and subsequent cerebral edema. It is important to assess the ability to clear the airway. Blood or mucus from injuries may block the airway, or the patient may have vomited and suctioning may be necessary. Inability to clear the airway can lead to airway obstruction, as well as aspiration pneumonia. Oxygen should be given to the patient with a head injury, and if the patient cannot clear the airway an endotracheal tube should be used. Arterial blood gas levels are checked frequently to determine whether respiratory exchange is adequate. Suctioning should be done as necessary.

□ Rest and control of convulsions

The patient should be kept as quiet as possible. No vigorous effort should be made to "clean the patient up" during the first few hours after the accident. Side rails should always be on the bed because restlessness may come on suddenly or convulsions may occur. The head of the bed is usually elevated 30 degrees. Restlessness may be caused by the need for a change of position, pain, or the need to empty the bladder. Codeine or other analgesics that do not depress the respiratory system are used for pain control. Anticonvulsants may be given to prevent seizures.

□ Vital signs and temperature control

The blood pressure, pulse, and respiratory rate are taken frequently until they have stabilized and remain within safe limits. A sudden sharp rise in temperature, which may go to 42° C or higher, and a sudden drop in blood pressure indicate that the regulatory mechanisms have lost control. The prognosis is poor. Measures are used to reduce temperature to normal because hyperthermia increases brain metabolism, resulting in brain damage. These measures include the following:
1. Administration of aspirin
2. Tepid sponge baths
3. Ice bags to the groin and axilla
4. Reduction of temperature in patient's room
5. Electrically controlled cooling mattress

□ Prevention of infection

The patient's ears and nose are checked carefully for signs of blood and serous drainage, which would indicate that the meninges have been torn and that spinal fluid is escaping. No attempt should be made to clean out the orifices. Loose sterile cotton may be placed in the outer openings only. This procedure is performed with caution so that the cotton does not act as a plug to interfere with the free flow of fluid. The cotton should be changed whenever it becomes moist. If there is evidence of drainage of CSF from the nose, the patient should not cough, sneeze, or blow the nose. These activities may enable air to enter the cranial cavity where it may increase symptoms of increased ICP. If there is question about whether drainage from the nose is CSF, a Tes-Tape will show a positive sugar reaction.

Meningitis is a possible complication when communication with the nose and ears occurs. With basal skull fracture, antibiotics are commonly used because of the high rate of infection following this type of fracture.

□ Medications

Medications are used to reduce cerebral edema and increased ICP, which are common problems in patients with head injuries. These medications include the following:
1. Osmotic diuretics that penetrate the brain slowly
   a. 30% solution of urea
   b. 20% mannitol
2. Dexamethasone

If the patient is receiving one of the diuretics and is not alert, a Foley catheter should be inserted to enable accurate accounting of output. Large amounts of urine can be anticipated.

□ Electrolyte imbalance

Careful monitoring of electrolytes is necessary. Several types of imbalance may occur with a head injury including the following:
1. Natriuresis (increased urinary excretion of sodium)
2. Inappropriate ADH syndrome (increased plasma levels of ADH, serum hyponatremia, and hypotonicity)
3. Hypernatremia
4. Cerebral sodium retention
5. Elevated plasma cortisol levels

□ Elimination

The patient's intake and output should be carefully measured and recorded. The specific gravity of the urine is also measured and can yield clues to electrolyte imbalance. In acute situations these measurements are done hourly.

The urinary output should be approximately 0.6 to 1 ml/kg of body weight/hour. If osmotic diuretics have been given, this amount will be greater. An indwelling catheter may be necessary; appropriate measures should be used to prevent infection. The person with cranial trauma should also be assessed for symptoms of diabetes insipidus, a common occurrence.

Bowel function is not encouraged for several days following a head injury. Mild bulk laxatives, bisacodyl suppositories, or oil-retention enemas may be used; a stool softener is often prescribed. The patient is taught not to strain at stool. When the patient is receiving dexamethasone or other steroids, it is important to check the stool for the presence of occult blood. This will also give a clue to the presence of stress ulcers, which are somewhat common after head injury. The ulcers are apparently caused by autonomic imbalances associated with the injury. Cimetidine (Tagamet) and antacids are routinely given if the patient with a closed head injury is receiving steroids.

□ Assisting with comfort and ADL
□ Emotional support

It is not uncommon that the patient with a head injury manifests loss of memory and loss of initiative. Behavioral problems associated with lack of judgment and restlessness may also occur. These patients need firm but gentle care, with specific guidelines for what behavior is allowed. It is not helpful to argue with the patient. It may be helpful to redirect their attention to another subject or task. Memory aids such as a log book or written schedule can be very useful in assisting with reorientation. The patient and family need to have gains in functioning pointed out, as it is easy to become frustrated and depressed when progress is slow.[14]

□ Resumption of activities

The length of convalescence will depend on the amount of brain damage and how rapid the recovery has been. Patients are usually urged to resume normal activity as soon as possible. Headache and dizziness may be present for some time following a head injury. Some persons require intensive and lengthy rehabilitation in a rehabilitation center. Many of these patients recover physically but will have behavioral and psychologic problems that make it difficult for them to function completely independently.[17,30]

Some patients are left with serious deficits that include hemiplegia. The nursing care of these patients is described in the section on patients who have had a stroke (p. 472).

□ Counseling and teaching

Patients with head injury may be seen in an emergency room but not admitted to the hospital. These patients need teaching about observations for complications. A sample set of instructions is found in the box below.

Teaching for the patient with a head injury who is left with deficits severe enough to require extended rehabilitation is similar to that for the patient with a motor problem. See p. 448 for a description of this teaching. In addition, the following points are important:
1. Causes of increased ICP
2. Factors that can increase or decrease intracranial pressure

a. No sneezing
b. No heavy lifting, bending, or straining
c. No straining at stool
3. Signs and symptoms to report to the physician

It is essential that the family be present at the teaching sessions.

✝ EVALUATION

Evaluation of the patient with a head injury is based on the expected patient outcomes. Questions to ask include the following:
1. Are there symptoms of increased ICP?
2. Does the patient have minimal difficulties in carrying out ADL?
3. Does the patient have a patent airway and effective breathing pattern?
4. Is the patient able to verbalize follow-up care and discharge regimen?
5. Is the patient taking medication accurately?
6. Is the patient functioning in a socially acceptable way?
7. Is the patient able to communicate in an effective way?
8. Is the patient continent of bowel and bladder?
9. Is the patient free of pain?
10. Is the patient afebrile?
11. Is the patient practicing safety techniques?
12. Is the patient's mobility functioning at optimal levels?
13. Is the patient demonstrating a positive self concept?
14. Is the patient compensating for sensory-perceptual difficulties?
15. Is the patient able to swallow safely and maintain an adequate diet?
16. Is the patient's skin intact?

Instructions for the patient with a head injury

Patient should be awakened periodically through the first 24 hours to be sure he or she can wake up easily.
Also, for the first 24 to 48 hours, the family should watch carefully for the following warning signs:
1. Vomiting—often with force behind it
2. Unusual sleepiness, dizziness, and loss of balance or falling
3. Complaint of seeing two of everything or blurry objects, jerking movement of the eyes
4. Bleeding or discharge from nose or ears
5. A slight headache may be expected; however, if it gets worse and the patient complains of feeling even worse when moving about, it should be reported
6. Convulsions (fits)—any twitching or movements of arms or legs that the patient is not able to stop
7. Any behavior or symptom that is not normal for the individual
Call a doctor at once if any of these signs are observed by the family.
Call either your personal physician or the emergency services.

Courtesy Department of Nursing, University Hospitals of Cleveland, Cleveland, Ohio.

■ Spinal cord trauma

Spinal cord injury from accidents is a common and increasing cause of serious disability and death in the United States. Approximately 10% of traumatic injuries to the nervous system involve the spinal cord. It has been estimated that over 100,000 persons in the United States are paralyzed as a result of spinal cord injury and that 10,000 more are injured every year. Most persons involved with spinal cord injuries are males between the ages of 18 and 25.[48] Automobile, motorcycle, diving, surfing, and other athletic accidents and gunshot wounds are major causes of spinal cord injuries. The largest number of spinal cord injuries are caused by vehicular accidents.

The most common sites of injury are the lower cervical region and the junction of the thoracic and lumbar region.

■ PATHOPHYSIOLOGY

The spinal cord may be damaged by lesions arising outside the cord or by lesions within the cord itself. The latter are a less common cause and are usually the result of tumors. Trauma to the spinal cord can result in *concussion, contusion, laceration, complete* or *partial transection, hemorrhage,* or *loss of blood supply to a part of the cord* (Fig. 19-38).

The soft tissue of the spinal cord is protected by the vertebral column. This column can be injured by various mechanisms, including the following:

1. Hyperextension—also called whiplash. These occur most often in the cervical region and result from the

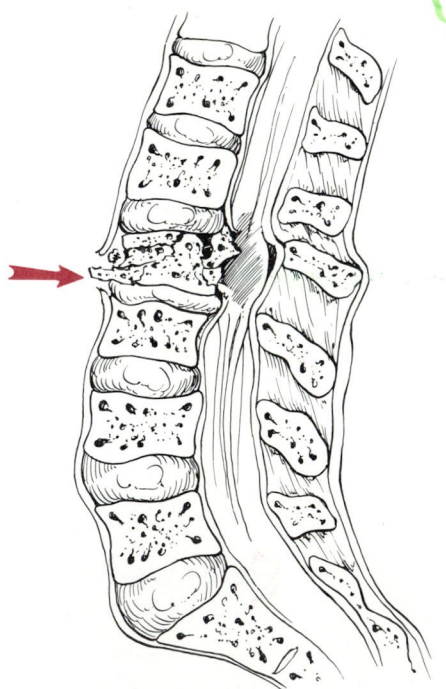

Fig. 19-38   Damage to spinal cord and distortion of adjacent structures that may occur in traumatic injuries to spine.

forces of acceleration-deceleration and the reduction of diameter of the spinal cord.
2. Hyperflexion—results in overstretching, compression and deformity of the spinal cord.
3. Vertical compression—primarily occurs in the area of T12 to L2. Injuries result from a force applied downward from the cranium that often results in a burst vertebra.
4. Rotation injury—can involve all parts of the vertebrae.

Injuries that occur to the vertebrae include the following types:

1. Simple fracture—single break affecting the spinous or transverse process. The spinal cord is not usually compressed and the alignment of the vertebrae is not altered.
2. Compressed or wedged fracture—occurs when the vertebral body is compressed anteriorly. Cord compression may be present.
3. Comminuted or burst fractures—vertebral body shatters into many fragments, any of which may injure the cord.
4. Dislocation of vertebrae—may result in nonalignment of vertebral column with injury to the spinal cord. Partial dislocation is called subluxation.

Severe traumatic lesions of the spinal cord may result in total transection of the spinal cord or a tearing of the cord from side to side at a particular level, with a complete loss of spinal cord functions. This total transection is also referred to as a "complete cord injury." With the complete injury all voluntary movement below the level of the lesion is lost. A partial transection or "incomplete injury" involves a partial transection or injury of the cord. Quadriplegics are patients who sustain injuries to one of the eight cervical segments of the spinal cord. Paraplegics are those whose lesions are confined to the thoracic, lumbar, or sacral regions of the spinal cord. The symptoms of incomplete injuries can vary depending on the nature of the injury and the resultant syndrome. Resultant syndromes can include the following:

1. Anterior cord syndrome
2. Central cord syndrome
3. Brown-Séquard syndrome
4. Herniated disc syndrome

The anterior cord syndrome most often results from a flexion injury to the cervical vertebrae. It is the most common type of cord syndrome and damages the anterior spinal artery, as well as the spinal cord. Upper and lower motor function is lost. The central cord syndrome results from flexion or hyperextension injuries. There is resultant compression of the anterior horn cells and edema of the central spinal cord, causing mixed upper and lower motor neuron loss and spasticity below the level of the injury. Usually more impairment occurs in the upper extremities.

Another syndrome is the Brown-Séquard syndrome, which results from rotation-flexion injuries where subluxation or dislocation of the fracture fragments occurs. There is ipsilateral paresis, loss of proprioception, and contralateral loss of pain and temperature sensation.

Muscle function after spinal cord injury

Spinal cord injury	Muscle function remaining	Muscle function lost
Cervical above C4	None	All, including respiration
C5	Neck	Arms
	Scapular elevation	Chest
		All below chest
C6-C7	Neck	Some arm, fingers
	Some chest movement	Some chest
	Some arm movement	All below chest
Thoracic	Neck	Trunk
	Arms (full)	All below chest
	Some chest	
Lumbosacral	Neck	Legs
	Arms	
	Chest	
	Trunk	

The last syndrome is the herniated disc syndrome, which is very common. In this syndrome, there is displacement of discs with the escape of cartilage. It occurs spontaneously or in response to activity or slight injury.

All of these injuries are more common in older persons because of degenerative changes with aging. The lower lumbar and lumbosacral areas are affected most often.[48]

□ Spinal shock

Initially, in most spinal cord injuries there is a period of flaccid paralysis and a complete loss of reflexes below the level of the lesion. Sensory and autonomic functions are also lost. This is called spinal or neural shock, or areflexia, and it is a transitory event. Spinal shock results from the loss of inhibition of the descending tracts. During this period persons may require temporary respiratory assistance until recovery begins.

Within hours, days, or weeks the involved muscles gradually become spastic and hyperreflexic with the characterisic signs of an upper motor neuron lesion. These changes are thought to represent the release of the muscle stretch reflexes from the inhibitory influence of the damaged pyramidal tract, resulting in hyperactive responses.

The amount of disability that results from spinal cord injury is dependent on the level of injury. See the box above for specifics of muscle function following spinal cord injury.

□ Voiding

The center for micturition is located in the conus medullaris (S2-S4) and is linked to the detrusor muscle of the bladder by parasympathetic sensory and motor fibers that run in the pelvic nerves. Levels above the conus result in a bladder that is capable of emptying itself reflexly or involuntarily after the spinal shock phase. The bladder is hypertonic and it is variously known as an "upper motor neuron bladder" and "reflex neurogenic bladder." The emptying occurs spontaneously or automatically. The patient has no control over the act of micturition. Voiding may occur at intervals of 3 to 4 hours; there may be frequency, urgency, and incontinence. The reflex arc is intact in this type bladder. When the cord lesion is at or below the micturition center, the center or the sacral nerve roots are destroyed; the reflex arc is no longer intact. This type of bladder condition is known as a "lower motor neuron bladder" or an "autonomous neurogenic bladder." Contractions of the bladder muscle are the result of impulses transmitted through a mechanism within the bladder wall but are not of sufficient strength or duration to empty the bladder. Abdominal straining or manual compression is necessary for this to happen. Retention of urine and infection are common complications.

□ Autonomic dysreflexia

One complication of spinal cord injury that is extremely important to understand is *autonomic dysreflexia*, or hyperreflexia. It occurs in patients with cord lesions above the sixth thoracic vertebra and most commonly in patients with cervical injuries. (Fig. 19-39). Autonomic dysreflexia occurs as a result of abnormal cardiovascular response to stimulation of the sympathetic division of the autonomic nervous system. The clinical signs include the following:

1. Bradycardia
2. Paroxysmal hypertension
3. Sweating
4. "Goose flesh"
5. Severe headache
6. Nasal stuffiness

Patients tend to develop individual symptoms of this condition and are soon able to recognize them.

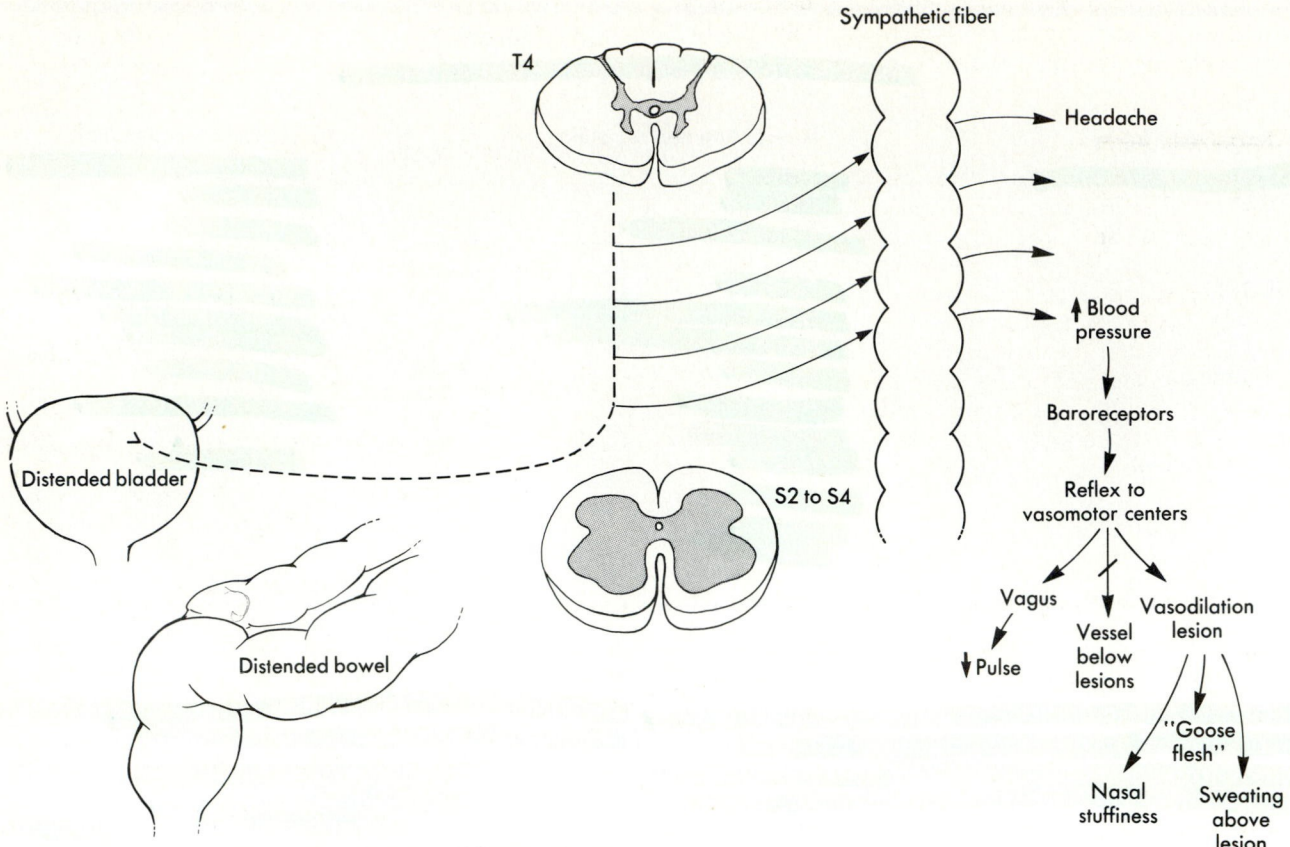

Fig. 19-39 Pictorial diagram of cause of automomic hyperflexia and results.

The most common cause is visceral distention, which can include a distended bladder or impacted rectum. It is a medical emergency that requires immediate treatment, because it can lead to cerebrovascular accident, blindness, or death. Treatment is discussed later in this chapter (p. 498).

Sexual function

In most cases, men experience impotence, decreased sensation, and difficulties with ejaculation. Impairment of fertility is common. The act of erection is under the control of sensory and parasympathetic fibers, while ejaculation requires sympathetic and parasympathetic innervation. Lesions above S2 leave the parasympathetic reflex arc intact; patients may be able to have an erection, but ejaculation is not usually possible. Lesions in the S2 to S4 area usually prevent erection and ejaculation. The higher the level of injury, the more likely a man with complete cord injury is able to perform sexually. The experience of orgasm is described as different than before the injury. Women with spinal cord injury are able to continue to perform sexually, although perception of sexual pleasure is usually altered.[52,67]

ASSESSMENT

Assessment of the patient with spinal cord injury includes both subjective and objective data.

Subjective data

1. Patient's understanding of injury and resulting deficit
2. Information about nature of injury—how it happened
3. Presence of dyspnea
4. Unusual sensations (paresthesias, and so on)
5. History of loss of consciousness
6. Presence of pain
7. Absence of sensation—sensory level

Objective data

1. Respiratory status
2. Level of alertness and consciousness
3. Orientation
4. Pupil size, equality, and reactivity
5. Proper alignment of body in neutral alignment
6. Motor strength
7. Temperature, blood pressure, and pulse
8. Skin integrity
9. Bowel and bladder status and distention
10. Presence of other injuries

As with the patient with a head injury, the patient with a spinal cord injury should be assessed carefully for the presence of other injuries, primarily fractures or head injury.

☐ Diagnostic tests

It is most important to first detect if there has been any cervical vertebra fracture or displacement. X-ray films are always taken to detect any fracture-dislocations. These often occur before the patient is moved from the backboard or stretcher. A spinal tap or myelography may also be done to detect blockage. It can be carried out also without moving the patient if the dye is injected at the junction between the first cervical vertebra and the base of the skull. CT scanning may also be very helpful in ruling out spinal cord injury. The MRI can detect spinal cord compression and edema. These procedures were discussed earlier in this chapter.

➡ DATA ANALYSIS: NURSING DIAGNOSES

Nursing diagnoses are determined from assessment of patient data. Possible nursing diagnoses for the person with spinal cord injury may include, but are not limited to, the following:

Diagnostic title	Possible etiologies
Impaired adjustment	Disability requiring change in lifestyle, indequate support system, altered locus of control, incomplete grieving
Ineffective airway clearance	Tracheobronchial infection/obstruction, trauma
Anxiety	Threat to self-concept, threat/change in health status/role functioning
Body image disturbance	Loss of body functions, severe trauma, immobility, change in life-style
Ineffective breathing pattern	Neuromuscular impairment, musculoskeletal impairment
Ineffective individual coping	Situational crisis
Fear	Life-style changes
Impaired home maintenance management	Individual injury, inadequate support system
Hyperthermia	Decreased ability to perspire
Bowel incontinence	Neuromuscular impairment
Potential for injury: trauma	Sensorimotor deficits, lack of awareness of environmental hazards
Knowledge deficit	Lack of exposure/recall, unfamiliarity with information sources
Impaired physical mobility	Neuromuscular impairment, musculoskeletal impairment
Pain	Spinal cord injury, immobility, trauma/diagnostic tests
Powerlessness	Health-care environment

Diagnostic title	Possible etiologies
Feeding, bathing/hygiene, dressing/grooming, toileting self-care deficit	Neuromuscular impairment, musculoskeletal impairment
Sensory-perceptual alterations: tactile	Altered sensory reception/transmission/integration
Sexual dysfunction	Physiologic limitations
Potential impaired skin integrity	Mechanical forces, immobility
Altered tissue perfusion	Decreased blood flow, immobility, pressure
Altered patterns of urinary elimination	Sensorimotor impairment, urinary infection

⌶ PLANNING: EXPECTED PATIENT OUTCOMES

Expected patient outcomes for the patient with spinal cord injury may include, but are not limited to, the following:

1. Patient's airway is maintained.
2. Patient maintains an effective breathing pattern.
3. Patient's function is preserved to the extent possible with no increase in the level of injury.
4. Patient has minimal limitations in ADL.
5. Patient's skin is intact.
6. Patient can do skin inspection or direct the inspection of the skin.
7. Patient remains free of further injury.
8. Patient demonstrates an optimal level of mobility.
9. Patient verbalizes a positive self-concept.
10. Patient is able to direct own care and has involvement in plan of care.
11. Patient demonstrates minimal feelings of powerlessness.
12. Patient has a low level of anxiety.
13. Patient demonstrates minimal complications of bowel and bladder incontinence.
14. Patient evacuates bowel on a regular schedule without diarrhea or constipation.
15. Patient can carry out or direct own bowel and bladder program, including possible intermittent catheterization and use of suppositories and digital stimulation.
16. Patient remains infection free.
17. Patient has adequate spinal cord perfusion.
18. Patient can demonstrate exercises to maintain function.
19. Patient can explain the medication regimen (side effects, desired effects, time, dose, and route).
20. Patient can explain plans for follow-up care.
21. Patient can explain how to obtain community resources, including the Bureau of Vocational Rehabilitation.
22. Patient can explain importance of frequent position changes, including the use of the prone position and weight shifts in the wheelchair.
23. Patient can explain the need for assisted coughing if required and have caregiver demonstrate.

24. Patient remains free of respiratory complications.
25. Patient can explain autonomic dysreflexia, characteristic symptoms, and the actions to be taken when it occurs.
26. Patient remains sexually active, if so desired.
27. Patient demonstrates optimal coping skills.
28. Patient makes a reasonable choice for living arrangements.
29. Patient has minimal complications from sensory-perceptual deficit.
30. Patient has minimal discomfort.

IMPLEMENTATION

☐ **Assisting with achievement of therapeutic goals**
☐ *Immediate stage*

CERVICAL INJURIES. Immediate care after spinal cord injury is directed toward realignment of the cervical bony column in the presence of demonstrated fractures or dislocations. These measures include the following:
1. Simple immobilization
2. Skeletal traction
   a. Crutchfield tongs (Fig. 19-40)
   b. Halo traction
   c. Stryker or Foster frame
3. Surgery for spinal decompression

It is important to maintain strict body alignment, with the body kept straight and the head flat. Sandbags may be used to maintain alignment.

With Crutchfield tongs it is important to check the traction and orthopedic frame frequently (usually every 4 hours). The tongs should be secure and the weights should hang freely. The sites where the tongs enter the head are cleansed with hydrogen peroxide and povidine iodine solution is applied. Usually this is done every shift. When halo traction is used it is also important to check the pin sites and cleanse them as described above. The traction is attached to a fiberglass body jacket, which should be checked for proper fit. The nurse should be able to insert a finger between the cast and skin.

With the use of a frame (Foster or Stryker), it is important to check pressure points before and after the patient is turned. At least two persons should turn the patient and all bolts on the frame should be tightened securely before turning. Padding may be used for comfort, but care must be taken to maintain body alignment. It is important to assess the patient for any respiratory or cardiovascular difficulty when on the frame.

Often surgical decompression is not performed until after a period of skeletal traction. This allows the patient's condition to stabilize and some initial swelling of the cord to subside. The beginning spontaneous healing of the fracture site provides more stability. With the introduction of the anterior surgical approach to the cervical spinal column, surgical intervention is safer and can be attempted earlier in the hospitalization. The primary advantage of the anterior surgical approach is that it provides immediate stabilization of the spinal cord by techniques of interbody cervical fusion and the direct removal of any extruded disc materials. See the box on p. 497 for care of the patient who has had surgical decompression.

Intubation and respiratory assistance may be required

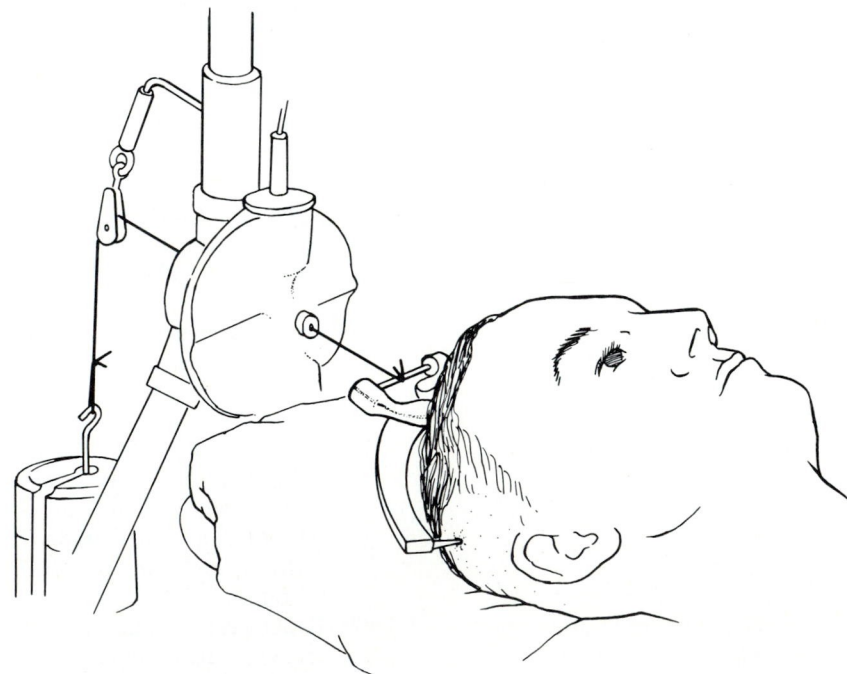

Fig. 19-40   Patient with Crutchfield tongs inserted into skull to hyperextend head and neck.

Nursing care of the patient undergoing spinal decompression

Preoperative care

1. Clarify patient's knowledge of surgery and expected changes.
2. Explain expected postoperative measures (including positioning, bed rest).
3. Encourage patient and family to verbalize fears.
4. Baseline neurologic and physiologic data should be assessed and recorded.

Postoperative care

1. Monitoring
   a. Assess ability to move legs; ask patient to do straight leg raises, dorsiflexion, and plantar flexion. Assess ability to move arms and hands if cervical decompression has occurred.
   b. Assess degree and character of drainage.
      (1) Amount of drainage and bleeding should be minimal.
      (2) Initial dressing can be reinforced as needed.
   c. Assess ability of patient to swallow; observe for swelling of neck.
2. Promoting mobility
   a. Patient can be turned side to side and onto back.
   b. If decompression is in lumbar area, sitting is usually not permitted.
   c. If decompression is in thoracic area, patient should not use arms to pull or push; no trapeze on bed.
   d. Patient is encouraged to do active range of motion and leg exercises such as quadriceps setting.
3. Promoting psychologic comfort
   a. Patient is encouraged to verbalize fears and reactions.
   b. Time should be spent with patient other than when giving direct care.
   c. Information about daily activities, tests, and procedures should be shared with patient.
   d. Medicate as needed for pain.
4. Preventing infection
   a. Incisional area kept clean and dry.
   b. Temperature checked frequently for first several days; report any elevation to physician.
   c. Report any redness, drainage, or hardness of wound.
   d. Incision often left open to air after first several days.

---

in the immediate stage following upper cervical cord injury. Any patient with a cord lesion at the C4 level probably will demand permanent ventilatory support. Careful monitoring of blood gas levels and regular pulmonary toilet are essential.

THORACIC AND LUMBAR INJURIES. Less immediate attention to thoracic and lumbar fracture immobilization is necessary for the patient with limited neurologic deficits. The patient is often treated with bed rest, hyperextension, and bracing. Stabilization of the spine may occur early in the recovery course or may be delayed until some healing has occurred.

MEDICATIONS. The use of adrenal corticosteroids for the prevention and alleviation of spinal cord edema is widespread. It is felt that the steroids assist in the reestablishment of membrane stability and in the control of central nervous tissue stability.

☐ Intermediate stage

Throughout all stages of hospitalization of the patient with a spinal cord injury, nursing and medical interventions are directed toward restoration of structural or body integrity. All efforts are taken to ensure that the following occur:

1. Skin is intact.
2. Contractures do not develop.
3. Range of motion is maintained to the greatest degree possible.
4. Muscle tone is consistent with pathologic condition.
5. Bowel and bladder function are maintained.

The reader is referred to the section on care of the patient with a motor dysfunction (p. 439). Most of the care described there applies to the patient with a spinal cord injury. Additional care is described below.

POSITION AND MOVEMENT. In addition to frequent positioning, the patient with a spinal cord injury is usually placed on a bed with a firm surface or may even be placed

☐ Counseling and teaching

Teaching of the patient with spinal cord injury encompasses all of the points covered in teaching the patient with

Early mobilization of the patient is important. When patients, especially quadriplegics, begin to sit up, it may be necessary to wrap their legs with elastic wraps to encourage venous return. Slowly increasing the angle of sitting is essential to prevent hypotension. For this reason a newly quadriplegic patient should use a recliner wheelchair until he or she is able to sit at a 90-degree angle for several hours.

Before the patient is permitted to be up following a spinal injury, a brace may be prescribed. All braces and corsets must be custom made; they are usually expensive, and the cost is dependent on the type of material used. The brace or corset should be applied before the patient gets out of bed. The patient should wear a thin, knitted undershirt next to the skin to keep the brace clean and to protect the skin. For some paraplegics, leg braces may permit them to stand and ambulate. Many find, however, that the effort to walk is not justified.

URINARY ELIMINATION. Since there is no sensation of needing to void in the patient with spinal cord injury, distention occurs easily. Usually a Foley catheter is inserted initially. Later, bladder training is started. Measures important in this training can be found in Chapter 32.

The presence of an indwelling catheter makes the patient highly susceptible to urinary infection, which can include bladder or kidney infections. These are major causes of death in patients with spinal cord injury, so it is imperative that infection be avoided, if at all possible. The best means of preventing infection is maintenance of fluid intake (3 to 4 L a day) and meticulous aseptic technique. Drinking cranberry juice several times a day has been found helpful in preventing infection, along with prophylactic antibiotic therapy such as nitrofurantoin or sulfamethoxazole and trimethoprim (Septra, Bactrim).

Autonomic dysreflexia is one complication associated with urinary elimination in the patient with spinal cord injury. It is a medical emergency, and the nurse should be aware of the actions to take in preventing and alleviating the symptoms. The care required with the presence of symptoms is outlined in the box below.

BOWEL ELIMINATION. Patients are started on a bowel program early in the recovery period. At first, bisacodyl (Dulcolax) suppositories are given at regular intervals—usually every other night. This is followed by digital stimulation to further stimulate peristalsis. The goal is to eliminate the need for the suppositories. Other aids to bowel programs are the use of adequate fluids, stool softeners, and prune juice.

RESPIRATORY FUNCTION. Generally, patients with cervical injuries below C4 are able to breathe without ventilatory support. However, they do not have normal control of chest muscles or the diaphragm, which makes them prone to respiratory complications. Care of the patient may include use of the inspirometer to increase tidal volume. Other breathing exercises may also be prescribed. The patient may require assisted coughing in which the caregiver exerts upward and inward pressure on the fleshy part of the stomach just below the diaphragm while the patient attempts to cough. This action is similar to the Heimlich maneuver but is done with less force. The patient should also be encouraged to avoid situations where respiratory infections may be transmitted. Respiratory infections are often the cause of death in patients with spinal cord injury, especially those with high cervical injury.

If a patient is ventilator dependent, attempts are made to have the patient use a portable ventilator, which allows for mobility. Diaphragmatic pacemakers may be inserted. This is still an uncommon procedure, but it has been effective in allowing patients time off the ventilator.

SKIN INTEGRITY. Another problem that occurs with spinal cord injury is decubitus ulcers. Every effort should be made to avoid skin breakdown, which is a major cause of morbidity in the patient with spinal cord injury.

□ **Counseling and teaching**

Teaching of the patient with spinal cord injury encompasses all of the points covered in teaching the patient with a motor dysfunction and sensory dysfunction (p. 448). In addition, the patient needs assistance in learning about the effects of the injury on sexual functioning (see the box on p. 499). The important thought to keep in mind is that most patients with a cooperative partner are able to engage in a satisfying sexual relationship. The limitation depends on the site of the lesion and whether the cord injury is complete or incomplete. Generally, the higher the lesion, the more normal sexual function is likely to be. Patients with sacral lesions are the only patients with spinal cord injuries who are not able to have an erection and ejaculate.

Nursing care of the patient with autonomic dysreflexia

1. Place patient in sitting position to decrease blood pressure.
2. Check patency of catheter for kinking. If catheter is plugged, insert new catheter immediately.
3. Check rectum for impaction.
4. If it is necessary to remove impaction, dibucaine (Nupercaine ointment) should be instilled in the rectum for its anesthetic effect.
5. Send urine for culture if no other cause is found; urinary infection can lead to symptoms of autonomic dysreflexia.
6. Administer ganglionic blocking agent such as hexamethonium chloride or a vasodilator such as nitroprusside (Nipride) if conservative measures are not effective.

Sexual functioning in patients with spinal cord injury

1. Reflexogenic erections occur not only as a result of stimulation of the genitalia, but also as a result of stimulation of "trigger points."
   a. Stroking the thigh
   b. Stimulating the rectum with a finger
   c. Manipulating the catheter
2. Male patients with catheters can either remove the catheter just before sexual activity or turn it back on the penis where it provides extra support.
3. Bowels should be emptied before intercourse to prevent incontinence.
4. Female patients who have a catheter can keep it in place if desired.
5. Female patients should realize that they maintain the ability to conceive—birth control should be practiced if pregnancy is not desired.

Education of the patient in terms of sexual function includes the points outlined here.

✚ EVALUATION

The evaluation of the care of the patient with spinal cord injury is the same as that for the patient with a motor dysfunction (p. 448) or sensory dysfunction (p. 449).

■ Peripheral nerve trauma

The peripheral nerves that lie outside the brain and spinal cord include the cranial nerves and spinal nerves and their branches and plexuses. The disorders involving the peripheral nerves are similar to those that affect the central nervous system and are the result of traumatic, degenerative, vascular, inflammatory, neoplastic, and metabolic causes. Important terms are listed in the box at right.

Traumatic causes of peripheral nerve injuries include gunshot and knife wounds, fragmented fracture wounds, and surgical transections, as in denervation surgery and amputation. They result in stretching, laceration, and compression of the peripheral nerve. The degree of injury is variable. Recovery is also variable—axons of peripheral nerves are capable of regeneration under favorable conditions.

■ PATHOPHYSIOLOGY

Following trauma (or disease) the axon undergoes secondary or *wallerian degeneration* distal to the lesion and for several segments proximal. The axon and myelin sheath degenerate and undergo fragmentation. The fragmented particles are completely ingested within several weeks; the axis cylinder remains. Schwann's cells and fibroblasts begin to proliferate, covering the degenerated fibers. During the regenerative phase, new axoplasm forms at the proximal edge of the injury and the regenerating fibers now grow distally and enter the empty neurolemmal sheath, which has in the meantime proliferated. Myelin then forms

Common terminology with peripheral nerve trauma

Neuropathies	Noninflammatory disorders
Mononeuro-pathy	Disorder affecting one peripheral nerve
Polyneuropa-thy	Disorder involving multiple nerves
Neuritis	Inflammatory disorder
Neuralgia	Painful nerve disorder

around the regenerated axon. When a nerve has been severely damaged and fibrous tissue is abundant, regeneration is interfered with by a tangled mass known as a traumatic neuroma; this may have to be removed surgically.

▦ ASSESSMENT

Assessment includes both subjective and objective data.

☐ Subjective data

1. Patient's understanding of condition
2. Alteration in sensation
   a. Pain
   b. Touch
   c. Temperature
   d. Proprioception
3. Site of sensory problem
4. Onset of problem
5. Presence of associated symptoms

☐ Objective data

1. Presence of motor alterations
2. The clinical signs and symptoms resulting from peripheral nerve lesions depend on the exact location of the lesion and the specific function of the involved nerve

or nerves. Because peripheral nerves contain both sensory and motor components, there may be deficits in both components distal to the site. Alterations will occur in pain, touch, temperature, proprioception, and stereognosis. Motor alteration includes lower motor neuron signs such as flaccid paralysis and muscle wasting in the muscles innervated by the affected nerves.

➡ DATA ANALYSIS: NURSING DIAGNOSES

The nursing diagnoses and expected patient outcomes are the same as those for the patient who has sensory (p. 448) or motor dysfunction (pp. 442-443).

▦ IMPLEMENTATION

Nursing care is specific on the areas of the body affected by the sensory and motor deficits. Plans for care include measures found in the section on motor dysfunction and sensory dysfunction. Promotion of good health habits in general assists in the creation of conditions favorable to nerve regeneration.

✚ EVALUATION

The evaluation for the patient with peripheral nerve dysfunction is the same as for the patient with motor (p. 446) and sensory problems (p. 449).

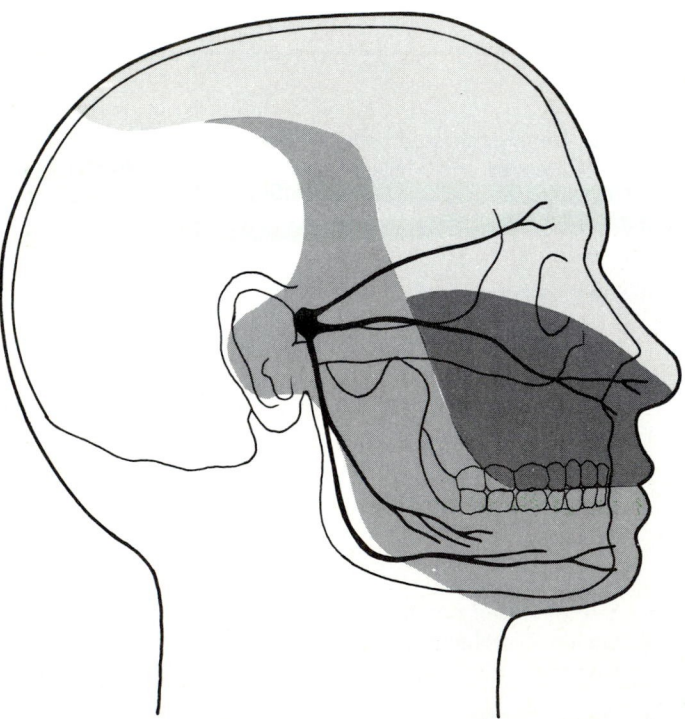

Fig. 19-41 Pathway of trigeminal nerve and facial area innervated by each of three main branches.

■ Trigeminal neuralgia

Trigeminal neuralgia is one specific kind of peripheral nerve problem. It is also called *tic doloreaux*. It usually affects persons in middle or late adulthood and is slightly more common in women.

▦ ASSESSMENT

Assessment is basically the same as for any patient with peripheral nerve trauma. Trigeminal neuralgia is characterized by excruciating, burning pain that radiates along one or more of the three divisions of the fifth cranial nerve (Fig. 19-41). The second and third divisions are most commonly affected. The pain typically only extends to the midline of the face and head, because this is the extent of the tissue supplied by the offending nerve. There are areas along the course of the nerve known as trigger points and the slightest stimulation of these areas may initiate pain. Persons with trigeminal neuralgia try desperately to avoid triggering them.

▦ IMPLEMENTATION

☐ **Assisting with the achievement of therapeutic goals**
☐ *Medication*

Carbamazepine (Tegretol) is the drug of choice for the treatment of trigeminal neuralgia pain. Drugs such as nicotinic acid, thiamine chloride, analgesics, and even cobra venom have been tried with little success. Absolute alcohol may be injected into the peripheral branches of the trigeminal nerve. This provides relief for weeks to months.[25]

Postoperative concerns for the patient with trigeminal neuralgia

1. Preservation of eye function (if the upper branch is completely severed the corneal reflex is lost)
   a. Eye shield to prevent dust or lint from getting into the cornea
   b. Avoidance of contact with eye while bathing
   c. Eye baths with methylcellulose solution
   d. Inspection of eye several times a day
2. Promoting mouth function (lower branch of fifth cranial nerve)
   a. Avoidance of hot food
   b. Food should be placed in unaffected side of mouth
   c. Mouth care after each meal
3. Safety concerns
   a. Electric razor should be used for shaving

□ *Surgery*

Permanent relief of pain is obtained only by surgery that consists of either inserting a fine needle through the cheek or by surgical resection of the sensory root of the trigeminal nerve. This is not always successful. Preoperative care includes the following:

1. Measures of comfort
2. Allowing patient to voice questions or concerns
3. Education about procedure and what to expect

Postoperative care includes the measures listed in box on p. 500.

Within 24 hours after a fifth nerve resection, many patients develop herpes simplex (cold sores) about the lips. Usually the lesions heal in about a week.

□ **Assisting with comfort and ADL**

It is not uncommon for patients with trigeminal neuralgia not to have eaten properly for some time, since eating causes pain. They may be undernourished and dehydrated. They may not have washed or shaved or combed the hair for some time. Oral hygiene often has been neglected.

**Comfort measures for patients
with tic doloreaux**

1. Keep room free of drafts
2. Avoid walking briskly to bedside of patient
3. Place bed out of traffic area to prevent jarring of bed
4. Avoid touching the patient's face
5. Patients should not be urged to wash or shave the affected area or to comb the hair
6. Avoid hot or cold liquids that trigger pain
7. Diet may have to be pureed and lukewarm and taken through straw

---

**Teaching for the patient
with trigeminal neuralgia**

1. Eye care—frequent inspection and washing with methylcellouse
2. Good oral hygiene
3. Avoidance of hot or cold food or liquids
4. Importance of seeing dentist at frequent intervals—dental caries will not cause pain
5. Wearing of glasses outdoors to protect eye from dust or flying particles

---

Measures to increase comfort preoperatively or of patients being treated nonsurgically are found in the box at left.

□ **Counseling and teaching**

Teaching for the patient with trigeminal neuralgia is found in the box at left, below.

■ Bell's palsy (peripheral facial paralysis)

■ PATHOPHYSIOLOGY

Bell's palsy is thought to be caused by an inflammatory process involving the facial nerve (VII) anywhere from the nucleus in the brain to the periphery. Other theories of origin include local ischemia and edema or emotional trauma with resultant vasoconstriction. Any of the three branches of the facial nerve may be affected. The disorder can be unilateral or bilateral. Most patients (80%) recover spontaneously over a period of a few weeks, although recovery may take as long as a year.

ASSESSMENT

Subjective and objective data are the same as for the patient with peripheral nerve trauma (p. 499). With Bell's palsy there is usually an abrupt onset of numbness or a feeling of stiffness or drawing sensation of the face. Unilateral weakness of the facial muscles usually occurs, resulting in inability to wrinkle the forehead, close the eyelid, pucker the lips, or retract the mouth on that side. The face appears asymmetric with drooping of the mouth and cheek.

Other symptoms that may occur with Bell's palsy include the following:

1. Loss of taste
2. Reduction in saliva on affected side
3. Pain behind the ear
4. Ringing in ear or other hearing loss

DATA ANALYSIS: NURSING DIAGNOSES

See appropriate sections in the discussion of the patient with peripheral nerve trauma (p. 499).

IMPLEMENTATION

There is no specific therapy for Bell's palsy. Electrical stimulation or warm moist heat along the course of the nerve may help. Steroids given early in the course may speed recovery. Protection of the eyes when the eyelid does not close is important. Massage of the affected areas is sometimes recommended. Exercises may be prescribed for 5 minutes three times a day. These include wrinkling the brow and forehead, closing the eyes, and puffing out the cheeks.

INTERFERENCE WITH FUNCTION BECAUSE OF TUMORS

Intracranial tumors

PATHOPHYSIOLOGY

Intracranial tumors include both benign and metastatic lesions. All areas and structures of the brain can be affected. Primary intracranial tumors, or neoplasms, arise from the intrinsic cells of brain tissues and the pituitary and pineal glands. Second or metastatic tumors are also a frequent contributing type of intracranial tumor. The prognosis for patients with an intracranial tumor is dependent on early diagnosis and treatment because as the tumor grows it exerts pressure on vital centers and causes brain damage and death. Although approximately one half of all tumors are benign, they may also cause death by exerting pressure on vital centers.

Brain tumors are named for the tissues from which they arise. The more frequently encountered ones are described in Table 19-7. The brain, in addition, is also a frequent site for secondary tumors from other organs.

The symptoms of intracranial tumors result from both local and general effects of the tumor. Locally, the effects are from infiltration, invasion, and destruction of brain tissues at a particular site. Direct pressure is also exerted on nerve structures, causing degeneration and interference with local circulation. Local edema develops, and ICP increases. The increased ICP is then transmitted throughout the brain and the ventricular system. Eventually, the ventricular system is distorted and displaced sufficiently to cause partial ventricular obstruction (Fig. 19-42). Papilledema results from the general effects of the increased ICP. Death is usually from brainstem compression resulting from herniation.

ASSESSMENT

It is important to assess both subjective and objective data in the patient with an intracranial tumor. The box on p. 503 contains a comparison of the symptoms of tumors in specific brain lobes.

☐ **Subjective data**

1. Patient's understanding of diagnosis
2. Changes in personality or judgment
3. Presence of abnormal sensations (paresthesia or anesthesia)
4. Visual problems—loss of visual acuity or diplopia
5. Complaints of unusual odors (often accompanies tumors of temporal lobe)
6. Presence of headache
7. Hearing loss
8. Inability to carry on daily activities

Table 19-7 Type of brain tumor

Type	Incidence	Pathology
Glioma	Accounts for one half of brain tumors	Arises in any part of the brain connective tissue. Infiltrates primarily the cerebral hemisphere tissue. Not so well outlined as to be incised completely. Grows rapidly—most persons live months to years. Tumors assigned grade from 1 to 4, with 4 the most malignant. Different gliomas are as follows: 1. Astrocytomas 2. Oligodendrogliomas 3. Ependymomas 4. Medulloblastoma 5. Glioblastoma multiforme—most malignant
Meningioma	13% to 18% of all primary tumors in intracranial cavity	Arise from the meningeal coverings of the brain. They are usually benign but may undergo malignant changes. Usually encapsulated, and surgical cure is possible. Recurrence is possible.
Pituitary tumor	Occurs in all age groups but more often in women	Arise from a varied number of tissues. Surgical approach is usually successful. Recurrence is possible.
Neuroma (schwannoma, neurofibroma)	Acoustic neuroma is most common	Arises from Schwann's cells inside the auditory meatus on the vestibular portion of cranial nerve III. Usually benign but may undergo cellular change and become malignant. Will regrow if not completely excised. Surgical resection is often difficult because of location.
Metastatic tumors	From 2% to 20% of all patients with cancer have metastasis to the brain	Cancer cells spread to the brain via the circulatory system. Surgical resection is very difficult; even with treatment prognosis is very poor. Survival beyond a year or two is uncommon.

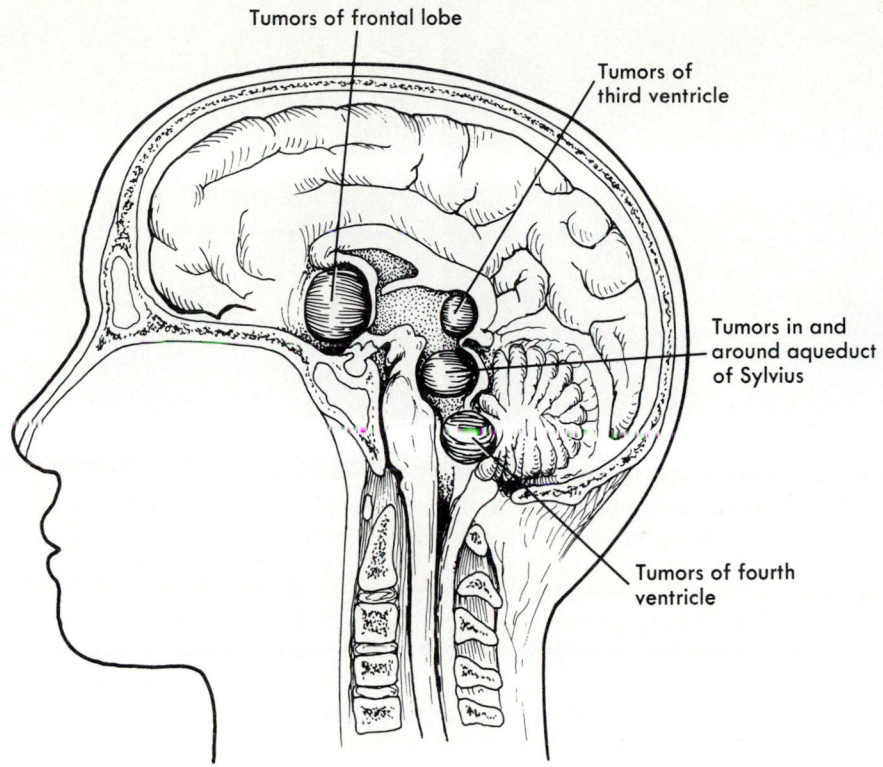

Fig. 19-42 Sites of brain tumors adjacent to ventricular system. Note how developing tumor at varied sites with extension distorts, compresses, and obstructs ventricular system at some point so that increased intracranial pressure occurs early. (From Yahr, WD: Hosp Med 9:8, 1973.)

Comparison of symptoms of tumors found in specific brain lobes

Area of the brain	Symptoms
Frontal lobe	Personality disturbances (range from subtle personality changes to frank psychotic behavior)
	Inappropriate effect
	Indifference of bodily functions
Precentral gyrus	Jacksonian seizures
Occipital lobe	Visual disturbances preceding convulsions
Temporal lobe	Olfactory, visual, or gustatory hallucinations
	Psychomotor seizures with automatic behavior
Parietal lobe	Inability to replicate pictures
	Loss of right-left discrimination

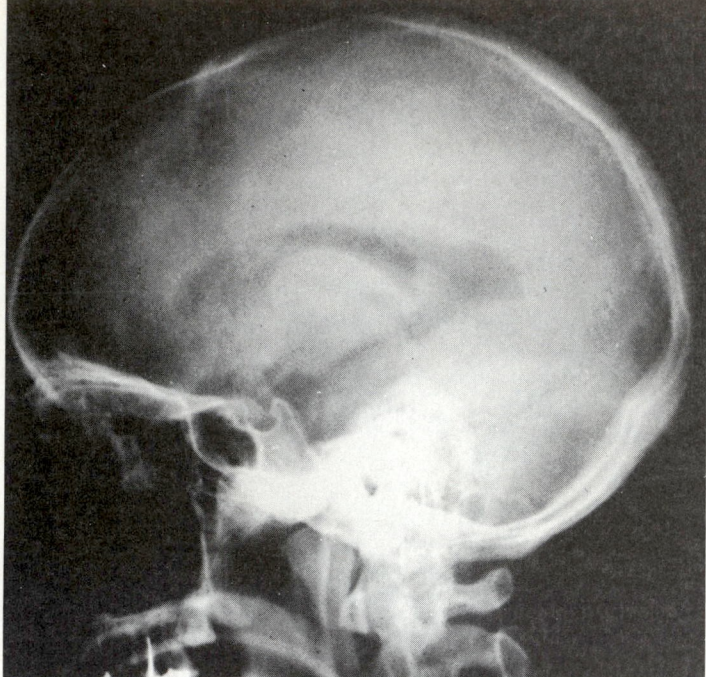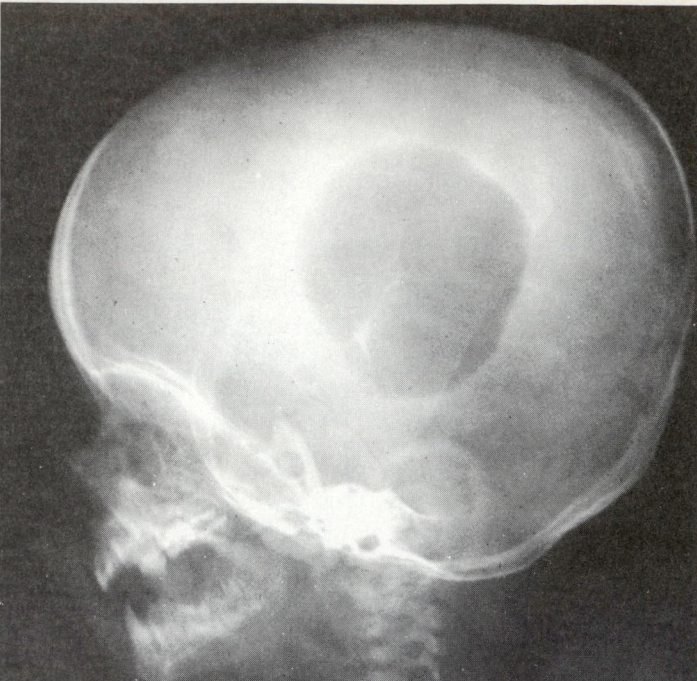

Fig. 19-43 Pneumoencephalogram. **A,** Lateral view showing outline of normal ventricle. **B,** Lateral view showing marked distention of ventricle with cerebrospinal fluid (caused by hydrocephalus).

Pneumoencephalogram

Purpose

To detect lesions of the ventricles and cisternal system using air as contrast.

Preparation of patient

1. Prepare as if for surgery.
2. Permit must be signed.
3. Sedative may be given evening before procedure and just before test.
4. General anesthesia may be used.
5. Patient teaching:
   a. Explain procedure.
   b. Time: approximately 2 hours.
   c. Sensation: patient is usually very uncomfortable. Headache is usually severe during procedure; nausea and vomiting are common.

Procedure

1. Patient is positioned as for lumbar puncture or cisternal tap (p. 422).
2. After the tap is done and pressure measured, the contrast medium (air or oxygen) is injected in amounts of 25 to 30 ml. Patient is watched carefully for headache, nausea, vomiting, or any change in vital signs or color.
3. Head of the table is gradually raised, and head may be rotated to assist air in filling ventricles.

After procedure

1. Patient is placed in bed with head flat. May be in bed 24 to 48 hours.
2. Constant attention with frequent vital signs and neurologic checks is needed until the patient is awake and alert.
3. Severe headache is common and may last for 48 hours.
4. Seizure precautions should be maintained if patient has history of seizures.
5. Tracheostomy set at bedside.
6. Reactions to procedure may be severe and include vomiting, shock, respiratory difficulty, and other signs of increased ICP.

Other

Pneumoencephalogram is now used less frequently because of the availability of the CT scanner. It is never done in the presence of increased ICP because of the danger of herniation.

☐ Objective data

1. Motor strengths
2. Gait
3. Level of alertness and consciousness
4. Orientation
5. Pupils: size, equality, and reactivity
6. Vital signs
7. Fundoscopic examination for evidence of papilledema
8. Presence of seizures
9. Speech abnormalities
10. Cranial nerve abnormalities
11. Symptoms of increased intracranial pressure

Seizures occurring for the first time after middle age are very suggestive of a brain tumor in the cerebrum or its coverings. Intracranial tumors occurring within the cerebral lobes present disturbances that can be related to the function of the specific part of the brain.

Signs and symptoms of increased ICP resulting from intracranial tumors usually occur after localized signs and symptoms have been present for varying periods. See the previous discussion of increased ICP. Headache is at first transitory and later becomes constant; it increases in intensity with straining, coughing, stooping, and change of position. The headache is present in the morning and often awakens the person from sleep. Nausea and vomiting usually occur as the headache increases.

☐ Diagnostic tests

No one procedure is entirely diagnostic of brain tumors, but the CT scan is often the basis of the diagnosis. Other tests that may be done include the brain scan and the EEG. These are discussed on p. 426 and p. 452. Another test that is used less frequently since the introduction of the CT scanner is the pneumoencephalogram (Fig. 19-43). See the box on p. 504 for details about a pneumoencephalogram.

Other tests that may be helpful in locating the tumor are *arteriography* or *ventriculography* (see the box below for details about a ventriculogram). Arteriography is described on p. 470. The ventriculogram is used when the suggested diagnosis is such that a spinal or lumbar puncture is contraindicated because of the presence of increased ICP. Fig. 19-44 shows an aneurysm found on a cerebral angiogram.

→ DATA ANALYSIS: NURSING DIAGNOSES

Nursing diagnoses are determined from assessment of patient data. Possible nursing diagnoses for the person with an intracranial tumor may include, but are not limited to, the following:

Ventriculogram

Purpose

To detect pathology within the ventricular and cisternal system.

Preparation of patient

1. Procedure is performed in the operating room.
2. Surgical permit must be signed.
3. Patient is prepared as if for surgery.
4. Top or back of head is partially shaved.
5. Intravenous or general anesthesia is commonly used.
6. Patient teaching
   a. Explain procedure.
   b. Time: variable. Often patient has craniotomy for tumor removal immediately after test.
   c. Sensation: none during procedure because of anesthesia.

Procedure

1. Patient is positioned, usually supine.
2. Trephine openings (burr holes) are made into the lateral ventricles.
3. Air is introduced directly via the ventricles.
4. X-ray films of the brain and ventricles are taken at intervals.

After procedure

1. Same as for pneumoencephalogram.
2. Observe site of burr hole for bleeding or drainage.
3. Observe for signs of neurologic deterioration that would indicate formation of intracerebral clot.

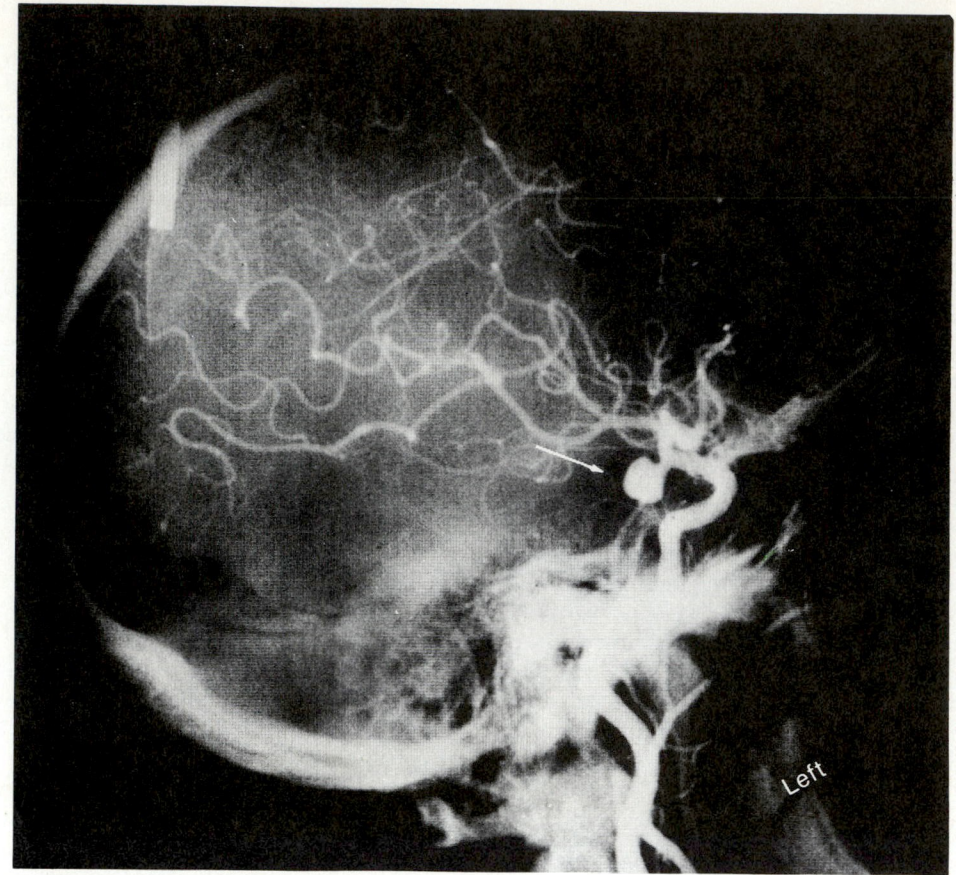

Fig. 19-44 Cerebral angiography showing location of aneurysm at posterior communicating artery. (From Tortorici, M: Fundamentals of angiography, St. Louis, 1982, The CV Mosby Co.)

Diagnostic title	Possible etiologies
Anxiety	Threat of death, change in health status
Pain	Brain tumor, immobility
Impaired verbal communication	Aphasia
Anticipatory grieving	Potential loss of life
Knowledge deficit	Lack of exposure/recall, cognitive limitation
Impaired physical mobility	Pain/discomfort, perceptual/cognitive impairment
Sensory/perceptual alterations: visual, auditory, kinesthetic, gustatory, tactile, olfactory	Altered sensory reception/transmission/integration
Altered thought processes	Neurologic disorders
Altered cerebral tissue perfusion	Decreased blood flow, pressure

These diagnoses reflect the patient's initial diagnosis. Patients with brain tumors that have caused significant problems may initially have nursing diagnoses indicative of increased intracranial pressure or motor dysfunction.

PLANNING: EXPECTED PATIENT OUTCOMES

Expected patient outcomes for the person with an intracranial tumor may include, but are not limited to, the following:

1. Patient verbalizes minimal anxiety.
2. Patient maintains communication, even if it is non-verbal.
3. Patient demonstrates appropriate grieving and coping mechanisms.
4. Patient maintains optimal mobility.
5. Patient is able to compensate for deficits in thought processes.
6. Patient compensates for sensory-perceptual deficits.
7. Patient maintains adequate cerebral perfusion.
8. Patient can explain prescribed therapy.
9. Patient can state signs and symptoms to report to the physician.

10. Patient can explain the medication regimen (dose, side effects, route and times).
11. Patient can explain plans for follow-up care.
12. Patient can verbalize fears and concerns related to the diagnosis.

▦ IMPLEMENTATION

☐ Assisting with the achievement of therapeutic goals

The general methods of treatment for intracranial tumors include surgical removal when feasible, radiotherapy, and chemotherapy. The choice of therapy is determined by the tumor type and site of the tumor. A combination of methods is often necessary.

When gliomas are located in areas that are not critical to vital functions, they are usually removed surgically. Most gliomas, however, infiltrate and are difficult to completely excise and treat. Surgery is often combined with radiotherapy and chemotherapy. When the tumor is located in a more critical area where removal would leave the patient with impaired function, a biopsy of the tumor is performed, it is "debrided" if possible, and the patient is treated with radiotherapy or chemotherapy.

Meningiomas are commonly treated by complete excision of the tumor (and overlying bone if infiltrated), because they are usually located in areas that permit removal. Meningiomas are often encapsulated, which aids in their removal.

☐ Surgery

Intracranial surgery is commonly done for all types of pathologic conditions of the brain, including the relief of increased ICP and removal of tumors.

A surgical opening through the skull is known as *craniotomy*. It is a basic preparatory procedure for intracranial surgery. A series of burr holes is made first, and then the bone between the holes is cut with a Gigli saw to permit removal of the bone. Bone is then removed in such a way that it can be replaced if desired. Brain surgery may be done with the patient under hypothermia to lessen bleeding during the procedure. Drugs of hypotension may be used, such as norepinephrine bitartrate (Levophed). Patients may also be placed in a barbiturate coma during the surgery and for several days following it to lessen brain activity, metabolism, and oxygen needs. This may help to prevent worsening of deficits because of hypoxia.

When the brain lesion is in the supratentorium (above the tentorium or in the cerebrum), the incision is usually made behind the hairline. When the incision is into the infratentorium (below the tentorium or in the brainstem and cerebellum), it is made slightly above the nape of the neck.

Following craniotomy and removal of the bone, an incision is made into the meninges and the tumor is removed or other cranial surgery performed. The removed bone is carefully saved or preserved and may be replaced at the end of the surgery if there is no indication of infection or increased ICP. If it is not replaced, a bone prosthesis may later be placed over the deficit. The removal of part of the skull without replacement is called *craniectomy*. *Cranioplasty* is the repair of a cranial defect through use of a substitute bone material such as plastic or methylmethacrylate cement.

Tumors involving the pituitary gland that do not extend outside the sella turcica are usually removed using a transsphenoidal approach. After the surgery, packing is placed inside the nose and remains for 3 to 4 days. A muscle graft from the thigh is used to close the defect in the dura. With this type of surgery, recovery is relatively rapid and the patient has no loss of hair or external cranial incision.[34]

Preoperative preparation of both the patient and family is important. They both are usually very threatened by the prospect of brain surgery. Specific fears may be related to those of a permanent change in appearance, dependency, or both. Preoperative care includes the points listed in the box below.

During the postoperative period the patient is observed regularly for signs of increased ICP. The frequency of making and recording specific observations depends on the patient's condition. A device to measure ICP is often inserted during the surgery (p. 437). Any change in the pa-

---

Preoperative care of the patient undergoing intracranial surgery

1. Baseline data of neurologic and physiologic status should be recorded.
2. Patient and family should be encouraged to verbalize fears.
3. Treatments and procedures are explained fully, even if unsure whether patient understands.
4. If head is shaved, it is usually done in the operating room.
5. Antiseptic shampoo may be ordered night before surgery and may be repeated in morning.
6. If hair is shaved, it is saved and given to patient or family.
7. Prepare family for appearance of patient following surgery.
   a. Head dressing
   b. Edema and ecchymosis of face common
   c. Temporary decreased mental status (possible).

tient's vital signs, state of consciousness, pupillary response, or ability to move muscles is reported at once. Restlessness, often secondary to tissue hypoxia, may be the first warning of increased ICP. See pp. 432-439 for specifics about ICP.

Postoperative care is determined by the patient's condition. Most patients spend at least 1 or 2 nights in an intensive care unit, where arterial monitoring and close nursing observation is possible. Other details of postoperative care are found in the section on intracerebral hematomas.

☐ Hydrocephalus

Occasionally a catheter is placed in a ventricle of the brain to drain excess spinal fluid and to prevent hydrocephalus and increased ICP. The catheter is usually attached to a drainage system. The tubing and drainage receptacle should be sterile, and care must be taken to prevent kinking of the tubing. If drainage seems to have stopped, the neurosurgeon should be notified. At times, the nurse may adjust the level of the drainage device to facilitate drainage. This is only done with specific parameters for drainage, which are ordered by the physician. For example the physician may order that the patient should drain 30 ml every 4 hours. The catheter is usually left in place for 24 to 48 hours and then is removed by the surgeon.

Hydrocephalus of a more permanent nature also occurs in the presence of intracranial tumors and is manifested by symptoms of increased ICP. Hydrocephalus can be communicating or noncommunicating. In communicating hydrocephalus an obstruction exists outside the ventricular system. The ventricles contain an excessive amount of CSF because fluid is not adequately absorbed from the cerebral subdural space. In noncommunicating, or intraventricular hydrocephalus CSF is accumulated secondary to a blockage of the normal flow at some point in the ventricular system. The cerebral ventricle proximal to the blockage then dilates.

Treatment consists of a shunting procedure. The different types of shunt procedures are named for their point of origin and termination and include the following:

1. Cyst to peritoneal
2. Lumbar-peritoneal
3. Ventricular-jugular
4. Ventricular-peritoneal

In this type of surgery excessive CSF is shunted away from the central nervous system and into either the periotoneal cavity (where it is absorbed) or into the jugular vein. At times a Ryckham reservoir is placed through a burr hole into the ventricle. This device can easily be palpated through the skin. Some of the shunts have an on-off valve, as well as a part that may be pumped to facilitate drainage. Valves that are inserted can be set for a pressure with some control over the amount of fluid drained.

Preoperative care is the same as for any patient having intracranial surgery. Key points of postoperative care are listed in the box below.

Two other types of hydrocephalus do not result in ICP:

Postoperative care of the patient with a shunt

1. Monitoring
   a. Assess neurologic status frequently for any decrease in mental status.
   b. Observe for symptoms of subdural hematoma, one of the possible side effects of the surgery.
   c. Monitor for symptoms of overdrainage, as evidenced by headache, especially when patient is sitting upright or standing.
   d. Assess degree and character of drainage.
      (1) Amount of drainage and bleeding should be minimal.
      (2) Reinforce dressing as needed.
      (3) Often incisional areas are left open to air after several days.
2. Maintain gastrointestinal status
   a. Check frequently for signs of paralytic ileus, because the manipulation of the bowel that occurs with the placement of the peritoneal part of the shunt can predispose the patient to this.
   b. Patient is usually kept NPO for first day, and then clear liquids are started.
   c. Regular diet is resumed as soon as good bowel sounds are present and patient tolerates liquids.
3. Maintaining comfort
   a. Patient may need more frequent pain medication because of involvement of abdominal area.
   b. Keep pressure off incisional sites.
4. Promoting mobility
   a. Turning to either side is permitted.
   b. Raise head of bed gradually when mobilizing patient.
   c. Patient is encouraged to ambulate as much as possible to encourage adaptation to decreased ICP.

(1) hydrocephalus, which occurs as ventricles dilate to fill spaces caused by decreasing brain mass, and (2) normal pressure hydrocephalus (NPH). Persons with NPH have dilated ventricles with normal tissue mass and a normal intracranial pressure. The cause is unknown.

□ Radiation therapy and chemotherapy

In some patients with intracranial tumors surgery may not be possible or indicated. In these cases radiation therapy and/or chemotherapy may be used. They are also used at times after intracranial surgery. See Chapter 12 for the care of the patient undergoing these treatments. One new and experimental chemotherapeutic treatment for brain tumors uses mannitol given via the arterial approach to open the blood-brain barrier. The chemotherapy is then given directly into the tumor area of the brain.

□ Assisting with comfort and ADL

Some patients who have had cranial surgery will have residual physical and mental limitations. The patient may have hemiplegia, aphasia, and personality changes. The rehabilitative care and planning are the same as for other patients with chronic and permanent neurologic disease (see sections on the patient with motor dysfunction and the patient with a stroke). Regardless of the eventual prognosis and the diagnosis of the tumor, each patient should be helped to be as independent as possible for as long as possible.

✠ EVALUATION

Evaluation of the patient with an intracranial tumor involves both the patient and the family. It is based on the expected patient outcomes. Pertinent questions to ask include the following:

1. Is the patient able to carry on ADL?
2. Can the patient explain the therapy and why it is occurring?
3. Can the patient state signs and symptoms to report to the physician?
4. Can the patient explain the medication regimen?
5. Is the patient taking medication as ordered?
6. Are any incisional areas healing?
7. Can the patient explain plans for follow-up care?
8. Can the patient explain how to obtain community support?
9. Is the patient carrying out prescribed exercises?
10. Is the patient verbalizing feelings and fears?

■ Intravertebral tumors

■ PATHOPHYSIOLOGY

The pathologic condition that results from spinal cord tumors is caused by spinal cord destruction and infiltrates, displacement and compression of the cord, and disruption of the blood supply or CSF circulation. The severity of symptoms depends on the degree of compression and the speed with which it develops. Adaption can occur with slow-growing tumors. Eighty-five percent of spinal cord tumors are benign.

Primary neoplastic tumors occur either extramedullary (outside the cord) or intramedullary (within the cord). Secondary or metastatic tumors may also involve the spinal cord, its coverings, and the vertebrae.

Extramedullary tumors of the intradural type may at first cause subjective nerve root pain. With tumor growth there will be motor and sensory deficits related to the level of the root and spinal cord involvement. As the tumor enlarges, it compresses the cord. Eventually, the patient loses all motor and sensory function below the level of the tumor.

An intramedullary tumor, beginning within the spinal cord, often initially appears as a central cord syndrome including segmental loss of pain and temperature function. In addition, anterior horn cell function is often lost, especially in the hands. Most of the central long tracts next to the gray matter become dysfunctional. Loss of pain and temperature sensations and motor weakness is gradual, progressive, and descending. Caudal motor and sensory functions are the last to be lost, including loss of bowel and bladder function.

⊞ ASSESSMENT

The subjective and objective data for the patient with an intravertebral tumor are the same as for the patient with spinal cord injury (p. 494).

⊞ IMPLEMENTATION

□ Assisting with the achievement of therapeutic goals
□ Surgery

A spinal decompression is commonly done even when complete removal of the tumor is not considered possible. As much of the tumor as possible (and possibly bone) is removed to reduce the obstruction for a time. It can be done at any level of the vertebral column and may include several vertebrae. The operation is sometimes palliative. Care of the patient undergoing spinal decompression is found in the section on spinal cord injury (p. 497).

□ Assisting with comfort and ADL

Convalescent care and rehabilitation depend entirely on the type of tumor and whether it has been succesfully removed. The decompression operation may give relief of symptoms for months and sometimes for years. If the tumor is a slow-growing one, radiation therapy may be given while the patient is in the hospital and continued after discharge.

✠ EVALUATION

The evaluation of the care of the patient with an intravertebral tumor is the same as for the patient with a motor dysfunction (p. 446).

■ SUMMARY

1. The neuron is the basic structural and functional unit of the nervous system.
2. Afferent neurons are sensory neurons that conduct impulses from the periphery to the central nervous system, and efferent or motor neurons transmit impulses from the CNS to the periphery.
3. Impulses travel across neurons as a result of action potentials.
4. Contacts between neurons occur at synapses, where neurotransmitters are released.
5. The nervous system is divided into two major divisions—the central nervous system and the peripheral nervous system.
6. The brain is composed of the cerebrum, the brainstem, and the cerebellum, each of which has specific functions.
7. Systemic circulation favors the CNS overall, balancing parts to assure a constant supply of nutrients to the brain.
8. The general sensory system is made up of receptor neurons, posterior roots of the afferent or posterior sensory nerves, ascending sensory tracts in the spinal cord and brain, and the sensory area of the cerebral cortex.
9. The descending motor systems include the corticospinal system (pyramidal tracts), the extrapyramidal system, and the cerebellar system.
10. Normal changes that occur in the nervous system cannot be equated with senility, Alzheimer's disease, or organic brain disease.

Putting knowledge to practice

- What four functions does the nervous system accomplish?
- What are the four cerebral lobes and what are their functions?
- What structures are located in the brainstem and what are the functions of each?
- What are the two major connecting arteries in the brain and what areas do they supply?
- What purpose does the Circle of Willis serve?
- What is the difference between efferent and afferent nerves?
- What are the normal characteristics of cerebrospinal fluid?
- What are the six major components of the neurologic assessment?
- What are the definitions of the following terms?
  - a. Paresthesia
  - b. Hyperalgesia
  - c. Hypoalgesia
  - d. Analgesia
  - e. Dysesthesia
  - f. Referred pain
  - g. Causalgia
  - h. Local pain
- What are nursing interventions that increase and decrease increased intracranial pressure?
- How is the CT scan done and what is it effective in diagnosing?
- What are four preventive factors that can help prevent neurologic disease?
- What is one contraindication to lumbar puncture?
- What is Cushing's response and what does it indicate?
- What rehabilitative nursing measures are important in persons with increased intracranial pressure?
- What are the classic signs of increased intracranial pressure?
- Why is mannitol given with increased intracranial pressure and what does it do?
- What is the difference between an upper motor neuron lesion and a lower motor neuron lesion?
- What is an aura?
- Why is it sometimes difficult to diagnose multiple sclerosis?
- What types of drugs cause drug-induced parkinsonian syndromes?
- What is the most common disease of the nervous system?
- Why is the incidence of bacterial meningitis higher in the fall and winter?
- What type of isolation is necessary for the patient with disseminated herpes zoster and why?
- What are the general effects of moderate to severe head injuries?
- Why is it important to immobilize the spine of the patient with spinal cord injury in the initial period?
- Why does hydrocephalus develop and what can be done for it?
- What is autonomic hyperreflexia and what nursing actions are important?
- What are the meanings of the following terms?
  - a. Coup-contrecoup injuries
  - b. Acceleration-deceleration injuries

11. The Glasgow Coma Scale is one tool that is useful in standardizing observations of neurologic patients.

12. The source of headache should be determined through careful assessment because it may be a symptom of serious neurologic pathology.

13. The CT scan is an important diagnostic tool in the assessment of brain pathology.

14. The lumbar puncture is not done if there is a question of increased intracranial pressure because it may result in brain herniation.

15. Drugs commonly prescribed for patients with migraine headache include ergotamine tartrate, propranolol hydrochloride (Inderal), and methysergide maleate (Sansert).

16. It is extremely difficult to evaluate neurologic pain objectively.

17. Any increase in the volume of one of the cranial contents (brain tissue, vascular tissue, and cerebrospinal fluid) results in increased intracranial pressure because the cranial vault is rigid, closed, and nonexpandable.

18. As intracranial pressure rises, it is first compensated for by venous compression and cerebrospinal displacement.

19. Classic signs of increased intracranial pressure include restlessness, disorientation, headache, contralateral hemiparesis, an ipsilaterally dilated pupil, and visual changes that include blurring of vision or diplopia.

20. Nursing care measures can significantly influence intracranial pressure.

21. Mannitol is given in the presence of acute increased intracranial pressure.

22. Three types of intracranial monitoring devices include the ventricular catheter, the subarachnoid bolt or screw, and the epidural sensor.

23. Lower motor neuron (LMN) lesions result in flaccid muscle weakness, loss of reflex activity, loss of muscle tone, and atrophy confined to the involved muscles.

24. Upper motor neuron (UMN) lesions result in spasticity and paresis of voluntary muscle tone, hyperreflexia, late atrophy from disuse, and increased muscle tone.

25. Epilepsy is a transitory disturbance in consciousness or in motor, sensory, or autonomic functions with or without loss of consciousness caused by sudden, excessive, and disorderly electrical discharges of the brain.

26. The aura is a set of symptoms that occurs before a seizure and varies from person to person.

27. The mouth of a person having a seizure should never be pried open to insert an airway or tongue blade.

28. Respiratory complications are common in patients with myasthenia gravis.

29. Early symptoms of multiple sclerosis are usually transitory.

30. The use of adrenocorticotrophic hormone (ACTH) and corticosteroids has shown favorable results in the treatment of multiple sclerosis.

31. Drug-induced parkinsonian syndromes occur with drugs that interfere with the synthesis or storage of dopamine or interfere with the striatal dopamine receptors.

32. Death usually occurs within 5 years from the diagnosis of amyotrophic lateral sclerosis (ALS) because of respiratory problems or bulbar paralysis.

33. Alzheimer's disease is a degenerative disorder, usually of older adults, that affects the cells of the brain and causes impairment of intellectual functioning.

34. Neurofibromatosis is a genetic disorder transmitted as an autosomal dominant trait that causes numerous fibromas of the spinal or cranial nerves and skin, café au lait spots on the skin, and developmental disorders of bone, muscle, and viscera.

35. Cerebrovascular accident (CVA) is the most common disease of the nervous system and can be caused by thrombus, embolus, or hemorrhage.

36. The incidence of bacterial meningitis is higher in fall and winter, when upper respiratory infections are common.

37. More than half of the persons affected with Guillain-Barré syndrome have had a nonspecific infection 10 to 14 days before the onset of the disease.

38. Repiratory isolation is necessary for the patient with herpes zoster until drainage from the lesions stops.

39. Approximately 40% of AIDS patients have neurologic symptoms that result from infection from HIV itself or from associated infections.

40. General effects of moderate to severe head injury include cerebral edema, sensory and motor deficits, and increased intracranial pressure (ICP).

41. Injuries to the brain result from direct or indirect trauma to the head.

42. Direct trauma to the head causes acceleration-deceleration injuries.

43. Contusion or laceration directly below the site of the cranial impact is called a coup lesion, whereas one opposite the impact site is called a contrecoup injury.

44. Subdural hematomas can occur from hours to months after the initial head injury.

45. Many patients with head injury may recover physically, but they will have behavioral and psychologic problems that make it difficult for them to function completely independently.

46. The amount of disability that results from spinal cord injury is dependent on the level of injury.

47. Autonomic dysreflexia is a complication of spinal cord injury that occurs as a result of abnormal cardiovascular response to stimulation of the sympathetic division of the autonomic nervous system and is considered a medical emergency.

48. The symptoms of intracranial tumors result from both local and general effects of the tumor.

49. A surgical opening through the skull is called a craniotomy, the removal of part of the skull without replacement is called a craniectomy, and the repair of a cranial defect through the use of substitute bone material is called cranioplasty.

50. Increased intracranial pressure (ICP) is one of the most common complications of intracranial surgery.
51. Hydrocephalus may occur after intracranial surgery; it can be treated with a shunt.
52. The pathologic conditions that result from spinal cord tumors are caused by spinal cord destruction and infiltrates, displacement and compression of the cord, and disruption of the blood supply or CSF circulation.

REFERENCES AND SUGGESTED READINGS
Contemporary

1. *Ake, J, and Perlstein, L: AIDS: impact on neuroscience nursing practice, J Neuroscience Nurs 19:300-304, 1987.
2. *Anderson, M: Assessment under pressure: when your patient says "my head hurts," Nurs 84 14:34-42, 1984.
3. Arnason, B: Multiple sclerosis: current concepts and management, Hosp Pract 82:81-89, 1982.
4. Arsenault, L: Selected postoperative complications of cranial surgery, J Neurosurg Nurs 17:155-163, 1985.
5. *Beckham, M, and Rudy, R: Acquired immunodeficiency syndrome: impact and implications for the neurological system, J Neuroscience Nurs 18:5-10, 1986.
6. *Blanco, K, and Cuomo, N: From the other side of the bedrail: a personal experience with Guillain-Barre syndrome, J Neurosurg Nurs 15:355-359, 1983.
7. *Boss, B: Dysphasia, dyspraxia, and dysarthria: distinguishing features, Part I, J Neurosurg Nurs 16:151-160, 1984.
8. *Boss, B: Dysphasia, dyspraxia, and dysarthria: distinguishing features, Part II, J Neurosurg Nurs 16:211-216, 1984.
8a. Boss, B: Memory impairment: forgetfulness vs. amnesia, J Neurosci Nurs 20:151-158, 1988.
9. Chase, M, and Whelan-Decker, E: Nursing management of a patient with a subarachnoid hemorrhage, J Neurosurg Nurs 16:23-39, 1984.
10. Connolly, R, and others: Update: head injury, J Neurosurg Nurs 13:195-201, 1981.
11. Conway-Rutkowski, B: Carini and Owen's neurological and neurosurgical nursing, ed 8, St. Louis, 1982, The CV Mosby Co.
12. Daly, B: Intensive care nursing, ed 2, Garden City, NY, 1985, Medical Exam Publishing Co.
12a. Delgado, J, and Byllo, J: Care of the patient with Parkinson's disease—surgical and nursing interventions, J Neurosci Nurs 20:142-150, 1988.
13. Devenport-Fortune, P, and Dunnum, L: Professional nursing care of the patient with increased intracranial pressure: planned or "hit or miss," J Neurosurg Nurs 17:367-370, 1985.
13a. Doolitle, N: Stroke recovery—review of the literature and suggestions for future research, J Neurosci Nurs 20:169-173, 1988.
14. *Elliott, J, and Smith, D: Meeting family needs following severe head injury: a multidisciplinary approach, J Neurosurg 17:111-113, 1985.
15. *Findley, L: Altered consciousness, Nursing 84 2:663-664, 666, 1984.

15a. Fode, N: Subarachnoid hemorrhage for ruptured intracranial aneurysm, Am J Nurs 88:673-680, 1988.
15b. Friedman, D: Taking the scare out of caring for seizure patients, Nurs 88 18(2):52-60, 1988.
16. Garrett, E: Parkinsonionism: forgotten considerations in medical treatment and nursing care, J Neurosurg Nurs 14:13-18, 1982.
17. Haberman, B: Cognitive dysfunction and social rehabilitation in severly head-injured patients, J Neurosurg Nurs 14:220-224, 1982.
18. *Hart, G: Strokes causing left versus right hemiplegia: different effects and nursing implications, Geriatric Nurs 4:39-43, 1983.
19. *Hendrickson, S: Psychological care of the patient with neurological dysfunction, J Neurosurg Nurs 16:202-207, 1984.
20. Hollans, N, and others: Overview of multiple sclerosis and nursing care of the multiple sclerosis patient, J Neurosurg Nurs 14:28-33, 1982.
21. Horvath, M: Myasthenia gravis: a nursing approach, J Neurosurg Nurs 14:7-12, 1982.
22. *Howard, M, and others: Psychological after effects of halo traction and a review of acute care, Am J Nurs 2:1839-1843, 1982.
23. *Johnson, L: If your patient has increased intracranial pressure: your goal should be no surprises, Nurs 83 15:58-64, 1983.
23a. Johnston, K, and Olson, E: Application of Bobath principles for nursing care of the hemiplegic patient, Rehab Nurs 9(2):18-25, 1980.
24. Kirk, E, and Bradford, L: Effects of alcohol on the CNS: implications for the neuroscience nurse, J Neuroscience Nurs 19:326-335, 1987.
25. Kirkland, J, and others: Trigeminal neuralgia: approach to nursing care, J Neurosurg Nurg 15:149-153, 1983.
26. Konikow, N: Alterations in movement: nursing assessment and implications, J Neurosurg Nurs 17:61-65, 1985.
27. *March, K: Look into my eyes: assessing the neurologic patient, J Neurosurg Nurs 15:213-221, 1983.
28. Martin, N, and others: Comprehensive rehabilitation nursing, New York, 1981, McGraw-Hill Book Co.
29. Mauss-Clum, N: Bringing the unconscious patient back safely makes the critical difference, J Neurosurg Nurs 14:32-43, 1982.
29a. Mauser, G: Neuromuscular respiratory failure—what the nurse knows makes a difference, J Neuroscience Nurs 20:110-117, 1988.
29b. McBride, EV, and DiStefano, K: Explaining diagnostic tests for MS, Nurs 88 18(2):68-72, 1988.
30. McClelland, P: Behavioral problems after closed head injury, Top Emerg Med 4:42-50, 1983.
31. Mitchell, P, and others: Moving the patient in bed: effects of increased intracranial pressure, Nurs Res 30:212-218, 1981.
32. Mitchell, S, and Yates, R: Extracranial-intracranial bypass surgery, J Neurosurg Nurs 17:288-292, 1985.
33. Monson, R: Autonomic dysreflexia: a nursing challenge, Rehabil Nurs 6:18-19, 1981.
34. Nemeroff, D: Transphenoidal hypophysectomy, J Neurosurg Nurs 13:303-312, 1981.

*References preceded by an asterisk are particularly well suited for student reading.

35. Nicholson, C: Cranial bypass: a case study, J Neurosurg Nurs 15:165-168, 1983.
36. *Norman, E, and others: Seizure disorders, Am J Nurs 81:983-1000, 1981.
37. *Norman, S: The pupil check, Am J Nurs 82:588-591, 1982.
38. Perlstein, L, and Ake, J: AIDS: an overview for the neuroscience nurse, J Neuroscience Nurs 19:296-299, 1987.
39. Price, M, and DeVroom, H: A quick and easy guide to neurological assessment, J Neurosurg Nurs 17:313-320, 1985.
40. *Reinisch, E: Quick assessment for hemiplegic's functioning, Amer J Nurs 81:102-104, 1981.
41. Rhodes, M, and others: Complications of posterior fossa craniotomy, J Neurosurg Nurs 15:19-21, 1983.
42. Rudy, E: Advanced neurological and neurosurgical nursing, St. Louis, 1985, The CV Mosby Co.
43. Rudy, E: Magnetic resonance imagery: new horizons in diagnostic testing, J Neurosurg Nurs 17:331-337, 1985.
43a. Santilli, N, and Sierzant, T: Advances in the treatment of epilepsy, J Neuroscience Nurs 19:144-157, 1987.
43b. Schaefer, S: Relieving pain—an analgesic guide, Am J Nurs 88:815-827, 1988.
44. Shpritz, D: Craniocerebral trauma, Crit Care Nurs 3:49, 52, 55-56, 1983.
45. *Smith, S: Continuous intracranial monitoring: implications and applications for critical care, Crit Care Nurs 3:42-51, 1983.
46. Spielman, G: Metabolic complications associated with severe diffuse brain injury, J Neurosurg Nurs 17:83-88, 1985.
47. Stevens, M: Post concussive syndrome, J Neurosurg Nurs 14:239-244, 1982.
47a. Stone, N: Amyotrophic lateral scleroses: a challenge for constant adaptation, J Neuroscience Nurs 19:166-173, 1987.
48. Thompson, J (editor): Clinical nursing, St. Louis, 1986, The CV Mosby Co.
49. Wahlquist, G: A great nursing challenge: recovery and effective management of the patient with herpes simplex encephalitis, J Neurosurg Nurs 13:220-225, 1982.
50. *Walleck, C: A neurologic assessment procedure that won't make you nervous, Nurs 82 12:50-57, 1982.
51. Warren, J, and Peck, E: Factors which influence neuropsychological recovery from severe head injury, J Neurosurg Nurs 16:248-252, 1984.
51a. Whitney, F: Relationship of laterality of stroke and emotional and functional outcome, J Neuroscience Nurs 19:158-165, 1987.
52. *Woods, N: Human sexuality in health and illness, ed 3, St. Louis, 1984, The CV Mosby Co.
53. Woodward, E: The total patient: implications for nursing care of the epileptic, J Neurosurg Nurs 14:166-169.
54. *Young, M: A bedside guide to understanding the signs of increased intracranial pressure, Nurs 81 11:59-62, 1981.

Classic

55. *Bartel, M: Dialogue wih dementia: nonverbal communication in patients with Alzheimer's disease, J Gerontol Nurs 5:21-31, 1979.
56. Blount, M, and others: Management of the patient with amyotrophic lateral sclerosis, Nurs Clin North Am 14:157-171, 1979.
57. Brunnstrom, S: Movement therapy in hemiplegia, New York, 1970, Harper & Row, Publisher.
58. *Burnside, J: Alzheimer's disease: an overview, J Gerontol Nurs 5:14-20, 1979.
59. *Carlson, C: Psychological aspects of neurologic disability, Nurs Clin North Am 15:309-320, 1980.
60. *Donahue, R: Symposium on care of the patient with neuromuscular disease, Nurs Clin North Am 14:95-106, 1979.
61. Doolittle, N: Arteriovenous malformation: the physiology, symptomatology, and nursing care, J Neurosurg Nurs 11:222-226, 1979.
62. Felder, L: Neurogenic bladder dysfunction, J Neurosurg Nurs 11:91-104, 1979.
63. *Mitchell, P, and Maus, N: Intracranial pressure: fact and fancy, Nurs 76 6(6):53-57, 1976.
64. Jones, S: Glasgow coma scale, Am J Nurs 79:1551-154, 1979.
65. *King, R, and others: Symposium on rehabilitative nursing: rehabilitation of the patient with spinal cord injury, Nurs Clin North Am 15:225-243, 1980.
66. *Kolb, D: Understanding aphasia and the aphasic, J Neurosurg Nurs 9:15-18, 1977.
67. Levitt, R: Understanding sexuality and spinal cord njury, J Neurosurg Nurs 12:88-89, 1980.
68. Mitchell, P: Intracranial hypertension: implication of research for nursing care, J Neurosurg Nurs 12:145-154, 1980.
69. Mitchell, P, and Irvin, N: Neurological examination: nursing assessment for nursing purposes, J Neurosurg Nurs 9:23-38, 1977.
70. Mitchell, P, and Maus, P: Relating of patient's nursing activities to increased pressure variations: a pilot study, Nurs Res 27:4-10, 1978.
71. *Olsen, E, and others: The hazards of immobility, Am J Nurs 67:779-797, 1967.
72. Patient assessment: neurological assessment I, Am J Nurs 75:1511-1535, 1975.
73. Patient assessment: neurological assessment II, Am J Nurs 75:2037-2057, 1975.
74. Patient assessment: neurological assessment III, Am J Nurs 76:609-633, 1976.
75. Plank, N: Multiple sclerosis: an update and review, J Neurosurg Nurs 11:44-47, 1979.
76. Polhopek, M: Stroke: an update on vascular disease, J Neurosurg Nurs 12:81-87, 1980.
77. Ross, AJ, and others: Neuromuscular diagnostic procedures, Nurs Clin North Am 14:107-121, 1979.
78. Samond, R: Guillain-Barre syndrome: helping the patient in the acute stage, Nurs 80 10:34-41, 1980.
79. Taylor, J, and Bellinger, S: Neurological dysfunction and nursing interventions, New York, 1980, McGraw-Hill Book Co.
80. Terzian, M: Neurosurgical intervention for the management of chronic intractable pain, Top Clin Nurs 1:75-88, 1980.
81. Webb, P: Neurological deficit after carotid endarderectomies, Am J Nurs 79:654-658, 1979.
82. Wheeler, P: Care of the patient with a cerebellar tumor, Am J Nurs 77:263-266, 1977.
83. Wing, S: Cervical spine injuries: treatment and related nursing care, J Neurosurg Nurs 9:138-140, 1977.

20

The Patient with Eye Problems

BARBARA C. LONG

CHAPTER OBJECTIVES

After studying this chapter, the student should be able to:

- Describe measurement and alterations in visual acuity and types of corrective lenses.
- Identify eye safety measures.
- Identify nursing interventions for the newly blind person.
- Describe major eye inflammations and appropriate nursing interventions.
- Explain the nature of cataracts, glaucoma, and retinal detachment and appropriate interventions.
- Describe the care of the person having eye surgery.

■ ANATOMY AND PHYSIOLOGY

■ Accessory eye structures

The eye is protected from dirt and foreign bodies by the eyebrow, eyelashes, and eyelids. The *conjunctiva* is a thin membrane that lines the eyelids (palpebral conjunctiva) and most of the anterior portion of the eye (bulbar conjunctiva) except for the pupil. The palpebral conjunctiva folds back on itself where it joins the bulbar conjunctiva, forming a saclike recess (conjunctival sac). Although the conjunctiva is transparent, the palpebral portion appears pink, reflecting the underlying blood vessels. Small blood vessels may be noted in the bulbar conjunctiva over the sclera of the eye. The conjunctiva protects the eye and prevents it from drying. Inflammation of the conjunctiva (conjunctivitis, p. 528) gives a reddened appearance to the eye.

The *lacrimal gland* is located above and lateral to the eyeball (Fig. 20-1). Lacrimal fluid (tears) is secreted by the lacrimal gland. The tears provide moisture to lubricate the cornea; excessive secretion drains into the lacrimal sac, on the nasal side of the eye, and through the nasolacrimal ducts into the nose. Eye medications that are dropped into the inner canthus rather than the conjunctival sac drain out into the nose and thus lose their effectiveness on the eye (p. 530).

■ Eyeball

■ LAYERS OF THE EYE

The eyeball is composed of three coats or layers of tissue: the sclera, the choroid, and the retina (Fig. 20-2). The tough outer coat, or *sclera,* is opaque (white) but becomes transparent anteriorly over the iris and pupil to form the *cornea.* The middle layer, the *choroid,* contains blood vessels and is modified anteriorly into the ciliary body, which is attached to the suspensory ligament and to the iris. The inner coat, the *retina,* which does not have an anterior portion, contains the photoreceptors (rods and cones). These photoreceptors synapse in the retina with bipolar neurons and then with ganglion neurons, and these become the fibers of the optic nerve. The cones, which are less numerous than the rods, are found mostly near the center of the retina and are considered to be the receptors for bright daylight and color vision. The rods, found mostly in the periphery of the retina, are receptors for dim or night vision. Rods contain rhodopsin, a photosensitive protein that becomes rapidly depleted in bright light. The slow regeneration of rhodopsin, which is dependent on the presence of vitamin A, explains the time needed for the eyes to adjust from bright to dim light. Vitamin A deficiency affects night vision.

■ CHAMBERS OF THE EYE

The interior of the eyeball is divided into two cavities, the anterior and the posterior. The *anterior cavity,* in front of the lens, is further subdivided into two *chambers,* an anterior chamber (between the cornea and the iris) and a posterior chamber (between the iris and the lens). The anterior cavity is filled with a clear liquid, the aqueous humor, which is produced in the ciliary body, drains into the posterior chamber, passes through the pupil into the anterior chamber, and drains out the canal of Schlemm at the junction of the iris and cornea (anterior chamber angle). Obstruction of this drainage leads to glaucoma (p. 536) The *posterior cavity* of the eye is filled with a clear gelatinous substance, the vitreous humor, which helps maintain eye body. If vitreous humor is removed, the eye collapses.

■ IRIS AND LENS

The iris is a colored, ring-shaped membrane containing involuntary dilator and sphincter muscles that control pupillary size. The pupil is the space in the center of the iris. The size of the pupil varies in response to light intensity and to focusing from far to near objects (accommodation) to enhance visual acuity; the pupil constricts with bright lights or for near vision. The pupil also responds to autonomic nervous stimulation; pupils dilate with stress to permit more light to enter to see better during the "fight or flight" response.

The lens of the eye is a crystalline, transparent biconvex structure behind the iris, separating the anterior and posterior chambers. The lens is composed of epithelial cells and is covered by an elastic membrane (capsule). It is held in place by fibers from the ciliary body. Because of its elasticity, the lens can change shape, becoming more or less convex. The more convex the lens, the greater the refraction (see below). If the lens becomes cloudy and opaque, it is called a *cataract* (p. 533).

■ MUSCLES OF THE EYE

Eye muscles are of two types, extrinsic and intrinsic. The extrinsic voluntary muscles outside the eyeball control extraocular movement. The intrinsic involuntary muscles within the eye are the ciliary body, which controls the shape of the lens, and the iris, which controls pupil size.

■ Physiology of vision

Light rays entering the eye bend (*refraction*) as they pass over the curved surfaces of the cornea and through various structures of the eye (cornea, aqueous humor, lens, vitreous humor), which have different densities, to focus on the retina. When light rays do not focus on the retina, it is called a refractive error.

The eyes adjust (*accommodation*) so as to see objects at various distances by flattening or thickening of the lens. Near vision requires contraction of the ciliary body, which decreases the distance between the edges of the ciliary body, thus relaxing the suspensory ligament attached to the lens. The lens then bulges to bend the light ray more acutely so that the rays focus on the retina. Continual close vision may produce eye strain through constant con-

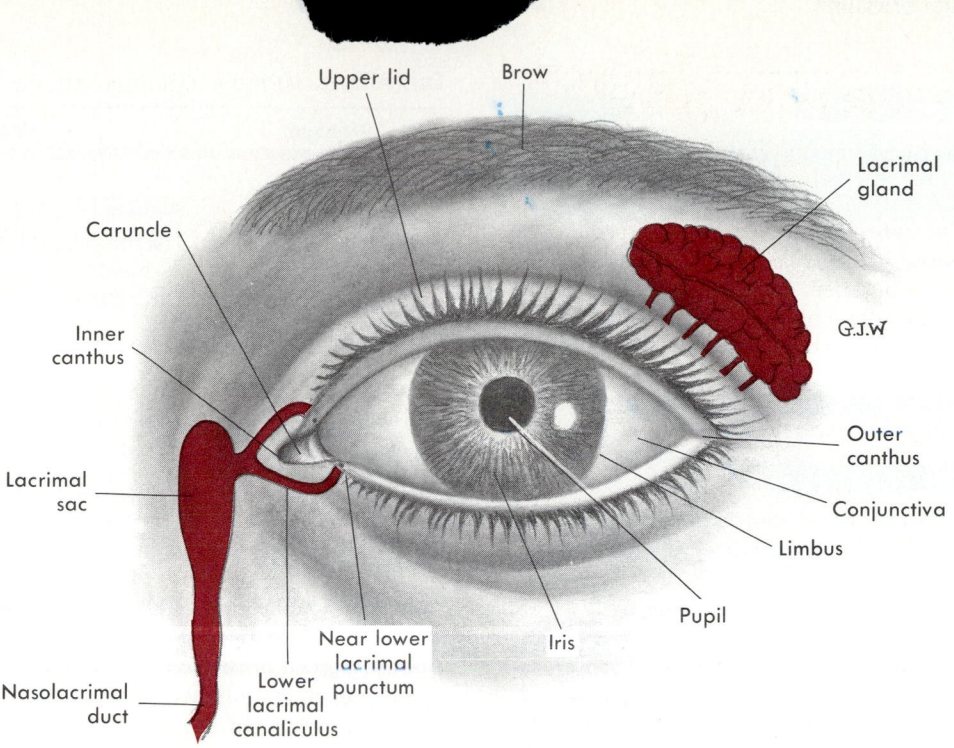

Upper lid

Brow

Lacrimal gland

Caruncle

Inner canthus

G.J.W

Outer canthus

Lacrimal sac

Conjunctiva

Limbus

Pupil

Nasolacrimal duct

Lower lacrimal canaliculus

Near lower lacrimal punctum

Iris

Fig. 20-1 External eye structures. (From Thompson, JM, and others: Clinical nursing, St. Louis, 1986, The CV Mosby Co.)

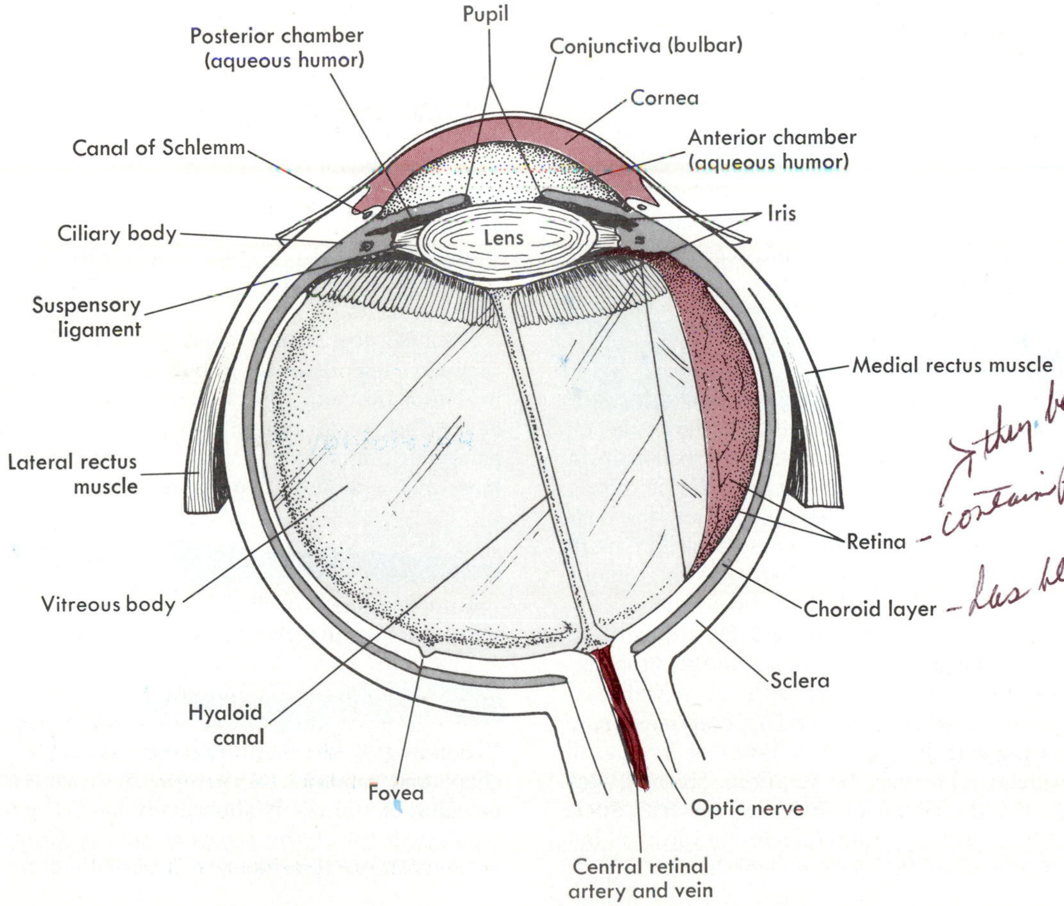

Posterior chamber (aqueous humor)

Pupil

Conjunctiva (bulbar)

Cornea

Canal of Schlemm

Anterior chamber (aqueous humor)

Ciliary body

Iris

Suspensory ligament

Lens

Medial rectus muscle

Lateral rectus muscle

Retina

Vitreous body

Choroid layer

Sclera

Hyaloid canal

Fovea

Optic nerve

Central retinal artery and vein

they become fibers of optic nerve

– contain photoreceptors (rods & cones)

– has bld. vessels

receptors color for dim & nyte vision

bright daylight

↓

Rhodopsin needs Vit A

Fig. 20-2 Horizontal section through left eyeball.

traction of the ciliary muscle; this can be relieved by frequent shifting of the eyes to distant objects. Accommodation is also facilitated by changing the size of the pupil. With near vision the iris constricts the pupil to force light rays to pass through the shortened but thicker lens.

Light rays are absorbed by the photoreceptors on the retina and are changed to electrical activity to transmit the image to the cortex. The fibers of the optic nerve (cranial nerve II) divide at the optic chiasm, the medial portion of each nerve crosses to the opposite side, and the impulses are then transmitted to the visual cortex (see Fig. 20-5). Bilateral vision provides depth perception.

■ Intraocular pressure

Intraocular pressure (IOP) is maintained by the balance between the production and drainage of aqueous humor. Drainage can be impeded by blockage of the trabecular meshwork (which filters the aqueous humor as it enters the canal of Schlemm) or by increasing pressure in the episcleral veins into which the canal of Schlemm empties.[25] Some aqueous humor may also drain into ciliary muscle spaces, then into the suprachoroidal space. The trabecular meshwork and entrance to the canal of Schlemm can be blocked by the iris. The Valsalva maneuver, which increases venous pressure, increases the pressure in the episcleral veins, permitting less aqueous humor to drain out and thus increasing IOP.

The normal range of IOP is 10 to 21 mm Hg, with a mean value of 16mm Hg. The pressure may vary up to 5 mm Hg as a result of diurnal changes. Temporary increases in IOP may occur with emotional stress.

■ Physiologic changes with aging

Visual acuity declines rapidly, often by the middle 40s or early 50s. By age 70 most persons use visual aids. Structural changes occur in the retina, pupil, lens and cornea; the retina loses cells, the pupils decrease in size, the lens becomes less elastic and may become more opaque, and the cornea flattens (Table 20-1). Farsightedness results from the decreased elasticity of the lens (presbyopia). Astigmatism may occur from the irregular curvature of the flattened cornea. The smaller pupil permits less light to reach the retina and, in addition to a decrease in rhodopsin in the rods, night vision is decreased. Older people, therefore, require more light for seeing objects, especially for near vision, than do younger persons. The lens also yellows with age, leading to increased difficulty distinguishing among colors, especially at the blue end of the spectrum.

Peripheral vision decreases with age. It is uncertain, however, which of the above factors leads to this problem.

Secretions of the eye also decrease with age. Fewer tears are produced and those that do tend to evaporate more quickly, producing a feeling of scratchiness or dryness of the eyes. Artificial tears may be required. Tearing may occur, despite the decreased quantity, if the tear ducts become blocked. Aqueous production is diminished, but because the anterior chamber becomes smaller, a relatively

Table 20-1 Physiologic eye changes with aging

Problem	Etiology
Farsightedness	
Astigmatism	Flattened cornea
Decreased vision, especially at night	Decreased pupil size, decreased rhodopsin
Decreased peripheral vision	Cause unknown
Difficulty distinguishing colors	Yellowed lens
Dryness and scratchiness of eyes	Decreased tear production
Corneal gray ring	Corneal fat deposits

stable intraocular pressure is maintained.[17] Older persons, however, have an increased chance of developing glaucoma from increased pressure in the anterior chamber (p. 536).

A common eye change noted in older persons is a hazy gray ring around the periphery of the cornea resulting from fat deposits.

■ PREVENTION AND HEALTH EDUCATION

Vision is one of the most important senses. It orients us to the world around us. It provides pleasure through beautiful sights. It provides data to promote safety and effective interaction with others. Vision also contributes to our self-concept and feeling of personal worth and well-being. People should therefore be encouraged to have their eyes tested for any problems encountered with visual acuity when young, about every 5 years as a young adult, and every 2 years after age 40. The box on p. 519 differentiates among eye specialists.

Because nurses have contacts with persons of all ages, they have opportunities to become involved in many activities that promote good vision and help to prevent injury or further impairment. This is accomplished by participation in promotion of visual acuity, promotion of safety measures, and detection of possible eye disorders.

■ Promotion of visual acuity

Interference with visual acuity may result from refractive errors or disturbances in visual fields.

■ REFRACTIVE ERRORS

Bending of the light ray (refraction) depends on the shape and condition of the eye. If the anteroposterior dimension of the eye is abnormally long, the light rays will focus in front of the retina (myopia). Conversely, if the anteroposterior dimension is abnormally short, the rays will

Persons who specialize in eye problems or corrective lenses	
Ophthalmologist	Physician who specializes in diagnosis and treatment of eye diseases; may also prescribe lenses
Oculist	Same as ophthalmologist
Optometrist	Professional with special preparation in assessment of vision and in treatment of visual problems (e.g., prescribes lenses, visual training, or orthoptic exercises); is not a physician and does not treat eye diseases
Optician	Person who grinds and fits lenses according to prescriptions written by ophthalmologist or optometrist

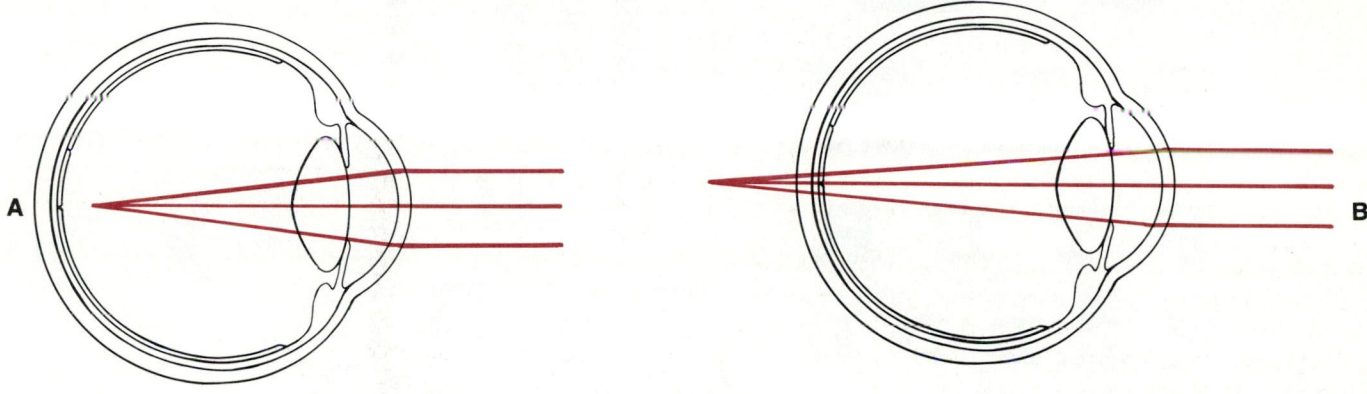

Fig. 20-3   **A,** Myopia (nearsightedness); image is focused in front of retina. **B,** Hyperopia (farsightedness); image is focused behind retina.

focus behind the retina (hyperopia) (Fig. 20-3). As noted earlier, decreased elasticity of the lens occurring with age (presbyopia) also produces hyperopia. The curvature of the cornea may also be asymmetric or irregular so that rays in the horizontal and vertical planes do not focus at the same point (astigmatism). Refractive errors account for the largest number of impairments of good vision.

MEASUREMENT OF VISUAL ACUITY

Distance vision is usually determined by use of a *Snellen chart* (Fig. 20-4). The person sits or stands 20 feet from the chart, covers one eye with a piece of stiff paper or a plastic occluder, and reads the line as specified by the examiner. The eyes are tested with and without distance lenses.

Visual acuity is expressed as a fraction; a reading of 20/20 is considered normal. The upper figure refers to the distance at which the person can read the chart, and the lower figure indicates the distance at which a normal eye can read the line. For example, if an individual is able to read at 20 ft only the line that should be readable at 70 ft, he or she has 20/70 vision in the eye tested.

Near vision is tested by reading small print, such as newsprint, held 35 cm (14 in) from the eye. Any person with vision less than 20/30 in either eye is referred to an ophthalmologist or optometrist for further testing.

Some terms related to acuity are defined in the box on p. 520.

VISUAL FIELDS

The visual field is that portion of the environment that the eye can perceive. The field of vision thus includes peripheral vision or indirect vision. Normality depends on intactness of all parts of the visual pathways of the eye. Lesions of the retina, optic pathways, and central nervous system affect sections of the field of vision. Damage to the optic disk (retina) or to the optic nerve anterior to the optic chiasm, as seen with glaucoma, affects only the field of the *involved* eye (Fig. 20-5, *B1*). Lesions at the chiasm or posterior to it produce bilateral visual field defects of a wide variety. For example, a pituitary gland tumor compressing the optic chiasm damages the crossing fibers from the nasal retina and classically causes bitemporal hemianopsia, or the loss of vision in the temporal halves of each eye (Fig. 20-5, *B2*). Loss of vision in the corresponding halves of both visual fields produces homonymous hemianopsia (Fig. 20-5, *B3*) and can be further designated as right or left. For example, patients with *right* cerebrovas-

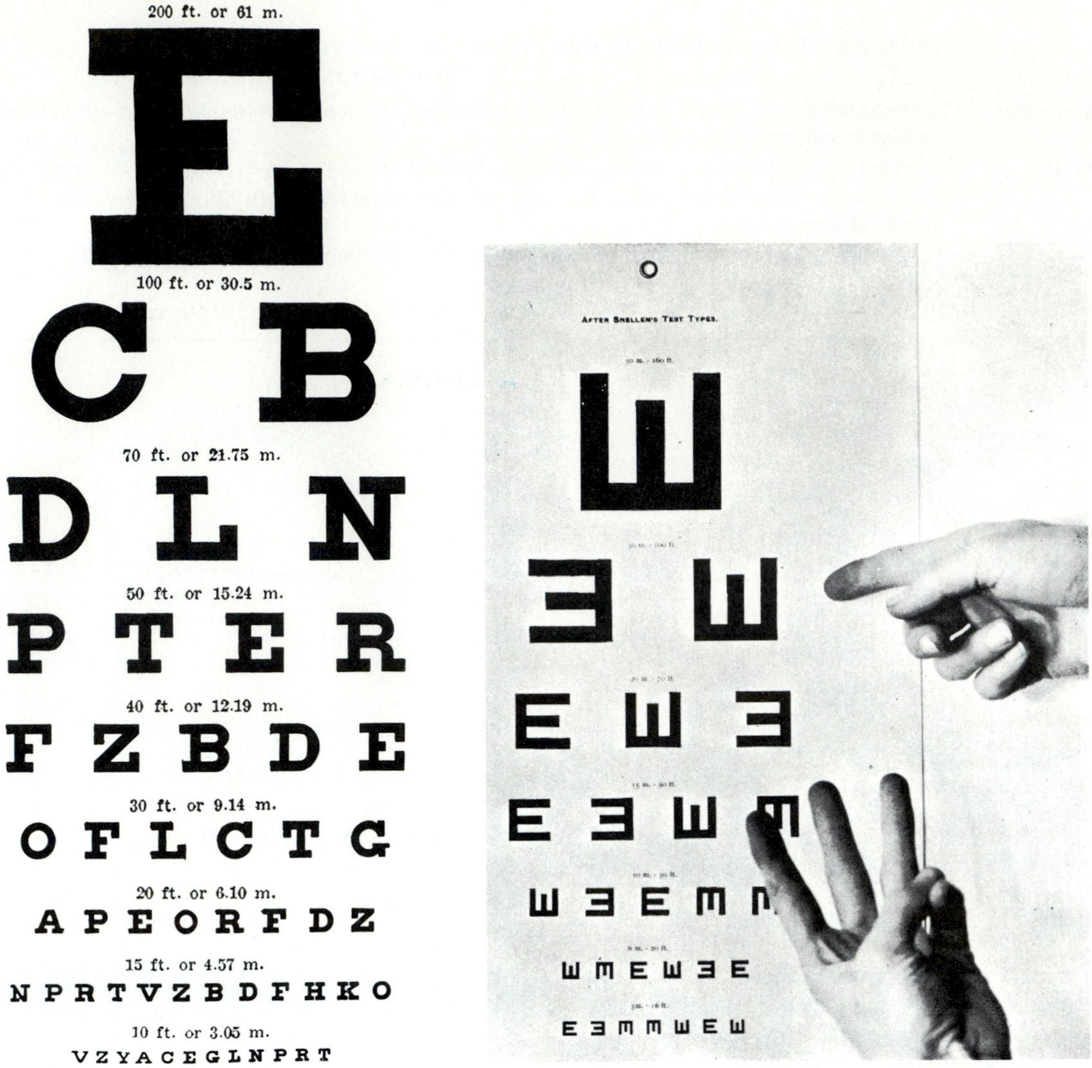
200 ft. or 61 m.
E
100 ft. or 30.5 m.
C B
70 ft. or 21.75 m.
D L N
50 ft. or 15.24 m.
P T E R
40 ft. or 12.19 m.
F Z B D E
30 ft. or 9.14 m.
O F L C T G
20 ft. or 6.10 m.
A P E O R F D Z
15 ft. or 4.57 m.
N P R T V Z B D F H K O
10 ft. or 3.05 m.
V Z Y A C E G L N P R T
AFTER SNELLEN'S TEST TYPES.

A B

Fig. 20-4 **A,** Snellen chart used in testing vision. **B,** Modified Snellen chart, called "E" game, for testing vision of small children and persons unfamiliar with English alphabet.

Terms describing visual acuity

Accommodation	Ability to adjust for far and near objects
Emmetropia	Normal eyesight; light rays focus on retina
Ametropia	Refractive error; light rays do not focus on retina
Myopia	Nearsightedness; light rays focus in front of retina (Fig. 20-3)
Hyperopia	Farsightedness; light rays focus behind retina
Presbyopia	Hyperopia from loss of lens elasticity because of age
Astigmatism	Irregular curvature of cornea; light rays do not focus at same point

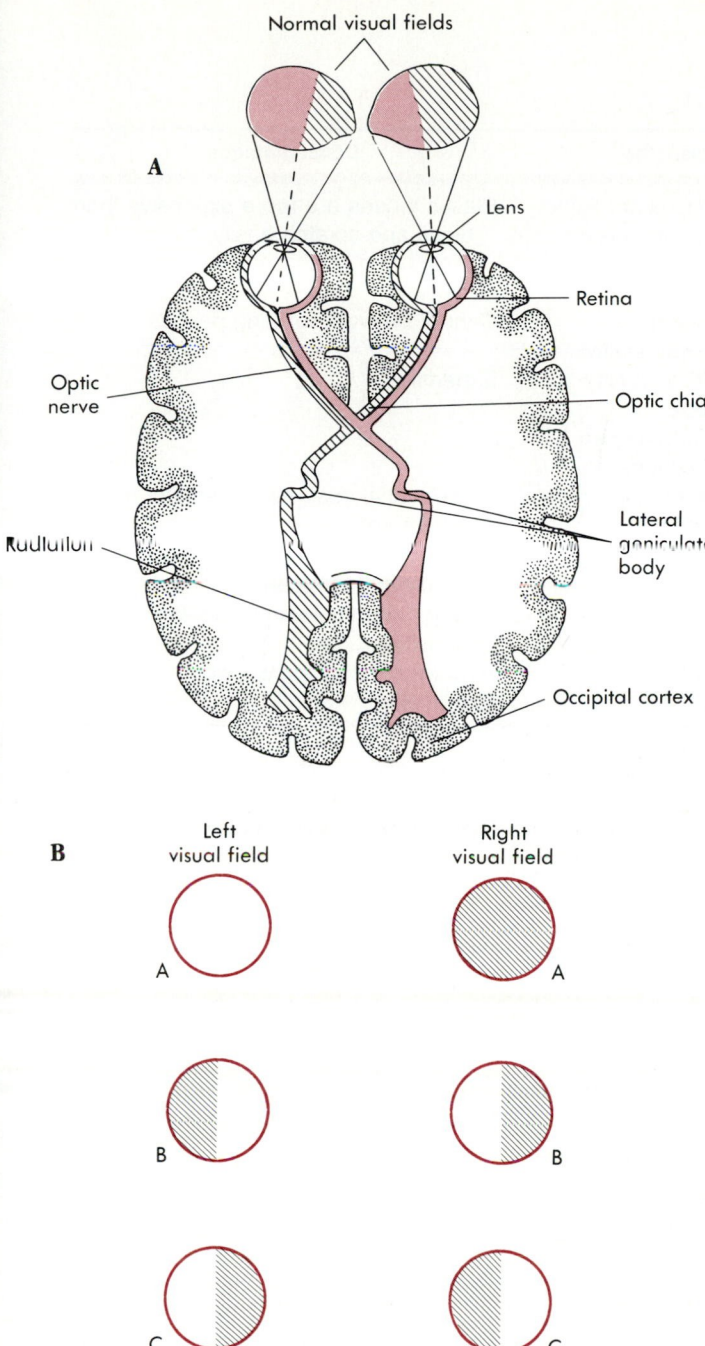

Fig. 20-5 **A,** Visual pathways showing partial decussation at optic chiasm. Normal visual fields show reversal of light rays from the temporal and nasal sides to receptors in the retina. **B,** Abnormal visual fields. *1,* Normal left field of vision with loss of vision in right field as a result of complete lesion of right optic nerve. *2,* Loss of vision in temporal half of both fields as a result of lesion of optic chiasm. This is called bitemporal hemianopsia. *3,* Loss of vision in nasal field of right eye and temporal field of left eye caused by lesion of the right optic tract. This is called homonymous hemianopsia.

cular accidents often experience hemianopsia with *left* field loss.

☐ Measurement of visual fields

Visual fields can be tested by various means. One method (confrontation test) is to ask the person to cover one eye and focus on a point directly ahead. An object, such as a pencil, is placed peripherally beyond the person's vision, then advanced centrally until the person first indicates that the object is seen. Normally, the person should see about 60 degrees nasally, 90 degrees temporally, 50 degrees superiorly, and 70 degrees inferiorly.

■ TYPES OF LENSES

Lenses may be worn as glasses or contact lenses (Table 20-2). Glasses may have one focus (for near or far vision), *bifocal* (upper part for distance, lower part for near vision) or *trifocal* (for distance, intermediate, and near vision).

Contact lenses are usually chosen for cosmetic reasons or for sports activities because they do not fog or break easily. Persons who have lenses removed because of cataracts (but without lens implants) achieve better vision with contact lenses than with glasses. Some industrial occupations prohibit use of contact lenses because of irritation of the cornea by dirt or dust trapped under the lens.

Contact lenses are small corrective lenses made of different types of ground plastic worn over the cornea of the eye or between the cornea and sclera (scleral lens). The lenses may be of various types: rigid, gas permeable (rigid), soft, or extended wear (soft) (Table 20-2). The rigid lenses are commonly used because they are cheaper and easier to maintain; they cannot be worn for long periods (usually not over 12 to 24 hours).

The disadvantages of soft-type lenses may include a higher initial cost and more frequent replacement. They are also more difficult to clean and maintain. Extended wear soft contact lenses have increased in use in the United States. Although some of these lenses can be left in place for as long as a month, the current trend is to limit wear to 1 week before removal for cleaning and disinfection. Persons who use extended wear lenses must be educated and prepared for the extra care required for these lenses. Scleral lenses are more difficult to wear than corneal lenses and are less frequently prescribed.

Newer contact lenses with the optical qualities of the rigid lenses and the comfort of the soft are now becoming available. Because of their special properties, along with specially developed contact lens solutions, some of the complications associated with both the rigid and soft lenses can be avoided.

Contact lenses are inserted after being cleaned thoroughly and immersed in a wetting agent such as methylcellulose. Conjunctival secretions provide the lubrication needed for the lenses to be worn in comfort. The lenses are held in place by capillary attraction and by the upper lid. If the person is injured or unconscious, the nurse removes the contact lenses (see the box on p. 522). Lenses are stored separately in special containers, labeled left or

Table 20-2 Types of corrective lenses

Lens	Characteristics	Benefits	Disadvantages
Glasses	Impact-resistant material (plastic or glass)	Plastic lenses are lighter in weight than glass	Plastic lenses are more expensive than glass and scratch easily
Contact lenses			
Rigid	Hydrophobic, rigid plastic Usually tinted Covers only the cornea	Least expensive Easy to clean Good optical quality	Easily lost Cannot be worn for long periods
Gas permeable	Rigid plastic, permeable to oxygen and other gases Covers only cornea	Good optical quality Comfortable Can be worn longer than hard lenses	Expensive
Soft	Hydrophyllic, flexible plastic Covers cornea and part of sclera	Can be worn longer (up to 18 hours) Comfortable	Higher initial cost, need frequent replacement Must be kept wet to prevent damage More difficult to clean Absorb atmospheric pollutants
Extended wear	Same as soft lenses but contain more water	Can be worn continuously for several weeks	Expensive Require medical supervision Tear easily

---

Removal of contact lenses

Rigid lens

Method 1
  a. Place finger at outer canthus of eye.
  b. Pull skin obliquely upward, then straight down.
  c. Lens will appear on lower lashes as the upper lid moves downward.
  d. If lens moves off center, reposition it by gentle pressure on lid or lens itself.

Method 2
  a. Place finger or thumb of each hand at base of eyelashes (upper and lower).
  b. Bring eyelids together, trapping the lens (the lens will eject).
  c. If lens moves off center, reposition it by gentle pressure on lid or lens itself.

Method 3
  a. Using eye irrigation set, gently flush eye with sterile normal saline solution.
  b. Retrieve lens in curved basin.

Method 4
  a. Use small suction device shaped like a miniature "plumber's helper."
  b. Place over center of lens and pull lens off gently.

Soft lens

  a. Pull upper lid up with one thumb.
  b. Be sure lens is in place before attempting removal.
  c. Move lens over conjunctiva before grasping it, if possible. If lens does not move freely, put several drops of sterile saline solution in eye, close lid, and wait 1 minute before trying again.
  d. Grasp lens with thumb and forefinger or other hand and pinch the soft lens (it will pop off).

right lens. Soft lenses are kept wet at all times with special solution or sterile saline solution.

Lenses should not be worn longer than the prescribed length of time. Overwearing can cause edema and abrasion of the cornea. All contact lenses can cause problems; most problems are minor and can be handled by changes in routine or lenses. However, problems should not be ignored, since they may lead to or be indicative of more serious difficulties.

Promotion of eye safety

Everyone should know how to protect their eyes from injury (see the box below). Many people keep unused eye medications and then use them for self-treatment at a later date. This is hazardous because it not only may lead to eye injury but may delay necessary treatment. Ophthalmic drugs may deteriorate, become more concentrated from evaporation of liquid, or become contaminated with bacteria or fungi.

Preventive goggles and break-resistant corrective lenses are available for persons who engage in very active physical activities such as sports and selected occupations. Prompt and appropriate care of an injured eye may prevent serious vision impairment or loss of the eye (Table 20-3).

Secondary prevention

Early detection of eye disease is imperative for protection of vision. Inflammations of the eye are more easily detected than other eye disorders; the person usually complains of discomfort, and redness and discharge are easily observed. Glaucoma is the greatest threat to vision in older persons; the permanent vision loss it causes is preventable if the condition is identified early. Mass screening programs for glaucoma detection have been instituted in many communities, and everyone is urged to participate in these programs. All persons with symptoms suggestive of eye disease (Table 20-4) are urged to seek medical assistance.

Eye safety measures

1. Avoid frequent rinsing of eyes with unprescribed solutions.
2. Discard any ophthalmic solution that is cloudy, discolored, has been open for ≥3 months, or contains particles.
3. Avoid self-treatment of an eye inflammation with a medication prescribed for a previous eye disorder.
4. To avoid eye strain:
   a. Use a good light for reading or doing work that requires careful visual focus.
   b. When reading or focusing eyes for long periods, look at distant objects for a few minutes at repeated intervals to rest eyes.
5. Avoid rubbing eyes.
6. Wash hands before touching eyes.
7. Wear safety glasses when engaging in activities that could injure the eyes.
8. Wear dark glasses for prolonged exposure to very bright light (such as sunlight on snow or water)
9. Flush eyes with copious amount of water when any irritating substances are accidentally introduced.
10. Do not attempt to remove foreign bodies from the cornea; cover eye and seek medical attention.
11. If a speck of dust blows in eye, pull upper lid over lower lid and let the tears wash the speck to the inner canthus or lower lid, where it may be safely removed.

Table 20-3 First aid for eye injuries

Injury	Interventions
Burns: chemical, flame	Flush eye immediately for 15 minutes with cool water or any available nontoxic liquid; seek medical assistance
Loose substance on conjunctiva: dirt, insects	Lift upper lid over lower lid to dislodge substance, produce tearing; irrigate eye with water if necessary; do not rub eye; obtain medical assistance if above interventions fail
Contact injury: contusion, ecchymosis, laceration	Apply cold compresses if no laceration present; cover eye if laceration present; seek medical assistance
Penetrating objects	Do not remove object; place protective shield over eye (e.g., paper cup); cover uninjured eye to prevent excess movement of injured eye; seek medical assistance

Table 20-4 Symptoms suggestive of eye disease

Symptom	Eye disease
Conjunctival redness	Conjunctivitis, blepharitis, sty
Crusting discharge	Conjunctivitis, blepharitis, sty
Ocular pain	Foreign body, sty, acute lid infection, glaucoma, keratitis, uveitis
Foreign body sensation	Foreign body, corneal erosion, blepharitis, chronic conjunctivitis
Blepharospasm	Keratitis, corneal ulcer
Multiple spots ("floaters")	Retinal detachment, intraocular hemorrhage, diabetic retinopathy
Photophobia	Uveitis, keratitis, glaucoma, corneal abrasions
Vision changes	
Blurred vision	Refractive error, cataract, glaucoma, uveitis, retinal detachment
Double vision	Strabismus
Halos around lights	Glaucoma
Blind spots	Hemorrhage, choroiditis
Sudden vision loss	Central retinal artery or vein occlusion

Table 20-5 Eye manifestations of systemic disorders

Disorder	Effect on eye
Diabetes mellitus	Senile cataracts occur earlier and progress more rapidly
	Diabetic retinopathy; retinal changes lead to decreased vision
	Vitreous hemorrhages
	Retinal detachment
Persistent systemic hypertension	Retinal hemorrhage, retinal edema, and retinal exudate lead to loss of sight
Cerebral vascular accident	Loss of sight in one half of visual field (hemianopsia)
	Emboli may occlude retinal vessel
Demyelinating neurologic disorders (e.g., multiple sclerosis)	Nerve damage to eye
Increased intracranial pressure	Papilledema (swelling of optic disc)
Nutritional disorders	
Lack of vitamin A and B	Changes in conjunctiva, cornea, and retina
	Tears reduced
	Eyes and lids become reddened and inflamed
	Night blindness
Excess of vitamin A	Retinal damage

Diseases of other parts of the body may also affect the eye (Table 20-5). Early detection and treatment of these diseases can help to prevent loss of vision.

■ VISUAL IMPAIRMENT: BLINDNESS

Vision is essential to most employment and necessary in countless experiences that make life enjoyable and meaningful. Yet in the United States there are an estimated 1 million legally blind persons. Approximately 1.5 million Americans are so visually handicapped that they cannot read ordinary newsprint even with the aid of corrective lenses. In underdeveloped countries there is a high incidence of blindness from preventable causes such as malnutrition and eye infections. The visually impaired population includes not only those who are legally blind. There are well over a million people who, although unable to see well enough to read a newspaper, have vision better than 20/200. Also, there are over 3 million who are monocularly blind, with a small proportion having a defective but not blind second eye.[24] Most persons in this visually impaired but not legally blind population are between the ages of 25 and 64.

Although there has been a reduction of blindness in the United States from infections and certain diseases and injuries, blindness from diseases that occur most frequently among older persons, including diabetic retinop-

Report of the National Advisory Eye Council, US Department of Health, Education and Welfare, no. (NIH) 75-664, 1975.

Legal criteria of blindness

A person is considered legally blind when either of the following conditions exist:
1. Visual field no greater than 20 degrees
2. Central distance vision in better eye 20/200 or less with use of corrective lenses (eye can see at 20 ft what the normal eye can see at 200 ft)

---

athy, glaucoma, cataract, and retinal degeneration, has increased. It is likely that the incidence of blindness will continue to increase because of the steady growth in the number of persons aged 65 and older.

Impaired vision

Vision impairment ranges from refractive errors correctable with lenses to total blindness, in which the person may not even be able to perceive light. For legal purposes blindness is defined very precisely in order to determine eligibility for assistance of various kinds (see the box above). Although many nonseeing persons now prefer to be called *visually handicapped,* the term blindness is still in common usage.

Responses to loss of vision

IMPACT OF VISUAL LOSS

People who are born blind or develop blindness very early in life and who are raised as children who can see, neither overprotected or rejected, frequently are self-confident persons leading active productive lives.

Loss of vision may affect the self and the ability to interact with others and with the environment. The adult in whom blindness develops fairly rapidly usually has greater difficulty adjusting to the handicap. The impairment may cause a decrease in feelings of self-confidence and in the self-concept. Communication with others is affected, and a sense of isolation may develop. Familiar hobbies that require vision, such as reading, sewing, or crafts, may no longer be possible. Even listening to television creates problems when gaps in sound occur. Mobility or ability to carry out activities of daily living may be restricted or at least modified. Career options, job opportunities, and financial security may be affected. Blindness may influence the person's ability to remain independent, to feel socially adequate, or to feel that he or she is an esteemed contributing member of society.

Limitations in the range and variety of experiences are related to the fact that a person who cannot see must use touch and kinesthetic experience to gain knowledge of the world. Objects too large or too small to handle are not perceivable. Many blind persons feel that the restriction in mobility resulting from blindness is its most serious effect. Blind persons cannot move about as quickly, as securely, or as easily as sighted persons. These individuals need to rely on aids or other persons, particularly in unfamiliar areas.

COPING WITH VISUAL LOSS

After a person has been told that blindness will result, there is a normal reaction described as a period of mourning for the "dead" eyes. Grief and mourning over the loss of vision can cause emotional reactions such as denial, anger, guilt, resentment, hopelessness, helplessness, loneliness, and depression. These strong emotional feelings interfere with the blind person's ability to plan new ways of accomplishing tasks of living.

Fluctuating vision, a common occurrence for many visually impaired persons, leads to frustration and difficulties in planning or implementing tasks. Fears and uncertainties about the progression of visual impairment can lead to concern about the ability to cope with further deterioration of vision or the necessity of preparing for the future.

The ability to cope with the loss depends on the extent and duration of the handicap, the age at which it occurs, how the person has successfully coped in the past, and the presence of available support systems (family and friends).

Over time, persons with visual losses appear to be able to compensate for their deficit by an increase in sensitivity of the other senses. For example, some blind people compensate by increasing auditory acuity, tactile acuity, sense of smell, or kinesthetic awareness.

Nursing activities for the newly blind

COUNSELING

Newly blind persons who are trying to cope need an opportunity to talk about their feelings, concerns, and anxieties about the future. Once they have identified these feelings and concerns, they can be helped to identify their strengths and resources and to consider different approaches to dealing with tasks of everyday living. Alternate forms of recreation and pleasurable activities can also be explored. For example, the person who enjoyed reading may be interested in learning Braille or in using "talking books."

Some persons need assistance in developing a new self-image. It is not unusual for the person to reject initially any aids that officially identify them as "blind," such as the white cane. Patience is required; it sometimes takes a long time to change the self-image.

Persons who become blind do not develop impaired hearing or intelligence, yet some sighted persons insist on speaking loudly. Communication should be done naturally (see the box on p. 526).

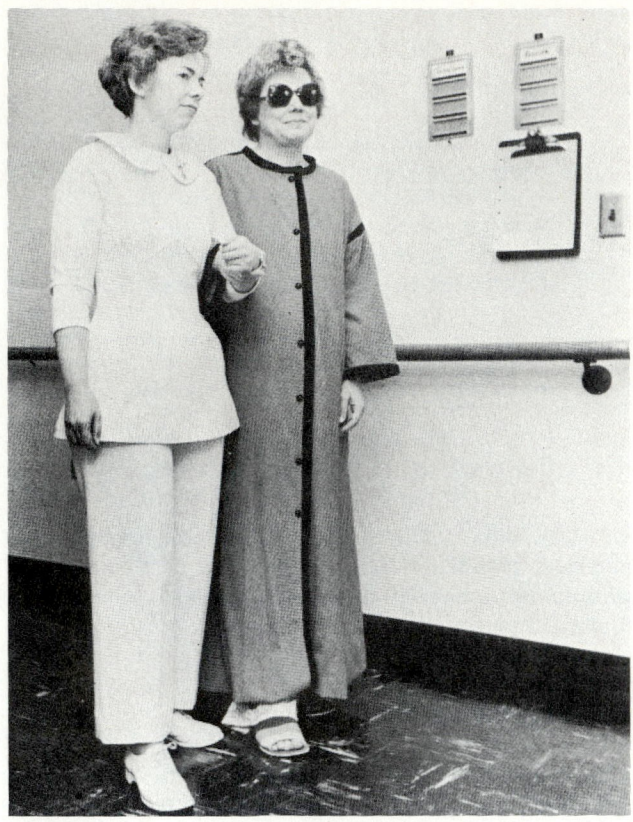

Fig. 20-6 Ambulation of patient who cannot see. Note that patient holds nurse's arm and is led without being held.

■ ASSISTANCE WITH ADL

Given time, most blind persons develop ways of coping with activities of daily living (ADL) (see the box below). One elderly blind lady was able to take her many medications accurately by devising a system using rubber bands and strings around the medication bottles to provide clues to when they were to be taken.

■ COMMUNITY SERVICES

Many federal, state, and local agencies provide services to persons with severe visual impairment. The health professional can refer these persons and their families to a social worker familiar with services and facilities available in their home area. Community health nurses often have this information readily available. Services to visually impaired persons include mobility training, personal counseling, vocational rehabilitation, relearning independent self-care, special education, and financial compensation in some instances. "Talking books" and tapes are available from public libraries, as well as from organizations for the blind.

■ GOVERNMENT ASSISTANCE

Legal blindness entitles a person to certain federal assistance based on need. Blind persons are entitled to an extra personal deduction in reported income. Counseling and placement services are available through the Social and Rehabilitation Service (SRS) of the U.S. Department of Health and Human Services.

Major health problems of the eye

The most common disorders of the eye in adults include the following:

1. Inflammatory disorders of the eyelid, conjunctiva, cornea, choroid, ciliary body, and iris
2. Cataracts: opaqueness of the lens
3. Glaucoma: increased intraocular pressure
4. Retinal detachment

■ INFLAMMATORY EYE DISORDERS

Inflammations and infections may occur in any of the eye structures (Table 20-6), and account for more than half of eye disorders.

■ Pathophysiology

Most eye inflammations are caused by microorganisms, mechanical irritation, or sensitivity to some substance. Fortunately, a large percentage of inflammations are self-limiting, with no permanent scars. Severe corneal inflammation or ulceration can damage the cornea, causing visual

Table 20-6 Inflammatory disorders of the eye

Disorder	Description	Signs and symptoms	Medical therapy
Hordoleum (sty)	Staphylococcal infection of gland at eyelid margin	Localized abcess at base of eyelash, edema of lid, pain	Hot compresses to hasten pointing of abcess, topical antibiotic
Chalazion	Cyst from obstruction of sebaceous gland at eyelid margin	Initial edema and discomfort; later, painless mass in lid	Warm compresses and topical antibiotic initially; surgical removal if large and pressing on cornea
Blepharitis	Inflammation of lid margins, usually by staphylococci	Itching, redness, lid pain, lacrimation, photophobia; crusting ulceration; lids become glued together during sleep	Warm compresses followed by erythromycin or bacitracin eye ointment; steroid eye drops may be prescribed
Conjunctivitis (pink eye)	Inflammation of conjunctiva by viruses, bacteria (highly infectious), chlamydia, allergy, trauma (sunburn)	Redness of conjunctiva, lid edema, crusting discharge on lids and cornea of eye; itching with allergies	Cleansing of lids and lashes, warm compresses; topical antibiotics; steroid eye drops for allergies (contraindicated for herpes simplex virus); no eye patch
Keratitis	Inflammation of cornea by bacteria, herpes simplex virus, allergies, vitamin A deficiency	Severe eye pain, photophobia, tearing, blepharospasm, loss of vision if uncontrolled	Warm compresses; topical antibiotics for bacterial infections; atropine sulfate; idoxuridine for herpes simplex; eye patch, rest; corneal grafting if cornea injured
Corneal ulcer	Necrosis of corneal tissue from trauma, inflammation; may be superficial or may penetrate deeper tissue	Pain and blepharospasm may occur; ulcer may be outlined by fluorescein dye	Superficial ulcer: antibiotic eye drops, eye patch Deep ulcer: topical and systemic antibiotics, atropine sulfate, warm compresses, eye patch; cauterization; corneal transplant if necessary
Uveitis	Inflammation of iris and ciliary body (anterior) or choroid (posterior); the cause is often unknown	*Anterior:* eye pain, photophobia, lacrimation, blurred vision, small pupil *Posterior:* blurring, decreased vision, mild eye discomfort	Scopolamine or atropine to dilate pupil (rests pupil, prevents adhesions), moist eye compresses, corticosteroids

impairment. Complications from uveitis can lead to formation of adhesions, secondary glaucoma, and loss of vision.

The most common eye inflammations are styes and conjunctivitis. Styes are relatively mild infections of the follicle of an eyelash or gland at the lid margins. Staphylococci are often the infecting organisms. These infections tend to occur in crops because the infecting organism spreads from one hair follicle to another. Poor hygiene and excessive use of cosmetics may be contributing causes. Persons should be taught not to squeeze styes because the infection may spread and cause cellulitis of the lids.

Conjunctivitis is the most common eye disease and may be acute or chronic. Acute bacterial conjunctivitis is usually transmitted by direct contact; the person touches the eyes following finger contact with contaminated objects such as towels or tissues. The most common infecting organisms are staphylococci and adenoviruses. Simple conjunctivitis is usually self-limiting.

Infection by *Chlamydia trachomatis* leads to *trachoma*, a form of conjunctivitis that is rare in the United States, but is the leading cause of blindness worldwide, particularly in low-income persons living in the dry, hot Mediterranean countries of the Far East. Following the acute conjunctivitis stage in trachoma, the eyelids become scarred, and granulations form on the inner surface of the lids and invade the cornea. The entire cornea may eventually become involved with subsequent loss of vision. Secondary bacterial infection is common. Hygienic measures are important in the prevention and treatment of trachoma. Corneal scarring may require corneal transplantation.

Allergic conjunctivitis is commonly associated with hay fever. It is usually chronic and recurrent.

Assessment

■ SUBJECTIVE DATA

Persons with inflammations of the eye may complain of itching, pain (mild to severe), lacrimation, sensitivity to light (photophobia), or spasms of the eyelids (blepharospasms).

■ OBJECTIVE DATA

The external structures of the eye are routinely inspected during the physical examination (Chapter 3). Inflammations are identified by the presence of redness, edema of the lids, and pus or discharge. When considerable discharge is present, the lids may become glued together during sleep.

Corneal ulcers may be identified by instilling sterile fluorescein, a yellow-green harmless dye. Because fluorescein harbors the growth of microorganisms such as *pseudomonas*, only a new, unopened bottle should be used. Also available are single-use fluorescein-impregnated paper strips that are gently touched to the inside of the lower lid. The ulcer is then assessed by shining a penlight obliquely across the eye from the side. If pain and blepharospasm interfere with

examination, a drop of anesthetic such as 0.5% proparacaine can be used.

→ Data analysis: nursing diagnoses

Nursing diagnoses are determined from assessment of patient data. Possible nursing diagnoses for the person with an eye inflammation may include, but are not limited to, the following:

Diagnostic title	Possible etiologies
Potential for infection: spread to nonaffected eye	Lack of knowledge
Pain: eye	Edema of the eye, secretions, photophobia

▥ Planning: expected patient outcomes

Expected patient outcomes for the person with an eye inflammation may include, but are not limited to, the following:

1. Patient states pain is decreased.
2. Infection does not spread to opposite eye.
3. The patient can:
   a. State name, dosage, and frequency of eye medication to be taken and the need to destroy unused ophthalmic medications after therapy.
   b. Describe method and frequency of eye compresses to be used.
   c. Describe measures to prevent spread of infection to the uninvolved eye and to others in the household.
4. If corneal grafting has been performed, the person can:
   a. Describe the medication program.
   b. Describe activities and movements to be avoided.
   c. Describe the need for medical follow-up.

▦ Implementation

Nursing interventions for the person with an eye inflammation consist primarily of giving eye treatments and medications to hasten healing and decrease pain, and helping prevent the spread of infection (see the box on p. 529).

■ ASSISTING WITH ACHIEVEMENT OF THERAPEUTIC GOALS

☐ Eye compresses

Warm moist compresses (see the box on p. 529) help relieve pain, promote healing, and help to cleanse the eye, which is normally cleansed by tears. Treatment is repeated two to four times a day.

Cold moist saline compresses may be ordered to prevent or control edema and severe itching of the eyes and to help control bleeding immediately after eye injury. A small basin of sterile solution may be placed in a bowl of chipped ice at the bedside. Sterile forceps are used to wring out and apply the compress. If the compress does not need to be sterile, a washcloth or compress may be placed on pieces

---

Nursing care of the patient with an eye inflammation

1. Apply warm moist compresses as prescribed for healing and to decrease pain.
2. Irrigate eye, if prescribed, to remove discharge.
3. Administer prescribed eye medications.
4. Use eye pads only for inflammations without infection.
5. Dim bright lights if photophobia is present.
6. Give prescribed analgesics for pain.
7. Prevent spread of infection by:
   a. Using separate medication bottles or tubes for each eye if infection is present.
   b. Washing hands before touching eye.
   c. Using washcloths and towels only once if infection is present.

Guidelines for application of warm moist eye compresses

1. Use sterile technique when infection or ulceration is present; clean technique may be used for allergic reactions.
2. Use separate equipment for bilateral eye infections.
3. Wash hands before treating each eye.
4. Temperature of compresses should not exceed 49° C (120° F).
5. Change compresses frequently over 10 to 20 minutes.
6. Do not exert pressure on eyeball.
7. Sterile petrolatum may be used on skin *around* eyes, if desired, to protect skin.
8. If sterility is not necessary, moist heat may be applied by means of a clean wash cloth.

---

of ice in a basin. A rubber glove or small plastic bag packed with finely chipped ice may be applied to the eye and requires fewer compress changes.

☐ **Eye irrigation**

Irrigation is used to remove secretions, discharge, foreign bodies, and chemical irritants from the eye (see box on p. 530). Physiologic saline solution or lactated Ringer's solution is commonly used because these isotonic solutions do not remove the electrolytes necessary for normal eye action. If only a small amount of fluid is needed, sterile cotton balls may be used to drip fluid into the eye.

☐ **Eye pads**

Eye pads are contraindicated in general eye infections because they enhance bacterial growth. They may be used for photophobia when the inflammation is *not* caused by bacteria and to protect the eye when corneal ulceration is present.

☐ **Eye medications**

Accuracy and safety in the administration of eye medications is essential to prevent irreparable damage to the eye. The correct eye to receive the medication must be identified. Labels must be checked carefully, and all medications with labels that are smeared or obliterated are discarded. Solutions that have changed color, are cloudy, contain sediment, or are outdated are also discarded. Elderly persons are particularly susceptible to side effects of medications.

Ophthalmic medications may be instilled as eyedrop solutions or ointment (see the box on p. 530).

All patients should have their own bottles of eyedrops or tubes of ointment to prevent cross-infection. If an eye infection is being treated with an antibiotic and the same drug is being given prophylactically in the other eye, separate bottles or tubes are used. Methods for instilling eyedrops and ointments are described in the box on p. 530.

Different types of drugs are used for treatment of eye diseases (Table 20-7). The most commonly used drugs for eye inflammations are antibiotic, steroid, and cycloplegic drugs (Tables 20-8 and 20-9).

Drugs applied topically to the eye can be absorbed and may cause systemic side effects. To avoid undesired systemic reactions, care should be taken with topically applied medications to give exactly what is ordered and no more.

1. Place patient lying toward side to be irrigated to prevent fluid from flowing into other eye.
2. A plastic squeeze bottle is used unless very large amounts of fluid are needed.
3. Direct the irrigating fluid along the conjunctiva from the *inner* to the outer canthus (Fig. 20-7).
4. Avoid directing a forceful stream onto the eyeball.
5. Avoid touching any eye structures with irrigation equipment.
6. A piece of gauze may be wrapped around the index finger to raise upper lid for better cleaning if heavy discharge is present.
7. Place an emesis basin at side of face to collect irrigating fluid.

Forms of eye medications

Ophthalmic solutions

1. Easily instilled
2. Do not interfere with vision
3. Cause few skin reactions
4. Do not interfere with mitosis of corneal epithelium
5. Disadvantage: do not remain in contact with eye for very long

Ophthalmic ointments

1. Remain in contact with eye for extended periods
2. Do not cause discomfort when instilled
3. Less absorption into lacrimal passageways
4. More stable than solutions
5. Disadvantages:
   a. Produce film across eye, which may interfere with vision
   b. May cause contact dermatitis
   c. May inhibit mitosis of corneal epithelium

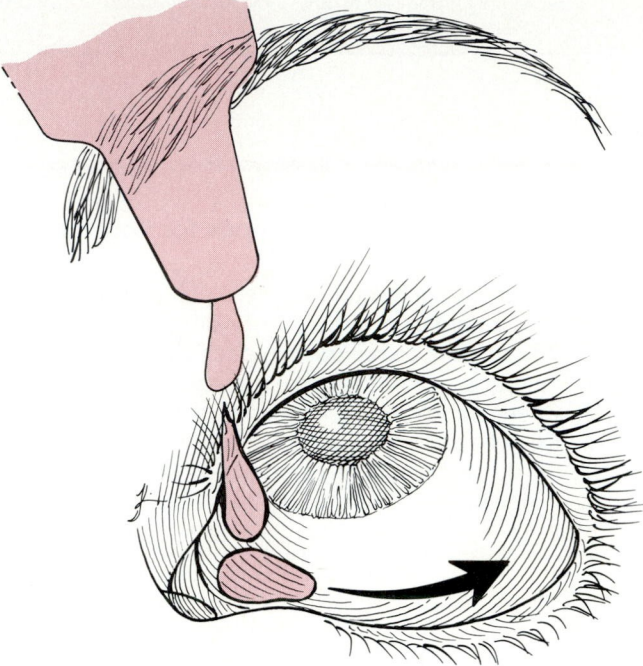

Fig. 20-7   Irrigating the eye. Fluid is directed along conjunctiva and over eyeball from inner to outer canthus.

Guidelines for instilling eye medications

Eyedrops

1. Wash hands before touching eyes.
2. Clean eyes before instilling eyedrops if crusting or discharge is present.
3. Ask patient to tilt head back and look up (Fig. 20-8).
4. Evert lower lid by pulling down gently on skin below eye.
5. Approach eye from side (not directly from front).
6. Place drops on *center* of conjunctival sac of lower lid.
7. Avoid touching eye with tip of dropper.
8. Ask patient not to squeeze eye shut (loss of medication down cheek).
9. Provide patient with a tissue.

Ointment

1. Follow steps 1 through 4 above.
2. Press the ointment from the tube directly onto exposed conjunctival sac.
3. Avoid touching eye tissue with tube.

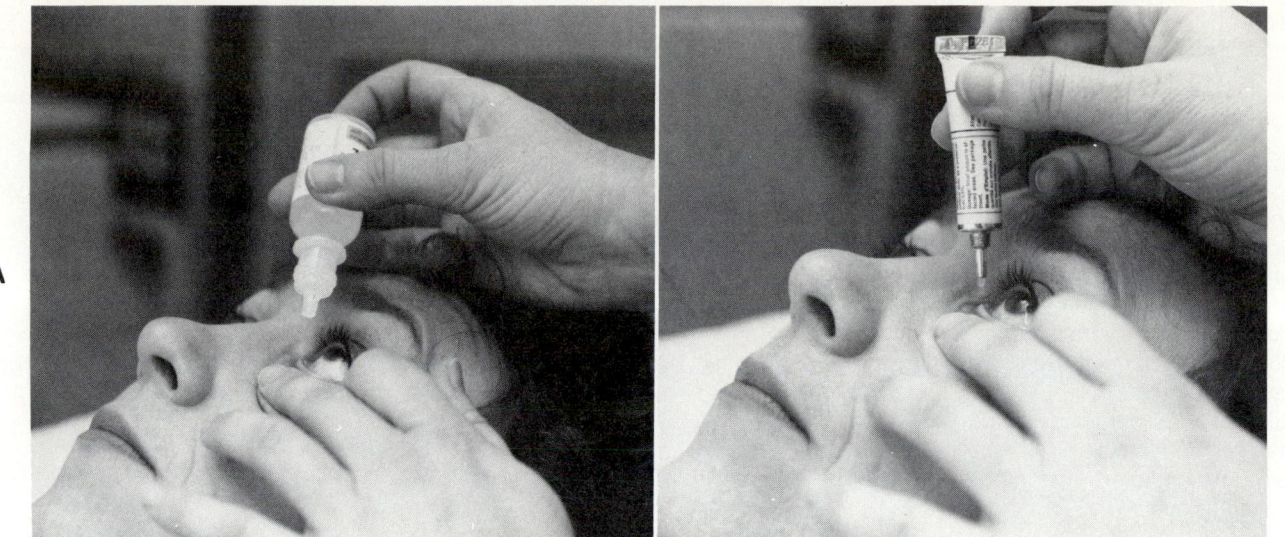

Fig. 20-8   **A,** Ophthalmic solution is dropped onto conjunctiva of lower lid. **B,** Ophthalmic ointment is squeezed onto conjunctiva of lower lid.

Table 20-7   Types of ophthalmic drugs

Type	Action	Uses
Mydriatic	Dilates pupil	Examination of interior of eye Prevents adhesions of iris with cornea in eye inflammations
Cycloplegic	Dilates pupil Paralyzes ciliary muscle and iris	Decreases pain and photophobia and provides rest in inflammations of iris and ciliary body and diseases of cornea Eye examinations
Miotic	Contracts pupil Permits better drainage of intraocular fluid	Glaucoma
Osmotic	Decreases intraocular pressure	Acute glaucoma Eye surgery
Secretory inhibitor	Decreases production of intraocular fluid	Glaucoma
Topical anesthetic	Decreases sensation (pain)	Surgery, treatments Eye inflammations
Topical antibiotic	Antiinfective	Eye inflammations
Steroid	Antiinflammatory	Eye inflammations and allergic reactions

Table 20-8   Mydriatic and cycloplegic drugs

Drug	Maximal effect	Duration
Mydriatic action		
Phenylephrine (Neo-Synephrine)	20 min	3 hr
Epinephrine (Epitrate)	3 to 5 min	—
Cycloplegic and mydriatic action		
Atropine sulfate (Atropisol, Isopto-Atropine)	30 to 120 min	2 wks
Cyclopentolate (Cyclogyl)	15 to 45 min	2 days
Homatropine (Isopto-Homatropine)	10 to 90 min	2 to 3 days
Scopolamine hydrobromide	15 to 45 min	5 to 7 days
Tropicamide (Mydriacyl)	20 to 35 min	4 to 6 hrs

Table 20-9 Other ophthalmic drugs

Ophthalmic drug	Use and effect
Antiinfectives	
Polymyxin B, neomycin, bacitracin (Neosporin) Neomycin sulfate (Myciguent) Gentamicin sulfate (Garamycin) Chloramphenicol (Chloromycetin, Chloroptic) Erythromycin (Ilotycin) Tetracycline hydrochloride (Achromycin) Chlortetracycline hydrochloride (Aureomycin) Sulfacetamide sodium (Sodium Sulamyd, Isopto-Cetamide) Sulfisoxazole diolamine (Gantrisin) Natamycin (Natacyn) Idoxuridine (Herplex, Dendrid, Stoxil) Acyclovir (Zovirax)	Antibiotic agents may be given for acute inflammatory conjunctivitis, styes, eyelid infections, keratitis, and uveitis; natamycin is antifungal; idoxuridine and acyclovir are antiviral, especially for herpes simplex eye infections
Adrenocorticoids	
Dexamethasone (Decadron phosphate) Fluorometholone (FML Liquifilm) Hydrocortisone (Hydrocortone, Cortamed) Medrysone (HMS Liquifilm) Prednisolone (Pred Forte, Pred Mild, Metimyd)	Topical ophthalmic steroid therapy is indicated for allergic conjunctivitis, nonpyogenic eye inflammations, and for eye trauma (burns, foreign body penetration); chronic therapy may cause increased IOP, susceptibility to fungus infections, glaucoma, and cataracts
Tears substitutes	
Hydroxypropyl methylcellulose (Tears Naturale, Isopto-Tears, Tearisol)	Artificial tears provide lubrication when tears are deficient (age, heredity, connective tissue disorders, environment); also used for lubrication with contact lenses and artificial eyes

☐ Corneal surgery

When the cornea is so damaged from corneal inflammation (keratitis) or from a corneal ulcer, corneal transplantation (keratoplasty) may be performed. Corneal grafts are taken from healthy donor eyes, preferably from young donors (ages 25 to 35) who have died from an acute disease or from injury.[25] The corneas need to be obtained within 5 hours of death. For best results the donor cornea must be used within 48 hours (preferably 24).[30] Transplants preserved for longer periods may be used for lamellar grafts. Presons wishing to donate their eyes for use in keratoplasty may write the Eye Bank Association of America* for information. Some states use driver's licenses for potential donors to signify their intent. Nurses need to be alert to situations where corneas may be obtained and to offer the suggestion to the family of a recently deceased person.

Either total or partial replacement of the cornea may be performed (Fig. 20-9). The total penetrating graft is the most frequently used type and is the most effective. A second transplant may be performed if the first is unsuccessful.

Keratoplasty may be performed with local or general anesthesia or a combination of both. The new cornea is

sutured in place, and an antibiotic is injected subconjunctivally. An eye shield is applied, remains in place until the day after surgery, and is reapplied at night to prevent inadvertent injury during sleep. Postoperative care for eye surgery is discussed on p. 535. Glasses may be worn during the day to protect the eye and the patient can expect that some vision will be restored immediately. Vision improves over the following 6 to 12 months.

Corneal grafts heal very slowly because of the lack of blood vessels in the cornea. The patient is advised to avoid bending, lifting, or straining for 1 month to prevent increased intraocular pressure or suture strain; strenuous activities should be avoided for 3 months.

The graft is never totally integrated into the eye; therefore, the person must check the eye for the remainder of life for signs of rejection (redness, photosensitivity, pain, vision loss).[34] Any symptoms that persist or increase in severity in a 24-hour period are reported to the physician.

■ ASSISTING WITH COMFORT

Pain from eye inflammations can be reduced by applying warm moist compresses several times each day and by instilling prescribed eyedrops (particularly the cycloplegic drugs, which put the iris and ciliary body at rest). If pho-

---

*1511 K Street NW, Suite 830, Washington, DC 20005-1401.

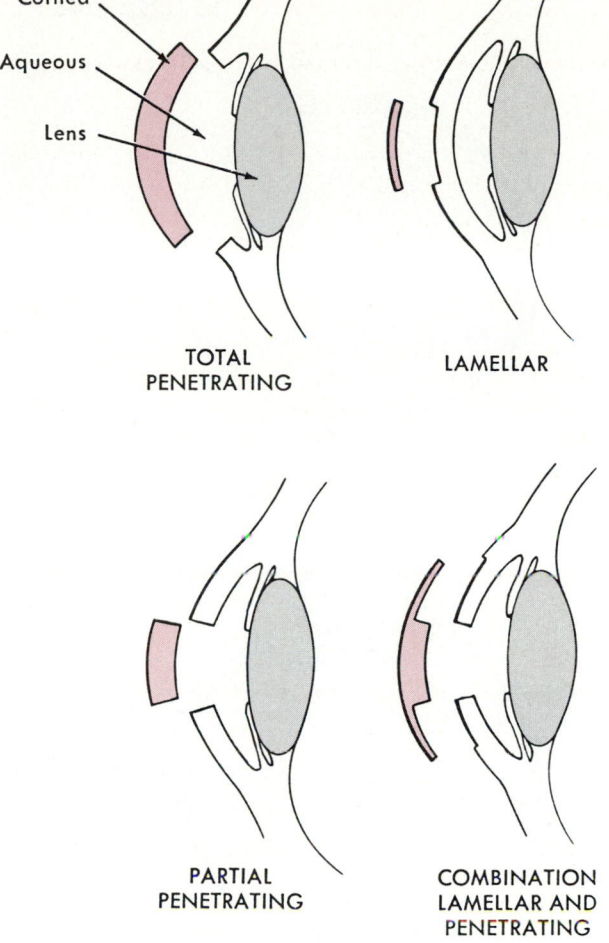

Fig. 20-9 Types of corneal grafts now being used. Note that in lamellar graft, defect does not penetrate entire thickness of cornea.

tophobia creates discomfort, bright lights can be dimmed. Mild analgesics such as aspirin or acetaminophen (Tylenol) usually suffice, but if pain is severe (as may occur with uveitis) a narcotic may be required.

■ CONTROL OF ENVIRONMENT

When a highly infectious eye condition, such as acute bacterial conjunctivitis, is present, precautions need to be taken to prevent the spread of infection to others. Individual washcloths and towels should be used. Hands should be washed after any contact with the infected eye.

✚ Evaluation

When providing care for the patient with an eye inflammation or infection, consider the following:
1. Is the patient comfortable?
2. Is the uninvolved eye free of signs of infection?
3. Does the patient know how to carry out prescribed treatments after discharge?

4. If corneal surgery has been performed, does the patient know about activity limitations and need for continued medical follow-up?

■ CATARACT

A cataract is a clouding or opacity of the lens that leads to gradual painless blurring of vision and eventual loss of sight (Fig. 20-10). The most common cause of cataract formation is aging (senile cataract); other causes include trauma, other eye diseases (for example, uveitis), systemic diseases (diabetes mellitus), or congenital defects (either hereditary or as a result of prenatal viral infections such as German measles).

■ Pathophysiology

The lens of the eye is normally transparent, so that light rays can pass through. Biochemical changes may occur within the lens, or trauma may cause fiber changes that cause the lens to become cloudy and finally opaque, thus blocking the light rays from reaching the retina. A *mature cataract* is a developed cataract that separates easily from the lens capsule. It was previously thought that a cataract had to be mature ("ripe") before it could be extracted. Now cataracts are removed whenever the decreased vision interferes with activities of daily living. Cataracts may develop in both eyes, such as with senile cataracts, but usually at different rates.

▦ Assessment

Acquired cataracts, either from aging or disease, usually develop gradually. Blurring of vision may occur immediately after trauma. The predominant symptom is progressive loss of vision; the degree of loss depends on the location and extent of the opacity. Persons with an opacity in the center portion of the lens can generally see better in dim light, when the pupil is dilated. The person with pres-

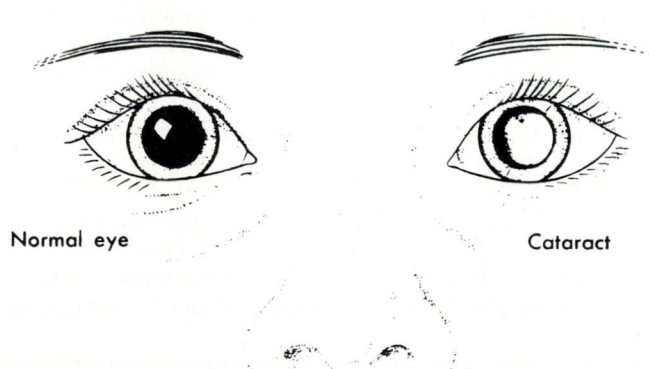

Fig. 20-10 Cataract visible in left eye as white opacity of lens seen through pupil.

byopia may find that reading without glasses is possible in the early stages because of resulting myopia.

▪ Cataract surgery

Surgery is the only method for treating cataracts, although only a small percentage of senile cataracts progress to the point where surgery is required. Patients of any age, even in their nineties, can be operated on with good results. The decision to remove the cataract depends on the degree of visual impairment, general health, and the use made of the eyes.

Because surgery is usually indicated only for advanced cataracts, elderly persons may believe they should wait until vision loss is far advanced before consulting an ophthalmologist. Delaying medical examination of the eye can lead to permanent vision loss if there is glaucoma, either alone or in combination with cataracts.

▪ SURGICAL PROCEDURE

Cataract surgery has changed in recent years as a result of the use of the operating microscope, better instrumentation, improved suture material, and refinement of the intraocular lens.[35] There are two methods of cataract extraction, extracapsular and intracapsular. the more commonly used procedure now used is the *extracapsular*, consisting of removal of the lens and anterior capsule leaving the posterior capsule intact. The *intracapsular* method removes the lens with all of its capsule. With the extracapsular technique, the lens may be removed by phacoemulsification, which breaks up the lens and flushes it out in small pieces. Only a small incision is required; thus healing is more rapid. Either cryoextraction or a small suction cup may be used to remove an intact lens.

A complication of extracapsular lens extraction is a developing opaqueness of the posterior capsule (called after-cataract). An after-cataract may be treated with laser therapy to improve vision.

▪ CORRECTIVE LENSES

☐ Intraocular lens

Over 75% of cataract surgery in the United States now involves intraocular lens implantation at the time of surgery.[35] The intraocular lens provides binocular vision and better optical results than external lenses. There are different styles of lenses, but all the lenses consist primarily of two parts, the lens (usually made of polymethylmethacrylate) and the attached flexible loops to hold the lens in position. The lenses may be implanted in the *anterior* chamber in front of the iris or in the *posterior* chamber behind the iris (Fig. 20-11). The posterior lens implant, suitable for an extracapsular lens extraction, is used in the majority of patients.

☐ External lenses

If an intraocular lens is not inserted during surgery, the person must wear an external lens (Table 20-10). The

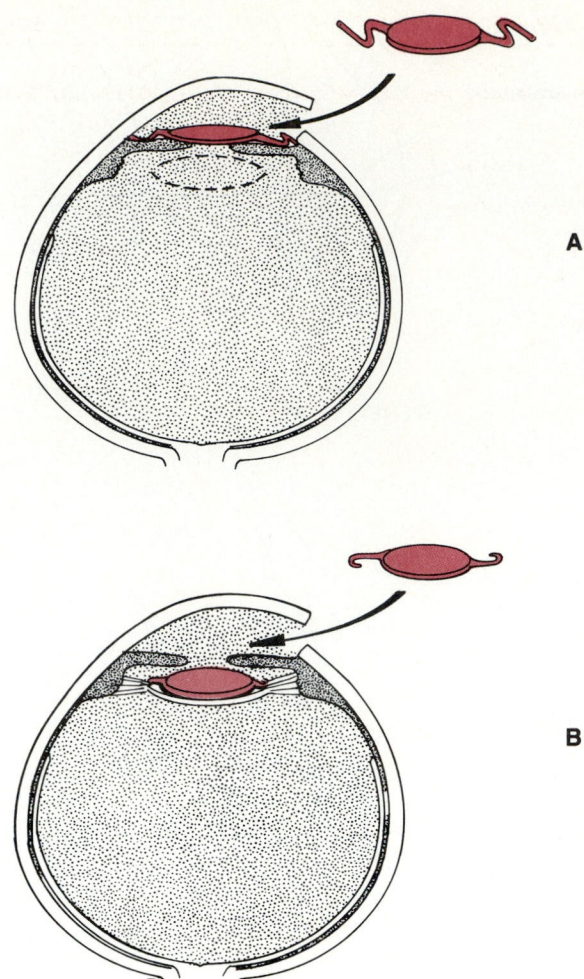

Fig. 20-11 Intraocular lens. **A,** Anterior lens implant in front of iris. **B,** Posterior lens implant behind iris.

cataract glasses are the least desirable but are used if the person cannot use contact lenses. Loss of depth perception and some peripheral vision make walking difficult. The final pair of glasses is not prescribed until vision has stabilized several months after surgery.

Contact lenses correct some of the problems encountered with cataract glasses but not entirely.[25] The extended wear soft contact lens (p. 520) is commonly used. Interruption of the nerve supply to the cornea from surgery usually facilitates the wearing of a contact lens.[25] Persons with rheumatoid arthritis, hemiplegia, parkinsonism, or Alzheimer's disease may have difficulty inserting and maintaining contact lenses.

▪ Eye surgery

Most eye surgery is now being performed as ambulatory surgery except when complications are present preoperatively. Local anesthesia is used for most of the procedures in adults; a general anesthetic (such as Pentothal Sodium) may be used briefly for initial eye injections and incision.

Table 20-10 Corrective lenses after cataract surgery

Type	Advantages	Disadvantages
Lens implant	Cannot be lost or broken Better binocular vision No handling required	Possible complications: vitreous loss, inflammation
Contact lenses	Better visual correction than glasses Better cosmetic appearance Better binocular vision if only one lens removed	Awkward for some elderly persons to manage Easy to lose Difficult adjustment for some persons May cause irritation
Cataract glasses	More acceptable to some elderly persons No physical complications	Magnify objects by 25%; objects appear closer than they actually are Distort peripheral images and colors Heavy lenses May cause visual distortion if poorly positioned

Because the pupil is widely dilated during surgery, the patient can see only light but not the surgeon's actions. The patient's head is positioned during surgery to avoid movement.

■ PREOPERATIVE CARE

Preparation of the eye includes instillation of eyedrops, such as a mydriatic/cycloplegic and a local anesthetic (tetracaine, proparacaine) on the day of surgery. An anti-anxiety agent or mild sedative may also be prescribed. If a topical anesthetic is given in advance of surgery, the eye can be protected by an eye pad or glasses.

■ POSTOPERATIVE CARE

The goals of postoperative care are to *prevent* (1) increased intraocular pressure, (2) stress on the suture line, (3) hemorrhage into the anterior chamber, and (4) infection. When intraocular pressure (IOP) is increased, pressure is put on the suture line and bleeding may occur. Anterior flexion of the head not only increases IOP but also may cause anterior synechia (adhesion of the iris to the cornea) because of decreased fluid in the anterior chamber and inflammation from the trauma of surgery. Thus activities that increase IOP, such as straining and leaning over, are contraindicated after surgery. Protection (eye shield, glasses) of the eye from sudden pressure prevents

Teaching the patient following eye surgery

1. Sleep on unaffected side for the prescribed time (3 to 4 weeks) to prevent pressure on operated eye.
2. Wash hands before instilling eye drops (p. 530) or changing eye pad.
3. If an eye pad is required:
   a. Use two oval eye pads, to provide snug but gentle pressure to prevent blinking against resistance.[34]
   b. Apply tape (paper or silk) diagonally from above nose to lower cheek.
4. Apply metal eye shield at night to protect eye.
5. Use glasses indoors and sunglasses with side sections outdoors to protect eyes from foreign substances and ultraviolet light until healing occurs.
6. Avoid rubbing or pressing on the eye (creates pressure and may dislodge sutures).
7. Avoid showers and shampooing hair (soap may irritate eye) for specified period as instructed; the time period differs from 1 day to up to 2 weeks.
8. Avoid bending at the waist or lifting heavy objects for at least 1 month to prevent increased IOP or adhesions of the iris.
   a. To pick up objects from floor, kneel while keeping head erect.
   b. To put on stocking or to tie shoes, sit and raise foot to reach hand while keeping head erect.
   c. Long pick-up "forceps" can facilitate picking up small objects from the floor without having to bend over.
9. Avoid straining with bowel movements or with other activities and avoid violent coughing (increases IOP).
10. Limit reading (back and forth movement may loosen stitches); television is usually permitted.
11. Report signs of swelling, discharge, or pain to physician (may indicate infection or hemorrhage).

stress on the suture line. Infection is prevented by the correct use of eye drops and eye pads; topical antibiotics may be given prophylactically.

Specific instructions regarding activities to avoid, eye drops to be instilled, and symptoms to be reported are provided to the patient by the surgeon and nurse. The instructions may include those listed in the box on p. 535.

GLAUCOMA

Glaucoma is a group of eye disorders characterized by increased intraocular pressure. It is a major cause of blindness in the United States, and the incidence is increasing as the number of older persons increase. Glaucoma may be either primary or secondary to other eye disorders. Primary glaucoma has a genetic predisposition. Primary open-angle glaucoma (the most common form) is more common in blacks than whites; in persons age 45 to 64, the incidence in blacks is 15 times that of whites.[35] Because early signs may be absent in some forms of glaucoma, many persons are unaware that they have glaucoma until loss of vision occurs. Early diagnosis and treatment are essential to prevent loss of vision.

Pathophysiology

Intraocular pressure is maintained by ongoing production and drainage of aqueous humor in the anterior cavity (p. 518) (Fig. 20-12, A). Glaucoma results when there is interference with the outflow of aqueous humor, leading to an increase in IOP. If the pressure remains elevated, eye damage occurs. The optic nerve degenerates at its origin (has a "cupping" appearance) and the ganglionic and nerve cells of the retina degenerate. These changes produce loss of vision, first peripheral vision, then eventual blindness if the condition is untreated.

The two major types of glaucoma are primary in origin, open-angle and angle-closure (closed-angle). *Secondary* glaucomas may result from eye disorders that block aqueous outflow or increase vitreous pressure (lens changes, uveitis, melanoma of the uveal tract), eye trauma or surgery, or long-term topical steroid therapy.

OPEN-ANGLE GLAUCOMA

Most glaucomas (90% to 95%) are primary open-angle glaucomas. Both eyes are involved. The onset is insidious and the disorder is slowly progressive. It is termed *open-angle* because the aqueous humor has open access to the trabecular meshwork. However, drainage is impeded by degenerative changes in the trabecular meshwork, canal of Schlemm, and adjacent canals.[35] Degenerative changes in the optic nerve may also occur. Early signs are usually absent, but the disorder can be diagnosed by the increased IOP and the normal anterior chamber angle. The pressure may eventually lead to dull eye pain (Table 20-11).

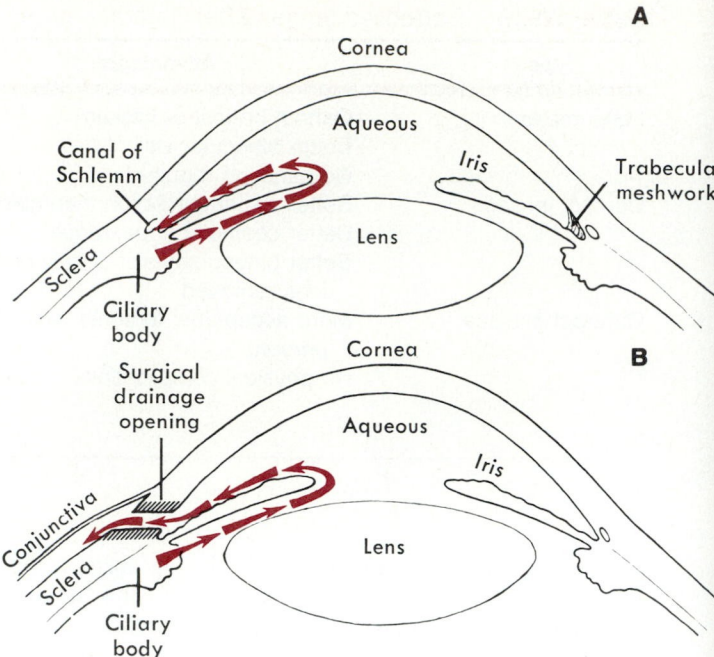

Fig. 20-12 **A,** Originating from ciliary processes, aqueous flows through pupil into anterior chamber and normally leaves eye by way of canal of Schlemm. **B,** In glaucoma, normal aqueous outflow is blocked. Purpose of glaucoma surgery is to create new channel through which aqueous can leave eye. (From Havener, WH: Synopsis of ophthalmology, ed 5, St. Louis, 1979, The CV Mosby Co.)

ANGLE-CLOSURE (CLOSED-ANGLE) GLAUCOMA

Closed-angle glaucoma usually occurs as an acute episode, although it may be subacute or chronic. It is termed *angle-closure* because the anterior chamber is anatomically narrow allowing the iris to be pushed forward, adhering to the trabecular meshwork and impeding aqueous humor flow to the canal of Schlemm. The forward movement of the iris may result from increased vitreous pressure, buildup of fluid in the posterior chamber, or thickening of the lens with age. IOP is normal when the angle is narrow but open and the drainage is not blocked. Symptoms result from sudden closure, with an increase in IOP, and include severe eye pain, blurred vision, and halos seen around lights. The adhered iris produces a dilated pupil. If untreated, a blind painful eye results.

Assessment

DIAGNOSTIC TESTS

Intraocular pressure is measured by means of *tonometry*. In an ophthalmologist's office, an applanation tonometer is generally used. With the use of a slit lamp, a small area of the cornea is flattened to counterbalance a spring-loaded measuring device that measures the pressure (Fig. 20-14).

Table 20-11 Types of glaucoma

Type	Characteristic	Manifestations	Treatment
Open-angle (chronic, simple)	Most common type (90%) Usually caused by obstruction in trabecular meshwork	Frequently no signs or symptoms in early stages Slow loss of vision Peripheral vision lost before central (Fig. 20-13) Tunnel vision Persistent dull eye pain Difficulty adjusting to darkness Failure to detect color changes Later: headache, pain, blurred vision, halos around lights	Medical: miotics, β-blockers, carbonic anhydrase inhibitors Surgical: trabeculectomy, trabeculoplasty
Angle-closure (narrow-angle, acute)	Outflow impaired as result of narrowing or closing of angle between iris and cornea Intermittent attacks, pressure normal when angle open; if persistent, acute ocular emergency	Acute: severe prostrating pain, decreased vision, pupil enlarged and fixed, colored halos around lights, eye red, steamy cornea Permanent blindness if marked increase in IOP for 24-48 hours	Medical: osmotic diuretics, carbonic anhydrase inhibitors, miotics Surgical: peripheral iridectomy, iridotomy
Congenital	Abnormal development of filtration angle Can occur secondary to other systemic eye disorders Rare (0.05%)	Enlargement of eye, lacrimation, photophobia, blepharospasm	Goniotomy (incision into region of trabecular meshwork) Trabeculotomy
Secondary	Can result from ocular inflammation, blood vessel changes, trauma	May be similar to open-angle and angle-closure, depending on cause	Directed at cause as well as decreasing the IOP

A less accurate direct method, but useful because the instrument if cheaper and portable, is the Schiøtz tonometer. The eye is anesthetized and the tonometer is placed directly on the cornea (Fig. 20-15). The amount of indentation that the instrument plunger makes on the cornea is measured on the attached scale. Noncontact tonometers measure IOP by deformation of light reflex from the cornea from a puff of air.[25] Readings greater than 24 mm Hg may suggest glaucoma.

The anterior chamber angle can be visualized using a contact lens and special lens (*gonioscopy*). This technique distinguishes open-angle from closed-angle glaucoma. Visualization of the optic disk by ophthalmoscopy will show cupping of the disk; visual field testing may show decreased peripheral vision.

■ NURSING ASSESSMENT

Nursing assessment consists of identifying any changes in vision and assessing discomfort.
1. Vision: note changes
   a. Visual acuity: Snellen chart if available, reading distant signs, close reading
   b. Visual fields: confrontation test (p. 521)
   c. Report of halos around lights

2. Discomfort
   a. Eye pain: dull, severe
   b. Headache: severity
   c. Nausea and vomiting

▶ Data analysis: nursing diagnoses

Nursing diagnoses are determined from assessment of patient data. Possible nursing diagnoses for the person with glaucoma may include, but are not limited to, the following:

Diagnostic title	Possible etiologies
Potential for injury	Decreased peripheral vision, blurred vision
Knowledge deficit	Lack of exposure/recall, information misinterpretation
Pain: headache	Acute glaucoma, stress, spasms

Planning: expected patient outcomes

Expected patient outcomes for the person with glaucoma may include, but are not limited to, the following:
1. Patient states discomfort is decreased.
2. Vision is not decreased further.

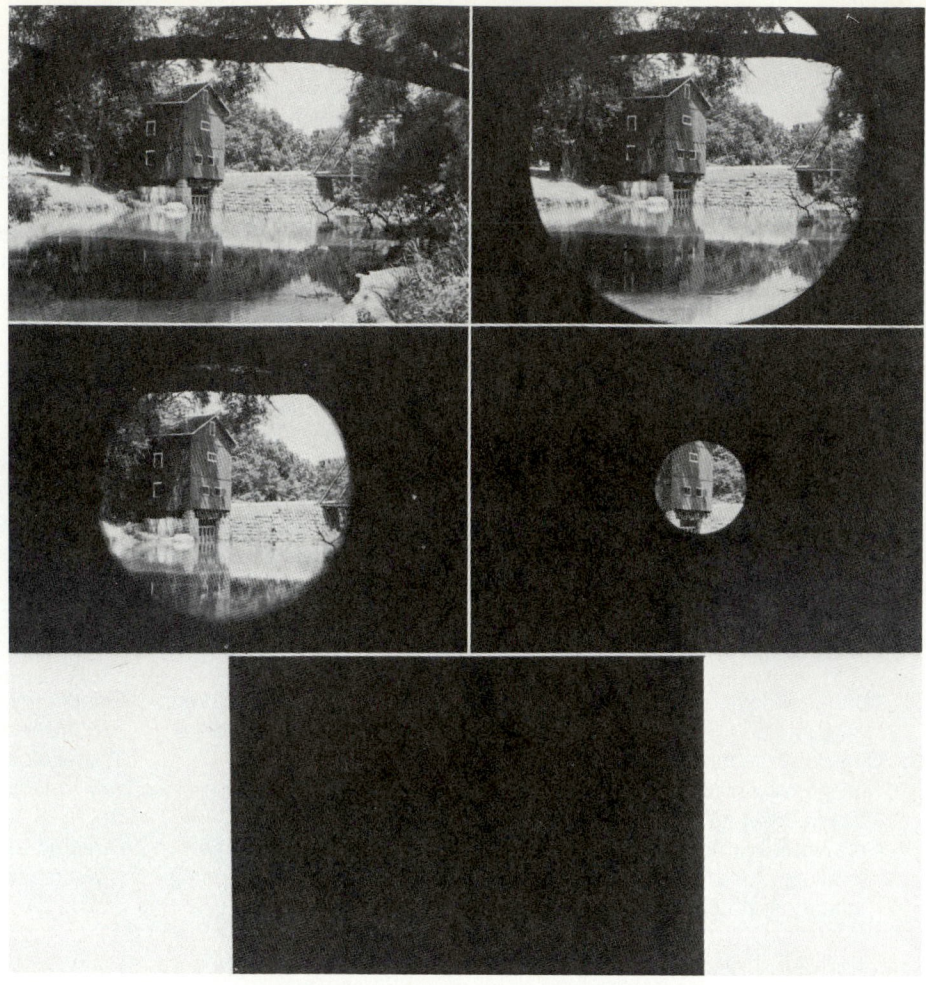

Fig. 20-13 Gradual loss of sight from glaucoma so insidiously destroys vision that person is unaware of impending blindness until extensive and irreversible damage is already present. (From Saunders, WH, and others: Nursing care in eye, ear, nose, and throat disorders ed 4, St. Louis, 1979, The CV Mosby Co.)

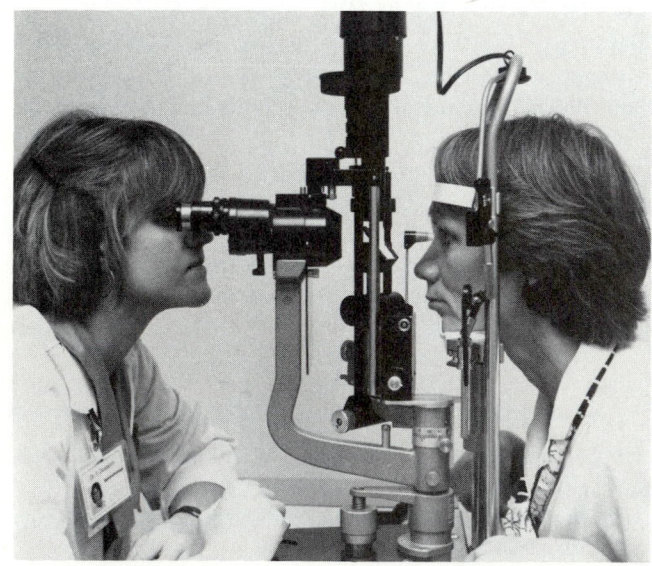

Fig. 20-14 Measurement of intraocular pressure with applanation tonometer.

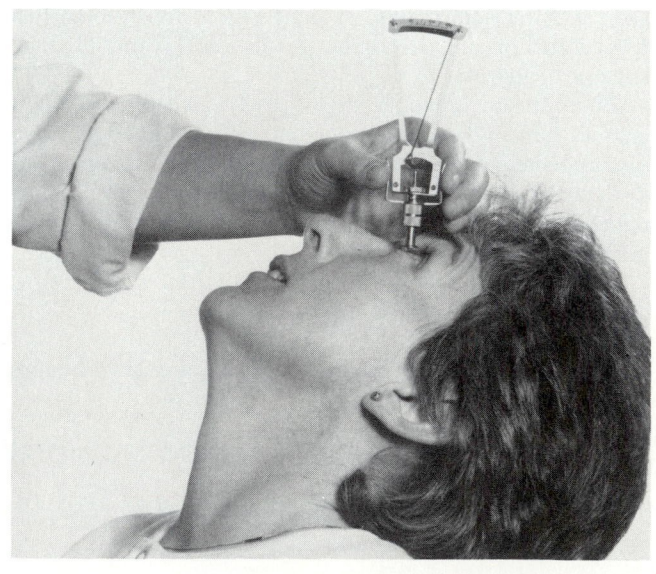

Fig. 20-15 Measurement of intraocular pressure with Schiøtz tonometer.

3. Patient can state recognition of lifetime need for eye medication.
4. Patient can state name, dosage, frequency, and side effects of prescribed eye medications.
5. Patient can describe measures to prevent complications.
6. Patient can list signs indicating need to report immediately to ophthalmologist.

Implementation

ASSISTING WITH ACHIEVEMENT OF THERAPEUTIC GOALS

Medications

It is vital in the control of glaucoma that eye medications be given as prescribed. Drugs used in treatment of glaucoma are listed in Table 20-12. The purpose of pharma-cologic therapy is to keep the pupil constricted to permit better drainage of the aqueous humor and to decrease the amount of aqueous humor produced.

Pilocarpine is the miotic drug of choice in the treatment of open-angle glaucoma. Pilocarpine may be given in solution (eye drops) or by membrane-controlled delivery system (Ocusert). The Ocusert is placed in the upper or lower conjunctival sac, preferably at night so the miotic effect reaches a stable level by morning; the effect lasts for 1 week. A pilocarpine gel, Piloplex, decreases the need for the more frequent insertion of pilocarpine eye drops. Miotics frequently decrease vision for 1 to 2 hours after instillation and may cause eye spasms in younger persons.

Beta-adrenergic blocking agents can be used alone or in combination with other drugs. The newer drug, Betaxolol, has an added advantage of decreased pulmonary side effects. Pressing the lacrimal duct for 1 minute after inser-

Table 20-12 Drugs used in treatment of glaucoma

Drug*	Effect with glaucoma
Cholinergic agents (miotics)	
Pilocarpine Carbachol (Carbacel)	Stimulates cholinergic receptors; contracts iris muscle constricting pupil and decreasing resistance to aqueous humor outflow; also constricts ciliary muscle to increase accommodation
Cholinesterase inhibitors (miotics)	
Physostigmine (Eserine) Isoflurophate (Floropryl) Demecarium bromide (Humorsol) Echothiophate iodide (Phospholine iodide)	Inhibits destruction of acetylcholine producing same effects as cholinergic drugs. DO NOT USE CHOLINESTERASE DRUGS WITH ANGLE-CLOSURE GLAUCOMA (increases pupillary block)
Beta-adrenergic blockers	
Timolol maleate (Timoptic) Betaxolol hydrochloride (Betoptic) Levobunolol hydrochloride (Betagan)	Blocks the adrenergic (sympathetic) impulses which normally produces mydriasis; mechanism by which the IOP is decreased is unclear
Adrenergic agents	
Epinephryl borate (Eppy) Epinephrine hydrochloride (Glaucon, Epifrin) Epinephrine bitartrate (Epitrate, Murocoll) Dipivefrin (Propine)	Decreases production of aqueous humor and increases aqueous outflow. DO NOT USE FOR ANGLE-CLOSURE GLAUCOMA
Carbonic anhydrase inhibitors	
Acetazolamide (Diamox) Ethoxzolamide (Cardrase) Dichlorhenamide (Daranide) Methazolamide (Neptazane	Slows production of aqueous humor
Osmotic agents	
Glycerine (Glycerol, Osmoglyn) Mannitol (Osmitrol) Urea (Ureaphil, Urevert)	Increases blood plasma osmolarity, enhancing fluid flow from aqueous humor into the plasma

*NOTE: The miotics, beta blockers, and adrenergic agents are given by eye drops; carbonic anhydrase inhibitors and osmotic agents are given orally or intravenously (as appropriate).

NURSING CARE PLAN

Person with open-angle glaucoma

DATA: Mr. Miller is a 76-year-old man with a history of open-angle glaucoma. His peripheral vision is markedly decreased. He was admitted for prostate surgery, but his primary nurse elicited the following information during the admission history: he has prescribed eye drops (pilocarpine 1% qid, timolol 0.5% bid) which he uses periodically. He states the drops blur his vision. He knows that his "eye pressure is high" but says he thinks it's getting better because his eyes don't bother him. His wife notes that he bumps into objects more frequently.

Nursing diagnosis: Knowledge deficit: related to lack of recall and information misinterpretation

Expected patient outcomes	Nursing interventions	Rationale
Patient describes chronicity of glaucoma and need for continued treatment	Ask patient to explain understanding of glaucoma: What it is Result if untreated Symptoms to be reported Need for medical followup	Start teaching at patient's level of knowledge. Since glaucoma is a chronic condition, he needs to know the effects of nontreatment (painful blind eye) and how to prevent it
Patient states symptoms requiring reporting to physician	Teach him about glaucoma and need for lifetime eye medication	
Patient demonstrates correct installation of eye drops	Ask him to demonstrate instilling eye drops; correct his technique as necessary	If his vision is decreasing, he may be having difficulty instilling his eye drops

Nursing diagnosis: Noncompliance with medications: related to drug side effects and lack of knowledge

Expected patient outcomes	Nursing interventions	Rationale
Patient states plans to take eyedrops at correct times	Explore other reasons for not taking the eyedrops	He may have difficulty reading the labels or remembering
	Ask his wife to bring in the eyedrop vials and role play with him use of vials and how to remember to take the eye drops	Role playing will help to identify problems he may be having reading the labels
	Enlist him and his wife in developing a plan to help remember how and when to take the eyedrops (such as after meals and at bedtime)	Client participation in planning ensures greater probability of carrying out plan; connecting the eyedrops with an activity helps the person remember
	Explain relationship of blurred vision with pilocarpine; suggest he consult physician and not plan specific activities for about 1 hr after instilling eyedrops	Blurred vision is a side effect of pilocarpine; it usually improves in 1 to 2 hrs

Nursing diagnosis: Potential for injury: related to decreased peripheral vision

Expected patient outcomes	Nursing interventions	Rationale
Patient describes measures to prevent injury	Explain nature of decreased peripheral vision and relate it to bumping into objects	Knowledge of rationale may increase probability of actions to prevent injury
	Suggest he turn head to see each side	Increases field of vision
	Suggest couple consider clearing wider walk areas in living quarters	Reducing clutter will decrease chance of injury

tion of eye drops helps to prevent rapid systemic effects.

In severe acute conditions, osmotic agents are given to lower IOP by drawing fluid from the eye. If the oral osmotic agent is ineffective or produces nausea, mannitol is given intravenously.

Mydriatics and cycloplegic agents are *contraindicated* in persons with glaucoma because these drugs may further restrict drainage of aqueous humor.

☐ Surgery

For open-angle glaucoma, surgery is indicated when conservative measures fail to control the rise in IOP. The procedure of choice is *laser trabeculoplasty* in which an argon laser beam is directed toward the trabecular meshwork to change the meshwork pattern and open drainage for the aqueous humor. The procedure is performed as ambulatory surgery; the person usually remains at the surgical center for 3 to 4 hours to monitor IOP, which may rise initially. Most persons need to continue taking antiglaucoma medications after surgery.

Angle-closure glaucoma usually requires surgery. Different procedures may be used. Peripheral *iridotomy* or *iridectomy* may be performed for open- or closed-angle glaucoma as a hope for permanent cure. Lasers are now used to destroy a small wedge of the iris and open a permanent drainage system between the posterior and anterior chambers. This procedure may also be done as ambulatory surgery.

Filtering procedures are done when other procedures fail to halt the rise in IOP. The procedure of choice is usually a *trabeculectomy* in which an opening is made between the anterior chamber and the subconjunctival space (Fig. 20-12, *B*). Trabeculectomy usually requires hospitalization. The care of the postoperative patient is described on p. 535.

■ ASSISTING WITH COMFORT

Pain usually decreases as the IOP decreases. Analgesics may be prescribed. Cold eye compresses may be helpful for painful eye spasms.

■ COUNSELING AND TEACHING

Glaucoma is a chronic condition, and the patient with newly diagnosed glaucoma needs assistance in understanding and learning to live with the disease. Despite explanations from the physician, the person frequently hopes that an operation will provide a cure, that no further treatment will be necessary, and perhaps that the lost sight will be restored. It should be explained that *lost vision cannot be restored* but that further loss can usually be prevented and normal activities can be pursued if the person continues medical care. There usually is no restriction on the use of the eyes (see the box below).

✣ Evaluation

Evaluation is based on the expected patient outcomes. Questions to ask include the following:
1. Is the patient comfortable?
2. Does the patient know the chronic nature of the disease and treatment?

■ RETINAL DETACHMENT
■ Pathophysiology

The retina is the part of the eye that perceives light; it coordinates and transmits impulses from receptor nerve cells to the optic nerve. It consists of two layers.

Teaching the patient with glaucoma

1. Medical supervision will be required for the rest of life.
2. Eye drops *must* be continued as long as prescribed, even in the absence of symptoms
   a. Blurred vision decreases with prolonged use
   b. Avoid driving for 1 to 2 hours after administration of miotics.
3. To prevent complications:
   a. Press lacrimal duct for 1 minute after eye drop insertion to prevent rapid systemic absorption
   b. Have reserve bottle of eyedrops at home
   c. Carry eyedrops when away from home
   d. Carry card identifying glaucoma and the eyedrops solution prescribed.
4. Bright lights and darkness are not harmful.
5. There is no apparent relationship between vascular hypertension and ocular hypertension.
6. Report any reappearance of symptoms immediately to ophthalmologist.
7. If admitted to hospital for a different medical condition, alert the staff of continued need for prescribed eyedrops.
8. Avoid the use of mydriatic or cycloplegic drugs (for example, atropine) that dilate the pupils.

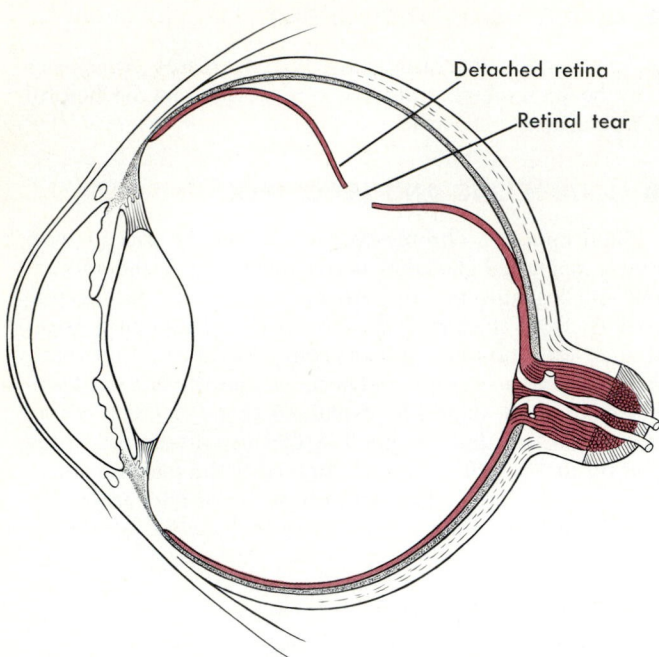

Detached retina

Retinal tear

Fig. 20-16   Retinal detachment.

Retinal detachment occurs when the two retinal layers separate as a result of accumulation of fluid or traction produced by contraction of the vitreous body (Fig. 20-16). As the detachment extends and becomes complete, blindness results. Myopic degeneration, trauma, aphakia (absence of the crystalline lens) are the most frequent causes of retinal detachment. Detachment may follow sudden severe physical exertion, especially in persons who are debilitated. Most often, however, there is no apparent cause.

Assessment

Retinal detachment may occur suddenly or develop slowly. The person first notices flashes of light, followed by floating spots before the eye and progressive loss of vision. The floating spots are blood and retinal cells that are freed at the time of the tear and cast shadows on the retina as they seem to drift about the eye. The area of visual loss depends entirely on the location of the detachment. Usually there is a superior retinal detachment with inferior visual loss. When the detachment is extensive and occurs quickly, the patient may have the sensation that a curtain has been drawn before the eyes. The diagnosis is confirmed by ophthalmoscopic examination.

Ongoing nursing assessment includes the patient's subjective statements concerning changes in vision and observations related to signs of anxiety. The person with both eyes bandaged is assessed for ability to carry out activities of daily living.

Data analysis: nursing diagnoses

Nursing diagnoses are determined from assessment of patient data. Possible nursing diagnoses for the person with retinal detachment may include, but are not limited to, the following:

Diagnostic title	Possible etiologies
Anxiety	Threat of loss of vision, threat to self-concept, threat of change in role functioning
Potential for injury	Decreased vision
Knowledge deficit	Lack of exposure/recall, information misinterpretation, lack of interest in learning

Planning: expected patient outcomes

Expected patient outcomes for the person with retinal detachment may include, but are not limited to, the following:
1. Anxiety is decreased.
2. No further vision loss occurs.
3. Patient can describe
   a. Correct use of eye medications
   b. Signs and symptoms indicating further retinal detachment
   c. Extent of limitations on activity

Implementation

ASSISTING WITH ACHIEVEMENT OF THERAPEUTIC GOALS

Immediate care for the person with detachment of the retina includes keeping the eye at rest and in position to prevent further detachment until surgery can be done to repair the detachment. Bed rest with monocular or bilateral eye patches is usually prescribed. The head is positioned so the retinal hole is in the most dependent position (gravity may help prevent the first retinal layer from pulling further away from the second coat).

Although most surgeons do not use binocular patches, some do patch both eyes preoperatively and for 2 or 3 days postoperatively. Safety precautions, such as side rails, are essential if binocular patching is used. Call signals are placed within easy patient reach. Activities that facilitate communication with blind persons are employed (p. 526).

COUNSELING

Anxiety frequently results from concern over possible loss of vision and feelings about having eyes bandaged. Generally, the person has lost vision rapidly and is afraid of losing more vision. Patients need an opportunity to dis-

Table 20-13 Surgical procedures for retinal detachment

Purpose	Procedure	Method
Removal of fluid from sub-retinal space	Drainage	Needle insertion
Sealing of retinal tear by creating inflammation to adhere retina to choroid	Cryosurgery	Supercooled probe applied to scleral surface over tear
	Diathermy	Application of diathermy (heat) to scleral surface over tear
	Photocoagulation	Strong light focused through pupil onto retinal tear
	Laser	Laser beam focused through pupil onto retinal tear
Splinting of choroid to retina until choroidal scar can seal tear	Scleral buckling	Tuck taken in sclera (to indent sclera and choroid) and sutured; buckle held in place with a piece of silicone held by a strap (Fig. 20-17)

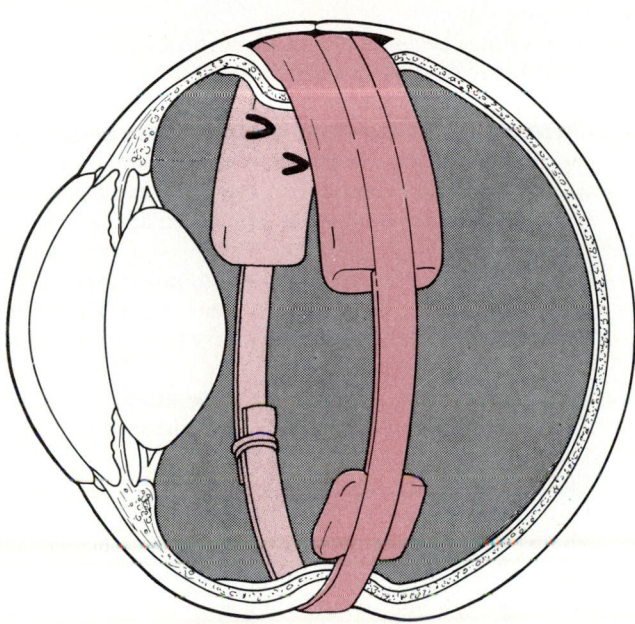

Fig. 20-17 Scleral buckle.

cuss their concerns. Although the promise of restoration of vision cannot be made, it can be comforting to the person to know that with care most retinal detachments can be repaired by surgery.

■ RETINAL SURGERY

□ Surgical procedures

Surgery is done under either local or general anesthesia. Although subretinal fluid may be removed by perforating the choroid through the sclera, the fluid usually reabsorbs if the retinal layers are rejoined.[25] Surgery consists of producing an area of inflammation in the defect to close the opening and seal the retinal layers together. The sealing process may be done by cold (cryosurgery), heat (dia-

thermy), light (photocoagulation), or by laser (Table 20-13). Cyclopentolate or phenylephrine is used to keep the pupils widely dilated during surgery so that the tears in the retina can be identified.

A scleral buckling procedure (Fig. 20-17) may be done to hold the retina and choroid together until the choroidal scar can form to permanently seal the hole or tear. The choroid is pushed into contact with the retinal tear during healing, and vitreous adhesions that have exerted a pull on the retinal break are relaxed as the size of the scleral shell is decreased.

□ Postoperative care

1. Position patient as instructed.
2. Avoid jerking movements of the head (combing hair, sneezing, coughing, vomiting); give prescribed anti-emetics or cough medications as necessary.
3. Assist with activities of daily living as necessary to prevent jerking or excessive head movements.
4. Tell patient to limit reading to prevent excess movements of eyes; television is permitted.
5. Apply cold compresses as prescribed to reduce swelling and promote comfort.
6. Instill prescribed eyedrops (mydriatics, cycloplegics, steroids, antibiotics).

□ Patient teaching

Patients need to know about activity restrictions, correct instillation of eye medications, and signs and symptoms indicating further retinal detachment to report to the ophthalmologist (see the box on p. 544).

✚ Evaluation

Evaluation is based on expected patient outcomes. Questions to ask may include the following:
1. Is patient comfortable?
2. Has further detachment been avoided?
3. Has patient had opportunities to express concerns?
4. Does patient know expectations after discharge?

Teaching the patient with retinal detachment

1. Return to sedentary activity in 2 weeks; no heavy lifting or active physical activity for 6 weeks, or as instructed by physician.
2. Check with physician concerning shampooing of hair.
3. Limit reading for 3 weeks (or as instructed by physician).
4. Use correct technique for administration of eye medications (p. 530).
5. Report to ophthalmologist any signs of further detachment (flashes of light, increase in "floaters," blurred vision).
6. Report for medical follow-up visits as instructed.

■ SUMMARY

1. Ophthalmologists (oculists) are physicians who treat eye diseases and may prescribe lenses; optometrists prescribe lenses and provide visual training; opticians make eyeglasses and contact lenses.
2. With hyperopia (farsightedness) light rays focus behind the retina; with myopia (nearsightedness) the rays focus in front of the retina; with astigmatism the rays do not focus at the same point because of irregular curvature of the cornea.
3. 20/40 vision means that the person is able to read at 20 feet only what should be readable at 40 feet.
4. Contact lenses may be rigid (including gas permeable) or soft (including extended wear lenses); there are advantages and disadvantages of each type.
5. Eye safety measures include early medical care of eye problems, avoidance of use of previously prescribed eye medications, protecting eyes against foreign objects or bright lights, and removing nonembedded foreign objects immediately by rinsing with water or by carefully removing from the conjunctival sac.
6. Activities for the newly blind person consist of facilitating their independence in ADL and providing counseling to facilitate coping.
7. Inflammation of the eye can occur in the external structures, cornea, and uvea (iris, ciliary body, and choroid); the most common inflammations are styes and conjunctivitis.
8. Treatments for eye inflammations include eye compresses, eye irrigations, and ophthalmic antibiotics (steriods may be given for allergic inflammations but not pyogenic).
9. If the cornea becomes damaged, corneal grafts (keratoplasty) may be performed using donor corneal tissue.
10. A cataract is an opacity of the lens. A cataract that interferes with vision may be removed either extracapsularly (leaving the posterior capsule intact) or intracapsularly (lens and entire capsule). Most persons now have an intraocular lens implanted at the time of surgery.
11. Most eye surgery is performed as ambulatory surgery. Preoperative care includes insertion of mydriatic or cycloplegic (dilates pupil and relaxes ciliary muscle) and local anesthetic eye drops.
12. Postoperative care centers on preventing increased IOP, stress on the suture line, hemorrhage into the anterior chamber, and infection.
13. The characteristic sign of glaucoma is increased IOP. Most glaucomas are of the primary open-angle type in which aqueous outflow is blocked because of degenerative changes in the trabecular meshwork, canal of Schlemm, and adjacent channels; the disorder is insidious in onset, slowly progressive, and usually lacks symptoms in the early stage.

Putting knowledge to practice

■ Examine the chart of a patient with an eye problem. Explain the rationale for the drug therapy.

■ Write a care plan for a patient with limited vision. How would a care plan for a person who has recent loss of vision compare with that of a person blinded from childhood?

■ Consider bandaging your eyes for one day and carry out all your usual activities. What problems did you encounter? What did you find helpful?

■ Describe how you would respond to a person who says, "I don't see as well as I used to. I don't have to go to an eye doctor; he'll only tell me I need glasses, and I already have a pair."

■ What services and facilities are available to persons in your community who have limited vision? How are these financed?

■ Pretend for 2 days that you have had eye surgery and are instructed not to bend at the waist or lift any heavy objects or to strain with any activity. What problems did you encounter? Now consider that your knees are crippled with arthritis: how would that affect an activity such as putting on pantyhose, given the same restrictions?

14. Closed-angle glaucoma occurs in a person with a narrow anterior chamber when the iris falls forward, blocking entrance to aqueous fluid outflow; it is often sudden in onset and requires immediate medical attention; symptoms include severe eye pain, blurred vision, and halos seen around lights.
15. Conservative treatment for glaucoma includes medications to decrease the IOP (miotics and beta-blockers that constrict the pupil, adrenergic agents and carbonic anhydrase inhibitors that decrease production of aqueous humor, and osmotic agents that enhance fluid flow out of the eye). Surgery consists of opening up the trabecular meshwork, opening a channel between the anterior and posterior chambers, or opening a channel between the anterior chamber and subconjunctival space.
16. Persons with glaucoma require continued treatment for life to prevent buildup of IOP; lost vision cannot be restored.
17. Retinal detachment results when the two retinal layers separate, interfering with vision; symptoms include flashes of light, floating spots before the eye, and progressive loss of vision. Persons with retinal detachment require immediate medical treatment.
18. Surgery is performed to return the retina to its original position and adhere the first layer to the bottom layer by means of an inflammatory process. Postoperative care includes avoiding jerking movements of the head and limiting exertional activities until healing has occurred; eyedrops are required during this period to rest the eye and prevent infection.

REFERENCES AND SELECTED READINGS

1. American Foundation for the Blind: Directory of agencies serving the visually handicapped in the United States, New York, 1983, The William Byrd Press.
2. Andreason, MEK: Color vision defects in the elderly, J Gerontol Nurs 6:383-384, 1980.
3. Boruchoff, SA: Ophthalmic surgery: risks and benefits, Emerg Med 19(11):59-62, 1987.
4. Boyd-Monk, H: Examining the external eye, I, Nurs 80 10(5):58-63, 1980.
5. Boyd-Monk, H: Examining the external eye, II, Nurs 80 10(6):58-63, 1980.
6. *Boyd-Monk, H: Retinal detachment and vitrectomy: nursing care, Nurs Clin North Am 16:433-451, 1981.
7. *Boyd-Monk, H, and Starita, RJ: Surgical intervention to stop glaucoma, JONT 4(3):12-15, 1985.
8. Capeno, D and others: The elderly patient with cataracts, Hosp Pract 22(3):19-24, 1987.
9. *Conrad, FL: Tips for treating corrosive burns, Nurs 83 13(4):55-57, 1983.
10. Contact lens allergy: the new conjunctivitis, Am J Nurs 87:11-12, 1987.
11. *Carver, J: 630, 1987.
12. *Ehrenberg, M: 1987.
13. *Gallagher, MA: Co 81:1845, 1981.
14. Gottsch, JD and others: Ca Hosp Med (suppl) 23(4):21-29,
15. *Hayes, PL: Treatment and nurs Nurs Clin North Am 16:383-392, 1.
16. *Herget, M: For visually impaired di 83:1557-1560, 1983.
17. Kapperud, MJ: The aging eye: a guide for n al, 1983, The Minnesota Society for the Prevention ness and Preservation of Hearing.
18. *Kilroy, JL: Care and teaching of patients with glaucoma, Nurs Clin North Am 16:393-404, 1981.
19. Kopak, CA: Sensory loss in the aged: the role of the nurse and family, Nurs Clin North Am 18:373-384, 1983.
20. *Lent-Wunderlich, E, and others: Helping your patient through eye surgery, RN 49(6):43-47, 1986.
21. Lindstrom, RL: Advances in corneal transplantation, New Eng J Med 315(1):57-59, 1986.
22. Mason, G, and others: Postanesthesia care of the ophthalmic patient, J Post Anesth Nurs 1:23-25, 1986.
23. Misuse of steriod eye medications, Nurses' Drug Alert, Am J Nurs 87:71, 1987.
24. National Society to Prevent Blindness, Operational Research Analysis, New York, 1980, The Society.
25. Newell, F: Ophthalmology: principles and practice, ed 6, St. Louis, 1986, The CV Mosby Co.
26. *Osguthorpe, NC: If your patient has contact lenses, Am J Nurs 84:1255-1256, 1984.
27. *Resler, MM, and Tumulty, G: Glaucoma update, Am J Nurs 83:752-756, 1983.
28. *Shadick, MH: I feel I'll be able to serve my patients more effectively because of my blindness, Occup Health Nurs 29(2):16-18, 1981.
29. Smith, S: Day-care cataract surgery: the patient's perspective, J Ophthalmic Nurs Technol 6(2):50-56, 1987.
30. Soll, DB, and others: Drugs and glaucoma, Am Fam Phys 34(1):181-185, 1986.
31. *Stern, EJ: Helping the person with low vision, Am J Nurs 80:1788-1790, 1980.
32. *Sullivan, N: Vision in the elderly, J Gerontol Nurs 9:228-235, 1983.
33. *Todd, B: Using eye drops and ointments safely, Geriatric Nurs 4:53, 56-57, 1983.
34. *Tooke, MC, Elders, J, and Johnson, DE: Corneal transplantation, Am J Nurs 86:685-687, 1986.
35. Vaughan, D, and Asbury, T: General ophthalmology, ed 11, Los Altos, Calif, 1986, Lange Medical Publications.
36. West, K: ABC's of cataract surgery preparation: assessment, briefing, and counseling, J Ophthalmic Nurs Technol 6:156-158, 1987.
37. *Wong, EK: Cataract surgery: providing total patient care, Nurs 83 13(4):65-69, 1983.

*References preceded by an asterisk are particularly well suited for student reading.

21

The Patient with Ear Problems

BARBARA C. LONG

CHAPTER OBJECTIVES

After studying this chapter, the student should be able to:

- Describe the mechanics of sound waves and hearing.
- Describe measures to prevent hearing loss.
- Describe the pathophysiology and nursing requirements for persons with ear infections.
- Describe the pathophysiology and care of the person with a balance disorder.
- Describe care of the person having ear surgery.
- Differentiate conductive and sensorineural hearing loss and describe methods of assessment.
- Describe methods of aural rehabilitation and communication with hearing impaired persons.

The ear is the organ of hearing and equilibrium. Sound is transmitted to the inner ear where it is converted to neural activity and transmitted to the brain for interpretation. Interference with this process leads to impaired hearing. In addition, structures in the inner ear maintain an individual's sense of equilibrium; interference with this mechanism leads to vertigo, producing dizziness and loss of balance.

The root word for the ear is *oto-*, such as in *otology* (science of the ear) or *otosclerosis* ("hardening of the ear"). In some instances the second "o" is dropped, such as in *otitis* (inflammation of the ear).

Nurses are involved primarily in prevention and detection of hearing and vestibular disorders. In addition, nurses participate in health teaching for hearing-impaired persons, in facilitating communication when hearing-impaired persons are hospitalized, and in providing care for persons receiving treatment for disorders of the ear.

■ ANATOMY AND PHYSIOLOGY

The ears are normally placed on each side of the head at eye level; an imaginary line parallel to the floor can be drawn from the outer canthus of the eye to the top of the outer ear. A lower placed ear may indicate chromosomal or congenital renal abnormalities. The ears are located in the temporal bone, which provides protection for the organs of hearing and equilibrium. Each ear is divided into three parts: the external ear, the middle ear and mastoid, and the inner ear.

■ External ear

The external ear consists of two parts, the pinna (auricle) and the external auditory canal. The *pinna* is composed primarily of cartilage and skin with little subcutaneous fat except for the lobule (lower tip). The external ear is innervated by cranial nerve V (trigeminal), a branch of cranial nerve X (vagus), and by cervical nerves.

The ear canal provides a channel along which sound travels to the eardrum. The canal is an S-shaped curve about 2.5 cm (1 inch) long through the temporal bone in an inward, forward, and downward slope in an adult. There are constrictions in the canal close to the midpoint and the eardrum. The canal and outer ear drum are covered by thin sensitive skin. Numerous fine hairs protect the canal from foreign debris, and sebaceous glands in the distal third of the canal provide cerumen (wax) for lubrication.

The *tympanic membrane* (eardrum) separates the external ear from the middle ear. The eardrum is a thin, tough, translucent membrane, nearly oval in shape and directed obliquely downward. The malleus ossicle of the middle ear generally can be seen through the membrane. The tym-

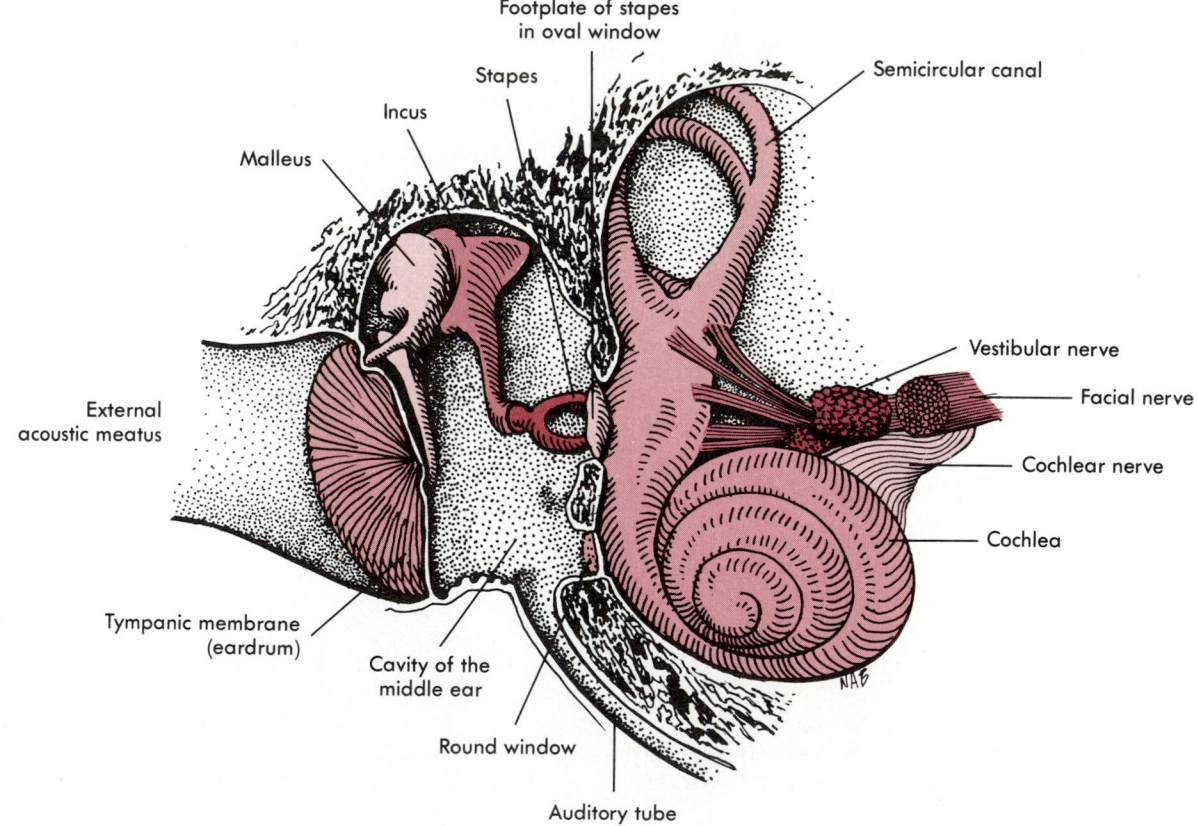

Fig. 21-1 Structures of the ear.

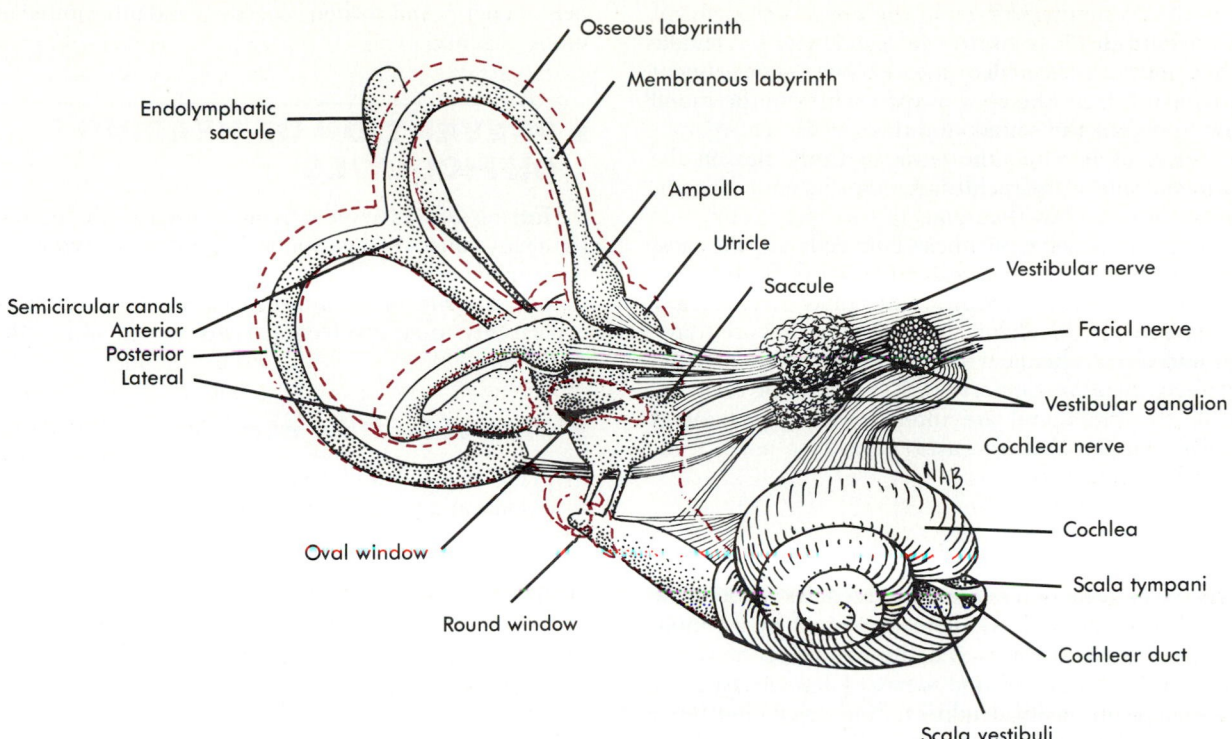

Endolymphatic
saccule

Osseous labyrinth

Membranous labyrinth

Ampulla

Utricle

Saccule

Vestibular nerve

Facial nerve

Vestibular ganglion

Cochlear nerve

Semicircular canals
Anterior
Posterior
Lateral

NAB.

Cochlea

Scala tympani

Cochlear duct

Oval window

Round window

Scala vestibuli

Fig. 21-2   Structures of the inner ear.

panic membrane protects the middle ear and vibrates with incoming sound waves for hearing.

■ Middle ear

The middle ear lies directly behind the eardrum and is a small air-filled space located in the petrous portion of the temporal bone (toward the face). It contains the ossicles, oval and round windows, and the eustachian tube (Fig. 21-1). The *ossicles* are three movable small bones that transverse the middle ear; these three bones are called the *malleus* (hammer), *incus* (anvil), and *stapes* (stirrup) because of their shapes. The malleus is attached at one end to the tympanic membrane and at the other end to the incus. The stapes connects the incus to the oval window in direct contact with the perilymph of the inner ear. The ossicles mechanically transmit sound vibrations to the fluid in the inner ear. The *oval window* is not a true window because it is covered by the footplate of the stapes. The *round window* provides an exit for sound vibrations from the inner ear.

The *eustachian tube* (auditory tube) is a channel extending from the middle ear into the nasopharynx. It allows air to enter and leave the middle ear to equalize pressure on both sides of the eardrum. Swallowing or yawning can move air in and out of the middle ear to change air pressure in the middle ear. Portions of the facial nerves that control movement of the face and supply taste to the tongue are located in the middle ear.

The *mastoid* portion of the temporal bone is located pos-

terior to the external ear and includes the mastoid air cells and mastoid antrum (cavity) that connects to the middle ear. Because of this direct connection infection of the middle ear may lead to mastoiditis. The mastoid process is a conical-shaped portion of mastoid bone that protrudes behind the lower portion of the pinna. The mastoid assists the middle ear in adjusting to pressure changes and lightens the mastoid bone.

■ Inner ear

The inner ear (labyrinth) contains both the organs for hearing (cochlea) and the organs of balance (semicircular canals and vestibule) (Fig. 21-2). The bony labyrinth is a rigid capsule. The membranous labyrinth (consisting of three semicircular canals, vestibule, and cochlea) lies within the bony labyrinth but does not completely fill it. Position and balance are maintained by the semicircular canals (rotational movement) and by the membranous utricle and saccule in the vestibule (linear movements).

Two separate fluids are found in the labyrinth, the *perilymph* between the bony and membranous labyrinths and the *endolymph* within the membranous labyrinth. The endolymph is in a contained closed system; the perilymphatic spaces connect to the subarachnoid space containing cerebrospinal fluid.

The *cochlea* is a spiraling bony tube resembling a snail shell. The tube is separated into two compartments by a membranous tube called the *cochlear duct*, which contains endolymph and the organ of Corti. The two compartments of the cochlea contain perilymph; the upper compartment (scala vestibuli) leads from the oval window of the middle ear to the apex of the cochlea, and the lower compartment (scala tympani) from the apex of the cochlea to the round window to permit the sound vibrations to escape.

The organ of hearing, the *organ of Corti,* lies on the basilar membrane of the cochlear duct for its entire length. The organ of Corti has thousands of tiny "hair cells" that project into the endolymph; these hair cells are the most fragile elements in the ear and are crucial for hearing. Sound waves enter the cochlear duct and mechanically bend the hair cells. Mechanical sound vibrations are transformed into electrochemical impulses that are then transmitted along the acoustic nerve (CN VIII) to the temporal cortex of the brain and are interpreted as meaningful sound. Destruction of the acoustic nerve by a tumor leads to loss of hearing.

■ Sound waves and hearing

Sound is a form of energy generated by a vibrating source. Pure tones such as those generated by a tuning fork are simple sound waves. The human voice, however, produces more complex sound waves. Characteristics of sounds include intensity, loudness, frequency, and pitch (see the box below).

Speech that is comfortably loud to a person with normal hearing ranges in intensity from approximately 40 to 65 decibels. The decibel levels of various environmental sounds and situations are found in Fig. 21-3.

A sound with a low frequency is perceived as a tone low in pitch, whereas a sound with high frequency is perceived as a high-pitched tone. A child or young adult with normal hearing can often hear frequencies ranging from 20 to 20,000 Hz. Hearing is most sensitive for frequencies of 500 to 4000 Hz.

Sound reaches the inner ear by one of two ways: air conduction or bone conduction. Air conduction is the most sensitive. In air conduction sound waves pass through the ear canal to the ossicular chain to the inner ear (Fig. 21-4). In *bone conduction* hearing is caused by sound being transmitted through the bones of the skull to the inner ear. Sound energy is transformed in the inner ear into

neural energy and is then "decoded" and interpreted by the brain as sound.

■ PREVENTION OF HEARING DIFFICULTIES

Hearing difficulties may begin at any age. Understanding the many causes of hearing loss is important for all health team members in all settings. Because nurses occupy a unique position in the health care system, they have the opportunity to be involved in many aspects of health care of the ear.

■ Care of healthy ears

A certain amount of cerumen (ear wax) in the ear canal is normal, and persons who have no wax have itching and scaling in the ear canal. Usually it is not necessary to clean the ears to remove wax. Occasionally, when the wax be-

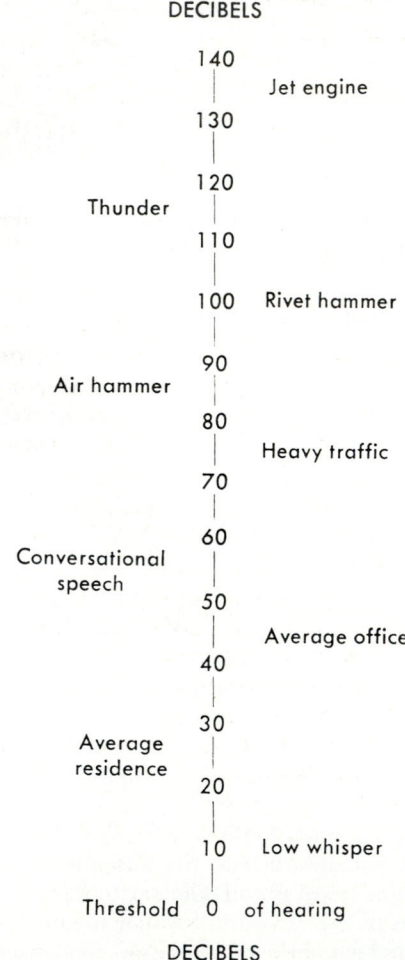

Fig. 21-3 Intensity range of human hearing. Intensity levels of various environmental sounds and situations. (From Saunders, W.H., and others: Nursing care in eye, ear, nose, and throat disorders, ed 4, St. Louis, 1979, The CV Mosby Co.)

Characteristics of sound

Intensity	Pressure exerted by a sound measured in decibels (db)
Loudness	Sensation of sound intensity experienced by a person
Frequency	Number of sound waves emanating from a source per second; expressed in hertz (Hz)
Pitch	Sensation of sound frequency experienced by a person

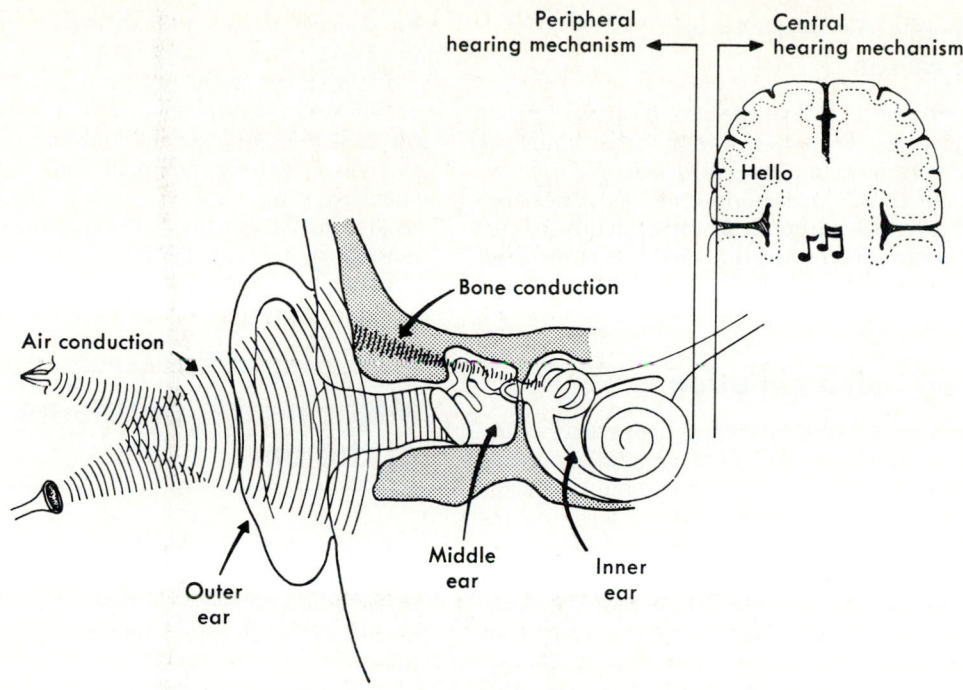

Peripheral hearing mechanism

Central hearing mechanism

Hello

Bone conduction

Air conduction

Middle ear

Inner ear

Outer ear

Fig. 21-4 Schema depicting functions of hearing mechanism as it translates sound waves into meaningful sensations. (From Saunders, WH, and others: Nursing care in eye, ear, nose, and throat disorders, ed 4, St. Louis, 1979, The CV Mosby Co.)

comes impacted and causes pain or temporary deafness, it must be removed by the physician or person instructed in the procedure.

The outer ear may be washed with soap and water during bathing, although this is often unnecessary as the ear canal is generally self-cleaning. If necessary, a cotton-tipped applicator moistened with alcohol may be inserted into the ear canal *only the length of the cotton tip,* which is more than enough to clean the short external canal without causing further problems.

■ Prevention of ear disease/trauma

During upper respiratory tract infections, the nose should be blown with both nostrils open. Excessive pressure from nose blowing can force infected secretions up the eustachian tube into the middle ear, leading to middle ear infection.

Persons having ear pain, swelling, drainage, prolonged feelings of plugged ears, or decreased hearing are referred to a physician for treatment. Chronic problems such as perforated ear drums and necrotic ossicles may result from inattention to early signs of ear disorders.

The following activities may lead to ear infection or trauma and should be *avoided:*

1. Inserting foreign objects into the ear (such as a hard object to remove wax or to scratch the ear canal if itching)
2. Swimming in stagnant water or in water identified as polluted
3. Instilling outdated medicated solutions into the ear

Selected ototoxic drugs

Antibiotics

Streptomycin
Dihydrostreptomycin
Gentamicin (Garamycin)
Neomycin
Kanamycin
Vancomycin
Polymyxin B/Colistin
Chloramphenicol (Chloromycetin)
Capreomycin

Diuretics

Ethacrynic acid (Edecrin)
Furosemide (Lasix)
Acetazolamide (Diamox)

Salicylates

Acetylsalicylic acid (aspirin)

Other drugs

Quinine
Chloroquine
Nitrogen mustard
Bleomycin
Quinidine

■ Monitoring side effects of ototoxic drugs

Some drugs are ototoxic (see the box on p. 551); that is, they have adverse effects on the cochlea, vestibule, or acoustic nerve. Persons taking ototoxic drugs need to know the side effects of these drugs to prevent loss of hearing. If symptoms of dizziness, decreased hearing acuity, or tinnitus (ringing in the ears) occur, the next dose of the drug is omitted and the physician is consulted. Audiometric testing may be necessary.

■ Monitoring noise pollution

A major cause of hearing loss is occupational hearing loss. Exposure to *industrial noise* levels greater than 85 to 90 db for months or years causes cochlear damage. Some 9 million workers are exposed daily to noise levels on the job that are potentially hazardous to hearing. Health team members in industry can help prevent deafness caused by noise of high intensity by teaching employees why they should wear earplugs. Courses are available to familiarize nurses with industrial hearing conservation requirements.

The Occupational Safety and Health Administration (OSHA) has established acceptable levels of noise in work environments. *Unprotected* exposure to noise levels in excess of 90 db over an 8-hour day is considered excessive and should be avoided (Table 21-1).

Other causes of noise-induced hearing loss include *firearms* and *high-intensity music*. With an M16 rifle or sport rifle, hearing loss tends to be greater in the ear opposite the dominant hand. With revolvers, hearing loss is equal in both ears. A person firing guns who notices tinnitus, sensation of fullness in the ear, or temporary hearing loss should stop firing guns or wear suitable ear protectors.

Sound in front of a rock band can reach up to 120 db, and hearing losses of up to 50 db have been measured in some members of rock bands. In the early stage, there is a loss of hearing *at* or *near* frequencies of 4000 Hz. Later

Table 21-1 Permissible noise exposures

Duration per day (hr)	Sound level (dbA, slow)
8	90
6	92
4	95
3	97
2	100
1½	102
1	105
½	110
¼	115

From US Department of Labor, Occupational Safety and Health Administration: Noise: the environmental problem, a guide to OSHA standards, Washington, DC, 1979, US Government Printing Office.

the damage extends to both higher and lower tones, with the lower tones affected least.

If proximity to the high noise level cannot be avoided, *ear protectors or earplugs* should be worn. The earplugs are inserted into the external auditory canal and can reduce the noise reaching the middle ear by 10 to 30 db. Usually standard plugs are effective, but custom-made plugs molded to the person's ear canal may be obtained. If the noise level is extremely high (sound levels may reach 140 db or higher), individuals are not adequately protected with earplugs alone and must wear *ear muffs.*

Major health problems of the ear

Ear disorders may occur in any part of the ear. The more common ear disorders are discussed in this chapter under three headings because of the commonalities in the required care. Disorders included in each category are as follows:

1. Infections of the external/middle ear
   a. External otitis
   b. Otitis media: serous, purulent (acute, chronic)
   c. Chronic mastoiditis
2. Disorders affecting balance
   a. Labyrinthitis
   b. Menière's disease
   c. Acoustic neuroma
3. Disorders affecting hearing
   a. Conductive hearing loss: otosclerosis
   b. Sensorineural hearing loss
   c. Presbycusis

■ EXTERNAL/MIDDLE EAR INFECTIONS

The most common disorders of the external and middle ear are infections (Table 21-2). Although many of these infections occur in children, they may also occur in adults.

■ Pathophysiology

Organisms may enter the external ear by way of the external orifice or the middle ear via the eustachian tube, resulting in infections. Infection of the labyrinth (inner ear) may result from extension of middle ear infections, but the effect there is primarily on balance (p. 557).

Infections of the external ear, *external otitis*, are primarily bacterial (staphylococci or gram-negative organisms) or fungal. A form of seborrheic dermatitis (Chapter 39) may result from extensive use of objects such as earphones. Infection develops in the skin lining the ear canal, and swelling and debris may lead to closure of the canal. Furuncles (boils) may also develop. Pain results from pressure

Table 21-2   Infections of the external/middle ear

Disorder	Description	Signs and symptoms	Medical therapy
External otitis	Inflammation of the external ear; may be acute or chronic	Pain with movement of auricle, redness, scaling, itching, swelling, watery discharge, crusting of external ear	Cleaning to remove debris; antibiotic drops or ointment, systemic antibiotics if necessary
Serous otitis media	Collection of sterile serum in middle ear; may be acute or chronic	Sense of fullness in ear, hearing loss, low-pitched tinnitus, earache	Removal of eustachian obstruction by aspiration or insertion of tubes for drainage
Acute purulent otitis media	Infection of middle ear, usually by pneumococci, streptococci, staphylococci, or *Haemophilus influenzae*	Sense of fullness in ear, severe throbbing pain, hearing loss, tinnitus, fever	Antibiotics If severe, bed rest, analgesics, nasal vasoconstrictors Myringotomy if necessary
Chronic otitis media	Chronic inflammation of middle ear; sequela of acute otitis media	Deafness, occasional pain, dizziness, chronic discharge from ear	Local debridement; topical and systemic antibiotics; mastoidectomy and tympanoplasty may be necessary
Chronic mastoiditis	Spread of infection into mastoid from repeated otitis media	Middle ear drainage	Mastoid irrigation; antibiotics; may need mastoidectomy

on the sensitive skin lining and can be severe because there is no room for expansion in the bony canal. Activities leading to water retention in the ear such as swimming, especially in contaminated water, promote external otitis.

Infection of the middle ear, *otitis media,* is the most common disorder of the middle ear. The infection may be serous or purulent and acute or chronic. *Serous otitis media* develops from collection of sterile serum in the middle ear when the eustachian tube becomes blocked because of previous infection or allergy (Fig. 21-5). *Purulent otitis media* develops from bacterial infection and may be acute or chronic. Chronic infection may spread into the mastoid

(chronic mastoiditis) or cause necrosis of the tympanic membrane or ossicles, leading to hearing loss. Acute mastoiditis is rare because of antibiotic treatment of acute otitis media. With chronic mastoiditis, a *cholesteatoma* (benign growth) may develop. It is a skin-lined sac with debris and is often infected. The cholesteatoma may recur when removed.

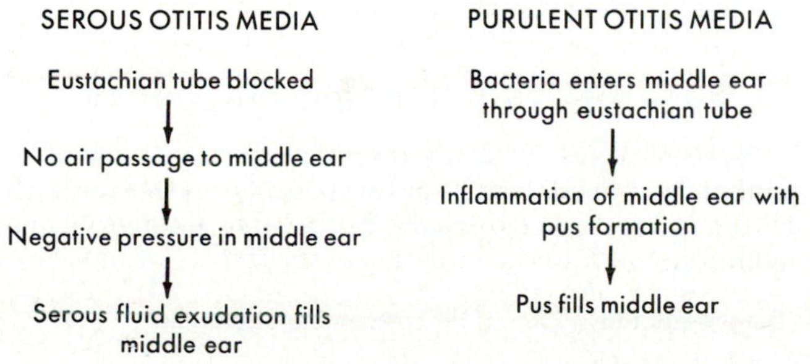

Assessment

A person with an ear infection is usually diagnosed and treated on an ambulatory basis. Early detection and treatment are important to prevent development of chronic infections with subsequent loss of hearing.

■ SUBJECTIVE DATA

The major symptoms of external and middle ear infections are *pain* and *loss of hearing,* and data are collected about the onset, duration, and severity of these symptoms. Pain results from pressure on the sensitive skin lining the external canal or pressure on the eardrum from fluid buildup in the middle ear. A blocked external canal or fluid in the middle ear interferes with passage of sound waves leading to decreased hearing. Persons with ear infections should be questioned about knowledge of preventive measures.

SEROUS OTITIS MEDIA

Eustachian tube blocked

↓

No air passage to middle ear

↓

Negative pressure in middle ear

↓

Serous fluid exudation fills middle ear

PURULENT OTITIS MEDIA

Bacteria enters middle ear through eustachian tube

↓

Inflammation of middle ear with pus formation

↓

Pus fills middle ear

Fig. 21-5   Pathogenesis of otitis media.

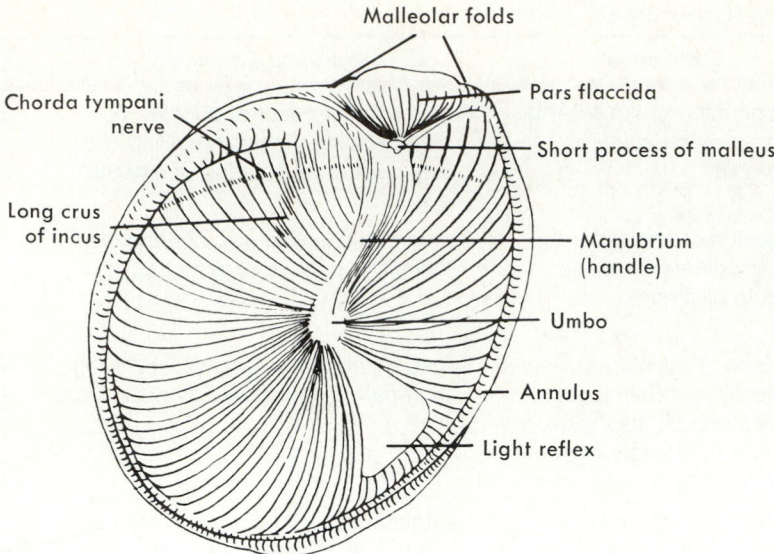

Malleolar folds

Chorda tympani
nerve

Pars flaccida

Short process of malleus

Long crus
of incus

Manubrium
(handle)

Umbo

Annulus

Light reflex

Fig. 21-6 Right tympanic membrane. (From Prior, JA, and Silberstein, JS: Physical diagnosis: the history and examination of the patient, ed 5, St. Louis, 1977, The CV Mosby Co.)

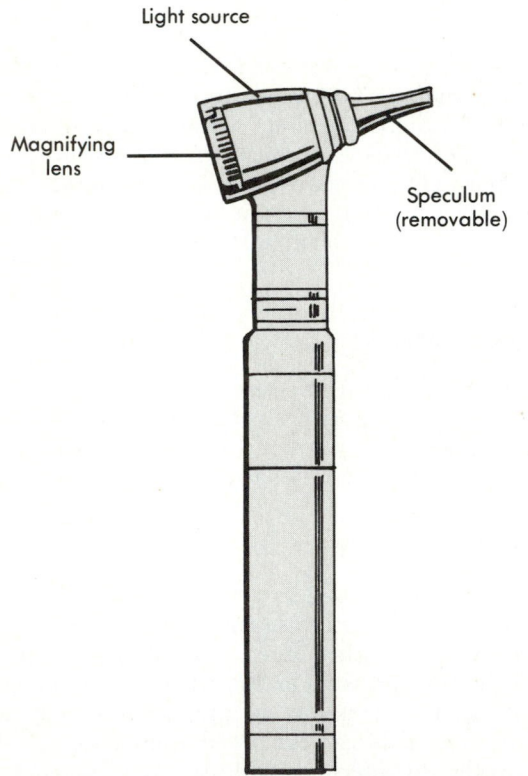

Light source

Magnifying
lens

Speculum
(removable)

Fig. 21-7 Otoscope.

■ OBJECTIVE DATA

The outer ear is inspected for *drainage,* which is described in terms of type (serous, purulent, bloody) and extent of crusting. Pain with palpation of the external ear occurs with external otitis but not usually with otitis media.

☐ Assessment of the external ear canal and eardrum

The eardrum is important in physical assessment of the ear because it serves as a translucent window through which disease processes in the middle ear can be inferred. The normal tympanic membrane has a wide range of colored hues, the most common being pearly gray. Located in the membrane or seen through it are certain landmarks (Fig. 21-6). For visualization of the external ear canal and eardrum, an otoscope (Fig. 21-7) is used; it has an ear piece (speculum) that can be placed into the ear canal, has illumination to visualize the eardrum, and may have magnification for a more accurate assessment. Otoscopy is performed by persons (including nurses) who are specially prepared to use an otoscope.

➡ Data analysis: nursing diagnoses

Nursing diagnoses are determined from assessment of patient data. Possible nursing diagnoses for the person with an ear infection may include, but are not limited to, the following:

Diagnostic title	Possible etiologies
Knowledge deficit	Lack of exposure/recall, information misinterpretation
Pain: ear	Inflammation

Planning: expected patient outcomes

Expected patient outcomes for the person with an ear infection may include, but are not limited to, the following:
1. Patient states ear discomfort is decreased
2. Patient describes preventive measures and symptoms requiring medical attention

Implementation

ASSISTANCE WITH ACHIEVEMENT OF THERAPEUTIC GOALS

Manipulation of the ear during treatments requires gentle handling to maintain comfort. Cross-contamination is prevented by good medical asepsis, including washing hands before and after treatments.

Ear wash

A solution of boric acid and alcohol (which can be obtained at the drugstore) may be used to clean the external ear and provide a drying effect. A small (2 to 3 oz) syringe is used to instill the fluid, and the solution is warmed to body temperature to prevent discomfort or dizziness. The person places the affected ear upward. The pinna is pulled up, back, and out, and the tip of the syringe is placed in the ear canal. The solution is pumped vigorously and repeatedly in and out of the canal. The patient then leans over and lets extra solution run out. An ear wash is usually prescribed for twice a day until the ear stops draining. Dryness is checked by inserting a cotton-tipped applicator into the ear canal (no farther than the cotton tip).

Ear irrigation

The ear may be irrigated to remove wax, drainage, or debris. A larger amount of solution is used than for an ear wash. Irrigations are avoided if the eardrum is perforated (causes further inflammation) or if the foreign body to be removed is of vegetable origin or an insect (moisture will cause object or insect to swell). Tap water is generally used; hydrogen peroxide may be used to help dislodge wax. A large syringe is used, but the technique for insertion of the syringe tip is similar to an ear wash. The person's clothes are protected, and a kidney-basin is placed below the ear to catch the solution. The fluid is directed in a steady stream along the upper wall of the ear canal (Fig. 21-8).

Ear wicks

Ear wicks are used to promote drainage or for instillation of eardrops if the external canal is occluded. A bayonet forcep is used to insert the wick gently into the ear canal. Commercially prepared wicks or a single piece of ¼-inch gauze about 2 cm long may be used.

Eardrops

Antibiotics and antiinflammatory agents may be prescribed locally as eardrops, especially for external otitis. Guidelines for instillation of eardrops are listed in the box on p. 556.

Ear ointment

Use a cotton-tipped applicator to apply ear ointment. Insert the applicator no farther than the cotton end, and use a new one for each application.

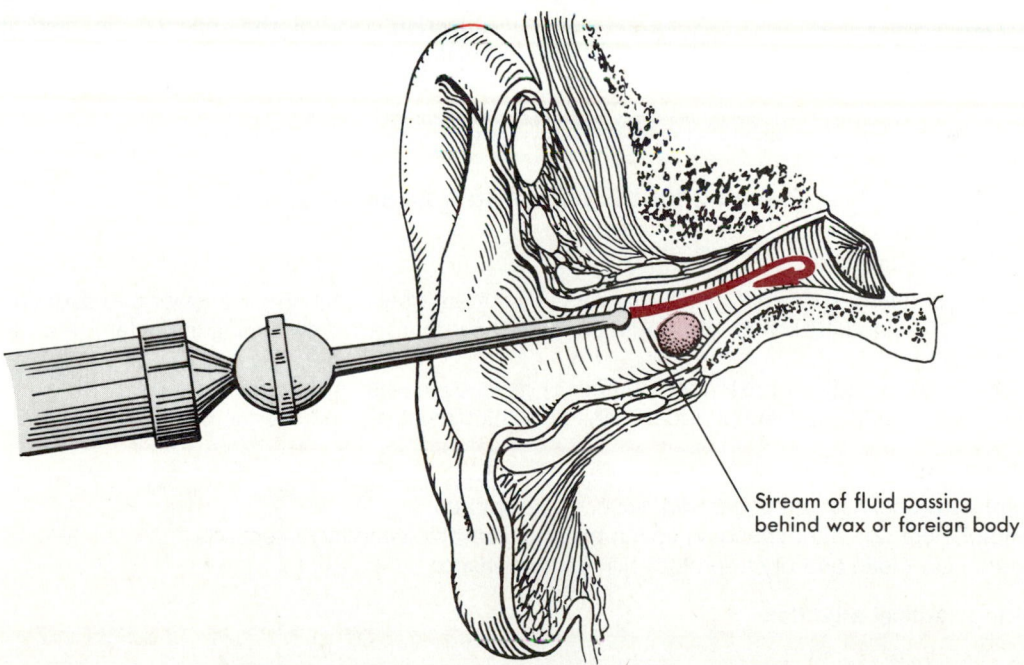

Stream of fluid passing behind wax or foreign body

Fig. 21-8 Ear irrigation. Note that fluid is directed toward upper canal wall so that stream will pass behind the wax or object.

Guidelines for instillation of eardrops

1. Warm solution to body temperature (no more than 38° C); vertigo may result from high or low temperatures. (Warm vial by holding in hand for a few minutes or placing in warm water.)
2. Have patient tilt head so ear is uppermost.
3. Straighten ear canal by pulling up and back (adults).
4. Instill drops to run along canal wall to prevent air entrapment.
5. Have patient hold head in position for 2 to 3 minutes.
6. Dry external ear thoroughly to prevent skin irritation.
7. Place cotton in ear only if desired.

Table 21-3 Surgeries of the eardrum, middle ear, and mastoid

Type of surgery	Description
Myringotomy	Removal by suction of middle ear fluid through an incision made in eardrum
Myringoplasty	Repair of a tympanic membrane perforation
Tympanoplasty (ossiculoplasty)	Reconstruction of ossicles of middle ear
Mastoidectomy	
Simple (closed)	Removal of mastoid air cells
Radical (open)	Removal of mastoid air cells, ossicles, eardrum, wall of ear canal, and middle ear mucosa
Modified (open)	Less extensive than radical mastoidectomy; preserves middle ear structures

■ SURGERY

Surgery may be performed on the eardrum to relieve fluid pressure or to repair a perforation (Table 21-3). If it is desirable to keep the eardrum open for fluid drainage, transtympanic tubes can be inserted in a myringotomy incision; the tubes usually drop out by themselves in several months. Surgery of the ear is performed under high power magnification. If mastoidectomy is indicated, a simple procedure is preferred, if possible, as this maintains hearing. Tympanoplasty may follow mastoidectomy if the ossicles are removed. Care of the person following ear surgery is described on p. 559.

■ ASSISTING WITH COMFORT

Because ear pain results from the fluid exudate of the inflammatory process, pain usually begins to subside with adequate antibiotic therapy and drainage measures. Analgesics may be helpful.

■ PATIENT TEACHING

Ear infections may recur and become chronic; therefore, persons with ear infections need to know how to prevent chronic infection. Teaching includes prevention of further infection, care of the infected ear, and signs requiring further medical attention (see the box below).

Teaching for the patient with an ear infection

Prevention of further infection

1. Protect ear canal during showers (cotton with petrolatum in external canal; use a shower cap over ears).
2. Avoid swimming during infection or following a perforated eardrum; avoid swimming in contaminated water when infection is healed.
3. Continue antibiotic therapy for prescribed number of days, even when symptoms disappear.
4. Get adequate and early treatment of upper respiratory tract infections and allergic conditions.

Care of infected ear

1. Use correct eardrops insertion or ear irrigations, as prescribed.
2. Wash hands before and after changing cotton plugs to prevent secondary infection.
3. Keep external ear clean and dry to protect skin from drainage.

Signs requiring medical attention

Fever
Return of ear pain or drainage

✠ Evaluation

Evaluation is based on expected patient outcomes. Questions to ask may include the following:
1. Is the patient comfortable?
2. Can the patient describe care required at home?
3. Can the patient describe measures to prevent recurring infection?

■ DISORDERS AFFECTING BALANCE

■ Pathophysiology

Disorders of the inner ear usually affect the semicircular canals, causing *vertigo* (the sensation of the body or objects spinning in the room). "Dizziness" is commonly used synonymously with vertigo but is actually incorrect because dizziness refers mainly to "light-headedness" but not necessarily a spinning sensation. Vertigo may also be caused by disturbances in CNS pathways because of the many interconnections of the vestibular nuclei within the CNS.[30] There may also be an idiopathic positional vertigo that is associated with specific head positions (different to dizziness caused by orthostatic hypotension).

Labyrinthitis is the most common cause of vertigo. Virus infection may spread into the inner ear from an upper respiratory tract infection. Certain drugs, especially streptomycin, can destroy the vestibular portion of the inner ear, and foods can also cause labyrinthitis (Table 21-4). There is usually complete recovery without the hearing being affected.

Menière's disease is thought to result from an excess of endolymph. As the volume of endolymph increases, the membranous labyrinth ruptures and the endolymph mixes with the perilymph.[30] The rupture produces the disease symptoms (Table 21-4). The person usually has recurrent attacks at varying intervals. During an attack, the person is unable to sit or walk and must lie with the head in a fixed position to prevent further vertigo. In most cases, Menière's disease is unilateral and loss of hearing is progressive until deafness results in that ear. There is no cure for the disease, but control is possible.

An *acoustic neuroma* is a slow-growing, benign tumor on the vestibular portion of cranial nerve VIII causing tinnitus and vertigo. The neuroma can be removed easily without side effects if identified early. If allowed to grow, however, it encroaches on the brain and more extensive surgery is necessary with loss of hearing.

▥ Assessment

■ SUBJECTIVE AND OBJECTIVE DATA

Subjective data are collected initially from a patient subject to vertigo. Data include knowledge of the disorder, patterns of the episodes (frequency, duration), accompanying symptoms, and safety measures taken. Because of the discomfort of vertigo, many persons are fearful of the attacks; therefore, the persons's feelings concerning the vertigo are explored. Initial objective data include an assessment of the person's hearing ability (p. 562) because of the close relationship between balance and hearing in the inner ear.

During a vertiginous attack, the following additional data are collected:
1. Onset and duration of the attack.
2. Presence of nystagmus (involuntary jerky movements of the eyeballs); note if nystagmus occurs in one eye or both eyes and the rapidity of the movement.
3. Reports of tinnitus (ranges from buzzing sounds to painful, loud ringing noises).
4. Color and moisture of skin (pallor and diaphoresis from an autonomic response).
5. Occurrence of vomiting (autonomic response).

Table 21-4   Disorders affecting balance

Disorder	Etiology	Signs and symptoms	Medical therapy
Labyrinthitis	Viruses Drugs: streptomycin Food: shellfish Tobacco, alcohol	Vertigo, tinnitus, nausea Hearing often unimpaired	Bed rest if symptoms are severe Antimotion drugs and histamines Sedation
Menière's disease	Overaccumulation of endolymph in inner ear	Recurrent episodes of vertigo, nausea, and vomiting and diaphoresis Tinnitus in affected ear; sense of fullness Progressive deafness	No specific therapy Diuretics, low-salt, diet Antihistamines, vasodilators, antivertiginous drugs (meclizine [Antivert], dimenhydrinate [Dramamine]) Surgery may be necessary
Acoustic neuroma	Slow-growing, benign tumor of cranial nerve VIII in inner ear	Tinnitus initially; vertigo, hearing loss; facial weakness in later stage	Surgical removal

■ DIAGNOSTIC TESTS

Specific diagnostic tests include *electronystagmography* (ENG) and a caloric test. ENG is a test used to measure nystagmus. It records the position and movement of the eyeball by recording the changes in the electrical field around the eye when there is a change in position of the eye. Electrodes are placed on the face around the eye; no discomfort is involved.

In the *caloric test,* cold water or air is irrigated in the external auditory canal. When labyrinthine function is normal, the person experiences vertigo and nystagmus. In labyrinthine disorders, the response is hyperactive or absent.

Audiometric testing (p. 562) is performed to identify concurrent hearing loss. With many labyrinthine disorders, the test initially reveals low-tone sensorineural hearing loss. Neurologic consultation is usually obtained to rule out neurologic disease.

⭢ Data analysis: nursing diagnoses

Nursing diagnoses are determined from assessment of patient data. Possible nursing diagnoses for the person with a balance disorder may include, but are not limited to, the following:

Diagnostic title	Possible etiologies
Anxiety	Concern over future attacks
Potential for injury	Loss of balance
Knowledge deficit	Lack of exposure/recall, information misinterpretation
Sensory/perceptual alteration: auditory	Inner ear disorder

◪ Planning: expected patient outcomes

Expected patient outcomes for the person with a balance disorder may include, but are not limited to, the following:
1. Signs of anxiety are decreased
2. Injury from loss of balance does not occur
3. The person describes:
   a. The nature of the disorder
   b. Circumstances that precipitate an attack and what to do when an attack occurs
   c. Safety precautions to take
   d. Prescribed medication regimen
   e. Symptoms requiring medical intervention

◪ Implementation

■ ASSISTING WITH ACHIEVEMENT OF THERAPEUTIC GOALS

Most persons with a vertiginous disorder receive therapy on an ambulatory basis. Medications may be prescribed to decrease the incidence or severity of the vertigo and consist primarily of *antivertiginous drugs,* such as meclizine (An-

tivert), demenhydrinate (Dramamine), or diphenhydramine (Benadryl). A *diuretic* such as ammonium chloride or hydrochlorodiazide (Hydrodiuril) may be prescribed to help decrease fluid volume of the endolymph. A *low-salt diet* is usually prescribed for the same reason as a diuretic. A *vasodilator* such as nicotinic acid is helpful for some persons.

■ PROMOTING COMFORT AND SAFETY

During a vertiginous attack, the person either feels as though the room were spinning around or that he or she is spinning in a stationary room. To prevent falling and to decrease the vertigo sensation, the person has to lie down, avoiding all head movements that aggravate the spinning sensation. If tinnitus is severe, the person may cover the ears in an attempt to lessen the sound. Measures must be taken to protect the person from falling at the onset of the attack. The acute manifestations may last from 1 to 3 hours.[30] After an attack the person is exhausted and requires rest and sleep.

Measures that help reduce vertigo or dizziness include the following:
1. Stand directly in front of person when speaking so person does not have to turn head
2. Encourage person to move *slowly*
3. Avoid bright, glaring lights
4. If bed rest is prescribed:
   a. Assist with ADL as needed
   b. Keep side rails up
5. Assist with ambulation as needed to prevent falls

Teaching for the patient with vertigo

1. Nature of the disorder
   a. Physiologic basis for the vertigo
   b. Avoidance of any known precipitating factors
   c. Rationale for a low-salt diet
2. Actions to take during an attack
   a. Lie down immediately and call for help if necessary at the first signs of an attack
   b. If driving when an attack occurs, pull over immediately to the curb
   c. Lie immobile and hold head in one position until vertigo lessens
3. Ask for assistance when ambulating if dizzy
4. Take prescribed medications as instructed, even if no recent attacks have occurred; check with physician before discontinuing any medication
5. Symptoms requiring medical attention: changes in symptoms or nature of attacks

6. If vertigo occurs when person is ambulating, have person lie down immediately and hold head still

■ COUNSELING AND TEACHING

The threat of vertigo often leads to anxiety. The person may dread the experience of an attack or may be embarrassed by the concurrent side-effects such as vomiting. Give the person opportunities to explore feelings and concerns. Anxiety may be decreased by awareness of measures to decrease vertigo occurrences or to minimize the effects.

Teaching for the patient with vertigo includes the nature of the disorder, actions to take during an attack, measures to prevent injury, the prescribed medication regimen, and symptoms requiring medical attention (see the box on p. 558).

■ Surgery of the ear

■ TYPES OF SURGERY

Surgery may be performed for Menière's disease if the attacks are incapacitating and cannot be controlled by medication. About 5% to 10% of persons with the disorder require surgery. The types of surgery are described in Table 21-5.

Surgery is required for removal of acoustic neuromas. A translabyrinthine or mastoidectomy approach is preferred, although a suboccipital approach may be needed. Very large tumors may require resection of the facial nerve.

■ PREOPERATIVE CARE

Ear surgery is often performed with local anesthesia, with the person receiving sedation to relieve anxiety and provide relaxation. The following instructions are given about what to expect in the postoperative period:
1. Minor earache can be expected, but pain is not usually a problem
2. Hearing is decreased because of the ear packing
3. Noises such as crackles or pops may be heard
4. Swelling of the ear will occur
5. Extent of postoperative vertigo depends on the nature of the procedure (more extensive with inner ear surgery)

■ POSTOPERATIVE CARE

1. Position patient with operative ear up for 4 hours after surgery
2. Medicate as necessary for discomfort or vertigo
3. Keep side rails up when patient is in bed (when vertigo is present)
4. Supervise patient during ambulation if vertigo/dizziness is present
5. Monitor patient for:
   a. Changes in hearing, tinnitus, or vertigo
   b. Headache
   c. Bleeding (rare)
   d. Signs of facial paralysis if extensive inner ear surgery is performed (asymmetry when frowning, smiling, closing eye, baring teeth, or blowing through lips)

Table 21-5   Surgery for Meniére's disease

Type	Description	Residual	Postoperative care
Surgical destruction of labyrinth	Extraction of membranous labyrinth by suction; access to inner ear through external canal (stapes and incus removed)	Destroys remaining hearing	Bedrest and NPO until vertigo subsides in 1 to 3 days Avoid sudden movement of head for 1 to 2 weeks Take action to prevent falls from unsteadiness for 1 to 3 weeks
Endolymphatic subarachnoid shunt	Insertion of drain tube from endolymphatic sac into subarachnoid space; access through mastoid	Preserves hearing in 60% to 70% of patients	Monitor for dizziness (rare)
Cryosurgery	Application of intense cold to lateral semicircular canals to decrease sensitivity or to create an otic-perotic shunt; access through mastoid	Preserves hearing in 80% of patients	Monitor for dizziness for 2 days Take action to prevent falls from unsteadiness for 2 to 3 weeks
Vestibular nerve section	Dissection of cranial nerve VIII (vestibular portion); access through mastoid or through cranial drilling over roof of internal auditory canal	Preserves hearing in 90% of patients	Same as for surgical destruction of labyrinth

---

Teaching for the patient after ear surgery

1. Change cotton in ear daily as prescribed
2. Open mouth when sneezing or coughing and blow nose gently one side at a time for 1 week (to prevent increased ear pressure and infection)
3. Keep ear dry for 6 weeks (to prevent infection)
   a. Do not wash hair for 1 week
   b. Protect ear when outdoors using two pieces of cotton (use petroleum jelly on outer ball)
   c. Protect ear with shower cap when bathing
4. Wear ear protectors as necessary for exposure to loud noises
5. Follow activity guidelines
   a. No physical activity for 1 week
   b. No exercises or active sports for 3 weeks
   c. Return to work in 1 week (3 weeks for strenuous work)
6. Avoid exposure to persons with upper respiratory tract infections
7. Avoid airplane flights for at least 1 week (to prevent effects of pressure changes)

---

6. Instruct patient to keep mouth open if sneezing or coughing and to blow nose gently one side at a time, if necessary (prevents increased middle ear pressure and transmission of organisms into middle ear)

Most ear surgeries require only a cotton ball in the ear after surgery because only small amounts of serosanguineous drainage are expected. Dressings may be used for surgeries other than transcanal approaches. Hospital stays range from 1 to 4 days. Guidelines for patient teaching are listed in the box above.

⊞ Evaluation

Evaluation is based on the identified patient outcomes. Questions to ask may include the following:
Have signs of anxiety decreased?
Has injury from falls been prevented?
Does the person know the nature of the disorder, the medication regimen, and what to do if an attack occurs?
Does the patient ask for assistance in ambulating if dizziness is present or if vertigo is imminent?
Does the patient plan for ongoing medical supervision?

■ HEARING LOSS

Most ear disorders interfere with hearing to a lesser or greater extent. Inflammations may plug the ear canal or fill the middle ear with fluid, interfering with transmission of sound waves. If the ossicles become fixed, they are less able to transmit the sound vibrations. Inner ear disorders also interfere with the sound vibrations reaching the organ of Corti. Growth of acoustic neuromas places pressure on the cochlear division of the eighth cranial nerve.

■ Implications of impaired hearing

More than 13 million people in the United States have some kind of hearing impairment. Of these persons, 6 million are seriously handicapped, and more than 1.7 million are totally deaf.

Hearing is as important as speech in our daily lives. Sound helps keep us in touch with reality and our environment; it adds esthetic pleasure, as well as warnings of danger, to our world. The sense of hearing is critical to normal development and maintenance of speech. Infants learn to speak by imitating others and listening to the sounds they make in relationship to the sounds of others. Congenitally deaf persons lack aural stimulation, which affects their development of speech and conceptual ability. This severe handicap can affect both personality development and responses on intelligence tests.

As hearing diminishes, the impact of not understanding others and not being understood may make people withdraw from social situations, and they may become anxious and insecure. Fear of inadequacy and inferiority may make them suspicious and depressed. When hearing is completely gone, they may find the silent world almost intolerable.

People who are hard of hearing or deaf are not easily recognized; they appear quite normal. When they fail to respond or respond inappropriately to oral communication, their actions are interpreted as slow or odd, and the speaker may withdraw. This withdrawal response of others may be perceived as rejection by the aurally handicapped person and may further increase isolation and withdrawal. The person who is hard of hearing or deaf may experience varying degrees of stress, depending on personality, the extent and type of loss, the age at onset of loss, and the reaction of family and friends to the loss of hearing.

■ Classification of hearing loss

■ CONDUCTIVE HEARING LOSS

Any interference with conduction of sound impulses through the *external ear canal*, the *eardrum*, or the *middle ear* produces a conductive hearing loss. The inner ear is not involved and sound amplification will reach the inner ear. Causes of conductive hearing loss are listed in the box on p. 561.

Otosclerosis is a bony disorder of the middle ear in which excess spongy bone is formed with fixation of the stapes footplate. It is a familial disease, more common in whites and women, and begins insidiously in the third or fourth decades of life. The number of persons with otosclerosis is decreasing. The disorder is correctable by surgery with a prosthetic replacement.

■ SENSORINEURAL HEARING LOSS

Sensorineural hearing loss results from interference with hearing occurring in the *inner ear* or its *neural pathways*. The hearing loss may result from a known disorder (see the box below), but it is often a functional hearing loss (no organic lesion found) and may be a result of aging. Hearing loss may fluctuate initially, but further progressive hearing loss occurs. Most disorders of the inner ear produce some hearing loss, and a characteristic of severe loss is the inability to discriminate words. Amplification of sounds often causes sound distortion and increases the hearing problem.

Cochlear implants are now available for persons with complete hearing loss. An external device consisting of a small computer changes spoken words to electrical impulses. The impulses are transmitted across the skin to an implanted coil that carries the impulses to an electrode inserted through the round window into the cochlea (Fig. 21-9). Single channel implants are available, but newer multichannel implants are being employed that increase speech discrimination.

Causes of specific types of hearing loss

Conductive hearing loss

Impacted cerumen
Foreign body in external auditory canal
Thickening, retraction, scarring or perforation of eardrum
Otosclerosis

Sensorineural hearing loss

Arteriosclerosis
Infectious diseases (mumps, measles, meningitis)
Ototoxic drugs
Neuromas of cranial nerve VIII
Blows to head or ears
Noise of high intensity
Old age (presbycusis)

■ OTHER TYPES OF HEARING LOSS

Mixed hearing loss is a combination of both sensorineural and conductive hearing loss. Both elements of air and bone conduction hearing loss occur.

Central hearing loss is a form of sensorineural hearing loss resulting from some type of damage to the brain's auditory pathways or auditory center, such as with a cerebral vascular accident. Sounds may be conducted normally through the ear to the neural pathways, but the person is deaf.

Presbycusis is the term used to describe hearing loss resulting from aging. Changes in the delicate labyrinthine structures cause a hearing loss, primarily in the higher frequencies. It may be accompanied by tinnitus (ringing in the ears). The amount of hearing loss in presbycusis has familial differences and can start in middle age. The hearing of most people eventually decreases during the aging process. Presbycusis cannot be treated, but hearing can be improved by hearing aids.

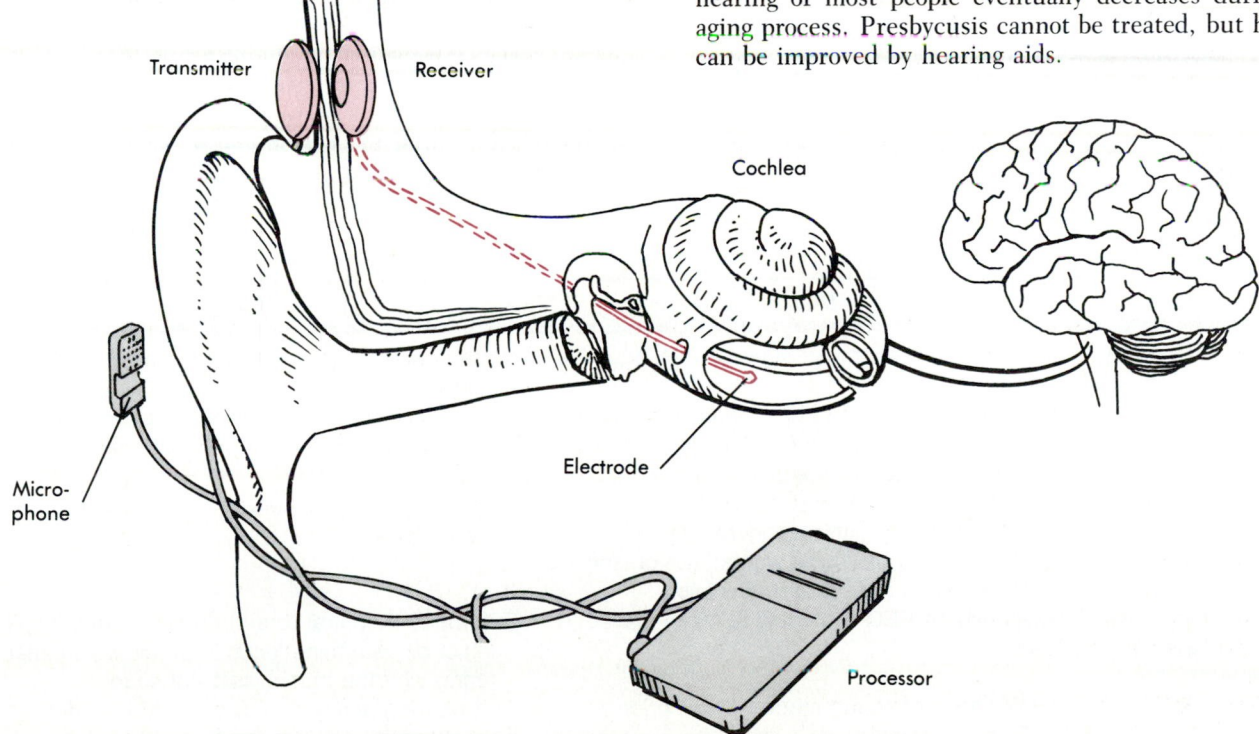

Fig. 21-9 Cochlear implant.

⊡ Assessment

The extent of assessment of auditory acuity by nurses depends on the nurse's preparation and focus of care. All nurses, however, should be prepared to carry out an inspection of the outer ear and at least a gross assessment of hearing ability for all persons entering a health care setting, regardless of the presenting problem (see Chapter 3). Gross assessment of hearing may be accomplished by evaluating the logical sequences of replies during the admission history. One method is to turn ones' head away from the individual when asking a simple question that cannot be answered by a yes or no response.

■ SUBJECTIVE DATA

If the person has been identified as having hearing loss, the following data are obtained:

1. Onset, nature and progression of the hearing loss
2. Noticed differences in hearing in right or left ear
3. Any family history of hearing loss
4. Presence of other ear symptoms: pressure or pain in ears (middle ear), or ringing in ears or dizziness (inner ear)
5. History of head trauma or exposure to noise (past, present)
6. Current medications with known ototoxic effects (p. 551)
7. Any neurologic symptoms, including visual or speech disorders

■ OBJECTIVE DATA

The person who begins to have difficulty hearing usually demonstrates some behavioral clues indicating that hearing is decreased (see the box above, right). Persons who exhibit any of these behavioral clues should have their ears examined by an otolaryngologist, who will perform a complete evaluation.

Behavioral clues indicating difficult hearing

Any adult who
  Is irritable, hostile, hypersensitive in interpersonal relations
  Has difficulty in hearing upper frequency consonants
  Complains about people mumbling
  Turns up volume on television
  Asks for frequent repetition and answers questions inappropriately
  Loses sense of humor; becomes grim
  Leans forward to hear better; face serious and strained
  Shuns large- and small-group audience situations
  May appear aloof and "stuck-up"
  Complains of ringing in the ears
  Has an unusually soft or loud voice
  Repeatedly states, "What did you say?"

■ AUDIOMETRIC TESTING

Functional examination for sensitivity (ability to hear sounds) and for speech discrimination (ability to distinguish different speech sounds) is done by audiometry. The graph of the hearing levels of both of these is called an *audiogram*. *Hearing threshold* is defined as the lowest intensity of sound at which an auditory stimulus can be heard.

Audiologists (specialists in administering hearing tests) have developed audiometric tests to determine not only whether a hearing loss is present, but also the frequency of the loss, how well the person can understand speech, and whether the problem site is in the middle ear (con-

---

Table 21-6 Types of audiometric testing

Test	Method	Use
Pure-tone audiometry	Person wears earphone; signals when sound is heard	General screening to identify persons requiring further testing
Impedance audiometry	Probe inserted in ear canal; measurements of middle ear pressure are obtained; does not require response from person	Assess presence or absence of abnormality of conductive mechanism of middle ear
Speech audiometry	Speech reception threshold: lowest intensity level in decibels at which person can correctly repeat selected bisyllabic words 50% of time; also a test of speech discrimination	Determine how well person can hear and understand speech
Electrocochleography; evoked-response audiometry	Response on EEG recording to clicks played to ear	Determine if central (brain) portion of hearing is intact or determine location of the lesion interfering with the transmission of sound
Tuning fork tests	Identification of sound made by tuning forks placed on head	Test hearing acuity and discriminate conductive vs sensorineural hearing losses

ductive loss) or inner ear or auditory nerve system (sensorineural loss) (Table 21-6).

Pure-tone audiometry must be performed in a specially constructed soundproof booth for best results. To test the sound intensity by air conduction, persons wear earphones and are instructed to signal (usually with a finger) when they first hear the tone and when they no longer hear it. The middle frequencies are tested first, and the operator alternately increases and decreases the intensity of the sound until the dial setting is found at which the person being tested can just perceive sound (threshold). In audiometric testing the frequencies 125, 250, 500, 1000, 2000, 4000, and 8000 Hz are commonly employed to assess the hearing sensitivity of an individual.

Hearing loss is identified as the number of decibels reached before the person hears the sound for each specific frequency. Zero loudness is calibrated for that sound barely heard by a person with normal hearing. Up to a 20 db loss is considered to be within the normal range.

→ Data analysis: nursing diagnoses

Nursing diagnoses are determined from assessment of patient data. Possible nursing diagnoses for the hard-of-hearing person may include, but are not limited to, the following:

Diagnostic title	Possible etiologies
Ineffective individual coping	Situational crises, personal vulnerability
Knowledge deficit	Lack of exposure/recall, information misinterpretation
Sensory/perceptual alteration: auditory	Altered sensory transmission

⌇ Planning: expected patient outcomes

Expected patient outcomes for the person with hard of hearing may include, but are not limited to, the following:
1. Person actively seeks aural rehabilitation, if necessary
2. Person can explain:
   a. The basis for the hearing loss and any appropriate therapy
   b. Care of hearing aid, if appropriate
   c. Available community resources
3. Person understands oral communications

▤ Implementation

Activities for the hearing impaired person include facilitation of communication and aural rehabilitation. It is not uncommon for persons who are beginning to lose their hearing to deny that changes are occurring and that an evaluation of hearing and follow-up of rehabilitative methods are important. Much support and encouragement to explore methods to improve hearing may be needed.

■ FACILITATING COMMUNICATION WITH THE HEARING-IMPAIRED PERSON

Specific actions to facilitate hearing or speech-reading for persons with impaired hearing are listed in the box below.

Additional activities can be used if the person is hospitalized. Patients are helped to use visual cues by placing them in a bed where they can observe activity and antic-

---

Facilitating communication for persons with impaired hearing

1. Get the person's attention by raising an arm or hand.
2. Start with the light on your face; this will help the person speech read.
3. Face the person when speaking.
4. Speak clearly, but do not overaccentuate words.
5. Speak in a normal tone; do not shout. Shouting overemploys normal speaking movements and may cause distortion and be too loud for the person with sensorineural damage. If the person has conductive loss only, sometimes making the voice louder without shouting is helpful.
6. If the person does not seem to understand what is said, express it differently. Some words are difficult to "see" in speech reading, such as *white* or *red*.
7. Move closer to the person and toward the better ear if the person does not hear you.
8. Write out proper names or any statement that you are not sure was understood.
9. Do not smile, chew gum, or cover the mouth when talking to a person with limited hearing.
10. Observe for inattention that may indicate tiredness or lack of understanding.
11. Use phrases to convey meaning rather than one-word answers. State the major topic of the discussion first and then give details.
12. Do not show annoyance by careless facial expression. Persons who are hard of hearing depend more on visual clues for acceptance.
13. Encourage the use of a hearing aid if the person has one; allow the person to adjust it before speaking.
14. If in a group, repeat important statements and avoid asides to others in the group.
15. Avoid the use of the intercommunication system as this may distort sound and cause poor communication.
16. Do not avoid conversation with a person who has hearing loss.

Adapted from Conover, M, and Cober, J: Nurs Clin North Am 5:497, 1970.

ipate others approaching them. They will be easily startled if people suddenly enter the unit if the vision is obscured. Because hearing-impaired persons are often sensitive to light changes, they can easily be awakened by turning on a light. Many patients feel less isolated if the nurse touches them lightly on the arm to gain attention and wakes them by touching them on the arm. Special efforts must be made to communicate information about hospital routines and diagnostic tests.

■ AURAL REHABILITATION

If hearing loss is irreversible and not amenable to surgery, aural rehabilitation may make it possible for the individual to understand and communicate with others again. The purpose of aural rehabilitation is to maximize the hearing-impaired person's communication skills.

The person's acceptance of the hearing impairment, desire to seek help, and use of the facilities available, along with motivation, perseverence, and patience contribute to the success of aural rehabilitation. Rehabilitation is affected by severity of impairment. For people who, although hard of hearing, have normally acquired communication skills, efforts are geared toward correcting, restoring, complementing, and maintaining those skills. For deaf persons who have not developed communication skills, efforts are made to teach language and speech skills by special methods.

□ Hearing aids

Hearing aids are commonly used by both hearing-impaired persons and deaf persons. Hearing aids are instruments through which sounds are amplified in a controlled manner. They are used to increase the intensity of the sound reaching the ear. Hearing aids do not improve the ability to hear, but they make the *sound louder*. Persons who have difficulty with speech discrimination benefit less from a hearing aid. Persons with a conductive hearing loss benefit most from wearing a hearing aid because their ability to understand speech is usually not impaired if the speech is loud enough.

□ *Types of hearing aids*

There are several types of hearing aids, differing in size and location to be worn (Table 21-7). Most hearing aids consist of the following parts:
1. Microphone to receive and convert speech into electric signals
2. Amplifier to increase signal strength
3. Receiver to convert electric signals back to sound
4. Energy supply (battery)

All hearing aids except for the body-worn type have all components housed in a small case connected to an earmold (Fig. 21-10). The body-worn type is usually placed in a shirt pocket or in a special pocket sewn into underclothing. The body-worn aid should not be covered by heavy clothing that can muffle sound.

During the next few years, it is anticipated that microchip technology will be used in the development of hearing

Table 21-7 Types of hearing aids

Type	Location
Postauricular aid	Behind ear
Within-ear aid	Totally in ear canal (least noticeable)
Eyeglass aid	In eyeglass temple
Body-worn aid	Placed in a shirt or specially made pocket (most powerful)

aids. According to Lee,[20] the new digital aids will do the following:
1. Have specific programming for the user's hearing loss
2. Automatically monitor and adjust volume on a consistent basis
3. Enhance clarity of speech sounds

□ *Assisting the person with a hearing aid*

Persons with hearing aids should know how to care for the aid and what to do if the aid fails to work (see the box on p. 565). The aids have adjustable tone and volume controls, and several adjustments may have to be made before the aid is correctly set for the person's needs. Because a hearing aid is not selective when amplifying sounds, the amplified background sounds can often be annoying to the individual.

Persons who are reluctant to wear their hearing aids (often for cosmetic reasons) need counseling about the benefits of wearing the aid and the improvements in their ability to speak more distinctly. The aid may also serve to

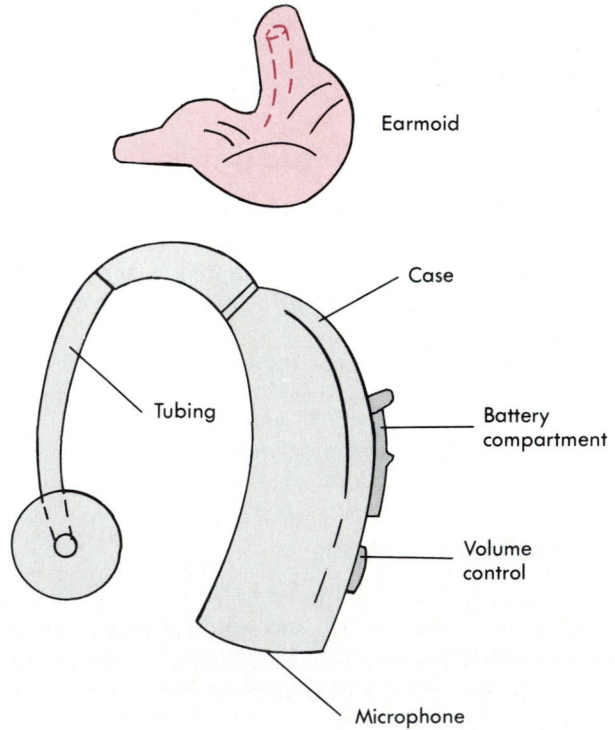

Fig. 21-10 Parts of a hearing aid.

Care of hearing aid

1. Wash earmold or plug daily in mild soap and water using a pipe cleaner to cleanse the cannula.
2. Dry earmold or plug thoroughly before reconnecting it to the receiver.
3. Keep an extra battery and cord available at all times.
4. When hearing aid is not in use, turn aid off and open battery compartment.
5. If hearing aid whistles, reinsert earmold.
6. If hearing aid fails to work:
   a. Check the on-off switch
   b. Inspect earmold for cleanliness
   c. Examine battery for tightness of fit
   d. Examine cord plug for tightness of insertion
   e. Examine cord for breaks
   f. Replace battery and/or cord

notify others to speak more distinctly. When a person with a hearing aid is hospitalized, it is important to encourage use of the aid during hospitalization and its safe storage when not in use.

□ Assistive hearing devices

Other types of technologies are available to assist the hearing-impaired or deaf persons who do not have hearing aids. One type of assistive hearing device is a hand-held amplifier attached to headphones. The speaker holds the amplifier when communicating to the hearing-impaired person wearing the headphones.

Special amplifiers can also be placed in telephones to magnify the sound for hearing-impaired persons; these amplifiers are obtained from the telephone company.

□ Other types of aural rehabilitation
□ *Auditory training*

Auditory training is used to encourage those who are hard of hearing to use their residual hearing more effectively. The training consists of helping the affected person to develop *listening skills*. It helps the hard of hearing person to do the following:

1. Establish attitudes of critical listening
2. Develop an awareness of the kinds of listening errors that are most likely to be made in view of the nature of the hearing impairment
3. Compensate for these errors by using other special clues that are still heard correctly
4. Improve listening habits and skills in general

□ *Speech-reading*

Speech-reading (commonly known as lipreading) is taught to *supplement the hearing function*. It includes the following:

1. Lipreading
2. Study of facial expressions
3. Study of gestures and body movements used in speech
4. Use of environmental clues that facilitate hearing

□ *Speech training*

Speech training is given to *conserve, develop, or prevent deterioration of speech skills*. Clearness, pitch, quality, and rate of speech may deteriorate with loss of hearing and are the focus of speech training.

■ COMMUNITY SERVICES

Special services for persons with a hearing loss are offered by audiology clinics sponsored by universities, hospitals, community programs, local or state departments of

Agencies providing services for the hearing-impaired

American Annals of the Deaf, 5034 Wisconsin Ave., N.W., Washington, DC 20016. The April issue every year lists a directory of programs and services for the deaf available by state.

American Federation of the Physically Handicapped, Inc., 1370 National Press Building, Washington, DC 20004. Provides counseling and information.

American Speech and Hearing Association, 10801 Rockville Pike, Rockville, MD 20852. Provides information on hearing aids, hearing loss in the elderly, and list of certified audiologists by state.

Gallaudet College, 7th and Florida Ave., Washington, DC 20002. The only liberal arts college in the world for the deaf.

National Association of Hearing and Speech Agencies, 919 18th St., N.W., Washington, DC 20006. Provides counseling and information.

Self-Help for Hard-of-Hearing People (Shhh), 4848 Battery Lane, Dept. E, Bethesda, MD 20814. National organization for the hard-of-hearing; publishes a bimonthly magazine with helpful information.

State Office of Vocational Rehabilitation (in each state). Provides vocational training and placement services.

Veterans Administration. Provides audiology clinics and rehabilitative services for veterans.

Putting knowledge to practice

- Walk around for a day with earplugs in your ears. Describe your reactions. How do you think you would feel if you were told you would never hear well again?
- Visit a speech and hearing clinic. What types of services are offered? How do the clients get referred to the clinic? What are the costs?
- What agencies are available in your community that provide services for the hard-of-hearing or deaf persons?

---

health and education, or the Veterans Administration. National organizations are available to give information and counseling (see the box on p. 565).

☷ Evaluation

Evaluation is based on expected patient outcomes. Questions to ask may include the following:
1. Has the person obtained appropriate aural rehabilitation?
2. Does the person know (1) the nature of the disorder, (2) care of the hearing aid (if worn), and (3) where to seek appropriate assistance?
3. Does the person respond appropriately during interactions?

■ SUMMARY

1. Sound reaches the inner ear by air conduction through the ear canal and ossicles of the middle ear and by bone conduction through the skull bones to the inner ear. In the cochlea of the inner ear the sound waves are transformed into neural energy and transmitted to the brain for interpretation.
2. Disorders that plug the outer ear, add fluid to the middle ear, make the ossicles unmovable, destroy the hair cells of the organ of Corti, or interfere with nerve stimulus transmission over the acoustic nerve will lead to decreased hearing.
3. Hearing can be preserved by preventing infection or trauma of the ear, by using ototoxic drugs with caution and seeking medical attention if symptoms occur, and by preventing frequent exposure to loud noises (or using ear protection for constant loud noises).
4. Ear infections are the most common disorders of the external and middle ears; pain results from pressure by fluid buildup within the enclosed spaces.
5. Serous otitis media develops from collection of serous fluid in the middle ear when the eustachian tube becomes blocked. Purulent otitis media develops from bacteria entering the middle ear through the eustachian tube; pus collects in the middle ear.
6. Ear infections are treated with antibiotics, given by eardrops, ear ointments, or systemically. Treatments to remove drainage may include ear wash, ear irrigation, or surgery of the eardrum.

7. The person with an ear infection should avoid getting water in the ear (care during showering and shampooing and avoiding swimming).
8. Vertigo is the major symptom of disorders (such as labyrinthitis, Menière's disease, acoustic neuroma) affecting the semicircular canals of the inner ear. Tinnitus (ringing in the ears) often accompanies vertigo. Potential for injury is a major problem for the person with vertigo.
9. The uncomfortable sensation of vertigo can be minimized by lying down and holding the head still.
10. Most ear surgeries are microsurgeries performed through the ear canal. Following surgery, hearing will be temporarily decreased because of the swelling and ear packing; crackling noises may be heard. The patient is instructed postoperatively to avoid actions that may increase intraaural pressure or that may lead to infection.
11. Conductive hearing loss, a problem of decreased amplification, is the result of problems of the external or middle ear; it responds well to aural rehabilitation. Otosclerosis (immobility of the ossicles) produces conductive hearing loss.
12. Sensorineural hearing loss results from interference with hearing in the inner ear or neural pathways; it may result from a known disorder or be idiopathic. Presbycusis (hearing loss resulting from aging) is a form of sensorineural hearing loss. The hearing loss is primarily that of sound discrimination, and amplification may further distort the sound.
13. Aural rehabilitation includes the use of hearing aids or other assistive hearing devices, auditory training (improving listening skills), speech-reading (lipreading), or speech training (improving speech clarity).

REFERENCES AND SELECTED READINGS
Contemporary

1. Becker, G, and Nadler, G: The aged deaf: integration of a disabled group into an agency serving elderly people, Gerontologist 20:214-221, 1980.
2. Berger, KW: The hearing aid: its operation and development, ed 3, Livonia, Mich, 1984, The National Hearing Aid Society.

---

*References preceded by an asterisk are particularly well suited for student reading.

3. *Caruso, VG: When the patient has otitis externa, Geriatrics 35(5):35-42, 1980.

4. Chung, DY, and Gannon, RP: Hearing loss due to noise trauma, J Laryngol Otol 94:419-423, 1980.

5. Conklin, JM, and Subtelny, JD: Effect of speech training upon speech-reading in hearing-impaired adults, Am Ann Deaf 125:442-448, 1980.

6. *Connolly, P: Growing up with deafness, Comm Outlook 9:290-293, 1980.

7. *DeBlase, R, and Kucler, M: Assistive hearing device aids patient-staff communication, Geriatr Nurs 6:223-224, 1985.

8. DeWeese, DD, and Saunders, WH: Textbook of otolaryngology, ed 7, St. Louis, 1987, The CV Mosby Co.

9. *Else, D: Hearing protection: who needs training? Occup Health 33:451-453, 1981.

10. Fountain, D: Hearing aids and their care, Geriatr Nurs Home Care 7(2): 12-14, 1987.

11. Healy, GB: Hearing loss and vertigo secondary to head injury, N Engl J Med 306:1029-1031, 1982.

12. *Heller, BR, and Gaynor, EB: Hearing loss and aural rehabilitation of the elderly, Top Clin Nurs 3(1):21-29, 1981.

13. *Holder, L: Hearing aids: handle with care, Nurs 82 12 (4):64-67, 1982.

14. *How to test your patient's hearing acuity, Nurs 80 10 (7):60-61, 1980.

15. Hughes, GB: Textbook of clinical otology, New York, 1985, Thieme-Stratton, Inc.

16. *Hughes, JL: Audiometry, Nurs Times 78:635-637, 1982.

17. *Jackson, J: Don't shout nurse!: hearing problems in the elderly, Geriatric Nurs (Oxford) 6(3):12-13, 1986.

18. *Kamenir, S, and Fothersill, R: Hands on skills for dealing with hearing aids, Can Nurs 78(11):44-45, 1982.

19. *Koch, KJ: The deaf and hard of hearing: some hints, Nurs. Times 77(32): Suppl. 19-20, 1981.

20. Lee, JC: Deafness: the next ten years, J Rehabil 51(4):79-83, 1985.

21. *Levene, B: Sorry nurse, I can hear you but I can't understand you, Nurs 85 (Oxford) 2(41):1221-1225, 1985.

22. *Makliewicz, J: The fine art of giving a physical: how to assess the ears and test hearing acuity, RN 45(3):56-63, 1982.

23. *McCormick, GP, and others: Artificial speech devices, Am J Nurs 82:121-122, 1982.

24. Mitchell, VL: Cochlear implantation: a nursing perspective, J Soc Otorhinolaryngol Head Neck Nurses 5(2):11-15, 1987.

25. Riley, MA: Nursing care of the client with ear, nose, and throat disorders, New York, 1987, Springer Publishing Co.

26. Rubin, W: Noise-induced deafness: major environmental problem, Hosp Med 23(7):19-21, 25-27, 1987.

27. Tortora, ML: Noise-induced hearing loss: prevention in the work environment, AAOHN J 35:271-273, 1987.

28. Ward, RR: Treatment of elderly adults with impaired hearing resources, outcomes, and efficiency, J Epidemiol Commun Health 34:65-68, 1980.

29. Wilson, WR, and Nadol, JR: Quick reference to ear, nose and throat disorders, Philadelphia, 1983, JB Lippincott Co.

30. Wolfson, RJ, and others: Vertigo, Clin Symp 38(6):2-32, 1986.

Classic

31. *Conover, M, and Cober, J: Understanding and caring for the hearing impaired, Nurs Clin North Am 5:497-506, 1970.

22

The Patient with Musculoskeletal Disorders

WILMA J. PHIPPS and GRACE McCARTHY HARLAN

CHAPTER OBJECTIVES

After reading this chapter, the student should be able to:

- Describe measures to prevent musculoskeletal dysfunction.
- Describe conservative health measures for persons with joint and muscle disorders.
- Describe the pathophysiologic changes and therapy for rheumatoid arthritis, SLE, degenerative joint disorders, and scoliosis.
- Explain the nature of and describe the care of the patient undergoing total hip and total knee replacement.
- Describe the care of the patient undergoing spinal fusion.
- Identify different types of fractures and their treatment.
- Explain the pathophysiology of bone healing.
- Describe problems that may occur with immobilization.
- Describe care of the patient following closed and open reduction of hip fractures (including cast care and traction).

■ ANATOMY AND PHYSIOLOGY

Among the characteristics that distinguish man as a species is the ability to maintain an erect posture and to move about. The individual's posture and movements depend on the proper functioning of the musculoskeletal system. The *musculoskeletal system* is composed of bones, muscles, cartilage, ligaments, tendons, fascia, bursae, and joints.

■ Components of the musculoskeletal system

■ BONES

Bones are composed of both living cells and nonliving intracellular material. They are derived from embryonic hyaline cartilage that undergoes *osteogenesis* to become bone. This process is accomplished by cells called *osteoblasts*. The hard quality of the bone is the result of the deposits of calcium salts.

The functions of the bones are as follows:
1. *Support* body tissues and provide the skeletal framework of the body
2. *Protect* body organs (for example, the bony casing of the skull protects the brain)
3. Provide for *movement* (muscles are attached for contraction and motion)
4. Be a *storehouse* for mineral salts (for example, calcium)
5. Provide for *hematopoiesis* (formation of red blood cells in red bone marrow)

Bones are classified into four groups according to their shape:
1. *Long bones* (femur, humerus) consist of a shaft and two epiphyses (see Fig. 22-1). The shaft is formed mainly of *compact* bone tissue. The epiphyses are formed from spongy (cancellous or trabecular) bone. Trabecular bone provides strength to bone while reducing its weight.
2. *Short bones* (carpals) are irregularly shaped and have an inner core of *cancellous* (spongy) bone with an outer layer of compact bone.
3. *Flat bones* (skull) consist of two outer plates of compact bone with an inner layer of cancellous bone.
4. *Irregular bones* (vertebrae) are similar to short bones.

■ MUSCLES

Muscles are divided into three major groups, with the principal function to contract and produce movement of parts of the body or of the entire body. The grouping of muscles is as follows:
1. *Skeletal (striated)* muscle: found in the skeletal system; provides controlled movement, maintains posture, and produces heat
2. *Visceral (smooth)* muscle: found in the digestive tract, urinary tract, and blood vessels; innervated by the autonomic nervous system; contractions not under voluntary control

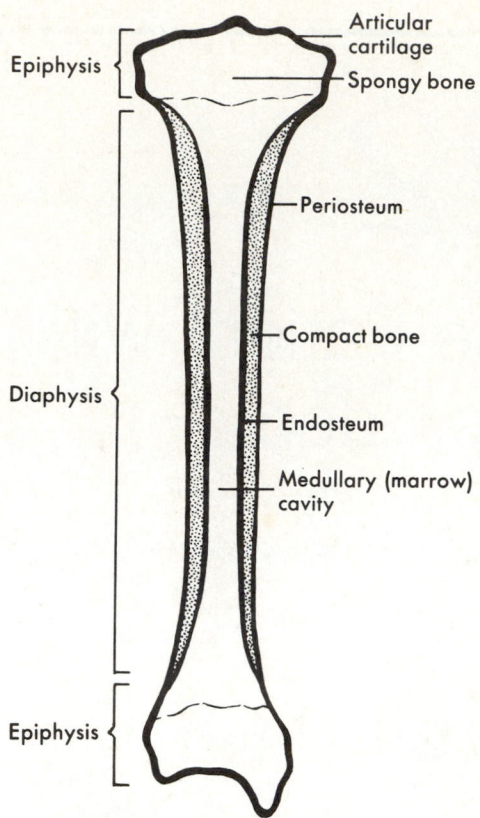

Fig. 22-1   Structure of bone. (From Anthony, CP, and Thibodeau, GA: Textbook of anatomy and physiology, ed 12, St. Louis, 1987, The CV Mosby Co.)

3. *Cardiac* muscle; found only in the heart; contractions not under voluntary control

Skeletal muscles are organs; they vary in size and shape from long and thin to broad and flat, or they may form bulky masses. Skeletal muscles contract only if they are stimulated. The energy for muscle contraction is supplied by the breakdown of adenosine triphosphate (ATP) and the action of calcium. Fig. 22-2 illustrates the mechanism of skeletal muscle contraction. Muscle fibers that are adequately oxygenated will contract more forcefully than those not adequately oxygenated.

Movements are produced by muscles pulling on bones that serve as levers and joints that serve as fulcrums.

Skeletal muscle is highly vascular. During muscle contraction chemical changes occur, resulting in the formation of waste products. Muscle fatigue and pain result when insufficient oxygen is delivered to the muscle and when waste products are not removed.

■ CARTILAGE

Cartilage is composed of fibers embedded in a firm gel. It is strong but flexible, and it is avascular. Nutrients reach the cartilage cells by the process of diffusion through the gel from capillaries located in the *perichondrium* (fibrous

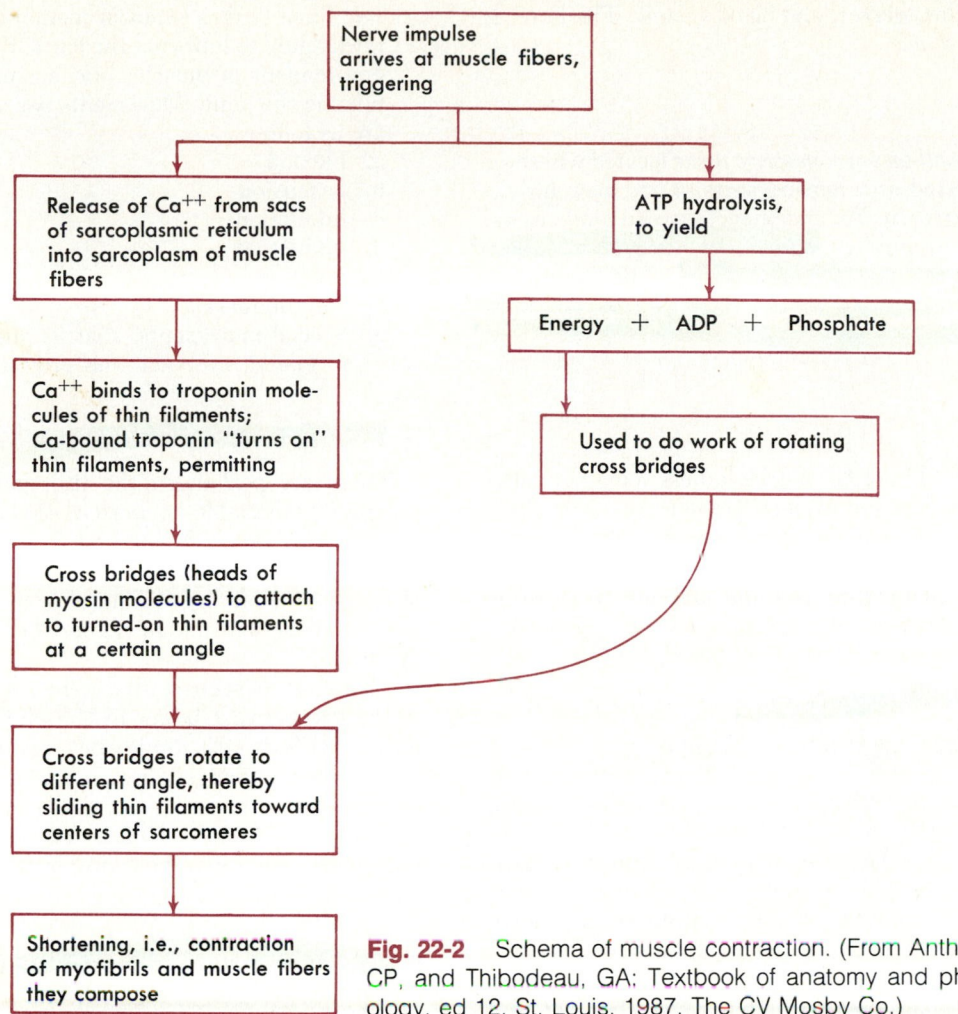

Fig. 22-2 Schema of muscle contraction. (From Anthony, CP, and Thibodeau, GA: Textbook of anatomy and physiology, ed 12, St. Louis, 1987, The CV Mosby Co.)

covering of the cartilage) or, in the case of articular cartilage, through the synovial fluid. The number of collagenous fibers found in the cartilage will determine its type: *fibrous, hyaline, or elastic*. *Fibrous* (or fibrocartilage) has the most fibers and therefore the greatest tensile strength. Fibrocartilage composes the intervertebral disks. *Articular* (hyaline) cartilage—smooth, white, shiny, and resilient—covers the articular surfaces of the bone and serves as a cushion. *Elastic* cartilage has the fewest fibers and may be found in areas such as the external ear.

◼ LIGAMENTS

Ligaments are *bands of dense fibrous connective tissue* that are flexible and tough. They connect the articular ends of bones and provide stability. Examples are the medial and lateral collateral ligaments of the knee, which provide mediolateral stability to the knee joint, and the anterior and posterior cruciate ligaments within the joint capsule of the knee, which provide anteroposterior stability. Ligaments may also attach to soft tissue to suspend structures. An example of this is the suspensory ligament of the ovary that passes from the tubal end of the ovary to the peritoneum.

◼ TENDONS

Tendons are *bands* of *dense fibrous tissue* that form the termination of a *muscle* and serve to *attach it to a bone*. The tendon is an extension of the fibrous sheath that envelops each muscle and is continuous with the periosteum at its other end. *Tendon sheaths* are tubular structures of connective tissue that enclose certain tendons, especially in the wrist and ankle. These sheaths are lined with synovial membrane that provides lubrication for easy movement of the tendon.

◼ FASCIA

Fascia is a *sheet of loose connective tissue* that may be found directly under the skin as *superficial fascia* or as a sheet of dense, fibrous connective tissue making up the sheath of muscles, nerves, and blood vessels. The latter is known as *deep fascia.*

■ BURSAE

Bursae are *small sacs of connective tissue* located wherever pressure is exerted over moving parts. They may, for example, occur between skin and bone, between tendons and bone, or between muscles. Bursae are lined with *synovial membrane* and contain synovial fluid. They serve as cushions between moving parts. Such a bursa, the *olecranon bursa,* is located between the olecranon process and the skin.

■ JOINTS

Movement would not be possible unless some flexibility was provided within the skeletal framework. This flexibility is provided by *joints,* or places where the bones come together. The shape of the joint will determine the amount and type of movement that is possible, and the classification of joints is based on the amount of movement they allow.

■ Classification of joints

There are three major classes of joints:
1. *Synarthroses* or *immovable joints:* Bones connected by fibrous tissue or cartilage, such as the bones of the skull that allow no movement.
2. *Amphiarthroses* or *slightly movable joints:* Joints that allow little movement (for example, intervertebral joints). There is no joint cavity, but tissue (fibrous, cartilage, or bone) is found between the articular surfaces.
3. *Diarthroses* or *freely movable joints:* These include most joints in the body, such as the hip, knee, shoulder, and elbow. The adjacent ends of the bones are covered with hyaline cartilage and surrounded by a fibrous *joint cap-*

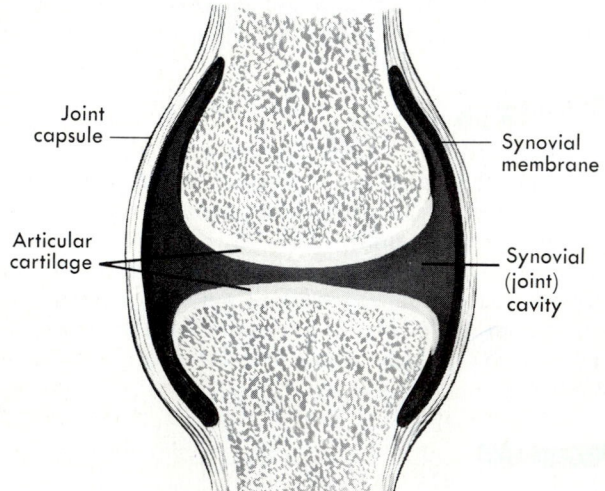

Joint capsule
Articular cartilage
Synovial membrane
Synovial (joint) cavity

Fig. 22-3 Joint capsule. (From Anthony, CP, and Thibodeau, GA: Textbook of anatomy and physiology, ed 12, St. Louis, 1987, The CV Mosby Co.)

sule lined with a synovial membrane that secretes synovial fluid to lubricate the joint (Fig. 22-3). Ligaments and tendons of muscles play an important part in stabilizing the joint. Movements permitted by these joints are as follows:
a. Flexion
b. Extension
c. Adduction
d. Abduction
e. Rotation
f. Circumduction
g. Special movements, that is, supination, pronation, inversion, eversion, and protraction

■ Physiologic changes with aging

There are periods in the life span when individuals are most vulnerable to musculoskeletal changes. These changes may occur during childhood and adolescence because of rapid growth and development or from the onset of maturity to old age. Changes in musculoskeletal structure and function vary among individuals during the aging process.

Changes that occur with aging constitute a continuation of the decline that began in the middle years. The total number of body cells diminishes, resulting in evident connective tissue changes, decrease in the amount and elasticity of subcutaneous tissue, and loss of muscle bulk, tone, and strength. Total body fat is decreased and redistributed from the periphery to the center of the body and especially on the abdomen.

■ COMMON PHYSIOLOGIC CHANGES

1. There is a general decrease in stature of 6 to 10 cm from onset of maturity to old age.
2. Shoulder width decreases.
3. Flexion occurs at the knees and hips.
4. A narrowing of the intervertebral disk causes diminished size of the intervertebral and intercostal spaces.
5. The following occurrences are common:
   a. Compression fractures of the vertebrae.
   b. Increased curvature of the thoracic spine (senile kyphosis, dowager's hump, or widow's hump).
   c. Backward tilting of the head and a shortening of the neck to compensate for the kyphosis deformity.
   d. Greater arm span than height, thus giving the older person a "gangly" appearance.
   e. Unsteady gait, with changes in the muscles and motor function.

■ PREVENTION AND HEALTH EDUCATION

■ Persons at risk and risk factors

Whatever the nature of the musculoskeletal disability, there are factors of prevention and teaching that must be considered.

■ NONPREVENTABLE FACTORS

Many of the diseases that affect the musculoskeletal system have at this time an unknown cause. Rheumatoid arthritis and the diffuse connective tissue diseases are but a few examples. Although these diseases are not now preventable, complications of the diseases are preventable—contractures, atrophy, skin breakdown, and others. In these instances, prevention depends on teaching the patient about the disease process and how to employ preventive measures. These preventive measures will be covered in this chapter.

■ PREVENTABLE FACTORS

Polio vaccine, screening of school-aged children for scoliosis, and screening tests for streptococcal infections with early treatment of the infection to prevent rheumatic fever are examples of preventive measures that can be employed on a community-wide basis in combating illnesses that cause musculoskeletal disability. Early attention to posture; good dietary habits; genetic counseling for individuals with sickle cell anemia and hemophilia; teaching of good body mechanics for individuals whose jobs entail lifting or carrying heavy objects; and concern and attention to the recommendations of the National Safety Council to help avoid accidents at home, on the job, and on the road are all examples of preventive measures that may be employed to decrease musculoskeletal disability within the general population.

■ Preventive health teaching

■ PROMOTION OF SAFETY

For those individuals who have limitations of motion or mobility, a variety of precautions and protective or safety devices can be employed in the hospital or the home. Examples would be grab bars that can be mounted on a wall near a tub or toilet, safety arms that fit around a toilet, and rails that fasten onto the side of a bathtub. These devices provide the person with both a stable place to hold onto and a point of leverage for assuming a standing or sitting position. Throw rugs and obstacles should be removed from areas used by individuals with ambulatory difficulties, and floors should not be highly waxed. Wheelchairs should have adequate locking devices, and patients who must use wheelchairs should be taught how to lock and unlock the chair. Nurses should know where in the community needed equipment can be obtained.

■ PREVENTION OF MUSCLE AND JOINT COMPLICATIONS

□ Maintenance of joint mobility

For the individual with limited motion or mobility, range of motion exercises should be carried out to prevent joint stiffness or contracture from disuse. Whenever it is possible, except in conditions where acute joint inflammation is present, range of motion exercises should be performed several times a day. *Active range of motion* is most beneficial for the patient. Encouraging patients to do as much of their own care as they are able to do within the restrictions of their disability will often satisfy active range of motion requirements.

Several precautions should be mentioned. *Passive range of motion* exercises should not be performed past the point of the complaint of pain. Particularly in individuals with pathologic skeletal conditions (gross deformity, osteoporosis), fractures can result if a joint is forced through "normal" range of motion. Also, acutely inflamed, painful, or septic joints should be rested, because harm can be done by moving the joint before inflammation has subsided. The person who has pain is also likely to resist movement to avoid further pain.

□ Maintenance of posture

Although maintenance of good posture is important for all persons, it is especially important for the patient with chronic arthritis. Poor posture exerts further strain on already damaged joints and not only may cause pain and fatigue but predisposes to increased deformity.

The person who must remain in bed for a long period of time in traction or in a cast should be in a bed with a firm mattress, and a bed board should be placed under the mattress. A firm bed lessens pain by preventing motion and consequent pull on painful joints and helps to keep the spine in good alignment. Boards should be long enough and wide enough to rest firmly on the main side and end rails of the bed, not on the bedsprings. The person with arthritis should either use no pillow or should use one small pillow that fits well down under the shoulder so that forward flexion of the cervical spine is not encouraged. Knees should not be flexed on pillows, and all patients who must be confined to bed most of the day should lie prone with a pillow under the abdomen for a part of each day to relieve supine pressure areas (inferior scapular areas, sacrum, coccyx, and ischial tuberosities) (Fig. 22-4).

Careful positioning with *trochanter rolls* (rolled towels or bath blankets to brace an extremity in the desired position), supportive pillows, attention to avoiding extreme flexion of joints, and care to avoid compressing nerves or arteries (the result of which can be neurologic or circulatory compromise) are all important considerations for both skin care and general maintenance of the patient.

The unaffected foot (or feet) should rest against a footboard at least part of the day. This helps to maintain the foot in a neutral position for a more normal walking position, prevents the weight of bedclothes from contributing to foot-drop, and provides a firm surface against which the person can do resistive foot exercises. Patients should be taught to check the position of their lower limbs when at rest. If their problem is nonneurologic, they should "toe in" to prevent external rotation contracture of the hip and pronation of the foot. These complications cause serious difficulty when walking is resumed.

For the general public, it should be remembered that *poor posture* throughout life may contribute to *hypertrophic arthritis*. Molding the pelvis correctly with a posterior pelvic tilt will help prevent increased curvature of the lower back

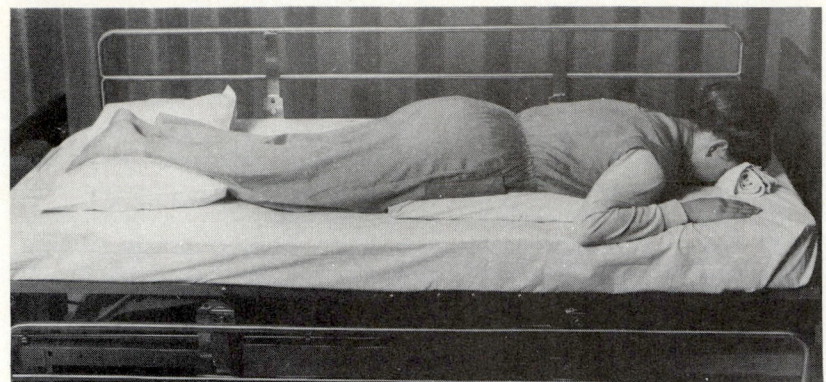

Fig. 22-4 Prone position. (From Rantz, M, and Courtial, D: Lifting, moving, and transferring patients: a manual, ed 2, St. Louis, 1981, The CV Mosby Co.)

with its resultant strain on muscles and joints. Holding the head up with the chin in takes a great deal of strain from the joints of the upper spine. It is surprising how many older persons can benefit from posture improvement even though damage may date from childhood. Nurses should teach patients good body mechanics to prevent muscle strain that could pull a joint out of alignment just enough for musculoskeletal changes to develop or to cause symptoms.

Conservative measures of health teaching

The following are primarily for individuals with joint and muscle disorders. They can be restorative, preventive, or analgesic in nature.

ACTIVITY

Because many musculoskeletal disorders are problems of activity limitation, nursing care is directed toward improving activity. Absolute rest of a limb, joint, or part of the body may be ordered to prevent further tissue destruction and pain. As symptoms subside, activity will be gradually increased.

Clues such as pain, tiredness, and progressive loss of dexterity are helpful in recognizing the need for rest. The most frequent indicator that the patient has overused or misused a joint is an increase in pain or fatigue. Joint protection techniques that can be helpful, particularly for chronic inflammatory joint disorders, are as follows:

1. *Energy conservation techniques:* Examples are sliding rather than lifting objects and moving dishes, utensils, or equipment on a cart rather than carrying them.
2. *Avoiding positions of possible deformity:* Because flexor muscles are stronger than extensor muscles, joints tend to become deformed in a position of flexion. For example, avoid sitting for long periods, keeping the knees or elbows bent to avoid pain, and twisting motions to turn doorknobs or remove a jar lid.
3. *Learning to avoid holding muscles or joints in one position for a long time:*
   a. Activities need to be varied (as just mentioned).
   b. Active range of motion exercises are encouraged.

4. *Learning to use the strongest joints for activities:*
   a. Use good posture when sitting and standing.
   b. Work at a comfortable height.
   c. Stoop and use the knees and not the back when lifting objects.

ASSISTIVE, SUPPORTIVE, AND SAFETY DEVICES

Although the occupational therapist may recommend specific assistive devices and teach the patient how to use them, the nurse needs to understand the need for them and encourage their use in self-care activities.

Supportive devices or ambulatory aids (walkers, canes, crutches) permit part of the person's weight to be transferred to the upper extremities. The physical therapist determines the specific device that is needed. Physical therapists generally select and teach the person how to use ambulatory devices. However, nurses may be called on to do this teaching. They must, in any case, know how to supervise the person who uses ambulatory aids. The most common gait patterns that may be used with a walker, cane, or crutches are the *three-point gait,* the *two-point gait,* and the *four-point gait.* These gait patterns are covered in Chapter 26.

Examples of *safety devices* used include the following:
1. Grab bars around toilets, tubs, and showers
2. Elevated toilet seats
3. Skid-proof mats or adhesive strips on tub floors
4. Hand rails along hallways and staircases
5. Nonskid wax applied to floors

USE OF HEAT AND COLD

1. Moist heat is often used for relaxation of muscles and for sedative and analgesic effects.
2. Cold is often used to reduce or prevent swelling after trauma and to reduce pain and stiffness in some cases.
3. Precautions when using heat or cold:
   a. Apply with care to persons with decreased sensation.
   b. Check skin frequently for evidence of redness or burning.
   c. Moist compresses must be left on for 15 to 20 minutes to achieve maximal effectiveness.

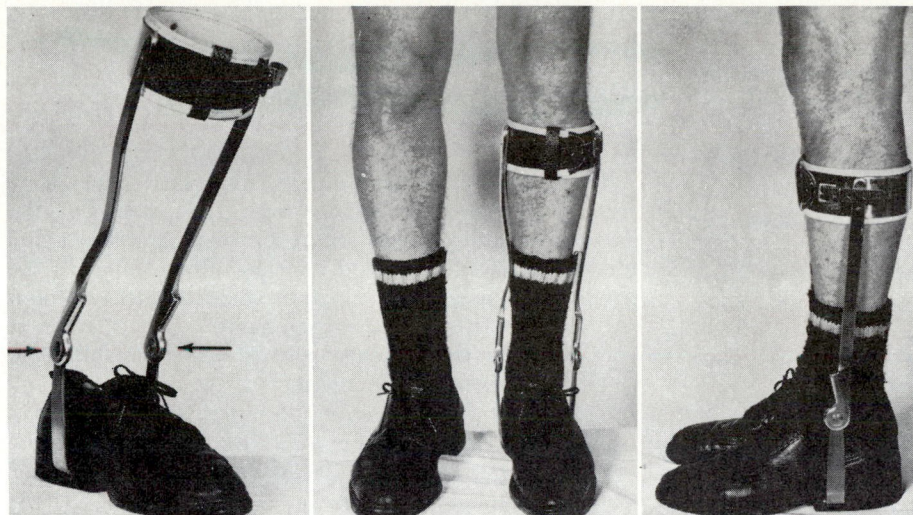

Fig. 22-5 Spring-loaded brace. (From Brashear, H, and Raney, R: Shand's handbook of orthopaedic surgery, ed 10, St. Louis, 1986, The CV Mosby Co.)

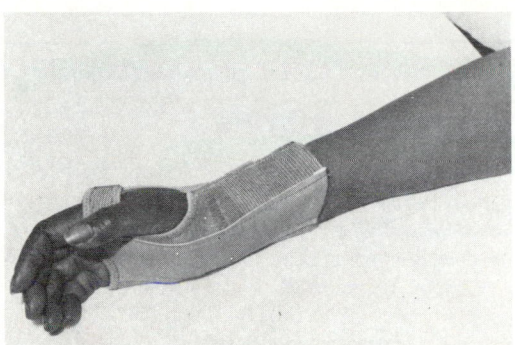

Fig. 22-6   Resting splints.

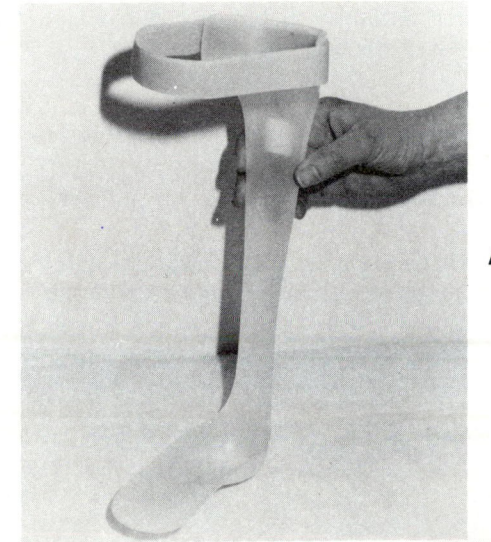

A

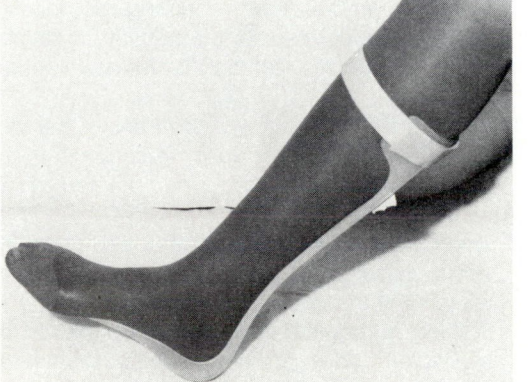

B

Fig. 22-7   Functional splints.

d. Dry heat must have a control device to regulate the heat at a low level.
e. Do not use heat on joints that are or may be *infected*.
f. Ice packs must be wrapped in toweling to protect the skin.

■ **SPLINTING AND BRACING**

Splints and braces (orthoses) are used to stabilize or support a joint to protect it from improper use or external trauma.

1. *Spring-loaded braces* are designed to oppose the action of unparalyzed muscles and to act as partial functional substitutes for the paralyzed muscles (Fig. 22-5).
2. *Resting splints* are designed to maintain a limb or joint in a functional position while permitting the muscles around the joint to relax (Fig. 22-6). They are used by the patient with rheumatoid arthritis to decrease muscle spasms that contribute to joint deformity.
3. *Functional splints* maintain the joint or limb in a usable position such as in the case of a drop wrist or foot-drop (Fig. 22-7).

Special considerations for splinting and bracing include the following:

1. Corrective shoes may be ordered for the feet to provide support and safety. These should be oxford type with laces.
2. Observations of the patient's skin should be made after an orthosis has been worn, even for short periods, for areas of skin irritation. Adjustment may be needed by the *orthotist* (brace maker).
3. Patients must learn how to apply and remove braces or splints and how to care for them.
   a. Metal braces should be stored upright.
   b. Splints of molded materials should be stored away from sources of heat.
   c. Leather materials should be treated with Neatsfoot Compound or other leather preservative to prevent drying and cracking.
4. The brace should be adjusted if there is a change in weight (loss or gain).

■ MOVING THE PATIENT

The student is referred to sources that are available regarding proper transfer techniques. A few basic guidelines are given in the box below.

Guidelines for moving the patient

1. If one side of the body is stronger than the other, *the patient should always be moved toward the strong side.* This guideline correlates with the principle that it is easier to move objects by pulling them than by pushing them. If the patient moves toward the strong side, the strong side is being used to pull the weak side through the required movement. The person assisting with the move should *support the strong side* to make it more effective.
2. If there is any question regarding the patient's ability to cooperate with the transfer, a second person should be standing by for assistance if needed.
3. If the person helping with the transfer has any doubt about his or her ability to accomplish the transfer safely, help should be obtained before attempting it.
4. The transfer should be accomplished using the strong muscles of the legs rather than the weak muscles of the back.
5. If lifting is required, adequate help should be available. If adequate help is not available, the transfer should not be attempted at that time.
6. Whenever possible, pull sheets should be used to move the patient rather than trying to slide the patient (for example, from bed to cart).

Major health problems of the musculoskeletal system

The disorders and injuries of the musculoskeletal system are vast in scope. They range from those that cause the patient minor discomfort and inconvenience to those that are life threatening. Listed here are some common musculoskeletal disorders that will be covered in this chapter.

1. *Inflammatory disorders:* rheumatoid arthritis, systemic lupus erythematosus, polymyositis (dermatomyositis), ankylosing spondylitis
2. *Nonarticular rheumatism:* bursitis, carpal tunnel syndrome, Dupuytren's contracture
3. *Degenerative disorders:* degenerative joint disorder and degenerative joint disorder of the spine
4. *Restrictive disorders:* scoliosis
5. *Other disorders:* gout, bacterial arthritis
6. *Trauma:* fractures of bone and soft tissue injuries

■ INFLAMMATORY DISORDERS

■ Rheumatoid arthritis

The etiology, signs and symptoms, and medical therapy for rheumatic disorders appear in Table 22-1.

Rheumatoid arthritis is a chronic, systemic, progressive inflammatory disorder that is more prevalent in women (3:1 over men) between 25 and 35 years of age.

■ PATHOPHYSIOLOGY

The inflammation begins in the synovial joints with edema, vascular congestion, fibrin exudate, and cellular infiltration. Continued inflammation leads to thickening of the synovium, particularly where it joins the articular cartilage. At these junctures, granulation tissue forms a *pannus*, or mantle, that covers the surface of the cartilage. The pannus also invades subchondral bone. As the amount of granulation tissue from inflammation increases, it interferes with normal nutrition of the articular cartilage. The cartilage becomes necrotic. The degree of erosion of the articular cartilage will determine the amount of articular disability. If large areas of cartilage are destroyed, adhesions form between the joint surfaces, and fibrous or bony union (ankylosis) develops between what were previously articulating surfaces. Destruction of cartilage and bone, in addition to some weakening of tendons and ligaments, may lead to subluxation or dislocation of joints. Invasion of the subchondral bone may cause eventual regional osteoporosis (increased bone porosity).

The course of rheumatoid arthritis varies greatly from person to person. It is marked by periods of exacerbation and remission. Some individuals have been known to recover from a first attack and never suffer a recurrence. For others, particularly those in whom the rheumatoid factor is found (seropositive rheumatoid disorder), the disorder tends to be chronically progressive. In a small number

Table 22-1   Inflammatory disorders

Disorder	Etiology	Signs and symptoms	Medical therapy

Rheumatoid arthritis	Cause unknown
	Theories of causation:
	1. Immune mechanisms (antigen-antibody) such as interaction of the IgG class of immunoglobins with the rheumatoid factor (RF)
	2. Metabolic factors
	3. Infection with attention to viruses
		Local signs and symptoms:
		1. Generalized joint aching with stiffness and limitation in motion
		2. Gradual swelling, warmth, redness, and tenderness
		3. Changes in appearance of hands
		  a. Fusiform or spindle-shaped swelling of fingers
		  b. Swan-neck deformities of fingers
		  c. Ulnar deviation of the hands
		4. All joints can become involved: hips, knees, wrists, elbows, shoulders, and jaw
		Systemic signs and symptoms:
		Fatigue, malaise, fever, tachycardia, weakness, loss of weight, anemia; gradual bilateral, symmetric polyarthritis of small and large joints in all extremities
			Rest: complete bed rest during acute periods; otherwise 2 to 4 hr daily; rest for joints with splints
			Physical therapy:
			1. Active-assistive exercises to regular program of active exercises to preserve function
			2. Moist heat packs or baths for muscle relaxing and relief of pain
			Medications: Table 22-2 lists medications prescribed in the treatment of the disorder
			Reconstructive surgery may be necessary

of individuals the disorder may be rapidly progressive, marked by unremitting joint destruction and diffuse vasculitis. Exacerbations can be triggered by physical or mental stress.

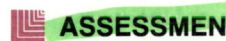 **ASSESSMENT**

☐ **Subjective data**

The early manifestations of the disorder may lead the person to describe the location of aching and stiffness "in my arms," "in my hands," or "in my legs" as opposed to naming specific joints. This kind of discomfort may be present for some period of time before the person begins to see and feel the joint changes.

☐ **Objective data**

1. Inspection and palpation: check same joints on *both sides of body* for symmetry, skin color, size and shape, tenderness, and swelling
2. Evaluate passive range of motion of synovial joints
   a. Note any deviation form normal (limited joint movement most important)
   b. Note presence of crepitation (*crepitus*), which is an audible grating sound made by movement of bony surfaces within the joint
   c. Note pain with range of motion

3. Inspect and palpate skeletal muscles bilaterally
   a. Note atrophy, tone, and tenderness
   b. Test muscle strength by resistive movements

☐ **Diagnostic tests**

1. Serologic tests
   a. Erythrocyte sedimentation rate: will be elevated
   b. Red and white blood cell count: will reveal anemia and leukocytosis
   c. Rheumatoid factor (RF) (present in 50% to 90% of patients, depending on duration and severity of disease): serum will show presence of large antibody-like protein molecules
   d. Latex fixation test is positive
2. Roentgenographic examinations
   a. Periarticular osteoporosis: joint surface erosion
   b. Later: narrowing of joint space, subluxation, and ankylosis
3. Joint aspiration: samples of synovial fluid from within the joint cavity will determine the presence of an aseptic inflammatory process; synovial fluid is cultured and examined microscopically

➡ **DATA ANALYSIS: NURSING DIAGNOSES**

Nursing diagnoses are determined from assessment of patient data. Possible nursing diagnoses for the person with

Table 22-2 Medications prescribed in the treatment of rheumatoid arthritis

Medication	Action	Side effects/toxic effects	Precautions
Salicylates			
Examples: acetyl-salicylic acid, choline salicy-lates	Analgesic, antipyretic, an-tiinflammatory	Gastric irritation; dose related salicylism; skin rash; hyper-sensitivity	Take with food, milk, or antacid; space q 4-6 hr to maintain antiin-flammatory effect
Nonsteroidal antiinflammatory agents (NSAIAs)*			
Indomethacin (In-docin)	Analgesic, antiinflammatory	Headache; dizziness; insom-nia; confusion; gastrointes-tinal irritation	Take with food, milk, or antacid; dis-continue if CNS symptoms develop and notify physician
Ibuprofen (Motrin)	Same as indomethacin	Same as indomethacin but believed less irritating to GI tract; fluid retention	Delayed absorption if taken with food
Tolmetin sodium (Tolectin)	Same as ibuprofen	Same as ibuprofen	Take with food or milk
Naproxen (Napro-syn)	Same as ibuprofen	Same as ibuprofen; also drowsiness	Take with food, milk or antacid; avoid driving until dosage effect estab-lished
Fenoprofen calcium (Nalfon)	Same as ibuprofen	Same as naproxen	Delayed absorption if taken with food; avoid driving until dosage ef-fect established
Sulindac (Clinoril)	Same as ibuprofen	Same as ibuprofen; also skin rash	Take with food, milk, or antacid; not to be used with acetylsalicylic acid
Diflunisal (Dolobid)	Analgesic, antiinflammatory	Gastric irritation; headache; dizziness; skin rash; tinni-tus; fluid retention	Take with food or milk; not to be used with salicylates or other an-tiinflammatory medications
Piroxicam (Fel-dene)	Analgesic, antiinflammatory	Gastric irritation; anemia; skin rash; fluid retention; dizzi-ness; headache	Take with food or antacid
Potent antiinflammatory agents			
Adrenocortico-steroids (for ex-ample, Predni-sone)	Interfere with body's normal inflammatory response	Fluid retention, sodium reten-tion, potassium depletion; hypertension; decreased healing potential; increased susceptibility to infection; gastrointestinal irritation; hir-sutism; osteoporosis; fat de-posits; diabetes mellitus; myopathy; adrenal insuffi-ciency or adrenal crisis if abruptly withdrawn	Take with food, milk, or antacid; dos-age not to be increased or de-creased without physician supervi-sion; take in morning if taken on a once-a-day basis
Phenylbutazone (Butazolidin)	Antiinflammatory; analgesic at subcortical site in brain	Gastrointestinal irritation; he-matologic toxicity; hyperten-sion; impaired renal function	Used for a short term (7-10 days); take with food or milk
Slow-acting antiinflammatory agents†			
Antimalarials			
Hydroxychloroquine (Plaquenil)	Antiinflammatory (mecha-nism unknown); effect not expected to be noted for 6-12 mo after begin-ning therapy	Gastrointestinal disturbances; retinal edema that may re-sult in blindness	Eye examination before beginning therapy and every 6 mo thereafter
Chloroquine (Ara-len)	Same as hydroxychloro-quine	Same as hydroxychloroquine	Same as hydroxychloroquine
Quinacrine (Ata-brine)	Same as hydroxychloro-quine	Same as hydroxychloroquine but may be better tolerated; yellow discoloration of skin	May be stopped periodically to pre-vent deepening of skin discolor-ation

*Acetylsalicylic acid (aspirin) is the drug of choice in the initial treatment of rheumatoid arthritis. NSAIAs are aspirin-like drugs. They may produce less gastric irritation, and some need to be taken only once or twice a day.

†It should be noted that the immunosuppressive agents azathioprine (Imuran), cyclophosphamide (Cytoxan), chlorambucil (Leukeran), and methotrexate have been used on an investigational basis in patients with severe disease that has not responded to the conventional medications. These are used with great care because of their severe side effects and the attendant risks of the development of neoplasms.

Table 22-2   Medications prescribed in the treatment of rheumatoid arthritis—cont'd

Medication	Action	Side effects/toxic effects	Precautions
Gold salts—IM			
Gold sodium thiomalate (Myochrysine) Gold thioglucose (Solganal)	Antiinflammatory; effect not noted for 3-6 months after beginning therapy	Renal and hepatic damage; corneal deposits; dermatitis; ulcerations in mouth; hematologic changes	Urinalysis and CBC before each injection; report dermatitis, metallic taste in mouth, or lesions in mouth to physician
Gold—oral Auranofin (Ridaura)			Oral gold may produce fewer side effects than injectable, but periodic laboratory tests are required
Others			
Penicillamine (Cuprimine)	Antiinflammatory (mechanism unclear); effect not expected to be noted until several months after beginning treatment	Fever, skin rash; nephrotic syndrome; hematologic changes; gastrointestinal irritation; lupuslike syndromes; allergic reactions (33% probability if allergic to penicillin); retarded wound healing	Urinalysis, CBC, differential, hemoglobin and platelet count at least weekly for 3 mo, then monthly; report skin rash, fever to physician; food interferes with absorption—take on empty stomach between meals

rheumatoid arthritis may include, but are not limited to, the following:

Diagnostic title	Possible etiologies
Body image disturbance	Change in body appearance, swollen, deformed joints, change in posture
Potential for injury	Loss of muscle strength, pain and stiffness in joints
Knowledge deficit	Unfamiliarity with information sources
Pain: joints	Pathologic changes caused by rheumatoid arthritis
Bathing/hygiene, dressing/grooming, toileting self-care deficit	Musculoskeletal impairment, inability to use certain joints/limitations in motion

PLANNING: EXPECTED PATIENT OUTCOMES

Expected patient outcomes for the person with rheumatoid arthritis may include, but are not limited to, the following:

1. Patient is more comfortable.
2. Patient has improved active joint range of motion.
3. Patient demonstrates improved ability to perform ADL.
4. Patient has a more positive self-concept.
5. Patient can explain the disease process and follow-up care including prescribed therapy (exercises, medications) and plans established for follow-up by the physician.

IMPLEMENTATION

☐ **Assisting with achievement of therapeutic goals**

1. Give prescribed medications on time and in prescribed doses (Table 22-2).
2. Assist with selection of foods; assist with feeding if necessary; encourage small, frequent meals.
3. Encourage patient to maintain normal weight.
4. Encourage and assist with range of motion exercises to increase mobility and muscle strength.

☐ **Assisting with comfort and ADL**

1. Keep patient free of pain with prescribed medications.
2. Apply heat to joints as ordered by physician.
3. Assist with self-care while promoting independence as much as possible.
4. Promote frequent position changes.
5. Provide for adequate periods of rest.
6. Encourage use of resting splints.

☐ **Counseling and teaching**

When teaching persons about rheumatoid arthritis (and other rheumatic diseases) nurses may find it helpful to use some of the patient teaching material that has been prepared by the Arthritis Foundation.* Booklets, such as *Arthritis: the basic facts,* are written in such a way that most patients can understand and learn from them.

---

*3400 Peachtree Dr. N.E., Atlanta, GA 30326.

Patient teaching should include information about the following[8]:
1. Proper balance of rest and activity
2. Joint protection and energy conservation techniques
3. Proper use of medications—names of drugs, dosages, precautions in administration, and side effects or toxic effects
4. Plans for implementation of exercise program prescribed by the physician or physical therapist
5. Proper application of heat and/or cold packs
6. Proper use of walking aides and other assistive devices
7. Safety measures to prevent injury
8. Application of appropriate use of, and care of splints, braces
9. The basics of good nutrition and the importance of avoiding weight gain
10. The importance of regular follow-up with the physician
11. The risks of following programs that promise a "cure"
12. Information about local arthritis support groups and programs, services of the Arthritis Foundation

✚ EVALUATION

Evaluation is based on the expected patient outcomes. Questions to be asked include the following:
1. Is patient comfortable?
2. Is the potential for injury lessened?
3. Can the patient explain the need for follow-up care?
4. Can the patient explain the program of exercises?
5. Can the patient explain the importance of alternating rest and activity?

■ RECONSTRUCTIVE SURGERY

When rheumatoid arthritis is progressive or has caused severe joint destruction, surgery may be indicated to relieve pain and improve function.

The common types of surgery and the indications for each are outlined below.

Synovectomy: The early removal of synovial tissue to arrest the course of rheumatoid arthritis in a particular joint, to maintain joint function, and to prevent recurrent inflammation. The knee and the wrist are the joints most often subjected to this procedure.

Arthrotomy: Opening into a joint. The procedure is used to accomplish the following:
1. Explore the joint to determine the presence of a disease process
2. Drain the joint
3. Remove damaged tissue or foreign bodies within the joint
4. Most often performed on the knee

Arthrodesis: Surgical fusion of a joint. Commonly performed on knee, wrist, or ankle. The procedure is used to accomplish the following:
1. Eliminate painful motion
2. Provide stability

Arthroplasty: Resurfacing of one or both sides of a diseased joint.
1. Purposes
   a. Restore motion of the joint
   b. Relieve pain
   c. Correct deformity
2. Types
   a. Replacement of part of the joint with a prosthesis made of metal or other material such as the "cup" or "mold" arthroplasty of the hip joint.
   b. Surgical reshaping of the bones of the joint, which are then covered with soft tissue used as an interposition device.

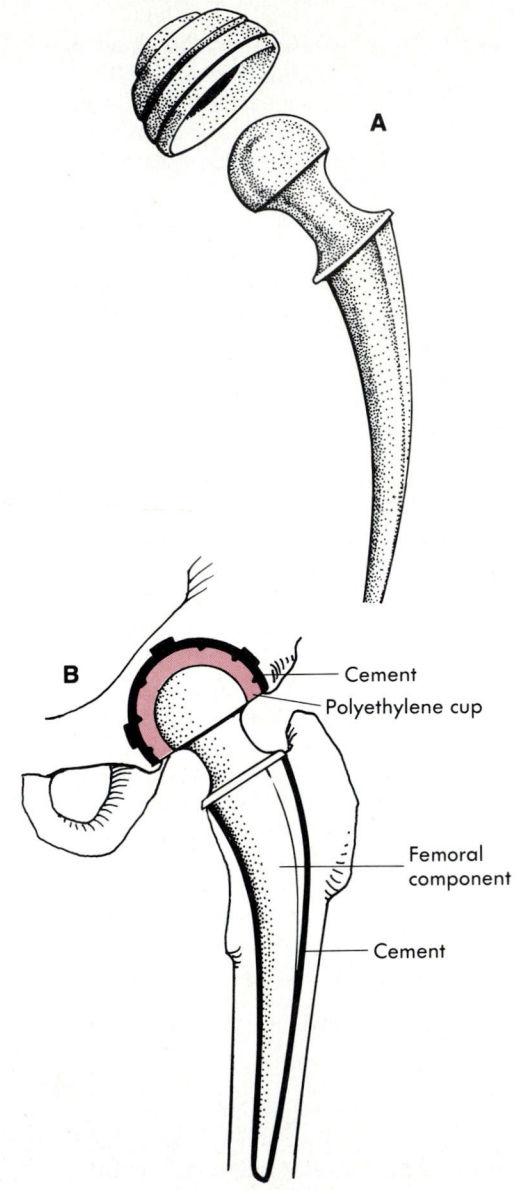

Fig. 22-8 **A,** Acetabular and femoral components of total hip prosthesis. **B,** Total hip prosthesis in place.

Nursing care of the patient undergoing total hip replacement

Preoperative care

1. Skin care
   a. Preparation of the skin will follow the hospital's written procedure or the surgeon's written orders.
   b. The area must be kept free of contamination.
   c. The patient's environment must be as free as possible from potential sources of contamination.
2. Reassurance and education
   a. Patient needs to understand about the surgical procedure, postoperative care, and expectations after discharge.
   b. Patient is to sign the operative permit and have an understanding of its importance (informed consent).

Postoperative care

1. Positioning
   a. Position will depend on the design of the prosthesis and the method of insertion.
   b. Restrictions designed to avoid dislocation of the prosthesis usually include the following:
      (1) Flexion limited to 60 degrees for 6-10 days, then 90 degrees for 2-3 months
      (2) No adduction beyond midline for 2-3 months, therefore no sidelying on operative side. Leg is maintained in abduction when lying supine or on the nonoperative side.
      (3) No extreme internal or external rotation.
2. Wound care: Drains are placed in the wound to prevent formation of a hematoma.
   a. Maintain constant suction through the self-contained vacuum of the Porto-Vac.
   b. Note amount and types of drainage.
   c. Keep area free of contamination. (Infection at the site of the prosthesis results in total failure of the surgery.)
3. Activity
   a. Observe flexion restrictions when elevating head of bed.
   b. Encourage periodic elevation and lowering of head of bed to provide motion at hip.
   c. Instruct patient in use of overhead trapeze to shift weight and lift for bedpan, change of linen.
   d. Encourage active dorsi-plantar flexion exercise of ankles, quadriceps and gluteal setting exercises to promote venous return, prevent thrombus formation, and maintain muscle tone (see Chapter 18).
   e. Patient may be turned to unoperative side with operative leg maintained in abduction and extension.
   f. Begin ambulation about the third or fourth postoperative day.
      (1) Observe flexion and adduction restrictions.
      (2) Observe weight-bearing restrictions prescribed by surgeon (usually partial weight bearing assisted with walker or crutches).
      (3) Increase amount of walking each day according to patient's tolerance.
   g. Begin sitting when patient demonstrates sufficient control of leg to sit within flexion restrictions (usually requires elevation of sitting surfaces, including use of raised toilet seat).
4. Medications
   a. Prophylactic anticoagulant drugs (acetylsalicylic acid, low dose heparin, or coumadin) may be prescribed to decrease risk of thrombus formation.
   b. Initial pain control with positioning; narcotics, gradually tapered to nonnarcotic analgesics according to patient's tolerance.
5. Discharge instructions
   a. Patient must use ambulatory aid, avoid adduction, and limit hip flexion to 90 degrees for about 2 months.
   b. A raised toilet seat is to be obtained and used at home until flexion restrictions are removed.
   c. Patient may need a long-handled shoe horn and reacher to facilitate ADL within flexion restriction.
   d. Patient must be made aware of the life-long need for antibiotic prophylaxis to protect the prosthesis from bacterial infection during dental work, intrusive procedures, or surgery.

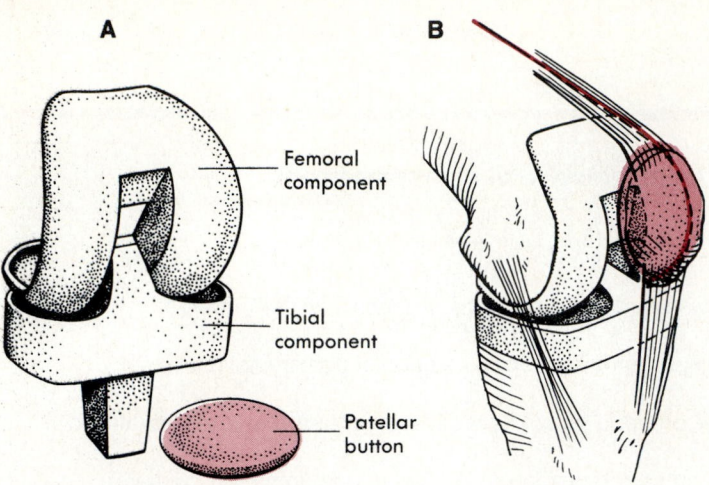

A

Femoral
component

Tibial
component

Patellar
button

B

Fig. 22-9 **A,** Tibial and femoral components of total knee prosthesis. Patellar button, made of polyethylene, protects posterior surface of patella from friction against femoral component when knee is moved through flexion and extension. **B,** Total knee prosthesis in place.

Nursing care of the patient undergoing total knee replacement

Preoperative care

Same as for total hip replacement.

Postoperative care

1. Positioning
   a. The operative leg is elevated on pillows to enhance venous return for the first 48 hours. Pillows are placed with caution not to flex the knee (Fig. 22-10).
   b. The patient may be turned from side to back to side.
2. Wound care
   a. Care of drains as for total hip replacement.
   b. Patient is assessed for systemic evidence of loss of blood (hypotension, tachycardia) if bulky compression dressing is used as it may hold large quantities of drainage before drainage is visible.
   c. Bulky dressings are removed before the patient begins active flexion.
3. Activity
   a. Passive flexion in a continuous passive motion machine (CPM) within prescribed flexion-extension limits may be started in the recovery room. Patient's leg should remain in machine as much as tolerated (up to 22 hours per day) to facilitate even healing of tissue.[31]
   b. Patient is encouraged to perform active dorsi-plantar flexion of the ankles, quadriceps setting, and, after the drain is removed, straight leg raising exercises.
   c. Patient begins active flexion exercises three to four times a day about the fifth postoperative day.
   d. Light weight bearing with an assistive device may be started as early as the first postoperative day and increased as the patient tolerates.
   e. Sitting in a chair with the leg elevated may be started on the first postoperative day.
   f. Patient is encouraged to wear a resting knee extension splint (immobilizer) on the operated leg until able to demonstrate quadriceps control (independent straight leg raising).
4. Pain control
   a. Initial control of pain with narcotics, positioning; gradual decrease of medication to nonnarcotic analgesics as patient tolerates.
   b. Patient is encouraged to use ice to knee for 20-30 minutes before and after active flexion exercise.
5. Discharge instructions
   a. Patient must observe partial weight-bearing restriction and use ambulatory aid for approximately 2 months following discharge.
   b. Patient should continue active flexion and straight leg raising exercises at home.
   c. Patient must be made aware of the life-long need for antibiotic prophylaxis (see p. 581).

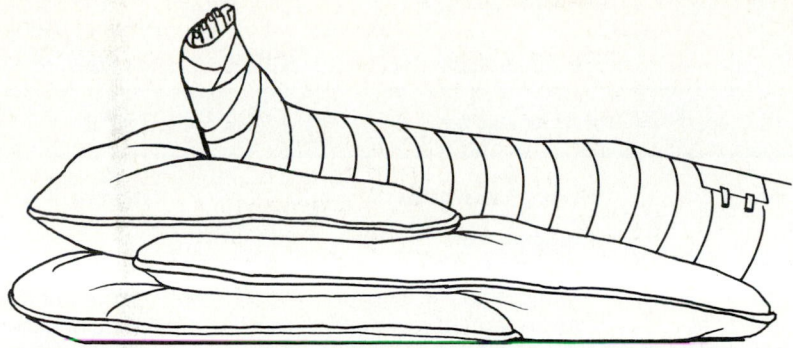

Fig. 22-10   Leg properly elevated on pillows, avoiding knee flexion.

c. Total joint replacement where both sides of the joint are replaced by metal or polyethylene implants.

Replacement arthroplasty

Replacement arthroplasty is available for the shoulder, wrist, elbow, phalangeal joints of the fingers, hips (Fig. 22-8), knee (Fig. 22-9), and ankle. Because the hip and knee are the most commonly replaced, the discussion that follows will be limited to these two joints.

Rheumatoid arthritis, degenerative joint disease, and avascular necrosis are the major reasons for performing total joint or replacement arthroplasty. *Avascular necrosis of the bone,* or bone death, is caused by inadequate blood supply. It can be a *complication of bone fractures,* as well as corticosteroid treatment for rheumatoid arthritis and systemic lupus erythematosus. Pain (even at rest), restricted motion, and gait disturbances are characteristic. Surgery in the form of total joint replacement is performed to alleviate pain and increase motion.

The hip prosthesis consists of an acetabular portion (cup) and a femoral component. The designs of the various prostheses vary in size of the femoral head, shape and length of the femoral shaft, and design of the acetabular component. The care of the patient undergoing total hip or total knee replacement is outlined in the box on p. 582 and in the Nursing Care Plan below.

◻ PLANNING: EXPECTED PATIENT OUTCOMES

Expected patient outcomes for the person undergoing surgery for a rheumatoid condition may include, but are not limited to, the following:

1. Patient continues with activities and weight-bearing restrictions for period recommended by surgeon.
2. Patient uses assistive devices as prescribed.
3. Incision heals without infection.

NURSING CARE PLAN

Person with total knee replacement

DATA: Mr. Kathcarb is a 59-year-old married office manager with osteoarthritis of the right knee. Over the past 8 months he has had increased pain in his knee with only minimal relief from the nonsteroidal antiinflammatory medications prescribed by his internist. He reports that he must now ambulate with a cane when his pain is severe. He can no longer participate in many activities he used to enjoy because of his discomfort and limited mobility. After consulting his internist and an orthopaedic surgeon he has decided to undergo elective total knee replacement. Mr. Kathcarb is admitted to the nursing division the afternoon before he is scheduled for surgery.

The nursing history identified the following:
1. He and his wife reside in a two-story colonial house with the bedroom upstairs.
2. He plans to return home after this hospitalization and has received a 6-week leave of absence from his job.
3. He is not prescribed any medications other than his "arthritis pills" and has no other preexisting medical problems.
4. He was last hospitalized 18 years ago for a cholecystectomy.

Nursing diagnosis: Knowledge deficit: related to lack of exposure to total knee replacement surgery

Care Plan by Kyle Paskert, MSN, RN.   *Continued.*

NURSING CARE PLAN

Person with total knee replacement—cont'd

Expected patient outcomes	Nursing interventions	Rationale

Patient states he understands the teaching provided by the nurse
 	
Patient will have less anxiety related to fear of the unknown and/or misconceptions regarding the surgery and recovery period
	Preoperative:
	Assess need for instruction and provide as necessary
	Provide written materials pertaining to total knee replacement (TKR) surgery available in the institutions
	Review preoperative instruction with patient and family before the surgery
	Evaluate patient's understanding of the information taught
	Postoperative:
	By discharge the patient should be instructed and able to demonstrate:
	  Independent ambulation on level surfaces with appropriate ambulatory aid, and independent stair climbing
	  Exercises to be performed at home and frequency (straight leg raising and active flexion)
	  Activity restrictions to be observed for approximately 2 months until follow-up with physician. These include no kneeling or jarring activities
	  Rationale for antibiotic prophylaxis for dental procedures and procedures requiring instrumentation or surgery
	  Use of knee immobilizer as resting splint
		Understanding about surgical procedure and postoperative care should lessen anxiety and promote desired behaviors for recovery from surgery

Nursing diagnosis: Impaired home maintenance management: potential for, related to numerous discharge needs

Expected patient outcomes	Nursing interventions	Rationale
Patient and family will express satisfaction with arrangements made to manage self-care at home	Discuss with the patient and family their plans upon discharge from the hospital Determine with them information needed to be taught and learned for home care (refer to knowledge deficit, post-operative) Determine the type of equipment needed, for example, crutches, walker, elevated toilet seat, and consult appropriate department or agency for securing these supplies	Adequate discharge planning will foster successful completion of rehabilitation at home

Person with total knee replacement—cont'd

Collaborative nursing actions after surgery include those to identify possible complications of the surgery. Immediate reporting of and treatment of early signs may prevent serious effects. Nursing actions include monitoring for the following:

a. Neurocirculatory compromise—perform neurocirculatory checks q 2h for the first 24 to 48 h; notify physician of any changes from preoperative status

b. Dislocation of the prosthesis—notify physician if patient complains of sudden onset of increased (severe) pain, joint deformity

c. Impaired skin integrity and/or incision healing—monitor pressure areas for signs of redness; monitor temperature; assess incision for signs or symptoms of infection and excessive drainage

d. Atelectasis/respiratory infection—monitor breath sounds until ambulatory

e. Problems with elimination—assess for urinary stasis and constipation

f. Fluid and electrolyte imbalance—monitor input and output until patient is taking oral fluids equal to at least 1200 ml output; monitor IV fluid flow; assess patient for fluid volume excess or deficit

The following nursing diagnoses are especially pertinent for persons who have undergone TKR surgery. Implementation and evaluation of the related nursing interventions will help to prevent postoperative complications.

Nursing diagnosis: Pain: related to total knee replacement surgery

Expected patient outcomes	Nursing interventions	Rationale
Patient states feeling more comfortable Patient is able to perform necessary postoperative routines/exercises because pain is adequately managed	Assess patient's pain and evaluate response to comfort measures provided	Subjective and objective data are important in ascertaining the nature of the patient's postoperative pain and in determining its management It is usually necessary to administer a narcotic the first 48-72 h after surgery
	Administer prescribed analgesics (usually narcotic) at timely intervals during the initial postoperative period	Analgesics have a greater effect if they are administered before pain becomes severe
	Teach relaxation techniques as appropriate	Relaxation facilitates rest and may modify the response to pain
	Use other pain-relieving techniques as pertinent, for example, back rubs, repositioning, ice to knee for 30 minutes before and after active flexion exercises	A change in type of cutaneous stimulation may result in pain relief. Ice packs can reduce inflammation
	As pain decreases use milder analgesics	As pain lessens in severity it may be controlled by less potent analgesics (with fewer untoward side effects)

Nursing diagnosis: Impaired physical mobility: related to alterations in lower limb S/P TKR surgery

Expected patient outcomes	Nursing interventions	Rationale
Patient will demonstrate optimal level of mobility with adaptive devices by time of discharge No injury has occurred during hospitalization	Cough and deep breathe with incentive spirometer q 1-2 h until fully ambulatory	If carried out correctly and at appropriate intervals, pulmonary exercises can effectively prevent atelectasis and pneumonia
	Turn the patient side to back to side q 2 h and prn while bedrest is prescribed	Turning and repositioning frequently provides for better ventilation of the lungs

Continued.

NURSING CARE PLAN

Person with total knee replacement—cont'd

Expected patient outcomes	Nursing interventions	Rationale
	Encourage the patient to perform active dorsi-plantar flexion, iso-metric quadricep sets, and after the drain is removed, straight leg raises q 2 h until ambulatory, then qid	Exercises of the lower extremities will prevent venous stasis and promote muscle-strengthening
	Elevate the operative leg on pillows in bed and in chair for the first 48 h. Place the pillows under the calf to avoid knee flexion	Elevation of the operative leg on pillows enhances venous return. Flexion contracture is to be avoided
	Sitting in a chair with the leg ele-vated may be started as early as the first postoperative day	The exercise of getting in and out of bed is one means of increas-ing activity in the early postoper-ative period; the patient accrues numerous physiologic benefits from such activity
	Transfer the patient out of bed to chair bid-tid once initiated	
	Begin light weight-bearing ambula-tion with assistive device when patient can straight leg, raise in-dependently, and flex operative leg to 45 degrees (may be started first postoperative day) Increase frequency and distance of ambulation as tolerated	Early ambulation is a significant factor in hastening recovery and preventing postoperative compli-cations
	If continuous passive motion ma-chine (CPM) is used, patient's leg should remain in the machine as tolerated (up to 22 h/day) within the prescribed extension-flexion limits	Passive flexion of the knee may prevent excessive swelling and bruising around the prosthesis and promote greater ease with active flexion
	Begin active flexion exercises ap-proximately fifth postoperative day, qid	Active flexion of the knee is neces-sary to promote return of func-tion; it is desired that the patient achieve approximately 90 de-grees of flexion before discharge from the hospital
	Patient should wear knee immobi-lizer on operative leg until able to demonstrate quadriceps control (independent straight leg raising) except when flexing; the knee immobilizer should also be worn at night as resting splint	The knee immobilizer provides support of the operative leg and prevents incorrect positioning

Table 22-3 Inflammatory disorders

Disorder	Etiology	Signs and symptoms	Medical therapy

Systemic lupus erythematosus (SLE)	Cause unknown
	Theories of causation:
	1. Aberration of the immune system causes immune complexes containing antibodies to be deposited in tissue, thus damaging the tissue
	2. Viral infections caused by or resulting from some immunologic abnormality
	3. Both of above combine to produce the disease
	4. Some drugs cause lupus-like syndromes
	  a. Procainamide (Pronestyl)
	  b. Isonicotinic acid hydrazide (INH)
	  c. Penicillin
		General complaints: Moderate to severe—fever, weakness, fatigue, weight loss, sensitivity to sun, erythematous rash ("butterfly" pattern over bridge of nose and cheeks)
		Polyarthralgia and arthritis with pain and swelling
		Polyserositis (pleurisy and pericarditis)
		Anemia, thrombocytopenia and renal, neurologic, and cardiac abnormalities
		Alopecia (hair loss) possible during periods of active systemic disease
			Rest: when disease active
			No specific treatment; therapeutic program is ordered for the specific problems of the patient
			Medications (Table 22-2): adrenocorticosteroid therapy to control active manifestations of SLE; salicylates for joint pains; antimalarial drugs (Chloroquine) for cutaneous lesions; cytoxic agents if other drug fails

Systemic lupus erythematosus

Systemic lupus erythematosus (SLE) is a chronic inflammatory disorder that affects women, particularly adolescent and young adults, eight to ten times more often than it affects men. The name of the disorder means "red wolf," after its characteristic rash, "likened to the damage wrought by a hungry wolf."

Once thought to be relatively rare and always fatal, the disorder has been found to be fairly common, and its course can be controlled by corticosteroids. Some patients may eventually die as a result of vascular lesions affecting the kidneys, central nervous system, or other vital organs; others may die of complicating secondary infections.

The etiology, signs and symptoms, and medical therapy are presented in Table 22-3.

PATHOPHYSIOLOGY

Pathologic manifestations of the disease include the following:
1. Synovial involvement as a fibrous villous synovitis
2. Severe vasculitis with necrosis of the walls of the small arteries
3. Renal involvement with thickening of the basement membrane of the glomerular tufts and necrosis of the glomerular capillaries
4. Lymph node necrosis
5. Development of small white spots in the retina called *cytoid bodies*
6. Lesions of the nervous system

The initial manifestation of SLE is often arthritis. In many instances the joint symptoms are transient and respond to treatment. Weakness, fatigue, and weight loss may be present. The patient may complain of sensitivity to the sun, developing a rash and at times fever or arthritis on exposure to sunlight. Erythema, usually in a butterfly pattern, appears over the cheeks and bridge of the nose. The margins of these lesions are bright red, and the lesions may extend beyond the hairline with partial alopecia (loss of hair) above the ears. Lesions may also occur on the exposed part of the neck. Lesions spread slowly to the mucous membranes and other tissues of the body, or they may originate there. These lesions do not ulcerate but cause degeneration and atrophy of tissues.

Depending on the organs involved, the patient may have findings of glomerulonephritis, pleuritis, pericarditis, peritonitis, neuritis, or anemia. Renal and neurologic manifestations are among the more serious manifestations of the disease.

ASSESSMENT

Subjective data

1. Note that patients may express vague symptoms or simply say that they are "always tired."
2. Question patients about generalized weakness, loss of appetite, loss of weight, skin rashes, and specific joint discomfort (even at rest).
3. Identify the presence and extent of discomfort or stiffness of muscles or joints.
4. Identify the presence of sensitivity of eyes and skin to the sun.
5. Question patients regarding hair loss, which occurs during acute episodes.

□ Objective data

1. Observe for erythema over the cheeks and bridge of the nose, above the ears, on exposed part of the neck, and over other body areas
2. Examine for loss of hair or partial loss at normal hairline
3. Check for muscle strength and range of motion of joints

□ Diagnostic tests

As mentioned above, many organs may be involved. Laboratory findings may be specific to the organs involved, as with proteinuria, abnormal cerebrospinal fluid, or roentgenographic evidence of pleural reactions. A positive lupus erythematosus (LE) cell reaction and immunofluorescent studies to identify the antibody responsible for LE cell reaction are helpful in making the diagnosis of the disease. Laboratory findings may also show the presence of anemia, thrombocytopenia, leukocytosis, or leukopenia. A *skin biopsy* is taken of the rash and studied for histopathologic evidence of the disorder.

➡ DATA ANALYSIS: NURSING DIAGNOSES

Nursing diagnoses are determined from an assessment of patient data. Possible nursing diagnoses for the patient with systemic lupus erythematosus may include, but are not limited to, the following:

Diagnostic title	Possible etiologies
Activity intolerance	Fatigue/weakness, painful joints
Anxiety	Change in health status; uncertainty about outcome; change in status/role/lifestyle
Knowledge deficit	Lack of information, unfamiliarity with information source/not a commonly known disease
Altered nutrition: less than body requirements	Weakness/fatigue make eating difficult, loss of appetite
Pain	Joint pain

⌊⌉ PLANNING: EXPECTED PATIENT OUTCOMES

Expected patient outcomes for the person with systemic lupus erythematosus may include, but are not limited to, the following:

1. Patient maintains skin integrity.
2. Appetite improves and nutrition is improved.
3. Patient has less fatigue and weakness and activity tolerance is improved.
4. Patient states feeling more comfortable and pain is under control.
5. Patient can explain prescribed therapy and plans for follow-up care.

⌊⌉ IMPLEMENTATION

□ Assisting with achievement of therapeutic goals

1. Medications: administer as prescribed
   a. Antiinflammatory analgesics to control arthritic pain
   b. Antimalarial drugs, particularly if rash is extensive
   c. Corticosteroids for severe neurologic and renal involvement
   d. Cytotoxic agents if other drugs fail
   e. Ointments or skin creams for rash
2. Nutrition: encourage well-balanced diet consisting of all major food groups
3. Activity: encourage planned program of exercises and joint range of motion
4. Kidney dialysis or transplant for uncontrolled lupus nephritis (Chapter 32)
5. Total hip replacement for avascular necrosis consequent to high dose steroid therapy (p. 581)

□ Assisting with comfort and ADL

1. Administer medication for pain of joints and muscles
2. Prevent skin lesions by protecting skin while in sunlight.
3. Help patient with gradual independence in ADL.
4. Provide rest periods as necessary.

□ Counseling and teaching

1. The nature, course, and treatment of the disease
2. Appropriate balance of rest and activity
3. Appropriate exercise
4. How to avoid exposing skin to sunlight; for example, wearing long sleeved blouses or dresses, slacks, broad brimmed hats, cotton gloves
5. Appropriate use of prescribed medications—dose, frequency, precautions, potential side effects
6. Application of cosmetics (hypoallergenic, approved by physician) to mask skin lesions, and/or wigs to mask hair loss
7. Information about lupus support groups (if available in patient's area)

⌗ EVALUATION

Evaluation is based on the expected patient outcomes. Questions to be asked include the following:

1. Has skin integrity been maintained?
2. Can the patient explain the need for rest periods alternating with periods of activity?
3. Can the patient explain the disorder and the need for continued follow-up care?
4. Can the patient explain how to maintain adequate diet?
5. Is the patient more comfortable?

■ Polymyositis (dermatomyositis)

Polymyositis (dermatomyositis) is a diffuse inflammatory disorder of the *striated* (voluntary) muscles. Females are affected twice as commonly as males. The disorder can

Table 22-4 Inflammatory disorders

Disorder	Etiology	Signs and symptoms	Medical therapy
Polymyositis (dermatomyositis)	Cause unknown Theories of causation: 1. Reaction of the autoimmune system, perhaps triggered by a virus 2. Related to malignant tumors	Activities involving movement and lifting become difficult or impossible: 1. Climbing stairs 2. Arising from a chair 3. Combing the hair 4. Getting out of bathtub Weakness can lead to contractures and atrophy Difficulty with swallowing and presence of reflux esophagitis Decreased peristalsis Pulmonary function tests: may indicate impaired gas exchange, decreased vital and total lung capacity Muscle tenderness, transitory joint pain Dusky-red, patchy rash over elbows, dorsum of hands, knees, face, neck, shoulders (dermatomyositis) Weight loss	Symptomatic treatment Medications (Table 22-2): corticosteroids and mild analgesics Physical therapy to prevent contractures, preserve muscle strength Frequent small meals Antacids for reflux esophagitis May need complete bed rest with head of bed elevated on blocks Treatment of underlying malignancy if present

occur at any age. The etiology, signs and symptoms, and medical therapy are listed in Table 22-4.

■ PATHOPHYSIOLOGY

Pathologic findings on histologic studies of biopsied muscle vary, but the alterations found, in order of their frequency, are the following:

1. Primary degeneration of muscle fibers, either focal or extensive
2. Basophilia of some fibers with central migration of the sarcolemmal nuclei
3. Necrosis of parts or entire groups of muscle fibers
4. Inflammation of blood vessels supplying the muscles
5. Interstitial fibrosis varying in severity with the duration and, to some extent, the type of the disease
6. Variation in the cross-sectional diameter of fibers.[56]

The disease usually runs a course of exacerbations and remissions. Often it is first noted in proximal muscles, in particular the pelvic and shoulder girdles. Climbing stairs, arising from a chair, and other activities that involve lifting the body become increasingly difficult or impossible. Lifting the arms becomes progressively more difficult, and combing the hair may be impossible. Other muscles (neck flexors, the muscles of swallowing) may also become involved. Muscle pain or tenderness is present in some instances in the early stages. The presence of a rash marks the disease as *dermatomyositis*. A dusky red lesion may be found in the periorbital region, along with periorbital edema. This dusky red rash may extend over the face, forehead, neck, upper shoulders, chest, and upper back. Lesions on the arms and legs commonly affect the extensor surfaces. These patches are sometimes scaly.

The weakness of myositis, if it persists, can lead to contractures and atrophy. Individuals with the dermatomyositis form of the disease, particularly if they are over 40 years of age, have a 40% to 50% greater chance of having evidence of a malignant neoplasm found during the first 5 years of illness than the population at large. Some physicians believe that routine yearly examinations should be performed to define or exclude the presence of neoplasms in these patients during that 5-year period.

■ ASSESSMENT

□ Subjective data

Polymyositis may vary in its mode of onset and in the rate of progression of symptoms, whether muscular, dermal, or articular. The clinical course may be one of spontaneous remissions and exacerbations.

1. Because muscular weakness is present in nearly all patients and particularly in the lower extremities, the patient is asked to describe the weakness and effect on ADL.
2. Questions are asked about joint and muscle pain, gastrointestinal problems, appetite, and weight loss.

□ **Objective data**

1. Weakness of myositis can lead to contractures and atrophy. Test strength of upper and lower extremities against resistance.
2. Observe patient for respiratory difficulty, because diaphragm may be affected by weakness.
3. Palpate muscles and joints for pain or tenderness.
4. Examine for dusky-red, patchy rash over elbows, dorsum of hands, knees, forehead, neck, shoulders, and chest (dermatomyositis).

□ **Diagnostic tests**
□ *Manual muscle tests*

Manual muscle tests are used to determine the degree of muscular weakness from the disorder. They are used also in cases of injury or muscle disuse. The physical therapist rates the strength of muscles in relation to gravity and applied resistance. Muscle testing is helpful in determining which muscle should be chosen for biopsy. When muscle-strengthening exercises are indicated, the test will indicate the group of muscles that requires the most therapy.

□ *Muscle biopsy*

Biopsy is performed to aid in the diagnosis of specific myopathic disorders. The muscle tissue may reveal degeneration, inflammatory reactions, or involvement of specific fibers.

A muscle biopsy is an operative procedure usually performed by a surgeon. A local or general anesthetic may be used. Following the procedure the patient will have minor to moderate discomfort in the form of stiffness or pain at the operative site. The patient is encouraged to resume range of motion activity to avoid undue stiffness.

□ *Electromyography*

Electromyography measures the electrical activity of muscles; an *electromyogram* (EMG) is a recording of the electrical potential detected by a needle electrode inserted into skeletal muscle. The electrical activity can be heard over a loudspeaker and viewed on an oscilloscope and graph. Normal muscles at rest give off no electrical activity.

The EMG provides evidence of *lower motor neuron disease, primary muscle disease,* and *defects in the transmission of electrical impulses* at the neuromuscular junction, such as in myasthenia gravis. The test cannot be used to differentiate *specific* muscle disorders. There is no specific preparation of the patient, except to reassure the patient that the electrode needles will not cause electric shock and the procedure is not dangerous.

□ *Serum enzyme tests*

Serum glutamic-oxaloacetic transaminase (SGOT), creatine phosphokinase (CPK), and aldolase levels are elevated in the presence of active polymyositis or dermatomyositis.

□ *Twenty-four hour urine tests*

These urine specimens are used to determine if there is an abnormal creatine/creatinine ratio.

DATA ANALYSIS: NURSING DIAGNOSES

Nursing diagnoses are determined from an assessment of patient data. Possible nursing diagnoses for the person with polymyositis may include, but are not limited to, the following:

Diagnostic title	Possible etiologies
Activity intolerance	Generalized weakness because of muscle involvement
Fear	Loss of ability to carry out ADL as in past
Potential for infection	Related to autoimmune response to disease
Potential for injury: muscle weakness	Motor deficits caused by muscle involvement
Knowledge deficit	Lack of exposure to information about a disease that is not commonly understood
Impaired physical mobility	Musculoskeletal impairment
Altered nutrition: less than body requirements	Difficulty in swallowing; in some difficulty lifting head and holding up
Personal identity disturbance	Change in mobility/musculoskeletal involvement may result in changes in life-style
Self-care deficit	Musculoskeletal impairment

PLANNING: EXPECTED PATIENT OUTCOMES

Expected patient outcomes for the person with polymyositis may include, but are not limited to, the following:

1. Patient performs ADL without fatigue or discomfort.
2. Patient has increased energy for physical activities and self-care.
3. Patient maintains nutritional status.
4. Patient understands disease and need for continuing with prescribed therapy and follow-up medical care.

IMPLEMENTATION

□ **Assisting with achievement of therapeutic goals**

1. Promote mobility
   a. Elevate sitting surfaces to facilitate transfers
   b. Provide appropriate ambulatory device to facilitate comfortable walking
   c. Provide for frequent changes of position and range of motion to prevent contractures
   d. Encourage patient to gradually resume independent ADL as symptoms subside
2. Prevent skin breakdown
   a. Reposition patient frequently
   b. Avoid pressure over bony prominences with appropriate protective devices

□ **Assisting with comfort and ADL**

1. During acute episodes, assist with frequent changes of position.

2. Administer prescribed analgesics.
3. Assist with ADL.
4. Provide adequate rest.

☐ **Counseling and teaching**

1. Instruct patient, family in nature and course of disease.
2. Instruct patient in appropriate balance of rest, activity.
3. Instruct patient in use of selected ADL devices to enhance function; for example, long-handled comb.
4. Instruct patient in appropriate use of prescribed steriods—how to take them, dosage, side effects, precautions.

⌗ EVALUATION

Evaluation is based on the expected patient outcomes. Questions to be asked include the following:

1. Does the patient have more energy?
2. Can the patient perform ADL with greater ease?
3. Is the patient maintaining nutritional status?
4. Is the patient able to describe the nature of the disorder and prescribed therapy and why there is a need for continued professional help?

■ Ankylosing spondylitis

Ankylosing spondylitis is a chronic and usually progressive disorder of the sacroiliac and hip joints, the synovial joints of the spine, and the adjacent soft tissues leading to spinal fusion. It affects both sexes, with males being more severely affected. The onset is usually between ages 10 and 30. The progression of the disorder usually decreases after age 50, but limitation of movement of the spine persists. Fusion of the sacroiliac joints and spine up through the cervical vertebrae may occur over periods of 10 to 20 years.

The etiology, signs and symptoms, and medical therapy can be found in Table 22-5.

■ PATHOPHYSIOLOGY

Spondylitis means inflammation of the spine. As a result of inflammation, the bones of the spine grow together, or ankylose (fuse). Inflammation usually begins around the sacroiliac joints, eventually obliterating articular cartilage of the affected bones. The cartilage is replaced by new bony growth. The inflammatory process progresses up the spine, eventually resulting in fusion of the entire spine.

Initial symptoms may include low back pain or aching; pain and swelling of the hips, knees, or shoulders; mild fever; loss of appetite; and fatigue. Low back pain flares and subsides intermittently. Over a period of time, pain subsides and motion of the back becomes restricted. Fusion of the sacroiliac joints and spine up through the cervical vertebrae may occur over a period of 10 to 20 years; as a result, the patient may present either a "poker-back" deformity or a kyphosis at the cervicodorsal junction (Fig. 22-11). Knees are flexed as the person attempts to move the head into an upright position.

Table 22-5 Inflammatory disorders

Disorders	Etiology	Signs and symptoms	Medical therapy

Ankylosing spondylitis	Unknown
	Strong genetic link with the genetic marker HLA-B27; it is thought that there is a link between HLA-B27 and some form of trigger (such as an infection), which sets off a reaction in the immune system leading to the inflammatory response
		Initial symptoms: mild with early morning stiffness and aching
		Later: intermittent pain and restricted motion of the back
		Extraspinal symptoms include:
		1. Pleuritic-like chest pain
		2. Achilles tendonitis
		3. Peripheral arthropathy (especially hips)
		4. Nonspecific symptoms include:
		  a. Weight loss
		  b. Malaise
		  c. Fatigue
		  d. Mood change
		5. "Poker-back" deformity or kyphosis at the cervicodorsal junction
			Postural exercises
			Lying prone (extension) three to four times a day for 15 to 30 minutes
			Rest
			Heat
			Antiinflammatory analgesics
			1. Salicylates
			2. Nonsteroidal antiinflammatory agents
			3. Potent antiinflammatory for short term (phenylbutazone)
			Spinal osteotomy or arthroplasty for severe symptoms

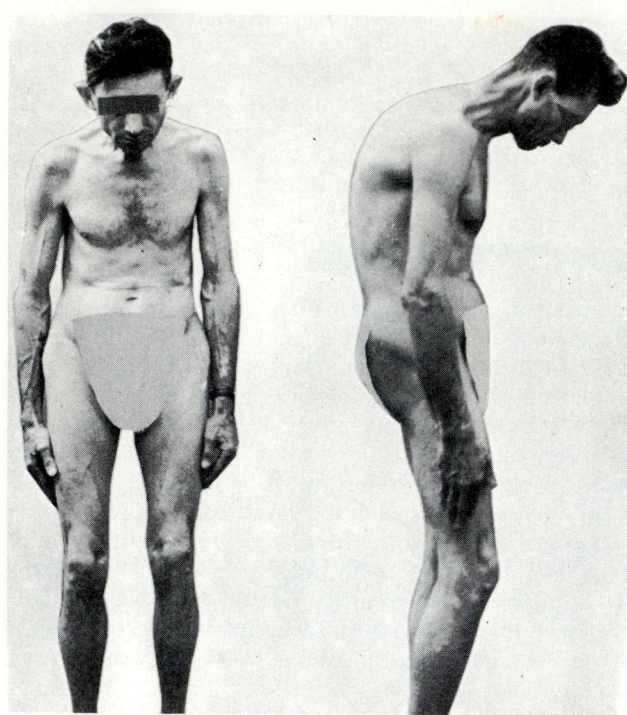

Fig. 22-11 Ankylosing spondylitis in 46-year-old man with ankylosis of entire spine in faulty position. (From Brashear, H, and Raney, R: Shand's handbook of orthopaedic surgery, ed 10, St. Louis, 1986, The CV Mosby Co.)

ASSESSMENT

☐ Subjective data

Many persons with ankylosing spondylitis remain undiagnosed. The patient complains of low backache, stiffness, and alternating or bilateral "sciatica" that lasts for a few days at a time and subsides. Later the symptoms become more persistent and begin to include evidence of ankylosis of joints, particularly of the spine. The patient should be questioned about changes in body shape and any loss in height.

☐ Objective data

1. Observe for pain on assuming or maintaining an erect position.
2. Examine patient's posture: patient appears bent forward at the waist, often compensating to achieve an erect position by flexing hips and knees.
3. Palpate for tenderness over the spine and sacroiliac region.
4. Note pain on motion and limitation in turning and bending upper body.

☐ Diagnostic tests

Roentgenograms are most helpful in delineating the disorder. Changes in the sacroiliac joints are the earliest and most diagnostic. There is blurring of the bony margins, then sclerosis, and later ankylosis. Bony growths, called *syndesmophytes*, that bridge the adjacent vertebrae give the appearance of a "bamboo spine." The presence in the serum of HLA-B27 helps to establish the diagnosis.

➡ DATA ANALYSIS: NURSING DIAGNOSES

Nursing diagnoses are determined from the assessment of patient data. Possible nursing diagnoses for the person with ankylosing spondylitis may include, but are not limited to, the following:

Diagnostic title	Possible etiologies
Body image disturbance	Change in body appearance/immobility, change in lifestyle
Impaired gas exchange	Changes in the spine and in posture change the chest cavity and decrease chest excursion
Knowledge deficit	Lack of exposure to information
Impaired physical mobility	Intolerance to activity because of pain/fatigue and musculoskeletal impairment
Pain	Inflammation of the spine causing pain

PLANNING: EXPECTED PATIENT OUTCOMES

Expected patient outcomes for the person with ankylosing spondylitis may include, but are not limited to, the following:
1. Patient states that pain is improved.
2. Patient is able to perform ADL with less fatigue and discomfort.
3. Patient has minimal interference with breathing capacity.
4. Patient knows course of disease, prescribed therapy, and plans for follow-up care.

IMPLEMENTATION

☐ Assisting with achievement of therapeutic goals

1. Maintain alignment of the spine.
   a. Mattress should be firm.
   b. Bed board may be used.
   c. Patient should sleep flat without pillow.
   d. A back brace may be necessary for support.
2. Postural and breathing exercises
   a. Extension exercises should be performed to maintain erect posture and normal height and to strengthen paraspinal muscles.
   b. Abdominal lying should be done three to four times a day for 15 to 30 minutes.
   c. Breathing exercises will help increase breathing capacity.

3. Give antiinflammatory analgesics as prescribed.
4. Provide for rest periods alternating with activity.
5. Provide care for the patient who may have a spinal osteotomy or hip arthroplasty (p. 588).

☐ **Assisting with comfort**

1. Apply heat to painful joints.
2. Apply hydrotherapy to entire body; this is best if done just before postural and deep breathing exercises.

☐ **Counseling and teaching**

1. Nature and course of disease
2. Prescribed postural exercises
3. Appropriate use of prescribed medications
4. Methods of applying heat to back and hips

⊞ EVALUATION

Evaluation is based on the expected patient outcomes. Questions to be asked include the following:

1. Is the patient able to perform ADL with less discomfort?
2. Is the patient more comfortable?
3. Is the patient able to maintain adequate breathing capacity?
4. Can the patient explain prescribed therapy and plans for follow-up care?

■ NONARTICULAR RHEUMATISM

Nonarticular rheumatic diseases include those disorders in which the supportive structures and structures located near the joints are inflamed, but the joints themselves are not involved except by the limitations imposed by the supportive structures. Some of these disorders are fibrositis, tenosynovitis, bursitis, and carpal tunnel syndrome.

■ Bursitis

Bursitis is inflammation of a bursa, a small fluid-filled saclike cavity between two articular soft tissue layers. The bursa facilitates joint movements and acts like a pad to cushion joints. The joints affected are the shoulders, elbows, hips, knees, and ankles. In some instances the inflammation of the bursa is preceded by tendonitis, that is, inflammation of a tendon, or by tenosynovitis, which is inflammation of a tendon and the tendon sheath.

Bursitis may be acute or chronic. It is usually caused by trauma, strain, and overuse of the joint with which the bursa is associated. The shoulder bursa is most often affected. The etiology, signs and symptoms, and medical therapy are listed in Table 22-6.

■ PATHOPHYSIOLOGY

The synovial lining of the bursal sac becomes inflamed, more fluid is secreted, and the bursa swells. Occasionally, large calcium deposits are present. The swelling is accompanied by pain and limited ability to move the associated joint or the entire extremity.

⊞ ASSESSMENT

☐ **Subjective data**

1. Ask patient to describe location and severity of pain and what preceded present shoulder pain.
2. Is patient being treated for inflammation of joints resulting from a known cause for the pain?
3. Does the patient have a history of rheumatoid arthritis?
4. Is the patient able to use the joint?

☐ **Objective data**

1. Palpate the joint for tenderness and swelling of the soft tissues. The swelling will feel "boggy."
2. Observe degree of limited mobility of affected joint.

Table 22-6 Nonarticular rheumatism

Disorder	Etiology	Signs and symptoms	Medical therapy
Bursitis	Repeated trauma, strain, and overuse of joint	Deep-seated pain in area of bursa Pain on movement of involved extremity Passive and active range of motion limited in adjacent joint	Antiinflammatory agents are given (Table 22-2) Adrenocorticosteroids may be injected into bursa Rest of involved area Cold compresses during acute phase to help relieve discomfort Heat is avoided because it increases fluid exudate in the bursa during inflammatory phase Surgical removal of calcium deposits

□ **Diagnostic tests**

Affected joint is x-rayed to determine extent of involvement.

➡ DATA ANALYSIS: NURSING DIAGNOSES

Nursing diagnoses are determined from an assessment of patient data. Possible nursing diagnoses for the person with bursitis may include, but are not limited to, the following:

Diagnostic title	Possible etiologies
Pain	Inflammation of joint space
Knowledge deficit	Lack of information about cause and prevention of bursitis

PLANNING: EXPECTED PATIENT OUTCOMES

Expected patient outcomes may include, but are not limited to, the following:
1. Patient will be free of pain.
2. Patient will be able to move affected joint freely.

IMPLEMENTATION

□ **Assisting with achievement of therapeutic goals**

1. Medications are given as prescribed for inflammation and discomfort:
   a. Salicylates
   b. Phenylbutazone
   c. Indomethacin
   If the above are not effective in relieving pain, the physician may inject adrenocorticosteroids into the bursa.
2. Rest for the involved area may be necessary during the acute phase.
3. Modified joint and extremity exercises may be prescribed to prevent "frozen shoulder," for example.
4. *Cold* (not heat) is applied during acute phase; heat is avoided, as this increases the fluid exudate (additional fluid in the bursa). Heat may be used later.

■ SURGERY

Roentgenographic study may disclose a calcific mass in the subdeltoid area that may need to be removed.

✛ EVALUATION

Evaluation is based on the expected patient outcomes. Questions to be asked include the following:
1. Is area free of pain?
2. Is full joint range of motion possible?

■ Carpal tunnel syndrome

Carpal tunnel syndrome is caused by pressure being exerted on the median nerve of the wrist. The condition

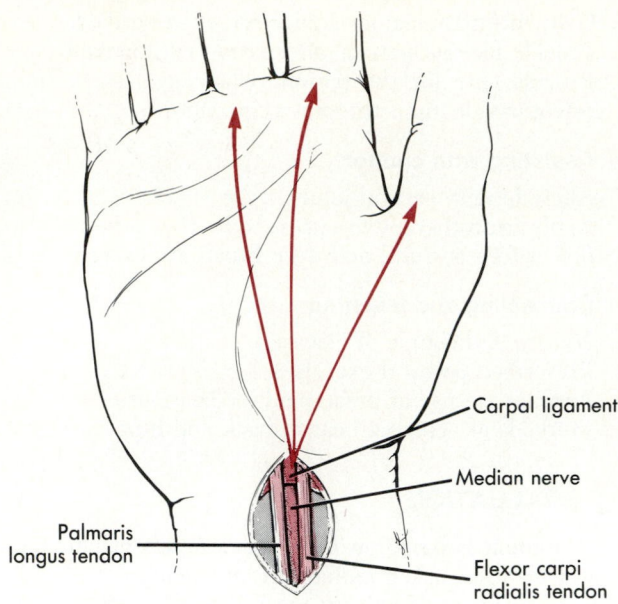

Fig. 22-12 Carpal tunnel syndrome. Volar aspect of wrist retracted to demonstrate position of median nerve. Distribution of median nerve is to thumb annd first two fingers. (Adapted from Compere, EL: Orthopaedic surgery, Chicago, 1974, Year Book Medical Publishers, Inc.)

is most common in middle-aged and often obese women and may occur as a result of trauma or of swelling of tendon sheaths caused by processes such as rheumatoid arthritis.

The person will complain of dysesthesia, paresthesia, and hypesthesia of the thumb, index, and middle fingers. Complaints will usually increase when there has been forced flexion of the hand for long periods, such as when typing. The symptoms can be elicited by tapping the median nerve at the wrist (Tinel's sign). The patient may feel that the hand is swollen and may complain of clumsiness when using the hand, especially when grasping or holding onto small objects. Referred pain to the upper extremity is common. Atrophy of the thenar eminence (the padded area of the palm below the base of the thumb) may be present late in the disease.

■ PATHOPHYSIOLOGY

The median nerve passes through a tunnel bounded by the carpal bones dorsally and the transverse carpal ligament volarly (Fig. 22-12). Flexor tendons run through the tunnel parallel to the median nerve. Inflammation and swelling of the synovial lining of tendon sheaths narrow the space available and cause compression of the median nerve.

ASSESSMENT

□ **Subjective data**

The symptoms that the patient describes are from the compression of the median nerve and include the following:

1. Episodes of burning pain or tingling in the hands that the patient says are relieved by vigorous shaking or exercising of the hand
2. Numbness (hypesthesia) affecting the thumb, index, and ring fingers, particularly after prolonged or forced flexion of the wrist, as in knitting or holding a book
3. Feeling of "swelling" in the affected hand
4. Complaint of difficulty grasping or holding onto small objects; "feels clumsy"

□ **Objective data**

1. There is no swelling in the hand, wrist, or fingers.
2. There is a wasting or depressed appearance of the soft tissue at the base of the thumb on the palmar surface (thenar eminence).

□ *Diagnostic tests*

Motor nerve velocity studies, which demonstrate a conduction block at the wrist, confirm the diagnosis.

DATA ANALYSIS: NURSING DIAGNOSES

Nursing diagnoses are determined from assessment of patient data. Possible nursing diagnoses for the person with carpal tunnel syndrome may include, but are not limited to, the following:

Diagnostic title	Possible etiologies
Knowledge deficit	Lack of exposure to information
Impaired physical mobility	Inflammation and swelling causing compression of the median nerve

PLANNING: EXPECTED PATIENT OUTCOMES

Expected patient outcomes for the person with carpal tunnel syndrome may include, but are not limited to, the following:
1. Patient will have maximum function of hand, thumb, and finger.
2. Patient will be free of discomfort.
3. Patient will be free of infection throughout the surgical site.

IMPLEMENTATION

□ **Assisting with achievement of therapeutic goals**

1. Rest
2. Splinting of the wrist
3. Local injections of corticosteroids

■ SURGERY

Decompression by surgical release of the transverse carpal ligament and removal of tissues that may be compressing the median nerve.

□ **Postoperative care**

1. Promoting comfort, circulation
   a. Elevate hand and arm for 24 hours.
   b. Encourage active thumb and finger motion within limits imposed by dressing.
   c. Administer prescribed analgesic as necessary.
2. Promoting safety
   a. Check fingers for circulation, sensation, and movement q1-2h for 24 hours.
3. Promote self-care
   a. Encourage patient to use hand in normal ADL 2 to 3 days after surgery.

EVALUATION

Evaluation is based on the expected patient outcomes. Questions to be asked include the following:
1. Is the patient able to use the hand and fingers with normal range of motion?
2. Is the patient free of discomfort in the hand?
3. Is the patient free from infection?

■ Dupuytren's contracture

■ PATHOPHYSIOLOGY

Dupuytren's contracture is a common problem, particularly in men past middle age. The disorder is caused by a thickening and shortening of the palmar fascia on the ulnar side of one or both hands causing flexion of the ring finger and sometimes the small finger. The bands shorten, and the fingers are pulled into fixed flexion. The skin of the hand is drawn down, forming tight puckers and nodules. Joints, muscles, tendon, or nervous or vascular tissue do not appear to be involved.

ASSESSMENT

□ **Subjective data**

The patient complains of a gradual decrease in the ability to extend the ring and small fingers.

□ **Objective data**

The most obvious appearance of the patient's hand is the flexed position of the ring finger and possibly the small finger. The skin of the palm is drawn down, forming tight puckers and nodules. The condition starts in one hand but often occurs in both hands. The patient cannot actively extend the fingers.

DATA ANALYSIS: NURSING DIAGNOSES

Nursing diagnoses are determined from the assessment of patient data. Possible nursing diagnoses for the person with Dupuytren's contracture may include, but are not limited to, the following:

Diagnostic title	Possible etiologies
Impaired physical mobility	Musculoskeletal impairment/ thickening and shortening of palmar fascia

PLANNING: EXPECTED PATIENT OUTCOMES

Expected patient outcomes for the person with Dupuytren's contracture may include, but are not limited to, the following:
1. Patient will have full use of fingers and hand.
2. Patient will not develop an infection in surgical site.

IMPLEMENTATION

□ Assisting with achievement of therapeutic goals

1. Soak patient's hand in warm water while having patient actively perform finger extension exercises.
2. Teach patient to avoid activities that require grasping an object.
3. Prepare patient for surgery.

SURGERY

The major therapy is surgical removal of the involved palmar fascia. Postoperative care is listed below.
1. Elevate hand to control swelling.
2. Apply ice packs as ordered.
3. Give analgesics to relieve pain.
4. Check fingers for sensation, circulation, finger movements.
5. Encourage patient to extend fingers.
6. In 2 to 3 days patient may use hand in daily activities.

EVALUATION

Evalution is based on the expected patient outcomes. Questions to be asked include the following:
1. Does the patient have full use of hand and fingers?
2. Is the patient free of infection?

DEGENERATIVE DISORDERS

Degenerative joint disease

Degenerative joint disease, also known as *osteoarthritis, hypertrophic arthritis, osteoarthrosis,* or *senescent arthritis,* is an extremely common disease that is probably as old as civilization. Almost everyone past 40 years of age has hypertrophic changes in the joints. Although symptomatic degenerative joint disease is usually noted in the 50- to 70-year age group, it has been observed as early as age 20. It is estimated that 17 million people in the United States have osteoarthritis serious enough to cause pain. There are two forms of osteoarthritis: *primary,* for which the cause is unknown, and *secondary,* a result of trauma, infections, previous fractures, another type of arthritis (such as rheumatoid arthritis), the stress put on weight-bearing joints from long-term obesity, or the "wear and tear" on joints associated with some occupations (for example, coal mining and boxing). There may also be a genetic predisposition to the development of osteoarthritis.[15,29] See Table 22-7 for etiology, signs and symptoms, and medical therapy.

PREVENTION

Factors to be considered in the prevention of osteoarthritis are the following:
1. Avoidance of obesity
2. Avoidance of repeated trauma to joints
3. Practice of joint protection techniques in occupations that put joints at risk

PATHOPHYSIOLOGY

Degenerative joint disease (DJD) is a disease of the articular cartilage. Normally this cartilage is white, translucent, and smooth. When affected by the disease, it becomes yellow and opaque. Areas of cartilage soften and the surface becomes rough, frayed, and cracked. This process is thought to occur as a result of digestion of the cartilage by enzymes and alteration of the nutrition of the cartilage. Eventually the cartilage is destroyed, and the underlying subchondral bone goes through a remodeling process. *Osteophytes,* or spurs of new bone appear at the joint margins and at the sites of attachment of supporting structures. These may break off and appear in the joint cavity as "joint mice." Unlike rheumatoid arthritis (RA), DJD affects only the joints and their surrounding tissue. It is not a systemic disease.

Individuals with DJD have pain in the movable joints, particularly the large weight-bearing joints (hips, knees), and the joints of the hand. Inflammation is usually not present, and tenderness is mild; however, the joints may become enlarged. Crepitation may be present on movement, and alignment of the extremity may be changed. The patient usually has stiffness after periods of rest.

ASSESSMENT

□ Subjective data

The person with degenerative joint disorder is usually in good health. Questions that are asked include the following:
1. When does pain occur?
2. What measures give relief?
3. What joints are involved?
4. What modifications in ADL have been made because of pain or restricted mobility?

□ Objective data

Because signs and symptoms are usually local, inspection and palpation are the best evaluators.

Table 22-7 Degenerative disorders

Inflammatory disorder	Etiology	Signs and symptoms	Medical therapy

Degenerative joint disorder (DJD)	Cause of degeneration of articular cartilage is unknown
	Theories of causation:
	1. Digestion of cartilage by enzymes and alteration of cartilage nutrition
	2. Predisposition to excessive "wear and tear" of affected joints (chronic irritation)
	3. Obesity and excessive weight on joints
	4. Metabolic disturbances (for example, acromegaly)
	5. Repeated joint hemorrhages
	6. Trauma
	7. Genetic predisposition
	8. Congenital problems (for example, hip dislocations)
	9. Stress on joints with aging process
	10. Certain occupations such as coal mining and boxing
		Pain in the movable joints, particularly on weight bearing
		Mild tenderness to aggravated pain on overuse of joint
		Joints become enlarged with loss of motion
		Crepitation
		Changes in alignment of affected part with flexion deformity
		Stiffness following periods of rest
		Changes in certain joints:
		1. *Heberden's nodes*—bony protuberances on dorsal surface of distal interphalangeal joints of fingers (Fig. 22-13)
		2. *Bouchard's nodes*—on proximal interphalangeal joints of fingers
		3. *Coxarthrosis*—a degenerative change presenting with pain in hip with weight bearing; may progress to include groin and medial side of knee
		4. *Knee involvement*—varus, valgus (Fig. 22-14), flexion deformity, limited range of motion
			1. Salicylates and nonsteroidal antiinflammatory agents
			  a. Aspirin
			  b. NSAIAs
			  c. Intraarticular injection of steroids for severe pain
			  d. Adjunctive analgesics (Tylenol, Darvon)
			2. Assistive devices to unload weight bearing on joints (canes, walkers, crutches)
			3. Rest
			4. Exercise
			5. Joint protection
			6. Surgery
			  a. Arthroscopy to remove bits of broken cartilage or bone
			  b. Realignment (osteotomy)
			  c. Fusion (arthrodesis)
			  d. Joint replacement

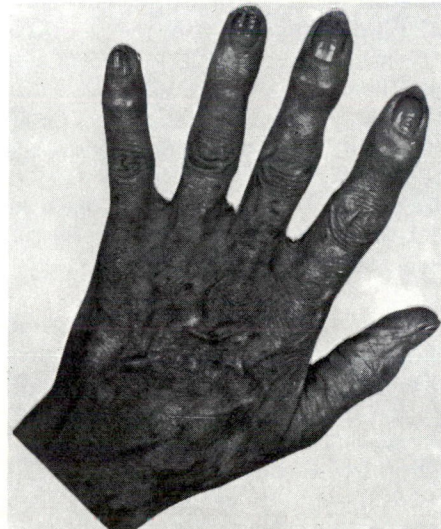

Fig. 22-13 Osteoarthritis of hand. Note enlargement of distal joints of index, middle, and little fingers (Heberden's nodes). (From Brashear, H, and Raney, R: Shand's handbook of orthopaedic surgery, ed 10, St. Louis, 1986, The CV Mosby Co.)

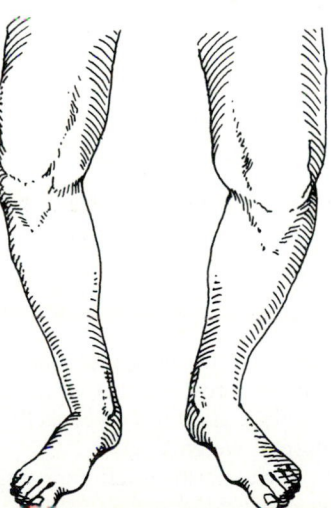

Fig. 22-14 Characteristic valgus deformity (bowing) of knees in degenerative arthritis. This deformity can be corrected by tibial osteotomy or total knee replacement

1. Affected joints may appear normal.
   a. Check for tenderness, grating, and crepitus.
   b. Palpate for enlargement or irregularity in size of joint and flexion or lateral deformities.
2. Observe the person walking. Is there a limp?
3. Evaluate range of motion of major joints.
4. Assess the vertebral column for limitation in cervical or lumbar areas.
5. Does the person have difficulty standing for periods of time or difficulty in arising from chair (particularly one without arms) after sitting for a period of time?

□ Diagnostic tests

1. X-ray films may be normal if pathologic changes are mild.
2. Progressive changes include the following:
   a. Narrowing of joint spaces
   b. Marginal osteophyte formation
   c. *Eburnation* (sclerosis) of subchondral bone
3. Serologic and synovial fluid examinations will be essentially normal.

➡ DATA ANALYSIS: NURSING DIAGNOSES

Nursing diagnoses are determined by assessment of patient data. Possible nursing diagnoses for the person with degenerative joint disease may include, but are not limited to, the following:

Diagnostic title	Possible etiologies
Activity intolerance	Restricted mobility caused by joint involvement
Knowledge deficit: DJD	Lack of exposure to sources of information
Impaired physical mobility	Musculoskeletal impairment caused by degeneration of affected joints
Altered nutrition: more than body requirements	Excessive intake in relation to metabolic needs
Pain: in affected joints	Degeneration in affected joints
Self-care deficit: ADL	Pain and limited joint movement

▢ PLANNING: EXPECTED PATIENT OUTCOMES

Expected patient outcomes for the person with degenerative joint disease may include, but are not limited to, the following:

1. Patient is feeling more comfortable.
2. Patient is able to be more physically active.
3. Patient balances rest and activity.
4. Patient is able to state reason for achieving and maintaining normal weight.
5. Patient is able to perform self-care activities with less difficulty.
6. Patient is able to explain disease process, treatment measures, and plans for follow-up medical care.

▦ IMPLEMENTATION

Measures to relieve pain and discomfort and to promote mobility and increased ability to accomplish ADL are the same as those for the person who has rheumatoid arthritis.

□ Counseling and teaching

The teaching plan would include the following:
1. Attention to posture
2. Weight reduction, prevention of weight gain
3. Use of ambulatory aids such as canes, crutches, or walkers to remove weight from painful joints
4. Alteration in ADL to avoid painful activities
5. Use of external measures such as local heat, prescribed exercises, and use of traction (if this is prescribed)

■ SURGERY

Surgical intervention may be necessary to remove damaged bone or cartilage from the joint, realign or change the weight-bearing surfaces of the joint, or to resurface the joint. The objectives of surgery are to (1) relieve pain, (2) restore joint function (if possible), and (3) prevent disability or further progression of the disease. Surgery to the knee and hip are most common, but shoulder surgery is becoming more practical and effective. Specific surgeries are:

1. *Debridement* (usually by arthroscopic surgery or arthrotomy): See p. 580.
2. *Arthrodesis:* Through fusion of the joint, pain is relieved, joint motion is lost, but weight-bearing function is maintained. See p. 580.
3. *Osteotomy:* Bone is cut to change alignment, thereby correcting deformity in the bone or adjacent joint. The procedure corrects angulation of rotational deformities or alters the weight-bearing surface in a diseased joint (Fig. 22-15). Osteotomy may be thought of as a surgical or intentional fracture, and the extremity is treated the same as following a fracture with the exception that weight bearing may be started earlier. Immobilization of the extremity and nursing interventions are similar to those employed following a fracture (p. 614).
4. *Arthroplasty:* The two types of arthroplasty are:
   a. Interposition—resurfacing of one side of the joint with metal or other inert material or soft tissue such as fascia.
   b. Replacement—resurfacing of both sides of the joint with metal or polyethylene implants. Replacement implants are available for the hip (see Fig. 22-8), knee (see Fig. 22-9), shoulder, ankle, elbow, wrist, and interphalangeal joints of the fingers. Replacement prostheses may be either *cemented* (held into bone with polymethylmethacrylate) or *uncemented* (treated with a special porous coating that promotes in growth of bone). Care of the patient having an arthroplasty is discussed on p. 583.

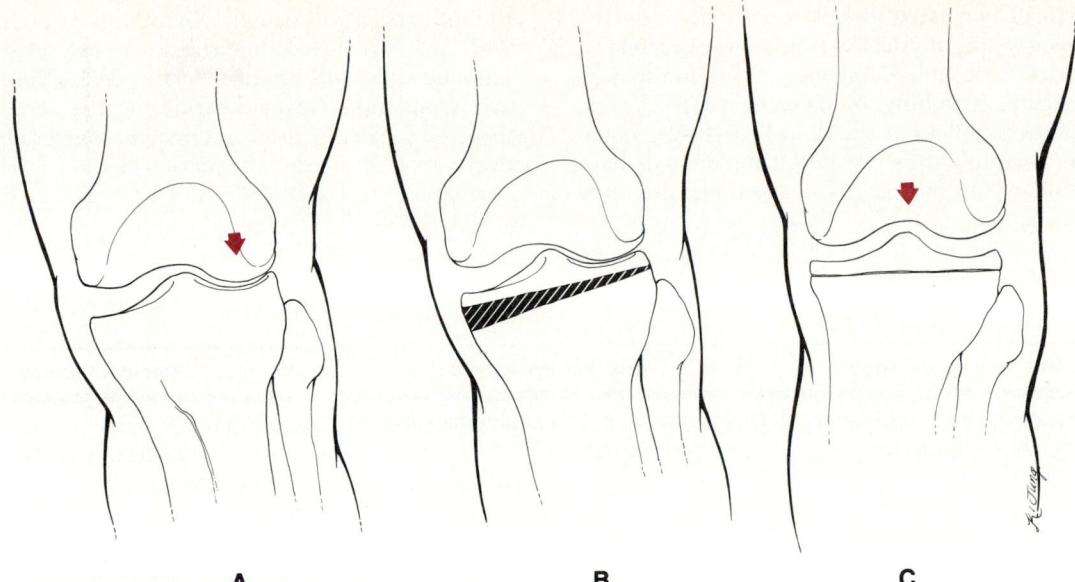

A   B   C

Fig. 22-15 Osteotomy of tiba. Genu valgum (anterior view of left knee). **A,** Weight-bearing force is concentrated on one compartment of knee. **B,** Wedge of bone is removed from tibia. Amount of bone removed is determined by how much correction in angulation is necessary. **C,** Distal portion of tibia is swung to proximal portion. Correction of angulation obtained allows weight-bearing forces to be more evenly distributed through both compartments of knee. (Adapted from Hollander, JL, and McCarty, DR, Jr: Arthritis and allied conditions, ed 8, Philadelphia, 1972, Lea & Febiger.)

✚ EVALUATION

Evaluation is based on the expected patient outcomes. Questions to be asked include the following:
1. Is the patient more comfortable?
2. Is the patient able to be more physically active?
3. Is the patient able to perform self-care activities with less difficulty?
4. Can the patient discuss the reason for achieving and maintaining ideal weight?
5. Is the patient able to explain disease process, treatment measures, and follow-up care?
6. Is the patient able to perform prescribed exercises independently?

■ Degenerative disease of the spine

Degenerative disease of the spine is a common but difficult problem that merits special consideration. The etiology, signs and symptoms, and medical therapy are listed in Table 22-8.

■ PATHOPHYSIOLOGY

The spine has 23 intervertebral disk joints and 46 posterior facet joints (Fig. 22-16), all of which are subjected to stresses and strains in holding the human body upright and moving it about. The vertebrae in the spinal column are articulated in a series of "couplets" that are able to move through an intervertebral disk joint and two posterior facet joints. The intervertebral disks are composed of an outer layer of cartilage called the *anulus fibrosus* and an inner layer of cartilage called the *nucleus pulposus*. Several common problems arise with these structures in degenerative disease of the spine. They are the following:

1. *Herniated nucleus pulposus* (HNP)—Degeneration and dehydration of the cartilage composing the anulus and the nucleus results in a loss of elasticity. As the disk loses its resiliency, a strong force exerted across it can result in herniation of the nucleus through the anulus, either posteriorly or laterally. This results in compression of a spinal nerve root and subsequent pain (Fig. 22-17).
2. *Osteophyte* formation along the vertebral column can cause fusion of vertebrae with consequent limitation of motion, usually in the lumbodorsal region.
3. *Spinal stenosis,* or narrowing of the intervertebral foramina at any level of the spine, creates pressure on nerve roots in the involved area, resulting in neurologic symptoms including pain.
4. Degenerative and/or rheumatoid involvement of the hyaline articular surfaces of the facet joints results in pain and limited motion. Rheumatoid involvement with consequent loss of vertebral stability is particularly troublesome in the cervical spine.

The *diagnosis* of herniated disk is usually made on the basis of the history and physical examination. A history of low back pain relieved by recumbency and aggravated by flexion of the trunk, coughing, or sneezing is typical. The patient will often complain of sciatic pain radiating down the leg. Some persons, after the initial injury, will have sciatic pain but no pain in their back. Deep pressure over the interspace will usually elicit pain. Straight leg raising with the hip flexed and the knee extended (a positive Lasegue sign) will produce sciatic pain. Neurologic signs and symptoms help in determining the level of the disk involved because sensory and motor changes depend on the nerve root involved. The most common sites of lumbar herniation are L3-4, L4-5, and L5-S1.

Table 22-8 Degenerative diseases

Disorder	Etiology	Signs and symptoms	Medical therapy

Degenerative joint disease of spine	A wide variety of disorders	Chief complaint: low back pain relieved by recumbency
		a. Occasionally pain radiates to buttocks
		b. There may be sciatic pain radiating down leg
		c. Pain follows overactivity
		d. Pain aggravated by flexion of trunk, coughing, and sneezing
			Conservative
			1. Rest (complete or modified) depending on symptoms
			2. Heat
			3. Medications
			  a. Analgesics and/or antiinflammatory agents
			  b. Muscle relaxants (for example, diazepam)
			4. Traction to relieve muscle spasm
			  a. Bilateral Buck's traction (Fig. 22-18)
			  b. Pelvic traction
			5. Corset may be prescribed to support spine

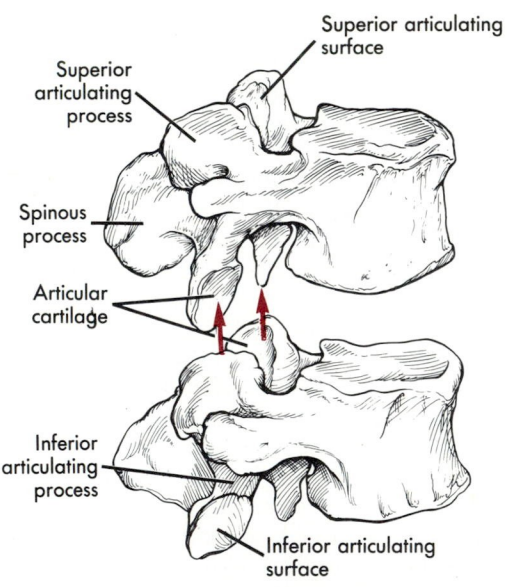

Fig. 22-16 Posterior facet joints of lumbar vertebrae. Each vertebra has four surfaces by which it articulates with its adjacent vertebrae: two on its superior aspect and two on the inferior. Superior articulating surfaces are medially located; the inferior, laterally. These joints are diarthrotic, having a joint capsule with a synovial lining.

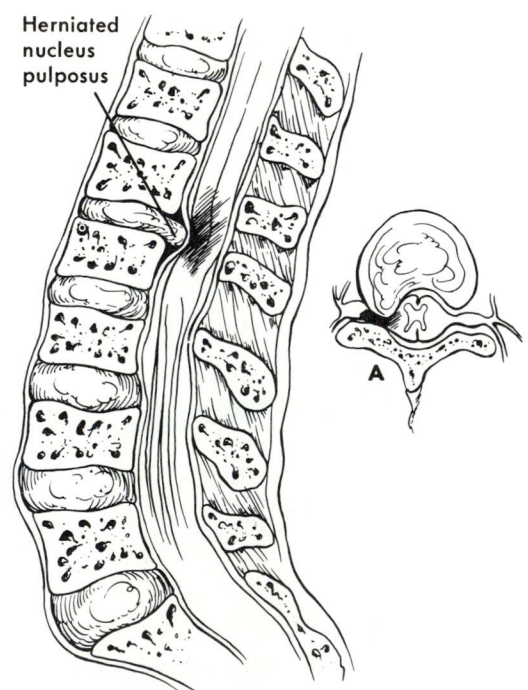

Fig. 22-17 Compression of spinal cord caused by herniation of nucleus pulposus into spinal cord. **A,** Pressure on nerves as they leave spinal canal.

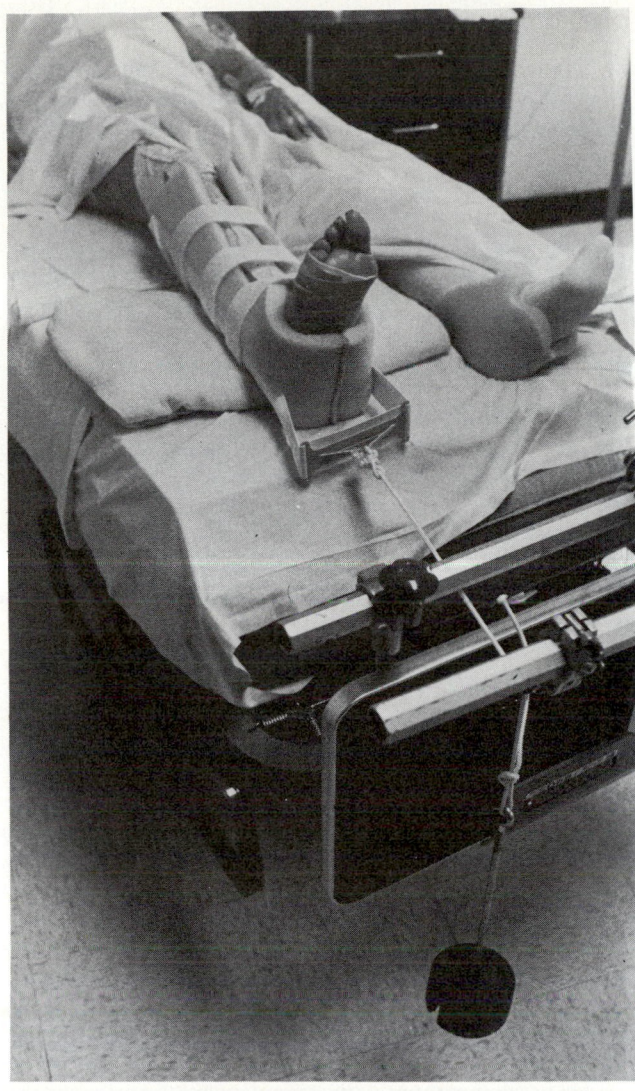

Fig. 22-18 Buck's extension.

■ SURGERY

Surgery may be necessary to relieve pressure on nerve roots and to stabilize the spine. See the box above for types of spine surgery. Care of patients who are treated surgically is discussed on p. 602.

Compression of nerve roots from other causes—stenosis, vertebral instability, osteophyte formation—will also cause neurologic signs and symptoms relative to the level of the nerve root(s) involved. Signs and symptoms may include the following:

1. Numbness, tingling, and/or decreased motion in one or more extremities
2. Pain
3. Weakness of one or more extremities
4. Muscle wasting in one or more extremities
5. Partial or complete loss of bowel and bladder control

Types of spine surgery

Procedure	Description
Laminectomy	Removal of a portion of the lamina
Diskectomy	Removal of all or part of a herniated intervertebral disk
Foraminotomy	Widening of the intervertebral foramen to allow free passage of the spinal nerve
Spinal fusion	Fusion of two or more vertebrae by insertion of bone grafts with or without the addition of metal rods or wires to achieve vertebral stability
	Thoracic and cervical sugeries require fusion because of mobility of the spine in these areas

▦ ASSESSMENT

☐ Subjective data

The patient seeks help because of pain and inability to walk or to carry on normal activities. Answers to the following questions should be sought:

1. Is low back pain relieved by recumbency?
2. Is pain aggravated by flexion of the trunk, coughing, or sneezing?
3. Is there a history of injury followed by back pain?

☐ Objective data

1. Observe movements and walking.
   a. Patient appears to guard hips and back.
   b. Patient seeks frequent position changes.
2. Straight leg raising flexing the hip with the knee extended may produce sciatic pain.
3. Palpate for tender areas and spasm of the paravertebral muscles and posterior superior iliac spine.
4. Observe relief of discomfort when patient is supine with head elevated a few degrees and knees flexed.
5. Observe for muscle atrophy; if back problem has been long-standing, changes will be seen in affected leg.

☐ Diagnostic tests
☐ *Neurologic examination*

1. Neurologic signs and symptoms will help in determining the level of vertebrae involved. Sensory and motor changes depend on the nerve root involved.
2. Roentgenographic evaluation
   a. For those patients whose symptoms are of short duration, the x-ray examination may fail to reveal any abnormality.
   b. For those patients with long-standing disorders, the x-ray examination may show significant narrowing of the disk space.

c. Myelography, valuable in localizing the lesion, is reserved for confirmation of physical findings before surgery or to exclude conditions such as tumors.
d. CAT scanning or magnetic resonance imaging (MRI) may be used for diagnosis.

➡ DATA ANALYSIS AND PLANNING: EXPECTED PATIENT OUTCOMES

Nursing diagnoses and expected patient outcomes are similar to those for degenerative joint disease (p. 598).

IMPLEMENTATION

☐ **Assisting with the achievement of therapeutic goals**

For the patient being treated conservatively, the following measures are appropriate:
1. Promoting comfort
   a. Encourage slight elevation of head of bed and flexion of the knees when supine.
   b. Roll patient onto bedpan rather than lifting onto pan.
   c. Use fracture bedpan or small bedpan.
   d. Apply heat as patient desires and tolerates.
   e. Remove skin traction for periods of time if it causes patient discomfort.
   f. Provide analgesics, antispasmodics at regular intervals as necessary.
2. Promoting circulation
   a. Encourage patient to perform active dorsi-plantar flexion of the ankles at regular intervals.
   b. Report any difficulty with brace to physician immediately.
   c. Do not drive a car during period that brace must be worn.

☐ **Counseling and teaching**

1. Patients should learn to turn in bed in a *logrolling* fashion to maintain good spinal alignment: *cross the arms over the chest, bend the uppermost knee to the side to which they wish to turn, and then roll over as a unit.*
2. Constipation may be a problem.
   a. Urge patient to drink 3000 ml of fluids daily.
   b. Increase amount of roughage eaten; bran and fresh fruit are helpful.
   c. Give a mild laxative if necessary.
3. If brace or corset is ordered to provide external support for the spine, explain its need and application.
4. Teach principles of body mechanics.
   a. Avoid movements and positions that cause poor alignment of the spinal column and put strain on an injured nerve.
   b. Use a straight chair, not an overstuffed one.
   c. Avoid crossing the legs at the knees.
   d. Elevate the feet but flex the knees.
   e. During acute episodes, avoid stretching of the legs, such as driving a car or climbing stairs.

f. In picking up items off the floor, bend the knees and keep the back straight.
5. When the acute episode subsides, the physician will order exercises designed to strengthen the back and abdominal muscles.

✚ EVALUATION

Evaluation is based on the expected patient outcomes, which are the same as for degenerative joint disease (see p. 599).

■ SURGERY

A laminectomy and/or spinal fusion may be performed. The nursing care for persons with lumbar, thoracic, or cervical spinal fusion is discussed next.

Care following spinal surgery (lumbar, thoracic, cervical) focuses on positioning and mobility, wound care, and patient comfort. Changing position in bed following *lumbar* surgery must be performed by logrolling; assistance is given as necessary, but patients can learn to do this for themselves. Because patients tolerate sitting less well than walking or lying, sitting is avoided until the person can tolerate it.

Thoracic spinal surgery may involve entering the chest cavity; if so, nursing care will include postoperative measures following chest surgery (Chapter 24). Mobility restrictions are more prolonged than with lumbar surgery because the thoracic spine is more mobile; consequently, there is greater risk of dislodging grafts through improper motion.

Persons with *cervical* spinal surgery may require tong or halo traction (Chapter 19) or a halo brace. The person has edema of the throat in the early postoperative period, requiring attention to the person's ability to breathe and swallow.

The care of patients undergoing spinal fusion is discussed below.

■ NURSING INTERVENTIONS FOR PATIENTS WITH LUMBAR SURGERY[14,19]

☐ **Preoperative care**

1. Instruct patient in logrolling and performance of dorsi-plantar exercises
2. Instruct patient about the surgical procedure, postoperative care, and expectations at discharge

☐ **Postoperative care**

1. Positioning
   a. Head of bed is kept flat.
   b. Patient is encouraged to logroll when changing position from side to back to side.
   c. Use of a turning sheet (Fig. 22-19) is advised until patient can assist with turning.
2. Wound care: drains may be placed in wound to prevent hematoma formation.

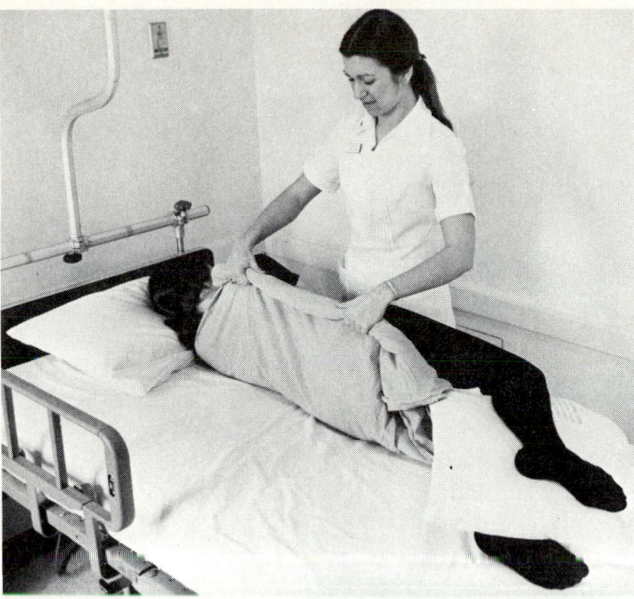

Fig. 22-19 Positioning a patient after back surgery by means of turning sheet extending from shoulders to thighs.

a. Maintain constant suction through drain if required.
b. Maintain drain free of contamination.
c. Inspect surgical area frequently for evidence of excess drainage or formation of hematoma (bulging of tissues surrounding surgical site).
d. If a spinal fusion, inspect donor site (usually iliac crest) for drainage or hematoma.
3. Promoting comfort
a. Reposition patient frequently.
b. Narcotics are used initially, then nonnarcotic analgesics as patient tolerates.
c. Use fracture bedpan or small bedpan.
4. Promoting mobility
a. Patient with a *simple laminectomy* may be out of bed on the first day after surgery.
b. Patient with a *laminectomy and fusion* may not be able to be out of bed for 3 to 5 days following the surgery.
c. Two persons will be required to help patient out of bed. This patient should sit as little as possible while getting up.
(1) If the patient has a brace or corset, it is applied *before* the patient gets out of bed.
(2) Assist patient in moving to edge of the bed before turning on side.
(3) Instruct patient to push off the bed with the uppermost hand and lowermost elbow.
(4) One person guides the patient's trunk, the other assists the patient's legs over the side of the bed.
(5) The process is reversed in getting patient back in bed.

d. Patient may walk as much as tolerated; an assistive aid such as cane may be necessary.
e. Patient is encouraged to participate in ADL within prescribed limits of mobility.
5. Discharge instructions
a. May not lift or carry anything heavier than 5 lbs. (2.25 kg).
b. May not drive car until permitted by surgeon.
c. Should avoid twisting of the trunk.

■ NURSING INTERVENTIONS FOR PATIENTS WITH THORACIC SPINE SURGERY

☐ Preoperative care

This care is the same as for lumbar surgery.

☐ Postoperative care

This care is the same as for lumbar surgery, with the following *additions or exceptions:*
1. Positioning
a. Head of bed may often be elevated to 30 degrees.
2. Wound care
a. If pleural cavity is entered, a chest tube will be inserted and must be managed after surgery (see Chapter 24).
3. Promoting comfort
a. Assist patient in splinting chest while coughing.
4. Promoting mobility
a. Encourage and assist patient in vigorous pulmonary toileting.
b. Assist patient in maintaining bedrest for 2 to 4 weeks or longer with strict attention to avoidance of twisting or bending motions to prevent dislodging grafts.
c. Discourage patient from vigorous pulling or pushing with the arms, because placing weight on them may dislodge the graft.
d. Brace is routinely prescribed and must be applied before patient is mobilized.
e. Permit patient to perform whatever activities are comfortable within the limitations of the brace.
f. Encourage participation in ADL within prescribed limits of mobility.
5. Discharge instruction
a. Teach patient to apply and remove the brace before getting out of bed for the first time.
b. Teach patient to wear the brace whenever out of bed.

■ NURSING INTERVENTIONS FOR PATIENTS WITH CERVICAL SPINE SURGERY

☐ Preoperative care

1. General instructions are the same as for any spine surgery.
2. If tong or halo traction or halo brace is to be used after surgery, familiarize patient with the apparatus before surgery.

□ **Postoperative care**

1. Positioning
   a. Keep head of bed elevated 30 to 45 degrees, particularly if anterior surgical approach was used, to decrease swelling in throat.
   b. If patient is in cervical brace, position is not restricted except by patient's tolerance.
   c. If patient is in cervical traction, may be turned side to back to side as tolerated.
2. Wound care
   a. Inspect surgical area, including iliac crest donor site, frequently for evidence of excess drainage or formation of hematoma.
   b. If tong or halo traction is being used, pin care may be required (see Chapter 19).
3. Promoting comfort
   a. Provide ice chips to soothe sore throat.
   b. Progress diet slowly because patient will have difficulty swallowing and will be afraid of choking. Full liquids (ice cream, custards, jello, nectars) are often better tolerated than clear juice or broth.
   c. Medicate with analgesics as for any spine surgery. Donor sites often cause more discomfort than cervical site.
   d. May require aerosol treatments or humidification of air to loosen mucous secretions, facilitate their removal, and make breathing more comfortable.
4. Promoting mobility
   a. If patient is in traction, encourage to perform ankle dorsi-plantar flexion exercises and quadriceps-setting 3 times daily to promote circulation, maintain leg strength.
   b. If patient is in brace, may be out of bed and walk as soon as tolerated.
   c. Walker may be necessary if donor site pain restricts mobility.
   d. Encourage participation in ADL to greatest extent possible.
5. Promoting safety
   a. Keep suction equipment and tracheostomy set in patient's room until swelling in throat subsides and patient is swallowing and breathing normally.
   b. Check adjustment screws and straps on brace frequently to ensure there is no loosening of the brace.
   c. When edema decreases brace will need to be readjusted by physician or orthotist.
6. Discharge instruction
   a. Teach patient to wear brace at all times.

■ RESTRICTIVE DISORDERS

■ Scoliosis

Lateral deviation of the spine from the midline is known as scoliosis. The classifications of scoliosis are the following:[12]

Congenital	Present at birth
Acquired	Not present at birth; develops at a later time
Idiopathic	Most common type, usually develops in adolescence
Functional	Postural or nonstructural—develops from temporary postural influences; easily correctable
Structural	Changes in structures of spine from various causes
Paralytic	Develops following neurologic disease such as poliomyelitis

Scoliosis may be present in both children and adults. Table 22-9 lists the etiology, signs and symptoms, and medical therapy for scoliosis.

■ PREVENTION

Screening programs for school-age children are effective in identifying early indications of scoliosis. Attention to good posture may be effective in preventing the disorder in both children and adults.

■ PATHOPHYSIOLOGY

Scoliosis may develop in localized areas of the spinal column or involve the whole spinal column. Curves may be S-shaped or C-shaped. The degree of rotation of the curve is important because it determines the amount of impingement on the rib cage. Significant cardiac and pulmonary restrictions may be imposed by curves with a large degree of rotation. The balance of the curve is also important because it affects the stability of the spine and mobility of the trunk. Significant deviations in balance of the curve affect gait patterns.

■ DIAGNOSIS

The individual may initially have slight, mild, or severe deformity. Early deformity may not be obvious except on specific examination. Deformity will increase with growth and age. In the early stages, individuals may note that clothing does not fit correctly or hang evenly. The height of the shoulders is uneven. Pain is not usually an accompanying factor. In advanced scoliosis, when the cardiorespiratory system is impaired, respiration is restricted and cardiac output is compromised.

▦ ASSESSMENT

□ **Subjective data**

1. Clothing does not fit correctly or hang well.
2. Patient is unable to breathe comfortably or take a deep breath (pain may not be a problem).
3. Patient complains of progressive difficulty with ambulation.
4. Patient may state negative feelings about appearance.

□ **Objective data**

Observation and palpation are most important. Observe the gait, posture, and ability to rise from a chair; compare

height of the shoulders. Palpate the spinal column with the patient in an upright position and bending forward. Palpate chest expansion on deep inspiration.
1. Visible curvature of spine when patient bends forward from waist
2. Notable limp

→ **DATA ANALYSIS: NURSING DIAGNOSES**

Nursing diagnoses are determined from assessment of patient data. Possible nursing diagnoses for the persons with scoliosis may include, but are not limited to, the following:

Table 22-9   Restrictive disorders

Disorder	Etiology	Signs and symptoms	Medical therapy

Scoliosis	Rickets
	Neuromuscular disorders
	Vertebral disorders
	Congenital
	Idiopathic (cause unknown)
		Lateral deviation of spine away from midline (in thoracic spine region)
		One shoulder is higher than other
		Movement of chest is restricted on deep inspiration
		May complain of shortness of breath or difficulty in taking deep breath
			1. Early or postural scoliosis may be amenable to:
			  a. Postural exercise
			  b. Exercise combined with traction (for example, Cotrel's traction)
			2. In scoliosis where the curve is flexible (less than 40 degrees) and the patient is cooperative, bracing in combination with exercise may be sufficient to correct the deformity
			  a. Milwaukee brace
			  b. Risser cast
			  c. Halofemoral or halopelvic traction
			3. Corrective surgery (realignment of vertebrae and fusion) when curve exceeds 40 degrees and/or bracing has failed; usually accomplished with bone grafting and instrumentation
			  a. Harrington rod instrumentation—series of rods and hooks that apply compression to the posterior spinal elements
			  b. Dwyer instrumentation—titanium cables passed through heads of titanium screws imbedded in the vertebral bodies (Fig. 22-20)
			  c. Luque instrumentation—two L-shaped rods and a series of wires that apply transverse traction to the vertebral bodies

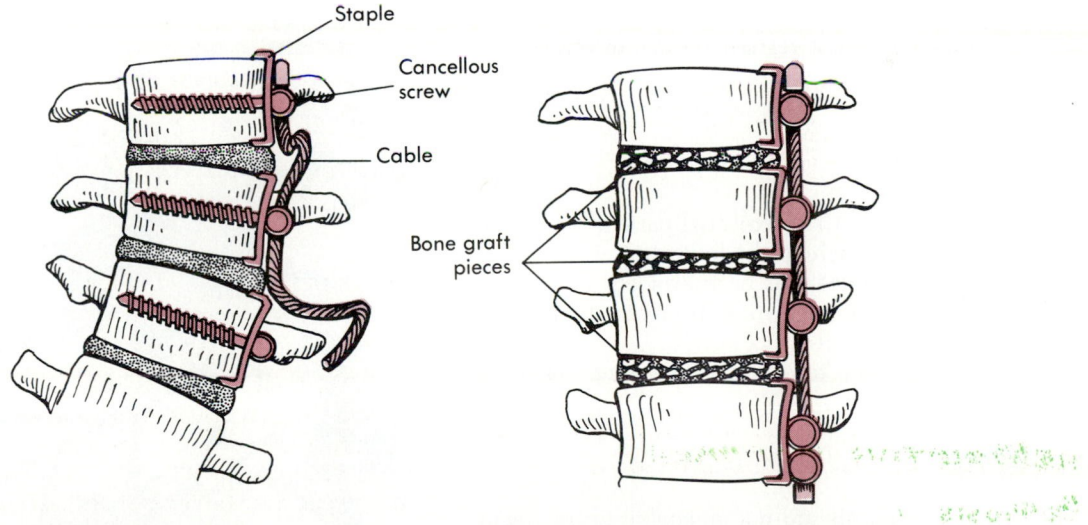

Fig. 22-20   Scoliosis fusion with Dwyer instrumentation. Cable is passed through openings in heads of screws that are imbedded in vertebral bodies. Spaces between vertebrae are filled with bone chips as grafting material. Cable is pulled taut to secure and maintain correct alignment of vertebrae.

Diagnostic title	Possible etiologies
Potential activity intolerance	Musculoskeletal impairment
Body image disturbance	Scoliosis/change in body image
Ineffective breathing pattern	Musculoskeletal impairment/ change in shape of thoracic cavity
Knowledge deficit	Lack of exposure to newer methods of treatment
Impaired physical mobility	Musculoskeletal impairment/ scoliosis
Pain: back	Musculoskeletal impairment/ scoliosis

▣ PLANNING: EXPECTED PATIENT OUTCOMES

Expected patient outcomes for the person with scoliosis being treated conservatively may include, but are not limited to, the following:
1. Patient avoids potential complications.
2. Patient maintains maximal functioning and independence.
3. Patient participates in long-range planning of his or her care.

▣ IMPLEMENTATION
□ Conservative therapy
□ *Assisting with achievement of therapeutic goals*

1. Assist patient with postural exercises
2. Assist patient in applying brace
3. Assist patient in doing prescribed exercises

□ *Counseling and teaching*

1. How to apply, remove, and care for brace
2. Selection of loose fitting, attractive clothing that conceals brace
3. Wearing brace need not restrict normal or desired activities
4. Postural and other prescribed exercises

▣ EVALUATION

Evaluation is based on the expected patient outcomes. Questions to be asked include the following:
1. Have spinal complications been avoided?
2. To what degree has the patient been able to function without back support?
3. Is the patient able to describe long-range plans of care?

■ SURGERY

Some forms of scoliosis are not amenable to treatment with bracing or body cast; surgery may be performed to correct the scoliosis. Most commonly, lumbar fusion is performed through a posterior incision, with the bone for the graft being taken from the iliac crest. Scoliosis fusions involve internal devices such as those listed in Table 22-9.

Following surgery, the patient may be immobilized in a cast that extends from neck to pelvis. The cast remains on for 6 months. The care of the patient in a cast is covered on p. 617.

Care of the person following spinal fusion for scoliosis is outlined below. The risk of postoperative pulmonary complications as a result of immobilization is high; therefore, preventive measures are important. Paralytic ileus is a common complication, and nasogastric suction is commonly employed in the first 24 to 72 hours after surgery. Patients with major *spinal procedures* also tend to retain fluid; therefore, they are *at risk for fluid overload* in the early postoperative period.

□ **Nursing care of the patient undergoing scoliosis fusion**
□ *Preoperative care*

1. Instruct the patient regarding pulmonary function studies.
2. Instruct the patient regarding the surgery, postoperative care, and expectations after discharge.

□ *Postoperative care*

1. Promote comfort
   a. Medicate with narcotic analgesics as necessary; gradually decrease to nonnarcotic analgesics as patient tolerates.
   b. Turn and position frequently.
   c. Use a small or a fracture bedpan.
2. Positioning
   a. Bed is kept flat from 1 to 14 days, depending on the surgical technique used.
   b. Position patient side to back to side with use of a turning sheet (see Fig. 22-19) and pillows between the legs (Fig. 22-21) to maintain alignment.

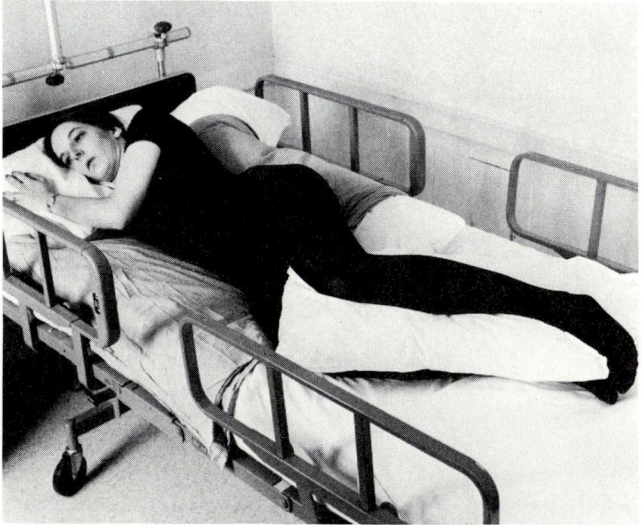

Fig. 22-21 Pillows behind the back provide support. Pillows between legs maintain anatomic alignment and decrease pull on lower back.

3. Promote safety
   a. Monitor vital signs, motor function and sensation in the lower extremities frequently.
   b. Monitor closely for respiratory impairment.
4. Promote mobility
   a. Encourage leg exercise as for other spinal surgery.
   b. Encourage participation in ADL to extent possible within limits imposed by surgery and/or brace, cast.
   c. Begin activity out of bed, in brace or cast if prescribed, as soon as surgeon permits. (Commencement of activity is dependent on surgical technique.)
5. Prevent complications
   a. Encourage breathing exercises
   b. Delay administration of oral food and fluid until patient is actively passing flatus.
   c. Monitor intravenous intake and urine output closely to prevent fluid overload until patient has postoperative diuresis (usually 3 to 4 days).
6. Wound care—same as for any spine surgery
7. Discharge instruction
   a. Care of brace or cast if required
   b. Use of bed board at home
   c. Plans for follow-up with physician

EVALUATION

Evaluation is based on the patient outcomes. Questions to be asked include the following:
1. Have complications of surgery been avoided?
2. Can the patient explain the nature of the surgery that has been performed?
3. Can the patient perform prescribed exercises correctly?
4. Is the patient functioning at the highest possible level?
5. Does the patient understand the reason for the physician's follow-up program?

OTHER DISORDERS

Gout

Gout or gouty arthritis is a metabolic disorder that affects men eight to nine times more frequently than women. It can occur at any age, the peak age of onset occurring in the fifth decade. Eighty-five percent of all persons with gout have a genetic or familial tendency to develop the

Table 22-10 Other disorders

Disorder	Etiology	Signs and symptoms	Medical therapy

Gout	Metabolic disorder in synthesis of purines, or poor renal excretion of uric acid leading to chronic hyperuricemia	Acute: rapid onset of severe pain in inflamed joints—most frequently large toe
		Presence of swelling and tenderness, malaise, headache, and fever
		Chronic: always present in those who have familial tendency
		Acute exacerbations occur when not diagnosed or not treated
		Deposits of *tophi* (deposits of monosodium urate in tissues) most noticeable in ears, on knuckles, and on great toe
			1. Medications—acute attack
			  a. Colchicine (0.6 mg)—oral administration of 2 tablets initially, then 1 tablet each hour until nausea, vomiting, or diarrhea, or joint symptoms subside; limit is 6.0 to 8.0 mg
			  b. Colchicine 1.0 to 3.0 mg in saline intravenously over a 10-minute period
			  c. Phenylbutazone (Butazolidin)
			  d. Indomethacin (Indocin)
			2. Absolute rest of the joint
			Preventive therapy consists of reduction of the body pool of urates by one of two methods:
			1. Enhancing uric acid excretion
			  a. Probenecid (Benemid)—0.5 g daily for 1 week, then increased by 0.5 g weekly until serum uric acid is in normal range, then 0.5 g daily
			  b. Sulfinpyrazone (Anturane)—used for patients who do not tolerate Benemid
			2. Decreasing uric acid formation
			  a. Allopurinol (Zyloprim)—100 mg twice a day initally, increased by 100 mg every 2-4 weeks until serum uric acid level is normal; then 500 mg daily

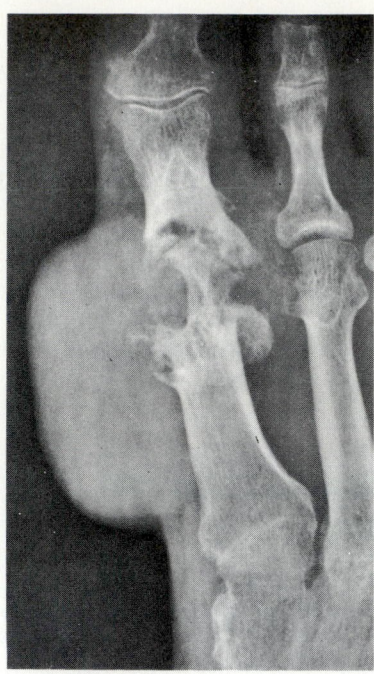

Fig. 22-22   Gout.

disease. Gout develops as a result of prolonged hyperuricemia (elevated serum uric acid) caused by problems either in synthesizing purines or by poor renal excretion of uric acid. The etiology, signs and symptoms, and medical therapy are listed in Table 22-10.

■ PATHOPHYSIOLOGY

Urate crystals form in the synovial tissue, causing severe inflammation. The inflammatory process is extremely rapid, occurring over a few hours, Acute symptoms are extreme pain, swelling, and erythema of the involved joints. Typically the great toe is involved (the first metatarsophalangeal joint), but other joints, such as the heel, ankle, and knee, may also be affected. Pain is so severe that the patient may not tolerate even the weight of a sheet over the joint. Renal damage may occur, especially if recurrent uric acid stones have been present. Between attacks of gout, the patient may be asymptomatic, but repeated attacks can occur with gradually increasing frequency if the disease is untreated. Patients with gouty symptoms may develop *tophi*, or deposits of monosodium urate in their tissues. These consist of a core of monosodium urate with a surrounding inflammatory reaction. Patients with tophaceous deposits (Fig. 22-22) tend to have more frequent and more severe episodes of gouty arthritis.

▨ ASSESSMENT

☐ Subjective data

1. Acute episodes: chief complaint will be severe pain in great toe or other joints.

2. Question patient about previous episodes and what brought relief.
3. Has there been weight gain?
4. Is there a history of gouty arthritis in the family?
5. Does the patient take medication for gout?

☐ Objective data

1. Patient cannot tolerate touching the joint and will display guarding of the affected joint.
2. The joint is swollen and red (first metatarsal, tarsal joints, ankle, knee, or elbow) (see Fig. 22-22).
3. A low-grade fever is present.
4. Nodular swelling may be visible in the subcutaneous tissues overlying the joints or in the cartilage of the helix of the ear.

☐ Diagnostic tests

1. Serum uric acid level will be elevated (hyperuricemia).
2. The 24-hour urinary uric acid level may be elevated.
3. Synovial fluid from the joint shows presence of monosodium urate crystals.
4. Sedimentation rate will be elevated.
5. X-ray examination will reveal soft tissue swelling.

▶ DATA ANALYSIS: NURSING DIAGNOSES

Nursing diagnoses are determined from an assessment of patient data. Possible nursing diagnoses for the person with gout may include, but are not limited to the following:

Diagnostic title	Possible etiologies
Potential for injury: damage to joints or kidneys	High urinary levels of uric acid/uric acid stones, urate crystals in synovial tissues
Knowledge deficit	Lack of exposure to information about gout
Pain: joint	Inflammation of joints with deposits of urate crystals in synovial tissues

▧ PLANNING: EXPECTED PATIENT OUTCOMES

Expected patient outcomes for the person with gout may include, but are not limited to, the following:
1. Patient is free of discomfort.
2. Patient avoids subsequent attacks of gout.
3. Patient understands need to take medication as prescribed. Most patients take uricosuric agents daily for life.

▨ IMPLEMENTATION

☐ Assisting with achievement of therapeutic goals

1. Give medications as prescribed.
2. Ensure that prescribed fluid intake is met.
3. Promote comfort
   a. Provide absolute rest until pain of acute attack subsides.
   b. Avoid touching joint or moving affected extremity until acute pain subsides.

☐ Counseling and teaching

1. Instruct patient in nature of disease.
2. Instruct patient in proper use of prescribed medications.
3. Encourage patient to lose weight if overweight.
4. Encourage patient to take in sufficient fluid to ensure daily *output* of 2000 to 3000 ml.

⊞ EVALUATION

Evaluation is based on the expected patient outcomes. Questions to be asked include the following:
1. Is the patient free of joint pain?
2. Is the patient able to discuss medications and follow-up care to avoid attacks of gouty arthritis?

■ Bacterial arthritis

Bacterial arthritis is inflammation of the synovial tissues caused by bacterial agents. The joint cavity may become involved. The etiology, signs and symptoms, and medical therapy are listed in Table 22-11.

■ PATHOPHYSIOLOGY

Synovial tissues respond to bacterial invasion by becoming inflamed. If the joint cavity becomes involved, pus will be present in the synovial membrane and the synovial fluid. If allowed to progress, the infection will cause abscesses in the synovium and subchondral bone, eventually destroying cartilage. Ankylosis of the joint may result.

▤ ASSESSMENT

☐ Subjective data

1. Ask patient to describe the onset of pain and changes noted in the joints.
2. Is patient being treated for another infection?

3. Is there a history of recent surgery or trauma?
4. Is there a history of recent sexual contact with a carrier of gonorrhea?

☐ Objective data

1. Monitor the affected joint: it will be swollen and warm to touch.
2. Observe patient's resistance to movement.
3. Monitor body temperature; fever may be present.
4. Observe for contractures that may be present if infection is of long duration.

☐ Diagnostic tests

1. Joint may be aspirated to obtain synovial fluid for culture and sensitivity.
2. Joint fluid white cell count will be elevated, and glucose content will be reduced.
3. Roentgenograms may show loss of joint space and lytic changes in bone.

➡ DATA ANALYSIS: NURSING DIAGNOSES

Nursing diagnoses are determined from assessment of patient data. Possible nursing diagnoses for the person with bacterial arthritis may include, but are not limited to, the following:

Diagnostic title	Possible etiologies
Activity intolerance	Immobility; infection of joint
Pain	Infection in joint capsule
Knowledge deficit	Lack of exposure to information

▤ PLANNING: EXPECTED PATIENT OUTCOMES

Expected patient outcomes for the person with bacterial arthritis may include, but are not limited to, the following:
1. Patient's pain is lessened.
2. Infection is responding to antibiotic therapy.

Table 22-11 Other disorders

Disorder	Etiology	Signs and symptoms	Medical therapy
Bacterial arthritis	1. Invasion of synovial membrane by micoorganisms: a. Gonococci b. Meningococci c. Staphylococci d. Coliforms e. Salmonella f. *Haemophilus influenzae* 2. Predisposition: a. Susceptibility of the patient b. Recent joint surgery or trauma c. Intraarticular injections d. Rheumatoid arthritis	Pain Swelling Tenderness of joint	Rest or immobilization Antibiotics specific for the organism Surgical drainage may be necessary Resumption of acitve range of motion when infection subsides

3. Patient understands need to take medication as prescribed after discharge.
4. Patient understands need to rest joint as prescribed.
5. Patient demonstrates ability to care for own cast or other joint-immobilizing device after discharge.
6. Patient can state plans for follow-up care.

IMPLEMENTATION

☐ **Assisting with achievement of therapeutic goals**

1. Antibiotics are given as prescribed; reactions to drugs are monitored.
2. Surgical drainage or system of irrigation and drainage may be employed. Drainage is monitored for amount and color.
3. As soon as infection subsides, encourage the patient to move the affected joint to prevent contracture.

☐ **Assisting with comfort and ADL**

1. Give pain medication as prescribed.
2. During the acute stage, assist patient in resting and immobilizing the joint to help control pain and prevent deformity.
3. Assist patient with self-care.

☐ **Counseling and teaching**

1. Instruct patient in care of cast or other joint-immobilizing device.
2. Encourage active joint motion when motion is permitted.
3. Instruct patient in proper administration of antibiotics if therapy is to be continued after discharge.
4. Assure that patient is aware of plans for follow-up with physician.

EVALUATION

Evaluation is based on the expected patient outcomes. Questions to be asked include the following:
1. Has infection of the joint subsided?
2. Can patient demonstrate joint range of motion without discomfort?
3. Can the patient care for cast or other joint-immobilizing device?
4. Can patient state plans for follow-up care?

TRAUMA

The person who has suffered trauma to the musculoskeletal system has sustained an interruption in the integrity of one or more components of that system. Musculoskeletal trauma is most frequently manifested as bone fracture, but it may also include injury to soft tissue, muscle, ligament, meniscus, tendon, or joint.

Trauma to bone

FRACTURE OF BONE

Fracture of bone usually occurs as a result of a blow to the body, a fall, or other accident. However, fracture may occur during normal activity or following a minimal injury if the bone is weakened by a disease such as primary or metastatic cancer or osteoporosis. This is called a *pathologic fracture,* or a collapse of the bone. Bone may also fracture when the muscles associated with it are unable to absorb energy as they usually do. This type of fracture is called a *fatigue* or *stress fracture.* Fracture can occur at any age, although older persons, persons with balance or mobility problems, persons who work at high-risk occupations (for example, steelworkers, race car drivers), and persons with chronic degenerative or neoplastic diseases are at higher risk for injury. The etiology, signs and symptoms, and immediate medical therapy are listed in Table 22-12.

☐ **Prevention**

One approach to preventing fracture is to make the environment safer. Examples of measures that can be taken include the following:
1. Mounting grab bars on the wall next to a tub or toilet
2. Attaching safety arms around a toilet
3. Removing throw rugs and obstacles from areas used by individuals with locomotor difficulties
4. Assuring that wheelchairs have adequate locking devices
5. Teaching individuals who must use ambulatory devices and wheelchairs how to use them properly

A *second* approach is to continue to educate the public regarding the following:
1. The dangers of drinking and driving
2. The advisability of using seat belts
3. Attending to safety precautions when climbing ladders, using power tools or heavy equipment
4. Wearing recommended protective clothing (for example, steel-toed shoes, hard hats) for hazardous work at home or on the job
5. Wearing proper protective clothing while engaging in sports (for example, protective padding, well-fitting running shoes)

A *third* approach is to continue to educate women regarding the problem of *osteoporosis.* Individuals most at risk to develop osteoporosis are small-framed, nonobese, menopausal white females. Contributing factors are diets low in calcium throughout life, smoking, excessive coffee intake, too much protein in the diet, and a sedentary lifestyle. Measures that can be taken to retard osteoporosis include the following:
1. Increasing calcium intake
2. Stopping smoking
3. Decreasing coffee intake
4. Decreasing excess protein in the diet
5. Engaging in some regular moderate activity such as walking
6. Exploring with one's physician the advisability of estrogen replacement at menopause

Table 22-12 Fractures

Etiology	Signs and symptoms	Therapy

Blow or injury (fall, accident)
Pathologic fracture: weakened by disease such as cancer or osteoporosis
Fatigue fracture: a bone fractures when muscles involved are unable to absorb energy, such as on long foot marches
	Complete fracture
	Pain immediate and severe and aggravated by movement and pressure at site
	Loss of function of injured part
	Obvious gross deformity when compared to normal extremity
	Loss of rigidity of injured part—motion at site
	Movement produces grating sound (crepitus) of bone fragments
	Soft tissue edema—localized swelling and ecchymosis (may not be apparent for several hours)
	Shock caused by severe injury, pain, and blood loss into damaged tissues
	NOTE: Symptoms may be absent in linear compacted fractures.
	There may be little or no swelling
	Pain is present only when pressure is applied to fracture site or on use of limb or body part
		Management objectives
		Reduction of fracture
		Maintenance of fragments in correct alignment
		Prevention of excessive loss of joint mobility and muscle tone
		Immediate management
		Provide splint before moving patient or maintain support above and below fracture site until patient can be moved and immobilization applied with splints for transportation
		Elevate extremity to minimize edema
		Transport patient for emergency treatment
		Observe injured part at frequent intervals for local changes in color, sensation, or temperature
		Tetanus immunization is given if compound fracture is present
		Cold applications are given to reduce hemorrhage, edema, and pain
		Medication for pain (aspirin or narcotics) is given
		
		Secondary management
		Simple fracture
		1. Optimal reduction (replacing bone fragments in their correct anatomic position
		  a. Manual manipulation: moving the bone fragments into position by applying distraction and pressure to the distal fragment
		  b. Traction
		  c. Open reduction: surgical intervention that may incorporate use of an internal fixation device
		2. Immobilization
		  a. External fixation: cast or splint
		  b. Traction
		  c. Internal fixation: pins, plates, screws, wires, prostheses
		  d. Combination of the above
		Compound fracture
		1. Surgical debridement of wound to remove dirt, foreign material, devitalized tissue, and necrotic bone
		2. Administration of tetanus toxoid
		3. Culture of wound
		4. Packing of wound
		5. Treatment with antibiotics
		6. Observation for signs of osteomyelitis, tetanus, or gas gangrene
		7. Closure of wound when there is no sign of infection
		8. Reduction of fracture
		9. Immobilization of fracture
		Treatment of complications is discussed in Table 22-14

Classification of bone fractures

A. Classification according to types of fractures
 1. *Complete* fracture: complete separation of the bone producing two fragments
 2. *Incomplete* fracture: a partial break in the bone without separation of the bone
 3. *Simple* or *closed* fracture: bone is broken; skin is intact
 4. *Compound* or *open* fracture: the fracture parts extend through the skin
 5. *Fracture without displacement:* bone is broken; bone fragments are in alignment in normal position
 6. *Fracture with displacement:* bone fragments have separated at the point of fracture
 7. *Comminuted fracture:* the bone has broken into several fragments
 8. *Impacted* ("telescoped") fracture: one bone fragment is forcibly driven into another bone fragment

B. Classification according to line of fracture (Fig. 22-23)
 1. *Greenstick:* splintering of one side of the bone (occurs most often in children with soft bones)
 2. *Transverse:* break across the bone
 3. *Oblique:* line of fracture at an oblique angle to the bone shaft
 4. *Spiral:* line of fracture encircles the bone

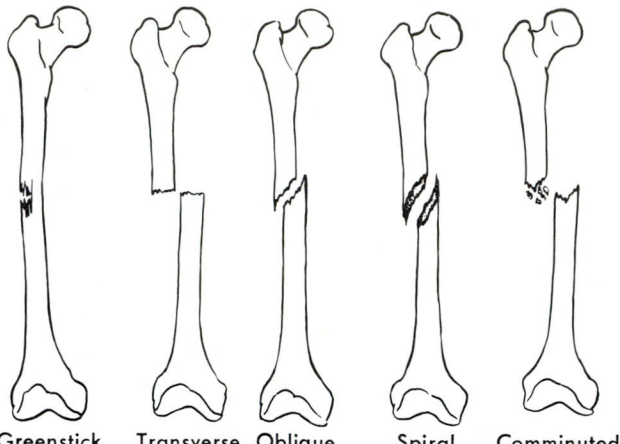

Greenstick Transverse Oblique Spiral Comminuted

Fig. 22-23 Types of fractures.

□ **Pathophysiology and bone healing**

A bone is said to be *fractured* or *broken* when there is an interruption in bone continuity. Commonly, a fracture is accompanied by *soft tissue* injury to surrounding tissues, that is, ligaments, muscle, tendons, blood vessels, and nerves.

The classification of bone fractures is given in the box above.

Immobilization of a bone that is fractured is necessary for bone healing. Immobilization takes place by the following means:

1. *Physiologic splintage.* This form of splintage will occur naturally, since guarding, avoidance of use, and muscle spasm will occur as a result of pain on movement.
2. *External orthopedic splintage.* This is accomplished with devices such as plaster casts and traction.

3. *Internal fixation.* In this method the opposing ends of the fracture are held in place by screws, plates, or rods.

Once immobilization is accomplished, new bone called *callus* begins to form by the following stages of growth (Fig. 22-24):

1. *Hematoma formation.* Because blood vessels are injured, bleeding occurs at the site of the fracture. The blood collects and fastens the broken ends together.
2. *Fibrin meshwork.* The hematoma becomes organized as fibroblasts invade the area, forming the fibrin meshwork. White blood cells wall off the area, localizing the inflammation.
3. *Invasion by osteoblasts.* The osteoblasts enter the fibrous area to help hold the union firm. Blood vessels develop, establishing a source of nutrients for building collagen. Collagen strands begin to incorporate calcium deposits.
4. *Callus formation.*
 a. Osteoblasts continue to lay the network for bone buildup.
 b. Osteoclasts destroy dead bone and help to synthesize new bone.
 c. The collagen strengthens and continues to incorporate calcium deposits.
5. *Remodeling.* In this final step, excess callus is reabsorbed and trabecular bone is laid down along lines of stress.

Factors that impede or prevent callus formation include the following:

1. *Delayed healing or delayed union.* Delayed union occurs when the fracture does not heal within the usual time for healing.
 a. Reasons:
 (1) Callus is broken or torn apart by too much activity.
 (2) Edema at the fracture site impedes flow of nutrients to the area.
 (3) Immobilization is inefficient.
 (4) Infection is present at fracture site.
 (5) Patient is in poor nutritional state.

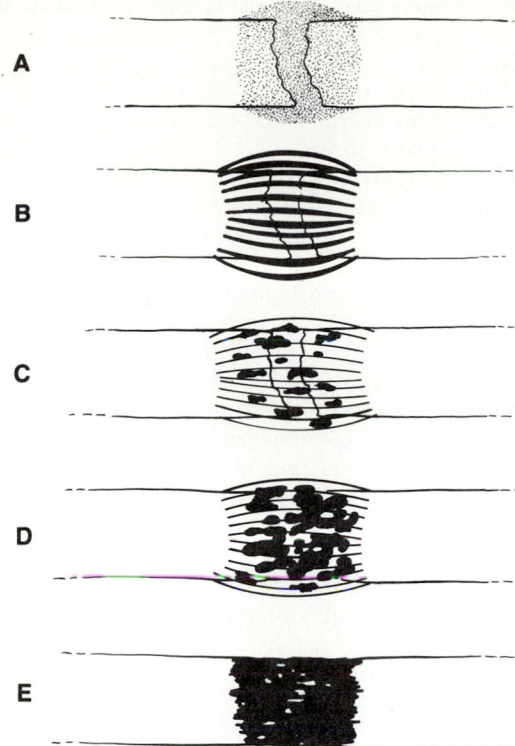

Fig. 22-24 Bone healing (schematic representation). **A,** Bleeding at broken ends of bone with subsequent hematoma formation. **B,** Organization of hematoma into fibrous network. **C,** Invasion of osteoblasts, lengthening of collagen strands, and deposition of calcium. **D,** Callus formation: new bone is built up as osteoclasts destroy dead bone. **E,** Remodeling is accomplished as excess callus is reabsorbed and trabecular bone is laid down.

b. Correction: More complete immobilization or open reduction for surgical measures.
2. *Nonunion.* Nonunion is the term used when healing does not occur even in a much longer period of time.
  a. Reasons:
    (1) Too much bone loss at time of injury to permit bridging of bone fragments.
    (2) Bone necrosis has occurred because of lack of blood supply.
    (3) Anemia, endocrine imbalance, or other systemic conditions are present.
  b. Correction:
    (1) Crutches may have to be used indefinitely.
    (2) A brace may be worn to support the limb.
    (3) Surgery may be performed to unite bone fragments with a bone graft.

ASSESSMENT
□ Subjective data
1. Pain at site of injury
2. Loss of sensation or movement of affected part
3. Description of how trauma occurred

4. Understanding of injury sustained (may report having heard bone snap)

□ Objective data
1. Warmth, edema, and/or ecchymosis over and surrounding the injured part
2. Obvious deformity
3. Loss of normal function in the injured part
4. Immobilization device(s) applied to the injured part
5. Signs of systemic shock
6. Signs of circulatory, motor, or sensory impairment to the injured part (see Table 22-13)
7. Indicators of apprehension or fear

□ Diagnostic tests
Radiographs of site to determine extent of injury.

DATA ANALYSIS: NURSING DIAGNOSES

Nursing diagnoses are determined from assessment of patient data. Possible nursing diagnoses for the person with a fractured bone may include, but are not limited to, the following:

Diagnostic title	Possible etiologies
Potential for infection	Trauma/exposure to nosocomial organisms
Potential for injury: trauma	Motor deficits
Knowledge deficit	Lack of exposure, unfamiliar situation
Impaired physical mobility	Trauma/fracture
Altered nutrition: potential for less than body requirements	Trauma/pain/immobility
Pain	Trauma/fracture
Powerlessness	Helplessness because of trauma/immobility
Self-care deficit	Trauma/immobility because of treatment
Impaired skin integrity	Trauma/fracture/immobility

PLANNING: EXPECTED PATIENT OUTCOMES

Expected patient outcomes for the person with a fractured bone may include but are not limited to the following:
1. Pain is reduced.
2. Healing occurs.
3. Complications are avoided.
4. The patient or significant other is able to explain the nature of the injury and the course of treatment that must be followed.
5. The patient or significant other is able to explain the limitations of motion and restrictions of activity to be observed and how long they must continue.
6. The patient is able to demonstrate how to perform or modify ADL within the limitations of activity and motion that must be observed.
7. The patient or significant other is able to explain how to care for cast, pins, or other immobilization devises (if applicable).

8. The patient is able to demonstrate safe use of an ambulatory or other ADL assistive device (if necessary).

9. The patient or significant other is able to demonstrate safe technique in carrying out wound care (if necessary).

10. The patient or significant other is able to demonstrate techniques appropriate to prevent skin breakdown, swelling, and neurocirculatory impairment.

11. The patient or significant other is able to explain measures that can be taken for relief of pain or discomfort.

12. The patient or significant other is able to explain how to use prescribed medications.

13. The patient or significant other is able to explain plans for follow-up care.

IMPLEMENTATION

☐ *Assisting with the achievement of therapeutic goals*

POSITIONING

The purpose of positioning is to promote comfort and prevent complications. Knowledge needed before positioning includes the following:

1. Where is the fracture?
2. What is the nature of the fracture?
3. Has the fracture been reduced?
4. What method was used to reduce the fracture?
5. What are the tolerances of the method used to reduce the fracture?
6. Is the fracture stable?
7. Has the orthopedist requested special precautions?

After this information is obtained, positioning should be carried out with careful attention to the following:

1. Avoid altering the alignment of the fracture
2. Avoid changing the direction of the pull of traction
3. Avoid compromising the integrity of the cast
4. Avoid placing undue stress on the internal fixation device

5. Avoid changing position of patient before fracture has been reduced or splinted
6. Once fracture is reduced or splinted, assist patient in changing position at *least* every 2 hours
7. Provide overhead frame and trapeze to assist patient in moving about in bed

NEUROCIRCULATORY MONITORING

Monitoring for neurocirculatory compromise must be carried out every hour in the initial stages of fracture. Damage to blood vessels and/or nerves may occur at the time of the fracture or subsequent to the fracture or its reduction. Some swelling of a fractured extremity may be expected and is often well controlled by elevating the extremity. However, unrelieved swelling of an extremity that is in a cast or compression dressing can result in tissue damage and/or neurologic impairment. Evidence of impaired circulation or sensation must be reported to the physician immediately. Frequency of neurocirculatory checks can usually be reduced if there is no evidence to compromise within 48 hours of the fracture or reduction of the fracture (See Table 22-13).

Monitoring neurocirculatory status of the injured part includes the following:

1. Palpation for warmth
2. Observation of color
3. Application of moderate pressure to the nail bed and subsequent observation of speed of capillary refill
4. Questioning the patient regarding pain or paresthesias in the injured part
5. Touching the injured part to test the patient's ability to discriminate sensation
6. Observation of patient's ability to voluntarily move body part distal to fracture

PRESERVING STRENGTH AND MOBILITY

Encourage the patient to do the following:

1. Move about to the greatest extent possible within the restriction of the fracture reduction and the immobilizing devices
2. Accomplish as much of own self-care as possible

Table 22-13 Observations for signs and symptoms of neurocirculatory impairment

Observation	Interpretation
Tissue color white	Decreased arterial blood supply
Tissue color blue	Venous stasis and poorly oxygenated tissue
Color slow to return to nail bed after application of moderate pressure	Decreased arterial blood supply
Edema	Fluid accumulating in tissues; poor venous return
Tissue cold or cool to touch	Decreased arterial blood supply
Patient unable to move parts distal to cast	Pressure on nerves innervating parts distal to cast
Patient complaint of heightened or decreased sensation or paresthesia in part underlying or distal to cast	Pressure on nerves innervating parts underlying or distal to cast
Patient complaint of extreme pain unrelieved by elevation, analgesic, or repositioning	Pressure on nerve endings in parts underlying or distal to cast

NOTE: Comparison of tissue should be made with contralateral tissue to determine extent of deviation from normal

3. Perform muscle toning (isometric) exercises on a regular basis: quadriceps setting, gluteal setting
4. Follow through with exercise programs (including ambulation) prescribed by the physician and taught by the physical therapist
5. Resume normal functioning for all ADL (within limits of immobilization or fixation device) as soon as possible; for example, using bedside commode or toilet instead of bedpan

MAINTAINING SKIN INTEGRITY

1. Early identification of skin areas at risk, particularly areas over bony prominences (for example, heels, sacrum, elbows, ischial tuberosities)
2. Application of a skin toughening agent, such as tincture of benzoin, two to three times a day to areas identified as being at risk
3. Regular (at least every 8 hours) inspection for signs of pressure (erythema, induration)
4. Regular turning (at least every 2 hours) within the limits of the system of fracture immobilization
5. Turning the patient with a turning sheet (see Fig. 22-19)
6. Moving the patient from one surface to another with a pull sheet or roller board
7. Rolling the patient onto his or her side or lifting them to place them on a bedpan rather than sliding the pan under them
8. For patients who cannot be fully turned because of traction or other limiting factors, consideration should be given to using one or more of the following:
   a. Sheepskin pads
   b. Flotation pads
   c. Alternating air pressure mattress or alternating air pressure system, such as the Lapidus system
   d. Foam mattress
   e. Foam heel and/or elbow pads
   f. Special beds, such as the CircOlectric, Clinitron, or Mediscus bed
   g. Turning frames, such as the Foster or Stryker frames
9. Regular inspection of skin areas in contact with cast edges or traction apparatus and taking appropriate measures to eliminate chafing or rubbing in those areas
10. Assisting the patient with keeping skin clean and dry, especially under casts, slings, traction apparatus

PROMOTING WOUND HEALING

1. Strict attention to aseptic technique during dressing changes
2. Attention to drains to maintain their placement and patency
3. Caring for pin site as ordered
4. Encouraging to eat a well-balanced diet

PROMOTING NUTRITION

1. Encourage patient to eat regular meals
2. Give the patient plenty of time to eat
3. Encourage self-feeding, but assist the patient or provide special assistive utensils as necessary
4. Attend to the patient's need for roughage and fluid as noted, and encourage protein intake of 150-300 g per day

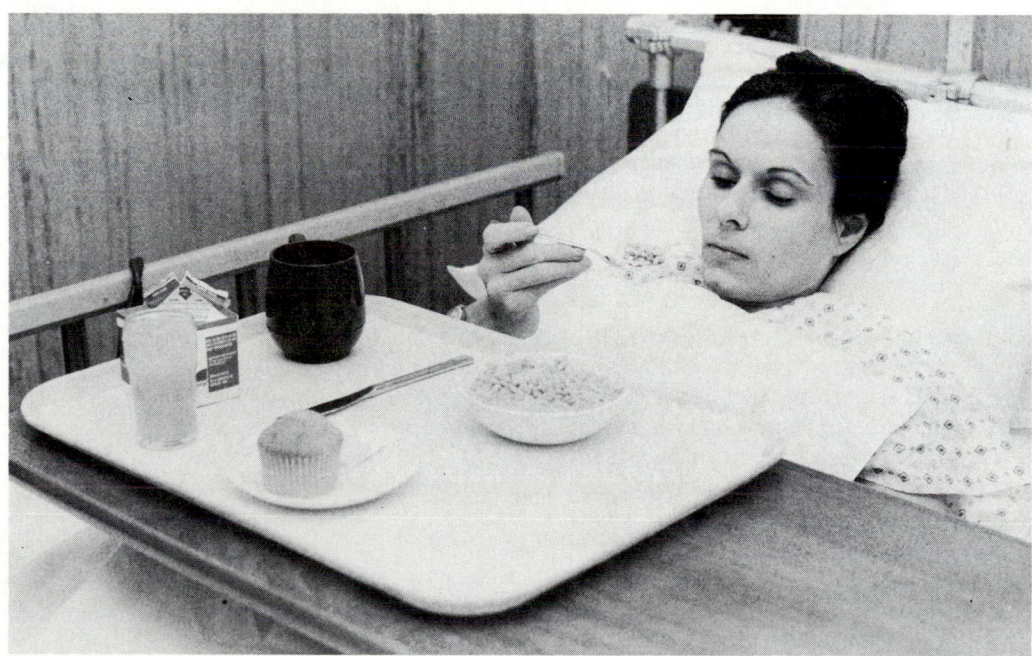

Fig. 22-25 Patient who can neither sit up nor lie on one side to eat meals can still be made comfortable with some elevation of the head and shoulders on pillows. Additional means of elevating patient to a more upright position is to put frame of bed in reverse. Trendelenburg's position.

5. Position the patient to facilitate comfortable intake of food and fluid (Fig. 22-25)

MAINTAINING IMMOBILIZATION OF THE
REDUCED FRACTURE

The purpose of immobilization is to hold the broken bone fragments in contact with each other until healing takes place. Immobilization can be accomplished in the following ways:

1. Externally with
   a. Cast
   b. Splint
   c. Brace
   d. Cast brace
   e. Traction
2. Internally with
   a. Metal plates, pinc, screws, nails
   b. Bone grafts with addition of metal plates, pins
   c. Prosthetic implants
3. Externally and internally with combinations of the above

□ *Assisting with comfort and ADL*

MANAGING PAIN. The person with a fracture will most often have severe pain at the fracture site, pressure from edema in damaged soft tissues adjacent to the fracture, and spasm of muscles in the fracture area. Continued pain and the muscle spasm accompanying it can put undue stress on the fracture fragments and retard efforts both to reduce and to maintain reduction of the fracture. Patients who are in severe pain will resist efforts to assist them in carrying out measures designed to prevent complications. If the fracture is repaired by open reduction and internal fixation, the patient will have operative pain.

Measures the nurse can take to help reduce pain include the following:

1. During the initial stages of treatment, administer prescribed narcotic and nonnarcotic analgesics in appropriate dosages at timely intervals
2. Administer prescribed agents such as diazepam (Valium) to reduce muscle spasm
3. Apply ice compresses, as ordered, to affected part
4. Reposition the patient frequently within the restrictions of the prescribed treatment
5. Instruct the patient how to use relaxation techniques (deep breathing, imagery) to reduce tension
6. As pain subsides, negotiate with the patient a reduction in the strength and/or frequency of analgesics

It is important, in using analgesics, to try to strike a balance between having the patient comfortable enough to perform required exercises and other activities, but not so overly medicated as to risk potential damage through overextending activity or being heavily sedated.

□ *Monitoring for complications*

The complications of bone fractures, mechanism, signs, onset, and treatment are listed in Table 22-14.

Table 22-14 Complications of fracture

Complication	Mechanism	Signs	Onset	Treatment
Fat embolism	Pressure changes in interior of fractured bones force molecules of fat from marrow into systemic circulation, resulting in respiratory and central nervous system problems	Chest pain Pallor Dyspnea Prostration Confusion Petechial hemorrhage of skin and conjunctivae	2-3 days following injury	Supportive measures; that is, high Fowler's position, oxygen therapy, blood transfusion to relieve hypovolemic shock, digitalization for heart failure Diuretics Bronchodilators Corticosteroids Proper immobilization and careful handling may help prevent occurrence
Ischemic paralysis (contracture)	Arterial flow is interrupted to injured part by trauma or pressure	Coldness, pallor, cyanosis, pain, swelling distal to injury or cast	At injury or after cast application	Treatment of fracture Release of cast or constricting bandages
Osteomyelitis	Bacteria introduced through wound or from another site in body (for example, boils) Infection of marrow spaces, haversian canals, and subperiosteal space with subsequent destruction of bone by proteolytic enzymes	Hyperemia, edema, pain, pus		Culture and sensitivity testing, antibiotics, surgical drainage, and debridement Prevention: use of aseptic technique when caring for open wound

⊞ EVALUATION

Evaluation is based on the expected patient outcomes. Questions to be asked include the following:

1. Is the patient comfortable?
2. Have complications been avoided?
3. Does the patient know how to care for the cast?
4. Does the patient know how to care for the limb after the cast is removed?
5. Does the patient know how to perform ADL within any limitations?
6. Can the patient explain plans for follow-up care?

■ Treatment of fractures with external fixation devices

■ CASTS

Casts are the most common external fixation device. They are made of plaster of Paris, fiberglass, and plastic, which are available in the form of rolled bandages that are applied over the part to be immobilized in much the same manner as an Ace bandage. *Plaster,* which has to be moistened before application, dries very slowly, is heavy, and loses its strength and integrity if it becomes wet. If a plaster cast requires revision, it generally must be removed and a new one reapplied. However, plaster is less expensive than fiberglass or plastic.

Fiberglass and *plastic* dry quickly, are light in weight, and may be immersed in water without losing their strength. Plastic casts may be reheated and remolded if revision is necessary. Disadvantages include the fact that some types of fiberglass require drying under special ultraviolet lights, and persons wearing fiberglass or plastic casts may suffer maceration of the skin under the cast following immersion in water unless they dry the skin thoroughly with a warm air dryer. Specific discussions regarding the advantages and disadvantages of various cast materials can be found in orthopaedic texts.

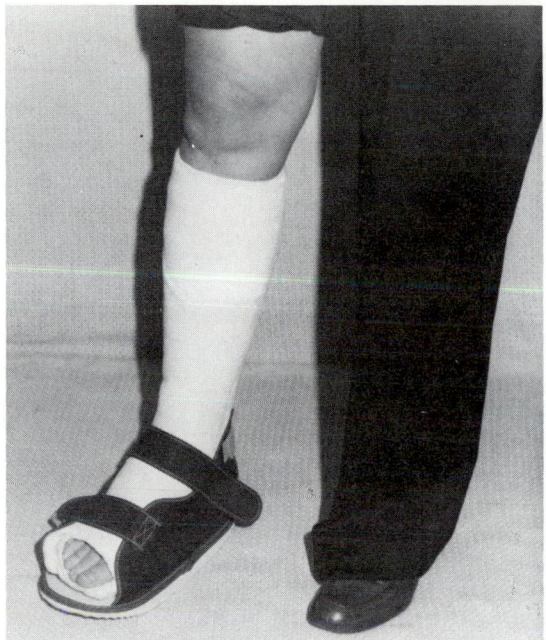

Fig. 22-26   Short leg walking cast with cast shoe.

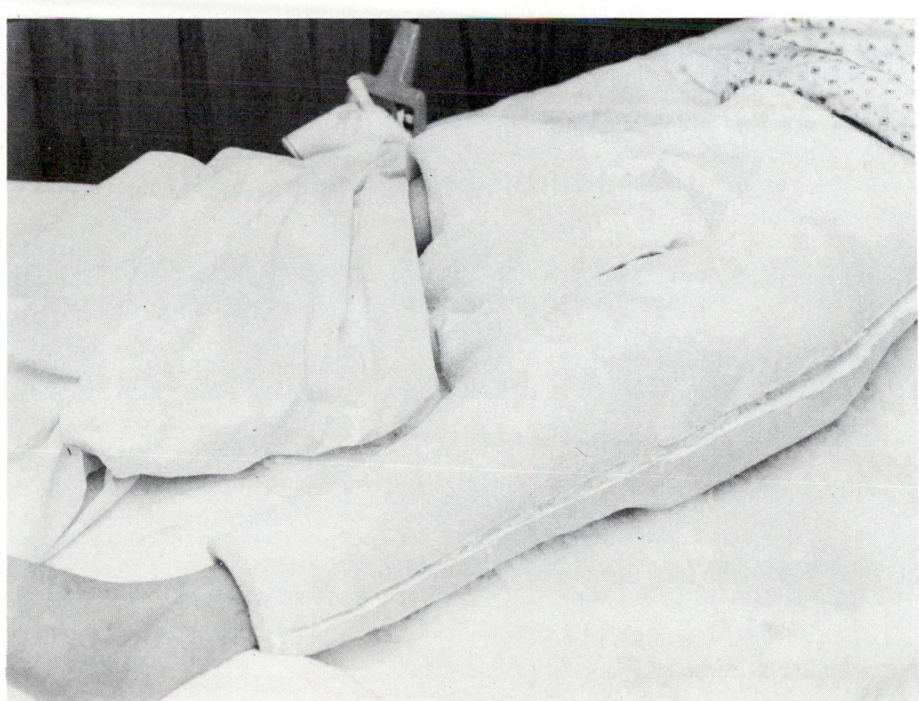

Fig. 22-27   Bivalved cast.

Nursing care of the patient in a cast

1. Patient education
   a. Explain why the cast is being applied and how it will be applied
   b. Advise the patient that the plaster cast will feel warm as it dries
   c. Explain the extent of immobilization
   d. Explain care of the cast and expectations after discharge
   e. Instruct patient not to insert sharp objects (coat hangers or pencils) under the cast as these may abrade the skin and lead to infection
2. Handling the new cast
   a. Support wet cast with the flat of the hands or on pillows to avoid indentations that will cause pressure on underlying skin
   b. Place cotton blankets or other absorbent material under the cast to aid drying
   c. Expose the cast to air as much as possible to aid drying
   d. Turn the patient frequently to aid drying
   e. Use a cast dryer or hair dryer on a warm, not hot, setting to circulate air over the cast
   f. Do not apply paint, varnish, or shellac to the cast; plaster is a porous material that allows air to circulate to the skin
3. Skin care
   a. Inspect skin at edges of cast and underlying cast for redness or irritation; apply petal-shaped strips of adhesive tape or moleskin around rough edges of cast
   b. Remove plaster crumbs from skin with a washcloth moistened with warm water
   c. Use creams and lotions sparingly as they may soften the skin and cause the cast to stick to the skin
   d. Apply waterproof material around perineal area to prevent soiling of and damage to cast and irritation of the skin
   e. Attend to patient's complaint of pain under the cast, particularly over bony prominences, as this may indicate pressure on the skin. If discomfort is not relieved by repositoning, report to physician. Cast pressure may need to be relieved by windowing or bivalving (cutting cast into two halves)
4. Turning—turning to any position is generally permitted so long as the integrity of the cast is not compromised and the patient is comfortable
5. Toileting—for a long leg or hip spica cast
   a. Use a fracture pan with blanket roll or padding as support under the small of the back
   b. Elevate the head of the bed, if permitted, or place the bed in reverse Trendelenburg's position
6. Abdominal discomfort—cast may be "windowed" (an opening cut into it) to provide relief of abdominal distention or a port for checking bladder distention
7. Mobilization
   a. Weight bearing is at the discretion of the physician, and the amount of weight bearing will be prescribed
   b. A cast shoe (Fig. 22-26) or a walking heel incorporated into a lower extremity cast will permit weight bearing without damaging the cast
8. Prevention of neurocirculatory problems
   a. Perform neurocirculatory checks every h for at least 24 hours after cast application to detect difficulty from swelling or pressure of cast on nerves or vessels. Notify physician of color changes, alterations in sensation, or motion unrelieved by position change. Cast may need to be bivalved (cut in two) to relieve pressure (Fig. 22-27)
   b. Elevate affected extremity on pillows until danger of swelling is over (usually 24-48 hours)
   c. After mobilizaton of patient with lower extremity or upper extremity cast, avoid keeping extremity in dependent position for prolonged periods
   d. After lower extremity cast is removed, encourage patient to wear elastic stocking and elevate affected leg at rest until full mobility is regained

Before a cast is applied, the skin is cleansed and inspected for cuts or abrasions that may become infected. Skin lesions are treated with disinfectant. Before the cast is applied, normal skin may be treated with tincture of benzoin, then wrapped with cotton padding or stockinette. Bony prominences are padded with sheet wadding or felt to protect them from pressure. For specific techniques of cast application, consult specialized texts.

A cast is removed by splitting it with an electric cast saw. The saw is very noisy; but if it is used properly, it will not damage the skin beneath the cast. Skin enclosed in a cast for a period of time will be covered with an exudate of built-up secretions and dead skin. To remove this exudate, oil is applied, followed by numerous soaks and bathing with warm water. This process may take several days, but attempts to remove the exudate more rapidly may result in uncomfortable skin irritation.

Special considerations in caring for the patient in a cast are outlined in the box on p. 618.

■ TRACTION

Traction is the mechanism by which a steady pull is placed on a part or parts of the body. Traction may be used to accomplish the following:
1. Reduce a fracture
2. Maintain correct position of bone fragments during healing
3. Immobilize a limb while soft tissue healing takes place
4. Overcome muscle spasm
5. Stretch adhesions
6. Correct deformities

Countertraction is a force that counteracts the pull of traction. *Suspension* is the use of traction equipment—frames, splints, slings, ropes, pulleys, weights—to suspend a body part but not exert a "pull" on that part. To suspend the part correctly and continuously, the suspension has to be balanced by weights. Suspension is often referred to as *balanced suspension*. Balanced suspension is often used in conjunction with traction.

There are two types of traction: skin traction and skeletal traction.

□ Skin traction

Skin traction is achieved by applying wide bands of moleskin, adhesive, or commercially available devices directly to the skin and attaching weights to them. The pull of the weights is transmitted indirectly to the involved bone. Buck's extension and Russell traction are the two most common forms of skin traction used for injury to the lower extremities.

□ Buck's extension

Buck's extension is the simplest form of skin traction and provides for straight pull on the affected extremity (Fig. 22-18). It is often used to relieve muscle spasm and to immobilize a limb temporarily; for example, following hip fracture before open reduction and internal fixation. If adhesive substances are to be used, the skin of the leg is shaved and tincture of benzoin is applied to protect the skin. Adhesive tape or moleskin is then placed on the lateral and medial aspects of the leg and secured with a circular gauze or elastic bandage. The adhesive material should not cover the malleoli, since skin breakdown would occur over these bony prominences. The tapes are attached to a spreader bar sufficiently wide to pull the tapes away from the malleoli. Rope is attached to the spreader, passed through a pulley on a crossbar at the foot of the bed, and suspended with weights. The maximal weight that should be applied by skin traction is 3.6 kg (8 lb). Greater amounts of weight can cause skin damage. Commercial foam rubber Buck's traction splints are also in wide use and are applied simply with Velcro straps. Contraindications to placing a patient in Buck's traction are stasis dermatitis, arteriosclerosis, allergy to adhesive tape, severe varicosities or varicose ulcers, diabetic gangrene, or marked overriding of bone fragments that would require more than 3.6 kg of weight to reduce the fracture.

□ Russell traction

Russell traction is sometimes used because it permits the patient to move somewhat freely in the bed and it permits flexion of the knee joint (Fig. 22-28). It requires an overhead frame attached to the bed and preparation of the leg as for Buck's traction. A footplate with pulley attachments is used instead of a spreader bar. The knee is suspended in a sling to which a rope is attached. The rope is directed upward to a pulley that has been placed on the overhead frame directly above the tibial tubercle of the affected extremity. The rope is then passed downward through a pulley on a crossbar at the foot of the bed, back through a pulley on the footplate, back again to another pulley on the crossbar, and then suspended with weights. This arrangement effects a double pull from the crossbar to the footplate, so the traction is equal to approximately double the amount of weight used. Usually the foot of the bed is elevated on blocks (or the bed put in Trendelenburg position) to provide countertraction.

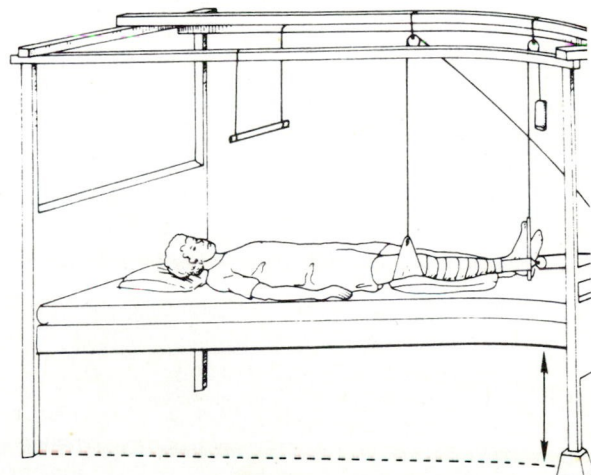

Fig. 22-28   Russell traction. Note that Balkan frame is attached to bed, leg is supported on pillows, and heel extends beyond pillow.

NURSING CARE PLAN

Person with fractured hip

DATA: Mrs. West is an 81-year-old widowed, retired secretary. This evening she tripped and fell on an icy step when leaving her niece's home. She complained of immediate, severe pain in her left hip and was unable to move her leg. Emergency Medical Services was phoned, and Mrs. West was brought to the hospital accompanied by her niece and her niece's husband. In the emergency room it was noted that her left leg was shorter than her right leg and externally rotated. Her vital signs were stable and the neurocirculatory status of the left leg was intact. Radiographic studies revealed a femoral neck (intracapsular) fracture. Intravenous fluids were initiated. An ECG, urinalysis, and bloodwork were obtained. She was transferred to the nursing division with physician's order for morphine sulfate 4-6 mg q 3-4 h prn for pain. Buck's extension traction was applied. Consent was obtained for surgical repair in the morning. Replacement of the femoral head and neck with regular stem *Austin Moore* prosthesis is planned.

The nursing history identified the following:
1. Mrs. West lives alone in her own apartment in a senior citizen complex.
2. She has no children but has nieces and nephews in the area who see her regularly. They assist with shopping and other errands.
3. She would like to return to her own apartment upon discharge from the hospital but is worried that she might need help at home. Her family is considering hiring a home health aide.
4. She takes no medications other than aspirin for occasional "stiffness" upon awakening.
5. She has never been hospitalized and last saw a physician 2 years ago for "the flu."

Nursing diagnosis: Knowledge deficit: related to lack of exposure to surgery

Expected patient outcomes	Nursing interventions	Rationale

Patient states she understands the teaching provided by the nurse
Patient will have less anxiety related to fear of the unknown and/or misconceptions regarding the surgery and recovery period
	Preoperative:
	  Assess need for instruction and provide by the nurse
	  Provide written materials pertaining to the surgery if available in the institution; review preoperative instruction with patient and family before surgery; evaluate patient's understanding of information taught
	Postoperative:
	  By discharge the patient should be instructed and able to demonstrate:
	  Independent ambulation on level surfaces with appropriate ambulatory aid, and independent stair climbing
	  Activity restrictions to be observed for approximately 2 months until follow-up with physician; these include no flexion of affected hip beyond 90 degrees, no adduction of affected leg beyond midline, no elevation of leg when sitting, and maintenance of partial weight-bearing status
	  Independent ADL with assistive devices
	  Rationale for antibiotic prophylaxis
		Understanding about surgical procedure and postoperative care should lessen anxiety and promote desired behaviors for recovery from surgery

Care Plan by Kyle Paskert, MSN, RN.

Continued.

Person with fractured hip—cont'd

Nursing diagnosis: Improved physical mobility: related to alterations in lower limb S/P surgical repair of hip fracture

Expected patient outcomes	Nursing interventions	Rationale
Patient will demonstrate optimal level of mobility with adaptive devices and within prescribed limit-actions by time of discharge No injury has occurred during hospitalization	Cough and deep breathe with incentive spirometer q1-2h until fully ambulatory	If carried out correctly and at appropriate intervals, pulmonary exercises can effectively prevent atelectasis and pneumonia
	Encourage patient to perform active dorsiplantar flexion, isometric quadriceps and gluteal sets, and active ROM of unaffected limbs q2 h until ambulatory, then qid	Exercises promote venous return and prevent thrombus formation and help to maintain muscle tone
	Determine from surgeon the limits of motion and weight bearing permitted: Hip flexion is limited to 60 degrees for 6-10 days, then 90 degrees for 2-3 months. Patients are usually permitted 90 degrees by time of discharge No adduction is permitted beyond midline for 2-3 months Usual weight-bearing restriction is *partial* weight-bearing assisted with walker or crutches	Specific restriction will depend on the design of the prosthesis and method of insertion; restrictions are designed to avoid dislocation of the prosthesis
	Turn patient side to back q2h and prn while bedrest is prescribed. Avoid positioning patient on operative side and observe flexion restrictions when elevating the head of the bed; avoid extreme internal or external rotation of the leg	Turning and repositioning frequently provides for better ventilation of the lungs and prevents skin breakdown
	Assist patient in turning by holding operative leg in abduction; use pillows to maintain 30 degrees of abduction while lying in bed	
	Assist patient in ambulating within weight-bearing restriction when permitted (about third postoperative day) using ambulatory aid; increase frequency and distance of ambulation as tolerated	Early postoperative activity including ambulation can hasten recovery and prevent postoperative complications
	Begin sitting when patient demonstrates sufficient control of leg to sit within flexion restrictions (60 degrees at operated hip initially); transfer the patient out of bed to chair bid-tid once initiated	
	Elevate sitting surface with pillows to keep angle of hip within prescribed limits	

Continued.

Person with fractured hip—cont'd

Nursing diagnosis: Impaired home maintenance management: potential for, related to numerous discharge needs

Expected patient outcomes	Nursing interventions	Rationale
Patient and family will express satisfaction with arrangements made to manage self-care at home	Discuss with the patient and family their plans upon discharge from the hospital Determine with the patient the information needed to be taught and learned for home care (Refer to knowledge deficit, postoperative) Determine the type of equipment and services needed, for example, crutches, walker, elevated toilet seat; homemaker, companion, Meals on Wheels Consult appropriate department or agency for these arrangements	Adequate discharge planning will foster successful completion of rehabilitation at home

Postoperatively, collaborative nursing actions include those to identify possible complications of the surgery. Immediate reporting of and treatment of early signs may prevent serious complications. Nursing actions include monitoring for the following:

a. Neurocirculatory compromise—perform neurocirculatory checks q2h for the first 24-48 h; notify physician of any changes from preoperative status
b. Dislocation of the prosthesis—notify physician if patient complains of sudden onset of increased (severe) pain (especially groin pain), deformity, or external rotation
c. Impaired skin integrity and/or incision healing—monitor pressure areas for signs of redness; monitor temperature; assess incision for sign or symptoms of infection and excessive drainage
d. Atelectasis/respiratory infection—monitor breath sounds until patient is ambulatory
e. Problems with elimination—assess for urinary stasis and constipation
f. Fluid and electrolyte imbalance—monitor input and output until patient is taking oral fluids equal to at least 1200 ml output; monitor IV fluid flow; assess patient for fluid volume excess or deficit

The following nursing diagnoses are especially pertinent for persons who have undergone surgical repair of a hip fracture. Implementation and evaluation of the related nursing interventions will help to prevent postoperative complications.

Nursing diagnosis: Pain: related to surgical procedure

Expected patient outcomes	Nursing interventions	Rationale
Patient states feeling more comfortable Patient is able to perform necessary postoperative routines and exercises because pain is adequately managed	Assess patient's pain and evaluate response to comfort measures provided Administer prescribed analgesics (usually narcotic) at timely intervals during the initial postoperative period Teach relaxation techniques as appropriate Use other pain-relieving techniques as pertinent, for example, back rubs, repositioning As pain decreases give milder analgesics	Subjective and objective data are important in ascertaining the nature of the patient's postoperative pain and in determining its management It is usually necessary to administer a narcotic q 3-4 h for the first 48-72 h after surgery Analgesics have a greater effect if they are administered before pain becomes severe Relaxation facilitates rest and may modify the response to pain A change in type of cutaneous stimulation may result in pain relief As pain lessens in severity it may be controlled by less potent analgesics (with fewer untoward side effects)

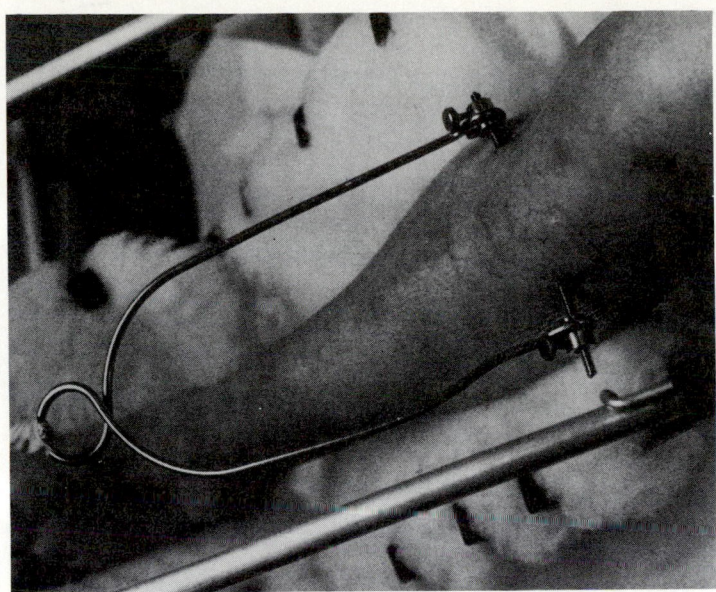

Fig. 22-29 Skeletal traction.

Russell traction is used in the treatment of intertrochanteric fracture of the femur when surgery is contraindicated. Bilateral Russell or Buck's traction may be used to treat back pain because they partially immobilize the patient and reduce muscle spasm.

□ Skeletal traction

Skeletal traction is traction applied directly to bone. Under local or general anesthesia, a Kirschner wire or Steinmann pin is inserted through bone distal to the fracture (the site of insertion varies with the type of fracture) (Fig. 22-29). The pin protrudes through the skin on both sides of the extremity, and the ends of the pin are covered with corks or metal protectors. Small sterile dressings are usually placed over the entry and exit sites of the pin. A metal U-shaped spreader or bow is attached to the pin, and the rope on which the traction weights are hung is tied onto the spreader. Skeletal traction can be used for fractures of the tibia, femur, humerus, and cervical spine. Skeletal traction to the cervical spine is achieved through use of tongs applied to the skull (Fig. 22-30).

When a balanced suspension apparatus is used in conjunction with skin or skeletal traction, the patient is able to move about in bed more freely without disturbing the line of pull of the traction. The use of a balancing apparatus facilitates nursing measures such as bathing, skin care, and placing the bedpan. A full or half-ring Thomas or Hodgen splint (Fig. 22-31) is frequently used for suspension of the lower extremities. Straps of canvas, muslin, or synthetic lamb's wool are placed over the splint and secured to provide a support for the leg. The areas under the popliteal space and heel are left open to prevent pressure on these parts. If it is desirable to have the knee flexed or to permit movement of the lower leg, a Pearson attachment is clamped or fixed to the Thomas splint at the level of the knee.

Special considerations in caring for the patient in traction are described in the box on p. 624.

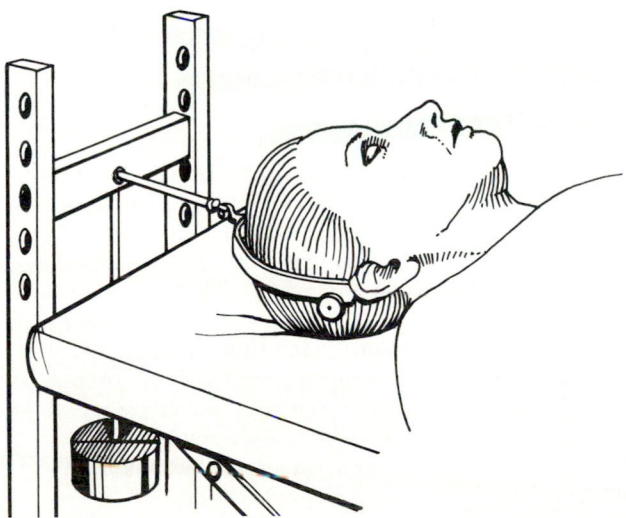

Fig. 22-30 Traction to the cervical spine can be maintained through the use of Crutchfield tongs inserted into the skull.

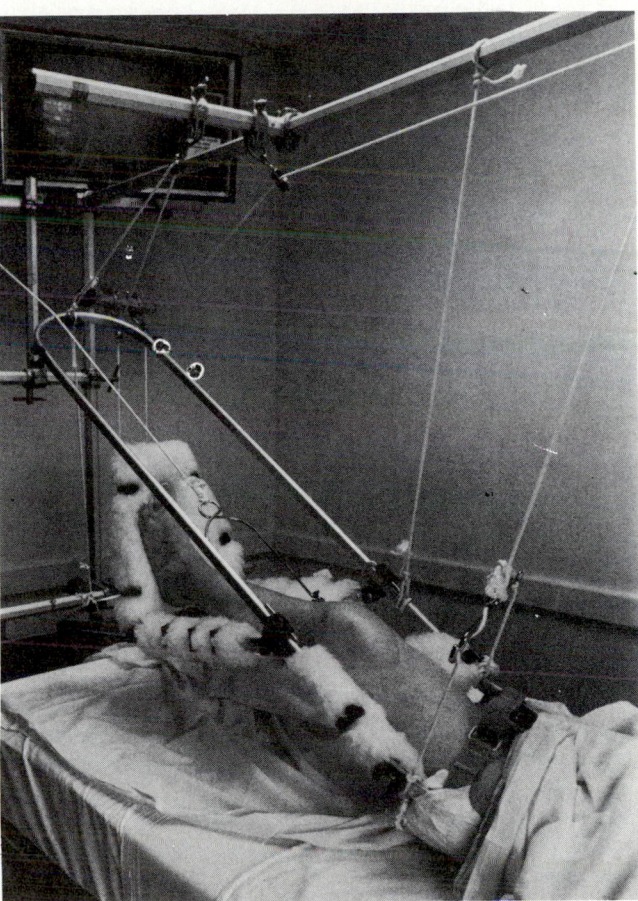

Fig. 22-31 Pearson attachment and Thomas splint.

Nursing care of the patient in traction

1. Patient education
   a. Explain traction in relation to fracture and physician's plan of treatment
   b. Explain amount of movement permitted and how to achieve it (for example, how trapeze can be used to assist with movement)
   c. Explain correct body positioning
2. Maintaining the traction
   a. Inspect traction apparatus frequently to assure that ropes are running straight and through the middle of the pulleys; that weights are hanging free; that bedclothes, the bed, or the frame and bars on the bed are not impinging on any part of the traction apparatus
   b. Check ropes frequently to be sure they are not frayed
   c. Avoid releasing weights from or altering the line of pull of the traction
   d. Avoid adding weight to the traction
   e. Check the position of the Thomas splint frequently; if the ring has slid away from the groin, readjust the splint to its proper position without releasing traction
   f. Avoid bumping into or jarring the bed or traction equipment
   g. Be sure weights are securely fastened to their ropes
   h. Avoid manipulation of pins
3. Skin care
   a. Encourage the patient to turn slightly from side to side and to lift up on the trapeze to relieve pressure on the skin of the sacrum and scapulae; have the patient lift up for routine skin care
   b. Avoid padding the ring of the Thomas splint as this will create dampness next to the skin. Bathe the skin beneath the ring, dry it thoroughly, and powder the skin lightly
   c. Inspect skin frequently to be sure it is not being rubbed, contused, or macerated by traction equipment; readjust splints or the extremity in the splint to free the skin from pressure
   d. Keep skin areas around pin sites clean and dry; direct care to pin sites (that is, cleansing with cotton applicators and hydrogen peroxide or alcohol) is *controversial,* so check with patient's physician to determine if pin care is to be done routinely and what method the physician prefers
4. Toileting
   a. Use a fracture pan with blanket roll or padding as support under the small of the back
   b. Protect the ring of the Thomas splint with waterproof material when female patients are using the bedpan

□ Other types of external immobilization

Other devices for external immobilization of fractures include the following:
1. Braces made of rigid plastic material
2. Plaster or plastic braces that incorporate metal struts attached to pins inserted into bone (for example, a halo brace) (Fig. 22-32)
3. Metal struts attached to pins inserted into bone (for example, the various types of Hoffman or Charnley external fixation devices) (Fig. 22-33).

Devices such as the Hoffman or Charnley may be used in conjunction with plaster or alone. All of these devices provide extremely rigid fixation while allowing the patient some degree of mobility. It is quite possible for the patient in a halo brace to ambulate. The patient with an external fixator on the lower leg can be out of bed in a wheelchair, or even ambulate without bearing weight on the affected leg.

Nursing care for patients in these devices is essentially the same as for patients in casts and/or skeletal traction, with the exception that they may be mobilized earlier.

■ Treatment of fractures with internal fixation devices

■ OPEN REDUCTION

Open surgical reduction of fractures has the advantage of allowing visualization of the fracture and surrounding tissues. It is particularly indicated when soft tissue is caught between bone fragments or when known damage to nerves or blood vessels exists. The disadvantages of internal fixation are that it requires anesthesia and it carries the risk of infection at the time of surgery. Internal fixation is carried out under the most vigorous aseptic conditions, and patients may receive a short course of prophylactic intravenous antibiotics after surgery.

The internal fixation devices available include the following:
1. Plates and nails such as the Neufeld nail and the Kuntschner nail (Fig. 22-34)
2. Transfixion screws (Fig. 22-35)
3. Intramedullary rods (Fig. 22-34, *B*)

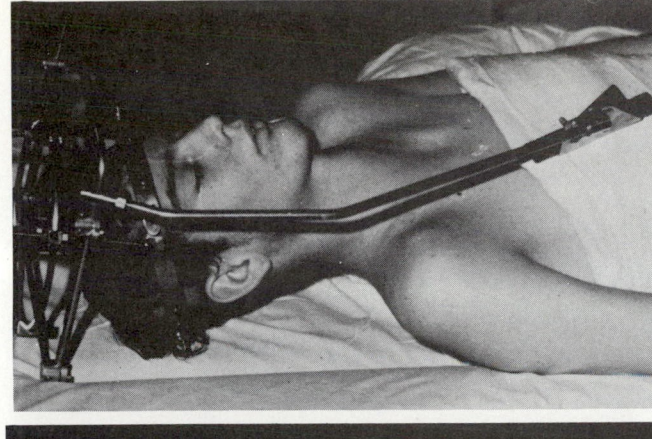

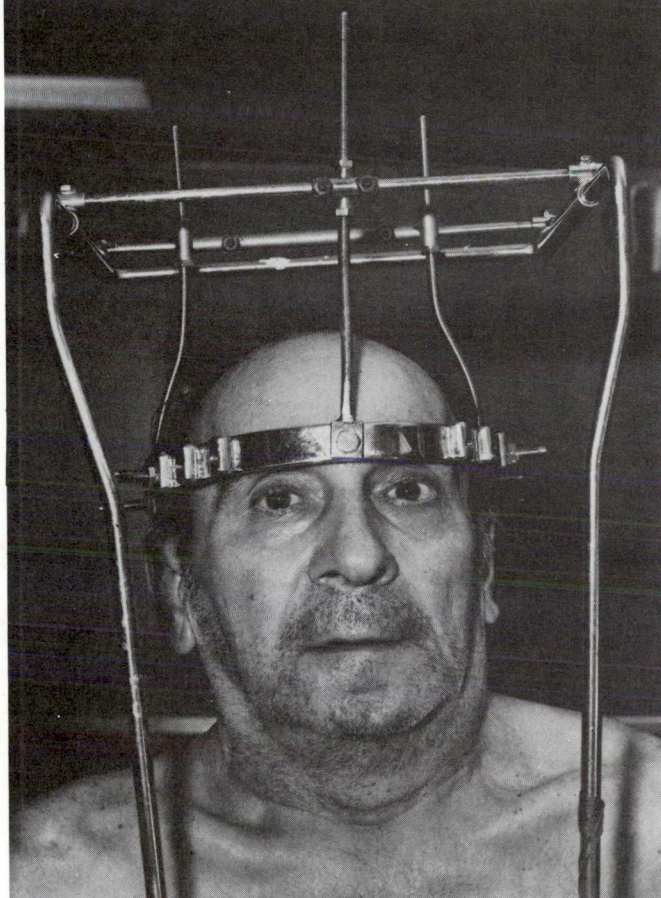

Fig. 22-32 **A,** Halo attached to body cast. Metal strut will be anchored firmly into body cast with additional plaster. **B,** Metal ring, or halo, that attaches to skull. (Courtesy Dr. Henry Bohlman, Cleveland, Ohio.)

4. Prosthetic implants such as the Austin Moore prosthesis (Fig. 22-36), which are used when proximal fragment of the fracture is jeopardized

It should also be noted that *bone grafts,* either *autograft* (the patient's own bone) or *allograft* (cadaver bone), may be used either in conjunction with internal fixation devices when excessive bone is lost at the fracture site, or alone, as in spine surgery. It should also be noted that fixation

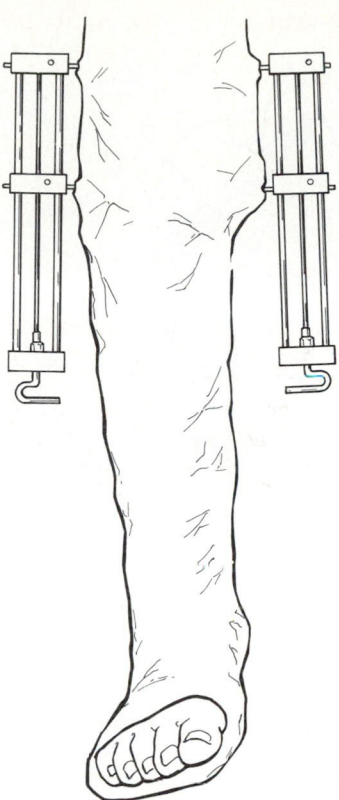

Fig. 22-33 Example of an external fixator, in this case a Charnley compression apparatus. Skeletal pins through bone above and below the area of fracture or repair attach to the external metal supports to maintain rigid fixation. This particular device is equipped with hand screws that allow the pins to be brought closer together, thus providing increased compression.

with internal devices does not preclude additional fixation with external devices (casts, braces, or traction), particularly in cases of very complicated fracture or multiple trauma.

In general, the major objective of care is to protect the fixation until healing takes place. Metal that can fatigue and break cannot be expected to substitute for intact bone. If the fixation device breaks, healing of the fracture will be disrupted. However, mobilization of patients who have had an internal fixation is usually much faster than for those who have had external fixation. Nursing interventions for patients with *internal fixation* include the following:

1. Patient education
   a. Prepare the patient for general anesthesia
   b. Explain the surgical procedure and general nursing care after surgery
   c. Postoperatively, explain the limits of motion and weight bearing on the affected part
2. Promoting mobility
   a. Determine, in consultation with the physician, the limits of motion and weight bearing permitted

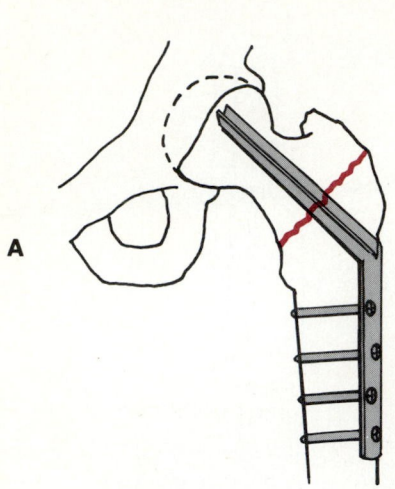
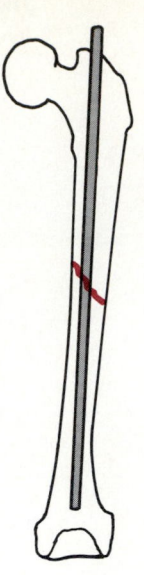

Fig. 22-34 **A,** Neufeld nail and screws, used in repair of intertrochanteric fracture. **B,** Kuntscher nail (intramedullary rod) used in repair of mid-shaft femoral fracture.

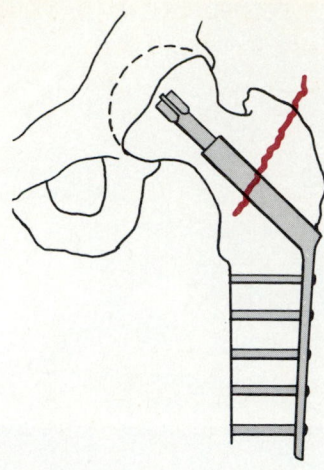

Fig. 22-35 Ken sliding nail used in repair of intertrochanteric fracture. Sliding nails will usually permit the patient to weight bear to some degree as they will "give" slightly when subjected to weight bearing forces without shifting their placement or "cutting out" (penetrating) through the femur.

b. Assist the patient with turning within the prescribed limits

c. Assist the patient in transferring and ambulating within the prescribed limits (may be up as early as first postoperative day)

3. Prevention of neurocirculatory problems
   a. Perform neurocirculatory checks every hour for the first 24 to 48 hours; notify physician of any change from preoperative status that may indicate pressure from *swelling, constriction of bandages, or damage to nerves or vessels* during surgery
   b. Maintain elevation of affected extremity

4. Maintenance of immobilization of fracture; considerations for care are the same as for patients in casts (p. 618) or traction (p. 624) if these devices are used

■ Fracture of the hip

Hip fractures are perhaps the most common fracture seen in the hospital. They occur more frequently in women than in men. Some factors explaining this follow:

1. Women have a wider pelvis with a tendency to coxa vara
2. Women have postmenopausal hormonal changes often accompanied by an increased incidence of osteoporosis
3. Women's life expectancy is greater than that of men

The following is a review of the hip joint for a clearer understanding of what is involved in a fracture in this area. The hip joint is a ball-and-socket joint formed by the acetabulum, a deep round cavity in the innominate bone, and the rounded upper portion of the femur. The upper part of the femur is composed of a head, neck, greater and lesser trochanter, and shaft. The distal part of the femur ends in two condyles. The head of the femur fits into the

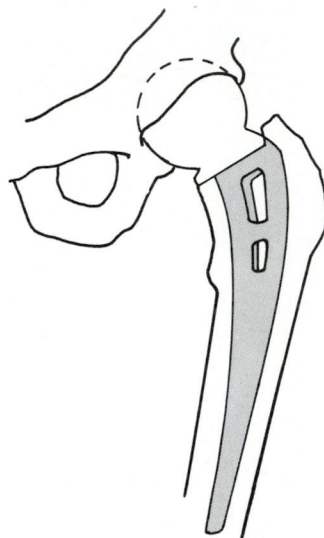

Fig. 22-36 Regular stem Austin Moore prosthesis, commonly used to replace the femoral head and neck in hip fractures when the vascular supply to the femoral head may eventually be compromised.

acetabulum. The hip joint is surrounded by a fibrous capsule, ligaments, and muscles. The greater trochanter serves as a point of insertion for the abductor muscles and short rotator muscles of the hip, whereas the lesser trochanter serves as a point of insertion for the iliopsoas muscle.

■ PATHOPHYSIOLOGY

Fractures of the hip may be classified into two general categories (Fig. 22-37):

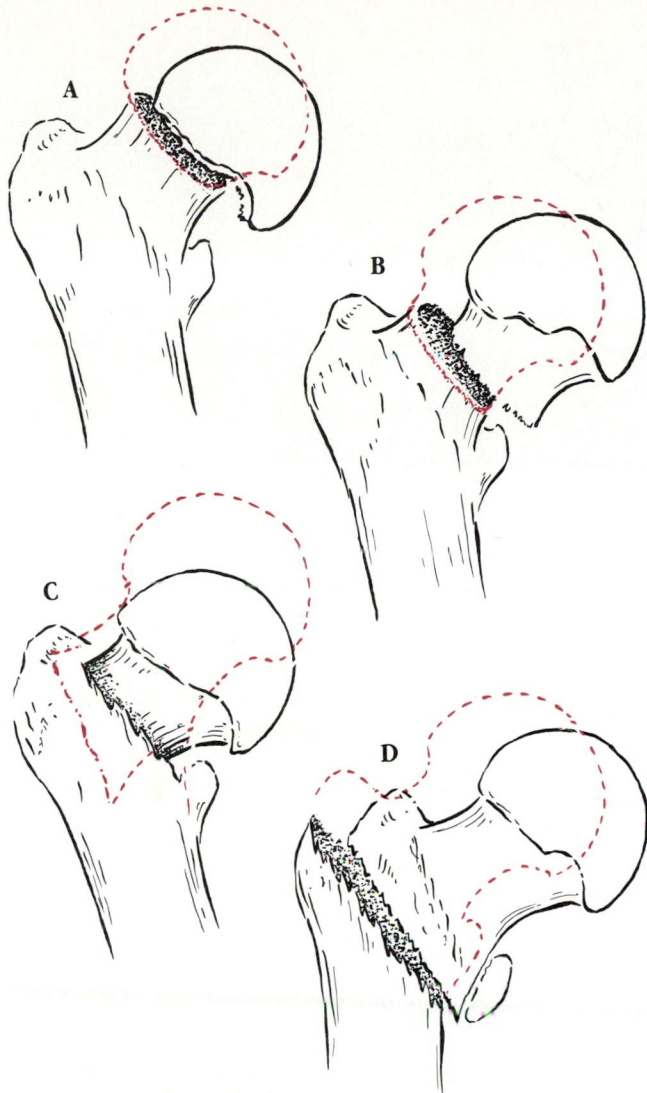

Fig. 22-37   Fractures of hip. **A,** Subcapital fracture. **B,** Transcervical fracture. **C,** Impacted fracture of base of neck. **D,** Intertrochanteric fracture.

1. *Intracapsular*—occurring within the hip joint and capsule; these include
   a. Subcapital fracture
   b. Transcervical fracture
   c. Basal neck fracture
2. *Extracapsular*—occurring outside the hip joint and capsule to an area 5 cm (2 in.) below the lesser trochanter; these are called *intertrochanteric* fractures

The blood supply to the femoral head is of paramount importance in fractures in or about the hip joint. The blood supply to the femoral head varies with age. The chief source of blood supply to the femoral head in adults is the posterior retinacular artery (Fig. 22-38). The nutrient and periosteal vessels of the femoral shaft extend into the trochanteric region and lower part of the neck.

Blood supply to the head of the femur comes up through

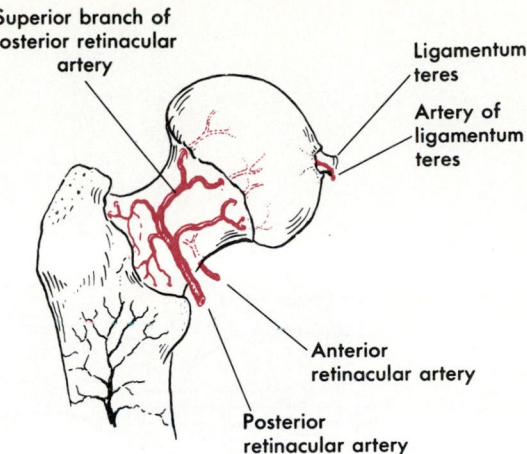

Fig. 22-38   Posterior view of the blood supply to head of femur.

the neck of the femur and is often disrupted in an intracapsular fracture. When blood supply is interrupted, death (*avascular necrosis*) of the femoral head may occur.

■ ASSESSMENT

Signs and symptoms of hip fracture include the following:
1. Severe pain at the fracture site
2. Inability to move the leg voluntarily
3. Shortening and external rotation of the leg
4. Other signs and symptoms consistent with signs and symptoms of any fracture

■ MEDICAL INTERVENTIONS

The choice of fixation device depends on the location of the fracture, the potential for avascular necrosis of the femoral head, and the personal preference of the surgeon. An *impacted intracapsular fracture without displacement* may be treated with bedrest alone. Common choices include the following:
1. Stable plate and screw fixation; implies non–weight-bearing status for 6 weeks to 3 months
2. Telescoping nail fixation; implies minimal to partial weight-bearing status for 6 weeks to 3 months
3. Prosthetic implant, usually Austin Moore prosthesis or Bi-Polar prosthesis, to replace femoral head and neck; implies some position restrictions for 2 weeks to 2 months and partial weight-bearing restrictions for up to 2 months
4. Closed reduction and external fixation if general medical condition precludes surgery

■ NURSING INTERVENTIONS

Nursing interventions should include those already noted for general care of patients with fractures with specific attention to interventions for persons with internal fixation. Special consideration should be taken in regard

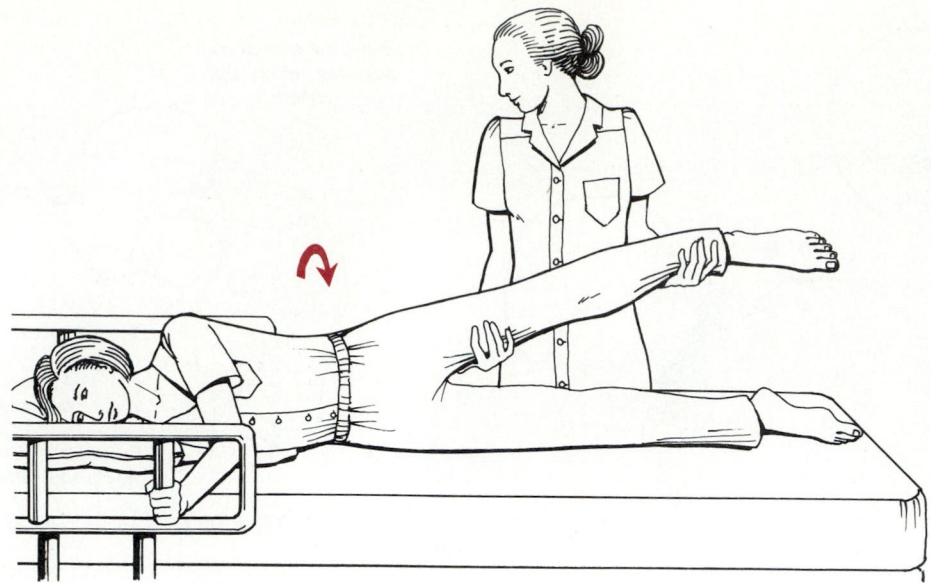

Fig. 22-39 Assisting patient in turning while maintaining abduction of the hip. Leg is supported at the thigh as well as just above the ankle to avoid putting undue stress on the hip.

to persons who have had a prosthetic implant in that, unless they have external fixation as well, there will be specific position restrictions. These include the following:

1. Avoidance of hip flexion beyond 60 degrees for approximately 10 days
2. Avoidance of hip flexion beyond 90 degrees from the tenth day to 2 months
3. Avoidance of adduction of the affected leg beyond midline for 2 months
4. Maintenance of partial weight bearing status for approximately 2 months

Suggestions for nursing care are:

1. Instruct the patient regarding the limits of motion to be observed
2. Avoid positioning the patient on the operative side in bed
3. Assist patient in maintaining abduction of hip (Figs. 22-39 and 22-40)

4. Carefully monitor the patient's position through transfer, standing, and sitting
5. Provide a chair with a firm, nonreclining seat and arms; elevate the sitting surface as necessary with pillows or foam cushions to keep the angle of the hip within the prescribed limits when the patient is sitting

In general, patients who have had *any* kind of internal fixation for fractured hip should avoid elevation of the operated leg when sitting in a chair as this puts excessive strain on the fixation device.

■ Fractures of the spine

Spinal, or vertebral, fractures occur as the result of falls, diving accidents, blows to the head or body by heavy objects, or with increasing frequency, as the result of osteoporosis and metastatic lesions of the spine. Spine fracture can occur at any age.

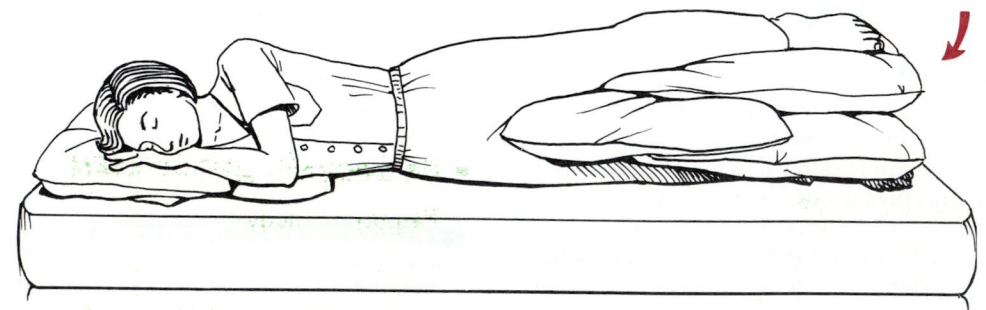

Fig. 22-40 Pillows are staggered in a wedge-shaped arrangement to maintain abduction of the hip.

PATHOPHYSIOLOGY

Vertebral fracture may occur with displacement or without displacement. If fracture fragments are displaced, they may place pressure on spinal nerves or injure the spinal cord itself. Such pressure will result in partial or complete dysfunction of the body parts innervated from the level of injury. Depending on the extent of injury to the nervous system structures, dysfunction may be permanent, partially permanent, or temporary. Fracture can occur at any level of the spine, from occiput through the sacrum.

ASSESSMENT

Signs and symptoms of vertebral fracture include the following:
1. Pain at the site of injury
2. Partial or complete loss of mobility or sensation below the level of injury
3. Evidence of fracture/fracture dislocation on routine x-ray film, myelography, and/or high resolution CAT scans

MEDICAL INTERVENTIONS

Objectives in management will be stabilization of the fracture, reduction of the fracture, and decompression (that is, removal of pressure from spinal nerves or the spinal cord).

☐ Immediate management

1. Immobilization of the patient with backboard; cervical collar
2. Immediate transport to a hospital

☐ Surgical management

1. Decompression of nerve structures through laminectomy (see Chapter 19) or appropriate reduction of the fracture and removal of fracture fragments
2. Reduction of the fracture through operative procedures, or in some cases, traction (for example, cervical traction through application of tongs to the skull)
3. Stabilization of the fracture with bone grafting and/or internal fixation devices such as Harrington, Jacobs, or Luque rods.
4. Maintenance of stabilization with external fixation devices such as casts, corsets, or braces as necessary
   NOTE: Compression fractures of the spine may be treated with bed rest until the patient's pain subsides, then the patient is gradually mobilized, sometimes with stabilization by a corset or brace.

NURSING INTERVENTIONS

Many of the nursing interventions required by the patient with spinal fracture are identical to those outlined for the patient with spinal cord injury in Chapter 19. Of special concern are interventions designed for the following purposes:

1. Maintaining the stability of the fracture fixation
   a. Pay strict attention to logrolling the patient for position changes (Fig. 22-41)
   b. Position the patient with pillows between the legs (see Fig. 22-40) and at the back when side lying to prevent strain on the back
   c. Observe proper technique when turning the patient on a Stryker frame or Foster bed, (CircOlectric beds are often contraindicated for patients with spine fracture as they load [put weight through] the spine when the patient is in the vertical position
   d. Avoid elevating the head of the bed beyond the prescribed level (usually only 30° and only on the physician's order)
   e. When the patient is to be mobilized, apply prescribed corsets or braces *before* getting the patient out of bed
2. Preventing neurocirculatory problems
   a. Perform neurocirculatory checks every hour in the first 24-48 hours after surgery; report decrease in neuromotor function to the physician
   b. Perform passive range of motion to involved extremities at least qid
   c. Encourage patient to actively and frequently move noninvolved extremities to the extent possible
3. Promoting comfort—in addition to usual comfort measures
   a. Reposition the patient frequently
   b. Wait a few minutes to ascertain the patient's comfort, because small adjustments may be necessary and may not be immediately recognized
4. Promoting psychologic comfort
   a. Recognize that the patient may have feelings of powerlessness, anger, and/or fear about the situation, particularly if there is neuromotor deficit
   b. Encourage the patient to express such feelings
   c. Encourage the patient to take advantage of psychologic and or social counseling where it is available
   d. If long-term rehabilitation is indicated, prepare the patient for care in a rehabilitation setting

Other nursing interventions are similar to those for any patient who has a fracture, including interventions for individuals in casts or traction.

Effects of immobilization

Persons who are immobilized after a fracture may have complications related to their immobility. An outline of the effects of immobilization on the various body systems, pathophysiology, nursing assessment, and nursing interventions follows.

CARDIOVASCULAR SYSTEM

☐ Pathophysiology

The common problems associated with the cardiovascular system are as follows:
1. Increased incidence of deep vein thrombosis (DVT) and pulmonary embolus (PE)
2. Increased work load on the heart

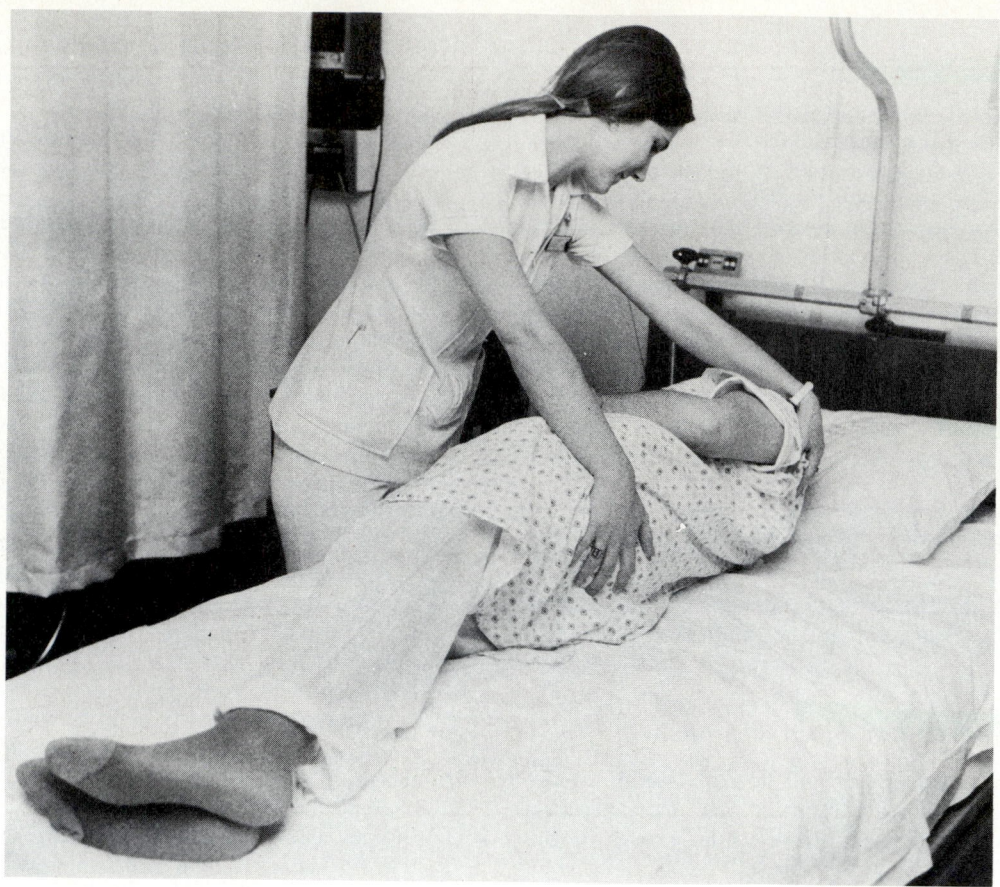

Fig. 22-41 Logrolling patient. Patient crosses arms over chest, holds legs in extension and feet together. Nurse supports patient at level of shoulders and buttocks.

Failure of the vessels in the legs to assume or maintain vasoconstriction results in the pooling of venous blood, decreased venous return, and diminished cardiac output.

☐ **Nursing assessment**

1. Palpate peripheral pulses.
2. Monitor blood pressure and heart rate and force.
3. Observe for signs and symptoms of DVT (pain in leg) and PE (chest pain, cough).

☐ **Nursing intervention**

1. Assist patient with active and passive range of motion and isometric exercises of extremities.
2. Reposition patient frequently within limitations as directed by physician's orders.

■ **RESPIRATORY SYSTEM**

☐ **Pathophysiology**

Decreased movement, decreased stimulus to cough, and decreased depth of ventilation all contribute to the pooling of secretions in the bronchi and bronchioles.

☐ **Nursing assessment**

1. Observe for inability to cough and raise secretions.
2. Auscultate for sounds of moisture in the chest.

☐ **Nursing interventions**

1. Reposition frequently within prescribed limitations.
2. Encourage active range of motion exercises of unaffected joints.
3. Prevent hypostatic pneumonia by having patient cough and deep breathe at regular intervals (at least every 2 hours).

■ **SKIN INTEGRITY**

☐ **Pathophysiology**

Loss of skin integrity (abrasions, decubitus ulcers) is caused by friction, pressure, or tissue layers sliding on each other. The process of restricted circulation and tissue ischemia is intensified by infection, trauma, obesity, sweating, and poor nutritional state.

☐ **Nursing assessment**

1. Observe for *areas of pressure* and *irritation,* as may occur from the plaster cast or traction equipment or from pressure on the sacrum, elbows, and heels.

2. Monitor *body temperature for elevation,* which may indicate infection.

☐ **Nursing interventions**

1. Prevent decubitus ulceration by keeping skin clean and dry, especially sacrum, elbows, and heels.
2. Turn the patient as physician permits to change points of pressure at frequent intervals. Some patients cannot be fully turned, for example, patients in traction. In this instance, other methods must be provided, such as the following:
   a. Flotation pads that distribute pressure equally over large skin areas.
   b. Air pressure mattresses that alternate pressures on the skin.
   c. Sheepskin pads that decrease friction, distribute pressure, and reduce moisture.
   d. Elbow and heel pads.
3. Special beds may be necessary to turn the patient from supine to prone positions.
   a. The Stryker or Foster frame permits movement in a horizontal direction to two positions—supine and prone.
   b. The CircOlectric bed permits more position changes. Movement is vertical and can be stopped at any angle while good body alignment is maintained.
4. If decubitus ulcer results, follow hospital policy for special nursing measures.

■ **GASTROINTESTINAL SYSTEM**

☐ **Pathophysiology**

Constipation is the most frequent complication of immobility. The change in normal dietary habits and fluid intake, lack of activity, and having to use a bedpan are contributing factors.

☐ **Nursing assessment**

1. Ask the patient about daily habits of evacuation.
2. Observe appetite and foods the patient selects.
3. Monitor the fluid intake.
4. Ask the patient what is normally taken for constipation.

☐ **Nursing interventions**

1. Encourage the patient to be as active as possible within the limitations (turning, moving).
2. Encourage fluid intake to 2500 to 3000 ml/day unless contraindicated.
3. Assist the patient in selecting foods that have roughage or fiber content.
4. Give stool-softening agents and suppositories as prescribed.

■ **URINARY SYSTEM**

☐ **Pathophysiology**

Increased urinary calcium from bone destruction, increased urinary pH (alkaline), increased citric acid (which causes the precipitation of calcium salts), stasis of urine in the bladder, and infection can all cause urinary problems.

☐ **Nursing assessment**

1. Observe quantity of fluid intake. Ask the patient about normal fluid intake.
2. Has the patient a history of urinary problems?
3. Ask the elderly male patient about urinary problems before admission. Some men will describe hesitancy and frequency because of an enlarged prostate gland.

☐ **Nursing interventions**

1. Encourage fluid intake.
2. Limit calcium intake (milk) to dietary orders.
3. Monitor urinary output and report difficulties to the physician. (Potential is present for bladder infection and formation of renal stones.)

■ **MUSCULOSKELETAL SYSTEM**

☐ **Pathophysiology**

Atrophy and weakness of the muscles will occur because of disuse. Bone growth (*osteoblastic*) and bone destruction (*osteoclastic*) activity is disrupted by immobility. The osteoclastic activity takes precedence, with the result that bone matrix is destroyed and calcium is released. The end result is *osteoporosis* and renal stones.

☐ **Nursing interventions**

1. Encourage active and isometric exercises of unaffected limbs.
2. Have patient demonstrate prescribed exercises.
3. Do passive exercises when patient is unable to do active movement.

☐ **Nursing assessment**

1. Ask patient to demonstrate prescribed exercises.
2. Ask patient to demonstrate movement of unaffected limbs.

■ **SUMMARY**

1. Bones have several functions. These include the following: (a) *supporting* body tissues *and* providing the *skeletal framework,* (b) *protecting* body organs, (c) *providing* for *movement,* (d) serving as a *storehouse* for mineral salts and, (e) providing for *hematopoesis.*
2. There are four types of bones; *long* bones (femur, humerus); *short* bones (carpals); *flat* bones (skull); and *irregular* bones (vertebrae).
3. Bursae are lined with synovial membrane and serve as cushions between moving parts.
4. Joints provide flexibility at places where bones come together.
5. There are 3 major classes of joints: (a) synarthroses, or immovable joints, (b) amphiarthroses, or slightly movable joints, and (c) diarthroses, or freely movable joints.

6. Joints permit the following movements:
   a. Flexion
   b. Extension
   c. Adduction
   d. Abduction
   e. Rotation
   f. Circumduction
   g. Special movements such as supination, pronation, inversion, eversion, and protraction.
7. Preventive health teaching requires knowledge about safety devices such as grab bars and safety arms around toilets that can be used by patients in their own homes.
8. Both heat and cold are prescribed in treating persons with musculoskeletal problems, and precautions must be observed with both.
9. Rheumatoid arthritis is more common in women than in men.
10. The cause of rheumatoid arthritis is unknown but immune mechanisms are considered to be a strong etiologic factor.
11. Persons with rheumatoid arthritis can benefit from being involved in a support group.
12. The major group of drugs used to treat rheumatoid arthritis are the nonsteroidal antiinflammatory agents.
13. Replacement arthroplasty can be used to replace a variety of joints. The most commonly replaced joints are the hip and the knee.
14. Restrictions on movement necessary to prevent dislocation of a prosthesis are prescribed by the surgeon and depend on the design of the prosthesis and method of insertion.
15. Persons with joint replacements are vulnerable to bacterial infections and must be taught to take prophylactic antibiotics before dental work, intrusive procedures, or surgery.
16. Persons with joint replacements will have a prescribed exercise program, which should be followed after discharge.
17. The course of systemic lupus erythematosus (SLE) is believed to be caused by an aberration of the immune system.
18. Polymyositis (dermatomyositis) is an inflammatory disorder of striated muscles of unknown causation.
19. Persons with polymyositis have exacerbations and remissions of their disease.
20. Ankylosing spondylitis causes the bones of the spine to grow together and the patient may have a "poker-back" deformity or scoliosis.
21. Persons with ankylosing spondylitis may have impaired gas exchange because of change in the chest cavity and decrease in chest excursion.
22. Bursitis refers to inflammation of a bursa. The shoulder joint is the most commonly affected.
23. Bursitis is usually caused by trauma, strain, or overuse of a joint. It is often treated by injection of corticosteroids into the affected joint capsule.
24. Carpal tunnel syndrome causes episodes of burning pain or tingling in the hands. Numbness (hypesthesia) affecting the thumb, index, and ring fingers occurs after prolonged flexion of the wrist, as in typing.
25. Degenerative joint disease (DJD) is also known as osteoarthritis, hypertrophic arthritis, osteoarthrosis, or senescent arthritis.
26. DJD is very common in persons between 50 and 70 years of age.
27. Prevention of DJD centers around (a) avoiding obesity, (b) avoiding repeated trauma to joints, and (c) protecting joints in occupations that put joints at risk.
28. Treatment of DJD includes agents to relieve pain, assistive devices to unload weight on weight-bearing joints, rest, exercise, and surgery including arthroplasty.
29. A herniated disk is an example of degenerative disease of the spine.
30. Sciatic pain is common in persons with a herniated disk.
31. Persons with a herniated disk can be treated conservatively with rest, heat, analgesics, muscle relaxants, and sometimes traction to relieve muscle spasm.
32. When conservative therapy is not successful in treating a herniated disk, surgery may be necessary to relieve compression on nerve roots.
33. Patients who have spinal surgery must be taught to do logrolling when turning from side to side.
34. Scoliosis causes a visible curvature of spine when the patient leans forward from the waist.
35. Corrective surgery to realign vertebrae and fusion are used to treat scoliosis when the curve of the spine exceeds 49 degrees.
36. Scoliosis surgery usually involves bone grafting and the use of instrumentation such as Harrington rods, Dwyer instrumentation, or Lugue instrumentation.
37. Gout is a metabolic disorder involving the joints.
38. Treatment of gout involves preventive therapy with uricosuric agents, which either enhance uric acid excretion (probenecid [Benemid]) or decrease uric acid formation (Allopurinol [Zyloprim]).
39. Fracture of bones is treated with immobility by splinting, bracing, casting, traction, or surgery.
40. A major complication of fracture is fat embolism, which can be life-threatening and is manifested by chest pain, pallor, dyspnea, prostration, confusion, and petechial hemorrhage of skin and conjunctivae.
41. Monitoring for neurocirculatory status in a patient with a cast includes palpation for warmth, observation of color, application of moderate pressure to nail bed, touching the injured part to test sensation, observing patient's ability to move body part distal to fracture, and questioning patient about pain or decreased or increased sensation distal to the cast.
42. A wet cast is handled with the flat of the hands or on a pillow to avoid indentations and pressure on underlying skin.
43. Because a plaster cast is porous, paint, varnish, or shellac should not be applied to the cast because this will interfere with circulation of air to the skin.
44. Traction is a mechanism that provides a steady pull on part or parts of the body.
45. Traction is used to reduce a fracture, maintain correct position of bone fragments during healing, immobilize

<h2 style="text-align:center;">Putting knowledge to practice</h2>

- Describe the anatomic structure of bones and the purposes of the skeletal system.
- Discuss the importance of the synovial joint and the composition of the joint.
- Review the range of motion through which a joint such as the shoulder would be exercised.
- Describe the complications that may occur from immobilization of the joint; the complications that may arise from total body immobilization.
- Select a patient who has a form of "arthritis." Outline a plan of care based on the patient's defined nursing problems.
- Outline the care of the patient immobilized in a spica hip cast.
- What precautions must be taken in the care of a patient in traction?
- What precautions must be taken in the care of a patient with a total hip replacement?

a limb while soft tissue healing takes place, overcome muscle spasm, stretch adhesions, and correct deformities.

46. Maintaining traction requires that ropes run straight and through pulleys, weights hang free, and nothing impinges on any part of the traction apparatus.

REFERENCES AND SELECTED READINGS

Contemporary

1. Agee, BL, and Herman, C: Cervical logrolling on a standard hospital bed, Am J Nurs 84:315-318, 1984.
2. *Allard, JL, and Dibble, SL: Scoliosis surgery: a look at Luque rods, Am J Nurs 84:609-611, 1984.
3. Anderson, LP: Carpal tunnel syndrome, Orthop Nurs 5(4):40-42, 1986.
4. Bailey, RW, and others (editors): The cervical spine, Philadelphia, 1983, JB Lippincott Co.
5. *Barden, RM: Osteonecrosis of the femoral head, Orthop Nurs 4(4):45-51, 1985.
6. Blaha, JD, and Pickett, JC (editors): Controversy on total knee arthroplasty, Clin Orthop Related Res 192S:2-112, 1985.
7. Blake, SA: Non-cemented femoral prostheses: intraoperative focus, Orthop Nurs 4(1):40-42, 1985.
8. Bluestone, R, (editor): Rheumatology, Boston, 1980, Houghton Mifflin Professional Publishers.
9. *Brunner, NA: Orthopedic nursing: a programmed approach, ed 4, St. Louis, 1983, The CV Mosby Co.
10. Burgess, S, and others: Systemic lupus erythematosus and renal insufficiency, ANNA J 13(3):168-171, 1986.
11. *Cave, L: Lowering the uncertainties of arthritis with a nurse-led support group, Orthop Nurs 3(5):39-42, 1984.
12. Cochran, S: Action stat! Open fracture, Nurs 87, 17(5):33, 1987.
13. *Cohen, S, and Viellion, G: Patient assessment: examining joints of the upper and lower extremities, Am J Nurs 81:763-768, 1981.
14. Dickinson, GR, and Gorman, TK: Adult arthritis: the assessment, Am J Nurs 83:262-265, 1983.
15. *Doheny, MO: Porous coated femoral prosthesis: concepts and care considerations, Orthop Nurs 4(1):43-45, 1985.
16. Doheny, MO, and Sedlak, CA: Body image considerations, for adult scoliosis patient having spinal fusion surgery, Orthop Nurs 6(6):18-22, 1987.
17. Edmonson, AS, and Crenshaw, AH (editors): Campbell's operative orthopaedics, ed 6, St. Louis, 1980, The CV Mosby Co.
18. Enis, JE: Total hip arthroplasty in the geriatric patient, Hosp Med (suppl.) 23(4):44-48, 1987.
19. Farrell, J: Illustrated guide to orthopedic nursing, ed 2, Philadelphia, 1982, JB Lippincott Co.
20. *Farrell, J: Orthopedic pain. What does it mean? Am J Nurs 84:466-469, 1984.
21. Falkenburg, SA: Choosing hand splints to aid carpal tunnel syndrome recovery, Occup Health Saf 56(5):60-64, 1987.
22. Flatt, AE: Care of the arthritic hand, ed 4, St. Louis, 1982, The CV Mosby Co.
23. Fractured femur with internal fixation (pictorial), Orthop Nurs 6(2):38-41, 1987.
24. Gardine, A: Not another fractured hip, Can Nurse 82(6):34-36, 1986.
25. *Hausman, KL, and others: Percutaneous lateral disectomy: another approach for the treatment of a herniated nucleus pulposus, Orthop Nurs 3(6):9-17, 1984.
26. Hennig, LM, and others: Keeping up on arthritis meds, RN 49(2):32-38, 1986.
27. *Hilt, NE (editor): Assessment and fracture management of the lower extremities, a monograph, 1984, Anthony J Jannetti, Inc.
28. Hines, NA, and Bates, MS: Discharging the patient in skeletal traction, Orthop Nurs 6(4):21-24, 1987.
29. Ignatavicius, DO: Meeting the psychosocial needs of patients with rheumatoid arthritis, Orthop Nurs 6(3):16-21, 1987.
30. Ivey, M, and Clark, R: Arthroscopic debridement of the knee for septic arthritis, Clin Orthop Related Res 199:201-206, 1985.
31. *Johnson, C (editor): Symposium on orthopedic nursing, Nurs Clin North Am 16(4):707-766, 1981.
32. Karlin, L: Musculoskeletal trauma, Emerg Care Q 3(1):57-60, 1987.

*References preceded by an asterisk are particularly well suited for student reading.

33. *Karn, MA, and Crawford, AH: Postoperative nursing management of the patient following posterior spinal fusion, Orthop Nurs 3(2):21-25, 1984.

34. *Koerner, ME, and Dickenson, GR: Adult arthritis, Am J Nurs 83:253-278, 1983.

35. Koffler, D: Immunology of systemic lupus erythematosus and related rheumatic diseases, Clin Symp 39(2):2-36, 1987.

36. *Kushner, I, and others (editors): Understanding arthritis, New York, 1984, Arthritis Foundation, Charles Scribner's Sons.

37. Lambert, VA, and others: Coping with rheumatoid arthritis, Nurs Clin North Am 22:551-558, 1987.

38. *Ledo, KM: Diagnostic overview: ankylosing spondylitis, Orthop Nurs 2(6):39-40, 1983.

39. *Levy, RN, and others: Progress in arthritis surgery: with special reference to current status of total joint arthroplasty, Clin Orthop Related Res 200:299-321, 1985.

40. *Liddel, DR: An in-depth look at osteoporosis, Orthop Nurs 4(3):23-28, 1985.

41. Lin, P (editor): Posterior lumbar interbody fusion, Clin Orthop Related Res 193:2-132, 1985.

42. McCarty, DJ (editor): Arthritis and allied conditions: a textbook of rheumatology, ed 10, Philadelphia, 1984, Lea & Febiger.

43. *McFarland, MB: Encircling cast drainage: is it valuable? Orthop Nurs 3(2):41-43, 1984.

44. Maher, AB: Early assessment and management of musculoskeletal injuries, Nurs Clin North Am 21:717-727, 1986.

45. Malasanos, L, and others: Health assessment, ed 3, St. Louis, 1985, The CV Mosby Co.

46. *Marchette, L, and Marchette B: Back injury: a preventable occupational hazard, Orthop Nurs 4(6):25-29, 1985.

47. Moskowitz, RW: Clinical rheumatology: a problem oriented approach to diagnosis and management, ed 2, Philadelphia, 1982, Lea & Febiger.

48. Moskowitz, RW, and others: Osteoarthritis: diagnosis and management, Philadelphia, 1984, WB Saunders Co.

49. *Mourad, L: Nursing care of adults with orthopedic conditions, New York, 1980, John Wiley & Sons, Inc.

50. *Nordby, EJ: A comparison of discectomy and chemonucleolysis, Clin Orthop Related Res 200:279-283, 1985.

51. Osborne, LJ, and DiGiacomo, I: Traction: a review with nursing diagnoses and interventions, Orthop Nurs 6(4):13-18, 1987.

52. *Panush, RS: Controversial arthritis remedies, Bulletin on the Rheumatic Diseases 34(5):1-10, 1984.

53. *Pigg, J, Driscoll, P, and Caniff, R: Rheumatology nursing: a problem-oriented approach, New York, 1985, John Wiley & Sons, Inc.

54. *Phillips, KF: The use of gold therapy with rheumatoid arthritis, Orthop Nurs 2(4):31-34, 1983.

55. Rodman, G, and Schumacher, H: Primer on the rheumatic diseases, ed 8, Atlanta, Arthritis Foundation, 1983.

56. Rodts, MF: Surgical intervention for adult scoliosis, Orthop Nurs 6(6):11-17, 1987.

57. *Salmond, SW: Trauma and fractures: meeting your patient's nutritional needs, Orthop Nurs 3(4):27-33, 1984.

58. Schoen, DC: Assessing a fractured hip, Nurs 87, 17(3):97-98, 1987.

59. *Spindler, CE: Audiovisual preoperative teaching for the total hip patient, Orthop Nurs 3(1):30-40, 1984.

60. *Sproles, KJ: Nursing care of skeletal pins: a closer look, Orthop Nurs 4(1):11-20, 1985.

61. *Strang, EL, and Johns, JL: Nursing care of the patient treated with continuous passive motion following total knee arthroplasty, Orthop Nurs 3(6):27-32, 1984.

62. *Swinson, DR, and Swinburn, WR: Rheumatology, New York, 1980, John Wiley & Sons.

63. *Walsh, CR, and Wirth, CR: Total knee arthroplasty: biomechanical and nursing considerations, Orthop Nurs 4(1):29-34, 1985.

64. *Wittert, D, and Barden, R: Deep vein thrombosis, pulmonary embolism, and prophylaxis in the orthopaedic patient, Orthop Nurs 4(4):27-37, 1985.

Classic

65. *Olson, EV (editor): The hazards of immobility, Am J Nurs 67:780-797, 1967.

UNIT VI
Gas Transport Problems

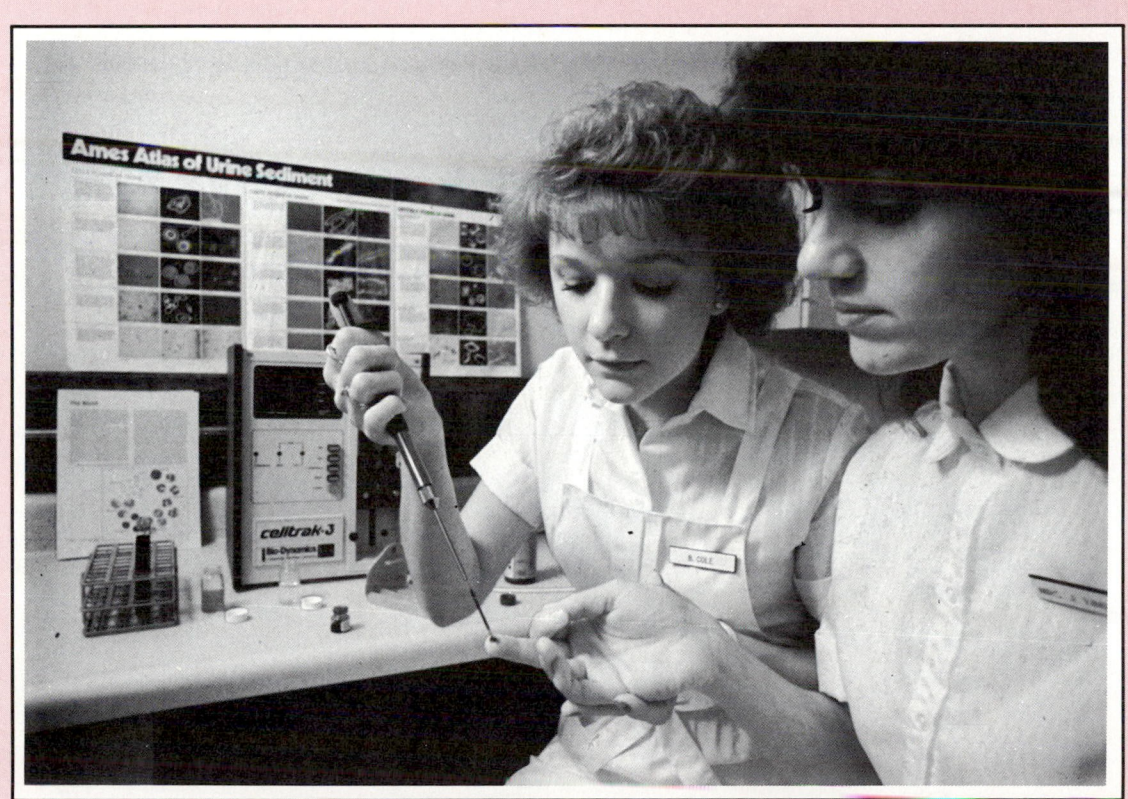

23

The Patient with Nose and Throat Problems

WILMA J. PHIPPS and LINDA ANNE BROSEMAN

CHAPTER OBJECTIVES

After studying this chapter, the student should be able to:

- Describe pathophysiologic bases of upper respiratory infections and therapeutic modalities.
- Describe nursing care of persons having nose and sinus surgery and tonsillectomy.
- Describe etiology and interventions for nosebleeds.
- Describe etiology and symptoms of cancer of the larynx and postoperative care following surgery.

Disorders of the nose and throat are very common, and nurses in particular are often asked to give advice about these problems. To be effective, nurses need a basic understanding of the structure and function of the organs of the upper airway, as well as knowledge of the medical and nursing regimens for problems affecting the upper airway.

ANATOMY AND PHYSIOLOGY

Nose and sinuses

The nose is supported by the nasal bones, the nasal processes of the maxillary bones, the cartilaginous and bony parts of the septum, and the upper and lower nasal cartilages. The septum, which divides the nares, is rarely straight in adults because at some time it has been injured.

The nasal cavities are located between the roof of the mouth and the frontal, ethmoid, and sphenoid bones. Three projections, which are lined with mucous membrane and called the *turbinate bones*, are located on the lateral walls of each nasal cavity (Fig. 23-1). Their purpose is to increase the mucous membrane surface over which air passes as it travels to the nasopharynx, thus allowing for precipitation of inhaled particles and warming and moistening the inhaled air.

The mucous membrane posterior to the vestibule (anterior part) of the nose contains cilia that beat in a constant wavelike motion to carry mucus into the nasopharynx. Trapped in the mucus are bacteria, dust, and other foreign matter entering the nose. The olfactory epithelium is located in a small area superiorly and provides the end organ of smell.

There are four sets of paranasal sinuses located on either side of the head (Fig. 23-2). These sinuses are air-filled spaces in the skull that serve to lighten the head. They drain into the nasal cavities through openings behind the turbinates. The maxillary sinuses are the largest and most accessible. The sinuses are lined with mucous membrane continuous with that of the nose.

Upper throat: pharynx and tonsils

The pharynx is the space behind the oral cavity that extends from the base of the skull to the larynx. The pharynx can be considered in three parts: the nasopharynx, the oropharynx, and the hypopharynx (Fig. 23-3). It is lined with mucous membrane.

The adenoids are located in the nasopharynx, the palatine tonsils anterior to the oropharynx, and the lingual tonsils in the hypopharynx. The adenoids and tonsils are lymphoid tissue that help to filter the circulating lymph of bacteria or other foreign matter that penetrate the body, especially by way of the nose or mouth.

Lower throat: larynx and hypopharynx

The larynx forms the upper extremity of the trachea. The framework of the larynx is made up of several cartilages held together by muscle and ligaments (Fig. 23-4). The cartilaginous framework protects the vocal cords and affords a stiffness that permits an airway. The thyroid cartilage, the "Adam's apple," is the largest cartilaginous

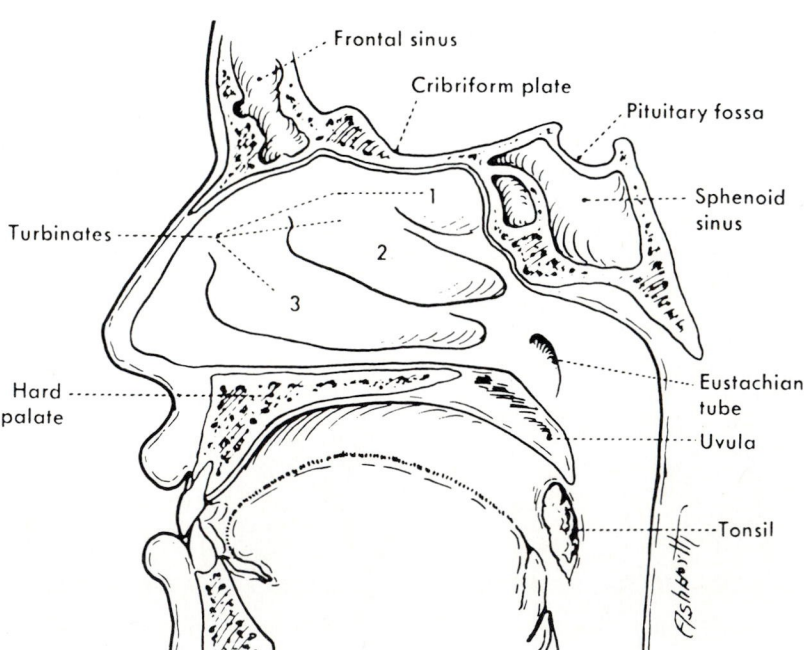

Fig. 23-1 Turbinates of nose: *1,* superior; *2,* middle; *3,* inferior. (From DeWeese, DD and Saunders, WH: Textbook of otolaryngology, ed 7, St. Louis, 1987, The CV Mosby Co.)

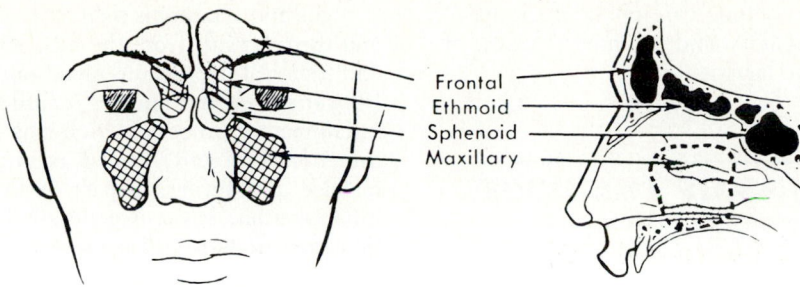

Fig. 23-2   Location of sinuses.

Frontal
Ethmoid
Sphenoid
Maxillary

element in the larynx and protects the inner structures. The hyoid bone forms an attachment for the larynx and tongue. The larynx is lined with mucosa continuous with that of the hypopharynx and trachea. The vagus nerve innervates the larynx.

The chief function of the larynx is to serve as an airway between the pharynx and trachea. A leaf-shaped lid of fibrocartilage (epiglottis) protects the glottis by covering the entrance to the larynx during swallowing to prevent aspiration of food or fluids. The closing of the glottis also allows for an increase of intrathoracic pressure, which is needed, for example, in coughing or lifting. This increased pressure increases the use of the muscles of the shoulder and thorax.

In addition, a most important function of the larynx is phonation. The larynx creates sounds as a result of vocal cord vibrations that are formed into speech patterns by the movement of the pharynx, palate, tongue, teeth, and lips.

Major health problems of the nose and throat

Most disorders of the nose and throat may be categorized as inflammatory, obstructive, or malignant as follows:
1. Inflammatory disorders include rhinitis, sinusitis, pharyngitis, tonsillitis, peritonsillar abscess, and laryngitis.
2. Obstructive disorders include a deviated septum, hypertrophy of the turbinates, nasal polyps, foreign bodies, fractures (nasal, maxillary, zygomatic), and epistaxis.

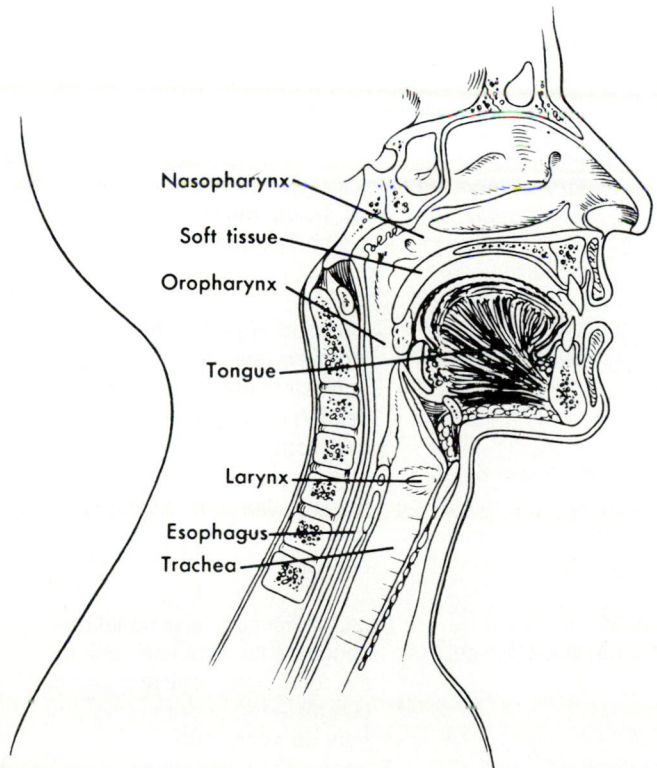

Nasopharynx
Soft tissue
Oropharynx
Tongue
Larynx
Esophagus
Trachea

Fig. 23-3   Sagittal section of head showing pharynx and larynx.

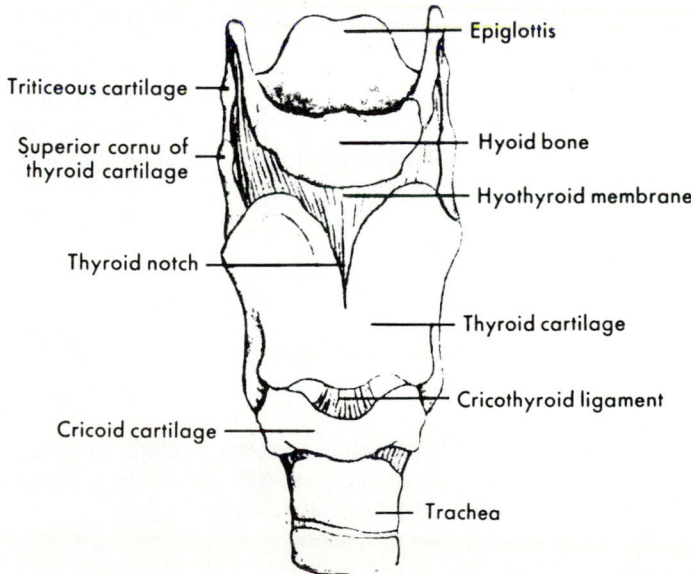

Triticeous cartilage
Superior cornu of thyroid cartilage
Thyroid notch
Cricoid cartilage
Epiglottis
Hyoid bone
Hyothyroid membrane
Thyroid cartilage
Cricothyroid ligament
Trachea

Fig. 23-4   Anterior aspect of larynx. (From Francis, CC: Introduction to human anatomy, ed 6, St. Louis, 1975, The CV Mosby Co.)

3. Malignant disorders include carcinoma of the naso-pharynx, of the maxillary and ethmoid sinuses, of the tonsil, and of the larynx.

■ INFLAMMATIONS OF THE NOSE AND THROAT

Inflammations may develop in the nose and sinuses (Table 23-1). A more detailed discussion of these conditions follows.

■ Pathophysiology

Inflammations of the upper airway structures may result from numerous viruses and bacteria. Many filtrable viruses (such as the more than 30 identified rhinoviruses, adeno-virus, echovirus, influenza and parainfluenza viruses, and coxsackievirus) may serve as etiologic agents of inflammations. Bacteria include primarily streptococci, staphylococci, and pneumococci.

Inflammations of the upper respiratory tract, primarily in the nose and sinuses, are often an allergic reaction to pollens of grasses and flowers, dust, animal dander, wool, and certain foods. Maxillary sinusitis may also occur as an extension of infection from abscessed teeth and tooth extraction, because the apices of many of the upper teeth roots are in close contact with the mucosal lining of the sinus.

Signs and symptoms seen with inflammations of the nose and throat result from the inflammatory process. Redness and edema of the mucous membrane occur early. Discharge from the nose and sinuses include fluid exudate from the inflammatory process (which may be serous or purulent if infection is present), as well as mucous secretions. General malaise and fever are part of the systemic response to inflammation. Fever is generally low in acute viral infections and higher with acute bacterial infections.

■ INFECTIONS OF THE NOSE AND SINUSES

■ Infections of external tissues around the nose

The skin around the external nose is easily irritated during acute attacks of rhinitis or sinusitis. Furunculosis (boils) and cellulitis (see Chapter 39) occasionally develop. Infections around the nose are extremely dangerous because the venous blood supply from this area drains directly into the cerebral venous sinuses. Septicemia, therefore, can occur easily, and for this reason no pimple or lesion in the area should ever be squeezed or "picked." Hot packs may be used. If any infection in or around the nose persists or shows even a slight tendency to spread or increase in severity, a physician should be consulted.

Table 23-1 Infections of the nose and sinuses

Disorder	Etiology	Signs and symptoms	Medical therapy
Rhinitis (coryza, common cold)	Filterable virus	Initial: dryness of mucous membranes, chills, general malaise 12-24 hrs: profuse watery discharge, sneezing, tearing of eyes	Rest, fluids, moist inhalations, antihistamines and decongestants
Allergic rhinitis (hay fever)	Pollens or other allergens	Sneezing, nasal obstruction, watery nasal discharge, frontal headache, itching of eyes and nose	Separation of person from sensitizing allergens, desensitization, antihistamines; submucous resection or polypectomy may be necessary
Chronic rhinitis	Follows repeated acute infections, allergy, or vasomotor rhinitis	Stuffiness and pressure in the nose; nasal discharge, which may be serous, mucopurulent or purulent; polyp formation; frontal headache; vertigo; sneezing	Antibiotics, avoidance of the offending allergens, antihistamines, polypectomy may be necessary
Sinusitis			
Acute	Streptococcus, staphylococcus, pneumococcus, *Haemophilus influenzae*	Constant severe headache, pain over sinuses, orbital edema, nasal discharge, fever	Rest, analgesics, oral nasal decongestants, systemic antibiotics, local heat, topical nasal decongestants; antrum puncture may be necessary
Chronic	Same as above	Chronic purulent nasal discharge, dull sinus headache, loss of ability to smell	Surgery; sinus irrigations

Correct administration of nose drops

1. Wash hands.
2. Assume a position that will facilitate flow of medication.
   a. Sit in chair and tip head well backward, or
   b. Lie down with head extended over edge of bed, or
   c. Lie down with pillow under shoulders and head tipped backward
3. Turn head to side that will receive the drops.
4. Place no more than 3 drops of solution into each nostril at one time (unless otherwise prescribed).
5. Remain in position with head tilted backward for 5 minutes to permit solution to reach posterior nares.
6. If marked congestion is still present 10 minutes after nose drop insertion, another drop or two of solution may be administered (constriction of nasal membranes from first insertion may facilitate additional drops reaching posterior nares).

■ RHINITIS

Rhinitis refers to inflammation of the mucous membrane of the nose. It may be acute or chronic.

Acute rhinitis (coryza, common cold) is an inflammatory condition of the mucous membranes of the nose and accessory sinuses caused by a filtrable virus. It affects almost everyone at some time and occurs most often in the winter, with additional high incidence in early fall and spring. Some of the known causes of the common cold are more than 30 identified rhinoviruses, adenoviruses, echoviruses, influenza and parainfluenza viruses, and coxsackievirus. The common cold is spread by droplet nuclei from sneezing and the condition is contagious for the first 2 to 3 days. Secondary invasion by bacteria may complicate the cold, possibly causing pneumonia, bronchitis, sinusitis, and otitis media.

Allergic rhinitis (hay fever) can be acute and seasonal when caused by the pollens of grasses and flowers, or it may be chronic and perennial when associated with numerous allergens, such as house dust, animal dander, wool, and certain foods.

Chronic rhinitis is a chronic inflammation of the mucous membrane caused by repeated acute infections, by an allergy, or by vasomotor rhinitis. The cause of vasomotor rhinitis is unclear, but this condition may result from an instability of the autonomic nervous system caused by stress, tension, or some endocrine disorder. Often it is mistaken for nasal allergy, but the allergen cannot be identified. Formation of nasal mucus is increased, leading to a runny nose. Rhinitis can also be caused by the overuse of nose drops *(rhinitis medicamentosa);* a rebound phenomenon occurs after the immediate effect of the nose drops with the return to congestion. Discontinuing use of the nose drops usually clears up this condition within a week or two. The correct administration of nose drops is listed in the box at left.

In all forms of rhinitis sneezing, nasal discharge with nasal obstruction, and headache are present, but the form of these symptoms varies with the type of rhinitis (Table 23-2). Acute rhinitis also includes signs of acute inflammation (early chilliness followed by "feverishness" and malaise). A painful throat is not always associated with a cold. However, the pharynx may feel sore because of early dryness followed by irritation from postnasal drainage. If uncomplicated, the cold is usually self-limiting and lasts for about 1 week.

In chronic rhinitis, acute symptoms are absent. The chief complaint is nasal obstruction accompanied by a feeling of stuffiness and pressure in the nose. Polyp formation (p. 648) may occur and vertigo may be present.

■ SINUSITIS

The sinuses are air-filled cavities lined with mucous membrane. Any inflammation of the mucous membranes of the sinuses is called *sinusitis*. Sinusitis is a frequent disorder, although it is less common since the advent of antibiotics. Often patients who complain of sinusitis do not have sinus infection but some other disorder. When an otolaryngologist refers to sinusitis, a bacterial invasion of the mucous membrane is implied. Sinusitis may be acute or chronic.

The most common cause of *acute sinusitis* is the obstruction of the paranasal sinuses that blocks the egress of secretions from the sinuses. These secretions become infected, giving rise to acute sinusitis. Sinusitis may follow acute or allergic rhinitis or other respiratory diseases such

Table 23-2 Symptoms of rhinitis

	Acute rhinitis	Allergic rhinitis	Chronic rhinitis
Nasal discharge	Initially watery, then mucoid	Thin, watery	Serous, mucopurulent, or purulent
Eyes	Tearing during early phase	Tearing, itching	No tearing
Turbinates	Edematous	Pale, edematous, mucoid	Enlarged
Nasal polyps	No	Yes	Yes
Headache	Generalized	Frontal	Frontal

Location of pain with sinusitis

Sinus	Pain location
Maxillary	Under eyes, front of face, dental, or eyes
Frontal	Over eyebrow
Ethmoid	Periorbital and frontal
Sphenoid	Retroorbital, occipital, or top of head

---

as pneumonia or influenza. Streptococci, staphylococci, pneumococci, or anaerobic bacteria are the infecting organisms. Abscessed teeth or tooth extraction may cause acute maxillary sinusitis because the apices of many of the upper teeth roots are in close contact with the mucosal lining of these sinuses. In *chronic sinusitis,* the mucous lining of the sinus becomes thickened from prolonged or repeated irritation and infection.

☐ Acute sinusitis

The patient with acute sinusitis often complains of a constant, severe headache or of pain over the infected sinus (see the box above). The patient may have the sensation of "pain in the bone" when even slight pressure is applied over the affected sinus. Occasionally there may be notice-

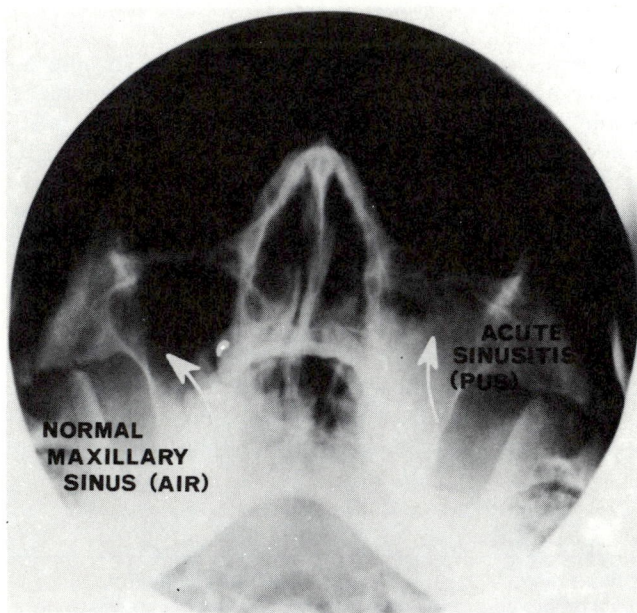

Fig. 23-5 Roentgenogram of maxillary sinus showing normal sinus on left and acute sinusitis on right. (From Saunders, WH, and others: Nursing care in eye, ear, nose, and throat disorders, ed 4, St. Louis, 1979, The CV Mosby Co.)

able swelling over the maxillary or frontal sinuses, or there may be orbital edema. Nausea, purulent nasal discharge, low-grade fever, and general malaise may be present. Fever is proportional to the amount of obstruction present and the virulence of the infecting organism. If the sinus is abscessed, the temperature may be as high as 40° C (104° F). The throat may be sore because of irritation from postnasal drainage. Complications of severe untreated sinusitis include osteomyelitis in the adjacent bone, abscesses that may involve the brain, venous sinus thrombosis, orbital cellulitis, orbital abscess, and septicemia.

☐ Chronic sinusitis

The patient with chronic sinusitis usually has a chronic purulent nasal discharge, a chronic cough caused by postnasal drainage, and a chronic dull sinus headache that characteristically starts during the late morning hours and gradually subsides during the evening hours. The varied positions and movements of the head during the day help to drain the sinuses and to diminish the headache. *Anosmia* (loss of smell) or *parosmia* (a perverted sense of smell) may be a result of the nasal blockage.

▊ ASSESSMENT

☐ Subjective data

1. Obstruction of nares
   a. History of mouth breathing—time of day or night when it occurs, duration and frequency
   b. History of nasal surgery or injury to nose
   c. Use of nasal drops or spray—type, amount, frequency, and duration of use
2. Nasal discharge
   a. Color, amount, and consistency of discharge
   b. Nasal bleeding (epistaxis)—one or both nares
   c. Presence of nasal crusting or pain
3. History of sinusitis
   a. Headaches—location and severity
   b. Relationship of sinusitis to certain seasons or types of weather
4. Other general symptoms such as malaise

☐ Objective data

1. Fever and drainage (serous, mucopurulent, purulent)
2. Polyps (pale, soft, edematous out-pouching of nasal or sinal mucosa)—may be present and are usually bilateral in inflammations of the nose and sinuses
3. Redness and edema of mucous membrane

☐ Diagnostic tests

1. Culture of nose or throat for causative organism
2. Roentgenograms of sinuses are used to determine the presence and extent of the disease and whether there is involvement of the bony walls (Fig. 23-5). When an infection is present, the film appears cloudy. In persons with chronic sinusitis the sinus roentgenograms demonstrate thickening of the mucous membrane and diffuse cloudiness.

➡ DATA ANALYSIS: NURSING DIAGNOSES

Nursing diagnoses are determined from assessment of patient data. Possible nursing diagnoses for the person with rhinitis or sinusitis may include, but are not limited to, the following:

Diagnostic title	Possible etiologies
Knowledge deficit	Lack of exposure to information
Pain: headache, throat, sinus	Inflammation in nose or sinuses

▦ PLANNING: EXPECTED PATIENT OUTCOMES

Expected patient outcomes for the person with rhinitis or sinusitis may include, but are not limited to, the following:

1. Symptoms (headache and nasal stuffiness) are improved.
2. Patient can prevent further attack by doing the following:
   a. Avoiding crowds during high-incidence periods of infection
   b. Avoiding allergens
   c. Getting adequate rest
   d. Eating a well-balanced diet
3. Patient demonstrates the correct use of nose drops.
4. Patient can state how to use prescribed medications and what over-the-counter medications should be avoided.
5. Patient states plans for follow-up care.

▦ IMPLEMENTATION

☐ Medical interventions

Management of acute sinusitis is directed at pain relief and establishment of sinus drainage. Aspirin is usually avoided as a pain medication because it may be associated with nasal polyposis. Acetaminophen is a good substitute for aspirin, and occasionally codeine or another narcotic may be necessary to relieve pain.

Medications include systemic broad-spectrum antibiotics and nasal decongestants (for example, phenylephrine [Neo-Synephrine]) by nose drops or by spray inhalation. Forced air pressure of the atomizer breaks the large droplets of fluid into a fine mist. If a nebulizer is used, the solution is usually forced through the apparatus by oxygen or compressed air. Antibiotics are less effective for chronic sinus infections than for acute sinus infections.

Antral irrigation is used when conservative methods have failed to resolve a maxillary sinusitis. Anesthesia may be obtained with 4% xylocaine (topical), 1% Neo-Synephrine with epinephrine, or 4% cocaine. After insertion of a trocar through the nose into the sinus, a 20 ml syringe is used to withdraw any pus or fluid that may be present. If no pus is found, sterile saline is injected, withdrawn, and sent for culture and sensitivity (and cytology if indicated).

Antral irrigations are sometimes used to ensure better sinus drainage in persons with chronic sinusitis.

☐ Nursing interventions
☐ *Assisting with the achievement of therapeutic goals*

1. Give medications as prescribed (antihistamines, decongestants, antibiotics).
2. Provide an allergen-free environment.

☐ *Assisting with comfort and ADL*

1. Apply local heat as prescribed.
2. Provide moist inhalations as prescribed.

☐ *Counseling and teaching*

1. Avoid factors that contribute to the sinusitis.
   a. Avoid chilling and cold, damp atmospheres.
   b. Avoid air conditioning when outside air is warm and moist, if this precipitates sinus irritation.
   c. Avoid smoking (further irritates damaged mucous membranes).
   d. Avoid fatigue.
   e. Try to avoid upper respiratory tract infections.
   f. Protect nose during swimming; avoid diving.
   g. Inform dentist of chronic sinus condition before tooth extraction.
2. If allergens are a contributing factor, prepare an environmentally controlled bedroom (Chapter 38).
3. Use acetaminophen rather than aspirin for pain relief; apply moist heat over sinus.
4. During an acute sinus infection, get additional rest and drink 2 to 3 L fluids per day.
5. Take antibiotic for prescribed time period, even if symptoms abate.
6. Keep room temperature constant (changes in room temperature aggravate sinusitis).

■ SURGERY OF THE SINUSES

Treatment for chronic sinusitis may be surgical. Removal of nasal deformities, such as a deviated nasal septum, hypertrophied turbinate bones, or nasal polyps that are obstructing the sinus openings may give relief. If the patient has recurrent attacks of sinusitis, it may be necessary to provide better drainage by permanently enlarging the sinus openings or by making a new opening and removing the diseased mucous membrane. Surgery usually is performed during the subacute stage of infection. General or local anesthesia may be used. Incisions for sinus surgery may be made intranasally, under the upper lip, or externally depending on the location and extent of surgery (Table 23-3).

☐ Caldwell-Luc surgery

The Caldwell-Luc procedure of the maxillary sinus is performed through an incision under the upper lip (Fig. 23-6) and is indicated as partial treatment for chronic sinusitis. An opening is made in the anterior wall of the sinus, and the infected contents of the sinus are stripped

Table 23-3 Sinus surgery

Surgery	Procedure	Use
Antral irrigation	Insertion of trocar intranasally and withdrawal of fluid; irrigation with normal saline	Acute maxillary sinusitis not relieved by conservative methods
Caldwell-Luc	Cleaning out of maxillary sinus through incision under upper lip	Chronic maxillary sinusitis
Ethmoidotomy, sphenoidotomy	Incision into ethmoid or sphenoid sinus for drainage; incision is intranasal for sphenoid sinus and external through eyebrow incision for ethmoid	Chronic sinusitis of ethmoid or sphenoid sinus
Ethmoidectomy	Excision of ethmoid tissue	Extensive ethmoiditis, nasal polyps
Osteopathic flap	Complete removal of diseased mucosa of frontal sinus with obliteration of sinus; space is packed with subcutaneous fat obtained from abdomen	Chronic frontal sinusitis

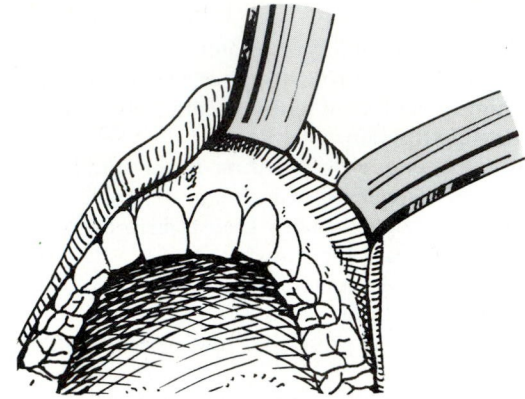

Fig. 23-6 The incision into the maxillary sinus (Caldwell-Luc surgery) is made under the upper lip.

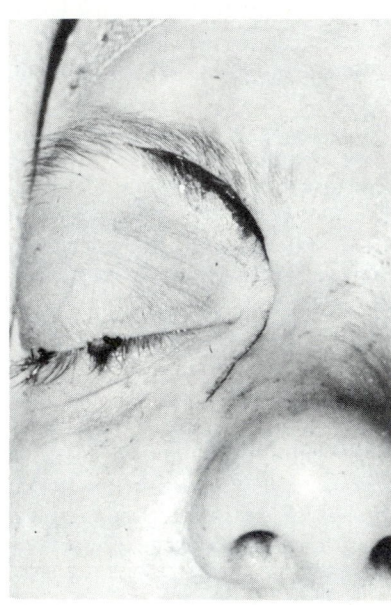

Fig. 23-7 Incision in inner half of eyebrow to expose ethmoid and frontal sinuses. Almost no visible scar results. (From DeWeese, DD, and Saunders, WH: Textbook of otolaryngology, ed 6, St. Louis, 1982, The CV Mosby Co.)

out. An antrostomy (window in the anterior portion of the middle third of the inferior turbinate) is performed as part of the Caldwell-Luc procedure to promote normal drainage and better aeration.

The sinus is packed with petrolatum or antibiotic impregnated gauze for about 48 hours. Numbness of the upper lip and upper teeth may be present for several months after a Caldwell-Luc operation because some nerves to these structures pass through the site of the incision. Interference with eating will occur initially. Only liquids will be given for at least 24 hours, followed by a soft diet for several days.

In addition to general care of the patient following sinus surgery, patient teaching specific to Caldwell-Luc surgery includes the following:
1. No chewing on affected side until incision heals
2. Use caution with oral hygiene to avoid injury to the incision
3. Avoid wearing dentures for about 10 days
4. Avoid blowing nose for about 2 weeks after packing has been removed

☐ Ethmoidotomy and ethmoidectomy

The external approach is preferred for ethmoid surgery because it allows better visualization and reduces the risks of complications such as damage to the optic nerve and central spinal fluid leak. Ethmoidotomy is an opening made for drainage, whereas an ethmoidectomy entails removal of ethmoid tissue (Table 23-3). The incision is made in the inner half of the eyebrow downward along the side of the nose (Fig. 23-7).[25,42] Ethmoidectomy is performed for correction of nasal polyps and for ethmoiditis because nasal polyps frequently originate in the ethmoid cells.

☐ Osteoplastic flap surgery

The advent of the osteoplastic flap operation makes frontal sinus surgery different from that performed on the other sinuses. Surgery of the other sinuses basically provides for an open, well-drained cavity, which in the past proved inadequate for the frontal sinuses because recurrence of disease was common. The osteoplastic flap operation allows for complete removal of diseased mucosa of the frontal sinus and for obliteration of the sinus so that it is no longer functional or in continuum with the inner nose.

The osteoplastic flap procedure is performed through a "gull-wing" or "cross-bow" incision.[20] In men, the incision extends along the eyebrows and connects along the bridge of the nose. In women, where baldness is not a problem in later life, the incision connects both temporal areas a few centimeters posterior to the hairline. Both incisions give excellent postoperative cosmesis and are extended to the periosteum of the bone overlying the frontal sinus.

The skin overlying the sinus is reflected, and a radiograph of the frontal sinus (obtained preoperatively) is used as a template for sawing the lateral and superior borders of the anterior frontal bone. The anterior bone is then reflected inferiorly, thus exposing the entire contents of the frontal sinus. The mucosa is removed under direct vision, and an operating microscope is used to ensure that all fragments of mucosa are removed. An incision is then made in the left-lower-abdominal quadrant and subcutaneous fat obtained for placement into the frontal sinus cavity. The bony flap and skin are then repositioned. Nasal packs are not required.

Postoperatively, pain in the frontal area is not significant after 24 hours. Pain in the abdominal area, however, often lasts several days and serous drainage from this area is common after the drain is removed. Sutures are removed about the fifth postoperative day. Because nasal packs are not used, special oral hygiene care is not needed.

☐ Postoperative care for sinus surgery

Care of the patient following sinus surgery is described in the box below, left. Gauze packing is usually inserted into the nares and removed after 48 hours. The patient thus breathes through the mouth, with subsequent dryness of mouth and lips. Mouth care is required and warm or cool vapor inhalations often are prescribed. If there is an oral incision, mouth care is given before meals to improve appetite and after meals to decrease danger of infection. Antibiotics may be prescribed prophylactically. For 1 or 2 weeks swelling or ecchymosis may be present around the nose and eyes. Ice compresses will constrict blood vessels, decreasing oozing and edema, and help relieve pain.

⊞ EVALUATION

Evaluation is based on the expected patient outcomes. Questions to be asked include the following:

1. Is the patient comfortable?
2. Can the patient describe the required care at home?
3. Can the patient describe measures to prevent further infection?
4. Can the patient demonstrate the correct use of nose drops and other medications?
5. Can the patient state plans for follow-up care?

■ INFECTIONS OF THE PHARYNX AND LARYNX

■ Acute pharyngitis

Acute pharyngitis is the most common throat inflammation. It may be caused by hemolytic streptococci, staphylococci, or other bacteria or viruses. There is an increased incidence of gonococcal pharyngitis caused by the gram-negative diplococcus *Neisseria gonorrhoeae*. The disease is increasingly found in both men and women who engage in oral-genital sex. When gonorrhea is suspected, a throat culture is indicated.

A severe form of acute pharyngitis often is referred to as *strep throat* because of the frequency of streptococci as the causative organisms.

Symptoms usually precede or occur simultaneously with

Postoperative care for surgery of the sinuses

1. After general anesthesia, position patient on side to prevent swallowing or aspirating bloody drainage.
2. Encourage mid-Fowler's position when patient is fully awake to promote drainage and decrease edema.
3. Apply ice compresses over nose (or ice bag over maxillary or frontal sinuses) in the early postoperative period.
4. Monitor the patient for:
   a. Excessive bleeding from nose (may be evidenced by repeated swallowing)
   b. Decreased visual acuity, especially diplopia, indicating damage to optic nerve or muscles at globe of eye
   c. Complaints of pain over the involved sinus may indicate infection or inadequate drainage
5. Give frequent mouth care.
6. Change nasal pad when it becomes soiled.
7. Encourage liberal fluid intake.
8. Teach patient
   a. Avoid blowing nose for at least 48 hours after packing is removed
   b. Report signs of infection (fever) to surgeon
   c. Expect stools to be tarry from swallowed blood
   d. Avoid constipation (Valsalva maneuver can initiate bleeding)

Table 23-4 Infections of the pharynx and larynx

Disorder	Etiology	Signs and symptoms	Medical therapy
Pharyngitis Acute	Gram-positive bacteria or viruses Gram-negative diplococci	Redness and soreness of throat, difficulty in swallowing, fever Hacking cough	Hot saline gargles, ice collar, aspirin, moist inhalations, antibiotics, anesthetic lozenges may be given
Tonsillitis Acute follicular	Usually streptococcus	Sudden onset of sore throat, dysphagia, fever, chills, malaise	Rest, fluids, warm saline gargles, ice collar, antibiotics, analgesics; tonsillectomy may be performed
Laryngitis Acute	Extension of inflammation from rhinitis, excessive use of voice, excessive smoking, irritating fumes, changes in temperature	From slight huskiness to total voice loss, sore throat, dry harsh cough	Symptomatic treatment, voice rest; steam inhalations; avoidance of smoking and being near those who are smoking

the onset of acute rhinitis or acute sinusitis. Pharyngitis can occur after the tonsils have been removed because the remaining mucous membrane can become infected. Pharyngitis is also a common manifestation of infectious mononucleosis.

Table 23-4 summarizes the etiology, signs and symptoms, and therapy for infections of the pharynx and larynx.

▦ IMPLEMENTATION

☐ Assisting with the achievement of therapeutic goals

1. Give medications as prescribed. Penicillin or erythromycin may be prescribed prophylactically to prevent superimposed infections, especially in persons with a history of rheumatic fever or bacterial endocarditis.
2. If the diagnosis is gonococcal pharyngitis, the patient will need instruction in how to avoid reinfection (see Chapter 35).
3. Provide moist inhalations and ice collar if ordered.
4. Provide a liquid diet with at least 2-3 L of fluids.
5. Bedrest if temperature is elevated; otherwise, extra rest.

☐ Counseling and teaching

The major points to be taught are outlined in the box on p. 647.

▦ EVALUATION

Evaluation is based on the expected patient outcomes. Questions to be asked include the following:

1. Are patient's signs and symptoms relieved?
2. Can the patient describe how to provide an environmentally controlled room that is allergen free?
3. Can patient state how to avoid future infections?
4. Can patient correctly instill nose drops?
5. Can the patient describe how to use prescribed medications?
6. Can the patient state plans for follow-up care?
7. If patient has gonococcal pharyngitis, can patient explain treatment and how to avoid reinfection?

■ ACUTE FOLLICULAR TONSILLITIS

Acute follicular tonsillitis is an acute inflammation of the tonsils and their crypts. It is usually caused by the *Streptococcus* organism. It is more likely to occur when the person's resistance is low and is very common in children. (See Table 23-4 for summary of signs and symptoms and medical therapy.)

Complications of untreated tonsillitis include heart and kidney damage, chorea, and pneumonia. Incidence of these complications is decreasing with the widespread use of penicillin and early diagnosis. Most physicians believe that persons who have recurrent attacks of tonsillitis should have a tonsillectomy. This procedure is usually performed from 4 to 6 weeks after an acute attack has subsided.

Because the person with acute tonsillitis is usually cared for at home, the nurse should help in teaching the general public the care that is needed, which is the same as that described in Table 23-4 for the person with pharyngitis. The office nurse, the clinic nurse, the nurse in industry, the school nurse, and the community health nurse have many opportunities to do this teaching.

■ Tonsillectomy

Tonsillectomy for the adult may be performed under local or general anesthesia. Hemorrhage may occur postoperatively. The physician may be able to control minor postoperative bleeding by applying a sponge soaked in a solution of epinephrine to the site. The person who is bleeding excessively often is returned to the operating room for ligation or cauterization of the bleeding vessel. If sutures must be used, the person will have more pain and discomfort than following a simple tonsillectomy. The patient may not be able to take solid food for several days. Some surgeons no longer prescribe aspirin for pain after tonsillectomy, as it increases the tendency to bleed. Acetaminophen or another aspirin substitute is usually ordered.

Teaching for the patient with an infection of the nose or throat

1. Get additional rest (hastens recovery)
2. Drink at least 2 to 3 L of fluid every day
3. Medications
   a. Antihistamines are effective primarily during the initial period only; care should be taken when driving or working with heavy machinery when taking antihistamines
   b. Take prescribed antibiotics for bacterial infections for the prescribed period of time
   c. If using nose drops
      1. Place no more than 3 drops of solution in each nostril at one time (unless otherwise prescribed)
      2. Keep head tilted back for about 5 minutes to permit solution to reach posterior nares
      3. Insert 1 to 2 additional drops after 10 minutes if marked congestion is still present
   d. If using atomizer:
      1. Occlude opposite nostril with finger pressure to prevent entrance of air
      2. Administer no more than 3 sprays of solution in each nostril at one time
4. Promote throat comfort through use of the following:
   a. Warm saline gargles
   b. Ice collar
   c. Throat lozenges
   d. Moist inhalations
5. Avoid further upper respiratory infections
   a. Avoid direct exposure to others with respiratory infections, if possible
   b. Teach all persons to cover nose and mouth with tissue when coughing or sneezing
   c. Wash hands after disposing of tissues
6. Rationale for prophylactic antibiotics for persons with a history of rheumatic fever or bacterial endocarditis
7. Symptoms of recurrence requiring medical attention (fever, excessive pain, dysphagia, expectoration of pus)

Postoperative care for tonsillectomy

1. Side-lying position until awake, then mid-Fowler's
2. Monitor for signs of hemorrhage
   a. Repeated swallowing
   b. Vomiting of bright red blood
   c. Increased pulse rate while sleeping
3. Diet
   a. Offer fluids when vomiting has ceased
   1. Encourage patient to take large swallows (more comfortable than small sips)
   2. Avoid using a straw (suction may cause bleeding)
   3. Ice-cold fluids better tolerated
   b. Offer bland nourishment
      1. Ice cream, cold custards, cream soups, and bland juices (for example, pear) offered initially
      2. Refined cereal and soft-cooked egg usually better tolerated morning after surgery
      3. Avoid citrus juices, hot fluids, rough or highly seasoned foods for 1 week
   c. Relieve throat discomfort
      1. Apply ice collar if desired
      2. Give prescribed analgesic (avoid aspirin)
   d. Teach patient about the following:
      1. Avoid vigorous exercise, coughing, sneezing, clearing throat, and vigorous nose blowing for 1 to 2 weeks
      2. Report signs of bleeding immediately to physician
      3. Drink fluids (2 to 3 L/day) until mouth odor disappears
      4. Stools may be tarry for several days from swallowed blood
      5. Throat discomfort may increase slightly between fourth and eighth postoperative day (membrane separation)

A tough, yellow, fibrous membrane that forms over the operative site begins to break away between the fourth and eighth postoperative days, and hemorrhage may occur. The separation of the membrane accounts for the throat being more painful at this time. Pink granulation tissue soon becomes apparent, and by the end of the third postoperative week, the area is covered with mucous membrane of normal appearance.

Postoperative care is outlined in the box on p. 647.

■ Laryngitis

■ SIMPLE ACUTE LARYNGITIS

Simple acute laryngitis is an inflammation of the mucous membrane lining the larynx accompanied by edema of the vocal cords. It may be caused by a cold, by sudden changes in temperature, or by irritating fumes. Symptoms vary from a slight huskiness to complete loss of voice. The throat may be painful and feel scratchy, and a cough may be present. (See Table 23-4 for etiology, signs and symptoms, and therapy.)

■ CHRONIC LARYNGITIS

Some people who use their voices excessively, who smoke a great deal, or who work continuously where there are irritating fumes develop a chronic laryngitis. Hoarseness usually is worse in the early morning and in the evening. There may be a dry, harsh cough and a persistent need to clear the throat.

Treatment may consist of removal of irritants, voice rest, correction of faulty voice habits, steam inhalations, and cough medications. The physician may order spraying of the throat with an astringent antiseptic solution such as hexylresorcinol (S.T. 37). To carry out this procedure properly the patient must use a spray tip that turns down at the end so that the medication reaches vocal cords and is not dissipated in the posterior pharynx. The spray tip is placed in the back of the throat with the bent portion behind the tongue. The patient should then take one or two deep breaths and spray the medication on inhalation. This procedure may cause temporary coughing and gagging. Many medications used as throat sprays are now sold in plastic squeeze bottles with tube and spray tip attached.

■ OBSTRUCTIVE DISORDERS OF THE NOSE AND THROAT

Trauma or polyps in the nose, nasal bones, turbinates, maxillary bones, and zygomatic bones may cause obstruction (Table 23-5). Many persons with obstructions of the nose may be diagnosed and treated on an ambulatory basis.

■ PATHOPHYSIOLOGY

Obstruction may be caused by a deviated septum, either congenital or, more commonly, as a result of trauma. Allergy and chronic sinusitis may lead to the development of nasal polyps, grape-like growths of mucous membrane and loose connective tissue in the sinus mucosa. Fractures of e nasal, maxillary, and zygomatic bones may result from

---

Common causes of nosebleeds

Local irritation of superficial blood vessel

Trauma
Chronic infection
Lack of humidity in air breathed
Violent sneezing or noseblowing
Nose picking (most common cause)

Systemic causes

Hypertension
Blood dyscrasias (for example, leukemia)
Deficiency in vitamin K

Table 23-5 Obstructions of the nose

Disorder	Etiology	Signs and symptoms	Therapy
Deviated septum	May be congenital but is usually the result of injury	Noisy, difficult breathing; postnasal drip; dry mucosa and crusts	Submucous resection or septoplasty
Hypertrophy of turbinates	Inflammation of inferior turbinates	Nasal obstruction	Aerosols containing corticosteroids; cryosurgery or electric fulguration may be used
Nasal polyps	Irritation to mucous membranes from allergy or chronic sinusitis	May cause anosmia, obstruction of breathing, blockage of sinus drainage	Aerosol sprays or polypectomy
Foreign bodies	Objects in nose	Nasal obstruction, discharge, bleeding	Topical vasoconstrictors; extraction of foreign body

falls, motor vehicle accidents, and fights. Displaced fragments from the fractures obstruct passage of air. Malignant growths may also cause obstruction.

Nosebleeds, epistaxis, may result from a number of causes (see the box on p. 648). When the bleeding stops, some nasal obstruction may occur from the blood clot until the mucosa heals. In adulthood, nosebleeds are more common in men than in women.

ASSESSMENT

Subjective data

Symptoms of nasal obstructions include the following:
1. Noisy, difficult breathing
2. Dry mucosa
3. Postnasal drip
4. Nasal discharge
5. Anosmia (loss of sense of smell)
6. Bleeding from nose

If nasal trauma is present, additional symptoms include displacement of the bones, cosmetic deformity, pain, and ecchymosis around the eyes or jaw.

Objective data

1. Inspection for deformity or asymmetry
2. Some septal deviation is common in adults (Fig. 23-8) and is asymptomatic
3. Check for abnormal findings in nose
   a. Excessive redness
   b. Edema
   c. Exudate
   d. Bleeding

DATA ANALYSIS: NURSING DIAGNOSES

Nursing diagnoses are determined from an assessment of patient data. Possible nursing diagnoses for the person with obstruction of the nose and throat may include, but are not limited to, the following:

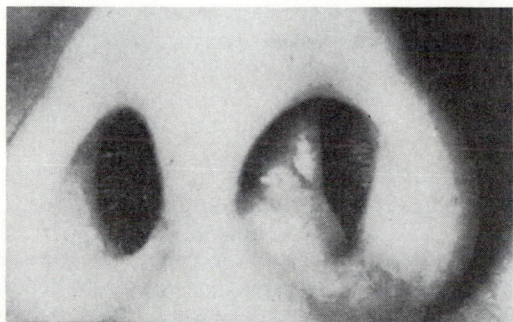

Fig. 23-8 Septal deviation. Anterior end of septal cartilage is dislocated and projects into nasal vestibule. (From Saunders, WH, and others: Nursing care in eye, ear, nose, and throat disorders, ed 4, St. Louis, 1979, The CV Mosby Co.)

Diagnostic title	Possible etiologies
Body image disturbance	Severe trauma/disfiguring surgery
Pain	Trauma/obstruction
Knowledge deficit	Lack of exposure to information
Sensory/perceptual alterations: olfactory	Trauma/surgery

PLANNING: EXPECTED PATIENT OUTCOMES

Expected patient outcomes for the person with an obstruction of the nose or throat may include, but are not limited to, the following:
1. Patient is feeling comfortable.
2. Patient can state care required after surgery and discharge from hospital.
3. Patient knows how to prevent nosebleeds or to treat them if they occur.

IMPLEMENTATION

Assisting with achievement of therapeutic goals
Nasal bleeding

Nosebleeds from the tiny blood vessels in the anterior part of the septum are usually controllable by compressing the soft tissue of the nose against the septum with a finger. Firm pressure should be maintained for at least 5 to 10 minutes, and it may be necessary for as long as 30 minutes. The person should breathe through the mouth during this time. Ice compresses may be applied over the nose; however, the primary benefit of the application of ice is that it requires the patient to remain still.

Bleeding may also be controlled by placing a cotton ball soaked in a topical vasoconstrictor such as phenylephrine (Neo-Synephrine) in the nose and applying pressure. Other first-aid measures include having the person sit quietly with the head up and inclined slightly forward to prevent blood from entering the pharynx and causing gagging or swallowing of blood. The person is instructed not to blow the nose for several hours after a nosebleed.

If these measures do not control bleeding, the help of a physician should be sought. After identifying the site of bleeding, the physician may cauterize the bleeding vessel with a silver nitrate stick or electrode cautery.

Bleeding from the posterior part of the nasal septum is more common in elderly persons and is more likely to be severe. If the bleeding point cannot be seen and cauterized, a postnasal pack may be inserted (Fig. 23-9). Because this procedure is extremely painful and sometimes causes faintness, patients may be admitted to the hospital. Pain medication, antibiotic therapy, and sedation may also be ordered for a person with posterior packing. Sedation may be ordered, because bleeding tends to be increased by apprehension and restlessness. The pack is left in place for 2 to 5 days and then gently removed.

Severe bleeding results in a drop in blood pressure, which may cause the bleeding to stop; therefore, exsan-

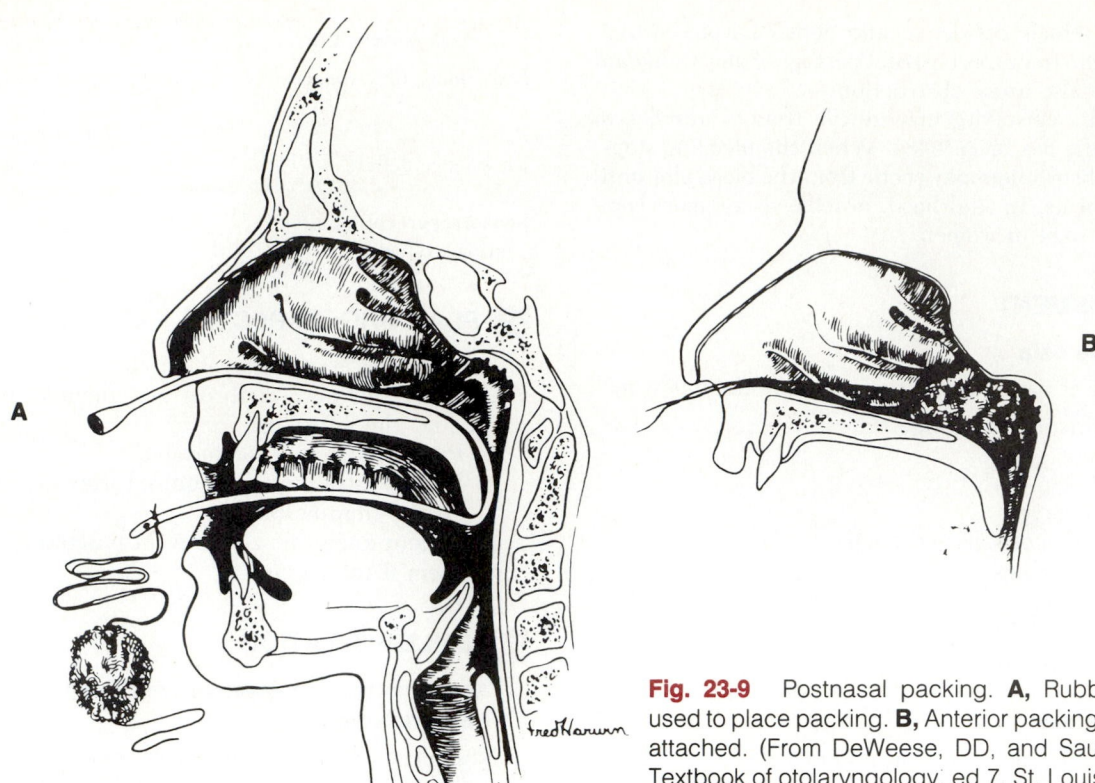

Fig. 23-9 Postnasal packing. **A,** Rubber catheter used to place packing. **B,** Anterior packing with strings attached. (From DeWeese, DD, and Saunders, WH: Textbook of otolaryngology, ed 7, St. Louis, 1987, The CV Mosby Co.)

guination from the usual nosebleed is rare. To prevent recurrent hemorrhage, the person is warned not to blow the nose vigorously and to avoid dryness of the nose. This can be accomplished by using saline or nasal lubricants.

Persistent or recurrent profuse epistaxis, especially posterior epistaxis, may require surgical ligation of the external carotid artery, the ethmoid artery, or the internal maxillary artery, all of which supply blood to the nose.

□ Surgery

Surgery is performed when obstruction occurs and consists of either a submucous resection or nasoseptoplasty (see Table 23-6). *Submucous resection* usually is performed under local anesthesia. An internal incision is made on one side of the nasal septum from top to bottom. The mucous membrane is elevated away from the bone, the

obstructive parts of the cartilage and bone are removed, and the mucous membrane is sutured back into place. Packing is placed in both nostrils to prevent bleeding and to splint the operative area (Fig. 23-9). Commonly used gauze packs are ½ inch petrolatum-impregnated gauze, Adaptic gauze, iodoform gauze with bacitracin, and Cortisporin-impregnated gauze. The latter is particularly effective in reducing nasal pack odor. Nasal packing can be left in place from 24 to 48 hours depending on the extent of surgery and the surgeon's preference.

Nasoseptoplasty involves reconstruction of the septum and is becoming more widely used to treat deviated nasal septum. Reconstruction of the external nose (*rhinoplasty*), often done for cosmetic reasons (Chapter 39), is often combined with septoplasty. It is usually performed under local anesthesia. With rhinoplasty, the nasal bones or car-

Table 23-6 Surgeries to relieve nasal obstruction or trauma

Procedure	Description	Comments
Nasal polypectomy	Removal of polyps from nose	Local anesthesia given; nasal packing for 24 hours
Submucous resection	Removal of obstructive parts of cartilage and bone from nasal septum	Local anesthesia given; both nostrils packed to provide splinting
Nasoseptoplasty	Reconstruction of nasal septum	Same as for submucous resection
Rhinoplasty	Reconstruction of external nose following trauma or for cosmetic reasons	Often combined with septoplasty following nasal trauma; nose splinted after surgery; nasal packing

tilaginous framework of the nose are altered. The nose is usually protected with a plaster-of-Paris splint, adhesive tape dressing, or plastic mold following a plastic procedure on the nasal bones. Firm healing develops on about the tenth day. Usually only the surgeon changes a septoplasty or rhinoplasty dressing.

☐ *Postoperative care for nasal surgery*

Nursing diagnoses for the patient undergoing nasal surgery are determined from assessment of patient data. Possible nursing diagnoses may include but are not limited to the following:

Knowledge deficit

Comfort, alteration in

Injury, potential for (hemorrhage)

Nutrition, alteration in: less than body requirement

Following nasal surgery, the patient is placed in mid-Fowler's position to decrease local edema, and ice compresses are usually applied to the nose to lessen the discoloration, bleeding, and discomfort. Patients can usually apply their own ice compresses.

The patient is monitored for signs of hemorrhage (see the box at right). Some oozing on the dressing below the nose (Fig. 23-10) is expected and this dressing may be changed as necessary. If bleeding becomes pronounced, the surgeon is notified and material for repacking the nose is prepared. This material consists of a hemostatic tray containing gauze packing, umbilical tape for posterior packing, a few small gauze sponges, small catheter (used for inserting a postnasal plug), packing forceps, tongue blades, and scissors. The surgeon may require a head mirror, good light, epinephrine 1:1000 or other vasoconstrictor, 4% topical lidocaine (Xylocaine) or 4% cocaine solution, applicators, nasal speculum, and suction.

Postoperative care for nasal surgery

1. Assessment
   a. Monitor for hemorrhage
      (1) Excessive blood on nasal dressing
      (2) Bright red vomitus
      (3) Repeated swallowing (use penlight to check back of throat for blood running down throat)
      (4) Rapid pulse
   b. Monitor for infection: fever, elevated WBC
2. Discomfort
   a. Mid-Fowler's position to decrease local edema
   b. Ice compresses over nose for 24 hours prn
   c. Support and sedation for patient apprehension because of difficulty in breathing caused by blockage of nasal passages
   d. Frequent oral care
   e. Change dressing under nose prn
3. Nutrition
   a. Food as tolerated
   b. Encourage increased fluid intake
4. Patient teaching
   a. Avoid blowing nose for 48 hours after packing removed
   b. Avoid constipation (Valsalva maneuver) and vigorous coughing until healing occurs (can initiate bleeding)
   c. Expect stools to be tarry for several days
   d. Expect face to be discolored around eyes and nose for several days
   e. Cosmetic effect from nasal surgery cannot be judged for 6 to 12 months (time for tissue to return to normal and for scar resolution)

Because packing blocks the passage of air through the nose, a partial vacuum is created during swallowing, and the person may complain of a sucking action when attempting to drink. Postnasal drainage, the presence of old blood in the mouth, dryness of the mouth from mouth breathing, and loss of the ability to smell often lead to anorexia. Antihistamines may be prescribed to reduce nasal secretions, and frequent mouth care is important. Postoperative care is described in the box above.

☐ Counseling and teaching

Persons with trauma to the nose should be encouraged to seek medical attention, even if obstruction is not present, since a broken nose can lead to chronic problems (chronic sinusitis) if not treated.

Teaching the person who has had nasal surgery is described above. If deformities are present, the person may be disturbed about body image because of the high

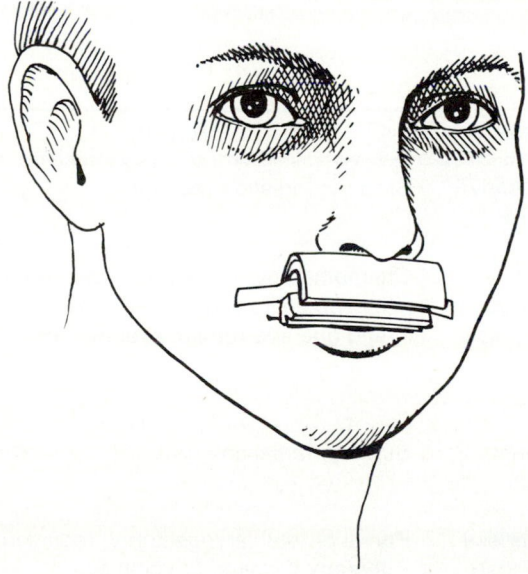

Fig. 23-10 Dressing placed under nose for nasal drainage.

visibility of the face. These persons need an opportunity to talk about their feelings and are encouraged to talk to the physician about possible long-term positive changes through plastic surgery (see Chapter 39).

✠ EVALUATION

Evaluation is based on expected patient outcomes. Questions to ask may include the following:
1. Is the patient comfortable?
2. Can the patient describe care required at home following surgery?
3. Can the patient describe ways to prevent nosebleeds?
4. Can the patient describe the expected time frame for positive cosmetic effects following rhinoplasty?

■ MALIGNANCIES OF THE NOSE AND THROAT

Malignancies may develop in the nasopharynx, sinuses, tonsils, and larynx (Table 23-7).

■ Pathophysiology

Nasopharyngeal carcinomas obstruct the nose; they metastasize early to the neck. Carcinomas of the maxillary and ethmoid sinuses may erode the adjacent nasal walls and bleed easily. Carcinoma of the maxillary sinus causes dental problems initially; other effects may include nasal obstruction, nosebleeds, and displacement of the eye. Carcinoma of the ethmoid sinus causes outward displacement of the eye, disturbance of the sense of smell, and nosebleeds. The prognosis is grave.

■ Malignancy of the tonsils

Malignancy of the tonsils can be one of three types: carcinoma, lymphoepithelioma, or lymphosarcoma. Carcinomas are more common in men, possibly related to the longer smoking history of some men. The carcinomas spread upward into the soft palate and usually metastasize early to the neck. Local ulceration and otalgia (earache) are early symptoms. Lymphoepitheliomas often remain small and do not ulcerate, but neck metastasis occurs early. Lymphosarcomas produce large tonsils, usually without ulceration or pain, and metastasize early to the neck.

Medical interventions for all tonsillar malignancies always include radiation in conjunction with an extensive surgical procedure to remove all the malignant tissue. Chemotherapy may be used also, but it is still being tested for effectiveness. The cure rate is improved using this combined technique.[10] Recurrence often occurs locally or with distant metastasis.

■ Malignancy of the larynx

■ PATHOPHYSIOLOGY

Squamous cell carcinoma of the larynx is increasing in frequency. It is estimated that in the United States there are over 12,100 new cases and over 3800 deaths every year.[1] Cancer of the larynx limited to the true vocal cords grows slowly because of the limited lymphatic supply. Elsewhere in the larynx (epiglottis, false vocal cords, and pyriform sinuses) lymphatic vessels are abundant, and cancer of these tissues often spreads rapidly and metastasizes early to the deep lymph nodes of the neck.

Cancer of the larynx is five times more common in men than in women, and it occurs most often in persons over

---

Table 23-7 Malignant disorders of nose and throat

Disorder	Description	Signs and symptoms	Therapy
Nasopharyngeal carcinomas	Carcinomas that obstruct nose first on one side then the other	Nasal obstruction, early metastasis to neck, bleeding	Surgery; radiation therapy
Carcinoma of maxillary and ethmoid sinuses	Relatively uncommon	Loosening of upper teeth; nasal obstruction, nosebleeds, displacement of eye, anosmia, tearing and diplopia	Chemotherapy; radiation; surgery that removes entire upper jaw (maxillectomy) and one eye (orbital exenteration)
Cancer of tonsil	May be carcinoma, lymphoepithelioma, or lymphosarcoma	Local ulceration, enlarged tonsil, pain	Surgery; radiation
Carcinoma of larynx	Squamous cell carcinoma of vocal cords and surrounding tissue	Progressive hoarseness that lasts longer than 2 weeks	Partial or total laryngectomy; radiation therapy if limited to vocal cord

60 years of age. There appears to be some relationship between cancer of the larynx and heavy smoking, alcohol, chronic laryngitis, vocal abuse, and family predisposition to cancer. Because of the number of women who continue to be heavy smokers, the incidence of carcinoma of the larynx has increased in this group.

Any person who becomes progressively hoarse or is hoarse for longer than 2 weeks should be urged to seek medical attention at once. Hoarseness is an early symptom of cancer of the vocal cords. If treatment is given when hoarseness appears (caused by the tumor's preventing the complete approximation of the vocal cord), a cure usually is possible. Signs of metastases of cancer to other parts of the larynx include a sensation of a lump in the throat, pain in the Adam's apple that radiates to the ear, dyspnea, dysphagia, enlarged cervical nodes, and cough. The diagnosis of cancer of the larynx is made from the history, from visual examination of the larynx with indirect laryngoscopy, and from a biopsy and microscopic study of the lesion.

ASSESSMENT

☐ Subjective data

Persons with carcinomas of the nose, sinuses, tonsils, or larynx can have a variety of symptoms, which include the following:

1. Nasal obstruction, either unilateral or bilateral
2. Bleeding from the nose
3. Dental problems, for example, loosening of the upper teeth, or poorly fitting dentures
4. Disturbance of the sense of smell
5. Eye problems: displacement, tearing, diplopia
6. Local ulceration of the tonsil with or without pain
7. Hoarseness

Hoarseness is an early symptom of cancer of the vocal cords. If treatment is given when hoarseness first appears (caused by the tumor's preventing the complete approximation of the vocal cord), a cure usually is possible.

☐ Diagnostic tests

The nose may be examined by the physician by direct inspection using a nasal speculum. A laryngeal mirror is used to visualize the larynx. Roentgenograms of the sinuses may help to establish the diagnosis.

☐ *Direct laryngoscopy*

A direct laryngoscopy is performed on all persons with suspicious lesions of the larynx. It is usually performed with the patient under local anesthesia with 10% cocaine or under general anesthesia. A sedative (for example, secobarbital, meperidine, or other narcotic) and atropine sulfate (to decrease secretions) are given 1 hour before the examination. The person is placed in a reclining position with the head in a head holder or with the head extended over the edge of the table and manually supported by a physician or nurse. The laryngoscope is inserted through the mouth and hypopharynx, making the interior of the larynx easily visible. Minor surgical procedures, such as a biopsy, may be performed through the laryngoscope.

If local anesthesia has been given, the patient should not eat or drink anything until the gag reflex returns, usually within 2 hours. The gag reflex can be tested by touching the back of the throat with a tongue blade or applicator. After the gag reflex returns, the patient should first try to drink water, because if it is accidentally aspirated into the trachea or lungs, it is the fluid least likely to cause aspiration pneumonia.

IMPLEMENTATION

☐ Surgery

The treatment for metastatic disease of the nose and throat is primarily surgical. Radiation therapy may also be indicated.

☐ *Maxillectomy and orbital exenteration*

Surgery for malignancies of the sinuses often consists of removal of the entire upper jaw (maxillectomy) and one eye (orbital exenteration). Split-thickness skin grafts (see Chapter 40) are usually applied to the operative area. Postoperatively, the deformity of the jaw is managed with a dental prosthesis, which closes off the defect in the mouth. Several different prostheses may be needed before a final one fits because of shrinking of the cavity as healing progresses. Radical surgery is required because of the danger of recurrence.

Postoperative care includes the following:

1. Monitor for signs of meningitis (fever, headache, neck rigidity).
2. Provide care related to nasogastric intubation (see Chapter 31).
3. Provide tracheostomy care, if indicated (see Chapter 24).
4. Provide mouth care.
   a. Use a gentle spray or oral irrigation.
   b. Use saline with hydrogen peroxide, weak sodium bicarbonate, or prescribed antibiotic solution.
   c. Aspiration of drainage may be necessary (care is taken to prevent trauma from suction tip).
5. Provide pain medication as needed.
6. Give prescribed prophylactic antibiotics.
7. Encourage early ambulation.
8. Provide emotional support.

Persons who undergo radical surgery of this type have a number of emotional adjustments to make.[61,62] The alteration in their physical appearance is readily visible; the person feels conspicuous and different. In addition to disfigurement, the person has all the normal fears of surgery and of cancer. Fear, anger, and grief are normal reactions to the situation. Fear is focused on concerns about the future, the ability to live normally, and also of being rejected. Anger and grief are common responses to the loss and the helplessness to control the loss. Oral communication also may be a problem immediately following surgery, and every effort is made to allow the person to express needs and feelings by writing if necessary. Conveying compassion and concern to the person is important.

□ *Laryngectomy*

PARTIAL LARYNGECTOMY

If the tumor is limited to portions of the vocal cords or areas just above them, a partial laryngectomy may effect a cure. Patients suitable for partial laryngectomy have only one diseased vocal cord and both cords are completely mobile. The most common technique is a *laryngofissure* (Table 23-8). Scar tissue fills the defect where the diseased cord was removed and becomes a vibrating surface for speech. A *supraglottic* partial laryngectomy is performed for carcinoma of the epiglottis and adjacent structures above the level of the true vocal cords. The postoperative rehabilitation of persons following hemilaryngectomy or supraglottic partial laryngectomy is more arduous than for a laryngofissure.

Following partial laryngectomy, a temporary tracheostomy tube is inserted and removed when edema in the

---

NURSING CARE PLAN

Person with laryngectomy

DATA: Mr. Knox, a 68-year-old man, had noted progressive hoarseness for several months. Indirect laryngoscopy and biopsy confirmed cancer of the larynx and he was admitted for a total laryngectomy. His wife accompanied him to the hospital and planned to be with him as much as possible during his hospitalization. She was attentive and supportive.

The following pertinent data were identified on admission:
1. He was visibly apprehensive (pacing the floor, restless, asking repeated questions).
2. His major concerns centered on the extent of the cancer and on communication problems following the surgery.
3. Height 175 cm (5 ft 10 in), weight 68 kg (150 lb).
4. He wears glasses; near vision is poor without glasses.

Before surgery, Mr. Knox's primary nurse spent time with him, encouraging him to express his concerns and providing information about what to expect in the postoperative period and care that would be provided. Following the interaction, Mr. Knox's restlessness decreased and he was observed talking quietly with his wife and watching TV.

During surgery the larynx was removed; a permanent tracheostomy was performed with insertion of a temporary laryngectomy tube. A nasogastric tube was inserted, to be removed after Mr. Knox was swallowing well. During the first postoperative day, Mr. Knox again appeared apprehensive (restlessness, pointing frequently to his tracheostomy, pulling on wife's hand and pointing to call cord to call the nurse). Breath sounds in the upper lobes were clear but were absent in the lower lobes. Codeine and acetaminophen were prescribed for pain.

Nursing diagnosis: Anxiety (related to breathing difficulties and inability to communicate)

Expected patient outcomes	Nursing interventions	Rationale
Patient rests quietly, does not call frequently for suctioning	Explain suctioning procedure to patient and carry out regular suctioning of tracheostomy	If patient knows tube will be suctioned frequently, fear of possible asphyxiation should decrease
	Develop a means of communication (such as cards with needs printed clearly, a magic slate, or paper for writing); be sure patient wears glasses	If patient can communicate needs, anxiety should decrease; his glasses are needed for visual communication
	After initial period and if wife is willing and able, teach her to help with suctioning tracheostomy	Participating in husband's care may assist wife in feeling she is helping, thus decreasing her anxiety (anxiety can be transmitted to patient)
	Encourage patient to care for own tracheostomy when feasible	Self-care enhances feelings of control of situation

NURSING CARE PLAN

Person with laryngectomy—cont'd

Nursing diagnosis: Ineffective airway clearance: related to secretions in upper airway and laryngectomy tube

Expected patient outcomes	Nursing interventions	Rationale
Respirations are effortless, quiet, and at baseline rate	Place patient in semi-Fowler's position	Position uses gravity to help expand thorax and decrease pressure on lower lobes
Breath sounds are clear at all lobes	Suction laryngectomy tube as often as needed as evidenced by noisy respirations, increased pulse and respiratory rate, and restlessness (may be as often as every 5 min initially)	Air blowing through secretions produces noisy respirations; pulse and respirations are increased when oxygen intake is decreased; restlessness may indicate decreased oxygenation
	Provide tracheostomy care	Keeping tube patent will facilitate air interchange
	Provide air humidification	Humidity will help keep secretions liquid for easier removal
	Encourage deep breathing and coughing	Deep breathing will help aerate lower lobes; coughing will help expel secretions

Nursing diagnosis: Altered nutrition: less than body requirements related to difficulty in swallowing

Expected patient outcomes	Nursing interventions	Rationale
Weight is not less than 5 lb from baseline	Give prescribed tube feedings via N/G tube until patient can swallow well	Tube feedings provide more adequate nutrients than IV fluids; swallowing is impaired initially from postoperative edema of lower pharynx
	When N/G tube is removed, give fluids only until patient is swallowing well	Fluids are easier to swallow than solid food until edema subsides
	Explain anatomic changes to patient (no connection between esophagus and tracheostomy)	May help to decrease patient's concern of choking
	Stay with patient during initial eating of semisolid and solid foods	He may fear choking and not be willing to swallow initially; encouragement by nurse with assurance of suctioning if necessary may give patient more confidence
	Use measures to encourage eating as necessary (tray for wife so they can eat together, selection of desired foods, and so forth)	Return to usual eating patterns may encourage patient to eat
	Encourage him to monitor weight 2 to 3 times a week until baseline weight is regained	Participating in monitoring own weight may motivate him to eat

Continued.

NURSING CARE PLAN

Person with laryngectomy—cont'd

Expected patient outcomes	Nursing interventions	Rationale

Nursing diagnosis: Pain: related to surgery

Expected patient outcomes	Nursing interventions	Rationale
Patient is relaxed and signals feeling comfortable	Give prescribed analgesic	Analgesics will decrease transmission and interpretation of pain stimuli
	Encourage other pain-relieving measures such as relaxation exercises or distraction	Help to minimize pain perception
	Provide nose and mouth care while N/G tube is in place	Tube may irritate nose; mouth becomes dry and uncomfortable from open mouth breathing and decreased lubrication (unable to swallow fluids)

Nursing diagnosis: Impaired verbal communication: related to laryngectomy

Expected patient outcomes	Nursing interventions	Rationale
Patient communicates with others	Encourage him to communicate via an established system (such as hand signals, writing) during initial period	With larynx removal, sounds cannot be made by previous method of vibrating vocal cords
Patient begins speech rehabilitation	Support activities of speech therapist: Encourage him to practice burping as instructed	Burping provides air movement; esophageal tissue folds act as vibrating surface
	Monitor for gastric flatus or gastric discomfort; explain that this may be caused by muscle strain or nervous tension	Excessive air may be swallowed when practicing burping and may discourage him from further practice; discomfort will decrease with practice
	Discuss availability of mechanical devices for speech or telephone use	Until esophageal speech is perfected, mechanical devices can help the person communicate verbally

Nursing diagnosis: Knowledge deficit: related to lack of exposure/recall

Expected patient outcomes	Nursing interventions	Rationale
Patient describes self-care	Teach patient description of anatomic changes	Providing own care will give him self-confidence; care is needed to keep the tracheostomy open for air exchange
	Teach patient care of stoma including self-suctioning	
	Teach patient methods to protect stoma	
	Advise patient of availability of community resources	He may be interested in the Lost Chord Club for sharing of experiences

Table 23-8 Laryngectomy surgery for cancer

Type	Description	Voice result
Partial laryngectomy		
Laryngofissure	Opening into larynx through thyroid cartilage with removal of diseased vocal cord	Husky but acceptable
Hemilaryngectomy	Same approach as for laryngofissure with removal of diseased false cord, arytenoid, and one side of thyroid cartilage	Hoarse voice
Supraglottic partial laryngectomy	Horizontal incision passes above true cords (left intact) with removal of epiglottis and diseased tissue	Normal voice
Total laryngectomy	Removal of epiglottis, thyroid cartilage, and 3 or 4 tracheal rings; closure of pharynx with trachea; permanent tracheostomy	No voice

surrounding tissues subsides. The person is not on absolute voice rest but is not permitted to use the voice until the surgeon gives specific approval (usually 3 days postoperatively). Only whispering is then permitted until healing is complete, after which time the person usually adjusts quite readily to relatively minor limitations of speech. The main problems encountered by persons undergoing partial laryngectomy are those of swallowing and aspiration.

TOTAL LARYNGECTOMY

When cancer of the larynx is advanced, total laryngectomy may be performed. This includes removal of the epiglottis,

thyroid cartilage, hyoid bone, cricoid cartilage, and three or four rings of the trachea. The pharyngeal opening to the trachea is closed, the anterior wall of the hypopharynx is closed, and the remaining trachea is brought out to the neck wound and sutured to the skin. It forms an opening (permanent tracheostomy) through which the patient breathes (Fig. 23-11).

RADICAL NECK DISSECTION

Radical neck dissection often accompanies total laryngectomy because of the possibility of metastases to the neck from carcinoma of the larynx. It is always indicated when cervical nodes are palpable at the time of surgery. The

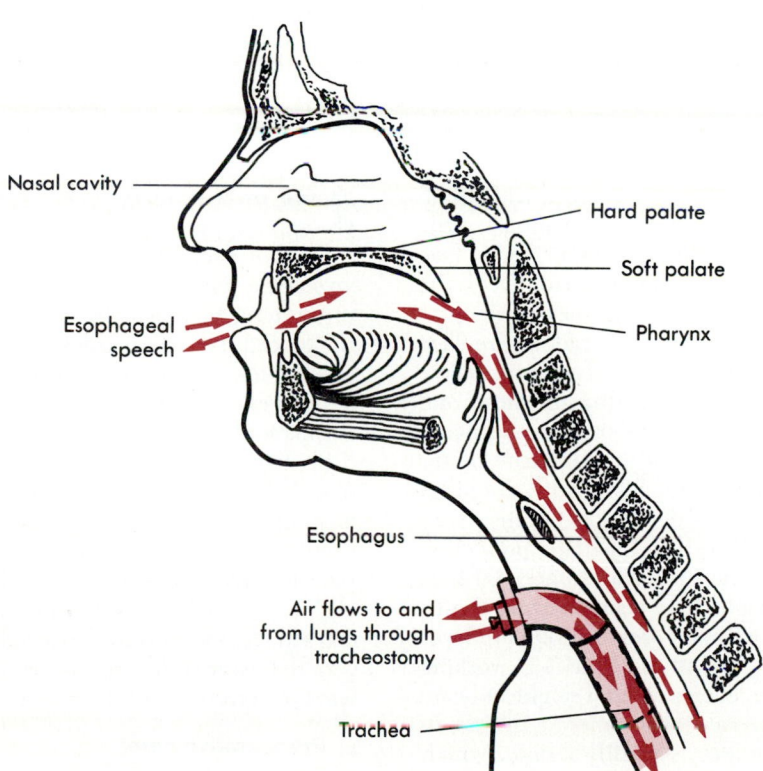

Fig. 23-11 Permanent tracheostomy: no connection exists between trachea and esophagus.

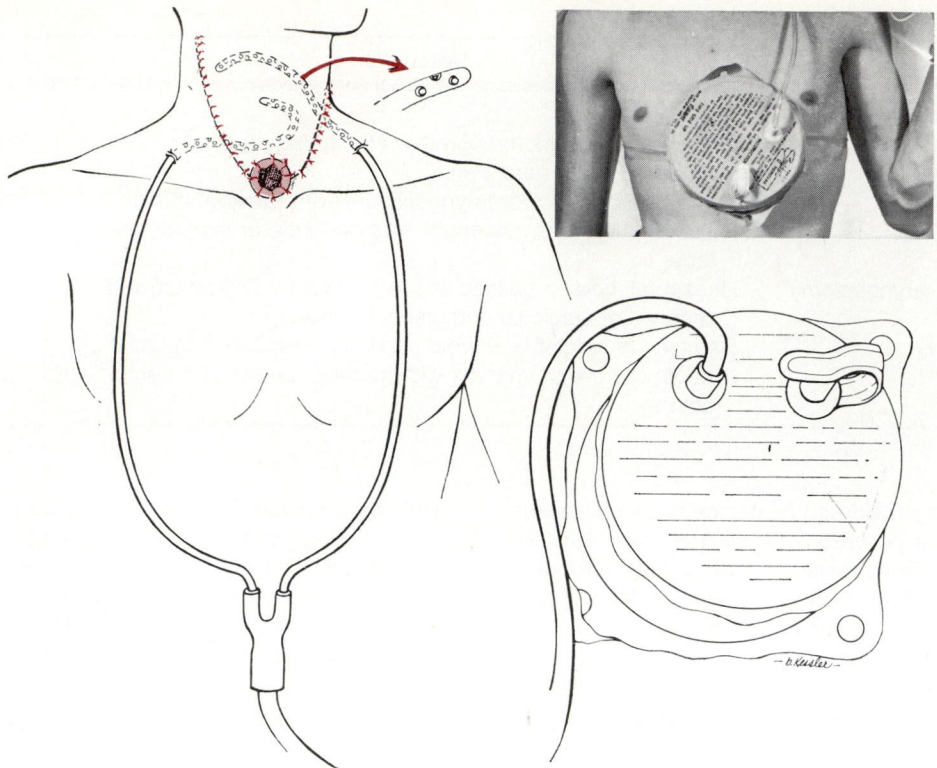

Fig. 23-12 Hemovac apparatus for constant closed suction. In this system of wound drainage, suction is maintained by plastic container with spring inside that tries to force apart lids and thereby produces suction that is transmitted through plastic tubing. Neck skin is pulled down tight, and no external dressing is required. Container serves as both suction source and receptacle for blood. It is emptied as required, and drainage tubes are left in neck for 3 days. (From DeWeese, DD, and Saunders, WH: Textbook of otolaryngology, ed 7, St. Louis, 1987, The CV Mosby Co.)

surgery is aimed primarily at removing the cervical lymph nodes. To do that, the sternocleidomastoid muscle, the internal jugular vein, and the spinal accessory nerve have to be sacrificed. These resections cause atrophy of the trapezius muscle, and the shoulder drops on one side.

Patients can be taught to do exercises to gradually replace the function of the lost muscles with that of other muscles. A patient may have some difficulty lifting the head and can achieve this by placing the hands behind the head. The patient is more comfortable and can breathe better when placed in mid-Fowler's position. Pressure dressings are best avoided in radical neck dissection because they compromise the blood supply to the skin flaps protecting the vital neck structures. The Hemovac (Fig. 23-12) is currently the best device available to keep constant drainage from the neck wound without pressure on the flaps. The Hemovac must be checked to see that it is working properly and that there is no edema, which might indicate hematoma.

Some alteration of appearance is readily visible, which may cause the person to feel somewhat conspicuous. Anger, grief, or denial may be part of the normal response to the change in body image. (For further information on psychologic support, refer to Chapter 12.)

Radical neck dissection can be performed without laryngectomy for persons whose primary malignant lesion is in the tongue, tonsil, lip, nasopharynx, or thyroid. Often the procedure accompanies other procedures and is termed a *composite* resection. Composite resections may include either radical neck dissection in addition to the removal of the mandible; removal of the mandible and resection of the floor of the mouth; or removal of the mandible, floor of the mouth, and the tongue. The nursing care for these patients is similar to the care given for maxillectomy and orbital exenteration (p. 653). Emotional reactions to this type of radical surgery may be profound. Disfigurement is readily visible, and reactions to the change in body image are marked. In addition to the usual fears of surgery and cancer, the patient having a composite resection may have fears of rejection and fears concerning the future.

☐ *Preoperative care*

The person who is to have a laryngectomy is told by the physician that breathing will occur through a special opening made in the neck and that normal speech will not be possible. This is often depressing to the patient because it threatens economic status, as well as life. In some instances, it is helpful to receive a visit from another person who has made a good recovery from laryngectomy and who has undergone rehabilitation successfully. In other instances, this visit may depress the patient further. Careful assessment must be made to determine if the person will benefit from such a visit and whether the visit should be made preoperatively, immediately after surgery, or later in the recovery period.

Often no one else can give a person the reassurance that speech can be regained as well as a fellow patient. Many large cities have a "Lost Chord Club" or a "New Voice Club," and the members are willing to visit hospitalized patients. Information regarding these clubs may be obtained by writing to the International Association of Laryngectomees.* Local speech rehabilitation centers may supply instructive films and other resources. The local chapter of the American Cancer Society and the local health department also have information available. If possible, the family also should learn about the method of esophageal speech that the person will learn to use.

→ DATA ANALYSIS: NURSING DIAGNOSES

Nursing diagnoses are determined from an assessment of patient data. Possible nursing diagnoses for the person undergoing total laryngectomy may include, but are not limited to, the following:

Diagnostic title	Possible etiologies
Ineffective airway clearance: potential	Surgery
Anxiety	Threat to self-concept, threat of death, threat to socioeconomic status
Potential for aspiration	Presence of laryngectomy tube
Body image disturbance	Disfiguring surgery
Impaired verbal communication	Surgery/loss of ability to speak normally
Altered nutrition: less than body requirements	Swallowing difficulty
Altered oral mucous membrane	Surgery
Pain: postoperative	Surgery

☐ *Postoperative care*

Postoperative care of the person is essentially the same as that described for tracheostomy (Chapter 24) except that these persons will have a *laryngectomy tube* in place, a tube that is shorter and wider in diameter than a tracheostomy tube. Some patients may not have a tube in the stoma after the operation because the stoma is a permanent one kept

*American Cancer Society, 777 Third Ave., New York, NY 10017.

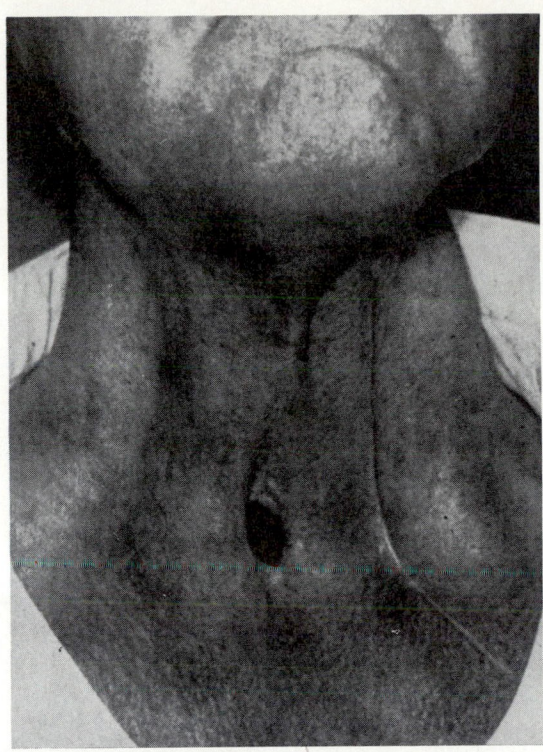

Fig. 23-13　After laryngectomy. Note scars of bilateral radical neck dissections. (From DeWeese, DD, and Saunders, WH: Textbook of otolaryngology, ed 6, St. Louis, 1982, The CV Mosby Co.)

open initially by the sutures and because their surgeon believes that there is less tissue reaction and a better stoma if no tube is used. If a laryngectomy tube is used, it will remain until the wound is healed and a permanent fistula has formed, usually in 2 to 3 weeks (Fig. 23-13). Frequent suctioning is necessary in the early postoperative period to keep the trachea free of secretions.

A *nasogastric tube* is usually inserted during the surgical procedure for the instillation of food and fluids at regular intervals postoperatively for about 10 days (Fig. 23-14). The use of the tube to give food is thought to minimize contamination of the pharyngeal and esophageal suture lines and to prevent fluid from leaking through the wound into the trachea before healing occurs. The nasogastric tube is removed as soon as the person can safely swallow. The person then needs careful attention in the first attempts to swallow. There may be the sensation of choking, as well as severe coughing, that is frightening and painful. Aspiration cannot occur because the trachea no longer communicates with the esophagus.

The sense of smell is affected after laryngectomy because breathing through the nose is impossible, therefore, the patient does not receive olfactory sensations.

SPEECH REHABILITATION

Esophageal speech is the primary speech method used following total laryngectomy (see the box on p. 660). It is

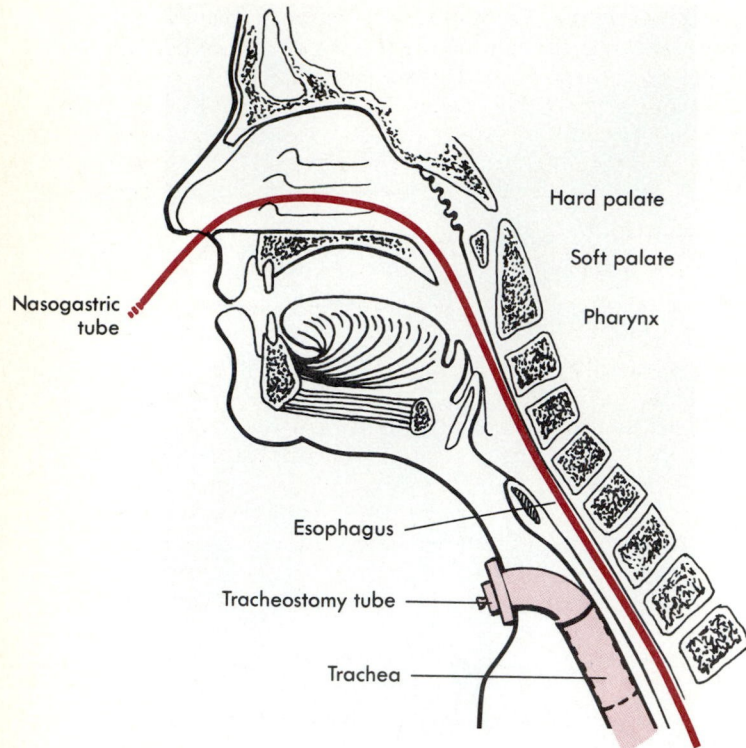

Nasogastric tube

Hard palate

Soft palate

Pharynx

Esophagus

Tracheostomy tube

Trachea

Fig. 23-14 Position of tracheostomy tube and nasogastric tube following total laryngectomy.

started as soon as the esophageal suture line is healed. To learn esophageal speech, the patient must first practice burping. This provides the moving column of air needed for sound, while folds of tissue at the opening of the esophagus act as the vibrating surface. The patients must learn to coordinate articulation with esophageal vocalization made possible by aspirating air into the esophagus. The new voice sounds are natural, although somewhat hoarse. The qualities of speech provided by the use of the naso-

Speech methods following total laryngectomy	
Esophageal speech	Speech produced by expelling swallowed air (burping) across constricted tissue in the pharyngoesophageal segment
Tracheal-esophageal prosthesis	Formation of a tracheal-esophageal fistula with insertion of a silicone prosthesis that produces a sound in the esophagus
External speech aids	Mechanical devices, such as a vibrator or electronic artificial larynx, used externally

pharynx are still present. The patient may have digestive difficulty while learning to speak; this is caused by swallowing air during practice, by unusual strain on abdominal muscles, and by nervous tension. Digestive difficulties usually abate with proficiency in speaking.

Most patients learn esophageal speech best at a special clinic. Although some individuals may need to go to a nearby city for this instruction, they usually must remain away from home for only 1 or 2 weeks. Motivation and persistent effort are essential in learning this kind of speech; encouragement and support from the professional staff and the patient's significant others are important to the patient's morale. About 75% of all patients who have their larynx removed master some sort of speech, and the average person can return to work 1 or 2 months after leaving the hospital. Information on esophageal speech can be obtained from the American Speech and Hearing As-

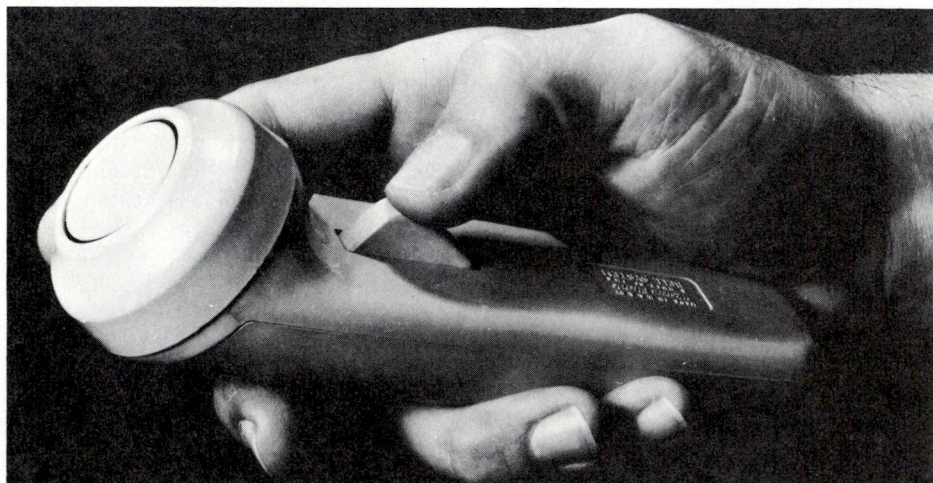

Fig. 23-15 Battery-powered electronic artificial larynx for patient who has total laryngectomy and cannot learn esophageal speech. (Courtesy Illinois Bell Telephone Co.)

Patient teaching following total laryngectomy

1. Wear a scarf or shirt with closed collar of porous material (to warm and screen air over stoma).
2. Use caution while taking a bath or shower (to prevent aspiration of water in stoma).
3. Check with surgeon concerning swimming or boating; if swimming is permitted, use a special snorkle device designed for tracheostomies.
4. Use available community resources for support and speech rehabilitation as necessary (for example, laryngectomee clubs, American Cancer Society).
5. Seek immediate medical attention for respiratory tract infection or signs of stomal bleeding.
6. Continue medical follow-up per physician instructions.

---

sociation,* the International Association of Laryngectomees, and the American Cancer Society.

If a person is unable to learn esophageal speech in 60 to 90 days after surgery, a *speech aid* such as a vibrator or an electronic artificial larynx (Fig. 23-15) may be prescribed. Various mechanical devices are available, and the new ones permit a natural type of speech, providing pitch inflections and volume control. The local chapter of the American Cancer Society or the local telephone company can provide information about the purchase of these devices.

Several surgical and prosthetic techniques are being refined, one of which is a *tracheal-esophageal prosthesis* inserted in a surgical tracheal-esophageal fistula. The fistula can be created during the laryngectomy or postoperatively, usually after 2 to 3 months to allow for good wound healing, especially if radiation was used preoperatively. Insertion of the "duck-bill" prosthesis permits exhaled air to pass into the esophagus and exit through the mouth. Pharyngoesophageal or cricopharyngeal muscles are used to produce sound, and words are formed by the mouth in the usual manner. The stoma must be blocked during speech, either by a finger placed over the stoma or by a special tracheostomal valve inserted after the person has learned to use the prosthesis. The person is taught to remove, clean, and reinsert the prosthesis following its blockage by mucus.[9]

DISCHARGE TEACHING

Persons with laryngectomies must take special precautions because of the permanent tracheostomies (see the box above). Usually by the time of discharge, patients with laryngectomies do not need suctioning of the tracheostomy,

*10801 Rockville Pike, Rockville, MD 20852

but can cough up secretions. If suctioning is deemed necessary, patients or their families need to be told where to secure the necessary suction equipment and how to care for themselves. Suction equipment can be rented for home use or obtained in many communities through the local chapter of the American Cancer Society.

■ SUMMARY

1. The major infections of the nose and sinuses are rhinitis (common cold), allergic rhinitis (hay fever), chronic rhinitis secondary to repeated infections or allergy, and sinusitis caused by a bacteria or virus.
2. Persons with allergic rhinitis (hay fever) are usually sensitive to pollen of grasses such as ragweed (see Chapter 38).
3. It is important for persons who are allergic to know which allergens they are allergic to and to avoid these allergens if at all possible. For this reason, they need to know how to prepare an environmentally controlled bedroom (see Chapter 38).
4. Persons with acute sinusitis usually have a severe headache and pain over the infected area. Fever is common and is related to the amount of sinus obstruction. If the sinus is abscessed, fever may be as high as 40° C (104° F).
5. Subjective assessment of the person with a nose or sinus problem includes a careful history of previous infections, how they were treated and self-treatment by the person including the use of over-the-counter medications.
6. Acetaminophen is recommended instead of aspirin in persons with nasal problems because aspirin may be associated with nasal polyposis.
7. There are six surgical procedures that may be used to treat chronic sinusitis. These are antral irrigation, Caldwell-Luc procedure, ethmoidotomy, sphenoidotomy, ethmoidectomy, and osteopathic flap.
8. Postoperative care for persons having sinus surgery includes the following:
   a. Place patient in side-lying position until reacted from anesthesia and then mid-Fowler's position.
   b. Place ice compresses over nose or ice bag over maxillary or frontal sinuses.
   c. Monitor for bleeding and for decreased visual acuity such as diplopia, which indicates damage to the optic nerve.
   d. Provide frequent mouth care.
   e. Change nasal pad when soiled.
   f. Teach patient not to blow nose for at least 48 hours *after* packing is removed.
   g. Instruct patient to avoid constipation because Valsalva maneuver can cause bleeding.
9. The most common throat inflammation is acute pharyngitis. Hemolytic streptococci, staphylococci, and other bacteria and viruses may be the source of infection. Pharyngitis caused by *Neisseria gonorrhoeae* is being seen more commonly in both men and women.

Putting knowledge to practice

- Review the anatomy of the nose and throat.
- How do your mouth and throat feel when your nose is blocked and you are mouth breathing? What can you do to keep the mucous membranes moist?
- What actions can you take to prevent spreading a cold to others?
- What resources are available in your community to assist persons who have had a total laryngectomy?

---

10. To obtain material for culture and sensitivity, a throat culture is taken to identify the organism and determine appropriate antibiotic therapy.
11. To prevent superinfection, prophylactic antibiotics are often prescribed for persons with pharyngitis who have a history of rheumatic fever or bacterial endocarditis.
12. Obstructions of the nose, such as a deviated septum, are often treated surgically by submucous resection or septoplasty.
13. Postoperative care following nasal surgery includes the following:
    a. Monitor for hemorrhage.
    b. Place patient in mid-Fowler's position to decrease local edema.
    c. Place ice compresses over the nose for 24 hours and as needed.
    d. Provide food and fluids as tolerated.
    e. Provide frequent oral care.
    f. Change dressing under nose as needed.
    g. Teach patient to avoid blowing nose for 48 hours after packing is removed to prevent bleeding.
    h. Teach patient to avoid constipation and vigorous coughing until healing occurs because coughing and Valsalva maneuver may initiate bleeding.
    i. Explain that stools may be tarry for several days.
14. Progressive or persistent hoarseness that lasts longer than two weeks requires medical evaluation for cancer of the larynx.
15. Carcinoma of the larynx is treated with a partial or total laryngectomy.
16. Partial laryngectomy may be achieved by laryngofissure, hemilaryngectomy, or supraglottic partial laryngectomy after which the person will be able to speak.
17. Total laryngectomy is necessary when cancer of the larynx is far advanced. Persons with total laryngectomy are unable to speak.
18. Radical neck dissection is commonly performed along with total laryngectomy because of the possible metastasis to the neck.
    a. Postoperatively the person will have a laryngectomy tube and a nasogastric tube in place.
    b. Communication is impaired because of the loss of ability to speak and the person will require speech rehabilitation.
    c. Esophageal speech, which requires expelling swallowed air (burping), is the most commonly used speech method.
    d. For the person who is unable to learn esophageal speech after 60 to 90 days, a speech aid such as electronic larynx may be prescribed.
19. Persons with a total laryngectomy will have a permanent tracheostomy and need to be taught certain precautions including the following:
    a. Wear a scarf or shirt with a closed collar of porous material.
    b. Use caution when showering or bathing to prevent aspiration of water in stoma.
    c. Check with surgeon concerning swimming or boating. A special snorkel device for use with a tracheostomy is available.
    d. Support groups, such as laryngectomee clubs, exist.

REFERENCES AND SELECTED READINGS
Contemporary

1. American Cancer Society: 1987 Cancer facts and figures, New York, 1987, The Society.
2. Anderson, S, and Bouwens, E: Chronic health problems: concepts and application, St. Louis, 1981, The CV Mosby Co.
3. Annvas, AA, and others: Groningen prosthesis for voice rehabilitation after laryngectomy, Clin Otolaryngol 9:51-51, 1984.
4. Argawal, MK, and others: Fibrosarcoma of nose and paranasal sinuses, J Surg Oncol 15:53-57, 1980.
5. Baker, KH, and Feldman, JE: Cancers of the head and neck, Cancer Nursing 10(6):293-299, 1987.
6. Burke, RH: A simplified nasal packing, J Oral Maxillofac Surg 43:555, 1985.
7. Carroll, PF: Laryngospasm, Nurs 86 16(5):33, 1986.
8. Causes of stuffy nose: external nasal deformity, Hosp Med 21:(5):194-198, 1985.
9. Chisholm, S, and others: Duck-bill prosthesis: words of hope for the laryngectomy patient, Nurs 86 16(3):29-31, 1986.
10. DeWeese, DD, and Saunders, WH: Otolaryngology, head and neck surgery, ed 7, St. Louis, 1987, The CV Mosby Co.
11. Ebersole, P, and Hess, P: Toward healthy aging, ed 2, St. Louis, 1985, The CV Mosby Co.
12. Eichel, B: Ethmoiditis: pathophysiology and medical management, Otolaryngol Clin North Am 18(1):43-53, 1985.

---

*References preceded by an asterisk are particularly well suited for student reading.

13. Estelle, R, Simons, R, and Simons, KJ: Pharmacologic treatment of rhinitis, Clin Rev Allergy 2:237-253, 1984.

14. Feinstein, D: What to teach the patient who's had a total laryngectomy, RN 50(4):53-57, 1987.

15. Fosso, BA: Sore throat, antibiotics and rheumatic fever, Fam Pract 2:101-107, 1985.

16. *Gannon, EP: Giving your patient meticulous mouth care, Nurs 80 10(3):70-75, 1980.

17. Griffin, CW, and Lockhart, JS: Learning to swallow again, Am J Nurs 87:314-317, March 1987.

18. Harris, LL, and Kraege, J: After T-E puncture: relearning to speak, Am J Nurs 86:55-58, 1986.

19. Harold, ML: Rehabilitation of the dysphagic client following ablative surgery for laryngeal cancer, J Soc Otorhinlaryngol Head Neck Nurses 5(2):16-18, 1987.

20. Hassard, AD, and Holness, RO: The "crossbow" incision and nasal flap: its blood supply and clinical application, Head Neck Surg 7:135-138, 1984.

21. Hendrickson, FR: Radiation therapy treatment of larynx cancers, Cancer 55:2058-2061, 1985.

22. Holt, JE: Orbital blowout fractures, Ear Nose Throat J 62:346-351, 1983.

23. *Hutton, B, and Hutton, J: Living with facial prosthesis: a guide to patient care, Am J Nurs 84:50-52, 1984.

24. Innes, AJ, and Gates, N: ENT surgery and disorders, with notes on nursing care and clinical management, London, 1985, Faber & Faber.

25. Jafek, BW: Intranasal ethmoidectomy, Otolaryngol Clin North Am 18(1):61-67, 1985.

26. Johnson, JT, Neman, RK, and Olson, JE: Persistent hoarseness: an aggressive approach for early detection of laryngeal cancer, Postgrad Med 67:122-126, 1980.

27. *Kane, KK: Carotid artery rupture in advanced head and neck cancer patients, Oncolog Nurs Forum 10(1):14-18, 1983.

28. Kennedy, DW, and others: Endoscopic sinus surgery: ambulatory surgery, AORN J 42:932-936, 1985.

29. *Key, G: Stopping nosebleeds in the elderly: pressure, cautery, or packing? Geriatrics 36:74-80, 1981.

30. Knegt, PP, and others: Carcinoma of the paranasal sinuses: results of a prospective pilot study, Cancer 56:57-62, 1985.

31. Konda, M, and others: Prognostic factors influencing relapse of squamous cell carcinoma of the maxillary sinus, Cancer 55:190-196, 1985.

32. Konrad, HR: Carcinoma of the larynx, Hosp Med 20(8):165-179, 1984.

33. Krupp, MA, Chatton, MJ, and Werdegar, D: Current medical diagnoses and treatment, 1985, Los Altos, Calif, 1985, Lange Medical Publications.

34. Larson, GL: Rehabilitation for the patient with head and neck cancer, Am J Nurs 82:119-120, 1982.

35. *Lyons, RJ: Surgical implants: voice prosthesis, AORN J 37:1369-1373, 1983.

36. *Lyons, RJ: The head and neck patient, AORN J 40:751-760, 1984.

37. Mack, RM: Lessons from living with cancer, N Engl J Med 311:1640-1644. 1984

38. Mandel, JH: Pharyngeal infections: causes, findings, and management, Postgrad Med 77:187-193, 1985.

39. McCormick, GP, and others: Artificial speech devices, Am J Nurs 82:121-122, 1982.

40. Minx, SM, and others: Carcinoma of the parasinus: perioperative nursing responsibilities, AORN J 42:671-681, 1985.

41. Moore, JC: Establishment of an outpatient ENT clinic, AORN J 31:620-626, 1980.

42. Neal, GD: External ethmoidectomy, Otolaryngol Clin North Am 18:55-60, 1985.

43. Norante, JD: Surgical management of sinusitis, Ear Nose Throat J 63:155-162, 1984.

44. Norris, JL: Fiberoptic endoscopy: where to go from here, laryngoscopy, AANA J 52:611-613, 1984.

45. *Patry-Lahey, R: Doing it better: helping a laryngectomy patient go home, Nurs 85 15(3):63-64, 1985.

46. Richardson, JL: Vocational adjustment after total laryngectomy, Arch Phys Med Rehabil 64:172-175, 1983.

47. Romm, S: Cancer of the larynx: current concepts of diagnosis and treatment, Surg Clin North Am 66:109-118, 1986.

48. Schweiger, J: Oral assessment, Am J Nurs 80:654-657, 1980.

49. Segal, C, and others: Adenotonsillectomies on a surgical day-clinic basis, Laryngoscope 93:1205-1208, 1983.

50. Singer, MI, Blom, ED, and Hamaker, RC: Voice rehabilitation after total laryngectomy, J Otolaryngol 12:329-334, 1983.

51. *Stephens, DJ: An information guide for patients receiving head and neck irradiation, Oncol Nurs Forum 11(5):75-80, 1984.

52. Ulbricht, GF: Laryngectomy rehabilitation: a woman's viewpoint, Women Health 11:131-136, 1986.

53. Weingrad, DN, and Spiro, RH: Complications after laryngectomy, Am J Surg 146:517-520, 1983.

54. Wetmore, SJ, and others: Long-term results of the Blom-Singer speech rehabilitation procedure, Arch Otolaryngol 111:106-109, 1985.

55. Wyngaarden, JB, and Smith, LH: Cecil textbook of medicine, ed 17, Philadelphia, 1985, WB Saunders Co.

56. Yarington, CT: The Caldwell-Luc operation revisited, Ann Otol Rhinol Laryngol 93:380-384, 1984.

Classic

57. Baker, DC: Intranasal steroid injections: indications, technique, results, complications, Laryngoscope 89:998-1003, 1979.

58. Fiumara, NJ: Pharyngeal infection with Neisseria gonorrhea, Sex Transm Dis 6:264-266, 1979.

59. Lucente, FE: Psychological problems in otolaryngology, Laryngoscope 83:1684-1689, 1973.

60. McCaffrey, TV, and Kern, EB: Clinical evaluation for nasal obstruction: a study of 1000 patients, Arch Otolaryngol 105:542-545, 1979.

61. *Oser, J: Oral cancer: coping with the changes, Am J Nurs 79:1418-1419, 1979.

24

The Patient with Pulmonary Problems

WILMA J. PHIPPS and MARY KAY LEHMAN

CHAPTER OBJECTIVES

After studying this chapter, the student should be able to:

- Differentiate between restrictive and obstructive pulmonary disorders
- Describe the nature of viral respiratory infections and methods of assisting effective coughing.
- Compare classic, atypical, aspiration, and hematogenous pneumonia.
- Describe measures to promote oxygenation, facilitate breathing, and provide ventilation and hydration.
- Describe incidence, preventive measures, and therapeutic approaches to tuberculosis.
- Compare fungal infections of the respiratory tract.
- Explain the pathophysiology of adult respiratory distress syndrome (ARDS).
- Describe incidence, prevention, and therapy for lung cancer.
- Describe types of chest surgery and the care of the patient undergoing chest surgery (including patients with chest tubes).
- Describe the pathophysiologic conditions of chest trauma (for instance fractured ribs, penetrating wounds, and pneumothorax).
- Explain the pathophysiologic conditions and interventions for chronic obstructive pulmonary disease.
- Describe the nature of respiratory insufficiency and the care of the patient with an artificial airway or mechanical ventilation.

■ ANATOMY AND PHYSIOLOGY OF THE RESPIRATORY TRACT

The main purpose of respiration is to provide oxygen to body cells and to remove excess carbon dioxide from them. For respiration to take place there must be a way to deliver oxygen (O_2) to the body and a circulatory system to carry it to the cells and to remove carbon dioxide (CO_2) from them. The transport of O_2 is accomplished through the upper and lower airway.

The upper airway consists of the nose and nasopharynx, the mouth and oropharynx, and the larynx. The lower airway is made up of the trachea, mainstem bronchi, bronchioles, and alveolar ducts, which lead to the alveoli themselves. The airway, in addition to providing a passageway for air, serves three functions: *filtering*, *warming*, and *humidifying* air.

Air inspired through an intact respiratory tree is cleansed of all particles larger than 2 μm in diameter before reaching the alveoli. The removal of this particulate matter, such as dust and bacteria, preserves the sterility of the alveolus. Foreign material is filtered through several mechanisms. *Goblet cells* in the epithelial layer of the airway secrete copious amounts of a thick mucopolysaccharide substance, mucus, which coats the airways and entraps particles. *Cilia*, which are found as far into the respiratory tree as the bronchi, then propel the mucus and foreign material up into the pharynx where it can be expelled by coughing or sneezing.

The *warming* and *humidifying* functions are made possible by the rich capillary blood supply in the submucosal layer of the airways. During inspiration, air is heated to body temperature, and up to 1000 ml of water is used per day to raise the humidity of inspired air to at least 80%. On expiration some of this water is reabsorbed, thus conserving fluid; an average of 300 ml of water per day is lost in normal respiration.

The basic gas exchange unit of the respiratory system is the alveolus. Alveoli, which number over 300 million in the healthy adult, are minute sacs that arise from alveolar ducts. The ducts are composed of smooth muscle that is capable of expanding and contracting; the alveolus itself is composed of a single layer of squamous epithelium and an elastic basement membrane. These two layers, in addition to the endothelial and basement layers of the adjacent capillary, form the *alveolar-capillary membrane* or *interface* (Fig. 24-1). It is across this membrane, a distance of less than 1μm, that gas exchange takes place.

The lungs themselves are subdivided into lobes (Fig. 24-2). The right lung has three lobes: upper, middle, and lower. The left lung has two lobes: upper and lower. Air is conducted to each lobe through lobar bronchi that branch off the mainstem bronchus. An important difference between the right and left lungs is the size of the airways leading to them. The right bronchus is significantly wider and shorter and extends at a straighter angle from the trachea, making it the more likely lodging point for aspirated material. The left bronchus is narrower and extends

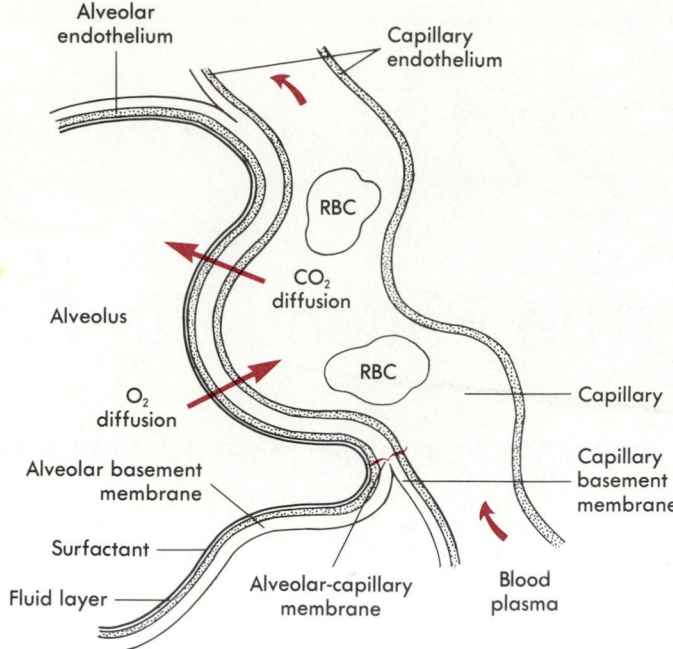

Fig. 24-1 Alveolar-capillary membrane.

at more of a right angle off the trachea, making it more difficult to suction secretions from the left lung.

The lungs lie in and are protected by the thoracic cavity. This bony cage is composed of the sternum and ribs anteriorly and the ribs, scapulae, and vertebral column posteriorly. On the anterior surface, the apices of the lungs lie just above the clavicle and extend posteriorly to the eleventh or twelfth rib.

The thoracic cavity is lined with pleurae. The pleura is a continuous *serous* membrane, one surface of which lines the inside of the rib cage (parietal pleura), while the other surface (visceral pleura) covers the lungs. The space between the two surfaces is known as a *potential space*. It normally contains a few milliliters of *serous fluid* that prevents friction rub when the two surfaces come together.

There are three processes involved in respiration. These are ventilation, perfusion, and diffusion. *Ventilation* involves the movement of air in and out of the tracheobroncheal tree, thereby delivering oxygen to the alveoli and removing carbon dioxide. *Perfusion* refers to the blood flow in the capillary bed in the lung. Fear or an injection of adrenalin increases perfusion, whereas vagal stimulation or acetylcholine decreases it. During *diffusion* there is movement of gases (O_2 and CO_2) across the alveolar-capillary membrane, with the flow being from the area of greater concentration to that of lesser concentration, resulting in alveocapillary equilibrium.

■ Pulmonary ventilation

Air moves in and out of the lungs as a result of the principle of fluid flow; that is, movement is from an area

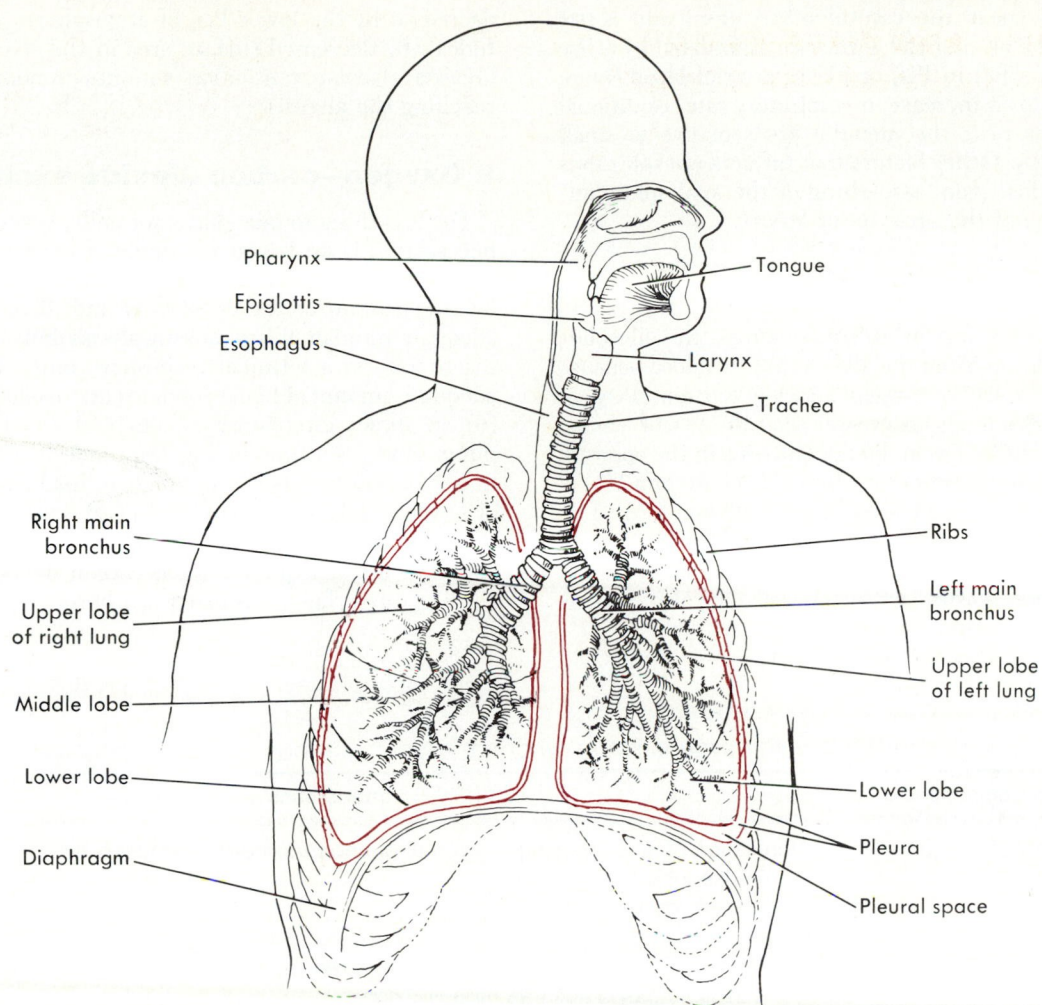

Pharynx

Epiglottis

Esophagus

Tongue

Larynx

Trachea

Right main bronchus

Ribs

Left main bronchus

Upper lobe of right lung

Upper lobe of left lung

Middle lobe

Lower lobe

Lower lobe

Diaphragm

Pleura

Pleural space

Fig. 24-2 Anatomy of the thorax and lungs.

of greater pressure to an area of lower pressure. At the start of inspiration the atmospheric air pressure is greater than alveolar pressure; therefore air moves through the respiratory passageway into the alveoli. When the alveolar pressure exceeds atmospheric pressure, expiration occurs, and air moves out of the lungs into the atmosphere.

The pressure gradient between the alveoli and the atmosphere is established by changes in the size of the thorax cavity. As the size of the thorax increases, pressure decreases, and air flows into the lung. Thoracic size is increased by contraction of the diaphragm and the external intercostal muscles. The diaphragm descends as it contracts and flattens, increasing the longitudinal diameter of the thorax. The external intercostal muscles pull the ribs up and out, elevating the sternum and increasing both the anteroposterior and lateral diameters of the chest. The accessory muscles (scalene, sternocleidomastoid, trapezius, and pectoralis) are active only in labored respiration.

As the thorax expands, it pulls the lungs with it because of cohesion between the moist surfaces of the lungs and chest wall. Expiration is normally a passive process that results from the elastic recoil of the lungs and thoracic muscles. Any condition that interferes with contraction of the diaphragm or intercostal muscles decreases pulmonary ventilation.

■ Control of respiration

Breathing is an automatic process, but it may also be controlled voluntarily; that is, although humans do not have to think about breathing, they can breathe slower or faster at will. Voluntary control of respiration is centered in the cerebral cortex, from which impulses are sent to innervate the muscles of respiration.

Automatic control of respiration is centered in the medulla and pons. The pons is responsible for maintaining rhythmicity of respirations. The respiratory center that is located in the medulla is controlled primarily by the carbon dioxide tension (P_{CO_2}), oxygen tension (P_{O_2}), and acidity (pH) of arterial blood (p. 721). Chemoreceptors in the carotid bodies (near the carotid bifurcation) and aortic bodies (near the arch of the aorta) are stimulated by a rise in Pco_2 or by a fall in Po_2 or pH of arterial blood (more acid), leading to an increase in respiratory rate. Additional chemoreceptors near the medulla are sensitive to small changes in Pco_2. Other factors that influence respirations include emotions, pain, stretching of the anal sphincter, and stimulation of the pharynx or larynx.

■ Gas exchange in the lung

In the alveoli, oxygen diffuses across the alveolar-capillary membrane from the alveoli into the blood because the partial pressure of oxygen (oxygen tension, Po_2) of *alveolar air* (100 mm Hg) is greater than the Po_2 of venous blood (40 mm Hg). Carbon dioxide diffuses in the opposite direction because the Pco_2 of *venous blood* (46 mm Hg) is greater than the Pco_2 of alveolar air (40 mm Hg). The pulmonary diffusion capacity for carbon dioxide is much greater than the capacity for oxygen, and thus carbon dioxide diffuses more easily. Diffusion capacity of oxygen is decreased by the lower Po_2 of atmospheric air (high altitudes), by decreased surface area in the alveoli, or by decreased alveolar ventilation volumes (amount of oxygen reaching the alveoli).

■ Oxygen—carbon dioxide exchange

For breathing to take place normally, several factors are necessary: (1) an adequate supply of oxygen in the environment, (2) a patent airway, (3) a normally functioning bellows motion of the chest wall and diaphragm, (4) an adequate number of functioning alveoli and capillaries that together form a terminal respiratory unit (TRU), (5) an adequate amount of hemoglobin to carry oxygen to the cells, (6) an intact circulatory system and an effective heart pump, and (7) a functioning respiratory center. Problems in one or more of these can result in inadequate exchange of oxygen and carbon dioxide and, if severe enough, can cause death. Table 24-1 lists some of the conditions that can lead to inadequate oxygen-carbon dioxide exchange. Each of these factors is discussed here.

Table 24-1 Factors interfering with oxygenation and normal oxygen—carbon dioxide exchange

Necessary component	Interference
Adequate supply of oxygen	Inhalation of air containing oxygen at subnormal pressure caused by: Smoke inhalation Carbon monoxide poisoning High altitudes Dilution of inspired air with inert gases (nitrogen, helium, hydrogen, methane, or anesthetic gases such as nitrous oxide)
Patent airway	Interference with the passage of oxygen from air through tracheobronchial tree to alveolar-capillary membrane caused by mechanical obstruction such as drowning or foreign bodies in tracheobronchial tree: Children (aspiration of objects such as pennies, pins, or jacks) Unconscious adults (tongue obstructing airway, aspirated vomitus, or loose dentures) Mucus plug resulting in atelectasis Allergic reactions resulting in bronchoconstriction, increased mucus secretions, and increased capillary permeability
Normally functioning bellows	Trauma to chest wall with possible sequelae of paradoxical breathing, pneumothorax, and mediastinal shift Muscle or nerve trauma or impairment (quadriplegia, paraplegia, poliomyelitis, myasthenia gravis, Guillain-Barré syndrome, Landry's ascending paralysis, and muscular dystrophy)
Adequate functioning alveoli and capillaries (TRU)	Pulmonary edema Adult respiratory disease syndrome (interstitial edema) Physiologic shunts Damage to alveolar-capillary membrane secondary to conditions such as pulmonary emphysema
Adequate amount of hemoglobin	Severe anemia Carbon monoxide poisoning Methemoglobinemia
Intact circulatory system and pump	Congestive heart failure Hemorrhage
Functioning respiratory center	Depression of respiratory center by drugs (heroin, morphine, barbiturates, alcohol, or a combination of alcohol with a tranquilizer or barbiturates) Increased intracranial pressure (head injury or disease such as meningitis)

■ MAINTAINING AN ADEQUATE SUPPLY OF OXYGEN IN THE ENVIRONMENT

High altitudes do not change the composition of the air, but the oxygen pressure (PO_2) decreases.[43] Persons exposed to high altitudes, such as pilots, astronauts, mountain climbers, and those moving to high altitudes, have various reactions depending on the rate at which hypoxia develops, the degree of oxygen requirements as determined by physical exertion, and the duration of exposure.[43]

The initial reaction to high altitudes results in the same signs and symptoms seen in anyone experiencing oxygen lack. Headache, dizziness, breathlessness, weakness, nausea, sweating, palpitation, dimness of vision, partial deafness, and sleeplessness occur with moderate hypoxia.[43] With exertion, dyspnea and other symptoms worsen. These signs and symptoms have been referred to as *mountain sickness* because they are evident as persons drive or take a train through altitudes higher than those to which they have been accustomed.

These symptoms gradually disappear over days or weeks depending on the altitude, and the person is eventually able to carry out more activities without becoming short of breath. This is known as *acclimatization* and is caused in part by an increased capacity for supplying oxygen to the tissues and in part by overcoming the consequences of hypocapnia produced by excessive breathing.[43]

The factors involved in acclimatization include: (1) a sustained increase in alveolar ventilation, (2) adjustment in the acid-base composition of the blood and other body fluids, (3) an increase in oxygen-carrying capacity, and (4) an increase in cardiac output.[43]

Persons moving to higher altitudes, such as mountain climbers, are advised to allow time for their bodies to adjust to changes in various altitudes. Trained climbers, especially those ascending to very high altitudes, allow themselves weeks or even months at base camps at various altitudes in preparation for their ascent.[43]

■ MAINTAINING A PATENT AIRWAY

Several measures may be used to ensure a patent airway. The most basic measure involves simply positioning the person in such a way as to prevent obstruction of the airway. This is most relevant in resuscitation or in caring for an unconscious person. The position of choice is supine or side-lying with the neck hyperextended. Persons who are unconscious or very lethargic may suffer airway obstruction if the tongue should fall back and cover the glottis; the side-lying position prevents this from happening.

When a person has a mechanical obstruction of the airway and is expected to be unconscious for some time, it may be necessary to use an artificial airway (p. 739).

■ MAINTAINING BELLOWS FUNCTION OF THE CHEST WALL AND DIAPHRAGM

Whenever there is interference with the bellows function of the chest wall, there are changes in breathing pattern. The major cause of disruption of the bellows function is trauma to the chest involving fractures of the ribs or penetrating chest wounds (p. 715). These conditions and their sequelae of paradoxic breathing and pneumothorax are discussed on p. 715.

■ MAINTAINING AN ADEQUATE NUMBER OF TERMINAL RESPIRATORY UNITS

The individual with pulmonary disease may have impaired ability to aerate alveoli. The impairment may be related to several factors. These include (1) inability to move adequate amounts of air in and out of the lungs, (2) interference with alveolar expansion secondary to an accumulation of secretions resulting in collapse of portions of the lungs (*atelectasis*), and (3) restriction of lung expansion by mechanical factors such as air in the pleural space (*pneumothorax*) or fluid or blood in the pleural space (*pleural effusion* or *hemothorax*). An increase in respiratory rate and pulse rate indicates that the body is trying to compensate for hypoxia. Patients who must make a conscious effort to breathe become very tired. They also become anxious because of shortness of breath and hypoxia.

■ MAINTAINING TRANSPORTATION OF OXYGEN AND ADEQUATE OXYGENATION OF TISSUES

For oxygen to be supplied to the cells there must be (1) an adequate amount of hemoglobin available to transport oxygen and (2) an effective heart pump and circulatory system to deliver the oxygen to the tissues. The amount of oxygen delivered to body tissues each minute equals the cardiac output in liters per minute times the number of milliliters of oxygen contained in 1 L of arterial blood. In the resting state this is about 5×200, or 1000 ml O_2/min. About one fourth of this is used by the tissues, and three fourths returns to the heart in mixed venous blood. During exercise the amount of oxygen contained in 1 L of arterial blood does not increase, but the cardiac output does increase. With a cardiac output of 24 L/min, the oxygen delivered would be 24×200, or 4800 ml/min. The tissues would use three fourths of this amount, and only one fourth would be returned to the heart in mixed venous blood.[99]

An inadequate amount of hemoglobin (such as occurs in anemia), an inadequate heart pump, or a problem with the circulatory system can all have a deleterious effect on the delivery of oxygen. In these situations the basic problem is treated in an attempt to increase the amount of available hemoglobin, to strengthen the heart pump and thus increase the cardiac output, or to improve the circulatory system. As can be seen in Table 24-1, severe anemia, carbon monoxide poisoning, methemoglobinemia, congestive heart failure, and hemorrhage are possible interferences that must be corrected before an optimal amount of oxygen is available to the tissues.

If hypotension is present secondary to hemorrhage or a failing heart pump, there may be several sequelae. These include (1) anginal pain, because the coronary vessels that normally extract almost the maximal amount of oxygen uptake to meet their needs and (2) changes in sensorium and behavior secondary to cerebral anoxia. If this situation continues and there is inadequate oxygenation of tissues, respiratory or cardiac arrest may result. If an arrest occurs, cardiopulmonary resuscitation (CPR) must be instituted. CPR is discussed in detail in Chapter 25, and the reader is referred there for details.

■ MAINTAINING A FUNCTIONING RESPIRATORY CENTER

Hypoventilation or apnea can occur if there is depression of the respiratory center by general anesthesia, morphine, heroin, barbiturates, or alcohol. Diseases of the central nervous system, such as bulbar poliomyelitis or meningitis, also depress the respiratory center, as does an increase in intracranial pressure. In these situations the patient's respirations must be assisted until the patient is able to maintain his or her own breathing. Intubation with an endotracheal tube, supplemental oxygen, and artificial respiration with a ventilator may all be required. The conditions causing depression of the respiratory center need to be identified and treated while the person's ventilation is being maintained. Details of management of patients in respiratory failure are discussed on p. 737.

■ PHYSIOLOGIC CHANGES WITH AGING

Several changes occur in the lungs and other parts of the respiratory tract with aging.

Structural alterations in the thorax may limit lung expansion. Ribs do not move as freely because of cartilage calcification and partial contraction of respiratory muscles.[21] Kyphosis (hunchback) decreases the transverse measurement of the thorax. The lungs become more rigid and less elastic. There is an increase in residual capacity and a decrease in vital capacity secondary to a decrease in the strength of the inspiratory and expiratory muscles. The result is incomplete lung expansion and basilar lung collapse. These changes may *not* cause an obvious decrease in lung performance unless there is an increase in activity or stress when dyspnea and other symptoms occur.[21]

As a result of these changes the aged are very vulnerable to respiratory problems if they develop a pulmonary infection or other illness that places stress on their already compromised respiratory system. For instance, changes in the thorax and altered muscle strength cause a decreased ability to clear the airway and cough effectively.

■ PREVENTION AND HEALTH EDUCATION

Disorders of the respiratory tract are probably the most common health problems for most persons in the Western world.

The objectives of health education in relation to pulmonary diseases are the same as for other diseases. Prevention, early diagnosis, prompt and often continued treatment, limitation of disability, and rehabilitation should be emphasized for all persons. Early symptoms of respiratory diseases are probably those most often ignored by the general population. Perhaps this is because, with the exception of influenza and some types of pneumonia, respiratory diseases often develop slowly and progress without the individual's awareness.

Because of the deleterious effects of cigarette smoking on the cardiopulmonary systems, a concerted effort is indicated to teach persons about the hazards of smoking. In recent years many organizations, most notably the American Lung Association (ALA), the American Cancer Society (ACS), the American Heart Association (AHA), and the federal government, have launched campaigns to reduce cigarette smoking in the United States. A major emphasis has been on preventing children and teenagers from beginning to smoke. These campaigns have been somewhat successful, and it is now estimated that only one third of the adult population in the United States smokes. However, the number of women smokers has increased, and this is reflected in the ever-rising increase in morbidity and mortality from lung disease, especially cancer of the lung and chronic obstructive pulmonary diseases, among women.

■ Primary prevention: prevention of disease

Because the cause of many respiratory disorders is known, prevention is possible. The major emphasis is on avoiding respiratory infections and educating the public about the risks of cigarette smoking. Health practices helpful in preventing infection are outlined in the box below.

Prevention of respiratory infections

Preventing spread of infection

1. Isolate the infected person.
2. Teach the infected person to cover nose and mouth when coughing or sneezing so that droplet nuclei are not released into the air.

Maintaining resistance to infection

1. Eat a balanced diet.
2. Get adequate rest and sleep.
3. Avoid crowds during periods of prevalent respiratory infections.
4. Receive annual influenza immunization and pneumonia vaccine every 3 to 5 years if over age 65 or if younger with chronic heart, lung, or renal disease.

Guidelines for early detection of major pulmonary disorders

1. Signs or symptoms requiring immediate medical follow-up
   a. Chronic cough
   b. Sputum
   c. Dyspnea (shortness of breath)
2. American Cancer Society recommendations for screening for cancer of the lung
   a. Yearly chest x-ray examination for men over age 40
   b. Yearly examination for heavy cigarette smokers over age 50, for persons who started smoking at age of 15 or younger, and for smokers working in or near asbestos

---

■ Secondary prevention: early detection

Medical attention should be sought for respiratory symptoms that do not subside within 2 weeks. Guidelines for early detection are listed in the box above.

Major health problems of the respiratory system

There are several ways to classify disorders affecting the lung and respiration, but one of the most useful and commonly used is to divide them into restrictive and obstructive diseases.

In *restrictive lung disease*, there is a restriction in lung volume and a reduction in lung compliance. As a result there is a reduction in total lung capacity (TLC) and a decrease in vital capacity (VC) to less than the predicted norm.

In contrast, in *obstructive lung disease*, there is an increase in airway resistance resulting in prolonged exhalation. This results in an increase in residual volume (RV) while TLC may be normal or increased. Thus pulmonary function tests are necessary to establish the diagnosis. A comparison of the characteristic changes in pulmonary function tests for restrictive and obstructive disease is shown Table 24-2.

There are several conditions that can cause restrictive pulmonary disease and not all of these are discussed here. Some of the conditions that are *not* discussed include atelectasis; fluid or air in the pleural space; changes in the bony thorax, such as kyphoscoliosis, limitation of thoracic mobility from abdominal tumors, ascites, or paralytic ileus; neuromuscular depression from disease or drugs, that is, Guillian-Barré syndrome, poliomyelitis, myasthenia gravis, and CNS depression from heroin or morphine.

Conditions that result in restrictive or obstructive pulmonary disease that are discussed in this chapter are the following.

1. Restrictive pulmonary disorders
   a. Infectious diseases of the pulmonary tract
      (1) Viral: acute bronchitis
      (2) Bacterial: pneumonia, tuberculosis
      (3) Fungal: histoplasmosis, coccidiomycosis, blastomycosis
   b. Occupational lung disease
      (1) Inhalation of inorganic dust: silicosis
      (2) Inhalation of organic dust: allergic alveolitis (farmer's lung)
   c. Adult respiratory distress syndrome (ARDS)
   d. Carcinoma of the lung
2. Obstructive pulmonary disorders
   a. Chronic bronchitis
   b. Pulmonary emphysema
   c. Asthma

Table 24-2 Comparison of pulmonary function test results in restrictive and obstructive disease

Test	Restrictive	Obstructive
FVC	Decreased	Decreased or normal
RV	Decreased	Increased
TLC	Decreased	Normal or increased
RV/TLC	Normal or increased	Significantly increased
$FEV_{1.0}$/FVC	Normal or increased	Decreased
$FEV_{3.0}$/FVC	Normal or	Decreased

From Morrissey, W: Respiratory diseases. In Kaye, D, and Rose, LF, editors: Fundamentals of internal medicine, St. Louis, 1983, The CV Mosby Co.

Lung defense mechanisms

I. Upper airway defenses against pulmonary infection
  A. Removing particulate matter from inspired air
    1. Particles greater than 20 μm settle back on surfaces
    2. Particles 5-10 μm deposited in nose
    3. Particles 0.1-10 μm remain suspended in air for long periods and are then inhaled
    4. Particles 1-5 μm deposited in tracheobronchial tree
      a. Droplet nuclei 2-4 μm (dried particles from sneezing, coughing, talking)
      b. May contain viruses or bacteria
      c. Spread organisms from person to person
  B. Minimizing the microbial population on membranes of upper respiratory tract
    1. Mucocillary transport
      a. Posterior two thirds of nasal cavity, sinuses, and nasopharynx lined by *ciliated epithelium* covered with thin layer of mucus
      b. Dense concentration of small blood vessels present beneath ciliated epithelium and mucous layers
      c. Mucus and fluid produced = 1000 ml/24 hr in normal persons
      d. Mucus and fluid carried at rate of 5-10 mm/min back into hypopharynx by beating action of cilia
      e. Substances in secretions inhibit microbial growth and prevent organisms from sticking to mucous membranes
        (1) Immunoglobulins (secretory IgA)
        (2) Lysozyme
        (3) Complement
  C. Minimizing possibility of aspiration
    1. Motor function of upper airway
      a. Laryngeal mechanism—closes glottis when swallowing to protect larynx
        (1) Gag reflex also closes glottis
        (2) Clearing throat, spitting, clear upper airway
    2. Contamination of lower respiratory tract
      a. Impaired clearance of particles in upper airway = spread of bacteria
      b. Accumulation of debris and microbes → penetration of tissues = sinusitis, otitis media
      c. Accumulation of debris and microbes → aspiration into traches; lung abscess caused by anaerobic bacteria secondary to severe gingival disease
      d. Intoxication or distraction → aspiration
      e. Normal sleep → minor aspiration
      f. Aspiration of pharyngeal contents → lung → bacterial pneumonia
II. Lower respiratory tract clearance mechanisms
  A. Pulmonary reflex
    1. Cough—an involuntary reflex elicited by stimulation of irritant receptors in subepithelium of hypopharynx, larynx, and tracheobronchial tree: mediated by vagus nerve
      a. Facilitator of mucociliary clearance
      b. Aids in dealing with gross contamination from above larynx
    2. Bronchoconstriction—reflex response to airway irritants
      a. Decreased size of bronchus and forced expiration and cough propel debris toward mouth
      b. Excessive bronchoconstriction (asthma) = decreased expiratory airflow, air trapped in lung, effective cough difficult
  B. Mucociliary clearance
    1. Mucus secreted by epithelial goblet cells from submucosal glands; 0.10-100 ml passes up trachea into hypopharynx and is swallowed; amount and nature of mucus secreted are controlled, in part, by parasympathetic nervous system affected by neurohumoral stimulation (adrenergic or cholinergic) and by direct mucosal irritation
    2. Cilia (200 cilia/each cell surface) beat rhythmically 1200 beats/min mouthward beginning at terminal bronchioles → larynx; beating of cilia → overlying mucous layer → mouthward at rate of 0.5 mm/min in small airways to about 10 mm/min in major bronchi

Adapted from Light, B: Respiratory infections. In Kryger, MH, editor: Pathophysiology of respiration, New York, 1981, John Wiley & Sons, Inc.

Lung defense mechanisms—cont'd

3. Clearance increased by:
   a. Bronchodilator drugs
      (1) β-Adrenergic agents (ephedrine) stimulate transport of water and salt into mucus = ↓ viscosity of mucus
      (2) Methylxanthines (aminophylline) → ↑ mucous production and ciliary activity
4. Ciliary function depressed by:
   a. Chronic exposure to airway irritants—cigarette smoke and other irritants
   b. Pharmacologic agents—100% O_2, anticholinergic agents, alcohol
   c. Infection such as viral bronchitis
5. Mucous production increased by:
   a. Chronic irritation of respiratory tract → increase in number of mucus-secreting gobler cells = ↑ mucus
   b. Inflammatory response to irritation → ↑ numbers of phagocytic cells and amount of cellular debris in mucus (especially DNA) = ↑ viscosity of mucus, which is less readily moved along by ciliary action
6. Immotile cilia—congenital impairment
   a. *Kartagener's syndrome*—sinusitis, recurrent lung infection and sinusitis
   b. *Cystic fibrosis*—infection, chronic imflammatory increases in respiratory mucous volume and viscosity = impaired lung clearance and progressive lung damage

III. Intrapulmonary detoxification mechanism
   A. Phagocytes
      1. Alveolar macrophage
         a. Phagocytosis of particles—inhaled particulate debris, bacteria, or cell constituents
         b. Kills most microbes
      2. Polymorphonuclear neutrophil present in blood (normally only small number in lung)
         a. Avid phagocyte—kills microbes
         b. Defends against established infectious processes
         c. Infection—products of inflammation attract neutrophils to site of infection (chemotaxis)
      3. Factors interfering with phagocytosis
         a. Inhibition of alveolar macrophage function
            (1) Cigarette smoke
            (2) Other inhaled pollutants—ozone, nitrogen dioxide, oxygen
            (3) Drugs—corticosteroids, antineoplastic and antiinflammatory cytoxic agents, and ethanol (alcohol)
            (4) Metabolic derangements—uremia, hyperglycemia of diabetes mellitus
            (5) Acquired granulocytopenia—bone marrow depression from cytoxic drugs
   B. Immunoglobulins
      1. IgG and IgA—most important for lung defense; present in secretions of respiratory tract as well as in blood
         a. IgA antibodies—specific for viral antigens; neutralize viruses and prevent infection
         b. IgG predominates in terminal lung units; antigen-specific IgG contributes to local defense against bacterial infections (important in neutralizing highly pathogenic encapsulated bacteria [especially *Streptococcus pneumoniae* and *Hemophilus influenzae*], which are resistant to phagocytosis)
   C. Cell-mediated immunity (CMI)
      1. One half of lymphocytes in and around airways are rhymus-derived lymphocytes, or *T cells*
         a. Found in lymphoid aggregates adjacent to bronchi (bronchus-associated lymphoid tissues, or BALT)
         b. T cells important in:
            (1) Resistance to some viral infections
            (2) Resistance to most fungal infections
            (3) Infections by organisms that survive and multiply inside host cells: *Mycobacterium* tuberculosis, *Brucella*, *Listeria monocytogenes,* and *Pneumocystis carinii*
      2. Impaired CMI = ↑ susceptibility to infection
         a. Deficient T cell function (anergy) associated with:
            (1) Neoplasms—lymphoma
            (2) Cytotoxic or corticosteroid therapy
            (3) Systemic diseases—sarcoidosis, malnutrition
         b. Some lung infections occur almost exclusively with severely impaired CMI—pneumonia caused by cytomegalovirus, herpes zoster, aspergillus species, or *Pneumocystis carinii*

■ RESTRICTIVE PULMONARY DISORDERS

■ Infectious diseases of the pulmonary tract

For an infection of the lung to occur, pathogens must be able to enter the lower respiratory tract. This means that the defense mechanisms of the lung must be overcome in some manner. There are many lung defense mechanisms including upper airway defenses, lower respiratory tract clearance mechanisms, and intrapulmonary detoxification mechanisms. These mechanisms are outlined on pp. 672-673.

■ VIRAL INFECTIONS

Many respiratory diseases are probably caused by viral infections. Presently, over 30 diseases have been found to be directly related to viral infections, and there are probably many more. Some diseases may be caused by one virus, different viruses may cause the same symptoms.

If specific signs are not evident, the clinical illness is termed a common cold, viral infection, fever of unknown origin (FUO), or acute respiratory illness. The most common specific respiratory diseases caused by the various viruses are epidemic pleurodynia (Bornholm's disease), acute laryngotracheobronchitis, viral pneumonia, and influenza. Most adults have developed antibodies for the more common viruses, and most viral infections are relatively mild. However, they are frequently complicated by secondary bacterial infections. When new strains of the influenza virus develop, severe epidemics may ensue, and many people may die from secondary infections such as pneumonia.

□ Acute bronchitis
□ *Pathophysiology*

Bronchitis can be acute or chronic. Acute bronchitis is an inflammation of the bronchi and sometimes the trachea (tracheobronchitis). It is often caused by an extension of upper respiratory tract infection such as the common cold and is therefore communicable. It also may be caused by physical or chemical agents such as dust, smoke, or volatile fumes. As air pollution increases, the incidence of acute bronchitis increases.

▦ Assessment

SUBJECTIVE DATA
1. Onset and duration of symptoms (see Table 24-3)
2. Medications taken for cough and their effectiveness

OBJECTIVE DATA
1. Vital signs—temperature may be elevated; tachypnea frequent with severe bronchitis
2. Rasping cough with mucoid sputum
3. Chest percussion—normal
4. Auscultation—vesicular breath sounds, vocal fremitus normal, adventitious sound—localized rales and sibilant rhonchi

→ *Data analysis: nursing diagnoses*

Nursing diagnoses are determined from assessment of patient data. Possible nursing diagnoses for the person with acute bronchitis may include, but are not limited to, the following:

Diagnostic title	Possible etiologies
Ineffective airway clearance	Tracheobronchial infection, obstruction, or secretion
Ineffective breathing pattern	Decreased energy, fatigue
Knowledge deficit	Lack of exposure
Pain	Rib or muscle trauma from coughing

▦ *Planning: expected patient outcomes*

Expected patient outcomes for the person with acute bronchitis may include, but are not limited to, the following:
1. Patient demonstrates effective cough with adequate sputum production.
   a. Both cough and sputum production decrease within 72 hours of treatment initiation.
   b. For persons with chronic lung disease, sputum becomes clear and thin (return to prebronchitis status).
2. Patient demonstrates effective breathing patterns.
3. Patient demonstrates prebronchitis vital signs.
4. Patient reports that chest pain is decreased.

Table 24-3 Signs and symptoms and medical therapy for acute bronchitis

Etiology	Signs and symptoms	Medical therapy
Any of 30 different viruses	Chills, malaise, muscular aches, headache, dry scratchy throat, hoarseness, cough, tightness and soreness in chest after coughing	No specific therapy, therapy directed to relief of symptoms, i.e., cough medicine, vaporizer; fluid intake 3-4 L/day Bland diet Antibiotics for elevation in temperature Rest Avoiding exposure to further infection

5. Patient describes the cause and factors contributing to the occurrences of acute bronchitis and names common symptoms of it.

Implementation

ASSISTING WITH ACHIEVEMENT OF THERAPEUTIC GOALS
Assist the patient to cough effectively. Coughing is normally a mechanism that aids in the removal of inhaled foreign materials. When an infection is present the throat becomes dry and irritated and there is an increase in mucus production as part of the lung defense mechanisms.

Receptors for the cough reflex are located in the tracheal and bronchial mucosa with the largest concentration of them being found in the larynx, carina, and bifurcations of the large and medium-sized bronchi. When these receptors are stimulated, impulses are transmitted primarily via the afferent nervous pathways (vagus, phrenic, and spinal motor nerves) to expiratory musculature (larynx, tracheobronchial tree, diaphragm, and the abdominal wall).[32]

To produce an effective cough there must be a deep inspiration followed by maximum expiratory effort against a closed glottis. This results in a tremendous increase in intrathoracic pressure. As the glottis opens, mucus and inhaled particles are forced out of the airways at a high velocity.[59]

Persistent coughing can be very annoying and tiring to the patient and those around her or him. Complications of persistent coughing include insomnia, exhaustion, vomiting, urinary incontinence, rib or muscle trauma, pneumothorax, or fainting. If cough is present, give prescribed medication. Table 24-4 lists commonly used medications and their desired effects.

Assist with coughing as necessary by supporting chest (front and back) as patient coughs. Teach patient to cough effectively to maintain a clear airway and collect required specimens. Tell patient to take a deep breath, force the air out down to residual volume, contract the diaphragm, and exhale forcefully.

Additional assistance in achieving therapeutic goals includes the following:
1. Provide for good drainage of tracheobronchial secretion.
2. If antibiotics are prescribed, give on time to maintain therapeutic blood levels.
3. If steam vaporization is prescribed, administer it using precautions described on p. 680.

ASSISTING WITH COMFORT AND ADL
1. Place patient in position of comfort; semi-Fowler's or high-Fowler's position may be helpful.
2. Assist with ADL as necessary during acute phase of illness.

COUNSELING AND TEACHING
The patient should be taught to avoid persons with upper respiratory infections. If respiratory infection does occur, the patient should seek medical attention.

If the patient smokes cigarettes, he or she should be encouraged to quit smoking. Group programs are helpful to some persons and the local branches of the American

Table 24-4 Medications used to treat cough

Desired effect	Medications prescribed
↑ Secretions	Expectorants 　Ammonium chloride 　Ammonium carbonate 　Sodium iodide 　Potassium iodide (saturated solution; SSKI) 　Ipecac 　Terpin hydrate
↓ Secretions	Anticholinergic agents 　Atropine
Thin secretions	Mucolytic agents 　Acetylcysteine (Mucomyst) 　Desoxyribonuclease (Dornavac)
Depress cough reflex	Antitussives 　Narcotic 　　Codeine 　Nonnarcotic agents 　　Benzonatate (Tessalon) 　　Noscapine (Nectadon) 　　Dextromethorphan hydrobramide (Romilar) 　　Carbetapentane citrate (Toclase) 　　Levopropoxyphene napsylate (Novrod) 　　Chlophedianol hydrochloride (Ulo)

Lung Association or American Heart Association can supply the names of local programs to assist persons to stop smoking.

Evaluation

Evaluation is based on patient outcomes. Questions to be asked include the following:
1. Have the patient's cough and sputum production decreased?
2. Has the patient's chest pain decreased?
3. Is the patient breathing effectively?
4. Can the patient list common symptoms and describe the cause of and factors contributing to acute bronchitis?

■ BACTERIAL INFECTIONS

□ Pneumonia
□ *Pathophysiology*

Pneumonia is an inflammatory process in which there is consolidation caused by exudate filling the alveolar spaces. Gas exchange cannot take place in consolidated areas, and blood is shunted around the nonfunctioning alveoli. *Hypoxemia* may occur depending on how much lung tissue is involved.

About 60% of patients with pneumococcal pneumonia have some degree of pleural effusion. Empyema may also occur in some patients with pneumonia.[28]

Acute pneumonias are responsible for 10% of hospital admissions in the United States. Pneumonia can occur in any season but is most common during winter and early spring. Persons of any age are susceptible, but pneumonia is more common among infants and the elderly. Pneumonia is often caused by aspiration of infected materials into the distal bronchioles and alveoli. Certain individuals are especially susceptible. This includes persons whose normal respiratory defense mechanisms are damaged or altered (those with chronic obstructive pulmonary disease, influenza, and tracheostomy, and those who have recently had anesthesia); persons who have a disease affecting antibody response (those with multiple myeloma, hypogammaglobulinemia, and so on); and alcoholics in whom there is increased danger of aspiration and persons with delayed white blood cell response to infection. Increasingly, nosocomial pneumonia (acquired in the hospital) is a cause of morbidity and mortality. This is the direct result of an increase in the number of patients with impaired defenses resulting from certain types of therapy and of an increase in the number of patients whose lives are being prolonged with life support therapy.

Pneumonia is a communicable disease; the mode of transmission is dependent on the infecting organism. Pneumonia is classified according to the offending organism rather than the anatomic location (lobar or bronchial) as was the practice in the past. A classification of pneumonia and its causative organisms in adults is presented in the box below, left.

□ Typical or classic pneumonia

Typical or classic pneumonia occurs in both males and females of any age. It is found both in persons without underlying disease and in those with diminished defense mechanisms. Commonly, there is a history of alcoholism, recent respiratory tract infection, or viral influenza.

▦ Assessment

SUBJECTIVE DATA
1. Onset and duration of cough, fever, and shaking chills
2. Color and consistency of sputum
3. Therapy used since onset of infection
4. See Table 24-5 for common signs and symptoms of pneumonia

OBJECTIVE DATA
1. Tachypnea
2. Guarding and restricted motion of the chest on the affected side
3. Palpation of chest to check for limited expansion and increased tactile fremitus on the affected side
4. Percussion of chest to check for dull to flat sounds
5. Auscultation to check for
   a. Breath sounds increased in intensity; bronchovesicular or bronchial breath sounds over affected area
   b. Vocal fremitus—increased bronchophony, egophony, and presence of whisper pectoriloquy
   c. Adventitious sounds—inspiratory rales, terminal third of inspiration

DIAGNOSTIC TESTS. The diagnosis of bacterial pneumonia is made from the patient's history, parenchymal infiltrates on the chest film, leukocytosis (increase in number of neutrophils), and sputum culture. Hypoxemia and respiratory acidosis may also be present.

A chest roentgenogram showing lobar consolidation is most common with pneumococcal or *Klebsiella* organism infections. Multiple infiltrates are more common with *Staphylococcal* and *Haemophilus* organism infections.[28]

Sputum specimens are collected for microscopic examination and for culture and sensitivity. The best sputum specimens are obtained from a deep, spontaneous cough. The sputum specimens are removed as soon as possible,

---

Organisms causing infectious pneumonia in adults

I. Typical or classic pneumonia syndrome
   A. Bacterial pneumonia
      1. Common
         a. *Streptococcus pneumoniae*
      2. Uncommon
         a. *Haemophilus influenzae*
         b. *Staphylococcus aureus*
II. Atypical pneumonia syndrome
   A. Common
      1. *Mycoplasma pneumoniae*
      2. Viral
   B. Uncommon
      1. *Legionella pneumophila*
      2. *Pneumocystis carinii*
III. Aspiration pneumonia syndrome
   A. Hospitalized, debilitated, or antibiotic-treated patients
      1. Mixed anaerobic/aerobic pharyngeal flora
      2. *Staphylococcus aureus*
      3. *Klebsiella pneumoniae*
      4. *Pseudomonas aeruginosa*
      5. *Serratia marcescens*
      6. *Acinetobacter* species
      7. Enteric gram-negative aerobes (*Escherichia coli* and *Enterobacter* and *Proteus* organisms)
   B. Outpatients with normal pharyngeal flora
      1. Mixed anerobic/aerobic pharyngeal flora
IV. Hematogenous pneumonia syndromes
   A. *Staphylococcus aureus*
   B. *Escherichia coli*
   C. Enteric/pelvic anaerobes

Adapted from Frame, PT: Basics RD 10:1-8, 1982.

Table 24-5 Etiology, signs and symptoms, and pharmacotherapy of pneumonia

Pneumonia	Etiology	Risk factors	Signs and symptoms	Pharmacotherapy
Typical syndrome	Streptococcus pneumoniae; uncomplicated Streptococcus p.; complicated (empyema, metastatic infection)	Sickle cell disease Hypogammaglobulinemia Multiple myeloma	Sudden onset with shaking, chill Fever (39° to 49° C), pleuritic chest pain, productive cough Sputum—green and purulent and may be blood tinged; "rusty" Respirations—rapid and shallow with "grunting" at end of each breath Nasal flaring, intercostal rib retraction, use of accessory muscles, and cyanosis may be present	Drugs of choice Penicillin G procaine, IM Aqueous crystalline penicillin G, IV Penicillin V Other effective drugs Erythromycin, clindamycin, cephalosporins, other pencillins, trimethoprim with sulfamethoxazole
	Haemophilus influenzae Staphylococcus aureus	Advanced age COPD Alcoholism Recent influenza		Penicillin G Ampicillin Other effective drugs Chloramphenicol, cefamandole, trimethoprim with sulfamethoxazole, nafcillin Other effective drugs Methicillin, oxacillin, cefazolin, cephalothin, vancomycin, clindamycin Vancomycin, IV Cafazolin, IV, plus gentamicin or tobramycin
Atypical syndrome	Common cause: Mycoplasma pneumoniae Viral pathogens	Childhood, young adults	Onset gradual over 3-5 days Malaise, headache, sore throat, dry cough May have chest wall soreness from coughing	Drug of choice: Erythromycin Other effective drugs: Tetracycline None
	Uncommon cause: Legionella pneumophilia	Recent URI; influenza	Above plus abdominal pain and diarrhea Temperature 49° C or greater Shaking chills Respiratory distress Renal failure, hyponatremia, hypophosphatemia, elevated creatine phosphokinase	Drug of choice: Erythromycin Other effective drugs Rifampin, gentamicin
	Pneumocystic carinii	Renal transplantation Autoimmune disease Immunologic deficiency Debilitation	Gradual onset with increasing dyspnea, dry cough, tachypnea, hypoxemia X-ray film—diffuse interstitial involvement	Trimethoprim Pentamidine

Continued.

Table 24-5 Etiology, signs and symptoms, and pharmacotherapy of pneumonia—cont'd

Pneumonia	Etiology	Risk factors	Signs and symptoms	Pharmacotherapy
Aspiration	Aspiration of: gram-negative bacilli; *Klebsiella, Pseudomonus, Serratia, Enterobacter, Escherichia, Proteus;* gram-positive bacilli *Staphylococcus* Gastric acid aspiration Aspiration of inert substances: water, barium, nutritional supplements	Alcoholism Debilitation Hospitalization (i.e., nosocomial infection) Altered consciousness	Mixed anerobic: At first gradual onset Low-grade fever, cough Sputum—increased production, foul smelling Chest x-ray film—interstitial involvement in dependent portion of lung Gram negative or positive infection: may present same clinical picture as classic pneumonia Sudden onset of respiratory distress, severe dyspnea, cyanosis, coughing, hypoxemia, followed by signs and symptoms of secondary infection	Antibiotic therapy dependent on pathogen causing infection
Hematogenous	Occurs when pathogens are spread to lungs via the bloodstream: Staphalococcus, *E. coli,* Enteric anerobes	Infected intravascular catheter Endocarditis, IV drug abuse Intraabdominal abcess Pyonephrosis Empyema of gallbladder	Pulmonary symptoms minimal compared with the symptoms of septicemia Nonproductive cough and pleuritic pain similar to that seen in pulmonary embolism are most common complaints	*Drugs of choice* Nafcillin IV; ampicillin IV; plus gentamicin or tobramycin Clindamycin IV; plus gentamicin or tobramycin

labeled, and sent to the laboratory. Oral hygiene is provided after a patient has expectorated sputum.

Microscopic examination of sputum can help establish a diagnosis. Constituents indicative of infection include polymorphonuclear neutrophils (pus cells) and ciliated bronchial epithelial cells, which are an index of damage to bronchial epithelium.

Color of sputum is not always an accurate diagnostic tool but is sometimes helpful (see box above). Microscopic examination is essential to distinguish between allergic and infected sputum. Allergic sputum (asthma) usually contains an increased number of eosinophils. Consistency of sputum is described as being thick, thin, or tenacious.

➡ Data analysis: nursing diagnoses

Nursing diagnoses are determined from assessment of patient data. Possible nursing diagnoses for the person with bacterial pneumonia may include, but are not limited to, the following:

Diagnostic title	Possible etiologies
Ineffective airway clearance	Tracheobronchial infection or secretion
Ineffective breathing pattern	Musculoskeletal impairment, decreased energy, fatigue
Pain: chest	Rib or muscle trauma
Impaired gas exchange	Ventilation or perfusion
Knowledge deficit	Lack of exposure
Altered nutrition: less than body requirements	Anorexia

⌐ Planning: expected patient outcomes

Expected patient outcomes for the person with bacterial pneumonia may include, but are not limited to, the following:

a. Patient demonstrates effective cough with adequate sputum production. (Both cough and sputum production decrease within 72 hours of treatment initiation. Patient with chronic lung disease returns to prepneumonia status.)
2. Patient reports absence of chest pain.
3. Patient demonstrates improved ventilation and adequate oxygen of tissues.

a. pH returns within normal limits.
b. PaO₂ during active disease—60 to 80 torr; after resolution of disease, process PaO₂ within normal limits.
4. Patient describes the cause and factors contributing to the occurrence of pneumonia and names common symptoms indicating pneumonia.
5. Patient maintains prepneumonia body weight.

⊞ Implementation
ASSISTING WITH ACHIEVEMENT OF THERAPEUTIC GOALS
MEDICATIONS

1. Before beginning administration of prescribed antibiotic, sputum is collected for culture. If blood culture is ordered, blood is also drawn before therapy is begun.
2. Antibiotic blood levels are monitored by giving antibiotics at scheduled times. (Table 24-5 lists the antibiotic therapy currently employed in treating pneumonia.)
3. Give medication prescribed to relieve pain. Codeine may be prescribed to relieve pain because it is less likely to inhibit the cough reflex than more potent narcotics.

OXYGEN THERAPY

Oxygen by mask or cannula (Figs. 24-3 and 24-4) is usually ordered when PO₂ is less than 60 mm Hg.[28] When supplemental oxygen is necessary it may be administered by nasal prongs or by mask. The method used depends on the patient's condition and the concentration of oxygen required. The nurse should be familiar with the various devices used to administer oxygen, and when oxygen is in use the nurse should check the equipment frequently to be sure that it is working properly.

When the patient is having difficulty exchanging oxygen and carbon dioxide, such as occurs in pulmonary edema, oxygen may be given under positive pressure. In some situations, such as chronic obstructive pulmonary disease, low-flow rates of oxygen are indicated. The use of low-

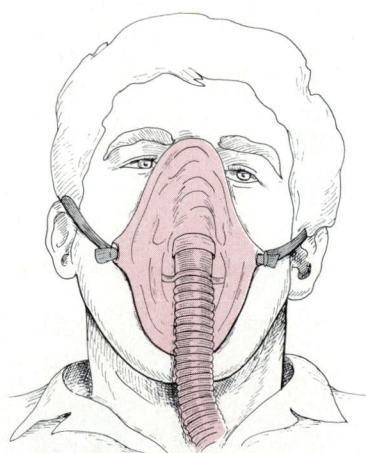

Fig. 24-3　Simple face mask. (From Abels, LF: Mosby's manual of Critical Care, St. Louis, 1979, The CV Mosby Co.)

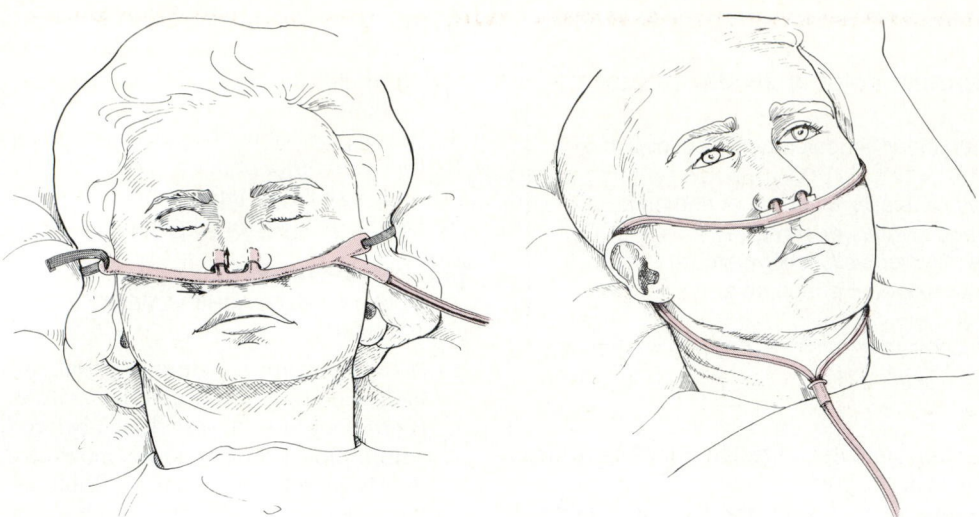

Fig. 24-4   Two types of nasal cannulas. (From Abels, LF: Mosby's manual of critical care, St. Louis, 1979, The CV Mosby Co.)

flow oxygen is discussed on p. 737. In all situations, the nurse should remember that a patient suffering from hypoxemia may not be breathless or cyanotic because cyanosis does not occur until there is 5 g or more of deoxygenated hemoglobin. In a person with anemia, all the available heme is completely saturated with oxygen and thus these patients are never cyanotic even though they may be hypoxemic. For this reason an increase in the pulse rate may be the first indication that the patient is experiencing hypoxemia. When patients are receiving oxygen therapy they are monitored by arterial blood gas studies. These studies are explained on p. 721.

FACILITATING BREATHING

Assist the patient to breathe deeply and expand the chest to increase ventilation.
1. Place patient in position to facilitate breathing—usually upright or semi-upright position (Fig. 24-5).
2. A pillow may be placed lengthwise at patient's back to provide support and thrust thorax slightly forward, allowing freer use of the diaphragm.
3. The patient who must be upright to breathe may find it restful to rest head and arms on a pillow placed on an overbed table (Fig. 24-6).

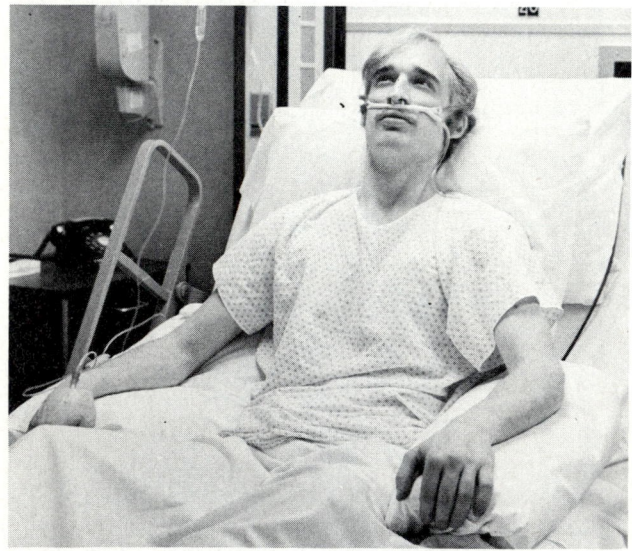

Fig. 24-5   Patient sitting upright with pillows under head and each arm to promote chest expansion and comfort.

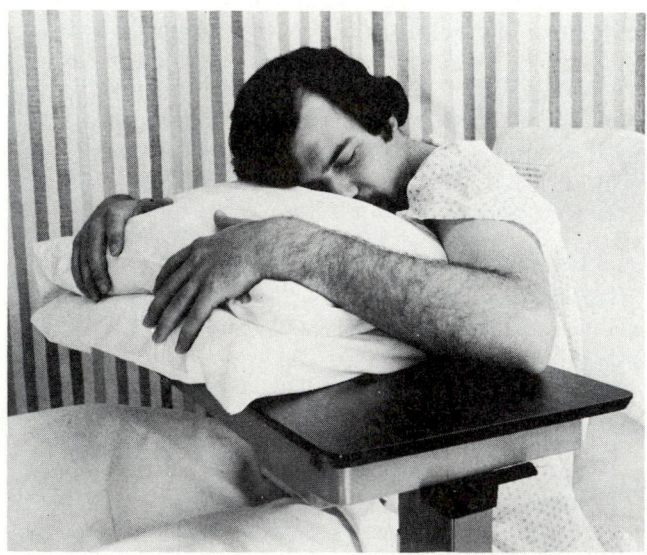

Fig. 24-6   Pillows placed on over-bed table provide comfortable support for the patient who must sleep in a sitting position.

Precautions when using a humidifier

1. Use only a direct *heated* humidifier or nebulizer with a bacterial filter. Cold vapor or cool mist humidifiers are not recommended because they cannot withstand daily sterilization.
2. Use only sterile water in the humidifier and drain remaining water each time the humidifier is refilled, or at least every 24 hours. Tap water is not safe to use because it is frequently contaminated with *Pseudomonas, Flavobacterium, Acinetobacter,* or other organisms.
3. Establish a routine maintenance schedule.
4. Set medical guidelines to determine which patients should receive humidification and which should not. It may not be advisable to use humidifiers for immunosuppressed patients.
5. Do not send humidifying unit home with patients because of the concern about transporting highly resistant hospital organisms into the community.

---

4. For the patient with severe hypoxemia, safety side rails should be in place. Patient can use them to assist in moving about in bed.
5. Some patients may breathe best when sitting up in a large armchair while leaning on a smaller chair placed in front of them. This chair is blocked to prevent it from slipping.

PROVIDING VENTILATION, HUMIDITY, AND A COMFORTABLE TEMPERATURE

1. Most patients are most comfortable if air is cool and not too humid. An air-conditioned room may make the patient more comfortable.
2. If patient has nose, throat, or bronchial irritation, warm moist air from a *humidifier* or *vaporizer* may be helpful.
3. Because of concern about cross-infection from room humidifiers, the precautions listed in the box above are recommended by the Centers for Disease Control (CDC).

Vaporizers. Small electric vaporizers can be purchased at most local drugstores. However, when a patient cannot afford to purchase one, the nurse can assist in improvising equipment for inhalation and for proper humidity. An empty coffee can or a shallow pie tin can be filled with sterile water and placed on an electric plate in the person's room to increase humidity. If the inhalation is to be directed, an ordinary steam kettle or a tea kettle with a longer improvised paper spout may be used. The paper should be changed frequently. A few drops of menthol or oil of eucalyptus can be put into the water. Benzoin causes corrosion in the kettle, which is exceedingly difficult to remove. The kettle and electric plate should be placed a safe distance from the face so the medicated steam can be breathed freely, and yet the person cannot be burned by accidentally tipping the kettle or by touching the hot plate. After the 25- to 30-minute treatment, equipment should be removed from the bedside.

Hydration. Dehydration results in thick, tenacious secretions. The best liquefying agent is water, and it is preferable to adequately hydrate the patient rather than attempt to loosen secretions with mist therapy. If the patient does not have cardiovascular disease requiring fluid restriction, a fluid intake of 3 to 4 L/day should be provided.

ASSISTING WITH COMFORT AND ADL
1. Place patient in position of comfort—patients are usually most comfortable with head of bed elevated 45 to 90 degrees.
2. Support the patient's chest during coughing.

CONTROL OF ENVIRONMENT
1. Respiratory isolation is required for patients with staphylococcal pneumonia. Other forms of pneumonia do not require isolation.
2. Hand washing is the most important way to prevent spread of pneumonia from one patient to another via the hands of hospital personnel.

COUNSELING AND TEACHING
The major emphasis is on prevention.
1. Two vaccines are now available to prevent respiratory infections: influenza vaccine and pneumococcal vaccine.
2. Persons at high risk for developing complication of influenza (pneumonia) should be immunized unless they are allergic to eggs or egg products or had a previous reaction to vaccine.
   a. Influenza vaccine given yearly.
   b. *Pneumonia polysaccharide* vaccine given only every 3 to 5 years.[28]
3. Attention needs to be paid to reducing the likelihood of gram-negative colonization of patients. For this reason many hospitals have instituted tighter control policies on the use of antibiotics except in situations where a review panel of physicians approves their use. A reduction in use of antibiotics also reduces the incidence of antibiotic-resistant hospital flora, which are the source of many nosocomial infections. (See Chapter 11.)

COMPLICATIONS OF PNEUMONIA
With the advent of antibiotics and better diagnostic measures such as x-ray procedures, complications during or following pneumonia are rare in otherwise healthy persons. Atelectasis, delayed resolution, lung abscess, pleural effusion, empyema, pericarditis, meningitis, and relapse are

complications that were common in the past. The fact that pneumonia and influenza rank fifth as a cause of death in the United States is an impressive reason for strict adherence to the prescribed medical treatment. Careful and accurate observation as well as sufficient time for convalescence also helps to ensure the average patient has a smooth recovery. Aged persons and those with a chronic illness are likely to have a relatively long course of convalescence from pneumonia, and there is a greater possibility of their developing complications. There has been an increase in the incidence of staphylococcal pneumonia subsequent to influenza. Consolidation of lung tissue, pleural effusion, and empyema frequently occur soon after onset of this type of pneumonia and may cause death.

⊞ Evaluation

Evaluation is based on patient outcomes. Questions to be asked include the following:
1. Are the patient's signs and symptoms improved?
2. Have the patient's PaO_2 and pH returned to within normal limits?
3. Can the patient state the cause of and factors contributing to pneumonia?
4. Can the patient state the common symptoms of pneumonia?
5. Can the patient state when influenza or pneumonia vaccines should be taken?

☐ Atypical pneumonia
☐ Epidemiology

The most common form of atypical pneumonia in adults is caused by *Mycoplasma pneumoniae*. *Legionella pneumophila* is an uncommon cause of atypical pneumonia. It occurs more commonly in older adults and in persons who smoke or have abnormal pulmonary defenses.[28] *Legionella pneumophila* is the agent causing Legionnaires' disease (legionellosis). It is three times more common in men than in women. A number of conditions are felt to predispose one to legionellosis. These include chronic renal disease, chronic bronchitis or emphysema, diabetes, cancer, immunosuppressive medications, and smoking. It is estimated that about 25,000 cases of Legionnaires' disease occur each year.[118]

Both epidemics and sporadic cases of Legionnaires' disease occur. Epidemics have been associated with common source exposures such as air conditioning, water-cooling towers, and excavation sites. *Legionella pneumophila* has been isolated from soil and fresh water and from shower heads in hospitals.

Fine inspiratory rales may be present, but there is no evidence of consolidation. A roentgenogram of the chest shows patchy segmental infiltrates, which may progress from unilateral to bilateral. Pleural effusion is uncommon. Patients with legionellosis may have renal failure, hyponatremia, hypophosphatemia, and an elevation of creatine phosphokinase.

☐ Medical therapy

The usual treatment for both *Mycoplasma pneumoniae* and *Legionella pneumophila* pneumonia is erythromycin (Table 24-5). If a patient is seriously ill with Legionnaires' disease, rifampin may be added to the treatment with erythromycin. Rifampin should never be used alone because of the great likelihood of resistant organisms developing during monotherapy. Because relapses have occurred within 1 to 2 weeks of therapy, it is recommended that treatment for Legionnaires' disease be continued for 3 weeks.

The overall mortality of Legionnaires' disease is almost 15%. Most of this is attributed to respiratory failure.

When *Mycoplasma* pneumonia is untreated, the fever and malaise generally resolve in 1 to 2 weeks. Serious systemic complications are quite rare, although hemolytic anemia, disseminated intravascular coagulation (DIC), thrombocytopenic purpura and renal failure, myocarditis and pericarditis, meningoencephalitis and other neurologic syndromes, arthritis, and hepatitis have been reported.[111] The mortality for *Mycoplasma* pneumonia is less than 1%.[28]

☐ Pneumocystis carinii

For approximately 40 years, *Pneumocystis carinii* has been recognized as a cause of pneumonia in immunosuppressed patients. *Pneumocystis carinii* is the most common life-threatening infection to persons with acquired immunodeficiency syndrome (AIDS). Malaise, fever, nonproductive cough, and dyspnea are the usual symptoms. A roentgenogram of the chest shows diffuse bilateral pulmonary infiltrates, although the infiltrates may be found only in upper or lower lobes.[13]

Medical treatment includes the intravenous administration of trimethoprim-sulfamethoxazole. Pentamidine isethionate may be used in place of trimethoprim-sulfamethoxazole in persons intolerant to it. The relapse rate of *Pneumocystis carinii* in persons with AIDS is estimated at approximately 20% to 30%. Failure to respond to therapy, the necessity of mechanical ventilation, and repeated episodes of *Pneumocystis carinii* are all associated with a poor prognosis.[13] (See Chapter 38 for further discussion of AIDS.)

☐ Aspiration pneumonia

The common factor in all forms of aspiration pneumonia is the aspiration of material into the airways. Aspiration pneumonia can occur while the patient is in the hospital, but diligent nursing care may prevent it. The types of aspiration pneumonia are listed in the box on p. 683.

☐ Hematogenous pneumonia

Bacterial infections of the lung can also occur when pathogenic organisms are spread to the lungs through the blood stream. See Table 24-5 for etiologic factors, signs and symptoms, and medical therapy of this type of pneumonia.

☐ Tuberculosis

In 1900 tuberculosis was the leading cause of death in the United States. It remained a major cause of death until the introduction of antituberculosis drug therapy in the late 1940s and early 1950s. The most effective of these agents is isoniazid, which first became available clinically

---

Types of aspiration pneumonia

Noninfectious aspiration pneumonia

1. Aspiration of gastric acid
   a. Only a small quantity of aspirated gastric acid causes severe respiratory distress within a few seconds.
   b. Bacterial superinfection, if it does occur, does not become evident for 48 to 72 hours.
2. Aspiration of large quantities of inert substances
   a. Common substances include water, barium, tube-feeding liquids, and nonacid gastric contents.
   b. Aspirated substances obstruct airways, causing respiratory distress.
   c. Secondary bacterial infection may occur in lung segments that have obstructed airways.
3. Noninfectious aspiration syndrome is witnessed or identified from suctioning of foreign material from lungs.

Bacterial aspiration pneumonia

1. High-risk persons
   a. Persons with disorders of consciousness (for example, anesthesia, coma, seizures, or alcoholism).[28]
   b. Persons with poor cough mechanisms (for example, laryngeal dysfunction or respiratory muscle paralysis).
2. Mixed anerobic and aerobic flora of the upper respiratory tract is most common cause.

---

in 1952. The use of isoniazid in combination with two agents introduced earlier, streptomycin and para-aminosalicylic acid, resulted in a striking decrease in tuberculosis mortality rates. It also made it possible for patients with tuberculosis to be treated on an outpatient basis. However, some patients still have to be hospitalized during their illness, and most nurses will care for a patient with tuberculosis at some time in their careers.

Although tuberculosis is now considered a preventable and curable disease, it still is a disease requiring public health attention. In 1984 there were 22,225 cases of tuberculosis reported to the Centers for Disease Control (CDC).[14] Since 1986 the case rates have been increasing, after remaining at about 20,000 cases yearly for several years. These new cases were not evenly distributed throughout the population, however, and some differences bear mentioning.

The highest case rates are in California, New York, Texas, and Florida. These states have the highest numbers of immigrants, many of whom come from countries where tuberculosis is endemic. These states also have the largest numbers of AIDS patients. According to the CDC, there seems to be evidence that HIV infection, in the absence of AIDS itself, is responsible for an increase in tuberculosis in New York City. The CDC believes that this may also be true in other parts of the country.

During the last decade, the highest case rates were among persons 65 years and older. Recently, the highest case rate has been among those between 25 and 44 years of age, with an increasing proportion being attributed to AIDS.

Tuberculosis is caused by bacillus, *Mycobacterium tuberculosis,* or the tubercle bacillus, a gram-positive and acid-fast organism. If microscopic study of a slide prepared from the sputum of an individual reveals tubercle bacilli, the individual is said to have positive sputum; and this confirms the diagnosis of tuberculosis. However, some persons with tuberculosis will not have positive sputum on smear, and a positive sputum culture is necessary to confirm the diagnosis. Patients who have a positive culture and negative smear are less infectious than are those with both a positive smear and culture.

When a person with tuberculosis speaks, coughs, sneezes, or sings, minute droplets fall to the ground; the smaller ones evaporate, leaving *droplet nuclei* that remain suspended indefinitely in the air and are carried on air currents. Droplet nuclei are *1 to 10 μm* in size and are small enough to be inhaled into the alveoli. Thus it is by inhalation of tubercle-laden droplet nuclei that tuberculosis is transmitted.

☐ *Pathophysiology*

When an individual with no previous exposure to tuberculosis (negative tuberculin reactor) inhales a sufficient number of tubercle bacilli into the alveoli, tuberculosis *infection* occurs. The body's reaction to the tubercle bacilli depends on the susceptibility of the individual, the size of the dose, and the virulence of the organisms. Inflammation occurs within the alveoli (parenchyma) of the lungs, and natural body defenses attempt to counteract the infection. Lymph nodes in the hilar region of the lung may be involved as they filter drainage from the infected site. The inflammatory process and cellular reaction produce a small, firm, white nodule called the *primary tubercle.* The center of the nodule contains tubercle bacilli. Cells gather around the center, and usually the outer portion becomes fibrosed. Thus blood vessels are compressed, nutrition of the tubercle is interfered with, and necrosis occurs at the center. The area becomes walled off by fibrotic tissue around the outside, and the center gradually becomes soft and cheesy in consistency. This latter process is known as *caseation.* This material may become calcified (calcium deposits), or it may liquefy and is known as *liquefaction necrosis.* The liquefied material may be coughed up, leaving a *cavity* or hole in the parenchyma of the lung. The cavity or cavities are visible on chest x-ray films and result in the diagnosis of *cavitary* disease. Most individuals who are exposed to tuberculosis and develop a tuberculosis infection (confirmed by a positive tuberculin test) do not develop an active case of tuberculosis. The only x-ray evidence of their tuberculosis infection is a calcified nodule known as the *Ghon tubercle.* The evidence on x-ray film of enlarged hilar lymph nodes and a Ghon tubercle is sometimes referred to as the *primary complex.*

Persons who have been exposed to the tubercle bacillus become sensitized to it, and this is confirmed by a positive tuberculin test. Sensitization, once developed, usually remains throughout life unless something interferes with the immune response. Recent evidence suggests that about 50% of tuberculin reactors who take isoniazid for 1 year convert back to negative test results. A positive tuberculin test does not mean that one has tuberculosis, however, and nurses should explain this fact to persons who are having the test.

Tuberculosis infection is unlike other infections. Usually, other infections disappear completely when overcome by the body's defenses and leave no living organisms and generally no signs of infection. However, a person who has been infected with tubercle bacilli harbors the organism for the remainder of his or her life. Tubercle bacilli remain in the lungs in a dormant, walled-off, or so-called resting, state. When a person is under physical or emotional stress, these bacilli may become active and begin to multiply. If body defenses are low, active tuberculosis may develop. Most persons who have active tuberculosis developed it in this manner. However, it is generally accepted that only 1 out of 20 persons with a positive tuberculin test ever develop active tuberculosis, and the incidence is expected to be much lower among those who receive preventive therapy with isoniazid.

□ *Classification*

The classification used by states and territories of the United States when reporting morbidity statistics to the CDC of the Public Health Service is outlined in Table 24-6. The six basic classifications cover the total child and adult population, those unexposed to tuberculosis, those uninfected even though exposed, those with evidence of tuberculosis infection without disease, those with current disease, those with evidence of tuberculosis without current disease, and those in whom tuberculosis is suspected (diagnosis pending).

□ *Prevention*

To eliminate tuberculosis, the organism must be prevented from being transmitted from one person to another. Preventive measures are directed toward the recommendations described under classification. Preventive therapy emphasis is on (1) finding all persons who have tuberculosis and getting them adequate treatment, (2) identifying persons who should be on preventive chemotherapy and getting them treatment (see the box on p. 685), and (3) locating persons who had tuberculosis in the past and who did not receive adequate treatment with chemotherapy and treating them.

Persons over 35 years of age without the risk factors listed here are not given preventive chemotherapy because of the risk of isoniazid-associated hepatitis. Although the risk is small, it is age related and increases from less than 0.2% in those under age 20 to up to 2.3% in those 50 to 64 years of age.

If isoniazid-associated hepatitis occurs, the symptoms are mild, nonspecific, and resemble those of any viral illness. (See Chapter 30 for a discussion of viral hepatitis.)

Contraindications to the use of isoniazid preventive therapy are (1) previous isoniazid-associated liver disease; (2) severe adverse reactions to isoniazid, including fever, chills, rash, and arthritis; and (3) *acute* liver disease of any cause.

Persons receiving isoniazid preventive chemotherapy should be seen monthly by a health care provider for the purpose of reinforcing the necessity of taking the chemotherapy regularly and to monitor the patient for any serious side effects.

Table 24-6 Classification of tuberculosis

Class	Description	Therapy
0	No TB exposure, not infected	None
1	TB exposure, no evidence of infection	Preventive chemotherapy may be given for persons converting their tuberculin test from negative to positive
2	TB infection, no disease	Isoniazid (INH) for 1 year (preventive chemotherapy) for *positive reactors* under age 35
3	TB: current disease (persons with completed diagnostic evidence of TB: both a significant reaction to tuberculin skin test and clinical and/or x-ray evidence of TB)	Antituberculosis drugs: at least 2 of the first-line drugs (INH, ethambutol, rifampin, streptomycin)
4	TB: no current disease (persons with previous history of TB or with abnormal x-ray films but no significant tuberculin skin test reaction or clinical evidence)	No new therapy (persons may still be receiving chemotherapy)
5	TB: suspect (diagnosis pending); Used during diagnostic testing of suspect persons, for no longer than a 3-month period	Preventive chemotherapy may be instituted

Persons who should be considered for preventive chemotherapy

1. Persons known to be exposed to tuberculosis who may be in the process of converting their tuberculin test (recent converters under 35 years of age)
2. Household contacts of persons diagnosed as having tuberculosis, especially children under age 5
3. Positive reactors to the tuberculin test under age 35
4. Tuberculin reactors over age 35 who are at special risk:
   a. Those receiving corticosteroid therapy
   b. Those receiving immunosuppressive therapy
   c. Those having a disease that impairs the immune response
5. Persons with:
   a. Leukemia or lymphoma
   b. Silicosis
   c. Diabetes difficult to control
   d. Gastrectomy

VACCINATION. Efforts continue in the search for a more satisfactory tuberculosis vaccine. Presently, BCG (bacille Calmette-Guérin) vaccine is in use in many countries throughout the world. This vaccine contains attenuated tubercle bacilli that have lost their ability to produce disease. It is administered only to persons who have a negative reaction to the tuberculin test. It is not widely used in the United States because of disagreements among physicians as to its safety and effectiveness. Also, vaccination with BCG induces hypersensitivity to tuberculin in vaccinated persons. Thus the tuberculin test loses its value as a diagnostic tool for these persons, which is one of the major objections to its use in the United States.

The vaccine should be given only by persons who have had careful instruction in the proper technique. A multiple-puncture disk is used. When there is a positive reaction to skin testing with tuberculin, when acute infectious disease is present, or when there is any skin disease, BCG vaccine is not given. Possible complications following vaccination are local ulcers, which occur in a relatively high percentage of persons vaccinated, and abscesses or suppuration of lymph nodes, which occur in a small percentage.

In countries where living conditions are such that transmission of tuberculosis is to be expected, BCG vaccine is given early in life and then repeated after 12 to 15 years. The intradermal method is used to administer the vaccine so that a uniform controlled dose can be given. BCG vaccine is not generally recommended for use in the United States, although some highly susceptible groups such as migrant workers may be immunized.

Assessment

SUBJECTIVE DATA

It is important to determine whether the patient was exposed to a person with active tuberculosis. Often the cause of the infection is unknown and may never be determined. At the same time, close contacts of the patient need to be identified so that they may undergo examination to determine if they have active disease or have a positive tuberculin test.

OBJECTIVE DATA
1. Presence of cough
2. Afternoon temperature elevation
3. Night sweats

DIAGNOSTIC TESTS

TUBERCULIN SKIN TESTING

Tuberculin skin testing provides evidence of whether the individual tested has been infected by tubercle bacilli. It is based on the fact that a hypersensitivity reaction develops to certain products of *Mycobacterium tuberculosis*. This cell-mediated or delayed hypersensitivity reaction is manifested by induration caused by cellular infiltration at the site of the injection in persons who have been sensitized to the tubercle bacillus. Such persons are called "reactors." In the past the terms *negative* and *positive* were used to describe the results of tuberculin testing. In 1981 the American Thoracic Society (ATS), the medical section of the American Lung Association, suggested that the terms positive and negative are not the most accurate way to describe the results of tuberculin skin testing.[6] They recommend that the number of millimeters of induration be recorded and then interpreted appropriately.

Two substances may be used for tuberculin skin testing: OT (old tuberculin), which is prepared from dead tubercle bacilli and contains their related impurities; and PPD (purified protein derivative), which is a highly purified product containing protein from the tubercle bacilli.

The tuberculin test that gives the most accurate results is the *Mantoux test,* or intracutaneous injection of either PPD or OT. A tuberculin syringe and a short (½-inch), sharp, 24- to 26-gauge needle are used. With the skin (usually the inner forearm is used) held taut, the injection of 0.1 ml of PPD or OT is made into the superficial layers, and it produces a sharply raised white wheal. Weak dilutions are used first. If there is no reaction, stronger dilutions are used. This precaution prevents severe local reactions that might occur in highly sensitive individuals if the higher dilutions were used initially. The most frequently used strength of PPD is an intermediate strength of 0.0001 mg/dose, or 5 tuberculin units (5 Tu). PPD is also available in first- and second-strength dilutions. For broad-screening and case-finding purposes, a single test of intermediate strength is recommended. Interpretations of the test are made after 48 hours. A tuberculin reaction may begin after 12 to 24 hours with an area of redness and a central area of induration, but it reaches its peak in 48 hours. The area of induration (not the erythema) indicates how positive the test is. Induration should be examined in a good light and palpated gently. Tuberculin reactions should always be measured and recorded in millimeters at the largest diameter of the induration. When successive dilutions are being used, it is advisable to have tests read by the same person so that individual variation in interpretation can be prevented. If the test is negative, there may be no visible reaction or there may be only slight redness with no induration.

One of the most important steps in tuberculin testing is the accurate measurement of reaction. A reaction is considered to be significant when it is 10 mm or more in diameter. Reactions between 5 and 9 mm are considered to be doubtful reactions and are more likely to indicate infection with atypical acid-fast bacilli than with *Mycobacterium tuberculosis*, except in persons who are suspects or close contacts of persons with tuberculosis. In this instance a reaction of 5 mm or more is considered significant.[8]

ROENTGENOGRAPHIC EXAMINATIONS

Persons with positive tuberculin tests undergo chest x-ray examinations to determine if there is evidence of active tuberculosis. Standard posteroanterior and lateral chest films are usually ordered. Body-section roentgenograms (planography, tomography) also may be ordered. These views are helpful in defining nodules, cavities, cysts, calcification and vascular details in the parenchyma of the lung.

Tuberculosis lesions usually occur in the apical and posterior segments of the upper lobe or in the superior segment of the lower lobe.

Pleural effusion may be the only x-ray finding evident with pleural tuberculosis.

SPUTUM EXAMINATION

For the diagnosis of tuberculosis to be made there must be microscopic identification of *M. tuberculosis* (acid-fast bacillus).

Tests to be done on sputum are explained to the patient so that a suitable specimen is obtained. The patient is instructed to collect only sputum that has come from deep in the lungs. When instructed inadequately, patients often expectorate saliva rather than sputum. They are likely to exhaust themselves unnecessarily by shallow, frequent coughing that yields no sputum suitable for study and that affords them little relief from discomfort. *The first sputum raised in the morning is usually the most productive of organisms.* During the night, secretions accumulate in the bronchi, and just a few deep coughs will bring them to the back

---

---

of the throat. If patients do not know this fact, on awakening they may almost unconsciously cough, clear their throats, and swallow or expectorate before attempting to produce the specimen.

The patient should be supplied with a wide-mouthed container and instructed to expectorate directly into it. Because the sight of sputum is often objectionable to the patient and to others, the outside of a glass container is covered with paper or other suitable covering. Usually 4 ml of sputum is sufficient for necessary laboratory tests and examinations. Guidelines for sputum collection are listed in the box above.

Occasionally patients have difficulty producing sputum for examination. Inhalation of a hypertonic solution such as 10% saline in distilled water is used to temporarily stimulate sputum collection. Other methods to collect sputum include: (1) endotracheal aspiration with a suction catheter and special sputum collection container, (2) transtracheal aspiration—insertion of a needle with a catheter through the cricothyroid cartilage, and (3) fiberoptic bronchoscopy (p. 699).

GASTRIC WASHINGS

Gastric aspiration is occasionally used to collect gastric contents, which may contain swallowed sputum. It is usually done when the diagnosis or suspected diagnosis is tuberculosis. Because most patients swallow sputum when coughing in the morning and during sleep, an examination of gastric contents may reveal causative organisms. The procedure requires the following steps:

1. Breakfast is withheld before aspiration.
2. A nasogastric (NG) tube is passed into the stomach (see Chapter 31).
3. A large syringe is connected to the NG tube and a specimen of stomach contents is gently withdrawn.
4. The specimen is placed in a covered container.
5. The NG tube is withdrawn.

ESTABLISHING THE DIAGNOSIS OF TUBERCULOSIS. Results of roentgenograms and sputum examinations will either rule out the possibility or confirm a diagnosis of tuberculosis. Bacteriologic confirmation of the presence of *M. tuberculosis* is necessary to establish the diagnosis of tuberculosis. Because it is impossible to differentiate between typical and atypical acid-fast bacilli by a sputum smear, cultures are obtained on all persons. Cultures are also used for antimicrobial susceptibility (sensitivity) studies. *Despite the introduction of improved culture media, the tubercle bacillus grows slowly on artificial media, and culture reports are not available for 3 to 6 weeks.*

Blood-streaked sputum in the absence of pronounced coughing may be the first indication to the person that anything is wrong. Pathologic changes may have occurred in the lungs, but sputum examination may not show tubercle bacilli. However, if the nodules produced in the parenchyma of the lung become soft in the center and then caseated and liquefied, the liquefied material may break through and empty into the bronchi and be raised as sputum. Cavities in the lung may appear on x-ray film and may be present in more than one lobe of the lung.

Data analysis: nursing diagnoses

Nursing diagnoses are determined from assessment of patient data. Possible nursing diagnoses for the person with tuberculosis may include, but are not limited to, the following:

Diagnostic title	Possible etiologies
Ineffective airway clearance	Decreased energy, fatigue
	Tracheobronchial infection or secretion
Knowledge deficit	Lack of exposure to information

Planning: expected patient outcomes

Expected patient outcomes for the person with tuberculosis may include, but are not limited to, the following:

1. Patient can explain how tuberculosis is spread and those measures necessary to prevent spread (for instance, continuing chemotherapy and covering mouth and nose when coughing or sneezing).
2. Patient can state name, dosage, actions, and side effects of prescribed medications.
3. Patient can state why at least two chemotherapy agents must be taken uninterruptedly.
   a. Patient can explain drug-resistant organisms and relate this to the need to take chemotherapy uninterruptedly.
   b. Patient can explain why the health care provider should be notified immediately if for any reason chemotherapy cannot be taken (for example, because of side effects).
4. Patient can state where to receive new supply of chemotherapy and date it is to be obtained.
5. Patient can state plans for follow-up care.
   a. Patient can list signs and symptoms that indicate need for immediate medical care (increased cough, hemoptysis, unexplained weight loss, fever, night sweats).
   b. Patient can state when next sputum test or roentgenogram is to be taken and where.

c. Patient is able to state plans for ongoing follow-up care.

Implementation
ASSISTING WITH ACHIEVEMENT OF THERAPEUTIC GOALS
MEDICATIONS

Medical treatment is antituberculosis drug therapy. The drugs used to treat tuberculosis, their classification, side effects, and tests for side effects can be found in Table 24-7.

At least two drugs are given together to prevent the development of resistant strains of the tubercle bacillus. The most commonly prescribed drugs for the initial treatment of active tuberculosis are isoniazid (INH) and rifampin (RIF). The latest schedule of therapy recommends dosages of 300 mg of INH and 600 mg of RIF daily for 30 days; then 15 mg/kg of INH and 600 mg of RIF twice weekly for 8 weeks.

When drug resistance develops, other drugs to which the patient's organisms are sensitive are prescribed.

Some persons are infected with resistant strains of the tubercle bacillus. Resistance is most common to isoniazid and streptomycin. There are race or ethnic differences in rates for primary drug resistance. Asians and Hispanics have the highest rates, followed by blacks, whites, and American Indians.[14] Primary drug resistance rates vary widely in the United States and Canada, and nurses need to know the local resistance rates for areas where they are working. It can be assumed that resistance rates are highest in those areas where large numbers of Hispanics and Asians are living.

CONTROLLING THE ENVIRONMENT TO PREVENT CONTAMINATION OF AIR WITH DROPLET NUCLEI

Preventing contamination of air with tubercle bacilli is accomplished by: (1) treating the patient with antituberculosis drugs and (2) preventing contamination of air with tubercle bacilli. The most effective way to achieve both of the above is by patient teaching (see the box on p. 688).

Evaluation

Evaluation is based on patient outcomes. Questions to be asked include the following:

1. Does patient cover nose and mouth when coughing, sneezing, or laughing?
2. Are the patient's sputum cultures negative, indicating that antituberculosis drugs are effective and are being taken as prescribed?
3. Can the patient state name, dosage, and side-effects of prescribed antituberculosis drug therapy?
4. Can the patient explain why two or more drugs are prescribed and why they must be taken without interruption?
5. Can the patient state the signs and symptoms that indicate a need for immediate medical care?
6. Can the patient state the dates of the next sputum and x-ray examinations?
7. Can the patient state the date of the next medical appointment?

Table 24-7 Drugs used to treat tuberculosis

Drug	Classification	Common side effects	Tests for side effects
Isoniazid (INH)	Bactericidal	Peripheral neuritis, hepatitis, rash, fever	SGOT, SGPT (not as routine)
Rimfampin (RIF)	Bactericidal	Hepatitis, febrile reactions, thrombocytopenia (rare)	SGOT, SGPT, platelet count (not as routine)
Ethambutol (EMB)	Bacteriostatic	Optic neuritis (reversible with discontinuation of drug; very rare at 15 mg/kg skin rash)	Visual acuity; red-green color discrimination
Pyrazinamide (PZA)	Bactericidal	Hyperuricemia, hepatitis, arthralgia	Uric acid, SGOT, SGPT
Streptomycin (SM)	Bactericidal	8th cranial nerve damage (vestibular); nephrotoxicity	Vestibular function, angiograms; creatinine level determined before therapy started

---

Patient teaching to prevent transmission of tuberculosis

1. Patient must take antituberculosis drugs as prescribed.
   a. Drugs are always taken in combination of two or three drugs.
   b. Drugs must be taken uninterruptedly.
   c. Both of the above are necessary to prevent development of resistant strains of *M. tuberculosis*.
2. Preventing contamination of air with *M. tuberculosis*.
   a. Cover nose and mouth with disposable tissues when coughing, sneezing, or laughing.
   b. Place used tissues in paper bag, which will be burned.

■ FUNGAL INFECTIONS

There are three major fungal infections of the lungs: *histoplasmosis*, *coccidioidomycosis*, and *blastomycosis*. They are classified as deep mycoses because there is involvement by the parasite of deeper tissues and internal organs.[91] The incidence and prevention of these fungal (mycotic) infections are discussed in Table 24-8.

□ Histoplasmosis
□ *Pathophysiology*

The spores are inhaled and phagocytized by alveolar macrophages within which they germinate. They form yeast cells and multiply by budding. In persons previously uninfected there is a primary or initial infection that resembles the infection in primary tuberculosis with involvement of regional lymphatics and early dissemination via lymphatics and blood to other organs. Yeast cells spread hematogenously and are phagocytized by reticuloendothelial cells in the liver, spleen, and bone marrow. The process in the lung is similar to that seen in tuberculosis with necrosis and healing by fibrosis encapsulation. Eventually, the areas show calcification in the original parenchymal foci in the lung and in the hilar lymph nodes. Usually the initial infection is self-limiting and does not require antifungal chemotherapy. However, some persons, such as infants and adults with immunologic incompetence

(lymphoma), may develop a rapidly progressive primary infection that can be fatal without antifungal therapy.

Reinfection histoplasmosis and *progressive histoplasmosis* can also occur. Reinfection with histoplasma causes an illness resembling the initial infection. Since some degree of immunity to histoplasmosis is conferred by the initial infection, the extent of disease is modified by the degree of fungal immunity.[2] Heavy inoculation may cause *pneumonitis*, which is usually self-limiting over days to weeks. The onset is acute with nonproductive cough, fever, malaise, and dyspnea. Some persons who are fully immune may develop a hypersensitivity-like pneumonitis with small, discrete granulomatous foci that may give a *miliary* appearance on x-ray examination. This means that the infection is spread throughout the lung, giving the appearance of the presence of small millet seeds throughout the lung.

Progressive histoplasmosis is usually chronic; chronic pulmonary histoplasmosis is the most frequently encountered symptomatic form of the disease. It develops almost exclusively in middle-aged white men who have chronic obstructive pulmonary disease. There are recurrent episodes of necrotizing segmental or lobar granulomatous pneumonitis, which have a tendency to cavity formation, contraction, fibrosis, and compensatory emphysema.

Progressive disseminated histoplasmosis usually occurs as a consequence of the initial infection in persons with very

Table 24-8   Incidence and prevention of fungal infections

Type of infection and source	Incidence	Prevention
Histoplasmosis		
Soil contaminated with fowl excreta. Bats may be infected and areas they inhabit (caves, attics, hollow trees) can be extremely infectious.	Quite high in United States. Endemic areas in Missouri, Kentucky, Tennessee, Southern Illinois, Indiana, and Ohio.	Locate areas where soil is infected with fowl excreta. Teach public to avoid inhalation of dust from infected soil. Infants and the elderly are especially susceptible.
Coccidioidomycosis		
Soil contaminated with spores. Heavy rainfall in the desert enhances growth of the fungus—sunlight inhibits it. Liberation of dust in the spring disperses anthrospores, which are inhaled.	Endemic to well-defined areas in southwestern United States, Mexico, and South America. In United States, endemic in San Joaquin Valley, Southern Arizona, New Mexico, and Southwestern Texas.	Wearing of masks by persons working in desert dust; archeologists, construction workers.
Blastomycosis		
Soil contaminated with spores that are carried on air currents and inhaled by humans and animals. Dogs can acquire the disease. Not believed to be spread from animals to man; believed that both humans and animals are infected by inhaling spores.	Most prevalent in the United States and Canadian valley areas surrounding the Mississippi, Missouri, Ohio, and St. Lawrence rivers. Also present in Africa, South America, and Mexico.	Avoid inhalation of spores in areas where cases have been identified.

low resistance to the infection (for instance, infants and persons with immunologic incompetence). Rarely, it can occur in adults of both sexes and all ages with no known immune disorder. These persons have fever, weakness, weight loss, hepatosplenomegaly, leukopenia, and mucous membrane ulceration involving the oropharynx, tongue, or larynx. Adrenal insufficiency occurs in about 50% of these persons.[2]

☐ **Coccidioidomycosis**
☐ *Pathophysiology*

The process following inhalation of spores is believed to be very similar to that described under histoplasmosis. The arthrospores reach the alveoli, where they are phagocytized. If the disease becomes disseminated, there is marked hilar adenopathy, and fungi can be isolated from lymph nodes. A pneumonic disease with necrosis and cavitation may occur after development of delayed hypersensitivity.[91] The disease process is controlled and resolved in most persons as the result of cell immunity to infection. Thus progressive disseminated coccidioidomycosis or progressive pulmonary disease is found only in those persons whose ability to resist infection or develop immunity has been compromised in some way. Susceptibility to infection is in part genetically determined. Coccidioidomycosis is 50 times more common in Filipino men and 10 times more common in black men than it is in white men.[91] This increased susceptibility to progressive disease in these groups of men parallels their susceptibility to tuberculosis. The increased susceptibility of some races to diseases such as coccidioidomycosis and tuberculosis is believed to be the result of a genetically determined impairment of their capacity to develop cellular immunity to infection.[91]

Skin testing with coccidioidin, 1:10 or 1:100, is available to test for the disease. The test is read in 48 hours. It takes 3 to 6 weeks after exposure for the test to become positive. In severe disseminated disease the test may be negative, indicating that the patient's immune system is no longer able to respond.

Roentgenograms of the chest may exhibit pneumonic infiltrate, hilar adenopathy, pleural effusion, or a cavitary lesion.[42] About 5% of persons with primary pulmonary involvement have residual lung lesions such as cavities or nodules. Only about 0.5% of infected individuals go on to develop a severe, progressive mycosis.

Extrapulmonary dissemination of coccidioidomycosis can occur. One of the most frequent sites of dissemination is the meningeal surfaces of the brain. If there is any indication of involvement of the central nervous system, a lumbar puncture is performed. A positive complement fixation titer in the spinal fluid is diagnostic of meningitis.[42]

Dissemination can also occur to skin, soft tissue, and bones, and the patient is monitored by physical examination of the skin, gallium scanning of soft tissues, and bone scans. A bone scan should be performed before starting amphotericin B therapy.

Surgical intervention for localized lesions may involve either excision or drainage to facilitate healing.

☐ **Blastomycosis**
☐ *Pathophysiology*

Although skin lesions are the first evidence of blastomycosis, it is believed that the initial site of infection is in the lung. It is assumed that spores are inhaled and phagocytized in the alveoli as part of the primary infection. Thus the pathogenesis of blastomycosis is similar to that of tuberculosis, histoplasmosis, and coccidioidomycosis. The infection is spread by the lymphatics and spread throughout the body. The skin lesions represent metastatic infection from the primary pulmonary disease.[91]

Acute pulmonary blastomycosis in the form of a self-limited pneumonia can occur. Otherwise, blastomycosis is a chronic progressive disease with a mortality of about 90% when untreated. For this reason it is recommended that every person in whom the diagnosis is established be treated.[61]

Assessment

SUBJECTIVE DATA
1. Onset and duration of signs and symptoms. (See Table 24-9 for common signs and symptoms.)
2. History of exposure to soil contaminated with spores

OBJECTIVE DATA
1. Palpation of chest to check for limited expansion
2. Percussion of chest to check for dull to flat sounds
3. Auscultation to check for type of breath sounds or adventitious sounds

DIAGNOSTIC TESTS
1. Direct demonstration of intracellular yeasts in smears of bone marrow and biopsy of lymph nodes, liver, and spleen; cultures of bone marrow, blood, or sputum.
2. Serologic tests. Agglutination, precipitation, and complement-fixation tests are used to help establish diagnosis of histoplasmosis and coccidioidomycosis. Serologic tests become positive about 1 month after the primary infection. Titers of serial tests are used to determine activity of the infection.
3. Skin testing. Skin test for histoplasmosis is only used for screening purposes. In endemic areas, between 90% and 95% of young adults have positive test results. The person should be tested with histoplasmin, tuberculin, blastomycin, and coccidioidin because of the likelihood of cross-reaction. The strongest reaction indicates the likely cause of the infection.
4. In histoplasmosis and coccidioidomycosis, chest x-ray films demonstrate a nodular infiltrate similar in appearance to tuberculosis. In blastomycosis, chest x-ray films may be nonspecific.
5. White blood cell count is usually normal but in acute causes may increase to 13,000 mm².
6. Leukopenia and anemia may be present in persons with disseminated disease.

Data analysis: nursing diagnoses

Nursing diagnoses are determined from assessment of patient data. Possible nursing diagnoses for the person with severe mycotic infection may include, but are not limited to, the following:

Diagnostic title	Possible etiologies
Ineffective airway clearance	Tracheobronchial infection and secretions
Ineffective breathing pattern	Musculoskeletal impairment
Pain	Rib or muscle trauma
Impaired gas exchange	Ventilation and perfusion impairment
Knowledge deficit	Lack of exposure

Planning: expected patient outcomes

Expected patient outcomes for the person with *severe mycotic infection* may include, but are not limited to, the following:
1. Patient demonstrates cough with adequate sputum production.
2. Patient states that chest pain is reduced.
3. Patient demonstrates improved ventilation and adequate oxygenation of tissues.
4. Temperature returns to normal.
5. Patient knows source of infection and can teach others to avoid infected areas (Table 24-9).
6. Patient states plans for follow-up care.

Implementation

ASSISTING WITH ACHIEVEMENT OF THERAPEUTIC GOALS
1. Place patient in position to facilitate breathing.
2. Administer medications as prescribed and monitor patient for side effects.
   a. Amphotericin B (Fungizone Intravenous) is the standard therapy for mycotic infections. The dose and length of therapy are determined by the difficulty in eradicating the infection and the likelihood of relapse.[2] The therapy may last 2 to 3 weeks or 2 to 3 months.
   b. Amphotericin B must be given intravenously and has many toxic properties, including local phlebitis, systemic reactions, renal toxicity, hypokalemia, and anemia. In rare instances anaphylaxis, bone marrow suppression, and cardiovascular and hepatic toxicity develop.
   c. Systemic toxicity (chills, fever, aching, nausea, and vomiting) can be lessened by premedication with 600 mg of aspirin along with 25 to 50 mg of diphenhydramine (Benadryl) or promethazine (Phenergan) or 10 mg of prochlorperazine (Compazine) orally.[2] Heparin and hydrocortisone succinate (Solu-Cortef) are sometimes added to the infusion to minimize phlebitis.
   d. A reversible azotemia occurs regularly when amphotericin B is administered. The level of azotemia is monitored by biweekly BUN and serum creatinine determinations. A BUN of greater than 40 or a creatinine nearing 3.0 indicates a need to temporarily reduce or stop the drug. Therapy is not continued until the azotemia is improved.[2] Serum potassium levels are checked biweekly, and hypokalemia is treated with oral potassium. Anemia is common, and

Table 24-9 Signs and symptoms and medical therap...

Type of infections	Etiologic factors	Signs a...	
Histoplasmosis	Inhalation of spores of *Histoplasma capsulatum*	*Severe infections* Acute onset with fever, c... pnea, prostration, weight loss... spread pulmonary infiltrates, hep... megaly, and splenomegaly. Some p... sons show no symptoms; others have... benign acute pneumonitis	
Coccidioidomycosis (Valley fever, San Joaquin Valley fever)	Inhalation of spores of *Coccidioidoides immitis*	Asymptomatic upper respiratory tract infection in about 60% of those who inhaled spores; 40% have symptoms ranging from flulike illness to frank pneumonia	The... of th... mainde... remission
Blastomycosis	Believed to be inhalation of *Blastomyces dermatitidis*	Skin lesions that appear as small papular or pustular lesions on exposed parts of the body such as hands and face Lesions develop peripherally, may become raised and do *not* itch	Amphotericin B...

the hematocrit level usually stabilizes at 25% to 35%.[2]

e. Ketoconazole (Nizoral) is a newer drug, administered orally, that is effective in the treatment of systemic mycotic infections. It is given daily for a minimum of 6 months. Toxicity appears to be minimal; pruritus, minor gastrointestinal intolerance, and liver function abnormalities have been reported. It is not known whether late relapses of histoplasmosis will occur in persons treated with ketoconazole, since the drug has been in use for only a short time.

f. Resectional pulmonary surgery is seldom required, and it is reserved for patients with adequate pulmonary reserve and residual cavities who are not able to tolerate amphotericin B.

ASSISTING WITH COMFORT AND ADL

1. Take measures to reduce fever (if present) by cool sponge baths, and so on.
2. Maintain room temperature desired by patient.

COUNSELING AND TEACHING

1. Review precautions for preventing reinfection (avoid infected areas).
2. Assist patient with plans for recuperation after leaving hospital.

⊞ *Evaluation*

Evaluation is based on patient outcomes. Questions to be asked include the following:

1. Is patient comfortable?
2. Are the patient's signs and symptoms improved?
3. Is the amphotericin infection site free of complications?
4. Can the patient identify the source of his or her infection and teach others to avoid infected areas?
5. Can the patient state plans for follow-up care?

■ Occupational lung diseases

■ EPIDEMIOLOGY AND ETIOLOGY

Many pulmonary diseases are believed to be caused by substances inhaled in the work place. They are more common (1) in blue-collar workers than in white-collar workers, (2) in industrialized areas than in rural areas, and (3) in small and medium-sized businesses than in larger industrial plants.

In some instances it is debatable whether a persons' lung disease is clearly occupation specific. This is especially so in cases of bronchitis, asthma, emphysema, or cancer because all of these conditions can be caused or aggravated by several factors found in many different occupations and by nonoccupational factors such as smoking and pollution of the atmosphere.[94]

Millions of Americans are believed to be suffering from job-related diseases. Because these diseases are not reportable, exact statistics do not exist. The Department of Health and Human Services has estimated that 400,000 persons develop job-related diseases each year. They also estimate that there are 100,000 deaths each year from occupational diseases. The National Heart, Lung, and Blood Institute stated in a 1977 report that lung diseases cause more than half of these deaths.[94] Over $5 billion a year is paid out in workers' compensation for job-related illnesses and injuries.[94]

■ PREVENTION

Occupational lung diseases are preventable. However, there must be a concerted effort by the public, governmental agencies, and industry if these diseases are to be prevented.

Governmental action has been slow and has only oc-

...rican Lung Association believes that several
... to be done to reduce the incidence of occu-
...ed diseases: (1) education of the public about
...nship between polluted air in the work place
...diseases; (2) general commitment to reducing,
..., or avoiding air pollution of the work place;
...limination of the most prevalent and notorious

...y for fungal infections

The patient with pulmonary problems 691

...d symptoms

Medical therapy

Drug(s) of choice
Amphotericin B
(Fungizone intravenous)
Newer drug
Ketoconazole (Nizoral)

...est pain, dys-
...wide-
...ato-
...er-

Amphotericin B IV
...rapy required for only 10%
...se with symptoms, re-
...have spontaneous

...logic conditions	Signs and symptoms
...lated in tissue → ...ction with whorl- ...odules throughout	Breathlessness with exercise
...WP: dust accumulation ...visible on x-ray film; ...ars piles up and respi- ...ronchioles are dilated ...focal emphysema)	Simple CWP: no symptoms, no respiratory difficulty

...sures; 10%-30%... miners develop simple form of the disease; more prevalent in miners of anthracite, or hard coal; other minerals found in miner's lung (silica, koalin, mica, beryllium, copper, cobalt, and others); unknown whether these minerals contribute to development or progression of CWP

| Complicated CWP or progressive massive fibrosis (PMF) | 3% of persons with simple CWP develop complicated form; more often occurs in miners with heavy deposits of coal dust in lungs; may appear suddenly years after miner has left the mines; can stop suddenly for no discernible reason; smoking seems to have no affect on development of CWP, but smoking has adverse effect on miners' health; miners who smoke have 5-6 times more lung obstruction than nonsmoking miners; cigarette smoking causes chronic bronchitis and emphysema as in nonminers | Fibrosis develops in some dust-laden areas; fibrosis spreads and fibrotic areas coalesce, eventually most of lung is stiffened and useless; silica plays some role in fibrosis but despite international research, role of silica in CWP is not understood | PMF shortens life span; may die from respiratory failure, cor pulmonale, or superimposed infection Prevention: dust control; reduced levels of coal dust can lower simple CWP and reduce number of miners who develop complicated CWP |

From American Lung Association: Occupational lung diseases: an introduction, New York, 1979, The Association.
*Also known as "dust in the lungs."

Continued.

Table 24-10   Major occupation-related lung diseases—cont'd

Type	Etiologic and epidemiologic factors	Pathophysiologic conditions	Signs and symptoms
Asbestos-related lung disease†	Asbestos is one of the most dangerous occupational hazards; can cause both fibrosis and cancer in asbestos workers; also a general environmental hazard because of its extensive use before health hazards were recognized; most dangerous to those who mine the ores and process the crude material into pure form; no asbestos mines in United States, but it is processed and used in United States; federal agencies and state governments moving to tighten controls on use of asbestos; lung cancer associated with all types of asbestos; 20-25% of deaths of workers with heavy exposure are from lung cancer; cancer is related to degree of asbestosis and to cigarette smoking, which enhances carcinogenic properties of asbestos; asbestos worker who smokes is 90 times as likely to get lung cancer as smoker who never worked with asbestos	Asbestos occurs in several different forms or ores; commercially important ores are chrysolite, crocidolite, and amosite; most hazardous medically are crocidolite and amosite; fibrosis caused by asbestos is called *asbestosis;* asbestos fibers accumulate around terminal bronchioles; body surrounds fibers with iron-rich tissue = asbestos body with characteristic picture on x-ray film; more asbestos bodies as more fibers are inhaled; after 20-30 yr of exposure, fibrosis begins in lungs; if heavy exposure, fibrosis appears in 4-5 yr	After fibrosis begins, cough, sputum, weight loss, increasing breathlessness; most die within 15 yr of first symptoms
	Mesothelioma (cancer of the pleura) accounts for 7%-10% of deaths of asbestos workers; inoperable and always fatal; can occur after very little exposure to crocidolite; has been reported in wives of asbestos workers and in persons living near asbestos plants; cigarette smoking not a contributing factor; only a few fine, straight crocidolite fibers are necessary; asbestos workers have a higher incidence of other cancers (esophagus, stomach, and intestines); swallowing of asbestos-contaminated sputum responsible for these cancers	Occurs in persons exposed to crocidolite fibers of a certain size; a few cases involve amosite fibers; needlelike shape of crocidolite fibers enables them to pass through lung tissue to pleura	Prevention: number of asbestos-related diseases has been increasing despite recognition of hazards and dust-control measures; much tighter controls are needed; some countries have taken such steps; there is need for massive efforts to educate general public of danger of asbestos
Hypersensitivity diseases	Hypersensitivity diseases fall into occupational category when antigen is found primarily in work place; lung hypersensitivity can occur in bronchi; bronchioles, or alveoli; coarse dust causes bronchial reactions; fine dust provokes small airway and alveolar reactions		

†Asbestos is a fire-proofing and insulating agent.

Continued.

Table 24-10 Major occupation-related lung diseases—cont'd

Type	Etiologic and epidemiologic factors	Pathophysiologic conditions	Signs and symptoms
Occupation-related asthma	More common in the 10% of the population who are atopic (genetic tendency to develop an allergy); nonatopic persons can also become sensitized; substances with antigenic properties include detergent enzymes, plantinum salts, cereals and grains, certain wood dusts, isocyanate chemicals used in polyurethane paints and other products, agents used in printing and some pesticides	Hypersensitivity reaction mediated by histamine → bronchoconstriction and ↑ mucus production; repeated attacks if cause unrecognized and asthma is untreated may lead to permanent obstructive lung disease; asthmatic response that is well established can be provoked by other factors (house dust, cigarette smoke) and by fatigue, breathing cold air, and coughing	Wheezing is major symptom Prevention: total elimination of antigen, desensitization not successful
Allergic alveolitis (farmer's lung)	Hypersensitivity disease caused by fine organic dust inhaled into smallest airways: cause of farmer's lung is moldy hay; other dusts can cause allergic alveolitis: these include moldy sugar cane and barley, maple bark, cork, animal hair, bird feathers and droppings, mushroom compost, coffee beans, and paprika; often disease is named for cause (mushroom worker's lung, etc.); fungus spores growing in the apparent antigen are thought in many cases to be real cause of the disease	Alveoli are inflamed, inundated by WBCs, sometimes filled with fluid; if exposure is infrequent or level of dust low, symptoms are mild; if treatment not sought, chronic form develops over time; eventually, fibrosis occurs, and fibrosis may be so well established that it cannot be arrested	Symptoms begin some hours after exposure to offending dust and include fatigue, shortness of breath, dry cough, fever, and chills; symptoms may be severe enough to require emergency treatment and hospitalization; acute attacks treated with steroids; recovery may take 6 wk and patient may suffer residual lung damage; real cure is permanent separation of patient and antigen Prevention: Properly dried and stored farm products (hay, straw, sugar cane) do not cause allergic alveolitis; presumably fungi only grow in moist conditions
Byssinosis (brown lung)	Occupation-related disease occurring in textile workers; mainly in cotton workers but also afflicts workers in flax and hemp industries; cause is found in bales of raw cotton that contain not only cotton fibers but fragments of cotton plant; something in plant matter, rather than pure cotton, is cause	Chronic bronchitis and emphysema develop in time; constriction of bronchioles in response to something in crude cotton; symptoms of asthma and allergy persist as long as there is exposure to cotton antigen	Tightness in chest on returning to work after a weekend away (Monday fever); strong relationship between amount of dust inhaled and symptoms; persistent productive tight chest with chronic bronchitis and emphysema; person leaves industry as respiratory cripple Prevention: dust control measures; pretreating bales of cotton by washing with steam and other agents may inactivate causative agent; try to detect persons who are likely to become sensitized to cotton dust and keep them out of high-risk areas

lung hazard, cigarette smoke. (The reader is referred to reference 94 for more information.)

Education of the public includes not only employers and employees but also engineers and planners who design operations; buyers and purchasers who select ingredients, cleaning agents, and equipment; and physicians who see persons with occupation-related diseases. Many times, workers who are instructed about the hazards involved in certain occupations and work places are helpful in deciding what preventive measures need to be taken to combat or minimize the effects of hazards. The commitment to reduce, eliminate, or avoid pollution of work place air requires full consideration of possible health effects whenever operations are planned and improvement of conditions whenever possible.

It is well documented that smokers get occupation-related lung diseases more often than nonsmokers and that smokers' lungs are more vulnerable to the effects of these diseases than are nonsmokers' lungs. The combined effects of cigarette smoke and industrial pollutants are very great. The risk of developing chronic bronchitis, emphysema, lung cancer, and heart disease is much increased when a worker smokes.[94] Some of these risks, such as lung cancer in asbestos workers who also smoke, are becoming more commonly known.

Occupation-related lung diseases can be divided into several categories. The major ones are (1) the pneumoconioses, including silicosis and coal miner's pneumoconiosis (black lung disease); (2) asbestos-related lung disease; and (3) hypersensitivity diseases, including occupation-related asthma, allergic alveolitis (farmer's lung), and byssinosis (brown lung disease). The etiology, pathophysiologic conditions, signs and symptoms, and prevention of these diseases are listed in Table 24-10.

The medical therapy and nursing care of these patients is dependent on the patient's signs and symptoms and complications. The reader is referred to other sections of this chapter for discussion of these topics.

The major role of nurses is to be knowledgeable about the etiology and prevention of these diseases so that appropriate information and teaching can be presented to the public.

■ Adult respiratory distress syndrome

Adult respiratory distress syndrome (ARDS) was first described by T.L. Petty in 1967. ARDS is often fatal and is characterized by severe dyspnea, hypoxemia, and diffuse bilateral pulmonary infiltrations following lung injury in previously healthy persons. Before 1967, what is now known as ARDS was known by several other names including pump lung, traumatic wet lung, shock lung, progressive pulmonary congestion, and Da Nang lung.

The etiology, signs and symptoms, and medical therapy for ARDS are summarized in Table 24-11. The clinical conditions that are associated with ARDS are listed in the box on p. 696.

■ PREVENTION

Prompt treatment of the underlying cause of ARDS is the major focus of preventive care. Additionally, judicious use of the mechanical ventilator and oxygen therapy are required to avoid inducing ARDS as an untoward complication of these treatment modalities.

■ PATHOPHYSIOLOGY

Several changes occur in ARDS. First, there is damage to the alveolar-capillary membrane. The damage can be on either the alveolar or capillary side of the membrane. Second, as a result of damage to the alveolar-capillary membrane, there is an increase in vascular permeability, and fluid may leak into the interstitial space and alveoli, causing pulmonary edema. Fluid and red blood cells can be found in the interstitial space and in the alveoli. Later, hyaline membranes (made up of proteins, mainly fibrinogen) that have leaked into the alveoli are seen.[65] The alveolar-capillary damage and the presence of interstitial and pulmonary edema impair gas exchange between the alveoli and the capillaries, and ventilation-perfusion abnormalities result (p. 704). Third, surfactant is inactivated resulting in an increase in surface tension and collapse of alveoli, especially smaller ones that are more dependent on surfactant to reduce their surface tension and keep them open. As

Table 24-11 Etiology, signs and symptoms, and medical therapy of ARDS

Etiology	Signs and symptoms	Medical therapy
Shock, trauma, infection, drug overdoses, and pulmonary infections See box on p. 696 for summary of clinical conditions associated with ARDS	Latent period of 18 to 24 hours after time of lung injury until symptoms develop Tachypnea, labored breathing, air hunger, and cyanosis Dry cough and fever develop over a few hours; fine crackles in lung fields; altered sensorium	Oxygen—100% with nonrebreathing face mask Mechanical ventilator support with volume-cycled ventilator attached to endotracheal or tracheostomy tube with positive-end expiratory pressure (PEEP) Drug therapy to treat specific symptoms such as shock and infection

Clinical conditions associated with ARDS

1. Shock
   a. Septic
   b. Hemorrhagic
   c. Cardiogenic
   d. Anaphylactic
2. Trauma
   a. Pulmonary contusion
   b. Nonpulmonary, multisystem
3. Infection
   a. Pneumonia
      (1) Viral
      (2) Bacterial (staphylococcal or strepto-coccal)
      (3) Legionellosis
   b. Miliary tuberculosis
4. Disseminated intravascular coagulation (DIC)
5. Fat emboli
6. Near-drowning
7. Aspiration: highly acid gastric contents (pH < 2.5)
8. Inhaled toxic agents
   a. Smoke
   b. Phosgene
   c. Oxides of nitrogen
9. Pancreatitis
10. Oxygen toxicity
11. Narcotic drug abuse
    a. Heroin
    b. Methadone
    c. Propoxyphene (Darvon)
12. Radiation pneumonitis
13. Drugs
    a. Ethchlorvynol
    b. Salicylates

Adapted from Petty, TL: Adult respiratory distress syndrome. In Kryger, M: Pathophysiology of respiration, New York, 1981, John Wiley & Sons, Inc.

areas of the lung become atelectatic, it is more difficult to inflate them with each breath, compliance decreases, and the work of breathing increases. The atelectasis also further increases the ventilation-perfusion disparity. The result of these processes is severe hypoxemia, which is resistant to oxygen therapy. These changes are summarized in Fig. 24-7.

There are many similarities between infantile respiratory distress syndrome (IRDS) and ARDS. For example, deficient surfactant plays a major role in IRDS. In both ARDS and IRDS there is congestive atelectasis, alveolar debris, and hyaline membrane formation. The approach to treatment is comparable in IRDS and ARDS.[65]

Chest x-ray films show diffuse, bilateral, and usually symmetric interstitial and alveolar infiltrations. These x-ray findings are commonly described as a "wet snowstorm."

Nursing care of patients with ARDS depends on the patient's signs and symptoms. If the patient is critically ill, he or she requires care in an intensive care unit. Airway management and ventilator support are usually necessary. These are discussed under respiratory failure (p. 737).

ASSESSMENT

Nursing assessment of the patient with ARDS needs to be tailored to maximize information obtained without increasing respiratory distress.

□ Subjective data

Background information and history of present illness can be obtained from significant others, because the patient is usually too ill to give details.

□ Objective data

The process of gathering objective data is the same as that described for respiratory failure (see p. 737).

DATA ANALYSIS: NURSING DIAGNOSES

Nursing diagnoses are determined from assessment of patient data. Possible nursing diagnoses may include, but are not limited to, the following:

Diagnostic title	Possible etiologies
Anxiety	Threat of death
Impaired gas exchange	Ventilation and perfusion imbalance
Altered nutrition: less than body requirements	Fatigue or difficulty in chewing and swallowing
Altered cardiopulmonary tissue perfusion	Decreased blood flow (physiologic shunting)

PLANNING: EXPECTED PATIENT OUTCOMES

Expected patient outcomes for the person with ARDS may include, but are not limited to, the following:
1. Patient will have improved ventilation and oxygenation.
   a. PaO_2 is maintained at 50 to 60 torr during the acute phase of illness.
   b. Upon resolution of ARDS, PaO_2, pH, and PCO_2 return to acceptable baseline limits.
   c. Sensorium returns to preillness level.
   d. During acute phase of illness, patient is able to tolerate mechanical ventilatory assistance.
   e. Inspiratory to expiratory ratio = 5:10 seconds.
   f. Respiratory rate and tidal volume are within normal limits.
   g. Patient does not complain of dyspnea

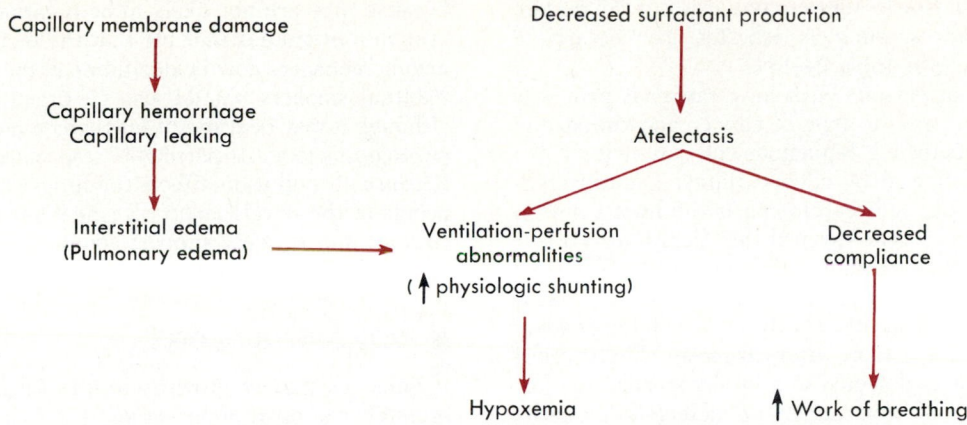

Fig. 24-7 Pathophysiologic events in adult respiratory distress syndrome.

2. Patient will have adequate tissue perfusion.
   a. Pulmonary capillary wedge pressure (measure of pulmonary capillary pressure) is maintained within established range (usually below 18 torr).
   b. Urinary output is at least 30 ml per hour.
   c. Peripheral pulses are present, and extremities are warm to the touch.
3. Patient will have increased physiologic and psychologic comfort.
   a. Patient tolerates ventilator and artificial airway.
   b. Patient communicates personal needs effectively with staff and family.
   c. Patient cooperates and assists with care.
4. Body weight stabilizes within normal range.

IMPLEMENTATION

Patients with ARDS are critically ill and are best cared for in an intensive care unit. Care for these patients centers around the following measures:
1. Maintaining adequate gas exchange
   a. Oxygenation
      (1) Maintain oxygen therapy as ordered.
      (2) Monitor for signs of hypoxemia (p. 736).
   b. Ventilatory support
      (1) Maintain a patent airway.
      (2) If artificial airway is present (endotracheal tube or tracheostomy):
         (a) Secure tube to avoid movement either in or out of established position.
         (b) Position patient for optimal oxygenation (see p. 680).
         (c) Auscultate lungs hourly to assess placement of endotracheal tube (which may slip into right mainstem bronchus).
      (3) Suction tube as needed.
      (4) Administer bronchodilators as ordered.
      (5) Check ventilator settings frequently.

2. Maintaining adequate tissue perfusion
   a. Monitor pulmonary capillary wedge pressure.
      (1) Notify physician if pressure is above or below established range.
      (2) If pressure is below established range, administer plasma volume expanders or hypotensive medications as ordered.
      (3) If pressure is high, administer diuretics or vasodilators as ordered.
   b. Assess urine output, vital signs, and extremities hourly.
3. Maintaining adequate nutrition
   a. Nutritional interventions for patients are the same as those for the patient with chronic obstructive pulmonary disease (see p. 731).

EVALUATION

Evaluation is based on patient outcomes. Questions to be asked include the following:
1. Is the patient able to maintain adequate gas exchange? Are arterial blood gases within normal limits?
2. Is the patient's urine output within normal limits?
3. Is the patient able to maintain nutrition by eating an adequate diet?

Cancer of the lung

During the last 50 years there has been a startling increase in the incidence of cancer of the lung. The American Cancer Society estimates that there were 150,000 new cases in 1987 and 136,000 deaths. Also in 1986, cancer of the lung surpassed breast cancer to become the number one cancer killer of women. Thus lung cancer is now the leading cause of death from cancer in both men and women.

The increase in death rates for both men and women is directly related to cigarette smoking. A history of smoking, especially for 20 years or more, is considered to be a prime risk factor. Other risk factors include exposure to certain industrial substances, such as asbestos, particularly in those who smoke (see Table 24-13).

The mortality of persons with lung cancer is primarily dependent on the specific type of cancer and the size of the tumor when detected. Squamous cell carcinoma is the most common, followed by adenocarcinoma; undifferentiated small cell (oat cell) carcinoma is the least common and has the lowest 5-year survival rate (less than 1%). If the tumor is of the squamous cell type and is detected while still small and localized (less than 3 cm), the 5-year survival rate is as high as 40%. Only 13% of all lung cancer patients live 5 years or more after diagnosis. The survival rate is 40% for cases detected in a localized stage. Unfortunately, only 20% of lung cancers are detected that early. Survival rates have improved only slightly over the past 10 years.[4] Most people who develop the disease are over 50 years of age. Some of the factors believed to be involved in the increased incidence of cancer of the lung include an increase in smoking among women, more accurate diagnosis, and tendency to name the lung as the primary site.

Cancer of the lung may either be metastatic or primary. Metastatic tumors may follow malignancy anywhere in the body. Metastasis from the colon and kidney is common. Metastasis to the lung may be discovered before the primary lesion is known, and sometimes the location of the primary lesion is not determined during the person's life.

■ PREVENTION

The cause of cancer of the lung is closely related to cigarette smoking. Table 24-12 shows the extreme increase in mortality from lung cancer in those persons who smoke. Prevention is the best protection against cancer of the lung because early detection of the disease is difficult, and at the present time only about 1 person in 9 (9%) is "cured" (living at the end of 5 years following diagnosis and treatment). From available research data it seems evident that curtailing smoking is a primary preventive measure. The nurse should be active in teaching the dangers of smoking. It is especially important that teenagers be given specific facts concerning the dangers involved in cigarette smoking,

because they are not likely to be habitual smokers at that age. Recent studies indicate that the incidence of smoking among teenagers may be declining. People who are already habitual smokers should also be urged to stop smoking, although it may be difficult for them to do so. Various types of programs to assist persons to stop smoking are available. Because air pollution affects the lungs and may predispose people to the development of cancer the nurse should encourage and actively support community programs to decrease the amount of air pollution.

■ PATHOPHYSIOLOGY

Since most new growths in the lungs arise from the bronchi, the term *bronchogenic carcinoma* is widely used. The symptoms that a patient has depend on whether the neoplasm is located peripherally or centrally. Peripheral lesions may not cause any symptoms and may be discovered only on routine chest roentgenograms. If peripheral lesions perforate into the pleural space, there will be *pleural effusion* (fluid in the pleural space), and direct invasion of the ribs and vertebral bodies may follow. If this occurs, the pain may be severe.

Centrally located lesions arise from one of the larger branches of the bronchial tree. They cause obstruction and ulceration of the bronchus with subsequent distal suppuration. Symptoms include cough, hemoptysis, dyspnea, chills, and fever. Unilateral wheezing may be heard on auscultation.

In the later stage of the disease, weight loss and debility usually indicate metastases, especially to the liver. Cancer of the lung may metastasize to nearby structures such as the prescalene lymph nodes, the walls of the esophagus, and the pericardium of the heart or to distant areas such as the brain, liver, or skeleton.

▦ ASSESSMENT

☐ **Subjective data**

1. Onset and duration of signs and symptoms (See Table 24-13 for common signs and symptoms of bronchogenic carcinoma.)
2. What the patient understands about why he or she is hospitalized
   a. For diagnostic tests
   b. For chest surgery
3. Whether the patient states that carcinoma of the lung is present or suspected
4. Smoking history

☐ **Objective data**

1. Presence of cough and whether or not productive of sputum
2. If sputum is present whether it is blood-streaked, indicating hemoptysis
3. Obvious shortness of breath when talking or on exertion
4. Unilateral wheezing on auscultation

Table 24-12 Deaths caused by lung cancer, according to smoking habits

	Deaths per 100,000 population
Nonsmokers	3.4
10-20 cigarettes per day	54.3
20-40 (1-2 packs) per day	143.9
More than 40 (2 packs) per day	217.3

From American Cancer Society: Cancer facts and figures, New York, 1976, The Society.

Table 24-13 Epidemiologic conditions, signs and symptoms, and medical therapy of bronchogenic carcinoma

Epidemiology	Signs and symptoms	Medical therapy
Cigarette smoking	*Bronchopulmonary*	Surgical excision by lobectomy or pneumonectomy—50% of patients inoperable when first seen by physician
Four to ten times more common than in nonsmokers	10% of patients are asymptomatic and are identified by chest x-ray	
Fifteen to thirty times more common in heavy smokers than nonsmokers	Cough present in 75% of patients	Radiation therapy for palliation in inoperable patients
Asbestos workers	Hemoptysis present in 50% of patients	Chemotherapy with alkylating agents
Six to ten times more common than in population at large	Local unilateral wheeze	
	Shortness of breath	
Genetic and immunologic factors	*Extrapulmonary intrathoracic*	
	Pleura	
Some evidence of genetic predisposition	Pain on breathing	
	Friction rub	
	Pleural effusion	
	Superior vena cava	
	Edema of face and neck	
	Generalized	
	Fatigue	
	Clubbing of fingers	
	Weight loss	

□ Diagnostic tests

In addition to x-ray films of the chest, the procedures used to diagnose bronchogenic carcinoma include bronchoscopy, mediastinoscopy, cytologic examination of sputum, bronchial washings and pleural fluid, and scalene node biopsy.

Time is very important in the treatment of lung cancer. If cancer is detected while it is still confined to a local area, immediate surgery, with removal of all or part of a lung (pneumonectomy or lobectomy), may be successful. Unfortunately, most patients are not seen by a surgeon early enough. It is estimated that one half of patients are inoperable on exploratory thoracotomy. Of those who are operable, the surgical mortality is 10% for pneumonectomy and 2% to 3% for lobectomy. The nursing care of the patient following surgery of the lung is discussed on p. 706.

Palliative treatment (irradiation, chemotherapy, or both) may be used for those persons who cannot be treated surgically, particularly when there is obstruction of an airway, obstruction of major vessels, severe pain, or recurrent pleural effusion. Presently, about one third of the patients who have surgery experience tumor spread. Radiation and chemotherapy are frequently prescribed for these patients.[4] Experimental studies with immunotherapy as an adjuvant to surgery and radiotherapy are also under way.

Efforts to detect malignant lesions of the lung early, while curative treatment may be possible, must be continued. The nurse should urge all persons over 40 years of age to have an x-ray examination of the chest periodically, in addition to a yearly physical examination. As a result of various public education media, many people have become more conscious of early signs of pulmonary cancer, but there is still a great need for them to learn about diagnostic tests that are available, including x-ray examinations, bronchoscopic examinations, and cytologic studies of sputum. The nurse should know of available cancer detection clinics in the community and should assist patients to secure proper medical supervision (see Chapter 12).

□ *Bronchoscopy*

A *bronchoscopic examination* is performed by passing a bronchoscope into the trachea and bronchi. Bronchoscopy is used to diagnose or treat conditions of the trancheobronchial tree. Diagnostic purposes include visualizing the source of hemoptysis; detecting the cause of atelectasis or the source of localized wheezing, that is, from an obstruction; and obtaining a specimen and assessing tracheal damage in an intubated patient. Therapeutic indications include lavaging patients with retained secretions, removing foreign bodies, draining a lung abscess, and removing food particles in aspiration pneumonia.

A bronchoscope is a long, slender, hollow instrument through which light can be reflected and visual examination of the branchings can be made. There are two types of bronchoscopes, the rigid metal or open-tube bronchoscope (Fig. 24-8) and the fiberoptic or flexible tube (Fig. 24-9). The *fiberoptic bronchoscope,* because of its flexibility, allows for greater visualization with passage into segmental and subsegmental bronchi. It has been employed with increasing frequency particularly for diagnostic examinations. The use of this instrument is also associated with less discomfort for the patient as compared to the rigid metal bronchoscopy.

Local anesthesia is applied by aerosal spray, transpharyngeal injections, ultrasonic nebulization or by cotton pledgets soaked in the anesthetic solution. The most commonly used anesthetic agents are cocaine, tetracaine hydrochloride, and lidocaine hydrochloride. The patient is closely monitored in the operating room for signs of toxic effects of these agents. Preparation of the patient for bronchoscopy

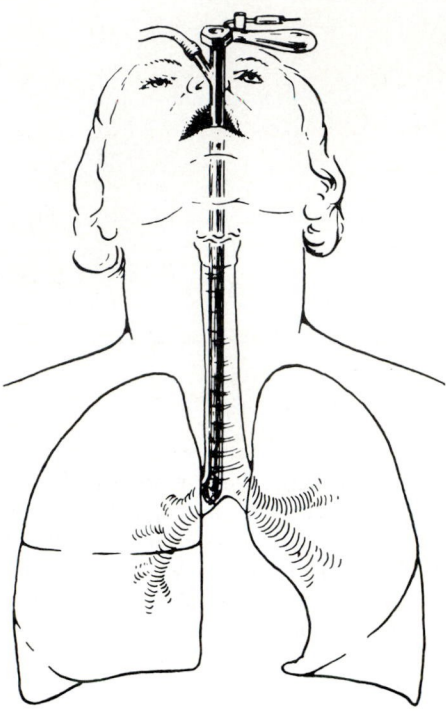

Fig. 24-8 Bronchoscope inserted through trachea into bronchus. (From DeWeese, DD, and Saunders, WH: Textbook of orolaryngology, ed 6, St. Louis, 1982, The CV Mosby Co.)

and care after the procedure is presented in the boxes on p. 701.

☐ *Mediastinoscopy*

In mediastinoscopy a *mediastinoscope,* which is an instrument much like a bronchoscope, is inserted through a small incision in the suprasternal notch and advanced into the mediastinum where inspection and biopsy of the lymph nodes can then be carried out.

➡ DATA ANALYSIS: NURSING DIAGNOSES

Nursing diagnoses are determined from assessment of patient data. Possible nursing diagnoses for the person with bronchogenic carcinoma may include, but are not limited to, the following:

Diagnostic title	Possible etiologies
Ineffective airway clearance	Decreased energy, fatigue
Anxiety	Threat of death
	Threat of or change in health status/threat to socioeconomic status/threat to role functioning and environment
Pain	Pleuritic chest pain (if pleura involved)
Impaired gas exchange	Ventilation and perfusion impairment
Knowledge deficit	Lack of exposure or unfamiliarity with information sources

⧉ PLANNING: EXPECTED PATIENT OUTCOMES

Expected patient outcomes for the person undergoing thoracic surgery may include, but are not limited to, the following:
1. Patient or significant other can explain recommended changes in ADL.
   a. Which usual activities to limit and for how long
   b. Exercise program

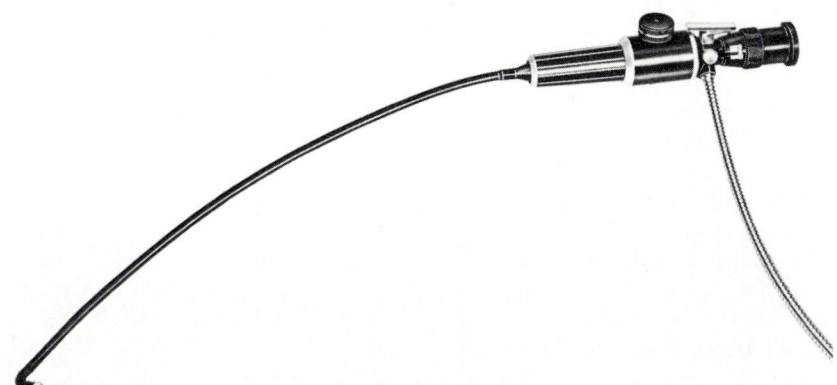

Fig. 24-9 Fiberoptic bronchoscope. Because of its flexibility it allows better visualization of bronchi. (Courtesy American Cystoscope Makers, Inc., Pelham, NY)

Preparation of patient for bronchoscopy

1. Physician should explain procedure to patient and obtain patient signature on informed consent form.
2. Patients are advised not to smoke for at least 24 hours.
3. Dentures are removed. Loose teeth are noted and called to physician's attention.
4. Preanesthetic medications are administered 30 to 60 minutes before procedure. Commonly prescribed are the following:
   a. Morphine sulfate, 5 to 15 mg IM, to suppress cough and relieve pain and anxiety. Demerol 50 to 100 mg IM is used in persons who have asthma or bronchospasm.
   b. Diazepam (Valium), 5 to 10 mg IM, for sedation and to protect against convulsive reactions to local anesthetic agents.
   c. Atropine sulfate, 0.4 to 1.0 mg IM, to reduce vasovagal reflex and decrease oral secretions.

---

2. Patient or significant other can explain any changes required in life-style (reason and plans for changes in occupation and habits such as smoking, activity level, and so on).
3. Patient can state name, dosage, action, and side effects of medications ordered.
   a. How and when to use prn medications
   b. Schedule for other medications and how to take them
4. Patient or significant other can describe professional and community resources necessary for structuring an environment compatible with convalescence.
   a. Plans for obtaining assistance of agencies such as Visiting Nurses Association
   b. Plans for necessary modifications of home

5. Patient or significant other can describe plans for follow-up care.
   a. Signs or symptoms requiring immediate medical assistance
   b. State plans for ongoing medical care

■ SURGICAL TREATMENT

When cancer of the lung is diagnosed or suspected, diagnostic tests are completed as soon as possible so that there is no delay in scheduling the patient for resectional surgery. The goal in surgery for cancer of the lung is the same as for other pulmonary diseases, to remove all the diseased tissue while preserving as much as possible of functional nondiseased lung.

Nursing care of the patient who has undergone bronchoscopy under local anesthesia

1. Patient lies flat or is placed in semi-Fowler's position based on physician's preference.
2. Lying on the side facilitates removal of secretions. Usually large amount of secretions are produced. All sputum is saved for culture and cytologic examination unless otherwise ordered.
3. Patient may be hoarse and complain of sore throat. Lidocaine (Xylocaine) is often helpful in reducing discomfort.
4. Vital signs are monitored for several hours.
5. Nothing is given by mouth for at least 2 hours or until gag reflex returns.
6. Patients may receive oxygen by mask or cannula for 4 hours after bronchoscopy to improve arterial blood oxygen levels, which may become lowered during the procedure.
7. Patients are monitored for complications including the following:
   a. Massive hemoptysis (blood-tinged sputum is normal for several hours after procedure)
   b. Bronchospasm: lungs should be auscultated when vital signs are taken. If bronchospasm is present, it may be treated with aminophylline intravenously or by bronchodilator administered by aerosol.
   c. Pneumothorax: if pneumothorax is present, a chest tube is inserted and connected to water-seal drainage.
   d. Laryngeal edema and airway obstruction: shortness of breath and laryngeal stridor are symptoms. The physician should be notified immediately.
8. Patient should not smoke for several hours. Smoking may cause coughing and start bleeding.
9. Sputum may be blood streaked for a few days. Pronounced bleeding should be reported at once.

Table 24-14 Types of thoracic surgery and indications for their use

Procedure	Indications
Exploratory thoracotomy	To confirm suspected diagnosis of lung or chest disease, especially carcinoma; to obtain a biopsy
Pneumonectomy (removal of a lung)	Bronchogenic carcinoma when lobectomy will not remove all of lesion; tuberculosis when other surgery will not remove all of diseased lung
Lobectomy (removal of lobe of lung)	Bronchogenic carcinoma confined to a lobe, bronchiectasis, emphysematous blebs or bullae; lung abscess, fungal infections, benign tumors; tuberculosis
Segmental resection (segmentectomy); (removal of one or more lung segments)	Bronchiectasis; lung abscess or cyst; metastatic carcinoma
Wedge resection (removal of pie-shaped section from surface of lung)	Well-circumscribed benign tumors, metastic tumors, or localized inflammatory disease such as tuberculosis
Decortication (removal of a fibrinous peel from the visceral pleura)	Chronic empyema

Table 24-14 lists the types of thoracic surgery and indications for their use. A brief explanation of each of these procedures follows.

☐ **Operative procedures**
☐ *Exploratory thoracotomy*

An exploratory thoracotomy is an operation used to confirm a suspected diagnosis of lung or chest disease. The usual approach is by a posterolateral parascapular incision through the fourth, fifth, sixth, or seventh intercostal space. Occasionally, an anterior approach is used. The ribs are spread to give the best possible exposure of the lung and hemithorax. The pleura is entered and the lung examined, a biopsy usually is taken, and the chest closed. This procedure may also be used to detect bleeding in the chest or other injury following trauma to the chest. Because the pleural space was entered, a chest tube and water-seal drainage are necessary.

☐ *Pneumonectomy*

A pneumonectomy, the removal of an entire lung, is most commonly used to treat bronchogenic carcinoma (Fig. 24-10, *B*). It may also be used to treat tuberculosis. However, a pneumonectomy is only performed when a lobectomy or segmental resection *will not* remove all the diseased tissue. A thoracotomy incision is made in either the posterior or anterior chest using the method described under exploratory thoracotomy. Before the lung can be removed, the pulmonary artery and vein are ligated and then cut. The mainsteam bronchus leading to the lung is clamped, divided, and sutured, usually with black silk. To ensure an airtight closure of the bronchus, a pleural flap is placed over it and sutured into place. The phrenic nerve on the operative side is crushed, causing the diaphragm on that side to rise and reduce the size of the remaining space. Because there is no lung left to reexpand, *drainage tubes are not used*. Ideally, the pressure in the closed chest is slightly negative. The pressure is taken postoperatively

using a pneumothorax apparatus, and air can be instilled or withdrawn to attain the desired pressure. The fluid left in the space will consolidate in time, helping to prevent the remaining lung and heart from shifting toward the operative side (mediastinal shift).

☐ *Lobectomy*

In a lobectomy one lobe of the lung is removed (Fig. 24-10, *C*). It is used to treat bronchiectasis, bronchogenic carcinoma, emphysematous blebs or bullae, lung abscess, benign tumors, fungal infections, and tuberculosis. For a lobectomy to be successful the disease must be confined to one lobe and the remaining lung tissue must be capable of overexpanding to fill up the space. Two chest tubes are connected to water-seal bottles for postoperative drainage.

☐ *Segmental resection (segmentectomy)*

In a segmental resection one or more segments of the lung are removed. This operation is used in an attempt to preserve as much functioning lung tissue as possible. It is a very taxing operation for the surgeon, because the dissection between segments must be done very carefully and slowly, and the identification of the segmental pulmonary artery and vein and bronchus is more difficult than when a lobe is involved. Since there are ten segments in the right lung and eight segments in the left lung, only a portion of a lobe or lobes may need to be removed. The most common indication for segmentectomy is bronchiectasis. It is also used to treat the other conditions listed in Table 24-14. Chest tubes and water-seal drainage are necessary postoperatively. Because of air leaks from the segmental surface, the remaining lung tissue may take longer to reexpand.

☐ *Wedge resection*

In a wedge resection a well-circumscribed diseased portion is removed without regard to the segmental planes. The area to be removed is clamped, dissected, and sutured.

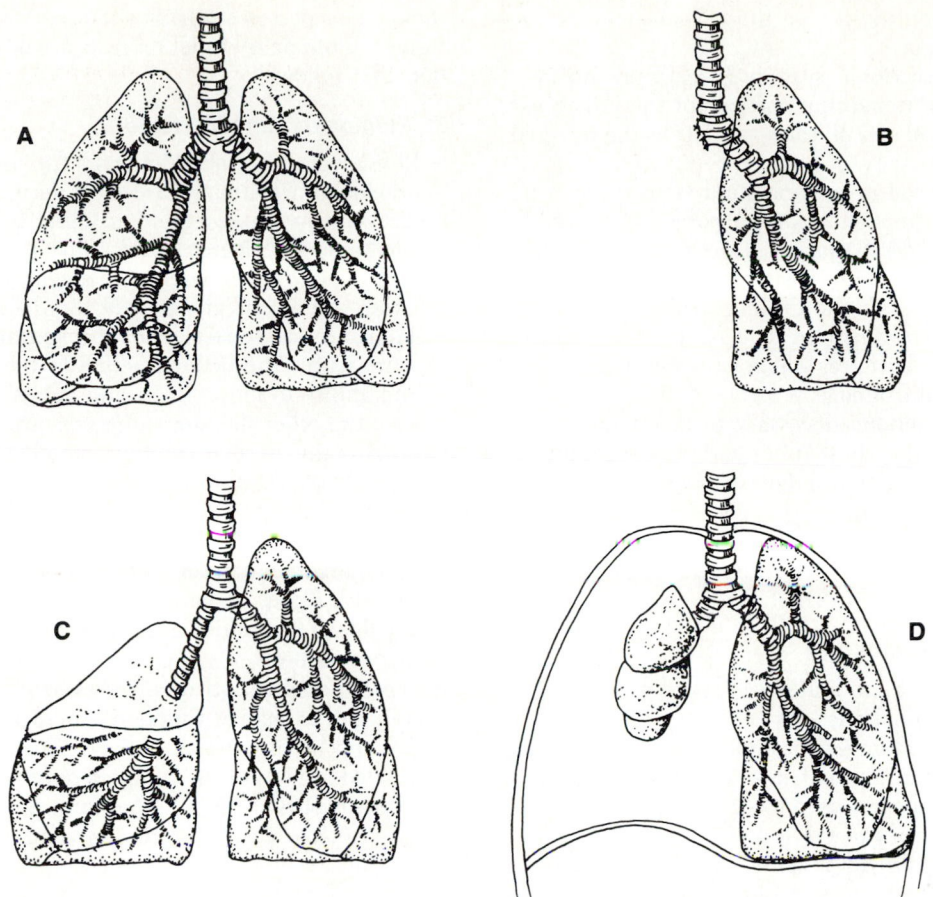

Fig. 24-10   **A,** Normal lungs. **B,** Surgical absence of right lung following a pneumonectomy. **C,** Surgical absence of the right upper lobe following a lobectomy. **D,** Complete
collapse of the right lung due to air in the pleural cavity (pneumothorax).

Chest tubes and water-seal drainage are used postoperatively.

□ Decortication

In a decortication, a fibrinous peel is removed from the
visceral pleura, allowing the encased lung to reexpand and
obliterate the pleural space. This procedure is discussed
further under the treatment of empyema (p. 712). Chest
tubes and chest suction are used to facilitate the reexpansion of the lung. If the lung has been encased for a long
time, it may be incapable of reexpanding following decortication. In this situation thoracoplasty may be necessary.

□ Principles of resectional surgery

1. Endotracheal anesthesia is used for surgery involving
   the lung in which the pleural space is entered.
2. With endotracheal anesthesia it is possible to keep the
   uninvolved ("good") lung expanded and functioning
   when the chest is opened and atmospheric pressure
   enters the pleural space.
3. To understand resectional surgery and the purpose of
   chest tubes and water-seal drainage an understanding
   of the following is necessary.

a. *Physiology of breathing*
   (1) The pressure in the pleural space (the space
       between the visceral and parietal pleura) is
       subatmospheric (less than 760 mm Hg) and is
       referred to as negative.
   (2) The pressure in the pleural space is usually 756
       mm Hg and goes down to 751 mm Hg before
       inspiration. This change in pressure allows air
       (atmospheric pressure) to enter the lungs.
   (3) When the pleura is entered surgically or by
       trauma to the chest wall, atmospheric pressure
       (760 mm Hg) enters the pleural space and the
       lung collapses.
b. *Purpose of chest tubes and water-seal drainage*
   (1) After resectional surgery of the lung (except
       pneumonectomy), two drainage tubes are in-
       serted into the pleural space and each tube is
       connected to a water-seal drainage bottle con-
       taining 1 to 2 cm of sterile water.
   (2) The tip of each tube is under water. This "seals"
       the chest tube, allowing air and fluid to drain
       from the pleural space into the water-seal bottle

and preventing air or fluid from entering the pleural space.

(3) In all resectional surgery (except pneumonectomy) the remaining portions of the lung must overexpand and fill the space left by the resected portion.

(4) The removal of air and fluid from the pleural space accomplishes two purposes. These are to (1) *aid in the expansion of the remaining portion of the lung* as air (positive pressure) and fluid escape through the drainage tubes, and (2) to *reestablish negative pressure in the pleural space.* These are basic reasons for the chest tubes and water-seal drainage.

(5) Nursing actions necessary to maintain the integrity of the chest tubes and water-seal drainage are discussed under postoperative care.

□ Preoperative evaluation

Special tests are required by a patient having chest surgery. These are discussed in the following sections.

□ *Radiologic procedures*

1. Posteroanterior (PA) and lateral chest films
2. Other x-ray examinations
   a. Laminograms (tomograms, planograms)—in this x-ray technique, special layers of lung tissue are visualized. They are used to study neoplasms, cavities, and densities of the lung.
   b. CT scanning provides more accurate information than laminography in some instances.

□ *Bronchoscopy*

Bronchoscopy (p. 699) is performed before any thoracic surgery. For the patient being considered for pneumonectomy, the evaluation is even more precise, because it must be determined if the uninvolved lung will be able to maintain the patient's respiration after the diseased lung is removed. Pulmonary function tests are usually used to determine the patient's ability to withstand pneumonectomy. In one center, patients who are being considered for pneumonectomy are evaluated on the basis of their forced expiratory volume in the first second (FEV_1) as follows:

1. If the FEV_1 is greater than 70% of the predicted normal level (approximately 2.5 L of flow), the patient's lung function is essentially normal and the patient should be able to tolerate a pneumonectomy as long as cardiac status and arterial blood gas levels are acceptable.
2. If the FEV_1 is less than 35% of the predicted normal level (less than 1.1 L of flow), there is severe ventilatory impairment, and surgical resection is not feasible.
3. If the FEV_1 is between 35% and 70% of the predicted normal level (1.2 to 2.4 L of flow), there is mild to moderate ventilatory impairment, and further studies will be necessary to determine the maximal amount of lung tissue that can be resected.[53]

The nurse should be sure that the patient understands what tests are to be performed and the preparation for them. The person's significant others also should be informed. Pulmonary function tests are described in the section that follows.

□ *Pulmonary function tests*

Physiologic tests of pulmonary function are performed to provide information regarding abnormalities in function, progression or improvement in clinical status, effects of medication, and degree of disability present. These tests cannot be used by themselves to diagnose specific diseases, but they are an integral part of the diagnostic process.

There are two general kinds of respiratory function tests. One measures the bellows action of the chest and lungs, or the ability to move air in and out of the alveoli (*ventilation*); the other measures *diffusion*, the movement of the gas across the alveolar-capillary membrane, and *perfusion*, the supply of blood to the lungs.

For the lung to perform gas exchange efficiently, the ventilation-perfusion ratio (V/Q ratio) must be balanced. That is, areas that receive ventilation should be well perfused with blood, and areas that receive blood flow should be capable of ventilation. Although in the normal lung with its many millions of gas exchange units, some imbalance in ventilation and perfusion exists, this has little effect on overall gas exchange function. In fact, adaptive mechanisms appear to exist that divert blood flow to the best-ventilated regions of the lungs or redirect ventilation away from nonperfused areas to maintain a normal ratio in the range of 0.8 to 1.0. Alteration in ventilation-perfusion relationships (either overall or in circumscribed areas of lung tissue) is largely responsible for the *hypoxemia* or *hypercapnia* seen in clinical practice. The nurse should be familiar with pulmonary function tests to be able to explain them to the patient. The total gas content of the lungs can be subdivided into volumes and capacities as defined in the box on p. 705.

MEASUREMENT OF PULMONARY VOLUMES AND CAPACITIES. To determine the functional capacity of the lungs, basic ventilation studies are performed by using a spirometer. Some measurements, such as the *residual volume,* cannot be measured directly and are calculated mathematically.

A spirogram giving the normal volumes and lung capacities is shown in Fig. 24-11. These volumes and capacities vary with age, sex, weight, and height. Two ventilatory studies are of particular clinical significance. They are the *forced expiratory volume* (FEV), or *timed vital capacity,* and the *maximal voluntary ventilation* (MVV), or *maximum breathing capacity* (MBC). The FEV measures the volume of air expired forcefully at 1, 2, and 3 seconds after a full inspiration. The FEV at *1 second* is the most useful of the three values, particularly when it is compared with the vital capacity (FEV_1/VC ratio). The MVV measures the volume of air exchanged per minute with maximal rate and depth of respiration. FEV and MVV can be affected by lung *compliance* (distensibility of the lung) because of the increased muscular effort required. FEV and MVV are decreased in obstructive lung disease and may be normal or decreased in restrictive lung disease.

The patient is usually instructed in how to participate

Definitions of lung volumes

Definitions of lung volumes (nonoverlapping measures)

Tidal volume (TV)	Volume of gas inspired and expired with a normal breath
Inspiratory reserve volume (IRV)	Maximal volume that can be inspired from the end of a normal inspiration
Expiratory reserve volume (ERV)	Maximal volume that can be exhaled by forced expiration after a normal expiration
Residual volume (RV)	Volume of gas left in lung after maximal expiration

Definitions of lung capacities (combinations of various volumes)

Inspiratory capacity (IC)	Maximal amount of air that can be inspired after a normal expiration (TV + IRV)
Functional residual capacity (FRC)	Amount of air left in lungs after a normal expiration (ERV + RV)
Vital capacity (VC)	Maximal amount of air that can be expired after a maximal inspiration (TV + IRV + ERV)
Forced vital capacity (FVC)	Maximal amount of air that can be expelled with a maximal effort after a maximal inspiration
Total lung capacity (TLC)	Total amount of air in lungs after maximal inspiration (TV + IRV + ERV + RV)

Volume/time relationships

Minute volume (MV)	Volume inspired and expired in 1 min of normal breathing
Forced expiratory volume in 1 sec FEV$_1$)	Amount of air expelled in the first second of the forced vital capacity maneuver
FEV$_1$/VC ratio	Amount of air forcefully expelled in 1 sec compared to total amount forcefully expelled
Maximal voluntary ventilation (MVV) (also termed *maximal breathing capacity* [*MBC*])	Amount of air exchanged per minute with maximal rate and depth of respiration

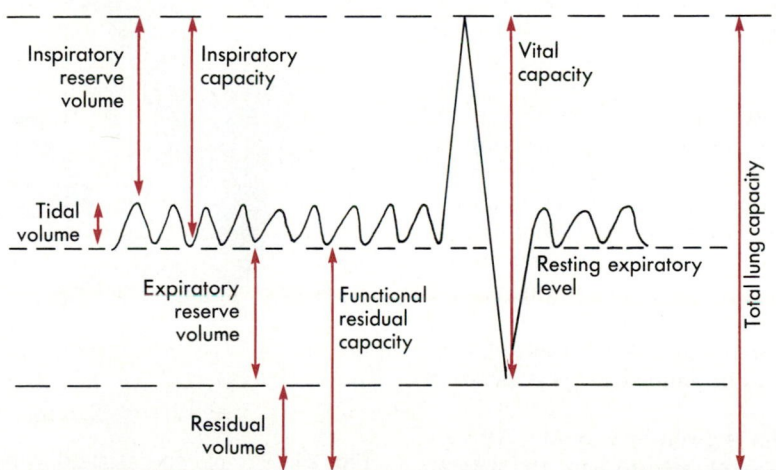

Fig. 24-11   Lung volumes and capacities illustrated by spirography tracing. (Adapted from Wade, JF: Respiratory nursing care, ed 3, St. Louis, 1982, The CV Mosby Co.)

in the tests by the physician or the technician in the testing laboratory. For all these tests the patient must breathe only through the mouth. A recording device and a spirometer are used. When the patient breathes through the mouthpiece and connecting tube, a noseclip is usually used so that the patient cannot breathe through the nose. Although a noseclip may seem like a small, harmless piece of equipment, the patient often becomes apprehensive about it. Time should be allowed for the patient to adjust to the clip. Fear of cutting off the air supply, particularly when a person has a breathing limitation, may cause anxiety. Because these tests are dependent on patient effort and can also be very exhausting to a patient with respiratory disease, rest both before and after the testing is necessary. If the patient is receiving regular bronchodilator treatments, these are withheld for 4 hours before testing if a part of the examination is to include measurements taken before and after the use of nebulized bronchodilators. Nurses can allay some of the patient's apprehension by giving clear and confident explanations.

☐ Care of patient having surgery
☐ *Preoperative care*

1. Determine patient's knowledge of procedure.
2. Explain expected postoperative measures including site of incision, oxygen, and chest tubes.
3. Provide opportunity for patient to ask questions or express concerns about diagnosis or the outcome of surgery.
4. Teach patient how to cough and explain postoperative coughing and deep breathing routine.
5. Teach patient arm exercises and explain postoperative expectations regarding arm exercises.
6. In some hospitals nurses from the operating room, the recovery room, or the intensive care unit assist in the preoperative teaching of the patient. It is the responsibility of the floor nurse caring for the patient preoperatively to determine what the patient understands about the impending surgery and to ensure the preoperative teaching is complete.

☐ *Postoperative care*

The care of the patient after thoracic surgery centers on promoting ventilation and reexpansion of the lung by maintaining a clear airway; promoting comfort by pain relief; promoting reexpansion of the lung by proper maintenance of the water-seal drainage system; promoting arm exercises to maintain full use of the patient's arm on the operated side; promoting nutrition; and monitoring the incision for bleeding and subcutaneous emphysema.

In most hospitals the patient goes from the recovery room to the intensive care unit. The immediate postoperative care is outlined below:

1. *Oxygen therapy.* Oxygen is given by cannula. An oxygen mask is not used because of need to have the patient cough and raise secretions frequently.

2. *Position of patient in bed.* The patient is kept flat in bed or with head elevated slightly (20 degrees) until blood pressure is stabilized to preoperative levels. Once blood pressure is stabilized, the patient can usually breathe best in semi-Fowler's position with a pillow under the head and neck but not under the shoulder and back because of the subscapular incision.

3. *Monitoring vital signs.* Vital signs are taken every 15 minutes until the patient is well reacted from anesthesia and then every hour until his or her condition has stabilized. It is not unusual for blood pressure to fluctuate during the first 24 to 36 hours, and close monitoring of it is essential. A persistently low blood pressure should be reported to the surgeon.

4. *Initiating coughing and deep-breathing exercises.* The patient should be assisted to cough as soon as conscious. If the blood pressure is stable, the patient is assisted to a sitting position and the incision is supported anteriorly and posteriorly by the nurse's hands. Firm, even pressure over the incision with the open palm of the hands is a most effective method. The nurse's head should be behind the patient when the patient is coughing (Fig. 24-12). The patient is encouraged to breathe deeply, exhale, and then cough. Sips of fluids, especially warm ones such as tea or coffee, often facilitate coughing. Mist therapy may be used to loosen secretions. Coughing *keeps the airway patent, prevents atelectasis,* and *facilitates reexpansion of the lung.* The patient should be assisted to cough every hour for the first 24 hours, and then every 2 to 4 hours. The patient should cough until the chest sounds clear. Otherwise, secretions will accumulate in the tracheobronchial tree.

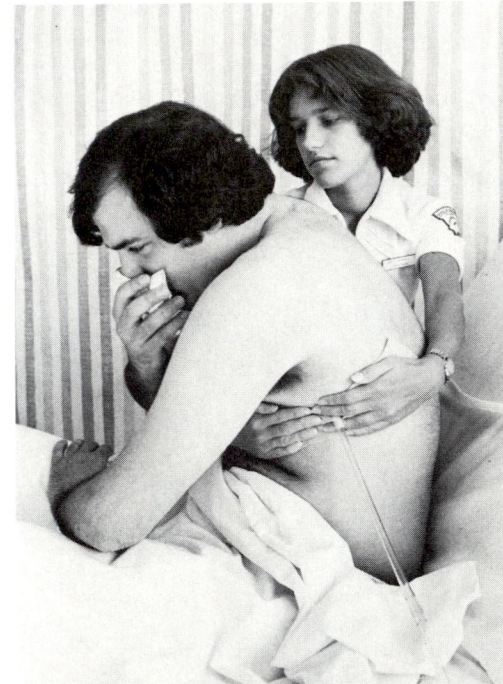

Fig. 24-12 Nurse assists patient to cough by splinting incision with firm support from hands. This lessens muscle pull and pain as patient coughs. Note that nurse keeps her head behind patient while he coughs, and patient uses tissue to cover mouth.

Abdominal breathing exercises such as those described on p. 725 are a valuable adjunct to the care of the patient with chest surgery because they improve ventilation without increasing pain and assist in coughing more effectively. The exercises should be taught preoperatively so that the patient has time to practice them before surgery. *The patient can cough most effectively 20 to 30 minutes after receiving pain medication*, and this should be capitalized on by the nursing staff. Patients who cannot raise secretions on their own may have to be suctioned.

5. *Promoting comfort by pain relief.* Morphine or meperidine hydrochloride is usually ordered for pain. Medication for pain should be given as needed and may be required as often as *every 3 to 4 hours during the first 48 to 72 hours*. The patient is extremely uncomfortable and will not be able to cough or turn unless there is relief from pain. In some instances the dose of the narcotic is decreased so that it may be given more often and yet not depress respirations. The tubes in the chest cause pain, and the patient may attempt rapid, shallow breathing to splint the lower chest and avoid motion of the catheters. This impairs ventilation, makes coughing ineffective, and causes secretions to be retained. Thus it is *a nursing responsibility to do all that is possible to make the patient comfortable, since this facilitates deep breathing and coughing.* If, despite all possible efforts, the patient's discomfort is interfering with adequate chest excursion, an intercostal nerve block may be performed.

6. *Monitoring the incision for bleeding or subcutaneous emphysema.* Dressings are checked periodically for evidence of bleeding. *Blood on the dressings is unusual* and should be reported to the surgeon at once. The time and amount of blood is recorded in the patient's record. The surgeon may reinforce the dressing, and in the rare instance when bleeding persists the patient may be taken back to surgery. The chest will be reopened and the source of bleeding located and ligated.

Subcutaneous emphysema is not unusual after chest surgery. In subcutaneous emphysema, air leaks from the pleural space through the thoracotomy incision or around the chest tubes into the soft tissues. When palpating the chest the presence of air under the skin is readily detected and has been described as feeling like *"tissue paper"* or *"Rice Krispies"* under the skin. Subcutaneous emphysema is most notable in the neck and chest, and if considerable air is leaking, the patient's face and neck become considerably enlarged. Small amounts of air reabsorb over time and cause no problem; but if subcutaneous emphysema is worsening, the chest tube may be changed by the surgeon and a larger one inserted, since air is leaking into the tissues faster than it is being removed by the tube. Additional suction may also be applied to the chest tube(s) in an attempt to remove air more rapidly. Rarely a patient will need to return to surgery for closure of air leaks.

The patient with a pneumonectomy should have only a small amount (if any) of subcutaneous emphysema. *Progressive subcutaneous emphysema after pneumonectomy is very serious and should be reported to the surgeon immediately*, since it could indicate a major leak in the bronchial stump. This also is a rare occurrence, requiring return of the patient to surgery for reclosure of the bronchial stump.

7. *Promoting arm exercises.* Passive arm exercises are usually started the evening of surgery. The purpose in putting the patient's arm through range of motion is to prevent restriction of function. Most patients are reluctant to move the arm on the operative side, but with proper preoperative instruction and postoperative follow-through they do so readily. It is important for both the patient and nurse to understand that the longer the arm is unexercised, the stiffer it becomes. The patient should put both arms through active range of motion two or three times a day within a few days after surgery. The recommended exercises are similar to those done following mastectomy (Chapter 36). The exercises are best done when the patient is upright or lying on his or her abdomen. Exercises such as elevating the scapula and clavicle, "hunching the shoulders," bringing the scapulae as close together as possible, and hyperextending the arm can only be done in these positions. Because lying on the abdomen may not be possible at first, these exercises are done with the patient sitting on the edge of the bed or standing.

8. *Promoting nutrition.* The patient is encouraged to take fluids after surgery and to progress to a general diet as soon as it is tolerated. Forcing fluids helps to liquefy secretions and makes them easier to expectorate. A diet adequate in protein and vitamins (especially vitamin C) facilitates wound healing.

9. *Ambulation.* There is no contraindication to ambulating with a chest tube in place. As long as the water-seal bottle remains below the level of the chest, the patient may assume any position of comfort in bed or may be out of bed in a chair or walk about.

10. *Maintaining chest tubes and drainage.* All patients who have resectional surgery of the lung, except those having a pneumonectomy, require drainage of the pleural space by chest tubes connected to closed drainage. Usually two tubes are used. One catheter is inserted through a stab wound in the anterior chest wall above the resected area. This is referred to as the *anterior* or *upper tube*. It is used to remove air from the pleural space. The second tube is inserted through a stab wound in the posterior chest and is referred to as the *posterior* or *lower tube*. It is primarily for the drainage of *serosanguineous* fluid that accumulates as the result of the operative procedure. The lower tube may be of a larger diameter than the upper tube to prevent it from becoming plugged with clots. Fig. 24-13 shows the placement of tubes within the pleural space.

When initiating chest tube drainage, a 2-liter clear glass bottle is usually used, although other commercial devices, such as the PleureVac system (Fig. 24-14) are available. Approximately 300 ml of sterile water, or enough to fill the bottle 1 to 2 cm from the bottom, is then added. If considerable drainage accumulates in the bottle, this increases the amount of *subatmospheric (negative) pressure* in the system, and it is more difficult for the patient to expel air and fluid from the pleural space. In this instance the glass rod may be pulled up so that less of it is under water or the surgeon may order the drainage bottle to be changed.

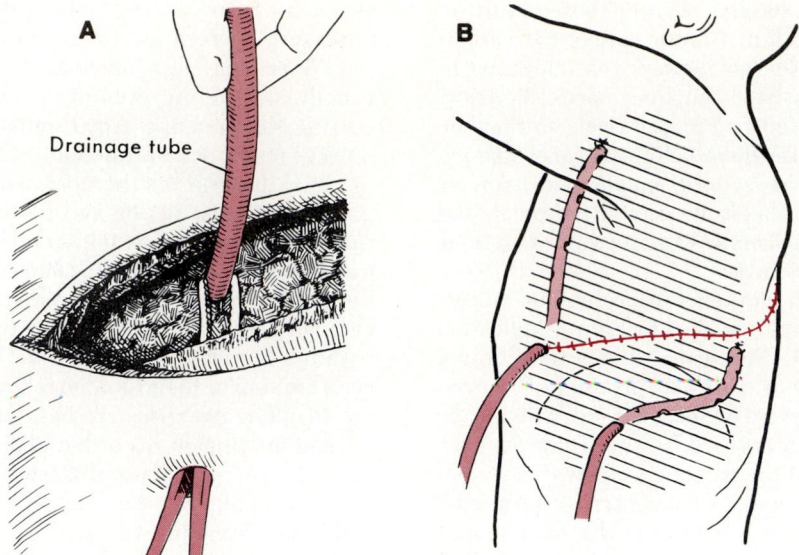

Fig. 24-13 **A,** Drainage tube inserted into pleural space. **B,** Note that upper and lower tubes are placed well into pleural space (From Johnson, J, MacVaugh, H, III, and Waldhausen, JA: Surgery of the chest, a handbook of operative surgery, ed 4, Copyright © 1970 by Year Book Medical Publishers, Inc., Chicago. Used by permission).

Fig. 24-14 Pleurevac—one of several available brands of chest drainage systems. The system functions like a three-bottle system in that the unit collects drainage, maintains a seal to prevent air from entering the pleural cavity, and prevents excessive build-up of negative pressure. (From Abels, LF: Mosby's manual of critical care, St. Louis, 1979, The CV Mosby Co.)

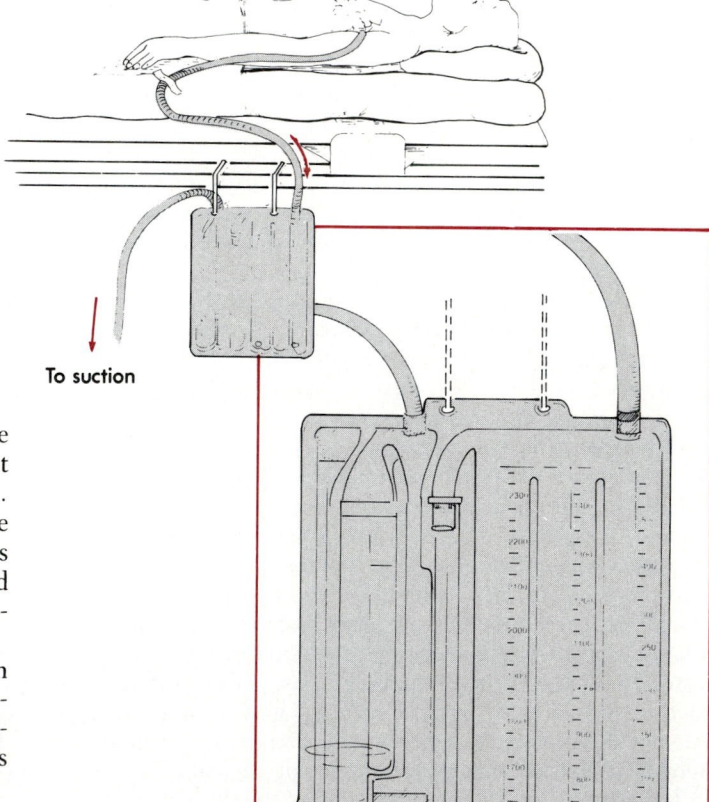

To suction

In this case a sterile setup is prepared. When the sterile bottle with sterile water and the tubing are ready, the chest tubes is clamped as close to the patient's chest as possible. The chest tube is then disconnected from the drainage tubing, the new setup is connected, and the chest tube is unclamped. The amount of drainage in the bottle should be measured and usually is sent to the laboratory for examination.

As the patient breathes, there is movement of fluid in the glass tube that is under water. This is known as *fluctuation* or *oscillation*. The column moves up when the patient inhales or coughs, and it falls when the patient is exhaling.

Some thoracic surgeons wish to have the chest tubes "milked" or "stripped" every hour to prevent formation of clots that could plug the tubes. Recently, questions have been raised about routinely stripping chest tubes, because the practice increases the negative pressure exerted on the pleural space. A study by two nurse–clinical specialists revealed the following: (1) the pressure generated by stripping was considerably higher than the suction pressures of −15 to −20 cm of water commonly applied to chest drainage systems; (2) the amount of pressure was directly related to the length of the tubing stripped; and (3) even stripping only a few centimeters produced pressures near −100 cm of water, and stripping the entire tube produced pressures exceeding −400 cm of water. They also found that higher negative pressures resulted when a roller was used to strip the tubes rather than hands.[20]

Undesirable side effects of increased levels of negative pressure reported in the literature include (1) lung entrapment in the thoracic tube eyelets and focal tissue infarction and (2) persistent pneumothorax. The persistent pneumothorax occurs when the pleural surface of lung, which normally has air leaks at the close of the operative procedure, does not "seal off." Usually fibrin seals the air leaks; however, the presence of an increased amount of negative pressure may prevent the air leaks from sealing off and may even increase the size of the air leaks. This is the reason why some thoracic surgeons do not attach additional suction to the water-seal drainage system for the first 24 hours or so after surgery. They believe that this amount of time is sufficient in most instances to allow the pleural surface to seal off.

In view of these findings, the nurse should consult with the thoracic surgeon about the desirability of routinely stripping chest tubes. Because the anterior (upper) tube usually evacuates mainly air, there is less reason to believe that this tube will clot off. Posterior tubes, which are commonly inserted lower in the chest, usually drain more fluid and blood and are more likely to clot off. However, gentle squeezing of the tube is usually sufficient to move the bloody drainage along in the tubing. Special caution should be used in stripping tubes of patients with a known history of fragile tissue, such as occurs in emphysema.[20] The nursing measures necessary in maintaining chest tubes and closed drainage are listed in box below.

ADDITIONAL SUCTION

Suction is usually used to speed reexpansion of the lung after surgery, using either wall suction or an Emerson suction machine (Fig. 24-15, *B*). Commonly −10 to −30 cm of suction is applied, according to the surgeon's pref-

---

Maintaining chest tubes and closed chest drainage

1. Mark water level in bottle with strip of adhesive tape so that amount of drainage can easily be determined. Write date and hour on tape.
2. Fasten tubing to the bed so that there are no dependent loops between the bottles and the bed (Fig. 24-15). Dependent loops allow fluid to collect in tubing and impede removal of air and fluid from pleural space.
3. Be sure that tip of chest tube is 1 to 2 cm under water so that if the bottle accidently tips over, the tube will remain under water.
4. Check the tubes for fluctuation frequently. If the column of water is not fluctuating:
   a. Be sure patient is not lying on tubes.
   b. Check connections to be sure chest tube system is airtight.
   c. Ask patient to cough or change position to see if fluctuation is restored.
   d. Fluctuation will stop when lung is reexpanded.
5. Milk or strip chest tubes as ordered (sometimes every hour). This is accomplished by gently exerting pressure along the chest tube with the right hand while holding the chest tube firmly with the left hand. Holding the tube with the left hand prevents tugging on it while the tube is being milked or stripped. See p. 708 for precautions about milking tubes.
6. Keep two hemostats at the bedside so that the chest tube can be clamped if a bottle is accidently broken. When a bottle is broken, the chest catheter should be clamped and then reconnected to a sterile bottle as soon as possible. Sterile water should be used in the bottle. As soon as the system is reconnected with the tip of the tube under water, the clamp should be removed. Except in case of an emergency, such as a broken bottle, most thoracic surgeons prefer that tubes not be clamped, and a specific order is written if clamping is desired.
7. Never clamp chest tubes unless a bottle breaks (a rare occurrence) or without written order. When chest tubes are clamped, air (positive pressure) may be trapped in the pleural space and further collapse the lung. If a patient is being transported from one place to another, such as to the x-ray department, tubes should not be clamped unless for only a few minutes.
8. Never lift chest tube bottles above the level of the patient's chest, because this allows fluid to be pulled into the pleural space.
9. The water-seal bottles should be placed on the floor so that they will not be broken by a lowered side-rail. When a Hi-Lo bed is being used, care should be taken not to lower the bed onto the bottles.

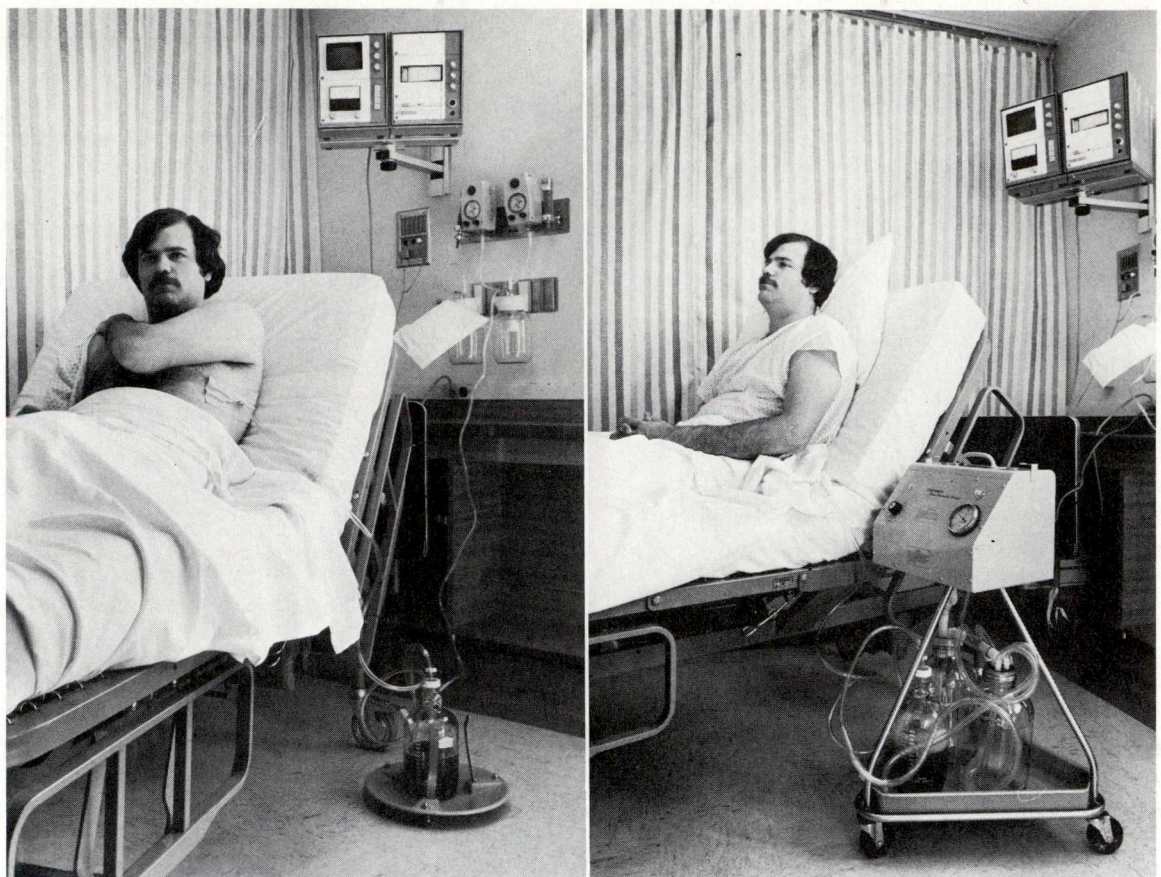

Fig. 24-15   Chest tube with water-seal suction. **A,** Wall outlet provides source of suction. Note holder used to secure bottle in upright position. **B,** Emerson suction machine as source of vacuum.

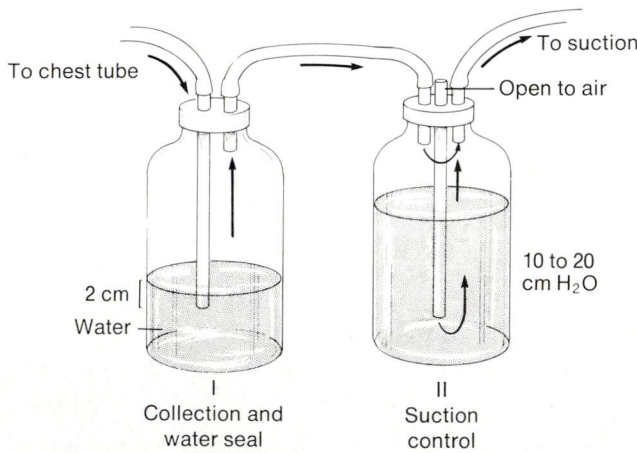

Fig. 24-16   Two bottle drainage system showing water-seal bottle connected to suction control ("breaker") bottle. Note that glass rod in suction control bottle is open to the air. This bottle regulates the amount of suction exerted on the pleural space. (From Abels, LF: Mosby's manual of critical care, St. Louis, 1979, The CV Mosby Co.)

erence. When it is particularly important to regulate the exact amount of suction used, a control or "breaker" bottle is added to the system between the suction source and the patient's drainage bottle. The use of a control or "breaker" bottle controls the amount of suction that is applied to the water-sealed bottle and thus to the patient's pleural space. The stopper in the control bottle has three openings. One in connected to the water-seal bottle, one is connected to the suction source, and the third contains a glass rod that is under water and open to the outside (Fig. 24-16). The amount of suction produced is determined by the distance between the surface of the water and the tip of this tube. When the suction source is turned on, the level of water in the open tube sinks in proportion to the amount of negative pressure in the system. Thus if there is 15 cm of water between the surface of the water and the tip of the tube, the amount of negative pressure in the system will be 15 cm of water pressure. Because the water is at the bottom of the tube when this amount of pressure is reached, any increase in negative pressure causes air to be drawn in from the outside, *breaking* the suction at this level. Therefore, it can be expected that the water in the control bottle will bubble almost continuously. If it fails to bubble at all, the desired level of suction is not being attained. When the water in the control bottle is not bubbling, the tubing should be checked for air leaks. If there are no leaks and bubbling still does not occur, the surgeon should be notified at once because the air leak in the pleura may be so great that the amount of negative pressure is not sufficient to overcome it. In this instance water may be added to the control bottle to increase the distance between the surface of the water and the tip of the tube, thereby increasing the amount of negative pressure being exerted on the pleural space.

The distance the tube is placed under water in the control bottle is determined by the surgeon. A bottle and suction may be attached to one or both tubes. Most commonly it is attached to the upper tube, since this is where air is most likely to be leaking from the pleural surface. A small empty trap bottle is usually attached by tubing between the control bottle and the suction source. The pur-

pose of this bottle is to protect the suction motor from becoming wet should the control bottle overflow.

REMOVAL OF THE CHEST TUBE

Chest tubes are removed when there is no fluctuation of fluid in the tubing, and when roentgenograms confirm the full reexpansion of the lung. The patient should receive medication for pain 30 minutes before removal of the tube. The exact procedure used to remove the tube may vary, but generally a sterile scissors, 4-inch × 4-inch gauze squares, and adhesive tape are the materials required. The suture holding the tube in place is cut, the patient is asked to exhale deeply, and the tube is removed. Some physicians cover the site with a Telfa dressing instead of gauze squares to ensure an airtight dressing. The dressing is covered securely by three strips of 2-inch adhesive tape. If a purse-string suture was used, it is retied and a dry sterile dressing is placed over the site.

Special care following pneumonectomy

1. Chest tubes are not necessary since there is no lung left to reexpand on the operative side.
2. Patient may lie on back or *operated side only*. Patient is not allowed to lie with operative side uppermost because of fear that the sutured bronchial stump may open, allowing fluid to drain into the unoperated side and drown the patient.
3. Pressure in the operative side is checked in the operating room after the chest is closed. A pneumothorax apparatus (which can instill or remove air) is used to check the pressure in the operative space, and air is removed or instilled as necessary to bring the pressure to slightly negative (slightly less than 760 mm Hg).
4. The surgeon palpates the patient's trachea at least daily to determine if it is in midline. Deviation of the trachea toward either the operated or unoperated side is a sign of *mediastinal shift.* If pressure builds up in the operated side, the trachea will deviate toward the unoperated side. The treatment is to remove air (positive pressure) with a pneumothorax apparatus. Mediastinal shift toward the "good" lung can seriously comprise ventilation and needs to be treated promptly. Deviation of the trachea toward the operated side indicates that more pressure (air) needs to be instilled into the empty space.
5. The patient with a mediastinal shift resembles the patient in congestive heart failure. Neck veins are distended, the trachea is displaced to one side, pulse and respirations are increased, and dyspnea is present.
6. Serous drainage collects in the operated space and over time congeals to the consistency of axle grease. This is often sufficient to keep the mediastinum from shifting toward the operative side. Persistent mediastinal shift toward the operative side may have to be treated with *thoracoplasty* (removal of ribs) to reduce the size of the remaining space and assist in maintaining the mediastinum in midline. Thoracoplasty is described on p. 712.
7. It usually takes 2 to 4 days for the remaining lung to adjust to the increase in blood flow. For this reason the amount of fluids and blood given intravenously is monitored closely to prevent fluid overload. CVP monitoring is common. Rales are commonly heard over the base of the remaining lung and vascular markings are more prominent on x-ray films. Any increase in rales, in pulse or blood pressure, and in dyspnea may indicate circulatory overload and should be reported immediately. Treatment may include diuretics and/or digitalization along with discontinuance of intravenous fluids.
8. Deep breathing, coughing, and arm exercises are the same as described earlier (p. 706).
9. Patients who have had a lung removed may have a lowered vital capacity, and exercise and activity should be limited to that which can be done without dyspnea. Because the body must be given time to adjust to having only one lung, the patient's return to work may be delayed.
10. If the diagnosis is cancer, radiation therapy is usually given, and it may be started before the patient leaves the hospital (See Chapter 12 for further discussion on nursing care for patients receiving radiation therapy.)
11. The patient who has had a pneumonectomy for cancer is urged to report to the physician at once if hoarseness, dyspnea, pain on swallowing, or localized chest pain develop, because these symptoms may be signs of complications.

□ *Care following pneumonectomy*

The postoperative care discussed above applies to all patients with resection surgery except those having a pneumonectomy. The special care required following pneumonectomy is outlined in the box on p. 711.

□ *Thoracoplasty*

A thoracoplasty is an extrapleural procedure involving the removal of ribs. By removing ribs it is possible to reduce the size of the chest cavity. Before the widespread use of resectional surgery, thoracoplasty was the basic surgical treatment for tuberculosis. Today thoracoplasty is used (infrequently) primarily to prevent or treat the complications of resectional surgery. When it is felt that a patient's lung may not be able to expand sufficiently after a resection to fill the space, a thoracoplasty is done 2 or 3 weeks before the resection. It also may be done before pneumonectomy, since this reduces the chance of mediastinal shift after surgery. This type of thoracoplasty is often called a *preresection* or *tailoring* thoracoplasty; that is, the chest wall is tailored to reduce its size.

If the remaining portions of the lung fail to reexpand sufficiently after resection or if another complication (such as empyema) occurs, a thoracoplasty is performed. In general, it is employed when there is a space in the chest that cannot be obliterated by other means. Usually no more than three ribs are removed, and therefore paradoxical motion following thoracoplasty is seldom seen anymore. Paradoxical motion is discussed under chest injuries (p. 714).

□ *Complications of chest surgery*

There are two major complications that are specific to chest surgery, empyema and bronchopleural fistula. The patient may have empyema with or without bronchopleural fistula. The signs and symptoms and treatment of these complications are outlined in Table 24-15.

□ *Evaluation for the patient having resectional surgery*

Evaluation is based on patient outcomes. Questions to be asked include the following:
1. Is the patient able to ambulate independently?
2. Does the patient have full use of the arm and the operative side?
3. Is the surgical wound free of infection?
4. Does the patient understand prescribed follow-up therapy such as radiation or chemotherapy?
5. Is the patient able to express concerns regarding diagnosis of cancer and his/her future?
6. Does the patient know signs and symptoms that indicate the need for immediate medical follow-up?

■ Chest trauma

■ EPIDEMIOLOGY AND ETIOLOGY

Trauma to the chest is a major problem most often seen first in the emergency department. Injury to the chest may affect the bony chest cage, pleurae and lungs, diaphragm, or mediastinal contents. Injuries to the chest are broadly classified into two groups—blunt and penetrating. *Blunt,* or nonpenetrating, injuries damage the structures within the chest cavity without disrupting chest wall integrity. *Penetrating* injuries disrupt chest wall integrity and result in alteration in intrathoracic pressures.

The leading cause of blunt chest injuries in the United States is motor vehicle steering wheel impaction in the person not wearing a seat belt. Blows to the chest with

Table 24-15 Empyema and bronchopleural fistula

Complications	Signs and symptoms	Treatment
Empyema		
Pus in the pleural space is a dreaded complication of thoracic surgery. Pus may drain from chest tube(s) or if chest tubes are already removed can be removed by thoracentesis (insertion of a needle attached to a syringe with a three-way stopcock used to remove fluid, blood, or pus from pleural space).	Unexplained elevation in temperature Evidence of pleural exudate on x-ray film	*Dependent drainage* by thoracentesis, intercostal chest tube, or open drainage with rib resection. Chest tube may be connected to water-seal bottle or cut off and allowed to drain into chest dressings. Water-seal no longer necessary if empyema space has a thick wall and there is no danger of lung collapse. Over time, as empyema drains out the tube, the space becomes smaller and fills in with granulation tissue. If space persists a thoracoplasty will be necessary.
Bronchopleural fistula		
Opening in the sutured bronchus that permits communication with pleural space. Space usually becomes infected and empyema develops.	Fever, leukocytosis, anorexia, expectoration of purulent sputum, and evidence of pleural exudate on x-ray film	Chest tubes connected to water-seal since there is a direct communication between bronchus (positive pressure being inspired) and the pleural space. A persistent bronchopleural fistula is treated by thoracoplasty and a muscle implant to seal off the bronchus.

Table 24-16 Types of penetrating and nonpenetrating (blunt) chest injuries

Penetrating	Blunt
Open pneumothorax (sucking chest wound)	**Closed pneumothorax**
Hemothorax	Tension pneumothorax
Tracheobronchial injury	Tracheobronchial injury
Pulmonary contusion	Flail chest
Diaphragm rupture	Diaphragm rupture
Mediastinal injury	Mediastinal injury
	Fractured ribs

blunt objects or as a result of a fall also cause nonpenetrating chest injury. Penetrating wounds usually result from gunshot or stabbing injuries.

Both penetrating and blunt chest injuries can be fatal. The common chest injuries and their sequelae are classified as primarily penetrating or nonpenetrating chest wounds in Table 24-16.

■ **PREVENTION**

Nurses can promote prevention of chest trauma through public education programs focused on safe practices in vehicle usage and in the work place. The major preventive measure is the use of seat belts when operating a motor vehicle.

■ **CHEST CAGE INJURIES**

☐ **Rib fractures**
☐ *Pathophysiology*

Rib fractures are the most common chest injury. Ribs 3 through 10 are most often fractured because they are less protected by the chest muscles. The ribs usually fracture at the point of maximal impact but may fracture at a distant site from impact. Fractures of the ribs are caused by blows, crushing injuries, or strain caused by severe coughing or sneezing spells. If the rib is splintered or the fracture displaced, sharp fragments may penetrate the pleura and the lung, resulting in a hemothorax or pneumothorax.

Common signs and symptoms of rib fracture include the following:

1. Pain at the site of injury, increasing on inspiration
2. Localized tenderness and crepitus on palpation
3. Patient splinting the chest and taking shallow breaths

■ **TREATMENT**

Treatment is individualized, based on the patient's age, whether there is preexisting chronic pulmonary disease history, and the number and location of ribs fractured. Medical treatment includes the following:

1. Stabilization of the fracture site with a rib belt or Ace bandage
2. Analgesics as needed
3. For severe pain, performance of a regional nerve block

▨ **ASSESSMENT**

☐ **Subjective data**

Subjective data include the nature of the injury and when it occurred. If patient is unable to answer questions, data are obtained from those with the patient.

☐ **Objective data**

1. Pain at site of injury that increases on inspiration
2. Area tender to the touch
3. Patient splints chest and takes shallow breaths

☐ **Diagnostic tests**

Fractures are confirmed by chest x-ray findings.

▶ **DATA ANALYSIS: NURSING DIAGNOSES**

Nursing diagnoses are determined from assessment of patient data. Possible nursing diagnoses for the person with rib fracture may include, but are not limited to, the following:

Diagnostic title	Possible etiologies
Ineffective airway clearance	Pain/trauma to rib cage
Anxiety	Threat to change in health status
Ineffective breathing pattern	Pain, musculoskeletal impairment
Pain	Trauma to rib cage
Knowledge deficit	Lack of exposure to information

▨ **PLANNING: EXPECTED PATIENT OUTCOMES**

Expected patient outcomes for the person with fractured ribs may include, but are not limited to, the following:

1. Pain is improved.
2. Patient is breathing effectively.
3. Patient maintains a patent airway.
4. Patient is less anxious.
5. Patient understands follow-up therapy.
6. Patient understands that physician is to be notified if shortness of breath, hemoptysis, or temperature elevation occur.

▧ **IMPLEMENTATION**

☐ **Assisting with achievement of therapeutic goals**
☐ *Initial care for fractured ribs*

If ribs are fractured and the rib has not penetrated the pleura, the chest is strapped with adhesive tape or an Ace bandage or chest binder is applied.

1. Check strapping to be sure it is secure.
2. Give analgesics as ordered.

□ **Assisting with comfort and ADL**

1. Place patient in position of comfort. May be able to breathe easier in Fowler's or semi-Fowler's position.
2. Give prescribed analgesics.
3. If pain persists despite analgesics, notify the physician, who may infiltrate the intercostal spaces above and below the fractured rib(s) with 1% procaine.

‡ EVALUATION

Evaluation is based on patient outcomes. Questions to be asked include the following:

1. Is the patient's pain improved?
2. Is the patient able to breathe effectively?
3. Is the patient less anxious?
4. Can the patient state plans for follow-up care?
5. Can the patient state the signs and symptoms (shortness of breath, hemoptysis, or elevated temperature) that require immediate medical attention?

■ FLAIL CHEST

□ **Pathophysiology**

When multiple ribs or the sternum are fractured in more than one place, a portion of the chest wall becomes separated from the chest cage, resulting in a *flail chest*. That is, the chest wall no longer provides the rigid bony support that is necessary to maintain the bellows function required for normal ventilation. This causes *paradoxical respiratory* movement. On inspiration the dislocated segment is pulled inward by the subatmospheric intrapleural pressure. During expiration the dislocated segment bulges outward as intrapleural pressure becomes less negative (Fig. 24-17, *A-D*).

Flail chest usually causes localized atelectasis secondary to decreased ventilation, resulting in hypoxemia. Because of the increased work of breathing, the individual may also develop hypercapnia and respiratory acidosis.

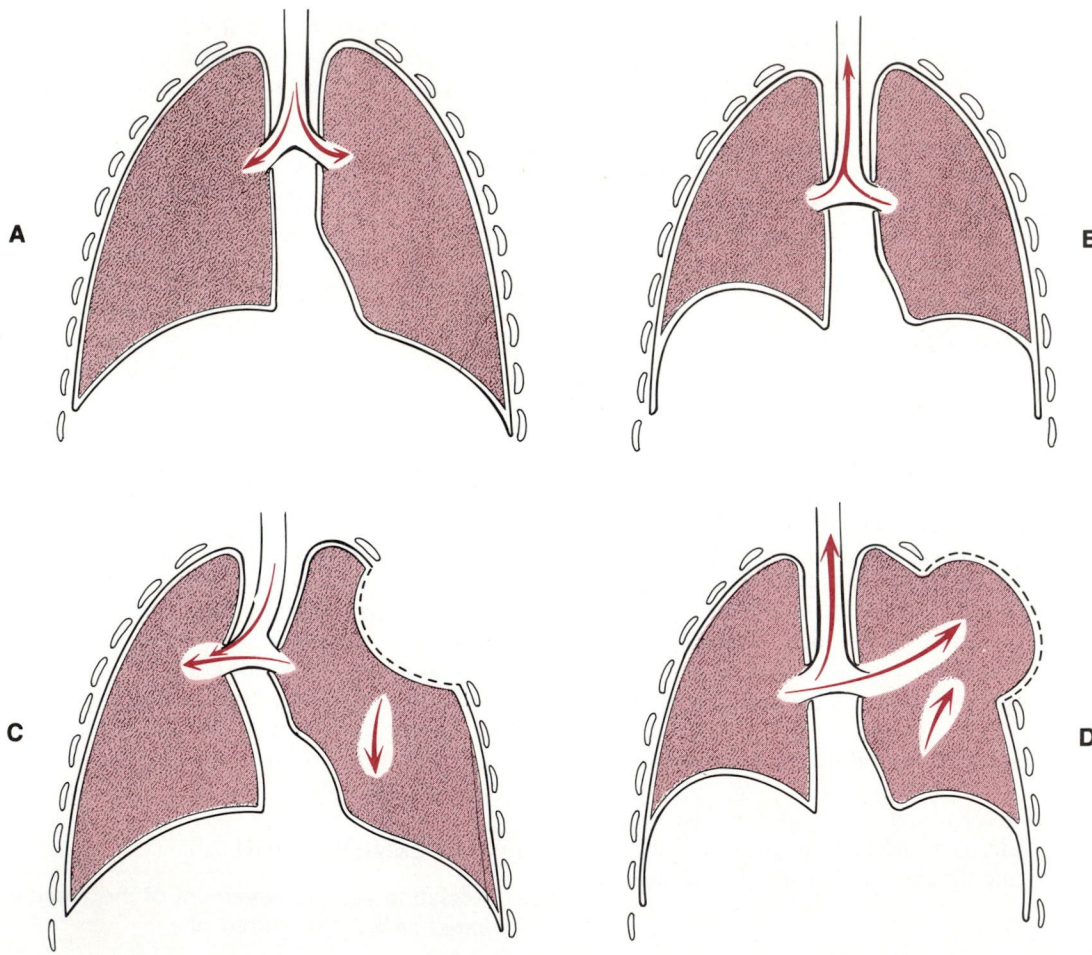

Fig. 24-17 Normal respiration. **A,** Inspiration; **B,** expiration. *Paradoxical motion:* **C,** inspiration, area of lung underlying unstable chest wall sucks in on inspiration. **D,** Same area balloons out on expiration. Note movement of mediastinum toward opposite lung on inspiration.

Assessment

☐ *Subjective data*

Data to be collected includes the nature of the injury and when it occurred. Often the patient is too badly injured to answer questions, and data are obtained from those accompanying the patient.

☐ *Objective data*

1. Pain is severe and increases with each respiratory movement.
2. Mediastinum oscillates, or "flutters," with each respiration.
3. Decreased breath sounds on auscultation.
4. If there is severe interference with cardiac function, neck veins will be distended.
5. Vital signs: increased pulse and respiratory rate. Blood pressure will fall if paradoxical motion is not relieved.

☐ *Diagnostic tests*

1. Chest x-ray examination to determine extent of trauma.
2. Arterial blood gasses to determine PaO_2 and $PaCO_2$.

☐ **Treatment for flail chest**

Treatment includes the following:
1. Stabilize the flail segment. After initial stabilization the individual is usually intubated and placed on a *volume-controlled ventilator*. Positive-pressure mechanical ventilation provides internal stabilization of the chest, decreases the work of breathing, and initiates the bellows function normally provided by the intact bony chest cage. If prolonged ventilatory support is required, a tracheostomy is performed.
2. Provide supplemental oxygen.
3. Correct acid-base imbalance. Mechanical ventilation is used to correct respiratory acid-base imbalance.
4. Provide analgesics for pain control.

■ PENETRATING CHEST WOUNDS

☐ Pathophysiology

When a knife, bullet, or other flying missile enters the chest, a penetrating wound occurs. The major problem in penetrating injury is not injury to the chest wall but injury to the structures within the chest cavity. Penetration of the lung is associated with leakage of air from the lung into the pleural cavity (pneumothorax) (Fig. 24-18, *B*). Blood may also leak into the pleural cavity (hemothorax). As the air or fluid accumulates in the pleural cavity, it builds up positive pressure, which causes the lung to collapse and may even cause a mediastinal shift. This compresses the opposite lung and interferes with cardiac action. The person then has serious difficulty in breathing and may go into shock.

Assessment

☐ *Subjective data*

Subjective data to collect include the nature of the injury and when it occurred. If the patient is too badly injured to answer questions, data is obtained from those accompanying the patient.

☐ *Objective data*

1. Signs of shock—weak and thready pulse, falling blood pressure, and cold and clammy skin
2. Severe shortness of breath
3. Check for mediastinal shift—trachea deviated from midline

☐ *Diagnostic tests*

1. Chest x-ray examination to determine extent of injury
2. Arterial blood gases to determine PaO_2 and $PaCO_2$

▦ Implementation

☐ *Initial care for penetrating chest wounds*

If an open sucking wound of the chest has been sustained, it should be covered immediately to prevent air from entering the pleural cavity and causing a pneumothorax. Several thicknesses of nonporous material such as plastic food wrap may be used, and these are anchored with wide adhesive tape, or the wound edges may be taped tightly together. If an object such as a knife is still in the wound, it is *not* removed until a physician arrives. Its presence may prevent the entry of air into the pleural cavity, and its removal may cause further damage. The person who sustained a penetrating wound of the chest should be placed in an upright position and taken to the nearest emergency room.

Emergency treatment is directed toward sustaining oxygen exchange and correcting circulatory failure. Usually the patient is intubated with an endotracheal tube and then is checked for air or blood in the pleural cavity. An emergency thoracentesis is done, and air and fluid are removed by syringe. Usually a catheter is inserted into the pleural space and connected to water-seal drainage (p. 707). If the lung fails to reexpand with this treatment or there is evidence of internal bleeding, surgical exploration may be necessary and will be done as soon as shock and other complications are under control.

To monitor the patient for hypovolemia, a central venous pressure (CVP) line is inserted. This line can also be used to administer intravenous fluids and blood as necessary. The CVP is a very effective way to monitor for cardiac tamponade. A pressure above 15 cm of water or a rising CVP in a patient in shock with penetrating trauma in the region of the heart often indicates cardiac tamponade.[47] If it is suspected that cardiac injury and tamponade may be present, a *pericardiocentesis* will be done.

■ PNEUMOTHORAX

☐ Pathophysiology

In pneumothorax air enters the pleural space between the lung and the chest wall. It can occur spontaneously or as a result of penetrating or nonpenetrating injuries.

A *closed pneumothorax* is caused by a blunt injury resulting in fractured ribs piercing the pleural membranes

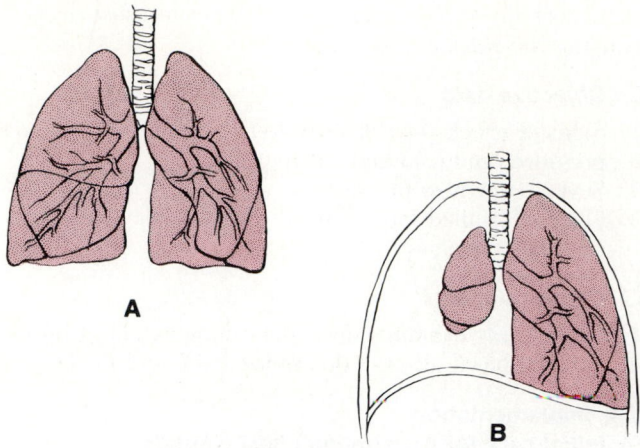

Fig. 24-18 **A,** Normal expanded lungs. **B,** Complete collapse of right lung caused by air in pleural cavity (pneumothorax).

or by a sudden compression of the rib cage. Air enters the pleural space, increasing intrapleural pressure, which collapses the lung (Fig. 24-18, *B*). A variant of a closed pneumothorax is a *spontaneous pneumothorax* that can result from the rupture of an emphysematous bleb on the lung surface or that may follow severe bouts of coughing in persons with a chronic pulmonary disease such as asthma. Frequently, it occurs as a single or recurrent episode in an otherwise healthy young person. If large enough and left untreated, a closed pneumothorax can become a tension pneumothorax.

A *tension pneumothorax* occurs when air leaking into the intrapleural space cannot escape during expiration. Although usually a result of a closed pneumothorax, a tension pneumothorax can be caused by a penetrating chest injury. The accumulating air builds up positive pressure in the chest cavity, resulting in (1) lung collapse on the affected side, (2) mediastinal shift toward the unaffected side, and

Table 24-17 Signs and symptoms and medical management of pneumothorax

Pneumothorax	Signs and symptoms	Medical management
Closed	Small or slowly developing pneumothorax may produce no symptoms	Observation on an outpatient basis
	Larger or rapidly developing pneumothorax results in:	
	Sharp pain on inspiration	Supplemental oxygen
	Increasing dyspnea	Needle aspiration of air from pleural space
	Increasing restlessness	Insertion of chest catheter connected to water-sealed drainage system
	Diaphoresis	
	Hypotension	
	Tachycardia	
	Absence of chest movement on affected side	
	Breath sounds absent on affected side	
	Hyperresonance on affected side	
Spontaneous	Sudden, unexplained shortness of breath	If there are frequent recurrences, silver nitrate is instilled into the pleural space to cause adhesions between the pleurae; if this procedure fails, lung portion with defect is resected and parietal pleura is abraded
Tension	Severe dyspnea	Same as open pneumothorax
	Agitation	
	Trachea deviated from midline toward unaffected side	
	Jugular venous distension	
	Absence of chest movement on affected side	
	Hypotension, tachycardia	
	Breath sounds absent on affected side	
	Hyperresonance on affected side	
	Diminished heart sounds	
Open	Sucking sounds at wound site with respiration	Occlude open wound
	Tracheal deviation (trachea moves toward unaffected side during inspiration and returns toward midline with expiration)	Same as closed pneumothorax

(3) compression of mediastinal contents (heart and great vessels), resulting in decreased cardiac output and decreased venous return.

An *open pneumothorax* occurs when a penetrating chest wound opens the intrapleural space to atmospheric pressure. Each time the patient inspires, air is sucked into the intrapleural space increasing intrapleural pressure. An open pneumothorax is also called a sucking chest wound because the wound makes a sucking sound on inspiration and expiration. Blood also may leak into the pleural cavity creating a *hemothorax.*

The signs and symptoms and medical management of the various types of pneumothorax are presented in Table 24-17.

Assessment

□ *Subjective data*

1. The nature of the injury
2. When injury occurred

□ *Objective data*

1. Sudden, sharp pain in chest
2. Dyspnea, anxiety, diaphoresis, weak and rapid pulse
3. Cessation of normal chest movements on affected side
4. Trachea deviated toward unaffected side
5. Hyperresonance on percussion
6. Breath sounds decreased or absent
7. Vocal fremitus depressed or absent
8. No adventitious sounds

□ *Diagnostic tests*

1. Chest x-ray examination
2. Arterial blood gas determinations of PaO_2, $PaCO_2$, and pH.

Data analysis: nursing diagnoses

Nursing diagnoses are determined from assessment of patient data. Possible nursing diagnoses for the person with a pneumothorax may include, but are not limited to, the following:

Table 24-18   Nursing diagnoses and interventions for pneumothorax

Pneumothorax type	Nursing diagnoses	Nursing interventions
Closed (spontaneous)	Knowledge deficit	For the outpatient or patient who has had chest tube removal, instruct patient to: 1. Report any increased dyspnea to physician 2. Avoid strenuous exercise or activity that increases rate and depth of breathing 3. Avoid holding breath 4. Follow physician's instructions about resuming normal activity
	Gas exchange, impaired	1. Place in a semi-Fowler's position 2. Administer oxygen 3. Monitor vital signs 4. Obtain a thoracentesis tray and water-sealed drainage equipment. See p. 707 for care of the patient with chest tubes.
Tension	Knowledge deficit	Same discharge instructions as for patient with closed pneumothorax.
	Gas exchange, impaired	A tension pneumothorax is a life-threatening event. It is imperative that interventions be carried out immediately to relieve the increased intrapleural pressure. Interventions are the same as those listed for closed pneumothorax.
	Cardiac output, decreased	1. Monitor vital signs frequently. 2. Observe for cardiac arrhythmias. 3. Palpate for subcutaneous emphysema in upper chest and neck.
Open	Knowledge deficit	Same discharge instruction as for closed pneumothorax.
	Gas exchange, impaired	1. Occlude wound with nonporous covering. 2. Same interventions as for closed pneumothorax.

Diagnostic title	Possible etiologies
Ineffective airway clearance	Trauma to pleura
Decreased cardiac output	Changes in intrathoracic pressure
Impaired gas exchange	V/Q abnormality
Knowledge deficit	Lack of exposure

Planning: expected patient outcomes

Expected patient outcomes for the person with a pneumothorax may include, but are not limited to, the following:
1. Lung is reexpanded and cardiac output is normal.
2. Patient is able to clear airway without difficulty.
3. Patient has arterial blood gases within normal limits.
4. Patients states plans for follow-up care.

Implementation
Assisting with achievement of therapeutic goals

INITIAL CARE FOR SPONTANEOUS PNEUMOTHORAX

When a spontaneous pneumothorax is suspected, a physician should be summoned immediately. The patient should not be left alone, should be reassured, and should be urged to remain still and not move about. Oxygen and equipment for a thoracentesis should be prepared. Air is immediately aspirated from the affected pleural space, and the intrapleural pressure is brought to normal if possible. If air continues to flow into the pleural space, a chest tube is inserted and connected to water-seal drainage (p. 708).

Vital signs are monitored every 15 minutes until stabilized and then every hour for the first 24 hours (see Table 24-18 for other nursing interventions).

Assisting with comfort and ADL

1. Place patient in upright position to facilitate breathing and comfort.
2. Assist patient to keep physical activity at minimum for 24 hours.
   a. Place call light and other necessary objects within easy reach of patient.
   b. Caution patient not to stretch, reach, or move suddenly.

Follow-up care for spontaneous pneumothorax

When air no longer is expelled from the pleural space through the underwater drainage system and a roentgenogram reveals that the lung has completely reexpanded, the chest tube is removed and the person is allowed out of bed. Strenuous exertion, which increases the rate and depth of respirations, should be avoided, but relatively normal activity may be resumed rather quickly. If there are frequent recurring episodes, some physicians instill silver nitrate into the pleural space to cause adhesions between the visceral and parietal pleurae. If this procedure is unsuccessful, the portion of the lung containing the defect may be resected and the parietal pleura abraded so that it adheres to the visceral pleura and obliterates the pleural space.

Counseling and teaching

See Table 24-18 for instructions for patients.

Evaluation

Evaluation is based on patient outcomes. Questions to be asked include the following:
1. Has the patient's lung reexpanded?
2. Has the patient's cardiac output returned to normal?
3. Are the patient's blood gases within normal limits?
4. Can the patient state plans for follow-up care?

OBSTRUCTIVE LUNG DISEASES

Chronic obstructive pulmonary disease

As mentioned on p. 671, *chronic obstructive pulmonary disease (COPD)* refers to diseases that produce obstruction of airflow and includes *asthma, chronic bronchitis*, and *pulmonary emphysema*. The disease spectrum associated with this diagnosis ranges from pure obstructive airway disease with the presence of bronchitis but no emphysema, through various combinations, to severe emphysema without bronchitis. The pathophysiologic processes that cause these changes are neither static nor are they necessarily progressive. Thus all stages are possible, from reversible abnormalities to relentlessly progressive cardiopulmonary insufficiency. There has been much confusion concerning the clinical use of the terms *chronic bronchitis, emphysema,* and *asthma;* therefore the term *chronic obstructive pulmonary disease* is now used rather than a designation of the specific disease. Frequently by the time the patient seeks medical attention, pathologic changes have occurred and symptoms are often moderately severe.

The incidence of COPD has increased spectacularly in recent years. Current statistics indicate that 17 million Americans suffer from emphysema, asthma, and chronic bronchitis.[7] Both the prevalence of COPD and the death rate attributed to it have reached epidemic proportions according to the American Lung Association. In 1984 COPD was the sixth leading cause of death following heart disease, neoplasm, strokes, accidents, and influenza-pneumonia.[4]

This increase in death rate from COPD is believed to be related to (1) the growing tendency of physicians to list it as a primary cause of death, (2) the greater use of pulmonary function testing, and (3) more emphasis in medical literature on the importance of this syndrome.[5] Despite these facts, it is believed that the mortality is even higher than reported because many persons who were reported to have died from pneumonia, asthma, or congestive heart failure probably had COPD. The major factors in this increase in mortality, in addition to improved reporting and the increased aging of the population, is a history of cigarette smoking.[5] These diseases are more prevalent among men than women, but death rates are now showing a higher percentage rate of increase in women than in men. This is believed to be directly related to the increase in smoking among women.

■ Chronic bronchitis

Chronic bronchitis is defined *symptomatically* by hypersecretion of mucus and recurrent or chronic productive cough for a minimum of 3 months per year for at least 2 consecutive years in patients in whom other causes have been excluded. It is characterized *physiologically* by hypertrophy and hypersecretion of bronchial mucous glands.

The etiologic factors, signs and symptoms, and medical therapy are outlined in Table 24-19.

■ PATHOPHYSIOLOGY

Persons with chronic bronchitis are susceptible to infection because of their inability to clear their bronchial tree of excess mucus. Bacteria proliferate in the mucous secretions in lumen of the bronchi. The most common infectious agents are *Streptococcus pneumoniae* and *Haemophilus influenzae*. As bacteria multiply, they exert a neu-

Table 24-19 Etiology, signs and symptoms, and medical therapy for chronic bronchitis and pulmonary emphysema

Bronchitis	Pulmonary emphysema
Etiology	
Inhalation of physical or chemical irritants or viral or bacterial infections	Not known. Believed that some change in the enzyme-inhibitor balance occurs allowing proteolytic enzymes to attack lung tissue
Most common inhaled irritant: cigarette smoke	Not known why some smokers develop bronchitis and others develop emphysema. A_1-antitrypsin deficiency occurs in some persons who develop severe, disabling emphysema early in life. Familial tendency for this type of emphysema
Signs and symptoms	
Early symptoms	Dyspnea on exertion indicating acute respiratory distress
Productive cough on awakening; often ignored by cigarette smokers who refer to it as their "cigarette cough"	Using accessory muscles to breathe; ruddy color
Later symptoms	Thin with a "barrel chest"
Significant physical incapacity; breathlessness even when walking on a flat surface; noticeable shortness of breath (SOB) and use of accessory muscles to breathe. Cyanosis is common. Ankle edema, bloated appearance, distended neck veins; sometimes referred to as "blue bloater"	Usually able to maintain resting Pao_2
	Cyanosis uncommon
	Sometimes referred to as "pink puffer"
	Late in disease
	$Paco_2$ ↑
Late in disease	Cor pulmonale and respiratory failure possible complications
Cor pulmonale (right ventricular hypertrophy), right-sided heart failure, and respiratory failure are frequent complications	
Pulmonary function test findings	
↓ Expiratory flow rates	↓ Expiratory flow rates, especially forced expiratory volume and maximal midexpiratory flow
↓ Vital capacity	↑ Total lung capacity
↑ Residual volume	↑ Residual volume
Total lung capacity usually within normal limits	Vital capacity may be normal or slightly reduced until late stages of disease. Change in FEV_1/VC ratio
Arterial blood gas findings	
Low resting Pao_2	Pao_2 normal or slightly reduced at *rest;* falls during exercise
Elevated $Paco_2$ (if obstruction severe)	Normal $Paco_2$
During exercise $Paco_2$ ↑ and Pao_2 may also ↑	Late in disease, elevated $Paco_2$

Table 24-19 Etiology, signs and symptoms, and medical therapy for chronic bronchitis and pulmonary emphysema—cont'd

Bronchitis	Pulmonary emphysema

Medical therapy

Medical therapy for chronic bronchitis and pulmonary emphysema is similar and is dependent on symptoms, pulmonary function test results, and blood gas findings. Therapy may include all or some of the modalities outlined here.

Supportive measures

Education of patient and family about:
  Avoidance of cigarette smoke
  Avoidance of other inhaled irritants
  Avoidance of persons with upper respiratory infections
  Control of environmental temperature and humidity
  Proper nutrition
  Adequate hydration

Specific therapy

Medications
  Bronchodilators (Table 24-21)
  Antimicrobials
    Tetracycline or ampicillin usually prescribed to treat respiratory tract infections
  Corticosteroids
    May be prescribed to alleviate acute symptoms. Prednisone most often used.
  Digitalis
    May be prescribed to treat left ventricular failure.

Respiratory therapy

Aerosol therapy
  Used to deliver bronchodilators through metered cartridge devices or hand-held nebulizers
Oxygen therapy
  Required for patients who are unable to maintain a Pa_{O_2} of 50 mm Hg or more at rest or who cannot carry out ADL without becoming short of breath; 1 to 2 L of O_2 given by nasal prongs (p. 680)

Physical conditioning

Relaxation exercises
  Progressive relaxation exercises are encouraged. Best practiced before meals or 2 hours or more after eating, since digestion seems to interfere with ability to relax (p. 732)
Meditation
  Meditation more widely used to assist patients to relax (p. 732)
Breathing retraining
  Pursed-lip breathing (Fig. 24-20)
  Leaning forward position for exhalation (Fig. 24-21)
  Abdominal breathing (p. 725)
  Inhalation-exhalation exercises (p. 727)
  Exhalation with exertion (p. 726)
Rehabilitation
  Muscle reconditioning programs specific for the patient (p. 727)

---

trophilic chemotaxis, and pus cells migrate from between bronchial epithelial cells to produce a mucopurulent exudate in the lumen, or it may progress to ulceration and destruction of the bronchial wall. When this occurs, granulation and fibrotic tissue replace the normal ciliated epithelium with flattened squamous epithelium.[103] The scarring in the airways leads to stenosis and airway obstruction. Small airways may be completely obliterated and others

may become dilated. This chain of events further traps secretions and promotes multiplication of bacteria. Airway obstruction occurs first in airways that are less than 2 mm in diameter.[103] Small airway obstruction can be detected only by pulmonary function tests, and this is why symptoms alone are not sufficient to establish the diagnosis.

Cor pulmonale (right ventricular hypertrophy, which develops as the result of increased pulmonary vascular resistance in response to hypoxemia and hypercapnia), failure of the right side of the heart, and respiratory failure are frequent complications of chronic bronchitis.

ASSESSMENT

☐ Subjective data

1. When productive cough was first noticed
2. Smoking history
3. Measures followed at home to improve breathing
4. Medications taken and their effectiveness in relieving symptoms

☐ Objective data

1. Edema of ankles and degree
2. Auscultation—bronchovesicular rhonchi, rales
3. Cough with copious production of yellow or green sputum
4. Epigastric fullness
5. Distended neck veins
6. Appears overweight
7. Appears slightly cyanotic

☐ Diagnostic tests

Diagnostic tests used in establishing a diagnosis of chronic bronchitis include sputum analysis, pulmonary function tests, and arterial blood gas levels.

☐ *Sputum analysis*

Sputum collection is discussed on p. 686. The type of cells present in the sputum helps to differentiate between allergic inflammation of the airways, as seen in bronchial asthma, and nonspecific inflammation, as seen in chronic bronchitis.[103] In chronic bronchitis polymorphonuclear leukocytes (neutrophils) are found. The sputum often changes color to green or yellow not from infection but from the action of the enzyme myeloperoxidase, which is associated with cellular breakdown under stasis from retained secretions.

The sputum specimen must be fresh and transported to the laboratory immediately for bacteriologic examination.

☐ *Pulmonary function tests*

Pulmonary function tests are explained on p. 704. The findings that are common in patients with chronic bronchitis can be found in Table 24-19. Pulmonary function tests results may improve slightly after the administration of bronchodilators.

☐ *Arterial blood gas levels*

Arterial blood gas studies have become a common tool to aid in physiologic diagnosis and therapeutic management of patients. These studies determine blood pH, carbon dioxide tension ($PaCO_2$), oxygen tension (PaO_2), and percent of oxyhemoglobin saturation (SaO_2). Blood gas studies are obtained to assess the adequacy of oxygenation and ventilation and to assess acid-base status. The blood sample is obtained from the radial, brachial, or femoral artery using a preheparinized syringe to prevent clotting. The syringe is capped after obtaining the blood sample to prevent contact with air and is placed in a container of ice water until analyzed. Pressure is maintained over the puncture site for at least 5 minutes after needle withdrawal to prevent bleeding.

Gas tensions refer to partial pressure, or that part of the total pressure exerted by a specific gas. For example, pressure exerted by the atmosphere at sea level is 760 torr. The amount of oxygen in air at sea level is 21%; that is, 21% of the total pressure is exerted by oxygen. Since 21% of 760 is approximately 159, the PaO_2 of air at sea level is 159 torr. Definitions of gas exchange functions and their normal values are given in the box below.

The measurement of oxygen values includes both the PaO_2 and SaO_2. The PaO_2 measures oxygen dissolved in the blood; however, the amount of oxygen carried in the blood in this form is small, since most oxygen is transported in chemical combination with hemoglobin. Oxyhemoglobin saturation refers to that percentage of the hemoglobin that is combined with oxygen. More than 90% of the oxygen-carrying capacity of blood is accounted for by oxyhemoglobin, with the partial pressure of oxygen acting as the driving force for this chemical combination. Therefore, both PaO_2 and SaO_2 levels must be examined to determine the adequacy of oxygenation of the tissues.

It is particularly important to understand the relationship of the PaO_2 to oxyhemoglobin saturation to assess adequacy of tissue oxygenation. This relationship is not directly linear; many factors affect the affinity of the heme molecule for oxygen. A sigmoid curve (Fig 24-19) represents the saturation percentages that occur at various PO_2 levels. Most significant of the factors that affect the ability of the blood to carry oxygen is the partial pressure of the oxygen itself in the blood. As can be seen in the oxyhemoglobin dissociation curve, in the upper portion of the curve, hemoglobin has an increased affinity for oxygen, so that large changes in PaO_2 levels can be tolerated without significantly changing the saturation. For example, at a

---

Definitions and normal values of gas exchange functions

pH	Acidity of blood	7.35 to 7.45
$PaCO_2$	Partial pressure of carbon dioxide in arterial blood	38 to 42 mm Hg
PaO_2	Partial pressure of oxygen in arterial blood	80 to 100 mm Hg
SaO_2	Percentage of available hemoglobin saturated with oxygen	95% to 98%

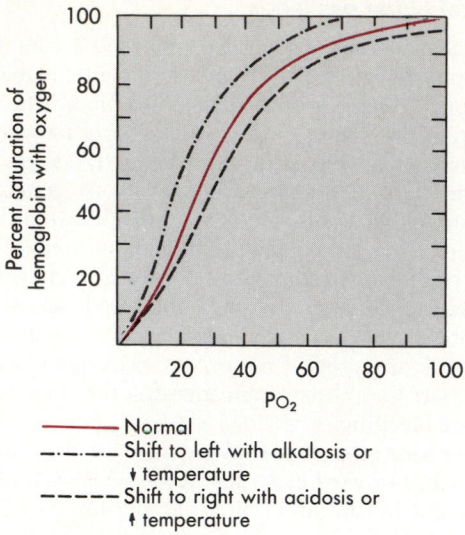

Fig. 24-19 Oxyhemoglobin dissociation curve. (Reproduced with permission from Comroe, JH, Jr: Physiology of respiration, ed 2, Copyright, 1974, by Year Book Medical Publishers, Inc., Chicago.)

PaO_2 of 100 mm Hg, hemoglobin saturation is almost total, 97%; even if the PaO_2 should fall to 70 torr, the saturation would only decrease to 94%. This serves as a protective mechanism that ensures adequate tissue oxygenation even when there is mild hypoxemia. It should be noted, however, that once the PO_2 level falls below 60 torr, saturation begins to decrease sharply, thus reducing the ability of the hemoglobin to transport oxygen.

Other factors that influence the oxygen affinity of hemoglobin are temperature, pH, and $PaCO_2$. At higher temperatures, increased levels of $PaCO_2$ (hypercapnia), and acidosis, the curve shifts to the right. This means that at any given PaO_2 the hemoglobin has less affinity for oxygen, and lower saturations will result. The converse of this is also true; with decreased temperature, decreased $PaCO_2$, and alkalosis, higher saturations occur with any given PaO_2.

The $PaCO_2$ is used as a measurement to determine the adequacy of ventilation and is dependent on the amount of carbon dioxide produced by the body and the ability of the lungs to eliminate it. *Hypoventilation*, therefore, is shown by an elevated $PaCO_2$, while *hyperventilation* is indicated by a decrease in $PaCO_2$ below normal levels.

The pH refers to the acidity of the blood and is an expression of the hydrogen ion concentration. Because pH is expressed as a negative logarithm, as hydrogen ion concentration increases and blood becomes more acid, the pH value falls. When hydrogen ion concentration decreases, the blood becomes more alkaline and the pH value rises.

The $PaCO_2$ is related to the pH because of the chemical reaction of carbon dioxide and water in the blood, which results in the formation of carbonic acid. Carbonic acid,

in turn, dissociates to form hydrogen and bicarbonate ions, as illustrated in the following equation:

$$CO_2 + H_2O \rightleftarrows H_2CO_3 \rightleftarrows HCO_3^- + H^+$$

The maintenance of a normal pH is dependent on a ratio of 20 bicarbonate ions to 1 hydrogen ion. It can be seen from the equation that the presence of an elevated $PaCO_2$ results in an excess of hydrogen ions. When this occurs, the pH falls and the patient is said to be in *respiratory acidosis*. Conversely, when $PaCO_2$ is decreased, the pH increases and the result is termed *respiratory alkalosis*.

➡ DATA ANALYSIS: NURSING DIAGNOSES

Nursing diagnoses are determined from assessment of patient data. Possible nursing diagnoses for the person with chronic bronchitis may include, but are not limited to, the following:

Diagnostic title	Possible etiologies
Ineffective airway clearance	Decreased energy, fatigue
	Tracheobronchial obstruction
Anxiety	Threat to self-concept
	Threat of death, unmet needs
Ineffective breathing pattern	Anxiety, decreased energy, fatigue
Fluid volume excess	Compromised regulatory mechanisms
Impaired gas exchange	Ventilation/perfusion imbalance
Knowledge deficit	Lack of exposure, unfamiliarity with information sources
Altered nutrition: potential for more than body requirements	Excessive intake in relation to metabolic needs
Self-care deficit	Intolerance to activity, fatigue
	Ventilation/perfusion imbalance
Sleep pattern disturbance	Discomfort, positioning
Altered cardiopulmonary tissue perfusion	Decreased blood flow
	Ventilation and perfusion imbalance

⊔ PLANNING: EXPECTED PATIENT OUTCOMES

In general the goals of treatment for the patient with chronic bronchitis are to (1) improve the patient's symptoms, (2) improve the ability to carry out ADL, and (3) reduce the progression of the disease when the disease is detected early.[103] Specifics of therapy are presented after the discussion of emphysema because the treatment for both of these diseases is similar (see p. 725).

Because it is often impossible clinically to determine if the patient has chronic bronchitis or pulmonary emphysema, and the patient often has some degree of both, the outcome criteria for COPD are presented after the discussion of pulmonary emphysema.

■ Emphysema

■ PATHOPHYSIOLOGY

Emphysema is defined *pathologically* by destructive changes in alveolar walls and enlargement of air spaces distal to the terminal nonrespiratory bronchioles. It is characterized *physiologically* by increased lung compliance, decreased diffusing capacity, and increased airway resistance. The etiology signs and symptoms, and medical therapy are outlined in Table 24-19.

Although it is not known when emphysema actually begins, there appears to be many years between the initial pathophysiologic changes and the onset of overt symptoms. Symptoms associated with emphysema usually appear in the fourth decade, and disability from disease usually occurs in the fifth or sixth decade of life. The typical individual with emphysema is a male of about 55 years of age with a history of cigarette smoking.

The cause of emphysema is not known; however, recent evidence suggests that *proteases* released by polymorphonuclear leukocytes or alveolar macrophages are involved in the destruction of the connective tissue of the lungs. *Connective tissue* in the lungs is primarily composed of *elastin, collagen,* and *proteoglycan,* which can be damaged and destroyed by enzymes such as proteases and elastase. It has been demonstrated that elastase (produced by alveolar macrophages) can destroy or damage the elastin in the connective tissue of the parenchyma of the lung.[103] Normally, inhibitors found in human serum, lung tissue, peripheral airways, and bronchial mucus protect the lung from the proteolytic enzymes. It is believed that some change in the enzyme-inhibitor balance occurs, which allows the proteolytic enzymes to attack lung tissue. It is not known, however, why some smokers develop bronchitis and others develop emphysema. Differences in susceptibility and the predominant type of disease are believed to be influenced by hereditary or environmental factors or those related to the patient's history.[103] It has been established, however, that there is familial tendency to develop alpha$_1$-antitrypsin deficiency and that relatives of persons with this type of emphysema should be screened and provided with counseling as discussed below.

■ PREVENTION

The cornerstone of prevention of emphysema is education. Public education must focus on the pulmonary health risks associated with inhaled irritants, regardless of their source. Increased public awareness of the vital role clean air plays in pulmonary health is essential for the success of any legislative actions promoting air quality standards. Individuals must also be educated to understand the importance of personal responsibility to decrease their own health risk through smoking cessation.

The diagnosis of emphysema is inferred from pulmonary function tests that show a decrease in airflow. The type of emphysema can be determined only by descriptive morphology. There are two principal types of emphysema morphologically—*centrilobular* emphysema (CLE) and *panlobular* emphysema (PLE). In CLE, there is distention and damage of the respiratory bronchioles selectively. Openings develop in the walls of the bronchioles; they become enlarged and confluent and tend to form a single space as the walls enlarge. The disease tends to be unevenly distributed throughout the lung but usually is more severe in the upper portions.

In PLE, there is a more uniform enlargement and destruction of the alveoli in the pulmonary acinus. PLE is usually more diffuse and is more severe in the lower lung. It is found in elderly persons who have no evidence of chronic bronchitis or impairment of lung function.[5] It occurs just as commonly in women as in men, but PLE is less frequent than CLE. PLE is a characteristic finding in persons with homozygous alpha$_1$-antitrypsin deficiency.[5]

Because of destruction of tissue, there is physiologic obstruction by collapse of airways on expiration. As a result, full exhalation is difficult, air trapping ensues, and the diaphragm becomes fixed in a flattened position.

▣ ASSESSMENT

☐ Subjective data

1. Onset and duration of symptoms
2. Measures followed at home to improve breathing
3. Use of supplemental oxygen at home during the day or during sleep
4. Medications taken and their effectiveness in relieving symptoms
5. Smoking history

☐ Objective data

1. Rapid respirations
2. Activities that cause patient to become dyspneic
3. Barrel chest
4. Palpation
   a. Diminished chest expansion
   b. Decrease in tactile fremitus
5. Percussion
   a. Resonant to hyperresonant
   b. Diaphragm moves very little
6. Auscultation
   a. Breath sounds exhibit decreased intensity, usually prolonged expiration
   b. Vocal fremitus is normal or decreased
   c. Adventitious sounds reveal occasional sonorous and/ or sibilant rhonchi, fine rales in late inspiration

☐ Diagnostic tests

Because patients with emphysema are very vulnerable to lung infections, sputum tests for culture and sensitivity are frequently ordered. Pulmonary function tests and arterial blood gas findings are necessary to determine the degree of impairment and therapy.

➡ DATA ANALYSIS: NURSING DIAGNOSES

Nursing diagnoses are determined from assessment of patient data. Possible nursing diagnoses for the person with pulmonary emphysema may include, but are not limited to, the following:

Diagnostic title	Possible etiologies
Activity intolerance	Imbalance between oxygen supply and demand
Ineffective airway clearance	Decreased energy, fatigue
	Tracheobronchial obstruction
Anxiety	Threat to self-concept
	Threat of death, unmet needs
Ineffective breathing pattern	Anxiety, decreased energy, fatigue
Impaired gas exchange	Ventilation and perfusion imbalance
Altered nutrition: less than body requirements	Anorexia
Self-care deficit	Intolerance to activity, fatigue
Personal identity disturbance	Immobility, change in life-style
Sleep pattern disturbances	Discomfort, positioning
Altered cardiopulmonary tissue perfusion	Decreased blood flow (arterial)

◳ PLANNING: EXPECTED PATIENT OUTCOMES

Expected patient outcomes for the person with chronic bronchitis, emphysema, or any combination of these two obstructive airway diseases may include, but are not limited to, the following:

1. Patient demonstrates an effective breathing pattern.
   a. Inspiratory to expiratory ratio = 5:10 seconds
   b. Pursed-lip breathing
   c. Appropriate use of leaning forward posture
   d. Diaphragmatic breathing (abdominal muscle breathing)
   e. Exhales with activity
   f. Respiratory rate within near normal limits, moderate tidal volume
2. Patient demonstrates improved ventilation and oxygenation.
   a. Arterial blood pH and PCO_2 that returns or stays within acceptable limits
   b. PaO_2 at optimal level for individual
   c. Explains how and when to use oxygen therapy
3. Patient demonstrates adequate airway clearance.
   a. Effective methods of coughing
   b. Appropriate use of nebulizers, humidifiers, mistometers, IPPB machine, and medications
4. Patient lists common signs and symptoms that require reporting to the health care provider.
   a. Change in sputum color, amount, and consistency
   b. Increased coughing
   c. Change in behavior
   d. Increased fatigue
   e. Increased dyspnea
   f. Weight gain
   g. Peripheral edema
   h. Elevated temperature
5. Patient explains the following aspects of home medication or treatment regimens:
   a. States name, dose, action, and side effects of each medication to be used at home
   b. How and when to use medications ordered on a PRN basis (for example, bronchodilators, antibiotics, steroids, and antacids)
   c. Techniques necessary for follow-up care (for example, segmental postural drainage, clapping and vibrating, and inhalation therapy treatments)
   d. How to obtain and maintain needed equipment or supplies such as oxygen, nebulizers, humidifiers, mistometers, IPPB, syringes, and medications
6. Patient demonstrates how to carry out the specific exercise program to be followed at home, including:
   a. Specific exercises to be completed daily
   b. Frequency of each exercise
   c. Criteria for monitoring physical response to exercises such as heart rate increase or perceived fatigue
7. Patient can list the names and telephone numbers of appropriate community support services such as the Visiting Nurse Association and a home medical equipment supplier.
8. Patient demonstrates comprehension of self-care activities:
   a. Explains health maintenance or therapeutic follow-up program
   b. Describes any home medication or treatment program
   c. Explains exercise program to be followed at home
   d. Describes how to obtain professional and community resources necessary to structure a satisfactory environment at home
   e. States plans for ongoing follow-up care
9. Patient maintains or works toward an optimal activity level:
   a. Pacing of activities
   b. Planning for simplification of activities
   c. Participating in planned muscle-conditioning program
10. Patient can explain dietary changes required after discharge:
    a. Food and fluid requirements and daily plan for achieving them
    b. Specific foods to be avoided (those that are perceived to produce "gas")
    c. Plan for frequent, small feedings that are soft and that do not require much chewing, and the need for increased time required for eating if indicated
    d. How to maintain optimal weight for height, age, and gender
11. Patient demonstrates activities to control stress response to symptoms:
    a. Muscle relaxation
    b. Meditation
    c. Participation in support group

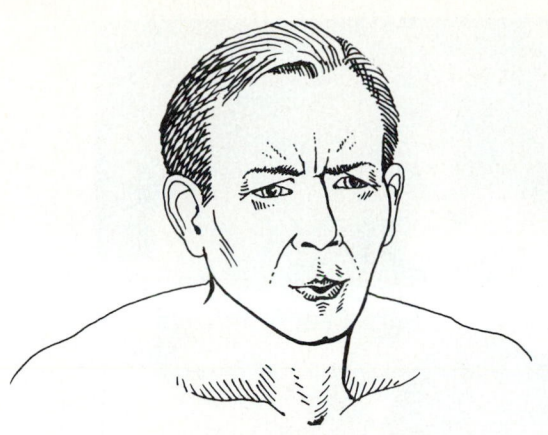

Fig. 24-20   Pursed-lip breathing.

IMPLEMENTATION

☐ Facilitating breathing

1. Teach patient to slow respiratory frequency and to breathe slowly and rhythmically.
2. Discourage patient from taking big gulps of air.
3. Teach patient to increase inspiratory:expiratory ratio so that expiration takes twice as long as inhalation.
   a. Teach patient to count in seconds and to concentrate on increasing time taken to exhale.
   b. Count to 5 on inhalation and to 10 on exhalation.

Teach pursed-lip breathing if the patient is not already using it (Fig. 24-20). Teach the forward-leaning position for exhalation. Using a forward-leaning position of 30 to 40 degrees with the head tilted at a 16- to 18-degree angle is a very effective way to improve exhalation (Fig. 24-21). As mentioned earlier, patients with emphysema have increased TLC and residual volume (RV) with the diaphragm in a fixed flattened position. For this reason, the diaphragm cannot assist in exhalation as it does normally. Leaning forward allows more air to be removed from the lungs on exhalation. The leaning-forward position can be achieved in either a sitting or standing position. For example, (1) the patient can sit on the edge of the bed or a chair and lean forward on two or three pillows placed on a table or overbed stand; (2) the patient can sit in a chair with the legs spread apart shoulder width (or wider, if obese) with the elbows on the knees and the arms and hands relaxed; or (3) the patient can stand with the back and hips against the wall with the feet spread apart and about 12 inches (30 cm) from the wall. The patient then relaxes and leans forward.[69] In these positions, the patient cannot use the accessory muscles of respiration, and the upward action of the diaphragm is improved.

☐ *Abdominal breathing and exercises*

Teach abdominal breathing, leg raising exercises, inhalation-exhalation exercises, and muscle reconditioning exercises.

Abdominal breathing improves the breathing efficiency of persons with COPD, because it assists the patient to elevate the diaphragm. Abdominal breathing can be taught in the sitting or lying position. In the sitting position, the patient sits on the side of the bed or in a chair and holds a small pillow or a book against the abdomen. The patient then exhales slowly while leaning forward and pressing

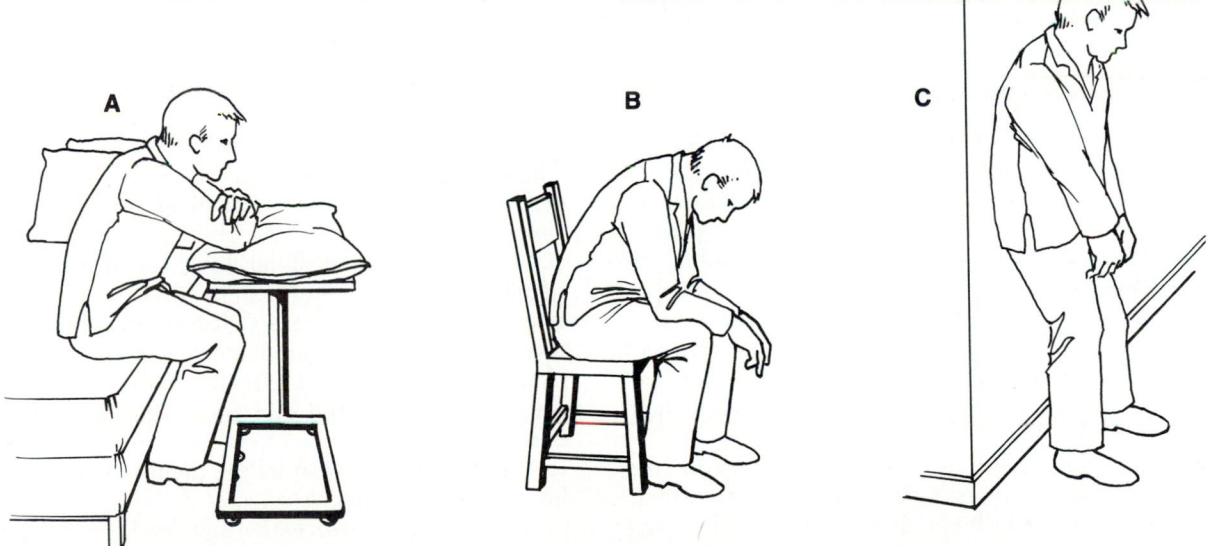

Fig. 24-21   Forward leaning position. **A,** Patient sits on edge of bed with arms folded on pillow placed on elevated bedside table. **B,** Patient in three-point position. Patient sits in chair with feet approximately 1 foot apart and leans forward with elbows on knees. **C,** Patient leans against wall with feet spread apart allowing shoulders to sag forward with arms relaxed.

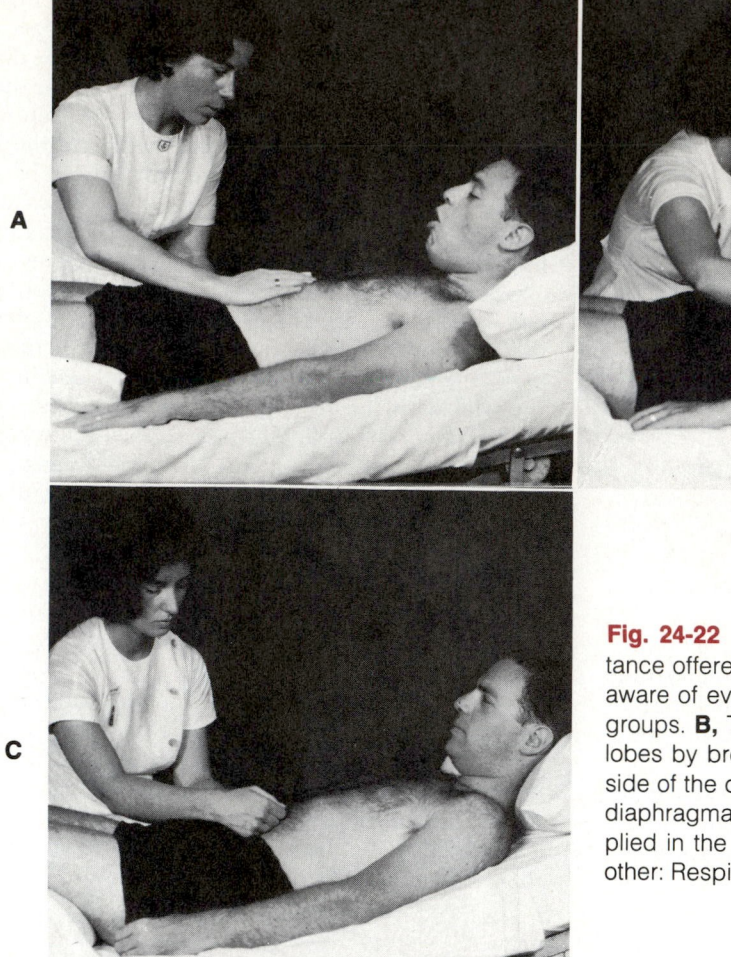

Fig. 24-22 **A,** When made to breathe against the resistance offered by the therapist's hands, the patient is made aware of every phase of his respiration and use of muscle groups. **B,** The patient learns how to fully expand his lower lobes by breathing against counterpressure applied to the side of the chest during inspiration. **C,** The patient is taught diaphragmatic control by breathing against a resistance applied in the costophrenic angle. (From Bendixen, HH, and other: Respiratory care, St. Louis, 1965, The CV Mosby Co.)

the pillow or book against the abdomen. In the lying position, a small pillow or a book is placed on the abdomen and the patient is asked to "puff out" the abdomen and raise the pillow or book as high as possible. The patient then exhales slowly through pursed lips while pulling in on the abdominal muscles. Manual pressure on the upper abdomen during expiration facilitates this maneuver (Fig. 24-22). In addition to abdominal breathing, exercises to strengthen the abdominal muscles assist patients to use their abdominal muscles more effectively in emptying their lungs.

This "controlled" breathing pattern is to be used while performing various activities of daily living—from sitting, standing, walking, and climbing stairs to more complex activities. As this pattern becomes natural, it will be used automatically during periods of increased shortness of breath. Persons who do not know how to use controlled breathing tend to increase their respiratory rate and their work of breathing when they are short of breath. As a result, physiologic obstruction increases, oxygen require-

ments increase, and effective ventilation decreases. Changing a person's respiratory pattern requires a great deal of effort by both the individual and those providing care.

This same method of teaching augmented abdominal (diaphragmatic) breathing can be used to teach the patient to cough. The difference is that expiration is forced down to residual volume. This maneuver often stimulates the cough reflex. If it does not, the person is taught to actively cough at the end of full expiration. Physiologically, forced expiration simulates the effects of a cough and is, therefore, more effective than telling the patient to take a deep breath and then cough.

Leg-raising exercises, with each leg being raised alternately as the patient exhales, is one way to strengthen abdominal muscles. Another way is to have the patient raise the head and shoulders from the bed while he or she exhales. Not all patients can do all exercises, but most can do some of them on a daily or twice daily basis. With practice and encouragement the patient can do the exercises 10 times each morning and evening after clearing the lungs as completely as possible of secretions.

Inhalation-exhalation exercises emphasize the need to prolong exhalation about four to five times longer than inhalation. Patients who walk can be taught to count in seconds and to concentrate on exhaling slowly and fully. While learning to *exhale with exertion,* the patient exhales during an activity such as bending over or sitting down.[69]

Muscle reconditioning refers to a variety of exercises that tone muscles. For patients who are able to be out of bed, walking, using a treadmill, or riding a stationary bicycle is helpful. The exercise period is started slowly with 10 minutes twice daily three time a week, increasing to 20 minutes twice daily three times a week. The patient needs to be assessed for his or her ability to carry out such an exercise program, and a staff member should be present during the exercise period.

☐ *Pulmonary physiotherapy*

The person who has difficulty in breathing may be taught how to increase the efficiency of his or her breathing pattern. Breathing exercises are usually a part of pulmonary physiotherapy, which may also include *segmental postural drainage, clapping,* and *vibrating.* Although pulmonary physiotherapy activities may be performed by a physical therapist, they are often part of a nurse's responsibility. Re-

gardless of where the primary responsibility lies, nurses must be familiar with the techniques so that they can demonstrate and reinforce them and ensure that the individual is doing them correctly. Also, the need for pulmonary physiotherapy may occur at a time when the physical therapist is not available to the patient.

☐ *Segmental postural drainage*

Segmental postural drainage with clapping and vibration is a technique used to combine the force of gravity with the natural ciliary activity of the small bronchial airways to move secretions upward toward the main bronchi and the trachea. From this point the patient can cough secretions up, or they can be suctioned. In the treatment of chronic obstructive pulmonary disease, drainage of all segments is usually accomplished by placing patients in various postural drainage positions (Fig. 24-23). Treatment may also be directed at draining specific areas of the lung. While the patient is in each position, *clapping* with a cupped hand is done over the area being drained. This maneuver helps to loosen secretions and stimulate coughing (Fig. 24-24). After clapping the area for approximately 1 minute, the patient is instructed to breathe deeply. *Vibrating* (pressure applied with a vibrating movement of the hand on the chest) is performed during expiratory phase of the deep breath (Fig. 24-25). This assists the patient

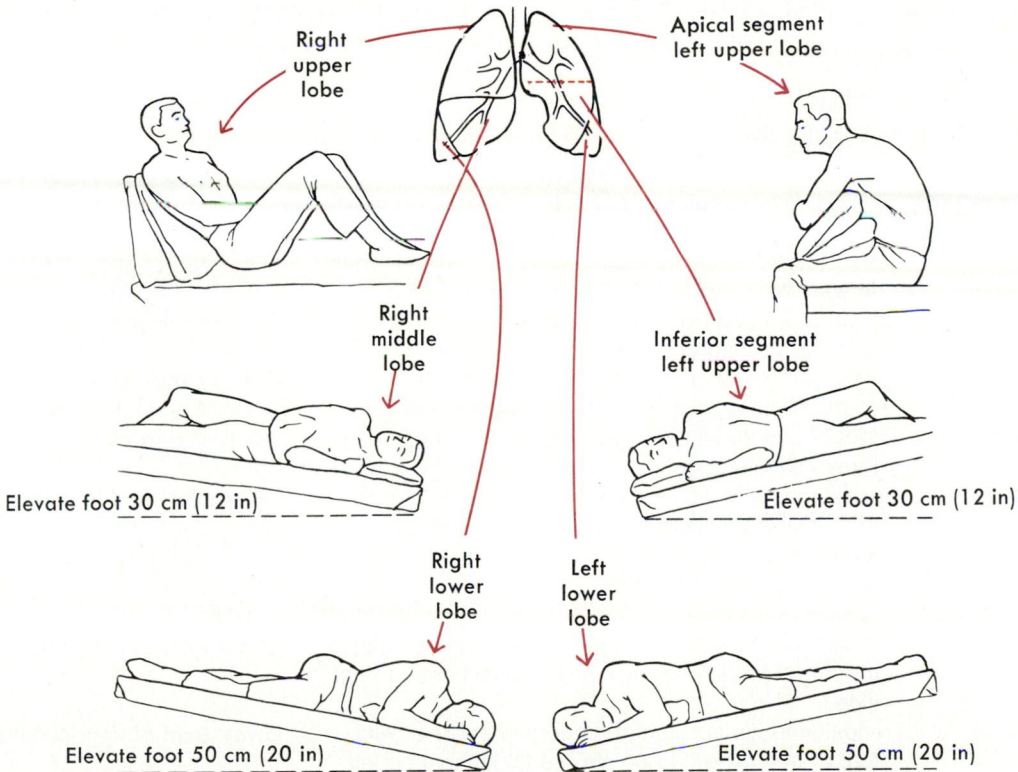

Right upper lobe

Apical segment left upper lobe

Right middle lobe

Inferior segment left upper lobe

Elevate foot 30 cm (12 in)

Elevate foot 30 cm (12 in)

Right lower lobe

Left lower lobe

Elevate foot 50 cm (20 in)

Elevate foot 50 cm (20 in)

Fig. 24-23 Postural drainage requires that the patient assume various positions to facilitate the flow of secretions from various portions of the lung into the bronchi, trachea, and throat so that they can be raised and expectorated more easily. Drawing shows the correct position to drain various portions of the lung.

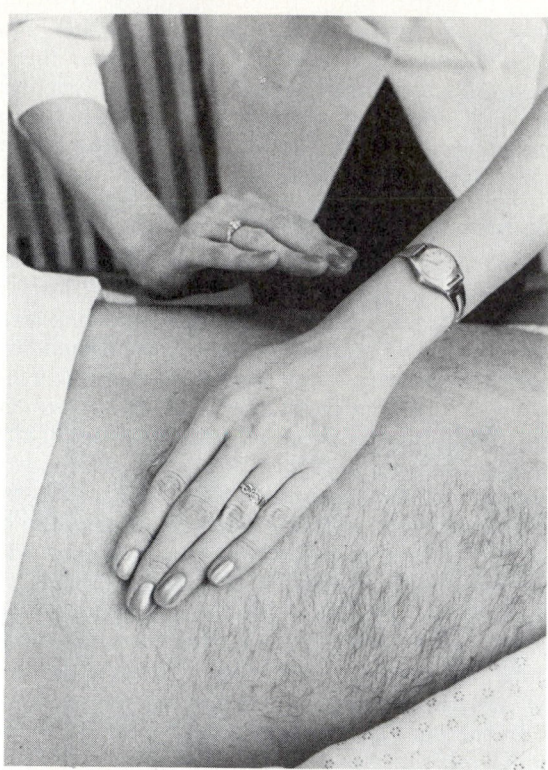

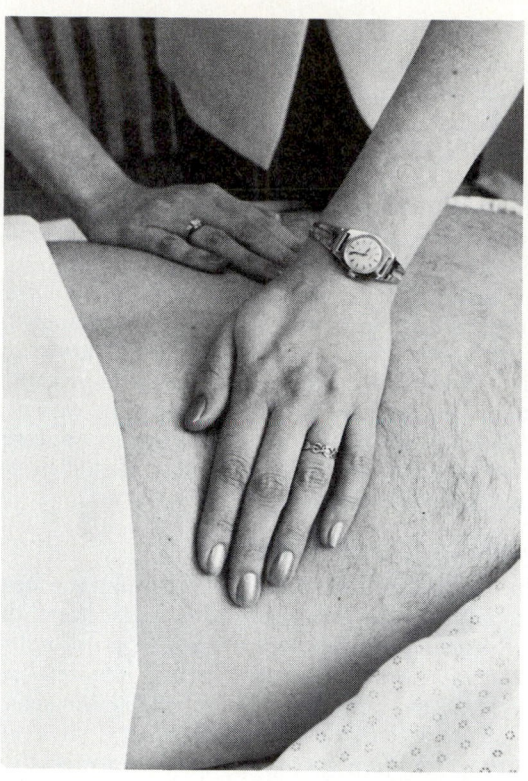

Fig. 24-24 Position of the hands for clapping the chest to loosen secretions.

Fig. 24-25 Position of the hands for vibrating the chest at the end of prolonged expiration.

Table 24-20 Positions for segmental postural drainage, clapping, and vibrating

Area of lung	Position of patient	Area to be clapped or vibrated
Upper lobe		
Apical bronchus	Semi-Fowler's position, leaning to right, then left, then forward	Over area of shoulder blades with fingers extending over clavicles
Posterior bronchus	Upright at 45-degree angle, rolled forward against a pillow at 45 degrees on left and then right side	Over shoulder blade on each side
Anterior bronchus	Supine with pillow under knees	Over anterior chest just below clavicles
Middle lobe (lateral and medial bronchus)	Trendelenburg's position at 30-degree angle or with foot of bed elevated 35-40 cm (14-16 inches), turned slightly to left	Anterior and lateral right chest from axillary fold to midanterior chest
Lingula (superior and inferior bronchus)	Trendelenburg's position at 30-degree angle or with foot of bed elevated 35-40 cm (14-16 inches), turned slightly to right	Left axillary fold to midanterior chest
Apical bronchus	Prone with pillow under hips	Lower third of posterior rib cage on both sides
Medial bronchus	Trendelenburg's position at 45-degree angle or with foot of bed raised 45-50 cm (18-20 inches) on right side	Lower third of left posterior rib cage
Lateral bronchus	Trendelenburg's position at 45-degree angle or with foot of bed raised 45-50 cm (18-20 inches) on left side	Lower third of right posterior rib cage
Posterior bronchus	Prone Trendelenburg's position at 45-degree angle with pillow under hips	Lower third of posterior rib cage on both sides

to exhale more fully. The procedure is repeated as necessary. When the patient cannot tolerate a head-down position, a modified position is used.

Positions that provide gravity drainage of the lungs can be achieved in several ways, and the procedure selected usually depends on the age and general condition of the person as well as the lobe or lobes of the lungs where secretions have accumulated. A young person usually can tolerate greater lowering of the head than an elderly person whose vascular system adapts less rapidly to change of position. A severely debilitated patient may only be able to tolerate slight changes in position.

Postural drainage can be achieved in several ways. Electric hospital beds can be tilted into a head-down position with little difficulty. If an electric bed is not available (for example, in the home), blocks can be placed under the casters at the foot of the bed or a hydraulic lift can be used under the foot of the bed. If these are not available, the foot of the bed can be supported on the seat of a firm chair to provide a position in which the head is lowered.

The nurse needs to know the part of the lung that is affected and how to position the patient to drain that portion of the lung. For example, if the right middle lobe of the lung is affected, drainage will be accomplished best by way of the right middle bronchus. The patient should lie supine with the body turned at approximately a 45-degree angle. The angle can be maintained by pillow supports placed under the right side from the shoulders to the hips. The foot of the bed is raised about 30 cm (12 inches). This position can be maintained fairly comfortably by most patients for half an hour at a time. On the other hand, if the lower posterior area of the lung is affected, the foot of the bed can be raised 45 to 50 cm (18 to 20 inches) with the patient assuming a prone position for drainage. A summary of the positions for segmental postural drainage is given in Table 24-20.

Postural drainage and percussion should be planned so as to achieve maximal benefit. The best time is generally in the morning soon after arising and at night before retiring. Frequency of treatments depends on each person's needs, but care should be taken to avoid exhaustion, which results in shallow ventilation and negates the positive effects of the treatment.

Patients having postural drainage of any kind are encouraged to breathe deeply and to cough forcefully to help dislodge thick sputum and exudate that is pooled in distended bronchioles, particularly after inactivity. Humidity, bronchodilators, or liquefying agents often are given 15 to 20 minutes before postural drainage is started, since they facilitate the removal of secretions. The patient may find that sputum can best be raised on resuming an upright position even though no drainage appeared while lying down with the head and chest lowered.

Because some patients complain of dizziness when assuming positions for postural drainage, the nurse stays with the patient during the first few times and reports any persistent dizziness or unusual discomfort to the physician.

Postural drainage may be *contraindicated* in some persons because of heart disease, hypertension, increased intracranial pressure, extreme dyspnea, or advanced age. However, most people can be taught to assume the positions for postural drainage and can proceed without help after being supervised once or twice.

Chest percussion (clapping) is *contraindicated* in patients with pulmonary emboli, hemorrhage, exacerbation of bronchospasms, or severe pain and over areas of resectable carcinoma. Often patients with a chronic pulmonary problem need to be taught to perform postural drainage independently so that they can continue it at home. The position usually is maintained for 10 minutes at first, and the period of time is gradually lengthened to 15 to 30 minutes as the patient becomes accustomed to the position. At first, elderly persons usually are able to tolerate these positions only for a few minutes. They need more assistance than other patients during the procedure and immediately thereafter. They should be assisted to a normal position in bed and required to lie flat for a few minutes before sitting up or getting out of bed. This helps to prevent dizziness and reduces the danger of accidents.

The patient may feel nauseated because of the odor and taste of sputum. Therefore, the procedure should be timed so that it comes at least 1 hour before meals. A short rest period following the treatment often improves postural drainage. Aromatic mouth washes should be available for frequent use by any patient who is expectorating sputum freely.

□ Oxygen therapy

Oxygen therapy is required for patients with COPD who are unable to maintain a PaO_2 of 50 torr or more at rest and for those who cannot carry out ADL (bathing, eating, dressing, toileting) without becoming very short of breath. In these instances, 1 to 2 L of oxygen is usually given via nasal prongs. In addition, some patients only require supplemental oxygen during sleep. Patients who complain of restlessness, insomnia, or headaches may be helped to sleep more comfortably if they receive low flow oxygen during the night. Because many patients with COPD have chronic carbon dioxide retention, they need to understand that the risk of high flow rates of oxygen to greater than 60 to 70 torr may remove the hypoxic drive and put them into respiratory failure. (See the discussion on respiratory failure, p. 736.)

Portable oxygen units are available that allow the patient to be up and about while receiving oxygen.

□ Medications

The types of medications that may be prescribed for persons with COPD include bronchodilators, expectorants, antimicrobials, corticosteroids, digitalis, diuretics, and psychopharmacologic agents.

BRONCHODILATORS. There are two basic categories of *bronchodilators*—sympathomimetic (adrenergic) agents and xanthine compounds. These bronchodilators act at different sites and appear to work synergistically when used

Table 24-21 Bronchodilators commonly used to treat COPD

Name	Mode of action
Methylxanthines	
Aminophylline Theophylline Dyphylline	Block action of phosphodiesterase and interfere with degradation of cyclic AMP, resulting in bronchodilation
Sympathomimetics*	

Beta$_1$-receptor sites
   Epinephrine (adrenaline HCl)
   Isoproterenol (Isuprel)
Beta$_2$-receptor sites
   Terbutaline (Brethine)
   Metaproterenol (Alupent)
   Isoetharine (Bronkosol)
	Activate adenylcyclase leading to increased production of cyclic AMP, resulting in relaxation of smooth muscle of airway; increase in cyclic AMP also inhibits release of chemical mediators that cause bronchospasm (histamine and SRS-A)

*Beta-adrenergic drugs.

together.[5] Table 24-21 lists the commonly used bronchodilators and their mode of action. Adrenergic agents that work at beta$_2$ sites located in smooth muscles of the airways have fewer cardiac side effects than do beta$_1$-agents whose receptor sites are in the myocardium. For this reason, isoetharine, metaproterenol sulfate, and terbutaline sulfate may be prescribed for patients with hypertension and those who have excessive palpitations or tachycardia from beta$_1$-agents.

AEROSOL THERAPY

Aerosol therapy is one of the most effective ways to deliver bronchodilators. There are several ways in which aerosolization of medications can be achieved. These include a Freon-propelled, metered-dosage cartridge inhalator; hand-held nebulizer; compressor pump; or IPPB machine. In general, metered-dosage cartridge inhalators and hand-held nebulizers are used more commonly than IPPB (see the box below). However, IPPB is still used to deliver aerosols to persons who cannot inhale repetitively to near TLC or in those persons who are unable to use a hand-held nebulizer because of lack of coordination or fatigue. When administering bronchodilators, the solution should be diluted with either water or saline. Some experts recommend that the diluent be water because saline solutions already contain a solute (NaCl) in water.[103] All bronchodilator solutions are high-molecular weight concentrated solutions and have a high solute content. When they are diluted with water, there is a maximal decrease in solute concentration; thus smaller particle size and deeper deposition of the aerosol in the smaller airways results.

Aerosol devices are excellent sites for bacterial growth, and patients using such equipment at home should be advised how to clean them appropriately.

EXPECTORANTS. Although expectorants are sometimes prescribed, some experts believe they do more harm than good.[103] Water is still considered to be the best expectorant, and adequate hydration without fluid overload should be encouraged. Usually 3.0 to 4.0 L of fluids daily are recommended unless the patient has *cor pulmonale* and is on fluid restriction.

ANTIMICROBIALS. Antimicrobials are prescribed to treat

Teaching patients to use a hand-held nebulizer

The steps to be followed in teaching a person to use a hand-held nebulizer:
1. Exhale fully.
2. Position nebulizer in mouth *without* sealing lips around it.
3. Take a deep breath through mouth while squeezing the bulb of the nebulizer *once*.
4. Hold breath for 3 to 4 seconds at full inspiration.
5. Exhale slowly through pursed lips.
Usually one inhalation is sufficient. Several inhalations of a bronchodilator may cause medication overdosage and result in side effects (for instance, tachycardia, palpitation, and nervousness).

respiratory tract infections in persons with COPD. The most commonly used ones are *tetracycline* and *ampicillin,* 1 to 2 g/day for 7 to 10 days. Some patients have a prescription on hand and self-administer the antimicrobial after telephone consultation with their physician. Antimicrobials should be started within 24 hours of the first sign of a respiratory infection (increased sputum production and purulence).[103] Patients who are febrile or have other signs and symptoms of infection that do not respond to the prescribed therapy should have a Gram stain and culture and sensitivity studies. When antibiotics are used inappropriately, especially in patients who are not adequately clearing their lungs of secretions, superinfection with bacteria or fungi may occur.[103]

CORTICOSTEROIDS. Corticosteroids may be prescribed for patients with intermittent bronchial obstruction and blood or sputum eosinophilia whose condition is not controlled by bronchodilators.[103] Usually a short course of corticosteroids is prescribed to alleviate acute symptoms. Prednisone is often prescribed for a total of 7 to 10 days. In some patients with asthma, a longer course of prednisone may be prescribed and some patients are on low-maintenance doses (5 to 10 mg/day) for several months or even years. Long-term corticosteroid therapy is usually not recommended for patients with chronic bronchitis or emphysema unless their disease is rapidly progressing.[103]

Persons who are on long-term steroid therapy should have a tuberculin test before initiation of therapy. Those with tuberculin reaction of 10 mm induration or more are candidates for isoniazid therapy (p. 685). The purpose of isoniazid therapy is to prevent reactivation of tuberculosis in persons receiving prolonged steroid therapy.

DIGITALIS. Digitalis may be prescribed for patients with COPD and left ventricular failure. The patient receiving a digitalis preparation should be carefully monitored for side effects (Chapter 25).

Patients with increased dyspnea secondary to pulmonary edema, or with right ventricular failure, or corticosteroid-induced fluid retention may benefit from *diuretics.* When diuretics are given, the patient should be carefully monitored for side effects. Those on thiazide diuretics need to be taught about eating foods high in potassium such as bananas, oranges, prunes, and raisins.

PSYCHOPHARMACOLOGIC AGENTS. Psychopharmacologic agents may need to be prescribed for some patients with severe emotional disturbances. The type of agent and size of dose are individually determined; but in general, the older the patient, the smaller the dose. When these agents are prescribed, a pharmacology book should be referred to for information about the side effects and precautions to be used in administering these agents.

□ **Maintaining adequate nutrition and fluid intake**

Persons with COPD may be very short of breath, and eating can become a real problem to the person who is breathless. The patient may be overweight early in the disease and will be urged to lose weight and keep it at normal or slightly below normal levels.

In later stages of COPD patients are often malnourished because of dyspnea and reduced energy levels. Suggestions to increase protein and caloric intake are listed in the box below.

□ **Assisting with comfort and ADL**

1. Place patient in position of comfort, usually Fowler's or high Fowler's.
2. Assist patient with progressive relaxation exercises and meditation (see boxes, p. 732).

□ **Assisting with control of environment**

Abrupt changes in weather or hot or cold environments can increase sputum production and bronchial obstruction.

□ *Temperature and humidity*

1. Humidity of 30% to 50% is ideal. This can be achieved by a humidifier as necessary.
2. An air conditioner may reduce dyspnea by controlling temperature and preventing pollutants from outside air from entering. The cost of an air conditioner is a medically deductible expense for persons with COPD.
3. Wearing a scarf over the nose and mouth in cold weather helps to warm the air and prevent bronchospasm. Masks for this purpose are also available.
4. Moving to another climate is usually not advised unless there is some other medical indication for doing so. Persons living at high altitudes may be advised to move

---

Foods to increase protein and caloric intake

1. Offer frequent small feedings of foods high in protein and calories, for example:
   a. Milk shakes
   b. Flavored gelatin or pudding with whipped cream
   c. Cream soups made with half and half
   d. Peanut butter spread on crackers, bananas, pears, or apples
   e. Crackers and cheese, nuts, dried fruits, and ice cream (readily available for snacks)
2. Avoid foods that are difficult to chew or to digest; patient usually indicates desires in this regard

---

Progressive relaxation exercises

1. Contract each muscle to a count of 10 and then relax it.
2. Do exercises in quiet room while sitting or lying in a comfortable position.
3. Do exercises to relaxing music, if desired.
4. Have another person serve as a "coach" by giving command to contract muscle, count to 10, and then give command to relax muscle.
5. Examples of exercises helpful to some persons with COPD:
   a. Raise shoulders, shrug them and then relax.
   b. Make a fist of both hands, squeeze them tightly for 5 seconds, and then relax them completely.
6. There are several articles in the nursing literature about relaxation techniques; the reader is referred to Broussard, P.: Using relaxation for COPD, Am J Nurs 69:1962-1963, 1969; and Richter, JM, and Sloan, R: A relaxation technique, Am J Nurs 79:1960-1964, 1979.

Meditation exercises

1. Sit or lie quietly with eyes closed and attempt to relax all muscles, beginning with feet and moving upward.
2. Breathe quietly and rhythmically through nose. If you cannot breathe through nose because of COPD, use pursed-lip breathing.
3. Meditate for 10 to 20 minutes once or twice daily.
4. Meditate before meals or 2 or more hours after eating, because digestion interferes with ability to relax.
5. Meditation at bedtime may help induce sleep.

---

to a lower altitude or use supplemental oxygen continuously.
5. Travel by airplane is possible. The airline needs to be informed in advance of the need for supplemental oxygen during the flight.

☐ *Avoidance of inhaled irritants*

Air pollution is a common problem in modern civilization and is a real threat to persons with COPD, who should observe the following:
1. Pay heed to announcements on radio and television regarding pollution alerts and avoid being outdoors when an alert is in effect.
2. Use an air conditioner or high-efficiency particulate air filter or electrostatic filter to remove particulate matter from air.
   a. Keep filters clean.
   b. Follow manufacturer's directions for use.
3. Use an activated charcoal filter if offending odors or gas pollutants are a problem.

☐ **Assisting with improving activity tolerance**

1. Allow ample time for activities; do not rush patient.
2. Provide oxygen as needed before and during activities.
3. Encourage gradual increase in activities such as walking.

4. Provide positive feedback on progress and encourage new endeavors when patient is ready.

☐ **Assisting with sleep pattern disturbance**

Persons with COPD usually only sleep for short periods of time. Most are most comfortable sleeping in an upright position in bed or in a lounge chair with foot rest.
1. Assist with relaxation exercises at bedtime.
2. Give backrub at bedtime and encourage family member to do so at home.
3. Provide relaxing music at bedtime and encourage same at home.
4. Ascertain preferred position for sleep, usually high Fowler's.
5. Establish regular bedtime to meet patient's usual schedule.
6. Give bedtime snack, if desired.

☐ **Assisting with anxiety reduction**

Persons who are short of breath are very anxious and frightened.
1. Encourage patient to talk about anxiety and fears with nurse and family members.
2. Take measures already discussed to improve airway clearance and breathing.

3. Do not leave patient alone during periods of breathlessness.
4. Explain to family reason for not leaving patient alone for long periods; assist them with securing community resources to assist as necessary (for instance, Homemakers, Visiting Nurses Association, and so on).

☐ Counseling and teaching

1. Stop or reduce smoking (if patient has not done so).
   a. Encourage attempts to reduce smoking.
   b. Make patient aware of resources to assist persons to stop smoking (p. 670)
   c. Encourage others not to smoke in presence of patient
2. Avoid persons with respiratory infections when respiratory infections are prevalent in the community
   a. Avoid crowds.
   b. Minimize contact with young children; they are common carriers of viruses that are uncommon to adults
3. Receive immunization for influenza and pneumonia (see the box on p. 670).

⌗ EVALUATION

Evaluation is based on patient outcomes. Questions to be asked include the following:

1. Is breathing improved?
2. Is patient able to do more without becoming breathless?
3. Is patient able to do breathing exercises and relaxation and meditation exercises by self?
4. Is patient able to give own aerosol treatments?
5. Is patient less anxious?
6. Is sleep improved?
7. Is patient able to plan a diet to meet nutritional needs?
8. Can the patient list signs and symptoms that require immediate contact with a health care provider?
9. Can the patient explain the dosages, actions, and side-effects of prescribed medications?
10. Can the patient state plans for follow-up?

■ Asthma

Asthma is discussed separately from bronchitis and emphysema because it results in intermittent rather than continuous airway obstruction. Its onset is sudden, as opposed to the slow insidious progression of symptoms seen in bronchitis and emphysema. Asthma is characterized by increased responsiveness of the trachea and bronchi to various stimuli with difficulty in breathing caused by narrowing of the airways.[5] The etiology, signs and symptoms, and medical therapy are outlined in the box on p. 734.

Persons who have asthmatic attacks usually seek medical care, because the attacks are both incapacitating and frightening. The individual must often make an attempt to reduce emotional stress and to control physical exertion because these factors are less amenable to management than are specific allergens. If the underlying cause of an allergy is obscure, if it is resistant to treatment, or if the

person has nonallergenic asthma, the recognition and control of secondary factors may be the main approach to treatment. *It is imperative to understand that even though psychologic factors may precipitate an attack, the response to it is physiologic and requires the same treatment as that prescribed for an attack precipitated by an allergen or any other factor.*

There is perhaps no disease in which knowing the patient well is more important than in asthma. Because sensitivity tests can be done with only a very small fraction of the substances with which the patient is in contact, the physician usually makes the diagnosis on the basis of a careful history. Knowing about the person's life-style such as the type of work and leisure-time activities and even food preferences may give useful clues as to what precipitates the asthmatic attack. Although the allergist urges persons to report seemingly trivial and insignificant details, they often hesitate to do so, because they are accustomed to reporting only physical changes within themselves. The alert nurse can be of help in learning the cause of an allergic reaction. It is often the nurse who may learn that a relative has just visited in the home and was accompanied by a cat or a dog. This information would be of great importance because animal dander is one of the most common allergens for individuals with atopic asthma.

The nurse may make observations regarding emotional stressors that appear to aggravate the patient's condition. Careful observation of relationships between the person and his or her significant others may give clues to sources of emotional stress. Some patients remain in the hospital during an acute episode and return home relieved of serious symptoms. However, unless life circumstances can be altered, family relationships and general socioeconomic conditions that cause stress may send that patient back to the hospital with another attack.

Patients with chronic asthma may gain a sense of security while in the hospital, and they may be reluctant to return home. Asthmatic attacks can be precipitated by plans for discharge, and the patient's stay may thus be prolonged. Patients with severe emotional problems may benefit from psychotherapy.

■ PATHOPHYSIOLOGY

An asthmatic attack is the result of an antigen-antibody reaction in which chemical mediators are released. The chemical mediators, which include histamine, slow-releasing substance of anaphylaxis (SRS-A), eosinophilic chemotactic factor of anaphylaxis (ECF-A), and perhaps others, cause three main reactions: (1) constriction of smooth muscles of both the large and small airways resulting in bronchospasm, (2) increased capillary permeability that contributes to mucosal edema and further narrows the airways, and (3) increased mucous glands secretions and increased mucus production. As a result, the person with an asthmatic attack struggles to breath through a narrowed airway, which is in spasm. Because breathing is labored, the person breathes through the mouth, which dries the mucus and further occludes the airway.

During an acute attack, the alveoli progressively distend

Etiology, signs and symptoms, and medical therapy for asthma

Etiology

Two basic types: immunologic and nonimmunologic

Immunologic or allergic asthma (formerly called extrinsic)

    Occurs in childhood.

    Often follows other allergic disease such as eczema—80% to 85% of children with eczema develop hay fever or asthma by 6 years of age. Persons with allergic asthma are considered to be atopic (see Chapter 38).

    Attacks are precipitated by contact with allergen to which person is sensitive.

Nonimmunologic or nonallergic (formerly called intrinsic)

    Usually develops in adults over 35 years of age.

    Attacks are frequently triggered by an infection in the sinuses or bronchial tree.

Some persons have *mixed asthma* in which attacks are initiated by viral or bacterial infections or by allergens.

    At different times, attacks may be precipitated by different factors.

In any type of asthma the airway is in a state of easy provocation.

Attacks may be precipitated by changes in temperature and humidity, irritating fumes and smoke, strong odors, physical exertion, and emotional stress. Some allergists refer to asthma in children as the "Christmas and birthday disease," because the excitement and stress of these days often precipitate an asthmatic attack.

Hypoxemia, hypercapnia, and overuse of bronchodilators may cause an asthmatic attack.

Signs and symptoms

Attacks frequently occur at night.

Patient wakens with feeling of choking.

Bronchospasm and narrowing of airways causes *wheezing* on exhalation.

Patient uses accessory muscles to breathe and may lean forward to breathe better.

Cyanosis may be present.

Attack usually subsides in 30 to 60 minutes.

Patient coughs up large quantities of thick, tenacious sputum.

Diaphoresis is common because of energy expenditure.

Exhaustion follows an attack.

Medical therapy

The management of asthma is directed toward symptomatic relief of attacks, control of specific causative factors, and general care for maintenance of optimal health. The chief aim of various medications is to afford the patient immediate and progressive bronchial relaxation. Following are some approaches to therapy*:

1. *Acute asthma*
   a. Moderate severity: treated safely on an outpatient basis when *no danger signs* are present.
      (1) Give nasal oxygen.
      (2) IV aminophylline in a loading dose or subcutaneous terbutaline or both may be given simultaneously.
      (3) Monitor FEV_1 and symptoms; when they improve, begin oral therapy.
      (4) Observe carefully for 48 hours and monitor for signs of relapse.
   b. Severe attack with *one or more danger signs:* vital capacity <1.0 L, FEV_1 < 0.5 L, Po_2 under 50 mm, increase in Pco_2, exhaustion, or disturbed consciousness.
      (1) Hospitalize; give supplemental oxygen; intubate if necessary.
      (2) Administer IV steroids (100 mg hydrocortisone [Solu-Cortef] or equivalent every 6 hours for four doses); begin prednisone, 60 to 80 mg every 24 hours until FEV_1 nears best previous value, then reduce dose over next 2 to 3 weeks; begin use of beclomethasone inhaler.
      (3) IV aminophylline in a loading dose and then in maintenance dose for 48 to 72 hours; monitor aminophylline blood levels.
      (5) IPPB may be used to deliver adrenergic agents and to facilitate bronchodilation.
2. *Chronic asthma*
   a. Mild to moderate or recurring
      (1) Theophylline compounds; cromolyn sodium may be tried; give adrenergic inhaler as needed.
      (2) Oral beta-2-adrenergic agents added in divided doses if above not effective.
   b. Moderately severe: add beclomethasone inhaler to items (1) and (2) above.
   c. Severe asthma causing interferences with work; give oral steroids every other day in addition to items listed above; keep steroids to minimal effective dose.

*Adapted from Jenne, JW: Basics RD 6:1-6, Sept. 1977.

as in emphysema; actually, acute emphysema exists. Unless relaxation of the bronchioles can be accomplished, insufficient oxygen passes through the alveolar-capillary membrane into the bloodstream (hypoxemia), and the person becomes progressively more cyanotic. At the same time, the person is usually hyperventilating and exhaling CO_2, and for this reason $PaCO_2$ is usually reduced. When the $PaCO_2$ becomes elevated and the person becomes hypercapnic, this is a danger sign because it indicates that the person is tiring and ventilatory efforts are becoming inadequate. Intubation and assisted ventilation may then be necessary. The person needs constant observation and support and should have everything done for him or her.

Some patients have *chronic mild asthma*. Symptoms are not noticeable when the person is at rest. However, after exertion such as laughing, singing, vigorous exercise, or emotional excitement, dyspnea and wheezing develop rapidly. These attacks are controlled with medications, and patients often can continue their usual mode of living with a few modifications and no serious lung changes. They are not hospitalized, but they sometimes come to outpatient clinics for medical supervision.

Persons who are severely affected with asthma and who have attacks that are difficult to control with the usual medications may develop *status asthmaticus*. In this case, the symptoms of an acute attack continue despite measures to relieve them. The patient is acutely ill. When admitted to the hospital, emergency treatment is begun. The patient is questioned as to medications already taken. Usually a bronchodilator has failed to relieve the attack, and that is why the patient is seeking medical assistance. The patient is often very anxious and may be in a near-panic state because of inability to relieve the symptoms. Aminophylline, 500 mg in an intravenous drip, is given over a 20-minute period. A prolonged attack causes exhaustion, and death from heart failure may occur. Oxygen is administered, and IPPB may be used intermittently. Blood gases are carefully monitored, and intravenous steroids are frequently given. Repeated attacks of status asthmaticus may cause irreversible emphysema, resulting in a permanent decrease in total breathing capacity.

◨ ASSESSMENT

☐ Subjective data

1. How long person has had history of asthma
2. What usually precipitates an attack
3. Medications taken daily
4. Medications taken to treat an acute attack

☐ Objective data during asthmatic attack

1. Tachypnea
2. Audible wheezing
3. Use of accessory muscles
4. Cyanosis
5. Tactile fremitus decreased on palpation
6. Hyperressonance on percussion
7. Breath sounds are distant, vocal fremitus is decreased and sibilant, rhonchi are the adventitious sounds on auscultation

☐ Diagnostic tests

Pulmonary function tests (p. 704) and blood gas analyses (p. 721) are used to determine degree of airway obstruction and effectiveness of therapy. Pulmonary function measurements are taken before and after use of a bronchodilator to determine therapeutic effectiveness.

▶ DATA ANALYSIS: NURSING DIAGNOSES

Nursing diagnoses are determined from assessment of patient data. Possible nursing diagnoses for the person with asthma may include, but are not limited to, the following:

Diagnostic title	Possible etiologies
Ineffective airway clearance	Tracheobronchial obstruction
Anxiety	Situational crisis
	Threat of death
Fatigue	Oxygen depriation
Impaired gas exchange	Ventilation/perfusion imbalance
Knowledge deficit	Lack of exposure
	Unfamiliarity with information sources

◨ PLANNING: EXPECTED PATIENT OUTCOMES

Expected patient outcomes for the person with asthma may include, but are not limited to, the following:

1. Patient or significant other can state the factors most likely to precipitate an asthmatic attack (for example, stress, allergens, and infections).
2. Patient or significant other can state the importance of keeping a diary of symptoms and medications (time and dose) during an asthma attack.
3. If the cause is allergic, state how to prepare an environmentally controlled bedroom (Chapter 38).
4. Patient or significant other can explain any home medication program.
   a. Give name, dose, action, and side effects of each medication.
   b. State conditions under which medications might be increased (for example, infection—start or increase antibiotics; increased stress or worsening of symptoms—increase corticosteroids).
5. Patient or significant other can demonstrate how to take inhaled medications (p. 730).
6. Patient or significant other can describe what to do when an acute attack occurs (for example, take medication and be quiet).
7. Patient or significant other can state signs and symptoms that indicate need for immediate medical attention (for example, asthmatic attack unrelieved by usual treatment).
8. If receiving corticosteroid therapy, patient can show card to be carried at all times giving data about the drug, dose, and name of physician; alternative is to wear Medic-Alert bracelet.
9. Patient can state plans for ongoing follow-up care including plans for desensitization if appropriate.

▓ IMPLEMENTATION

☐ **Assisting with achievement of therapeutic goals**

☐ *Medications*

1. Given medications as ordered. Monitor IV rates closely.
2. Monitor patient closely for side effects of medications.
   a. Epinephrine—increased heart rate, palpitations, increased blood pressure.
   b. Ephedrine—cerebral agitation especially if a barbiturate such as phenobarbital is not given with it. Often ephedrine is administered in a combination medication that contains a barbiturate. Some combination medications also contain theoplylline (aminophylline). Tedral and Bronkotabs, for example, contain all three medications.
   c. Terbutaline—increased heart rate, tremors, palpitations, sweating, headache, and cramps in hands and feet.
3. Recognize that sedatives should be given with caution during an asthmatic attack to avoid depressing respiratory center. Exception would be patient with severe attack who is intubated and on assisted ventilation.

☐ *Facilitating breathing*

1. Place in high Fowler's position.
2. Assist patient to cough up secretions. Mucous plugs are a common problem.
   a. Liquefying agents may be ordered.
   b. Humidification in form of aerosol may be necessary.
   c. Give fluids freely.

☐ **Assisting with comfort and ADL**

1. *Never leave patient alone during an asthmatic attack.* He or she may be frightened and need constant attention and reassurance.
2. At end of attack:
   a. Sponge patient and give backrub.
   b. Change patient's gown and bed which are often soaked because of diaphoresis.
   c. Stay with patient until he or she falls asleep.

☐ **Counseling and teaching**

1. Person with immunologic asthma
   a. Teach patient how to prepare an environmentally controlled bedroom (Chapter 38).
   b. Teach about avoiding allergens.
2. Persons with nonimmunologic asthma
   a. Teach how to avoid infections.
   b. Stress urgency of seeking immediate medical attention for upper respiratory infection.

▓ EVALUATION

Evaluation is based on patient outcomes. Questions to be asked include the following:

1. Can the patient state the names, dosages, and side-effects of prescribed medications?
2. Can the patient state what to do if he or she has an acute attack?
3. Can the patient state what to avoid to prevent an attack?
4. Can the patient describe how to prepare an environmentally controlled bedroom?
5. Can the patient demonstrate the correct way to use a hand-held nebulizer?
6. Can the patient identify factors that might precipitate an asthmatic attack?
7. Can the patient state plans for follow-up care?

■ RESPIRATORY INSUFFICIENCY AND RESPIRATORY FAILURE

■ Epidemiology and etiology

The term *respiratory insufficiency* is usually used to indicate that the exchange of oxygen and carbon dioxide is not adequate to meet the needs of the body during normal activities. *Respiratory failure* is said to occur when ventilation is not sufficient to achieve adequate gas exchange even at rest. Many disorders can lead to or are associated with both respiratory insufficiency and failure; these are listed in Table 24-22.

The diagnosis of respiratory insufficiency or failure is based on arterial blood gas studies, pulmonary function testing, and the clinical status of the patient. The criteria listed in the box below are generally used in defining a state of failure. However, it cannot be overemphasized that these parameters are only *guidelines* and must be applied in light of the individual's history, age, and overall condition.

■ Pathophysiology and clinical picture

Regardless of the underlying condition, the resultant events or processes that occur in respiratory failure are the same. With inadequate ventilation, the arterial PO_2 falls and tissues cells become hypoxic. The PCO_2 accumulates, leading to a fall in pH, and the patient becomes acidotic. The reader must keep in mind while working with the patient with COPD who has developed respiratory failure, that this patient normally exists in a compensated state with decreased PaO_2 levels and elevated $PaCO_2$ levels. Thus the parameters in the boxed material are not applicable; the pH level, however, is a useful guide in assessing the degree of insufficiency. When the pH begins to fall below

---

Criteria for diagnosis of respiratory failure

PaO_2 <50 mm Hg when breathing room air
$PaCO_2$ >50 mm Hg
Vital capacity <15 ml/kg
Respiratory rate >30/min or below 8/min

Table 24-22 Disorders associated with respiratory insufficiency and failure

Pulmonary disorders	Nonpulmonary disorders
Severe infection	CNS disturbance secondary to drug overdose, anesthesia, head injury
Pulmonary edema	Neuromuscular disorders (e.g., Guillain-Barré syndrome, myasthenia gravis,
Pulmonary embolus	multiple sclerosis, poliomyelitis, muscular dystrophy, spinal cord injury)
COPD	Postoperative reduction in ventilation following thoracic or abdominal surgery
Adult respiratory distress syndrome (ARDS)	Prolonged mechanical ventilation
Cancer	
Chest trauma	
Severe atelectasis	
Airway compromise secondary to trauma, infection, or surgery	

7.3, it is an indication that the patient is no longer able to compensate for the elevated $PaCO_2$ level.

Respiratory insufficiency and failure can result from a worsening in the condition of the patient with any of the disorders already mentioned.

■ Interventions

Intervention for the patient who has respiratory insufficiency or failure always begins with a recognition of the underlying disease state or cause of the disturbance in ventilation. Therapy is first directed at improving the underlying condition, such as sepsis, or by removing the cause, such as fluid overload.

The goals of intervention are to improve oxygenation and ventilation to restore the person's normal PaO_2 and $PaCO_2$ levels. The initial medical management can often be conservative if the diagnosis is made early enough.

■ OXYGEN

Particular care is needed in working with the patient who has chronic lung disease. As mentioned earlier, individuals with COPD normally exist with elevated $PaCO_2$ levels and have *lost the usual respiratory drive, carbon dioxide stimulation.* They no longer respond to increased carbon dioxide levels by increasing their rate and depth of respiration; rather, the elevated $PaCO_2$ depresses the respiratory center. Their respiratory drive is now derived from their low PaO_2 levels; therefore, even though these persons lack oxygen, it is extremely dangerous to raise their PaO_2 to normal levels. If the arterial PO_2 is normal and there is retention of carbon dioxide (*hypercapnia*), the person will have no respiratory drive. Hypoventilation becomes more severe and $PaCO_2$ continues to rise. This situation results in *carbon dioxide narcosis,* a markedly elevated carbon dioxide level that causes coma or semicoma. Persons with COPD are, therefore, treated with low flow or controlled flow oxygen; that is, inspired oxygen concentrations of 24% to 30%. These concentrations can easily be obtained by using a Ventimask (Fig. 24-26) or a two-pronged nasal cannula with a 1 to 2 L oxygen flow. This amount of oxygen

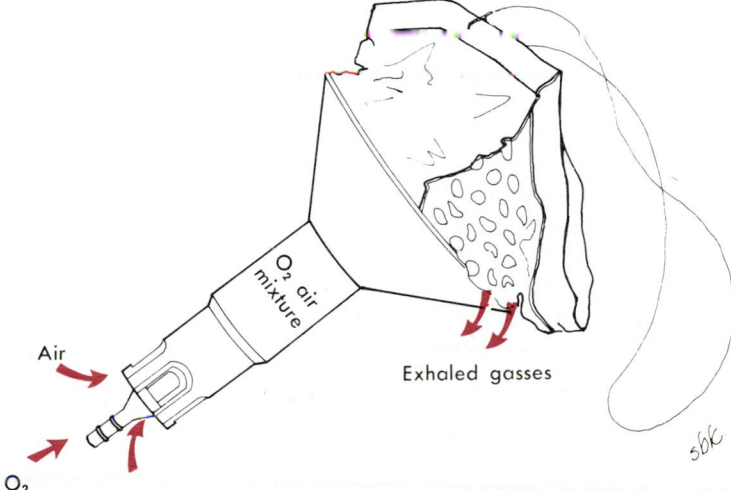

Fig. 24-26 Ventimask allows air to be mixed with oxygen to provide diluted oxygen to patient. (From Wade, JF: Comprehensive respiratory care, ed 3, St. Louis, 1982, The CV Mosby Co.)

can significantly increase the amount of oxygen carried by hemoglobin without a significant increase in arterial PO_2; therefore, the patient's blood carries much more oxygen even though hypoxemia is still present. The person continues to have respiratory drive, and the $PaCO_2$ does not rise.

By the use of low-flow oxygen, the amount of oxygen carried in the patient's blood can often be increased enough to maintain basic body functions without further reduction of ventilation. Persons who do not have COPD, who have a normal $PaCO_2$, but who are hypoxic are usually able to tolerate high flow rates of oxygen (5 to 10 L/min). Oxygen is an integral part of the therapy of patients with respiratory insufficiency and failure; however, some hazards are associated with prolonged use.

Oxygen toxicity is the term used to describe the damage to lung tissue that results from prolonged exposure to high concentrations of oxygen. Although the exact effects of

NURSING CARE PLAN

Person with COPD

DATA: Mrs. Davis is a 54-year-old housewife with a medical history of severe chronic obstructive pulmonary disease with cor pulmonale. She has a 75 pack year history of cigarette smoking and stopped smoking 2 years ago (husband still smokes). Patient states, "I am unable to walk back from the bathroom to the living room without a 30 to 60 minute rest." Lung sounds are diminished throughout. Chest x-ray examination indicates overinflation of the lungs. Pulmonary function tests show severe obstructive ventilatory dysfunction with hyperinflation. Arterial blood gases are: pH = 7.41; $Paco_2$ = 37; Pao_2 = 69; oxygen saturation = 94%. Current medications include metaproterenol inhaler, theodur, terbutaline sulfate, hydrochlorothiazide, potassium (K-lyte), and nitroglycerine sublingual tablets for chest pain prn. Patient has come in for outpatient rehabilitation, including muscle reconditioning and education.

Nursing diagnosis: Activity intolerance: related to tissue hypoxia associated with impaired gas exchange and fatigue

Expected patient outcomes	Nursing interventions	Rationale
Patient demonstrates increased tolerance for activity	Provide frequent rest periods Instruct patient in energy saving techniques Reinforce pursed-lip breathing Gradually increase activity	Improve activity tolerance

Nursing diagnosis: Impaired gas exchange: related to decrease in effective lung surface

Expected patient outcomes	Nursing interventions	Rationale
Dyspnea is decreased	Assess respiratory status Provide prescribed low-flow oxygen Provide breathing retraining Provide rest periods	Obtain baseline information Many persons with COPD depend on hypoxemia as stimulus to breathe Decrease work of breathing Improve tolerance

Nursing diagnosis: Potential for infection: related to increased secretions, decreased motility in lungs

Expected patient outcomes	Nursing interventions	Rationale
Infection are minimized	Restrict persons with URI Teach patient measures to prevent infections Encourage patient to get annual influenza immunization and pneumonia vaccine every 3 to 5 years	Decrease exposure

oxygen in any one individual may be dependent on the person's underlying pathologic condition, it is believed that exposure to greater than 60% oxygen for a period of more than 36 hours, or exposure to 100% oxygen for a period of more than 6 hours, results in atelectasis and alveolar collapse. Breathing very high concentrations of oxygen (80% to 100%) for prolonged periods (24 hours or more) is often associated with the development of ARDS. Thus it is a firm general principle that the lowest amount of oxygen that will achieve an acceptable Po_2 is the amount that should be used.

■ AIRWAY MANAGEMENT

In addition to providing supplemental oxygen, care of the person with respiratory insufficiency usually also includes aggressive airway management and attempts to improve ventilation. Suctioning, IPPB, ultrasonic mist ther-

NURSING CARE PLAN

Person with COPD—cont'd

Nursing diagnosis: Personal identity disturbance: related to changes in life-style, dependence on others

Expected patient outcomes	Nursing interventions	Rationale
Patient participates in necessary activities	Give patient opportunities to to express concerns about limitations	Allow for communication
	Provide rationale for necessary activities	Maintain sense of control
	Discuss with family and friends the need for patient to maintain role relationships	Increase self-esteem
	Assist patient to identify personal strengths	
	Provide information about community resources.	

Nursing diagnosis: Knowledge deficit related to lack of exposure/lack of recall

Expected patient outcomes	Nursing interventions	Rationale
Patient describes therapeutic regimen and health maintenance	Teach patient: Nature of COPD and need to follow prescribed therapy and activities Home medication and treatment plans Home exercise plans Avoidance of respiratory irritants and infections Signs requiring medical attention Professional and community resources	Increase self-care abilities and self-esteem

apy, and postural drainage with clapping and vibrating are all employed in an attempt to halt the progression of insufficiency. When the patient develops respiratory failure and can no longer maintain his or her own respirations, an artificial airway is necessary.

☐ Types of artificial airways

An endotracheal tube is usually chosen initially as a means of providing an airway; tracheostomy is only performed if airway maintenance is necessary for a prolonged period of time or if trauma to the airway prevents the use of an endotracheal tube. Although a tracheostomy has the *disadvantage* of a higher risk of infection, it is often elected for long-term airway management because it is much more comfortable than an endotracheal tube and allows the person to eat.

In endotracheal intubation a tube is passed through either the nose or mouth into the trachea, while in a tracheostomy an artificial opening is made in the trachea into which a tube is inserted (Fig. 24-27). These procedures are used (1) to establish and maintain a patent airway, (2) to prevent aspiration by sealing off the trachea from the digestive tract in the unconscious or paralyzed person, (3) to premit removal of tracheobronchial secretions in the person who cannot cough adequately, and (4) to treat the patient who requires positive pressure ventilation that cannot be given effectively by mask.[46] Whether an intubation or a tracheostomy is performed initially depends on the facilities available and the wishes of the physician. Most physicians now consider it safer to do an emergency endotracheal intubation and then perform a tracheostomy as a nonemergency procedure in the operating room if prolonged support of the airway is needed. In this instance the endotracheal tube is not removed until after the tracheostomy opening is made.

A tracheostomy is necessary when an endotracheal tube cannot be inserted or when it is contraindicated, as in severe burns or laryngeal obstruction caused by tumor,

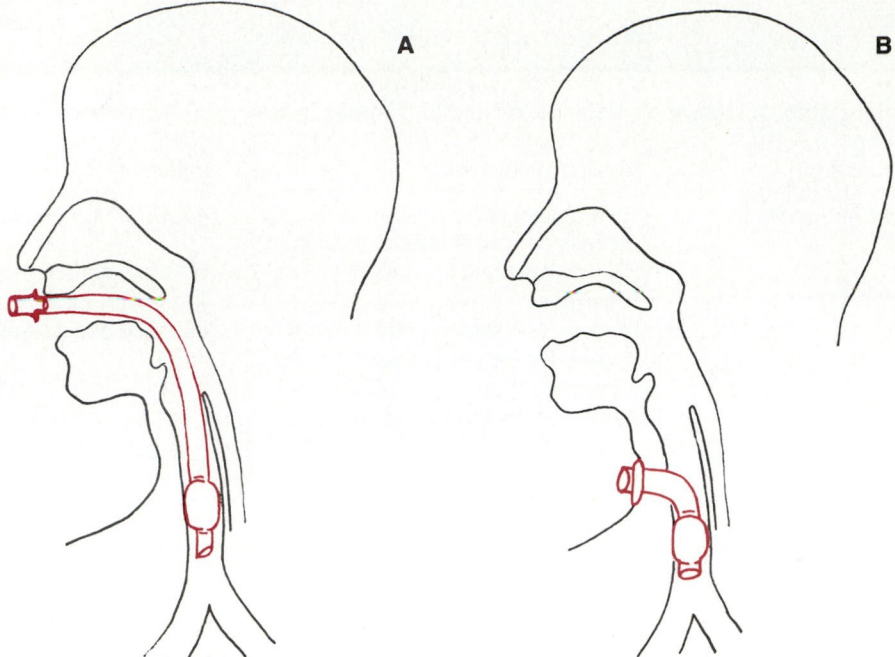

Fig. 24-27   **A,** Position of endotracheal tube. **B,** Position of tracheostomy tube.

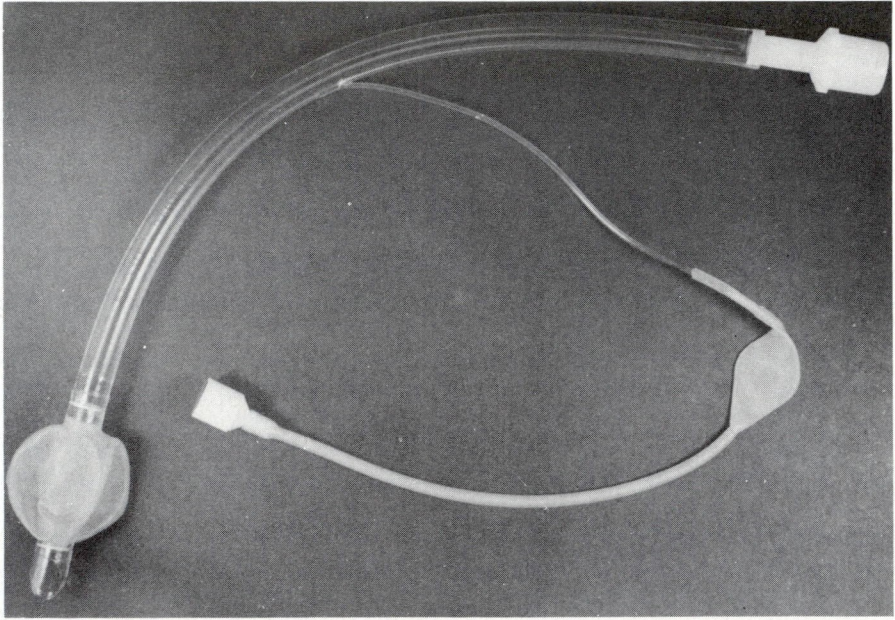

Fig. 24-28   Forregar high-volume, low-pressure cuffed endotracheal tube. Cuff shown here is not inflated. Low-pressure cuff is preferred because it is less likely to cause tracheal damage.

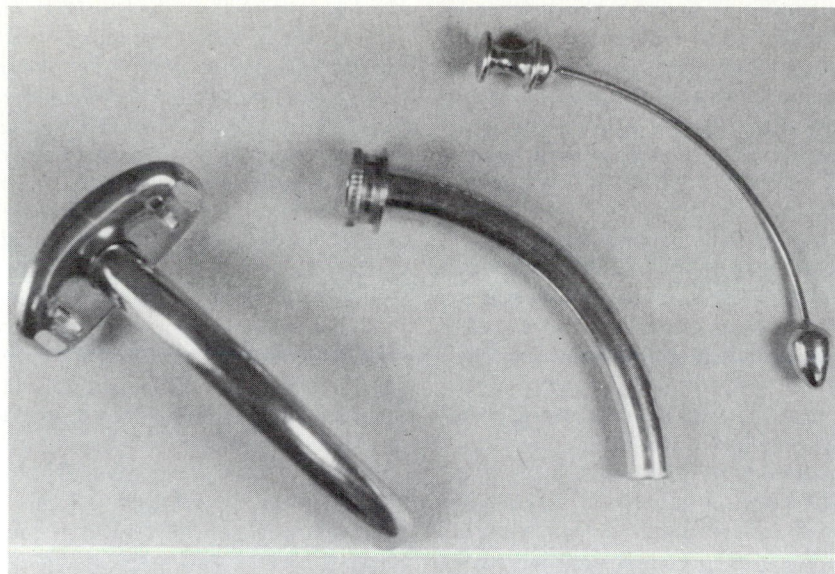

Fig. 24-29 Metal tracheostomy tube showing, from right to left, outer cannula, inner cannula, and obturator.

infection, or vocal cord paralysis.[46] Tracheostomy may also be required when a patient is conscious and cannot tolerate an endotracheal tube. Once the airway is secured either by intubation or by tracheostomy, secretions are aspirated and well-humidified oxygen is usually given. If the patient is unable to sustain respiration, a mechanical ventilator (for example, a Bennet or a Bird ventilator) is attached to either the endotracheal tube or the tracheostomy tube. When mechanical ventilation is required, a cuffed tube is used. Usually an endotracheal tube is not left in place longer than 5 to 7 days. If the patient is unable to maintain an open airway after this period of time, a tracheostomy is performed.

The endotracheal tube may be made of either plastic or rubber with an inflatable cuff so that a closed system with the ventilator may be maintained (Fig. 24-28). The tube is inserted via the mouth or nose through the larynx into the trachea. If an oral endotracheal tube is used, a rubber airway or bite block is often necessary to prevent the patient from biting down on the tube and obstructing the airway.

The tracheostomy tube is usually made of plastic, silver, or nylon. It may be either a single-lumen or double-lumen (Jackson) type (Figure 24-29). Both types of tubes may be cuffed, and the newer plastic tubes come with high-volume, low-pressure cuffs that are less likely to cause damage to the trachea (Fig. 24-30). Single-lumen tubes must be changed about every 72 hours, because they are more difficult to clean and more likely to become plugged than are double-lumen tubes.

Silver tubes are commonly available in sizes nos. 00 to 8 (no. 00 is used for the premature or newborn infant, while a no. 6 or 7 is used for most adults). The silver tracheostomy tube consists of two parts, an inner and an outer cannula. The outer cannula is removed only by the physician, whereas the inner cannula is removed regularly by the nurse for cleaning. The silver tracheostomy tube has a lock that must be turned to remove the inner cannula. The lock should be secured when the inner cannula is reinserted after cleaning. Twill tapes attached to either side of the tube are tied securely behind the neck to prevent the tube from becoming dislodged when the patient coughs or moves about.

Should the tube be coughed out, the opening may close

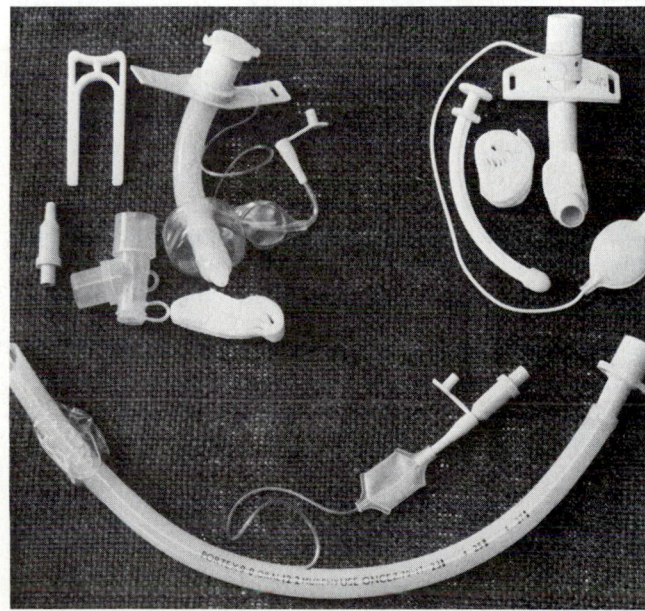

Fig. 24-30 *Top,* two types of high-volume low-pressure cuffed tracheostomy tubes. *Bottom,* Portex high-volume, low-pressure cuffed, endotracheal tube.

and the patient will be unable to breathe. Therefore, a tracheal dilator or curved hemostat is always kept at the bedside so that the opening can be held open if the tube is dislodged. Some surgeons prefer to place a retention suture on each side of the tracheostomy opening and tape the end of the suture to the skin. If the opening shows signs of closing, tension can be placed on the sutures to widen the opening.

The operative wound may be sealed with a plastic spray, or a small dressing may be placed around the tracheostomy tube. Although drainage should be minimal, the wound is inspected frequently for bleeding during the immediate postoperative period. The dressings are changed as they become soiled with drainage or mucus. Occasionally, young children require elbow restraints to prevent them from removing the tube or putting objects into it.

Immediately after insertion of the endotracheal tube and periodically thereafter the chest is auscultated to ensure that there are breath sounds on both sides. If a cuffed tube is inserted too far, it will slip into one of the mainstem bronchi (usually the right) and occlude the opposite bronchus and lung, resulting in atelectasis on the obstructed side. Even if the tube is still in the trachea, airway obstruction will reult if the end of the tube is located on the carina (area at lower end of trachea at point of bifurcation of mainstem bronchi). This causes dry secretions that obstruct both bronchi. Although these complications are more common with the use of an endotracheal tube, they can occur with a tracheostomy tube, especially in a small person with a short neck. In either case the tube is pulled back until it is positioned below the larynx and above the carina. The tube is then fastened securely in place. A replacement tube of the same size should always be kept at the bedside in the event that it is needed.

Depending on the patient's condition, a tracheostomy can be either temporary or permanent; the person who has a laryngectomy will require permanent tracheostomy. Any patient who has had a tracheostomy is apprehensive and is often fearful of choking. Thus when feasible, the procedure is thoroughly explained to the patient before surgery. Both patient and family need to understand that the patient will be unable to speak and that constant attendance will be provided until the patient can give self-care safely. The nurse should plan with the patient for some means of communication after the surgery. Hand signs such as the OK sign or a raised finger might be used as a means of expressing, for example, the need to void. The patient may want to write on a pad or a Magic Slate, or a word or picture chart can be used. The patient's ideas about means of communication should be considered. Patients should have their bell cords within reach, and a tap bell is reassuring to some patients.

□ Care of a person with a cuffed tube

The use of a cuffed endotracheal or tracheostomy tube has several implications for nursing care. Although the low-pressure cuffs have significantly lowered the incidence of tracheal erosion and necrosis from pressure on the wall of the trachea, there are still some hazards inherent in the use of artificial airways.

The cuff on the tube is used to maintain a closed system that permits positive-pressure ventilation. It is also used to prevent aspiration of secretions by the unconscious person. Sometimes the cuff is used to exert pressure on bleeding sites in patients who have undergone throat or neck surgery, such as a radical neck dissection. If none of these considerations apply, the cuff does not need to be inflated.

If the patient is being mechanically ventilated, the cuff should be inflated during the positive-pressure phase (inspiration) of the ventilator. Two different methods may be used to inflate the cuff, depending on the patient's condition and the preference of those responsible for care. In the first method, air is injected into the cuff until a full seal is attained. At this point a pressure-cycled respirator turns off and no air escapes around the tube or through the nose and mouth. The tubing leading to the cuff is then clamped. In the other method, air is injected until a full seal is attained, and then 0.5 ml of air is withdrawn and the tubing clamped. This latter method creates a partial leak for which the respirator can be set to compensate. The nurse should note the amount of air needed to inflate the cuff and use the smallest amount required to attain a seal. Overinflation of the cuff is extremely dangerous because it can lead to the development of tracheomalacia, tracheal stenosis, tracheosophageal fistula, or erosion through a major blood vessel.

In the past it was recommended that the cuff be routinely deflated for several minutes each hour to prevent tracheal necrosis. This is not necessary with low-pressure cuffs. It is sufficient to deflate the cuff and reinflate it once every 8 hours. This is necessary to ensure that the cuff is not overinflated and to check for tracheal dilation, indicated by the requirement of progressively larger amounts of air to obtain a seal.

It is important to remember that speaking is impossible with a cuffed tube in place because air does not pass directly through the larynx. The person is informed that speech will be normal when the tube is removed. Persons who are not informed of the change in function may believe that they have permanently lost their ability to speak.

Often the person with a tracheostomy tube can speak when the cuff is not fully inflated. Speech is still difficult because air must be forced around the tube and up through the larynx. For those who can tolerate it, it is often helpful to obstruct the opening of the tracheostomy tube while the cuff is deflated. This allows the person to breathe through the upper airway.

□ Suctioning the endotracheal tube

All persons with tubes require suctioning and should be suctioned as often as necessary. The frequency of suctioning is a nursing judgment. Many patients in respiratory failure have an infection and accumulation of secretions before intubation or tracheostomy is performed. Once the patient is intubated, the tube produces a natural route for introduction of bacteria into the lower airway, increasing the risk of infection. Much of the ability to produce an effective cough is lost, since it is impossible for the person to build up the pressure needed to create an expulsive cough. Because the patient has difficulty moving secretions up the tracheobronchial tree, it is important to suction as deeply as possible, using sterile technique. The depth to which a catheter can be inserted thorugh an *endotracheal tube* in an adult is approximately 45 to 55 cm (18 to 22 inches). Postural drainage with percussion and vibration (p. 727) is extremely helpful in moving secretions up to a point where they can be suctioned.

If the catheter cannot be inserted as far as usual, a mucus plug may be obstructing passage of the catheter. Instillation of approximately 5 to 10 ml of sterile saline solution often liquefies the obstructing secretions so they can be aspirated. When plastic suction catheters and plastic tubes are used, it is not uncommon for the surface of the catheter and tube to stick to each other, inhibiting passage of the catheter. Instilling 1 to 2 ml of sterile saline solution during insertion of the catheter usually prevents this problem.

To protect the suctioner, the CDC recommends that gloves, goggles, and a mask be worn. Persons with cuts or abrasions or severely chapped hands should not suction unless no one else is available. In this case, two pairs of gloves are recommended. A gown may be necessary to protect lesions on the arms.[48]

☐ Care of a person with a tracheostomy

Analgesics and sedatives are given judiciously so as not to depress the respiratory center. The patient is suctioned as often as necessary, possibly every 5 minutes during the first few postoperative hours. The need for suctioning can be determined by the sound of the air coming from the tracheostomy tube, especially after the patient takes a deep breath. When respirations are noisy and pulse and respiratory rates are increased, the patient needs to be suctioned. Patients who are conscious can usually indicate when they need to be suctioned. With any sign of respiratory distress, the tube should be suctioned. If mucus is blocking the inner cannula of a silver tube and cannot be removed by suctioning, the inner cannula is removed to open the airway. When the mucus is thick, the inner cannula should be cleaned and replaced at once because the outer tube may also become blocked. If, despite these measures, the patient becomes cyanotic, the physician should be summoned at once. A patient who is able to cough up secretions probably will require suctioning less frequently. The amount of mucus subsides gradually and the patient eventually may go for several hours without being suctioned. However, even when secretions are minimal, the patient is apprehensive and needs constant attendance.

The technique of suctioning needs to be carefully performed to prevent damage to the tracheobronchial mucosa. The purpose of the following section is to provide detailed guidelines about how to suction the tracheostomy tube efficiently and safely.

☐ *Suctioning the tracheostomy tube*

The aim in suctioning is to remove all secretions that have accumulated in the tracheobronchial tree since the last suctioning. In general, suctioning techniques are the same no matter what type of tracheostomy tube is in use.

However, silver tubes have both an inner and outer cannula, whereas plastic tubes have only one cannula. Physicians vary in their preference as to the type of tube used. When a double-lumen tube is used, the inner cannula can readily be removed for suctioning and cleaning, whereas tubes without an inner cannula may have to be completely removed and replaced should they become plugged with secretions. This can usually be prevented, however, by adequate humidification and frequent suctioning. The following guidelines apply to the suctioning of any type of tracheostomy tube:

1. The protective measures discussed under endotracheal suctioning are necessary. To protect the patient, sterile gloves and a sterile catheter are used.
2. The catheter must be of a small enough size that it does not occlude the cannula (one half to two thirds the diameter of the tube). Commonly, when a silver-tube is suctioned, a no. 8 or 10 catheter is used for children, and a no. 14 or 16 for adults.
3. A sterile catheter is used each time the tube is suctioned.
4. Before beginning suctioning, the patient is hyperoxygenated with 100% oxygen. An Ambu bag or anesthesia bag with attached oxygen is held lightly over the face, and the patient is instructed to take five or six deep breaths. Preoxygenation with 100% oxygen is necessary because oxygen will be removed during suctioning. If the PaO_2 falls in a patient with an already reduced PaO_2, cardiac arrhythmias such as ectopic beats and bradycardia may occur.
5. A fenestrated catheter with a whistle tip is attached to the suction machine. If a nonfenestrated catheter is used, it is connected to the suction machine with a Y tube. The catheter is always inserted without suction. Once the catheter is in place, suction is applied by placing the thumb over the fenestration in the catheter or over the open end of the Y tube. (Fig. 24-31)
6. The suction catheter is lubricated with water or a water-soluble lubricant and is inserted deep enough into the bronchus to stimulate coughing. Unless otherwise ordered, the recommended depth through the tracheostomy tube is 20 to 30 cm (8 to 12 in.), since this permits removal of secretions lying beyond the tip of the cannula. If the patient coughs, the catheter is removed because its presence obstructs the trachea and the patient must exert extra pressure to cough around it. As coughing occurs, the nurse or the patient should have tissues ready to receive mucus, which may be ejected with force. When the patient coughs, the tracheostomy tube is held in place, because it could come out with vigorous coughing.
7. If mucus is tenacious and difficult to remove, sterile saline solution may be instilled into the tube just before suctioning; 5 to 15 ml is commonly ordered.
8. Although some clinicians recommend that the patient's head and shoulders be turned to the right when suctioning the left bronchus and vice versa, there is no objective evidence that this technique

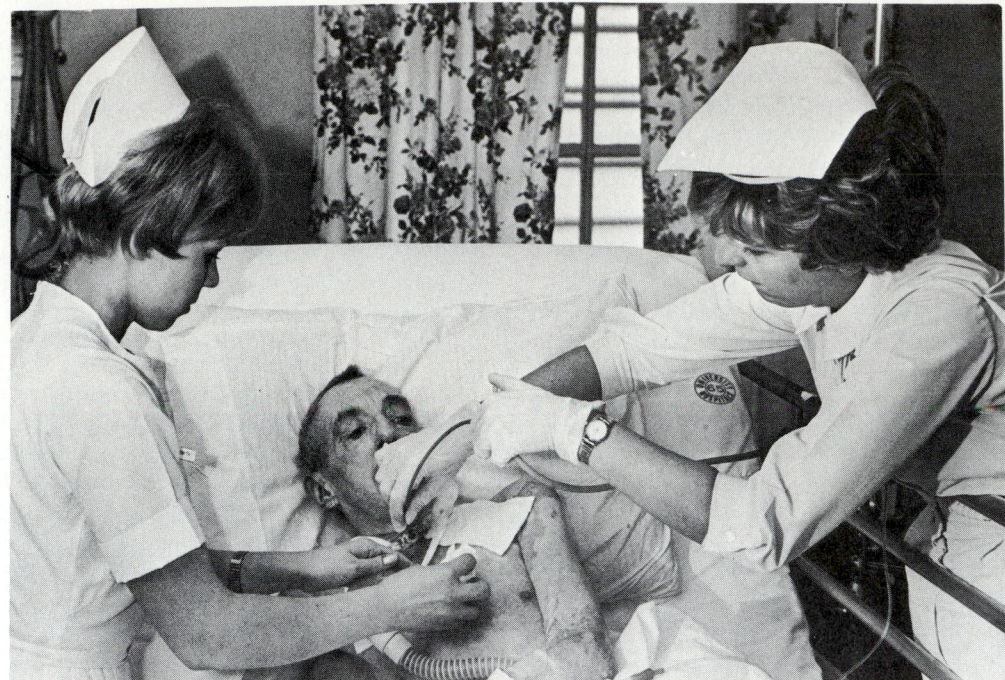

Fig. 24-31 Nurse is wearing sterile gloves and using Y tube attachment to suction patient's tracheostomy tube. (Courtesy Medical World News.)

improves suctioning the desired bronchus. In most patients the right mainstem bronchus is easier to enter anatomically and thus is suctioned more often than the left bronchus. The catheter is rotated as it is withdrawn with suction on.

9. To prevent hypoxia, the patient must *not* be suctioned longer than 10 to 15 seconds at a time, the patient should rest 3 minutes between aspirations, and 100% oxygen should be administered between suctionings. If secretions are interfering with breathing, suctioning may have to be more frequent.

10. The inner cannula of a silver tube is removed for cleaning every 2 to 8 hours, depending on the amount and consistency of secretions. If mucus collects and partially obstructs the lumen, it may be necessary to clean the inner cannula even more often than every 2 hours. Sterile water, detergent solution, pipe cleaners, and a small test-tube brush are used for cleaning. Hot water is not used because it coagulates mucus. The tube may be soaked in a solution of half-strength hydrogen peroxide to soften congealed secretions. The tube is inspected to see that all mucus has been removed. Gauze can be threaded through it to extract excess secretions and solution. Before reinserting the inner tube, the outer tube is suctioned.

☐ *Persons discharged with a tracheostomy*

Persons to be discharged with a tube in place are taught to care for and change the tube while in the hospital (Fig.

24-32). A mirror is necessary to do this procedure, which may be begun a few days after surgery.

Patients who go home with the tracheostomy tube in place must be provided with necessary supplies or with instructions as to where to secure them and with knowledge of how to care for themselves. They should have suction equipment. Suction machines can be rented for home use or obtained in many communities through the local chapter of the American Cancer Society. Suction can be provided by attaching a suction hose to a water faucet. Many hardware stores carry the necessary equipment. The amount of suction is controlled by the stream of water.

Persons who have a permanent tracheostomy must take some special precautions. They must not go swimming and must be careful while bathing or taking a shower that water is not aspirated through the opening into the lungs. They are advised to wear a scarf or a shirt with a closed collar that covers the opening, yet is of porous material. This material substitutes for some functions normally assumed by nasal passages, such as the warming of air and the screening out of dust and other irritating substances.

☐ *Air humidification*

Because the insertion of the endotracheal or tracheostomy tube bypasses the upper airway, the patient's ability to humidify and warm inspired air is lost. Therefore, whether the patient is on or off the repirator, the inspired air should be heated and humidified to prevent mucosal irritation and drying of secretions. *Large-bore* tubing is

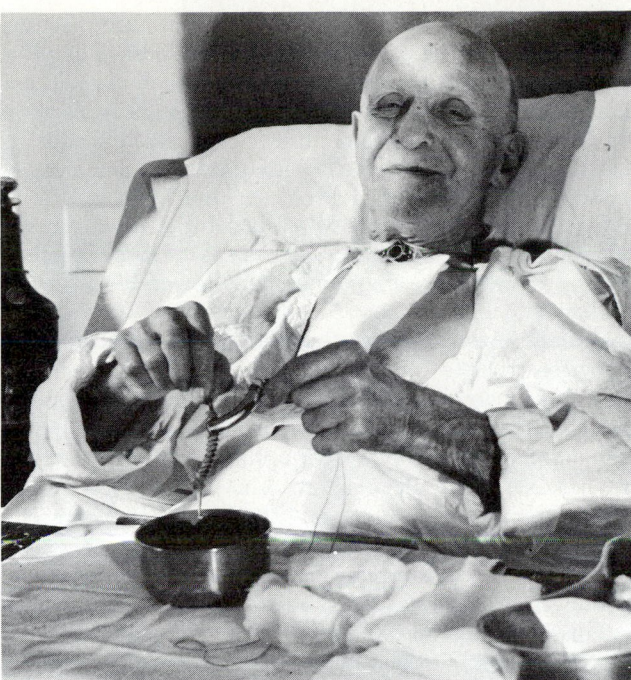

Fig. 24-32   This 82-year-old man cares for his own tracheostomy tube. He is about to clean inner tube with small tube brush. (From Anderson, HC: Newton's geriatric nursing, ed 5, St. Louis, 1971, The CV Mosby Co.)

needed to provide this mist, since water particles condense in *small-bore* tubing. A noticeable difference in the viscosity of secretions is evident in patients who do not receive mist for even as short a period as 30 minutes. Other important nursing care measures and observations vary with the route of intubation—via the larynx or from below the larynx. The patient who has an endotracheal tube in place usually has an increased volume of oropharyngeal secretions because of irritation from the tube. The patient also has great difficulty in swallowing (especially if an oral tube is used), necessitating frequent oropharyngeal suctioning.

□ Nourishment

The patient with an endotracheal tube is allowed nothing by mouth. Nourishment is given intravenously or by nasogastric tube feedings. The patient with a tracheostomy tube in place is usually able to swallow and have a normal oral intake. Some experts prefer that the cuff on the tracheostomy tube be inflated while the patient is eating to prevent aspiration. Others believe that the inflated cuff bulges into the esophagus and makes swallowing more difficult, and therefore, they prefer the cuff to be deflated. Nursing assessment determines which technique to use. In determining if the patient aspirates food, it is often helpful to feed the patient red gelatin. The consistency of gelatin makes it easier to swallow than water, and the red color makes it easy to detect if aspirated into the lower airway.

□ Complications

Both a tracheostomy tube and an endotracheal tube have a direct effect on the airway, but the potential damage of an endotracheal tube is more extensive than that of the tracheostomy tube. Movement with rubbing of the endotracheal tube may produce laryngeal erosion and damage to the vocal cords. There is also the danger of laryngeal edema when the tube is removed. The nurse must be alert to signs of laryngeal stridor and upper airway obstruction. If upper airway obstruction occurs, reintubation or tracheostomy is necessary. With both endotracheal and tracheostomy tubes, tracheal stenosis may result from irritation and scarring at the cuff site. Conscientious nursing care can often prevent this complication.

An additional consideration after the removal of a tracheostomy tube is assisting the patient to cough effectively. When an endotracheal tube is removed, the normal airway is restored and the patient is usually able to cough without difficulty. However, when a tracheostomy tube is removed, there is an air leak at the incision site. This air leak prevents the buildup of intrathoracic pressures high enough to produce an effective cough until the incision is healed. The patient can be taught to place two or three fingers firmly over the dressing that covers the tracheostomy site to reduce the air leak. If this is not successful in helping to generate a cough that clears the airway, the stoma can be suctioned. Frequent use of the stoma for suctioning, however, can delay closure and healing of the tracheostomy incision.

□ Mechanical ventilation

If the patient is unable to maintain ventilation (as indicated by a rising arterial P_{CO_2}), mechanical ventilation is necessary.

Many different kinds of respirators are available. In general, there are two kinds, pressure cycled and volume cycled. The Bird and Bennett (PR series) (Fig. 24-33) are pressure-limited ventilators, whereas the Emerson, Engstrom, Air Shields, Bennett MA-1, Bear, Siemen's Servo, and Ohio 560 are volume-limited machines (Fig. 24-34). Both types of machines can be used intermittently or continuously to assist or to control respiration. Table 24-23 lists the types of ventilators and their mode of function.

When a *pressure-cycled* ventilator is used, the machine is set to deliver a predetermined amount of pressure (usually 15 to 25 cm of water) with each breath. When this pressure is reached, the machine turns off and normal exhalation begins. The volume of gas delivered to the patient is not necessarily constant because it depends on the resistance of the entire system, including the patient's lungs. For this reason the expired tidal volume must be monitored frequently and adjustments made in the ventilator controls as needed.

With a *volume-controlled* machine, a *constant volume* of air is delivered with each breath. The volume is preset and is delivered to the patient at whatever pressure is necessary to attain that volume. A volume-cycled machine should have a pressure cutoff valve. Such a mechanism allows a pressure limit to be set. If the pressure required to deliver

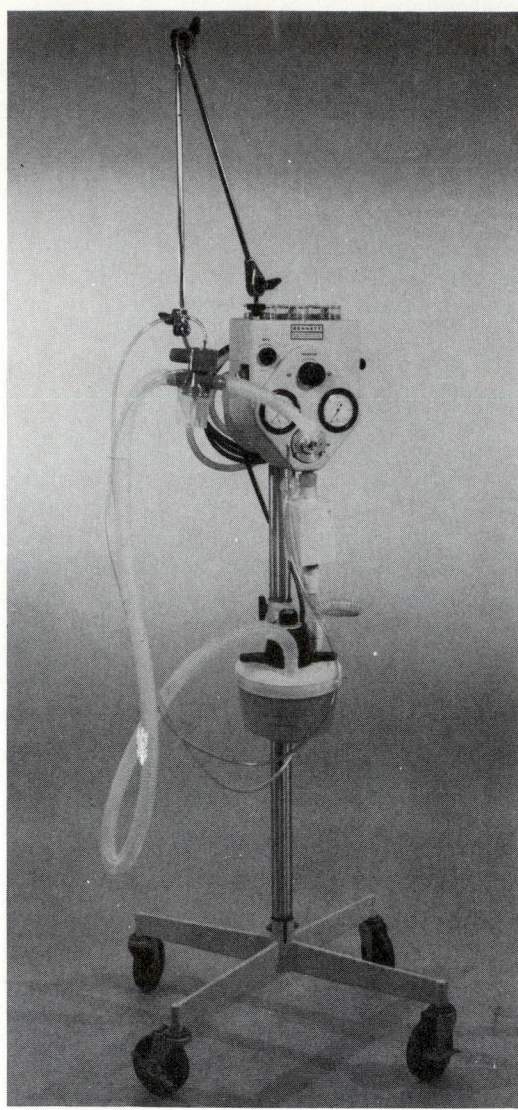

Fig. 24-33 Pressure-cycled ventilator, Bennett, PR-1. (From Abels, LF: Mosby's manual of critical care, St. Louis, 1979, The CV Mosby Co.)

the set volume exceeds the pressure limit, the machine turns off before the entire volume is delivered. The pressure limit on a volume-cycled machine usually has an audible alarm. The nurse can set the limit slightly above (5 cm of water) the pressure required to ventilate the patient. The alarm then goes off if the patient coughs, accumulates secretion, or starts to resist the machine.

Regardless of which type of ventilator is used, mechanisms for various regulations are necessary if the machine is to be adjusted to each patient. It is preferable to have a ventilator that can be used to assist or control the patient's breathing. "Assist" means that the patient's own inspiratory effort triggers (turns on) the machine. Most ventilators have a *sensitivity control knob* that can be adjusted to respond to weak inspiratory efforts. "Control" implies the use of automatic cycling. The patient may be apneic and the machine set at the desired rate; the patient's own respiratory rate may be too slow, and the automatic cycling can be used to force an increase in the rate; or the patient's own respiratory efforts can be ignored and an automatic rate used to ventilate the patient. (Some machines with automatic cycling do not allow for the latter adjustment.) It is also helpful to be able to regulate the flow rates at which the gas is delivered to the patient. For example, patients breathing at rapid rates and high volumes need faster flow rates than those breathing slowly and at moderate volumes. A final necessity is the ability to regulate the inspired concentration of oxygen from 20% (room air) to 100%.

All ventilators used for mechanical ventilation must do the following:
1. Provide for the heating and humidification of inspired air
2. Provide a means for measurement of expired volumes
3. Be dependable for long periods of use
4. Be easily cleaned

Any patient on continuous mechanical ventilation should be "sighed" (given a deep breath) several times an hour. Some ventilators automatically "sigh" the patient, whereas with others the patient is "sighed" manually using a self-inflating (Ambu) or anesthesia bag. This periodic deep breathing is necessary to prevent alveolar collapse and resultant atelactasis.

Table 24-23 Types of mechanical ventilators

Types	Basic function mode
Positive-pressure ventilator (requires intubation)	Types are based on how inspiratory phase is ended.
Pressure-cycled ventilator	Inspiration ends at a preset pressure limit; time and volume are variable.
Time-cycled ventilator	Inspiration is present for a given time interval; volume and pressure are variable.
Volume-cycled ventilator	Delivers a preset volume of air; time and pressure variable. However, these often have pressure-cycled and time-cycled capacities.
Negative-pressure ventilator (intubation not required)	Encapsulates, at least, the thorax. When ventilator expands, it creates negative pressure by pulling the thorax outward. Air rushes into the airways because of the pressure gradient created.
High-frequency ventilation (requires intubation)	Still under clinical investigation. There are several variants of this system. All use high respiratory rates to deliver small tidal volumes at low pressures.

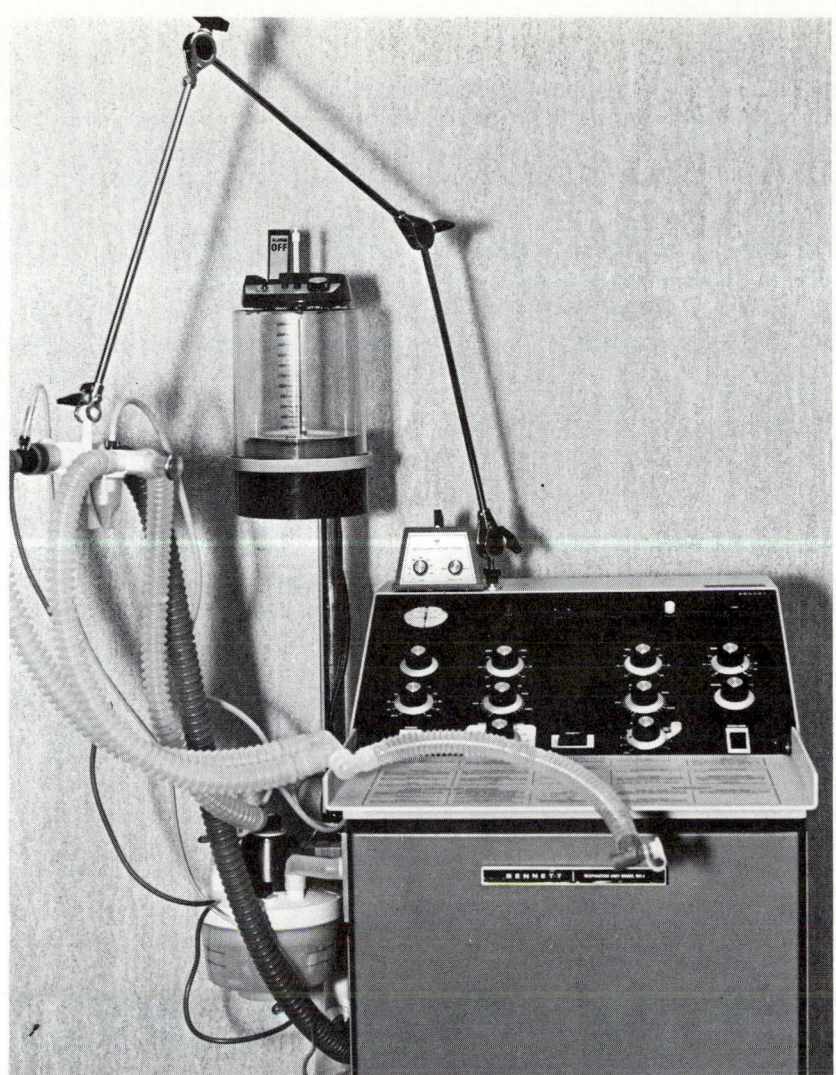

Fig. 24-34   Volume cycled ventilator, Bennett, MA-1. (From Abels, LF: Mosby's manual of critical care, St. Louis, 1979, The CV Mosby Co.)

□ *Positive-end expiratory pressure*

Positive end-expiratory pressure (PEEP) is ventilator mode that has been shown to increase the effectiveness of mechanical ventilation in certain patients. PEEP involves the maintenance of positive pressure, at the end of expiration, rather than allowing airway pressure to return to normal (atmospheric) as usually occurs. By maintaining positive pressure, alveoli that would otherwise collapse on expiration are held open, thus increasing the opportunity for gas exchange across the alveolar-capillary membrane. This is accomplished by the increase in functional residual capacity. The result is a decrease in physiologic shunting and the ability to achieve a higher level of PaO_2 with lower concentrations of delivered oxygen (FIO_2). PEEP has its greatest use in the treatment of ARDS, but is also used in treating any patient who would otherwise require unacceptably high concentrations of oxygen.

The hazards of PEEP are related to the increase in intrathoracic pressure. Most serious of the dangers related to this technique is the increased incidence of pneumothorax, particularly in those with friable lung tissue, as seen in persons with emphysema or lung cancer. The sudden disappearance of breath sounds on one side, in conjunction with signs of respiratory distress, in the patient being ventilated with PEEP *must be taken as an indication of a pneumothorax.* This can develop into a life-threatening episode if the pneumothorax is large, and the physician must be called immediately. Another less serious consequence of PEEP may be a reduction in venous return, which is impeded by the increased intrathoracic pressure, and a subsequent fall in cardiac output. This effect seems to be particularly common in patients who are relatively dehydrated and can sometimes be avoided by careful fluid administration.

NURSING CARE PLAN

Person on mechanical ventilation with PEEP

DATA: Mr. Rhodes is a 28-year-old married male admitted to the surgical intensive care unit after a motor vehicle accident. Injuries sustained included a ruptured spleen and liver laceration resulting in hypovolemic shock. Mr. Rhodes was taken to the operating room, where his injuries were repaired and blood losses were replaced. His early postoperative course was unremarkable. On Mr. Rhodes's third postoperative day, he began to experience some respiratory difficulties with a deterioration in his arterial blood gases. Because of severe hypoxemia, Mr. Rhodes was intubated. Chest x-ray examination revealed diffuse interstitial and alveolar infiltrates. Mr. Rhodes had developed ARDS and eventually required 16 cm H_2O of PEEP.

Mrs. Rhodes visited her husband daily and often attempted to communicate with him. She would reassure and calm him when he got anxious and resisted the ventilator. Mrs. Rhodes would ask the nurse many questions about her husband's status.

The nursing history identified the following:
1. Mr. and Mrs. Rhodes have been married 5 years; they have no children.
2. Mr. Rhodes has full hospitalization and medical coverage through insurance at work.
3. Mr. and Mrs. Rhodes come from large families that appear supportive.
4. Mr. Rhodes is a nonsmoker.

Collaborative nursing actions include those to assist in improving oxygenation through evaluating F_1O_2 and levels of PEEP as well as techniques used to wean Mr. Rhodes from the ventilator.

Nursing actions include:
1. Supporting oxygenation and ventilation to maintain Pao_2 over 60 torr and to maximize functional residual capacity
2. Weaning from F_1O_2 and levels of PEEP gradually, while monitoring arterial blood gases
3. Monitoring patient for signs of hypoxia

Nursing diagnosis: Impaired gas exchange: due to ARDS

Expected patient outcomes	Nursing interventions	Rationale
Patient will remain adequately oxygenated as evidenced by: 1. Pao_2 on blood gas > 75 mm Hg 2. Adequate color 3. Adequate peripheral circulation	Monitor arterial blood gases to determine Pao_2 Suction Mr. Rhodes only when necessary to prevent loss of PEEP secondary to disconnection from ventilator Monitor required levels of PEEP and F_1O_2 Assess peripheral circulation for pulses, color of extremities, and warmth Monitor mixed venous blood oxygen levels	ARDS is an acute lung injury that results in increased capillary permeability that permits proteins and fluids to leak out into alveoli and interstitial spaces, thus preventing normal gas exchange from occurring

Care Plan by Maria Takacs, MSN, RN.

☐ *Weaning from the ventilator*

The nurse plays an important role in weaning the patient from the ventilator. Both physiologic studies (blood gases, tidal volume) and clinical status determine the patient's readiness to breathe without mechanical assistance. Before weaning, the patient should have been taught breathing exercises. When the patient is taken off the ventilator, a nurse in whom the patient has confidence should be present. It is also helpful if the environment around the patient is calm. Much of the success of weaning is dependent on the interrelationship between the patient's physiologic and psychologic responses. If the patient becomes very anxious

NURSING CARE PLAN

Person on mechanical ventilation with PEEP—cont'd

Nursing diagnosis: Potential complications: related to use of PEEP

Expected patient outcomes	Nursing interventions	Rationale
Patient will not experience hemodynamic compromise related to PEEP	Monitor vital signs q1h and prn Monitor hemodynamic parameters for signs of decreased cardiac output, hypotension, elevated CVP, and oliguria Monitor intake and output Check peripheral circulation q 2 to 4 h and prn Elevate foot of bed 10 to 20 degrees to encourage venous return Perform passive range of motion exercises q 4 to 6 h to encourage venous return Administer adrenergic agents as ordered to improve cardiac output Notify physician of hemodynamic complications	PEEP may cause decreased cardiac output by increasing intraalveolar pressures, thereby decreasing venous return to the heart

Patient will not experience the following pulmonary complications secondary to PEEP:
1. Atelectasis
2. Pneumothorax
3. Pneumomediastinum
4. Subcutaneous emphysema
	Monitor respirations q1h and prn
	Assess breath sounds for adventitious findings
	Administer pulmonary toilet q2h and prn
	  a. Frequent turning
	  b. Chest physiotherapy
	Monitor for signs of pulmonary complications and respiratory distress:
	  a. Asymetric chest excursion
	  b. Sudden sharp chest pain
	  c. Cyanosis
	  d. Anxiety
	Assess for subcutaneous emphysema
	Keep chest tube setup at bedside
	Monitor arterial blood gases as needed
	Notify physician of respiratory complications
		When walls of alveoli cannot withstand the positive pressure from PEEP, perforation may occur; as a result, air leaks into the pleural space, mediastinum, or its subcutaneous space; result is a pneumothorax, pneumomediastinum, or subcutaneous emphysema, respectively

NURSING CARE PLAN

Person on mechanical ventilation with PEEP—cont'd

Nursing diagnosis: Altered nutrition: less than body requirements related to intubation

Expected patient outcomes	Nursing interventions	Rationale
Patient will receive adequate nutritional intake while intubated	Administer hyperalimentation or arterial feedings as prescribed Measure and record intake and output Record daily weights Administer albumin or volume expanders as prescribed Monitor serum albumin level	Nutritional status must be maintained to assist in weaning process; proteins and volume expanders increase serum colloidal osmotic pressure, thus maintaining fluid in the intravascular compartment

Nursing diagnosis: Anxiety: related to ARDS, intubation, and discomfort from PEEP

Expected patient outcomes	Nursing interventions	Rationale
Mr. and Mrs. Rhodes will exhibit behavioral signs of decreased stress and anxiety	Assess for signs of anxiety Explain ARDS to family, including rationale for mechanical ventilation and PEEP Allow Mr. and Mrs. Rhodes to express concern and fears Explain procedures to Mr. and Mrs. Rhodes before performing them Provide comfort measures Provide for a means of communication between Mr. Rhodes and his wife Attempt to anticipate their needs Administer light sedation/antianxiety medications if necessary, as ordered	ICU, mechanical ventilation, inability to communicate, and fear of the unknown all contribute to feelings of stress and anxiety for the patient in the ICU, as well as significant others
	Attempt to calm and reassure Mr. Rhodes if he begins to "buck" or resist the ventilator Provide Mr. Rhodes and his wife distraction from the ICU environment: soft music and TV for Mr. Rhodes; breaks from the ICU for Mrs. Rhodes	Positive pressure exhalation is often uncomfortable for the patient who frequently responds by resisting ventilator

and takes rapid, shallow breaths, being off the respirator will be poorly tolerated. If a pattern of controlled breathing can be maintained, success is more likely. Weaning is usually begun with short periods off the ventilator. The amount of time off the ventilator is increased according to the patient's tolerance. The nurse must carefully assess the adequacy of the patient's ventilation during the time off the ventilator. If, in the nurse's judgment, the patient cannot tolerate breathing on his or her own because of inadequate tidal volume, cyanosis, tachycardia, diaphoresis, or restlessness, mechanical ventilation should be reinstituted.

A more recent technique of weaning is the use of *intermittent mandatory ventilation* (IMV). This involves the addition of an oxygen reservoir with a one-way valve to the respirator circuit. The rate on the ventilator is reduced below the patient's normal rate. The ventilator then delivers the set minimum, and the patient spontaneously breathes several breaths in addition to that from the oxygen reservoir. For example, if the patient's natural respiratory rate is 16, the ventilator might be set to deliver 10 breaths per minute. The patient then takes an additional six breaths independently. In this way, the patient can gradually build up strength and gain respiratory independence without having to be taken completely off the ventilator.

Throughout the treatment of the patient in respiratory failure, ventilation should be carefully monitored by blood gas studies and simple spirometry (tidal volume, vital capacity). Alert nursing observation of the patient can determine the adequacy of ventilation. Meticulous attention is given to maintaining a patent airway, which is the prime nursing responsibility. (See specialized texts for further detail.[46,83,85,117])

☐ Rest

The patient who is subjected to many treatments can become excessively fatigued, further compromising ventilatory capacity. Frequent rest periods must be interspersed with treatments, and it is the nurse's responsibility to see that the patient has a quiet environment and is not disturbed by unnecessary interruptions at rest times. Unfortunately, persons who have severe insufficiency must have frequent treatments and interventions; it is *not* appropriate, although the person may be quite tired, to allow the patient to sleep through the night and to omit treatments. This inevitably leads to a worsened status.

Although persons with respiratory insufficiency are often anxious and frightened, sedation is contraindicated because it depresses respirations. Therefore, it is especially important the nurse be supportive of the patient and be skillful in assisting the patient to breathe effectively. The patient can be extremely demanding, and the nurse must understand the fear and anxiety that is often the basis for the patient's behavior.

☐ Monitoring

Aggressive, constant nursing care is essential for these patients. The nurse must be continually alert to clinical changes that represent changes in the patient's ventilation. Increasing confusion and behavioral changes often indicate an elevated $PaCO_2$. The behavioral changes may range from pugnacious, combative behavior to lethargy. Other clinical signs of *hypercapnia* are flushed skin color caused by reflex vasodilation, muscle twitching, and headache. Signs commonly seen in *hypoxia* include tachycardia, increased pulse rate, cyanosis, changes in blood pressure, and changes in behavior. In *early* stages of hypoxia, the blood pressure is elevated as a result of vasoconstriction and increased peripheral resistance. In *later* stages, the blood pressure falls to hypotensive levels and circulatory arrest can occur. It is important to point out that cyanosis is not an early sign of hypoxia, since it does not occur until arterial oxygen saturation is less than 85%; thus the nurse needs to be alert to the earlier signs of hypoxia mentioned previously.

■ SUMMARY

1. In restrictive lung disease, there is a restriction in lung volume and a reduction in lung compliance. In obstructive lung disease, there is an increase in airway resistance resulting in prolonged exhalation.
2. Acute bronchitis, pneumonia, tuberculosis, fungal infections, occupational-related lung diseases, adult respiratory distress syndrome, and cancer of the lung are examples of restrictive lung diseases.
3. Chronic obstructive lung disease refers to diseases that produce obstruction of airflow and includes asthma, chronic bronchitis, and pulmonary emphysema.
4. Primary prevention of respiratory infections includes prevention of the spread of infection by teaching the infected person to cover nose and mouth when coughing or sneezing so that *droplet nuclei* are not released into the air.
5. Histoplasmosis, coccidiodiomycosis, and blastomycosis are three major fungal infections of the lungs. Amphotericin B is the standard therapy for mycotic infection.
6. Adult respiratory distress syndrome is often fatal and is characterized by severe dyspnea, hypoxemia, and diffuse bilateral pulmonary infiltrations following lung injury in previously healthy persons.
7. The cause of cancer of the lung is closely related to cigarette smoking. From available research data, it seems evident that curtailing smoking is a primary preventive measure.
8. Efforts to detect malignant lesions of the lungs early, while curative treatment may be possible, are critical. The nurse should encourage all persons over the age of 40 to have an x-ray examination of the chest periodically in addition to a yearly physical examination.
9. Postoperative care of the patient after thoracic surgery centers on promoting ventilation and reexpansion of the lung by maintaining a clear airway; promoting comfort by pain relief; promoting reexpansion of the lung by proper maintenance of the water-seal drainage sytem; promoting nutrition; and monitoring the incision for bleeding and subcutaneous emphysema.
10. If an open sucking wound of the chest has been sustained, the wound should be covered immediately to prevent air from entering the pleural cavity and causing a pneumothorax.
11. Persons with chronic bronchitis are sometimes referred to as "blue bloaters." Persons with pulmonary emphysema are sometimes referred to as "pink puffers."
12. Hyperventilation is shown by an elevated $PaCO_2$ on arterial blood gas. Hypoventilation is indicated by a decrease in $PaCO_2$ below normal levels.
13. To facilitate breathing, the nurse teaches the person with COPD abdominal breathing, leg-raising exercises, inhalation-exhalation exercises, and muscle reconditioning.
14. The best time for postural drainage and percussion is generally in the morning soon after arising and at night before retiring.

Putting knowledge to practice

■ What is the quality of air in the community in which you reside? If air pollution is a problem, what are the major contributing factors (industries, automobile exhaust, and so on)? Are there community groups working to improve the problem? If so, what activities are they involved in and how might a nurse be helpful to their efforts?

■ Where is the branch of the American Cancer Society and the American Lung Association nearest your community? What services do they provide for health professionals and for patients?

■ What is the tuberculosis case rate in the area in which you live? Is this higher or lower than the national rate of 11/100,000 population? List the factors that contribute to a higher or lower case rate in your community.

■ List the services available in your community to assist persons who wish to stop smoking and to which you could refer patients or friends.

■ Design a teaching plan or project that you believe would help convince teenagers they should not smoke. Would you use a different approach for females than for males?

■ Plan a 3,000-calorie, high-protein diet for a 60-year-old man with pulmonary emphysema who is very short of breath and finds eating to be a chore.

---

15. Asthma results in intermittent rather than continuous airway obstruction.
16. Respiratory failure is said to occur when ventilation is not sufficient to achieve gas exchange even at rest.

REFERENCES AND SELECTED READINGS
Contemporary

1. *Ahrens, TS, and Rutherford, KA: The new pulmonary math, applying the a/A ratio, Am J Nurs 87(3):337-339, 1987.
2. Alford, RH: Histoplasmosis. In Conn, HF: Current therapy: 1982, Philadelphia, 1982, WB Saunders Co.
3. American Academy of Pediatrics: Report of the Committee on Infectious Diseases, ed 20, Evanston, Ill., 1986, The Academy.
4. American Cancer Society: Cancer facts and figures, New York, 1987, The Society.
5. *American Lung Association: Chronic obstructive pulmonary disease, New York, 1981, The Association.
6. American Lung Association: Diagnostic standards and classification of tuberculosis, New York, 1981, The Association.
7. American Lung Association: Facts in brief about lung disease, New York, 1983, The Association.
8. Bartlett, JG, and Garbach, SL: The triple threat of aspiration pneumonia, Chest 68:550-556, 1980.
9. *Burns, MR: Cruising with COPD, Am J Nurs 87:479-482, 1987.
10. *Callahan, M: COPD makes a bad first impression, but you'll find wonderful people underneath, Nurs 82 12:67-72, 1982.
11. *Cameron, TJ: Fiberoptic bronchoscopy, Am J Nurs 81:1462-1465, 1981.
12. *Carroll, PL: Cyanosis: the sign you can count on, Nurs 88 18(3):50, 1988.
12a. *Carroll, PL: Lowering the risks of endotracheal suctioning, Nurs 88 18(5):46-50, 1988.
13. Catterall, JR, Potasman, MD, and Remington, JS: *Pneumocystis carinii*: Pneumonia in the patient with AIDS, Chest 88:758-762, 1985.
14. Center for Disease Control: Annual summary 1983: reported morbidity and mortality in the United States, 32:54, 1983.
15. *Cohen, S: Pulmonary function tests in patient care: programmed instruction, Am J Nurs 80:1135-1161, 1980.
16. *D'Agostino, JS: Teaching tips for living with COPD at home, Nurs 84 14:57, 1984.
17. *D'Agostino, JS: You can breathe new life into your COPD patients, Nurs 83 13:72 and 74-77, 1983.
18. Daly, B: Intensive care nursing, ed 2, New York, 1985, Medical Examination Publishing Co.
19. DeVito, AJ: Rehabilitation of patients with chronic obstructive pulmonary disease, Rehab Nurs 10:12-15, 1985.
20. *Duncan, C, and Erichson, R: Pressures associated with chest tube stripping, Heart Lung 11:166-171, 1982.
21. Ebersole, P, and Hess, P: Toward healthy aging, ed 2, St. Louis, 1985, The CV Mosby Co.
22. *Einstein, HE: Coccidioidomycosis, Basics RD 9:1-6, 1980.
23. *Engelking, C: CE lung cancer therapy, Am J Nurs 87:1438-1439, 1987.
24. *Engelking, C: Teaching, counseling, and caring, Am J Nurs 87:1439-1440, 1987.
25. *Engelking, C: CE lung cancer: the language of staging, Am J Nurs 87:1434-1437, 1987.
26. Erickson, R: To cough or not to cough, Nurs 82 12:124-126, 1982.
27. Forouzesh, M, Price, JH, and Taylor, C: Pulmonary disease, Nurs Care 15:19-22, 1982.
28. *Frame, PT: Acute infectious pneumonia in the adult, Basics RD 10:3, 1982.
29. *Fuchs, PL: ARDS: physiology, signs, and symptoms, Nurs 83 13:52-53, 1983.

*References preceded by an asterisk are particularly well suited for student reading.

30. *Fuchs, PL: Asthma, signs, and symptoms, Nurs 83 13:36-37, 1983.

31. *Fuchs, PL: Before and after surgery: stay right on respiratory care, Nurs 83 13:47-50, 1983.

32. Gong, H: Evaluation and management of patients with cough, sputum, or hemoptysis. In Selecky, P, editor: Pulmonary disease, New York, 1982, John Wiley & Sons, Inc.

33. *Greenwood, BS: The before and after of good postop pulmonary care, Nurs 82 12:68-69, 1982.

34. Hanson, EI: Effects of chronic lung disease on life in general and on sexuality: perception of adult patients, Heart Lung 11:435-441, 1982.

34a. *Haylock, PJ: Radiation therapy, Am J Nurs 87:1441-1446, 1987.

35. Hodgkin, JE, and Petty, TL: Chronic obstructive pulmonary disease: current concepts, Philadelphia, 1987, WB Saunders Co.

36. Hudgel, DM, and Madsen, LA: Acute and chronic asthma: a guide to intervention, Am J Nurs 80:1791-1795, 1980.

36a. *Hoffman, LA: Airway management for the critically ill patient, Am J Nurs 87 17(1):39-43, 1987.

36b. *Hoffman, LA, and Maskiewicz, RC: The specifics of suctioning, Am J Nurs 87 17(1):44-53, 1987.

37. *Hughes, JM: Postoperative pulmonary care: past, present, and future, Crit Care Q 6:67, 1983.

38. *Hunter, PM: Bedside monitoring of respiratory function, Nurs Clin North Am 16:211-224, 1981.

39. Kamholz, SL, and Pinksker, KL: Bacterial pneumonia. In Conn, HF: Current therapy: 1982, Philadelphia, 1982, WB Saunders Co.

40. *Kirilloff, LH, and Tibbals, SC: Drugs for asthma: a complete guide, Am J Nurs 83:56-61, 1983.

41. *Kirkis, EJ: Infection consult: common error can cause pneumonia, RN 45:97-98, 1982.

42. Kravetz, HM: Coccidioidomycosis. In Conn, HF: Current therapy 1982, Philadelphia, 1982, WB Saunders Co.

43. Kryger, M, editor: pathophysiology of respiration, New York, 1981, John Wiley & Sons, Inc.

44. LaCamera, DJ, Masur, H, and Henderson, DK: The acquired immunodeficiency syndrome, Nurs Clin North Am 20:241-256, 1985.

45. *Landis, K, and Smith, S: The mechanically ventilated patient: a comprehensive nursing care plan, Crit Care Q 6:43, 1983.

46. Langston, HT, and Barker, WS: The adult thoracic surgical patient. In Neville, WE, editor: Intensive care of the surgical cardiopulmonary patient, ed 2, Chicago, 1983, Year Book Medical Publishers, Inc.

47. Leininger, BJ: Thoracic trauma, In Neville, WE: Intensive care of the surgical cardiopulmonary patient, ed 2, Chicago, 1983, Year Book Medical Publishers, Inc.

48. Mapp, CS: Trach care—are you aware of the dangers? Nurs 88 18(7):34-42, 1988.

49. McCauley, K, and Weaver, TE: Cardiac and pulmonary diseases: nutritional implications, Nurs Clin North Am 18:81-96, 1983.

50. *McNaull, FH: CE lung cancer: tobacconism in America, Am J Nurs 87:1430-1432, 1987.

50a. *McNaull, FW: CE lung cancer: What are the odds? Am J Nurs 87:1428-1429, 1987.

51. Miller, WC: Chronic bronchitis, bronchiectasis, and emphysema. In Conn, HF: Current therapy: 1982, Philadelphia, 1982, WB Saunders Co.

52. Mizuki, J.: There's no place like home, Am J Nurs 84:647, 1984.

53. Mountain, CF: Primary lung cancer. In Conn, HF: Current therapy: 1982, Philadelphia, 1982, WB Saunders Co.

54. Nielsen, L: Mechanical ventilation: patient assessment and nursing care, Am J Nurs 80:2191-2217, 1980.

55. Nursing Grand Rounds: Adult respiratory distress syndromes: a true test of nursing skills, Nurs 80 10:51-56, 1980.

56. Nursing Grand Rounds: Fighting the frustrations of status asthmaticus, Nurs 82 12:58-63, 1982.

57. *Nursing Grand Rounds: Teaming up to send the end-stage COPD patient home, Nurs 84 14:65-68, 1984.

58. Oermann, M, and others: Patient sensations following a tracheostomy: a discussion, Crit Care Q 6:53, 1983.

59. Ostrow, D: Symptoms and signs. In Kryger, M, editor: Pathophysiology of respiration, New York, 1981, John Wiley & Sons, Inc.

59a. *Openbrier, DR, Hoffman, LA, and Weismiller, SA: Home oxygen evaluation, Am J Nurs 88(2):192-197, 1988.

59b. *Openbrier, DR, Fuoss, C, and Mall, CC: What patients on home oxygen therapy want to know, Am J Nurs 88(2):198-202, 1988.

60. Pare, JA, and Fraser, RG: Synopsis of diseases of the chest, Philadelphia, 1983, WB Saunders Co.

61. Penn, RL: Blastomycosis. In Conn, HF: Current therapy: 1982, Philadelphia, 1982, WB Saunders Co.

62. Pennoyer, D, and Sheffer, AL: Asthma in adults. In Conn, HF: Current therapy: 1982, Philadelphia, 1982, WB Saunders Co.

63. Perdue, P: Urgent priorities in severe trauma: life-threatening respiratory injuries, RN 44:27-33, 1981.

64. *Petersen, GM: Application of oxygen therapy devices, Nurs Clin North Am 16:241-257, 1981.

65. Petty, TL: Adult respiratory distress syndrome. In Kryger, MH, editor: Pathology of respiration, New York, 1981, John Wiley & Sons, Inc.

66. Pfister, S: Respiratory arrest: are you prepared? Nurs 82 12:34-41, 1982.

67. *Rhodes, MK: Recognizing and caring for the patient with Legionnaire's disease, Nurs 80 10:104E, 1980.

68. *Rhodes, M: Update on chest trauma, Crit Care Q 6:59, 1983.

69. Rifas, EM: How you and your patient can manage dyspnea, Nurs 80 10:34-41, 1980.

70. Rifas, EM: Teaching patients to manage acute asthma: the future is now, Nurs 83 13:77-80, 1983.

71. *Risser, NL: Preoperative and postoperative care to prevent pulmonary complications, Heart Lung 9:57-67, 1980.

72. *Rokosky, JS: Assessment of the individual with altered respiratory function, Nurs Clin North Am 16:195-209, 1981.

73. Selecky, PA: Pulmonary disease, New York, 1982, John Wiley & Sons, Inc.

74. Shapiro, BA, Harrison, RA, and Trout, CA: Clinical application of respiratory care, ed 3, Bowie, Md, 1985, The Charles Press.

75. *Sjoberg, EL: Nursing diagnoses and the COPD patient, Am J Nurs 83:245-248, 1983.

76. Slonim, NB, and Hamilton, LH: Respiratory physiology, ed 5, St. Louis, 1987, The CV Mosby Co.

77. *Stevens, SA, and Becher, KL: Respiratory assessment, Nurs 88 18(1):57-63, 1988.

78. Straus, MJ: Lung cancer: clinical diagnosis and treatment, ed 2, New York, 1983, Grune & Stratton, Inc.

79. *Summer, SM, and Lewandowski, V: Guidelines for using artificial breathing devices, Nurs 83 13;54-57, 1983.

80. Symposium on respiratory care, Nurs Clin North Am 16:193-297, 1981.

81. Tellis, CJ: Clinical presentations of chronic obstructive pulmonary disease. Primary Care 12:227-237, 1985.

82. Thomson, PS, and Willis, JC: Compliance challenges in a black lung clinic, Nurs Clin North Am 17:513-521, 1982.

83. Traver, GA: Respiratory nursing: the science and the art, New York, 1982, John Wiley & Sons, Inc.

84. US Department of Health and Human Services/Public Health Service, Center for Disease Control: MMWR 31:10, 1982.

85. Wade, J: Comprehensive respiratory care; physiology and technique, ed 3, St. Louis, 1982, The CV Mosby Co.

86. *Weg, JG: Tuberculosis and other mycobacterial disease. In Conn, HF: Current therapy: 1982, Philadelphia, 1982, WB Saunders Co.

87. West, JB: Ventilation/blood flow and gas exchange, ed 3, Oxford, England, 1980, Blackwell Scientific Publications.

88. Woodin, LM: Your patient with pneumothorax: a patient in distress, Nurs 82 12:50-56, 1982.

89. Worthington, L: Hypoxemia: why giving oxygen isn't enough, RN 43:49-53, 1980.

90. Wyngaarden, J, and Smith, L: Cecil textbook of medicine, ed 17, Philadelphia, 1985, WB Saunders Co.

91. Youmans, GP, Patterson, PY, and Sommers, HM: The biologic and clinical basis of infectious diseases, ed 3, Philadelphia, 1986, WB Saunders Co.

Classic

92. Agle, DP, and Baum, GL: Psychological aspects of chronic obstructive pulmonary disease, Med Clin North Am 61:749-758, 1977.

93. American College of Chest Physicians: A report of the Committee on Emphysema: recommendations for continuous oxygen therapy in chronic obstructive lung disease, Chest 64:505-507, 1973.

94. *American Lung Association: Occupational lung disease: an introduction, New York, 1979, The Association.

95. American Thoracic Society: Treatment of myobacterial disease. Am Rev Respir Dis 115:185-187, 1977.

96. Brenner, DJ: Classification of the legionnaires' disease bacterium: an interim report, Curr Microbiol 1:71-75, 1978.

97. Carr, DT, and Rosenow, EC: Bronchogenic carcinoma, Basics RD 5:1-6, 1977.

98. *Cimprich, B, Gaydos, D, and Langan, R: A preoperative teaching program for the thoracotomy patient, Calif Nurs 1:35-39, 1978.

99. Comroe, JH: Physiology of respiration, ed 2, Chicago, 1974, Year Book Medical Publishers, Inc.

100. Eickhoff, TC: The current status of BCG immunization against tuberculosis, Ann Rev Med 28:411 and 423, 1979.

101. Fromm, C: Using basic laboratory data to evaluate patients with acute respiratory failure, Crit Care Q 1:43-52, 1979.

102. *Hanson, RR, and Kasik, JE: The pneumoconioses, Heart Lung 6:645-652, 1977.

103. *Hodgkin, JE: Chronic obstructive pulmonary disease, Park Ridge, Ill, 1979, American College of Chest Physicians.

104. Humidifiers: tips given on trimming infection hazards, Hosp Infect Control 8:24-26, 1979.

105. *Hunt, WJ, and Bespalec, DA: An evaluation of current methods of modifying smoking behavior, J Clin Psychol 30:431-438, 1974.

106. *Jacquette, G: To reduce hazards of tracheal suctioning, Am J Nurs 71:2362-2364, 1971.

107. Jones, RW, and Weill, H: Occupational lung disease, Basics RD 6:1-6, 1978.

108. Karetzky, MS, and Khan, AU: Review of current concepts in aspiration pneumonia, Heart Lung 6:321-326, 1977.

109. Keys, JL: Blood gas analysis and the assessment of acid-base status, Heart Lung 5:247-255, 1976.

110. *Koss, JA, and Cristoph, C: Oxygen therapy and other respiratory therapy in acute respiratory failure, Crit Care Q 1:53-63, 1979.

111. Levine, DP, and Lerner, M: The clinical spectrum of Mycoplasma pneumoniae infections, Med Clin North Am 62:961-978, 1978.

112. *Lynn, LJ: Psychosocial needs of patients with acute respiratory failure, Crit Care Q 1:65-74, 1979.

113. *Martini, N: Lung cancer—an overview, Calif Nurs 1:31-33, 1978.

114. Moorthy, SS, LoSasso, AM, and Gibbs, PS: Respiratory failure in patients following surgery and trauma, Crit Care Q 1:15-25, 1979.

115. *Nett, L, and Petty, TL: Oxygen toxicity, Am J Nurs 73:1556-1558, 1973.

116. *Petty, TL: A chest physician's perspective on asthma, Heart Lung 1:611-620, 1972.

117. *Phipps, WJ, Barker, WL, and Daly, BJ: Respiratory insufficiency and failure. In Meltzer, LE, Abdella, RG, and Kitchell, JF: Concepts and practices of intensive care for nurses specialists, ed 2, Bowie, Md, 1976, The Charles Press.

118. Rogers, BH, and others: Opportunistic pneumonia: a clinicopathological study of five cases caused by an unidentified acid-fast bacterium, N Engl J Med 301:959-961.

119. Stevens, PM: Positive and expiratory pressure breathing, Basics RD 5:1-6, 1977.

120. *Stewart, E: To lesson pain: relaxation and rhythmic breathing, Am J Nurs 76:958-959, 1976.

121. US Center for Disease Control—Tuberculosis branch: Tuberculosis statistics: cities and states—1976, Atlanta, 1977, The Center.

122. *Wagner, MM: Assessment of patients with multiple injuries, Am J Nurs 72:1822-1827, 1972.

123. Ziskind, MM: The acute bacterial pneumonias in the adult. In American Thoracic Society: Basics of RD, New York, 1974, The Society.

25

The Patient with Cardiovascular Problems

MARY A. (SANDY) WYPER and EILEEN WALSH

CHAPTER OBJECTIVES

After studying this chapter, the student should be able to:

- Differentiate between data obtained from a 12-lead ECG and data obtained from a cardiac monitor.

- Explain the differences between arrhythmias that are a disturbance of impulse initiation and those of impulse conduction, and identify life-threatening arrhythmias.

- Describe treatment modalities for cardiac arrhythmias.

- Identify risk factors for CAD.

- Explain the pathophysiologic basis, therapeutic modalities, and nursing interventions for angina pectoris and myocardial infarction, and congestive heart failure.

- Identify teaching needs of patients with angina, myocardial infarction, and congestive heart failure, and patients undergoing cardiac surgery.

- Describe the pathophysiologic bases for pulmonary edema and cardiogenic shock; relate the therapeutic modalities for these conditions to those for congestive heart failure.

- Explain the pathophysiologic bases for disorders of the various layers of cardiac tissue (pericardium, myocardium, epicardium), the cardiac valves, and the aorta.

- Describe surgical intervention for repair of cardiac valves and aortic aneurysms and the pre/postoperative nursing care required.

Heart disease remains the leading cause of death in the industrialized nations. In the United States alone, cardiovascular disease (CVD) is responsible for approximately 1 million deaths every year. Fortunately, during the past 2 decades cardiovascular research has significantly increased our understanding of the structure and function of the cardiovascular system in health and disease, and during the last 15 years there has been a steady decline in mortality from cardiovascular disorders. It is hoped that effective application of the increased knowledge of CVD and its risk factors will enable health care professionals to assist persons more effectively in achieving and maintaining optimal health.

■ ANATOMY AND PHYSIOLOGY

■ Basic structure of the heart

The heart is a small organ (about the size of a fist) located in the middle and slightly to the left of the mediastinum, where it is partially overlapped by the lungs. The heart is wider at the top (base) than at the bottom (apex) and is positioned in the chest such that the blunt tip of the apex projects forward and to the left. The lower border of the heart rests on the diaphragm.

The heart is enclosed by a loose, inelastic sac (*pericardium*) that consists of two layers: the inner layer (visceral pericardium) and the outer layer (parietal pericardium). The two pericardial surfaces are separated by a pericardial space that normally contains approximately 10 to 20 ml of thin, clear pericardial fluid. This lubricating fluid moistens the contacting surfaces of the pericardial layers and serves to reduce the friction produced by the pumping action of the heart. If too much fluid collects in the pericardial space (pericardial effusion), pressure is exerted on the heart muscle, leading to decreased pumping efficiency.

There are three layers of cardiac tissue:

Epicardium: Outer layer of the heart
   Same structure as the visceral pericardium
Myocardium: Middle layer of the heart
   Composed of striated muscle fibers
   Responsible for the heart's contractile force
Endocardium: Inner layer of the heart
   Consists of endothelial tissue
   Lines the inside of the chambers and covers the heart valves

■ CHAMBERS

The heart is divided into two halves by a muscular wall (septum) (Fig. 25-1). Each half has an upper collecting chamber (atrium) and a lower pumping chamber (ventricle). Oxygen-poor venous blood enters the right atrium, flows from the right atrium to the right ventricle (mainly by gravity) when the tricuspid valve is opened, and is pumped to the lungs through the pulmonary artery. Oxygen-rich blood returns from the lungs to the left atrium, enters the left ventricle when the mitral valve is opened,

and is ejected into the aorta for distribution to the peripheral tissues.

The overall workload of the right ventricle is much lighter than that of the left ventricle, because the pulmonary system is a low-pressure system. The left ventricle has thick walls, because it must contract against a high-pressure systemic circulation to deliver blood to the peripheral tissue.

■ VALVES

The four cardiac valves are flaplike structures that function to maintain unidirectional (forward) blood flow through the heart chambers. These valves open and close in response to pressure and volume changes within the cardiac chambers. The cardiac valves can be classified into two types: the atrioventricular (AV) valves, which separate the atria from the ventricles, and the semilunar valves, which separate the pulmonary artery and the aorta from their respective ventricles.

□ Atrioventricular valves

The AV valves are the *tricuspid* valve, located between the right atrium and the right ventricle, and the *mitral* (bicuspid) valve, located between the left atrium and left ventricle. The tricuspid valve contains three leaflets held in place by fibrous cords called the *chordae tendineae*, which in turn are anchored to the ventricular wall by the papillary muscles. The mitral valve on the left side of the heart has two valve cusps or leaflets. It is attached in the same manner as the tricuspid valve. The chordae tendineae are important, because they support the AV valves during ventricular systole to prevent valvular prolapse into the atrium. A degree of leaflet overlapping during closure of the AV valves helps prevent the backward flow of blood. Damage to the chordae tendineae or to the papillary muscles would permit blood to regurgitate (flow backward) into the atrium during ventricular systole. The AV valves are *closed during ventricular systole (contraction) and open during diastole (relaxation)*.

□ Semilunar valves

The semilunar valves include the *aortic* and *pulmonic* valves. The structural design of the semilunar valves is quite different from the AV valves; each consists of three cuplike cusps. They lie between each ventricle and the great vessel into which it empties. These valves are *open during ventricular systole* to permit blood flow into the aorta and pulmonary arteries and *closed during diastole* to prevent retrograde flow from the aorta and pulmonary artery back into the ventricle when it is relaxed.

■ CORONARY ARTERIES

The coronary arteries arise at the beginning of the aorta right behind the aortic valve (Fig. 25-2). The function of the coronary artery system is to provide an adequate blood supply to the myocardium.

There are two main coronary arteries, the left and the

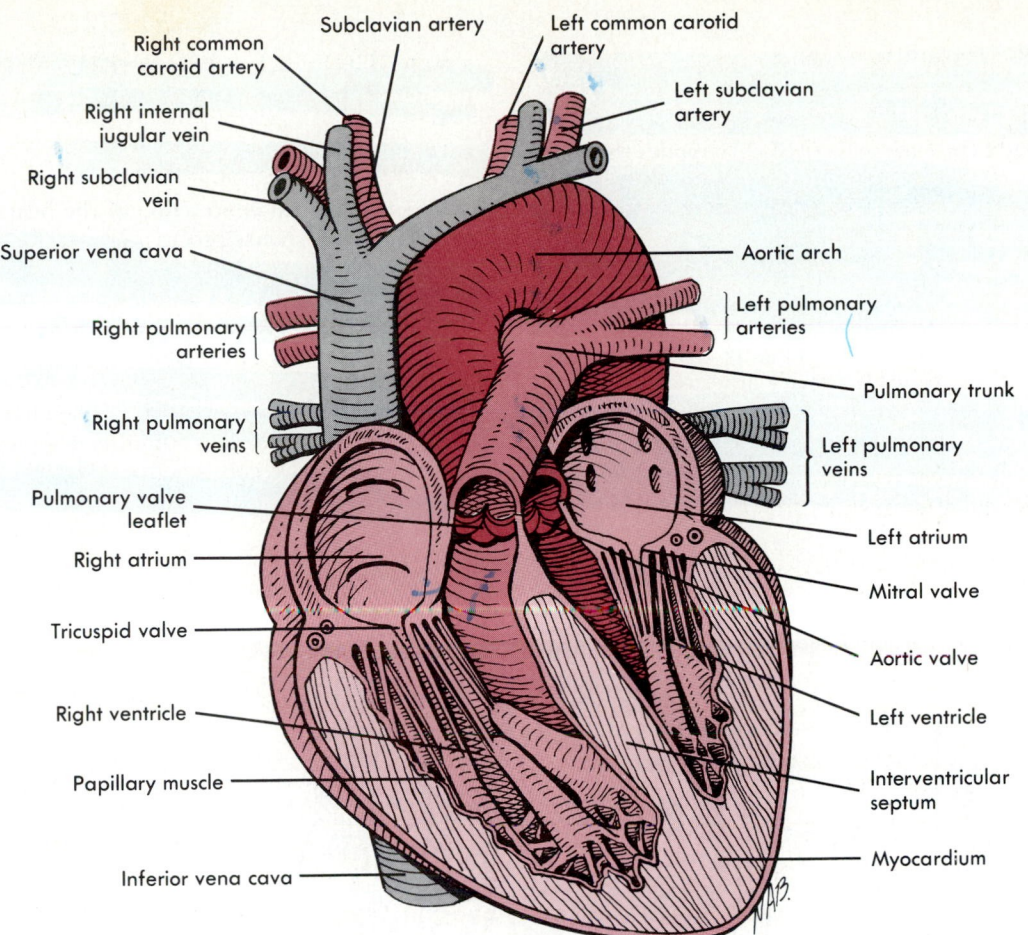

Fig. 25-1   Heart in frontal section.

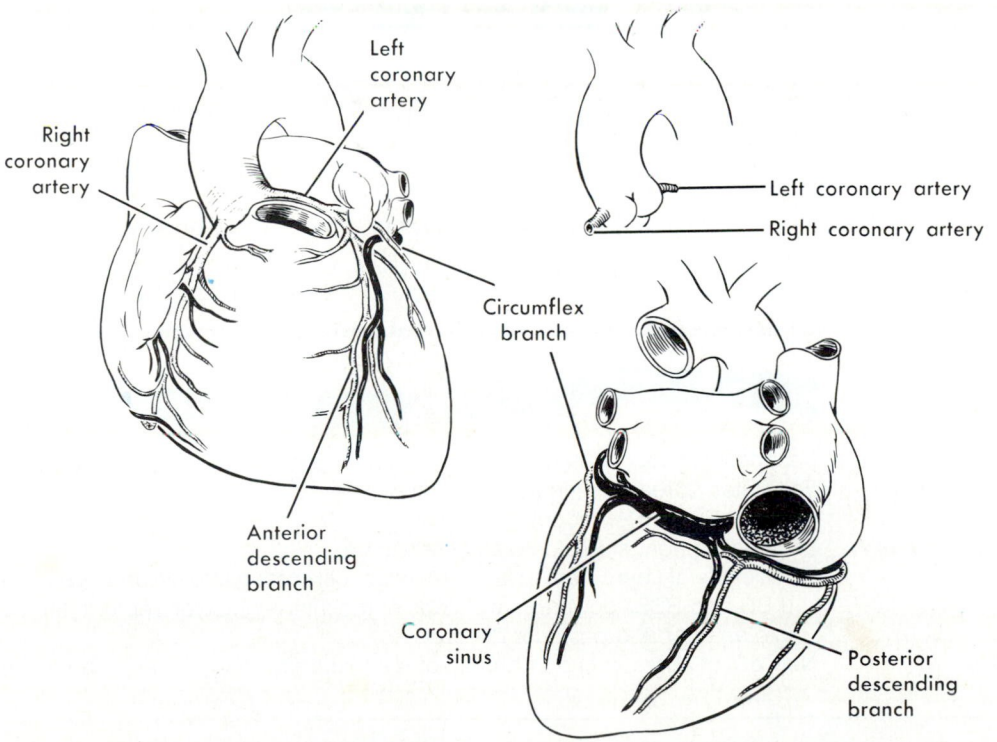

Fig. 25-2   Coronary blood vessels. (From King, OM: Care of the cardiac surgical patient, St. Louis, 1975, The CV Mosby Co.)

right. The left coronary artery, which supplies the left side of the heart, divides into two main branches, the *left anterior descending* (LAD) and the *circumflex coronary* arteries (CCA). The right coronary artery (RCA) supplies the right side of the heart. There are very few connections (anastomoses) between the main coronary arteries; therefore, blockage of a coronary artery or one of its branches will cause diminished blood flow (ischemia) to the portion of cardiac muscle supplied by that vessel and may result in angina pectoris or a myocardial infarction. Such blockages may be caused by clots or, more commonly, by fatty deposits in the walls of the arteries (coronary atherosclerosis).

The venous system of the heart has three subdivisions: the thebesian veins drain a portion of the right atria and right ventricular myocardium; the anterior cardiac veins drain a large portion of the right ventricle; and the coronary sinus and its branches drain the left ventricle (the greatest portion of the myocardial venous return).

■ Conduction system

The mechanical contraction of the heart is the product of a stimulus-response process. The resting myocardial cell has a membrane potential (that is, an electrical charge) as a result of the relative distribution of extracellular and intracellular sodium and potassium ions. Whenever the cell is stimulated, the membrane potential undergoes a change. A graphic record of this change forms the basis for an electrocardiogram (ECG). The change in electrical potential in response to a stimulus is known as the action potential. The two components of the action potential are *depolarization* (generation of the impulse) and *repolarization*

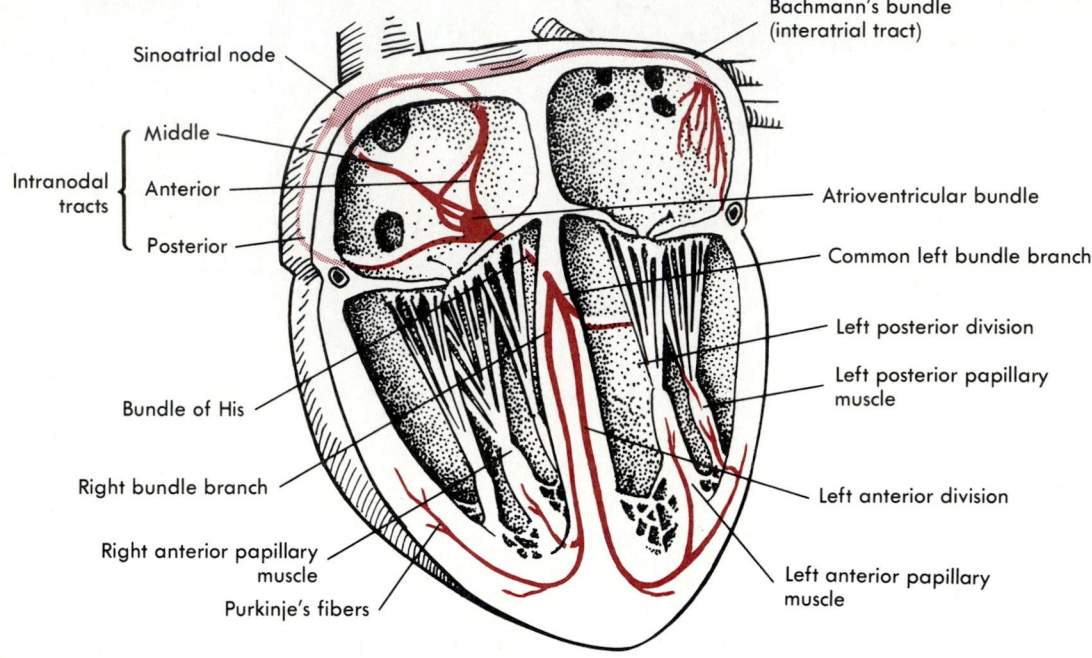

Fig. 25-3 Schematic diagram of heart illustrating the conduction system.

Structure of the conduction system of the heart

Sinoatrial (SA) node	Pacemaker node located in right atrium near opening of superior vena cava
Bachmann's bundle	Facilitates spread of impulse to left atrium
Internodal tracts	Connect SA and AV nodes
Atrioventricular node (AV)	Located on right side of interatrial septum
Bundle of His	Thick cable of fibers starting at the AV node, bifurcating into left and right bundle branches (LBB and RBB) down the two sides of the interventricular septum; the LBB bifurcates into anterior and posterior divisions
Purkinje fibers	Network of fibers at end of bundle of His that transmits impulse to both ventricular walls

(return of cell to resting state). The electrical current stimulates the release of calcium ions, which catalyze the reaction of myocardial contraction.

The primary structures of the conduction system are listed in box on p. 758 and illustrated in Fig. 25-3.

The sequence of cardiac activation is as follows:

1. Depolarization is initiated by an impulse from the SA node.
2. The impulse spreads through both atria.
3. The impulse reaches the AV node, which delays the impulse about 0.1 second.
4. The impulse is transmitted along the branches of the bundle of His to the Purkinje fibers, activating both ventricles almost simultaneously.
5. Activation of ventricular muscle proceeds from apex toward base of heart.

Cardiac cycle

The cardiac cycle has two phases, diastole and systole. Relaxation and filling of the chambers take place during diastole. Contraction and emptying occur during systole.

DIASTOLE

It is useful to envision the cardiac cycle starting at a point immediately after ventricular systole. At this time the AV valves are closed, and the atria are rapidly filling with blood (atrial diastole). Ventricular diastole is conceptualized in three phases:

1. *Isovolumetric ventricular relaxation:* ventricular muscle relaxed but not yet filling
2. *Rapid ventricular filling:* passive gravity flow of blood from atria to ventricles; starts when atrial pressure exceeds ventricular pressure and AV valves open
3. *Slow ventricular filling:* occurs as increasing blood volume causes ventricular pressure to rise, which slows further filling

SYSTOLE

Electrical activation (depolarization) precedes mechanical contraction of both the atria and the ventricles. Atrial systole occurs immediately after depolarization of the atria while the electrical impulse is delayed by the AV node. At this time the remaining blood in the atria is propelled into the ventricles. The ventricles are then depolarized, and ventricular systole begins. This process also has three phases:

1. *Isovolumetric ventricular contraction:* increase in myocardial tension and intraventricular pressure without change in blood volume; AV valves close
2. *Maximal ventricular ejection:* greater pressure in ventricles than in aorta or pulmonary artery forces open semilunar valves, and blood is pumped into pulmonary and systemic circulation
3. *Reduced ventricular ejection:* ventricles remain contracted and small quantity of blood is ejected from momentum built up by contraction; higher pressure

in aorta and pulmonary artery than in ventricles causes closure of semilunar valves, the end of ventricular systole

The familiar "lub-dub" heard when listening to the heart corresponds with the closure of the valves. The first sound results from closure of the atrioventricular valves at the beginning of ventricular systole. The second sound results from closing of the semilunar valves at the end of ventricular systole. (See Chapter 3 for auscultation of heart sounds.)

Cardiac output

The amount of blood ejected from the left ventricle into the aorta per minute is called *cardiac output* (CO). CO is equivalent to *stroke volume* (SV) (volume of blood ejected from the left ventricle with each contraction) multiplied by *heart rate* (HR) (number of heart beats per minute):

$$CO = SV \times HR$$

The average adult CO is 5.6 L/min. However, during periods of strenuous exercise the CO may reach 20 to 25 L/min.

CO is therefore dependent on the relationship between the stoke volume and the heart rate. Despite fluctuations in one of these two variables, CO can be maintained at relatively constant levels by compensatory adjustments made in the other variable. For example, if the heart rate slows, the time for ventricular filling (diastole) is lengthened. This allows for an increase in preload and a subsequent increase in stroke volume. Conversely, if the stroke volume fails, the heart rate can increase to compensate temporarily and to maintain cardiac output. Therefore, the actual determinants of cardiac output are the mechanisms regulating stroke volume and the heart rate.

CONTROL OF STROKE VOLUME

Three significant factors affecting stroke volume and thus cardiac output are preload, contractility, and afterload.

Preload

Starling's law of the heart states that myocardial fiber responds with a more forceful contraction when it is stretched. An example of this phenomenon is that of increasing the stretch of a rubber band to obtain a more forceful recoil when the rubber band is released. Myocardial fibers can be stretched by increasing the volume of blood delivered to the ventricles during diastole. The degree of myocardial stretch before contraction is expressed in terms of preload. *Preload is related to the volume of blood distending the ventricles at the end of diastole.* It is determined by the amount of venous return and the ejection fraction. The ejection fraction is the portion of the end-diastolic volume that is actually ejected (normally about two thirds). A decrease in the ejection fraction will result in a greater amount of blood left in the ventricle at the end of systole.

Since Starling's length-tension relationship is functional only within certain physiologic limits, it is important to note that prolonged, excessive stretching of the myocardial fibers will eventually lead to a *decrease* in cardiac output by reducing the stroke volume.

□ Contractility

Contractility refers to a change in the inotropic state (force of contraction) of the muscle without a change in myocardial fiber length or preload. Contractility can be increased by sympathetic stimulation or by the administration of substances such as calcium or epinephrine. Increased contractility improves ventricular emptying during systole, thereby increasing the stroke volume.

□ Afterload

Afterload is defined as *the amount of tension the ventricle must develop during contraction* to eject blood from the left ventricle into the aorta. The major impedance against which the left ventricle must pump is primarily determined by *peripheral vascular resistance*. Increase in pressure resulting from hypertension or vasoconstriction produces an increased resistance to pumping and will require an increase in ventricular tension to eject blood.

Ventricular tension is also directly proportional to ventricular size. Dilation of the ventricles resulting from increased ventricular volume will elevate ventricular tension and thus afterload. Excessive elevation of the afterload may impair ventricular emptying, thereby reducing stroke volume and cardiac output.

■ CONTROL OF HEART RATE

Under normal circumstances, heart rate is regulated by the activity of the sinoatrial (SA) node. The number of electrical impulses initiated per minute by this pacemaker is primarily the result of its innervation by fibers from both the sympathetic and the parasympathetic branches of the autonomic nervous system (ANS). Impulses from the sympathetic branch have a positive chronotropic effect (increase heart rate), and those from the parasympathetic branch have a negative chronotropic effect. Parasympathetic innervation occurs by way of the vagus nerve and is commonly thought to act as a "brake" that maintains resting heart rate at 65 to 75 beats/min. Some of the common conditions associated with increased or decreased impulse initiation by the SA node are listed in the box below, left. In addition to factors that influence the SA node, disturbances in the heart's conduction system and excitation of other pacemaker cells can affect heart rate. These will be discussed in more detail in the next section on cardiac arrhythmias (p. 769).

In summary, ventricular function and therefore CO are influenced by heart rate and stroke volume. Heart rate is primarily controlled by the ANS, and stroke volume is dependent on the three distinct variables of preload, contractility, and afterload.

■ Physiologic changes with aging

Age-related changes take place in the chemical composition, cells, and tissues of the heart and blood vessels and influence many aspects of cardiovascular functioning.[3,22] However, despite the physiologic changes of aging, the heart is able to meet the average day-to-day demands and function adequately. It is only under unusual circumstances or increased stress (such as sudden demands for more oxygen or the presence of cardiac pathologic conditions) that the deteriorating function of the heart is most apparent.

A number of physiologic factors reduce the efficiency of the heart as a pump as evidenced by a 30% reduction in cardiac output by age 65. Atrophy of muscle cells may lead to decreased muscle mass. Increased amounts of connective tissue add to myocardial stiffness and decrease cardiac compliance. The aorta and the major arteries also become less elastic, which compounds problems in filling and emptying the ventricles. The amount of subendocardial fat may increase, and the endocardium undergoes fibrosis, thickening, and sclerosis. In addition, delays may occur in the ability of myocardial cells to recover following electrical stimulation. The efficiency of the cardiac pump is also diminished because of decreased production of enzymes that influence the force and speed of ventricular contractions.

Increased amounts of connective tissue in the SA node, internodal tracts, AV node, and bundle branches may cause conduction defects and a less effective heart rate response to exercise. The heart rate tends to return to normal more slowly following any type of exertion. In addition, the elderly may be more prone to arrhythmias because of increased sensitivity to stimulation of the carotid sinus and an overall reduction in coronary blood flow.

The cardiac valves are also affected by the aging process. The mitral and aortic valves seem particularly vulnerable

---

Factors affecting sinus node

Increase heart rate

Emotions (fear, anger)
Pain
Decreased blood pressure
Increased body temperature
Exercise
Epinephrine

Decrease heart rate

Stimulation of baroreceptors in carotid sinus or aortic arch
Decreased body temperature
Increased intracranial pressure
Digitalis excess
Beta blockers

to fibrosis and calcification and can become somewhat rigid. Distortion of the aortic valve cusps can occur and may actually interfere with blood flow to the coronary arteries. These rigid valves can lead to audible systolic murmurs, usually of an ejection nature.

Confusion or decreased mental alertness may be early signs of a significant decrease in cardiac output in the elderly. These findings may mask other pertinent symptoms of decreased cardiac functioning, such as pain, fatigue, or dyspnea. Therefore, thorough evaluation of cardiovascular functioning should always be included in the assessment of changes in mental status.

■ CARDIAC ARRHYTHMIAS

Cardiac arrhythmias (abnormalities of heart rate or rhythm) are the result of disturbances in the initiation or conduction of electrical impulses within the heart. Some arrhythmias represent disturbances in both impulse initiation and impulse conduction.

The hemodynamic consequences of arrhythmias are extremely variable. Some cause no significant alteration in CO, although they may produce annoying symptoms such as a "fluttering" feeling in the chest or the sensation that the heart has "flipped over." Other arrhythmias cause reductions in CO that result in symptoms of decreased perfusion. This is particularly likely if the arrhythmia is associated with a very fast or very slow heart rate. Two arrhythmias, ventricular fibrillation and ventricular standstill, cause death if not promptly treated, because they result in *no* CO. There are many causes of arrhythmias,

some of which are not primarily related to a cardiovascular disease.

Accurate assessment of heart rate and rhythm and comparison of findings with baseline data will allow the nurse to detect some changes in the heart's electrical activity, but not all arrhythmias are easily noted by physical assessment. A visual display of cardiac electrical activity on the oscilloscope of a cardiac monitor or a graphic record such as an ECG is always required for definitive identification of cardiac arrhythmias.

■ Electrocardiogram (ECG)

An ECG is a graphic record of the electrical activity of the heart muscle. The recording is made at a standard speed on a grid that allows measurement of both the intensity of electrical events (voltage) and their duration. Intensity is measured on the vertical axis in millivolts (mV), and time is measured on the horizontal axis in seconds. Each small square on the grid is equivalent to a known unit of time (0.04 sec) and voltage (0.1 mV) that allows rapid calculation of both these parameters (Fig. 25-4).

The ECG may be recorded by a special technician or by health care professionals who have been trained in the procedure. It is essential that the patient be relaxed and cooperative, so the nurse must be able to explain both the purpose of this test and the procedure itself. An important point to emphasize is the fact that the ECG machine is merely *recording* electrical energy produced by the body and is not delivering any electrical current to the body. The patient's comfort and safety are maintained by preventing

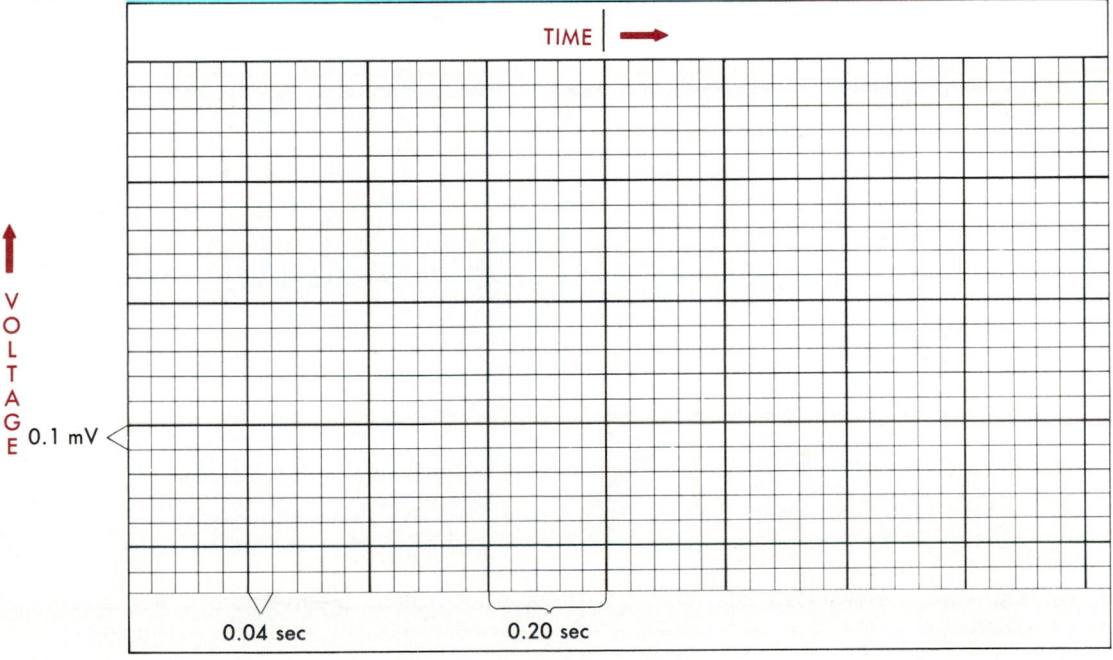

Fig. 25-4   Components of ECG paper.

unnecessary exposure and by ensuring adequate grounding of the ECG machine.

In brief, recording electrodes are placed on the patient's four extremities and on the anterior thorax. A conductive substance (jelly, paste, or a specially prepared disposable pad) is placed between the skin and the electrodes to facilitate achievement of a high-quality recording. The patient must sit or lie still during the procedure, which is not painful and takes less than 5 minutes. The operator controls the ECG machine, which is designed to record electrical activity in several different planes.

Typically, 12 different views are recorded, hence the term *12-lead ECG* (Fig. 25-5). The twelve typical views

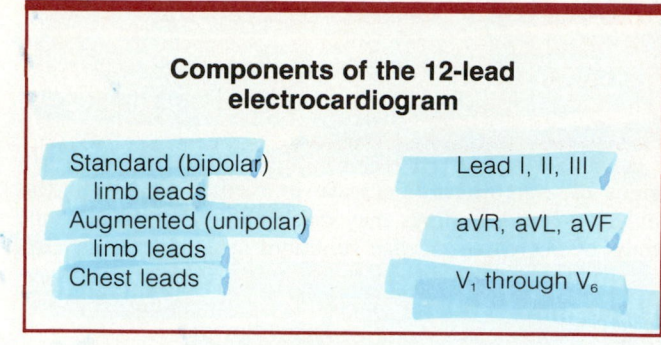

Components of the 12-lead electrocardiogram

Standard (bipolar) limb leads	Lead I, II, III
Augmented (unipolar) limb leads	aVR, aVL, aVF
Chest leads	V_1 through V_6

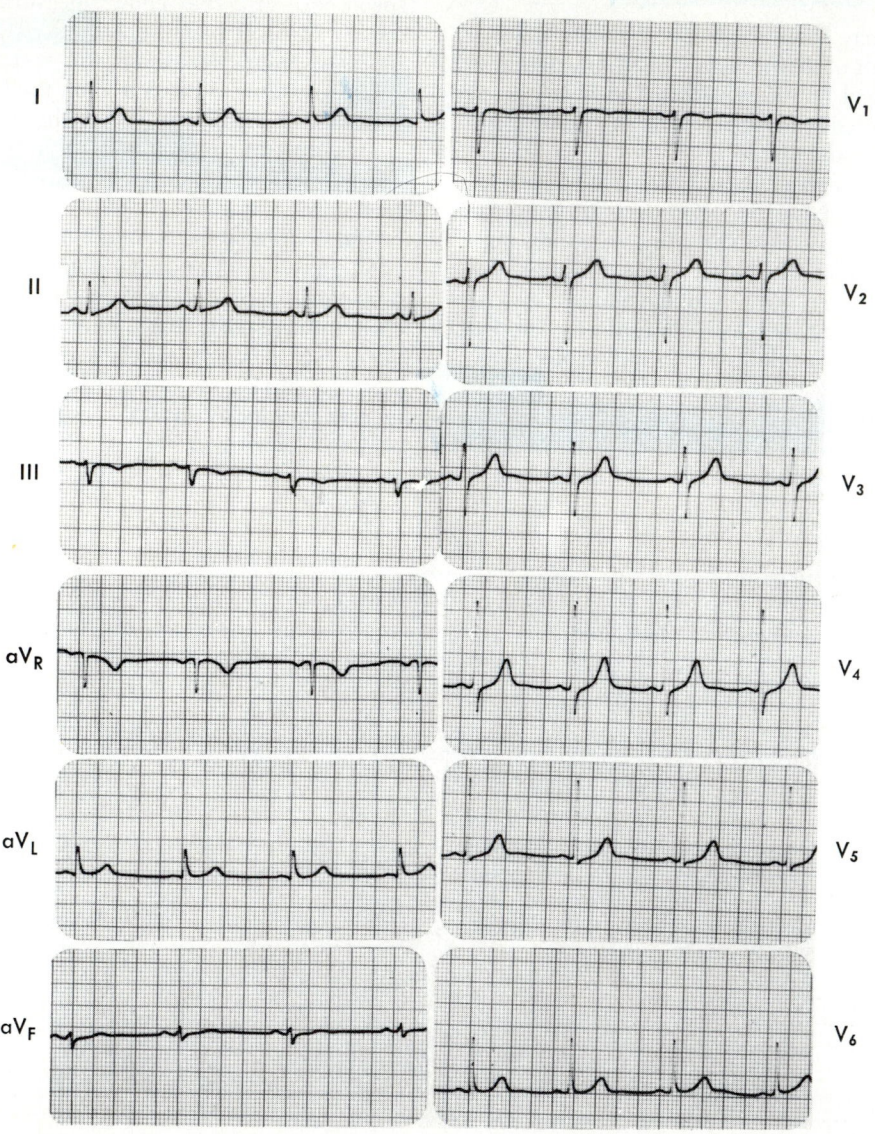

Fig. 25-5 Twelve-lead ECG showing normal sinus rhythm. (From Andreoli, KG, and others: Comprehensive cardiac care: a text for nurses, physicians, and other health practitioners, ed 5, St. Louis, 1983, The CV Mosby Co.)

Table 25-1 Normal cardiac electrical activity and resultant electrocardiographic findings

Cardiac electrical event	Electrocardio-graphic finding
Firing of SA node	Not recorded
Spread of impulse through the atria (atrial depolarization)	P wave
AV node delay	Isoelectric baseline between P and QRS
Atrial repolarization	Not recorded
Spread of impulse through the ventricles (ventricular depolarization)	QRS complex
Ventricular repolarization	T wave

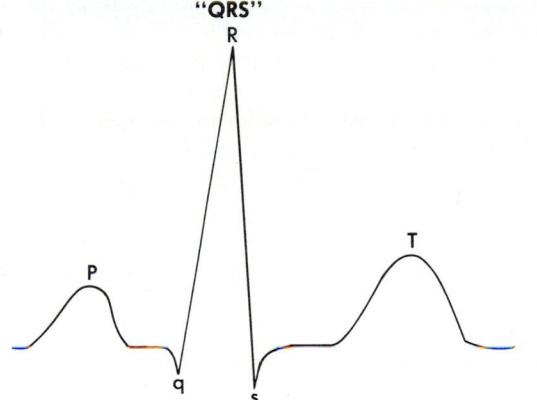

Fig. 25-6   Normal cardiac complex as seen in lead II.

of the heart's electrical activity actually represent three different methods of recording and provide information about activation on both the frontal (vertical) and horizontal planes. The subdivisions of the 12-lead ECG and the names of the leads are described in the box on p. 762.

Normal cardiac electrical activity as described earlier in the chapter and the resultant electrocardiographic findings are found in Table 25-1. When cardiac electrical activity occurs in a normal manner, a *cardiac complex* such as the one schematically depicted in Fig. 25-6 is produced. The voltage and major deflection (above or below the isoelectric baseline) of each component of the cardiac complex vary with the specific lead being recorded. A chest lead is compared with one of the standard leads shown in Fig. 25-7.

The nature of cardiac arrhythmias can be inferred by observing the presence, rate, and regularity of the various components of the cardiac complex and the relationship between the component parts. Ischemia, injury, or infarction of the myocardium, as well as an assortment of other conditions (some of which do *not* represent cardiac pathology), may alter the size, shape, or configuration of various components of the cardiac complex.

In summary, the ECG shows only the electrical activity of the heart, which may or may not be disturbed by a pathologic process. It does not show the actual physical state of the heart or indicate its ability to function as a pump. Its most important diagnostic uses are the interpretation of abnormal cardiac rhythms and the identification of coronary atherosclerotic heart disease.

■ Cardiac monitors

It is common practice to assess on a continuing basis the cardiac electrical activity of persons who are known or suspected to have arrhythmias or who are prone to develop arrhythmias. This assessment is carried out through the

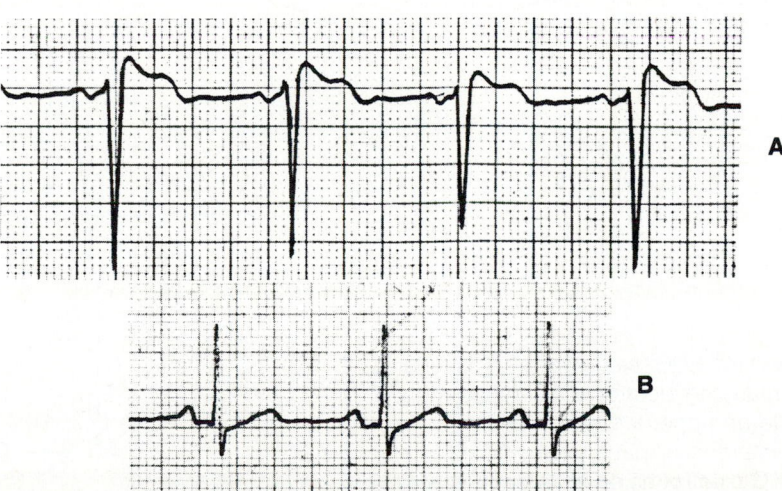

Fig. 25-7   **A,** Normal ECG in lead V$_1$. **B,** Normal ECG in lead II.

use of a cardiac monitor that displays information from *one* electrocardiographic lead on an oscilloscope. The lead chosen for display varies with the condition of the patient, but standard lead II or MCL₁ (a close facsimile of V₁) is frequently used. Fig. 25-8 shows the placement of electrodes on the chest for these two leads.

Most monitors provide a visual display of both cardiac electrical activity and the current heart rate. Preset alarms warn of heart rates that exceed or drop below limits considered acceptable for each specific patient. More sophisticated monitors are designed to detect and tentatively interpret arrhythmias through the use of a computer. Other physiologic parameters such as body temperature, systemic arterial pressure, and pulmonary artery pressures can also be monitored on a continual basis.

Acutely ill persons are monitored in intensive care settings, but the increased use of battery-powered ECG transmitters that do not require direct connection of the patient to the oscilloscope (*telemetry monitoring equipment*) has ex-

panded the use of such equipment to other patients as well. This development has resulted in the need for nurses working on general medical-surgical units to become familiar with monitoring equipment and to acquire some basic skills in rhythm interpretation.

Attachment to a cardiac monitor does not significantly alter a person's need for nursing care. Placement of the monitoring electrodes on the anterior thorax rather than the extremities leaves the patient relatively free to carry on usual activities. Special attention should be paid to the electrode sites to ensure a constant tight seal between the electrode and the skin and to note the development of any skin irritation. If a rash appears, the electrodes must be switched to alternate sites. Instructions supplied by individual electrode manufacturers guide the nurse in the application procedure and in necessary routine maintenance. Periodic checking of the monitoring system to ensure proper grounding and secure connection of all component parts is another general nursing responsibility.

■ Format for rhythm interpretation

A permanent graphic record of the heart's electrical activity can be obtained by either a standard ECG machine or a "write-out" component of a cardiac monitor. The monitor "write-out" is usually activated automatically when the monitor alarm sounds and can also be activated manually whenever a written record is desired for analysis. The record produced is commonly called a *rhythm strip* and should be at least 6 seconds long for proper interpretation. A long strip may be required if the heart rhythm is irregular.

Interpretation of a rhythm strip involves knowledge of normal electrophysiology and a measure of deductive reasoning. Systematic collection and analysis of the data listed

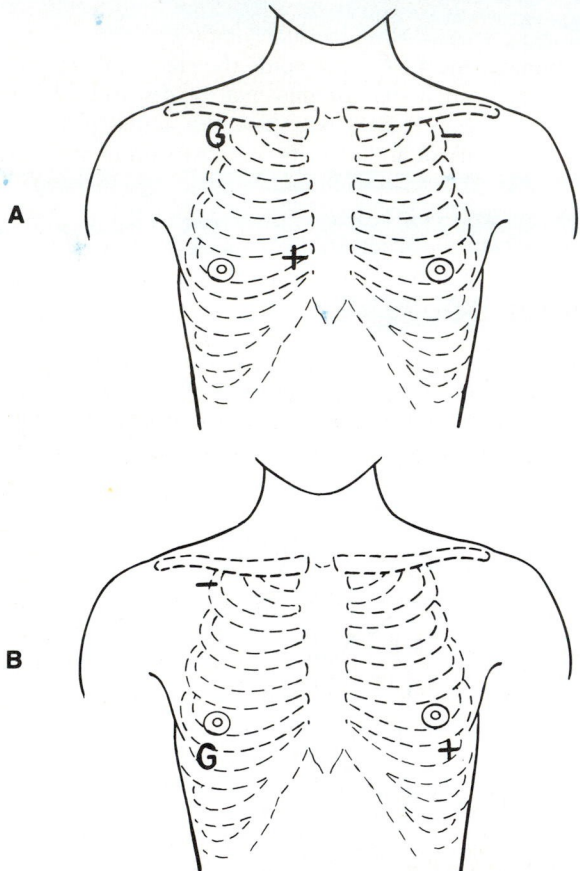

Fig. 25-8 **A,** Placement of ECG electrodes on anterior chest wall for lead V₁. Grounding electrode is on upper right chest, negative electrode on upper left chest, and positive electrode on right fourth intercostal space (along sternal border). **B,** Placement of ECG electrodes on anterior chest wall for lead II. Grounding electrode is on lower right chest, positive electrode on lower left chest, and negative electrode on upper right chest.

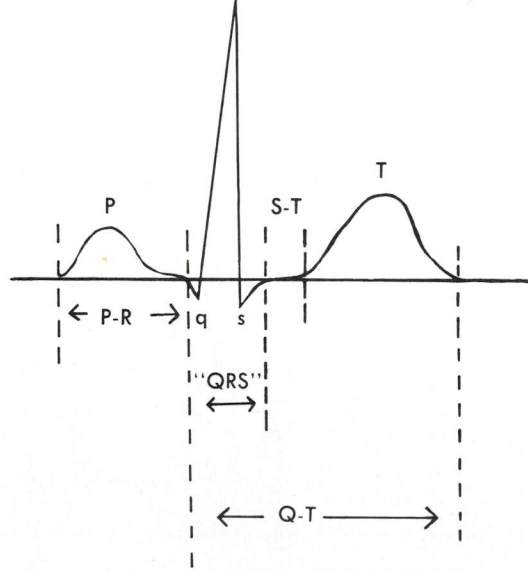

Fig. 25-9 Normal cardiac complex showing segments and intervals.

Rhythm strip analysis

1. **Heart rhythm.** Does this produce a pulse that is regular or irregular? Assess by noting whether the distance between QRS complexes (R-R) interval is consistently the same.
2. **Heart rate.** Number of ventricular contractions/min. Calculate by counting QRS complexes in 6 seconds and multiplying by 10 or by dividing number of small squares between two consecutive QRS complexes into 1500 (1500 × 0.04 sec = 60 sec). The latter method can be employed only if the rhythm is regular.
3. **Presence of P wave.** Indicates atrial depolarization.
   a. Do P waves occur regularly? The sinus node normally fires in a rhythmic fashion. Assess by noting whether P-P interval is consistent.
   b. Atrial rate: number of atrial contractions per minute. Calculate as with heart rate but use P waves.
   c. Is each wave followed by a QRS complex? If so, this verifies conduction of impulse from atria into ventricles; if not, a conduction defect is present.
4. **P-R interval.** Time from onset of atrial depolarization to onset of ventricular depolarization. It includes passage of impulse through the AV node.
   a. Length of P-R interval. Measure from beginning of P to beginning of QRS. Normal duration is 0.12 to 0.20 sec. Longer than 0.20 sec indicates a conduction delay in AV node.
   b. Is length of P-R interval consistent? If not, it may indicate lack of association between P and QRS.
5. **QRS duration.** Time needed for ventricular depolarization. Normal duration is 0.06 to 0.10 sec. Longer than 0.10 sec indicates abnormal ventricular depolarization.
6. **S-T segment and Q-T interval.** Assessment of these portions of the cardiac complex provides additional diagnostic information but is not required for rhythm interpretation.

---

in the box above is required. (The important segments and intervals of a single cardiac complex are schematically depicted in Fig. 25-9.)

Normal Sinus Rhythm

The term *normal sinus rhythm* implies that cardiac electrical activity is within normal limits as indicated by the following criteria (see Fig. 25-10).

1. P waves present and regular. If the SA node is initiating electrical activity in a rhythmic manner, atrial depolarization should occur in a rhythmic manner.
2. Atrial rate (P waves) between 60 and 100 beats/min. This represents the range of normal rates for SA node.

3. Each P wave is followed by a QRS complex. This verifies conduction of the impulse initiated by the SA node into the ventricles and implies that the heart rhythm is regular and the heart rate is also between 60 and 100 beats/min.
4. In addition, a normal P-R interval and QRS duration indicate normal functioning of all components of the conduction system.

Common arrhythmias

This discussion is intended as a brief introduction to the more common arrhythmias. Because of the complexity of this topic, some of the information is somewhat oversimplified. Nurses who are responsible for arrhythmia inter-

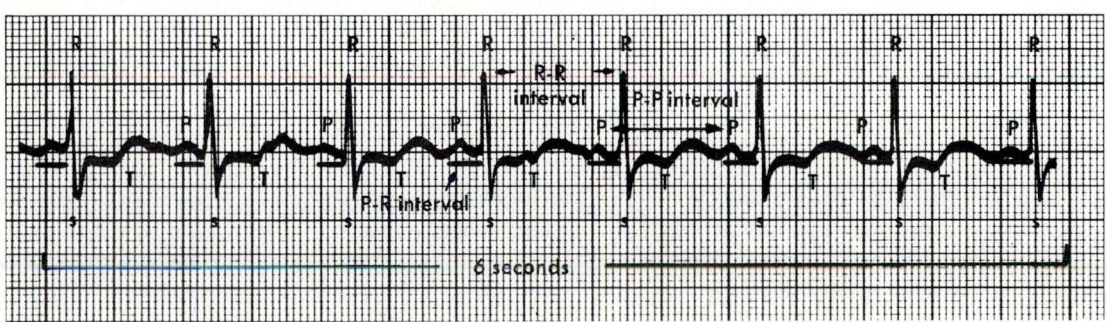

Fig. 25-10 Normal sinus rhythm showing R-R, P-P, and P-R intervals.

Table 25-2 Summary of selected cardiac arrhythmias

Arrhythmia category/name	Predisposing factors	ECG appearance	Significance/hemodynamic effects
Disturbances of impulse initiation			
Arrhythmias of the sinus node			
Sinus tachycardia	Increased metabolic demands: fever, exercise, excitement Compensatory response to blood loss, anemia, heart failure	Same as normal sinus rhythm except atrial and ventricular rates 100 to 150 beats/min	Increases cardiac output initially; prolonged episodes may lead to ↓ stroke volume
Sinus bradycardia	Peak cardiac efficiency (athletes) Parasympathetic stimulation, increased intracranial pressure, ↓ O_2 in sinus node	Same as normal sinus rhythm except atrial and ventricular rates 40 to 60 beats/min	Decreases cardiac output if not compensated by ↑ stroke volume
Sinus arrhythmia	Respiratory variation in impulse initiation by sinus node	Same as normal sinus rhythm except phasic shortening then lengthening of P-P (and consequently R-R) interval	Usually none
Ectopic arrhythmias			
Premature beats	Sympathetic stimulation, electrolyte imbalance, myocardial ischemia, chemical stimuli (caffeine, nicotine), distension of cardiac chambers, mechanical irritation (pacemaker catheter)	Cardiac complex comes "early" compared to normal rhythm *Artial:* complex has P wave and normal QRS *Ventricular:* complex has no P and wide, bizarre QRS	Serves as a warning of cardiac irritability; ventricular more serious than atrial Do not usually cause ↓ in CO unless very frequent
Ectopic tachycardias	Same as for premature beats; drug toxicity may also be a factor (especially digitalis and some antiarrhythmic agents)	Rapid heart rate—usually >150 beats/min Rhythm often irregular *Atrial:* P wave present (may merge into previous T wave); QRS usually normal *Ventricular:* no P wave before QRS; QRS wide and bizarre	May cause palpitations, dizziness Seldom seen in clients without heart disease; A serious arrhythmia CO ↓
Fibrillation Atrial	Same as for other ectopic rhythms; often associated with heart disease	Rhythm "irregularly irregular" No normal P waves seen QRS usually normal Heart rate variable	Loss of atrial contraction causes some ↓ in CO; situation worse if heart rate is rapid May persist as a chronic arrhythmia
Ventricular	Same as for other ectopic rhythms; often associated with acute myocardial infarction, electrocution	No recognizable QRS: pattern totally chaotic	Death-producing arrhythmia; no cardiac output Requires immediate termination

Continued.

Table 25-2   Summary of selected cardiac arrhythmias—cont'd

Arrhythmia category/name	Predisposing factors	ECG appearance	Significance/hemodynamic effects
Disturbances of impulse conduction ***Delays in impulse conduction***			
First-degree AV block	↓ O₂ in AV node Infections Drug effects (especially digitalis)	Same as NSR except P-R interval >0.20	Warns of impaired conduction
Bundle branch block	Degeneration or ischemia in conduction system; congenital anomalies; drug effects	Same as NSR except QRS duration >0.10	Same as first-degree block
Nonconduction of some impulses			
Second-degree heart blocks	Same as for first-degree or bundle branch blocks Often associated with myocardial infarction	P waves usually occur regularly at rates consistent with sinus node initiation Not all P waves followed by QRS: P-R interval may lengthen before nonconducted P wave or may be consistent QRS may be normal or prolonged	Hemodynamic effects depend on frequency of nonconduction and underlying sinus rate; significant ↓ in heart rate will cause ↓ in CO A serious arrhythmia
Nonconduction of all impulses			
Complete heart block (third-degree)	Same as for second-degree blocks	Ventricles controlled by subsidiary pacemaker; heart rate usually <70 beats/min; may be as low as 30 to 40 beats/min No relationship of P waves to QRS (P-R interval constantly varies) QRS often wide and bizarre	Usually associated with ↓ CO and requires prompt intervention
Ventricular standstill	Same as for second-degree blocks	Failure of even subsidiary pacemakers P waves often present No QRS complex	Death-producing arrhythmia Requires immediate intervention (cardiopulmonary resuscitation and other therapies)

pretation must undertake an in-depth study of electrophysiology and electrocardiography. Many continuing education courses enable the nurse to gain the specialized knowledge and skills required for this activity.

The arrhythmias will be discussed according to the two basic arrhythmia mechanisms: disturbances of impulse initiation and disturbances of impulse conduction. In addition to the description that follows, Table 25-2 summarizes the important features of each arrhythmia. Common treatment modalities are outlined in Table 25-3.

■ DISTURBANCES OF IMPULSE INITIATION

Most arrhythmias represent disturbances in impulse initiation. The disturbance may occur within the SA node or elsewhere in the heart (ectopic site).

□ Arrhythmias of the sinus node
□ *Sinus tachycardia*

Sinus tachycardia is the result of the SA node firing at a faster than normal rate (that is, greater than 100 beats/min). Any condition that increases the body's demand for oxygen may cause this arrhythmia, which is a normal response to exercise, excitement, and fever. Sinus tachycardia may also be a compensatory response to anemia, heart failure, and hemorrhage. The ECG appearance (Fig. 25-11) is the same as with normal sinus rhythm except for the faster atrial and ventricular rates (usually 100 to 150 beats/min). The general result of sinus tachycardia is an increased CO, although a prolonged episode may precipitate ventricular failure. When the underlying cause has been treated, the SA node returns to a normal rate.

Table 25-3 Summary of general treatment modalties for cardiac arrhythmias

Therapeutic aim/treatment	Indications for use
Increase heart rate	
Atropine	Sinus bradycardia (very slow rates)
Epinephrine, isoproterenol	Second- and third-degree heart blocks
Artificial pacemaker	Second- and third-degree heart blocks
	"Overdrive" of ectopic rhythms refractory to more usual therapy
Decrease heart rate	
Reduction of metabolic demands	Sinus tachycardia
Treatment of underlying cause of decreased stroke volume	Sinus tachycardia
	Ectopic tachycardias
Antiarrhythmic agents	Ectopic tachycardias
Verapamil	
Propranalol (Inderal)	
Suppression of ectopic impulse formation	
Antiarrhythmic agents	Premature beats
Bretylium tosylate (Bretylol)	Ectopic tachycardias and fibrillation
Disopyramide (Norpace)	
Lidocaine	
Quinidine	
Procainamide (Pronestyl)	
Verapamil	
Cardioversion	Ectopic tachycardias and atrial fibrillation
Defibrillation	Ventricular fibrillation

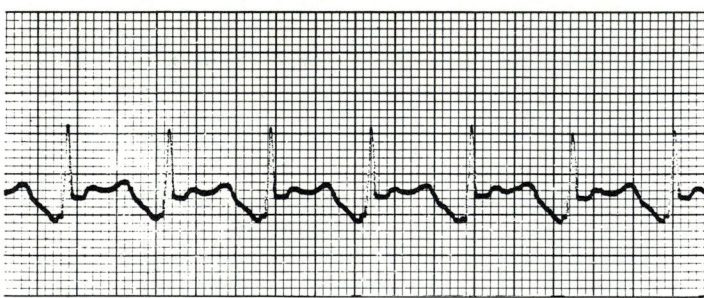

Fig. 25-11 Sinus tachycardia. Lead II showing heart rate of 115, regular rhythm, normal PR interval, and normal QRS duration.

□ *Sinus bradycardia*

Sinus bradycardia is the result of the SA node firing at a slower than normal rate (that is, less than 60 beats/min). This arrhythmia may be a normal finding in athletes or others whose heart muscles contract at peak efficiency. It may also be the result of stimulation of the parasympathetic nervous system, increased intracranial pressure, or lack of blood and oxygen in the SA node. The ECG appearance (Fig. 25-12) is the same as for normal sinus rhythm except for the slower atrial and ventricular rates (usually 40 to 60 beats/min). The general result of sinus bradycardia is a decreased CO, although the heart may compensate for the decreased rate by increasing stroke volume. If the person with sinus bradycardia shows clinical signs of decreased perfusion, atropine may be used to speed up the action of the SA node. On a long-term basis, a pacemaker may be required.

□ *Sinus arrhythmia*

Sinus arrhythmia is the term applied to irregularities in the rate of firing of the SA node that occur in a phasic, predictable manner. The rate alternately speeds up for a

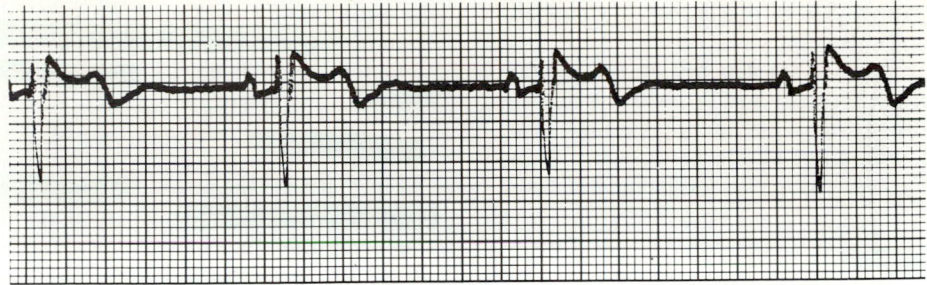

Fig. 25-12   Sinus bradycardia (lead V₁). P waves are present and regular. Atrial and ventricular rates are 44. Each P is followed by a QRS.

few beats and then slows down for a few beats. Assessment of the person's respiratory pattern reveals that the heart rate speeds up during inspiration and slows down during expiration. Except for the irregular P-P (and therefore, R-R) intervals, this meets the other criteria for normal sinus rhythm. Sinus arrhythmia is a benign condition and does not require treatment.

☐ Ectopic arrhythmias

Arrhythmias resulting from electrical impulse formation in ectopic sites can be classified according to the frequency with which the ectopic impulses occur. The frequency varies from occasional (premature beats) to one that exceeds the frequency of impulse initiation by the SA node (ectopic tachycardias and fibrillation).

☐ *Premature beats*

Premature beats may arise in the atria, the AV junctional region, or the ventricles. This arrhythmia causes the heart rhythm to be irregular because of the periodic early oc-

currence of an abnormal cardiac complex. In this instance, "early" means resulting in an R-R interval that is shorter than that between two consecutive normal cardiac complexes. The specific characteristics of the abnormal cardiac complex allow the interpreter to infer the location of the ectopic focus; for example, atrial premature beats have a P wave and normal QRS, whereas ventricular premature beats have no P wave and a bizarre, widened QRS (Fig. 25-13).

Premature beats represent the occasional firing of an ectopic focus that has been made irritable by the presence of a stimulus such as increased activity of the sympathetic nervous system, hypoxia, caffeine and nicotine ingestion, electrolyte imbalances, and distention of a group of cells by abnormally large blood volumes. This is not an all-inclusive list of potential stimuli but is intended to demonstrate the wide variety of possibilities. Ventricular premature beats are considered more serious than those arising above the ventricle, but as a group, premature beats do not generally cause significant alterations in CO. They

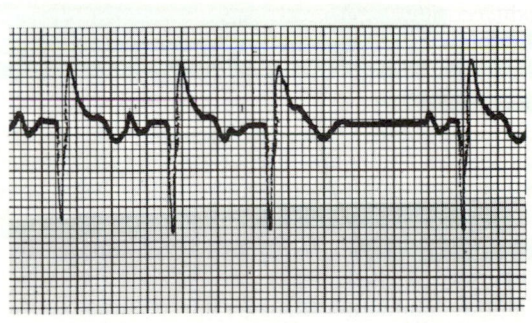

A

Fig. 25-13   **A,** Premature atrial beat (lead V₁). Third beat is premature atrial beat with abnormal early P wave followed by normal QRS complex. **B,** Premature ventricular beats (lead II). Fourth and tenth beats are premature with no P wave and wide, bizarre QRS. Different shapes of PVBs indicate two different ectopic sites in ventricles.

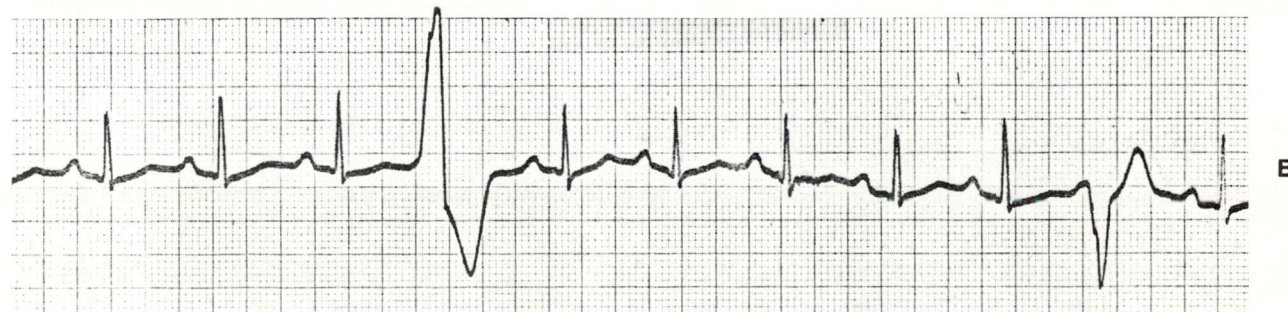

B

may be completely unnoticed by the person but may also be a cause of "palpitations."

Treatment of premature beats depends on the location of the ectopic focus, the frequency of occurrence, and the clinical condition of the patient. Frequent premature beats warn of increasing irritability of the ectopic focus, and treatment is aimed at preventing the development of more serious arrhythmias.

□ Ectopic tachycardias

Ectopic tachycardias arise from the same assortment of ectopic foci as premature beats but indicate much more severe irritability. These arrhythmias frequently start and end abruptly; therefore, the term *paroxysmal* is often included in the name, for example, *paroxysmal atrial tachycardia* (PAT) or *paroxysmal ventricular tachycardia*. An ectopic tachycardia may last a few seconds or as long as several hours, but regardless of its duration, it represents loss of control of the usual pacemaking function of the SA node. Initiation of cardiac electrical activity is regulated by the ectopic focus until the arrhythmia can be terminated.

General ECG characteristics of ectopic tachycardias include a rapid heart rate (often 150 beats/min or greater) and a regular rhythm. Those arising above the ventricles have normal cardiac complexes (that is, P waves preceding normal QRS complexes), whereas those initiated in the ventricles have wide, bizarre QRS complexes not preceded by P waves.

Paroxysmal atrial tachycardia can be precipitated by stress, excessive caffeine or alcohol intake, and distention of the atria related to heart failure or malfunction of one of the AV valves. An episode may be so brief as to make treatment unnecessary, but prolonged bouts may result in decreased CO because of decreased ventricular filling time. Stimulation of the parasympathetic nervous system by induced vomiting or pressure applied to the carotid sinus region by a physician frequently terminates this arrhythmia. Rapid-acting forms of digitalis or cardioversion (p. 777) may also be employed.

Paroxysmal ventricular tachycardia is a serious problem not commonly seen in persons who do not have heart disease of some type. It is a frequent complication of acute myocardial infarction. Because electrical activity is initiated in the ventricles and does not proceed in an orderly sequence, coordination of atrial and ventricular contraction is lost. Therefore, CO is almost always significantly decreased. Prompt treatment is essential and may take the form of intravenous lidocaine or procainamide. If the patient loses consciousness, immediate cardioversion is required.

□ Fibrillation

Fibrillation is the result of extremely rapid, chaotic firing of an ectopic focus. The hemodynamic consequences of this arrhythmia mechanism vary so drastically, depending on the site of the ectopic focus, that atrial and ventricular mechanisms must be discussed separately.

ATRIAL FIBRILLATION. Atrial fibrillation is a common arrhythmia. It is usually associated with organic heart diseases such as mitral stenosis or chronic heart failure, but it may also follow the injudicious use of alcohol, excessive smoking, or large meals. The atrial ectopic focus fires 350 to 600 times a minute, which again results in the SA node losing control of impulse initiation. Electrical impulses move through the atria so quickly that they are not depolarized as a unit (therefore, there are no normal P waves on the ECG), and they do not contract as a unit. Rather, individual muscle fibers contract and relax, giving an overall "twitching" effect. Loss of atrial contraction means that about 20% of the CO is never propelled into the ventricles. The other 80% falls into the ventricles because of the force of gravity and pressure changes within the chambers.

The AV node is incapable of conducting 350 or more impulses/min into the ventricles, so ventricular depolarization occurs in a more or less random fashion. The QRS complexes are normal, since the stimulus goes through the ventricular conduction system in the usual manner, but the rhythm is "irregularly irregular," that is, has no discernible pattern (Fig. 25-14). The irregular pattern of ventricular contraction results in varying amounts of blood being ejected with each beat. Some contractions are associated with so little output that no peripheral pulsations are produced. This creates an apical-radial pulse deficit. The heart rate of a person in atrial fibrillation should always be calculated from an apical pulse or from an ECG rhythm strip.

The hemodynamic consequences of atrial fibrillation depend largely on the heart rate of each specific episode. With more rapid heart rates (that is, 150 beats/min or greater), signs of decreased perfusion are likely to occur. Digitalis preparations are frequently employed to slow the ventricular rate. This occurs because of the delaying action of digitalis on conduction through the AV node. Once the

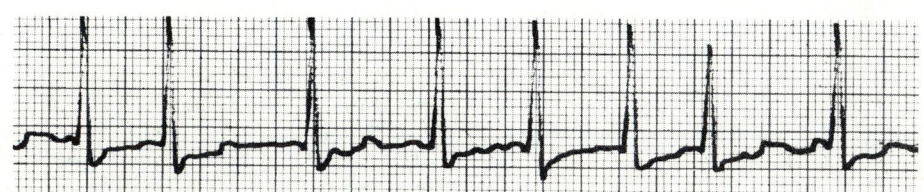

Fig. 25-14   Atrial fibrillation (lead II). Atrial rate is rapid with varying conduction to ventricles, rhythm is irregular, QRS complex is normal, no definite P waves are visible.

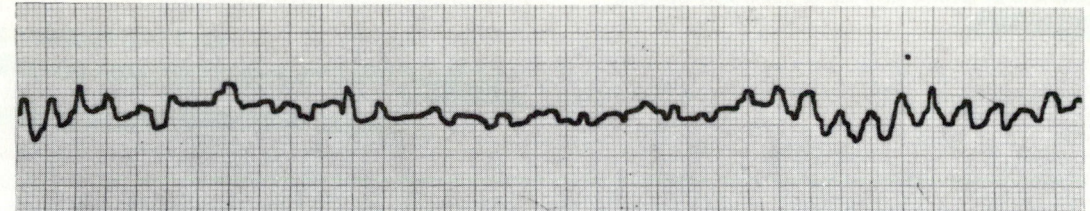

Fig. 25-15 Ventricular fibrillation (lead II). Tracing shows electrical chaos in myocardium. There are no QRS complexes and no definite P waves visible.

heart rate has been controlled, quinidine is usually given to suppress the irritability of the atrial ectopic focus. When treatment with quinidine is initiated, the patient is watched closely, since many persons are allergic to this drug. Flushing, ringing in the ears, syncope, or an increase in pulse rate are brought to the physician's immediate attention. Diarrhea is a common side effect of quinidine therapy and can usually be treated symptomatically for a day or so until the GI system adjusts to the drug.

Atrial fibrillation of recent onset may also be terminated electrically by cardioversion. If the underlying cause of this arrhythmia cannot be reversed, it may persist for months or years with little consequence to the person as long as the heart rate is not rapid. Long-standing atrial fibrillation is not likely to respond to cardioversion, since the SA node is not apt to resume its pacemaking role after a long period of dormancy.

VENTRICULAR FIBRILLATION. *Ventricular fibrillation* is the term given to rapid, chaotic electrical activity initiated by a ventricular ectopic focus. This death-producing arrhythmia may result from ischemia in the ventricles, electrocution, drowning, electrolyte imbalances, and toxic doses of digitalis or quinidine. As is the case in atrial fibrillation, extremely rapid firing of the ectopic focus causes the loss of coordinated depolarization and contraction. The important difference between atrial and ventricular depolarization, however, is that the ventricles contract normally in atrial depolarization, whereas in ventricular depolarization the ventricles do not contract at all. On the monitor, ventricular fibrillation is characterized by the absence of recognizable QRS complexes (Fig. 25-15).

The person with ventricular fibrillation has neither a palpable pulse nor detectable heart sounds and quickly loses consciousness. The definitive treatment for this arrhythmia is defibrillation (p. 777) performed by either a physician or a specially trained nurse. If a defibrillator is not immediately available, cardiopulmonary resuscitation (CPR) should be instituted to ensure perfusion of the brain, but this intervention does not reverse the arrhythmia.

■ DISTURBANCES OF IMPULSE CONDUCTION

Disturbances of impulse conduction may occur at the AV node or within the intraventricular conduction system (the right and left bundle branches). The most serious result of this type of arrhythmia is the failure of some or all of the impulses initiated by the SA node to reach the ventricles. Ventricular depolarization then occurs less frequently than it would if conduction were normal; heart rate decreases, and CO is likely to be diminished.

☐ Delays in impulse conduction

Conduction defects can be viewed as existing along a continuum. The less serious problems, first-degree AV block and bundle branch block, represent only delays in impulse conduction. In spite of the names applied to these conditions, no impulses are actually blocked from reaching the ventricles.

☐ *First-degree AV block*

First-degree AV block is the result of delayed impulse conduction through the AV node. It is manifested on the ECG by a prolonged P-R interval (greater than 0.20 sec). Decreased circulation of blood and oxygen to the AV node, infectious processes, and suppression of conduction by various drugs such as digitalis preparations are some of the common causes of first-degree AV block. Since this arrhythmia has no effect on heart rate, it has no hemodynamic consequences and is significant only as a warning of impaired conduction. There is usually no treatment.

☐ *Bundle branch block*

Bundle branch block is the result of a failure of impulse conduction in one division of the intraventricular conduction system. As long as only one major component is involved (the right or the left bundle branch), impulses continue to reach the ventricles and achieve depolarization, although by an abnormal route. This conduction abnormality is manifested on the ECG by QRS complexes whose duration exceeds the 0.10 sec upper limit of normal. The exact configuration of the QRS complex in selected leads of a 12-lead ECG determines the diagnosis of right or left bundle branch block.

Inadequate circulation to the intraventricular conduction system, congenital anomalies, degenerative diseases of the conduction system, and drug effects are some of the causes of bundle branch block. Although bundle branch blocks also have no hemodynamic consequences, they are considered a more serious problem than first-degree AV block because of their propensity to progress to more significant conduction disturbances.

☐ Nonconduction of some impulses (second-degree heart blocks)

Second-degree heart blocks are a group of conduction disturbances that result from the failure of some, but not all, of the impulses initiated by the sinus node to reach the ventricles. The site of conduction disturbance may be either the AV node or the intraventricular conduction system, and the frequency of nonconduction episodes may be only periodic or as often as every other cardiac cycle. The specific names given to second-degree heart blocks reflect both the frequency of nonconduction and the site of the pathologic condition. For example, a Mobitz I second-degree block indicates periodic nonconduction in the AV node. (The reader is referred to more specialized texts for an in-depth discussion of this topic.)

The absence of QRS complexes after some of the P waves initiated by the sinus node is the primary ECG characteristic of second-degree heart blocks. Unless there is also a disturbance in the sinus node, the P waves should occur regularly at a rate between 60 and 100 beats/min. The obvious result of this phenomenon is a heart (ventricular) rate that is *less than* the atrial rate. Whether or not the second-degree block creates a condition of decreased cardiac output depends on the following:

1. The rate at which the sinus node is firing (The more P waves there are, the less serious the consequences of occasional nonconduction)
2. The frequency with which nonconduction occurs
3. The ability of the ventricles to regulate stroke volume

Many episodes of second-degree heart block require therapeutic intervention to increase the heart rate. Atropine is used at times to improve conduction through the AV node, but the most dependable effective intervention is the installation of an artificial pacemaker (p. 773). It should be noted that interventions for conduction disturbances do not generally remove the underlying cause but merely serve to maintain an adequate heart rate.

☐ Nonconduction of all impulses (complete heart block)

Complete heart block, sometimes called *third-degree block*, occurs when no impulses initiated by the sinus node are conducted into the ventricles. The same causes discussed in relation to first- and second-degree blocks apply to this serious conduction defect. In the absence of stimulation from the sinus node, subsidiary pacemaking cells in the ventricles take over control of the electrical activity for this region of the heart. In effect, complete heart block represents activity of two independent pacemakers. The SA node controls electrical activity in the atria, and a slower, less dependable pacemaker controls the ventricles.

On the ECG, this is manifested by P waves occurring at one rate and QRS complexes occurring at a different, slower rate (usually 20 to 40 beats/min) (Fig. 25-16). Since the stimulus for ventricular depolarization arises in the ventricles and travels through the ventricles in a delayed, abnormal manner, the QRS complexes are likely to have a wide, bizarre contour. The lack of association between the P waves and the QRS complexes is shown by the lack of a consistent P-R interval.

Complete heart block is associated with both acute and chronic cardiovascular diseases. The slow heart rate that results almost always requires therapeutic intervention. Some persons with chronic degenerative diseases of the conduction system have periodic, transient episodes of complete heart block that produce symptoms known as *Stokes-Adams syndrome*. This condition is characterized by dizziness, fainting, and possible loss of consciousness resulting from a *sudden* decrease in heart rate and CO. Stokes-Adams attacks occur most often in elderly individuals and are of great concern, since they may lead to serious physical injury or death. Once the presence of Stokes-Adams syndrome has been detected, therapy in the form of a permanent pacemaker greatly improves the prognosis of these individuals. Temporary pacemakers are used in acute care settings to maintain the heart rate of persons with complete heart block until the condition either resolves or gives indication of requiring permanent therapy.

☐ Ventricular standstill

Failure of the ventricles to initiate their own electrical activity in the absence of stimulation from the SA node or any other supraventricular pacemaker is called ventricular standstill. This death-producing condition is characterized by no evidence of ventricular depolarization on the ECG, that is, no QRS complexes. P waves may be present, or the tracing may have a "straight-line" appearance.

The person with ventricular standstill has no peripheral pulse and no detectable heart sounds and loses consciousness. These signs are the *same* as those occurring with ventricular fibrillation; these two arrhythmias cannot be distinguished by clinical evidence. An ECG tracing is es-

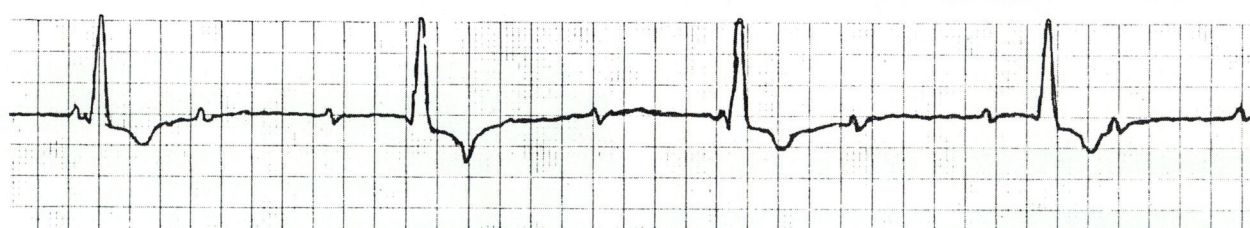

Fig. 25-16 Complete heart block (lead II). Atrial rate is 75; ventricular rate is less than 30. P waves have no consistent relationship to QRS complex.

sential in making a definitive diagnosis. CPR should be instituted at once for ventricular standstill, and cardiac stimulants such as epinephrine (Adrenalin) are administered intravenously or directly into the myocardium. Again, installation of a temporary pacemaker is often the only treatment that is effective over the long term. Prophylactic placement of temporary pacemakers has become common practice for individuals displaying evidence of progressive deterioration in cardiac conduction. The aim is to prevent the occurrence of ventricular standstill.

■ Treatment modalities

Three major treatment modalities are employed for cardiac arrhythmias:
1. Therapy aimed at relieving the underlying cause of the arrhythmia (see the box below)
2. Drug therapy aimed at suppression of impulse formation by ectopic sites or enhancement of impulse formation by the SA node
3. The use of electrical stimuli to suppress ectopic impulse formation or to initiate impulse formation in a regulated manner

---

Therapies to relieve underlying cause of arrhythmias

Oxygen to relieve hypoxia
Provision of depleted serum electrolytes (especially potassium)
Treatment of heart failure
Relief of anxiety
Removal of noxious stimuli (for example, caffeine)

■ ANTIARRHYTHMIC AGENTS

The list of *antiarrhythmic drugs* in current use appears to grow almost daily. The development of drugs that are effective and free of dangerous or annoying side effects has been a challenge to the pharmaceutical industry. The more common drugs are listed in Table 25-3; the reader is referred to pharmacology texts for specific information regarding antiarrhythmic agents.

■ PACEMAKERS

The use of various forms of electrical stimuli in the treatment of cardiac arrhythmias has a number of nursing implications; therefore, these modalities will be discussed in detail.

An artificial pacemaker is a mechanical device that electronically stimulates impulse initiation within the heart. The pacemaker system is composed of a battery-powered energy source (technically called a *pulse generator* but more commonly called a *pacemaker*) and a wire or catheter that delivers the electronic stimulus to a point of contact in the atrial or ventricular myocardium. The purpose of artificial pacing is control of heart rate.

Pacemakers are primarily used in the treatment of conduction defects, in which case the catheter is placed in the ventricle to ensure adequate depolarization beyond the site of impulse blockage (Fig. 25-17, A). These devices are also employed to remedy inadequate impulse initiation by the SA node and to suppress myocardial irritability that does not respond to antiarrhythmic therapy. In these instances the catheter may be placed in the atrium, since the underlying problem does not involve failure of the conduction system (Fig. 25-17, B). Atrial pacing has been technically difficult to achieve, although continual advances in catheter design will undoubtedly lead to increased use of this pacing mode in the future. Ventricular

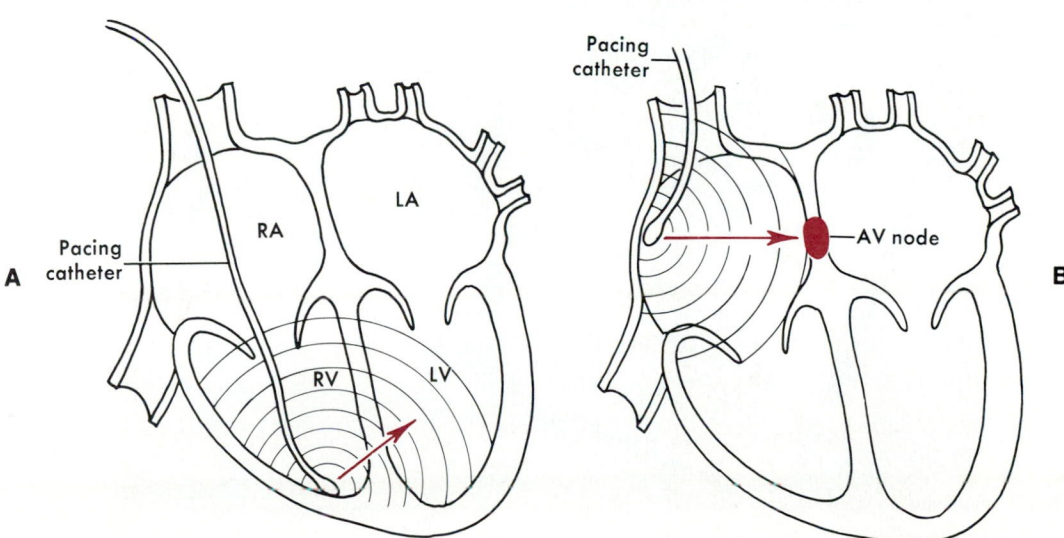

Fig. 25-17 **A,** Ventricular pacing. Impulses are initiated in ventricle. **B,** Atrial pacing. Impulses are initiated in atrium and travel to ventricles by normal conduction system.

pacing is "nonphysiologic," since it does not result in coordination between atrial and ventricular mechanical activity. The CO thus achieved, however, is adequate for the great majority of persons requiring pacemakers.

□ Pulse generators

The pulse generator has a number of controls that can be easily manipulated in a temporary system (Fig. 25-18) and that are more easily manipulated than has previously been the case in permanent systems because of improvements in technology. These controls include energy output, heart rate, and pacing mode (asynchronous or demand).

Energy output refers to the intensity of the electronic stimulus delivered to the myocardium. Output is measured in milliamperes (mA), and relatively low levels of energy (approximately 1.5 mA) are usually sufficient to cause depolarization if the catheter is in proper contact with the myocardium. Energy output is set by the physician at the time of pacemaker insertion after determination of the "threshold level" of stimulation, that is, the lowest output that will achieve depolarization. Because of continuous minor fluctuations in the threshold, energy output is usually set at twice the initial level.

Heart rate is set according to the clinical condition of the patient and the desired therapeutic aim. With rare exceptions, the rate is set between 70 and 80 beats/min when the aim is simple maintenance of adequate cardiac output. If the purpose of pacing is the suppression of myocardial irritability, the rate is set higher, often as high as 100 to 120. The heart rate setting reflects the *lowest* anticipated heart rate in a properly functioning pacemaker system.

There has been a considerable evolution in *pacing modes* since the original introduction of artificial pacemakers. The pacemaker may function in the atria, the ventricles, or both cardiac chambers. The mode may be asynchronous (stimulation at a preset fixed rate) or demand (stimulation only in the *absence* of specified electrical activity such as a P wave or a QRS complex). The combination of chamber, mode, type of programmability, and function during tacharrhythmias has become so complex that the Inter-Society Commission for Heart Disease (ICHD) has developed a code that allows easy identification of pacemaker function in a shorthand type of notation.[52]

An indepth discussion of the multiple pacing modes currently available is beyond the scope of this text. The reader is referred to specialized texts for more information. In general, the danger with *asynchronous* pacing is the possibility of competition between the pacemaker and naturally occuring electrical activity which, in the worst case, could result in ventricular fibrillation. Because of this hazard and the development of safer approaches to pacing, asynchronous pacing is rarely used today.

Demand pacing is the most frequently used mode and is characterized by stimulation of the myocardium *only* when the person's natural heart rate falls below the preset limit. This requires that the pulse generator perform two different functions. It must recognize the absence of natural electrical activity and stimulate the heart accordingly. In addition, the pulse generator must "sense" the presence of natural electrical activity that maintains the desired heart rate and withhold the pacing stimulus under those circumstances. These two functions are independent and must be assessed separately.

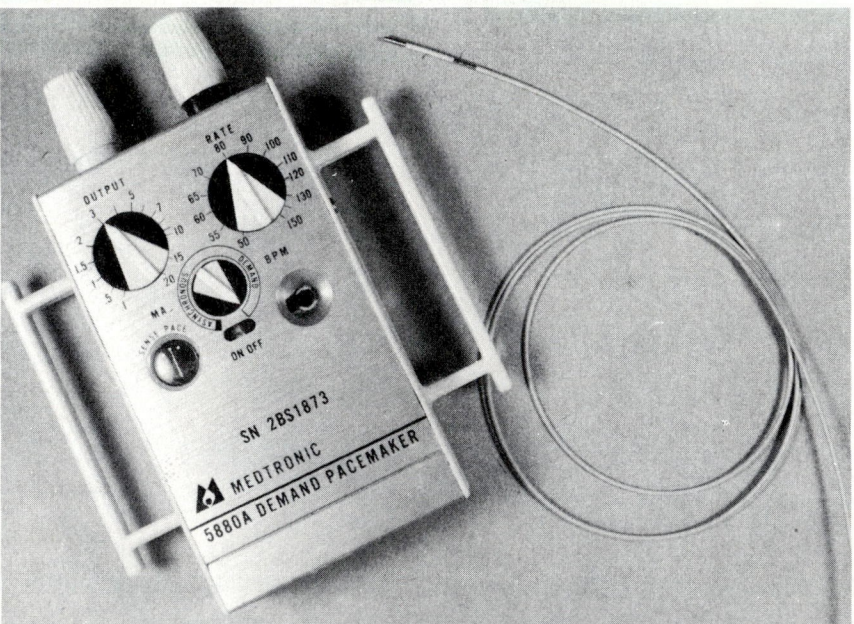

Fig. 25-18   Temporary (external) pacemaker. Pulse generator is battery powered. Electrode is passed into heart before being attached to pulse generator.

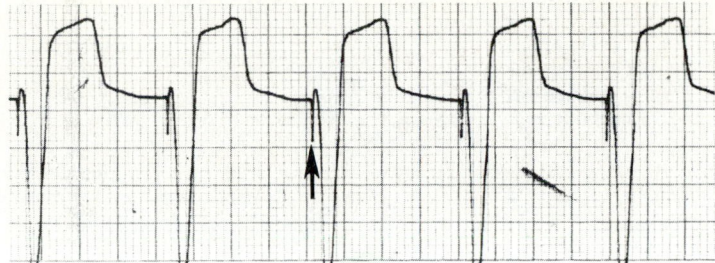

Fig. 25-19   Pacemaker ECG (lead V₁). Rate is 78, rhythm is regular. Pacing stimulus (arrow) followed by QRS. Pacing wire is in ventricle. QRS is wide and bizarre.

☐ **Temporary pacemakers**

Temporary pacemakers are used in the following situations:

1. Emergency treatment of ventricular standstill
2. Short-term treatment of conduction defects causing decreased CO
3. Prophylactic management of persons who are prone to the sudden development of complete heart block

A temporary pacing system is characterized by an *external* pulse generator attached to the distal end of the pacing catheter. The catheter may be advanced through the venous system to make contact with the endocardial surface of the heart, or it may be sutured directly to the epicardial surface. The transvenous approach can be employed at the bedside under ECG guidance or in a special procedure room under fluoroscopy. Direct suturing of the catheter to the epicardium is performed during cardiac or thoracic surgery.

If the patient is connected to a cardiac monitor, the presence of the pacing stimulus (a small vertical spike that indicates that the pulse generator has sent a stimulus to the heart) and evidence that the stimulus actually causes depolarization (either a P wave or a QRS complex immediately following the stimulus, depending on where the catheter has been placed) will be noted (Fig. 25-19).

The pulse generator may be secured to an arm if the antecubital fossa is the insertion site of the pacing catheter. If a subclavian site is used (an approach that has become more common because it leads to greater catheter stability), the pulse generator may be taped to the chest or placed in a chest pocket on specially prepared hospital gowns. Nursing care of patients with temporary pacemakers is summarized in the box below.

☐ **Permanent pacemakers**

Permanent pacemakers are used in the long-term treatment of persistent arrhythmias that are amenable to this type of therapy. The pacing system is totally implanted with the pulse generator generally placed in a subcutaneous "pocket" beneath the clavicle (Fig. 25-20). As with temporary pacing systems, the catheter may be placed in contact with the heart by either the transvenous or epicardial approach.

Permanent pacemakers (Fig. 25-21) are inserted in the operating room or in a special procedure room. The transvenous approach to insertion does not require general an-

---

Nursing care of the patient with a temporary pacemaker

1. Assessment of pacemaker function
   a. Monitor heart rate to verify that it has not dropped below the preset level
   b. If patient is connected to cardiac monitor, monitor presence of pacing stimulus and that a P wave or a QRS complex immediately follows the stimulus
2. Maintenance of system integrity
   a. Ensure that catheter terminals are securely connected to pulse generator
   b. Ensure that pulse generator is attached to person in such a way that accidental dislodgement of the system does not occur
3. Maintenance of patient safety and comfort
   a. Monitor for signs of infection at catheter insertion site
   b. Encourage range of motion in extremity to which pulse generator is attached, as permitted
   c. Ensure that patient avoids contact with any electrical machinery that is not properly grounded
   d. Give simple explanations concerning the purpose of the pacing system and any needed restrictions on activities to prevent anxiety

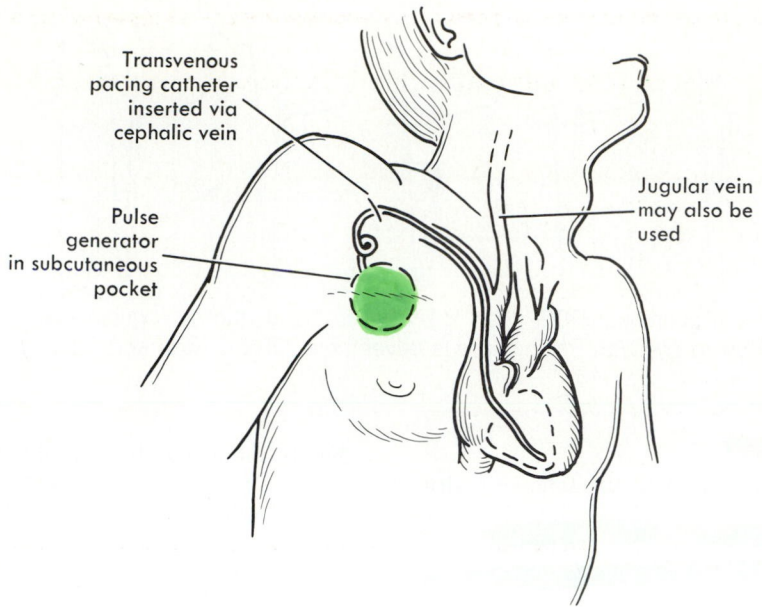

Fig. 25-20 Thoracic placement of a permanent pulse generator (pacemaker) and transvenous pacing catheter.

esthesia, a fact that decreases the risk of this procedure. The generator is powered by a battery that has an expected life of 4 to 6 years. Research is directed toward power sources that may function for 10 or more years.

Manipulation of heart rate and energy output has been difficult at best once the permanent unit was implanted; however, recent technologic advances have resulted in programmable pulse generators that allow variation in both the preset heart rate and the energy output. The latter manipulation has proved useful in reducing battery drain.

Immediate postinsertion care of a person with a permanent pacemaker includes relief of incisional discomfort, monitoring for infection, and assessment of the system's functioning. Attachment of the person to a cardiac monitor for 24 to 48 hours following insertion is the usual practice. Long-term follow-up of these persons is essential and is especially important within the last year of anticipated battery life. Pacemaker clinics have been established to faciliate follow-up, and in some instances, telecommunications systems allow telephone assessment of functioning. Literature published by pacemaker manufacturers and by the American Heart Association can be incorporated into teaching plans (see the box on p. 777) for persons with permanent pacemakers.

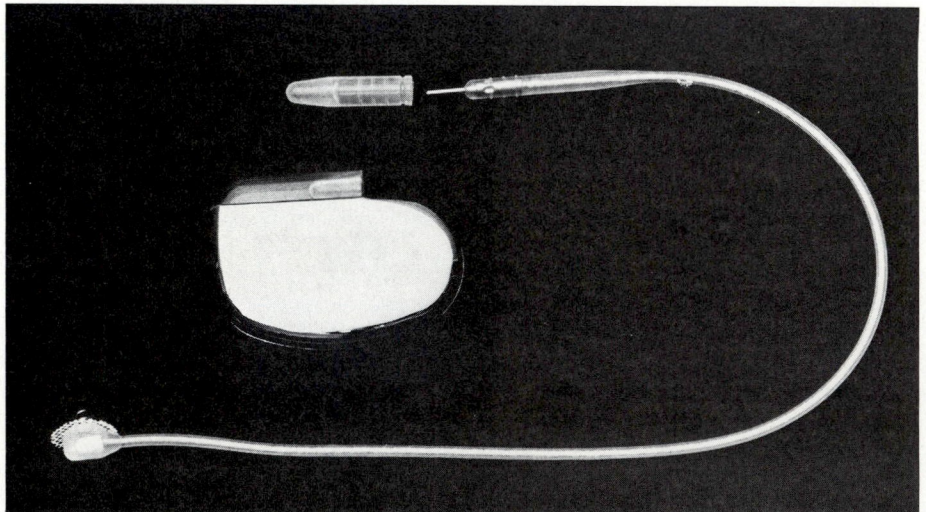

Fig. 25-21 One type of implantable pacemaker (pulse generator) usually implanted subcutaneously in right anterior chest below clavicle.

Teaching for the patient with a permanent pacemaker

1. Rationale for pacemaker insertion
2. Expected outcomes of treatment
3. Monitor pulse daily and report unusual changes to physician
4. Carry out usual physical activity (with avoidance of contact sports)
5. Use only electrical equipment that is in good working order
6. Show pacemaker identification to security officers at airport detector stations; request hand scanner to avoid false activation of metal detector
7. Carry identification card that states:
   a. Type of pacemaker and model number
   b. Heart rate and energy output settings
   c. Manufacturer's name and address
   d. Physician's name and phone number
8. Plan for regular medical follow-up

■ DEFIBRILLATION AND CARDIOVERSION

□ Defibrillation

Defibrillation operates on two electrophysiologic principles. The first is that electricity is a stimulus that can initiate depolarization. The second is that premature discharge of either a normal pacemaker or an ectopic focus can upset its rhythmicity and momentarily suppress its activity. The application of a large amount of electrical energy (400 joules) to the chest wall of a person in ventricular fibrillation allows enough current to reach the heart to cause depolarization of all the cells simultaneously. This serves to suppress the ectopic focus and, it is hoped, allows the SA node to regain control of cardiac electrical activity.

Defibrillation is achieved by placing the paddles from the defibrillator close to the sternum on the upper right chest and just below and lateral to the nipple line on the lower left chest along the "long axis" of the heart) (Fig. 25-22). Either conducting gel or saline-soaked pads (as pictured) must be applied between the paddles and the skin to ensure conductance of the electrical energy. The machine is triggered in such a way that the electrical energy is discharged simultaneously through both paddles.

Failure of defibrillation to achieve the desired results may be caused by profound myocardial ischemia, acidosis, or inadequate functioning of the SA node. Usual practice is to administer a second shock immediately and then proceed with adjunctive therapy if needed. An endotracheal tube is inserted so that adequate oxygenation can be achieved. Sodium bicarbonate is administered intravenously to reverse acidosis, and epinephrine may be used to stimulate the SA node. The American Heart Association Standards for Advanced Life Support serve as a guide for training health professionals to deal with life-threatening arrhythmias such as ventricular fibrillation and as criteria for evaluating their performance.

□ Cardioversion

Cardioversion differs from defibrillation in only one substantial respect. It is a synchronized procedure designed to deliver the electrical energy to the heart at a set time during the cardiac cycle. In brief, once the machine has been discharged, the shock is withheld until the next QRS complex occurs. The purpose of synchronization is to prevent ventricular fibrillation from occurring as the result of

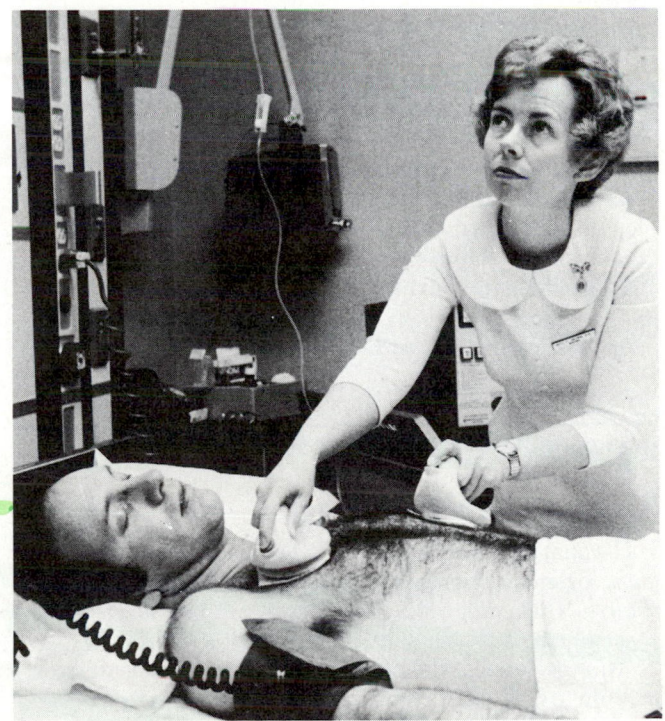

Fig. 25-22   Nurse defibrillating patient.

an improperly timed electrical stimulus. It is clear that cardioversion is *never* used to terminate ventricular fibrillation, since there are no QRS complexes to trigger the release of the electrical energy.

Cardioversion is largely an elective procedure that requires the person's consent. Exceptions would be made if the patient's clinical condition were deteriorating too rapidly to obtain consent. Premedication is given to allay the anxiety that naturally accompanies the thought of enduring an "electric shock." Diazepam (Valium) is frequently administered intravenously for this purpose because of its muscle relaxant and amnesic properties. An oral airway, oxygen, and emergency drugs should be available during this procedure.

Major health problems of the heart

Alterations in cardiovascular structure or function affect circulation and may therefore be life threatening. Disease of the heart and major blood vessels may be classified in a variety of ways such as congenital versus acquired, identification of the structure involved (valvular heart disease, myocarditis, endocarditis), etiology of the disease (inadequate coronary artery blood flow, hypertensive cardiovascular disease, rheumatic heart disease), disruption of cardiac physiology (arrhythmias), and disruption of cardiac function (heart failure, cardiogenic shock). The following common cardiac and aortic disorders are discussed in this chapter:

1. Interference with coronary blood flow: coronary artery disease (angina pectoris, myocardial infarction)
2. Failure of the heart as a pump: congestive heart failure, cardiogenic shock
3. Diseases of specific portions of the cardiac tissue: pericarditis, myocarditis, endocarditis
4. Diseases that are secondary to other diseases or conditions: cardiovascular syphilis, alcoholic cardiomyopathy, rheumatic heart disease
5. Inadequate valvular functioning: stenosis or insufficiency
6. Weakening of aortic wall: aortic aneurysms

■ CORONARY ARTERY DISEASE

■ Pathophysiology

Coronary artery disease (CAD) refers to a variety of pathologic conditions that obstruct blood flow through the arteries that supply the heart (see the box above). Atherosclerosis is the most common etiologic factor.

Atherosclerosis, the predominant type of arteriosclerosis in humans, is characterized by the accumulation of fatty materials (lipids) and fibrous tissue within the arterial walls. As these atherosclerotic changes progress, the lumen

---

Conditions that obstruct coronary blood supply

Atherosclerosis
Arteriosclerosis
Arteritis
Coronary artery spasms
Coronary thrombosis
Embolism

---

of the vessel becomes narrowed and blood flow is obstructed to those areas of the myocardium supplied by the artery. Since this is a form of arteriosclerosis, the arterial wall also loses its elasticity and becomes less responsive to changes in blood volume and pressure.

Although several theories have been postulated to explain the pathogenesis of atherosclerosis, the etiology of this condition remains unclear. Atherosclerotic lesions usually develop near the origin and bifurcation of the main coronary arteries (see Fig. 25-2). The left coronary artery is more often affected than the right coronary artery. The disease process is initially localized but then becomes diffuse with advancing coronary atherosclerosis.

The first lesion to form within the coronary arterial wall is called a fatty streak (Fig. 25-23). This lesion begins to appear in coronary vessels as early as 15 years of age. Lipid-filled cells or "foam cells" invade the intimal wall and produce a fatty streak. As the disease progresses, raised thick fibrous plaques form and with increasing size limit

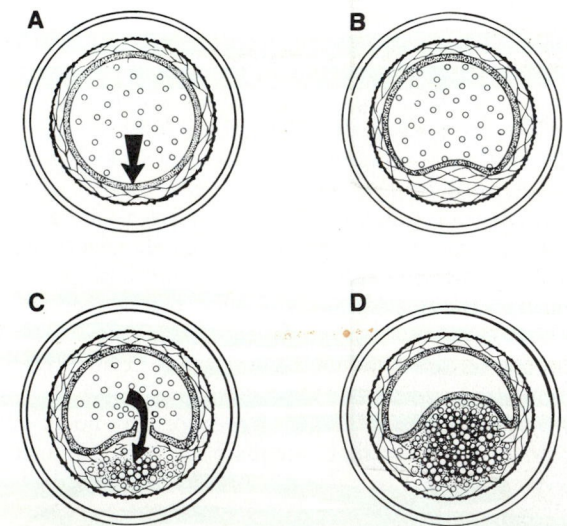

Fig. 25-23 Progressive development of coronary atherosclerosis. **A,** Injury to intimal wall. **B,** Lipoprotein invasion of smooth muscle cells. **C,** Development of fatty streak and fibrous plaque. **D,** Development of complicated lesion.

the luminal capacity of the vessel. These lesions are typically characteristic of advancing atherosclerosis.

An even more advanced stage of atherosclerosis is represented by a calcified fibrous plaque or complicated lesion. This calcified deposit can rupture and hence greatly increase the risk of spasm, thrombus formation, and embolization. It is this final type of atherosclerotic lesion that gives rise to the symptoms of CAD. The arterial lumen becomes so narrowed that a great imbalance exists between myocardial oxygen supply and myocardial oxygen demand. Manifestations of myocardial ischemia do not usually occur until the artery is about 75% occluded. They include the following:

1. Angina pectoris
2. Myocardial infarction
3. Sudden death

■ RISK FACTORS

The result of extensive clinical research has led to the identification of several contributing factors that place an individual at risk for the development of coronary artery disease. The cummulative effect of these risk factors accelerates the atherosclerotic process. Risk factors are grouped into two basic categories: those that cannot be altered by the individual (nonmodifiable) and those that the individual has the capacity to change (modifiable).

□ Nonmodifiable risk factors
□ Age

Both morbidity and mortality of coronary artery disease increase with age. Clinical symptomatology may be seen as early as the second decade of life, but the incidence of CAD steadily rises in the 30- to 50-year age group. About 55% of all heart attack victims are age 65 or older, and of those who die, almost four out of five are over 65.[2] Although

---

Risk factors for coronary artery disease

Nonmodifiable risk factors

Age
Sex
Race
Family history

Modifiable risk factors

Cigarette smoking
Hyperlipidemia
Diabetes mellitus
Hypertension
Obesity
Lack of exercise
Stress
Oral contraceptives

---

improvements in diet and reduction of other risk factors may alter this trend in the aged of the future, most persons in this risk category today are a reflection of yesterday's poor health practices.[22]

□ Sex

Men are at a greater risk for the development of CAD. Women are usually not affected by this disease until after menopause. The postmenopausal increase has been attributed to decreased levels of estrogens and rising blood lipids.

□ Race

Black Americans have a higher risk for CAD than do whites. One possible explanation for this finding is their increased incidence of hypertension (33% higher than in the white population).[2]

□ Family history

A familial tendency toward the development of CAD has been demonstrated. The presence of coronary atherosclerosis in a parent or sibling under 50 years old is associated with the same finding in another family member. The extent to which genetic and environmental factors contribute to this disorder, however, is still not known.

□ Modifiable risk factors
□ Cigarette smoking

Cigarette smoking is a major contributing factor of CAD. Cigarette smokers have a two to three times greater risk of death from CAD than nonsmokers. This risk is related to the number of cigarettes smoked per day; the more cigarettes smoked, the greater the risk. Individuals who quit smoking are at less risk than smokers.

Although the exact relationship between cigarette smoking and coronary atherosclerosis is unclear, it is thought to be associated with the effects of nicotine and the higher content of carbon monoxide produced by the smoker. Nicotine increases myocardial workload and subsequent oxygen demand. Carbon monoxide interferes with oxygen transport. The combination of these two factors may place an inordinate demand on a diseased heart.

□ Hyperlipidemia

Hyperlipidemia refers to the elevation of cholesterol and triglyceride levels within the blood. Cholesterol can be obtained directly from dietary sources or manufactured by the liver and intestine. Triglycerides are derived from fatty acids found in adipose tissue or the diet. Cholesterol and triglycerides are involved in the transportation, digestion, and absorption of fats.

Individuals with cholesterol levels in excess of 300 ml/dl have four times the risk of CAD of those with levels less than 200 mg/dl. There is also clinical evidence that high levels of a specific type of lipid-protein complex, the *low-density lipoproteins,* are indicative of CAD. These lipoproteins transport plasma lipids and contain approximately 50% cholesterol. In contrast, the high-density lipoproteins are thought to have an antiatherogenic effect.

A diet high in saturated fat, cholesterol, and calories is

thought to be a major factor in the development of hyperlipidemia. Dietary management, therefore, is an essential component in the prevention of this risk factor. Changes in long-established dietary patterns do not come easily, however. Awareness of the link between diet and the development of CAD is frequently not sufficient motivation for modifications in diet that require a great deal of determination and creativity.

□ Diabetes mellitus

Individuals with diabetes mellitus are at much greater risk for CAD. Coronary atherosclerosis has been found to be two to three times more prevalent in persons with diabetes, regardless of blood lipid levels. The mechanisms by which impaired glucose tolerance increases the risk for CAD is unclear. A predisposition to vascular degeneration has been noted in diabetics, and abnormal lipid metabolism may also play a role in the development of atheromas.[54] Adherence to a prescribed medical regimen for glucose regulation may diminish the effect of this risk factor and is within the realm of individual responsibility.

□ Hypertension

The relationship between high blood pressure and CAD has been attributed to acceleration of the process that results in coronary atherosclerosis. In addition, increased peripheral vascular resistance associated with hypertension increases afterload and the demand on the left ventricle. The result is an increased demand for myocardial oxygen in the face of a diminished supply. The effects of hypertension are potentially modifiable through adherence to a medical regimen for control of systolic and diastolic blood pressure.

□ Obesity

Obesity or excess body weight in relation to height increases the workload and hence the oxygen demand of the heart. Its effect as a risk factor is questionable, although obesity highly correlates with hypertension, hyperlipidemia, and diabetes. Specifically, obesity tends to be associated with increased caloric intake and elevated levels of low-density lipoproteins.

□ Lack of exercise

The lack of exercise has not been clearly linked to CAD. It has been demonstrated, however, that exercise can improve the efficiency of the heart by the reduction of heart rate and blood pressure. Other physiologic effects of regular exercise, such as decreased levels of low-density lipoproteins, lowered blood glucose levels, and improved cardiac output, have been associated with a lesser chance of CAD.[14] The psychologic benefits of exercise, reduced anxiety and depression, may also be of significance.

□ Stress

The effect of stress on the pathogenesis of CAD is controversial. Stress stimulates the cardiovascular system by the release of catecholamines, which in turn increase the heart rate and produce vasoconstriction. Stress also plays a major role in those individuals with type A behavior.

Behaviors including ambitiousness, aggressiveness, competitiveness, impatience, muscle tenseness, vigorous speech, and rapid pace in all activities are indicative of the type A behavior pattern.[15] These individuals are by virtue of their stressful life-style more likely to develop CAD.

□ Oral contraceptives

The use of oral contraceptives or birth control pills has been associated with an increased risk of CAD. The nature of the association is not clearly understood. It is possible that this risk factor acts synergistically with others.

■ Angina pectoris

■ PATHOPHYSIOLOGY

Angina pectoris or chest pain is a clinical syndrome produced by insufficient coronary blood flow. An imbalance exists between myocardial oxygen supply and myocardial oxygen demand, which creates transient myocardial ischemia. The underlying mechanism to account for the experience of pain is probably related to the change from aerobic to anaerobic metabolism. By-products from anaerobic metabolism, specifically lactic acid, may initiate sensory receptors and cause pain. The release of other substances from the ischemic cells may also produce pain in this manner. Since the basic problem in angina is an imbalance between oxygen supply and demand, the primary goals of therapy are directed to the restoration of this balance (Table 25-4).

Two subcategories of angina should be distinguished from the classic condition. These are unstable angina and variant angina. A brief description of these forms of angina is presented here. For further information, consult a cardiology text.

□ Unstable angina

Unstable angina is also referred to as preinfarction angina, crescendo angina, or intermittent coronary syndrome. This type of angina is characterized by an increase in the severity, frequency, or duration of symptoms without infarction.

□ Variant angina

Variant angina, or Prinzmetal's angina, is thought to develop from intermittent coronary artery spasm with or without atherosclerotic heart disease. This type of anginal pain can occur during normal activities and is not necessarily precipitated by exercise or stress. Anginal pain in this condition often develops at the same time of day or night, demonstrating a cyclic pattern. Some persons with variant angina may also have typical exertional angina.

■ ASSESSMENT

□ Subjective data

Data are collected concerning the person's knowledge about the disorder, presence of risk factors, and perception of the anginal pain. Specific data related to pain include the following:

Table 25-4   Coronary artery disorders

Disorder	Etiology	Signs and symptoms	Therapy
Angina pectoris	Atherosclerosis Coronary artery spasm Severe anemia Arteritis Aortic insufficiency	Chest pain (substernal, retrosternal), may radiate to neck, jaw, arm, back; usually brought on by exertion, emotional upsets; relieved by rest, nitroglycerine	Avoidance of precipitating factors Reduction of modifiable risk factors Medications: nitrates, beta-adrenergic blocking agents, calcium channel blockers Oxygen therapy ECG monitoring
Myocardial infarction	Atherosclerotic progression Coronary thrombosis Prolonged constriction of coronary arteries	Severe, crushing chest pain; may radiate as with angina; not relieved with rest, nitroglycerine May be associated with dyspnea, diaphoresis, apprehension, nausea	Relief of pain (O_2, morphine, other analgesics) ECG monitoring Reduction of O_2 demand (rest) Prevention of complications (stool softeners, anticoagulants) Treatment of complications (arrhythmias, CHF)

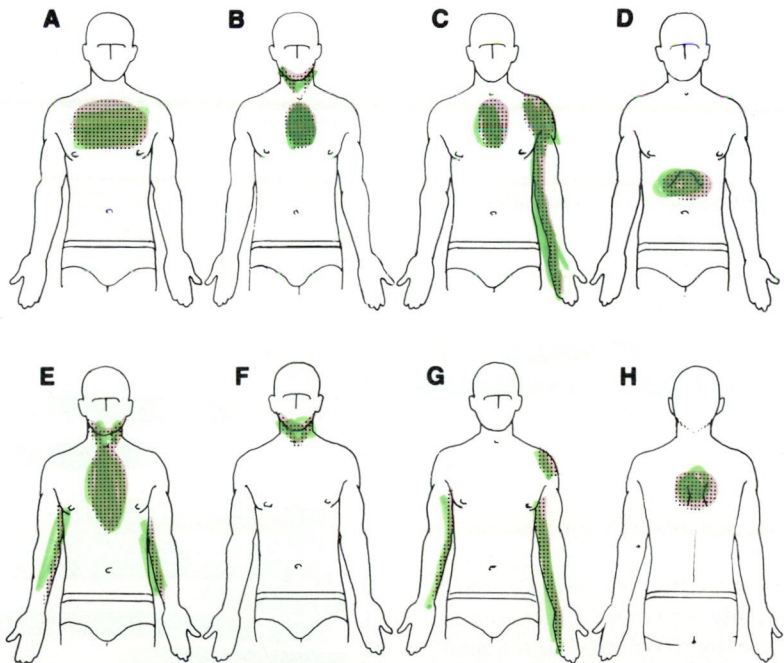

Fig. 25-24   Sites where ischemic myocardial pain may be referred. **A,** Upper chest. **B,** Beneath sternum radiating to neck and jaw. **C,** Beneath sternum radiating down left arm. **D,** Epigastric. **E,** Epigastric radiating to neck, jaw, and arms. **F,** Neck and jaw. **G,** Left shoulder, inner aspect of both arms. **H,** Intrascapular.

1. Location and radiation to other sites: the pain is most often substernal or retrosternal. Pain may radiate to other sites (Fig. 25-24) or may occur *only* in one of those sites.
2. Quality of the pain: the pain is frequently described as a tightness or heaviness in the chest. Pressure, or a squeezing sensation may also be part of the description. The person may complain only of a vague discomfort that is sometimes misinterpreted as indigestion. Angina is *not* usually described as a "sharp" pain.
3. Onset and duration of the pain: usually of brief duration.
4. Precipitating factors: often identified as exertion, exposure to extreme hot or cold, stress or emotional upset, or a heavy meal. *No* precipitating factor may be identified with variant angina.
5. Associated symptoms: apprehension, nausea, diaphoresis may be noted but are not common.
6. Relieving factors: angina is usually relieved by rest and/or nitroglycerin.

The nurse should be especially alert to reports of *change* in the frequency, severity, precipitating factors, or duration of anginal attacks.

☐ Objective data

1. Patient behavior: note presence of diaphoresis, apprehension. Persons with angina are sometimes seen pressing a fist against the sternum during an attack.
2. Changes in vital signs: increases in pulse rate, blood pressure, and respiratory rate may be noted.
3. Changes in cardiac rhythm.
4. Pattern of anginal attacks with particular attention to changes.

☐ Diagnostic tests

The diagnosis of ischemic heart disease is frequently made on the basis of the patient's history. Diagnosis of angina may also be facilitated by electrocardiogram (ECG) (p. 761), Holter monitor, coronary angiography, and stress testing.

☐ *Electrocardiogram*

Characteristic findings of ischemia, S-T segment depression, and T wave inversion may be seen during chest pain. The absence of ECG changes does not exclude the diagnosis of ischemia.

☐ *Holter monitor*

A Holter monitor is a small portable ECG monitor about the size of a large transistor radio. In nonacute situations, a patient can be connected to this monitor to evaluate chest pain during performance of daily activities. Two wires are attached to the patient's chest and connected to the monitor. The monitor is then worn for 24 hours, during which time the ECG tracing is recorded on tape and the patient maintains a log of daily activities, medications, and unusual sensations. The log is then compared with the corresponding segment of the ECG tracing.

Indications for stress testing

Evaluate symptoms of CAD.
Determine physical work capacity and aerobic capacity.
Determine functional capacity following a myocardial infarction.
Determine limitations for exercise programming.
Evaluate arrythmias that develop during exercise.
Screen patients over age 40 and at risk for CAD.
Evalute effect of pharmacologic agents on arrhythmias and angina.

☐ *Coronary angiography*

Selective coronary angiography may be carried out as part of a catheterization of the left side of the heart. Injection of contrast medium into the coronary arteries is followed by cineangiographic films to monitor the progression of the "dye." The contrast medium outlines the entire coronary circulation and enables the examiner to evaluate the anatomy of the coronary arteries, as well as note the location and nature of any lesions (that is, areas in which the arteries are narrowed or obstructed) and the presence of collateral circulation.

☐ *Stress testing*

Stress testing or exercise electrocardiography is a noninvasive test used to evaluate cardiovascular response to controlled physical work loads. The indications for performing a stress test are identifed in the box above.

During stress testing, the patient pedals a stationary bicycle or walks on a treadmill. Throughout the testing, the patient's blood pressure and ECG are recorded. Conditions that require termination of the testing are listed in

---

Conditions requiring termination of stress testing

Ventricular tachycardia
Marked decrease in peak systolic blood pressure
Marked decrease in heart rate
Vertigo
Frequent premature ventricular beats
Anginal pain
Severe dyspnea
Severe anxiety
Diagnostic ST segment depression on ECG

the box on p. 782. The risk of developing a myocardial infarction is less than 1 in 500; the risk of death is less than 1 in 10,000.[10]

Adequate patient preparation is extremely important. The patient should do the following:

1. Get adequate rest the night before the test
2. Avoid coffee, tea, and alcohol the day of the test
3. Avoid smoking and taking nitroglycerin during the 2-hour period immediately before the test
4. Eat a light breakfast or lunch at least 2 hours before the test
5. Wear comfortable, loose-fitting clothes; women need to wear a bra for support
6. Wear sturdy, comfortable walking shoes
7. Consult with the physician regarding the taking of medications before the test (Digoxin, propranolol, and vasodilators may affect the results of the stress test)
8. Inform the physician if any unusual sensations develop during the test (for example, chest pain, dizziness)
9. Rest after the test; do *not* take a hot shower; a warm bath 1 or 2 hours after the test is permitted

▶ DATA ANALYSIS: NURSING DIAGNOSES

Nursing diagnoses are determined from assessment of patient data. Possible nursing diagnoses for the person with angina may include, but are not limited to, the following:

Diagnostic title	Possible etiologies
Activity intolerance	Imbalance between oxygen supply and demand
Anxiety	Change in health status, diagnosis of pathology involving a major organ, threat to self-concept
Knowledge deficit: CAD risk factors, strategies to minimize symptoms, treatment regimen, diagnostic tests	Lack of exposure/recall, information misinterpretation, unfamiliarity with information resources
Pain: chest	Myocardial ischemia

▣ PLANNING: EXPECTED PATIENT OUTCOMES

Expected patient outcomes for the person with angina may include, but are not limited to the following:

1. Patient can describe the purpose, rationale, and preparation for diagnostic testing.
2. Patient can plan activity to balance myocardial oxygen demands with supply.
3. Patient can describe events that may precipitate anginal attacks and can state plans for avoidance of such events.

4. Patient can identify CAD risk factors present in own situation.
5. Patient can describe the prescribed medication regimen.
6. Signs and symptoms of anxiety are decreased.
7. Patient indicates plans for medical follow-up.

▦ IMPLEMENTATION

☐ Assisting with achievement of therapeutic goals

1. Administer medications as prescribed. If angina is present, give nitroglycerin sublingually. Repeat dosage in 5 minutes if pain does not subside. Repeat two or three times at 5-minute intervals.
2. Monitor for arrhythmias.
3. Administer oxygen per nasal cannula as prescribed.
4. Monitor effects of daily activities on cardiac status; occurrence of arrhythmias and need for oxygen.

☐ Assisting with comfort

1. Provide rest periods if fatigue present during daily activities

☐ Counseling and teaching

Measures are taken to reduce the increased myocardial demands for oxygen because of stress. Activities include the following:

1. Provide a calm environment to decrease stress and anxiety
2. Encourage expression of concerns regarding diagnosis, diagnostic tests, and prescribed changes in lifestyle

A major nursing intervention is teaching the patient about the following (see the box on p. 784):

1. Prescribed medications (see below)
2. Measures to minimize precipitating events (exertion, stress, overeating, exposure to cold or hot, humid conditions)
3. Effects of exercise on reduction of myocardial oxygen needs

☐ *Effect of medications*

Nitrates (nitroglycerin [Nitro-bid, Transderm], isosorbide) are given to dilate coronary arteries and collateral vessels of the heart and to dilate peripheral vessels, especially the veins. Specific patient instructions for taking nitrates are listed in the box on p. 784.

Beta (β) adrenergic blocking agents (propranolol, nadolol) lower oxygen demands during exercise and improve the oxygen supply/demand balance. They lower heart rate and blood pressure. Beta blockers should be withdrawn gradually.

Calcium channel blockers (nifedipine, diltiazem, verapamil) decrease the work load of the heart. They decrease heart rate and improve oxygen supply by dilating coronary arteries.

Teaching for the patient with angina pectoris

1. Use of nitrate medications
   a. Use nitroglycerin prophylactically to avoid pain known to occur with certain activities
   b. Burning sensation on tongue indicates nitroglycerin is activated
   c. Throbbing sensation in head and flushing may be felt
   d. Sit and stand slowly after taking nitroglycerin
   e. Place nitroglycerin tablets under the tongue at the onset of anginal pain; second tablet can be taken after 5 min and third tablet after another 5 min if pain is unrelieved
   f. Call physician if pain does not subside after third nitroglycerin tablet; go to nearest emergency department; do not drive yourself
   g. Always carry nitroglycerin
   h. Store nitroglycerin in dark bottle and keep in dry place
   i. Replenish nitroglycerin supply every 6 months or before expiration date
   j. Remove all old nitrate ointment just before application of new cream
2. Ways to minimize precipitating events
   a. Avoid overexertion
   b. Try to reduce stress and anxiety, which cause blood vessels to constrict
   c. Avoid overeating, as it places an increased work load on the heart
   d. Avoid cold weather (constricts coronary vessels to conserve body heat, hence anginal pain can develop more easily)
   e. Dress warmly in cold weather
   f. Avoid hot, humid conditions (increases work load of heart)
   g. Walk downhill and with wind since walking uphill and against wind increase work load of heart
3. Effects of exercise program in reduction of myocardial oxygen needs
   a. Engage in regular exercise program
   b. Exercise conditions heart muscle and can decrease oxygen demand during exercise
   c. Space exercise period with rest periods
   d. Take nitroglycerin before exertion
4. Need for regular medical follow-up

⊞ EVALUATION

Evaluation will be based on expected patient outcomes. Questions to ask may include the following:

1. Is patient able to control pain by use of prescribed medication?
2. Does the patient know action, usage, and side effects of prescribed medications?
3. Can patient describe ways to minimize events that may precipitate anginal pain?
4. Is patient engaged or planning to engage in a regular exercise program?
5. Does the patient know CAD risk factors that can be modified?

■ Myocardial infarction

■ PATHOPHYSIOLOGY

Myocardial infarction is a sudden complete blockage within a major coronary artery or one of its branches. The extent of myocardial damage is variable and depends on the size of the area perfused by the blocked artery. A myocardial infarction can cause necrosis with subsequent scar formation or fibrosis, or it can cause sudden death.

Prolonged ischemia lasting more than 35 to 45 minutes produces irreversible cellular damage and necrosis. The contractile properties of cardiac muscle within the necrotic areas become permanently impaired (Fig. 25-25). The final extent of the infarct is dependent on the ability of the surrounding ischemic tissues to recruit collateral circulation. Collateral circulation is the inherent development of new vessels within the heart to compensate for the damaged artery.

The clinical features of a myocardial infarct are determined by the site and extent of the disease process. An occlusion in the *left anterior descending* coronary artery (LAD) typically results in an *anterior wall infarction*. Depending on the exact site of the occlusion, the area involved may be limited or massive. Substantial loss of left ventricular muscle mass is associated with severe hemodynamic consequences.

An occlusion in the *right* coronary artery (RCA) may result in an *inferior* or *posterior* wall infarction. Although the loss of muscle mass may not be as extensive as in anterior infarctions, the person with an inferior infarction may be predisposed to arrhythmias and conduction defects

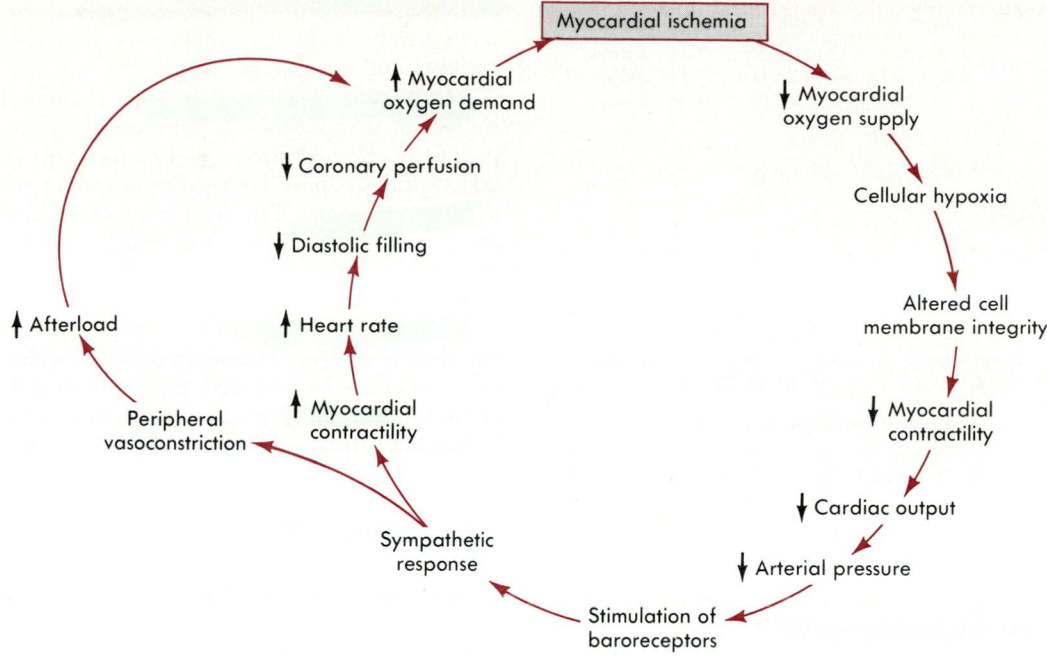

Fig. 25-25 Effects of prolonged myocardial ischemia.

because of the proximity of the RCA to the conduction system. A lateral wall infarction is usually caused by an occlusion of the *left circumflex* coronary artery. The etiology, signs, and symptoms, and medical therapies to curtail the complications of myocardial infarction are outlined in Table 25-4 (p. 781).

▦ ASSESSMENT

☐ Subjective data

Myocardial infarction can be equated with irreversible myocardial ischemia; hence many of the associated signs and symptoms are similar to those found with angina. Typically the symptoms are more severe and of longer duration than the person's usual angina attacks, although they may occur in a person who has never previously complained of angina. Symptoms are either absent or unreported in about 15% of all myocardial infarctions. Data to be collected include the following:

1. Patient's perception of the pain
   a. Location and radiation to other sites (Fig. 25-24)
   b. Quality of the pain: often described as crushing or viselike; often more severe than angina
   c. Onset and duration of pain: may be of sudden onset or may build up over a period of a few minutes; duration is longer than angina—may be several minutes to several hours
   d. Precipitating factors: often occurs with intense emotion or exertion but may also occur at rest
   e. Relieving factors: not relieved by rest, nitroglycerin, changes in body position
2. Associated symptoms: may include nausea, dyspnea, dizziness, weakness, and a sense of impending doom

☐ Objective data

1. Behavior: often very apprehensive
2. Changes in vital signs: pulse rate may increase in response to pain or diminished cardiac output; may decrease if conduction defects develop; blood pressure may decrease if the extent of myocardial damage is significant
3. Associated signs: may include diaphoresis, vomiting, pallor, cold clammy skin, cardiac arrhythmias, labored respirations
4. Breath sounds: no change may be noted, but if pulmonary edema develops, rales will be present
5. Presence of risk factors

☐ Diagnostic tests

Although the clinical picture of severe crushing chest pain, pallor, diaphoresis, and apprehension or a sense of impending doom is the classic description of a person having a myocardial infarction, it by no means describes *all* infarction patients. About 15% of myocardial infarctions occur without the characteristic signs and symptoms (called "silent infarctions") and individual variation in the symptoms is to be expected. A variety of diagnostic tests are used, therefore, to verify the diagnosis. These tests include blood tests that detect both nonspecific and specific changes caused by the infarction, ECG, and other procedures such as radionuclide imaging.

☐ *Blood tests*

A nonspecific reaction to myocardial injury is an elevation in white blood cell count (12,000 to 15,000/mm³). This increase begins a few hours after the onset of pain and lasts for 3 to 7 days. In general, high white blood cell

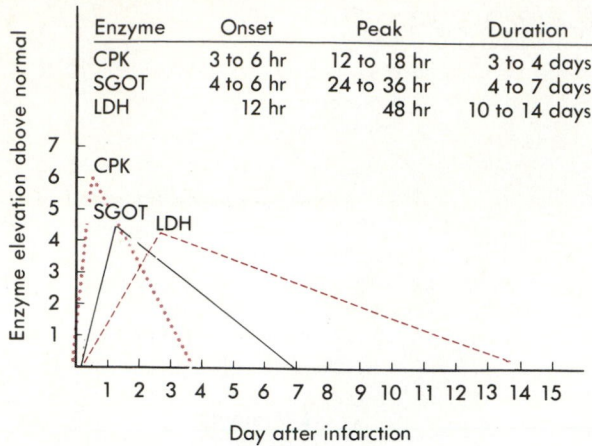

Enzyme	Onset	Peak	Duration
CPK	3 to 6 hr	12 to 18 hr	3 to 4 days
SGOT	4 to 6 hr	24 to 36 hr	4 to 7 days
LDH	12 hr	48 hr	10 to 14 days

Fig. 25-26   Patterns of serum enzyme levels following myocardial infarction.

counts are associated with larger infarcts. Also, the erythrocyte sedimentation rate (ESR) rises during the first week after the infarction and remains elevated for several weeks.

SERUM ENZYMES. As infarcted cardiac muscle cells die, cellular components are released into the vascular system. Some of these components are enzymes that can be evaluated by blood levels. Creatine phosphokinase (CPK), serum glutamic-oxaloacetic transaminase (SGOT) (also termed serum aspartate amino-transferase [AST]) and lactic dehydrogenase (LDH) are found to be elevated at varying times following a myocardial infarction (Fig. 25-26).

Since these enzymes are not exclusively found in the heart, measurements of enzyme fractions or *isoenzymes* are more diagnostic of myocardial insult. Isoenzymes levels of CPK are the most reliable indicators of cardiac damage. The CPK isoenzyme that contains the MB subunits, $CPK(MB)_1$, is elevated for 48 hours after a transmural infarction. LDH can be fractionated into five distinct isoenzymes. Of these, LDH_1 and LDH_2 are most important. LDH_2 is found more abundantly in serum, whereas heart muscle is rich in LDH_1. An elevation in serum LDH_1, therefore, is confirmation of a myocardial infarction.

Electrocardiogram

Characteristic findings of infarction include ST segment elevation in leads overlying the infarcted area (an early finding) and the development of pathologic Q waves (a later finding). As the infarction "evolves," the ST segments return to baseline and the T waves become inverted. The electrocardiogram is considered to be one of the most reliable tools for diagnosing a myocardial infarction, but occasionally the "typical" changes do not develop, and serum enzymes must be relied upon to a greater extent.

Radionuclide imaging

Radionuclide imaging is a noninvasive procedure that aids in evaluating the myocardium and coronary arteries. The two most commonly used techniques are pyrophos-

phate scanning and thallium scanning. Even though these scans involve radioactive materials, they are safe for both patients and hospital personnel.

PYROPHOSPHATE SCANNING. A radionuclide, technetium-99m pyrophosphate, is injected intravenously. The patient is scanned after 2 to 3 hours. This radionuclide is actively taken up by damaged myocardial tissue, producing a "hot spot" image. The scan takes 15 minutes to complete and is not painful. The scan will be negative during the first 12 hours after an infarction. Peak activity is evidenced at 36 hours.

THALLIUM SCANNING. Thallium-201 is an intracellular ion that is actively transported into normal cells. If the cell is ischemic or infarcted, the thallium will not be picked up and a "cold spot" image is produced. This radioisotope is injected intravenously with the patient at rest or during stress testing.

■ MEDICAL THERAPY

Medical therapy for the person with a myocardial infarction has traditionally been directed toward prevention of complications when possible. When complications are inevitable, the therapeutic aims are early detection and control. Healing of the myocardium is a natural process that is promoted by rest and reduction of myocardial oxygen demands. The trend toward early ambulation under carefully monitored conditions has reduced the incidence of complications, such as thromboembolic phenomena and psychologic manifestations of depression and hopelessness, that were largely related to a prolonged period of immobility.

In recent years, considerable attention has been directed toward therapies that limit the size of the infarcted area. One approach to this goal is reperfusion of the occluded coronary artery. To be effective, reperfusion must be attained within 3 to 5 hours following the onset of symptoms. Administration of fibrinolytic agents either systemically or directly into the coronary arteries activates mechanisms that lyse existing blood clots. Streptokinase, urokinase, and tissue plasminogen activator are currently used in reperfusion therapy. The use of laser angioplasty may also promote reperfusion and has the advantage of acting locally rather than initiating a more widespread fibrinolytic response.[54,57,60]

➡ DATA ANALYSIS: NURSING DIAGNOSES

Nursing diagnoses are determined from assessment of patient data. Possible nursing diagnoses for the person with myocardial infarction may include, but are not limited to, the following:

Diagnostic title	Possible etiologies
Activity intolerance	Imbalance between oxygen supply and demand
	Immobility in postinfarction period
Impaired adjustment	Disability requiring change in life-style, assault to self-esteem

Diagnostic title	Possible etiologies
Anxiety	Change in health status, threat of death, threat to self-concept situational crisis
Body image disturbance	Loss (or perceived loss) of body function, change in life-style
Constipation	Immobility in postinfarction period, opiate pain medications, possible reduced fluid intake, lack of privacy
Ineffective family coping: compromised	Inadequate information concerning CCU, patient, and other matters, situational crisis, need for role changes
Anticipatory grieving	Potential change in role(s), lifestyle
Knowledge deficit: CAD risk factors, diagnostic tests, pathophysiology of MI, treatment regimen, community resources for rehabilitation	Lack of exposure/recall, information misinterpretation, unfamiliarity with information resources
Pain: chest	Persistent myocardial ischemia
Self-care deficit	Intolerance of activity, fatigue, pain/discomfort, need for rest
Sexual dysfunction	Actual or perceived physiologic limitations, lack of knowledge of alternatives, fear

PLANNING: EXPECTED PATIENT OUTCOMES

Expected outcomes for the person with myocardial infarction may include, but are not limited to, the following:

1. Patient can describe the purpose, rationale, and preparation for diagnostic testing.
2. Patient can describe the nature of myocardial infarction and how the healing process relates to the treatment regimen.
3. Patient can plan activities to minimize frequency and severity of ischemic episodes (if any) in the postinfarction period.
4. Patient can identify CAD risk factors present in own situation.
5. Patient can describe the prescribed medication regimen and other measures necessary to reduce risk for additional infarctions.
6. Patient participates in a program of progressive activity.
7. Patient can describe plans for continuation of progressive activity and resumption of sexual activity (if appropriate).
8. Patient states plans for ongoing medical care and rehabilitation.
9. Other outcomes related specifically to the documented presence of nursing diagnoses listed previously.

IMPLEMENTATION

☐ **Assisting with achievement of therapeutic goals**

1. Administer medications as prescribed:
   a. Intravenous lidocaine is usually given prophylactically to prevent ventricular fibrillation
   b. Anticoagulants (heparin or coumadin) may be prescribed to decrease incidence of thrombophlebitis and pulmonary embolism
   c. *Avoid giving intramuscular injections* since these alter serum enzyme levels
2. Administer oxygen via nasal cannula to correct ventilation-perfusion abnormalities during the initial 24 to 48 hours; maintain oxygen therapy with persistent pain, hypotension, dyspnea, or arrhythmias
3. Monitor for cardiac arrhythmias (for example, premature ventricular beats, ventricular fibrillation)
4. Monitor for signs of other complications of myocardial infarction (See relevant sections in this chapter for an expanded discussion of these conditions.):
   a. Congestive heart failure (rales, tachycardia and tachypnea, dyspnea and increased respiratory effort, S_3 heart sound, weight gain, oliguria)
   b. Thromboembolic phenomena
   c. Pericarditis
   d. Mitral insufficiency
   e. Cardiogenic shock (decreased blood pressure, tachycardia, cold clammy skin, mental confusion, severe oliguria)
5. Maintain patient on prescribed low-cholesterol, low-salt diet without caffeine-containing beverages
6. Administer stool softener to prevent constipation effects of opiates and decreased mobility and to prevent Valsalva maneuver (see Chapter 31) when straining at stool
7. Maintain patient on prescribed bed rest for 24 to 48 hours; encourage progressive ambulation when permitted

☐ **Assisting with comfort**

1. Administer morphine intravenously to relieve pain and apprehension and to produce vasodilation
2. Administer prescribed tranquilizer (for example, diazepam [Valium]) to decrease anxiety and restlessness
3. Administer prescribed sleeping pill to promote sleep
4. Provide a calm environment
5. Answer patient's and family member's questions
6. Provide explanations for necessary monitoring and diagnostic tests
7. Plan patient care activites to minimize interruptions in rest

☐ **Counseling and teaching**

Education of the patient and family enables them to assume a more active role in the patient's health care. A great deal of anxiety and apprehension can be allayed by providing information about the cardiac condition and its management. Major points for teaching are outlined in the box on p. 788.

During the hospitalization, many patients experience

Teaching for the patient with a myocardial infarction

1. Effect of myocardial infarction, the healing process, and treatment regimen
2. Effect of medications in the treatment of myocardial infarction
3. Association between risk factors and coronary artery disease
   a. Identify nonmodifiable risk factors
   b. Identify modifiable risk factors (especially cigarette smoking)
4. Effect of dietary restrictions on CAD: low salt, low cholesterol, no caffeine, fluid restrictions
5. Effect of activity on heart and need to participate in a progressive activity plan
6. Resumption of sexual activity (if appropriate)
   a. Abstention of sexual intercourse as directed, usually for 4 to 6 weeks (sexual closeness, for example, cuddling, may be started earlier as desired)
   b. Reporting to physician the following symptoms occurring during or following intercourse
      1. Dyspnea or increased heart rate continuing for more than 15 min after intercourse
      2. Extreme fatigue
      3. Chest pain during intercourse
      4. Palpitations for more than 15 min after intercourse
      5. Insomnia after intercourse

---

denial, depression, and anxiety. Generally, patients tend to become more anxious on the second day of hospitalization after the immediate threat of death from infarction has passed. Depression may occur several days later and may continue after the patient is discharged. Most persons who have a myocardial infarction, however, adjust extremely well. Over 85% of all patients with uncomplicated myocardial infarctions are able to return to work. This, along with resuming normal sexual functioning, aids tremendously in the adjustment process.

The patients and their partners may need teaching and reassurance regarding resuming *sexual activities*. Many feel that their sex life is over after a myocardial infarction. Education should aim at supplying information and dispelling misinformation. Once patients with an uncomplicated myocardial infarction are capable of walking two flights of stairs without difficulty, they are generally able to perform sexual intercourse safely. Approximately 80% of all postcoronary patients will be able to resume sexual activity without serious risk. The other 20% need not totally abstain, but their sexual activity should be limited according to their cardiac capacity.

⌗ EVALUATION

Evaluation will be based on the expected patient outcomes. Some questions to ask may include the following:
1. Was chest pain decreased?
2. Was need for additional oxygen decreased?
3. Is activity tolerance increasing as evidenced by absence of fatigue, dyspnea, or discomfort with increasing activity?
4. Does the patient know the nature of the disorder, ways to decrease possibility of further ischemic attacks, activity prescription?

5. Has the patient made plans for follow-up medical care?

■ Cardiac surgery for myocardial ischemia

Surgical intervention is often necessary for patients with severe myocardial ischemia that is uncontrolled by medical therapy. Recommendation for surgery is based on the assessment of the expected benefits of the procedure and the inherent surgical risks. Patients with cardiomegaly, severe congestive heart failure, recent myocardial infarction, high left ventricular end-diastolic pressure, and an inadequate ejection fraction are at higher risk.

■ CORONARY ARTERY BYPASS GRAFT

Surgical correction of myocardial ischemia is usually done through a bypass procedure in which a graft is sutured above and below the area of blockage in the coronary artery. Any number of bypasses can be performed depending on the location and extent of the blockages. Blood flow to the ischemic areas of the heart is then conducted through the new grafts, thus "bypassing" the obstruction.

Bypass grafts are obtained from sections of the saphenous vein or the internal mammary artery. The saphenous vein is harvested from the inner thigh and sectioned. Removal of this vein does not compromise circulation in the leg, since there are numerous other vessels to assist in this function.

The heart is exposed through a median sternotomy or anterolateral thoracotomy; retractors are used to spread the chest wall. Saphenous vein sections are grafted from the aorta to the point beyond the blockage. The internal mammary artery remains attached proximally to the subclavian

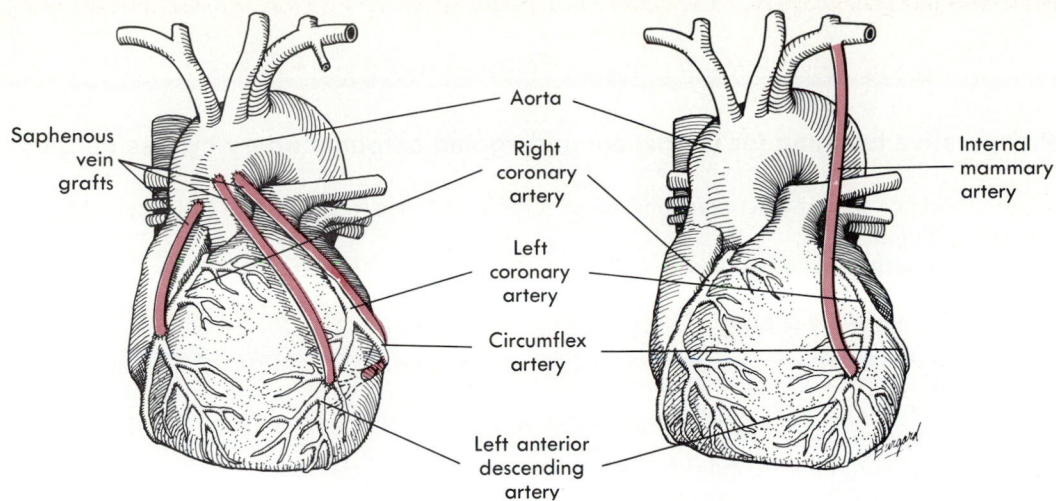

Fig. 25-27 Coronary artery bypass grafts.

artery. The distal portion is grafted to the coronary artery beyond the occlusion (Fig. 25-27). Cardiopulmonary bypass is often used during cardiac surgery to allow the surgeon easier access to the operative site while maintaining perfusion of vital organs.

Cardiopulmonary bypass

Most heart surgeries require partial or total cardiopulmonary bypass (Fig. 25-28). In *partial* bypass, pulmonary circulation is not interrupted. Oxygenated blood is drained

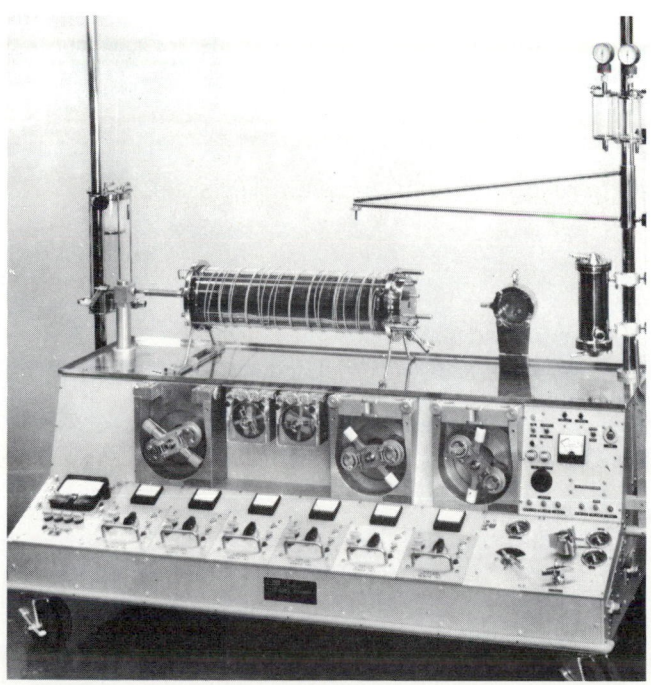

Fig. 25-28 Cardiopulmonary bypass machine used during heart surgery. (Courtesy, PEMCO, Inc, Cleveland, Ohio.)

from the left side of the heart, passed through a pulsatile pump, and returned through the descending aorta or common femoral artery. *Total* cardiopulmonary bypass involves both circulation and oxygenation of the extracted blood. Cannulas are placed in the right atrium to drain venous blood. The machine oxygenates this blood and pumps it back into the ascending aorta or femoral artery.

Besides the capability of the heart-lung machine to provide extracorporeal circulation, it also serves as a direct route for medication administration and systemic hypothermia. Cooling of the machine solutions and subsequent body cooling lowers oxygen consumption by decreasing cellular metabolism.

Types of equipment

Many different types of equipment are used during cardiac surgery. Some of these and their uses are described in the following list:

1. Endotracheal tube, ventilator: to maintain open airway, ventilation, and access to secretions
2. Cardiac monitor: to identify arrhythmias
3. Intravenous line: to replace fluids, monitor central venous pressure, administer medications
4. Arterial line: to monitor blood pressure, obtain arterial blood samples
5. Pulmonary artery catheter (Swan-Ganz): to monitor pulmonary artery pressure, capillary wedge pressure, and cardiac output
6. Chest tube: to drain blood and air from chest
7. Epicardial pacing wires: to facilitate temporary cardiac pacing, if necessary
8. Urinary catheter: to monitor fluid status

Preoperative care

Preoperative care consists of (1) altering medications, (2) preparing the operative site, and (3) providing patient teaching. Digitalis preparations are discontinued on the day of surgery. Diuretics are also withheld so that the

Preoperative teaching for the patient undergoing coronary artery bypass surgery

1. Simple explanation of anatomy of heart, function of coronary arteries, and effect of CAD (use of heart drawings and models is helpful)
2. Explanation of surgery
   a. Removal of saphenous vein
   b. Use of internal mammary artery
   c. Effect on cardiac function
3. Definition of terms: *bypass, graft*
4. Explanation of events on day of surgery
   a. Preoperative medications
   b. Length of time in surgery (depends on number of arteries to be bypassed)
   c. Length of time until able to see family
5. Explanation of the intensive care unit
   a. Description of physical facilities and layout
   b. Nurse will be available at all times
   c. Visiting hours for family
   d. Length of stay in unit (2 to 3 days)
6. Explanation of monitors
   a. Round patches on chest connected to cardiac monitor
   b. Beeping sounds from monitors may be heard
7. Explanation of lines
   a. Intravenous routes for fluid and medications
   b. Central venous line in chest or groin to monitor fluid status
   c. Faucetlike line to obtain blood samples without a needle prick
8. Explanation of drainage tubes
   a. Catheter draining urine from bladder
   b. Chest tube draining bloody fluid from incision (usually removed day after surgery)
9. Explanation of breathing tube
   a. Tube in windpipe connected to machine called ventilator
   b. Unable to speak with tube (can mouth words or write notes to communicate)
   c. Tube removed when patient is fully awake and stable
   d. Secretions in lungs or tube removed by nurse
10. Explanation and demonstration of activity and exercises
    a. Purpose of activity and exercises is to promote circulation, keep lungs clear, and prevent infection
    b. Activity will include:
       1. Turning from side to side in bed
       2. Sitting on edge of bed on night of surgery
       3. Sitting in chair day after surgery
    c. Range of motion exercises to arms and legs
    d. Effective deep breathing (use of sustained maximal inspiration, holding breath for 3 to 5 sec at end of deep inspiration)
    e. Effective coughing (coughing twice in succession with pillow splinting chest)
    f. Use of incentive spirometer (similar technique used to take deep breath)
11. Explanation of pain medication
    a. Pain will be present at chest incision and leg incision
    b. Medication reduces pain and makes activity and exercises easier
    c. Encourage use of pain medication
12. Explanation of diet
    a. After removal of breathing tube, will be given ice chips and water
    b. Clear liquids with gradual progression to regular diet

patient is adequately hydrated. Anticoagulants (coumadin, heparin) and other medications with anticoagulant effects (aspirin) are discontinued 48 hours before surgery.

In preparing the operative site, the patient showers with a special antimicrobial soap on the night before surgery. The chest and abdomen are shaved from neck to groin and from the left to the right midaxillary lines. If saphenous veins are needed for grafting, the inner aspects of the legs are also shaved.

Preoperative teaching is essential for a patient undergoing cardiac surgery. Involvement of the patient's family or significant others is also of importance in preparing the patient for surgery. The initial preoperative teaching is frequently done by nurses from the surgical intensive care unit. All nurses caring for the patient should be familiar with the content, however, so they may reinforce major points, be alert to areas of special concern, and answer questions posed by patients and family members. An outline of content specific to coronary bypass surgery is summarized in the box on p. 790.

☐ Postoperative care

Postoperative care includes the following goals: promotion of oxygenation and comfort, maintenance of fluid and electrolyte balance, and prevention or early detection of complications (thrombophlebitis, pulmonary embolus, cardiac tamponade, cardiac arrhythmias, and cardiac failure).

☐ *Promoting oxygenation*

1. Ventilate with supplemental oxygen
2. Turn from side to side
3. Keep head of bed elevated at least 10 to 20 degrees
4. Assess quality of breath sounds
5. Monitor arterial blood gases
6. Encourage performance of range of motion exercises
7. Encourage progressive activity level
8. Daily chest x-ray films will be obtained
9. Monitor patency and drainage from chest tube
10. Assist with deep breathing, coughing, and use of incentive spirometer

☐ *Maintaining fluid and electrolyte balance*

Crystalloid fluids are given intravenously to maintain adequate circulating blood volume. Colloids (whole blood, packed cells, plasma, or plasma expanders) are given depending on the hemoglobin and total protein concentrations. Potassium is frequently required after heart surgery, and the patient is monitored for signs of hypokalemia. Nursing activities include the following:

1. Maintain prescribed flow rate of parenteral fluids
2. Maintain patency of chest tube and urinary catheter
3. Record amount of drainage accurately
4. Assess for signs of fluid loss (dry skin, dry mucous membranes, decreased skin turgor) and fluid overload (peripheral edema, neck vein distention, moist respirations)
5. Monitor central venous pressure (CVP) readings
6. Monitor daily weight
7. Assess serum electrolytes (especially potassium) and hematocrit

8. Monitor Swan-Ganz parameters: pulmonary artery pressure, pulmonary capillary wedge pressure

☐ *Promoting comfort*

1. Administer narcotic analgesics (morphine sulfate or meperidine) on a fairly regular basis during first 48 to 72 hours to relieve severe pain
2. Provide frequent oral hygiene until patient is taking fluids regularly
3. Eliminate unnecessary environmental stimuli (noise, lights) that impair ability to rest/sleep
4. Change linens if profuse nights sweats occur; assure patient that this commonly occurs
5. Group daily activities to allow for periods of uninterrupted rest/sleep
6. Encourage use of splinting devices (pillow, blanket) during coughing
7. Provide explanations for activities, as necessary
8. Monitor patient for changes in behavior and encourage patient to express concerns

☐ *Preventing/detecting complications*

1. Thrombophlebitis/pulmonary embolism
   a. Encourage leg exercises until patient is ambulatory
   b. Encourage use of elastic stockings
   c. Encourage ambulation when permitted
2. Tamponade (compression of heart from accumulation of blood or fluid under pericardium)
   a. Monitor color and amount of chest tube drainage (change in color to bright red, sustained bleeding, or sudden cessation of drainage)
   b. Assess for increase in bleeding from midsternal incision
   c. Assess for other signs (restlessness, diaphoresis, hypotension, increased CVP, decreased urinary output)
3. Cardiac arrhythmias
   a. Maintain continuous ECG monitoring
   b. Assess cardiac rhythm
   c. Monitor daily electrolyte values (especially potassium)
   d. Medicate with antiarrhythmic drugs as prescribed
   e. Assist in treatment of other underlying causes of arrhythmias (decreased oxygenation)
4. Cardiac failure
   a. Monitor for signs of low cardiac output (hypotension, increased heart rate, restlessness, lethargy)
   b. Monitor CVP readings
   c. Monitor hourly urine output during initial period
   d. Monitor Swan-Ganz parameters
   e. Administer blood products and volume expanders as prescribed

☐ Discharge planning

The usual hospital stay is 7 to 10 days after surgery, barring any complications. Before discharge, the patient and family need specific guidelines for physical activity level. Activities are encouraged at a slow progressive pace unless overexertion occurs. Daily walking with a gradual increasing weekly distance is highly recommended. Patients are cautioned to avoid heavy lifting (greater than 30 pounds) and activities that require repetitive arm movements, such as vacuuming and playing golf. Patients are instructed not to drive a car or perform heavy labor until permitted by the physician.

Sexual intercourse can be resumed within the third or fourth postoperative week. Couples are cautioned to avoid sexual positions in which the patient would be supporting weight. Large meals or the consumption of alcohol should be avoided before sexual activity.

In summary, the following patient outcomes are expected:
1. Describe extent of permissible activity
   a. Describe plans for progressive return to physical activity as recommended by physician
   b. State awareness of when sexual activity may be resumed
   c. Describe criteria to use as a guide in determining if overexertion occurs (fatigue, dyspnea, pain)
   d. Describe plans to return to work if employed
2. Plan meals incorporating a balanced diet with any prescribed modifications
3. Describe any medication regimen
4. Describe plans for follow-up care
   a. Explain basis of any symptoms that may persist (dyspnea, pain, night sweats)
   b. Describe signs or symptoms requiring immediate medical attention (fever, increasing dyspnea, chest pain with minimal exertion)
   c. State plans for ongoing medical care

■ PERCUTANEOUS TRANSLUMINAL CORONARY ANGIOPLASTY

An alternative approach to coronary bypass surgery for selected patients with myocardial ischemia is percutaneous transluminal coronary angioplasty (PTCA). This procedure consists of dilating the coronary vessel wall by mechanical compression of the atheromatous plaque. PTCA is attractive because of a short recovery period, discharge within 3 days barring complications, and a shorter return-to-work time than with bypass surgery.[46]

Selection criteria for PTCA include persistent angina despite medical treatment and a lesion that is single, non-calcific, and located in a portion of a proximal vessel that does not involve a point of bifurcation. PTCA is not usually considered for lesions in the left main coronary artery. PTCA may also be used following thrombolytic therapy for myocardial infarction (see p. 786) and to dilate areas of stenosis in bypass grafts.

During PTCA a pacemaker catheter is inserted as a precautionary measure through the femoral vein, and a specially designed catheter is inserted in the femoral artery and advanced under fluoroscopy (similar to cardiac catheterization) to the site of the coronary obstruction. Once in position, a balloon on the catheter is inflated to provide compression and rupture the atheromatous plaque. Heparin is infused during the procedure, and anticoagulation may be continued for several months after the procedure. Following PTCA the patient may return to the general medical unit or may be admitted to an intensive care unit. In either case, nursing care includes immobilization of the legs for 6 to 12 hours, monitoring for bleeding at the catheter insertion sites, monitoring pedal pulses for indications of femoral artery thrombosis, and monitoring for chest pain that could be caused by an abrupt occlusion of the coronary vessel, restenosis of a dilated artery, coronary artery spasm, or pulmonary embolism. In the case of pulmonary embolus, the site of thrombus formation is usually the femoral vein puncture site. Chest pain requires an immediate ECG and the use of nitrates or calcium channel blockers as prescribed. ECG results may indicate the need for repeat PTCA or emergency coronary bypass surgery.

About 5% to 10% of patients who undergo PTCA have a major complication such as a myocardial infarction, the need for emergency coronary bypass surgery, or in-hospital death.[46,56] Minor complications include prolonged angina, bradycardia or transient ventricular arrhythmias, and excessive blood loss. Over the long term, restenosis of the vessel is a significant complication and occurs in about 25% to 30% of patients, usually within the first 8 months following the procedure.

■ Congestive heart failure

Heart failure (also known as cardiac insufficiency) is a state in which the heart is no longer able to pump an adequate supply of blood to meet the demands of the body. *Congestive heart failure* refers to a state of circulatory congestion resulting from heart failure and its compensatory mechanisms.[54] Heart failure may develop rapidly after a specific insult to the myocardium (such as an acute myocardial infarction) or may develop more gradually as response to a prolonged stress (such as hypertension). In the latter case, the person may initially seek medical at-

---

Causes of heart failure

1. *Direct damage to the heart* (reduction in contractile ability)
   Myocardial infarction, myocarditis, myocardial fibrosis, ventricular aneurysm
2. *Ventricular overload*
   a. Volume overload (increased preload): aortic regurgitation, ventricular septal defect
   b. Pressure overload (increased afterload): aortic or pulmonic stenosis, systemic hypertension, pulmonary hypertension
3. *Restriction to ventricular diastolic filling*
   Constrictive pericarditis or cardiomyopathy, rapid rate arrhythmias, cardiac tamponade, mitral stenosis

From Spann, JF, and Hurst, JW: The recognition and management of heart failure. In Hurst, JW: The heart, arteries and veins, ed 6, New York, 1986, McGraw-Hill Book Co.

Compensatory responses to inadequate cardiac output

Response	Initial effect
Stimulation of sympathetic nervous system	Increased rate and force of myocardial contraction
	Peripheral vasoconstriction—shunting of blood to vital organs, increased venous return, increased blood pressure
Activation of renin-angiotensin system	Increased reabsorption of sodium and water—increased blood volume;
	Peripheral vasoconstriction
Ventricular hypertrophy	Increased myocardial contractility

---

tention with milder symptoms because the circulatory system has had more time to adjust to the heart's decreased performance and the resultant compensatory responses.

■ ETIOLOGY

The causes of heart failure can be categorized to correspond to the three determinants of stroke volume: myocardial contractility, preload, and afterload (see p. 759). Heart failure can also be the result of conditions that reduce ventricular filling. Examples of specific etiologies of heart failure are summarized in the box on p. 792.

■ PATHOPHYSIOLOGY

□ Compensatory responses to inadequate cardiac output

Inadequate cardiac output triggers a number of compensatory responses that are geared toward maintaining adequate perfusion to vital body organs (see the box above). The initial response is stimulation of the sympathetic nervous system, which has two main effects: (1) increased rate and force of myocardial contraction and (2) peripheral vasoconstriction. Peripheral vasoconstriction shunts arterial blood away from less vital organs such as the skin and kidneys and toward more vital organs such as the brain. Constriction of the veins increases venous return to the heart, which increases cardiac volume and dilates the ventricles. The increased stretch of myocardial muscle fibers enhances contractility.

Initially these responses may result in improvements in cardiac output, but, in the long run, afterload and myocardial oxygen demands are also increased, and stretch of myocardial fibers moves beyond a point where contraction is enhanced. Unless the person was in a state of fluid depletion to start with, the increased ventricular volume aggravates preload and compounds the failure.

A second type of compensatory response involves activation of the renin-angiotensin system (Chapter 32). A decrease in renal blood flow and, subsequently, of glomerular filtration rate triggers the release of renin, which interacts with angiotensinogen to form angiotensin I. Conversion of angiotensin I to angiotensin II results in further peripheral vasoconstriction and increased reabsorption of sodium and water by the kidneys. These events increase fluid volume and maintain blood pressure in the short term but increase both preload and afterload in the long term.

A third type of compensatory mechanism involves changes in the structure of the myocardium itself. Over time, the ventricular myocardium thickens or hypertophies to improve contraction, but this too results in increased myocardial oxygen demands.

Initially, one side of the heart fails. Since the left ventricle is most often affected by coronary atherosclerosis and hypertension, heart failure usually begins there. However, since both ventricles are part of the same system, the right ventricle often becomes impaired as well. The symptoms of heart failure are the result of decreased cardiac output and congestion that involves the venous system or the pulmonary system or both. The symptoms are summarized in the box below. In general, the symptoms of heart failure

---

Signs and symptoms of congestive heart failure

Signs and symptoms caused by decreased cardiac output to systemic tissues

Fatigue	Oliguria
Angina	Decreased GI motility
Anxiety	Skin cool, pale
S₃ heart sound	

Signs and symptoms caused by congestion backward from left ventricle

Dyspnea	Pulmonary rales
Cough	X-ray evidence of pulmonary congestion
Orthopnea	

Signs and symptoms caused by congestion backward from right ventricle

Peripheral edema	Liver engorgement
Distended neck veins	Elevated central venous pressure

are considered relative to the amount of associated physical exertion. A classification scheme developed by the New York Heart Association ranges from "asymptomatic with ordinary physical exertion" (Class I) to "symptomatic at rest" (Class IV).[54]

Left ventricular failure

Failure of the left ventricle to pump adequate amounts of oxygenated blood to meet the demands of the body results in two major consequences: (1) signs and symptoms of decreased cardiac output (see general symptoms of heart failure) and (2) pulmonary congestion (sometimes called backward failure). The reduced ejection fraction leads to increased end-diastolic volume (preload) and increased left ventricular end-diastolic pressure (LVEDP). This increased pressure is reflected backward into the pulmonary circulation, which is normally a low pressure, high capacitance circuit. Ultimately, increased pressure in the pulmonary circulation causes fluid to be forced into the alveoli and interstitial tissue. In severe cases, fluid may reach the bronchioles or the pleural space. The symptoms may range from mild dyspnea to those of frank pulmonary edema (p. 802) or pleural effusion.

Dyspnea

Dyspnea, or labored breathing, is an early symptom of left ventricular failure. It is caused by interference with gas exchange as a result of the fluid in the alveoli. It may occur or become worse only on physical exertion, such as climbing stairs, walking up an incline, or walking against the wind, since these activities require increased amounts of oxygen.

Orthopnea

Difficulty in breathing when lying flat may be present, and persons often must sleep propped up in bed or in a chair. When the person is lying flat, ventilation is decreased and the blood volume in the pulmonary vessels is increased. Orthopnea is often described by the number of pillows required for the patient to rest comfortably when in bed, for example, "three-pillow orthopnea."

Although orthopnea may occur immediately after lying down, it often does not occur for several hours. At that time, it causes the person to wake with severe dyspnea and coughing. This condition is known as *paroxysmal nocturnal dyspnea* and results from the accumulation of fluid in the lungs as the person is lying in bed. The patient usually has a feeling of suffocation and often awakens in panic.

Apnea and hyperpnea (Cheyne-Stokes)

The patient with heart failure may have alternating periods of apnea and hyperpnea called Cheyne-Stokes respirations. Pulmonary congestion results in decreased oxygenation of the blood, and altered cardiac function may cause an abnormally long circulation time between the lungs and respiratory control centers in the brain. Periods of hyperpnea cause carbon dioxide levels to fall to such an extent that the respiratory center is not stimulated. A

period of apnea results that may last as long as 30 seconds. During this time the carbon dioxide levels build up again until respirations resume and another period of hyperpnea begins. This phenomena often begins as the patient goes to sleep and decreases as sleep deepens and ventilation decreases.

Cough

A persistent hacking cough is often a symptom of left-sided heart failure. It results from congestion of trapped fluid, which is irritating to the mucosal lining of the lungs and bronchi. The cough is usually productive of large quantities of frothy sputum, which is occasionally blood tinged. On auscultation *rales* may be heart. Rales are the moist popping and crackling sounds heard most often at the end of inspiration.

Right ventricular failure

Right ventricular failure occurs when this chamber is unable to pump effectively against increased pressure in the pulmonary circulation. Most often the increased pressure is the result of blood backing up from a failing left ventricle, but right ventricular failure can also be a consequence of chronic pulmonary disease and pulmonary hypertension.

Inability of the right ventricle to pump blood forward into the lungs results in congestion that is reflected backward into the systemic circulation. Increased venous volume and pressure forces fluid out of the vasculature into interstitial tissue (*peripheral edema*). This edema is first likely to appear in dependent areas of the body such as the feet, ankles, and sacrum. It is usually nontender and may become pitting (easily depressed by the pressure of an examiner's thumb). As right ventricular failure worsens, edema progresses up the legs into the thighs, external genitalia, and lower trunk. Extremely engorged tissue causes the skin to crack, and fluid may "weep" from the tissues.

The *liver* may also become engorged with intravascular fluid, resulting in enlargement and tenderness in the right upper abdominal quadrant. As venous stasis increases, pressure within the portal system becomes so great that fluid is forced through the blood vessels into the abdominal cavity (ascites). The ascitic fluid can reach volumes of more than 10 L, displacing the diaphragm and resulting in severe respiratory distress. A paracentesis (see Chapter 30) may be required to relieve the pressure on the diaphragm. *Distended neck veins* are a result of the increased systemic venous pressure and are usually observed when the patient is in a sitting position (see Fig. 9-2).

General symptoms of heart failure
Fatigue

Persons with heart failure commonly note fatigue following activities that ordinarily are not tiring. The fatigue results from impaired blood circulation to tissues as a result of the decreased CO. The reduction in tissue oxygen decreases the production of adenosine triphosphate (ATP), the immediate energy source for muscle contractions. In addition, the impaired circulation causes a decrease in the removal of metabolic waste products; the result of this is further decreased muscle function.

□ *Anginal pain*

Cardiac pain is *not* a typical symptom of heart failure; however, angina pectoris can occur from the decrease in CO. It is most likely to occur in patients with CAD, which increases the patient's sensitivity to a deficiency in the oxygen content in the circulating blood. As heart failure develops, the blood is less effectively oxygenated and angina occurs. As the fluid overload state is corrected, the chest pain resolves.

□ *Anxiety*

Most persons are aware of the importance of an effectively functioning heart. Awareness that one has signs and symptoms of heart failure may, therefore, be anxiety producing especially if the symptoms have occurred suddenly or are clearly getting worse. The frequent association of dyspnea with heart failure is another reason why anxiety is a common finding. Perceived difficulty with breathing can be a stressful experience, and anxiety may make the dyspnea worse. In extreme cases, anxiety may also increase oxygen demands on an already compromised heart.

▓ ASSESSMENT

□ Subjective data

Data are collected concerning the occurrence of signs and symptoms that may indicate the presence of heart failure, the person's ability to cope with the physical limitations, knowledge of the condition and treatment regimen, and ability to adhere to the treatment regimen. Patient concerns and anxieties are also elicited. Specific areas for assessment include the following:

1. Respiratory status—dyspnea, orthopnea (precipitating factors, severity, relieving factors)
2. Signs of fluid retention—recent weight gain, pedal edema (shoes too tight), skin feels tight
3. Ability to perform daily activities—fatigue, lack of endurance (precipitating factors, extent)
4. Comfort—anginal or abdominal pain
5. Knowledge of condition and treatment regimen
6. Ability to adhere to any prescribed treatment regimen; factors that make adherence difficult
7. Measures taken to compensate for physical limitations
8. Usual coping skills
9. Specific concerns related to condition

□ Objective data

1. Neck vein distention: presence, degree
2. Edema: site, degree of pitting
3. Abdominal distention
4. Daily weights: weigh on litter scale if severe heart failure present; weigh at same time of day (usually in morning after emptying bladder, before breakfast) and with same amount of clothing
5. Adventitious breath sounds
6. Gallop rhythm of heart on auscultation *S3*
7. Level of consciousness
8. Pulse changes and respiratory effort with activity

□ Diagnostic tests

Heart failure is typically diagnosed based on the clinical signs and symptoms and the presence of a precipitating cause. An electrocardiogram is usually done to determine the presence or absence of an acute myocardial infarction, to assess for arrhythmias, and to identify compensatory responses such as ventricular hypertrophy. Chest x-ray films are done to assess pulmonary congestion and cardiac enlargement. Actual cardiac output may be detemined by a variety of techniques, but this assessment is usually reserved for the more critically ill patient. A number of other tests have been devised to provide data about cardiac functioning and are discussed briefly below. They include echocardiograms, gated pool imaging, and pulmonary artery catheterization.

□ *Echocardiogram*

Information about the shape, size, and movement of the cardiac muscle and valves can be obtained through the use of ultrasonic sound waves directed to the heart. These waves are reflected by cardiac structures and can be visualized as an electronic wave form on an oscilloscope. The use of this noninvasive test to detect valvular abnormalities is discussed more fully on p. 812.

□ *Gated pool imaging*

This particular type of imaging involves the intravenous injection of technetium-99m. After 3 to 5 minutes, the patient is placed in a supine position, and computer outlines of the left side of the heart during all cardiac cycles are obtained. This procedure is used to evaluate left ventricular function and specifically to calculate the ejection fraction.

□ *Pulmonary artery catheterization*

The development of a balloon-tipped, flow-directed pulmonary artery catheter (commonly called a Swan-Ganz catheter in recognition of the physicians who developed it) has made possible significant advances in the diagnosis and treatment of cardiac failure. Specifically, its uses include the assessment of right and left ventricular function and evaluation of the effect of various cardiovascular drugs and other treatment modalities such as increasing or restricting intravenous fluids.

A flexible multilumen catheter (Table 25-5) is inserted into the antecubital vein by means of a cutdown. The catheter is threaded through the superior vena cava, the right atrium, right ventricle, pulmonary artery, and into a small branch of this artery (pulmonary wedge position) (Fig. 25-29).

Representative waveforms are viewed on an oscilloscope and pressure readings can be obtained from various cardiac chambers (see normal pressures on p. 814). Pulmonary wedge pressure is a reflection of left ventricular pressure

Table 25-5 Pulmonary artery catheter lumens

Type of lumen	Location	Purpose
Proximal	Right atrium	Administer intravenous fluids Obtain CVP readings
Distal	Pulmonary artery	Measure pulmonary artery pressure Measure pulmonary capillary wedge pressure (PCWP)
Balloon	Branch of pulmonary artery	Inflate balloon to obtain PCWP
Thermistor	Pulmonary artery	Measure CO

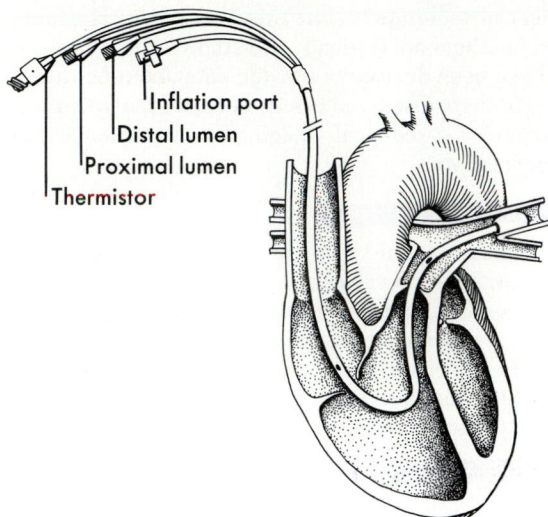

Inflation port
Distal lumen
Proximal lumen
Thermistor

Fig. 25-29 Placement of Swan-Ganz catheter.

and allows monitoring of preload. In addition, the thermistor port allows determinations of cardiac output.

⮕ DATA ANALYSIS: NURSING DIAGNOSES

Nursing diagnoses are determined from assessment of patient data. Possible nursing diagnoses for the person with heart failure may include, but are not limited to, the following:

Diagnostic title	Possible etiologies
Activity intolerance	Imbalance between oxygen supply and demand
Anxiety	Change in health status, threat to role functioning, situational crisis
Ineffective breathing pattern	Anxiety, decreased energy/fatigue, pulmonary congestion
Constipation	Enforced period of decreased mobility, possible fluid restriction, decreased perfusion of GI tract

Diagnostic title	Possible etiologies
Potential for disuse syndrome	Immobility
Knowledge deficit: pathophysiology of heart failure, diagnostic tests, treatment regimen	Lack of exposure/recall, information misinterpretation, unfamiliarity with information resources
Noncompliance (therapeutic regimen)	Patient value system, client-provider relationships, treatment side effects, complexity of regimen
Pain	Decreased perfusion of some organs (angina), congestion (abdominal, liver)
Self-care deficit	Activity intolerance/fatigue, pain/discomfort, anxiety
Impaired skin integrity	Immobility, decreased perfusion to skin, edema
Sleep pattern disturbance	Dyspnea, cough, pain/discomfort, anxiety, diuretics
Altered thought processes	Anxiety, inadequate oxygenation of cerebrum

▣ PLANNING: EXPECTED PATIENT OUTCOMES

Expected outcomes for the patient heart with failure may include, but are not limited to, the following:
1. Patient can breathe more comfortably.
2. Peripheral edema and signs of organ congestion are reduced.
3. Patient demonstrates relief from fatigue and other signs of decreased perfusion to skin and other organs.
4. Patient can describe and implement a plan for activity that will avoid fatigue or dyspnea.
5. Patient can describe the components of and rationale for the prescribed treatment regimen (diet and fluid restriction, medications, oxygen).
6. Patient can describe signs and symptoms that require medical attention.
7. Patient can state the plans for follow-up care.
8. Other outcomes that relate specifically to the documented presence of nursing diagnoses noted above.

Medical therapy for congestive heart failure

1. Reduction of oxygen requirements
   a. Treatment of precipitating causes
   b. Rest
2. Improvement of oxygen supply/reduction of congestion
   a. Oxygen therapy
   b. Positioning of patient to facilitate breathing
   c. Increase myocardial contractility (positive inotropic drugs)
   d. Reduce preload (sodium restriction, diuretics, venous dilating drugs)
   e. Reduce afterload (arterial dilating drugs, mixed arterial/venous dilating drugs, ACE inhibitors)

Implementation

☐ Assisting with achievement of therapeutic goals

Treatment of congestive heart failure has the overall aim of restoring a supply of blood and oxygen that is equal to the demands of bodily tissues. Approaches to treatment, therefore, may focus on increasing oxygen supply, decreasing oxygen demand, or both (see the box above). A second aim of treatment is the reduction of pulmonary and/or systemic congestion and the associated symptoms. Identification and treatment of the underlying etiology and factors that may have precipitated a particular episode of heart failure (that is, caused excessive demands on the heart) are important therapeutic goals.

At many acute care hospitals, patients with acute congestive heart failure are admitted to medical or cardiac intensive care units. Occasionally, the physician may elect to place the patient in the usual room accommodations, where the environment is less stressful and where family members can visit more routinely.

☐ *Promoting rest and activity*

Reducing the requirement for oxygen can best be effected by providing the patient with the degree of activity that does not compromise myocardial function, as demonstrated by the presence of symptoms. For mild heart failure, the patient may be treated on an ambulatory basis with only a regimen of less strenuous activity and more rest than usual.

For severe heart failure, a program of bed rest or limited activity may be necessary until symptoms abate. Permissible activity will be based on symptoms such as dyspnea and fatigue. A careful assessment must be made each day to determine the amount of rest required. If the patient

has difficulty relaxing because of apprehension or anxiety, a tranquilizer may be prescribed.

Ambulation is started slowly to avoid overloading the heart. The regimen varies depending on individual patient response. When a patient has been on restricted bed rest, activities progress slowly from dangling, to sitting, to walking increased distances under close supervision. If signs of dyspnea, fatigue, or increased pulse rate that does not stabilize readily occur, the patient is returned to bed. Oxygen is given for dyspnea, and the physician is notified.

The plan for increased activity is explained to the patient and family. They should understand that if activity tires the person excessively, it may be curtailed. Overactivity can produce physical and mental setbacks that delay ultimate recovery.

Rest to the heart is also promoted by preventing constipation, since straining at defecation places an extra burden on the heart. During straining against a closed glottis (Valsalva maneuver), venous return to the heart is decreased as a result of increased intrathoracic pressure. When this pressure is released after straining, a large amount of venous return creates an increased work load on the heart. The feces can be kept soft by stool softeners or bulk-forming laxatives. If an enema is necessary, it should be of low volume and given with a small rectal tube inserted only 3 to 4 inches.

☐ *Providing oxygenation*

In heart failure, the oxygen content of the bloodstream may be markedly reduced because of the less effective oxygenation of the blood as it passes through the congested lungs. The patient may be more comfortable and better able to rest when receiving oxygen, since it helps in reducing dyspnea and fatigue. Oxygen is usually administered by nasal cannula at 2 to 6 L/min. Baseline arterial blood gases are obtained at initiation of oxygen therapy and intermittently during therapy to assess effectiveness of the treatment.

Breathing is often made easier by maintaining the patient in semi-Fowler's or high Fowler's position. These positions maximize oxygenation by permitting greater lung expansion. The patient is often orthopneic and tends to breathe more easily sitting than lying in bed. If the patient is sitting in a chair, the feet are elevated to reduce pooling of fluid in the dependent limbs. When the patient is in high Fowler's position in bed, a pillow may be placed lengthwise behind the shoulders and back in such a manner that full expansion of the rib cage is possible. The arms may be supported on pillows to reduce the pull on the shoulder muscles (Fig. 25-30). An over-the-bed table may be placed close to the patient to allow resting of the head and arms.

☐ *Digitalis therapy*

Digitalis is the major therapeutic approach in the treatment of congestive heart failure. Digitalis and its derivatives usually are effective in improving myocardial function in persons with congestive heart failure (Fig. 25-31). The

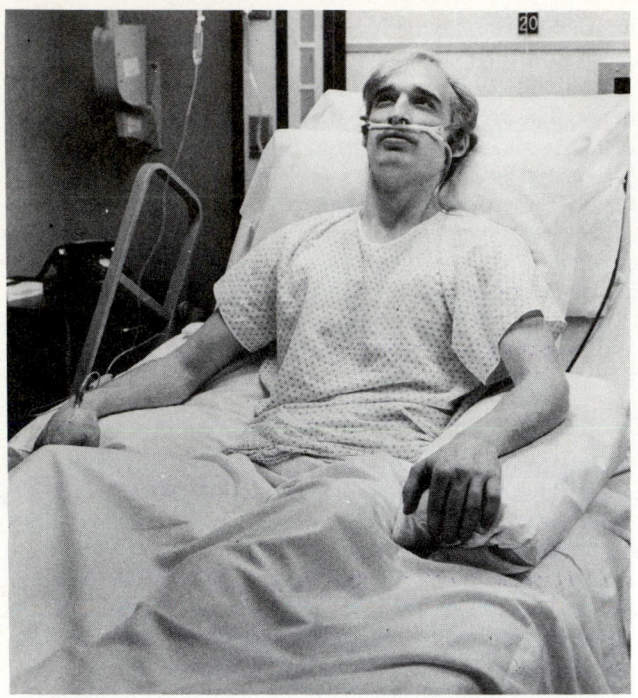

Fig. 25-30 Patient sitting upright with pillows under head and each arm to promote chest expansion and comfort.

positive inotropic action of digitalis preparations enhances mechanical performance by strengthening the force of myocardial contraction. This leads to increased CO and increased blood flow to the kidneys. Digitalis preparations also decrease heart rate (automaticity) and cardiac conduction velocity, which permits the ventricles to relax more to allow time for better filling of the ventricles with blood.

DIGITALIZATION. When acute congestive heart failure occurs, the physician usually orders an optimal therapeutic dose of a digitalis preparation to slow the ventricular rate and decrease symptoms. This larger dose given over a short period of time, usually 24 to 48 hours, is called a *loading* or *digitalizing* dose. In some instances the dose may approach the toxic level (see the box on p. 799). After the optimal therapeutic dose has been determined, the person is given a daily maintenance dose.

Numerous types of digitalis preparations may be used (Table 25-6). For rapid digitalization in emergency situations, deslanoside (Cedilanid-D) or ouabain is usually selected. Digoxin or digitoxin is most commonly used for maintenance drug therapy. Digoxin has a more rapid effect than digitoxin, yet it has sufficient duration for adequate maintenance therapy. Response to a digitalis preparation is evaluated on the basis of relief of symptoms.

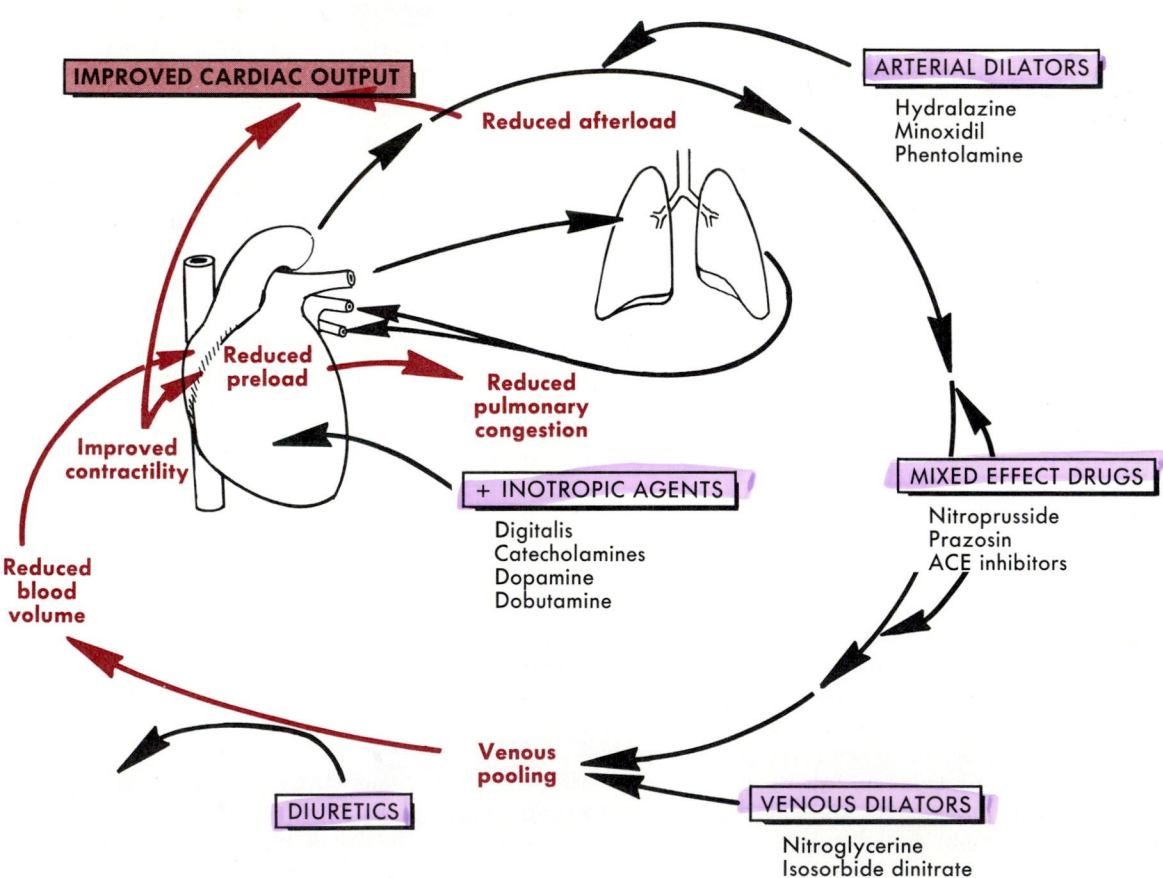

Fig. 25-31 Effect of medications used for severe congestive heart failure.

NURSING IMPLICATIONS
1. Take apical pulse before administering digitalis preparations; withhold medication and notify physician if pulse is below 60
2. Observe for signs of digitalis toxicity (see the box at right)
3. Monitor serum potassium blood levels (hypokalemia is the most common cause of digitalis toxicity)
4. Give potassium supplements (if prescribed)

□ **Diuretic therapy**

The purpose of diuretic therapy is to decrease circulating blood volume and thus reduce ventricular overload (preload) and symptoms of congestion. Most patients with heart failure eventually require diuretic therapy,[69] but this mode of treatment may be reserved until the effectiveness of digitalization and dietary sodium restriction can be evaluated.

Essential to proper initiation of diuretic therapy is determining how much fluid should be removed from the patient by establishing a "dry weight" or edema-free weight. This is accomplished by gradually removing fluid by use of diuretics and assessing the patient's blood pres-

---

Factors predisposing to digitalis toxicity

Hypokalemia: potentiates the effects of digitalis
Severe liver and kidney disease: the liver inactivates digitalis; the kidney excretes it
Primary myocardial disease: myocardium is more sensitive to the drug
Elderly persons: decreased tolerance from decreased metabolism

---

Signs and symptoms of digitalis toxicity

Cardiovascular effects

Bradycardia
Tachycardia
Bigeminy (double beats)
Ectopic beats
Pulse deficit (difference between apical and radial pulse)

Gastrointestinal effects

Anorexia
Nausea and vomiting
Abdominal pain
Diarrhea

Neurologic effects

Headache
Double, blurred, or colored vision
Drowsiness, confusion
Restlessness, irritability
Muscle weakness

Table 25-6 Digitalis preparations

Generic name	Trade name	Route	Onset	Duration
Purple foxglove				
(*Digitalis purpurea*)				
Powdered digitalis	Digifortis	Oral	Slow	Long
	Digiglusin			
Digitoxin	Crystodigin	IV	Slow	Long
	Purodigin	Oral		
	Digitaline Nativelle			
	Unidigin			
Gitalin	Gitaligin	Oral	Fast	Moderate
White foxglove				
(*Digitalis lanata*)				
Digoxin		Oral	Fast	Moderate
	Lanoxin	IV		
		IM		
Deslanoside	Cedilanid-D	IV	Fast	Short
		IM		
Lanatoside C	Cedilanid	Oral	Variable	Short
Acetyldigitoxin	Acylanid	Oral	Moderate	Short
Strophanthus gratus				
Ouabain		IV	Fast	Short

Table 25-7 Diuretics used in the treatment of heart failure

Type	Example	Onset/peak/duration	Side effects
Thiazide	Chlorothiazide (Diuril)	2 hr/4 hr/6-12 hr	Gastrointestinal upsets (can be minimized by taking medication with meals); hypokalemia; hyperglycemia
	Hydrochlorothiazide (Esidrix, Hydrodiuril)	2 hr/4 hr/6-12 hr	
Loop	Furosemide (Lasix)	1 hr/1-2 hr/6-8 hr	Similar to thiazide diuretics; also ototoxicity and blood dyscrasias
	Ethacrynic acid (Edecrin)	30 min/2 hr/6 hr	
Potassium-sparing	Spironolactone (Aldactone)	Gradual/3 days/2-3 days after therapy discontinued	Gastrointestinal irritation; hyperkalemia
	Triamterene (Dyrenlum)	Rapid/7-9 hr/12-16 hr	

sure. When the patient becomes hypotensive, particularly orthostatic, this signals the physician that too much fluid has been removed. The patient is then permitted to reaccumulate a small amount of fluid until hypotension no longer occurs. This weight is then considered the patient's dry weight.

Types of common diuretic drugs are listed in Table 25-7. Currently the *thiazides* are the diuretics of choice in the treatment of heart failure. The thiazides are inexpensive, easy to take, and effective when taken over a long time. Because these potent drugs can lead to electrolyte imbalance, serum chemistry levels are observed closely, particularly at the onset of therapy. The major complication is hypokalemia, which may produce ECG changes and cause digitalis toxicity. Foods high in potassium are encouraged, and potassium supplements may be prescribed.

If thiazides are ineffective, oral aldosterone antagonist, such as spironolactone (Aldactone) or triamterene (Dyrenium), may be given with the thiazide. These drugs work by competitive inhibition of aldosterone, resulting in retention of potassium and excretion of sodium and water.

The most potent diuretics currently available are furosemide (Lasix) and ethacrynic acid (Edecrin). These medications are reserved for severe congestive heart failure or when other forms of treatment are ineffective in relieving symptoms. These agents also increase renal blood flow and, therefore, may prove effective in treating heart failure when renal function is also impaired. Therapy is best initiated in the hospital setting so that electrolyte and acid-base balance may be monitored.

□ *Sodium-restricted diet*

Edema is often effectively controlled in patients with heart failure by restriction of sodium intake. The degree of restriction depends on the severity of the failure and the extent of diuretic therapy. The severely restricted sodium diet is rarely prescribed, because this diet is unpalatable and expensive, which results in poor patient compliance.

The amount of sodium in the normal diet is 3 to 10 g/day. Sodium restriction in persons receiving diuretics may not be dropped below 3 to 5 g/day because of the dangers of hyponatremia. In mild cardiac failure, sodium may be restricted to 1 to 2 g/day; this is known as a no-added salt (NAS) diet. It is essentially a normal diet, except that no extra salt is added to prepared foods and obviously salted foods such as potato chips are omitted. For moderate or severe heart failure, the amount of sodium permitted is specifically prescribed. Vitamin supplements are usually required when severely restricted sodium diets are prescribed.

Low-sodium diets can be made more appealing by adding salt substitutes to food in place of table salt. Since many salt substitutes contain potassium, the patient's need for potassium must be assessed. Often the increased potassium is beneficial when the patient is on diuretic therapy. The use of herbs often makes the food more appetizing.

Fluid restriction is less commonly instituted than in the past as long as the person is on a sodium-controlled diet and is receiving diuretics or digitalis. If fluids are restricted, the amount of fluid permitted is prescribed by the physician and a plan is made, in conjunction with the patient if possible, to space the fluids over the day.

□ **Assisting with comfort and ADL**

A careful assessment must be made each day to determine the extent to which the person can perform ADL such as eating and bathing. Most patients prefer to maximize their independence, and this is encouraged within the limitations of their symptoms.

Edematous skin is poorly nourished and very susceptible to breakdown. Edema of the sacrum is prevalent in patients with heart failure who are restricted to bed rest, and decubiti can develop quickly. Measures to prevent skin breakdown are instituted early.

□ **Counseling and teaching**

Since anxiety increases the symptoms of heart failure, measures are taken to help the person decrease anxiety. These measures include the following:

Nursing care of the patient with congestive heart failure

Assisting with achievement of therapeutic goals

1. Reinforce importance of conservation of energy and planning of activities to avoid fatigue
2. Provide diversional activity that will assist in conserving energy
3. Assist in maintaining an adequate nutritional intake while observing prescribed dietary prescriptions (sodium restrictions)
4. Monitor signs of fluid and electrolyte imbalance
5. Give medications as prescribed
   a. Careful and timely administration of diuretics
   b. Assess apical heart rate before administering digitalis preparations
   c. Observe patient for signs of digitalis toxicity
   d. Give pain medication or tranquilizer as indicated
6. Assess and record weight daily
7. Administer oxygen therapy as prescribed

Assisting with comfort and ADL

1. Assist with ADL as necessary
2. Encourage independence within the patient's limitations
3. Position patient carefully to promote comfort, ease of respirations, and venous return
4. Give meticulous skin care in patients with edema
   a. Careful washing of skin
   b. Frequent application of skin lotion
   c. Frequent repositioning
   d. Use of flotation mattress or waterbeds for severe edema
   e. Massage
5. Provide patient and family with opportunities to explore their concerns

Teaching

1. Need to monitor for signs and symptoms of congestive heart failure including daily weights, pedal edema, change in respiratory status
2. Need to avoid fatigue and plan for rest periods
3. Instructions for home oxygen therapy, if appropriate
4. Name, purpose, dosage, frequency, and side effects of prescribed medications (digitalis preparation, diuretic)
5. Dietary planning
   a. Rationale for sodium or fluid restrictions, as appropriate
   b. Foods to be avoided depending on diet prescription
   c. Small frequent feedings to decrease exertion and decrease GI blood requirements, which can tax the failing heart
6. Need for medical follow-up.

---

1. Identifying the feelings and the content related to these feelings
2. Identifying strengths that can be used for coping
3. Learning what can be done to decrease the anxiety, (for example, learning about measures to control heart failure and measures to reduce stress; see Chapter 7)

Working with family members in the same manner is also helpful to decrease their anxiety so they can be of greater support to the patient.

Patients who will be receiving oxygen therapy at home need to know how to manage the therapy. Instructions should include the following:

1. Indication for initiating oxygen therapy
2. How to initiate oxygen therapy
3. Mechanism for reordering oxygen supply
4. Precautions necessary when oxygen therapy is being used[23]

Teaching patients about their dietary restrictions, need for rest, and dietary regimen needs to be started early in the patient's hospitalization to permit time for learning and asking questions. The patient may need frequent interactions with the dietitian and nurse before being able to follow a prescribed sodium diet.

⊞ EVALUATION

Evaluation will be based on the expected patient outcomes. Questions to ask may include the following:

1. Is the patient breathing more easily?
2. Is the patient more comfortable?
3. Is peripheral edema decreased?
4. Is the patient less fatigued?
5. Does the patient know how to plan activities to prevent fatigue and dyspnea?
6. Can the patient describe components of the treatment regimen?
7. Can the patient explain the rationale for the treatment regimen?
8. Can the patient state plans for follow-up care?

■ PULMONARY EDEMA

Acute pulmonary edema is the rapid effusion of serous fluid from plasma into the pulmonary interstitial tissue and alveoli. It is a medical emergency that requires immediate

---

Signs and symptoms of pulmonary edema
Restlessness
Vague uneasiness
Dyspnea
Tachycardia
Pallor or cyanosis
Cough productive of large quantities of blood-tinged frothy sputum
Audible wheezing

---

care. The causes of pulmonary edema include the following:

1. Severe left ventricular failure
2. Inhalation of irritating gases
3. Rapid administration of intravenous fluids (whole blood, plasma, crystalloid fluids)
4. Barbiturate or opiate overdose

The signs and symptoms of pulmonary edema are listed in the box below, left.

□ Medical therapy

Treatment for acute pulmonary edema involves a number of simultaneous interventions to promote oxygenation, improve cardiac output, and reduce pulmonary congestion.[69] Whenever possible, the underlying cause is identified and remedied. The components of treatment are similar to those discussed for congestive heart failure but are applied more vigorously. Common interventions include patient positioning, morphine sulfate IV, oxygen, rapid digitalization, and aminophylline IV (see the box at bottom of page). Other measures to reduce circulating blood volume may include administering diuretics such as furosemide and ethacrynic acid, rotating tourniquets on three extremities, and performing a phlebotomy.

■ CARDIOGENIC SHOCK

Cardiogenic shock is a shock state of primary cardiac origin. It is most frequently caused by myocardial infarction but also may result from other cardiac disorders that lead to low cardiac output (see the box on p. 803).

■ Pathophysiology

Cardiogenic shock occurs when cardiac function is severely impaired and cardiac output is low. As the shock progresses, coronary artery perfusion is decreased, leading to development of cardiac muscle ischemia that leads to

---

Medical therapy for acute pulmonary edema

Intervention	Rationale
Patient in high Fowler's position or over side of bed with arms supported on bedside table	Promotes expansion of lungs; legs in dependent position causes venous pooling and reduction in venous return (preload)
Morphine sulfate, 5 to 10 mg, intravenously	Decreases anxiety; slows respirations; reduces venous return
Oxygen at 40% to 70% by face mask; intubation as needed	Promotes oxygenation; increased tidal volume also promotes removal of secretions from alveoli
Rapid digitalization if patient not previously taking digitalis	Improves contractility; increases CO and reduces heart rate; converts rapid rate arrhythmias such as atrial fibrillation
Aminophylline, 250 mg, given intravenously over approximately 30 min	Relieves bronchospasm and wheezing; acts as diuretic

Causes of cardiogenic shock

Myocardial infarction
Critical aortic stenosis
Intractable arrhythmias
Ruptured aortic aneurysm
Severe congestive heart failure
Massive pulmonary embolism
Cardiac tamponade

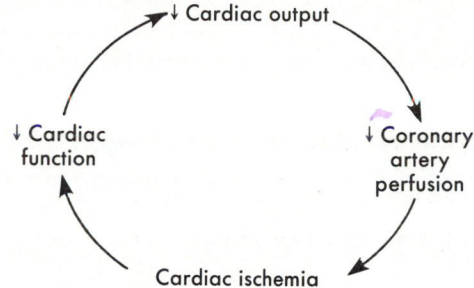

Fig. 25-32 Sequence of events in cardiogenic shock.

further decreased function (Fig. 25-32). Mortality is high. (See Chapter 9 for further discussion on shock.)

■ Medical therapy

Cardiogenic shock is a medical emergency that requires immediate intervention and constant attention to prevent irreversible cell damage and death. Therapy is aimed at correcting factors that contribute to decreased tissue perfusion, such as cardiac arrhythmias, hypoxemia, and pain.

Invasive monitoring lines that are usually placed include catheters in the pulmonary artery, systemic artery, and urinary bladder. The left ventricular end-diastolic pressure (LVEDP) is reflected in the pulmonary capillary wedge pressure, which is used as a guide to fluid therapy.

The following therapy may be initiated:

1. Vasopressors and cardiotonic agents (for example, dopamine, norepinephrine) to raise systemic arterial pressure without increasing cardiac work load; vasopressors are titrated to maintain systolic pressure, preferably about 90 mm Hg.
2. Hyperventilation and buffering agents (for example, sodium bicarbonate) to counteract lactic acidosis
3. Intravenous fluids if hypovolemia is present; care must be taken to prevent fluid overload with resulting pulmonary edema
4. Use of intraaortic balloon counterpulsation, if necessary (see discussion below)

General care of the patient in shock is described in Chapter 9.

■ INTRAAORTIC BALLOON COUNTERPULSATION

A counterpulsation device facilitates blood circulation by decreasing aortic pressure during systole and increasing it during diastole. The overall effects include the following:

1. Increase in coronary artery perfusion
2. Decrease in preload (degree to which the myocardium is stretched before contracting)
3. Decrease in afterload (resistance against which blood is expelled).

In addition to being used in the situations producing cardiogenic shock, the intraaortic balloon pump may be used in unstable patients with cardiac disease before and during open heart surgery and in assistance when removing these patients from cardiopulmonary bypass following surgery.

□ Technique

The intraaortic balloon is inserted percutaneously or by cutdown into the right or left femoral artery. It is advanced into the thoracic aorta and sutured into place at the insertion site after the balloon tip has been correctly positioned just distal to the left subclavian artery (Fig. 25-33).

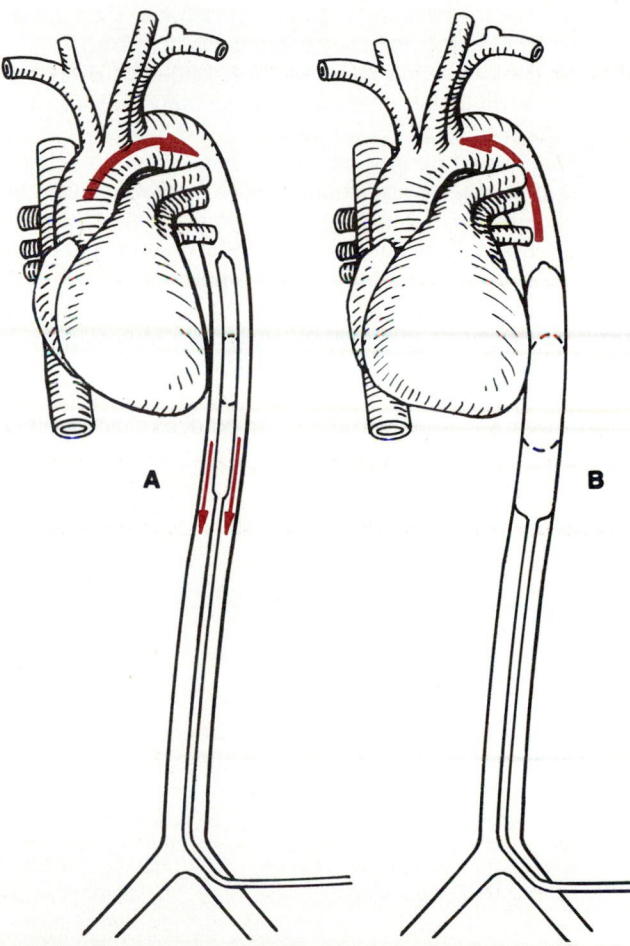

Fig. 25-33 Representation of intraaortic balloon positioned just distal to left subclavian artery. **A,** Balloon is deflated allowing forward blood flow during systole. **B,** Balloon is inflated to increase coronary perfusion during diastole.

NURSING CARE PLAN

Person with congestive heart failure

DATA: Mr. Green is a 59-year-old factory worker with a long history of hypertension. He has taken his antihypertensive medications only sporadically and frequently fails to keep follow-up appointments at the hypertension clinic. His blood pressure has never been under good control, and readings have typically been 160-190/96-100. Mr. Green has felt fatigued for several weeks and has noticed increasing difficulty with breathing, particularly when moving heavy equipment at work. At times he awakens during the night and feels like he is suffocating. He came to the clinic to get something to help him sleep better and was admitted to the hospital for evaluation. Tests revealed that he has hypertensive cardiovascular disease and congestive heart failure. Following loading doses of digoxin, he is being maintained on 0.25 mg po qd. He is also on a low-sodium diet and hydrochlorothiazide 50 mg po bid. His activity has been restricted to "up in room as tolerated."

The nursing history identified the following:

1. He and his wife have little understanding of the low-sodium diet that was prescribed years ago. He remembers the diet instructions as "not adding too much salt at the table." He frequently eats sandwiches of luncheon meat and cheese at work or has canned soup from the vending machine.

2. The episodes of nocturnal dyspnea have been very frightening to both Mr. Green and his wife. They have tried various preventive measures such as more fresh air, but nothing seems to work. Mrs. Green states that she is almost afraid to go to bed anymore.

3. He sees little need to take "medicine" if he doesn't feel sick. Now the doctor has prescribed more medicine for his heart when the trouble is his breathing.

4. He is reluctant to tell his boss about the dyspnea he encounters at work because he doesn't want to be labeled a "cry baby"—"It's better to just tough things out."

Collaborative nursing activites include those to assess (1) Mr. Green's response to the therapeutic regimen and (2) the presence of any complications associated with the regimen. Nursing actions include monitoring the following:

1. Response to exertion—especially heart rate and respiratory effort
2. Breath sounds—location and extent of adventitious sounds such as rales
3. Daily weights and intake/output
4. Blood pressure
4. Heart rate and rhythm; abnormal cardiac sounds such as an S_3 gallop
6. Serum electrolytes—especially potassium

Nursing diagnosis: Activity intolerance related to imbalance between oxygen supply and demand

Expected patient outcomes	Nursing interventions	Rationale
Patient complains of less dyspnea on exertion	Plan activities to conserve energy; allow for rest periods; provide assistance with aspects of physical care that are tiring; discuss ways to conserve energy at home and at work	Pacing of activities will lessen myocardial oxygen demand

Nursing diagnosis: Anxiety (Mr. Green and his wife) related to perceived change in health status (onset of frightening symptoms) and uncertainty regarding cause or measures to control

Expected patient outcomes	Nursing interventions	Rationale
Patient and wife express less anxiety about PND episodes	Explain basis for symptoms and expectations of therapeutic regimen; suggest sleeping with head of bed slightly elevated	Providing structure in a situation of uncertainty allows persons to gain control and feel less anxious

NURSING CARE PLAN

Person with congestive heart failure—cont'd

Nursing diagnosis: Knowledge deficit (low-sodium diet, pathophysiology of heart failure, rationale for therapeutic regimen) related to lack of recall and lack of exposure

Expected patient outcomes	Nursing interventions	Rationale
Patient and wife can describe CHF and explain the basis for symptoms	Teach about the heart as a pump and effect of hypertension; select an appropriate analogy from patient's home or work life regarding pumps and pressure	Learning is easier when content can be related to something familiar
Patient can explain rationale for low-sodium diet, diuretic, digoxin	Teach relationship between sodium, fluid retention, and hypertension; explain effect of digoxin on heart	Understanding of the rationale for therapeutic regimen may improve compliance
Patient and/or wife can describe basic elements of a low-sodium diet	Provide and discuss information on foods to avoid and foods that may be eaten liberally on this diet	Providing information on activities that are allowed, as well as those that must be avoided, gives persons resources for coping with restrictions

Nursing diagnosis: Noncompliance (previously) with therapeutic regimen possibly related to absence of physical symptoms or inability to cope with taking on any aspect of the "sick role"

Expected patient outcomes	Nursing interventions	Rationale
Patient adheres to therapeutic regimen	Explore previous noncompliance to determine reasons from patient's perspective; identify difficulties foreseen with new regimen; help patient explore acceptable alternatives	Data are insufficient to guide specific plan; patient's perceptions of difficulties with therapeutic regimen provide avenues for intervention by nurse

The end of the balloon catheter is attached to a pump console, which alternately inflates and deflates the balloon using either helium or carbon dioxide gas.

The timing of the inflation-deflation sequence is of the utmost importance in obtaining maximal counterpulsation effect. Using the ECG to trigger the pumping mechanism and the arterial waveform to determine the effectiveness of the counterpulsation, the balloon is timed to inflate just at the beginning of ventricular diastole, immediately after closure of the aortic valve. The balloon remains inflated during diastole and is then timed to deflate immediately before the next ventricular systolic ejection or just before the aortic valve reopens. Improper timing of the balloon not only defeats the purpose of counterpulsation, but also could directly damage the myocardium. This is particularly true in early inflation or late deflation, in which the heart would be ejecting blood against a partially inflated balloon.

Nursing management

1. Monitor vital signs and indices of cardiac function at frequent intervals as specified
2. Position patient:
   a. Head of bed elevated no more than 30 degrees to prevent balloon migration upward in aorta
   b. Reposition patient every 2 hours on alternate sides to prevent skin breakdown and other consequences of immobility
   c. Avoid hip flexion on catheterized side; restrain leg if necessary.
3. Monitor circulation of both legs before catheter insertion and hourly thereafter until balloon is removed
4. Keep dressing on balloon insertion site clean and dry; change every 24 to 48 hours using sterile technique
5. Administer prescribed heparin or low molecular weight dextran to prevent blood clotting or emboli

Considerable psychologic support is necessary for the patient and family during such critical therapy. Not only is the physical size and noise of the pump console very intimidating, but its presence only reinforces everyone's awareness of the frailty of the patient's heart and uncertainty about the future. Careful but simple explanations of the pump's action are necessary for patients who are alert enough to understand; it is important that they not get the mistaken idea that the pump is working instead of their heart. Some patients with this type of misunderstanding fear that they will die if the pump stops even momentarily. Such terrific fear makes them anxious and restless and further increases the body's demand for oxygen. Continuous reassurance and repeated simple explanations are essential. Some patients may benefit from mild sedation.

Table 25-8 Other heart disorders

Disorder	Etiology	Signs and symptoms	Medical therapy
Pericarditis	Infection (virus, bacteria), complication of systemic disease, trauma, neoplasm	*Acute:* Severe precordial chest pain referred to neck, shoulder, left arm; intensified when lying supine, coughing or breathing deeply or swallowing Pericardial friction rub Fever, leukocytosis, ECG changes Cardiac tamponade *Chronic:* Dyspnea, fatigue, congestive heart failure	*Acute:* Treatment of underlying condition Supportive care: salicylates, indomethacin, corticosteroids Pericardiocentesis for injection of antibiotic or sclerosing agent Pericardial fenestration *Chronic:* Digitalization, diuretics Low-sodium diet Pericardiectomy for severe cases
Myocarditis	Infection, drugs, chemicals, radiation, metabolic disorders	May be asymptomatic Nonspecific complaints of dyspnea on exertion, palpitations, precordial chest pain, fever, tachycardia	Antibiotics Corticosteroids for severe cases Antiarrhythmic drugs for arrhythmias
Endocarditis	*Streptococcus viridans,* staphylococci, enterococci; associated with rheumatic valvular disease and intrusive procedures; also seen in cases of drug addiction	Gradual onset: malaise, achiness, fever Splenomegaly, clubbing of fingers, Osler's nodes on fingers, petechiae in conjunctiva and mouth, cardiac murmur, anemia	Bed rest Antibiotics (IV) Prolonged antibiotic therapy Incision and drainage of abscesses Valve replacement
Rheumatic fever/ rheumatic heart disease	Unknown; seen in conjunction with group A beta-hemolytic streptococcal pharyngeal infections	Symptoms follow pharyngeal infection in 1 to 4 weeks Joint pain—recurrent Heart murmur, friction rub, cardiac arrhythmias, congestive heart failure	Antibiotics Antiinflammatory drugs (salicylates, corticosteroids) Early ambulation
Cardiovascular syphilis	Result of early syphilitic infection	Signs of aortic aneurysms, aortitis, aortic valve insufficiency, congestive heart failure	Penicillin Surgery for aneurysm or aortic valve insufficiency, if feasible Treatment of congestive heart failure, if it develops
Alcoholic cardiomyopathy	Chronic alcoholism	Gradual onset: fatigue, dyspnea on exertion Pulmonary rales, cardiac murmur, edema, hypertension, increased central venous pressure, congestive heart failure, thromboemboli	Symptomatic Treatment of congestive heart failure Vasodilators and prolonged bed rest are prescribed to decrease size of enlarged heart

---

Causes of pericarditis

Infection: viral, bacterial, fungal
Complications of systemic disease
   Rheumatoid arthritis
   Systemic lupus erythematosus
   Scleroderma
   Uremia
Trauma
   Closed chest trauma (for example, automobile accident)
   Myocardial infarction
Neoplasm: neoplastic infiltration, myxoma

Disorders associated with chronic pericarditis

Rheumatic heart disease
Congenital heart disease
Hypertensive heart disease
Systemic lupus erythematosus
Rheumatoid arthritis
Scleroderma
Myxedema
Renal failure

■ OTHER HEART DISORDERS

■ Pathophysiology

This section will discuss a group of cardiac conditions that are generally the result of inflammation or are the consequence of the long-term effect of toxins or pathogenic processes that are not primarily cardiac in origin. All cardiac tissues are susceptible to inflammation, and heart failure can be a serious and rapid result of the inflammatory process. The specific pathologic mechanisms are discussed below and are summarized in Table 25-8, along with signs and symptoms and medical therapy.

■ PERICARDITIS

Pericarditis is an inflammatory process of the visceral or parietal pericardium. It may result from infection, complication of systemic disease, trauma, or neoplasm (see the box above).

Symptoms of cardiac tamponade

Diminished or absent point of maximal impulse (PMI)
Diminished peripheral pulses
Distended neck veins (secondary to increased CVP)
Decreased blood pressure (secondary to ineffective pumping action)
Narrowing pulse pressure (difference between systolic and diastolic blood pressure)
Paradoxical pulse (decrease in pulse strength during inspiration)
Diminished heart sounds

Pericarditis may be acute or chronic, and infection may spread from or to the myocardium. *Acute pericarditis* is further classified as fibrinous or exudative. The exudate accompanying acute pericarditis may be serous, purulent, or hemorrhagic. When fluid accumulates in the pericardial sac, *cardiac tamponade* (compression of heart from blood or fluid) may occur with impairment of ventricular filling and emptying. If not diagnosed and treated promptly, the severe reduction in CO can result in shock and death. (See the box below, left).

Chronic pericarditis is referred to as chronic constrictive or adhesive pericarditis. It is three times more prevalent in men than women. It may result from fibrosing of the pericardial sac secondary to trauma or neoplastic disease. In the majority of cases, no specific pathogen can be identified as the causative agent. Chronic pericarditis is often associated with other disease processes (see the box above). If the pericardium becomes a constrictive band surrounding the heart, it will prevent adequate filling and emptying of the ventricles, thus decreasing CO and ultimately producing cardiac failure.

■ MYOCARDITIS

Myocarditis is an inflammatory disease of the myocardium. It may be classified as acute or chronic and can be either focal or diffuse in nature. Frequently, the inflammatory process develops secondary to acute endocarditis or pericarditis.

Infection may result in different ways:
1. Invasion by organisms of the myocardial tissue
2. Production of toxins (diphtheria)
3. Autoimmune reaction (rheumatic fever, systemic lupus erythematosus)

Worldwide, the more frequent infectious agents are rickettsiae, bacteria, protozoans, and metazoans. In North America, viral causes predominate, including Coxsackievirus, echovirus, and viral encephalitis, rabies, and herpes simplex.

■ ENDOCARDITIS

Endocarditis is an infection of the endocardium and most often of the heart valves. The more recent method of classificaton of infective endocarditis is on the basis of the causative organism, for example, enterococcal endocarditis or streptococcal endocarditis. It may occur in acute or subacute forms. Acute endocarditis occurs rapidly, often on normal heart valves, and if untreated may cause death within days or weeks. The subacute form develops more gradually, usually on previously damaged heart valves, and responds well to treatment.

The infecting organisms are carried by a turbulent blood flow and deposited on the heart valves or elsewhere on the endocardium. The turbulent blood flow occurs in areas of myocardial anomalies, such as prolapsed mitral valves or ventricular septal defects. The organisms bombard the heart valves, become embedded in the valve matrix, and result in vegetative growths that may scar and perforate the leaflets. Further risk results if the vegetative growths break free of the valves, enter the bloodstream, and cause emboli. If the vegetative emboli enter organs such as the spleen or kidney, abscesses may form.

■ RHEUMATIC HEART DISEASE

Rheumatic fever is an acute inflammatory reaction. It is important in the discussion of inflammatory heart disease, as it has tremendous potential for causing chronic heart problems. In the United States today approximately 1,750,000 adults and 100,000 children have rheumatic heart disease.[2] Symptoms of cardiac involvement usually follow a group A beta-hemolytic streptococcus pharyngeal infection. Ninety percent of the victims are between the age of 5 and 15.

Rheumatic fever may progress with mild symptoms and go undiagnosed, or the disease may be subclinical with no symptoms. The patient develops cardiac manifestations years later. On careful history taking, a recollection of a childhood illness confirming the likelihood of rheumatic fever is usually found.

The pathophysiology of rheumatic heart disease remains unclear. The pericardium, myocardium, or endocardium can be involved. The affected tissue develops small areas of necrosis (*Aschoff bodies*), which heal, leaving scar tissue. Myocardial changes are usually reversible. In the pericardium and endocardium, however, the disease process is usually not reversible and produces the disabling effects of rheumatic heart disease. The valves are typically most affected and become fibrous and incompetent. The leaflets of a valve may fuse during the healing phase.

■ CARDIOVASCULAR SYPHILIS

Cardiovascular syphilis usually occurs from 10 to 30 years after the primary syphilitic infection. Since the highest incidence of primary syphilis is among persons in their early twenties, persons with symptoms of cardiovascular syphilis are usually over 30 years of age.

Cardiovascular syphilis is an extremely dangerous complication of primary syphilis. The spirochetes attack the aorta, the aortic valve, and the myocardium. The ascending aorta is often affected. The wall of the aorta becomes weakened and an *aneurysm* (p. 817) develops. As the aneurysm grows, it may press on neighboring structures, such as the intercostal nerves, resulting in chest pain. An aneurysm may be present without symptoms. It may rupture as it increases in size. Because of this, the patient is encouraged to avoid strenuous activities that might cause a sudden increase in blood pressure.

Spirochetes may also attack the aorta more diffusely, causing *aortitis*. The aorta becomes dilated, and calcium plaques are laid down. The junction of the aorta with the coronary arteries becomes constricted, resulting in angina (p. 780). Thrombi may also develop in the aorta, leading to the development of emboli and resulting in myocardial infarction or cerebral emboli.

Spirochetes may also attack the aortic valve, resulting in scarring. Aortic insufficiency may develop. This is often complicated by heart failure.

■ ALCOHOLIC CARDIOMYOPATHY

When any form of ethanol (the chief substance in alcoholic beverages) is consumed in large quantities over a period greater than 5 years, it has a direct toxic effect on cardiac tissue. Additives in alcoholic beverages may also create their own toxic effects. Persons with alcoholic cardiomyopathy are usually well-nourished individuals; only 15% of these patients have thiamin deficiency as is seen in many alcoholics.

Alcohol cannot function as an adequate source of calories. The oxidation rate of alcohol cannot be accelerated to meet demands for increases in energy. In chronic alcoholism, these metabolic disturbances result in visceral fatty degeneration of heart tissue. In the early stages, the disease process may be totally reversed by abstinence from alcohol.

■ General management

Patients with the heart disorders described above generally have signs and symptoms of heart failure, so assessment and intervention are directed toward that entity. In addition, if the cardiac condition is the result of an acute inflammatory process, symptoms such as fever, pain, anorexia, and malaise may also be present. Intervention is aimed at treatment of the underlying condition (when possible), relief of symptoms, and management of the heart failure. Knowledge of measures that can be undertaken to prevent future episodes or sequelae of this condition (for example, prophylactic antibiotic therapy, good oral hygiene) is an important patient outcome.

■ VALVULAR HEART DISEASE

■ Pathophysiology

Valvular heart disease is a general term that refers to any one of a variety of conditions that affect the valves within the heart. Normal valves function to maintain a unidirectional flow of blood through the cardiac chambers by passively opening and closing in response to variant pressure gradients. The mitral and tricuspid valves (atrioventricular valves) prevent the backflow of blood from the ventricles into the atria during systole. Movement of the atrioventricular valves is facilitated by the chordae tendinae and papillary muscles (Fig. 25-1). Similarly, the aortic and pulmonic valves (semilunar valves) prevent the backflow of blood from the aorta and pulmonary artery into their respective ventricles during diastole.

The two basic problems that compromise the normal function of the valves are stenosis and insufficiency. *Stenosis* is a thickening of the valvular tissue, which causes a narrowing of the valvular orifice. *Insufficiency* refers to the inability of the valve to close completely. An insufficient or incompetent valve allows blood to flow in a retrograde or regurgitant manner.

The predominant etiologic factor in the development of a stenosed or insufficient valve is rheumatic fever. Throughout the course of this disease, large hemorrhagic and fibrinous lesions vegetate along the inflamed edges of the valves.[29] These lesions frequently develop on adjacent valve leaflets so that the edges adhere together. As the disease process progresses, the leaflets become so scarred there is permanent leaflet fusion and limited valvular movement of the normally free-flapping edges.

Since these underlying pathologic changes occur over a period of time, the clinical signs and symptoms of a stenosed or insufficient valve do not usually show up until 10 to 40 years after the onset of rheumatic fever. Furthermore, the extent of valvular damage is largely dependent on its normal degree of motion. Since the pressures and consequent valvular movement on the left side of the heart are greater than those on the right, the mitral and aortic valves are more susceptible. The tricuspid and pulmonic valves are much less frequently affected by rheumatic fever.

The etiology, signs and symptoms, and medical therapy of valvular heart disorders are outlined in Table 25-9 for each type of disorder. Additional information about specific valvular disorders is provided in the sections that follow.

Table 25-9 Valvular heart disorders

	Etiology	Signs and symptoms	Medical therapy
Mitral insufficiency	Rheumatic fever Papillary muscle dysfunction (for example, myocardial infarction, ventricular aneurysm) Ruptured chordae tendinae Floppy valve syndrome: prolapsed mitral valve Bacterial endocarditis Congenital abnormalities	Excessive fatigue, weakness, exhaustion Weight loss Exertional dyspnea, orthopnea, paroxysmal nocturnal dyspnea, rales Late stages: pulmonary edema, right-sided heart failure *Auscultation:* Palpable thrill at apex S_1 absent, soft, or buried in murmur Murmur: high pitched, blowing, swishing, throughout systole (at apex) S_3 low pitched	Activity limitations Sodium-restricted diet Diuretics Digoxin Treatment of atrial arrhythmias Surgery: valvuloplasty, valvular replacement, annuloplasty
Mitral stenosis	Rheumatic fever May be associated with congenital anomalies "Parachute" mitral valve	Excessive fatigue, weakness Dyspnea, exertional dyspnea, orthopnea, paroxysmal nocturnal dyspnea Dry cough, bronchitis, rales Pulmonary edema Recurrent pulmonary emboli Hemoptysis Right-sided heart failure *Auscultation:* Palpable thrill at apex S_1 snapping, increased, loud Murmur: soft, low pitched, rumbling, diastolic (at apex)	Sodium-restricted diet Diuretics Activity limitations Oxygen therapy Anticoagulant therapy Surgery: valvulotomy, valve replacement

Table 25-9 Valvular heart disorders—cont'd

	Etiology	Signs and symptoms	Medical therapy
Aortic insufficiency	Rheumatic fever Severe hypertension Bacterial endocarditis Syphilis Dissecting aortic aneurysm Traumatic valve rupture Marfan's syndrome Congenital anomalies	Palpitations, sinus tachycardia Exertional dyspnea, orthopnea, paroxysmal nocturnal dyspnea Excessive diaphoresis Angina Late stages: left- and right-sided heart failure *Auscultation:* Murmur: high pitched, blowing, diastolic (third intercostal space) Systolic ejection murmur at base	Digoxin Sodium-restricted diet Diuretics Nitroglycerin (angina) Penicillin therapy (if syphilis a cause) Surgery: valve replacement, valvuloplasty

Aortic stenosis	Congenital anomalies
	Acquired:
	   Rheumatic fever
	   Arteriosclerosis
	   Idiopathic hypertropic subaortic stenosis
	   Calcification of leaflets
		Angina
		Syncope
		Fatigue, weakness
		Exertional dyspnea, orthopnea, paroxysmal nocturnal dyspnea
		Pulmonary edema, rales
		Late stages: right-sided heart failure
		Auscultation:
		Murmur: low pitched, rough, rasping, systolic (at base or carotids)
		Systolic thrill at base of heart
			Activity limitations
			Sodium-restricted diet
			Diuretics
			Digoxin
			Nitroglycerin (angina)
			Surgery: valve replacement

Tricuspid stenosis	Rheumatic fever Carcinoid heart disease Fibroelastosis Endomyocardial fibrosis	Pulmonary congestion, dyspnea Right-sided heart failure Decreased CO: weakness, fatigue, weight loss, hypotension Late stages: cirrhosis, jaundice, malnutrition	Sodium-restricted diet Digoxin Diuretics Surgery: valvuloplasty, valve replacement
Tricuspid insufficiency	Rheumatic fever Bacterial endocarditis Trauma Carcinoid heart disease Endomyocardial fibrosis Infarction of right ventricular papillary muscle Congenital anomalies	Right-sided heart failure Decreased CO: weakness, fatigue, weight loss, hypotension *Auscultation:* Murmur: blowing, throughout systole (left sternal border, increases with inspiration)	Sodium-restricted diet Digoxin Diuretics Surgery: narrowing of annulus, valve replacement

MITRAL STENOSIS

Mitral stenosis is more often found in women than men. As rheumatic fever is the primary factor in its development, the progressive destruction of the valve occurs over a 20-year period. Mitral commissures (junctions between adjacent cusps) fuse and the valvular leaflets or cusps thicken and calcify. The chordae tendinae also become short and thick. These underlying changes result in a narrow mitral valve that impedes the normal flow of blood.

To accommodate the increased work load required to move blood through this narrowed orifice, the left atrium hypertrophies. The resultant left atrial pressure exerts further pressure onto the pulmonary vasculature, causing pulmonary hypertension and pulmonary congestion. Eventually these conditions result in right ventricular failure and right-sided heart failure.

Another common complication of mitral stenosis is atrial fibrillation. Structural changes in the atrial wall from the increased pressure predispose to this arrhythmia. The coupling of atrial fibrillation and pooling of blood in the atria increases the likelihood of thrombus formation and arterial embolization.

MITRAL INSUFFICIENCY

In contrast to mitral stenosis, mitral insufficiency is more commonly seen in men than women. Although the same pathologic processes occur as a result of rheumatic fever, several other acquired and congenital conditions can contribute to its development. The end result is that the mitral valve leaflets fail to close fully. Consequently, a variable amount of blood leaks back through the valve from the left ventricle into the atrium.

The left atrium dilates and hypertrophies to compensate for the increased volume and pressure. The left ventricle also hypertrophies in response to the increased preload (blood that was regurgitated into the atrium during systole is returned to the ventricle during diastole). In other words, the ejection fraction is reduced and the end-diastolic volume is increased.

AORTIC STENOSIS

Aortic stenosis constitutes 25% of all valvular heart diseases. Diseases of the aortic valve do not usually occur as a single entity; most often there is also involvement of the mitral valve. Aortic stenosis develops as a congenital or acquired condition. Clinical symptoms of aortic stenosis are not manifested until the size of the opening in the valve has been reduced to approximately one third of normal. This situation may not occur until many years after the inception of the disease process. The asymptomatic nature of this disease is largely caused by the tremendous compensatory abilities of the left ventricle.

The left ventricle must generate an abnormally high pressure to eject blood through the narrowed aortic orifice. This added pressure requirement results in ventricular hypertrophy with a concomitant increase in myocardial oxygen demand. The oxygen demand may exceed the sup-

ply because of reduced cardiac output and inadequate coronary artery perfusion. Classic symptoms of angina may result.

The progressive stenosis accompanied by ventricular hypertrophy in the presence of mitral valve disease causes a decrease in CO. Symptoms of pulmonary congestion and eventually right-sided heart failure ensue.

AORTIC INSUFFICIENCY

Rheumatic fever accounts for approximately 80% of all cases of aortic insufficiency. In this instance the valve fails to close completely, and this results in a retrograde blood flow from the aorta into the left ventricle during diastole. The ventricle hypertrophies to hold all the regurgitant blood. Over time, the left ventricle cannot withstand the added work load, leading to the development of decreased CO, left ventricular failure, and right-sided heart failure.

TRICUSPID STENOSIS

Tricuspid stenosis is a relatively uncommon valvular lesion that usually coexists with stenosis of the mitral or aortic valves. The major cause of this disease is rheumatic fever. The leaflets become thick and fuse together, and the chordae tendinae also become short and thick. Hence during diastole blood flow is reduced through the compromised valve. This blockage further causes a backflow of blood in the systemic circulation. Engorgement of the superior and inferior vena cava precede the development of right-sided heart failure.

TRICUSPID INSUFFICIENCY

Tricuspid insufficiency is a very rare disorder that is more prevalent in children than adults. The disease usually develops secondary to marked dilation of the right ventricle and tricuspid valve ring.[10] The valve itself widens and the leaflets are unable to close properly. Therefore, there is regurgitant blood flow to the right atrium during systole. The right atrium hypertrophies to accommodate the increased volume, but invariably the CO decreases with the concomitant decreased blood flow to the left side of the heart. Eventually the excess volume in the atrium causes right-sided heart failure.

PULMONIC VALVE DISEASE

Lesions of the pulmonic valve are extremely rare in adults. This valve is less likely to be affected by rheumatic fever and bacterial endocarditis. For a more detailed discussion of congenital pulmonic stenosis, refer to a standard pediatric text.

Assessment

Assessment data that the nurse obtains are essentially the same for any patient with valvular heart disease. Many of the symptoms are related to decreased CO.

■ SUBJECTIVE DATA

1. Ability to carry out ADL and other desired activities: changes in endurance, fatigue, weakness
   These symptoms result from inadequate CO with subsequent impairment in cellular oxygenation
2. Shortness of breath: occurrence, type
   The patient may have dyspnea on exertion (DOE), orthopnea, or paroxysmal nocturnal dyspnea (p. 794) depending on the degree of heart failure
3. Pain in chest (angina): occurrence, measures used to relieve pain
4. Palpitations: occurrence
   Palpitations are a sensation in the chest described as a bounding or pounding of the heart
5. Syncope: occurrence
   A patient may verbalize feelings of light-headedness, dizzy spells, or fainting; these symptoms can be associated with a decrease in CO
6. Peripheral edema: site, extent, time of day
   Swelling of legs during the day with decreased swelling at night when legs are elevated is usually reported
7. Body weight: perceived pattern of weight gain
8. Diet and medications: ability to carry out therapeutic regimen

■ OBJECTIVE DATA

1. History of rheumatic fever
2. Observation/inspection
   a. Position and comfort level of patient
   b. Character and rate of breathing
   c. Use of supplemental oxygen
   d. Skin color and temperature
   e. Nailbed color and blanching (capillary filling)
   f. Diaphoresis
3. Auscultation
   a. Cardiac rate and rhythm
   b. Presence or change in heart sounds (murmurs, S_3, S_4, friction rub)
   c. Character of heart sounds at all auscultatory sites (aortic, pulmonic, tricuspid, mitral)
   d. Character and distribution of breath sounds
   e. Presence of adventitious breath sounds (rales, rhonchi)
4. Palpation
   a. Warmth of extremities
   b. Equality and symmetry of pulses
   c. Presence of edema
   d. Signs of phlebitis (increased calf diameter, positive Homans' sign)
5. Change in body weight

■ DIAGNOSTIC TESTS

Four major diagnostic tests are used to determine the presence of valvular heart disease: chest radiograph, ECG, echocardiogram, and cardiac catheterization. Table 25-10

summarizes the findings that are indicative of each specific type of valvular disease.

□ Chest radiograph

A chest radiograph demonstrates the overall size and configuration of the heart and its chambers. Calcification in the pericardium, myocardium, valves, or large blood vessels is also evident on the film. Most cardiac abnormalities that are discernable on a chest radiograph can be detected with standard anterior-posterior and lateral views of the chest.

□ Electrocardiogram

An ECG (p. 761) is helpful in the diagnosis of valvular heart disease. Hypertrophy of either chamber, as well as specific arrhythmias, can be detected.

□ Echocardiography

Echocardiography is most useful in the detection of abnormalities in the mitral and aortic valves. It is some benefit in the diagnosis of tricuspid valve disease.

Echocardiography is a noninvasive technique that uses ultrasound to assess both the structures and motions within the heart. A small transducer is placed on the patient's anterior left chest and moved in various diretions to visualize specific cardiac areas. This small transducer functions as a transmitter and receiver. It transmits high-frequency sound waves to the heart and then receives the reflected or echoed ultrasonic beams from the patient's heart. The ultrasonic beam is converted into electrical energy so that lines and spaces are displayed on the oscilloscope. These lines and spaces represent bone, cardiac chambers, valves, the septum, and muscle. A representative copy of the echocardiogram is obtained on paper to become a permanent record of the findings.

Since echocardiography is a noninvasive procedure, it is safer than cardiac catheterization. Hence, whenever possible, it precedes the cardiac catheterizaton. No special preparation is required for the test. The patient can eat and take medications as usual. Most importantly, the patient should be told about the purpose and procedure of this test. The patient must be aware of the importance of lying still for approximately 30 to 60 minutes. After the test the patient may resume normal activities, since there are no adverse effects from this test.

□ Cardiac catheterization

Cardiac catheterization is an extremely valuable diagnostic procedure that provides information about the structure and the function of the cardiac chambers, valves, and vessels. Since this is an invasive procedure, it is usually performed after several other diagnostic tests. A catheterization is performed on either the right or left side of the heart depending on the suspected valvular dysfunction. The purpose and procedure of each type are outlined in the box on p. 814.

Normal pressure readings and oxygen concentrations for the chambers and great vessels are listed in Fig. 25-34.

Table 25-10   Findings in valvular heart disorders

Disorder	Chest radiograph	ECG	Echocardiogram	Cardiac catheterization
Mitral stenosis	Left atrial enlargement Mitral valve calcification Right ventricular enlargement Prominence of pulmonary artery	Left atrial hypertrophy Right ventricular hypertrophy Atrial fibrillation	Thickened mitral valve Left atrial enlargement	Increased pressure gradient across valve Increased left atrial pressure Increased PCWP Increased right heart pressures Decreased CO
Mitral insufficiency	Left atrial enlargement Left ventricular enlargement	Left atrial hypertrophy Left ventricular hypertrophy Atrial fibrillation Sinus tachycardia	Abnormal mitral valve movement Left atrial enlargement	Mitral regurgitation Increased atrial pressure Increased LVEDP* Increased PCWP Decreased cardiac output
Aortic stenosis	Left ventricular enlargement Aortic valve calcification May have enlargement of left atrium, pulmonary artery, right ventricle, right atrium	Left ventricular hypertrophy	Thickened aortic valve Thickened ventricular wall Abnormal movement of aortic leaflets	Increased pressure gradient across valve Increased LVEDP*
Aortic insufficiency	Left ventricular enlargement	Left ventricular hypertrophy Tall R waves Sinus tachycardia	Left ventricular enlargement Abnormal mitral valve movement Increased movement of ventricular wall	Aortic regurgitation Increased LVEDP* Decreased arterial diastolic pressure
Tricuspid stenosis	Right atrial enlargement Prominence of superior vena cava	Right atrial hypertrophy Tall peaked P waves Atrial fibrillation	Abnormal valvular leaflets Right atrial enlargement	Increased pressure gradient across valve Increased right atrial pressure Decreased CO
Tricuspid insufficiency	Right atrial enlargement Right ventricular enlargement	Right ventricular hypertrophy Atrial fibrillation	Prolapse of tricuspid valve Right atrial enlargement	Increased atrial pressure Tricuspid regurgitation Decreased CO

*Left ventricular end-diastolic pressure.

Cardiac catheterization

Right side	**Left side**
Purpose	
Confirm suspected valvular heart disease—congenital or acquired	Evaluate pressures on left side of heart Assess competency of valves Assess left ventricular function
Procedure	
Cutdown made in large vein in patient's arm	Cutdown made in large artery in patient's arm or groin
Catheter threaded via fluoroscopy through superior vena cava, right atrium, right ventricle, pulmonary artery and pulmonary capillaries	Catheter threaded via fluoroscopy through aorta, aortic arch, descending aorta, aortic valve, and left ventricle
Blood sample obtained to determine oxygen content and saturation	Blood sample obtained to determine oxygen content and saturation
Pressures recorded for each chamber/vessel	Pressures recorded for each chamber/vessel
	Pressure gradient measurement across valves obtained

The right side of the heart is a low-pressure system with less oxygen saturation, since the blood there is going to the lungs. In contrast, the left side of the heart is a relatively high-pressure system with full oxygen saturation, as the blood there is returning from the lungs. Any changes in normal pressures and oxygen saturation are significant. Abnormalities in pressure gradients across valve are also indicative of valvular heart disease.

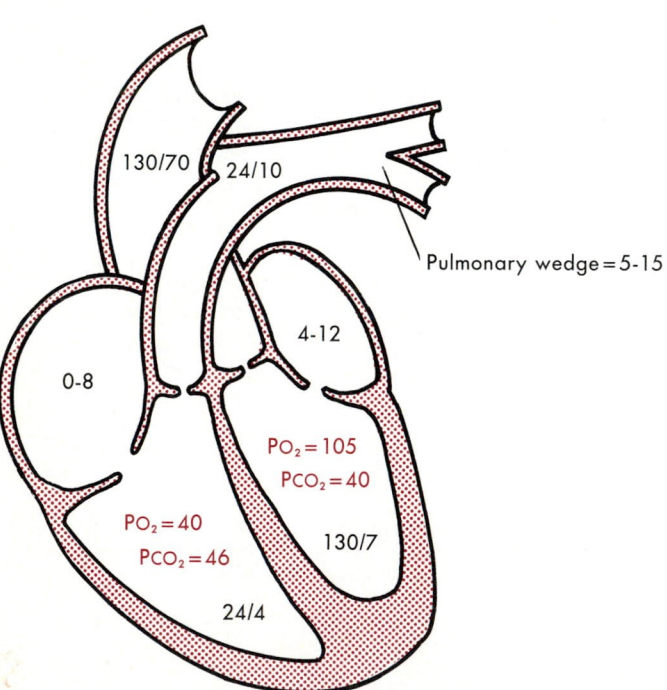

130/70   24/10

Pulmonary wedge = 5-15

4-12

0-8

$PO_2 = 105$
$PCO_2 = 40$

$PO_2 = 40$
$PCO_2 = 46$

130/7

24/4

Fig. 25-34   Pressure readings and blood gases in millimeters of mercury (mm Hg) in chambers of heart and major blood vessels.

➡ Data analysis: nursing diagnoses

Nursing diagnoses are determined from assessment of patient data. Possible nursing diagnoses for the person with valvular heart disease may include, but are not limited to, the following:

Diagnostic title	**Possible etiologies**
Activity intolerance	Imbalance between oxygen supply and demand
Knowledge deficit: pathophysiology of disorder, purpose of diagnostic tests, rationale for treatment regimen, strategies for conservation of energy	Lack of exposure/recall, information misinterpretation, unfamiliarity with information resources
Noncompliance: treatment regimen	Patient value system, treatment side effects
Pain	Angina, organ congestion
Sleep pattern disturbances	Nocturnal dyspnea, cough, anxiety

� Planning: expected patient outcomes

Expected therapeutic outcomes for the patient with valvular heart disease center around relief of symptoms and adequate cardiac functioning. Signs of pulmonary congestion and systemic venous congestion should be decreased, and improvement in cardiac output should be noted. The extent to which these outcomes are realized is dependent on the severity of the underlying problem, the presence or absence of other medical conditions, and the response of the patient to the treatment regimen. Outcomes related to the possible nursing diagnoses noted earlier may include, but are not limited to, the following:

1. Patient can state the purpose and procedure for diagnostic tests.
2. Patient can describe and implement a work, rest, and activity program to conserve energy.
3. Patient can describe the rationale for and components of the proposed treatment regimen (necessary dietary modifications, medications, surgery positioning to achieve comfort)
4. Patient can state plans for medical follow-up.

Implementation

ASSISTING WITH ACHIEVEMENT OF THERAPEUTIC GOALS

1. Administration of medications, as prescribed (diuretics, digoxin, antiarrhythmics)
2. Continued monitoring for signs of decreased CO
   a. Daily intake and output
   b. Daily weights
   c. Respiratory rate and rhythm
   d. Auscultation of breath sounds and heart sounds
   e. Condition of skin and mucous membranes
   f. Capillary perfusion
   g. Equality and strength of peripheral pulses
   h. Presence and extent of edema
   i. Blood pressure

ASSISTING WITH COMFORT AND ADL

1. Identify those activities of daily living which are fatiguing and for which patient may need some assistance
2. Design with patient a plan that will allow for completion of daily activities
3. Incorporate rest periods between activities
4. Maintain use of supportive oxygen therapy during activities, as necessary

TEACHING

1. Effect of a sodium-restricted or fluid-restricted diet on cardiac function, as appropriate
2. Effects of medications: diuretics, cardiac glycosides, anticoagulants
3. Prophylactic use of antibiotics before and after dental work
4. How to check for buildup of fluid in legs

5. Purpose and procedure for diagnostic tests (echocardiogram, cardiac catheterization)
6. Purpose and nature of surgical intervention, if appropriate

SURGERY

Surgical intervention is indicated for a patient whose life-style is severely compromised by valvular heart disease. If a patient has hemodynamically debilitating symptoms that are unsuccessfully managed by conventional medical therapies, surgery is then the recommended treatment modality. There are two basic surgical procedures: repair of the valve problem or replacement of the valve.

Repair of valve

Several terms are used to describe the specific anatomical structure undergoing repair (see the box below). Valvulotomy or commisurotomy can be done as a closed or open procedure. A closed approach involves the removal of a rib with a small incision into the left atrium. A dilator is then used to widen the narrowed valve and free the stenosed leaflet. The atrium is also palpated for thrombi. In the open technique, used also for valvuloplasty and annuloplasty, the thorax is incised and the heart completely exposed.

Replacement of valve

Many types of valves can be used for replacement. A valve is selected on the basis of location of the incompetent valve, the underlying pathologic changes, and the age of the patient. The size of the prosthetic valve is of major importance. Valves are grouped according to their design and function: caged-ball valves, tilting-disc valves, and biological valves (Fig. 25-35).

Caged-ball valves are the most durable. Their use, however, is restricted to patients with a large enough annulus and chamber to accommodate the cage itself. It is never used for tricuspid valve replacement because of the limited capacity of the right ventricle.

Tilting-disc valves require less space than caged-ball valves. The valve tilts when open and returns to flat position when closed. Similar to the caged-ball valve, the tilting-disc valve has a great potential for clot formation around the valve.

Biological valves are derived from animal cardiac tissue or human cadaver donors. Animal valves carry less risk for

---

Types of valve repair

Valvuloplasty	Repair of valve, suturing of torn leaflets
Annuloplasty	Repair of ring or annulus of incompetent valve, tightening and suturing of annulus
Valvulotomy/commissurotomy	Repair of a leaflet or commissure, fibrous band, or ring

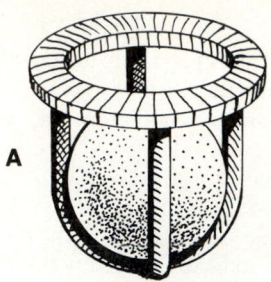 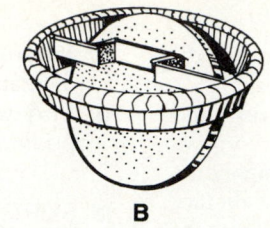 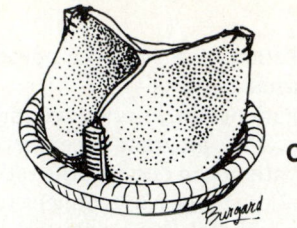

Fig. 25-35 Heart valve replacements. **A,** Caged-ball valve. **B,** Tilting-disc valve. **C,** Biological valve.

Nursing care of the patient undergoing valvular surgery

Preoperative care

1. Give medications as ordered
   a. Digitalis preparations and diuretics are often discontinued before surgery to avoid arrhythmias associated with digitalis toxicity that may be precipitated by cardiopulmonary bypass
   b. If the patient has been receiving anticoagulants, vitamin K may be administered before surgery to return prothrombin time to normal
   c. Antibiotics may be given to decrease incidence of postoperative endocarditis
2. Prepare patient for surgery by providing explanation of procedure and usual postoperative routines, addressing specific concerns of patient and family

Postoperative care

1. Administer anticoagulant therapy as prescribed (usually 5 to 7 days after valve replacement to prevent thrombus formation)
2. Assess apical heartbeat: a "click" sound is usually heard; reassure patient that this sound is normal; assess for development of murmur
3. Explain medication regimen to patient
   a. Need for antibiotics for approximately 1 month following valve replacement
   b. Need for cardiac glycosides to improve cardiac function and control arrhythmias for prescribed time (usually 3 to 6 months after surgery)

Table 25-11 Aneurysms

Type	Etiology	Signs and symptoms	Medical therapy
Abdominal aortic	Arteriosclerosis Hypertension Cystic medial necrosis Trauma Syphilis Other infections	Pulsating mass in mid-upper abdomen Systolic bruit over aorta Pain in mid-upper abdomen or in lower back or groin Long-standing cramps in buttocks, thighs, calves	Antihypertensive medications Pain medications Inotropic agents (for example, propranolol [Inderal]) Surgery: resection of aneurysm with graft replacement
Thoracic aortic	Arteriosclerosis Infection Congenital disorders causing cystic medial necrosis Trauma Syphilis Hypertension	*Ascending aorta:* Chest pain: deep, diffuse, aching *Transverse aorta:* Dyspnea, cough, hoarseness *Dissecting aneurysm:* Tearing sensation in chest, pain radiating to neck, shoulders, lower back, abdomen	Antihypertensive medications Negative inotropic agents (for example, propranolol [Inderal]) Surgery: Resection of aneurysm with graft replacement Aortic valve replacement (if aortic insufficiency)

thromboembolism; however, they tend to degenerate over time. Improvements in organ procurement and storage may make more human valves available in the future. These valves are less prone to infection and rejection than other replacements.

□ Preoperative and postoperative care

Nursing care for the patient undergoing valvular heart surgery is essentially the same as that for patients undergoing coronary bypass surgery (p. 788). Specific nursing care related to valvular surgery is listed in box on p. 816.

✠ Evaluation

Evaluation will be based on expected patient outcomes. Some questions to ask may include the following:

1. Can patient describe the nature of the valvular disorder?
2. Is patient able to describe a work, rest, and activity program to conserve energy?
3. Is patient able to explain any required dietary changes?
4. Can patient explain medication regimen?
5. Has patient made plans for continued medical follow-up?

■ ANEURYSMS

■ Pathophysiology

An aneurysm is a local or diffuse dilation of an artery. It occurs secondary to a variety of disease processes, although arteriosclerosis is the predominant etiologic factor (see Table 25-11). Regardless of the pathogenesis, the musculoelastic middle (media) layer of the artery becomes weakened, and it produces stretching of the inner (intima) and outer (adventitia) layers. Blood pressure within the vessel continues to weaken its walls and to enlarge the aneurysm.

The extent of arterial damage and clinical symptomatology vary greatly according to the type, size, and location of the aneurysm. An aneurysm is classified on the basis of its shape and subsequent damage to the affected artery (Fig. 25-36). The *fusiform aneurysm,* the most common type, assumes a spindle shape around the entire circumference of the vessel. In contrast, a *saccular aneurysm* affects only a part of the arterial circumference. This type of aneurysm appears as a unilateral sac or outpouching on the side of the artery. Also, a saccular aneurysm is more likely to rupture. A *dissecting aneurysm* develops from a split or tear in the intimal wall overlying a diseased media. This relatively uncommon occurrence leads to the accumulation of blood in a newly formed cavity between the vessel layers.

Although these types of aneurysms can develop in any artery, the major site for aneurysm formation is the aorta. Since the aorta has such a large diameter and is subject to great pressures, it is often the location for underlying

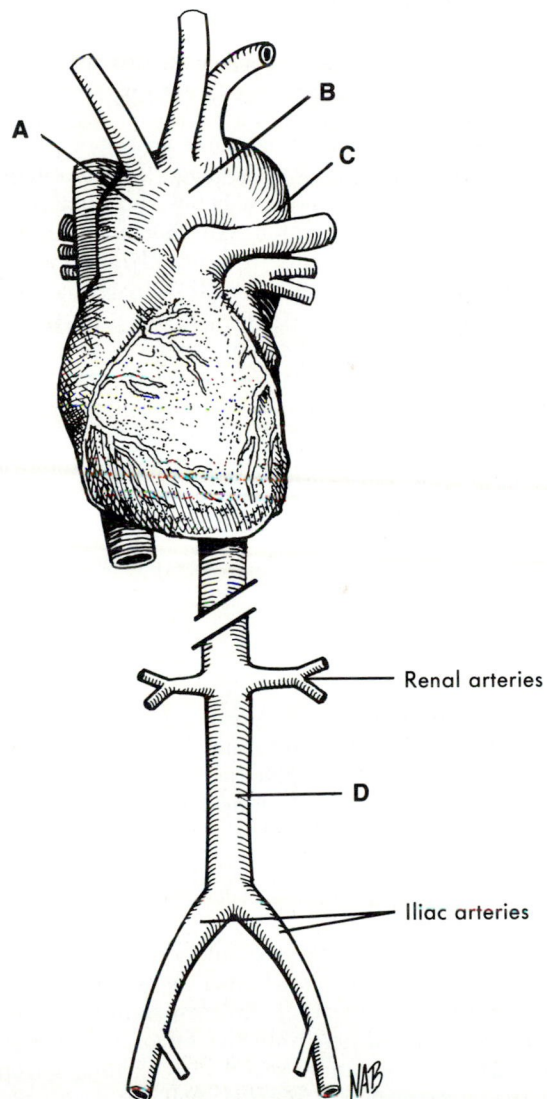

Renal arteries

Iliac arteries

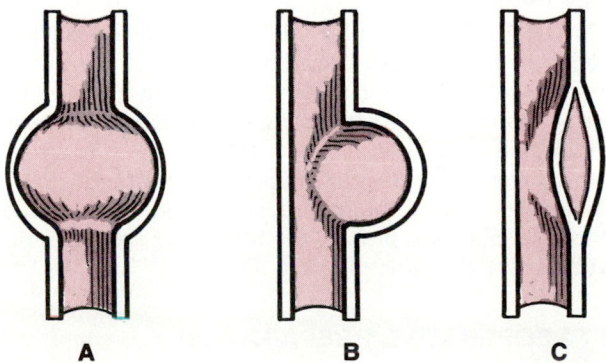

Fig. 25-36   Types of aneurysms. **A,** Fusiform. **B,** Saccular. **C,** Dissecting.

Fig. 25-37   Common sites of aortic aneurysms. **A,** Ascending aorta. **B,** Transverse aorta. **C,** Descending aorta. **D,** Abdominal aorta.

disease processes. Aortic aneurysms are found in the thoracic segment and, more commonly, in the abdominal portions (Fig. 25-37). Since there is some difference between aneurysms in these locations, they are discussed as separate entities.

■ THORACIC AORTIC ANEURYSMS

Aneurysms within the thoracic area can develop in the descending, ascending, or transverse section of the aorta. Hypertensive men between 50 and 70 years of age are typically subject to this disease.

Aneurysms in the *descending aorta* are usually fusiform and originate just distal to the left subclavian artery. A patient with this form of aneurysm is asymptomatic. Symptoms of chest pain are associated with aneurysms of the *ascending aorta*. Less frequent are aneurysms of the *transverse aorta* or aortic arch. Symptoms of this type directly relate to the aneurysms compression on surrounding structures, such as the lungs, trachea, and larynx.

■ ABDOMINAL AORTIC ANEURYSMS

Aneurysms of the abdominal aorta are more prevalent in hypertensive men over 60 years of age. The vast majority of these aneurysms develop just below the renal arteries but above the iliac bifurcation. An abdominal aneurysm grows slowly, hence the patient is usually asymptomatic. It can leak into the retroperitoneal or pelvic cavity, or dissect into the duodenum. As the aorta exceeds its normal 3 to 4 cm diameter at this point, there is an increased probability of rupture.

The prognosis for a patient with an abdominal aortic aneurysm depends not only on the size of the defect but, more importantly, on the extent of arteriosclerotic heart disease. More than half of those with untreated abdominal aneurysm die within 2 years of diagnosis; over 85% die within 5 years.

■ Diagnostic tests
■ RADIOGRAPHY

An aneurysm is most often detected accidentally by routine chest or abdominal radiograms, since symptoms are rarely manifested. Radiographic findings show widening of the aorta with a ring of calcification outlining the aneurysm and displacement of surrounding structures.

■ ANGIOGRAPHY

An aortogram reveals the size and location of an aneurysm. This test determines whether an aneurysm is leaking, expanding, or dissecting. An aortogram is performed by insertion of a catheter into the femoral, brachial, or axillary artery. The patient may feel a burning sensation when the contrast dye is injected. Following injection of the contrast material, a series of radiograms are taken at intervals to determine an accurate flow study.

After the procedure, the patient must remain resting in

bed for 6 to 12 hours with only minimal flexion of the cannulated joint. Vital signs are monitored every 15 minutes for 2 hours. Assessment of pulses, skin color, temperature, movement, and numbness distal to the site is also important. The injection site is inspected whenever vital signs are taken for the presence of bleeding, swelling, or hematoma.

■ SONOGRAPHY

Ultrasound is also helpful in determining the shape and location of the aneurysm. Special conducting gel is applied to the skin. The Doppler probe head is placed over the gel to intensify sounds of pulse vibration. Blood flow and presence of bruit are detected. Since this is a noninvasive procedure, there are no special precautions or posttest care.

■ Surgery

Surgery is the treatment of choice for patients with large or dissecting aneurysms or with those aneurysms that produce symptoms with a significant risk of rupture. Elective resection at the time of the first symptoms is often advised, since emergency surgery increases surgical risks. Complications of surgery include massive hemorrhage, injury to adjacent structures (duodenum, ureters, kidneys), myocardial infarction, renal failure, stroke, or graft infection.

■ PROCEDURES
□ Thoracic aorta

Surgical intervention for the patient with an aneurysm of the thoracic aorta is comparable to open heart surgery. A midline thoracic incision is made, and the aneurysm is exposed. Cardiopulmonary bypass (p. 789) is used to maintain tissue oxygenation during clamping of the aorta. Hypothermia may also be indicated to decrease the metabolic requirements of the tissues. While the aneurysm itself is being resected, cross-clamps are placed above and below the aorta to prevent blood flow into the operative area (Fig. 25-38). An artificial patch or tube (Teflon or Dacron) is grafted on the area.

□ Abdominal aorta

Surgical intervention for the removal of an abdominal aortic aneurysm is performed without use of heart and lung bypass, since arterial blood flow to lower extremities can be interrupted safely during the operative procedure. An abdominal incision is made, the aneurysm is opened, and any clots and debris are removed. A synthetic graft in the form of a patch or tube is sutured onto the tissues. Once the graft is replaced, the remaining arterial wall is sutured over the graft (Fig. 25-39).

■ PREOPERATIVE PREPARATION

The physician explains the surgical risks in obtaining informed consent for the surgery. The nurse provides support for the patient during the decision-making process,

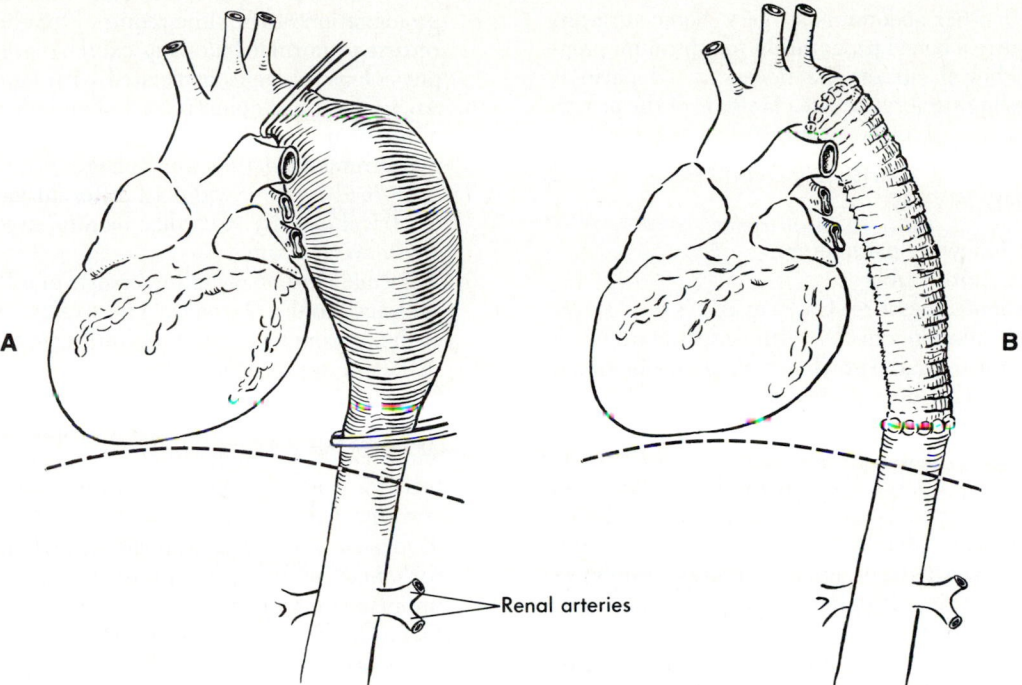

Renal arteries

Fig. 25-38 Aneurysm of descending thoracic artery. **A,** Resection of thoracic aorta with cardiovascular clamps in place. **B,** Permanent replacement graft after resection of aneurysm. (Redrawn from Bloodwell, RD, and others: Surg Clin North Am 46:901-911, 1966.)

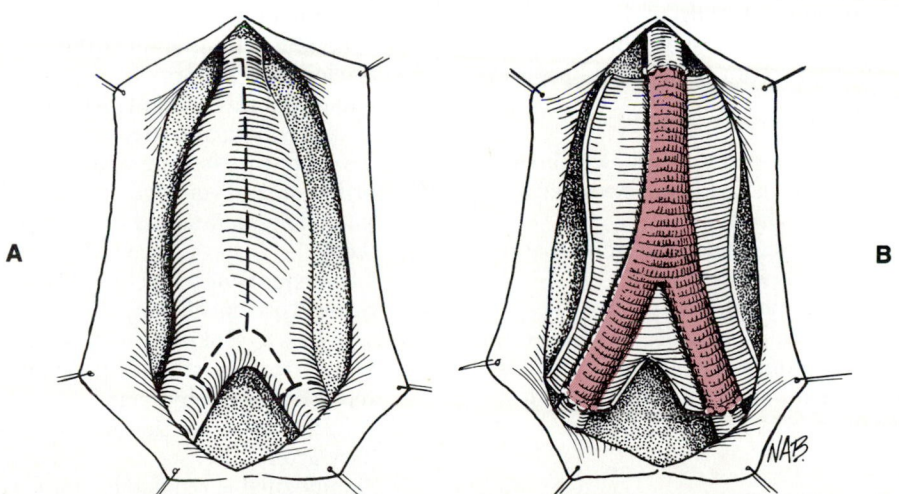

Fig. 25-39 **A,** Abdominal aneurysm of aorta and iliac arteries. **B,** Bifurcation graft used to replace excised aneurysm.

since the surgery is associated with some mortality and morbidity.

The preparation and postoperative care for resection of a thoracic aortic aneurysm are similar to that for cardiac surgery (p. 789). Resection of an abdominal aortic aneurysm is similar to other abdominal surgery. Some surgeons additionally require a bowel preparation for optimum preparation, should bowel surgery be necessary. Heparin is usually given during surgery, before clamping of the artery.

■ POSTOPERATIVE CARE (ABDOMINAL AORTIC ANEURYSM)

1. Monitor the following parameters:
   a. Vital signs until stable
   b. Central venous pressure (CVP) to assess fluid status
   c. Hourly circulation checks with assessment of all pulses distal to graft site (femoral, posterior tibial, posterior tibialis, dorsalis pedis)
      (1) Absent pulses more than 6 to 12 hours indicate arterial occlusion
      (2) Poor peripheral occlusion: marked decrease in blood pressure, weak thready pulses, cool skin temperature, diaphoresis
      (3) Advanced occlusion: pain, cramping, numbness in extremities; legs may be white or blue and cool to cold
   d. Renal function (since aorta was clamped during surgery, preventing blood flow to kidneys)
      (1) Hourly urine flow greater than 25 to 30 ml through indwelling catheter
      (2) Urine color (hematuria may occur with renal damage)
      (3) Daily blood urea nitrogen (BUN)
   e. Presence of back pain (indicative of retroperitoneal hemorrhage or thrombus at graft site)
2. Keep patient flat in bed without sharp flexion of hip and of knee to avoid pressure on femoral and popliteal arteries
3. Give medication for pain
4. Institute pulmonary ventilatory measures (deep breathing and coughing, and so on); use firm abdominal support to incision during coughing
5. Monitor for postoperative ileus and distention (patient may have an indwelling nasogastric tube)
6. Prevent postoperative thrombophlebitis
   a. Check for pain or cramps in calf, tenderness in specific areas of leg, redness along course of vein
   b. Encourage dorsiflexion and plantar flexion of feet
   c. Use elastic stockings

■ SUMMARY

1. Cardiac output is a function of heart rate and stroke volume.
2. Heart rate is generally under the control of the autonomic nervous system.
3. Stroke volume is determined by preload, contractility, and afterload.

4. Physiologic changes in cardiac functioning related to aging are most apparent in situations of increased stress on the cardiovascular system or in the presence of underlying cardiac pathologic conditions.
5. A less effective heart rate response to exercise and prolongation of the time required for the heart rate to return to normal following exercise are two common physiologic changes associated with aging.
6. An ECG is a graphic record of the electrical activity of the heart muscle. It is recorded on a grid that allows measurement of time and voltage.
7. A 12-lead ECG provides 12 different views of cardiac electrical activity; a cardiac monitor typically displays one view at a time.
8. A normal cardiac complex consists of a P wave, a QRS complex, and a T wave. The exact configuration of each component will vary according to the view or lead that is being recorded.
9. Normal sinus rhythm is characterized by a rhythm that is regular, a rate between 60 and 100 beats/min, and a cardiac complex that is within established criteria for configuration and duration of the components and intervals.
10. Two basic mechanisms of cardiac arrhythmias are disturbances of impulse initiation and disturbances of impulse conduction.
11. Disturbances of impulse initiation may occur in the sinus node or in an ectopic site (atrial or ventricular musculature). Premature beats and ectopic tachycardias are examples of disturbances in impulse initiation outside of the sinus node.
12. Disturbances of impulse conduction may prevent impulses initiated in the sinus node from being conducted into the ventricles or may result in altered conduction within the ventricles themselves.
13. Treatment for cardiac arrhythmias involves identification and elimination of the cause (if possible), drugs or electrical suppression of ectopic impulse initiation, and modalities to regulate heart rate (drugs, regulation of oxygen demand, and artificial pacemakers).
14. Two life-threatening arrhythmias are ventricular fibrillation and ventricular standstill. CPR must be initiated and maintained until definitive treatment is effective.
15. Components of a teaching plan for patients with permanent pacemakers include the rationale for insertion, activities to avoid, the method for monitoring the function of their particular pacemaker, and symptoms to report to their physicians.
16. Atherosclerosis is the most common etiology of coronary artery disease.
17. Nonmodifiable risk factors for CAD include advancing age, being of the male sex or Black race, and a positive family history of CAD.
18. Major modifiable risk factors for CAD include cigarette smoking, hyperlipidemia, diabetes mellitus, and hypertension. A diet high in cholesterol and saturated fats contributes to the risk factors.
19. Angina pectoris is chest pain caused by reversible myocardial ischemia. Treatment involves increasing myo-

cardial blood and oxygen supply (either with medications or surgical intervention) and reducing myocardial oxygen demands.

20. Teaching plans for patients with angina should include CAD risk factor identification and reduction, interventions to use when chest pain occurs, methods of reducing myocardial oxygen demands, and symptoms to report to the physician.

21. The most commonly used drugs for reduction or control of angina are nitrates, beta blocking agents, and calcium channel blockers.

22. A myocardial infarction is the result of prolonged myocardial ischemia that causes irreversible cellular damage and necrosis.

23. The clinical consequences of a myocardial infarction depend on the location of the coronary artery occlusion and the extent of necrosis.

24. Diagnosis of myocardial infarction is based on the clinical picture, ECG findings, elevation of serum enzyme levels, and other procedures that allow direct visualization of the area of myocardial damage.

25. Medical therapy for myocardial infarction includes measures to reduce the size of the infarcted area, to reduce myocardial oxygen demands, and to prevent or treat complications.

26. Possible nursing diagnoses for the patient with myocardial infarction include activity intolerance, self-care deficit, anxiety, knowledge deficit, and diagnoses related to psychosocial adjustment of the patient and the family.

27. The two most common complications of myocardial infarction are cardiac arrhythmias and left ventricular failure.

28. Teaching plans for patients with myocardial infarction should include content on the pathophysiology of myocardial infarction, the healing process, the treatment regimen, risk factors for coronary artery disease, the relationship between the treatment regimen and risk factor reduction, and resumption of activities (including sexual activity) following the acute phase of illness.

29. Coronary artery bypass graft (CABG) is one type of surgical intervention to improve coronary blood flow. This procedure involves grafting a blood vessel such as a portion of the saphenous vein from the aorta to a point beyond the occluson in a coronary artery.

30. Percutaneous transluminal coronary angioplasty (PTCA) is a newer procedure for improving coronary blood flow. This procedure involves insertion of a balloon-equipped catheter into a coronary artery and compressing or destroying an atherosclerotic plaque.

31. Heart failure is a state in which the heart is no longer able to pump an adequate supply of blood to meet the demands of the body.

32. Congestive heart failure (CHF) refers to a state of circulatory congestion resulting from heart failure and its compensatory mechanisms. Symptoms of conges-

---

Putting knowledge to practice

- Review the process of wound healing (see Chapter 18). How can this process be applied to a myocardial infarction?
- Examine the chart of a patient who has had a myocardial infarction. What ECG changes were noted? What changes occurred in the serum enzymes? What complications did the patient develop? What nursing diagnoses were identified? Are there classes for patients with myocardial infarction at your hospital? What content is included?
- What is being done in your community to increase the public's awareness of risk factors for CAD? How would you go about teaching the lay public about this health problem?
- How would you rate your own risk for CAD? (Contact your local branch of the American Heart Association for information on how to calculate risk.) Do you have any modifiable risk factors? What difficulties do you see in designing a program of risk modification for yourself?
- Examine the chart of a patient who has congestive heart failure. Compare and contrast the patient's symptoms with the usual symptoms of CHF. Did the patient have left-sided failure, right-sided failure, or both? What was the etiology of the failure in this patient? What data would indicate an improvement in the pumping capabilities of this patient's heart. What nursing diagnoses were identified?
- Examine the chart of a patient who has had coronary bypass surgery. Where were the lesions in the coronary arteries? What symptoms of CAD did the patient have before surgery? What therapeutic modalities had been employed before the surgery? How does the patient rate the "success" of the surgery at this point?
- Visit a clinic for patients with cardiac pacemakers. What kinds of problems do these patients have that nursing could help with?
- Examine the chart of a patient who has rheumatic heart disease. What can be noted about the development of the disease in this patient? Was rheumatic fever diagnosed in the past? When did the patient start to have symptoms associated with RHD? What is being done in your community to prevent rheumatic fever?
- Talk with the spouse of a patient who has had a myocardial infarction or coronary bypass surgery. What questions and concerns does the spouse have? What changes in family functioning does the spouse expect following this event?

tion may involve the pulmonary circulation, the systemic venous circulation, or both.

33. Signs and symptoms associated with CHF include those resulting from decreased cardiac output (forward failure) and those resulting from the subsequent congestion (backward failure).

34. Treatment for CHF involves improving oxygen supply to the tissues, decreasing oxygen demands on the myocardium, and relieving the symptoms of congestion. Common elements of treatment include oxygen, rest, positioning to facilitate optimal respiration, positive inotropic drugs, diuretics, sodium-restricted diet, and arterial/venous dilating drugs.

35. Teaching plans for patients with congestive heart failure include content on the pathophysiology of the condition, approaches to regulating and monitoring the effect of activity, avoidance of precipitating factors, rationale for the treatment regimen, approaches to implementing the treatment regimen, and signs and symptoms to report to the physician.

36. Pulmonary edema represents the most severe form of congestion resulting from left ventricular failure, and cardiogenic shock represents the most severe form of decreased cardiac output. Both conditions are medical emergencies and require immediate, intensive medical and nursing intervention.

37. Inflammation of the pericardium, myocardium, or endocardium may be a consequence of infectious diseases, neoplasms, and other metabolic disorders. Patients with these conditions have the usual signs and symptoms associated with the inflammatory process and may also develop heart failure. Measures to prevent further episodes are important aspects of the treatment regimen.

38. The two basic problems that compromise the normal functioning of the cardiac valves are stenosis and insufficiency. Stenosis causes a narrowing of the valvular orifice and impedes the forward flow of blood. Insufficiency causes imcomplete closure of the valve and allows blood to flow backward.

39. Cardiac murmurs are a common physical finding in patients with valvular heart disease. Depending on the severity of the disease, the patient may or may not develop clinical symptoms such as those associated with heart failure.

40. Diagnosis of the nature and extent of valvular heart disease is frequently based on the findings obtained from a cardiac catheterization. Pressure gradients between relevant cardiac chambers and O_2 content of the blood are two parameters that are measured with this procedure.

41. Treatment for cardiac valvular disease involves management of the clinical symptoms. Surgical repair of the valve or replacement of the valve with an artificial prosthesis may be necessary.

42. An aneurysm is a local or diffuse dilation of an artery. Atherosclerosis is a common cause of this problem. Aneurysms may be fusiform, saccular, or dissecting and may form in the thoracic or abdominal aorta.

43. Depending on the location and size of the aneurysm, surgical resection may be necessary. An artificial tube is grafted onto the resected area.

REFERENCES AND SELECTED READINGS
Contemporary

1. *Alpert, JS: The pharmacologic management of coronary artery disease in 1986, Heart Lung 15:558-561, 1986.
2. American Heart Association: Heart facts, Dallas, 1987, The Association.
3. Andreoli, KG, and others: Comprehensive cardiac care: a text for nurses, physicians, and other health practioners, ed 6, St. Louis, 1987, The CV Mosby Co.
4. Ayres, SM: The prevention and treatment of shock in acute myocardial infarction, Chest 93:17S-21S, 1988.
5. *Baggs, JG, and Karch, AM: Sexual counseling of women with coronary heart disease, Heart Lung 16:154-159, 1987.
6. *Baum, PL: Abdominal aortic aneurysm: the patient takes AAA care, Nurs 82 12(12):34-41, 1982.
7. Berne, RM, and Levy, MN: Cardiovascular physiology, ed 5, St. Louis, 1986, The CV Mosby Co.
8. Blowers, MG, and Smith, RJ: How to read an ECG: basic interpretation for nurses and other health workers, ed 3, Oradell, NJ, 1983, Medical Economics Co.
9. *Borders, CR: When the bypass patient returns home: problems your bypass patients face after discharge, Patient Care 19(13):65-76, 1985.
10. Braunwald, E, and others (editors): Harrison's principles of internal medicine, ed 11, New York, 1987, McGraw-Hill Book Co.
11. *Burden, LL, and Atwell, K: The treacherous waters of unstable angina pectoris, Nurs 83 13(12):50-55, 1983.
12. *Burgess, AW, and Hartman, CR: Patients' perceptions of the cardiac crisis, Am J Nurs 86:568-571, 1986.
13. *Campuzano, M: Self-care following coronary artery bypass surgery, Focus Crit Care 9:55-56, 1982.
14. *Cantwell, JD: Exercise and coronary heart disease: role in primary prevention, Heart Lung 13:6-13, 1984.
15. *Chesney, MA, and Rosenman, RH: Type A behavior: observations on the past decade, Heart Lung 11:12-18, 1982.
16. *Cohen, S: New concepts in understanding congestive heart failure. I. How the clinical features arise, Am J Nurs 81:119-142, 1981.
17. *Cohen, S: New concepts in understanding congestive heart failure. II. How the therapeutic approaches work, Am J Nurs 81:357-380, 1981.
18. Cohn, LH: Surgical treatment of acute myocardial infarction, Chest 93:13S-16S, 1988.
19. Conner, WE, and Bristow, JD: Coronary heart disease: prevention, complications, and treatment, Philadelphia, 1985, JB Lippincott Co.
20. Conover, MB: Understanding electrocardiography, ed 5, St. Louis, 1988, The CV Mosby Co.

*References preceded by an asterisk are particularly well suited for student reading.

21. *Crumlisch, CM: Cardiogenic shock: catch it early! Nurs 81 11(8):34-41, 1981.

22. Ebersole, P, and Hess, P: Toward healthy aging: Human needs and nursing response, ed 2, St. Louis, 1985, The CV Mosby Co.

23. *Ellmyer, P, and Thomas, N: A guide to your patient's safe home use of oxygen, Nurs 82 12(1):55-57, 1982.

24. *Fletcher, GF: Exercise and exercise testing: current state of the art, Heart Lung 13:5-6, 1984.

25. *Fletcher, GF: Long-term exercise in coronary artery disease and other chronic disease states, Heart Lung 13:28-46, 1984.

26. Giles, TD: Principles of vasodilator therapy for left ventricular congestive heart failure, Heart Lung 9:271-276, 1980.

27. Giving cardiac care, Nursing Photobook Series, Springhouse, Penn, 1983, Intermed Communications, Inc.

28. Gold, HK: Thrombolysis in acute myocardial infarction, Chest 93:10S-12S, 1988.

29. Guyton, AC, and others: Textbook of medical physiology, ed 7, Philadelphia, 1986, WB Saunders Co.

30. *Heger, JJ, and others: New drugs for the treatment of ventricular arrhythmias, Heart Lung 10:475-483, 1981.

31. *Jasinkowski, N: Aortic bypass: trimming the postop risks, RN 46:41-45, 1982.

32. *Johnson, GP, and Johanson, BC: β-Blockers: an expert's guide to what's on the market, Am J Nurs 83:1034-1043, 1983.

33. *Johnston, BL: Exercise testing for patients after myocardial and coronary bypass surgery: emphasis on predischarge phase, Heart Lung 13:18-27, 1984.

34. Joyce, NB: Care of the patient with cardiovascular disease. In Daly, BJ: Intensive care nursing, ed 2, New York, 1985, Medical Examination Publishing Co.

35. Kannel, WB, and Dawber, TR: Contributors to coronary risk: ten years later, Heart Lung 11:60-64, 1982.

36. *Klein, DM: Angina: physiology, signs and symptoms, Nurs 84 14:44-46, 1984.

37. *Kleinhenz, TJ: The inside story on preload and afterload, Nurs 85 15(5):50-55, 1985.

38. Kloosterman, ND: Prevention of ICU psychosis, Focus Crit Care 10:59-61, 1983.

39. Kovalesky, A: Mitral valve prolapse, Nurs 81 11(4):58-61, 1981.

40. *Kroncke, G, and others: What to do when your patient's pacemaker stops working, Nurs 81 11(10):74-78, 1981.

41. Levy, RI: Medicine for the laymen: heart attacks, US Department of Health, Education, and Welfare, DHEW publication no. (NIH) 81-1803, Washington, DC, 1981.

42. Litwak, R: Care of the cardiac surgical patient, New York, 1982, Appleton-Century-Crofts.

43. *Loan, T: Nursing interaction with patients undergoing coronary angioplasty, Heart Lung 15:368-375, 1986.

44. *Lovvorn, J: Coronary artery bypass surgery: helping patients cope with postop problems, Am J Nurs 82:1073-1075, 1982.

45. *Marinelli-Miller, D: What your patient wants to know about angiography, but may not ask, RN 46:52-54, 1983.

46. Martin, EG, and Hasselman, SJ: Surgical management and angioplasty for coronary heart disease. In Andreoli, KG, and others: Comprehensive cardiac care, ed 6, St. Louis, 1987, The CV Mosby Co.

47. McGill, HC Jr: The cardiovascular pathology of smoking, Am Heart J 115:250-257, 1988.

48. *Mickus, D, Monahan, KJ, and Brown, C: Exciting external pacemakers, Am J Nurs 86:403-405, 1986.

49. *Norsen, LH, and Fox, GB: Understanding cardiac output and the drugs that affect it, Nurs 85 15(4):34-41, 1985.

50. Pantaleo, N, and others: Thallium myocardial scintigraphy and its use in the assessment of coronary artery disease, Heart Lung 10:61-71, 1981.

51. *Parent, D, and others: Developing a cardiac teaching program, Can Crit Care Nurs 1(1):22-23, 1984.

52. Parsonnet, V, Furman, S, and Smyth, NPD: A revised code for pacemaker identification, PACE 4:400, 1981.

53. Porth, CM: Pathophysiology: concepts of altered health status, ed 2, Philadelphia, 1986, JB Lippincott Co.

54. Price, SA, and Wilson, LM: Pathophysiology: clinical concepts of disease processes, ed 3, New York, 1986, McGraw-Hill Book Co.

55. *Purcell, JA, and Burrows, SG: A pacemaker primer, Am J Nurs 85:553-568, 1985.

56. *Purcell, JA, and Giffen, P: Percutaneous transluminal coronary angioplasty, Am J Nurs 81:1620-1626, 1981.

57. *Rodriguez, SW, and Reed, RL: Thrombolytic therapy for MI, Am J Nurs 87:632-640, 1987.

58. *Rossi, LP, and Antman, EM: Calcium channel blockers: new treatment for cardiovascular disease, Am J Nurs 83:382-388, 1983.

59. *Runions, J: A program for psychological and social enhancement during rehabilitation after myocardial infarction, Heart Lung 14:117-125, 1985.

60. *Sakallaris, BR: Laser therapy for cardiovascular disease, Heart Lung 16:465-471, 1987.

61. Sanderson, RG, and Kurth, CL: The cardiac patient: a comprehensive approach, ed 2, Philadelphia, 1983, WB Saunders Co.

62. *Saul, L: Heart sounds and common murmurs, Am J Nurs 83:1679-1689, 1983.

63. Schlesinger, Z: An interdisciplinary approach to cardiac rehabilitation, Heart Lung 12:336-337, 1983.

64. *Scordo, KA: Hemodynamic monitoring: learning to read the waves, Nurs 85 15(7):40-42, 1985.

65. *Scordo, KA: Taming the cardiac monitor. I, Nurs 82 12(8):58-64, 1982.

66. *Scordo, KA: Taming the cardiac monitor. II, Nurs 82 12(9):60-69, 1982.

67. *Scordo, KA: This procedure called PTCA: your patient's CABG substitute? Nurs 82 12(2):50-55, 1982.

68. *Seger, U, and Schlesinger, A: Rehabilitation of patients after acute myocardial infarction: an interdisciplinary family-oriented program, Heart Lung 10:841-847, 1981.

69. Spann, JF, and Hurst, JW: The recognition and management of heart failure. In Hurst, JW: The heart, arteries and veins, ed 6, New York, 1986, McGraw-Hill Book Co.

70. *Summer, SM, and Grau, PA: Guidelines for running a 12-lead EKG, Nurs 85 15(12):30-33, 1985.

71. *Taylor, D: Congestive heart failure, Nurs 83 13(9):44-45, 1983.

72. Tirrell, BE, and Hart, LK: The relationship of health beliefs and knowledge to exercise compliance in patients after coronary bypass, Heart Lung 9:487-493, 1980.

73. *VanMeter, M: Balloon flotation catheters today: what they tell you, why they're vital, RN 46:36-41, 1983.

74. Waggoner, PC: Postoperative care of the patient undergoing cardiac valve replacement: a nursing perspective, Crit Care Q 4:57-65, Dec. 1981.

75. Walsh-Essig, ME: A restudy of structured repetitive preoperative teaching to coronary artery bypass patients master's thesis, Cleveland, 1982, Case Western Reserve University.

76. *Weiland, AP: A review of cardiac valve prostheses and their selection, Heart Lung 12:498-504, 1983.

77. Wenger, NK: Early ambulation physical activity: myocardial infarction and coronary artery bypass surgery, Heart Lung 13:14-18, 1984.

78. Wilhelmsen, L: Coronary heart disease: epidemiology of smoking and studies of smoking, Am Heart J 115:242-249, 1988.

79. Yusuf, S: The use of adrenergic blocking agents, IV nitrates, and calcium channel blocking agents, following acute myocardial infarction, Chest 93:25S-28S, 1988.

80. Zeluff, GW, Cashion, WR, and Jackson, D: Evaluation of the coronary arteries and myocardium by radionuclide imaging, Heart Lung 9:344-349, 1980.

Classic

81. American Heart Association: Living with your pacemaker, New York, 1979, The Association.

82. Barbarowicz, P: An active partnership for the health of your heart (after your coronary bypass surgery), Stanford, Calif, 1976, American Heart Association.

83. Conover, MB: Cardiac arrhythmias: exercises in pattern interpretation, ed 2, St. Louis, 1978, The CV Mosby Co.

26

The Patient with Peripheral Vascular Problems

EILEEN WALSH

CHAPTER OBJECTIVES

After studying this chapter, the student should be able to:

- Identify risk factors associated with the development of peripheral vascular disorders.
- Describe pathophysiology, nursing diagnoses, expected outcomes, and interventions for patients with arterial and venous disorders.
- Describe nursing interventions for patients having surgery for arterial and venous disorders.
- Describe the pathophysiology and nursing interventions for patients with leg ulcers and lymph disorders.
- Describe the pathophysiology and nursing interventions for persons with hypertension.

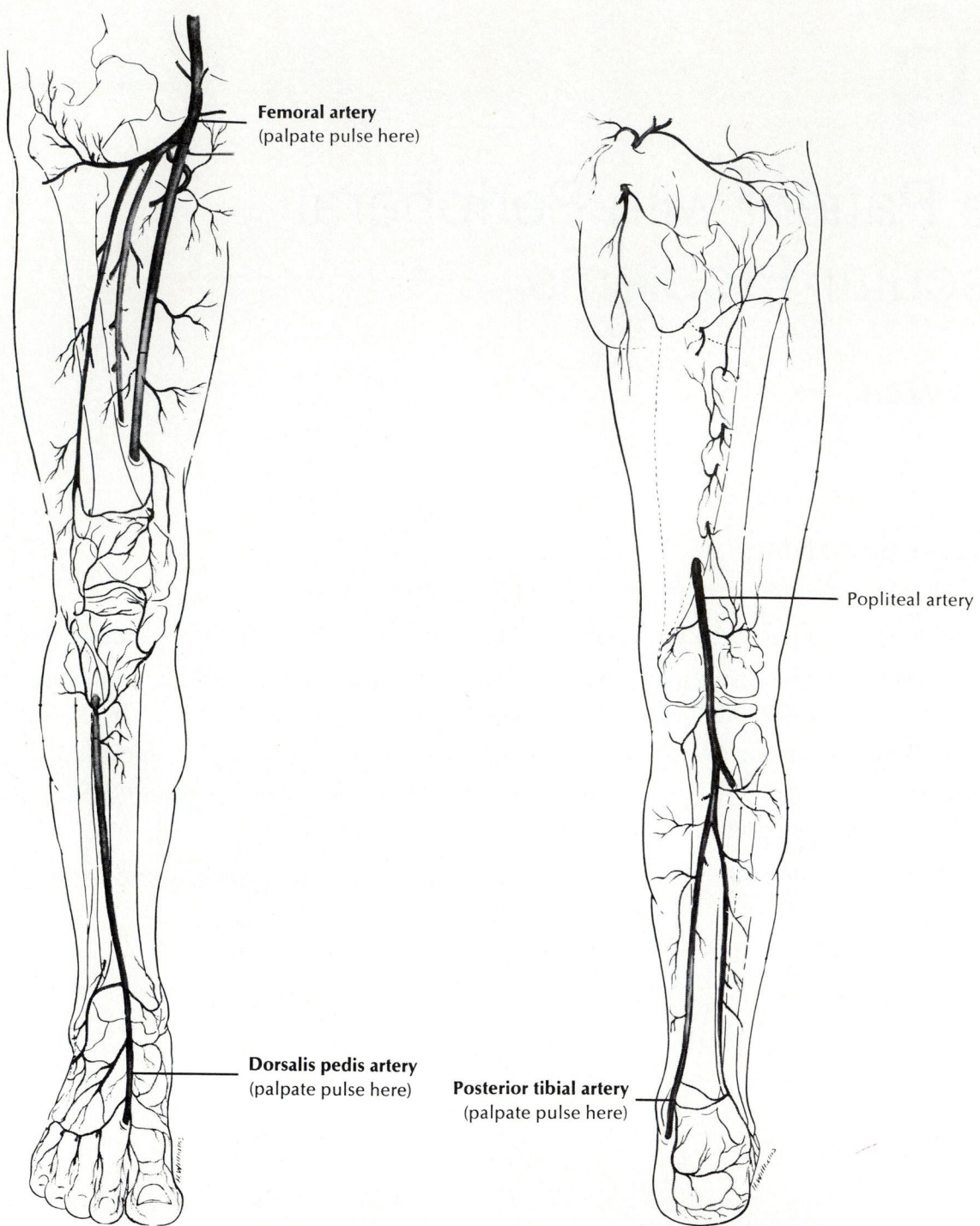

Femoral artery
(palpate pulse here)

Popliteal artery

Dorsalis pedis artery
(palpate pulse here)

Posterior tibial artery
(palpate pulse here)

Fig. 26-1 Arteries of the lower extremity. (Adapted from Francis, CC, and Martin, AH: Introduction to human anatomy, ed 7, St. Louis, 1975, The CV Mosby Co.)

Problems of the peripheral vascular system refer to a number of disorders that disrupt blood flow through the blood vessels. This classification generally excludes those conditions that affect the aorta and coronary arteries, which have a more direct relationship to the heart (see Chapter 25) and the cerebral vessels (Chapter 19). Specific alterations in arterial and venous blood flow in the lower and upper extremities are discussed in this chapter. Lymphedema is included because the lymphatic system complements the function of the vascular system. In addition, a section on hypertension is included because it is a major contributing factor to peripheral vascular problems.

■ ANATOMY AND PHYSIOLOGY

All the cells of the body are dependent on an intact and functioning vascular system. This vascular system is a closed circuit consisting of the systemic and pulmonary circulations. Blood circulates from the left side of the heart to the tissues and back to the right side of the heart. It then flows through the lungs and back to the left side of the heart. The main components of the vascular system are the arteries, capillaries, veins, and lymphatic vessels.

■ Arteries

Arteries are thick-walled vessels that transport oxygenated blood via the aorta away from the heart and to the tissues. As the arteries approach the tissues, they branch into smaller vessels called arterioles (Fig. 26-1). All arteries are composed of the following three basic tissue layers:

1. Inner layer of endothelium (intima)
2. Middle layer of connective tissue, smooth muscle, or elastic fibers (media)
3. Outer layer of connective tissue (adventitia)

The media comprises the major part of the vessel wall. In the large arteries the media is primarily composed of elastic and connective tissue, which enables the artery to respond to alterations of blood volume while maintaining a constant flow. There is much less elastic fiber in the smaller arteries and arterioles; these vessels have smooth muscle that contracts and relaxes through nervous, chemical, and hormonal factors.

■ Capillaries

The capillaries are minute, thin-walled vessels located in the tissues and are composed of a single layer of cells. The capillaries connect the arterioles to the smallest veins and venules and allow for the exchange of essential cellular products. Nutrients, oxygen, and regulatory substances move into the cells, whereas waste products, carbon dioxide, and cellular secretions move from the cells into the blood.

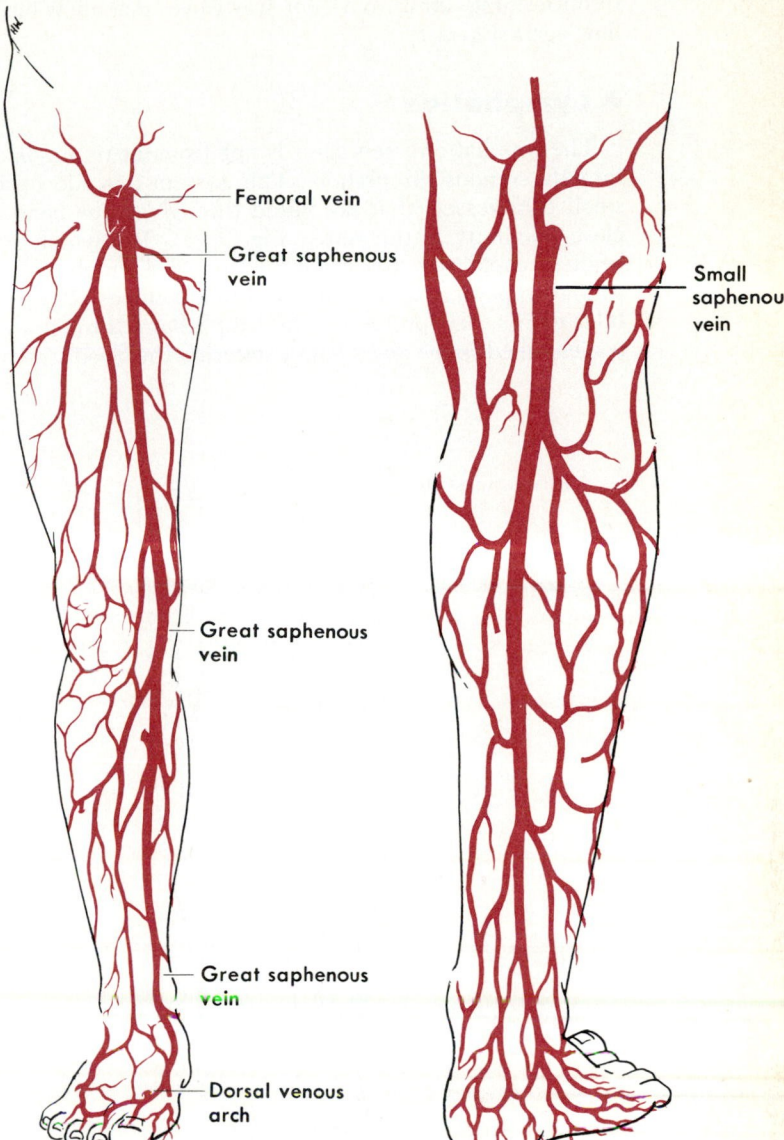

Fig. 26-2 Superficial veins of the leg and foot. (From Anthony, CJ, and Thibodeau, GA: Textbook of anatomy and physiology, ed 12, St. Louis, 1987, The CV Mosby Co.)

■ Veins

Veins are thin-walled vessels that transport deoxygenated blood from the capillaries back to the right side of the heart. They are composed of three layers: intima, media, and adventitia. These layers differ from arterial walls in that there is little smooth muscle and connective tissue. This makes the veins distensible and able to accumulate large volumes of blood. The sympathetic nervous system innervates the veins and causes venoconstriction, decreased venous volume, and increased circulating blood volume. Major veins, particularly those in the lower extremities (Fig. 26-2), have one way valves that allow blood flow against gravity.

■ Lymphatics

The lymphatic vessels carry lymph from the tissues back into the venous circulation. This system is made up of small thin vessels that are found throughout the body in close proximity to the veins (Fig. 26-3). The lymphatics begin as capillaries that drain the tissues of lymph (a fluid similar to plasma) and tissue fluid that contains cells, cellular debris, and proteins. The lymph flows through oval bodies called *lymph nodes* before entering the blood stream.

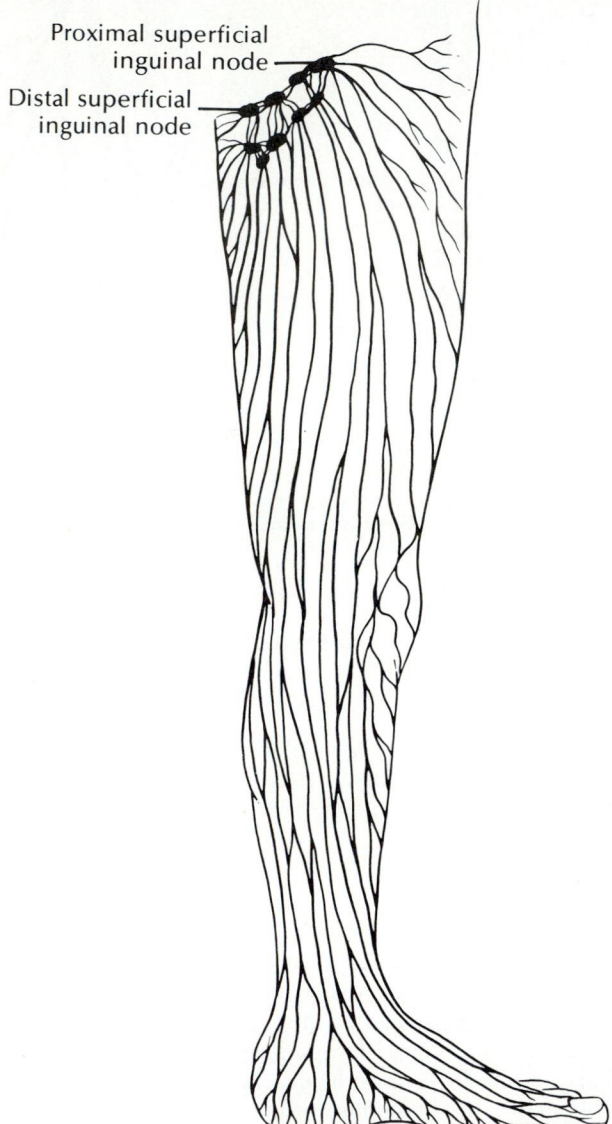

Proximal superficial inguinal node

Distal superficial inguinal node

Fig. 26-3 Superficial lymphatics of the medial aspect of the lower extremity (after Sappey). (From Francis, CC, and Martin, AH: Introduction to human anatomy, ed 7, St. Louis, 1975, The CV Mosby Co.)

The flow drains into the thoracic duct and the right lymphatic duct, which empty into the junction of the internal jugular vein and subclavian vein (Fig. 26-4).

■ Physiologic changes with aging

Degenerative changes occur in the vascular system as part of the normal aging process. These changes affect the walls of the blood vessels and predispose persons to problems in the transport of blood and nutrients to the tissues. There is an increased thickness in the intima wall resulting from fibrosis. Further wall stiffness is caused by an accumulation of collagen and calcium in the intima and media. The elastic fibers of the media become thin and calcified. These changes markedly decrease the elasticity and flexibility of the vessels and increase peripheral vascular resistance. As peripheral vascular resistance increases, there is less blood flow through the vessels and hence a decreased supply of oxygen and nutrients coupled with the accumulation of cellular secretions, waste products, and carbon dioxide. Blood pressure increases.

■ PREVENTION AND HEALTH EDUCATION

■ Risk factors

The risk factors that are associated with the development of peripheral vascular disorders are listed in the box below. These factors are similar to those that are correlated with the development of other forms of cardiovascular diseases (Chapter 25). Specific health teaching is discussed in the box on p. 846.

■ CIGARETTE SMOKING

Smoking is one of the major contributory factors in the development of peripheral vascular problems. Nicotine causes vasoconstriction and spasms of the arteries, thus reducing circulation to the extremities. The carbon monoxide inhaled in cigarette smoke reduces oxygen transport to the tissues.

Risk factors for peripheral vascular disorders

Cigarette smoking
Hypertension
Hyperlipidemia
Obesity
Physical inactivity
Emotional stress
Diabetes mellitus
Family history of atherosclerosis

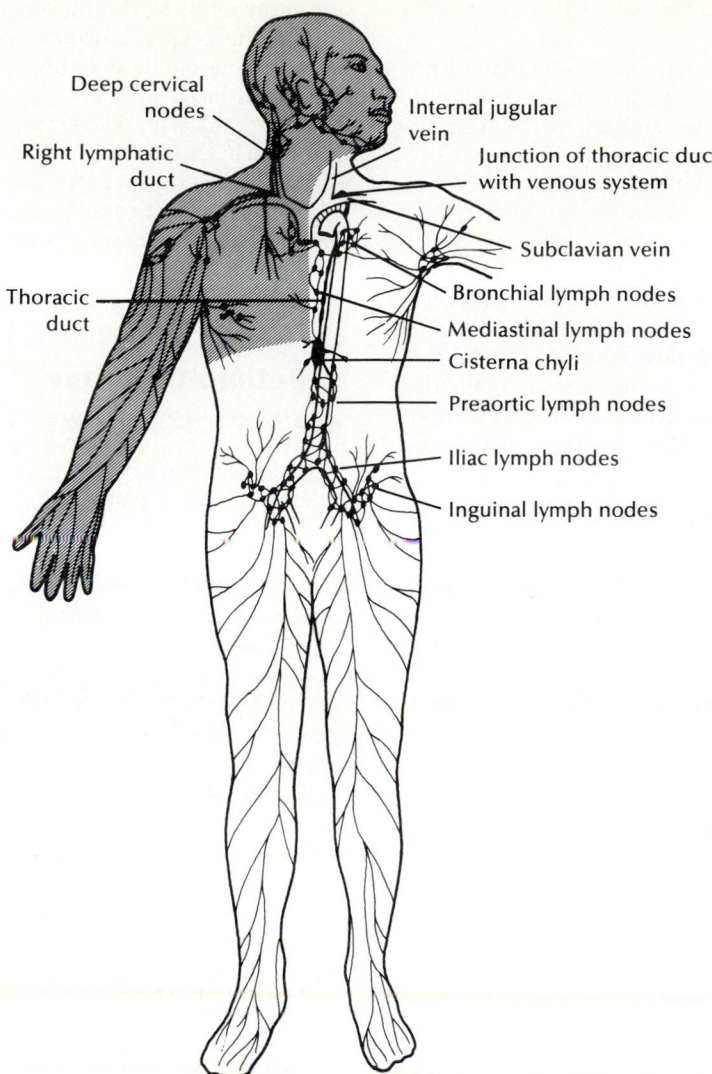

Deep cervical nodes

Right lymphatic duct

Thoracic duct

Internal jugular vein

Junction of thoracic duct with venous system

Subclavian vein

Bronchial lymph nodes

Mediastinal lymph nodes

Cisterna chyli

Preaortic lymph nodes

Iliac lymph nodes

Inguinal lymph nodes

Fig. 26-4   Lymph pathways of the lower-limb drain into the subclavian vein. (From Hamilton, WJ: Textbook of human anatomy, ed 2, St. Louis, 1976, The CV Mosby Co.)

■ HYPERTENSION

Hypertension causes the elastic tissue in the arteries to be replaced by fibrous collagen tissue. This makes the arterial wall less distensible and increases the resistance to blood flow (p. 856).

■ HYPERLIPIDEMIA

Hyperlipidemia refers to the elevation of lipids, such as cholesterol and triglycerides, within the blood. Cholesterol and triglycerides contribute to the development of atherosclerotic plaques in the vessels (see Chapter 25).

■ OBESITY

Obesity, or excess body weight in relation to height, places an added burden on the heart and blood vessels. Excess fat compromises blood vessels and contributes to increased venous congestion. Obese individuals are also more prone to physical inactivity, diabetes, hypertension, and hyperlipidemia.

■ PHYSICAL INACTIVITY

Physical activity promotes muscle contraction and relaxation. It improves the return of venous blood to the heart by the pumping of muscle on the veins and aids in the development of collateral circulation, which is useful for venous return when veins are blocked.

■ EMOTIONAL STRESS

Emotional stress stimulates the sympathetic nervous system and causes peripheral vasoconstriction. Stress can also cause increased cholesterol and platelet levels, decreased clotting time, and sustained high blood pressure.

■ DIABETES MELLITUS

The exact mechanism by which diabetes contributes to the development of peripheral vascular disorders is unknown. The changes in glucose and fat metabolism are thought to affect the atherosclerotic processes.

■ Prevention

Primary prevention is the most important means for reducing the incidence of peripheral vascular disorders. Nurses in all clinical settings can provide health education about the risk factors that affect development of peripheral vascular disorders. Because these disorders normally develop with advancing age, all individuals can benefit from this information, particularly those in the elderly age-groups.

Secondary prevention is also important because peripheral vascular disorders can become chronic and potentially disabling diseases. Persons with peripheral vascular disorders are subject to periods of exacerbation and complications such as infection, injury, thrombosis, and amputation. Persons with early symptoms are encouraged to seek medical care. Increasing the person's knowledge of the specific disorder and prevention of future occurrences is essential.

Major health problems of the peripheral vascular system

Changes in the peripheral vascular system may cause local arterial or venous disorders or may result in a systemic effect (for example, hypertension). Major peripheral vascular disorders that are discussed in this chapter include the following:
1. Arterial disorders
   a. Atherosclerosis
   b. Arteriosclerosis obliterans
   c. Thromboangiitis obliterans (Buerger's disease)
   d. Raynaud's disease
   e. Arterial embolism
   f. Arteriovenous fistula
2. Venous disorders
   a. Thrombophlebitis
   b. Varicose veins
3. Leg ulcers
4. Lymphedema
5. Hypertension

■ ARTERIAL DISORDERS

Any disturbance in the structure of the arteries interferes with transport of blood from the heart to the tissues. The result is diminished blood and decreased oxygen and nutrients to the tissues. The symptoms of arterial disease are not caused by the degree of obstruction or narrowing but by the degree to which the involved body part is deprived of circulation. This in turn is affected by such factors as blood pressure and presence or absence of collateral circulation. For example, occlusion of 50% of one artery may cause severe symptoms, whereas occlusion of 50% of another artery may cause no symptoms if collateral circulation is sufficient to provide oxygenation. The etiologic factors, signs and symptoms, and medical therapy for the various types of arterial disorders are listed in Table 26-1.

■ Pathophysiology
■ ATHEROSCLEROSIS

Atherosclerosis is generally viewed as a type of arteriosclerosis or as a part of the aging process. This disease involves the development of lesions on the intimal wall.

Three types of lesions have been identified: (1) fatty streaks, which consist of smooth-muscle cells and lipid deposits that are present in all individuals, although they do not necessarily progress to produce disease; (2) fibrous plaques, which involve a thickening of the intima and are surrounded by lipids, collagen, smooth muscle cells, and plasma components; and (3) the complicated lesion that is a large mass consisting of calcified fibrous plaques.

The result of atherosclerosis is narrowing of the artery, which progresses to obstruction, thrombosis, aneurysm development, and rupture. In addition, nutrients and oxygen to the tissues can be reduced, resulting in ischemic necrosis of the tissue cells.

■ ARTERIOSCLEROSIS OBLITERANS

Arteriosclerosis obliterans is a disorder in which there is segmented arteriosclerotic narrowing or obstruction of the intima and media of vessel walls. It is the most common cause of arterial obstructive disease in the extremities of persons over 30 years of age. This disorder affects men more than women with clinical symptoms evident between 50 and 70 years of age. The lower extremities are involved most often, and common sites include the femoral, iliac, and popliteal arteries. In individuals with diabetes mellitus, the disease becomes more progressive, affecting the smaller arteries primarily below the knee.

The primary lesion of arteriosclerosis obliterans is plaque formation on the intimal wall that causes partial or complete occlusion. There is calcification of the media and the gradual loss of elasticity that further weakens the arterial walls and predisposes the patient to aneurysm or thrombus formation.

As a result of these physiologic changes, the artery is unable to transport an adequate blood volume to the tissues during exercise or at rest. Symptoms appear when the blood vessels can no longer supply the tissues with required nutrients and remove wastes.

The most common symptom, *intermittent claudication,* occurs with exercise and is a pain that develops in a muscle

Table 26-1 Arterial disorders

Disease	Etiology	Signs and symptoms	Medical therapy
Atherosclerosis	Aging process Risk factors: physical inactivity, hypercholesteremia, hyper-triglyceridemia, obesity, emotional stress, cigarette smoking, diabetes, hypertension, family history of atherosclerosis	May not appear for 20 to 40 years Pain in lower limbs brought on by walking and exercise (intermittent claudication)	Regular exercise Drug therapy with vasodilators Low-fat, low-cholesterol diet Stop smoking, weight reduction, control of diabetes, control of hypertension
Arteriosclerosis obliterans	Advanced arteriosclerotic plaque formation Risk factors same as for atherosclerosis	Early: intermittent claudication, low skin temperature, diminished or absent arterial pulses distal to the obstruction, audible bruits Late: burning pain at rest, pallor or cyanosis, persistent reddish-blue discoloration, dry shiny skin, loss of hair on legs, deformed toenails, numbness and tingling, ulceration and gangrene of toes and foot	Cessation of cigarette smoking Regular exercise program Drug therapy with vasodilators (controversial) Weight reduction Low-fat and low-cholesterol diets, antilipemic medications Control of hypertension and diabetes Surgery: removal of occlusion, bypass of occlusion Percutaneous transluminal angioplasty
Thromboangiitis obliterans	Unknown cause Associated with: cigarette smoking, atherosclerosis, thrombosis and spasms, hypercoagulability of blood	Pain in digits at rest, sensitivity to cold, intermittent claudication in arm or hand, reduced or absent distal pulses, digits pale or persistently red, numbness and tingling, ulceration and gangrene of digits	Cessation of smoking Keep body warm Prevent injury to feet and hands Drug therapy with vasodilators (controversial) Surgery: sympathectomy to decrease arterial spasms, amputation of areas of ulceration and gangrene
Raynaud's disease	Cause unknown Associated with: emotional stress, sensitivity to cold, trauma from high-speed vibratory tools, occlusive arterial diseases, scleroderma, rheumatoid arthritis	Chronically cold hands and feet Vasospastic attack in digits: pallor, cyanosis, coldness, numbness, occasional pain After attack: intense redness, tingling, or throbbing Symptoms intensify to cold and emotional stress Ulcerations of fingertips in advanced cases	Protection against exposure to cold Cessation of cigarette smoking Drug therapy: calcium antagonists, vascular smooth muscle relaxants, vasodilators Biofeedback Surgery: sympathectomy, amputation of areas of ulceration and gangrene
Arterial embolism	Thrombi from heart chambers Associated with: atrial fibrillation, MI, infective endocarditis, CHF Associated with: immobility, anemia, dehydration	Sudden onset of pain, coldness, and numbness Burning or aching pain distal to occlusion Muscular weakness Diminished or absent pulses distal to occlusion Skin pallor or cyanosis Signs and symptoms of shock	Bed rest Drug therapy: anticoagulants, fibrinolytics (streptokinase) Treatment of shock Surgery: embolectomy
Aneurysm of the extremity	Atherosclerosis Associated with: arteriovenous fistula	May be asymptomatic Large pulsatile mass in area of artery Audible bruit Pain, coldness, and numbness distal to aneurysm	Drug therapy to control hypertension Surgery: removal of aneurysm
Arteriovenous fistula	Congenital anomaly Trauma	Pain at site of fistula Edema, varicosities, asymmetry of extremity Tortuous, dilated superficial veins Venous pulsations Audible bruit and palpable thrill	Relief of pain Support stockings Surgery: closure of fistula, ligation of artery or vein

that has an inadequate blood supply during exercise. It is described as a cramp that disappears within 1 or 2 minutes after the cessation of exercise. This pain is usually bilateral but may be unilateral. The muscles of the calf are more frequently affected because the femoral artery is often involved.

A gnawing or burning pain occurring at rest, especially at night, is indicative of severe disease. It is often accompanied by other signs of decreased circulation (for instance, feelings of coldness, numbness, and tingling). In advanced arteriosclerosis obliterans, the ischemia may lead to necrosis, ulceration, and gangrene, particularly of the toes and distal foot.

■ THROMBOANGIITIS OBLITERANS

Thromboangiitis obliterans (Buerger's disease) is characterized by inflammatory infiltration of vessel walls. It usually occurs in men aged 20 to 40. There is a strong association between this disorder and cigarette smoking. Although the cause of thromboangiitis obliterans is unknown, a hypersensitivity reaction to tobacco and alteration in cellular and humoral immunity have been suggested.

This disorder develops in the small arteries and veins in the feet and hands. Pain with exercise in the arch of the foot and instep claudication are typical and result from ischemic changes. Calf claudication is atypical because the femoral arteries are not usually involved. Other signs of decreased circulation may also be present.

■ RAYNAUD'S DISEASE

Raynaud's disease is a vasoconstrictive disorder characterized by episodic arterial spasms of the extremities, predominantly of the hands. Sluggish blood flow causes symptoms of coldness, numbness, cutaneous cyanosis, and pain. Raynaud's disease occurs mostly in young women between ages 16 and 40 and is more prevalent during winter months. Few pathologic changes occur in the early stages. With advancing stages, the intimal wall thickens and the medial wall hypertrophies. The exact cause is unknown.

Raynaud's phenomenon is a term used to denote a localized disorder, generally unilateral, affecting one or two digits. This phenomenon occurs secondary to other diseases, such as occlusive arterial diseases, immunologic and connective tissue diseases, trauma from occupational hazards, and neurogenic lesions.

■ ARTERIAL EMBOLISM

Arterial emboli are blood clots floating in the circulating blood. These clots most commonly originate in the heart as a result of atrial fibrillation, myocardial infarction, congestive heart failure, or vascular disease. The clot may be a fragment of an arteriosclerotic plaque loosened from the aorta. An embolus is carried into the arterial system, where it plugs an artery that is too small to allow it to pass. An embolus lodging at the bifurcation of any artery, a common site, is called a *saddle embolus*. Over half of the emboli to the lower extremity lodge in the femoral or popliteal arteries.

Abrupt onset of severe pain usually occurs from sudden cessation of circulation and is usually followed by other signs of decreased circulation. Pulses are absent distal to the site of occlusion. Detection of a bruit over the artery from turbulent blood flow is common when an ulcerated plaque or aneurysm is the source of the embolus. Signs of shock may also be present with a saddle embolus if a large artery is blocked because of the extent of circulation impairment.

■ ANEURYSM OF LOWER EXTREMITY BLOOD VESSEL

An aneurysm is an enlarged, dilated portion of an artery. Although it may follow trauma, such as an automobile accident, it is most commonly associated with atherosclerosis. The destruction of the medial layer leads to weakening of the artery wall and to the eventual formation of an aneurysm. Aneurysms of the arteries of the lower extremities, particularly in the popliteal area, are common in persons over age 60 who have pronounced arteriosclerosis (Fig. 26-5). Thrombi form at the site of the aneurysm, and emboli may travel and obstruct more distal portions of the artery.

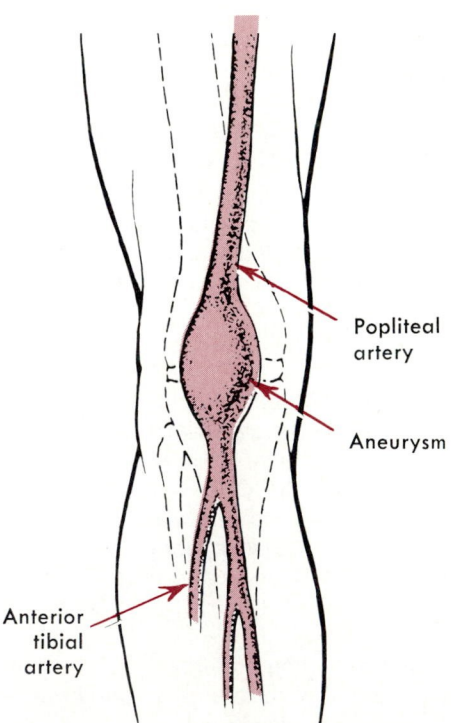

Fig. 26-5 Posterior view of the knee with an aneurysm of the popliteal artery. (From Anderson, HC: Newton's geriatric nursing, ed 5, St. Louis, 1971, The CV Mosby Co.)

■ ARTERIOVENOUS FISTULA

An arteriovenous fistula is an abnormal communication between an artery and a vein caused by a congenital anomaly or trauma. In an arteriovenous fistula the blood in the artery bypasses the capillary bed, which has a strong resistance to blood flow, and flows instead directly into the vein. Persistance of this high-pressure flow in the vein eventually results in venous dilation and may be associated with aneurysm formation.

Assessment

Data collection for the person with an arterial disorder focuses on noted changes in the circulation of the extremities and possible causative factors.

■ SUBJECTIVE DATA

1. Onset of symptoms: slow and progressive or sudden
2. Changes noted in skin color and temperature of extremities
3. Discomfort or pain in extremities: onset, location, quality, and occurrence with exercise or at rest
4. Effect on extremities of cold temperatures, cigarette smoking, or emotional stress
5. Effectiveness of measures used to relieve discomfort or pain
6. Presence of risk factors: cigarette smoking; physical inactivity; obesity; emotional stress; history of hypertension, hyperlipidemia, or diabetes; family history of atherosclerosis

■ OBJECTIVE DATA

1. Skin changes:
   a. Appearance: shiny, taut, absence of hair on extremities (indicates lack of tissue oxygen)
   b. Color: pallor, redness, cyanosis
   c. Temperature: coldness
   d. Presence of ulcerations or gangrene
2. Condition of nail beds: opaque, thickened, capillary refill >3 seconds
3. Peripheral pulses (Fig. 26-6): presence and quality (*Note:* compare bilaterally)
4. Presence of audible bruit or palpable thrill over artery
5. Symmetry of extremities
6. Sensation in extremities: numbness, tingling
7. Muscle tone: weakness, loss of tone
8. Effectiveness of prescribed medications

■ DIAGNOSTIC TESTS

Several tests may be used in the diagnosis of arterial disorders. Noninvasive diagnostic tests such as segmental limb pressure and pulse volume recordings are often used. Additional diagnostic tests are outlined in the box on p. 835.

□ Segmental limb pressure

Systolic pressure readings are obtained for each limb segment through the use of pneumatic pressure cuffs and a Doppler probe. The cuffs are applied to various parts of the extremities: ankle, below knee, thigh, groin, and upper arm. Differences between segmental pressure readings provide a useful index of arterial occlusion.

□ Pulse volume recordings

Pulse volume recordings are obtained to assess areas such as the foot and toes, which are not easily evaluated by segmental limb pressure, and to substantiate the diagnosis of arterial stenosis and occlusion. Pneumatic pressure cuffs are attached to the extremities. A pressure transducer records pressure changes as wave forms during cuff inflation and deflation.

Data analysis: nursing diagnoses

Nursing diagnoses are determined from assessment of patient data. Possible nursing diagnoses for the person with an arterial disorder may include, but are not limited to, the following:

Diagnostic title	Possible etiologies
Activity intolerance	Imbalance between oxygen supply and demand; immobility
Potential for infection	Lack of knowledge
Potential for injury	Sensorimotor deficits
Knowledge deficit: risk factors, medications, diagnostic tests, surgery	Lack of exposure/recall, information misinterpretation, unfamiliarity with information sources
Pain: extremities	Ischemic tissues and spasms
Potential impaired skin integrity	Immobility, hypothermia
Altered peripheral tissue perfusion	Decreased arterial blood flow

Planning: expected patient outcomes

Expected patient outcomes for the person with an arterial disorder may include, but are not limited to, the following:

1. Patient participates in activity, with a balance between rest and activity.
2. Patient states a reduction in discomfort and does not exhibit signs of uncontrolled pain.
3. Patient can describe potential for infection and injury and preventive measures.
4. Patient can describe risk factors that may compromise arterial circulation and plans to avoid these factors.
5. Patient can describe the prescribed medication regimen.
6. Patient can describe measures to increase peripheral tissue perfusion.
7. Patient can describe plans for ongoing medical care.

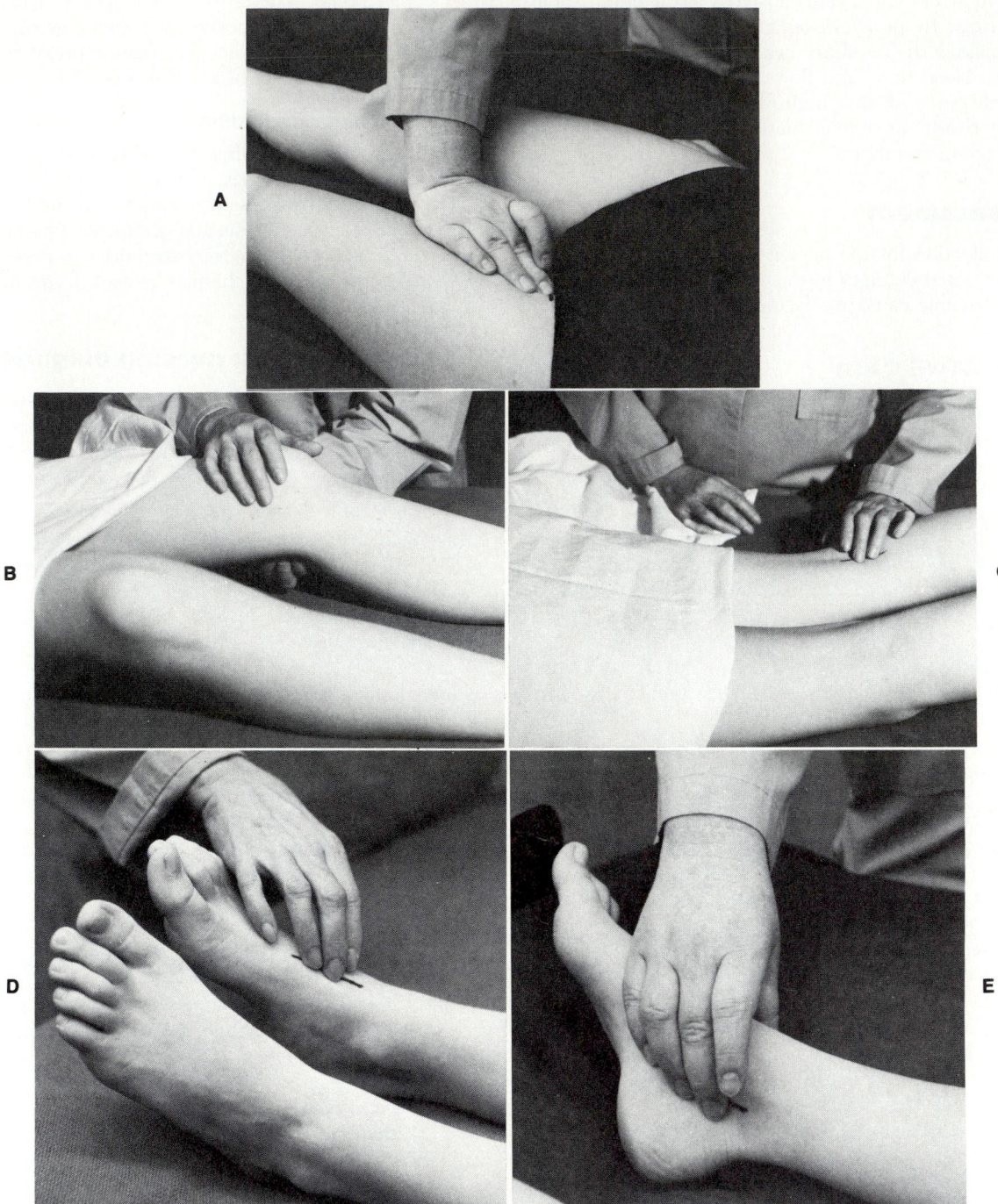

Fig. 26-6 **A,** Palpation of femoral pulse. **B,** Palpation of popliteal pulse with patient in the dorsal recumbent position. **C,** Palpation of popliteal pulse with patient in the prone position. **D,** Palpation of dorsal pedal pulse. **E,** Palpation of posterior tibial pulse. (From Malasanos, L, et al: Health assessment, ed 3, St. Louis, 1985, The CV Mosby Co.)

Diagnostic tests for arterial disorders

Peripheral vascular arteriography (angiography)
Purpose

1. Visualize the vascular system and detect changes in blood vessels.
2. Assess arterial blood flow.
3. Identify arterial obstruction, vascular abnormality, or aneurysm formation.
4. Diagnose arteriosclerosis, thromboangiitis obliterans, and arteriovenous fistulas.

Procedure

1. A radiopaque catheter is guided under fluoroscopy into the proximal iliac artery and through the aorta to the femoral artery on the affected side.
2. Radiopaque dye is inserted into the artery through the catheter.
3. A series of x-ray films is taken.

Nursing intervention

1. Explain the purpose and procedure (for example, transient flushing and burning sensations are felt when the dye is inserted).
2. Following the test, assess the following:
   a. Injection site for bleeding and hematoma
   b. Peripheral pulses distal to site every hour for 4 to 8 hours
   c. Allergic reaction to dye (dyspnea, flushing, hives, nausea, and vomiting).
   d. Sensation distal to site
3. Encourage patient to drink oral fluids to facilitate excretion of dye.

Digital subtraction angiography
Purpose

1. Visualize the vascular system.
2. Determine presence and extent of occlusion.

Procedure

1. Catheter is inserted into vein (usually antecubital vein).
2. Contrast medium is injected.
3. Images are displayed on TV monitor.

Nursing intervention

The nursing intervention for digital subtraction angiography is the same as that for arteriography.

Doppler ultrasonography
Purpose

1. Evaluate vascular network (that is, arteries, veins).
2. Measure blood flow through vessels.
3. Monitor status of bypass grafts.
4. Diagnose deep-vein thrombosis, arterial occlusion, and peripheral artery disease.

Procedure

1. Apply conductive jelly to skin.
2. Move the handheld transducer (which directs high-frequency sound waves to artery or veins) evenly back and forth across skin surface.
3. Obtain graphic recordings of blood flow.

Nursing intervention

1. Explain purpose and procedure to patient (for instance, no discomfort will be experienced).
2. Remove any excess lubricant from patient's skin.

Continued.

Diagnostic tests for arterial disorders—cont'd

Cold stimulation test
Purpose

1. Record temperature changes in patient's fingers before and after submersion in ice-water bath.
2. Diagnose Raynaud's phenomenon.

Procedure

1. Tape thermistor to each finger.
2. Submerge hand in ice-water bath for 20 seconds.
3. Obtain temperature recordings.

Nursing intervention

1. Explain purpose and procedure (for example, discomfort may be experienced from the cold water).
2. Have patient remove jewelry from hand.

Exercise testing
Purpose

1. Determine amount of exercise that precipitates ischemia and claudication.
2. Diagnose arteriosclerosis obliterans and thromboangiitis obliterans.

Procedure

1. Patient walks on treadmill for about 5 minutes at specific speed or until onset of pain in extremity.
2. Measurements made of ankle pressure, pulse volume, and blood pressure; comparison made to baseline.

Nursing intervention

1. Explain purpose and procedure.
2. Remind patient to stop exercise at onset of pain.

▥ Implementation

■ ASSISTING WITH ACHIEVEMENT OF THERAPEUTIC GOALS

☐ Medications

The most frequently used medications to treat arterial disorders include anticoagulants, fibrinolytics, and vasodilators.

☐ Vasodilators

The use of vasodilators in the management of arterial disorders is controversial; the majority of studies indicate that these drugs are not very effective. The drugs are used primarily for conditions causing vasospasm, such as Raynaud's disease.

☐ Anticoagulants

Anticoagulants are used to prolong the clotting time of blood and hence prevent extension of a clot and inhibit further clot formation. Heparin and warfarin sodium (Coumadin, Panwarfin) are the most commonly administered anticoagulants (Table 26-2). Patient teaching for persons taking warfarin sodium (Coumadin) includes the following:

1. Prevent bleeding.
   a. Use a soft toothbrush.
   b. Avoid the use of straight razors.
   c. Avoid intramuscular injections.
2. Recognize and report signs of bleeding: bleeding gums, nosebleeds, petechiae (pinpointlike red areas on skin), bruising, cuts that do not stop bleeding, red or brown urine, and red or black bowel movements.
3. At all times, carry an identification card or wear a MedicAlert bracelet containing the drug name, dosage, and physician's phone number.
4. Report for prescribed blood (prothrombin) tests as instructed to monitor effects of medication. (Medication may be adjusted on basis of blood test.)
5. Consult with physician before taking other medications (especially aspirin that has anticoagulant properties).
6. Do not stop taking an anticoagulant unless advised by physician.

☐ Fibrinolytics

Fibrinolytics, or thrombolytics, are useful in dissolving existing thrombi when rapid dissolution of the clot is re-

Table 26-2 Medications used in treatment of arterial disorders

Drug	Dosage	Mechanism of action	Nursing interventions
Anticoagulants			
Heparin	Intravenous: Loading dose at start of infusion: 5000 U Continuous drip: 20,000-30,000 U/day at 0.5 U/kg/min in 5% dextrose or NS *Intermittent:* Initially 5000 U; then 5000-10,000 U q4h	Antagonizes activation of pro-thrombin to thrombin Inhibits platelet aggregation Immediate action Duration 2 h	Hold pressure on venipuncture sites for 3 to 5 min. Control IV infusion accurately at desired units per hour. Assess skin for signs of bleeding, ecchymosis, petechiae, and hematoma. Check urine and stool for blood. Monitor partial thromboplastin time; desired effect is 1½ to 2 times normal level. Know that protamine sulfate is heparin antagonist. Avoid rectal temperature. Avoid IM route of injection.
	Subcutaneous: 5000 U 2 h before surgery and every 8 to 12 h thereafter Other: 10,000-12,000 U q8h 14,000-20,000 U q12h	Low-dose prophylaxis	Administer into subcutaneous tissue (abdominal fat pad). Use small gauge needle and 90-degree angle. Rotate injection sites. Do not aspirate. Do not massage tissue after injection.
Warfarin sodium (Coumadin, Panwarfin)	Oral 10 to 15 mg/day until pro-thrombin time within therapeutic range Then 2-10 mg/day	Depresses prothrombin activity Peaks in 36-72 h Action 2-5 days	Teach patient about warfarin. Monitor prothrombin time; desired effect is 2 to 2½ times normal level. Know that vitamin K counteracts anticoagulant effects of warfarin sodium.
Fibrinolytics			
Streptokinase (Streptase)	Intravenous Loading dose: 250,000 IU over 30 min Then 100,000 IU/hr for 24-72 h (arterial thrombosis) or 72 h (deep vein thrombosis)	Activates plasminogen	Monitor patient for bleeding. Assess patient for allergic reaction (for example, chills, bronchospasm, rash, and malaise). Have aminocaproic acid (a fibrinolysis inhibitor) available.
Urokinase (Abbokinase)	Intravenous Loading dose: 4400 IU/kg over 10 min Continuous: 4400 IU/kg/hr for 24 h	Direct activator of plasminogen	Refer to streptokinase.

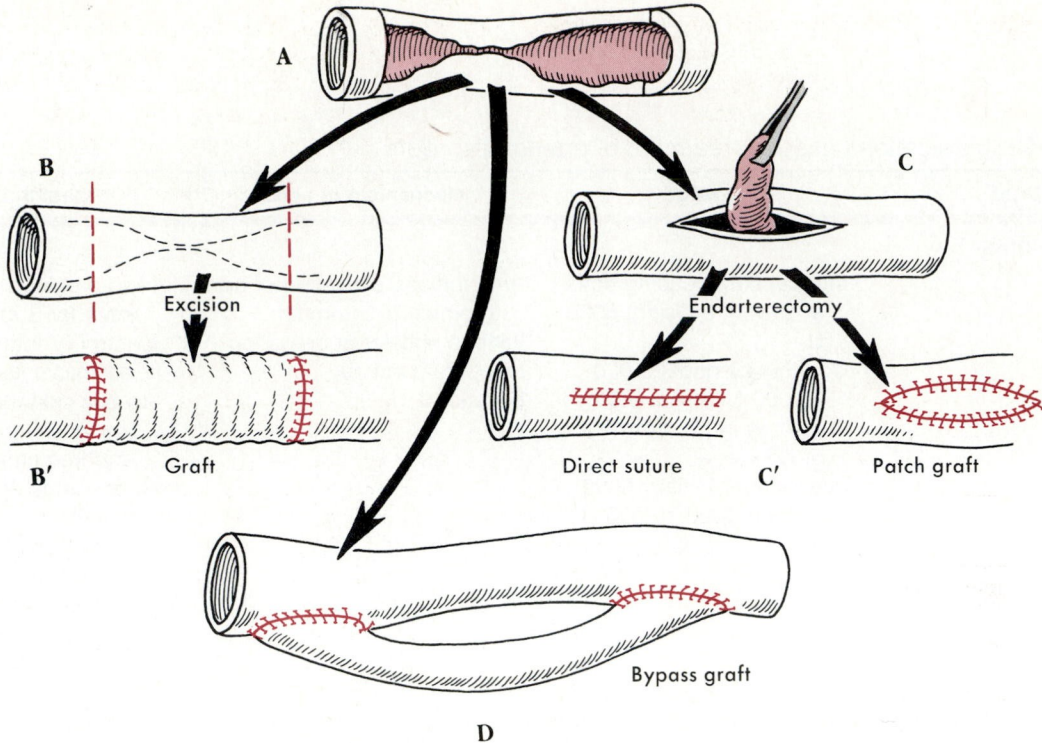

Fig. 26-7 **A,** Obstructed artery. Methods of restoring arterial blood flow include: **B,** excision; **B',** graft; **C,** endarterectomy; **C',** direct suture and patch graft reconstruction; and **D,** bypass graft. (Redrawn from Juergens, JL, et al: Peripheral vascular disease, Philadelphia, 1980, WB Saunders Co. By permission of Mayo Foundation.)

quired to preserve organ and limb function (Table 26-2). Streptokinase and urokinase impair hemostasis by increasing fibrinolytic activity. After infusion of fibrinolytics, the patient is started on heparin or oral anticoagulants to prevent extension of existing clots or formation of new clots.

☐ **Surgery**

Surgery is indicated for patients who have advanced arterial disease in which ischemic changes are present or for patients with severe pain that impairs their activities. These surgical procedures include arterial bypass surgery, embolectomy, percutaneous transluminal angioplasty, removal of aneurysm and closure of a fistula, sympathectomy, and amputation.

☐ *Arterial bypass surgery and reconstruction*

If *arteriosclerosis obliterans* is rapidly progressing and intermittent claudication has become gravely disabling, surgery to correct the obstruction is indicated. The most common procedure is a bypass of the obstructed arterial segment, using prosthetic material such as Teflon or Dacron or autogenous (the patient's own) artery or vein, such as the saphenous vein (Fig. 26-7). The bypass may involve the aorta itself, as with an aortofemoral bypass, or more distal vessels such as the femoral-popliteal bypass. Procedures that are performed either in conjunction with a bypass or by themselves include *patch grafting* (replacing a

damaged segment of the arterial wall with a vein patch) and *endarterectomy* (stripping arteriosclerotic plaques from the intima and inner media using balloon catheters or other instruments).

Nursing interventions for the patient undergoing arterial bypass and reconstruction include the following:
1. Monitor skin color and temperature distal to the graft site every hour.
2. Assess sensation and movement in the distal limb.
3. Assess peripheral pulses in the involved limb.
   a. Sudden absence of pulse may indicate thrombosis.
   b. Mark location of peripheral pulse with a pen to facilitate frequent assessment.
   c. Use a Doppler if pulses are difficult to palpate.
4. Monitor extremity for edema.
5. Check incision for redness, swelling, and drainage.
6. Monitor and immediately report signs of complication, such as increasing pain, fever, changes in drainage, absent or weakening pulse, change in skin color, limitation of movement, or paresthesia.
7. Promote circulation.
   a. Reposition patient every 2 hours.
   b. Tell patient not to cross legs.
   c. Use a footboard and overbed cradle to keep linens off extremity.
   d. Encourage progressive activity when permitted.
9. Avoid sharp flexion in the area of the graft.

☐ *Embolectomy*

An embolectomy is the removal of a blood clot and is most often used when large arteries are obstructed. The success of the surgery is dependent on the length of time the extremity was ischemic; surgery must be performed within 6 to 10 hours to prevent muscle necrosis and loss of the extremity. An endarterectomy may also be performed.

Nursing care of the patient undergoing an embolectomy includes the following:

1. Preoperative care
   a. Maintain bed rest.
   b. Keep affected extremity flat in bed (may be slightly dependent at 15 degrees to promote circulation).
   c. Monitor vital signs.
   d. Assess skin color and temperature and the quality of peripheral pulses.
   e. Keep extremity warm.
   f. Use overbed cradle to keep bed linens off affected extremity.
2. Postoperative care
   a. Assess surgical wound for redness, swelling, and drainage.
   b. Assess skin color and temperature and the quality of distal peripheral pulses.
   c. Monitor the patient for signs of bleeding secondary to anticoagulant therapy.

☐ *Percutaneous transluminal angioplasty*

Percutaneous transluminal angioplasty may be used as surgical treatment for atherosclerotic obliterans or in the removal of a stenotic arterial graft. A specially design cath-

eter is inserted under fluoroscopy and advanced to the site of the obstruction. The balloon tip of the catheter is inflated to provide compression and rupture the atherosclerotic plaque. Thrombosis may occur after treatment; therefore, anticoagulants are usually prescribed.

☐ *Removal of aneurysm and closure of fistula*

The blood vessel may be ligated unless the procedure is incompatible with the life of tissues distal to the lesion. Homografts or Teflon or Dacron grafts may be used in larger blood vessels of the extremities, either to replace the portion of the artery that contains the aneurysm or to bypass the abnormality. Fig. 26-8 illustrates the excision of an aneurysm and its replacement with a synthetic graft. Popliteal function is better at the flexion crease when the patient's own vein is used. Perioperative care is similar to that for the patient undergoing an embolectomy.

☐ *Sympathectomy*

A sympathectomy is the removal of the sympathetic ganglia or a division of their branches. This surgery may benefit patients with Raynaud's disease.

☐ *Amputation*

Although a partial or complete amputation of an extremity may be necessary as a result of sarcoma or trauma, most amputations are indicated for patients with advanced atherosclerosis and gangrene of the extremities. The majority of amputations are of the lower extremity; the toes are the most amputated part of the body. An amputation may also be offered as an option to improve functional ability with a prosthesis.

The surgical goal is to remove the least amount of tissue

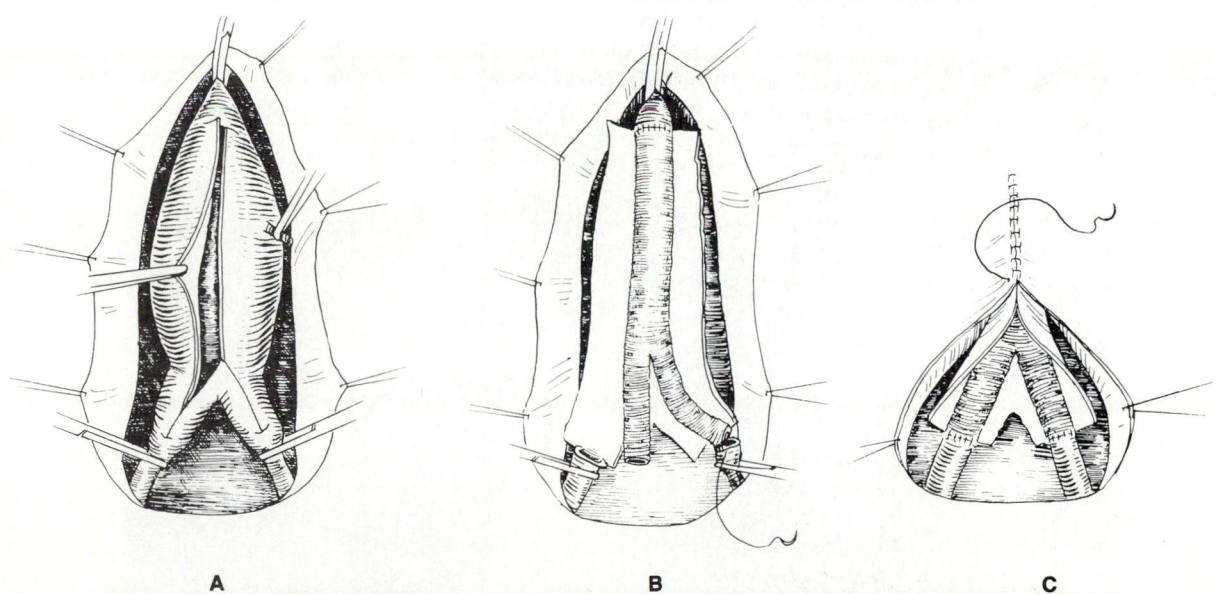

A **B** **C**

Fig. 26-8   Abdominal aneurysm. **A,** Aneurysm of the aorta and iliac arteries. **B,** Bifurcation graft used to replace the excised aneurysm. **C,** Closure of the posterior peritoneum over the graft and suture line. (Redrawn from Crawford, ES, et al: Surg Clin North Am 46:963-978, 1966.)

possible and to create a stump adequate for the fitting of a prosthesis. The specific level of amputation is determined by the extent of the disease process. Below-knee (BK) amputations maintain knee function and allow for greater stability with a prosthesis. A BK amputation is usually done in the lower third of the leg, leaving a 12 to 18 cm stump. An above-knee (AK) amputation may be made at any level, although it is frequently below the middle of the thigh to preserve an adequate stump for satisfactory use of a prosthesis. AK amputations are often performed after unsuccessful BK amputations.

Amputation involves loss of a body part; therefore, feel-

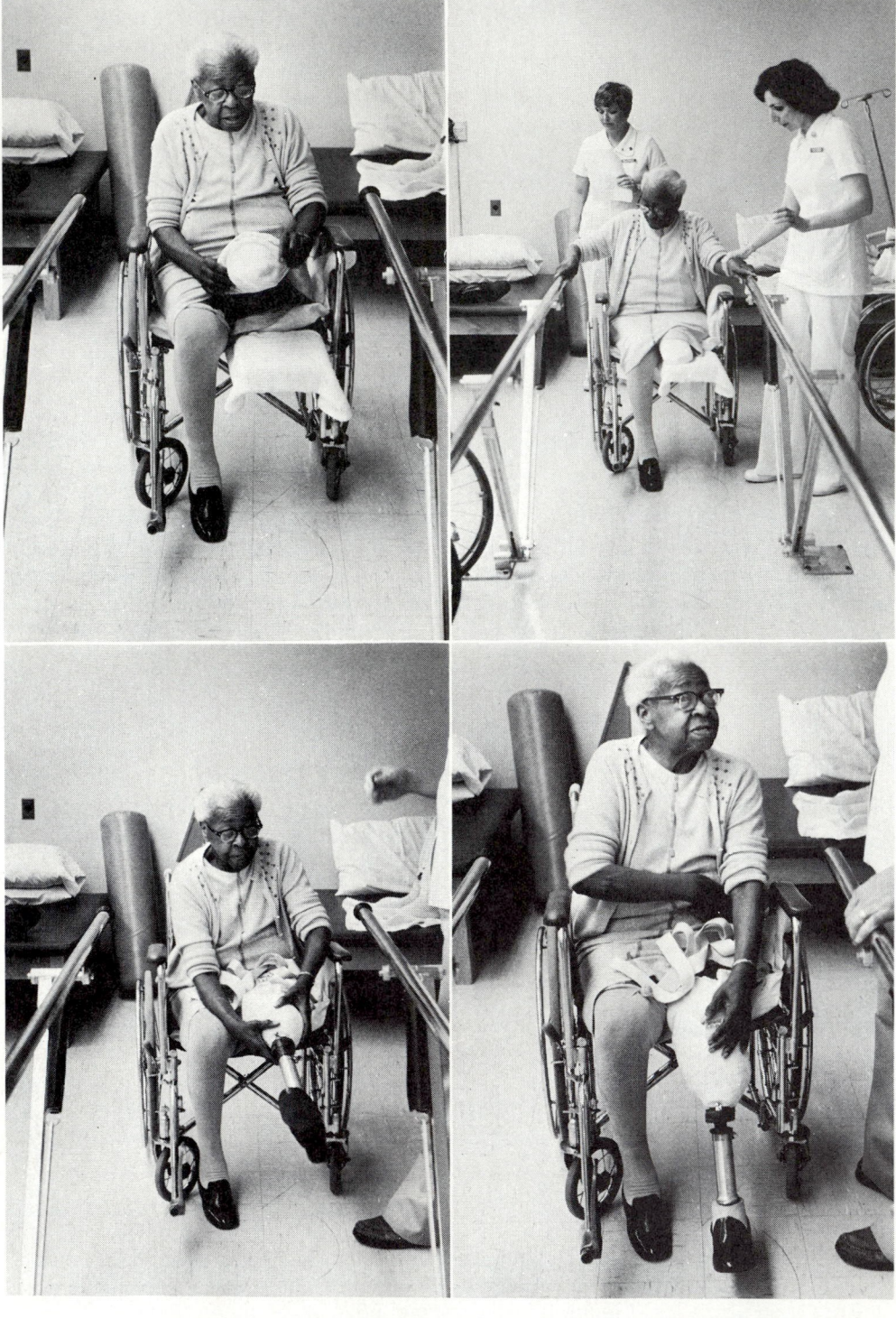

Fig. 26-9　Patient with cast on stump with metal pylon attached for weight bearing.

Continued.

ings of grief related to loss are usually experienced. (For further discussion on loss and grief see Chapter 15). Before and after surgery the patient should exercise to strengthen arm and leg muscles to promote movement and ambulation and to prevent knee and hip contractures.

Following surgery, most persons experience phantom sensations, or feelings related to the removed limb. About 10% of patients experience uncomfortable sensations (*phantom limb pain*) similar to the pain experienced before amputation or the sensation of a cramped or uncomfortable position. In most instances, this discomfort disappears with time, but the pain may become chronic for some persons.

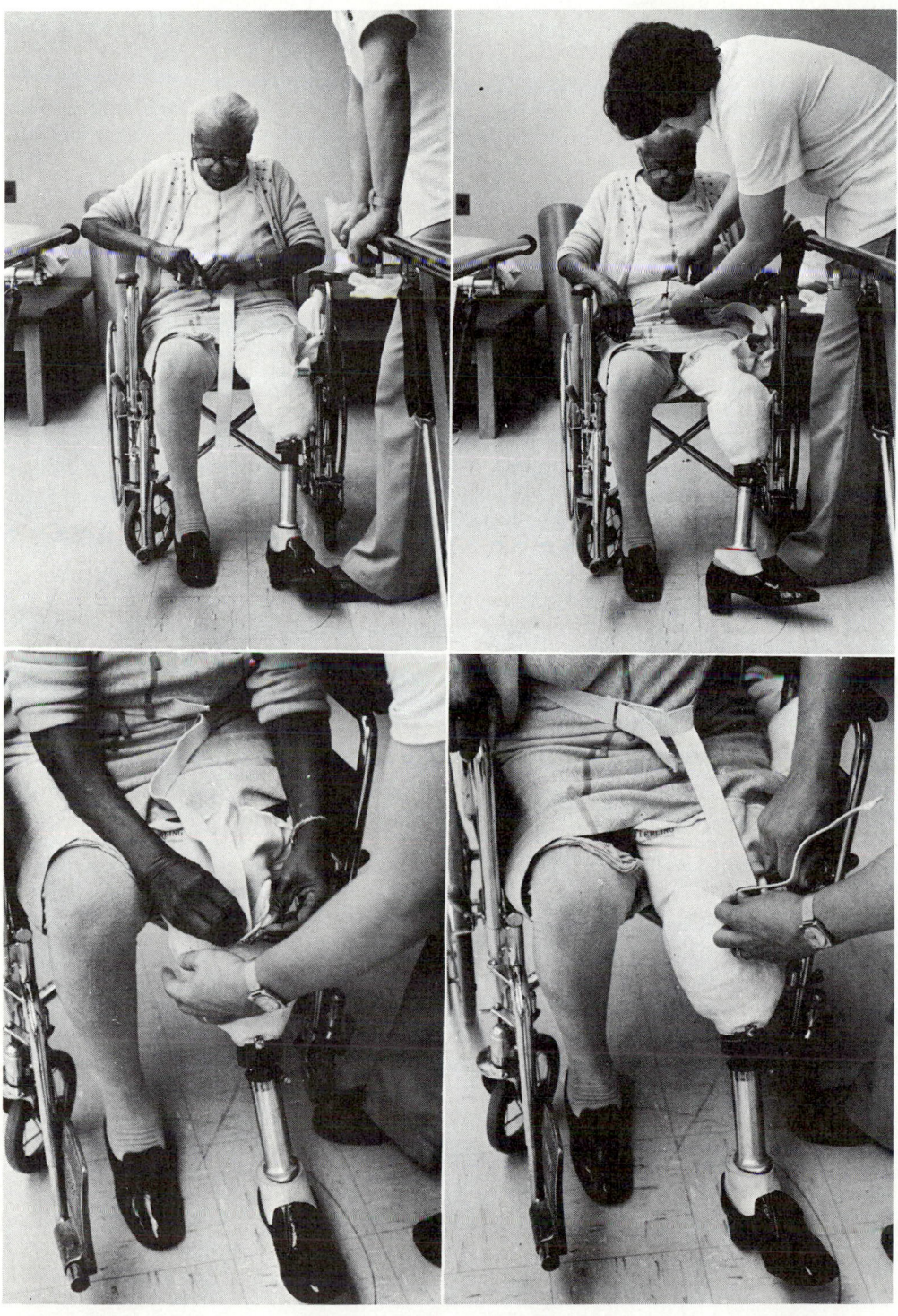

Fig. 26-9 cont'd.   Patient with cast on stump on metal pylon attached for weight bearing.

Even though the limb is removed, the pain is a real sensation and should not be dismissed as illusionary.

A *prosthesis* may be used immediately after or within 5 weeks of surgery. A cast may also be applied over the dressing to allow for attachment of a metal pylon prosthesis (Fig. 26-9). A permanent prosthesis is made 6 months after surgery to allow for stump shrinkage and molding.

A sample nursing care plan for a patient with an amputation is shown below, through p. 844. Care of the patient with a leg amputation includes the following:

1. Preoperative care
   a. Assist patient to express feelings, concerns, and fears; accept patient reaction of anger, discouragement, and grief.

   b. Discuss postoperative regimen with patient and family.
      1. Frequent positioning to promote circulation
      2. Exercises to strengthen arm muscles for the use of crutches: push-ups and weight lifting
      3. Exercises to strengthen leg muscles to prevent knee and hip contactures and to promote ambulation: ankle rotations, ankle pumps, and quadricep sets
   c. Teach crutch walking if appropriate (usually done by physical therapist).
2. Postoperative care
   a. Monitor stump and drainage catheter for color, amount of drainage; report signs of increased drainage.

NURSING CARE PLAN

Person with below-knee amputation

DATA: Mrs. Robins is a 65-year-old widowed, retired sales clerk with a history of diabetes and peripheral vascular disease. During the past 3 years she has been in and out of the hospital for treatment of recurrent infected leg ulcers. She was admitted to the hospital 2 days ago with ulcers on her right heel and toes, complaining of cramplike pain with activity and a burning pain at rest. Diagnostic findings from clinical examination and tests revealed severe arterial occlusions within her bypass grafts of one year. She underwent a below-knee amputation to prevent further progression of her disease and to improve her functional ability.

The nursing history revealed the following:

1. She has smoked one pack of cigarettes per day for 40 years despite recent efforts to quit smoking.
2. She is overweight for her height: 5 feet 4 inches and 155 pounds.
3. She takes 24U NPH insulin every day to control her diabetes of 10 years duration.
4. She has not been able to prepare meals, clean house, or visit friends because of pain and discomfort in her legs and a decreased ability to move around.
5. She has been unsuccessful in establishing a regular daily exercise program.
6. Before surgery she said that she was resigned to be a "gimpy" for life; she had been expecting that she would eventually lose her leg, but she was concerned about how she would manage at home with meals, cleaning, and other chores.
7. She returned from surgery with a below-knee stump; she will receive a prosthesis after the stump has healed.

Nursing diagnosis: Potential for injury: hemorrhage, infection, and contractures related to surgery (BK amputation)

Expected patient outcomes	Nursing interventions	Rationale
Hemorrhage, infection, contractures do not occur	Monitor stump and drainage catheter for amount of drainage; report signs of increased drainage	Bleeding may occur from surgery; purulent drainage may be noted with infection
	Monitor vital signs and signs of shock	Severe bleeding may cause shock
	Apply pressure bandage over stump dressing	Pressure decreases bleeding and prevents fluid collection
	Maintain aseptic technique when changing dressing	She is diabetic and has poor circulation; therefore, she is at higher risk for infection
	Elevate stump on pillow, avoiding flexion of knee; place a support along outer side	Elevation decreases edema (from the trauma of surgery); contractures from constant knee flexion and outward rotation of leg interferes with use of prosthesis

NURSING CARE PLAN

Person with below-knee amputation—cont'd

Nursing diagnosis: Pain: in stump related to removal of lower leg

Expected patient outcomes	Nursing interventions	Rationale
Patient states she is feeling better	Provide analgesics as needed during early postoperative period	Analgesics may relieve incisional pain. Phantom limb pain is real pain and needs to be accepted as such
	Reinforce explanation of phantom limb pain if this occurs	
	Use other forms of pain management (such as backrubs, distraction, and relaxation exercises)	Nonmedicinal forms of pain management can be useful adjuncts to analgesics in reducing pain

Nursing diagnosis: Body image disturbance: related to loss of leg and change in body appearance

Expected patient outcomes	Nursing interventions	Rationale
Patient expresses feelings about loss of leg	Be aware that initial reaction after surgery may include shock and denial	Mrs. Robins needs to work through grieving process; an expression of feelings and obtaining support from family, friends, and nurse are helpful in working through this process
	Be accepting of the patient's expression of frustration or anger	
	Continue to provide patient with opportunities to express feelings about the lost leg	
	Explain grief reactions if appropriate	
	Encourage supportive visits from family and friends	
	Encourage patient to look at stump when ready	Looking at stump is the first step toward incorporating lost leg into new body image
Patient carries out ADL	Encourage patient to move toward independence in ADL	Providing care to self and making decisions assist in regaining previous level of independent function and thus helps the patient feel better about self
Patient expresses confidence in self	Give patient opportunity to make decisions about care when appropriate	

Nursing diagnosis: Impaired physical mobility: related to decreased strength and endurance, pain, loss of leg

Expected patient outcomes	Nursing interventions	Rationale
Patient performs preparatory exercises	Encourage patient to do ROM of unaffected leg, biceps, triceps, and gluteal exercises	Active ROM exercises increase muscle strength and prevent contractures
Patient ambulates with crutches	Encourage patient to ambulate using correct crutch-walking technique	Exercises and early ambulation promote circulation and wound healing; ambulating helps patient begin to get a new sense of balance preparatory to using a prosthesis

Continued.

NURSING CARE PLAN

Person with below-knee amputation—cont'd

Nursing diagnosis: Constipation: related to immobility and opiates

Expected patient outcomes	Nursing interventions	Rationale
Stools are soft, formed, and at patient's normal frequency	Monitor stools for constipation	Immobility and opiates are high risk factors for constipation
	Encourage fluids and high-fiber diet	Fluids and fiber promote bowel motility
	Encourage maximum activity and ambulation	Activity promotes bowel motility

Nursing diagnosis: Impaired home maintenance management: related to impaired mobility

Expected patient outcomes	Nursing interventions	Rationale
Home is clean and balanced meals are available	Explore with patient ways in which housekeeping needs can be met	Encorporating patient in planning helps ensure results
	Enlist help of social worker in plans for use of community resources	Social workers have access to community resources

Nursing diagnosis: Knowledge deficit: related to lack of exposure or recall

Expected patient outcomes	Nursing interventions	Rationale
Patient demonstrates proper crutch walking	Reinforce teaching of crutch walking	Reinforcement of earlier teaching helps promote retention
Patient demonstrates stump care	Teach stump care and how to get supplies for care in the community	Patient needs to care for stump at home
Patient describes plans to stop smoking and to lose weight	Review effect of smoking, obesity, and uncontrolled diabetes on circulation	Patient is at high risk for arterial insufficiency in other leg
	Discuss previous efforts to discontinue smoking and losing weight; explore additional ways, expecially group programs	Programs that include group support are often more successful than individual efforts

b. Position patient with no flexion at hip or knee to avoid contractures.

c. Maintain patient in low-Fowler's or flat position following AK amputation.

d. Support stump with pillow for first 24 hours (according to physician preference and avoiding flexion); place rolled bath blanket along outer aspect to prevent outward rotation.

e. Encourage exercises to prevent thromboembolism.
1. Active ROM of unaffected leg, ankle rotations, and pumps
2. Use of overhead trapeze when moving in bed
3. Push-ups from sitting position and bed
4. Quadriceps sets (see Chapter 18)
5. Lifting stump and buttocks off bed while lying flat on back to strengthen abdominal muscles

f. Teach care of stump.
1. Inspect for redness, blisters, and abrasions.
2. Wash stump with mild soap, rinse with water, and pat dry.
3. Avoid use of alcohol, oils, and creams.
4. Remove stump bandage or stump sock and reapply as needed; use firm smooth figure-eight ace wrapping to reduce swelling and shape stump (Fig. 26-10).

g. Encourage patient to ambulate using correct crutch-walking technique.

h. Monitor patient's ability to use a prosthesis (Fig. 26-11).

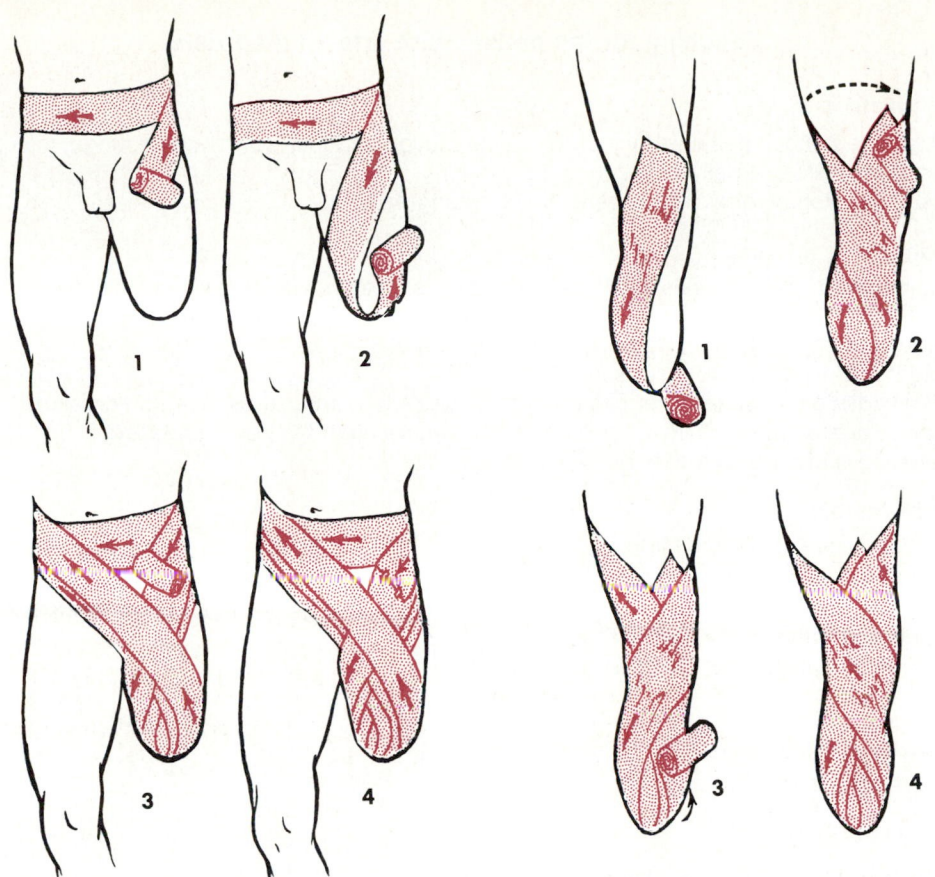

Fig. 26-10   Left, correct method of bandaging midthigh amputation stump. Note that the bandage must be anchored around patient's waist. Right, correct method for bandaging midcalf amputation stump. Note that bandage need not be anchored about waist.

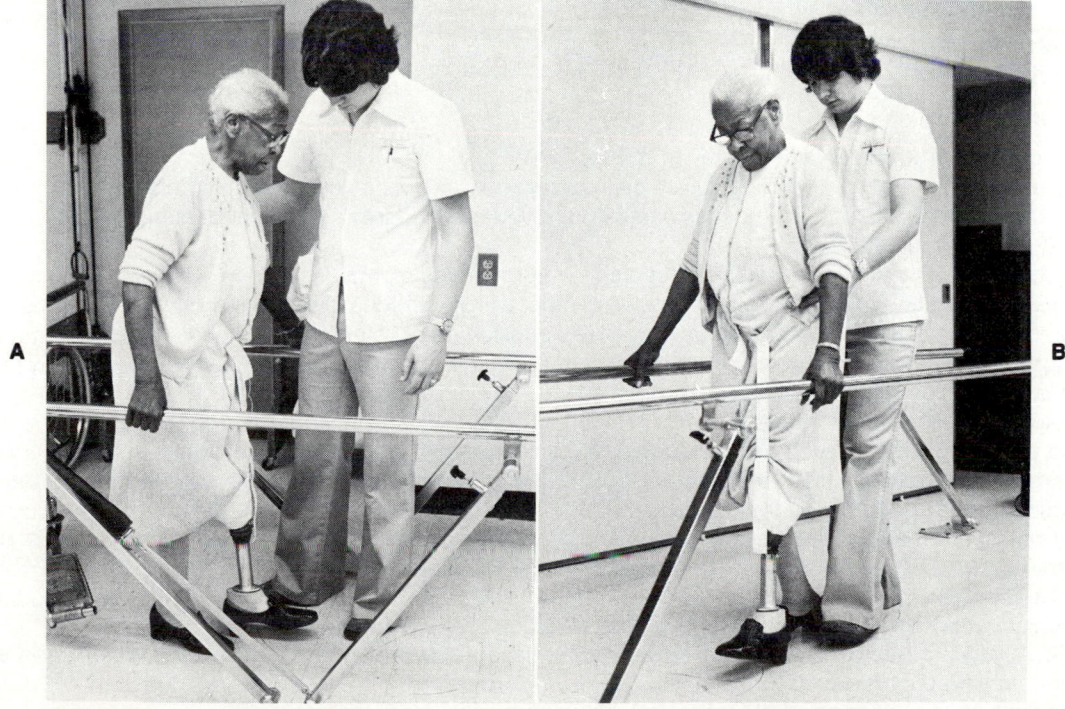

Fig. 26-11   **A,** Patient steps forward on the prosthesis while using the bars for stability. **B,** Walking behind the patient enables the therapist to assess her gait.

Teaching for the patient with arterial disorders

Prevention of infection

1. Avoid rubber-soled shoes because they prevent evaporation and thus contribute to fungal infection.
2. Assess skin condition on a daily basis.
3. Seek medical assistance for lesions, ulceration, and gangrene.

Prevention of injury

1. Wear comfortable protective shoes at all times; alternate shoes on a daily basis to allow for airing.
2. Trim nails carefully.
   a. Cut at regular intervals; soak in warm water to soften nails.
   b. Use straight nail clippers; avoid scissors.
3. Seek medical advice for thickened or deformed nails, blisters, corns, calluses, and ulcerations.
4. Check water temperature carefully, as ability to sense temperature may be decreased.
5. Avoid scratching and rubbing feet to prevent abrasion.

Alteration in risk factors

1. Maintain caloric intake desirable for height and weight.
2. Use vegetable fats rather than animal fats in cooking to decrease cholesterol intake.
3. Ensure intake of vitamins, especially B-complex (for maintenance of smooth muscle tone) and vitamin C (for tissue healing and prevention of hemorrhage).
4. Ensure adequate fluid intake to decrease blood viscosity.
5. Quit smoking.
6. Control diabetes.
7. Control hypertension.
8. Maintain physical activity.

Maintenance of skin integrity

1. Take a daily bath in tepid water (three baths per week if patient is elderly).
   a. Use a neutral pH soap.
   b. Wash gently; avoid scratching and vigorous rubbing.
   c. Dry skin gently.
   d. Lubricate skin with moisturizing agent; avoid alcohol.
2. Assess skin for intactness, dryness, redness, and lesions.
3. Take meticulous care of feet.
   a. Bathe each toe and dry well.
   b. Use only prescribed foot powders.
   c. Wear clean socks daily.
4. Avoid application of direct heat, such as hot water bottles or heating pads, to skin.

Increase tissue perfusion

1. Maintain warm environmental temperature of 21° C (70° F).
2. Avoid exposure to cold and chilling, which causes vasoconstriction; layer clothing in cold weather.
3. Avoid constrictive clothing that impedes circulation: rolled garters, socks with tight banding, girdles, tight waistbands, and tight shoelaces.
4. Avoid crossing legs at knees, which places pressure on arteries of legs.
5. Avoid sitting or standing for prolonged periods of time, which impedes circulation through venous congestion.
6. Place legs in slight *dependency* to promote tissue perfusion; avoid elevation of legs as it impedes arterial flow.
7. Engage in a regular exercise plan. Exercise stimulates collateral circulation and improves circulation by promoting muscle contraction and relaxation.
   a. Walk daily; allow time for rest periods.
   b. Do specific exercises such as rotation at ankle, ankle pumps, and extension at knee.
8. Quit smoking. Nicotine causes vasoconstriction and vasospasms; inhaled carbon monoxide reduces the oxygen-carrying capacity of the blood.
9. Avoid pressure on affected extremity; use padding for severe ischemia.
10. Avoid vigorous massage of extremities (may promote emboli formation).
11. Perform Buergen-Allen exercises.
    a. Lie flat in bed with legs elevated above heart level for 2 to 3 minutes.
    b. Sit on edge of bed for 2 to 3 minutes with legs relaxed and dependent; flex, extend, invert, and evert the feet, holding each position for 30 seconds.
    c. Lie flat with legs at heart level and cover with warm blanket for 5 minutes.
    d. Perform above exercises 4 times a day.

Table 26-3 Venous disorders

Disease	Etiology	Signs and symptoms	Therapy
Thrombophlebitis	Venous stasis from heart failure, shock, immobility, surgery (especially pelvic) Decreased venous return: pregnancy, malignant tumors, obesity Trauma: fractures, intravenous drugs or solutions Altered coagulability of blood: polycythemia, severe anemia, oral contraceptives Abrupt withdrawal of anticoagulants	Entire limb may be pale and cold Area along vein may be reddened and feel warm to touch Homan's sign: pain in calf on dorsiflexion Superficial veins feel hard and thready and are sensitive to pressure Difference in circumference of extremities	Bed rest during acute phase Warm moist heat to reduce discomfort and pain Elevation of extremity Elastic bandage Heparin and Coumadin Vasodilator to combat arterial spasms and improve circulation Fibrinolytics to resolve the thrombus Exercise program after acute phase

Varicose veins	Congenital valve defect or weakness of vein walls
	Prolonged standing
	Poor posture
	Pregnancy and abdominal tumors
	Chronic systemic disease: heart disease, cirrhosis
		Veins appear as darkened, tortuous, raised blood vessels; more pronounced on prolonged standing
		Feeling of heaviness in legs
		Fatigue
		Pain and muscle cramps
		Edema
			Conservative treatment:
			    Elevate legs at least every 2 to 3 hours
			    Wear elastic stocking
			    Avoid standing for long periods of time
			    Weight reduction if obese
			Surgery: venous ligation and stripping

■ COUNSELING AND TEACHING

Patient education is important in preventing exacerbations of symptoms of arterial disorders. Specific patient teaching is listed in the box on p. 846. This teaching includes prevention of infection, prevention of injury, alteration in risk factors, maintenance of skin integrity, and increase in peripheral tissue perfusion.

✣ Evaluation

Questions to ask in the evaluation of care of the person with an arterial disorder may include the following:
1. Is the patient able to tolerate activity and balance activity with rest?
2. Does the patient state that he or she is feeling more comfortable?
3. Have infection and injury been prevented?
4. Does the patient carry out daily physical activity?
5. Can the person describe risk factors to be avoided?
6. Can the person describe plans for daily activity?
7. Can the person describe the need to inspect skin of affected limbs on a regular basis and to give meticulous foot care?
8. Can the person describe avoidance of constrictive clothing and positioning?
9. Can the person describe plans for regular medical follow-up?

■ VENOUS DISORDERS

The thin walls of the veins allow for greater distensibility than do arteries. Veins of the extremities that carry blood against gravity are equipped with valves. Vascular distention or inefficient valves lead to venous stasis. The two major disorders of the venous system are thrombophlebitis and varicose veins (Table 26-3).

■ Pathophysiology
■ THROMBOPHLEBITIS

Thrombophlebitis or venous thrombosis is inflammation of the vessel wall with formation of a clot. Venous thrombosis is most frequent in the veins of the lower extremities in both deep and superficial veins. The most common veins affected are the saphenous, femoral, and popliteal veins and the small veins of the calf. If thrombophlebitis affects a deep vein, venous flow is obstructed and the extremity may become edematous. Thrombophlebitis in the superficial veins produces pain, tenderness, redness, and warmth along the course of the vein.

Thrombi in deep veins can grow larger with successive layering of platelets, fibrin, WBCs and RBCs. The greatest danger to the patient during the acute phase is of a portion of the thrombus breaking off, producing an embolus (Fig. 26-12). Emboli being carried back to the heart can lodge

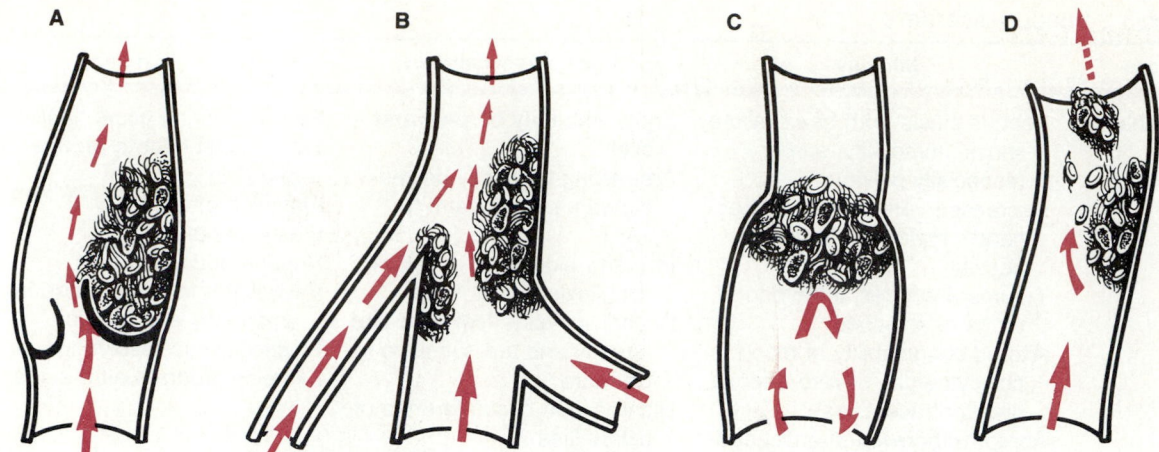

Fig. 26-12 Development of thromboemboli with arrows indicating direction of blood flow. **A,** Thrombus in a valve pocket of a deep vein with blood flowing beside thrombus. **B,** Thrombi tend to form at bifurcations of deep veins with some slowing of blood flow. **C,** Complete occlusion of vein by thrombus, forcing back flow of blood. **D,** Embolus that has broken off from thrombus and is floating in blood stream. Could migrate to lungs and cause pulmonary embolus.

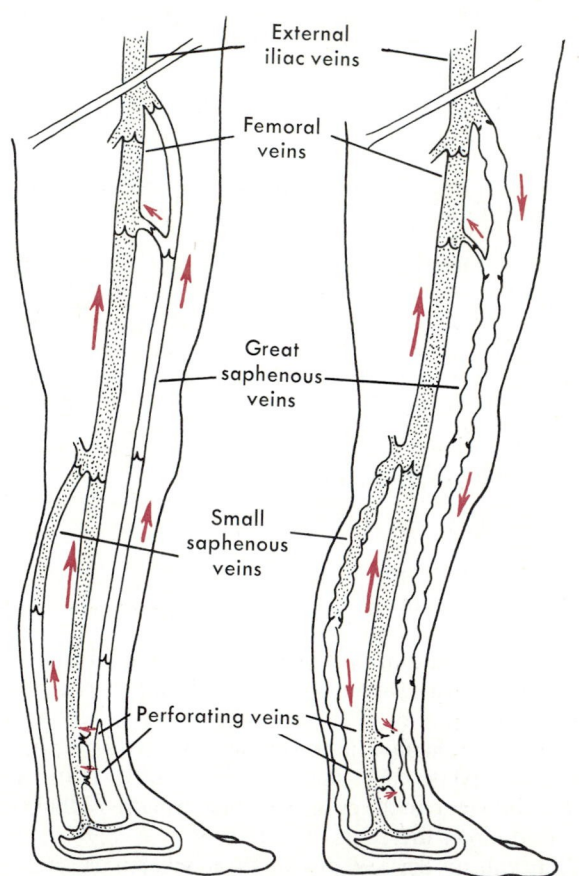

Fig. 26-13 Left, venous flow in normal veins. Right, venous flow in varicose veins. (Redrawn from Fairbairn, JF, Jurgens, JL, and Spittell, JA: Peripheral vascular disease, Philadelphia, 1972, WB Saunders Co.)

in the coronary arteries, but the most common site is the pulmonary vessels. Thrombi in the leg veins eventually become incorporated in the vessel wall and then no longer pose a threat for emboli. The vessel wall at the site of the inflammation, however, may become narrowed and present future circulatory problems for the patient.

■ VARICOSE VEINS

Varicose veins are abnormally dilated veins with incompetent valves, occurring most often in the lower extremities and lower trunk. In the lower limbs the great and small saphenous veins are most often involved (Fig. 26-13). At least 20% of the total population is affected by varicose veins. The highest incidence is in the third to fifth decades of life.

Varicose veins may be primary or secondary. *Primary varicose veins* have a gradual onset and affect the superficial veins. Often there are no accompanying symptoms except the appearance of darkened tortuous veins. Symptoms include dull aches, muscle cramps, pressure, heaviness, or fatigue. These symptoms arise from reduced blood flow to the tissues, resulting from venous pooling or stasis. *Secondary varicose veins* affect the deep veins and occur as a result of chronic venous insufficiency or venous thrombosis. Symptoms of edema, pain, changes in skin color, and ulcerations may occur from venous stasis.

The precipitating factor in varicose vein formation is simply a weakening of the vein wall. Because the vessel wall is weak, it does not withstand normal pressure and dilates with pooling of blood. As the vessel dilates, the valves become stretched and incompetent. This results in an inability to support a column of blood and more venous pooling occurs.

Assessment

Data are collected about the nature of the symptoms, appearance of the limbs, and circulatory involvement.

SUBJECTIVE DATA

1. Onset and duration of symptoms
2. Pain: onset, intensity, site, and activity that produces pain
3. Other discomforts: feeling of pressure, heaviness, and fatigue in legs
4. Daily activities that require extensive periods of sitting or standing

OBJECTIVE DATA

1. Appearance of legs: redness along a vein (thrombophlebitis) and darkened, tortuous veins (varicosities)
2. Presence of edema: pitting or nonpitting
3. Differences in size of extremities: measure and record
4. Peripheral pulses: presence and quality
5. Presence of Homan's signs (pain in calf on dorsiflexion of foot) seen with thrombophlebitis

DIAGNOSTIC TESTS

☐ Venography

Venography is used to assess the condition of the deep leg veins and to diagnose deep vein thrombosis. A radiopaque contrast dye is injected through a catheter placed in a foot vein. Serial films are obtained to detect filling defects. Injection of the dye can cause a brief inflammatory response or allergic reaction.

☐ Doppler ultrasonography

Doppler ultrasonography is used to measure flow through vessels. A probe or electronic stethoscope is placed over the patient's femoral and popliteal veins. The flow probe directs an ultrasound beam at the involved areas; the beam is reflected back off the red cells that circulate through the blood vessels. The reflection varies according to the rate of flow in the vessel. This change in the frequency of reflected sound according to velocity of the flow is referred to as a Doppler effect (Fig. 26-14). Both extremities are compared for diminished or absent readings over the veins.

☐ Impedance plethysmography

Impedance plethysmography is used to measure changes in venous volumes and to detect deep vein thrombosis. A pressure cuff is applied to the thigh and electrodes are attached to the patient's leg. A comparison of venous volume tracing during inflation and deflation of the cuff is made.

☐ Trendelenburg's test

Trendelenburg's test is a simple noninvasive diagnostic tool to assess the competency of the venous valves through measurement of venous filling time. The patient lies down

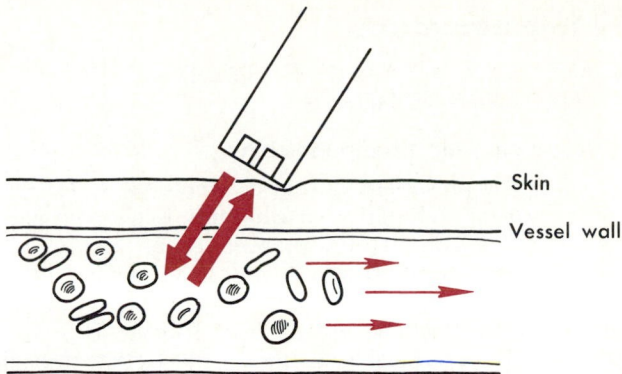

Fig. 26-14 Doppler effect showing red blood cells reflecting sound.

with the affected leg raised to allow for venous emptying. A tourniquet is then applied above the knee and the patient stands. The direction and filling time are recorded. The tourniquet is removed and the direction and filling time are noted again. Incompetent valves are present when the veins fill rapidly allowing backward blood flow.

Data analysis: nursing diagnoses

Nursing diagnoses are determined from the assessment of patient data. Possible nursing diagnoses for the person with a venous disorder may include, but are not limited to, the following:

Diagnostic title	Possible etiologies
Knowledge deficit: preventive measures, measures to enhance tissue perfusion	Lack of exposure/recall, information misinterpretation
Pain: leg	Inflammation, edema, venous stasis
Altered peripheral tissue perfusion	Decreased venous blood flow, immobility

Planning: expected patient outcomes

Expected patient outcomes for the person with a venous disorder may include, but are not limited to, the following:

1. Patient states that he or she experiences a reduction in pain.
2. Patient can describe rationale for activity limitations (thrombophlebitis).
3. Patient can describe medication regimen (thrombophlebitis).
4. Patient can describe measures to increase perfusion of lower extremities.
5. Patient can describe measures to prevent recurrences.

Implementation

ASSISTING WITH ACHIEVEMENT OF THERAPEUTIC GOALS

Acute care for thrombophlebitis

Bed rest is prescribed during the acute phase for *deep vein thrombosis.* The affected extremity is elevated periodically above heart level to prevent venous stasis and to reduce edema. Specific activity orders are dependent on physician preferences. When the patient begins to ambulate, elastic stockings or an elastic bandage is used to compress the superficial veins, increase blood flow through the deep veins, and prevent venous stasis. Anticoagulants are routinely given (p. 836), and vasodilators or fibrinolytics may also be prescribed.

Superficial thrombophlebitis is usually treated by rest; however, physicians differ in regard to the amount. Some physicians believe that complete immobilization is necessary to prevent emboli formation; others believe that clots are sufficiently adherent to vein walls and that mobility improves general circulation and prevents further venous stasis. Antiinflammatory drugs may be prescribed.

Surgery
Thrombophlebitis

Surgical intervention for venous thrombosis is indicated only when other conservative measures are unsuccessful. If the thrombosis is recurrent and extensive or if the patient is at high risk for pulmonary embolism, surgery may be necessary. A thrombectomy or a vena caval interruption

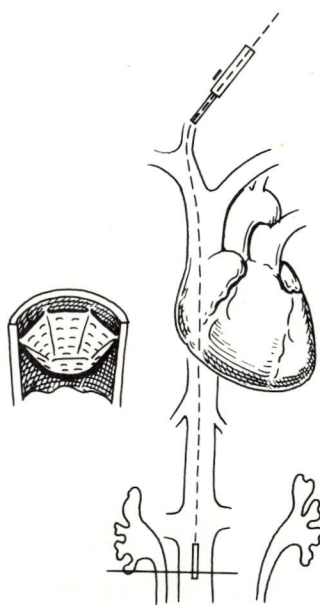

Fig. 26-15 Transvenous method of vena cava interruption using caval prosthesis of umbrella design. Insert illustrates open umbrella. (Redrawn from Fairbairn, JF, Jergens, JL, and Spittell, JA: Peripheral vascular disease, Philadelphia, 1972, WB Saunders Co.)

> **Nursing care of the patient who has undergone venous surgery**
>
> 1. Monitor for signs of bleeding, especially on first postoperative day; if incisional bleeding occurs, elevate the leg, apply pressure over the wound, and notify the surgeon.
> 2. Assist patient to ambulate as soon as permitted and elevate patient's leg when sitting to prevent venous stasis.
> 3. Check elastic bandage several times a day to maintain even pressure on leg veins.
> 4. Give analgesics as necessary for pain and discomfort.

may be performed. Vena caval interruption consists of transvenous placement of a grid or umbrella in the vena cava to block the passage of emboli (Fig. 26-15).

Preoperative care includes monitoring peripheral pulses and signs of bleeding from anticoagulant therapy and pulmonary emboli (for instance, sudden chest pain and cough). Postoperative nursing care is described in the box above.

Varicose veins

Surgical treatment for varicosities consists of ligation of the vein above the varicosity and removal of the varicosed vein distal to the ligation, provided the deep veins are able to return the venous blood satisfactorily (Fig. 26-16). The great saphenous vein is ligated close to the femoral junction if possible, and the great and small saphenous veins are then stripped out through small incisions at the groin, above and below the knee, and at the ankle. Sterile dressings are placed over the incisions, and an elastic bandage extending from the foot to the groin is applied firmly. Postoperative care is described in the box above. Postoperatively the patient should know that varicose veins may recur; large superficial collateral vessels may develop and in turn become varicosed.

ASSISTING WITH COMFORT

Analgesics reduce pain and discomfort in the person with acute thrombophlebitis. Antiinflammatory medication decreases the inflammation, thereby contributing to increased comfort. Warm moist heat, heating pads, or ice packs may be prescribed to enhance resolution of the inflammation.

COUNSELING AND TEACHING

The major emphasis of nursing interventions for the person with a chronic venous disorder is patient teaching. Important topics for teaching are measures to increase

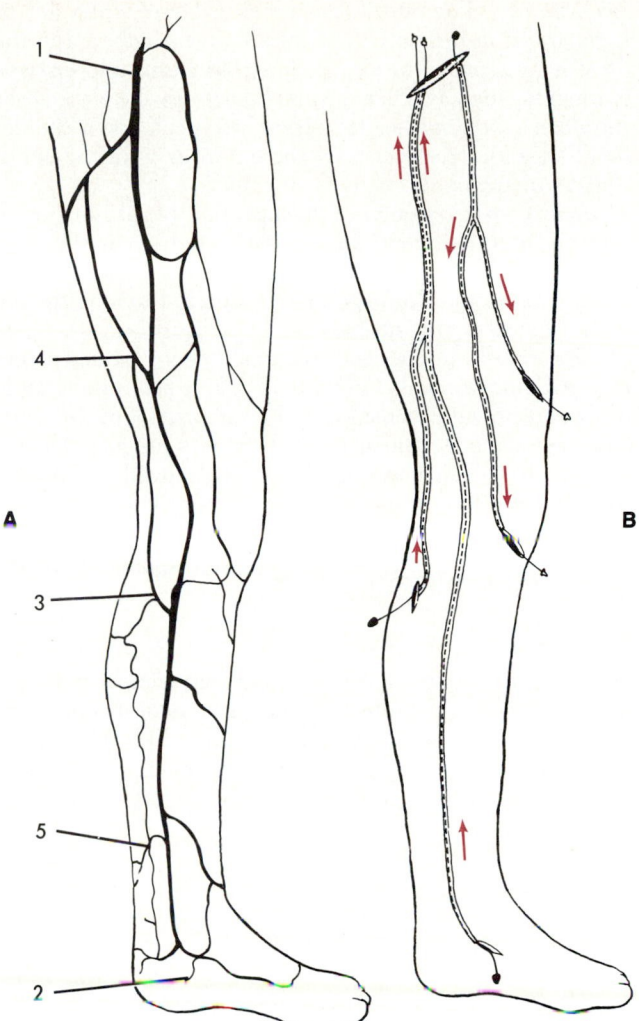

Fig. 26-16   A, Outline of incompetent great saphenous system, with numerals indicating main tributaries. **B,** Passing of strippers in preparation for removal of incompetent veins.

tissue perfusion by preventing venous stasis (and thereby preventing pain) and measures to prevent recurrences.
1. Prevention of venous stasis
   a. Avoid prolonged sitting or standing.
   b. Elevate legs when sitting.
   c. Avoid crossing the legs at the knee.
   d. Wear elastic stockings (see the box above).
   e. Avoid constriction on leg veins by tight bands (socks and garters).
   f. Carry out daily exercises and physical activity (for instance, promotion of blood flow by contraction of leg muscles).
      1. Practice dorsiflexion of both feet while sitting or lying down.
      2. Walk daily; increase distance as tolerated.
      3. Swim several times weekly if possible.
      4. Use stationary bicycle.

Teaching the use of elastic stockings

1. Use correct size (see instructions on box or consult medical supply person) and length (to knee or groin) as prescribed.
2. Apply stocking before getting out of bed.
3. For ease of application, turn foot of stocking inside out, slide foot into stocking, and pull stocking over leg.
4. Remove stocking at bedtime if desired; if leg aches at night, stocking may be of benefit if worn in bed.
5. Keep a second stocking on hand for use when the other is being laundered.

---

2. Prevent recurrence
   a. Maintain desired weight for height.
   b. Modify life-style (both at work and at home) as necessary to prevent long periods of standing or sitting.
   c. Follow activity program as described above.
   d. Take special precautions if pregnant (because extra pressure is placed on veins) or for any surgical procedure (especially pelvic surgery).

⊞ Evaluation

Questions to ask may include the following:
1. Is patient comfortable?
2. Can patient describe:
   a. Rationale for activity requirements?
   b. Measures to promote venous return and prevent recurrence of the disorder?

■ LEG ULCERS

■ Pathophysiology

A leg ulcer is an open necrotic lesion that results from inadequate exchange of oxygen and other nutrients within the vascular system. The majority of ulcers arise from chronic venous insufficiency caused by deep vein thrombosis or varicose veins. Less frequently, they develop from arterial insufficiency. Other causes include burns, leg traumas, and neurogenic disorders. Persons with diabetes are at high risk for development of leg ulcers because of vascular insufficiency.

Clinical signs vary, depending on the underlying problem. A *venous ulcer* is usually moderately painful and located on the medial aspect of the ankle. Edema and pigmentation are common around the area of ulceration. Most venous ulcers heal with therapy. An *arterial ulcer* causes more pain and has a more necrotic, pale gray base; it frequently develops on the heel, lateral malleolus, toes, and dorsum of the foot. Edema is infrequent, and peripheral pulses are diminished or absent.

Assessment

■ SUBJECTIVE DATA

1. Onset and duration of symptoms
2. Extent and characteristics of pain
3. Limitations in mobility and activity
4. History of deep vein thrombosis, varicose veins, arterial insufficiency, or diabetes

■ OBJECTIVE DATA

1. Appearance and temperature of the skin
2. Location and appearance of the ulcer
3. Presence and quality of all peripheral pulses
4. Presence of edema

Data analysis: nursing diagnoses

Nursing diagnoses are determined from the assessment of patient data. Possible nursing diagnoses for the person with leg ulcers may include, but are not limited to, the following:

Diagnostic title	Possible etiologies
Potential for infection	Lack of knowledge: decreased circulation
Knowledge deficit: ulcer care, prevention	Lack of exposure/recall, information misinterpretation
Pain: ulcer	Inflammation, necrosis
Altered peripheral tissue perfusion	Decreased blood flow (arterial or venous)

Planning: expected patient outcomes

Expected patient outcomes for the person with leg ulcers may include, but are not limited to, the following:
1. Ulcer shows signs of healing and absence of further breakdown.
2. Patient participates in ADL without discomfort or pain.
3. Patient can describe measures to prevent infection.
4. Patient can describe care of the ulcer.
5. Patient can describe measures to increase tissue perfusion.

Implementation

■ ASSISTING WITH ACHIEVEMENT OF THERAPEUTIC GOALS

□ Promotion of healing

The primary goal in treating leg ulcers is to promote wound healing and prevent infection. Necrotic tissue is debrided by mechanical, chemical, or surgical means. A wet-to-dry dressing may be applied to debride the wound

mechanically. The dressing is applied damp; when dry, it is removed, pulling off the debris that has adhered to the dressing. *Chemical* beads, such as Debrisan, and enzyme ointments, such as fibrinolysins (Elase), may be placed over the ulcer (avoiding healthy tissue) to break down the debris. Necrotic tissue can also be cut away with the aid of *surgical* instruments, usually a scalpel.

Topical and systemic *antibiotics* may be prescribed to prevent infection. Systemic antibiotic therapy is the most effective route in the treatment of leg ulcers. Periodic culture of wound drainage may be ordered to monitor the effectiveness of the antibiotics.

A *boot* may be applied to cover small, newly formed ulcers in ambulatory persons (Fig. 26-17). This boot protects the ulcer and provides constant and even support to the area. The boot is made from a special type of impregnated gauze (Unna paste) that hardens after it is wrapped around the patient's leg. The Unna boot is generally left on for 1 to 2 weeks, although it may be changed more often if there is copious drainage. Elastic bandages are applied to the leg after the ulcer has healed.

□ Surgery

Recurrent venous ulcers and nonhealing arterial ulcers may require surgical intervention. Ligation of incompetent veins may be necessary. Arterial bypass and reconstruction can be used to revascularize the artery and restore circulation (p. 838). Amputation may be required if less aggressive means are unsuccessful.

■ ASSISTING WITH COMFORT

The nurse can assist the patient in promoting comfort by doing the following:
1. Encourage the use of prescribed analgesics and antiinflammatory medication to reduce pain and inflammation.
2. Maintain proper body positioning to improve circulation by gravity.
   a. Elevate head of bed on 3- to 6-inch blocks for an arterial ulcer.
   b. Elevate lower extremities to decrease edema for a venous ulcer.
3. Use overbed cradle to protect leg from pressure of bed linens.
4. Remove obstacles from pathway if patient is ambulatory.
5. Use cotton between toes to prevent pressure on toe ulcer.
6. Medicate for pain 20 to 30 minutes before a dressing change.

■ COUNSELING AND TEACHING

Teaching includes prevention of infection, maintenance of skin integrity, and measures to increase peripheral tissue perfusion. The areas are outlined in the text under teaching for arterial and venous disorders (pp. 836 and 851). The patient is also taught how to change his or her own dressings, as appropriate.

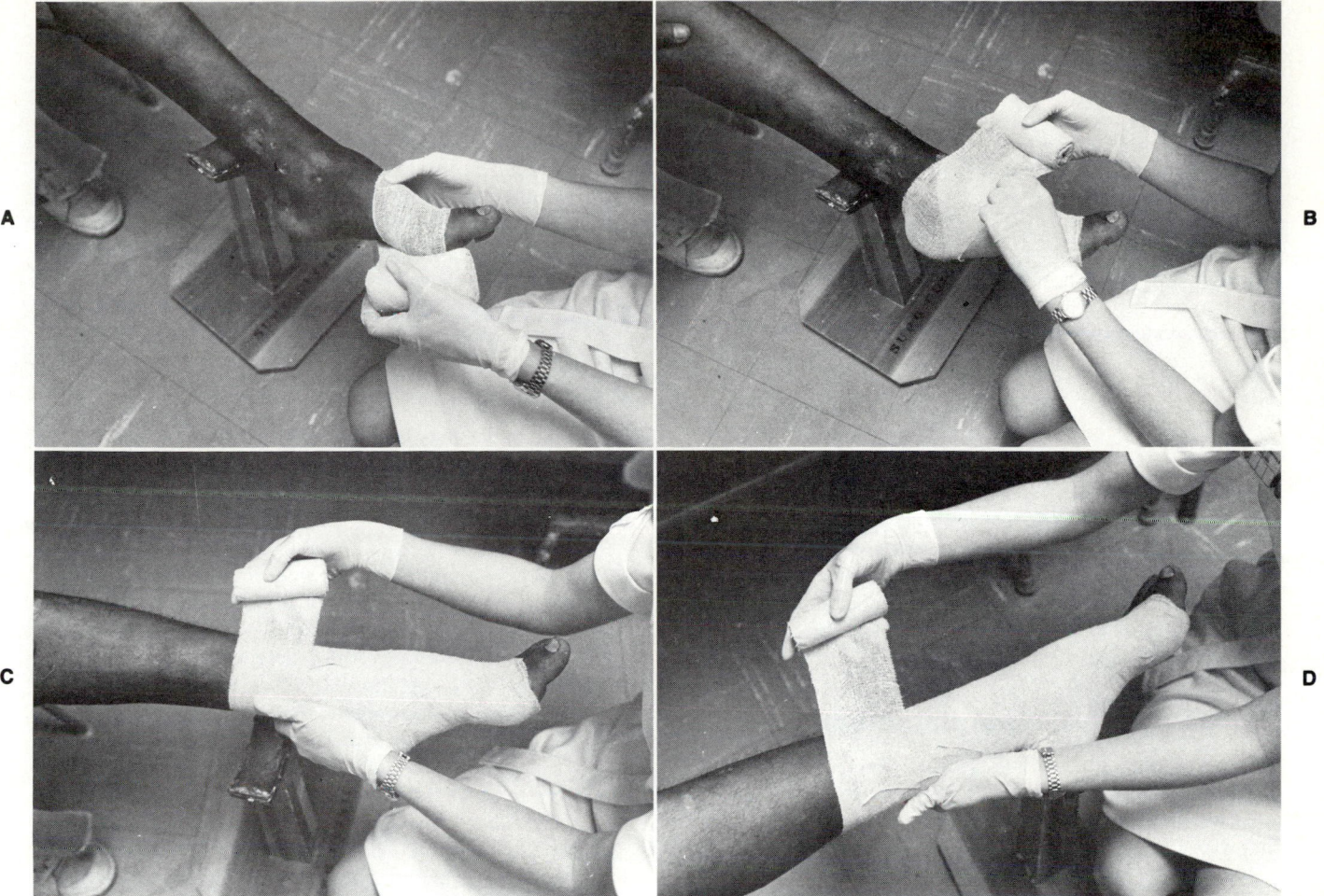

Fig. 26-17   Nurse applying Unna paste boot using specially impregnated gauze. Note ulcers on inferior aspect of patient's foot.

✚ Evaluation

Questions to ask may include the following:
1. Is the patient able to participate in ADL without pain?
2. Can the patient change the ulcer dressing correctly?
3. Can the patient describe measures to prevent infection and to increase tissue perfusion?

■ LYMPHEDEMA

■ Pathophysiology

Lymphedema is the chronic swelling of a part as a result of the collection of interstitial fluid secondary to an obstruction of the lymphatic vessels or lymph nodes. It may be primary (congenital or developing at puberty as a result of hypoplastic development of lymph vessels), or it may be secondary (see the box on p. 854).

Lymphedema of the lower extremities begins with mild swelling on the dorsum of the foot, usually at the end of the day, and gradually extends to involve the entire limb. The condition is aggravated by prolonged standing, pregnancy, obesity, warm weather, or menstruation.

🖳 Assessment

■ DATA COLLECTION

Subjective data include the following:
1. Onset of swelling in the affected extremity
2. History of secondary causes of lymphedema (see the box on p. 854)
3. Effectiveness of current therapy to reduce edema

Objective data include the following:
1. Observation of extremities for edema: unilateral, initially soft, and pitting, then progressing to firm, rubbery, and nonpitting
2. Comparison in size of extremities
3. Quality of peripheral pulses

Causes of secondary lymphedema

Obstruction
  Malignant tumors
  Postsurgical removal of lymph nodes
  Mechanical trauma
  Postirradiation
Inflammation
Infection (parasitic)

■ DIAGNOSTIC TESTS

Lymphangiography is the injection of a radiopaque contrast medium directly into the lymphatic vessels. This technique may be helpful in detecting the degree of lymph node involvement. An x-ray examination is made after the injection and at 24 hours. Periodic x-ray examinations can be made for up to 6 months because the dye remains in the lymph system.

➡ Data analysis: nursing diagnoses

Nursing diagnoses are determined from the assessment of patient data. Possible nursing diagnoses for the person with lymphedema may include, but are not limited to, the following:

Diagnostic title	Possible etiologies
Body image disturbance	Change in body appearance
Potential for infection	Decreased lymph drainage
Knowledge deficit	Lack of information/recall, information misinterpretation

▣ Planning: expected patient outcomes

Expected patient outcomes for the person with lymphedema may include, but are not limited to, the following:
1. Patient expresses confidence in self, despite change in appearance of extremity.
2. Patient can describe measures that will decrease infection, maintain intact skin, and improve lymph drainage.

▦ Implementation

■ ASSISTING WITH ACHIEVEMENT OF THERAPEUTIC GOALS

Therapy for lymphedema is conservative. The goal is to reduce edema and to maintain skin integrity. Therapy includes the following:

1. Passive and active exercises
2. Elevation of affected extremity
3. Elastic stocking to reduce edema of leg
4. Restriction of dietary sodium to reduce fluid retention and thereby decrease edema
5. Diuretic therapy to temporarily decrease limb size by decreasing total body fluid
6. Long-term antibiotic therapy to control recurrent cellulitis and infection

Most patients respond to conservative medical therapy and do not require surgical intervention. If indicated, surgery consists of removal of the edematous lymph tissues or reconstruction of the lymphatic drainage channels.

■ COUNSELING AND TEACHING

Lymphedema may cause a limb to become excessively large, which greatly alters the patient's appearance. Although the limb can be covered by clothing, the size cannot be hidden (except with a long skirt for women). The change in appearance can lead to a poor self-concept. The patient should be given opportunities to express feelings and encouragement to follow through on measures to decrease some of the edema. Positive attributes are emphasized. Patient teaching includes the following:
1. Take antibiotics as prescribed to prevent infection.
2. Take measures to promote skin integrity.
  a. Monitor skin for intactness, swelling, redness, and lesions.
  b. Seek medical assistance if skin changes occur.
3. Take measures to improve lymph drainage and decrease edema.
  a. Elevate affected extremity above level of heart.
  b. Elevate affected extremity when sitting.
  c. Avoid prolonged standing.
  d. Sleep with foot of bed elevated 4 to 8 inches.
  e. Massage affected extremity in direction of lymph flow.
  f. Wear elastic stockings.
  g. Avoid constrictive clothing.
  h. Exercise on a regular basis.
  i. Take diuretics as prescribed.
  j. Avoid excess intake of foods high in sodium.

✠ Evaluation

Questions to ask may include the following:
1. Does patient take antibiotics as prescribed?
2. Is patient able to discuss feelings about altered appearance of the extremity?
3. Does patient take measures to promote skin integrity and improve lymph drainage?

■ HYPERTENSION

Hypertension is often considered in conjunction with peripheral vascular disorders for several reasons. Both are disorders of the circulation; some of the same factors are

Table 26-4 Hypertension

Etiology	Signs and symptoms	Therapy

Primary (essential)
Risk factors
 	
Positive family history
Abnormal sodium retention and water retention
Sensitivity to the renin-angiotensin system, which regulates both vasoconstriction and sodium retention
Obesity
Hypercholesteremia and increased serum triglycerides
Smoking
Continuous emotional disturbances
 	
Secondary hypertension
 	
Coarctation of the aorta
Adrenal gland: pheochromocytoma, a catecholamine-secreting tumor; Cushing's disease
Kidney disease; chronic glomerulonephritis (most common known cause)
Toxemia of pregnancy
Thyrotoxicosis
Increased intracranial pressure from tumors or trauma
Collagen diseases
Secondary to the effects of certain drugs such as oral contraceptives
	In the early stages, hypertension is essentially asymptomatic. When symptoms do occur, they include:
	1. Headache: occipital and commonly present in the early morning
	2. Vertigo and flushed face
	3. Spontaneous epistaxis
	4. Blurring of vision or scotomas with retinal changes
	5. Nocturnal frequency caused by increased pressure and not by renal disorder
	6. Eventually as consequence of prolonged hypertension:
	  a. Coronary insufficiency and occlusion
	  b. Congestive heart failure
	  c. Renal failure
	  d. Cerebrovascular accident (stroke)
		Antihypertensive drugs (Table 26-6)
		Nutrition:
		1. Reduce caloric intake as necessary
		2. Reduce salt intake
		Weight control
		Exercise program

involved; and hypertension is a major risk factor in atherosclerosis, the largest cause of peripheral vascular disease.

Hypertension is generally considered to be present when a patient's *diastolic pressure* is consistently over 90 mm Hg. The World Health Organization (WHO) criteria for hypertension is blood pressures exceeding 160 mm Hg systolic and 95 mm Hg diastolic.[29] Hypertension may be *primary*, or it may be *secondary* to other conditions (Table 26-4). About 90% of hypertension is primary essential hypertension (having no known cause).

■ Prevention and health education

It is estimated that almost 60 million persons in the United States have elevated blood pressure requiring systematic monitoring or treatment.[42] Many of these persons are either unaware they have hypertension because of lack of symptoms or are not pursuing active treatment.

Hypertension is a major cause of cardiovascular disease (coronary artery disease and cardiac failure), strokes, and renal failure. *Primary prevention* for hypertension includes reducing factors that contribute to the development of hypertension (see Table 26-4).

Health education, therefore, includes teaching all persons to avoid excess sodium and saturated fats in their diet, maintain appropriate body weight, avoid smoking, and learn to cope effectively with stressors.

The major thrust of public health programs for hypertension is on *secondary prevention;* that is, identifying and controlling blood pressure elevations in high-risk persons, especially blacks (primarily young males), obese persons, and blood relatives of individuals with hypertension. Low-income persons are less likely to know they have hypertension because economic factors make them less likely to seek medical care. It is sometimes difficult to convince people to seek medical care for elevated blood pressure when they "feel good."

Some mass screenings for hypertension are conducted in places (such as malls or large-scale gatherings) where the environmental conditions contribute to inaccurate readings of blood pressure levels. In addition, some mass screenings are repeated in special centers that are frequented by the same people, often elderly persons looking for a social outlet. These types of screenings are not very cost effective. The present emphasis in organizing mass screenings, therefore, is on sites that include larger numbers of high-risk persons and better environmental con-

Table 26-5 Recommendations for follow-up of blood pressure findings

Range (mm Hg)	Recommended follow-up
Diastolic	
<85	Recheck within 2 years
85 to 89	Recheck within 1 year
90 to 104	Confirm within 2 months, then refer promptly to source of care
105 to 114	Evaluate or refer promptly to source of care within 2 weeks
≥115	Evaluate or refer immediately to a source of care
Systolic (when diastolic BP is <90)	
<140	Recheck within 2 years
140 to 199	Confirm within 2 months, then refer promptly to source of care
≥200	Evaluate or refer to source of care within 2 weeks

From US Department of Health and Human Services: The 1984 report of the Joint National Committee on Detection, Evaluation and Treatment of High Blood Pressure, NIH no 84-1088, Washington, DC, 1984, The Department.

ditions. Nurses can make important contributions to hypertension control by participating in screening and education programs. Table 26-5 gives recommended steps in the screening process.

■ Pathophysiology

Blood pressure is determined by two factors: flow and resistance. Blood flow is in turn determined by cardiac output (strength, rate, rhythm of heart beat, and blood volume [see Chapter 25]). The resistance to flow is primarily determined by the diameter of blood vessels and, to a lesser degree, by the viscosity of the blood. Increased peripheral resistance as a result of narrowing of the arterioles is the most common characteristic in hypertension.

Dilation and constriction of peripheral arterioles may be controlled by several mechanisms, particularly sympathetic nervous system stimulation and activation of the renin-angiotensin system. *Stimulation of the sympathetic nervous system* (such as by stressors) causes release of norepinephrine and epinephrine. Norepinephrine constricts blood vessels and increases peripheral resistance. Epinephrine increases the force of cardiac contractions while narrowing the passageway, causing the blood pressure to increase.

Renal regulation is an essential component of blood pressure control. Fig. 26-18 illustrates the normal steps in the *renin-angiotensin* system. Note that the action of angiotensin II is both vasoconstriction and sodium and water retention. Thus there is increased fluid in a smaller vascular system, causing the blood pressure to increase.

Age is a major factor in primary hypertension. Arterial

blood pressure rises gradually throughout a person's life span. After the age of 60, peripheral vascular resistance increases at about 1% per year. What constitutes normal blood pressure for the aged and what should be considered hypertension in the elderly continues to be debated. However, there is general agreement that, regardless of age, the higher the systolic or diastolic pressure the higher the morbidity and mortality.

■ COMPLICATIONS

With prolonged hypertension the elastic tissue in arterioles is replaced by fibrous collagen tissue. The thickened arteriole wall then becomes less distensible, offering even greater resistance to the flow of blood. The left ventricle must exert more force to empty completely; it becomes more distended as it fails to eject a normal stroke volume, and the muscle fibers stretch (hypertrophy) in an attempt to increase the strength of contraction. Inadequate blood supply through the coronary arteries may cause *angina pectoris*, or a *myocardial infarction* may occur. Eventually, the hypertrophy of the left ventricle results in *congestive heart failure*.

Outside the heart itself, the changes in the arteriolar walls may result in permanent damage to organs. The kidney is especially susceptible, and when fibrinoid necrosis occurs in the afferent arteriole, the glomerulus is deprived of its blood supply; permanent kidney damage and possible *renal failure* result. *Cerebral vessels* are also frequently affected; neurologic changes or frank *stroke* may result either from hemorrhage from a leaky vessel or from thrombosis.

Malignant hypertension refers to hypertension that is severe and rapidly progressive. It is most common in black men under age 40. Unless medical treatment is successful, the course is rapidly fatal, and most persons die within 2 years. Death is secondary to the changes that occur in the kidney, heart, or brain, and the patient dies from uremia, myocardial infarction, congestive heart failure, or cerebrovascular accident.

▥ Assessment

■ DATA COLLECTION

For the person with hypertension, subjective data are collected about the presence of any symptoms and the patient's knowledge of hypertension. Subjective data include the following:

1. History of headache, vertigo, flushed face, spontaneous epistaxis, or blurring of vision: onset and frequency
2. Weight changes
3. Dietary habits, especially intake of salt and saturated fats
4. Work and life stressors

Objective data consist of at least three blood pressure readings at approximately 5-minute intervals to determine a baseline average. The readings are preferably taken with

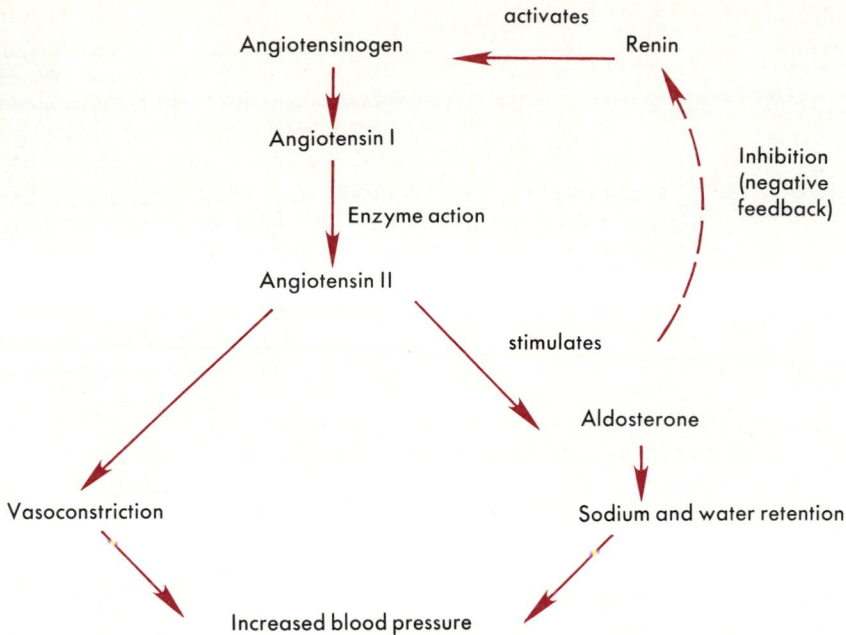

Fig. 26-18   Effect of renin-angiotensin system on blood pressure.

the person supine after a short rest period, to minimize the effects of exercise and stress.

■ DIAGNOSTIC TESTS

Diagnostic tests that may be performed when hypertension is present include the following:
1. Urinalysis, CBC, and serum electrolytes to determine severity of vascular disease and possible causes of hypertension
2. Chest x-ray examination to show cardiac size and pulmonary vasculature
3. ECG for cardiac function
4. Pheochromocytoma: urinary test for catecholamines
5. Cushing's syndrome urine test: 17 ketosteroids and serum corticoids

Data analysis: nursing diagnoses

Nursing diagnoses are determined from the assessment of patient data. Possible nursing diagnoses for the person with hypertension include, but are not limited to, the following:

Diagnostic title	Possible etiologies
Knowledge deficit	Lack of exposure/recall, information misinterpretation
Noncompliance: medications and ongoing medical care	Patient value systems, lack of knowledge, treatment side effects

Planning: expected patient outcomes

Expected patient outcomes for the person with hypertension may include, but are not limited to, the following:
1. Patient can describe the nature of hypertension.
2. Patient can demonstrate ability to take blood pressure measurement correctly, if applicable.
3. Patient can describe medication and treatment program.
4. Patient can explain dietary modification, including salt, cholesterol, and calorie restrictions as applicable.
5. Patient can describe plans for a regular exercise program.
6. Patient can define personal stress factors and ways to cope with them.
7. Patient can explain health maintenance program: stating symptoms that require immediate medical attention and plans for follow-up care with professionals.

Implementation

■ ASSISTING WITH ACHIEVEMENT OF THERAPEUTIC GOALS

Drug therapy is currently the only successful means of treating hypertension, with the exception of hypertension secondary to a cause such as coarctation of the aorta, in which surgery is the immediate recourse. Important drugs used for the control of hypertension are summarized

Table 26-6 Oral drugs used for treatment of hypertension

Drug	Action	Effects
Diuretics		
Thiazides		
Hydrochlorothiazide (Esidrix, Hydrodiuril) Chlorothiazide (Diuril) Quinethazone (Hydromox) Chlorthalidone (Hygroton)	Blocks sodium reabsorption in cortical portion of ascending tubule; water excreted with sodium, producing decreased blood volume. *Note:* thiazides ineffective in renal failure	Electrolytes changes: ↑ BUN, ↑ uric acid, ↓ potassium, ↑ blood glucose, ↑ calcium Potassium supplement suggested Possible postural hypotension in summer caused by sodium loss GI upset, dry mouth, thirst, weakness, muscle aches, fatigue, tachycardia
Loop diuretics		
Furosemide (Lasix) Ethacrynic acid (Edecrin)	Blocks sodium and water reabsorption in medullary portion of ascending tubule	Profound diuresis caused by rapid volume depletion Electrolyte depletion Thirst, skin rash, postural hypotension, nausea, vomiting
Potassium sparing agents		
Spironolactone (Aldactone) Triamterene (Dyrenium)	Inhibits aldosterone Sodium is excreted in exchange for potassium	Drowsiness, confusion Diarrhea—give drug after meals Hyperkalemia Gynecomastia with Aldactone
Drugs acting on CNS		
Adrenergic inhibitors (peripheral acting)		
Rauwolfia alkaloids Reserpine Guanethidine (Ismelin)	Depletion of catecholamines in sympathetic postganglionic fibers Blocks norepinephrine release from adrenergic nerve endings	Drowsiness, lethargy, depression—report manifestations Nasal congestion, gastric hyperactivity Caution about severe orthostatic hypotension Diarrhea and nausea Counsel about sexual dysfunction—impotence or loss of ejaculation
Adrenergic inhibitors (central acting)		
Methyldopa (Aldomet) Clonidine (Catapres)	Sympathetic nervous system activity decreased by displacing norepinephrine from receptor sites	Drowsiness, lassitude, mild orthostatic hypotension, positive Coomb's test, impotence Rebound hypertension with abrupt discontinuance of clonidine
Beta blockers		
Propranolol (Inderal) Metoprolol (Lopressor) Nadolol (Corgard) Atenolol (Tenormin)	Blocks β-adrenergic receptors of sympathetic nervous system, decreasing heart rate and blood pressure	Bradycardia, fatigue, insomnia, bizarre dreams, sexual dysfunction, occasional nausea, vomiting, and epigastric distress
Vasodilators		
Hydralizine (Apresoline)	Peripheral vasodilator that directly relaxes vascular smooth muscle	Headaches, tachycardia, nausea, vomiting, palpitations, fatigue, lupus syndrome—rare, occurs in high doses and prolonged therapy
Prazosin (Minipress)	Same as above, also may block post-synaptic α-adrenergic receptors	Warn patient of "first dose" syncope, orthostatic hypotension weakness, palpitations
Minoxidil (Loniten)	Peripheral vasodilation	Bloating, peripheral edema, rapid weight gain Fast or irregular heartbeat
Captopril (Capoten)	Reduces peripheral arterial resistance	Skin rash, dizziness, angioedema Fast or irregular heartbeat

in Table 26-6. A major therapeutic approach is to start with small doses of less potent drugs and then progress through the following steps until blood pressure control is reached.[45] The regimen is maintained at whatever step achieves control.

Step 1: Begin with less than a full dose of either a thiazide-type diuretic or a beta blocker.

Step 2: Add a small dose of either an adrenergic inhibiting agent or a thiazide-type diuretic; proceed to full dose if necessary; substitute other drugs as necessary.

Step 3: Add a vasodilator.

Step 4: Add guanethidine.

■ COUNSELING AND TEACHING

The major nursing strategy for the person with hypertension is counseling and teaching. The person is assisted in identifying possible daily stressors that could be decreased or avoided and to explore optional ways to cope with stress (see Chapter 7). Patient teaching is directed toward learning about hypertension, ways to decrease risk factors, and treatment programs, such as the following:

1. Nature of hypertension
   a. Meaning of systolic and diastolic blood pressures
   b. Effect on body of continued hypertension
2. Medication regimen:
   a. Dosage, frequency, and side effects
   b. Postural hypotension: causes and action to take (for instance, lie down with feet higher than head)
   c. Moderation in alcohol consumption which may potentiate effect of some antihypertensive drugs
   d. Reasons for continuing with prescribed drugs even though symptom free
3. Method of measuring blood pressure levels: whenever possible, the patient or a family member learns to measure blood pressure levels and to keep a record
4. Program of regular physical exercise, which increases cardiac output and decreases peripheral resistance

5. Diet: avoid adding salt to foods at table; avoid highly salted foods such as peanuts, potato chips, and hot dogs; limit "fast foods"; reduce saturated fats to minimize risk of cardiovascular disease
6. Effect of smoking on cardiovascular system (Chapter 25)
7. Need for follow-up care by professionals

♯ Evaluation

Questions to ask may include the following:
1. Is the patient keeping blood pressure level within "normal" range by taking medication and by maintaining dietary and exercise therapy?
2. Can the patient describe the nature of hypertension?
3. Can the patient or a significant other accurately measure blood pressure levels?
4. Is the patient coping effectively with life stressors?
5. Does the patient follow through with health supervision by professionals?

■ SUMMARY

1. Risk factors associated with the development of peripheral vascular disorders include cigarette smoking, hyperlipidemia, hypertension, obesity, physical inactivity, emotional stress, diabetes mellitus, and a family history of atherosclerosis.
2. Primary prevention through health education about risk factors is the most important means to reduce the incidence of peripheral vascular disorders.
3. Arterial disorders occur when any disturbance in the structure of the arteries causes diminished blood flow and decreased oxygen and nutrients to the tissues.
4. The symptoms of arterial disorders are not caused by the degree of obstruction but by the extent to which the involved body part is deprived of circulation.
5. Medical therapy for patients with atherosclerosis include: smoking cessation; low-fat, low-cholesterol diet; weight reduction; regular exercise; control of associ-

---

Putting knowledge to practice

■ Explain the physiologic basis for the difference in leg positioning for arterial and venous disorders.

■ Compare the similarities and differences in patient teaching for persons with arterial and venous disorders.

■ Examine the chart of a patient with an arterial disorder: What diagnostic tests were done and how would you explain these tests to a patient? What specific teaching is indicated for the patient? Is there notation of patient teaching on the chart?

■ Practice application of a stump bandage using an elastic bandage applied over another person's fist.

■ Practice teaching a person how to use crutches (review technique in a fundamentals of nursing text).

■ Observe a screening program for hypertension: What was the patient population? Did it include persons at high risk for hypertension? Did the clients ask any questions pertaining to hypertension? What patient teaching did the nurses initiate?

ated diseases (for example, diabetes and hypertension); and control of emotional stress.

6. Intermittent claudication is a symptom of arterial disorders. This term is used to describe a cramplike muscle pain that develops during exercise and is relieved after 1 to 2 minutes after stopping the exercise. It is usually unilateral and primarily affects the calf muscles.

7. Peripheral pulses may be absent or diminished in patients with arterial disorders.

8. Anticoagulants such as heparin and warfarin sodium (Coumadin) prolong clotting time, prevent extension of an existing clot, and inhibit further clot formation. Anticoagulants do not dissolve existing clots.

9. An important area to include in teaching a patient receiving Coumadin is the prevention of bleeding.

10. Protamine sulfate is a heparin antagonist, and vitamin K counteracts the effects of Coumadin.

11. Fibrinolytics such as streptokinase and urokinase dissolve existing thrombi.

12. Important nursing interventions for the patient undergoing arterial bypass surgery include: frequent assessment of peripheral pulses and the graft site, avoiding flexion in the area of the graft, and position changes to promote circulation.

13. Positioning a patient with an arterial disorder may include placement of the extremity flat in bed or in a slightly dependent (that is, 15 degree) position to promote circulation. Elevation is contraindicated in arterial disorders.

14. An important nursing intervention for the patient undergoing amputation surgery is to avoid flexion at the hip or knee to prevent contractures.

15. A teaching plan for a patient with arterial problems includes measures to prevent infection and injury, interventions to maintain skin integrity and to increase peripheral tissue perfusion, and methods to alter risk factors.

16. Thrombophlebitis can affect the superficial or deep veins. Thrombophlebitis in a deep vein can lead to a pulmonary embolus.

17. Deep vein thrombosis is treated by bed rest with periodic elevation of the affected extremity above heart level to prevent venous stasis and reduce edema.

18. Patients with chronic venous disorders such as varicose veins should be taught measures to increase perfusion. These include avoiding constrictive clothing, crossing legs at the knee, and long periods of sitting or standing, elevating legs when sitting, wearing elastic stockings, and using good posture.

19. Leg ulcers can develop secondary to arterial or venous disorders. The primary goal in treating these ulcers is to promote wound healing and to prevent infection.

20. Wet-to-dry dressings and debriding chemicals remove necrotic tissue from leg ulcers. A special protective boot (Unna paste boot) may be applied over ulcers for ambulatory patients. Arterial bypass surgery or amputation may be necessary for nonhealing chronic ulcers.

21. Lymphedema results from interference with the drainage of interstitial fluid from the tissues; the affected part becomes greatly edematous.

22. Counseling and teaching the patient with lymphedema includes elevation of the affected extremity, wearing elastic stockings, taking diuretics as ordered, and avoiding an excess intake of foods high in sodium.

23. Hypertension is generally considered to be present when blood pressure levels persistently exceed 140/90. Most hypertension is idiopathic. It is a major cause of coronary artery disease, cardiac failure, strokes, and renal failure.

24. Drugs to control hypertension include diuretics (especially thiazides), peripheral and central acting adrenergics, beta blockers, and vasodilators. Medications are added in steps, as necessary, to control the blood pressure within normal limits.

25. Persons with hypertension should monitor their own blood pressure, continue prescribed medication, exercise, avoid salty foods, stop smoking, and continue with follow-up health care.

REFERENCES AND SELECTED READINGS
Contemporary

1. *Baum, PL: Heed the early warning signs of peripheral vascular disease, Nurs 85 15:50-57, 1985.

2. Bartucci, MR, and others: Factors associated with adherence in hypertensive patients, ANNAJ 14:245-248, 1987.

3. *Beaver, BN: Health education and the patient with peripheral vascular disease, Nurs Clin North Am 21:265-272, 1986.

4. Cahill, M, and others: Cardiovascular system. In Diagnostics: the nurses reference library, Springhouse, Pa, 1981, Intermed Communications, Inc.

5. *Cornwall, JV: Guidelines to leg ulcer care, Nurs 83 13:37-39, 1983.

6. Crockett, F: Varicose veins as a cause of venous ulceration, Pract Cardiol 11:191-199, 1985.

7. Creager, MA: Preventing and treating deep-vein thrombophlebitis, Drug Ther 15:16-25, 1985.

8. Cunningham, SG: Nonpharmacologic management of high blood pressure, J Cardiovasc Nurs 23(4):18-22, 1987.

9. Dixon, MB, and others: Arterial reconstruction for atherosclerotic occlusive disease, J Cardiovasc Nurs 1(2):36-49, 1987.

10. *Doyle, JE: All leg ulcers are not alike: managing and preventing arterial and venous ulcers, Nurs 83 13:58-63, 1983.

11. *Doyle, JE: Treatment modalities in peripheral vascular disease, Nurs Clin North Am 21:241-253, 1986.

*References preceded by an asterisk are particularly well suited for student reading.

12. *Ekers, MA: Psychosocial considerations in peripheral vascular disease: cause or effect? Nurs Clin North Am 21:255-263, 1986.

13. *Fahey, VA: An in-depth look at deep vein thrombosis, Nurs 84 14:34-41, 1984.

14. Falotico, JB: Pulmonary embolisms, Crit Care Update 8:5-15, 1981.

15. *Finnerty, FA, Jr: Treatment of hypertensive emergencies, Heart Lung 10:275-284, 1981.

16. *Ford, RD, and others: Cardiovascular disorders, Springhouse, Pa, 1984, Springhouse Corporation.

17. *Foreman, MD: Arterial prosthetic graft infections: the pathophysiologic basis of nursing care, Focus Crit Care 12:23-28, 1985.

18. *Frank-Stromberg, M, and Stromberg, P: Test your knowledge of managing the patient with hypertension, Nurs 81 11:56-59, 1981.

19. *Galli, M: Promoting self-care in hypertensive clients through patient education, Home Health Care Nurse 2:43-45, 1984.

20. *Gerdes, L: Recognizing the multisystemic effects of embolism, Nurs 87 17(12):34-41, 1987.

21. Goldberg, K, editor: Vascular problems, Springhouse, Pa, 1986, Springhouse Corporation.

22. *Grim, CM: Nursing assessment of the patient with high blood pressure, Nurs Clin North Am 16:349-364, 1981.

23. Haimovici, H, editor: Vascular surgery, principles and techniques, ed 2, Norwalk, Conn, 1984, Appleton-Century-Crofts.

24. *Herman, JA: Nursing assessment and nursing diagnosis in patients with peripheral vascular disease, Nurs Clin North Am 21:219-231, 1986.

25. Hill, MN, and Foster, SB: High blood pressure, Nurs 82 12(2):72-75, 1982.

26. *Hudson, B: Sharpen your vascular assessment skills with the Doppler ultrasound stethoscope, Nurs 83 13(5):54-57, 1983.

27. *Ivancin, LA: Healing those frustrating stasis ulcers, RN 46:38-40, 1983.

28. Kaplan, NM: Hypertension. In Kaplan, NM, and Stamler, P, editors: Prevention of coronary heart disease, Philadelphia, 1983, WB Saunders Co.

29. Krupp, MA: Schroeder, SA, and Tierney, LM: Current medical diagnosis and treatment 1987, Norwalk, Conn, 1987, Appleton & Lange.

30. *Leech, JE: Psychosocial and physiologic needs of patients with arterial occlusive disease during the preoperative phase of hospitalization, Heart Lung 11:4422-4448, 1982.

31. *Loustau, A, and Blair, BJ: A key to compliance, Nurs 81 11:84-87, 1981.

32. *Massey, JA: Diagnostic testing for peripheral vascular disease, Nurs Clin North Am 21:207-218, 1986.

33. McCarthy, WJ, and Williams, LR: Femoral artery reconstruction, Crit Care Q 8:39-48, 1985.

34. *McMahan, BE: Why deep vein thrombosis is so dangerous, RN 51:20-23, 1987.

35. Miller, RA, and Evans, WE: Immediate postop prosthesis, Am J Nurs 87:310-311, 1987.

36. Moore, LD, and Pulliam CB: An on-the-spot guide to antihypertensive drugs, Nurs 86 16(1):54-57, 1986.

37. Moore, WS, editor: Vascular surgery: a comprehensive review, Orlando, Fla, 1986, Grune & Stratton, Inc.

38. *Peterson, FV: Assessing peripheral vascular disease at the bedside, Am J Nurs 83:1549-1556, 1983.

39. *Quinless, F: PVD: physiology, signs and symptoms, Nurs 84 14:52-53, 1984.

40. *Solid, R: Give venous leg ulcers the boot, Nurs 84 14:52-53, 1984.

41. Spittell, JA: Medical treatment of arteriosclerosis obliterans, Drug Ther 15:12-18, 1985.

42. Subcommittee on Detection and Prevalence of the Joint National Committee on Detection, Evaluation, and Treatment of High Blood Pressure: Hypertension prevalence and the status of awareness, treatment and control in the United States, Hypertension 7:457-468, 1985.

43. Swearingen, PL, editor: Manual of nursing therapeutics: applying nursing diagnoses to medical disorders, Menlo Park, Calif, 1986, Addison-Wesley Publishing Co.

44. *Turner, JA: Nursing interventions in patients with peripheral vascular disease, Nurs Clin North Am 21:233-240, 1986.

45. US Department of Health and Human Services: The 1984 report of the Joint National Committee on Detection, Evaluation and Treatment of High Blood Pressure, NIH no 84-1088, Washington, DC, 1984, The Department.

46. Vitello-Ciccio, J: Thrombolytic therapy: urokinase, J Cardiovasc Nurs 1(2):59-62, 1987.

47. Walter, J: Coping with leg amputation, Am J Nurs 81:1349-1352, 1981.

48. Wyngaarden, JB, and Smith, LH: Cecil textbook of medicine, ed 17, Philadelphia, 1985, WB Saunders Co.

Classic

49. *Adler, J, and Argondizzo, NT: Patient assessment: pulses, Am J Nurs 79:115-132, 1979.

50. *Eddy, ME: Teaching patients with peripheral vascular disease, Nurs Clin North Am 12:151-159, 1977.

51. *Engstrand, JL: Rehabilitation of the patient with a lower extremity amputation, Nurs Clin North Am 11:659-669, 1976.

52. *Fagin-Dubin, L: Atherosclerosis: a major cause of peripheral vascular disease, Nurs Clin North Am 12:101-108, 1977.

53. *Ryzewski, J: Factors in rehabilitation of patients with peripheral vascular disease, Nurs Clin North Am 12:161-168, 1977.

54. *Sexton, DL: The patient with peripheral arterial occlusive disease, Nurs Clin North Am 12:89-99, 1977.

27

The Patient with Hematologic Problems

ROSEMARIE M. HOGAN

CHAPTER OBJECTIVES

After studying this chapter, the student should be able to:

- Differentiate among the functions of red blood cells, white blood cells, platelets, and the lymphatic system.

- Compare and contrast different types of anemia in terms of pathophysiology, assessment, and interventions.

- Contrast bone marrow aspiration and biopsy, and describe the related care.

- Explain the genetic factors of sickle cell disease and describe sickle cell crisis.

- Compare and contrast disorders of coagulation (thrombocytopenia, hemophilia, DIC).

- Differentiate among the four types of leukemia and describe therapeutic modalities and nursing interventions.

- Differentiate between Hodgkin's disease and non-Hodgkin's lymphomas and describe treatment modalities and nursing interventions.

Disorders related to the hematologic system are usually the result of problems in the normal production, development, and function of the components of blood or alterations in the rate of blood cell destruction. The illness can be either chronic or acute or a combination of both.

■ ANATOMY AND PHYSIOLOGY

The hematopoietic system includes blood and its components as well as the reticuloendothelial system (RES), which is located throughout the body. The RES system's function is phagocytizing foreign materials and lysing (breaking down) red blood cells.

■ Components of the hematopoietic system

■ BLOOD

Blood is a suspension of particulate materials in an aqueous colloid solution. The aqueous component of blood (plasma) is 91% to 92% water and 7% to 9% solids such as proteins, inorganic substances such as sodium, potassium, and calcium, and organic constituents such as urea, uric acid and glucose.[35]

The cell components of blood include erythrocytes or red blood cells (RBC), leukocytes or white blood cells (WBC), and thrombocytes or platelets (Table 27-1). All normal cells are derived from a single stem cell located throughout the bone marrow. The stem cell can divide into lymphoid and blood stem cells, which in turn become progenitor cells that divide along a specific single pathway (Fig. 27-1). This process is known as *hematopoiesis* and takes place in the bone marrow of the skull, vertebrae, pelvis, sternum, ribs, and proximal epiphysis of long bones.

Production may take place in all the long bones during periods of increased demand, such as with hemorrhage or during blood cell destruction (hemolysis).

□ Red blood cells

An RBC is a nonnucleated biconcave disk that is soft and pliable. This property enables the RBC to change its shape during passage through the microcirculation. The RBC's major component is hemoglobin (Hb), a protein that transports oxygen and approximately 20% of carbon dioxide, and maintains normal pH through a series of intracellular buffers (see Chapter 8). The Hb molecule contains globin (two pairs of polypeptide chains) and four heme groups. Each heme group contains an atom of ferrous iron. Oxygen is loosely and reversibly combined with hemoglobin to form oxyhemoglobin. Each molecule of hemoglobin can carry four bound molecules of oxygen, one oxygen molecule to each of the four heme groups. At the tissue site, the oxygen is released into the plasma and diffuses into the tissue cells to supply their needs.

Maturation of RBCs requires adequate amounts and use of vitamin B_{12}, folic acid, proteins, enzymes, and minerals such as iron or copper. Erythropoietin, a glycoprotein hormone believed to originate in the kidney, appears to stimulate RBC production (erythropoiesis). Tissue hypoxia resulting from changes in oxygen stimulates erythropoietin production. The stem cells involved in RBC production then initiate formation and maturation of the erythrocytes.

RBCs circulate for 120 days. Their cell membranes become fragile and rupture during passage through tight spots in the circulation. Many RBC fragments in the spleen are phagocytized and digested by RES cells. Energy in the form of ATP is required to maintain cell membrane integrity and the relatively low sodium and high potassium content of the red cell, and for defense against oxidation and other environmental stressors.

Table 27-1 Normal values of cellular blood components

Type	Normal values
Red blood cells	Male: 4.6-6.2 million/mm³
	Female: 4.2-5.4 million/mm³
White blood cells	4000-10,000/mm³
Neutrophils	38%-70%
Eosinophils	1%-5%
Basophils	0%-2%
Monocytes	1%-8%
Lymphocytes	15%-45%
Platelets	150,000-400,000/mm³
Hematocrit	Male: 42%-53%
	Female: 38%-46%
Hemoglobin	Male: 13.4-17.6 g/100 ml
	Female: 12-15.4 g/100 ml
Mean corpuscular volume (MCV)	81-96 µm
Mean corpuscular hemoglobin concentration (MCHC)	30%-36%

Differential blood count—totals 100% (Neutrophils through Lymphocytes)

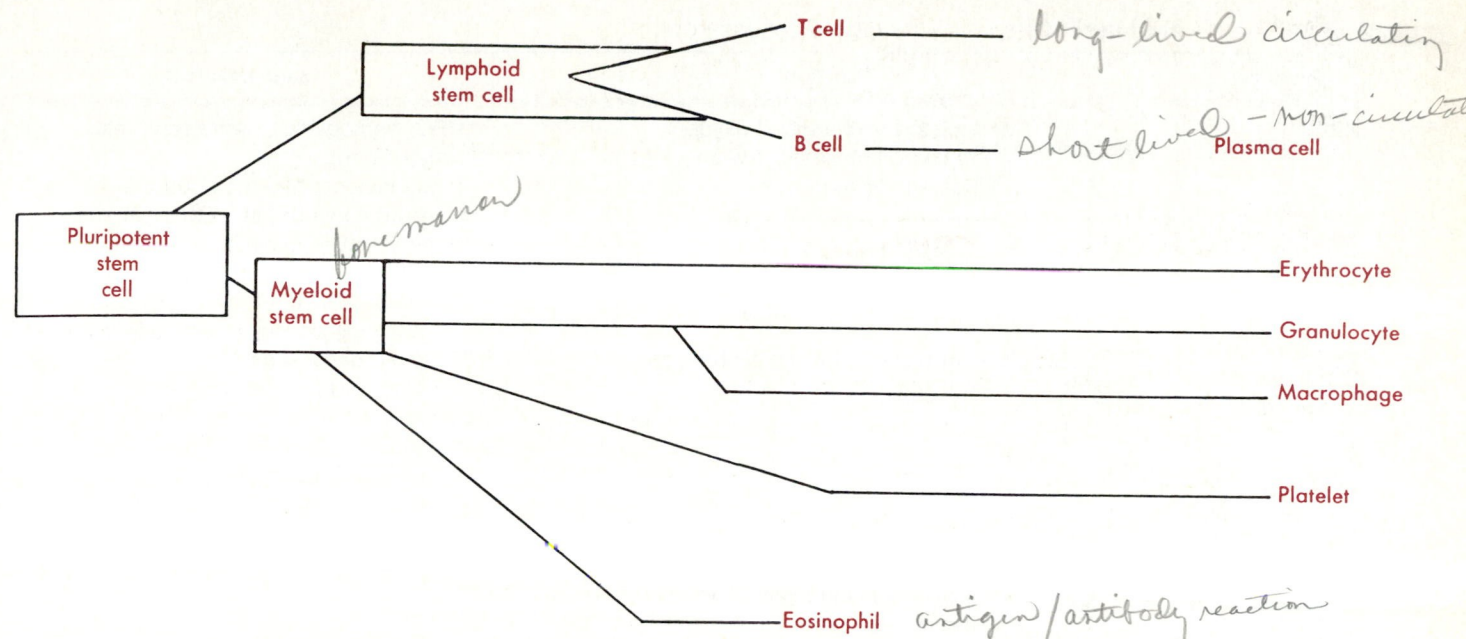

Fig. 27-1 Scheme of stem cell differentiation showing common progenitor cell for erythrocytes, granulocytes, and platelets. (Adapted from Clinc, M, and Golde, D: Blood 53:157-164, 1979).

□ White blood cells

WBCs may be classified into two groups: *granular leukocytes* (also called *polymorphonuclear* [PMN] *leukocytes*) consisting of neutrophils, eosinophils, and basophils; and *nongranular leukocytes* consisting of monocytes and lymphocytes. The granulocytes contain enzymes that kill and digest bacteria upon degranulation of the cells.

Eosinophils have a weak phagocytic action and function in antigen-antibody reactions. Levels are elevated in asthmatic attacks, drug reactions, and certain parasitic infections. The functions of basophils are poorly understood but they carry histamine and platelet-activating factors in their granules to inflamed tissues. Elevated basophil levels may be found in immunologic reactions and proliferative disorders of blood-forming cells.[35]

Neutrophils are present in the circulation or along the capillary walls (the margination pool). They move into the tissues and mucous membranes and serve as the body's primary defense against bacterial infection through the process of phagocytosis (see Chapter 37).

Monocytes are larger than neutrophils and have one large folded or indented nucleus. They leave the circulation and become tissue *macrophages,* which also have phagocytic action, removing dead and injured cells, cell fragments, and microorganisms.

Lymphocytes are mononuclear with a round or oval nucleus. They originate primarily in lymphoid tissue (lymph nodes) but also in the bone marrow. There are two types of lymphocytes, the long-lived circulating T lymphocytes (from the thymus) and short-lived noncirculating B-lymphocytes. T-lymphocytes initiate the cellular immune response, while B-lymphocytes (immunoglobulins) initiate the humoral immune response (see Chapter 37).

Laboratory tests have been developed to measure the amounts and functioning of all cellular components of the blood (Table 27-2).

□ Platelets

Platelets (thrombocytes) are not cells but are granular disk-shaped, nonnucleated cell fragments. One-third of the platelets are in the spleen as a reserve pool and the remainder in circulation. Platelets are derived from the stem cells that differentiate into the megakaryoblast, which in turn matures into megakaryocytes. These cells eventually break up into individual platelets that are essential to hemostasis and coagulation.

Hemostasis results from the adhesion and aggregation capabilities of platelets to plug small breaks in blood vessels. Platelets also release thromboplastin (factor III), which, in the presence of calcium ions, converts prothrombin into thrombin in the first step of the coagulation mechanism (Fig. 27-2). In the second step of the coagulation mechanism, thrombin promotes the conversion of fibrinogen (a soluble plasma protein) into fibrin (an insoluble strand). Step one requires coagulation factors IV, V, VIII, IX, X, XI, and XII; whereas step two requires factors IV and XIII (see the box on p. 867).

Clot resolution or fibrinolysis involves a sequence in which fibrin is split by plasmin (fibrinolysin) into fibrin degradation products, leading to dissolution of the clot. Plasminogen proactivators, circulating proteins in the presence of enzymes such as streptokinase, urokinase, tissue

Table 27-2 Laboratory tests for hematologic assessment

Blood cell	Function	Diagnostic test
RBCs	Mediate the exchange of oxygen and carbon dioxide between lungs and tissue	RBC, hemoglobin, hematocrit, reticulocyte count Blood indices: Mean corpuscular hemoglobin concentration (MCHC), mean cell volume (MCV), mean corpuscular hemoglobin (MCH) Red cell fragility Morphologic description in stained smear
Platelets	Platelet plug; promotion of thrombin production	Platelet aggregation Platelet count Bleeding time

WBCs
  Granulocytes
    Neutrophils
    Eosinophils
    Basophils
  Lymphocytes
  Monocytes
	
	Phagocytosis
	
	Allergic and immunologic responses
	Formation of immunoglobulins
	Phagocytosis
		WBC
		WBC with differential

kinase, and factor XIIa, are essential to the reaction. Plasmin splits fibrin and fibrinogen into fragments that interfere with thrombin activity, platelet function, and fibrin polymerization, leading to clot dissolution.[35]

■ RETICULOENDOTHELIAL SYSTEM

The RES, also called the monocyte-phagocyte system or macrophage system, includes circulating monocytes and their precursor cells in the bone marrow. It also includes more or less fixed mononuclear phagocytic cells found in blood channels in the spleen and liver (Kupffer cells), and in the lymphatic system, serosal cavities of the body, lungs, general connective tissue, and bone marrow.

The important function of the RES is phagocytosis, that is, cleaning the blood, lymph and intestinal spaces of foreign material, especially bacteria, that are removed in a few hours by macrophages (phagocytic cells) located throughout the body. This uptake of foreign materials is the first step—essential in the chain of events leading to the immune response (Chapter 37).

In addition to phagocytosis, the RES removes the Hg of RBCs that have reached the end of their life span, splitting Hb into an iron-containing substance and bilirubin (see Chapter 30).

■ Physiologic changes with aging

The effect of aging on hematopoiesis is still being studied with findings that are sometimes ambiguous. There is evidence from studies of mouse marrow that stem cells have a limited capacity to proliferate. Findings from animal studies suggest that changes related to aging do not have clinical significance.[46] The cellularity of human marrow decreases

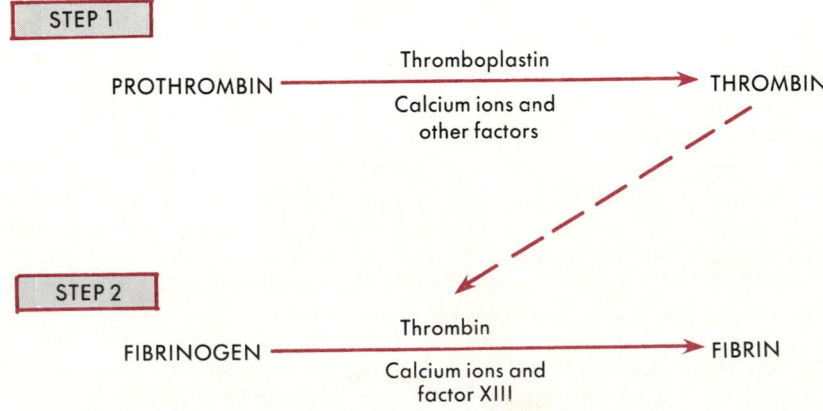

Fig. 27-2 Basic steps in coagulation process.

Coagulation factors	
Factor I	Fibrinogen
Factor II	Prothrombin
Factor III	Thromboplastin, tissue thromboplastin
Factor IV	Calcium
Factor V	Proaccelerin, labile factor
Factor VI	(Not assigned)
Factor VII	Serum prothrombin conversion accelerator (SPCA)
Factor VIII	Antihemophilic globulin (AHG) Antihemophilic factor (AHF)
Factor IX	Plasma thromboplastin component (PTG), Christmas factor — *Hemophilia B*
Factor X	Stuart factor
Factor XI	Plasma thromboplastin antecedent (PTA)
Factor XII	Hageman factor
Factor XIII	Fibrin-stabilizing factor

with age, but this may be the result of an increase in fat from osteoporosis rather than a decrease in hematopoietic cells.

In humans, the total number of leukocytes and differential counts show no variation through middle age and no gross changes in old age. In general the leukocyte count does not rise as high in response to infection, and studies suggest that the elderly have a diminished marrow granulocyte reserve.

The Hb level decreases after middle age although the decrease in women seems to be relatively less than that in men. Unexplained anemia in the elderly has been noted, but iron absorption is not impaired; however, use of orally administered iron is reduced. This anemia does not appear to be related solely to age.[46] Serum iron and iron-binding capacity decrease in the elderly, and low serum vitamin B_{12} and folic acid levels occur in a significant proportion of elderly people but without anemia.

No age-related changes in platelets have been reported. RBC sedimentation rate increases significantly, but this rate is of limited value in detecting disease in the elderly. Some of the plasma coagulation factors have been reported to increase with age (factors I, V, VII, and IX). Partial thromboplastin time may be shortened.[21]

◼ PREVENTION AND HEALTH EDUCATION

Exposure to certain chemicals and drugs place individuals at high risk for hematologic disorders, especially aplastic anemia and the leukemias. Individuals with inadequate dietary intake of iron and vitamins (for example, folic acid and B_{12}), alcoholics, and others with poor dietary habits because of inadequate knowledge or low income, are particularly susceptible to anemia. Women who have long-term blood loss because of heavy menstrual bleeding (menorrhagia) are also at risk for anemia, as are other persons with long-term slow blood loss.

Other diseases such as sickle cell anemia, the thalassemias, and hemophilia are hereditary; therefore, marriage between carriers of defective genes may result in children with the disease.

Health teaching involves identifying persons at high risk and ways in which the risk factors can be mitigated. Occupational health nurses are involved in identifying industrial chemicals or processes that place workers in danger and in working with companies to minimize those risks. Nurses in all settings teach about dietary needs for iron and other vitamins. An important facet of this teaching is helping those persons with low incomes to identify inexpensive sources of the vitamins and minerals necessary for hematologic health. Nurses also may become politically active in order to ensure that there is adequate government funding for food stamps and establishment or maintenance of other low-cost nutritional programs for those persons who have marginal incomes.

One of the most difficult and sensitive roles for nurses is that of genetic counselor, communicating to individuals with hereditary problems the risk factors involved and possibility of having children with severe hematopoietic disease. The persons are allowed to make their own decisions after information has been shared with them, a decision that can be devastating to the individual no matter what it is.

Major health problems related to blood and lymph systems

Disorders associated with the hematopoietic system are diverse in their underlying pathologic manifestations, disease course, and response to treatment. Most often, the symptoms manifested are the result of interference with the normal development and function of the blood components and with altered hematopoiesis (blood cell production). Normally homeostasis is maintained through a balance between the rate of production of normal blood cells and the rate of destruction. Disorders of the blood are manifested when this hemostatic balance is lost. Disturbances in the coagulation mechanism also result in blood disorders.

In addition to primary hematologic disorders, secondary effects from disease of another body system may also manifest themselves in abnormal hematologic findings. For example, the anemia that is associated with azotemia is the consequence of disease existing outside of the hematopoietic system. Major health problems include the following:

1. RBC disorders
   a. Anemias
   b. Erythrocytosis: polycythemia

Causes of anemia

1. Blood loss: acute or chronic
2. Impaired RBC production: aplastic anemia
3. Increased RBC destruction (hemolysis)
   a. Congenital: hereditary spherocytosis, sickle cell anemia, thalassemia, enzyme deficiency
   b. Acquired: autoimmune, drug induced
4. Nutritional deficiency
   a. Iron deficiency
   b. Megaloblastic anemia: B_{12} deficiency, folic acid deficiency

---

Descriptive cell characteristics in anemia

Size	Macrocytic (large)
	Normocytic
	Microcytic (small)
Hemoglobin	Normochromic
	Hypochromic (decreased)

---

2. Coagulation disorders
   a. Platelet disorders: thrombocytopenia, platelet function disorders
   b. Hemophilia
   c. Disseminated intravascular clotting (DIC)
3. WBC disorders: agranulocytosis, leukemia
4. Lymph systems disorders: lymphadenopathy, lymphomas (Hodgkin's and non-Hodgkin's)
5. Plasma cell dyscrasias: multiple myeloma

DISORDERS ASSOCIATED WITH ERYTHROCYTES

Anemia and erythrocytosis are the general categories of red cell disorders. *Anemia* refers to a deficiency of RBCs as reflected in a decreased Hb level, packed cell volume (hematocrit), and red cell count. Anemias may be divided into those that are the result of blood loss, impaired production of RBCs, increased destruction of RBCs, or nutritional deficiency (see the box at left).

Anemia may also be differentiated by examining the size of a red cell and the amount of Hb contained. The suffix *-cytic* refers to RBC size and *-chromic* refers to amount of hemoglobin (see the box above).

Anemia secondary to blood loss

PATHOPHYSIOLOGY

Anemia associated with blood loss may be acute or chronic. Acute anemia is the direct result of the decrease in a large amount of circulating RBCs. An adult of average build can lose 500 ml of blood (out of a total of 6000 ml) without serious or lasting effects. Losses of 1000 ml or more can cause acute consequences (Table 27-3). The severity of symptoms depends on the severity of blood loss and the resulting degree of hypoxia (inadequate tissue oxygenation); as the number of RBCs decreases, less oxygen is delivered to tissues. Sudden acute hemorrhage with loss

---

Table 27-3 Clinical significance of abnormal blood counts

	Increased values	Decreased values
RBC	Polycythemia (erythrocytosis)	Leukopenia
WBC	Neutrophilia	Leukopenia
	Leukemias	Aplastic anemia
		Neutropenias
Platelets	Polycythemia	Aplastic anemia
		Thrombocytopenia
		Disseminated intravascular clotting (DIC)
Hematocrit	Polycythemia	Anemias
		Hemorrhage
Hemoglobin	Polycythemia	Anemias
		Hemorrhage
Mean corpuscular volume (MCV)	Pernicious anemia	Iron deficiency anemia
	Folic acid deficiency	Chronic blood loss
Mean corpuscular hemoglobin concentration (MCHC)		Iron deficiency anemia
		Chronic blood loss

of 30% or more of blood volume causes symptoms of diaphoresis, restlessness, tachycardia, tachypnea, shortness of breath and, without intervention, shock. The body's compensatory responses to hypoxia include the following[47]:

1. Increased cardiac output and respirations increasing oxygen delivery to the tissues
2. Increased release of oxygen by hemoglobin
3. Expanded plasma volume by pulling fluid from tissue spaces
4. Redistribution of blood to vital organs.

Compensatory vasoconstriction to shunt blood to vital organs is responsible for some of the signs and symptoms of anemia, such as pallor, cold or clammy extremities. Cerebral hypoxia causes symptoms of mental confusion, bizarre behavior and drowsiness, headache, dizziness and tinnitus (ringing of the ears).

Chronic anemia secondary to blood loss is the most common cause of iron-deficiency anemia (p. 880). The body has remarkable adaptive powers and may adjust fairly well to a marked reduction in RBCs and Hb, provided the condition develops gradually. An individual may remain asymptomatic even though the total RBC count may drop to almost half of its normal level or the Hb level to below 7 g/100 ml. When blood loss is continuous and moderate in amount, the bone marrow may be able to keep up with the losses by increasing RBC production. If the cause of chronic blood loss is not found and corrected, eventually the bone marrow will not be able to keep pace with the loss, and symptoms of anemia will appear.

In addition to the previously listed symptoms, gastrointestinal symptoms (anorexia, nausea, constipation or diarrhea, stomatitis) may also occur as a result of chronic hypoxia. Poor oxygenation of muscles may cause weakness and fatigue.

ASSESSMENT

Subjective data include the patient's description of shortness of breath (dyspnea) if sufficient RBCs have been lost, and feelings of weakness or fatigue. Reports of dizziness or tinnitus are noted.

Objective data include the person's ability to respond to questions or other signs of confusion, vital signs, and color and temperature of the skin. Patients are monitored on a continuing basis for further signs of bleeding.

Decreased Hb and hematocrit serum levels are diagnostic tests of particular significance with acute anemia, although these signs will not be evident until several hours after the blood loss. With chronic anemia, RBC counts, Hb and hematocrit levels, mean corpuscular volume (MCV), and mean corpuscular hemoglobin concentration (MCHC) are usually below normal (see Table 27-1 for normal values).

DATA ANALYSIS: NURSING DIAGNOSES

Nursing diagnoses are determined from assessment of patient data. Possible nursing diagnoses for the person with anemia resulting from blood loss (exclusive of hypovolemic shock) may include, but are not limited to, the following:

Diagnostic title	Possible etiologies
Fatigue	Decreased tissue oxygenation
Impaired gas exchange	Ventilation/perfusion imbalance
Potential for injury	Weakness, fatigue
Altered cerebral tissue perfusion	Hypovolemia

PLANNING: EXPECTED PATIENT OUTCOMES

Expected patient outcomes for the person with anemia resulting from blood loss include, but are not limited to, the following:

1. Patient is alert and oriented.
2. Patient is relaxed and comfortable.
3. No injuries have occurred from falls.
4. Color and temperature of skin are normal.
5. Breathing is not labored (no shortness of breath).
6. Patient states feeling more rested, less fatigued.

IMPLEMENTATION

Nursing interventions for acute blood loss are the same as those for hypovolemic shock (Chapter 9). Since transfusion of whole blood may be used to replace both plasma and RBC loss, nurses are alert for signs of transfusion reactions (Chapter 38).

If patients are weak, dizzy, or in any way confused because of severe anemia, they are supervised in ambulation to prevent exertional dyspnea, fatigue, and falls. Rest periods are provided. If oral iron preparations are prescribed, patients are taught to take them with meals to avoid gastric irritation.

EVALUATION

Questions to ask may include the following:
1. Does the patient state that fatigue is controlled?
2. Is the patient comfortable?
3. Has the patient been free from falls?

Anemia secondary to impaired production of RBCs: aplastic anemia

PATHOPHYSIOLOGY

The defect leading to aplastic anemia is most likely injury or destruction of a common stem cell (Fig. 27-1), affecting all subsequent cell populations.

Causes of aplastic anemia may be antineoplastic or cytotoxic agents, drugs (certain antibiotics, anti-convulsants, thyroid medication, phenylbutazone, gold compounds), benzene, and viral infection. At times, no causative agent can be found (idiopathic aplastic anemia). It is characterized not only by impaired RBC production but also by depression or cessation of activity of all blood-producing elements. There is a decrease in white cells (leukopenia) and a decrease in platelets (thrombocytopenia).[18] Signs and symptoms and medical therapy for aplastic anemia are listed in Table 27-4.

Table 27-4 Disorders of red blood cells

Disorder	Etiology	Signs and symptoms	Medical therapy
Anemias			
Secondary to blood loss Acute	Hemorrhage	Hypovolemic and hypoxemic symptoms (weakness, stupor, irritability, cool moist skin, hypotension, tachycardia, ↓ Hb and Hct, pallor)	IV fluids, whole blood or packed cells; identify source of loss; administration of iron
Chronic	GI or other malignancy, slow bleeding ulcer, bleeding hemorrhoids, menorrhagia	Depends on degree of ↓ in Hb; if less than 8.0 g/dl: weakness, fatigue, ↑ pulse, pallor, exertional dyspnea	Packed cells, iron; identify source of loss
Aplastic anemia	Drugs, chemicals, radiation, chemotherapy, virus, congenital	As in chronic anemia plus those related to ↓ WBC and platelets (ecchymoses), petechiae, GI, GU, CNS bleeding, increased risk of infection)	Removal of causative agent; supportive care until bone marrow is regenerated: transfusions, laminar air-flow room, androgen to stimulate erythropoiesis, bone marrow transplantation, antilymphocyte-globulin therapy
Hemolytic anemia Congenital Sickle cell	Genetic	↓ Hb; ↓ Hct; pain (bones, joints, back): generalized, localized or migratory; vomiting; fever; infections; chronic leg ulcers; cardiomegaly; murmurs; CHF; delay in growth and sexual maturation; swollen hands and feet (dactylitis); jaundice	No specific therapy; analgesics, oxygen, adequate hydration, treatment of infection, polyvalent pneumococcal vaccine to prevent pneumococcal infections, antisickling agents (experimental), therapeutic apheresis
		Thrombotic crisis: severe pain in abdomen and musculoskeletal system	Adequate hydration, exchange transfusions (replacing person's blood with packed red cells, unit for unit)
		Aplastic crisis: rapid ↑ in anemia	
Thalassemia	Decreased synthesis of one of the globin chains of Hb	Thalassemia minor: mild anemia	No therapy required; transfusions with severe symptoms or to maintain Hb near normal
		Thalassemia major: severe anemia	
Enzyme deficiency	Genetic defect in pathways that metabolize glucose	Anemia when person exposed to oxidant drugs (aspirin, sulfonanmindes, antimalarial)	Cessation of causative drug
Acquired hemolytic anemia	Drug (alpha methyldopa, penicillin), autoimmune response, idiopathic or secondary to lymphocytic lymphomas or chronic lymphocytic leukemia	Same as with other anemias	Corticosteroids, splenectomy in those who do not respond to drug therapy
Nutritional anemia Iron deficiency anemia	Inadequate dietary iron, chronic blood loss	Gradual development; may have few signs; fatigue, exertional dyspnea, severe anemia, brittle spoon-shaped (concave) nails with longitudinal ridges, atrophy of tongue papillae, smooth shiny tongue, cheilosis (cracks in corner of mouth); low serum iron, pallor, weakness	Determine and correct cause Oral iron administration (ferrous sulfate); parenteral iron if oral not tolerated or not absorbed via GI tract; adequate balanced diet

Table 27-4   Disorders of red blood cells—cont'd

Disorder	Etiology	Signs and symptoms	Medical therapy
Megaloblastic anemia	Vitamin B_{12} deficiency caused by absence of intrinsic factor (pernicious anemia) or interference with absorption in ileum	Low serum B_{12} and folate levels, neurologic abnormalities (peripheral neuropathies, loss of balance), symptoms associated with underlying disease and anemia	
Erythrocytosis			
Polycythemia vera (primary)	Stem cell abnormality, cause unknown	Absent in early stages; headache, tinnitus, blurred vision, reddened skin, nosebleeds, ecchymoses, GI bleeding caused by platelet dysfunction, thrombosis, hepatomegaly, splenomegaly, ↑ total RBC volume, ↑ or normal plasma volume	Periodic phlebotomy (removal of blood), radioactive phosphorus, chemotherapeutic agents such as busulfan
Secondary polycythemia	Hypoxia, renal tumors, living at high altitudes	↑ RBC, ↑ Hct; symptoms may be similar to but less severe than those in polycythemia vera	Correct underlying condition
Pseudopolycythemia	Stress: occurs in middle aged, obese, highly anxious males; cigarette smoking exacerbates symptoms	As above; is self-limiting; symptoms are mild	Stress reduction

---

Drugs that may cause aplastic anemia

Chloramphenicol
Colchicine
Mephenytoin
D-Penicillamine
Phenylbutazone
Sulfonamides
Trimethadione

ASSESSMENT

Subjective data include the person's history of exposure to chemicals (insecticides, benzene) and drugs, plus the family history of any similar anemia. Physical examination is often normal. A hemogram characteristically reveals pancytopenia (a marked decrease in the numbers of all cell types). The reticulocyte count is low. The patient is monitored for signs of infection (from the leukopenia) and bleeding (from the thrombocytopenia).

Diagnostic tests include peripheral blood smears and bone marrow examination, which provides the definitive diagnosis. Examination of the peripheral blood smear allows for determination of the morphology of the cells (type, origin), the extent of cell maturity, and the ratio of the various cell types to each other.

☐ Bone marrow aspiration

Aspiration is the most common procedure for obtaining a bone marrow sample. The procedure is possible because normal bone marrow is soft and semifluid and can therefore be removed by aspiration through a needle. Bone marrow aspiration is also used in the diagnosis of acute leukemia and thrombocytopenia.

☐ *Procedure*

The skin surrounding the puncture site (Fig. 27-3) is shaved, if necessary, and cleansed with an antiseptic such as povidone-iodine complex (Betadine). Sterile towels are placed around the site. The skin and periosteum are anesthetized to avoid pain. First, the most superficial layer of the skin is infiltrated with procaine. After a few seconds the needle is further advanced until bone is touched. Procaine is then injected to anesthetize the periosteum. The marrow aspiration needle is inserted, and when the

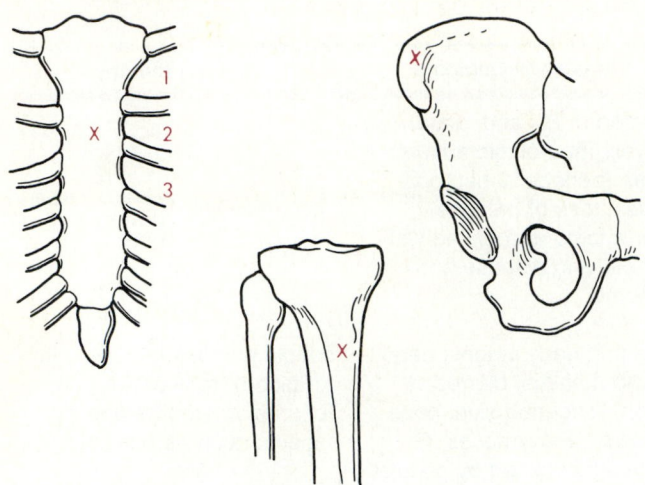

Fig. 27-3 Sites for bone marrow aspiration: sternum, iliac crest (most common), and tibia.

marrow cavity is entered, the marrow stylet is removed from the needle and a sterile syringe is attached. The syringe plunger is drawn back until marrow appears in the syringe. As the plunger is drawn back the person will experience a brief, sharp pain, sometimes described as a burning sensation. The pain is caused by the suction exerted as the plunger is pulled back. Some persons may complain of tenderness at the aspiration site for a few days. Most often no pain or discomfort is experienced following the procedure.

Attempts at bone marrow aspiration may yield a "dry tap" because of hypocellularity and a decrease in active marrow, and bone marrow biopsy is often necessary.

□ *Nursing care with bone marrow aspiration*

1. Explain procedure to patient, stating that there may be brief discomfort when the marrow is aspirated.
2. To prevent movement, place hands on patient's shoulders and instruct patient to remain still at the time of aspiration.
3. Apply pressure over aspiration site after needle is removed to prevent bleeding; apply pressure for 3 to 5 minutes if patient is thrombocytopenic.
4. Assess for bleeding from aspiration site.
5. Provide comfort measures to help patient relax.

□ **Bone marrow biopsy**

When a large sample of bone marrow is needed, a bone marrow biopsy may be performed. Persons also likely to undergo a bone marrow biopsy are those with pancytopenia, metastatic tumor, lymphoma, and multiple myeloma.

The most common site for bone marrow biopsy is the posterosuperior iliac spine, although the sternum may also be used. The initial steps in the biopsy procedure are similar to those outlined for bone marrow aspiration. The use of a Jamshidi needle allows for a core of marrow to be collected (Fig. 27-4). Nursing care following a bone marrow biopsy is similar to that of bone marrow aspiration.

From microscopic examination of the bone marrow, iron stores can be determined, as can the morphology of the progenitor cell. Megaloblastic (RBC precursor) changes

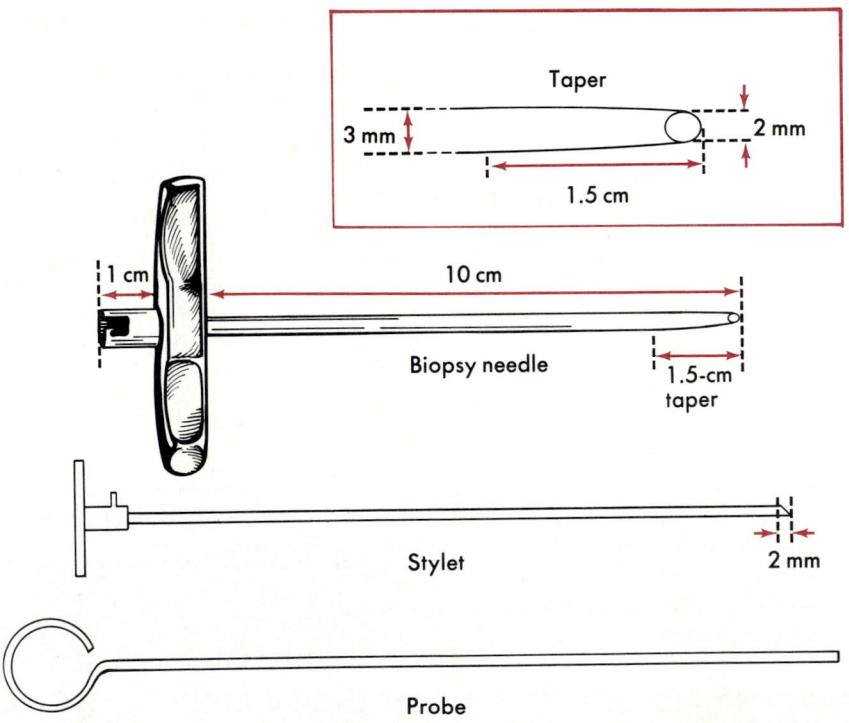

Fig. 27-4 Bone marrow biopsy needle showing shape and size.

and the absence of cells may be observed. Infiltration with leukemic cells may also be determined by bone marrow biopsy.

→ DATA ANALYSIS: NURSING DIAGNOSES

Because the levels of all of the blood cells are decreased, the individual is prone to severe and life-threatening complications, primarily infection and bleeding. (The nursing care of persons with decreased WBC and platelet count is discussed on pp. 885 and 889.)

Nursing diagnoses related to anemia from blood loss apply also to aplastic anemia, depending on the severity of the disease. Possible additional nursing diagnoses for the person with aplastic anemia may include, but are not limited to, the following:

Diagnostic title	Possible etiologies
Potential for infection	Lack of knowledge, decreased immune response
Potential for injury: bleeding	Impaired platelet production, lack of knowledge of environmental hazards
Knowledge deficit	Unfamiliarity with resources, lack of exposure/recall of information

⊏ PLANNING: EXPECTED PATIENT OUTCOMES

Expected patient outcomes for the person with aplastic anemia may include those for anemia from blood loss and also may include, but are not limited to, the following:
1. Patient is free from infection.
2. Bleeding is controlled or absent.
3. Patient can explain measures to prevent infection.

⊟ IMPLEMENTATION
☐ Assisting with implementation of therapeutic goals

Nursing care depends on the severity of symptoms. The patients may be critically ill. If bone marrow transplantation is attempted, prevention of infection while bone marrow elements are suppressed by radiation and chemotherapy is essential (p. 892). (See care of patients with leukemia and with clotting disorders, pp. 892 and 885). All people need to know how to protect themselves from infection and excessive bleeding, so teaching is of highest priority.

⌗ EVALUATION

Questions to ask may include the following:
1. Have infections been prevented?
2. Are breath sounds normal?
3. Are body secretions normal in color, odor, and consistency?
4. Has hemorrhage been prevented?
5. Does the patient know how to prevent infection and hemorrhage?

■ Anemia secondary to increased destruction of RBCs: hemolytic anemia

■ PATHOPHYSIOLOGY

Hemolytic anemia results when the red cells are destroyed at such a rapid rate that the bone marrow is unable to compensate for the loss. The severity of the anemia is determined by the degree of lag between the rate of RBC destruction (hemolysis) and the rate of bone marrow production of red cells (erythropoiesis). Hemolytic anemias may be congenital or acquired. The signs and symptoms and medical therapies for hemolytic anemias are listed in Table 27-4.

☐ Congenital hemolytic anemias

Congenital hemolytic anemias include hereditary spherocytosis, the hemoglobinopathies, thalassemia, and enzyme deficiency. *Hereditary spherocytosis*, an inherited autosomal dominant trait, is characterized by a membrane abnormality that leads to osmotic swelling of the red cell and susceptibility to destruction by the spleen. It is most commonly detected in childhood but may become manifest initially in adulthood. Diagnosis depends on observation of spherocytes on the peripheral blood smear and by demonstration of increased osmotic fragility of the red cells in the laboratory. It is almost invariably corrected by splenectomy.

Hemoglobinopathies refer to a group of diseases in which there is substitution of one or more amino acids in the globin chain of the Hb molecule, leading to the formation of abnormal Hb (for example, hemoglobins S and C). Their diagnosis and differentiation are facilitated by Hb electrophoresis. The most common hemoglobinopathy is Hb S disease, or sickle cell anemia.

☐ *Sickle cell anemia*

Sickle cell anemia occurs predominantly in the black population. Approximately 8% of American blacks are heterozygous for Hb S and therefore have *sickle cell trait* (Table 27-5). They produce both Hb S and normal Hb A. Sickle cell trait is a benign disorder, often asymptomatic, with no anemia and a normal life span. Genetic counseling and screening may be suggested to inform affected individuals that marriage to another person who is also heterozygous for Hb S may lead to offspring with sickle cell disease.

Table 27-5 Phenotypes for sickle cell

Genetic relationship	Hemoglobin alleles	Sickle cell disease
Homozygous dominant	Hemoglobin A Hemoglobin A	No disease
Heterozygous	Hemoglobin A Hemoglobin S	Sickle cell trait
Homozygous recessive	Hemoglobin S Hemoglobin S	Sickle cell anemia

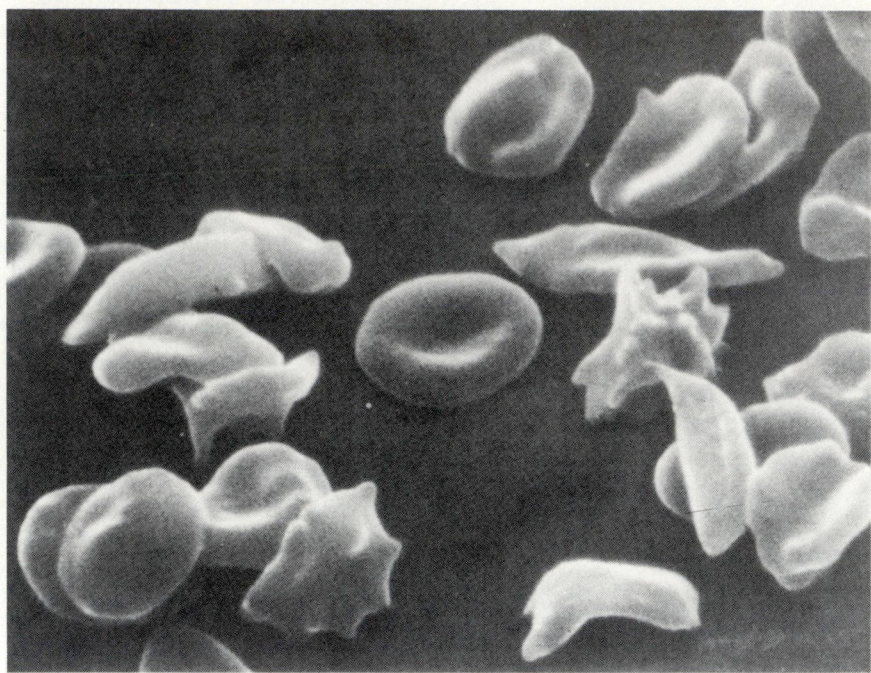

Fig. 27-5 Sickled red cells.

Individuals who are homozygous for Hb S can only produce the defective Hb S. It is these individuals who have sickle cell disease and are affected with a chronic hemolytic anemia, episodes of painful "crisis," and an anticipated shortened life span.

The basic abnormality lies within the globin (protein) fraction of the Hb, where a single amino acid is substituted for another in one of the polypeptide chains. This single amino acid substitution profoundly alters the properties of the Hb molecule. The tendency toward sickling is dependent on both the relative quantity of Hb S in the RBCs and the levels of oxygen tension within the tissues of the body.

The clinical manifestations of the disease result from the sickling phenomenon. Sickling occurs when red cells containing Hb S are deoxygenated; it is the result of the poor solubility of the Hb S, which crystallizes in the RBCs. The RBCs elongate and become rigid and crescent or sickle-shaped (tactoid formation) (Fig. 27-5). Sickling is always present to some extent in the person with sickle cell anemia. Because of increased RBC destruction, patients are often jaundiced and may develop gallstones (cholelithiasis secondary to increased bilirubin).

SICKLE CELL CRISES. Basically, any event that increases the body's need for oxygen or that alters the transport of oxygen may lead to the exacerbation of symptoms called *crisis*. Symptoms may be exacerbated by pregnancy, infection, surgery, trauma, and dehydration. Sickle cell crises are primarily thrombotic or aplastic.

Thrombotic crisis is the most common sickle cell crisis. Signs and symptoms occur as a result of occlusions in the microvasculature by sickled cells causing deoxygenation of tissues with pain and infarctions in organs such as the kidney, lung, bones, and central nervous system (Fig. 27-6). The sites most frequently affected in crises are the abdomen, back, chest, and joints.

Aplastic crisis, usually secondary to infection, involves cessation of bone marrow function and decrease in erythropoiesis and reticulocyte count. Signs of severe anemia are often present.

Megaloblastic crisis, the result of depletion of bone marrow stores of folic acid, is prevented or treated by folic acid administration. *Splenic sequestration crisis*, pooling of blood in the spleen, causes splenic enlargement and hypovolemia with signs of shock.

☐ **Thalassemia**

Thalassemia is an inherited disorder characterized by a decreased synthesis of one of the globin chains of Hb. The beta (β) chain is most often affected (β-thalassemia). As a result, there is a decreased synthesis of Hb as well as an accumulation in the erythrocyte of the unaffected globin chain. These alterations result in decreased red cell production and a chronic hemolytic anemia. The red cells are characteristically hypochromic (low MCH) and microcytic (low MCV). Hb electrophoresis is diagnostic.

There are two types of thalassemia, thalassemia minor, which is usually asymptomatic; and thalassemia major, which is characterized by severe anemia. Life span is significantly shortened, and frequent transfusion therapies may produce iron overload, a problem that can be ameliorated by use of an iron-chelating drug such as deferoxamine.

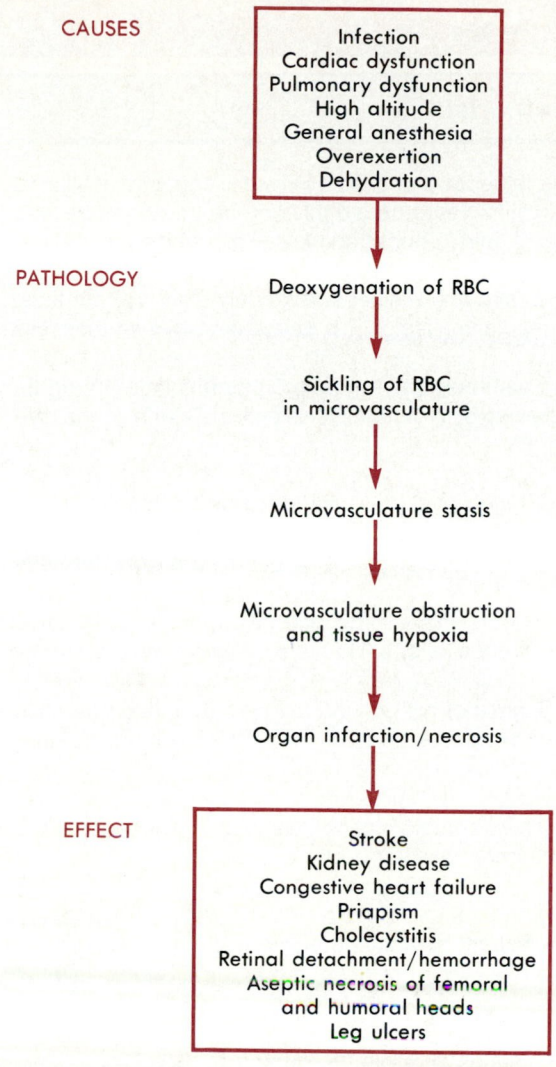

CAUSES

| Infection |
| Cardiac dysfunction |
| Pulmonary dysfunction |
| High altitude |
| General anesthesia |
| Overexertion |
| Dehydration |

PATHOLOGY

Deoxygenation of RBC

Sickling of RBC
in microvasculature

Microvasculature stasis

Microvasculature obstruction
and tissue hypoxia

Organ infarction/necrosis

EFFECT

| Stroke |
| Kidney disease |
| Congestive heart failure |
| Priapism |
| Cholecystitis |
| Retinal detachment/hemorrhage |
| Aseptic necrosis of femoral |
| and humoral heads |
| Leg ulcers |

Fig. 27-6 Pathology of sickle cell crisis.

☐ Enzyme deficiency

Deficiency of enzymes in the pathways that metabolize glucose and generate ATP frequently leads to premature red cell destruction. The most common clinically significant enzyme abnormality is that of *glucose-6-phosphate dehydrogenase*. This disorder is common in a mild form among the black population in the United States and in the Mediterranean area and may cause chronic hemolytic anemia. When an oxidant drug puts the cells under stress, acute hemolysis results.

☐ Acquired hemolytic anemia

Hemolytic anemia may be drug induced or may be caused by an autoimmune disorder. In the latter case an antibody develops that is directed against an antigen on the individual's own RBCs. The antibody-coated red cells are destroyed prematurely by reticuloendothelial cells, particu-larly in the spleen. Diagnosis is confirmed by demonstrating the presence of the antibody on the red cells (antiglobin or Coombs' test).

Drugs produce hemolysis in a variety of ways. Alpha methyldopa (Aldomet) is associated with production of an autoantibody and a positive Coombs' test in approximately 20% of patients. More rarely, high-dose penicillin produces hemolysis through production of an antibody that requires the presence of penicillin on the red cell membrane for its effects to occur. This disorder is often fatal, in part because transfusion is often made difficult and dangerous by the fact that the autoantibody reacts not only with the patient's red cells but also with all donor cells.

☐ ASSESSMENT

Data concerning knowledge about their disease and factors that appear to precipitate crisis or exacerbate symptoms are elicited from persons who have congenital hemolytic anemias. Fatigue may be reported by persons with severe anemia. Persons with sickle cell anemia are questioned about presence of pain and measures taken for pain relief.

Laboratory diagnosis is made by performing Hb electrophoresis. The basic concept of this test is that Hb molecules are electrically charged and will migrate in an electric field. Hb levels will be decreased; reticulocyte (immature RBCs) counts will be elevated; and in severe disease, mean corpuscular value will be decreased.[36]

☐ DATA ANALYSIS: NURSING DIAGNOSES

Nursing diagnoses are determined from assessment of patient data. Possible nursing diagnoses for the person with sickle cell disease may include, but are not limited to, the following:

Diagnostic title	Possible etiologies
Anxiety	Threat to self-concept, threat of death, situational crisis
Fatigue	Decreased metabolic energy production, discomfort
Impaired gas exchange	Ventilation/perfusion imbalance
Potential for infection	Knowledge deficit, tissue destruction, chronic disease, anemia
Knowledge deficit	Anxiety, poor motivation, cognitive limitations, lack of exposure to information, unfamiliarity with resources
Pain: joints and chest	Inadequate pain management techniques, decreased tissue oxygenation
Self-esteem disturbance	Loss of roles
Sexual dysfunction	Priapism, change in roles and relationships, pain
Altered renal, pulmonary, peripheral tissue perfusion	Interruption of arterial and/or venous flow, dehydration

Person with sickle cell crisis

DATA: Mr. Smith is a 24-year-old, married, black mail carrier, who is father of one child. He was diagnosed at age 10 as having sickle cell disease but has been largely asymptomatic until 2 years before this admission. When he was first admitted with symptoms of sickle cell crisis, he had severe joint pain in upper and lower extremities, moderate fever (38.1° C), shortness of breath.

PHYSICAL EXAMINATION: Coarse rales in both lower lobes, cyanosis of lips and nailbeds, dry scaly skin on both legs, 2+ pitting edema with a small (2 cm) reddened area over each medial malleolus. No hair was visible on toes. His Hb was 9 g/dl.

PHYSICIAN ORDERS: Oxygen by nasal cannula, 4L/min, bed rest with bathroom privileges, morphine sulfate 15 mg IM q3-4h prn. The patient was given two units of packed cells to be followed by IV fluids. Sickle cell crisis with congestive heart failure was diagnosed.

The nursing history identified the following:

1. The patient is very "worried" about the outcome of the hospitalization and his ability to "catch his breath."
2. He expresses concern about his ability to support his family and be a "father" to his son and especially to take part in athletic events: "I'm hardly a man." His wife has assumed responsibility for some of the yard work, formerly his responsibility.
3. He continues to exercise and jogs several times a week. He smokes one pack of cigarettes per day and states he has never been "a big fluid drinker," although he does have a beer a day. He states that he does not know what brings on the crisis.
4. He is concerned about his sexual relationship with his wife because of his general fatigue. They had one child before he was aware of the genetic nature of the disease and expresses concern about having other children who might inherit the disease.

Collaborative nursing action includes those to relieve pain, maintain fluid and electrolyte balance, and peripheral and pulmonary oxygen/carbon dioxide balance as well as to prevent further vascular occlusion.

Nursing actions include monitoring for the following:

1. Signs of infection: hyperthermia, abnormal fluid, positive blood and sputum cultures, tachycardia, tachypnea.
2. Signs of increased fluid/electrolyte imbalance, CHF and renal failure: hematocrit, electrolyte levels, intake and output, skin turgor; respiratory status (rate, depth of respiration, presence of rales, rhonchi, skin color, level of consciousness), renal function: creatinine, blood urea nitrogen.

Nursing diagnosis: Anxiety: related to threat to self-concept, health status and role functioning

Expected patient outcomes	Nursing interventions	Rationale
Signs of anxiety are decreased	Give patient opportunities to explore concerns about the effects of the disorder	Making the unknown known may decrease anxiety
	Assess patient's knowledge of sickle cell anemia and correct misunderstandings	
	Teach relaxation measures	Relaxation decreases the psychomotor responses to anxiety

Nursing diagnosis: Potential for infection: related to spleen dysfunction, inadequate primary defense (broken skin) and inadequate secondary defenses (decreased hemoglobin)

Expected patient outcomes	Nursing interventions	Rationale
Infection does not occur	Use good medical asepsis	Aseptic technique decreases patient's contact with pathogenic organisms; infection is predicted on type and number of organisms to which individuals are exposed and patient resistance to infection
	Restrict persons (staff/visitors) with any type of infection.	Restricting persons with infection decreases patient's contact with infectious agents

Person with sickle cell crisis—cont'd

Nursing diagnosis: Pain in joints and chest related to poor pain management techniques, lack of knowledge

Expected patient outcomes	Nursing interventions	Rationale
Patient states feeling comfortable	Give prescribed analgesics as necessary and evaluate effectiveness of medication: obtain orders for increased doses if necessary	Pain of sickle cell crisis is excruciating, large doses of medication may be required
	Identify measures patient has found helpful and include these measures in the care	Patients often have the most accurate information for their pain control
	Support joints gently when assisting patient to do ROM exercises	Improper support increases stress on joints and increases pain
	Use moist heat or massage, if helpful	Heat dilates blood vessels and increases circulation to the area
		Massage may increase circulation, relax tense muscles
	Use other pain-relieving measures; person with frequent crises may benefit from learning special techniques such as biofeedback or self-hypnosis	Biofeedback, self-hypnosis decrease the physiologic responses to pain (muscle spasm, increased pulse)

Nursing diagnosis: Impaired gas exchange: related to ventilation-perfusion imbalance

Expected patient outcomes	Nursing interventions	Rationale
No dyspnea occurs with activity Patient states feeling rested	Provide prescribed oxygen as needed	High concentration of O_2 in alveoli increases diffusion across membranes
	Limit activities and provide periods of rest	Decreased activity decreases O_2 needs of body
	Provide prescribed medications for fever/infection (antibiotics, antipyretics)	Antibiotics destroy pathogenic organisms and must be administered at times ordered to be effective
	Administer prescribed transfusion (packed red cells)	Packed cells increase the number of RBC available to carry O_2 to tissue cells in the anemic person

Nursing diagnosis: Potential sexual dysfunction: related to fatigue, pain, fear of pregnancy

Expected patient outcomes	Nursing interventions	Rationale
Patient and partner state the sexual relationship is satisfying	Discuss coital positions that require less energy for the person who becomes tired easily	Coitus requires energy, and involves neuromuscular activity; sidelying or male-inferior position is less demanding for male patient
	Suggest coitus at times of day when patient is less fatigued (morning, afternoon)	Fatigue increases with continued daily activities and demand on cardiovascular system
	Discuss genetic counseling and contraceptive methods for person fearful of having a child with sickle cell disease	Knowledge of and use of reliable methods to prevent pregnancy reduce fear that may cause sexual dysfunction

NURSING CARE PLAN

Person with sickle cell crisis—cont'd

Nursing diagnosis: Altered tissue perfusion: related to stasis and blockage of microcirculation by sickled cells

Expected patient outcomes	Nursing interventions	Rationale
Signs of thrombosis do not occur Leg ulcers, renal insufficiency and ocular microinfarction do not occur	Give prescribed IV fluids; because large amounts may be given, monitor patient for fluid overload	Increased hydration decreases blood viscosity and stasis and increases circulation to vital areas; renal failure decreases the kidney's ability to excrete water and sodium, causing fluid overload
	Encourage oral fluids, if permitted	Oral fluids are easier to administer with less discomfort to patient and less chance for septicemia resulting from long IV therapy
	Monitor for signs of thrombosis (pain in chest or abdomen, headache, decreased vision, oliguria, or low urinary specific gravity)	Stasis and blockage of vascular system may cause infarction of heart, abdominal vessels, brain, eye grounds
	Assess legs, especially medial malleoli for signs of skin breakdown; use measures to prevent skin dryness or injury from trauma	Prevention of skin breakdown due to inadequate blood supply requires frequent monitoring; dry skin and trauma to legs increases potential for injury

Nursing diagnosis: Self-esteem disturbance: related to loss of body function, change in life-style and masculine role

Expected patient outcomes	Nursing interventions	Rationale
Patient states satisfaction with life and self	Provide opportunities for patient to discuss feelings about inability to fulfill expected roles	Verbalization of concerns decreases their impact and assists in problem solving
	Assist patient to identify personal strengths	Focusing on strengths and positive factors provides the baseline for personal growth
	Assist patient to explore alternative ways to meet role expectations	Concern over losses may immobilize patient; assistance in exploring alternatives is a therapeutic role of the nurse
	Suggest joining a support group or obtaining counseling to minimize dependency behaviors	Research shows that increased social support from family and groups increases recovery from disease and disability and facilitates rehabilitation

NURSING CARE PLAN

Person with sickle cell crisis—cont'd

Nursing diagnosis: Knowledge deficit: related to lack of exposure/recall and unfamiliarity with information sources

Expected patient outcomes	Nursing interventions	Rationale
Patient/family describe the nature of the disorder and care requirements	Review with patient the basis of sickle cell disease and genetic effects	Knowledge of causes of disease is *one* factor in ensuring patient compliance with medical regimen and adherence to preventative measures
	Provide resources for family planning and genetic counseling	Individuals and groups with in-depth knowledge of family planning methods help patients identify a family planning method that conforms to the patient's cultural and religious values
	Teach patient to avoid situations that cause crises (see text)	(See first rationale and text)
	Teach patient to drink 4 to 6 quarts fluid daily	Dehydration is a primary cause of RBC sickling

PLANNING: EXPECTED PATIENT OUTCOMES

Expected patient outcomes for the person with sickle cell disease may include, but are not limited to, the following:
1. Signs of anxiety are decreased.
2. Patient states pain is relieved.
3. Blood gases are within normal limits for the patient, no dyspnea.
4. Oxygenation of tissues is adequate: no signs of thrombosis, renal and ocular occlusions.
5. No signs and symptoms of infection are present.
6. Patient and significant other state that the sexual relationship is satisfying.
7. Patient and family express feelings of self-worth and ability to carry out responsibilities.
8. Patient and family describe
   a. Basis of anemia
   b. Availability of genetic counseling
   c. Causes of sickle cell crisis

IMPLEMENTATION

☐ Assisting with achievement of therapeutic goals

Since there is no specific therapy for sickle cell anemia, treatment is symptomatic. Polyvalent pneumococcal vaccine is often advised because of the high risk for pneumococcal infections. When surgery is performed, special attention should be given to adequate ventilation, oxygenation, and hydration.

Therapeutic pheresis therapy may be instituted. This is a process of separating whole blood into its major components, RBCs (erythropheresis), WBCs (leukapheresis), platelets (plateletpheresis), and plasma (plasma exchange). The component that is causing disease is then removed, and the normal cells returned or replaced. Pheresis therapy is not a cure for the disease but a way of intervening with the pathophysiology. It is usually used when all conventional therapy has been tried and is a last resort effort.[28] It is also used for hemolytic anemia, leukemia, thrombocytosis, polycythemia vera, and autoimmune disease.

☐ Assisting with comfort

Pain management regimens, often including the use of narcotics, may be necessary with sickle cell anemia. Astute evaluation of the pain and its management are key nursing activities. Sickle cell patients may be labeled as malingerers because some of them demonstrate difficult behavior patterns that are influenced by their chronic illness and at times by drug abuse. Pain of sickle cell crisis is excruciating and medications must be given constantly; either orally, intramuscularly or intravenously.

☐ Promoting hydration

Because dehydration causes increased blood viscosity, persons with sickle cell crisis should drink at least 4 liters of fluid daily[38] and at least 6 to 8 liters during a crisis. If intravenous fluids are administered, small-bore needles (No. 23) are used and fluids are maintained as prescribed to prevent underhydration and further sickling or overhydration and congestive heart failure.

Nursing care of the patient with sickle cell anemia

1. Promoting adequate hydration
   a. Maintain intake of at least 4000 ml, unless contraindicated
   b. Maintain IV fluids as ordered
2. Maintaining tissue oxygenation
   a. Avoid overexertion by patient
   b. Maintain oxygen by mask or cannula as ordered
3. Preventing infection (same as for leukemia, p. 892)
4. Providing comfort
   a. Give pain medication as ordered
   b. Evaluate response to medication to determine if increased dosage is needed
   c. Do not discount severity of pain
5. Promoting psychologic comfort
   a. Encourage independence and productive life (refer to work classification clinic, if necessary)
   b. Be a good listener and give information to decrease anxiety

---

☐ Maintaining tissue oxygenation

Patients are taught to maintain a balance between rest and exercise to prevent increased oxygen expenditure, hypoxemia and sickle cell crisis. Oxygen by mask or cannula may be given during crisis to increase delivery to oxygen-deprived cells.

☐ Counseling and teaching

Counseling and the use of support groups are to be encouraged for patients with sickle cell disease so as to minimize behavioral dependency. Support is given to help the person be as independent and productive as possible, a difficult situation when sickle cell crises are frequent. In caring for this patient population it is helpful to maintain a sense of respect and consideration for persons who experience frequent crises and yet continue to try to live as normal a life as possible. Long-term counseling may be needed for severe psychosocial difficulties. Genetic counseling is indicated for persons with congenital hemolytic anemias.

Patients with congenital hemolytic anemias also need to know about their disease to dispel myths and misconceptions and to decrease anxiety. Important points to include in teaching these patients include the following:
1. Nature of sickle cell or other genetic disease
2. Avoidance of situations that cause crisis (infection, overexertion, emotional stress, alcohol, cigarette smoking)[36]
3. Importance of adequate fluid intake
4. Good hygiene practices (same as for aplastic anemia)
5. Family planning techniques, if desired

⌗ EVALUATION

Questions to ask the patient may include the following:
1. Is the patient free from signs of anxiety?
2. Is the patient comfortable?
3. Are blood gases within normal limits and is the patient breathing easily?
4. Is circulation adequate to extremities, is urine output and visual acuity adequate?
5. Is the patient free from signs of infection?
6. Does the patient verbalize satisfaction with life-style, sexual relationships, and role in the family?
7. Can the patient state the nature of the disease and situations that exacerbate symptoms?

■ Anemia secondary to nutritional deficiency

The nutritional anemias include iron-deficiency anemia and the megaloblastic anemias.

■ PATHOPHYSIOLOGY

☐ Iron deficiency anemia

Iron is a fundamental part of the Hb molecule, and its deficiency leads to production of red cells with a decreased amount of Hb and ultimately to a decreased number of red cells. The average adult body contains approximately 4 g of iron, 3 g of which are in Hb. Average daily loss of iron by the body is approximately 1.5 mg, which is compensated for by absorption from the diet of approximately that amount of iron daily. This tenuous balance may be compromised by chronic blood loss, which may be physiologic such as in menstruation or pathologic as in GI or other bleeding.

It is also common in menstruating women, pregnant women, and growing children. Aged individuals may eat an imbalanced diet because of limited income, mobility and isolation from those people who might help with preparation or purchase of food.

The anemia is characteristically hypochromic and microcytic (low MCHC and low MCH).

☐ Megaloblastic anemia

Megaloblastic anemia is characterized by the presence of megaloblasts (immature progenitors of abnormal RBCs) in the bone marrow. The red cells are macrocytic. There is a deficit in the nucleus of the maturing red cell as a result of interference with DNA synthesis from a nutritional deficiency, primarily vitamin B_{12} or folic acid.

☐ *Vitamin B_{12} deficiency*

Vitamin B_{12} requires the presence of an intrinsic factor from gastric secretion for absorption in the ileum. A vitamin B_{12} deficiency rarely results from a decreased intake but rather from decreased absorption. Two interferences with absorption include lack of intrinsic factor or direct interference with the transport of vitamin B_{12} across the membrane in the ileum. Intrinsic factor may be absent as a result of genetic factors (pernicious anemia) or from surgical resection of the stomach. Malabsorption in the ileum may result from malabsorption syndromes, small bowel diverticuli, intestinal inflammations, or intestinal resection.

Because vitamin B_{12} can be stored in the body, deficiencies may not produce symptoms for many years. Diagnosis of pernicious anemia is confirmed by an abnormal Schilling test, which demonstrates the inability to absorb vitamin B_{12} unless intrinsic factor is administered.

☐ *Folic acid deficiency*

Folic acid (folacin) is a vitamin of the B complex that is involved in the synthesis of amino acids and DNA and therefore in the maturation of RBCs. Folic acid deficiency results from inadequate dietary intake (often associated with chronic alcoholism), malabsorption syndromes, and certain medications that inhibit the enzyme involved in normal absorption of folate through the intestinal wall. Vitamin B_{12} deficiency and folic acid deficiency often occur together.

▊ ASSESSMENT

The following subjective data are collected from patients with nutritional anemias:
1. Knowledge of cause of anemia
2. Adequacy of diet

Food sources for nutrients required for RBC production

Iron	Liver, beef, egg yolk Dried fruits and legumes, dark green leafy vegetables Whole-grain products
Vitamin B_{12}	Liver, beef, eggs, chicken, milk
Folic acid	Liver, yeast, dark green leafy vegetables

---

3. Financial constraints on buying necessary foods
4. Ability to obtain and prepare food
5. Knowledge of food sources of deficient nutrient (see the box below)
6. Presence of fatigue, loss of balance, numbness, and tingling of feet

Objective data include skin color (pallor). A smooth inflamed tongue (glossitis) may be noted with pernicious anemia.

➡ DATA ANALYSIS: NURSING DIAGNOSES

Nursing diagnoses are determined from assessment of patient data. Possible nursing diagnoses for the person with anemia secondary to nutritional deficiency may include, but are not limited to, the following:

Diagnostic title	Possible etiologies
Activity intolerance	Generalized weakness resulting from decreased tissue oxygenation
Fatigue	Decreased metabolic energy production
Knowledge deficit	Lack of teaching resources
Altered nutrition: less than body requirements (iron, vitamin B_{12}, folic acid)	Knowledge deficit (balanced diet, effect of blood loss) economic limitations, inability to obtain or prepare food, social isolation

▊ PLANNING: EXPECTED PATIENT OUTCOMES

Expected patient outcomes for the person with nutritional anemias may include, but are not limited to, the following:
1. Patient describes causes and nature of anemias.
2. Patient plans menus and eats foods high in the deficient nutrient, if appropriate.
3. Patient explains need for replacement therapy and for medical follow-up.
4. Hemoglobin and hematocrit levels are within normal limits.
5. Feelings of fatigue are decreased.

▊ IMPLEMENTATION

Care of patients with nutritional anemias involves primarily teaching and counseling in relation to medications, diet, and need for medical treatment of conditions causing chronic blood loss.

The medical treatment for nutritional anemias is primarily drug replacement therapy (Table 27-4). Because iron may be irritating to the GI tract, ferrous sulfate should be taken after meals. The person should also be told that stools will be black and to report any symptoms of diarrhea or nausea to the physician. Vitamin B_{12} replacement therapy must be given parenterally because of the decreased oral absorptive capabilities. Life-long therapy is necessary for persons with pernicious anemia.

Poor diet is rarely the sole cause of iron-deficiency anemia, but it may be a contributing factor. It must be remembered that encouraging the intake of iron-rich foods for anemia is only effective *if the anemia is caused by an iron deficiency* and if the person can absorb the iron through the GI tract.

When indicated, follow-up through a clinic, home visits by a dietitian or community health nurse, and such community resources as Meals on Wheels can be effective ways of assuring the person of a well-balanced diet that includes the deficient nutrients. Persons who drink excessively may be referred to Alcoholics Anonymous.

⊞ EVALUATION

Questions to ask may include the following:
1. Can the patient explain the nature of the anemia and the correct method for taking the medication?
2. Is the patient eating foods rich in the deficient nutrient (if appropriate)?
3. Are hemoglobin and hematocrit levels increasing toward normal?

■ Erythrocytosis (polycythemia)

■ PATHOPHYSIOLOGY

Polycythemia, an abnormal increase in RBCs, may be primary or secondary. *Primary polycythemia (polycythemia vera)* is a proliferation disorder of unknown etiology. It is characterized by hyperplasia of the bone marrow; there is usually a simultaneous increase in WBCs and platelets.

Secondary polycythemia may result from cardiac, pulmonary, or renal disorders, or it may be stress related. Chronic hypoxia is a major cause of secondary polycythemia; it stimulates the production of the enzyme erythropoietin, which then stimulates the bone marrow to increase RBC production. More red cells are then available to carry oxygen.

The signs and symptoms of polycythemia are secondary to increased blood viscosity and total blood volume. Vasodilation occurs as a result of increased RBCs. There is also marked leukocytosis and thrombocytosis, which, along with the increased RBC count, predispose the person to thrombosis, tissue hypoxia and hemorrhage (Table 27-3).

▦ ASSESSMENT

Subjective data include reports of headache, blurred vision and fatigue. The person's knowledge about the nature of polycythemia is identified. Objective data include observations for signs of bleeding, such as nosebleeds or areas of ecchymosis. Principal laboratory tests to determine the nature of the erythrocytosis consist of determination of the arterial oxygen concentration, red cell volume, and plasma volume.

➡ DATA ANALYSIS: NURSING DIAGNOSES

Nursing diagnoses are determined from assessment of patient data. Possible diagnoses for the person with polycythemia include, but are not limited to, the following:

Diagnostic title	Possible etiologies
Knowledge deficit	Lack of exposure to pertinent information

⊞ PLANNING: EXPECTED PATIENT OUTCOMES

Expected patient outcomes for the person with polycythemia may include, but are not limited to, the following:
1. Patient explains the nature of the disorder, importance of continued medical care, and reason for therapy.
2. Patient learns foods to avoid.
3. Patient understands signs of thrombosis.

⊞ IMPLEMENTATION

Teaching the patient is the primary care for persons with polycythemia and includes the following:
1. Nature of the disorder
2. Importance of continued blood tests and medical care
3. Phlebotomy therapy
   a. Removal of 500 to 2000 ml blood per week until hematocrit level reaches 45%
   b. Repeat phlebotomy when hematocrit level rises over 50% (usually every 2 to 3 months)
4. Avoidance of foods high in iron content (liver, oysters, legumes)
5. Signs of extremity thromboses (swelling, redness, pain) requiring medical attention

⊞ EVALUATION

1. Can the person explain the nature of the disorder and rationale for therapy?
2. Does the person know signs of thrombosis requiring medical intervention?
3. Does the person describe plans to avoid iron-rich foods?

■ COAGULATION DISORDERS

Coagulation disorders may occur as a result of disturbance in the number or function of platelets or because of an absence of one or more clotting factors (p. 867). The 13 clotting factors, with the exception of tissue thromboplastin (III) and calcium ion (IV), are plasma proteins that circulate in the blood as inactive molecules. The clotting factors are activated by tissue injury. They also aid in clot dissolution (p. 865).

The coagulation process is thought to be activated when an enzyme splits off an inactive precursor (or precoagulant) of each factor. Each activated factor activates the succeeding procoagulant.[35] Two sequences of events have been identified: the extrinsic pathway and the intrinsic pathway. The *extrinsic* pathway requires tissue thromboplastin that is released by the vascular epithelium at the time of injury. The *intrinsic* pathway, activated by exposure to collagen within the damaged blood vessel, requires factors found within the plasma. In this sequence there is a "cascade" reaction, each factor being activated by the preceding type.

Table 27-6 Common bleeding/coagulation blood tests

[handwritten: Plat. last 10 days]

Test	Description	Normal value
Bleeding time	Evaluation of vascular and platelet factors—the time it takes for a small stab wound to stop bleeding	2 to 9 minutes
Clotting time	Time required for solid clot to form (less sensitive test than PTT)	5 to 10 minutes
Prothrombin time (PT)	Indicates rapidity of blood clotting (indicative of adequacy of extrinsic coagulation pathway; factors I, II, V, VII, X)	11 to 16 seconds; 100% as compared to control levels
Partial thromboplastin time (PTT)	More sensitive test than PT to evaluate adequacy of intrinsic coagulation pathway (fibrin clot formation)	60 to 90 seconds
Activated partial thromboplastin time (APTT)	Modified PTT; more sensitive; quicker to perform, frequently used to monitor heparin therapy and hemophilia	26 to 42 seconds

Both pathways appear to participate in hemostasis. Bleeding abnormalities can occur at any point in the coagulation process.

Coagulation disorders may be congenital or acquired. The most common *congenital* coagulation disorders are the hemophilias. Liver disease is the most common *acquired* coagulation disorder. The liver produces most of the clotting factors: II, V, VII, IX, X, and fibrinogen. Liver disease may produce impaired production of these clotting factors and an elevation of the prothrombin time (Table 27-6). A deficiency in vitamin K can also affect clotting since vitamin K is a cofactor in the synthesis of clotting factors II, VII, IX, and X. Approximately 50% of required vitamin K is obtained from a normal diet, and the remainder is produced by intestinal bacteria. Inactivation of intestinal bacteria by intestinal antibiotics can lead to vitamin K deficiency. DIC is also an acquired disorder of coagulation.

■ Platelet disorders— thrombocytopenia

Platelets are formed in the bone marrow. In the normal adult approximately 80% of the platelets are in free circulation and 20% are stored in the spleen. It is estimated that the normal life span of platelets is approximately 10 days. Laboratory values for a normal adult platelet count range from 150,000 to 400,000/mm³.

Changes in platelet function will interfere with coagulation. Altered platelet function may be congenital or acquired. Aspirin inhibits the release of intrinsic platelet ADP and produces a defect in platelet aggregation. The defect remains for the life of the platelet, and clot formation is inhibited.

Changes in circulating platelet numbers can also affect coagulation. *Thrombocytosis* (increase in number of circulating platelets) is usually seen in association with other diseases. The danger of thrombocytosis is that it may lead to thrombosis or abnormal bleeding (Table 27-7). Care of the patient is similar to that for persons receiving anticoagulation therapy. *Thrombocytopenia* (decrease in number of circulating platelets) leads to bleeding.

■ PATHOPHYSIOLOGY

Thrombocytopenia can be caused by decreased platelet production or increased platelet destruction. Decreased production is usually caused by drugs (see the box below) or bone marrow suppression from chemotherapy or radiotherapy.

The most common thrombocytopenia from increased platelet destruction is *idiopathic thrombocytopenia purpura* (ITP). It occurs most commonly in the second and third decades in life and is caused by production of an autoantibody (IgG), which is directed against a platelet antigen. It is manifested by excessive bleeding, which may be reflected in purpuric lesions on the skin or by visceral bleeding (Table 27-7).

▦ ASSESSMENT

Subjective data include eliciting a history of recent viral infection, as this may produce transient thrombocytopenia. A detailed history of drug and alcohol use is also obtained.

Objective data include observing the patient for the presence of ecchymoses (bruises or black and blue marks caused by bleeding into the subcutaneous tissues and skin) and petechiae (1 to 4 mm flat, round, purple-red hemorrhagic bruises in the skin), bleeding gums, vaginal bleeding, GI bleeding, or hematuria.

Drugs with thrombocytopenic effects

Alcohol
Nonsteroidal antiinflammatory agents (azathioprine, D-penicillamine, phenylbutazone)
Oral hypoglycemics
Quinidine
Salicylates
Sulfonamides
Thiazides

Table 27-7 Disorders of coagulation (platelets)

Disorder	Etiology	Signs and symptoms	Medical therapy
Idiopathic thrombocytopenia purpura (ITP)	Autoimmunity, infections	Petechiae, ecchymoses, easy bruising; platelet count below 10,000 cu/mm, prolonged bleeding time	Corticosteroids, splenectomy, transfusion with platelet concentration
Secondary thrombocytopenia	Aplastic anemia, acute leukemia, megaloblastic anemia, chemotherapeutic agents; conditions causing splenomegaly (cirrhosis, lymphomas), drugs	Same as above	Correct underlying cause
Altered platelet function	Drugs (aspirin, indomethacin, phenylbutazone), uremia	Same as above; symptoms mild	Correct underlying cause
Thrombocytosis	Myeloproliferative disorders; stress, hemorrhage, hemolytic anemia, splenectomy, iron deficiency anemia, tuberculosis	Bleeding (mucosal areas, especially GI tract); thrombosis (primarily venous, but may be arterial)	Cytotoxic drugs to decrease bone marrow activity; platelet pheresis, aspirin
Hemophilia	Genetic	Lifelong bleeding into any part of body, spontaneously or after trauma; may be into joints or retroperitoneal, intracranial areas; signs of blood loss	Replacement of deficient coagulation factor VIII or IX; topical coagulants (fibrin foam or thrombin); concentrated preparations of fibrinogen; plasma pheresis to remove antibody inhibitors against factor VIII
Disseminated intravascular clotting (DIC)	Massive tissue damage, endotoxins, postpartum, sepsis, shock	Diffuse bleeding into mucous membranes and tissues, wound sites; renal failure; prolonged prothrombin time	Correct underlying problem, cardiovascular support, platelet packs, cryoprecipitate, fresh whole blood; hemodialysis for renal failure

Diagnostic tests include laboratory studies and bone marrow examination (p. 871). Commonly used tests for assessment of platelets include platelet count, peripheral blood smear, and bleeding time, which is usually prolonged. The bone marrow is examined for the presence of *megakaryocytes* (precursors of platelets in the bone marrow). Their presence suggests that the thrombocytopenia is caused by peripheral platelet destruction, and their absence or decrease suggests a failure of thrombopoiesis.

DATA ANALYSIS: NURSING DIAGNOSES

Nursing diagnoses are determined from assessment of patient data. Possible nursing diagnoses for the person with thrombocytopenia may include, but are not limited to:

Diagnostic title	Possible etiologies
Potential for injury: hemorrhage	Inadequate clotting mechanism, knowledge deficit
Knowledge deficit	Lack of information

PLANNING: EXPECTED PATIENT OUTCOMES

Expected patient outcomes for the person with thrombocytopenia may include, but are not limited to, the following:

1. Injuries do not occur.
2. Patient can describe signs of decreased platelets.
3. Patient understands medication regimen.
4. Patient can describe measures to prevent injury.
5. Patient understands need for medical follow-up.

IMPLEMENTATION

The medical management of idiopathic thrombocytopenic purpura includes corticosteroid therapy and splenectomy. Steroids appear to decrease the autoantibody that is directed against the platelet antigen. Splenectomy removes the organ primarily responsible for destruction of the antibody-coated platelets. Danazol, gamma globulin, or immunosuppressive drugs also may be administered.

Teaching for the patient with thrombocytopenia

1. Nature of the disorder
2. Signs of decreased platelets (petechiae, ecchymoses, gingival bleeding, hematuria, menorrhagia)
3. Name dosage, frequency, side effects of prescribed medications (corticosteroids) and importance of not stopping corticosteroid medications suddenly
4. Measures to prevent injury/hemorrhage
   a. Use soft toothbrush or swab for mouth care
   b. Keep mouth clean and free of debris
   c. Avoid intrusions into rectum (for example, rectal medications, enemas)
   d. Use electric shaver
   e. Apply direct pressure for 5 to 10 minutes if any bleeding occurs
   f. Avoid contact sports, elective surgery, and tooth extraction
   g. Avoid picking or blowing nose forcefully
   h. Avoid trauma, falls, bumps, cuts; avoid contact sports
   i. Avoid use of aspirin or aspirin preparations
   j. Use adequate lubrication and gentleness during sexual intercourse
5. Need for follow-up medical care

Nursing care is primarily teaching the patient with thrombocytopenia. Of primary concern is the bleeding tendency and measures taken to prevent hemorrhage and injury (see the box above). Bleeding associated with trauma is likely with a platelet count less than 60,000/mm³. The need for avoidance of trauma is obvious. Spontaneous hemorrhage looms as a life-threatening possibility in individuals with a platelet count of less than 20,000/mm³. Teaching should also include signs of decreased platelets (petechiae, ecchymosis, hematuria, menorrhagia), and the need for continuous follow-up medical care.

✠ EVALUATION

Questions to ask might include the following:
1. Is patient free of injury and hemorrhage?
2. Is skin intact?
3. Can patient explain therapeutic measures, signs of decreased platelets, and measures to prevent injury?

■ Hemophilia

■ PATHOPHYSIOLOGY

Hemophilia is a hereditary coagulation disorder. Both hemophilia A (factor VIII deficiency) and hemophilia B, also called Christmas disease (factor IX deficiency), are inherited as sex-linked recessive disorders and are therefore almost exclusively limited to males. An example of the inheritance pattern of hemophilia is shown in Fig. 27-7.

The degree of bleeding is related to the amount of factor activity and the severity of injury. Spontaneous bleeding, joint bleeding (hemarthrosis) and deep tissue hemorrhage occur with factor levels less than one percent. Retroperitoneal and intracranial bleeding may also occur and may be life-threatening. Patients may experience bleeding after

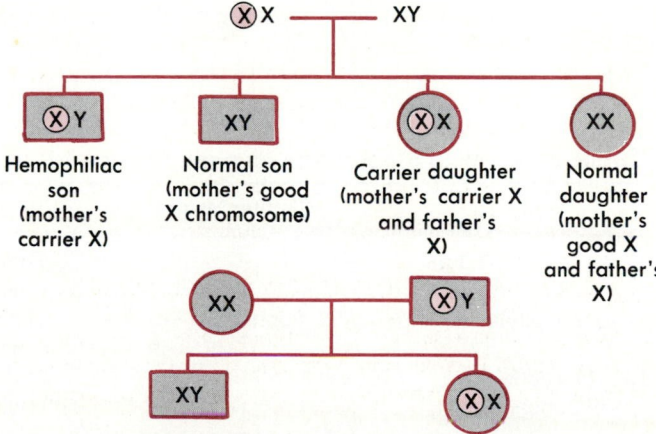

Defective gene is found on X chromosome. When faulty X chromosome is present in a male, the male will be a hemophiliac.

Ⓧ Y

When faulty X chromosome is present in a female, she will be a carrier of hemophilia.

Ⓧ X

In conception between a normal male and a carrier female, four possibilities arise:

In conception between a hemophiliac male and a normal female, son will be normal but daughter will be carrier.

Fig. 27-7 Pattern of inheritance of hemophilia.

tooth extraction, minor trauma, or during surgical procedures. Any body system may be affected.

ASSESSMENT

Subjective data include the patient's and family's knowledge of the disorder, measures taken to prevent injury, and coping mechanisms. If pain or bleeding are present, possible causes are explored to ascertain if these could have been prevented (data useful for teaching future prevention). *Objective data* include presence of bleeding or swelling of joints (indicating joint bleeding).

A diagnosis of hemophilia is made by specific assays for factors VIII and IX. The partial thromboplastin time (PTT) (Table 27-6) is prolonged in both types of hemophilia. The platelet count and prothrombin time are normal.

DATA ANALYSIS: NURSING DIAGNOSES

Nursing diagnoses are determined from assessment of patient data. Possible nursing diagnoses for the person with hemophilia may include, but are not limited to, the following:

Diagnostic title	Possible etiologies
Pain: joints	Swelling and hemorrhage
Ineffective individual and family coping	Situational crisis (hemorrhagic episodes)
Potential for injury	Knowledge deficit, environmental hazards
Knowledge deficit	Lack of exposure/recall, unfamiliarity with information resources

PLANNING: EXPECTED PATIENT OUTCOMES

Expected patient outcomes for the patient with hemophilia may include, but are not limited to, the following:
1. Patient states feeling comfortable.
2. Patient and family are able to problem solve.
3. Patient identifies and avoids possible sources of trauma.

4. Patient or family can describe signs and symptoms requiring immediate medical intervention.
5. Patient or family can describe ways to prevent excessive bleeding.
6. Patient or family state awareness of community resources for hemophiliacs and genetic counseling services.
7. Patient states plans to carry medical identification information.
8. Patient states plans for follow-up care.

IMPLEMENTATION

☐ **Assisting with achievement of therapeutic goals**

Bleeding disorders may require local treatment such as ice bags, manual pressure or dressings, immobilization, and elevation of a body part. Joint aspiration may be necessary. Muscle stretching exercises are begun after pain and bleeding have subsided (usually within 3 to 5 days). Active range of motion exercises are encouraged when swelling has subsided.

With major hemorrhages, careful monitoring is necessary to avoid fluid overload if large plasma volumes are given. Concentrates (Table 27-8) provide the deficient factors and prevent fluid overload and fewer side effects (such as urticarial or febrile reactions) in some patients. High cost and contamination with the virus of serum hepatitis are drawbacks, however, to the use of some of the concentrates.

Persons with hemophilia also have a higher risk of developing AIDS because of contamination of factor VIII concentrate with the HIV virus. Since 1983, donated blood from which the concentrate is extracted has been tested for the virus and the heat treatment now used for factor VIII concentrate will kill the virus.

Factor replacement therapy may be given on an outpatient basis, either in a clinic or in the home. Home infusion programs have gained interest and are seen as a way of controlling bleeding episodes more quickly, thereby decreasing the need for hospitalization and a long absence from school or work.

Table 27-8 Blood factor replacement therapy for hemophilia

Type	Clotting factors	Comments
Fresh frozen plasma	All	Thawed to 37° C before infusion; allergic reactions are common; fluid overload possible, especially in older persons
Cryoprecipitate	VIII, fibrinogen	Thawed to 37° C before infusion; occasional allergic reactions; low risk of hepatitis transmission, administer at 12-hour intervals
Lyophilized factor VIII concentrate	VIII	Stable at room temperature; possible hemolytic reactions for persons with blood types A, B, AB when given over prolonged period; allergic reactions rare
Vitamin K dependent complex	VII, IX, X, prothrombin	Keep refrigerated; higher risk of hepatitis transmission and thrombus formation (heparin usually given concurrently)

Teaching for the patient with hemophilia

1. Nature of the disease, genetic basis
2. Prevention of hemorrhage (p. 885)
3. Possibility of bleeding after dental extraction
4. Avoidance of contact sports
5. Importance of carrying a card or wearing a Medic-Alert tag with name, blood type, physician's name and phone number, and diagnosis
6. Community resources (National Hemophilia Foundation)
7. Family planning techniques if desired
8. Need for medical follow-up

A synthetic drug that is effective against mild hemophilia and von Willebrand's disease (deficiencies in factor VIII and in platelet adhesion) is desmopressin (DDAVP). It is administered intravenously and can cause a threefold to sixfold increase in factor VIII activity.

The outlook for the person with hemophilia has been greatly improved by the availability of transfusion therapy. In the past many people with factor VIII deficiency died in the first 5 years of life. Today people with moderate or mild hemophilia may live normal, productive lives.

☐ Counseling and teaching

Threat of spontaneous bleeding episodes and pain control are ongoing stressors the individual must confront.[38] Important points for teaching are listed in the box above. Those individuals who are able to meet the demands of their illness and adapt their life-styles accordingly are able to live productive lives as individuals, spouses, parents, and employees.

Genetic counseling, aimed at explaining the pattern of inheritance of hemophilia, may be of great value to adults contemplating parenthood. Such counseling can assist potential parents in evaluating realistically their ability to raise a child afflicted with hemophilia and to anticipate ways to meet the demands placed on both of them and the child.[21]

The National Hemophilia Foundation* is an organization established for persons with hemophilia and their families. The basic function of the national organization is hemophilia research. In addition, it publishes literature, produces films, and promotes health care legislation in Washington. Local chapter services include special camps for children with hemophilia, counseling and group therapy sessions, and a newsletter that reports on advances in hemophilic care. A chapter may function as a liaison agent between hospitals and families with insurmountable bills for blood.

*25 West 39th St., New York, NY 10018.

⊞ EVALUATION

Questions to ask the patient may include the following:
1. Is the person comfortable?
2. Is the person/family able to deal with the stresses associated with the disorder?
3. Can the patient state sources of injury, hemorrhage?
4. Can the patient describe signs and symptoms of hemorrhage?
5. Does the person know the nature of the disease, ways to prevent hemorrhage, available resources?

■ Disseminated intravascular coagulation

Disseminated intravascular coagulation (DIC) is a pathophysiologic response of the body's hemostatic mechanisms to disease or injury. DIC is a complicated and potentially fatal syndrome that is characterized initially by clotting and secondarily by hemorrhage.

It occurs in any condition where tissue thromboplastin is liberated subsequent to tissue destruction. One of the most common causes is abruptio placentae, premature separation of the placenta. Tumor products, crushing trauma, burns and leukemia, vasculitis, sepsis and shock, as well as surgery (especially prostatic, orthopedic or open-heart) may also initiate DIC.[35]

■ PATHOPHYSIOLOGY

DIC is essentially an imbalance between the processes of coagulation and anticoagulation. The normal balance of clotting factors and fibrinolytic factors, which under normal conditions prevent bleeding while maintaining the fluidity of the blood, are altered.

The primary disease or injury causes the initiation of the clotting process. This response is generalized and occurs throughout the vascular system, creating a state of *hypercoagulability*. The fibrinolytic processes, which normally operate to limit clot extension and dissolve clots, are then stimulated (Fig. 27-8). As clotting factors are depleted and fibrinolysis continues, a state of *hypocoagulability* develops.

The most common sequela of DIC is hemorrhage. This paradox is caused by decreased platelets and the depletion of clotting factors, II, V, VIII, fibrinogen and the production of fibrin degradation products (FDP) through fibrinolysis. The FDP acts as anticoagulants, which increase the hemorrhagic tendency.

▥ ASSESSMENT

The first signs and symptoms (Table 27-7) may be those of hemorrhage (oral, vaginal, rectal, after injection and venipuncture, petechiae, and ecchymosis). Pain may be present from joint bleeding.

Laboratory findings, which may be the only indications of the syndrome in the early stages, may include the following:

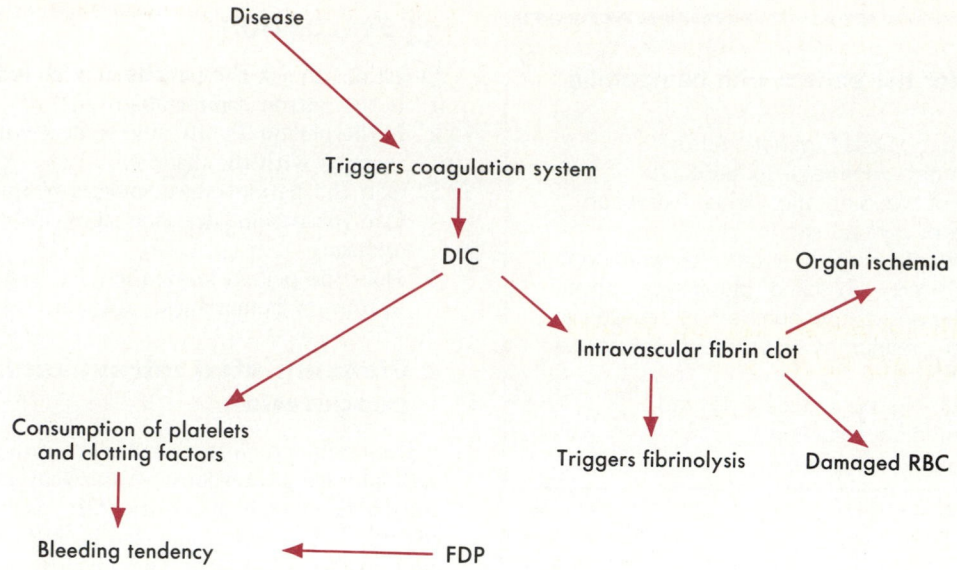

Fig. 27-8 Illustration of pathophysiology of disseminated intravascular coagulation, which may result in bleeding tendency, organ ischemia, and hemolytic anemia. (From Pagana, KD, and Pagana, TJ: Diagnostic testing and nursing implications, St. Louis, 1982, The CV Mosby Co).

1. Decreased circulating platelet count
2. Prolonged PT
3. Prolonged PTT
4. Decreased factors V and VIII
5. Decreased fibrinogen levels
6. Increased fibrin split products (fibrinolysis)
7. Abnormal RBCs on peripheral blood smear

➡ DATA ANALYSIS: NURSING DIAGNOSES

Nursing diagnoses include those related to fluid deficit.

PLANNING: EXPECTED PATIENT OUTCOMES

Expected patient outcomes are the same as those for acute blood loss (p. 869).

◼ IMPLEMENTATION

Medical management is aimed at correcting the underlying problem. Antibiotics, chemotherapeutic agents, and cardiovascular support may be used. Plasma factors with plasma and cryoprecipitate may be administered. The use of heparin is highly controversial; it is given to prevent tissue thromboplastin from activating the coagulation process and thus inhibiting the consumption of coagulation factors and fibrin deposition. The body is then able to produce enough plasma factor to stop the hemorrhage.

Nursing intervention in the care of the patient with DIC is extremely challenging. The person is critically ill and frequently has numerous sites of bleeding before DIC becomes evident. Frequently the patient is comatose, and the presence of purpura, numerous intravenous lines, and drainage tubes makes the patient's appearance especially

---

Nursing care of the patient with DIC

1. Monitor continually for bleeding sites or changes in amount of bleeding (especially if heparin therapy is given)
2. Assess and record amount of drainage from chest and nasogastric tubes and oozing from incisions
3. Monitor fluid rates; be alert for signs of fluid overload (increased pulse rate, distended jugular veins, and increased CVP)
4. Provide care for the critically ill patient (see Chapter 42)
5. Explain to family what is occurring and provide opportunities for expressions of feelings

upsetting to the family. Most of the primary conditions associated with DIC are of a sudden nature, and the family requires help in understanding this catastrophic occurrence and support during the long period of treatment.

Interventions for thrombocytopenia are applicable to the patient with DIC. The patient requires careful monitoring of fluid replacement therapy, renal function and fluid output, and signs and symptoms of further bleeding.

DISORDERS ASSOCIATED WITH WHITE BLOOD CELLS

Changes in number of white cells

NEUTROPENIA

Neutropenia is defined as a neutrophil count of less than 2000/mm³. It may occur as a primary hematologic disorder but is seen more often in association with other disorders, including malignant disease of the bone marrow, aplastic anemia, megaloblastic anemia, use of chemotherapeutic agents, starvation, and viral infections. Severe neutropenia can also occur as a reaction to drugs, particularly in the patient with aplastic anemia secondary to cytotoxic drugs. The degree of susceptibility to infection is in direct proportion to the degree of neutropenia. Individuals with marked neutropenia are at risk for contracting a life-threatening infection.

Agranulocytosis is an acute disease in which there is a sudden decrease in the number of WBCs, usually as the result of chemicals or drugs (sulfonamides, propylthiouracil, chloramphenicol, and bone marrow depressant drugs such as chemotherapeutic agents). Clinical signs include infection, malaise (discomfort, headache, lassitude, muscle aches), ulceration of mucous membranes, chills, and fever. A sepsis may develop, which may lead to death. Care is directed toward removal of the causative agents and resolving infection. If bone marrow is not destroyed, the prognosis for recovery is good.

Granulocyte transfusions may be used for the patient with severe neutropenia. Nursing interventions focus on prevention of infections (see the box above) and careful monitoring for early signs of infection so that prompt therapy can be begun. Because neutrophil count is low, some of the classic signs of infection and the inflammatory response (purulent drainage, abscess formation, sequestration of a local infection) may be absent (Chapter 37). Fever may also be absent because of a lack of the endogenous pyrogens that are produced by neutrophils in response to infection.

NEUTROPHILIA

Neutrophilia is defined as a neutrophil count greater than 10,000/mm³. Such an increase is a normal response to infections, primarily bacterial. It may also increase with strenuous exercise. Prolonged elevation of the neutrophil

---

Teaching for the patient with leukopenia to prevent infection

1. Use good handwashing technique.
2. Avoid contact with persons with infections.
3. Avoid sharing eating utensils and bath linens.
4. Take daily baths with meticulous perineal care.
5. Use good oral hygiene, avoiding gum injury.
6. Keep environment clean.
7. Monitor for signs of infection (if present) and report these to physician.
8. Avoid eating raw meats and fresh fruits and vegetables.

---

count, especially in the absence of an apparent cause, is a reason for a diligent search for the underlying cause. Persistent elevated neutrophil counts are associated with leukemia, polycythemia vera, myeloid metaplasia, and a variety of systemic and inflammatory disorders. Treatment consists of therapy for the primary condition.

Leukemia

PATHOPHYSIOLOGY

Leukemias are malignant disorders of the hematopoietic system involving the bone marrow and lymph nodes; they are characterized by uncontrolled proliferation of leukocytes and their precursors. The large number of cells accumulate first at the site of origin (granulocytes in the bone marrow, lymphocytes in the lymph nodes), then spread to hematopoietic organs, leading to organ enlargement (splenomegaly, hepatomegaly). The proliferation of one type of cell often interferes with the normal production of other hematopoietic cells, leading to the development of immature cells and to cytopenias (decreased numbers). The immaturity of the white cells leads to decreased immunocompetence with increased susceptibility to infections.

The cause of leukemia is unknown. An increased incidence of leukemia in siblings has led to hypotheses of genetic predispositions or viral origins. Radiation and chemicals (including antineoplastic drugs) have also been implicated.

CLASSIFICATION OF LEUKEMIAS

The leukemias are classified as acute or chronic and further subdivided according to cell type or maturity of the cell (Table 27-9).

Acute leukemias

Acute leukemias involve immature cells and are classified according to the predominant cell in the bone marrow,

Table 27-9 Characteristics of different leukemias

Type	Peak age (years)	WBC level	Bone marrow cell predominance
Acute lymphocytic leukemia (ALL)	2 to 4	Decreased (granulocytopenia)	Lymphoblasts (B) ↑ in abnorm. ones
Acute myelogenous leukemia (AML)	12 to 20; after 55	Normal or decreased	Myeloblasts
Chronic lymphocytic leukemia (CLL)	50 to 70 males	Increased 20,000 to 100,000	Lymphocytes
Chronic myelogenous leukemia (CML)	30 to 50 males	Increased 15,000 to 500,000	Granulocytes, Philadelphia chromosome — abnormality

either lymphoblasts (acute lymphocytic leukemia) or myeloblasts (acute myelogenous leukemia). Acute leukemias have a rapid onset and a short course, ending in death if untreated. The immaturity of the white cells leads to numerous infections, such as ulcerations of the mucous membranes, pneumonias, and septicemias. Early symptoms include fever, lymphadenopathy, pallor, and fatigue from anemia, and ecchymoses (Table 27-10). The WBC count may be normal or decreased.

□ *Acute lymphocytic leukemia (ALL)*

ALL arises from a single lymphoid stem cell (Fig. 27-1) with impaired maturation and accumulation of the malignant cells in the bone marrow. It is common to find different stages of lymphoid development in the bone marrow from very immature to almost normal cells. The degree of immaturity is a guide to prognosis; the more immature cells, the poorer the prognosis. Leukocytes in the blood-

Table 27-10 Leukemias

Type	Etiology	Signs and symptoms	Medical therapy
Acute lymphocytic leukemia (ALL)	Genetic predisposition; environmental factors (ionizing radiation); chemicals (benzene, arsenic, chloramphenicol, antineoplastic agents); immune deficiency states *WBC ↓*	Respiratory infections, anemia, bleeding of mucous membranes; proliferation of lymphoblasts in bone marrow, lymph nodes, spleen; hepatomegaly; splenomegaly; bone pain; CNS symptoms (headache, vomiting, seizures)	Combined chemotherapy, radiotherapy and immunotherapy; drugs: vincristine, prednisone, L-asparaginase
Acute myelogenous leukemia (AML) — *granulocytic WBC ↓*	Same as above	Same as above	Chemotherapy with daunorubicin, cytarabine, doxorubicin, 6-thioguanine
Chronic lymphocytic leukemia (CLL) *WBC ↑* *you have ↓ immune response*	Same as above	Painless and massive lymphadenopathy and splenomegaly; hepatomegaly with disease progression; anemia; thrombocytopenia; fatigue; weakness, pruritic vesicular lesions	Chemotherapy with alkylating agents (chlorambucil) and glucocorticoids (only when symptoms appear)
Chronic myelogenous leukemia (CML) *WBC ↑* *abn. stem cell → prolif. of granulocytic cells*	Same as above	Fatigue, weakness, anorexia, weight loss; blastic (accelerated) phase: anemia, thrombocytopenia, fever, adenopathy, splenomegaly with sensation of abdominal fullness	Chemotherapy with agents used in AML; also vincristine, busulfan

stream are predominantly in the blast form. The WBC count is often decreased but a blood smear will show immature lymphoblasts. It is primarily a disease of children, but adults may develop it.

□ Acute myelogenous leukemia (AML)

AML arises from a single myeloid stem cell (see Fig. 27-1) and is characterized by the development of immature myeloblasts in the bone marrow. The WBC count is usually in the low ranges of normal, and bone marrow aspiration reveals an increased number of myeloblasts. In the untreated patient or the person who is nonresponsive to therapy, the median survival time (MST) is approximately 2 to 3 months. Complete remission occurs in 50% to 75% of treated patients, and there is an MST of approximately 2 to 3 years. Approximately 20% of patients are in complete remission at 5 years and are capable of prolonged disease-free periods (remissions).

□ Chronic leukemias

Chronic leukemias are classified according to the predominant mature white cell, either lymphocytes (chronic lymphocytic anemia) or granulocytes (chronic myelogenous leukemia). Chronic leukemias have a more insidious onset and an MST of 3 to 4 years. Initially there are fewer infections than in acute leukemias because of the maturity of the white cells in the chronic disorder, but eventually infections of the skin and pneumonias result from decreased immunocompetence. Early signs of chronic leukemias include fatigue, weakness, anorexia, and weight loss characteristic of a hypermetabolic state. An enlarged spleen and liver can usually be palpated. The WBC count is usually elevated.

□ Chronic lymphocytic leukemia (CLL)

CLL is characterized by a proliferation of small, abnormal, mature B-lymphocytes, leading to decreased synthesis of immunoglobulins and depressed antibody response. The accumulation of abnormal lymphocytes begins in the lymph nodes, then spreads to other lymphatic tissues. There is a marked increase in the number of both leukocytes and mature lymphocytes. At the time of diagnosis the bone marrow is often filled by lymphatic infiltrations. The WBC count is elevated to a level between 20,000 and 100,000. Bone marrow biopsy shows infiltration of lymphocytes.

□ Chronic myelogenous leukemia (CML)

The primary defect in CML is an abnormal stem cell leading to an uncontrolled proliferation of the granulocytic cells. As a result of this proliferation, there is a marked increase in the number of circulating granulocytes. In most cases, a characteristic chromosomal abnormality, the *Philadelphia chromosome*, is present. Diagnosis of CML is made on the basis of an elevated WBC count of 15,000 to 500,000, granulocytes on the peripheral blood smear that range in maturity from blast cells to mature neutrophils, granulocytic hyperplasia in the bone marrow, and the presence of the Philadelphia chromosome.

ASSESSMENT

Subjective data include eliciting feelings of weakness and fatigue, and a history of predisposition to infection. The person's knowledge of the nature of leukemia and concerns related to the disease are also obtained. The type of objective data depends on the type of leukemia and may include monitoring for lymphadenopathy, splenomegaly, fever, and pallor. The mouth is examined for breaks in the mucous membranes. The person is also observed for behavioral signs of anxiety.

Laboratory tests include bone marrow biopsy or aspiration, and WBC counts for differentiation of the type of leukemia (Table 27-9).

DATA ANALYSIS: NURSING DIAGNOSES

Nursing diagnoses are determined from assessment of patient data. Possible nursing diagnoses for the person with leukemia may include, but are not limited to, the following:

Diagnostic title	Possible etiologies
Activity intolerance	Generalized weakness, bed rest
Anxiety	Threat of death, change in health status, situational crisis
Ineffectual individual and family coping	Situational crises, prolonged disability, ineffective problem solving
Potential for infection	Chemotherapy or radiation therapy, disease process, knowledge deficit of preventive measures
Potential for injury: hemorrhage	Trauma, disease process, chemotherapy
Knowledge deficit	Lack of exposure/recall of information
Altered oral mucous membrane	Ineffective hygiene, malnutrition, infection, chemotherapy
Altered nutrition: less than body requirements	Anorexia, nausea and vomiting
Sexual dysfunction	Change in roles, psychologic stress, fatigue, weakness

PLANNING: EXPECTED PATIENT OUTCOMES

Expected patient outcomes for the person with leukemia may include, but are not limited to, the following:
1. Patient can assume activities of daily living.
2. Patient is comfortable, not unduly concerned, exhibits no signs of anxiety.
3. Patient and family are able to problem solve and find satisfying solutions.
4. Patient is free of infection.
5. Patient does not hemorrhage.
6. Patient or family can state the nature of the disease, the chemotherapeutic program, symptoms requiring follow-up, and available community resources.

7. Patient gains weight to within 10% of his or her normal weight.
8. Oral mucous membranes are intact.
9. Patient and significant other express satisfaction with sexual relationship.

▮ IMPLEMENTATION

Many of the interventions for the listed nursing diagnoses are discussed in the chapter on cancer (see Chapter 12).

□ Assisting with achievement of therapeutic goals

Leukemia, by its nature, is a diverse illness. The varied courses and response or lack of response to treatment also add to the diversity. Complete remission of the disease is the goal of medical therapy since cure is not possible at this time. Complete remission exists when all tests are normal and all symptoms have disappeared. Partial remission occurs when symptoms have disappeared but the disease remains in the bone marrow.

Patients with leukemia are at high risk of infection as a consequence of neutropenia. They may suffer from recurrent perirectal abcesses, pneumonia, and septicemias. Thrombocytopenia results in bleeding evidenced by petechiae, ecchymosis (bleeding into the skin), epistaxis (nosebleeds), and gastrointestinal and urinary tract hemorrhage. Prevention of infection and hemorrhage are of highest priority.

□ *Preventing infection*

1. Place patient in a private room; avoid contact with visitors and staff who have infection.
2. Place patient in protective isolation or laminar airflow room (see Chapter 12), if necessary.
3. Provide meticulous hygiene, including daily bath, careful oral hygiene, and perineal care; use antiseptic creams.
4. Avoid catheterizations.
5. Use povidone iodine skin cleansing for one minute before parenteral injections (or other preparation as prescribed).
6. Maintain a clean environment.
7. Provide emotional support for anxiety when infection occurs.

□ *Preventing hemorrhage*

1. Assess all sites for bleeding.
2. Test urine (Hemastix) and stool (guaiac) for blood.
3. Keep venipuncture and intramuscular injections to a minimum.
4. Apply pressure to venipuncture sites for 5 minutes, arterial sites for 10 minutes.
5. Use soft toothbrush or swab for mouth care.
6. Keep mouth clean and free of debris with normal saline rinse if bleeding occurs.
7. Avoid taking rectal temperatures, administering rectal medications, or giving enemas.
8. Avoid invasive procedures.

Chemotherapeutic agents commonly used in leukemia therapy

L-Asparaginase	Melphalan
Busulfan	6-Mercaptopurine
Chlorambucil	Methotrexate
Cyclophosphamide	Prednisone
Cytarabine	6-Thioguanine
Daunorubicin	Vincristine
Doxorubicin	

□ *Chemotherapy*

Chemotherapy is the primary treatment modality. The first phase of chemotherapy is termed *induction chemotherapy* and consists of combination chemotherapy (use of more than one chemotherapeutic agent, see Chapter 12). Commonly used agents used in the treatment of leukemias are listed in the box above. Bone marrow studies are conducted 2 and 3 weeks following initiation of therapy. A different drug regimen will be given if evidence of disease in the marrow is still present after 3 weeks.

During induction therapy, the patient is at high risk for hemorrhage or infection. In addition to the interventions listed at left, nursing care of the patient during this phase includes the following:

1. Monitor vital signs every 4 hours
2. Use of bleeding precautions
   a. Use soft toothbrush or swabs for mouth
   b. No rectal temperatures, medications, or enemas
   c. Use of electric razor
   d. Avoidance of aspirin
3. Monitor for signs of bleeding (observation of skin, testing urine with hemastix and stool for guaiac)
4. Give antibiotics on time to maintain blood levels if fever occurs
5. Monitor administration of whole blood or blood component therapy, if given
6. Assess intravenous site of chemotherapy for redness, swelling, tenderness, extravasation of drugs (Chapter 12)
7. Provide immediate care of extravasation of chemotherapeutic drugs (discontinue infusion, apply ice to area, infiltrate subcutaneous area with sodium bicarbonate or steroids)[6]
8. Provide emotional support to patient and family
   a. Time for them to talk, share fears and concerns, ask questions
   b. Carefully explain therapy and planned activities
   c. Include family in all aspects of care

Maintenance therapy, the second phase of therapy, is usually required to maintain a complete remission. This therapy is often given on an outpatient basis. Appropriate duration of therapy in patients who continue free of disease varies, depending on the type of the disease and the patient's response to therapy. Chemotherapy is discussed in more detail in Chapter 12.

□ Bone marrow transplantation

Bone marrow transplantation, using HLA-identical bone marrow, has been used with increasing frequency and promises to have an increasing impact on the progress of AML. In addition to leukemia, bone marrow transplantation is being used for patients with lymphoma, aplastic anemia, thalassemia, and immunodeficiency disorders.

Pretransplant preparation is necessary for bone marrow transplantation. It has two goals, *immunosuppression* to allow acceptance of an immunologically nonidentical graft and *cytoreduction* to kill all tumor cells. This is accomplished by chemotherapy followed by total body irradiation.[16]

The procedure comprises taking 500 to 800 ml of blood and marrow cells from the donor, mixing it with heparin and tissue culture media, and then straining the mixture through a stainless-steel screen to break up marrow particles.[41] The marrow is then placed in a blood transfusion bag and administered intravenously through a Hickman catheter (see Chapter 12) at the same rate as RBC administration (about 4 hours).

About 40% to 50% of patients develop severe acute graft-vs-host reaction, which involves severe skin, liver, and GI symptoms and death[31] or veno-occlusive disease of the liver.[13] One approach being used to prevent graft-versus-host reaction is treatment of the donor marrow with monoclonal antibodies before transplantation; this removes mature T-cells, which cause the reaction, but leaves immature T-cells for prevention of infection (see Chapter 12).

Another method to prevent graft-versus-host reaction is *autologous* bone marrow transplant. Some of the *patient's* bone marrow is removed during a period of remission and frozen. It is stored for transplantation when needed by the patient.

Nursing care is focused on prevention of infection and on providing emotional support; skin care; and maintenance of fluid, electrolyte, and nutritional balance. Protective isolation (Chapter 12) may be used.

□ Counseling and teaching

Each individual with leukemia responds in a different way. It cannot be predicted for certain if an individual will respond to a prescribed treatment or how long a remission will last. Likewise, how the individual incorporates the illness into life is also unique to each person. Nursing has the key role in patient education. Of utmost importance in learning is the ability of the person to identify the body's signals that blood abnormalities exist. Bone pain, often severe, may signal blast crisis (acute proliferation of immature cells).

Individuals whose illness runs the course of several months to years often become very knowledgeable about their disease, blood components, related symptoms, and specific chemotherapeutic drugs. These persons sometimes discuss their progress in terms of changes in their blood

---

Teaching for the patient with leukemia

1. Nature of the disease process and its effects
2. Prevention of infection
3. Drug regimen: name, side effects (see Chapter 12)
4. Method of arranging for chemotherapy administration and periodic blood counts
5. Symptoms requiring immediate medical attention (fever, bleeding)
6. Available community resources (American Cancer Society, Leukemia Society*)
7. Need for continual medical follow-up

*211 East 43rd St. New York, NY 10017.

counts. Over time many individuals become attuned to how such changes affect them. For example, they often can predict their count by how they feel. Many such persons respond well to being included in their plan of care during hospitalization and in preparation for discharge.

Time set aside for patient teaching also allows for a sharing time with the individual. This time may provide the foundation for an honest nurse-patient relationship from which emotional support may be given.

✚ EVALUATION

Questions to ask the patient may include the following:
1. Is the patient knowledgeable about the disease, its effects, and the treatment regimen?
2. Can the patient describe symptoms that require medical intervention?
3. Can the patient state importance of and schedule for chemotherapy and periodic blood tests?
4. Are the laboratory tests showing improvement toward normal values with therapy?
5. Is the patient free from anxiety?
6. Do the patient and family say they are coping with the illness?
7. Are the patient's oral mucous membranes pink and free of lesions?
8. Has the patient gained or at least maintained his or her weight?

■ DISORDERS ASSOCIATED WITH THE LYMPHATIC SYSTEM

■ Lymphadenopathy

Lymph node enlargement (lymphadenopathy) may be caused by infection in the area drained by the lymph vessel containing the node or by systemic infection. Enlargement of the node, which in this situation is usually painful, is

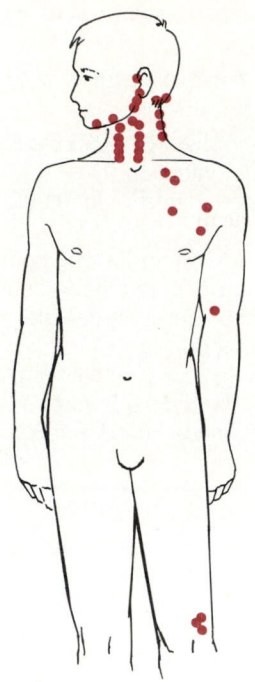

Fig. 27-9 Diagram of body areas where enlarged lymph nodes may be palpated.

a positive sign indicating immune responsiveness to the invading microorganisms. Lymphadenopathy may also occur when the node is invaded by cells normally not present (leukemic cells, cancer cells) and is a pathophysiologic sign with lymphomas, such as Hodgkin's disease. Some body areas where lymph nodes may be palpated are illustrated in Fig. 27-9.

Lymphangiography is a radiologic technique used for evaluation of lymph nodes to detect the presence of disease.

This procedure is especially valuable in the assessment of those nodes that are anatomically too deep to allow for evaluation by palpation. For this procedure a small incision is made on the dorsal surface of each foot so that the small lymph glands are made accessible. A dye is slowly instilled over several hours, filling all lymph chains and nodes. Radiographs are usually done immediately after the dye is absorbed and again at intervals of 24 and 48 hours after the procedure. In addition, because the dye remains in the lymph nodes for as long as 6 months after the initial study, disease status and response to therapy can be periodically evaluated with routine abdominal x-ray films.

■ Lymphomas

Lymphomas are malignant disorders of the lymph system. Hodgkin's disease is considered separate from other lymphomas (Table 27-11).

■ PATHOPHYSIOLOGY

□ Hodgkin's disease

Hodgkin's disease, which was considered fatal until fairly recently, is now potentially curable. Although the cause is unknown, it is thought that viruses may be implicated. The person has *defective cellular immunity (T-cell disease)* and is therefore at high risk for infections. Four pathologic variants of Hodgkin's have been recognized: *lymphocyte predominant, nodular sclerosis, mixed cellularity, and lymphocyte depletion*. The lymphocyte predominant and nodular sclerosis types have the best prognosis and lymphocyte depletion the worst. Hodgkin's disease is usually characterized by the presence of the Reed-Sternberg cell, a large machrophage-derived cell.

The most important prognostic indicator is the stage of disease at the time of diagnosis. Accurate staging (see the

Table 27-11 Disorders of the lymphatic system

Disorder	Etiology	Signs and symptoms	Medical therapy
Hodgkin's disease	Unknown	Lymph node enlargement (firm, nontender, painless), fever, weight loss, night sweats, pruritus, fatigue	Radiation therapy for stages IA and IIA, radiation and chemotherapy for stage IIIA, combination chemotherapy for stages IIIB and IVB
Non-Hodgkin's lymphoma	Unknown, viruses implicated	Nontender "bulky" lymphadenopathy, moderate hepatomegaly and splenomegaly, fever, night sweats, weight loss	Initial localized radiotherapy; total nodal radiation and chemotherapy for multifocal lesions
Multiple myeloma	Lymphoproliferative disorder of plasma cells (malignancy)	Severe disabling bone pain (especially in weight-bearing areas), hypercalcemia, renal failure, anorexia, CHF, bleeding tendency, coma	Radiation for bone pain, chemotherapy, hydration, ambulation, blood transfusions for anemia, analgesics

(handwritten annotation: presence of Reed-Sternberg cell)

Staging of Hodgkin's disease

TX cure rate 90% [handwritten]

Stage	Definition
I	Single abnormal lymph node
II	Two or more abnormal lymph nodes on *80% [handwritten]* the same side of the diaphragm
III	Abnormal lymph node regions on both sides of the diaphragm, which may also be accompanied by involvement of the spleen
IV	Diffuse or disseminated involvement of one or more extralymphatic organs or tissues with or without lymph node involvement

---

box) is crucial to the subsequent treatment regimen. All stages are subclassified further, as follows:

A: No symptoms
B: Presence of weight loss, fever, profuse night sweats

☐ Non-Hodgkin's lymphomas

Non-Hodgkin's lymphomas (NHL) include a broad spectrum of lymphoid malignancies with different histopathologies, disease courses, and responses to therapy. Accurate identification of the histopathology is crucial to the determination of the treatment plan. NHL can be categorized as *lymphocytic, histiocytic,* or *mixed cell types.* A lymphocytic cytology has the most favorable prognosis, and the histiocytic has the least favorable. Immature lymphocytes are produced, leading to impaired B-cell (humoral) immune response. These patients, therefore, are also at high risk for infections.

▨ ASSESSMENT

Subjective data include the following:
1. Knowledge of the disorder
2. Effect of fatigue on the ability to carry out ADL
3. Discomfort from night sweats or pruritus
4. Appetite and present nutritional status

Objective data include weight and condition of skin from scratching (for example, excoriations).

Diagnostic tests for lymphomas may include a chest x-ray film to identify a mediastinal mass and lymphangiography to evaluate the retroperitoneal nodes. The liver and spleen are evaluated by radionuclide scanning or by computed tomography (CT scan). A staging laparotomy may be performed to obtain a biopsy specimen of retroperitoneal lymph nodes and of both lobes of the liver and to remove the spleen. The diagnostic workup is often arduous and difficult, and explanation of the diagnostic procedures helps provide the patient with the emotional support so often needed during this time.

Slides are often sent to major cancer centers for con-

sultation regarding the classification of the disease. Once the diagnosis is made, the extent of the disease (staging) must be determined for planning the treatment regimen.

➡ DATA ANALYSIS: NURSING DIAGNOSES

Nursing diagnoses are determined from assessment of patient data. Possible nursing diagnoses for the person with lymphomas may include, but are not limited to, the following:

Diagnostic title	Possible etiologies
Potential for infection	Defective immune response
Knowledge deficit	Lack of exposure to or recall of information
Altered nutrition: less than body requirements	Hypermetabolism
Pain: pruritis, night sweats	Hypermetabolism
Potential impaired skin integrity	Scratching, trauma

▨ PLANNING: EXPECTED PATIENT OUTCOMES

Expected patient outcomes for the person with lymphomas may include, but are not limited to, the following:
1. Patient states feeling more comfortable without itching.
2. Patient is free from infection.
3. Patient can describe, the nature of the disorder, the therapeutic regimen, and identify resources in the community.
4. Skin breakdown from scratching is minimal.

▨ IMPLEMENTATION

☐ Assisting with achievement of therapeutic goals

Chemotherapy and radiation therapy are the primary treatment modalities for the lymphomas (Table 27-11). For Hodgkin's disease, treatment yields a cure rate of approximately 90% for stage I and 80% for stage II. Combination chemotherapy is the treatment of choice for stages IIIb and IV. The most commonly used combination is the MOPP regimen (see Chapter 12). It is administered in a 2-week course each month with prednisone added during the first and fourth course. The drugs are administered for at least 6 months or for two or three courses following the attainment of complete remission. Complete remissions are achieved in approximately 80% of these patients, and long-term, disease-free remissions and probable cures occur in half of this group.

When the nodal radiation is used, only those areas of the body to be irradiated are exposed; the other areas are protected by a mantle (Fig. 27-10).

Varying approaches are used for non-Hodgkin's lymphomas. Either single alkylating agents, such as chlorambucil, or combination chemotherapy may be used. Either local or total nodal radiation therapy may be given. Explanation of the treatment regimen is important to ensure patient un-

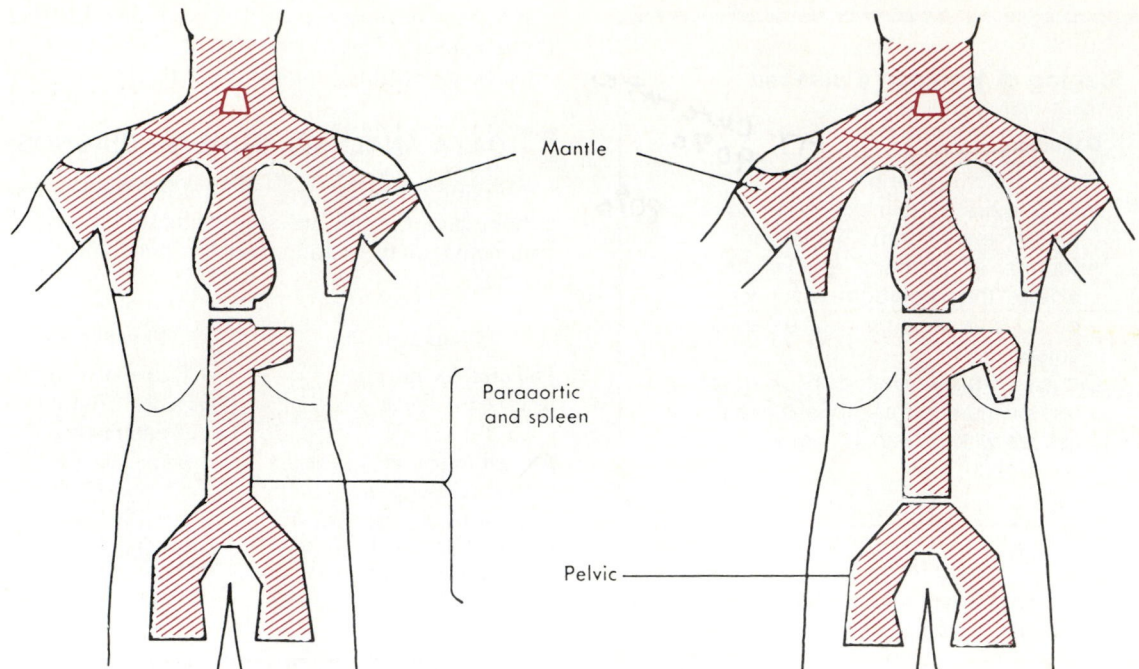

Fig. 27-10   Diagram of mantle and inverted Y fields used in total lymphoid radiotherapy of Hodgkin's disease. (From Rosenberg, SA, and Kaplan, HS, Calif Med 113:23, 1970).

derstanding and compliance to achieve the therapeutic goals.

□ Promotion of comfort and safety

Fever, pruritus, and profuse night sweats may lead to general discomfort. Comfort measures for pruritus (for example, baths, antipruritic medication [see Chapter 39]) may be instituted. Frequent changes of night clothing or bed linens may be necessary and high fluid intake is encouraged.

□ Counseling and teaching

Hodgkin's disease most often affects young adults, therefore special attention needs to be given to minimize the impact of the illness and its treatment on their lives, not only during the treatment period but beyond. Before the initiation of treatment, therapy-induced sterility should be discussed.[24] For young women receiving radiation therapy alone, surgical relocation of the ovaries outside the field of radiation may be performed. Sterility frequently occurs in association with chemotherapy. For women this is often temporary, and the ability to conceive and bear normal children often returns after therapy is completed. For men, sterility is more frequently permanent. For this reason the option of sperm banking should be discussed before beginning either radiation or chemotherapy.

To allow for work and career development, every effort should be made to schedule treatment at those times and days of the week that least interfere with work and other important events in the person's life. The nurse has a crucial role in assisting individuals to develop a realistic approach to the illness and in successfully meeting the demands and limitations imposed by the illness and its treatment.

Individuals with lymphomas may have periods of remission and recurrence. Such peaks and valleys are stressful and disruptive. Many patients describe subsequent courses of treatment following a recurrence as more stressful than the initial treatment. Comments include, "Is it worth it? I don't have the same faith." Other patients, realistically encouraged by the initial response to treatment, are able to express an optimistic outlook, "It worked the first time. It will work again." Recognition of the stress involved in therapy requires that support systems be available to the individual. The health care team can provide some of the needed support and guidance as the individual learns to incorporate the illness into daily life.

Teaching the patient includes the following:

1. Nature of the disorder
2. Importance of the extensive workup in identifying the treatment plan
3. Effects of therapy on sterility
4. Need for periodic blood counts
5. Side effects of radiation and chemotherapy and how to cope with them (see Chapter 12)
6. Need for continued medical follow-up
7. Community resources (American Cancer Society)

⌗ EVALUATION

Questions to ask may include the following:
1. Is the patient comfortable?
2. Is the patient infection free, with normal temperature and no abnormal discharges?
3. Can the patient describe the disease process, therapeutic regimen, and identify community resources?
4. Is the skin free from lesions and breaks in integrity?

■ PLASMA CELL DYSCRASIAS

■ Multiple myeloma

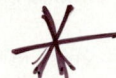

■ PATHOPHYSIOLOGY

Multiple myeloma is a lymphoproliferative disorder associated with plasma cells, the most mature form of activated B-lymphocytes that are responsible for immunoglobulin synthesis (see Chapter 37). This is a malignant neoplastic disease that arises in the bone marrow and involves bones primarily.

Plasma cell proliferation suppresses normal marrow elements resulting in "punched out" bone lesions that are visible on x-ray examination. Functionally abnormal immunoglobulin production suppresses formation of normal immunoglobulins needed to prevent infections.[35]

Because of changes in the bone, patients develop severe disabling bone pain, (especially in weight-bearing bones), pathologic fractures, neurologic symptoms from cord compression, hypercalcemia (because of bone destruction), with symptoms of renal failure, anorexia, confusion, and coma. Renal tubules may be damaged by myeloma proteins (Bence-Jones proteins).

Pneumonia, urinary tract infections and bacteremia occur because of the decrease in normal immunoglobulins. Expanded plasma volume may lead to congestive heart failure. Increased plasma viscosity leads to visual problems, headache, immobility, and confusion. Hemorrhage may occur because the myeloma proteins interact with plasma coagulation factors and also coat platelets, decreasing their function.

▣ ASSESSMENT

Subjective data include the presence of bone pain, anorexia, and neurologic symptoms such as numbness, tingling, and weakness. Objective data include skin color, urinary output, signs and symptoms of infection, level of consciousness, and signs of bleeding.

Diagnostic tests include x-ray evaluation of bones, hematologic studies (serum protein electrophoresis and immunoelectrophoresis), Bence-Jones proteins, and calcium levels.

➡ DATA ANALYSIS: NURSING DIAGNOSES

Nursing diagnoses are determined from assessment of patient data. Possible nursing diagnoses for the person with multiple myeloma may include, but are not limited to, the following:

Diagnostic title	Possible etiologies
Decreased cardiac output	Increased plasma volume, renal failure
Potential for infection	Decreased immune response
Potential for injury	Fragile bones, improper positioning and turning
Impaired physical mobility	Neuromuscular-skeletal impairment
Pain	Bone trauma, improper positioning

▣ PLANNING: EXPECTED PATIENT OUTCOMES

Expected patient outcomes for the person with multiple myeloma may include, but are not limited to, the following:
1. No signs of congestive heart failure are present (shortness of breath, dyspnea).
2. Patient states pain is absent or decreased.
3. Patient is free from infection.
4. No pathologic fractures occur.
5. Mobility is maintained within limits of the disease process.

▣ IMPLEMENTATION

Assisting with achievement of therapeutic goals includes careful monitoring of renal and cardiac function, administering of chemotherapeutic agents, and monitoring for infection and hemorrhage.

Pain control includes analgesic administration and careful handling of extremities when mobilizing or turning the patient. Because immobility increases bone demineralization and osteoporosis, it is essential that the patient maintain mobility to prevent fractures. Use of splints, braces, walkers may facilitate activity.

If the patient is prone to infection or bleeding, interventions are initiated to prevent their occurrence (see p. 892). Counseling and teaching about these side-effects are essential, as well as providing psychologic support for an individual with a chronic debilitating disease.

⌗ EVALUATION

Questions to ask may include the following:
1. Is the patient comfortable?
2. Is the patient free from respiratory distress?
3. Is the patient free of infection and bleeding?
4. Have pathologic fractures occurred?
5. Is the patient mobile and ambulatory?

■ SUMMARY

1. Major health problems of the hematopoietic system include RBC disorders (anemias, polycythemia), WBC disorders (leukemias), coagulation disorders (platelet

---

Putting knowledge to practice

- What are the normal cellular constituents of blood? Where are blood cells formed? How are they destroyed? What are the normal RBC count, WBC count, hemoglobin and hematocrit levels for men and women?
- What are blood coagulation factors? How are they involved in blood clotting process?
- From your knowledge of physiology, explain why the patient who is anemic may have dyspnea, tachycardia, and fatigue.
- Why does WBC count increase during infection? Why is a person with leukopenia (WBC count below 5000) more susceptible to infection?
- Why is the patient with leukemia and multiple myeloma at high risk of infection, even though WBC count may be elevated?
- What signs and symptoms would you look for in a patient who has been admitted after massive postpartum hemorrhage?

---

disorders, hemophilia, DIC), lymphatic system disorders (Hodgkin's disease, non-Hodgkin's lymphoma), and plasma cell disorders (multiple myeloma).

2. Anemia may be caused by blood loss, impaired RBC production, increased RBC destruction, or from nutritional deficiency.

3. Weakness and fatigue are major signs of anemia as a result of decreased oxygenation from lack of hemoglobin and increased energy needs required by increased RBC production.

4. Bone marrow samples may be obtained by aspiration or biopsy from the sternum, iliac crest, or tibia.

5. Sickle cell anemia is a hemolytic anemia with a genetic basis; a sickle cell crisis occurs when the RBC become deoxygenated, becme sickle-shaped, and cause stasis and obstruction of the microvasculature, leading to organ infarction and necrosis.

6. Ingestion of iron compounds is part of the therapy for iron-deficiency anemia only; it will not help the other types of anemias.

7. Thrombocytopenia is a decrease in the number of circulating platelets and leads to bleeding; persons with thrombocytopenia need to learn how to prevent injury and hemorrhage.

8. Hemophilia is a hereditary coagulation disorder; hemophilia A is a lack of coagulation factor VIII, and hemophilia B is a lack of factor IX; maintenance therapy consists of blood factor replacement therapy and prevention of injury.

9. Disseminated intravascular coagulation (DIC) is a coagulation disorder characterized initially by clotting and secondarily by hemorrhage, resulting from an alteration in the balance between clotting factors and fibrinolytic factors; the person is usually critically ill.

10. Persons with alterations of WBCs are at high risk of infection, because leukocytes are a major factor in the body's defense against invading microorganisms.

11. The leukemias are malignant disorders characterized by uncontrolled proliferation of WBCs and their precursors; the cause is unknown.

12. Leukemias may be lymphocytic or myelogenous, and acute or chronic. Acute leukemias have a rapid onset and a short course, if untreated; chronic leukemias have a more insidious onset and longer course. The major therapies for leukemias are chemotherapy and bone marrow transplantation.

13. Lymphomas are malignant disorders of the lymphatic system. Persons with Hodgkin's disease have defective cellular immunity and are therefore at high risk for infection. Non-Hodgkin's lymphoma is a group of lymphoid malignancies. Chemotherapy and radiation are the primary treatment modalities for lymphomas.

14. Multiple myeloma is a lympho-proliferative disorder associated with plasma cells (B-lymphocytes); it is a malignant disorder arising in the bone marrow and affects primarily bones. The person is at high risk for pathologic fractures.

REFERENCES AND SELECTED READINGS
Contemporary

1. Alcorn, R, and others: Fluid therapy and exercise in the management of sickle cell anemia, Phys Ther 64:1540-1522, 1984.

2. Barber, SM: Blood cell products in the supportive care of patients with acute leukemia, Nurs Times 76:152-154, 1980.

3. *Borley, D: Oncology nursing: leukemia and bone marrow transplant, Pt 3, Nurs Mirror 160(6):30-34, 1985.

4. Buetler, E: Iron. In Goodhart, R, and Shiels, M, editors: Modern nutrition in health and disease, ed 6, Philadelphia, 1980, Lea & Febiger.

5. *Brown, M: Standards of care for the patient with graft-vs-host disease post bone marrow transplant, CA Nurs 4:191-198, 1981.

6. *Campbell, VB, Preston, R, and Smith, KY: The leukemias: definition, treatment and nursing care, Nurs Clin North Am 18(3):523-542, 1983.

---

* References preceded by an asterisk are particularly well suited for student reading.

7. Carter, S, Glatstein, E, and Livingstone, R: Principles of cancer treatment, New York, 1982, McGraw-Hill Book Co.

8. *Cerrato, PS: Could you spot the other anemia? RN 49(10):63-64, 1986.

9. Coyle, MK: Organic illness mimicking psychiatric episodes, J Gerontol Nurs 13(1):31-35, 1987.

10. Curry, A: Protective isolation study: practice corner, Oncol Nurs Forum 8:42, 1981.

11. DeVita, V, Hellman, S, and Rosenberg, S: Cancer: principles and practices of oncology, ed 2, Philadelphia, 1985, JB Lippincott Co.

12. *Ford, R, McClain, RN, and Cunningham, BA: Veno-occlusive disease following marrow transplantation, Nur Clin North Am 18(3):563-568, 1983.

13. *France-Dawson, M: Sickle cell disease: implications for nursing care, J Adv Nurs 11(6):729-737, 1986.

14. *Gallagher, MT, and Wyland, N: Leukemia: when white cells run wild, RN 49(10):33-37, 1986.

15. Gibbons, PT: Transfusion therapy in sickle cell disease, Nurs Clin North Am 18(3):563-568, 1983.

16. *Gibson, L: Bone marrow transplant: the process, Nurs Times 83(3):36-38, 1986.

17. *Godwin, M, and Baysinger, MN: Understanding antisickling agents and the sickling process, Nurs Clin North Am 18(1):207-214, 1983.

18. Goldstein, M: Aplastic anemia, Hosp Pract 15:85-96, 1980.

19. Haskell, C: Cancer treatment, ed 2, Philadelphia, 1985, WB Saunders Co.

20. Herbert, C: Folic acid and vitamin B_{12}. In Goodhart, R, and Shiels, M, editors: Modern nutrition in health and disease, ed 6, Philadelphia, 1980, Lea & Febiger.

21. *Huckstadt, A: Hemophilia: the person, family and nurse, Rehab Nurs 11(3):25-28, 1986.

22. *Hutchinson, MM: Aplastic anemia: care of the bone marrow failure patient, Nurs Clin North Am 18(3):543-552, 1983.

23. Hutchison, MM, and King, AH: A nursing perspective on bone marrow transplantation, Nurs Clin North Am 18(3):511-522, 1983.

24. Kaempfle, S: The effects of cancer chemotherapy on reproduction: a review of the literature, Oncol Nurs Forum 8:11-18, 1980.

25. Kaye, D, and Rose, LF: Fundamentals of internal medicine, St. Louis, 1982, The CV Mosby Co.

26. Knobf, M, and others: Cancer chemotherapy treatment and care, Boston, 1981, GK Hall & Co.

26a. *Lakhani, AK: Current management of acute leukemias, Nurs 88 (London) 3:755-758, 1987.

27. Lamb, C: Managing sickle cell emergencies, Patient Care 19(1):92-95, 1985.

28. Lopez, JA, and Hausz, M: Therapeutic apheresis, Am J Nurs 82:1572-1578, 1982.

28a. Mauer, AM: Acute lymphoblastic leukemia in a young adult, Hosp Pract 22(9):145-156, 1987.

29. *McConnell, EA: Leukocyte studies: what the counts can tell you, Nurs 86 16(3):42-43, 1986.

30. *Moeller, KI: Suppressing the risks of bone marrow suppression, Nurs 87 17(3):52-54, 1987.

31. Nausef, WM, and others: A study of the value of simple protective isolation in patients with granulocytopenia, N Engl J Med 304:448-452, 1981.

32. Owen, H, and others: Bone marrow harvesting: nursing implications, CA Nurs 4:199-205, 1981.

33. Parker, N, and Cohen, R: Acute graft-vs-host disease in allogenic marrow transplantation, Nurs Clin North Am 18(3):569-578, 1983.

34. Post-White, J: Glucocorticoid-induced suppression in the patient with leukemia or lymphoma, CA Nurs 9(1):15-22, 1986.

35. Price, SA, and Wilson, LM: Pathophysiology, ed 2, New York, 1986, McGraw-Hill Book Co.

36. Refking, R, and others: Fundamentals of hematology, Chicago, 1981, Year Book Medical Publishers.

37. Rooks, Y, and Pack, B: A profile of sickle cell disease, Nurs Clin North Am 18(1):131-138, 1983.

37a. *Ross, MS, and others: Biotherapy with interferon in hematologic malignancies, Oncol Nurs Forum (suppl) 14(6):16-22, 1987.

38. *Rozzell, MS, Hijazi, M, and Pack, B: The painful episode, Nurs Clin North Am 18(1):185-199, 1983.

39. *Simonson, GM: Caring for patients with acute myelocytic leukemia, Am J Nurs 88:304-309, 1988.

40. *Terry, BA: Hodgkin's disease and non-Hodgkin's lymphomas, Nurs Clin North Am 20(1):207-217, 1985.

41. Thomas, ED: Bone marrow transplantation: present states and future expectations. In Isselbacker, KJ, and others, editors: Harrison's principles of internal medicine, ed 11, New York, 1987, McGraw-Hill Book Co.

42. *Trotta, P: Nursing assessment of symptoms associated with hyperviscosity syndrome, Oncol Nurs Forum 14(1):21-27, 1987.

43. *Varricchio, C: The patient on radiation therapy, Am J Nurs 81:334-342, 1981.

44. Victor, H: The nutritional anemias, Hosp Pract 15:65-89, 1980.

45. Walters, I, and others: Complications of sickle cell disease, Nurs Clin North Am 18(1):139-184, 1983.

46. *Williams, I, Earles, AN, and Pack, B: Psychological considerations in sickle cell disease, Nurs Clin North Am 18(1):216-230, 1983.

47. Williams, W, and others: Hematology, New York, 1983, McGraw-Hill Book Co.

48. Wyngaarden, JB, and Smith, LH: Cecil's Textbook of medicine, ed 17, Philadelphia, 1985, WB Saunders Co.

Classic

49. Bick, R: Disseminated intramuscular coagulation and related syndromes: etiology, pathophysiology, diagnoses and management, Am J Hematol 5:265-282, 1978.

50. Miller, VG: The sickle cell anemia patient in surgery, AORN J 30:1080-1090, 1979.

51. *Rossman, M, Slavin, R, and Taft, E: Pheresis therapy: patient care, Am J Nurs 77:1135-1141, 1977.

52. *Thomas, S: Transfusing granulocytes, Am J Nurs 79:942-945, 1979.

UNIT VII
Metabolic and Endocrine Problems

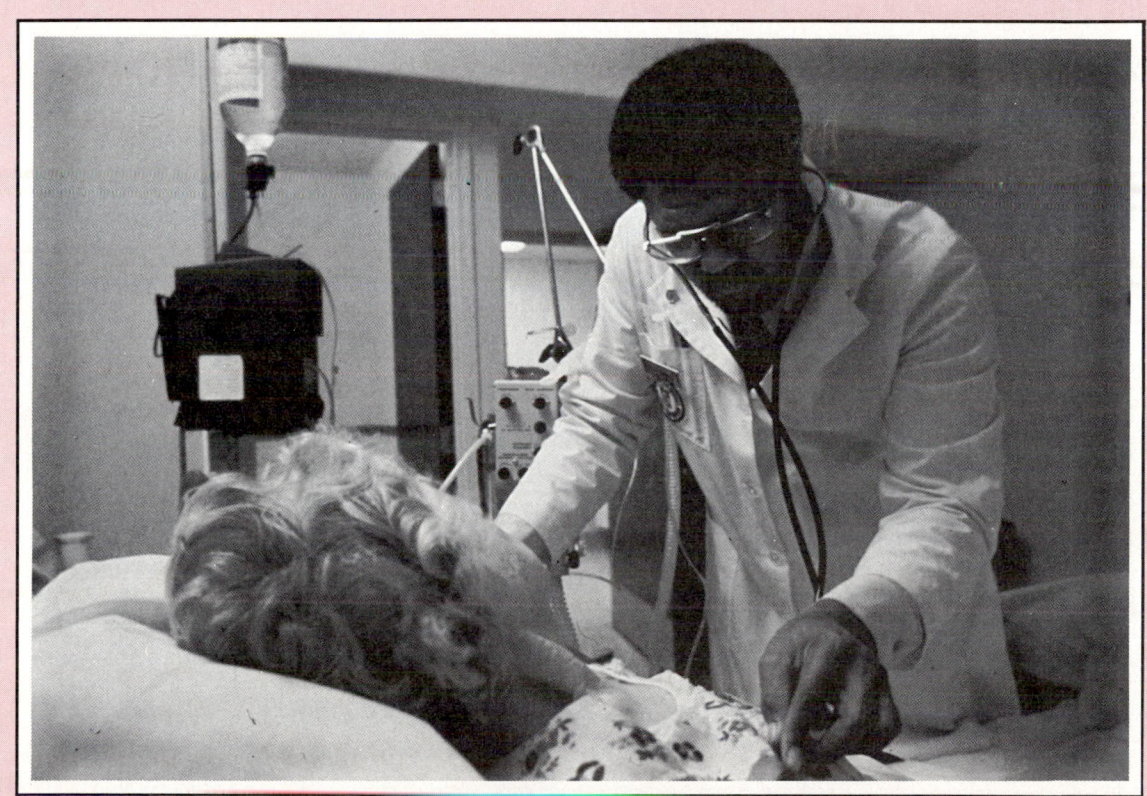

28

The Patient with Diabetes Mellitus

DOROTHY BLEVINS and VIRGINIA L. CASSMEYER

CHAPTER OBJECTIVES

After studying this chapter, the student should be able to:

- Differentiate between the two major types of diabetes mellitus (DM).

- Describe prevention and health education for DM.

- Explain the pathophysiologic bases for hyperglycemia, nonketotic coma, diabetic keto-acidosis, macrovascular and microvascular changes, neuropathy, and lower extremity changes.

- Identify assessment parameters of DM.

- Describe the dietary recommendations and systems for learning dietary requirements.

- Explain the role of exercise in DM.

- Describe medication regimens for DM.

- Describe therapy for correcting acute metabolic crisis.

- Explain the effect of surgery on the person with DM.

- Identify and describe the ten commandments of importance in teaching the patient with DM.

Diabetes mellitus (DM) is a complex chronic disease involving (1) disorders in carbohydrate, protein, and fat metabolism and (2) the development of macrovascular, microvascular, and neurologic complications. It is classified as an endocrine or hormonal disease because of its central feature of hyperglycemia, which results from a deficit in production or utilization of insulin.

■ ANATOMY AND PHYSIOLOGY

Persons with normal metabolism are able to maintain blood glucose levels of 70 to 110 mg/dl (euglycemia) under markedly different conditions of food intake. In nondiabetic persons, blood glucose levels may rise to 120 to 140 mg/dl after eating (postprandial), but these then rapidly return to normal, as excess glucose is extracted from the blood and stored as glycogen in liver and muscle cells (glycogenesis). Normal blood glucose levels are maintained during fasting states because glucose is released from these body stores (glycogenolysis), and new glucose is produced from amino acids, lactate, and glycerol derived from triglycerides (gluconeogenesis). The normalization of blood glucose is regulated by hormones.

■ Hormonal regulation of blood glucose

Of the five hormones involved in the regulation of blood glucose levels, the pancreatic hormone, *insulin,* is the only one that lowers blood glucose. (Glucagon, growth hormone, epinephrine, and glucocorticoids all raise blood glucose levels.) Research is ongoing to determine the effect of other hormones and neurotransmitters on insulin and blood glucose levels.

Insulin and glucagon are produced in the pancreas, which is both an exocrine and an endocrine gland. It lies retroperitoneally behind the stomach, with its head and neck in the curve of the duodenum, its body extending horizontally across the posterior abdominal wall, and its tail touching the spleen. More than 1 million islet cells are located throughout the organ.

The three types of endocrine cells are alpha (α), which secrete glucagon, beta (β), which secrete insulin, and delta (Δ), which secrete gastrin and pancreatic somatostatin.

Insulin is necessary for the transport of glucose, amino acids, potassium, and phosphate across cell membranes, especially those of adipose and resting muscle cells. Insulin is also needed to activate enzymes that promote intracellular metabolism. It seems to function by a fixed receptor model; that is, it combines with a receptor on the plasma membrane of the cell and initiates a sequence of postreceptor cellular activities that are coordinated by a second messenger, most probably cyclic guanosine 3,5-monophosphate (CGMP). (The reader is referred to a physiology text for further detail on the action of insulin.)

It should be apparent that when there is a deficit of insulin, as in diabetes mellitus, *hyperglycemia, increased fat metabolism,* and *decreased protein synthesis* occur.

See the box below for the actions of insulin that are hypoglycemic, antilipolytic, and anabolic.

Insulin has a major metabolic role during fed states whereas glucagon has a major role during fasting states. A small amount of insulin is secreted continually (basal secretion), and a bolus amount is secreted in response to intake of glucose and amino acids. Glucagon regulates the utilization of stored body fuels. It stimulates *glycogenolysis,*

Table 28-1   Glucose tolerance with aging (plasma glucose in mg/dl)

	Normal		
Age (yr)	Fasting	1 hr	2 hr
0-30	110	185	165
30-40	112	191	175
40-50	114	197	185
50-60	116	203	195
60-70	118	209	205
70-80	120	215	215

From Andres, R, adapted from Prout, TE: Diabetes mellitus, ed 4, New York, 1975, American Diabetes Association.

Actions of insulin

Hypoglycemic	Decreases blood glucose level overall
	Increases uptake and utilization of glucose by adipose and muscle cell
	Increases phosphorylation of glucose by liver
	Increases glycogenesis
Suppresses fat metabolism	Increases lipogenesis (antilipolytic)
Promotes protein synthesis	Increases amino acid incorporation into protein (anabolic)

gluconeogenesis, ketogenesis, and *lipolysis.* It inhibits the storage of glycogen. Excessive amounts of glucogon are present in diabetes mellitus and contribute to hyperglycemia and other metabolic derangements of the disease.

■ Physiologic changes with aging

Carbohydrate tolerance gradually declines as people age (Table 28-1). Glucose ingestion results in higher levels of blood glucose and longer durations of hyperglycemia in the elderly. After a loading dose of glucose, the 2-hour glucose blood level can be expected to increase 15 mg/dl for each decade of life.[5] The change in fasting blood glucose levels related to age is less marked, only 2 mg/dl per decade.

This age-related carbohydrate intolerance has been variously attributed to reduced insulin release from beta cells, a delay in insulin release, and/or a decrease in peripheral sensitivity to insulin.

A second physiologic change associated with aging that is important in diabetes management is a rise in the renal threshold for glucose above the average of 160 to 180 mg/100 ml blood glucose.

■ CLASSIFICATION OF DIABETES MELLITUS

The new classification system of glucose intolerance is described in Table 28-2. In addition to the five diagnoses of glucose intolerance shown, two others are specified:

1. Potential abnormality of glucose tolerance (in persons with known risk factors)
2. Previous abnormality of glucose tolerance (in persons who have had transient hyperglycemia)

This new system is designed to promote better comparison of research studies and to decrease the ambiguity of previously used terms. The reader needs to be familiar with older terms still in use by patients and health care providers (see the box on p. 906).

Table 28-2 Diagnoses of diabetes mellitus and other categories of glucose intolerance

Disorder	Description	Criteria for diagnosis
Diabetes mellitus Insulin dependent (IDDM), type 1	Insulin deficiency caused by islet cell loss; often associated with specific HLA types, predisposition to viral insulitis or autoimmune phenomenoa; *ketosis prone;* occurs at any age, common in youth	Unequivocal elevation of plasma glucose (≥200 mg/dl) and classic symptoms of diabetes (polydipsia, polyuria, polyphagia, weight loss) Fasting plasma glucose (FPG) ≥140 mg/dl on two occasions FPG <140 mg/dl and 2 hr plasma glucose ≥200 mg/dl with one intervening value ≥200 mg/dl after a 75 gm glucose load (OGTT)
Non–insulin dependent (NIDDM), type 2	*Ketosis resistant;* more frequent in adults, but occurs at any age; majority of patients overweight; familial tendency; may require insulin for hyperglycemia during stress	
Diabetes associated with certain conditions or syndromes	Hyperglycemia occurring in relation to other disease states: pancreatic disease, drugs or chemicals, endocrinopathies, insulin receptor disorders, certain genetic syndromes	
Impaired glucose tolerance	Abnormality in glucose levels intermediate between normal and overt diabetes; may progress to diabetes, improve to normal, or remain unchanged	FPG <140 mg/gl and 2 hr plasma glucose ≥140 mg/dl and <200 mg/dl with one intervening value ≥200 mg/dl after a 75 gm glucose load
Gestational diabetes (GDM)	Glucose intolerance with recognition of onset during pregnancy	Two or more of following plasma glucose concentrations met or exceeded using a 100 gm glucose load: FPG 105 mg/dl; 1 hr, 190 mg/dl; 2 hr, 165 mg/dl; 3 hr, 145 mg/dl

Adapted from Shuman, CR, and Spratt, IL: Office guide to diagnosis and classification of diabetes mellitus and other categories of glucose intolerance, Diabetes Care **4(2)**:335, 1981. With permission from the American Diabetes Association, Inc.

Older terms used to describe diabetes mellitus

Juvenile onset	*Usually* in younger individuals; IDDM (type 1)
Maturity onset	*Usually* in older persons; NIDDM (type 2)
Latent	No symptoms present, but hyperglycemia can be detected by laboratory examination
Subclinical	Under normal circumstances, results of fasting blood glucose tolerance test are normal; during stress, patient demonstrates impaired glucose tolerance
Secondary	Another disorder causes hyperglycemia

Table 28-3 shows a comparison of the essential features of the two types of diabetes mellitus: insulin dependent diabetes mellitus (IDDM) and non–insulin dependent mellitus (NIDDM).

A major characteristic of IDDM is the therapeutic need for insulin for survival. This insulin deficit is often termed absolute, in comparison with a relative deficit of insulin in NIDDM. Because of the complete dependency on exogenous insulin, persons with IDDM disease tend to have more severe and unstable glucose intolerance. In addition, they are prone to acute metabolic complications of ketosis and ketoacidosis (p. 911). Note that both forms of the disease may occur at any age; however, IDDM is more typically found in children, whereas NIDDM is more commonly associated with onset after age 25 years. Both forms of the disease are associated with vascular and neurologic complications; however, they differ in the organs most frequently affected. NIDDM can be associated with high levels of circulating insulin that is ineffective at the insulin receptor side and for postreceptor function.

Gestational diabetes mellitus (GDM) has its onset during pregnancy. If glucose tolerance remains impaired after the pregnancy, the disease is reclassified as IDDM or NIDDM. Pregnancy stresses glucose tolerance in all women, particularly in the latter half of pregnancy when growth hormones are secreted in increasing amounts. These hormones increase the supply of amino acids and glucose to the infant and diminish the effectiveness of insulin. There is a direct correlation between mean blood glucose levels and infant mortality and morbidity. The presence of any type of DM in pregnancy requires careful medical management if optimal health of the infant and mother is to be achieved. Close control of blood glucose is recommended before conception, as well as during pregnancy.

Glucose intolerance associated with certain conditions or syndromes is seen in persons who develop hyperglycemia as a complication of another disease or as a result of treatment. Commonly used drugs that can induce hyperglycemia include furosemide (Lasix) and thiazide diuretics, glucocorticoids, epinephrine, Dilantin, and nicotinic acid.

■ PREVENTION AND HEALTH EDUCATION

Diabetes mellitus is probably not a single entity but a heterogenous group of diseases with diverse causes that are incompletely understood.[16] Both genetic and environmental factors have been implicated and are under study. A combination of factors is most likely responsible for both IDDM and NIDDM. Although the same etiologic factors relate to both NIDDM and IDDM, the relative importance of individual factors differ. It is not possible at this time

---

Table 28-3 Comparison of insulin dependent and non–insulin dependent diabetes mellitus

	Insulin dependent DM (IDDM, type 1)	Non–insulin dependent DM (NIDDM, type 2)
Age of onset	More often in persons <40 years	More often in persons >40 years
Insulin	Absolute deficit	Relative deficit
Ketosis	Prone	Resistant
Serum insulin levels	Absent, low	Low, normal, or high
Insulin resistance	Occasional	Present
Complications	More often affects small blood vessels in eyes and kidneys	More often affects large blood vessels and nerves
Treatment	Insulin, diet, exercise	Diet and exercise; may be supplemented by hypoglycemic agents (about 30%)

Table 28-4   Heredity and diabetes mellitus

Evidence	IDDM	NIDDM
Concordance in monozygotic twins	Less than 50%	90%-100%
Autosomal dominant		Small subset of children with MODY (maturity-onset type of diabetes)
Presence of HLA antigens, DR3 and DR4	Increase the risk five-fold	
Prevalence rates in certain ethnic-cultural groups		American Indian tribes have rates of 1 in 3 compared to 1 in 20 for general population

to prevent the disease, but it is possible to modify some of the risk factors.

It has been long known that three factors increase the risk of diabetes: a *family history* of the disease, *obesity*, and, for the mother, the *birth of a large-weight baby* (over 9 lb). Table 28-4 shows that the evidence of *genetic transmission* of diabetes mellitus is stronger in NIDDM than in IDDM.

An *autoimmune* process is thought to be a major factor in IDDM, particularly when combined with genetic susceptibility. Islet cell antibodies are present in 85% of cases at onset of clinical diabetes.[5] In contrast, only 20% of patients with NIDDM have islet cell antibodies. Viral infection seems to play a major role in IDDM. The specific immunologic defect is unclear, but Fig. 28-1 shows a postulated interaction between viral agents and the beta cells.

■ Environmental factors

Epidemiologic studies have identified populations at high risk for NIDDM: the elderly, the poor, and the nonwhite. An association of acute viral infections and the occurrence of IDDM in communities has been noted. Certain viruses (Coxsackievirus B, rubella, and mumps) have been implicated in particular cases. The incidence of diabetes is decreased in populations with low food supplies and increased in those who undergo changes to food abundance.

About 80% of persons with NIDDM are obese; obesity is a high risk factor for NIDDM. It is known that the numbers of insulin receptors decrease with obesity and that weight loss, often as little as 20 pounds, may improve the glucose tolerance of obese patients with NIDDM.

■ Primary prevention

Currently, avoidance of obesity and, if necessary, reduction of weight under medical supervision are the major foci in primary prevention of NIDDM (type 2). Because of the strong association of NIDDM with hypertension, heart disease, and atherosclerosis, health practices that diminish risk factors for these diseases are recommended for the general population, for those identified at high risk

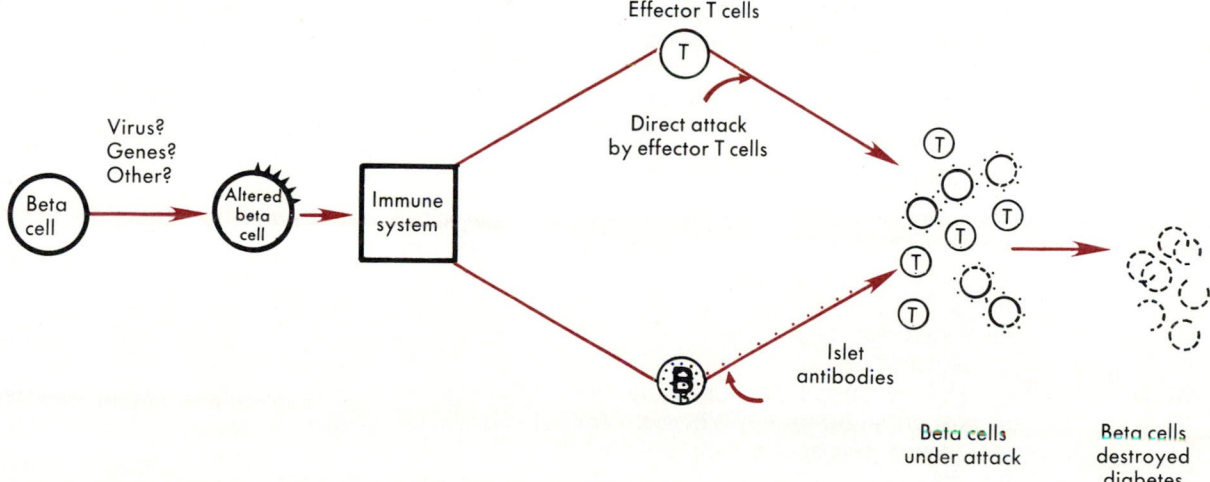

Fig. 28-1   Autoimmunity and diabetes.

for diabetes, and for persons with diagnosed diabetes (Chapter 29).

Genetic counseling is hindered by the current state of knowledge about modes of transmission. Persons with diabetes can be told that the rates of transmission from parent to child are low (2% to 5% for IDDM and 10% to 15% for NIDDM).[4]

Currently, researchers are exploring the effect of immunosuppressive agents on the clinical expression of diabetes mellitus in children newly diagnosed as having IDDM. Long-term side effects of such therapy (immunosuppression, malignancy) pose constraints upon the wide-spread use of these agents when other treatment options are available.

Table 28-5   Blood tests for diabetes mellitus

Test	Procedure and preparation	Interpretation
Fasting blood sugar (FBS) 70-110 mg/dl (venous plasma)	Fasting after midnight	Diagnostic criteria for DM: ≥ 140 mg/dl on at least two occasions or ≥ 140 mg/dl accompanied by classic symptoms of hyperglycemia; for IGT 115-140 mg/dl
2 hr postprandial blood sugar < 140 mg/dl	Blood sugar measured 2 hr after heavy meal or 2 hr after receiving loading of 100 gm of sugar	Used for screening or evaluation of treatment; it is not diagnostic
Random blood sugar < 140 mg/dl		Used for screening; it is not diagnostic
Oral glucose tolerance test (OGTT) FBS < 115 mg/dl; ½ hr, 1 hr, 1½ hr: < 200 mg/dl; 2 hr < 140 mg/dl	Fasting after midnight, FBS obtained, 75 mg glucose load taken; blood (and urine) samples collected at ½, 1, and 2 hr; sometimes at 3, 4, and 5 hr	Diagnostic criteria for DM: FBS < 140 mg/dl but both 2 hr and one other value > 200 mg/dl on two occasions. For IGT: FBS < 140 mg/dl; 2 hr value between 140 mg/dl and 200 mg/dl; and one other value ≥ 200 mg/dl. OGTT should be performed only in patients who have been on unrestricted diet and physical activity 3 days before test; not recommended for (1) fasting hyperglycemia; (2) persons taking thiazides, Dilantin, propranolol, Lasix, thyroid, estrogens, birth control pills, steroids; (3) hospitalized patients or acutely ill or inactive patients. The patient should remain seated and not smoke during the test.
Intravenous glucose tolerance test (IGTT)	Same as for OGTT	Performed when OGTT contraindicated (see OGTT) or in presence of gastrointestinal disorder that interferes with glucose absorption
Cortisone-glucose tolerance test	Performed similar to GTT except that cortisone is administered at start of test	Used when GTT results are inconclusive; cortisone causes an abnormal increase in blood glucose level and decreased peripheral utilization of glucose in persons predisposed to diabetes; blood glucose level of 140 mg/dl at end of 2 hr is considered positive result
Glycosated hemoglobin (hemoglobin AIC) 3.8-6.4 mg/dl	Blood sample drawn	Useful in monitoring average blood glucose levels over 3-month period; hemoglobin is linked to glucose in proportion to circulating glucose
C-peptide 1-2 mg/ml (fasting) 5-6-fold increase after glucose load	12 hr fasting blood sample drawn before ingestion of glucose and at 1 hr (may be combined with serum insulin test)	Measures proinsulin (biologically inactive byproduct) of insulin formation, thus can help determine insulin secretion
Serum insulin Fasting: 2-20 μU/ml Postglucose: up to 120 μU/ml	10-12 hr fasting blood sample drawn before ingestion of glucose and after 1 hr	Use is not clinically widespread; may be used in differential diagnosis of hypoglycemia or in diabetes research

■ Secondary prevention: detection of DM

The majority (90%) of persons with diabetes mellitus have NIDDM (type 2). It is estimated that more than 10 million persons in the United States have dibetes mellitus; 40% to 50% of these individuals have mild hyperglycemia and glucose intolerance and are relatively asymptomatic, and *the disease is undiagnosed*. However well they feel, they are at risk for developing more severe glucose intolerance and vascular and neurologic complications. NIDDM is a risk factor for heart disease, amputation, stroke, and hypertension. Although in some patients diabetes is diagnosed only when vascular or neurologic complications ensue, increasing evidence points to a relationship between the duration of the disease and metabolic control of blood glucose and the development of long-term complications of diabetes.[26]

■ SCREENING PROGRAMS

Screening programs are directed chiefly toward detection of NIDDM (type 2) for two reasons: (1) the incidence of NIDDM is greater, and (2) screening programs are not effective in identifying IDDM before the actual onset, which is very sudden and severe. Many authorities believe screening of high-risk populations (elderly, poor, nonwhite, pregnant women) to be a better use of resources than screening of entire populations.

A basic principle of screening programs is that adequate follow-up is available for persons with positive findings. Plans for screening for diabetes mellitus must take into consideration that the elderly, the poor, and the nonwhite populations are medically underserved; therefore, community or neighborhood screening programs must involve the local health care providers in planning for adequate follow-up.

Educational and case finding programs can be carried out in health departments, neighborhood clinics, outpatient clinics, physicians' offices, local diabetes associations, industry, or in the community at health fairs or in mobile health units.

■ SCREENING METHODS

Testing for hyperglycemia is a more reliable screening method for diabetes mellitus than is testing for glycosuria. The least reliable blood test is the random blood glucose level, collected without regard for whether the patient is fasting or fed. Table 28-5 lists other blood tests that may be used in screening programs. In the order listed, each succeeding blood test is more reliable but more costly and discomforting to patients. For screening purposes, Tes-Tape and Diastix urine tests are more reliable than Clinitest because they are specific for glucose, whereas Clinitest tablets show reactions to all sugars.

Table 28-2 explains how the various blood tests relate to the criteria used for diagnosis. A positive screening test is not sufficient for diagnosis.

> ### Recommended health behaviors for persons with diabetes mellitus
>
> Use dietary patterns to avoid hyperlipoproteinemia, obesity
> Develop pattern of consistent exercise
> Seek detection and control of glucose intolerance, hypertension
> Avoid cigarette smoking

■ SPECIFIC HEALTH TEACHING

Health behaviors recommended to modify the risk of diabetes mellitus and its complications are similar to those that modify the risk of cardiovascular disease (see the box above).

Because NIDDM is so underdiagnosed, the importance of screening and the symptoms (including asymptomatic disease) are basic components of public education about diabetes mellitus.

Education of the diagnosed patient will be discussed more fully later in the chapter.

■ PATHOPHYSIOLOGY

■ Hyperglycemia

Normally, when insulin is present, glucose intake (or glucose production) in excess of caloric needs is stored as glycogen in the cells of the liver and muscle. This process of glycogenesis prevents *hyperglycemia* (blood glucose concentrations > 110 mg/dl). When *insulin deficit* is present, four metabolic derangements lead to hyperglycemia:

1. Transport of glucose across cell membranes is diminished.
2. Glycogenesis is diminished and excess glucose remains in the blood.
3. Glycolysis is increased; thus glycogen stores are reduced and "liver" glucose is added to the blood continually rather than when needed.
4. Gluconeogenesis is increased and more "liver" glucose is added to the blood from the breakdown of amino acids and fat.

The classic signs of hyperglycemia include the following:

Polydipsia	Weight loss
Polyuria	Fatigue
Polyphagia	

■ CELLULAR STARVATION

Blood glucose concentration is high in uncontrolled diabetes mellitus, yet cells are subjected to starvation conditions. Insulin deficiency impairs the uptake of glucose in insulin-dependent peripheral tissues (skeletal muscle and adipose tissue). If glucose is not available, muscle cells metabolize their own glycogen supply, and in prolonged fasting, they may use free fatty acids and ketones. Brain cells are not insulin-dependent and must have a constant supply of glucose; they can utilize ketones for part of their energy requirement.

Similarly, the uptake of amino acids is impaired. Instead of protein synthesis, proteins are catabolized and the amino acids are used to provide the substrate necessary for gluconeogenesis in the liver. Fatigue, loss of weight, and loss of strength can occur, with stunting of growth in children. Insulin deficiency can lead to the increased mobilization and metabolism of fats. Instead of lipogenesis, lipolysis occurs when insulin deficiency is severe, as in IDDM. Increased fatty acids, triglycerides, and glycerol circulate and provide the liver with substrates for ketogenesis and gluconeogenesis. There is a resultant production of ketones (highly acidic, intermediate metabolites of fat). *Ketosis* is the condition of ketone excess in the blood. If severe enough, ketosis can lead to a form of metabolic acidosis and coma, *diabetic ketoacidosis* (p. 911).

In NIDDM ketosis is usually absent. There seems to be enough effective insulin to suppress the breakdown of fats and proteins, but not enough or not enough effective insulin to control blood glucose at normal levels.

■ INSULIN RESISTANCE

Insulin resistance is present when there is insensitivity to insulin of peripheral and liver tissue. Several factors contribute: decreased number of insulin receptors as in obesity and hyperglycemia, decreased insulin binding, and/or postreceptor defects. Insulin resistance is a major component of NIDDM and may be combined with a beta cell defect.[20]

An exogenous source of animal insulin leads to the development of insulin antibodies and is another reason for insulin resistance. Rarely, a *syndrome* of insulin resistance occurs in which insulin requirement exceeds 200u/24 hr.

■ HYPEROSMOLALITY

A major pathophysiologic alteration associated with hyperglycemia is hyperosmolality. Blood glucose concentrations of 60 to 100 mg/dl correlate with normal blood osmolarity values of 280 to 290 mosmols/dl. Hyperglycemia increases blood osmolality. Increases in blood glucose content and blood osmolality lead to *dehydration* by two mechanisms.

1. Glycosuria and osmotic diuresis ensue when blood glucose concentrations exceed the renal threshold. There can be losses of large amounts of calories, water, and electrolytes.
2. Fluid shifts from the intracellular compartment to the more highly concentrated extracellular compartment, resulting in intracellular fluid deficit.

The osmotic diuresis results in increased urine volume (*polyuria*). Thirst is stimulated, and the patient drinks large amounts of fluid (*polydipsia*). Because of the caloric loss

---

Signs of dehydration

Dry mucous membranes
Loss of skin turgor
Soft or sunken eyeballs
Red, parched lips and tongue
Tachycardia
Hypotension

---

and cellular starvation, the appetite is increased and the person eats more (*polyphagia*). When combined with *loss of body weight* and *fatigue,* the "three p's" (polyuria, polydipsia, and polyphagia) are the classic signs of hyperglycemia. These symptoms are usually less severe in NIDDM, but the risks of dehydration are still present. The signs of dehydration are listed in the box above.

■ Hyperglycemic, hyperosmolar, nonketotic coma (HHNC)

Table 28-6 compares the two major crises of diabetes mellitus that are acute and life threatening.

Blood glucose levels may exceed 1000 mg/dl, urinary glucose may be 5% to 10%, and serum osmolality may exceed 370 to 380 mosmols/dl in the absence of blood ketones. Coma in these circumstances is termed hyperglycemic, hyperosmolar, nonketotic coma (HHNC) and occurs in NIDDM. Most frequently, HHNC occurs in the elderly, debilitated, and those who have impairments of mobility or cognition. So long as persons with mild hyperglycemia and glycosuria can respond to thirst and replace fluids lost by glycosuria, the risk of HHNC is diminished.

If fluid intake is diminished and dehydration ensues, the risk becomes greater. Frequently an associated illness causes an increase in fluid losses (fever, diarrhea, vomiting) and an increase in insulin-antagonist hormones. Often, HHNC develops slowly over a period of days, and patients or caregivers may not identify the need for increased fluid intake. The elderly have less accurate thirst sensations, and they and persons who are acutely ill may not have access to fluids.

HHNC may also develop in nondiabetic persons receiving enteral or parenteral nutrition if hyperglycemia is induced. Adequate fluid intake and prompt recognition and treatment of hyperglycemia reduce the risk of HHNC in these persons. In some studies,[33] the mortality of HHNC is reported to be as high as 40% to 60%.

Blood hyperosmolality, marked dehydration, and resultant fluid shifts decrease intracellular fluid volume. Cerebral dysfunction reflects cell dehydration and is manifested by changes in neurologic parameters. (See the box on p. 911.) Laboratory findings reflect the fluid deficit and hyperosmolar state: normal to high serum sodium and chloride concentrations, elevated potassium concentration, and elevated blood urea nitrogen levels.

Table 28-6 Comparison of DKA and HHNC

Factors	DKA	HHNC
Mortality rate	About 10%	About 50% in elderly
Blood glucose levels	200-1000 mg/dl	600-2000 mg/dl
Ketonuria	Present	Absent
Metabolic acidosis	Present	Absent
pH 7.2	<7.2	
HCO₃	<15 mEq/L	
Kussmaul breathing	Present	
Flushed skin	Present	
Acetone odor to breath	Present	
Average fluid deficit	3-5 L	8-12 L
Abdominal pain	Frequent	Rare
Neurologic changes	Lethargy-coma	Lethargy-coma, but often accompanied by other neurologic deficits

---

Signs of hyperglycemic, hyperosmolar, nonketotic coma (HHNC)

Fluid deficit

Dehydration
Hypotension
Anuria
Circulatory collapse
Elevated body temperature

Neurologic changes

Sensory deficits
Motor deficits
Focal seizures
Aphasia
Coma

Signs of diabetic ketoacidosis

Dehydration
Lethargy leading to coma
Kussmaul breathing
Flushed face
Fruity breath odor
Nausea and vomiting

■ Diabetic ketoacidosis (DKA)

Diabetic ketoacidosis (DKA), a severe metabolic disorder, is characterized by hyperglycemia, hyperosmolality, and *metabolic acidosis*. This latter characteristic differentiates DKA from HHNC, as can be seen in Table 28-6. Six clinical signs are characteristic of DKA (see the box above, right).

DKA is considered preventable and treatable. Mortality of 100% in the preinsulin era has steadily decreased. It is most frequently seen in persons with IDDM but can occur in NIDDM. It is usually precipitated in the known diabetic by stressors that increase insulin needs, although it may occur when diabetes is out of control because of noncompliance with prescribed therapy.

The most frequent precipitating factor is an *infection,* such as those of the urinary or respiratory tracts. Other major stressors that can precipitate diabetic ketoacidosis are surgery, trauma, major illnesses, therapy with steroids, and emotional upset. Occasionally diabetic ketoacidosis is the initial symptom in adults with undiagnosed diabetes, and it is often the initial problem in children with diabetes.

Fig. 28-2 presents a schema of the major metabolic alterations of DKA. Increased lipolysis, oxidation of fats, and ketogenesis result in increased levels of organic acid (ketones) in body fluids. As ketones "use up" the body's alkali reserve for buffering, the pH of the blood decreases. Kussmaul breathing is stimulated to compensate for the metabolic acidosis. The osmotic diuresis is made worse by the ketonemia and from protein catabolism, which increases the protein load to the kidney. Ketones give the breath a fruity odor. Polyuria may decrease and anuria may be seen when the extracellular fluid deficit is severe.

The detection of symptoms of hyperglycemia, urinary ketones, sleepiness, "air hunger," nausea, and vomiting can alert diagnosed patients to seek medical help early so that prompt treatment can be given. (See the box above, right.)

■ Macrovascular changes

Diabetic persons develop *atherosclerotic changes* in larger arteries; these changes are the same as those seen in nondiabetics. It is well known, however, that diabetics are prone to develop atherosclerosis at an earlier age, that the disease progresses faster, and that it is more severe and extensive in diabetics than in nondiabetics. Persons with NIDDM develop macrovascular changes more frequently than do persons with IDDM. Diabetes is associated with

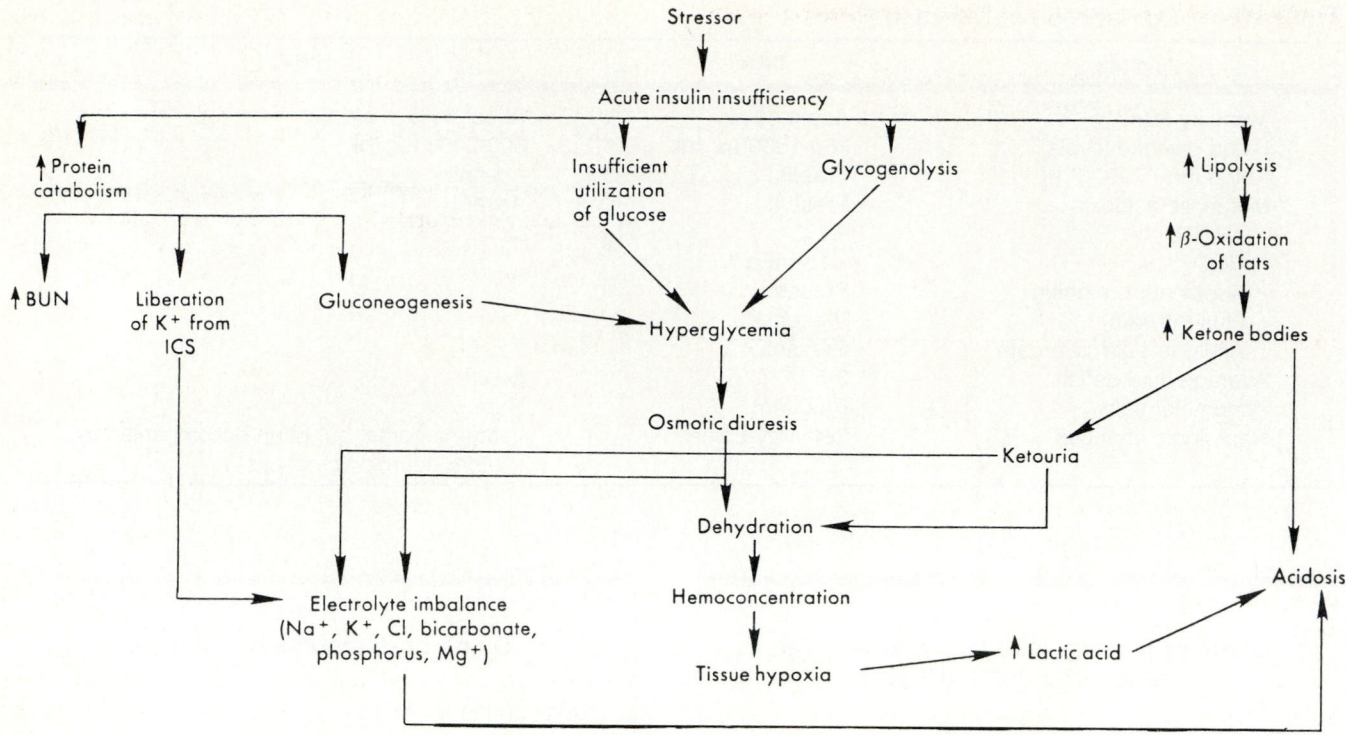

Fig. 28-2 Summary of metabolic alterations in diabetic ketoacidosis.

various atherogenic factors: abnormal lipid metabolism, changes in platelet adhesion, and hormonal changes (Chapter 29).

Insulin plays a major role in the metabolism of fats and lipids. *Lipid disorders* are frequently found in persons with diabetes mellitus. The hyperlipoproteinemia seen in diabetes is usually identified as type 4 or type 5 and is often the result of an excess of very-low-density lipoproteins. In addition, diabetes is considered to be a contributing factor in the development of *hypertension,* which can accelerate atherosclerosis.

Decreased lumens of large blood vessels compromise the delivery of oxygen to tissues and can cause tissue ischemia, resulting in *cerebrovascular disease, coronary artery disease, renal artery stenosis,* and *peripheral vascular disease.* Approximately three fourths of all cerebrovascular accidents are related to diabetes; and cardiovascular disease is the most common cause of death among older diabetics. The course and treatment in diabetics with these problems are the same as in nondiabetics; however, the underlying diabetes must be controlled for the best recovery from the cardiovascular complications. Likewise, the cardiovascular complications will make the diabetes more difficult to control.

■ Microvascular changes

Microvascular changes, characterized by thickening and damage to the basement membrane of the capillaries, are unique in diabetes. These changes occur most frequently in persons with IDDM and are responsible for diabetic nephrophathy and retinopathy. The causes of these changes are unknown but are thought to be related to uncontrolled diabetes. Various factors, such as the role of protein fractions, glycoproteins, lipids, and lipoproteins, have been studied. One theory proposes that capillary damage may be a result of increased sorbital content within cells. This occurs in hyperglycemia when the use of the alternative polyol pathway to metabolize glucose is increased. *Aldose reductase* regulates the conversion of glucose to sorbital. Sorbital is then slowly metabolized to fructose. Accumulations of sorbital within cells cause hyperosmolarity, edema, and, in the lens, opacities. Clinical trials are underway to investigate the effect of new agents, aldose reductase inhibitors, in preventing and reversing capillary damage.

■ NEPHROPATHY

One of the major results of microvascular changes is alterations in renal structure and function. Four types of lesions can occur: pyelonephritis, glomerular lesions, arteriosclerosis of the renal arteries and the afferent and efferent arterioles, and tubular lesions.

The progression of renal disease varies from person to person. An early sign of a glomerular lesion is *proteinuria* that gradually increases in severity. As renal insufficiency develops, the serum creatinine concentration and urea increase and other signs and symptoms of renal insufficiency and failure appear (Chapter 32).

Diabetes is present in approximately one fourth of all

**Factors accelerating renal disease
in persons with diabetes**

Uncontrolled hyperglycemia
Hypertension
Urinary tract infection
Nephrotoxic drugs
Radiologic contrast dyes

---

patients treated for end-stage renal disease in the United States. Each year about 4000 more diabetics require treatment for end-stage renal disease, at a cost of about $250 million. The incidence is much higher in patients who develop diabetes before age 20 years. After a duration of 20 years, the chance of a diabetic person developing renal disease is estimated at 50% in those with diabetes diagnosed before age 20 years, and 2% to 4% in those with diagnosis after age 20.[26] Attention is directed toward control or prevention of factors that are known to increase the progression of renal disease in diabetic persons. (See the box above.)

The treatment and nursing care of renal insufficiency in diabetes are similar to that in nondiabetics. It is important to remember that as renal insufficiency develops, the patient receiving insulin may require *less* insulin because it will be excreted more slowly. Renal transplantation is the treatment of choice, because diabetic complications progress rapidly in many patients who receive dialysis. At some centers pancreatic transplantation is also done at the time of kidney transplantation.

■ DIABETIC RETINOPATHY

Blindness in the diabetic person is most often a result of microvascular changes in the retina. After 10 years, half of all patients have some diabetic retinopathy. Diabetes is the leading cause of blindness in persons between the ages of 20 and 65 years. In addition to retinopathy, the diabetic person is also subject to increased *cataract* formation. Cataracts may be caused by prolonged hyperglycemia that results in swelling of the lens and opacity formation.

The early retinal lesion is a microaneurysm of the retinal vessels. Microinfarction and exudate formation follow. These early retinal changes may progress to a more serious stage, *proliferative retinopathy*, in which there is formation of new blood vessels on the retina (neovascularization). As these new vessels form, they shrink and cause traction on the retina. Retinal detachment and hemorrhage into the vitreous can result.

There are no symptoms of early retinal changes. Patients with diabetes are encouraged to have yearly eye examinations, preferably by an ophthalmologist. Efforts should be made to detect and control hypertension, because it is associated with increased incidence and rate of advance of diabetic retinopathy.[43]

Considerable evidence now indicates that *laser photocoagulation* controls retinopathy and decreases the risk of blindness. Photocoagulation uses thermal energy to seal capillary leaks, destroy new vessels, and cause adherence of the retina to the choroid. It is usually performed on an outpatient basis.

Vitrectomy, the removal of vitreous humor that has been infiltrated by hemorrhage, is another treatment for retinopathy. The removed vitreous humor is replaced by saline solution. Improved vision does not always result.

■ Neuropathy

Diabetes may affect peripheral nerves, the autonomic nervous system, the spinal cord, or the central nervous system. Multiple and varied symptoms may result, depending on the neurons involved. Sorbital accumulation and other metabolic alterations in myelin synthesis or functions related to hyperglycemia may result in altered nerve conduction. Neuropathy may only be involvement of one nerve, often a cranial nerve. The most common type of diabetic neuropathy, however, is *symmetrical peripheral polyneuropathy*. This is first seen in bilateral sensory loss in the distal lower extremities. Later, motor loss and upper extremity involvement can occur. The neuropathy can be painful also.

The diabetic may develop neuropathies that affect the autonomic nervous system. There may be gastric motility changes that lead to irregular food absorption, incontinence or impotence; or inability to detect early symptoms of hypoglycemia.

Nocturnal diarrhea and/or incontinence can be very disturbing to the patient and may not be revealed unless a specific question is asked. A complaint of excessive sweating on the upper body may be associated with anhydrosis on the lower body.

■ Lower extremity changes

The macrovascular changes, microvascular changes, and neuropathies all cause changes in the lower extremities. Diabetics develop gangrene considerably more often than nondiabetics. A significant change is anesthesia from loss of sensory nerve function; this contributes to minor trauma and undetected infections that result in gangrene. The infections start in cracks in hypertrophied skin, ingrown toenails, corns, and calluses, as well as in traumatized areas. Proper foot care could result in a reduction in the need for amputations.

A *neurotrophic ulcer* is one that is insensitive and often develops under corns or calluses. Pain in a neuropathic ulcer generally means infection with involvement of bone. The prognosis is not good.[25]

The interrelationships of vascular and nerve changes in diabetic foot lesions, which often result in amputation because of gangrene, are illustrated in Fig. 28-3. Gangrene may be dry or wet. *Dry gangrene* occurs when tissue death is not associated with inflammatory changes. Autoamputation (spontaneous detachment) of toes affected with dry gangrene is the treatment of choice. The area is kept dry

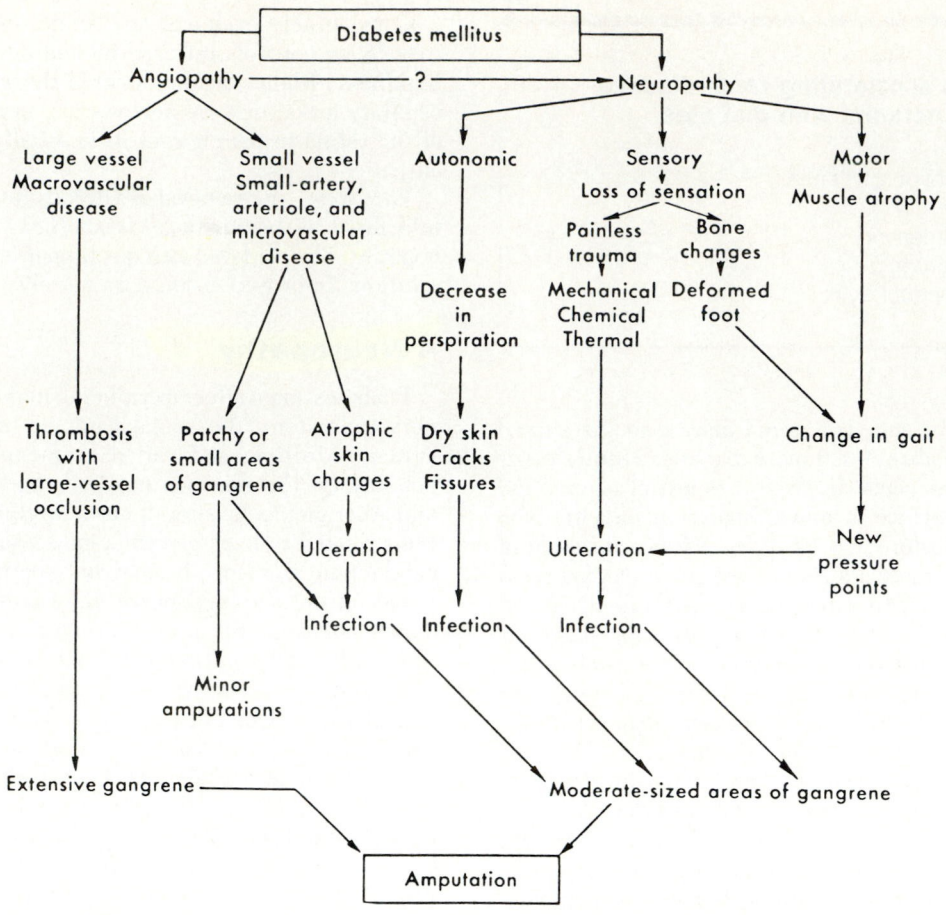

Fig. 28-3 How foot lesions of diabetes can lead to amputation. (Adapted from Levin, ME: Medical evaluation and treatment. In Levin, ME, and O'Neal, LW, (editor): The diabetic foot, ed 2, St. Louis, 1977, The CV Mosby Co.)

during the process. Close monitoring for signs of infection in proximal tissues is necessary.

Wet gangrene is gangrene coupled with inflammation. *Septicemia* and *septic shock* may occur. Bed rest, antibiotic therapy, appropriate cleansing and debridement, and continuous monitoring for signs of extension are the preliminary treatment. Various diagnostic tests to determine the extent of the lesion, status of circulation, and presence of bone involvement are done before amputation is considered (Chapter 26).

ASSESSMENT

■ Subjective data

If the patient is acutely ill, the priority assessment is focused on the extent of metabolic imbalance and its effects upon the patient's well-being. Does the patient complain of lethargy, air hunger, or the classic signs of hyperglycemia? Collect specific data about nausea, vomiting, abdominal pain, last food intake, and time and dosage of hypoglycemic agents.

A thorough history should be taken to determine whether any conditions are present that affect blood glucose concentrations:

1. Food intake in excess of caloric requirements
2. Infection or other acute illness
3. Stress related to psychologic or social factors
4. Drugs or other treatments that affect blood glucose
5. Omission of required insulin or oral hypoglycemic agent

Nursing assessment should not be limited to the determination of metabolic status. Also important to assess early after admission is the patient's knowledge and coping ability in diabetes management. Unless the patient is acutely ill, it is usually wise to complete a general nursing assessment before focusing on diabetes and its related care. There are two reasons for this. First, the nurse can learn a great deal about the patient's perspective of diabetes self-care during the general interview. Does the patient specify the disease, the regimen of therapy, and state special needs relating to diabetes? Is the patient concerned about how the plans for diet, activity, monitoring, medications, and foot care will differ from home schedules? A person well educated in diabetes management will be assertive in planning with the nurse how to minimize disruption of care while in the hospital.

The second reason to do a general assessment before focusing on diabetes is related to the reason for which the patient was admitted. Most newly diagnosed adults are not hospitalized; instead, they are treated in ambulatory settings. The primary concern at the time of hospitalization may be related to fears of blindness, amputation, heart attack or stroke, or a nondiabetes related medical problem. These concerns and expectations about treatment need to be explored before those of diabetes for the patient who believes diabetes problems to be secondary in importance.

How well the patient copes with this chronic illness can begin to be explored with questions such as: How difficult is it to stay on the diet? What is difficult about diabetes or its treatment for you? Asking the patient to describe a typical day (meal intake and times, sleep and work schedules, social activities, exercise and monitoring schedules) will help the nurse understand how the therapeutic regimen is incorporated into the patient's life-style and help identify areas of conflict and strengths of the patient.

Because education is an integral part of the treatment, the *learning needs* related to self-care of all patients who are diabetic are assessed. This assessment must be done early in the hospitalization in order to increase the time available for teaching. Unfortunately, many patients who have had diabetes for a long time may have inadequate knowledge, skills, or attitudes to manage their diabetes at optimal levels. The development of vascular or neurologic complications may require learning modifications of self-care measures. The last section of this chapter discusses the teaching needs of diabetic patients.

■ Objective data

Objective data to be collected include the following:
1. Level of consciousness
2. Blood and urinary glucose concentrations
3. Blood and urinary ketone concentrations
4. Blood urea nitrogen
5. Blood pressure, pulse, and respiratory pattern
6. Body temperature
7. Body weight
8. Urinary volume (per timed period)
9. Appearance of mucous membranes and skin
10. Skin turgor
11. Breath odor

When an acute metabolic crisis is suggested by the patient's clinical findings, further assessment is related to *metabolic acidosis* and *fluid imbalance* (p. 910). Table 28-6 is a comparison of signs and symptoms of the two metabolic crises: hyperglycemic, hyperosmolar, nonketotic coma (HHNC) and diabetic ketoacidosis (DKA).

Assessment of any adult patient with diabetes mellitus also includes data for identifying *abnormalities related to vascular or neurologic changes*. Measures directed toward prevention or treatment of these complications may be re-

quired. In addition, the patient often needs assistance with activities of daily living and modification of diabetes self-care activities. Assessment should always include attention to the *lower extremities, vision, cardiovascular-renal status,* and *neurologic status*.

➡ DATA ANALYSIS: NURSING DIAGNOSES

Nursing diagnoses are determined from assessment of patient data. Possible nursing diagnoses for the person with diabetes mellitus may include, but are not limited to, the following:

Diagnostic title	Possible etiologies
Fluid volume deficit: actual or potential	Polyuria, other fluid losses, decreased fluid intake, insulin deficit
Knowledge deficit (diabetes management)	Lack of exposure, poor recall, new diagnosis or new treatment, cognitive limitation
Noncompliance (with one or more aspects of diabetes regimen)	Cultural influences, established daily patterns of eating, activity, lack of resources
Altered nutrition: more than body requirements	Excessive intake in relation to metabolic needs, established eating patterns, knowledge deficit, noncompliance
Self-care deficit in one or more activities	Perceptual impairment (visual, sensory), motor impairment
Impaired skin integrity or potential impaired skin integrity	Pressure from ill-fitting shoes, lack of podiatry services, knowledge deficit about foot care

◳ PLANNING: EXPECTED PATIENT OUTCOMES

Expected patient outcomes for the person with diabetes mellitus may include, but are not limited to, the following:
1. Blood glucose level is at optimal level.
2. Ideal weight is maintained or achieved.
3. Hydration is adequate.
4. Patient has accurate information about diabetes mellitus and measures for its control.
5. Patient is able to perform required monitoring tests and interpret results.
6. Patient is able to implement self-care activities.
7. Patient can explain signs and symptoms of hypoglycemia and hyperglycemia and what to do when they occur.
8. Patient knows when to seek medical assistance.
9. Patient identifies one goal and states behavior necessary to achieve goal.

IMPLEMENTATION

Assisting with achievement of therapeutic goals

PROMOTING NUTRITION

Diet is considered to be the keystone of therapy in both IDDM and NIDDM with three nutritional goals[1]:
1. Control of blood glucose and blood fat levels
2. Achievement and maintenance of desirable body weight
3. Provision of adequate nutrition and balanced diet

Dietary recommendations

1. There should be sufficient calories to promote normal growth and activity in the child and to maintain *ideal* weight and activity in the adult.
2. Calorie intake should be provided as follows:
   a. Protein, 12% to 20% (0.8 g/kg body weight)
   b. Carbohydrate, 55% to 60%
   c. Fat less than 30%
3. The amount of carbohydrate is individualized and is dependent on the impact of carbohydrate on blood glucose and lipid levels and individual eating patterns.
4. No more than 10% of calories from fat should be from saturated fats and the remainder from unsaturated fats. Cholesterol should be restricted to less than 300 mg daily.
5. Foods with unrefined carbohydrates and foods with fiber should be incorporated in the diet. The amount of highly refined carbohydrates low in fiber should be reduced; the diet should include 25 to 30 gm plant fiber/1000 Kcal.
6. Consistency in timing and the distribution of calories, carbohydrates, protein, and fat for each meal is most important in IDDM.
7. Control of weight is more important in obese persons with NIDDM; balanced meals at consistent times will aid in achieving this goal.
8. Sodium intake should be limited to 1000 mg/1000 Kcal of total intake, not to exceed 3000 mg per day.
9. A variety of nutritive and nonnutritive sweeteners should be encouraged.
10. Alcohol should be used in moderation, if at all. Alcohol has 7 Kcal/gm when metabolized and must be included in calorie calculations.

Some evidence indicates that *water-soluble fiber* helps to reduce blood glucose levels in addition to reduction of blood lipids and enhancement of bowel function.[3] Fiber content should be increased gradually to prevent abdominal discomfort. Additional fluids should be recommended when fiber intake is increased. Foods containing water-soluble fiber include the following:
1. Legumes
2. Oats
3. Barley
4. Fruit

Individualization of dietary recommendations for a particular patient has always been a principle of dietary ther-

---

Glycemic index	
Glucose	100%
Rice, white	
Honey	
Potatoes	70%
Carrots	
Peanuts	
Lentils	<30%
Kidney beans	

From Franz, MJ: Evaluating the glycemic response to carbohydrates, Clin Diab 11:127-130, 1986.

---

apy. This principle has been reinforced by recent knowledge about the many factors that influence the effect of specific starches on blood glucose levels. Beginning research indicates that some starches (complex carbohydrates) may raise blood glucose more than previously thought.

The term *glycemic index* is used to describe the change in blood glucose levels from ingestion of specific foods compared with a standard glucose load.[14] (See the box above.)

Many factors, including the preparation of foods and the combination of foods, influence the glycemic index. Too little is known at this time to make generalized recommendations using the glycemic index. However, individual patients may use blood glucose monitoring to assess the effect of particular food intake. A second benefit of the knowledge gained by research in glycemic index is less reliance on *total* restriction of simple CHO. Small portions of foods containing sucrose can be eaten with meals, provided blood glucose levels are controlled.[14]

Patients may choose to include four "sweeteners" in their food. Aspartame and saccharin are nonnutritive sweeteners; fructose and sorbital are nutritive sweeteners, with a caloric value of 4 cal/g.

Principles of dietary planning

Should a nutritional history reveal that the patient's food intake and patterns of eating incorporate the above recommendations, few changes would be recommended. It is often said that the diet needed by a diabetic person is that needed by all persons. However, most Americans find it necessary to change dietary habits to reduce hyperglycemia and maintain ideal weight. Recommendations need to be made with awareness of the difficulty with which people change established eating habits.

Dietary planning should include considerations of the following factors:
1. The patient's personal, cultural, or religious food preferences
2. Life-style: working hours, family composition, financial resources

3. Activity: activity patterns; timing and level of exercise; periods of exercise, work, and sleep
4. Hypoglycemic drugs; onset, duration, and peak activity of insulin or oral hypoglycemic agents (p. 919)
5. Other modifications needed in consistency or nutrient content

Systems for learning dietary requirements

There are several systems by which dietitians and nurses help patients learn dietary requirements.[46] The simplest system is providing patients with *sample diet plans* for each meal that can be used until they are able to learn and choose more options. For example, the plan for breakfast could be as follows:

4 oz orange juice	1 C 2% milk
1 C cooked or dry cereal	Coffee
1 Slice toast with 1 tsp butter	

The *food exchange system* has been widely used throughout the United States because of its ease in teaching.[2] The exchange lists consist of six groups of food divided on the basis of similar amounts of *carbohydrates and fats*. Patients can learn to exchange foods within one list to obtain a variety of food intake. Some of the common foods in each of the food groups are listed in Table 28-7.

Information about the food exchange system is available from hospitals, clinics, and physicians' offices and in diabetic educational literature. Standardized diet plans have been developed for various levels of calorie intake and can serve as guides; however, these should not be used without attention to individual requirements. The dietitian translates the diet prescription into numbers of food exchanges and food distribution throughout the day that will meet the patient's nutritional requirements. An example of a meal plan for a day using a food exchange system is given in Table 28-8.

Table 28-7 Examples of food exchanges

Food product	CHO (g)	Fat (g)	Equivalents
Milk and milk products			
Skim	12	Trace	1 C skim or nonfat milk
Lowfat (2%)	12	5	1 C yogurt
Whole	12	8	½ C evaporated milk
Vegetable			
Nonstarchy	5	2	½ C asparagus, carrots, eggplant, collards, tomatoes, and such
Fruit	15	–	1 Apple (2 in across)
			½ C apple sauce
			½ Banana
			½ Grapefruit
Starch/bread	15	Trace	1 Slice bread
			½ Bagel
			1 Tortilla (6 in)
			½ Hamburger bun
			3 Graham crackers (2 × 2 sq)
			¾ C unsweetened cereal
Meat			
Lean	–	3	¼ C cottage cheese (dry)
			1 oz lean beef or fish
			¼ C tuna (water pack)
Medium fat	–	5	1 oz ground beef
			¼ C tuna (oil packed)
			½ C cottage cheese (creamed)
High fat	–	8	1 Tbsp peanut butter
			Pork ribs or deviled ham
			1 oz cheddar cheese
			1 oz frankfurter
Fats	–	5	1 tsp margarine or butter
			1 Strip crisp bacon
			2 tsp French dressing
Free food (cabbage, lettuce)	–	–	Calorie-free beverages, unsweetened gelatin, and such: as desired

Adapted from American Diabetes Association, Inc: American Diabetes Association and National Institutes of Health, US Public Health Service exchange lists for meal planning, Chicago, 1986, The Association.

Table 28-8　Sample of two menu plans using the exchange list*

Menu 1		Menu 2
Exchanges	**Breakfast**	**Breakfast**
1 Fruit	½ Glass orange juice	¼ Cantaloupe
1 Milk (skim)	1 Glass skim milk	1 Glass skim milk
1 Meat (medium fat)	1 Egg poached	1 Scrambled egg
3 Bread	2 Toast, ½ C oatmeal	1 English muffin, ½ C bran flakes
2 Fat	2 tsp margarine	2 tsp margarine
	Lunch	**Lunch**
1 Fruit	1 Peach	½ Banana
1 Milk (skin)	1 Glass skim milk	1 Glass skim milk
2 Meat (medium fat)	Tuna salad sandwich (¼ C tuna with celery, 2 slices	1 MacDonald's cheeseburger (2 bread, 2 meat)
2 Bread	bread, 3 tsp mayonnaise, and lettuce)	1 Lettuce salad with 2 Tbsp French dressing
3 Fat		
	Afternoon snack	**Afternoon snack**
1 Bread	6 Thin round crackers	Pretzels
1 Fruit	1 Apple	Grapes
	Dinner	**Dinner**
1 Fruit	1¼ C strawberries	¾ C pineapple
2 Vegetable	1 C green beans	Sliced tomatoes
4 Meat (lean)	4 oz round steak	4 oz chicken
1 Milk (skim)	1 Glass skim milk	1 Glass skim milk
2 Bread	1 Small baked potato	2 slices bread
	1 Roll	
3 Fat	1 Tbsp sour cream/2 tsp butter	1 tsp mayonnaise/2 tsp butter
	Evening snack	**Evening snack**
1 Bread	3 Rye wafers	6 Salt crackers
1 Meat	1 oz diet cheese	¼ C low-fat cottage cheese

Adapted from American Diabetes Association, Inc: American Diabetes Association and National Institutes of Health, US Public Health Service exchange lists for meal planning, Chicago, 1986, The Association.
*Diet distributed over three meals and two snacks. Diet based on 2000 calories with 45% CHO (225 g); 35% fats (78 g); and 20% proteins (100 g).

Additional nursing activities related to dietary control include the following:

1. Helping the patient eat according to the diet plan
2. Monitoring and recording food intake
3. Obtaining substitutes for foods not desired or refused
4. Coordinating care so that patient's food is not delayed or omitted

■ PROMOTING EXERCISE

Exercise is the second treatment modality of hyperglycemia in diabetes mellitus. Glucose can enter *active* muscle cells without the action of insulin and can then be oxidized to carbon dioxide and water in most patients; thus *exercise has a hypoglycemic action.* Exercise also decreases insulin resistance, perhaps by increasing the number of insulin receptors, and promoting weight loss in the obese diabetic. In patients with blood glucose levels above 300 mg/dl, exercise can increase the hyperglycemia and even promote ketosis. Very intense exercise, even in persons with well-controlled blood glucose, can increase blood glucose levels.

Before an exercise program is started, the patient should have a complete cardiovascular examination including a stress ECG if over age 40. Working capacity can be evaluated to determine the level of exercise that can be instituted safely. The person with diabetes mellitus should also be evaluated for the presence of retinopathy, neuropathy, and hypertension because particular types of exercises should be avoided in these conditions.[30] See the box on p. 919 for this information and for guidelines for exercise in persons with diabetes mellitus.

Those persons receiving insulin or orally administered hypoglycemic agents should understand that diet and medications are planned around the usual activity level and pattern of exercise. Changes in activity level require changes in diet or medication (Table 28-9).

Strenuous activity undertaken without a decrease in hypoglycemic agent or an increase in food is a common cause

---

Guidelines for exercise program of the person with diabetes mellitus

Exercise type: aerobic, start with light level

Exercise session: each session should include:
1. 5 to 10 minutes of warm-up stretching limbering exercises
2. 20 to 30 minutes of aerobic exercise with heart rate in target zone (75% to 80% of maximal heart rate)
3. 15 to 20 minutes of light exercise and stretching to cool down

Exercise frequency: three to five times

Special precautions for diabetic who is being treated with hypoglycemia agent
1. Carry an ID card or wear bracelet identifying wearer as having diabetes mellitus and what to do if person is observed as acting abnormally.
2. Monitor self during and after exercise for hypoglycemia (may include doing blood glucose self-monitoring at least at initiation of exercise program).
3. Carry a source of readily absorbable carbohydrate.
4. Avoid dehydration.
5. Consult professional (podiatrist) about footwear that is best for planned exercise.
6. Exercise when blood sugar is highest (1 to 3 hours after meals).
7. For regular, planned exercise, decrease insulin as prescribed.
8. Consume extra carbohydrate before, during, or after exercise; need is dictated by blood glucose self-monitoring, whether any reduction of insulin was instituted, length and level of exercise, presence of symptoms of hypoglycemia, and whether exercise was planned or spontaneous.

Precautions for selected persons
1. Persons with insensitive feet should avoid running and jogging and choose cycling or swimming.
2. Persons with proliferative retinopathy should avoid exercises associated with the Valsalva maneuver that cause jarring and jolting of head, and exercises associated with head in a lowered position.
3. Persons with hypertension should avoid exercises associated with the Valsalva maneuver; exercises involving intense exercise of the body and arms (exercises involving the lower extremities) are preferred.

Modified from Rifkin, H, editor: The physician's guide to type 2 diabetes (NIDDM): diagnosis and treatment, New York, 1984, American Diabetes Association.

---

of hypoglycemic reaction in patients receiving such medications. Patients are instructed to eat a quick-acting form of glucose just before an activity that is more strenuous than usual and to repeat this if the activity is lengthy (>1 hour). Such a glucose source should always be available for treatment if hypoglycemic reaction occurs.

There is greater chance of hypoglycemia when the peak action of the patient's insulin (or oral agent) and exercise coincide than when postprandial hyperglycemia and exercise coincide. Injections of insulin should be made into the abdominal tissue rather than the extremities before exercise of the legs and arms because exercise increases the speed of absorption.

■ MEDICATIONS

☐ Insulin

Insulin is necessary for the survival of patients with IDDM. It is also used to treat NIDDM in some patients in whom other measures have not achieved a desired level of blood glucose control.

The current trend in treatment is to achieve the best control of blood glucose possible for each individual, that is, to achieve blood glucose levels near normal limits if this can be done without significant hypoglycemia.

☐ *Properties of insulin*

Four properties of insulin preparations may comprise the prescription: (1) types of action, (2) strength, (3) species source, and (4) purity.

Table 28-9 Effect of exercise on need for medication and food

	Increased exercise	Decreased exercise
Hypoglycemic agent	Decreased need	Increased need
Food	Increased need	Decreased need

Table 28-10 Action of insulin preparations

Type of insulin	Time of onset (hr)	Peak of action (hr)	Duration of action (hr)	Insulin appearance
Rapid acting				
Regular	< 1	2-4	4-6	Clear
Crystalline zinc	< 1	2-4	5-8	Clear
Semilente	< 1	4-7	12-16	Cloudy
Intermediate acting				
NPH	1-2	8-12	18-24	Cloudy
Globin zinc	2-4	6-10	12-18	Clear
Lente	1-4	8-12	18-24	Cloudy
Slow acting				
Protamine zinc	4-8	16-18	36 +	Cloudy
Ultralente	4-8	16-18	36 +	Cloudy

TYPE OF ACTION. All insulins are hypoglycemic, but they differ in the speed with which they begin to act (*onset*), the period of time they have the strongest action (*peak*), and how long they act (*duration*). Insulins are classified as short, intermediate, and long acting. Table 28-10 gives the characteristics of eight standard insulin preparations. Nurses need to know the characteristics of each in order to coordinate food and activity with insulin action. This coordination is necessary so that (1) insulin is available when food is taken for optimal metabolism, and (2) food is available while insulin is acting to prevent hypoglycemic reactions.

Three principles are useful in coordinating food and hypoglycemic medications:

1. Food must be taken after insulin (or oral agent) within the time of onset; for example, with regular insulin, food must be taken within 1 hour after injection.
2. Intermediate- or long-acting insulins require that a supplemental feeding be given, timed to match the peak action of the insulin, for example, a 3:00 PM feeding if NPH insulin given at 7:00 AM.
3. With intermediate- or long-acting insulin a bedtime feeding is required so that glucose is available through the night.

STRENGTH. Insulin preparations vary in the concentration of insulin units in 1 ml volume. U-100 insulin, or 100 units/ml, is the strength most frequently used. A few patients requiring very small doses may use U-40 insulin because it is easier to measure small doses accurately. In *insulin resistance*, a rare condition in which daily insulin doses exceed 100 units, U-500 insulin may be ordered.

It is very important that the insulin concentration and the insulin syringe calibration match in units per milliliter to prevent errors in dosing (Fig. 28-4).

SPECIES. Insulin antigenicity can decrease insulin receptor effectiveness.[24] In the past, most insulin was prepared from a combination of beef and pork pancreas. Single-species insulin (usually pork) could be obtained for patients with beef-insulin allergy or antibodies. (Pork insulin most closely resembles human insulin and is considered the least antigenic animal insulin.) Recently several single-species pork or beef preparations have been marketed and used to decrease insulin antibody formation.

"Human" insulin is either porcine (pork insulin modified enzymatically to structurally resemble human insulin) or bacterially produced by recombinant DNA techniques. Human insulin has less antigenicity than animal insulin, and it greatly expands the insulin resources of the world. Human insulin may be prescribed to decrease antigenicity in persons with insulin resistance, lipoatrophy, occasional need for insulin, or newly diagnosed diabetes.[4] Table 28-11 shows the variety of short-acting insulins now available that differ according to species. A wide variety are also available in intermediate- and long-acting insulins.

PURITY. Over time, manufacturers have improved the purity of insulin preparations. Standard insulins (single-peak insulins) may contain small amounts of pro-insulin-like substances and other antigenic substances (for example, glucagonlike, pancreatic polypeptides). Insulins labeled "purified" contain less than 50 PPM (parts per million) or animal proinsulin. All standard insulins now contain less than 50 PPM; those labeled "highly purified" contain less than 10 PPM and may be prescribed to decrease formation of insulin antibodies.

Because of the many changes being made in insulin preparations, the nurse must clarify the insulin prescription if the type, strength, purity, or species is unclear. A change in any one of these properties may lead to significant differences in action. When the insulin prescription is changed, careful patient monitoring is necessary to identify the extent of clinical effect.

☐ Insulin administration

Increasingly, physicians are attempting to simulate the normal bodily secretion of insulin that occurs in nondiabetics, that is, a continuous basal level of insulin that rapidly increases with food intake. In addition, they try to mimic the tendency for glucose to reach its lowest peak between 3 AM and 4 AM and a tendency for basal insulin secretion to rise between 5 AM and 8 AM before breakfast

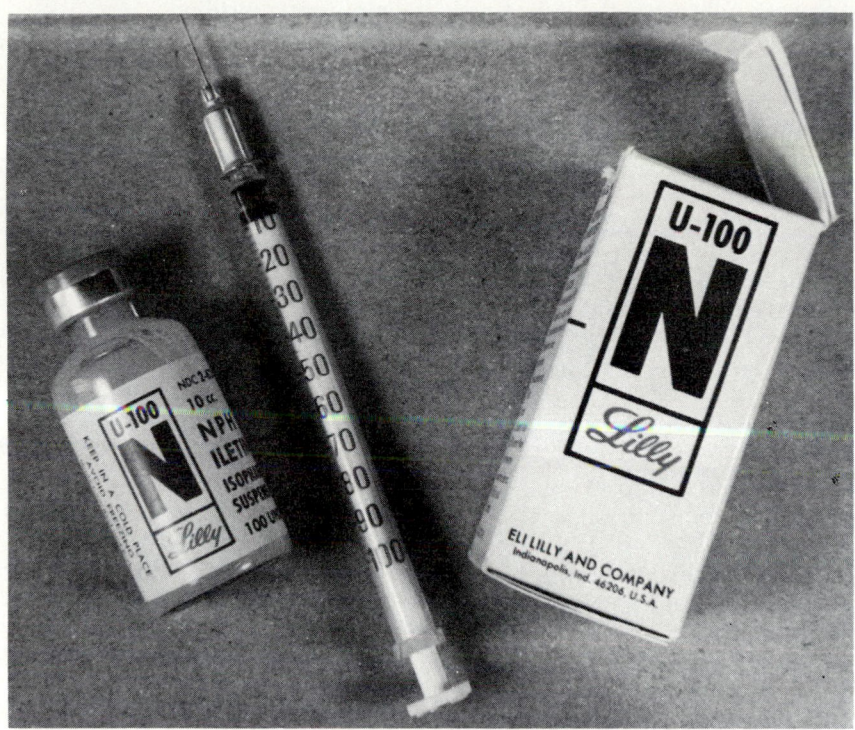

Fig. 28-4 U-100 insulin and disposable U-100 insulin syringe.

Table 28-11 Species of regular insulins

Product	Beef/pork	Beef	Pork	Human	
				Porcine	Recombinant DNA
Iletin II Regular (Lilly)		√	√		
Purified Pork R (Squibb/Nova)			√		
Velosulin (Regular) (Nordisk-USA)			√		
Purified Pork S (Squibb/Nova) (Semilente)			√		
Iletin I Regular (Lilly)	√				
Regular (Squibb/Nova)	√				
Iletin I Semilente (Lilly)					
Semilente (Squibb/Nova)		√			
Humulin Regular (Lilly)					√
Novolin R (Regular) (Squibb/Nova)				√	
Velosulin (Regular) (Nordisk-USA)				√	

(dawn phenomenon). A description of various regimens is presented in the box below; regimens 3-6 are designed to mimic the normal endogenous secretion pattern. These regimens are termed "intensive therapy" and are aimed at "tight control" of blood glucose. Obviously the risk of hypoglycemia is increased with intensive therapy.

Insulin therapy regimens

1. One injection of intermediate-acting insulin per day
   a. Most frequently used in persons with IDDM who are not controlled with diet and/or oral hypoglycemic agents
   b. Does not mimic the normal endogenous pattern
2. Two injections of intermediate-acting insulin per day
   a. Used mostly in persons with NIDDM
   b. Does not mimic the normal endogenous pattern
3. Split and mixed insulin regimen: injection of rapid-acting insulin and intermediate-acting insulin at breakfast and supper
   a. Used in many persons with IDDM
   b. Theoretically, the morning rapid-acting insulin covers breakfast and early morning, the morning intermediate-acting insulin covers lunch and afternoon, the evening rapid-acting insulin covers the evening meal, and the evening intermediate-acting insulin covers the bedtime snack and the *basal level needed* during the night
4. Split and mixed insulin regimens (similar to no. 3 above), except that the evening intermediate-acting insulin is given at bedtime instead of at supper time
   a. Used in persons with IDDM
   b. Theoretically provides better basal nighttime coverage and provides coverage for the natural prebreakfast elevation in glucose
5. Multidosage regimen: three injections of rapid-acting insulin, one before each meal; and one injection of intermediate insulin given at bedtime
   a. The rapid-acting insulin provides coverage for each meal
   b. The bedtime intermediate-acting insulin provides the nighttime basal level and coverage for the natural prebreakfast glucose elevation
6. Multidosage regimen: three injections of rapid-acting insulin, one before each meal; and an injection of long-acting insulin given at breakfast or at suppor or split between breakfast and supper (provides the same coverage as no. 5 above)

The insulin type and dosage is ordered in anticipation of food, activity, and other factors that balance or affect the insulin requirements. Regardless of the particular regimen, the following information is necessary before administering insulin:

1. Time of onset, peak, and duration of the insulin
2. Availability of food or adequate glucose at these times of action
3. Plans for treating hypoglycemia should it occur

Thus if a patient were ordered nothing by mouth for several hours, insulin should not be given until provision is made for an intravenous infusion of a dextrose solution. The box on p. 923 lists general guidelines for insulin administration.

ROTATION OF NEEDLE INSERTION SITES. The sites of injection must be rotated to assure proper absorption of insulin. Lipodystrophy can occur with repeated injections and can cause poor absorption of the medication. The major areas for injection of insulin are the arms, legs, buttocks, and abdomen. Each of these areas has multiple sites (Fig. 28-5).

Two forms of *lipodystrophy* can occur: hypertrophy and atrophy. *Hypertrophy* is thickening of an injection site because of the development of fibrous scar tissue from the repeated injections in the same site. A hypertrophic area is usually devoid of nerve endings, and the patient likes to reuse it because injections are painless. Absorption from this area is slow and erratic.

Atrophy is loss of subcutaneous fat. The cause is unknown. It is thought to result from repeated injections in

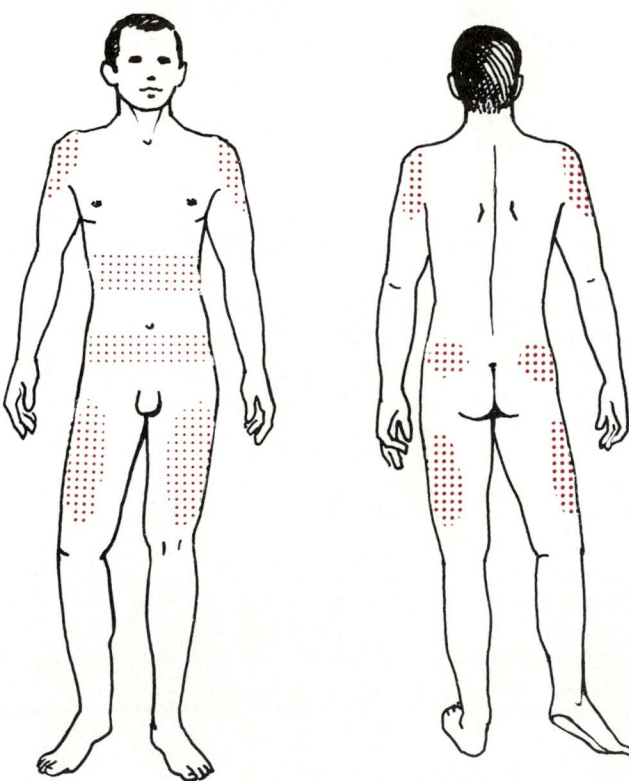

Fig. 28-5 Rotation of sites for insulin injection.

Guidelines for insulin administration

1. Always use an insulin syringe calibrated in the same units as the insulin.
2. Select insulin according to type, strength, species, purity, and brand name as specified by the prescription.
3. Rotate or gently roll the bottle if it is other than regular or globin insulin.
4. Do not inject cold insulin; allow it to come to room temperature before using.
5. Examine *intermediate-* and *long-acting* insulin vials for suspension of insulin (cloudy appearance); do not use if it is not cloudy.
6. Check for and remove any air bubbles after insulin is drawn into the syringe (do not use an air bubble to clear the needle after injection).
7. When mixing insulins, do not vary the sequence in which two insulins are drawn into the same syringe; usually air is injected into both bottles (regular and intermediate); the insulin is withdrawn first from the regular vial and then from the longer acting insulin vial.
8. Use an injection site that has not been used in the past month.
9. Insert the needle into fatty tissue *closer to muscle than to skin;* if there is little subcutaneous tissue, "pinch" up the skin and use a 45-degree angle and a ⅜ or ½ in needle; use a 90-degree angle when the fat pad is large.

---

the same site, faulty injection technique, or impurities in the insulin. Some researchers have successfully treated atrophy by injecting purified insulin into atrophic areas. A major nursing role is to ensure that the patient rotates the sites and gives the injections deep enough.

INSULIN PUMPS. Very close control of blood glucose can be achieved for some patients with IDDM by use of an insulin infusion pump. Insulin pumps, which are battery operated and portable, deliver regular insulin at a basal rate (continuously) and a bolus dose at meal times. The insulin is delivered from a reservoir through tubing to a needle placed in subcutaneous tissue (Fig. 28-6). Projected for the future is the closed-loop insulin delivery system, which will combine a pump, a blood glucose sensor, and a calculator to determine rate of delivery.

Insulin pumps now in use are open-loop systems. Although multiple insulin injections are avoided, patients must monitor blood glucose levels and manually set the insulin delivery rate. The pump is only disconnected to change the needle (every 2 or 3 days), while bathing or swimming, and during sexual activity.

About the same size as a small calculator, the pump can

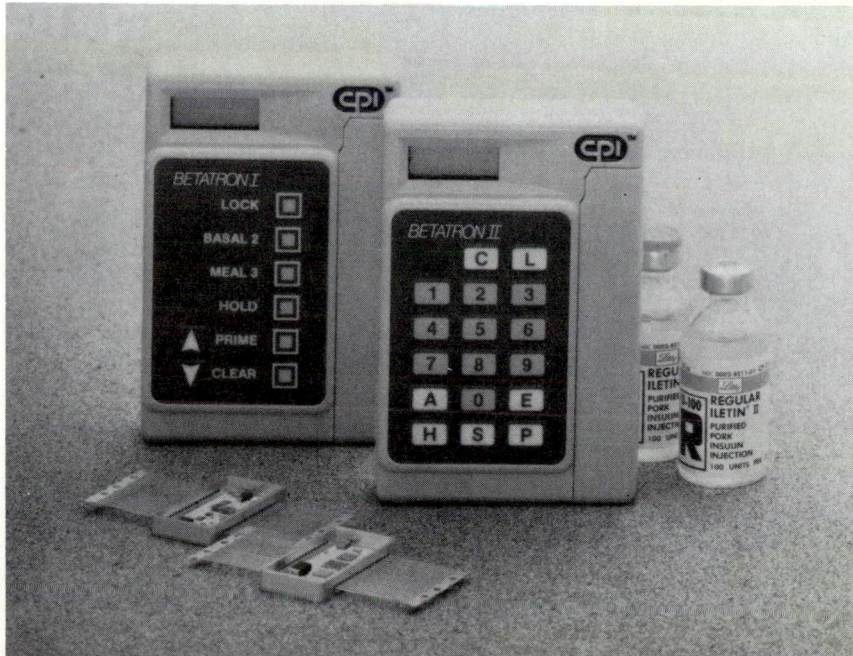

Fig. 28-6 Insulin infusion pumps. (Courtesy Cardiac Pacemakers, Inc, St. Paul, Minn.)

be worn on a belt at the waist or in a pocket. For each brand of insulin pump, the patient requires considerable education to ensure safe and effective insulin delivery. Complications include hypoglycemia, infection at the site of needle insertion, and rapid onset of ketoacidosis if the pump becomes disconnected.

Insulin pumps are expensive; however, insurance reimbursement of initial and maintenance costs is becoming more common. A policy statement by the American Diabetes Association[20] cautions that the use of portable infusion devices be prescribed and managed by diabetologists trained and skilled in their use.

☐ Oral hypoglycemic agents

Six orally administered agents are now available for use in controlling blood sugar levels in persons with diabetes mellitus; all are sulfonylurea compounds (Table 28-11). Glypizide (Glucotrol) and glyburide (Micronase) are more potent than the first-generation compounds, thus doses are smaller.[15] It is hoped there will be fewer drug-drug interactions, because they are not so easily displaced (unbound) from albumins by other drugs.

The sulfonylurea compounds increase the ability of the islet cells of the pancreas to secrete insulin, although other methods of action are being studied. With long-term use, they may increase the number of insulin receptors and correct defects in postreceptor insulin action.[29]

Complications of oral hypoglycemic agents are infrequent (see the box below). They differ in routes of excretion; the presence of liver or kidney dysfunction may increase the risk of complications. Hypoglycemia may be prolonged in use of chlorpropamide because of its long half-life (36 hours) and duration of action (24 to 60 hours). See Table 28-12 for information about the hypoglycemic agents.

Chlorpropamide is usually given in one dose per day; Tolbutamide has the shortest duration of action (6 to 12 hrs) and is ordered two to three times a day.

The drugs are not hormones, and it is a misnomer to refer to them as oral insulin.

Physicians vary in their use of these agents because of the controversial study conducted in the 1970s by the University Group Diabetes Program (UGDP). The FDA recommends that orally administered hypoglycemic agents be limited to persons with symptomatic adult-onset nonketotic diabetes mellitus that cannot be adequately controlled by

---

Table 28-12 Oral hypoglycemic agents

Agent	Proprietary name	Range of daily dose
Acetohexamide	Dymelor	250 mg to 1.5 g
Chlorpropamide	Diabinese	100 to 750 mg
Tolazamide	Tolinase	100 mg to 1 g
Tolbutamide	Orinase	0.25 to 3 g
Second generation		
Glyburide	Micronase	1.5 to 20 mg
Glipizide	Glucotrol	2.5 to 40 mg

---

diet or weight loss alone and in whom the administration of insulin is impractical or unacceptable. This recommendation was based on the report of the UGDP study that the death rate from cardiovascular disease was two and one half times higher in persons receiving tolbutamide as in those receiving a placebo. These results have been challenged by numerous groups.

The medications are most effective in older persons; they are not used to treat IDDM or in pregnant women. They are useless in the treatment of diabetic ketoacidosis. A few patients may be treated with a combination of insulin and oral agents in experimental trials to test the effectiveness in decreasing peripheral resistance.[29]

Persons taking oral hypoglycemic medications need to be as careful about taking the prescribed dosage, following the prescribed diet, maintaining the usual amount of exercise, testing the urine for sugar, and taking general health precautions as do persons taking insulin.

☐ Hypoglycemia

Hypoglycemia (plasma glucose level <60 mg/dl) occurs in at least two circumstances in diabetes mellitus. By far the most frequent occurrence is the patient receiving insulin or an oral hypoglycemic agent, when there is an insulin excess relative to food intake or energy expenditure. Hypoglycemia in this situation occurs for the following reasons:

1. Too large a dosage taken in relation to the need for insulin
2. Too little food taken (meals delayed or omitted) or delayed gastric emptying
3. Exercise excessive in relation to food intake and hypoglycemic agent
4. Emotional stress
5. Vomiting, diarrhea, or decreased food absorption

A less common instance is hypoglycemia occurring in the early phase of NIDDM, when a sluggish release of insulin allows peak insulin activity to occur hours after food has been ingested.

A *hypoglycemic reaction* can occur when hypoglycemia is present or when blood glucose level falls rapidly; that is, the blood glucose level may be >60 mg/dl, but the patient has the symptoms of hypoglycemia. Symptoms of hypogly-

---

Complications of oral hypoglycemic agents

Hypoglycemia
Allergic skin reactions
Gastrointestinal complaints
Hematologic disorders
Water retention and dilutional hyponatremia (with chlorpropamide)

Signs and symptoms of hypoglycemia

Sympathetic nervous system activity

Pallor	*Perspiration
Piloerection	Hunger
Tachycardia	Palpitation
*Nervousness	Irritability
*Weakness	Trembling

Central nervous system activity

Headache	Blurred vision
Diplopia	Incoherent speech
Emotional changes	Fatigue
*Mental confusion	Numbness of lips, tongue
Convulsions	Coma

*Four signs most commonly reported by patients.[24]

Carbohydrates (10 to 15 g) for relief of hypoglycemia

½ C fruit juice
½ C cola drink
½ C gelatin dessert
4 Cubes sugar
2 Packets sugar
2 Squares Graham crackers

---

cemic reaction can vary among patients and from time to time in one patient.

Symptoms of sympathetic nervous system (SNS) activity usually precede those of the CNS and are related to epinephrine action. Signs of cerebral dysfunction reflect hypoglycemia that interferes with the oxygenation of nerve cells. Repeated or prolonged attacks can cause brain damage.

For some patients, a disturbing development is a diminished ability to perceive hypoglycemic symptoms, particularly the early SNS symptoms. This dysfunction is associated with duration of disease, development of neuropathy, and use of certain drugs that affect the SNS (for example, beta blockers). Patients find this loss frightening because they no longer are able to intervene early in the reaction, but only when signs of cerebral dysfunction alert others or themselves to a more severe hypoglycemic reaction. If a hypoglycemic reaction is suspected, a blood glucose level should be obtained if it can be done quickly. For the patient who is not hospitalized, it may be done at home if the patient has been taught to measure blood glucose levels.

The treatment of hypoglycemia in a conscious patient is administration of a quickly absorbed sugar; 10 to 15 g carbohydrate should be given promptly (see the box above, right). With this amount of food, the patient usually feels better within 5 to 10 minutes. Should symptoms not decrease, another feeding should be given after this time. With unconsciousness or severe hypoglycemia, a bolus of 50% dextrose is given intravenously.

After recovery the patient should eat a snack consisting of complex carbohydrates and proteins (for example, milk and crackers) or eat the next meal if it is due. The reason for hypoglycemia should be ascertained if possible, and frequent monitoring should be carried out by the nurse until duration of the action of the hypoglycemic agent is completed.

The nurse should not hesitate to treat the patient if symptoms of hypoglycemia occur in a patient who has no prohibition on eating. Hospital protocols should clearly describe prompt treatment of hypoglycemia in patients who cannot take anything by mouth.

To facilitate prompt treatment for unconsciousness, diabetic persons should carry identification cards with the insulin or hypoglycemic agent and dosage listed. Medic-Alert bracelets or necklaces can also alert others to the diabetic status. Families can be taught to inject glucagon before transporting the patient to an emergency care facility.

□ **Somogyi phenomenon**

Some patients have great difficulty in stabilizing blood glucose levels. One cause of instability is the Somogyi phenomenon, a sequence of increasing peaks and valleys in blood glucose levels. It is often triggered by an insulin dosage in excess of true insulin requirements. The sequence of events is depicted in Fig. 28-7.

Very frequently the signs and symptoms are not obvious enough to be detected. In many instances the hypoglycemia occurs at night and is undetected. The hyperglycemia is not recognized until early morning, and it is assumed that the patient needs higher doses of insulin, but this treatment just makes the problem worse.

The signs and symptoms of the Somogyi phenomenon can be those normally seen with hypoglycemia, but frequently they consist only of nighttime sweats, nightmares,

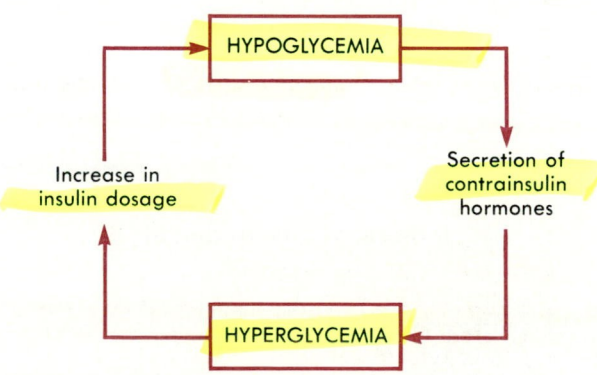

Fig. 28-7   Sequence of events in Somogyi phenomenon.

and a headache on arising. There may be weight gain in the presence of glycosuria, no glucose but ketone bodies in the urine (counterinsulin hormones stimulate lipolysis and beta-oxidation of fats), and wide fluctuations in blood and urine glucose levels unrelated to meals.

Treatment consists of decreasing the insulin dosage. A primary nursing role is to document complaints of hypoglycemia, glucose intake, and laboratory results, and in particular to look for complaints of night sweats, nightmares, and early morning headaches. Correlating these complaints and laboratory results with the time of meals will also help to identify the phenomenon.

■ CORRECTING ACUTE METABOLIC CRISES

Diabetic ketoacidosis (DKA) and hyperosmolar nonketotic coma (HHNC) are medical emergencies that require intensive nursing care. Therapy is directed toward correction of the hyperglycemia, dehydration, electrolyte imbalances, acidosis, and precipitating factors. All of these interventions are carried out simultaneously. Intense monitoring is necessary to evaluate the effects of treatment. Review Table 28-6 for the differences in symptoms of DKA and HHNC.

□ Insulin

Insulin replacement is based on one or a combination of several indices of insulin deficit (see box below).

Usually little insulin is needed to treat HHNC; in most instances patients are very sensitive to insulin and require small doses (5 to 15 units initially, with a total insulin dose of 25 to 50 units).

High-dose insulin therapy is the traditional treatment of DKA. It is effective and includes the use of subcutaneous or intravenous injections of regular insulin. *Regular insulin is the only insulin that may be given intravenously.* In this method, an adult patient with ketoacidosis might be given an initial dose of 50 to 150 units by bolus intravenously, then doses of 50 to 100 units every 1 to 2 hours until the acidosis is corrected. Or the patient might be given an initial bolus of 50 to 100 units of regular insulin intravenously and a similar dose subcutaneously, both of these doses repeated every 2 to 6 hours until the acidosis is corrected. Often adults may require 300 to 500 units of insulin in the first 24 hours of treatment. In children, dosage is more likely to be based on units per kilogram body weight.

In the last decade, a *low-dosage insulin* system of treatment has been used in DKA and is also effective. It may include the use of intramuscular or intramuscular and intravenous infusion of insulin. In this system, 0.2 U/ml regular insulin may be infused in 5% dextrose in water at a rate of 1 ml/min (10 to 12 U/hr). Often 10 to 12 U (50 ml) is injected in an intravenous bolus to initiate treatment.

Regardless of the method of insulin replacement, as blood glucose level decreases and nears 200 to 300 mg/dl, close attention must be given to preventing and detecting the onset of hypoglycemic reaction. The nurse should be more alert at this time for the symptoms of hypoglycemia and expect changes in insulin dosage that reflect the decreasing blood glucose levels.

□ Fluid and electrolyte replacement

The patient with HHNC may have a fluid deficit of 8 to 12 L, and the patient with DKA a deficit of 3 to 5 L. To correct the *dehydration and sodium deficit*, normal saline solution or 0.45% saline (half-strength normal saline) solution is given intravenously. Initially, the solution is infused rapidly and may be started at a rate of 1 to 3 L/hr or more in adults without cardiac or renal failure. When the urine output is 1 to 2 ml/min and the blood pressure is stable, the rate is reduced to 1 L in 2 to 4 hours. When the blood glucose level falls to 300 mg/dl, 5% glucose solutions are used. The patient must be monitored very carefully for signs of fluid overload.

Potassium is not initially added to the intravenous fluids because the patient's potassium serum level is usually *elevated* at the beginning of therapy, even though total body stores of potassium are depleted. With correction of the dehydration, acidosis, and insulin deficit, potassium moves back into cells and hypokalemia results. Potassium as potassium chloride is then added to the IV infusion. Serum potassium levels and ECG tracings are monitored continuously to determine the amount of potassium needed.

The administrations of fluids and insulin usually corrects the acidosis in DKA so that bicarbonate administration is seldom needed. Bicarbonate is not usually given unless the serum bicarbonate is 5 mEq/L and the blood pH is <7.

An additional electrolyte imbalance that may develop during ketoacidosis is *hypophosphatemia*. Without adequate phosphorus, decreased peripheral oxygen delivery and additional tissue anoxia may result. Phosphorus in the form of potassium phosphate may be given.

Nursing interventions planned for the patient depend on the severity of the clinical findings and the prescribed therapy. In all patients, careful and frequent monitoring of the following is necessary:
1. Vital signs
2. Level of consciousness
3. Intake and output
4. Resolution of other signs of dehydration and acidosis
5. Signs and symptoms of fluid overload
6. Urine and blood glucose and ketone bodies

The nurse must make sure that the specimens are collected as ordered and that the appropriate tests are done. It is important that the results of the tests be documented. The assessments made by the nurse and the results of laboratory

---

Indices of insulin deficit

pH value <7.35
Blood glucose level
Degree of ketonemia
Clinical findings, including degree of coma

tests will be used to make appropriate adjustments in therapy. A flow sheet with all pertinent laboratory and assessment data is instituted so that all changes in the patient's status are displayed in a readily comprehensible manner.

☐ Treatment of precipitating condition

As therapy of acute metabolic imbalance is begun (insulin, fluid and electrolyte replacement), attention is given to detecting and treating concurrent illness. Sometimes the precipitating factor is not determined until treatment is well under way and the patient is recovered from coma sufficiently to give a history of preceding events. Sometimes family members can give insight into possible etiology. A common cause of DKA is infection. Antibiotic therapy should begin after specimens for culture and sensitivity of urine, sputum, wound drainage, or blood are obtained.

Should lack of knowledge or of compliance be implicated in DKA, institution of a teaching plan is appropriate as soon as the patient has recovered enough to be comfortable and is feeling well enough to learn.

☐ Promoting safety and well-being

The patient with severe insulin deficit is critically ill and requires excellent nursing. Skilled care involves attending to the following:
1. Required monitoring (as discussed previously)
2. Prescribed therapeutic measures
3. Maintenance of airway in an unconscious patient
4. Frequent turning and skin care
5. Side rails and hand restraints if necessary to maintain intravenous lines
6. Attention to discomforts of abdominal pain, nausea, and vomiting usually present in the conscious patient
7. Maintenance of nutrition
   a. Fluids first when able to take something by mouth
   b. Solid foods as soon as possible to improve gastric tone
8. Maintenance of the flow sheet

■ MINIMIZING DISRUPTION OF DIABETES TREATMENT

Effective self-care of diabetes mellitus should be enhanced at every opportunity. Blood glucose control is increased when food intake, exercise, and medication are consistent from day to day. Mutual planning by patient and nurse can be done soon after admission if the patient is conscious. The following should be determined:
1. Self-care practices that will be continued by the patient
2. Practices that need to be done by the nurse
3. Timing of the administration of insulin and medications at home, so that a similar schedule can be established, if possible

■ CARE DURING SURGERY AND DIAGNOSTIC TESTS

When fasting is necessary, caution must be used to avert hypoglycemia in the person who takes insulin or an oral hypoglycemic agent. Orders must be clarified as necessary to ensure that glucose is available while insulin is acting. Sometimes insulin administration is delayed until the patient finishes a specific test.

It is routine to schedule diabetic patients early in the morning for diagnostic tests or surgery to minimize the amount of disruption in their regimen.

☐ Effects of surgery on the person with diabetes

Surgery is a physical and psychologic stressor for anyone. For the person with diabetes mellitus there are additional risks. The stress of surgery can result in disruption of metabolic control. Persons with diabetes are at increased risk for the following:
1. Decreased resistance to infection
2. Impaired wound healing
3. Age-related complications (many persons with diabetes are elderly)
4. Macrovascular and microvascular changes that may lead to postsurgical complications.

The person with diabetes mellitus is at risk for developing *hypoglycemia or hyperglycemia* during the perioperative period. During this period, patients usually are not given anything by mouth and are given fluids intravenously. This decreases total caloric intake and may also decrease insulin needs. However, the effects of surgery on contrainsulin hormonal changes may increase the need for additional insulin. The stresses of surgery cause the release of ACTH, glococorticoids, and catecholamines, all of which elevate serum glucose levels.

☐ Management of the diabetic person undergoing surgery

See the box on p. 928 for the modifications of therapy used during the perioperative period. To minimize the disruption in metabolic control, the patient's metabolism should be thoroughly regulated before surgery. The normal food, fluid, and medication routine is maintained until the night before surgery. After surgery, blood or urine checks are carried out on an every 4 to 6 hour schedule; the results are used to determine the amount of insulin needed. To prevent starvation ketosis, all diabetic persons should receive 125 to 250 gm carbohydrate/day until a normal diet is resumed.

■ Counseling and teaching

An integral part of the treatment of diabetes mellitus is education of patients so they can assume responsibility for required self-care, including seeking medical advice or treatment when needed. Teaching should begin at the time of diagnosis and continue until the patient is competent in maintaining on optimal level of wellness. The American Association of Diabetes Educators has proposed that 10 components comprise the educational program. (See the box on p. 929.)

The Association further proposes that educational programs for diabetic persons be planned in the following three phases:

Management of the person with diabetes during the perioperative period

1. Diabetics who receive insulin
   a. Preoperative
      1. Intravenous infusion of glucose on morning of surgery
      2. One-half usual insulin dose subcutaneously
   b. Intraoperative
      1. Monitoring of blood sugar levels if surgery is lengthy
      2. Additional insulin or glucose as needed
   c. Postoperative
      1. Intravenous infusion of glucose until food can be taken orally
      2. Insulin given subcutaneously in equally divided doses over 24 hours or added to intravenous fluids
      3. Urine or blood glucose monitored every 4 to 6 hours
      4. Additional insulin given if indicated from monitoring
2. Diabetics not normally given insulin
   a. Preoperative
      1. Intravenous infusion of glucose on morning of surgery
   b. Postoperative
      1. Blood sugar and urine glucose and ketone levels monitored every 4 to 6 hours
      2. Insulin given if indicated from monitoring
3. All diabetics
   a. 125 to 250 g CHO/day until normal diet resumed
   b. Normal regimen reinstituted as soon as possible before patient is discharged
   c. Continued monitoring of blood or urinary glucose and ketone levels even after usual diet resumed (increased insulin may be needed because of catabolism from surgery)

Table 28-13 Phases of diabetes education

Initial management	Home management	Improvement of life-style
Survival knowledge and skills	Self-sufficiency in daily management of diabetes	Enrichment of life by flexibility in management, insight, and self-determination
Objectives for the component—definition of diabetes		
States need for insulin in body	Lists symptoms of diabetes	Identifies significance of hyperglycemia in relation to other metabolic problems and long-term complications
Describes what happens in body when insulin is deficient	Explains relationship of symptoms to insulin deficiency	States significance of hyperglycemia and glycosuria, or vice versa, relative to changes in renal threshold
States simple working definition of diabetes	States how diagnosis of diabetes is made	Lists main differences between insulin-dependent and non–insulin-dependent diabetes
States role of food, activity, and medication in treatment of diabetes	IDDM: States relationship of undernutrition to insulin deficiency	States current knowledge of hereditary aspects of diabetes
	NIDDM: States relationship between state of overnutrition, inactivity, and relative insulin deficiency	Verbalizes concerns about diabetes in other family members

Diabetes Association.

Ten components of diabetes education

1. Definition of disease
2. Nutrition
3. Activity
4. Medication
5. Monitoring glucose control
6. Hypoglycemia
7. Illness
8. Psychologic adjustment
9. Hygiene and foot care
10. Follow-up

1. *Initial management,* in which the knowledge and skills needed to survive are emphasized
2. *Home management,* in which patients learn to be self-sufficient in the daily management of the disease
3. *Improvement of life-style,* in which patients learn how to enrich their lives by gaining flexibility in management, insight, and self-determination

The three phases of diabetes education are illustrated in Table 28-13. Each phase is specified by objectives and the requisite knowledges, skills, and attitudes. The nurse should begin teaching about initial management before introducing more complex home management content. Evaluation of learning and reinforcement should be part of the plan.

It is important that the nurse set priorities in teaching and begin with the most basic information. Too much information overwhelms patients, who often find the diagnosis emotionally disturbing. The resultant anxiety usually diminishes as patients learn they can perform the self-care measures and experience living with the disease and its treatment. Efforts are made that all those involved in the educational program have congruent goals and that plans are coordinated to avoid conflicts or discrepancies that confuse the patient and family.

Many diabetic patients are given initial instruction in the ambulatory setting, and further education is given at repeat visits. Initial instruction for a hospitalized patient with newly diagnosed diabetes should be planned with consideration of three factors:
1. Expected length of stay
2. Specific referrals for further teaching
3. Other concerns and teaching needs not related to diabetes self-care

■ NUTRITION

A dietary consultation should be initiated early in the educational program. The nurse and other health care professionals should not underestimate the difficulty with which persons change food habits. There is no substitute for a careful dietary history and mutual planning by patient and dietitian (or nurse) about those changes necessary to control blood glucose levels or weight. The nurse can assist the patient in selecting foods in the hospital, in planning menus for home, and in reinforcing the dietary instruction (see p. 916).

The diabetic diet does not require the use of special or dietetic foods. Persons with diabetes must be warned about being misled by the word *dietetic.* Dietetic may refer to low sodium content rather than to low sugar content. Dietetic candies and foods labeled light (or Lite) also must be used with care. Dietetic foods are not necessarily low in calories and may have high fat content. Sugar substitutes can be used and still are available despite the controversy about the possible carcinogenic effects of saccharin.

Some persons who develop diabetes are accustomed to having an alcoholic beverage daily. With approval of the physician, the diabetic may have small amounts of alcohol. Because alcohol is a high-calorie food, it must be exchanged for fat calories in the diet. The combination of alcohol and chlorpropamide should be avoided because of a severe Antabuse-like reaction.

Four strategies are useful in helping patients learn to manage blood glucose levels by diet:
1. Weighing of meat and measuring of other foods acquaint patients with portion size.
2. Written instruction should accompany verbal discussion of the meal plan.
3. The patient's record of food intake can be correlated with records of blood or urine, glucose tests, food intake, exercise, and medication.
4. Patients should be helped to apply dietary knowledge by doing exercises in which the person chooses foods from hospital and restaurant menus or from a variety of food items (models, pictures)

Participation in a behavior modification program for weight reduction and maintenance is highly recommended for obese persons with NIDDM. Teaching facts and principles about food intake and therapeutic requirements alone does not help the patient change eating behavior.

Special care must be taken to incorporate into the plan food preferences (ethnic, cultural, or vegetarian), as well as established eating patterns. The nurse can support the patient in identifying which changes in daily food patterns need to be made and in devising ways to make these changes.

■ ACTIVITY

All persons with diabetes benefit from regular exercise as part of treatment. Plans need to be reasonable and take into account previous activity level, cardiopulmonary status, mobility, and interests (see p. 918). For example, an elderly hemiplegic patient could be encouraged to do range-of-motion and leg-raising exercises, and a younger person with no disabilities could be encouraged to develop interest in a specific exercise or sports program. Sports that are contraindicated for patients receiving insulin include those in which the dangers of hypoglycemia increase the hazard of the sport (for example, scuba diving or sky diving).

In addition to stressing the importance of exercise, the nurse can assist the patient in planning how to incorporate regular exercise into the life-style after discharge. Optimal timing of exercise would be during periods of greater hyperglycemia when blood glucose is less than 300 mg/dl. A greater chance of insulin reaction occurs when peak actions of insulin coincide with unanticipated exercise in the patient receiving insulin or oral hypoglycemic agents. The benefits of exercise as part of the overall treatment should be emphasized to persons who are obese and have NIDDM (type 2) as well.

■ MEDICATION

□ Insulin knowledge

Patients should be able to name their prescribed type of insulin and the dosage (see p. 919.) They do not need to know all the insulin varieties, but they must be able to do the following:

1. Identify their prescribed insulin
2. Check the expiration date
3. Prepare and give the accurate dose
4. State that they will never change the insulin (type, purity, species, strength) without the physician's direction

□ Self-injection of insulin

Most persons are fearful of self-injection and would prefer to postpone learning this task; yet repeated practice is necessary if they are to safely administer an accurate dose with sterile technique. The nurse must teach this skill early and with attention to the patient's fear, whether that fear is or is not expressed.

One study supports the belief that adults can learn this skill most readily and cope best if the first self-injection is not delayed for practice with equipment.[10] The nurse should firmly encourage the patient to hold the syringe, cleanse and pierce the skin, and inject the ordered insulin (or an equivalent dosage of sterile saline) from the syringe previously prepared by the nurse. Verbal encouragement and a guiding hand may be necessary for the patient to self-inject successfully. After adults experience self-injection, they are better able to focus on preparation of the insulin syringe (see p. 923 for guidelines in insulin administration).

Most patients prefer disposable syringes and needles. Patients should be helped to determine the quantity of supplies needed for at least a month. Prescriptions are not necessary for insulin or for syringes and needles. Cotton balls purchased in bulk and a bottle of 70% ethyl alcohol, as compared with individually wrapped alcohol pledgets, can reduce costs (91% alcohol is recommended if skin redness or irritation develops).

Typical trays for injection at home can be set up for use in demonstrations and for patients to use in practice. The nurse can discuss boxes or trays that can be used at home to keep all equipment together. The equipment should be stored on a shelf or closet, out of reach of children and out of sight.

□ Storage of insulin

Patients should be taught to give insulin at room temperature to decrease the risk of lipodystrophy and to decrease the antigenicity of the insulin. The current practice is to keep the currently used vial at room temperature and refrigerate additional vials, even though insulin vial labels direct the refrigeration of all insulin. It is known that regular insulin will remain stable for 12 months at 37° C (modified insulins for 24 months). Travelers are taught to carry insulin with them rather than to pack it in baggage that might be subjected to extreme temperatures in car trunks or cargo compartments of planes or trains.

Refrigeration is recommended when prefilled syringes are used, to decrease the potential bacterial growth from contamination.

□ Measures to assist the visually impaired diabetic

Blind patients or those with hand disability may be able to self-inject if the syringes are prepared for them. Often a 1-week supply of syringes are prefilled by a family member or neighbor who has been taught by a home-care nurse. It is important that the patient gently rotate the prefilled syringe before administering the insulin and allow it to come to room temperature.

In addition to prefilled syringes, the visually impaired patient may be able to see the darker and larger markings on a "low dose" syringe (volume 0.5 ml, scale U-100). This syringe can only be used for doses of <50 units U-100 insulin. Similarly, a magnifier that clamps on the insulin syringe may aid the patient in withdrawing an accurate

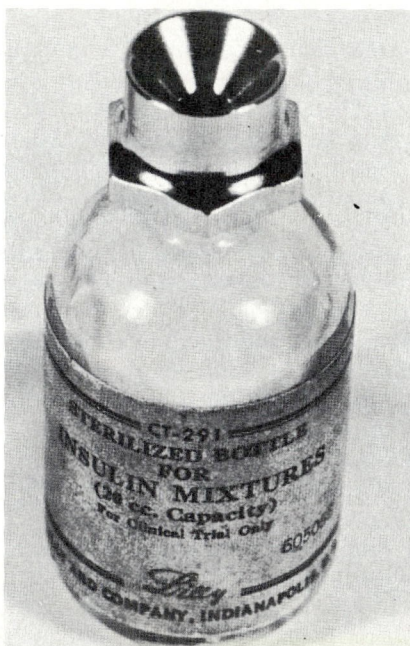

Fig. 28-8 Insulin needle guide that fits over top of insulin vial. Patient cleans stopper and guide with alcohol before placing guide on vial. Needle is laid in V of guide, and vial is pushed toward it. (Courtesy American Foundation for the Blind, Inc, New York, NY.)

dosage. Fig. 28-8 shows a needle insertion guide, which directs the needle into the rubber portion of the vial top.

Many other aids for the visually impaired diabetic are advertised in publications for diabetics or are available from the American Foundation for the Blind.* Special syringes with plunger locks or attachable devices for locking the plunger, and devices for measuring predetermined dosage can be purchased.

Persons with poor vision risk drawing air instead of insulin into the syringe. They must be cautioned to invert the bottle completely and to insert the needle only a short distance. Often they are advised to use only about two thirds of the bottle of insulin and to have on hand another full bottle. Some persons have a community health nurse or a friend withdraw the last doses in a bottle of insulin for them or they go to a clinic for the last few injections.

Table 28-14 Criteria for strict control of blood glucose level

Past criteria (mg/dl)	Current criteria	
	Ideal (mg/dl)	Acceptable (mg/dl)
Fasting 60-130	60-90	60-130
Before meals	60-105	60-130
After meals (1 hr) <200	≤140	≤180
After meals (2 hr) <140	≤120	≤150

From Skyler J, and others: Algorithms for adjustment of insulin dosage by patients who monitor blood glucose, Diabetes Care **4:**314, 1981. By permission of the American Diabetes Association, Inc.

■ **MONITORING GLUCOSE CONTROL**

The nurse can help patients understand that strict control of blood glucose levels offers the best chance of preventing the complication of diabetes. In the past, good to excellent control was defined by higher levels of blood glucose than is now thought to be ideal. Previously 5% to 10% of daily calorie loss through glycosuria was considered acceptable. Patients who received their diabetes education before 1980 may need reeducation about desired levels of control. Table 28-14 compares past and current criteria of blood glucose levels.[32]

☐ **Self-monitoring of blood glucose**

Increasingly, persons with diabetes mellitus are using home blood glucose monitoring techniques to determine their metabolic status rather than testing urine for glucose. Various types of tests for home blood glucose monitoring correlate well with laboratory measurement of blood glucose level. A reflectance meter adds to the cost and inconvenience of monitoring but gives a precise numerical value (Fig. 28-9). Some test strips (Chemstrip bG, Visidex) do not require a meter and indicate the *range* of blood glucose. For many patients, knowing the range is sufficient.

Self-monitoring has been found to facilitate attainment of glycemic control in insulin dependent diabetes (type 1) and in pregnant women. It is always used by those with multiple-injection schedules or infusion pumps. Self-monitoring can be used to validate subjective symptoms of hypoglycemia or hyperglycemia, and it allows more immediate feedback about the effects of food, activity, and medications.

*American Foundation for the Blind, Inc, 15 West 16th St, New York, NY 10011.

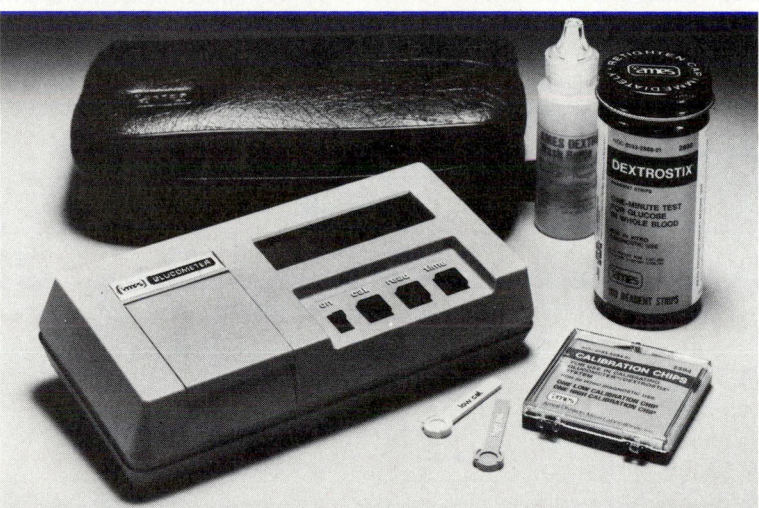

Fig. 28-9 Glucometer to measure blood glucose levels at home. Reflectance photometer to left, calibration chips, wash bottle, Dextrostix, and leatherette case. (Courtesy Ames Division, Miles Laboratories, Elkhart, Ind.)

Certain factors should be considered before recommending blood glucose monitoring to a particular patient. Those with neuropathy or vascular or inflammatory conditions of the fingers may be at risk for tissue injury from repeated pricking of the finger. Patients may not accept the expense, discomfort, and inconvenience of this technology. Visual acuity must be adequate to "read" the color changes of the test strips or to read the digital display of the meter. Those who believe that they have managed their diabetes well in the past with urine testing may have little incentive to do blood glucose monitoring. The most important factor, perhaps, is that the patient and the health care provider intend to use the information gained to achieve better blood glucose control than can be obtained with urine testing.

There is great variability in physicians' recommendations for frequency of testing. Some patients are advised to test before and after meals and at bedtime. For others who have established stable control, physicians may recommend testing frequently during one day of the week and whenever they feel ill.

To do the testing, the person sticks a finger and applies a drop of blood to a commercially prepared glucose oxidase stick. The timing for the reading and the preparation of the specimen are very important in obtaining accurate results. Self-monitoring of blood glucose is expensive, and not all insurance companies reimburse for this expense.

☐ Monitoring by Hb A$_{1C}$

Long-term control of diabetes mellitus is being monitored by Hb A$_{1C}$, which is a minor hemoglobin that results from the glycosylation of normal hemoglobin A.[23] Glycosylation results in the adherence of glucose to proteins; the amount of glycosylation directly correlates with the levels of blood glucose. Any protein can be measured; hemoglobin is chosen for convenience of sampling. The glycosylated hemoglobin accumulates during the 120-day life-span of red blood cells and reflects the *average* glucose level over several weeks. In normal persons the level of Hb A$_{1C}$ is 3% to 6%. The goal of therapy is for the person with

diabetes mellitus to be able to maintain Hb A$_{1C}$ no greater than one and one half times normal.

This test is the first measurement of how well patients have controlled blood glucose at home. It is also used in research studies of blood glucose control and to differentiate noncompliance from an acute illness that results in an elevated level of blood glucose. Findings can be summarized as follows:

1. Any level of blood glucose with a high Hb A$_{1C}$ value suggests poor compliance over several weeks
2. A high blood glucose level with a low Hb A$_{1C}$ value indicates recent onset of a hyperglycemic process, such as infection

☐ Urine testing

Many patients monitor glucose level by urine testing, even though the information obtained is imprecise and difficult to use in daily decision making about ways to achieve "strict" control. Nurses can help patients to understand that negative results of urine tests (in a patient with a renal threshold of 180 ≥mg/dl) may mask significant hyperglycemia. In contrast, some patients, often children, have low renal thresholds and can control blood glucoses at optimal levels with urine tests alone. Some patients combine urine testing with blood glucose testing to monitor blood glucose in time periods between blood tests.

Urine testing for the presence of ketone bodies should be encouraged for the following persons:

1. All patients with IDDM (type 1) on a routine daily basis
2. All diabetics who feel ill

The urine testing equipment used will depend on the stability of the disease, the degree of glycosuria anticipated, and the person's life-style, visual acuity, and physical limitations. Different urine testing products can give 0.5%, 2%, or 5% maximum readings of glycosuria. Some require accurate timing or an ability to measure drops of urine. The person may be able to distinguish shades of color more accurately on one specific color chart. (See Tables 28-15, 28-16, and 28-17.)

Table 28-15   Comparison of readings with various urine-sugar (glucose) tests

Product	\(^1\!/_{10}\)%	¼%	½%	¾%	1%	2%	3%	5%
				Glucose concentration				
Clinitest, 5-drop		Trace	+	+ +	+ + +	+ + + +		
Clinitest, 2-drop*			‡		‡	‡	‡	‡
Diastix	Trace	+	+ +		+ + +	+ + + +		
Clinistix†		Light (+)		Medium (+ +)		Dark (+ + +)		
Tes-Tape	+	+ +	+ + +			+ + + +		

*The 2-drop chart provides a "trace" color block without a percent value; a trace result only indicates less than ½%.
†Estimates relative presence of glucose, but cannot show percent amount.
‡Measures percent at these levels, but equivalent + signs not available.
NOTE: Blank spaces mean color blocks are absent for those concentrations.
From *Home urine testing for the diabetic*, Ames Company, Division of Miles Laboratories, 1976, Elkhart, Ind, p. 7.

Table 28-16 Urine tests for ketonuria

Test	Procedure	Interpretation
Acetest tablets	Use only whole tablets Place 1 drop on tablet; read after 30 sec Lavender-purple	Differentiates level of ketones: small, moderate, large
Ketostix	Dip test strip quickly in and out of urine; hold in air for reading; read after 30 sec Lavender-purple	Differentiates level of ketones: 0, trace, small, moderate, large
Keto Diastix		Also tests for glucose (see Table 28-15)
Kyotest UGK	Dip test strip quickly in and out of urine; hold in air for reading; read after 50 sec Lavender-purple	Differentiates level of ketones: under ¼%, ¼%, ½%, 1% +. Also for glucose (see Table 28-15)

Table 28-17 Urine tests for glycosuria

Test	Procedure	Interpretation
Clinitest tablets	Obtain freshly voided urine. Use only "fresh" whole tablets (off-white with blue specks) that completely dissolve. Use only the Clinitest dropper. Do not shake the tube during the reaction. Place required drops of urine (2 or 5) and 10 drops of *water* in a clean test tube. Drop 1 tablet into tube. Wait 15 sec after boiling has stopped to compare urine color with the proper color chart.	Clinitest is based on copper reduction of sugars, including glucose; thus false positive results can occur in the presence of other sugars. Other false positive results can occur if patient takes large doses of vitamin C, more than 6 tablets of aspirin per day, and certain drugs (gantrisin, levodopa, Benemid, Isonizid). Cephalosporins (for example, Keflex) may cause color reactions that make Clinitest results difficult to read.
2-drop method	Use 2 drops of urine and the 2-drop color chart. *Watch* the color reaction *during* the 15 sec waiting period.	Differentiates glucose content of 0.5%, 1%, 2%, 3%, and 5%. Large amounts of sugar may cause a "pass-through" reaction in which the color of the urine quickly changes from 5% to a lesser number.
5-drop method	Use 5 drops of urine and the 5-drop color chart.	Differentiates glucose content of 0.25%, 0.5%, 0.75%, 1%, and 2%.
Plastic, paper-impregnated strips and paper tape	All strips and tape should be held in air for reading; dip the test strip or tape quickly in and out of urine.	These strips and tapes show a reaction of urine and glucose oxidase, thus are specific for glucose. Inaccurate findings can occur if patients are taking ascorbic acid, pyridium, salicylates, or levodopa. More convenient and more costly than tablets.
Chemstrip uG	Read after 2 min: Block 1, yellow to green; Block 2, white to aqua.	Differentiates urine glucose content of ⅒%, ¼%, ½%, 1%, 2%, 3%, 5+%.
Chemstrip UGK		Also tests for ketones (Table 28-16).
Diastix	Read after 15 sec with proper color chart on container.	Differentiates urine glucose content of 0.1%, 0.25%, 0.5%, 1%, and 2%.
Keto Diastix		Also tests for ketones (Table 28-16).
Kyotest UGK	Read after 30 sec: shades of blue.	Differentiates urine glucose content of under ¼%, ¼%, ½%, 1% +; also tests for ketones (Table 28-16).
Clinistix	Read in 10 sec with Clinistix color chart.	Estimates glucose presence as light, medium, and dark, thus most imprecise of all tests.
Tes-Tape	Tear 1½ inch from Tes-Tape roll; dip in urine and *read in air* after 1 or 2 min: 1 min, yellow-green, 0.25% 2 min, dark green, ≥0.5%; 2 min, dark green, ≤0.5%; green-black, ≤2%.	Differentiates urine glucose content as 0.1%, 0.25%, 0.5%, and 2%.

NURSING CARE PLAN

Person with diabetes mellitus

DATA: Mrs. Toren is an obese, 52-year-old married woman with NIDDM diagnosed 3 years ago. She was referred to a short-term ambulatory diabetes education program by her physician for instruction on insulin administration, since blood glucose control had not been achieved with dietary measures.

The nurse history identified the following:

1. She saw referral as necessary but perceived it and inability to control weight and blood glucose as a personal failure.
2. She maintained inconsistent sleep/activity schedule. (Worked as an LPN 8 PM to 8 AM Saturday and Sunday with 2 to 4 hours sleep during day; arose at 8 AM and retired at 11 PM on other days.)
3. She had accurate knowledge about dietary modifications and had participated successfully in several weight reduction programs with 20- to 40-pound weight loss each time.
4. She does not exercise consistently.
5. She has performed blood glucose monitoring on others and once or twice on self.
6. She states that work is important to her; satisfactions were derived from work group socialization and it "keeps me busy."
7. She fears that her husband will die suddenly at home. Two years ago she had performed CPR when he had a cardiac arrest at home. Realizes that she maintains work schedule "to keep me from worrying about husband."

Objective data included blood glucose, 220 mg/dl; weight, 200 lb; BP 134/84; urine, glucose 2% with no ketones present.

Collaborative nursing actions include teaching Mrs. Toren those measures that would help her achieve control of blood glucose (insulin, diet, and exercise) and to detect, prevent, and treat hypoglycemic reactions. The nurse reported Mrs. Toren's work schedule to the physician and asked for insulin dosage alterations on weekends. The physician was unaware of her work schedule and stated that blood glucose control could not be optimum with this schedule.

Nursing diagnosis: Knowledge deficit: self-injections, self—blood glucose monitoring related to lack of exposure

Expected patient outcomes	Nursing interventions	Rationale
Patient will independently administer to self	Support patient as necessary to self-inject insulin	Adults who perform this task have minimal discomfort and realize they are capable of giving own insulin
Patient will perform blood glucose monitoring (BGM) accurately	Observe patient's skill in BGM; correct as necessary	Evaluation of patient technique is necessary to ensure accuracy
Patient will use measurements obtained by BGM to achieve blood glucose below 140 mg/dl	Review with patient the effect of activity, dietary intake, and insulin on blood glucose. Instruct patient on frequency and timing of BGM	BGM gives immediate feedback about previous behaviors and reinforces value of therapeutic measures
Patient can detect and treat hypoglycemia	Review with patient signs and symptoms and treatment measures	This knowledge assures that patient can safely give own insulin and decreases fear of a reaction
	Refer to dietician for modification of diet necessary with insulin, and for verification of diet knowledge	The dietician is the appropriate person to teach about diet

NURSING CARE PLAN

Person with diabetes mellitus—cont'd

Nursing diagnosis: Altered health maintenance: related to ineffective coping skill

Expected patient outcomes	Nursing interventions	Rationale
Patient will state at least one change that will improve blood glucose control	Teach patient effects of stress, lack of exercise, and activity pattern on blood glucose	If patient understands how stress impairs health, likelihood of change is more likely
	Explore with Mrs. Toren willingness and ability to change behaviors: sleep/activity, coping, and exercise	Goals are more likely to be achieved if patient makes realistic choices after considering cost and benefits
	Engage Mrs. Toren in mutual problem solving; refrain from prescribing	Increasing patients' sense of control can help with self-esteem and enhance attitudes toward change
	Explore sources for long-term support in learning more effective coping skills. Suggest support groups:	Changing life-style, eating behaviors, and coping skills are very difficult; support over long periods of time is usually required
	1. For spouses of patients with myocardial infarction	
	2. For weight loss *and maintenance* of weight loss	
	3. Available at work in health service program	
	Suggest to Mrs. Toren that she seek a trial period on day shift on weekends	Trial period can help person make informed choices about work schedule in attaining goals

Patients should record and report the extent of glycosuria by *percentage* rather than by plus signs ($+$, $++$, $+++$, $++++$) (Table 28-15); plus marks do not correlate with the same percentage of glycosuria on all urine tests. This can lead to errors in interpretation of the test results.

What the person does if the test results are abnormal depends entirely on the individual and the instructions that have been given. Instructions should be in writing and may include one or more of the following:

1. Do nothing, but repeat the test later in the day and keep a careful record of urine reactions
2. Increase or decrease insulin or oral drug dosage
3. Increase or decrease food intake
4. Notify physician immediately

Some physicians may want certain patients to show a trace or even 1% sugar in their urine once daily as evidence that the blood sugar concentration is not too low, whereas in most persons this would not be considered good control. The age of the individual, stability of disease, and renal threshold affect the physician's decision in advising a course of action. The nurse can assist the person in interpreting the urine test results and in understanding the rationale for the specific regimen.

☐ Hypoglycemia

Patients who are receiving insulin or orally administered hypoglycemic agents must know how to prevent, detect, and treat hypoglycemic reactions before discharge (see p. 925). The nurse provides and explains the following:

1. Written material describing symptoms and treatment
2. Written material describing exercise related to hypoglycemia
3. Diabetic identification card
4. Sample of quickly absorbed glucose to carry

Patients who have a hypoglycemic reaction during hospitalization are helped to identify those sensations for which glucose should be taken promptly.

In a recent study, patients reported the four most frequent symptoms of hypoglycemia: nervousness, weakness, sweating (all early symptoms), and mental confusion (late symptom). Thirty percent reported severe reactions with memory loss and unconsciousness. In addition, more than 60% reported night sweats.[28] It is suggested that these symptoms be emphasized in initial teaching and that patients be encouraged to treat early symptoms.[46] Patients are taught to take these actions if symptoms occur:

1. Take a quick-acting sugar for initial treatment
2. When symptoms have passed, take a snack of complex carbohydrates and protein (for example, cheese or peanut butter, crackers)
3. If the next meal is due, eat it instead of the snack

Some caregivers are supplied with a glucagon kit and taught to inject 1 mg glucagon in case of unconsciousness and to transport the patient to a medical facility.

■ ILLNESS

All illnesses influence the status of diabetes control. In most instances the person with diabetes needs increased insulin in the presence of a concurrent illness, especially infection. Yet many mistakenly believe that if they cannot eat they do not need to take the prescribed insulin or oral hypoglycemic agent. *Failure of patients with IDDM to take insulin when ill is a frequent cause of ketoacidosis.* These persons should take their insulin and *carbohydrate* in some form.

Guidelines for the diabetic person with an illness include the following:

1. Take prescribed dose of insulin.
2. Spread 50% of the daily CHO allowance over 24 hours.
3. Increase fluid intake.
4. Include food items with more simple sugars than regularly allowed, such as custard, nondiet soft drinks, gelatin.
5. Advance diet toward the normally prescribed diet as soon as possible.
6. Institute urine or blood glucose monitoring on a more frequent basis.

The person must know when to call the primary health care provider. Each person will receive individual instructions, but in general the primary health care provider should be called if any of the following occur:

1. A full day's urine glucose test results are at maximal readings or blood glucose levels are consistently elevated beyond a specified level, often 200 mg/dl
2. Ketone bodies persist in the urine
3. The person is not able to take *any* food or fluids for longer than 4 hours
4. The person is febrile

■ PSYCHOLOGIC ADJUSTMENT

The degree of diabetes control should be the optimal level that can be reasonably maintained considering the life-style of the person with diabetes. The degree to which persons participate in control of the disease depends on how well they have adapted emotionally to having diabetes and on their knowledge of the disease and motivation to pursue control measures. Helping the person cope with

the impact of the diagnosis and the necessary changes in daily living is a nursing care priority.

The emotional response to a diagnosis of diabetes is often severe and is not easily dealt with. Part of this may result from fear of disability and eventual death. Because diabetes is so widespread, many people have relatives or friends who have the disease and who have had an amputation or become blind. Perhaps an even greater cause of emotional upset is that diabetes affects the life-style in regard to food. Food and eating have meaning beyond the actual meeting of nutritional needs, and changes in eating habits are extremely difficult for some persons to accept.

Initiating a suitable plan of care for diabetes will often make a great difference in how the person continues with care. It can help the person and significant others avoid undue stress and concerns that may make it difficult to control the diabetes. Because most persons with diabetes now receive treatment in a physician's office or a hospital clinic, the community health nurse very frequently needs to help with the initial adjustment. Support groups sponsored by local chapters of the American Diabetes Association or Juvenile Diabetes Foundation may be helpful to patients and families.

Many diabetics are hospitalized because of complications of diabetes or for conditions other than diabetes. In these situations the nurse identifies during the initial interview the diabetic regimen being followed at home. Whenever possible, patients should continue this regimen in the hospital. This includes administering their insulin, monitoring their glucose status, and making personal food selections. Continuing to carry out their own regimen allows patients independence and promotes self-care. Sometimes, however, the patient cannot be independent, and the nurse makes judgments about when and how much self-care should be assumed by the patient.

■ HYGIENE

Persons with diabetes are more *susceptible to infection.* The effectiveness of the skin as a first line of defense is diminished. Uncontrolled diabetes leads to loss of fat deposits under the skin, loss of glycogen, and catabolism of body proteins. Protein loss can hamper the inflammatory response and wound healing. In addition, leukocyte function, migration of leukocytes to the site of infection, phagocytosis, and bacterial killing, all of which are involved in the ability of the body to combat infection, are impaired. Decreased circulation to a part can also delay healing.

The skin must be kept supple and as free of pathogenic organisms as possible. This is especially true in warm moist areas that encourage growth of the organisms (for example, between the toes, under the breasts, and in the axillae and groin). It is, therefore, very important that persons with diabetes carry out hygienic measures for prevention of infection.

□ Foot care

Prevention of ulcers, trauma, and infections of the lower extremities is the key to prevention of amputation. Ulcers, injured areas, and infections heal very slowly. The need

Guidelines for diabetic foot care

1. Wear well-fitting shoes and clean stockings at all times when walking, and never walk barefooted.
2. Bathe feet daily and dry them well, paying particular attention to area between the toes.
3. Do not self-treat calluses, corns, or ingrown toenails; a podiatrist should be consulted if these are present.
4. Bath water should be 29.5° to 32° C (85° to 90° F) and should be tested with a bath thermometer or the elbow before immersing the feet.
5. Heating pads and hot water bottles should not be used.
6. Measures that help increase circulation to the lower extremities should be instituted:
   a. Avoid smoking
   b. Avoid crossing legs when sitting
   c. Protect extremities when exposed to cold
   d. Avoid immersing feet in cold water
   e. Use socks or stockings that do not apply pressure to the legs at specific sites
   f. Institute a regimen of exercises (Chapter 6).
7. Inspect feet daily and report any cuts, cracks, redness, blisters, or other signs of trauma to health care provider so that early treatment can be instituted.
8. If feet are dry, use a lubricating lotion or cream; if moist use powder.

Summary of knowledge and skills for adequate self-care of diabetes mellitus

1. Basic understanding of diabetes mellitus and how metabolism is changed by it
2. Therapeutic regimen prescribed and how it works to keep the blood sugar level normal
3. Diet ordered (calories, CHO, and such), how to calculate diet requirements for each meal, ability to incorporate personal preferences
4. Exercise and its effect on caloric and insulin needs, and how to manage if exercise level is increased above usual
5. If receiving insulin:
   a. Type, amount, timing, method of administration
   b. Ability to give the insulin accurately
   c. Ability to care for equipment properly
6. If receiving oral hypoglycemic agents:
   a. Type, dosage, time schedule
   b. Potential side effects
   c. What to do if new or unexpected symptoms occur
7. Self-monitoring routine for glucose status (urine or serum glucose monitoring):
   a. How to do the tests accurately
   b. What to do if results show hyperglycemia, ketonuria, or hypoglycemia
   c. How to care for equipment and supplies
8. Signs and symptoms of hypoglycemia, how to treat them, and what to do if they occur frequently
9. Signs and symptoms of hyperglycemia and what to do when they occur
10. How to manage diabetes mellitus on days when usual diet cannot be eaten because of illness
11. Measures to prevent lower extremity trauma or injury
12. Type of follow-up care necessary and whom to contact with questions

for daily foot care, including inspection, cannot be overemphasized. A mirror can be used by the patient to examine soles of the feet. The nurse's effectiveness in teaching about foot care will be more effective if the patient has previously included foot care as a part of daily care. The upper box on p. 937 contains guidelines for instruction. Patients should also be taught to take shoes and stockings off at each medical visit and ask the physician to examine the feet. A podiatric evaluation is recommended for all diabetic patients; podiatric services are essential when there are vascular changes, neuropathy, or foot lesions such as callouses, corns, or bunions.

■ FOLLOW-UP

The many teaching needs of the person with diabetes mellitus have been discussed. Education is an integral part of therapy and must be planned over a period of time if the patient is to be capable of diabetes management. The knowledge and skills necessary for self-care are summarized in the lower box on p. 937. Teaching is usually begun at the time of diagnosis, but the nurse must be aware that everything cannot be learned during the first contact. Priorities need to be set: the person should be taught the skills necessary to meet immediate needs, and then be referred to an ambulatory setting or home health care agency. Follow-up might take place in a clinic, physician's or nurse's office, or in a program sponsored by the local diabetes association or a local hospital.

In addition to securing follow-up education appointments, the nurse can do the following:

1. Reinforce the value and need of continued learning
2. Encourage family members to participate
3. Give the patient written instructions and educational literature
4. Ensure that the patient has a resource person to call if assistance is needed before the next appointment

Written material should be selected carefully, for relative content, reading level, and ease in reading. Written material should reinforce prior instruction. The nurse may give the patient local sources of information, such as the public library and the local diabetes association, as well as specific appointment information.

♯ EVALUATION

Questions that guide the nurse's evaluation are derived from an understanding of potential effects of diabetes mellitus on physical well-being, the importance of education for self-management of blood glucose control, and the psychologic impact of this chronic disease and its treatment.

Specific goals or objectives for each patient identify the intended outcomes of health care.

1. What level of blood glucose control has been achieved?
2. Is the patient equipped with knowledge and skills to make decisions about food, exercise, medications, and when to seek medical advice?
3. Has the patient developed sufficient skill to be independent and safely carry out self-management of

the disease in terms of administration of insulin injections or oral hypoglycemic agents, treatment of hypoglycemic reactions, and foot care?
4. Is the patient committed to prevention of short- and long-term complications (follow-up, self-management)?
5. Is the patient coping with diabetes self-care measures, fears and concerns, and life-style changes?

■ SUMMARY

1. Diabetes mellitus is a complex metabolic disorder and may be clinically expressed as non–insulin dependent diabetes mellitus (NIDDM) and as insulin dependent diabetes mellitus (IDDM) in persons with onset before age 40.
2. Insulin deficit is a central feature of the disease; insulin deficit may be *absolute* when beta cells do not secrete insulin; or *relative,* when beta cell defect and peripheral resistance to insulin is present.
3. Glucagon excess and increase in other antagonists to insulin contribute to the hyperglycemia; these are increased in stress conditions.
4. Measures to prevent and treat obesity are the focus of primary prevention of NIDDM; screening to detect persons who are undiagnosed (50%) is the focus of secondary prevention.
5. Insulin deficit and hyperglycemia lead to many immediate alterations in metabolism: hyperosmolarity and osmotic diuresis, glycosuria, cellular starvation, calorie loss, and increased fat metabolism and catabolism.
6. Diabetic ketoacidosis (*DKA*) and hyperglycemic, hyperosmolar, nonketotic coma (*HHNC*) are two life-threatening situations that occur in diabetes mellitus.
7. The duration of hyperglycemia seems a major predictor of the development of microvascular lesions (nephropathy, retinopathy), macrovascular lesions (atherosclerotic disease), and neuropathy.
8. Amputation in diabetes mellitus can result as a consequence of alterations in blood vessels and nerves, tissue trauma, and infection occurring in persons with inadequate skin integrity and insensitivity to pain or pressure. Proper foot care can reduce the risk of amputation.
9. Because patients must be capable in diabetes management, nursing assessment must address the knowledge and coping skills of a patient early in hospitalization so that appropriate education and counseling can proceed.
10. A well-educated person with diabetes will be assertive in describing special needs relating to patterns of food intake, exercise, monitoring, medications, and foot care.
11. Assessment of the person with diabetes includes collecting objective data about metabolic status, cardiovascular-renal status, vision, and nerve function. The lower extremities should be carefully examined.

Putting knowledge to practice

- Use a standard initial assessment guide to collect data about the care needs of patients with diabetes mellitus. Assess whether there are knowledge deficits or inadequate coping skills related to diabetes management. What further information is needed?
- Develop a plan of care based on the data and identified nursing diagnoses.
- Price supplies needed for a month at a local drug store. The patient's therapeutic regimen follows: blood glucose testing qid; NPH insulin 100-U, 35 U bid; regular insulin 100-U, 10 U bid; ketone tests qid. What is the initial cost of a blood glucose meter? Automatic lancer?
- Review one or more patient charts for the presenting problem, precipitating factors, and treatment for DKA and HHNC.
- Evaluate the teaching materials available in one health care setting for relevancy to patients with NIDDM, reading level, and ease of reading.
- Select one or more components of diabetes education and develop objectives and content for initial "survival skills."
- What are policies and procedures for treating hypoglycemia in a hospital with which you are familiar?

12. Dietary recommendations in diabetes mellitus include the following: calorie distribution of CHO (55% to 60%), fat (20% to 30%) with restriction in saturated fat to 10%, and protein (20%); limitation of cholesterol, sodium, and refined simple CHO; and increased use of complex, unrefined CHO.

13. The three primary modalities of treatment of diabetes mellitus are diet, exercise, and hypoglycemic agents; education for self-management of these modalities is an integral part of treatment.

14. Exercise has a hypoglycemic action in most instances; it can increase hyperglycemia if blood glucose levels are above 300 mg/dl or if exercise is intense. Exercise also aids in cardiovascular fitness and weight reduction and weight maintenance programs, and it decreases peripheral resistance.

15. Nurses and patients must be careful to use prescribed insulin: strength, species, length of action, purity.

16. Oral hypoglycemic agents are used in NIDDM; they stimulate the pancreas and decrease peripheral resistance. They may induce hypoglycemia.

17. Self-monitoring of blood glucose is always used by patients using insulin pump therapy or multiple injections. This technology has made it possible to achieve normoglycemia in well-educated patients.

18. Hemoglobin A_{1C} measures the amount of glycosylation of normal hemoglobin A; it correlates with average blood glucose levels over the past 3 months.

19. The treatment of hypoglycemia must be prompt; 10 to 15 gm of simple CHO is given as soon as symptoms are detected. The first signs present are those of epinephrine excess; later signs are those of cerebral dysfunction.

20. Insulin or oral hypoglycemic agents should not be omitted when short illness occurs; about 50% of daily CHO intake should be distributed over 24 hours.

21. The impact of the diagnosis of diabetes mellitus and living with this chronic illness may be expressed by patients emotionally, in concerns about the future, in patient-family conflicts, and in noncompliance.

22. Treatment of DKA and HHNC requires replacement of insulin, fluids, and electrolytes, treatment of precipitating conditions, and monitoring and supportive nursing care of these acutely ill patients.

23. Patients fasting or undergoing surgery require modifications of insulin and food intake and increased monitoring of metabolic status.

24. Foot care includes daily inspection, measures to maintain integrity of skin, and prevention of injury. Referral to podiatric services is highly recommended.

25. Diabetes education must be individualized and planned over time. Initial instruction should be restricted to "survival skills" and beginning home management skills with referral for continued education.

26. An educational program for persons with diabetes mellitus has ten components: these components include knowledge, skills, and attitudes for effective diabetes management (p. 929).

27. Evaluation of nursing interventions includes assessment of whether the metabolic balance is improved, whether the patient has the requisite knowledge and coping skills for self-management, and whether appropriate referrals were made.

REFERENCES AND SELECTED READINGS
Contemporary

1. American Diabetes Association: Principles of nutrition and dietary recommendations for individuals with diabetes mellitus, 1986, Diab Care 10(1):126-132, 1987.
2. American Diabetes Association and American Dietetic Association Exchange lists for meal planning, Alexandria, Va, 1986, The Association.
3. Anderson, J, and Clark, JT: The promise of fiber, Diabetes Forecast 40:47-48,50,52, 1987.

References preceded by an asterisk are particularly well suited for student reading.

4. Andreoli, FE, and others, Cecil's essentials of medicine, Philadelphia, 1986, WB Saunders Co.

5. Benson, JW: In Metz, R, and Larson, E (editors): Blue book of endocrinology, Philadelphia, 1986, WB Saunders Co.

6. Bonheim, R: The second generation, Diab Forecast 36:29-31, 1983.

7. *Byrnes, CA: What's new in the diabetic diet, Nurs 87 17(8):58-59, 1987.

8. Cahill, G, and McDevitt, H: Insulin-dependent diabetes mellitus: the initial lesion, N Engl J Med 304:1444-1464, 1981.

9. *Callahan, M, and Bradley, DJ: Why you should teach your diabetic patients to chart, Nurs 88 18(3):48-49, 1988.

10. Carlyon, PE: Diabetic self-injections: analysis or two teaching/learning approaches, unpublished masters thesis, Kent, Ohio, 1980, Kent State University.

11. Danowski, TS, and others: Parameters of good control in diabetes mellitus, Diab Care 3:88-93, 1980.

12. Defronzo, RA, Ferrannine, E, and Kaivisto, F: New concepts in the pathogenesis and treatment of noninsulin dependent diabetes mellitus, JAMA 245:52-74, 1983.

13. *Dupuis, A: Assessment of the psychological factors and responses in self-managed patients, Diab Care 3:117-120, 1980.

14. Franz, MJ: Evaluating the glycemic response to carbohydrates, Clin Diab 11:129-130, 1986.

15. Gallaway, JA, and DeShazo, RD: The clinical use of insulin and the complications of insulin therapy, In Ellenberg, H, and Rifkin, H, editors: Diabetes mellitus: theory and practice, ed 3, Garden City, NJ, 1983, Medical Publishing Co.

16. Ganda, OP: Pathogenesis of macrovascular disease in the human diabetic, Diabetes 29:931-942, 1980.

17. Guthrie, DW, and Guthrie, RA: Nursing management of diabetes mellitus, ed 2, St. Louis, 1982, the CV Mosby Co.

18. *Hernandez, CM: Surgery and diabetes: minimizing the risks, Am J Nurs 87:788-792, 1987.

19. Heins, JM, Rosett, JW, and Davis, SG: The new look in diabetic diets, Am J Nurs 87:196-199, 1987.

20. Indications for use of continuous insulin delivery systems ands self-measurement of blood glucose: policy statement, American Diabetes Association, Diab Care 5(2):141-142, 1982

21. Jackson, JE, and Bressler, R: Clinical pharmacology of sulfonylurea hypoglycemic agent drugs, J Clin Pharmacol 22:211-245, 1981.

22. Johny, A: Glycosated hemoglobin test as an educational and motivational tool, Diabetes Educator 13:37-62, 1984.

23. Jovanovic, L, and Peterson, C: The clinical utility of glycosylated hemoglobin, Am J Med 70:331-338, 1981.

24. Kolterman, OG, Scarlet, JA, and Olefsky, JM: Insulin resistance in noninsulin-dependent type II diabetes mellitus, Clin Endocrinol Metab 11(2):363-388, 1982.

25. Levin, ME, and O'Neal, L (editors):The diabetic foot, St. Louis, 1983, The CV Mosby Co.

26. National Diabetes Advisory Board: The prevention and treatment of five complications of diabetes (monograph), Charles M Clark, Director, Diabetes Research and Training Center, Indiana University School of Medicine, Indianapolis, Ind.

27. Office guide to diagnosis and classification of diabetes mellitus and other categories of glucose tolerance, Diab Care 4(2):335, 1981.

28. Paulk, LH: Hypoglycemic reactions: from the diabetic's perspective, unpublished master's thesis, Kent, Ohio, 1983, Kent State University.

29. Peterson, CM, and others: Oral hypoglycemic agents, Diabetes Care 5:497, 1982.

30. Rifkin, H (editor): The physician's guide to type 2 diabetes NIDDM): diagnosis and treatment, New York, 1984, American Diabetes Association.

31. *Rossini, AA: Self against self, Diab Forecast 36:26-28, 1983.

32. Skyler, JS, and Cahill, G: Diabetes mellitus: progress and directions, Am J Med 70:101-104, 1981.

33. *Sneid, DS: Hyperosmolar hyperglycemic nonketotic coma, Crit Care Q 2:29-43, 1980.

34. Sulway, M, and others: New techniques for changing compliance in diabetes, Diab Care 3:108-111, 1980.

35. Symposium on home blood glucose monitoring, Diab Care 3:57-149, 1980.

36. US Department of Health and Human Services: The treatment and control of diabetes: a national plan to reduce mortality and morbidity, A report of the National Advisory Board, NIH Publication No. 81-2284, Washington, DC, 1980, US Government Printing Office.

37. Zinman, B, and Vranic, M: Diabetes and exercise, Med Clin N Am 69:145-157, 1985.

Classic

38. *Boyles, VA: Injection aids for blind diabetic patients, Am J Nurs 77:1456-1458, 1977.

39. *Christiansen, C, and Sasche, M: Home blood glucose monitoring, Diab Educator 6:13-21, 1980.

40. Gabbay, K, and O'Sullivan, J: The sorbitol pathway: enzyme localization and content in normal and diabetic nerve and cord, Diabetes 17:239-243, 1968.

41. Ganda, OP, and Soeldner, SS: Genetic, acquired, and related factors in the etiology of diabetes mellitus, Arch Intern Med 137:461-469, 1977.

42. Gerich, JE, and others: Characterization of the glucagon response to hypoglycemia in man, J Clin Endocrinol Metab 1:77-82, 1974.

43. Gerich, JE, and others: Clinical and metabolic characteristics of hyperosmolar nonketotic coma, Diabetes 20:228-238, 1971.

44. Graf, RJ, and others: Nerve conduction abnormalities in untreated maturity-onset diabetes: relation to levels of fasting plasma glucose and glyosylated hemoglobin, Ann Intern Med 90:298-303, 1979.

45. *Judd, S, and Sonksen, PH: Teaching diabetic patients about self-management, Diab Care 3:134-139, 1980.

46. Neville, J: Management by nutrition. In Blevins, D (editor): The diabetic and nursing care, New York, 1979, McGraw-Hill Book Co.

47. Siperstein, MD, and others: Control of blood glucose and diabetic vascular disease, N Engl J Med 296:1060-1063, 1977.

48. Skyler, JS, and others: Blood glucose control during pregnancy, Diab Care 3:69-76, 1980.

49. Unger, RH, and Orci, L: Role of glucagon in diabetes, Arch Intern Med 137:482-491, 1971.

29

The Patient with Endocrine Problems

DOROTHY BLEVINS and VIRGINIA L. CASSMEYER

CHAPTER OBJECTIVES

After studying this chapter, the student should be able to:

- Describe the nature of hormonal imbalances in terms of hyposecretion and hypersecretion.
- Identify specific endocrine gland disorders.
- Describe the pathophysiologic bases and signs and symptoms of dysfunction of the endocrine glands.
- Describe factors influencing hormonal replacement.
- Describe care of the patient undergoing surgery of specific endocrine glands.
- Specify learning needs of patients receiving hormonal replacement therapy.

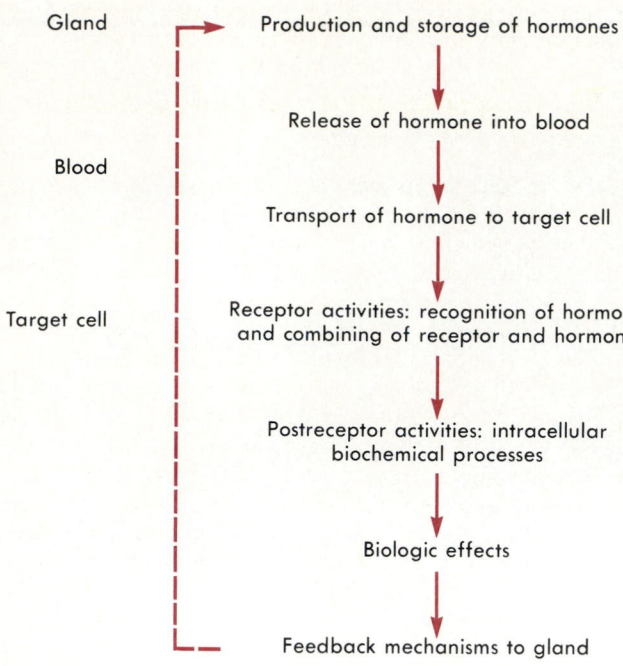

Gland → Production and storage of hormones

↓

Release of hormone into blood

Blood

↓

Transport of hormone to target cell

↓

Target cell

Receptor activities: recognition of hormone and combining of receptor and hormone

↓

Postreceptor activities: intracellular biochemical processes

↓

Biologic effects

↓

Feedback mechanisms to gland

Fig. 29-1 Processes of endocrine system.

The endocrine system functions as the regulator of multiple body processes, primarily through the actions of hormones. Hormones are chemical compounds that are synthesized in glands under genetic control and then secreted into the blood. They affect specific target cells in the body and control diverse physiologic functions. Alterations in the function of the endocrine glands, hormones, or target cellular activities usually result in a wide variety of effects. Many endocrine diseases have a slow and subtle onset of symptoms; yet, since many of the functions controlled by the endocrine system are vital, dysfunction can be serious and even fatal.

Research is advancing the knowlege of complex cellular activities that result from the presence of hormones. Fig. 29-1 illustrates a simple schema of the components of the endocrine system, that is, the series of processes that are now considered integral to the endocrine system. This chapter discusses the health problems related to the hormones of four endocrine glands: pituitary, adrenal, thyroid, and parathyroid. The endocrine functions of the pineal and thymus glands are poorly understood. The gonads are discussed in Chapter 34, and pancreatic dysfunction is discussed in Chapter 28.

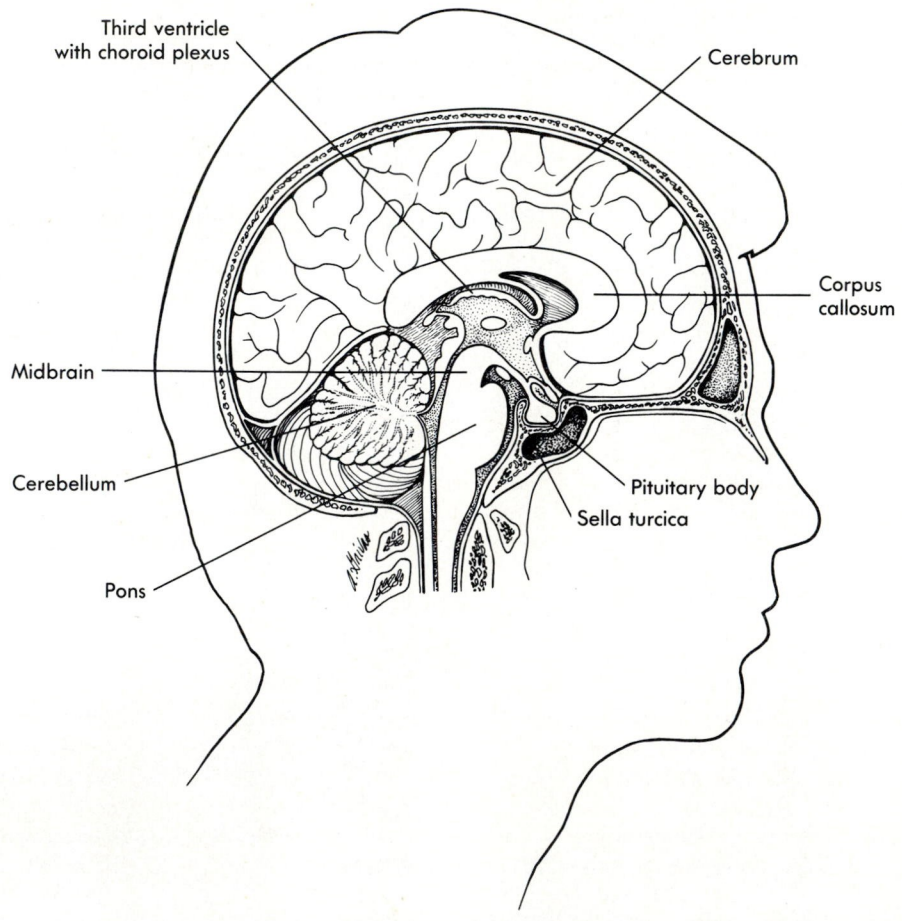

Fig. 29-2 Diagram of sagittal section of head.

■ ANATOMY AND PHYSIOLOGY

■ Pituitary gland

The pituitary gland (hypophysis) is approximately 1 cm in size and weighs 500 mg. It lies in the sella turcica of the sphenoid bone at the base of the skull and is separated from the oral cavity by the sphenoid bone (Fig. 29-2). The sella turcica is close to the optic chiasma. The pituitary gland is actually two glands, the larger anterior pituitary or adenohypophysis and the posterior pituitary or neurohypophysis. The small size of the pituitary gland should not be misleading. The anterior pituitary is often called the *master gland* because of its major influence on other glands and thus on the entire body. This influence is exerted by six hormones that are produced by differentiated cells of the anterior pituitary gland and by two hormones produced by the posterior pituitary gland. See Table 29-1 for the specific name and functions of each hormone.

Thyroid-stimulating hormone (TSH), adrenocorticotropic hormone (ACTH), and the gonadotropic hormones are called trophic hormones because they stimulate other glands to secrete active hormones, which effect changes on specific body cells. The other pituitary hormones exert their influence directly on body cells (non-trophic).

■ Relationship between hypothalamus and pituitary gland

The hypothalamus consists of numerous nuclei and serves as a vital link between the neurologic and hormonal regulatory mechanisms. The hypothalamus exerts control over the anterior pituitary gland and thus over other glands and body cells. The hypothalamus (located in tissues contiguous with the third ventricle) and the anterior pituitary lobe are connected by the hypothalamus-hypophyseal portal blood system, by which neurosecretory releasing factors (RF) and neurosecretory inhibiting factors (IF) are carried from the hypothalamus to the pituitary. It is believed that for each anterior pituitary hormone there is a RF and an IF that stimulates or inhibits the release of that hormone. As the chemical structure of an inhibitory or releasing factor becomes known, the term changes from *factor* to *hormone*. Fig. 29-3 summarizes the interactions between the hypothalamus, anterior pituitary gland, and other endocrine glands and target organs.

Table 29-1 Pituitary hormones

Hormone	Function	Hormone	Function
Anterior pituitary		**Anterior pituitary—cont'd**	
Growth hormone (GH)	Target organ: whole body, possibly works on most tissue through action of somatomedin	Adrenocorticoid-stimulating hormone (ACTH; corticotropin)	Target organ: adrenal cortex
	Concerned with growth of cells, bones, and soft tissues		Necessary for growth and maintenance of size of adrenal cortex
	Increases mitosis		Controls release of glucocorticoids (cortisol) and adrenal androgens
	Affects carbohydrate, protein, and fat metabolism		Minor role in release of mineralocorticoids (aldosterone)
	Increases blood glucose by decreasing glucose utilization; insulin antagonist		
	Increases protein synthesis	**Gonadotropins**	
	Increases free fatty acid levels, lipolysis, and ketone formation	Follicle-stimulating hormone (FSH)	Target organs: gonads
	Increases electrolyte retention and extracellular fluid volume	Luteinizing hormone (LH) (also previously called interstitial cell-stimulating hormone [ICSH] in males)	Stimulates gametogenesis and sex steroid production in males and females
Prolactin (PRL)	Target organ: breast and gonads		
	Necessary for breast development and lactation	**Posterior pituitary**	
	Regulator of reproductive function in males and females	Antidiuretic hormone (ADH)	Effects changes in kidney tubular membrane to increase water absorption; stimulates smooth muscle of intestines and blood vessels
Thyroid-stimulating hormone (TSH)	Target organ: thyroid		
	Necessary for growth and function of thyroid; controls all function of thyroid	Oxytocin	Stimulates uterine contractions and breast milk ejection

Dopamine Inhibits

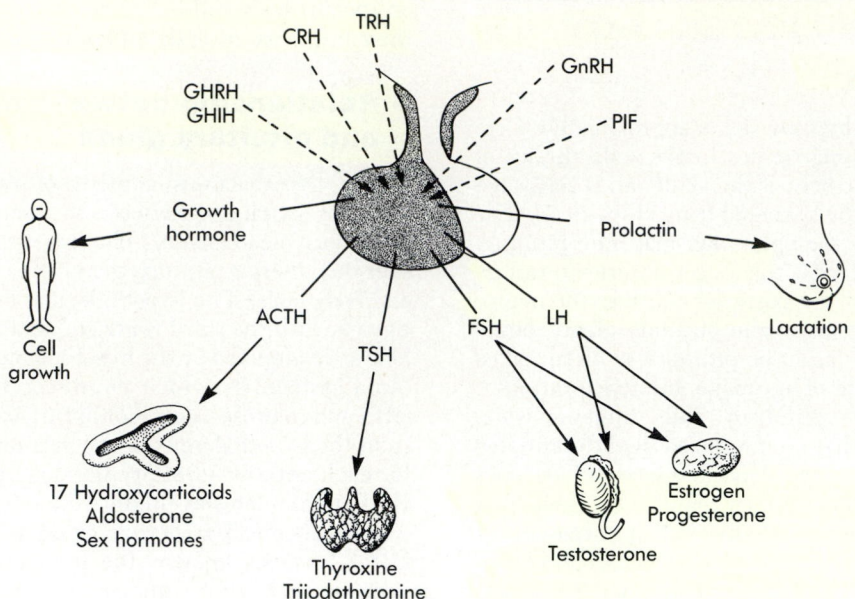

Fig. 29-3 Relationships between hormones of the hypothalamus, anterior pituitary gland, and target tissues are depicted. Only five releasing or inhibitory hormones have been chemically identified: growth hormone–releasing hormone *(GHRH)*; growth hormone–inhibitory hormone *(GHIH,* somatostatin); thyrotropin-releasing hormone *(TRH)*; corticotropin-releasing hormone *(CRH)*; and gonadotropin-releasing hormone *(GnRH)*. Dopamine is thought to be an inhibiting factor *(PIF)* for prolactin. Each anterior pituitary hormone is shown with its respective target tissues: body cells *(GH)*; adrenal cortex *(ACTH)*; thyroid *(TSH)*; testes and ovaries *(FSH* and *LH)*; and breasts (prolactin).

The hypothalamus also exerts control over the posterior pituitary gland to which it is structurally connected. ADH and oxytocin are actually produced in the hypothalamus in the paraventricular and supraoptic nuclei and are carried down neurons by axonal transport to the terminal branches that are located in the posterior pituitary lobe (Fig. 29-4). There they are stored and then released.

■ ADRENAL GLANDS

The two adrenal organs lie in retroperitoneal tissue, each capping the upper pole of a kidney. There are two glands in each adrenal organ: the adrenal cortex, or outer layer, and the adrenal medulla, or central portion. The *adrenal cortex* secretes two groups of hormones that are necessary for life: the *glucocorticoids* of which cortisol is the major hormone, and the *mineralocorticoids* of which aldosterone is the major hormone. The third group of hormones secreted by the cortex in both men and women are the two sex hormones, *androgen* and *estrogen*. The source of sex hormones is an important consideration in certain pathologic conditions or when treatments require the absence of a particular sex hormone.

Table 29-8 (p. 961) lists the specific effects of each adrenal hormone. Although the glucocorticoids have other important functions, they play a major role in *nutrition* (cortisol has hyperglycemic, catabolic, and lipolytic effects) and in *biologic defenses* (cortisol has antiinflammatory and immunosuppressive effects).

The secretion of cortisol is regulated by ACTH (a pituitary hormone) under the influence of corticotrophic-releasing hormone (CRH). Through a negative feedback system, serum levels of cortisol are the primary regulators for inhibition or stimulation of ACTH release (Fig. 29-5). Low serum levels of cortisol stimulate the release of ACTH and then, as a result, the release of cortisol. However, in stress states, hypothalamic stimulation (by CRH) of the pituitary results in increased ACTH secretion and stimulation of the adrenal gland that releases cortisol. This stress response overrides the usual feedback system.

Mineralocorticoid secretion is increased in stress states; however, the major regulator at all times is the renin-angiotensin system (see Chapter 32). An increased serum potassium level also stimulates the adrenal cortex to increase its release of aldosterone. Mineralocorticoids are necessary for the maintenance of sodium, potassium, and water balance; they act on the kidneys to increase the retention of sodium and water and the excretion of potassium.

The *adrenal medulla* secretes epinephrine and norepi-

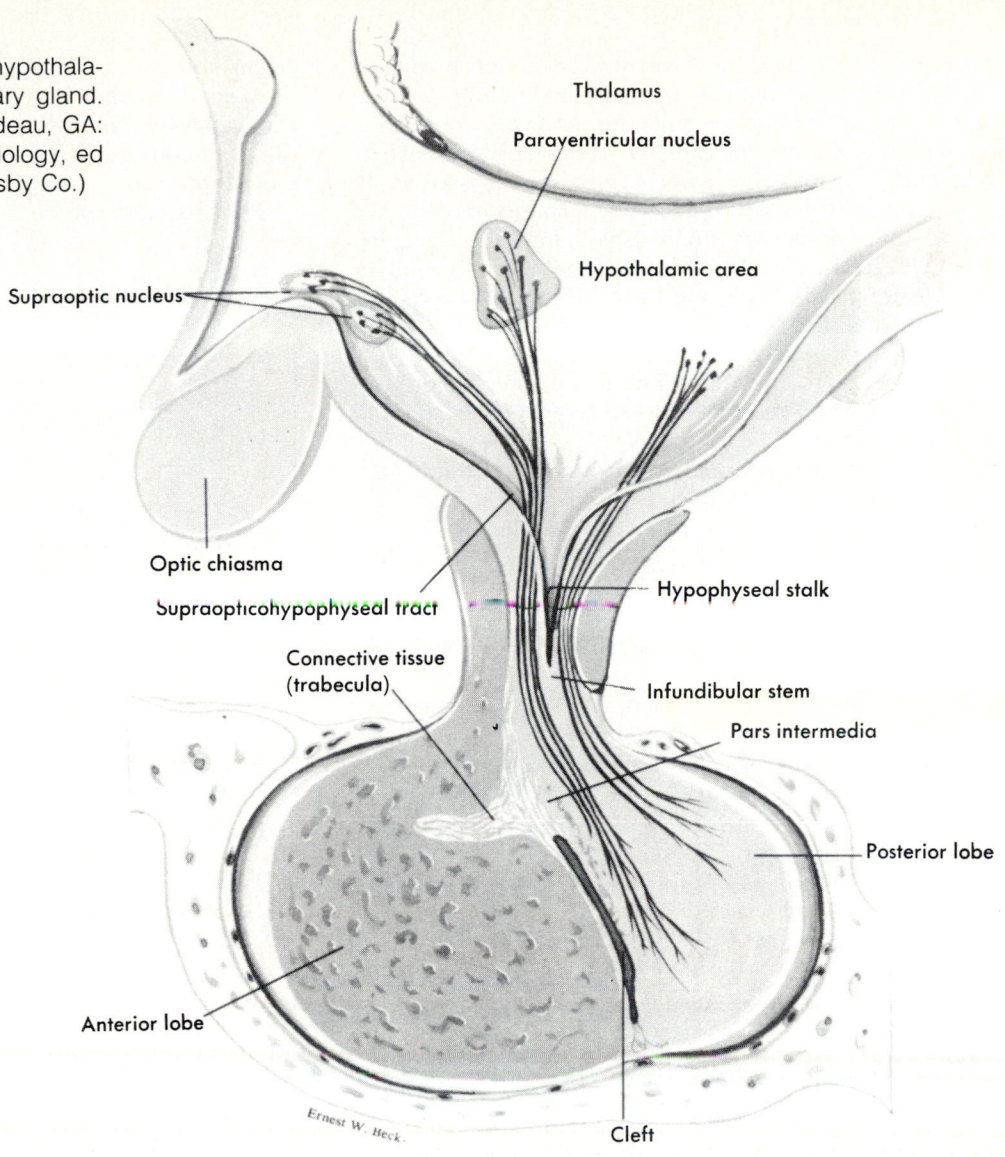

Fig. 29-4 Nerve tracts from hypothalamus to posterior lobe of pituitary gland. (From Anthony, CP, and Thibodeau, GA: Textbook of anatomy and physiology, ed 12, St. Louis, 1987, The CV Mosby Co.)

Thalamus

Paraventricular nucleus

Hypothalamic area

Supraoptic nucleus

Optic chiasma

Supraopticohypophyseal tract

Hypophyseal stalk

Connective tissue (trabecula)

Infundibular stem

Pars intermedia

Posterior lobe

Anterior lobe

Ernest W. Beck.

Cleft

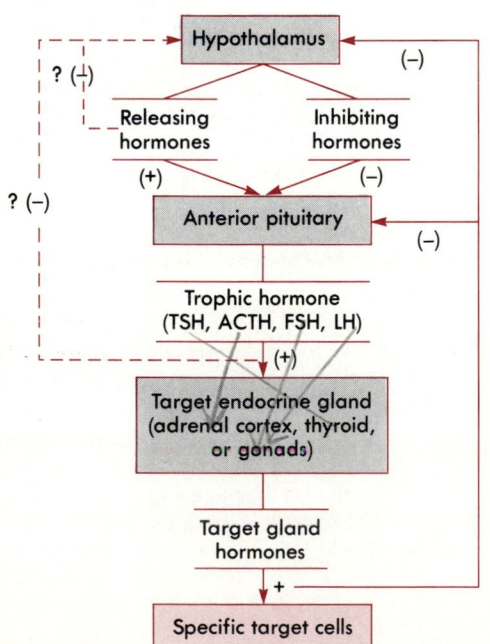

Fig. 29-5 Deficit amount of a target gland hormone allows development of more trophic hormone. This system controls the levels of some hormones secreted by the adrenal cortex (glucocorticoids), thyroid (T_3 and T_4), and the gonads. (Redrawn from Harvey, AM, and others: The principles and practice of medicine, ed 20, New York, 1980, Appleton-Century-Crofts.)

nephrine, which augment the neurotransmitters produced by the sympathetic nervous system. These *catecholamines* secreted by the adrenal medulla are not necessary for life but, in excess, are responsible for serious hypertension.

A small amount of the catecholamines is released at all times, but in stress states, excessive amounts are released as part of the *physiologic stress response*. Table 29-2 lists the multiple effects of increased adrenal-medullary stimulation. Different effects in the body are seen as a result of stimulation of different receptors on target organs. Receptors are classified as:

α-adrenergic (stimulated primarily by norepinephrine):
 α_1-adrenergic receptors are on target organs and are excitatory.
 α_2-adrenergic receptors are at presynaptic sites and are inhibitory.

β-adrenergic (stimulated primarily by epinephrine):
 β_1-adrenergic receptors are located primarily in the heart.
 β_2-adrenergic receptors are located elsewhere in the body.

■ THYROID GLAND

The thyroid gland is located in the anterior aspect of the neck and weighs about 20 g. It consists of two lobes connected by an isthmus and lies just below the larynx. The thyroid gland stores iodine and secretes the thyroid hormone and calcitonin. The thyroid hormone actually

consists of two hormones, thyroxin (tetraiodothyronine, T_4) and triiodothyronine (T_3). These hormones regulate the metabolic rate and the processes of growth and tissue differentiation. Calcitonin helps to maintain serum calcium levels.

The production of the thyroid hormone has several steps

Production of thyroid hormone

The steps in the production of thyroid hormones by follicular cells are as follows:
1. Uptake of iodide and oxidation of iodine
2. Production of thyroglobulin
3. Organification of thyroglobulin (iodine combines to tryosylmoieties in thyroglobulin) to form 3 monoiodotryosine and 3,5-diiodotyrosine
4. Coupling of mono-compounds and diiodo-compounds to form T_4 or T_3
5. Hormone stored in follicular cell attached to thyroglobulin
6. With appropriate stimulation, proteolysis clears T_4 and T_3 off thyroglobulin
7. T_3 and T_4 released and thyroglobulin recycled

Table 29-2   Effects of adrenal-medullary-sympathetic stimulation on body organs*

Organ	Effect	Organ	Effect
Heart	Increased conduction velocity, automaticity, contractility, rate, and stroke volume caused by β_1-stimulation	Gallbladder	Relaxation
		Kidney	Increased renin secretion caused by β_2-stimulation
Blood vessels		Urinary bladder	Relaxation of detrusor muscle and contraction of sphincter
Coronary vessels, brain, lungs	Dilation caused by β_2-stimulation and autoregulatory phenomena	Skin	Pilomotor muscle contraction and localized sweating
Skin, mucosa, abdominal viscera, renal and salivary gland vessels	Constriction caused by α-receptor stimulation; renal vessels also have dopaminergic receptors	Liver	Glycogenolysis and gluconeogenesis caused by β_2-stimulation
Veins	Constriction caused by α-stimulation	Pancreas	Decreased secretion of acini cells; β_2-stimulation causes increased secretion of islet β-cells but α-stimulation causes decreased secretion of islet cells; α-effect predominates
Bronchial muscles	Relaxation caused by β_2-stimulation		
Gastrointestinal tract	Inhibition of production of gastrointestinal secretions; decreased motility and contraction of sphincters caused by β_2-stimulation	Fat cells	Lipolysis
		Brain	Increased alertness, restlessness
		Eyes	Dilation of pupils and relaxation of ciliary bodies

*These total effects would be seen in the physiologic response to stress.

(see box on p. 946) and is under the control of thyroid-stimulating hormone (TSH) and thyroid-releasing hormone (TRH). The major regulator of T_4 and T_3 is the feedback system shown in Fig. 29-5. Calcitonin is primarily regulated by serum levels of calcium: elevated serum levels promote the release of calcitonin, and lowered levels inhibit its release.

The *parathyroid glands* consist of four minute glands that are variously located on the posterior aspect of each thyroid lobe. Occasionally extra glands are located on the thyroid, in the mediastinum, or behind the esophagus. Parathyroid hormone (PTH) regulates calcium and phosphorus metabolism by its effect on gastrointestinal absorption, kidney excretion, or bone resorption. A lowered serum calcium stimulates the release of PTH. The specific functions of PTH are listed in Table 29-12.

■ HORMONAL REGULATION

The amount of hormone available to receptors is critical for health. The amount is kept within definite limits by a number of factors. One factor, the closed-loop negative feedback system, is shown in Fig. 29-5. It is an important regulating mechanism for hormones secreted by the hypothalamus, anterior pituitary, thyroid, adrenal cortex, and gonads. This regulating mechanism for cortisol secretion is called the hypothalamic-pituitary-adrenal cortex (HPA) axis. A simpler and more direct feedback control is exerted by the level of a particular substance in the blood on a particular hormone's production or secretion. For example, a lowered serum calcium concentration stimulates the secretion of PTH, whereas hyperkalemia stimulates the secretion of aldosterone. Gland A produces tropic hormone X, which stimulates organ B to produce substance Y; substance Y then inhibits the secretion of hormone X by gland A. An extensive feedback loop exists between the hypothalamus, pituitary gland, and other endocrine glands.

Other factors influencing secretion patterns of hormones include sleep-wake patterns, age, and growth and development. Hormones are not secreted at a uniform rate or steady flow but are released in bursts. Some hormones have cyclic rhythmic patterns of secretions, and thus rhythmic patterns of serum hormone levels can be noted; for example, cortisol has a diurnal pattern and estrogen has a monthly cycle.

The rate of excretion or metabolic inactivation also affects the levels of circulating hormones. Usually hormones have a very short activity period before they are degraded and excreted by the liver or kidneys.

■ RECEPTOR ACTIVITY

It is hypothesized that hormones initiate cellular activity in one of two ways. In the *moblie receptor* method the hormones are thought to cross the plasma cell membrane and combine with receptors in the cytoplasm of the cell. They cross the nuclear membrane and react with particular proteins in the chromatin of the nucleus or bind with deoxyribonucleic acid (DNA). In general, steroid hormones, such as adrenal steroids, and androgen, estrogen,

and progesterone act in this manner. Thyroid hormone may also react in the same way.

In the second method or the *fixed receptor* method, the hormone combines with a receptor on the plasma membrane of a cell and initiates a sequence of events coordinated by a second messenger causing the cell to initiate whatever activity it is equipped to do. ACTH, TSH, glucagon, insulin, parathyroid hormone, and the catecholamines may initiate cellular activity in this manner.

■ HYPERSECRETION AND HYPOSECRETION

Regardless of the pathologic process involved, endocrine disorders are characterized by an alteration in *amount* of effective hormone, either an excess or a deficiency. Hormonal alterations may result from the following:
1. Change in the integrity of glandular tissue
2. Dysfunction of regulating mechanisms
3. Decrease in excretion or inactivation of hormones
4. Peripheral resistance to the action of the hormones

Etiologic factors of endocrine glandular disorders are classified as primary, secondary, or iatrogenic:

Primary: disorder of the gland

Secondary: disorder of a target gland because of disorder in the pituitary gland or the hypothalamus

Iatrogenic: disorder in a gland that occurs because of treatment

Hyposecretory states may occur when there is absence of glandular tissue or when there is hypoplasia. Atrophy and hypoplasia often occur together. Hypersecretory states may occur when there is hyperplasia or a tumor. For example, pituitary hyperplasia might be a response to hypothalamic stimulation. Hypertrophy is not always accompanied by an increased secretion of hormone. One pathologic cause of hypersecretory states is tissues secreting hormones in quantities not related to body needs. These tissues are not responsive to the regulating mechanisms, for example, to the negative feedback loops or to the trophic hormone stimulation or lack of stimulation. Tumors of hormone secreting cells commonly override the normal regulating mechanisms; they continue to secrete hormones in amounts excessive for the body's hormonal needs. The affected gland is said to be *autonomous* when this escape from regulation occurs. Ectopic glandular tissue (that is, tissue in an abnormal location) may also secrete hormones in amounts not controlled by the normal feedback mechanisms. Thyroid and adrenocortical dysfunctions are two

---

Terms denoting glandular changes

Hypoplasia	Decrease in amount of functioning tissues
Hyperplasia	Increase in active secreting cells
Hypertrophy	Increase in gland size
Atrophy	Decrease in gland size

examples in which early detection and treatment can minimize cardiovascular disease.

■ PHYSIOLOGIC CHANGES WITH AGING

Normal aging results in some changes in the endocrine system. Research is ongoing as health care professionals try to identify the changes that occur and the significance of these changes. The following changes have been reported[1]:

1. The most commonly seen change is decreased ovarian functioning, resulting in increased gonodotropins and decreased estrogens. No similar change is seen in males.
2. Basal levels of prolactin are decreased in females.
3. A decrease in growth hormones and somatomedins is seen.
4. Response to changes in serum osmolarity is increased, resulting in increased production of ADH. Elderly persons also have decreased renal sensitivity to ADH, so they are unable to concentrate urine as well as younger persons.
5. It is hypothesized that a decrease in serum calcium occurs, resulting in increased PTH. This finding has not been supported by all researchers.
6. The renin-aldosterone response to postural changes and volume depletion is depressed.
7. The clearance of blood glucose after meals is decreased, resulting in an elevated postprandial blood glucose. No change in insulin secretion is seen.

The above are explained more specifically in the sections describing dysfunction of each gland.

■ PREVENTION OF DISEASE AND HEALTH EDUCATION

■ Primary prevention

Few primary endocrine diseases can be prevented at this time. *Simple goiter*, a disease characterized by an enlargement of the thyroid gland, is an exception. This condition may occur because of a lack of ingested iodine. The nurse can participate in primary prevention by teaching the importance of eating foods that contain iodine, such as seafoods and leafy vegetables. In places where there is a known deficiency of iodine in the natural water (for example, the Great Lakes region), persons are encouraged to use iodized salt.

Although the relationship involved in hypernutrition and endocrine dysfunction are complex and not completely understood, prevention and control of obesity are helpful in reducing the risk of at least one endocrine disease, noninsulin dependent diabetes mellitus (Chapter 28).

Diseases similar to endocrine hypersecretory states may be caused by inappropriate use of hormones for nonmedical purposes. This abuse of hormones is termed *factitious* and is often concealed from health care providers. Primary prevention education programs should focus on the use of steroids and growth hormones by athletes and thyroid drugs by dieters.

■ Secondary prevention

Malignant tumors of the endocrine gland are less prevalent than other forms of cancer. The thyroid gland can be easily palpated, and people should be encouraged to have yearly physical examinations to help in early detection of thyroid carcinoma. This cancer appears in all age-groups and especially in those with a history of irradiation to the neck structures. In recent years, there has been a concerted search in the United States for adults who received irradiation of the thymus gland as children. These individuals are urged to seek medical attention for detection of thyroid cancer.

Heart disease can also be induced or aggravated by certain hormonal alterations. The nurse can assist in the early detection of these disorders by encouraging persons to seek medical attention for persistent vague complaints of decreased well-being that may include the following:

1. Fatigue
2. Altered nutritional intake
3. Changes in skin and hair appearance and condition
4. Changes in excretory patterns

Although endocrine disease is not the only cause of these symptoms, it is true that these are early symptoms of many endocrinopathies.

■ Tertiary prevention

A major contribution of the nurse to patients with diagnosed endocrinopathies is that of assisting them to learn self-management of their chronic diseases. The progression of many hormonal deficiency diseases can be halted or slowed by patients who are educated and motivated to follow prescribed regimens of hormonal replacement. Hormonal replacement, when necessary, is an important method of treatment that must be handled by the patient over a long period of time. It should be stressed that failure to maintain adequate hormonal replacement results in illness and death.

Major health problems of the endocrine system

The classifications of hyposecretion and hypersecretion of hormones helps organize the information in this chapter. Only those endocrine problems encountered most frequently are discussed; these are listed in Table 29-3. The most frequent endocrine disorder in the United States is diabetes mellitus, which is discussed in Chapter 28. The next most frequent disorder is hyperthyroidism. All of these disorders can lead to significant health problems in individuals.

Table 29-3   Health problems caused by imbalances in the endocrine system

Gland	Hyposecretion	Hypersecretion
Pituitary	Panhypopituitarism, hypopituitarism, dwarfism, pituitary Addison's disease, hypoprolactinemia, diabetes insipidus	Hyperpituitarism, acromegaly, gigantism, pituitary Cushing's syndrome, hyperprolactinemia, syndrome of inappropriate ADH secretion (SIADH)
Thyroid	Hypothyroidism, cretinism, myxedema	Hyperthyroidism, Graves' disease
Parathyroid	Hypoparathyroidism, tetany	Hyperparathyroidism
Adrenal cortex	Addison's disease	Cushing's syndrome, hyperaldosteronism
Adrenal medulla		Pheochromocytoma
Pancreas (endocrine)	Diabetes mellitus	Hypoglycemia

■ ANTERIOR PITUITARY DYSFUNCTION

The functions of the hormones of the anterior pituitary gland are listed in Table 29-1.

Hyposecretion or hypersecretion of these hormones produces different effects (Table 29-4). By comparing the information in Tables 29-1 and 29-4, the student can see the results of excessive or deficit amounts of hormonal secretion on normal body structure and function.

■ Pathophysiology

■ HYPERSECRETION

Hyperpituitarism is the oversecretion of one or more of the hormones secreted by the anterior pituitary gland. The most common cause of hyperpituitarism is pituitary adenomas.

Pituitary adenomas account for 5% of 10% of all intracranial tumors, and they most frequently arise in the anterior pituitary lobe. The factors responsible for their development is unknown. These adenomas have been classified according to the staining qualities of the cells of the tumors (chromophobic, acidophilic, or basophilic) and by the hormone-secreting characteristics of the cells. Approximately 75% of all anterior pituitary adenomas are of the chromophobic type, whereas basophilic tumors are the least common. Pituitary adenomas almost never secrete FSH or LH.

Pituitary tumors cause two clinical problems depending on the size, location, and secreting capacity of the tumor. These are (1) neurologic alterations resulting from pressure on surrounding nervous system structures; (2) hypersecretion of one or more anterior pituitary hormones; and (3), most common, hyposecretion because of compression of normal pituitary tissue.

Table 29-4   Anterior pituitary dysfunction

Alteration in secretion	Etiology	Signs and symptoms	Medical therapy
GH excess	*Primary* Pituitary tumors, pituitary hyperplasia	Gigantism in children; acromegaly in adults: growth of soft tissues, cartilages, bones; enlargement and coarsening of facial features; enlarged tongue; visceral enlargement; liver, spleen, heart, kidneys; warm, moist, coarse skin; husky voice; prominent muscle development; insulin resistance	Removal of tumor: adenectomy, hypophysectomy, irradiation; medications that suppress GH: estrogen, medroxyprogesterone, chlorpromazine, bromocriptine mesylate (Parlodel)
GH deficiency	*Primary* Pituitary or nonpituitary tumors; vascular lesions; hemorrhage, ischemia, or necrosis; *Secondary* Hypothalamic: GHRH deficiency	Dwarfism in children; sensitivity to insulin; fasting hypoglycemia; hypoglycemia	Growth hormone replacement in children

Continued.

Table 29-4 Anterior pituitary dysfunction—cont'd

Alteration in secretion	Etiology	Signs and symptoms	Medical therapy
ACTH excess	*Primary* Pituitary tumors; pituitary hyperplasia *Secondary* Cushing's disease; hyperplasia of pituitary related to increased CRH; ectopic tumors that secrete ACTH *Iatrogenic* Bilateral postadrenalectomy	Similar to Cushing's syndrome (adrenocortical excess) (Table 29-9)	Pituitary ablation: adenectomy, radiation, hypophysectomy; surgical removal of ectopic source of ACTH
ACTH deficiency	*Primary* Same as GH deficiency *Iatrogenic* Suppression of hypothalamic-pituitary-adrenal axis by exogenous corticosteriods; hypothalamic-pituitary ablation	Similar to Addison's disease (adrenocortical deficit) (Table 29-11); asthenia (weakness); nausea, vomiting; hypotension; hypoglycemia; hyponatremia; hyperkalemia	Cortisone or cortisone derivative (see Table 29-10 for other treatments)
TSH excess	*Primary* Pituitary tumor *Secondary* Hyperplasia of pituitary related to increased TRH	Same as hyperthyroidism (thyroid hormone excess) (Table 29-18)	Hypophysectomy
TSH deficit	*Primary* Same as GH deficit; hypothalamic: TRH deficiency *Iatrogenic* Hypothalamic-pituitary ablation	Same as hypothyroidism (thyroid hormone deficit) (Table 29-18); cretinism in newborn; myxedema in adult	Thyroid hormone replacement
Prolactin excess	*Primary* Pituitary tumor *Secondary* Hypothalamic dysfunction *Iatrogenic* Side effect of drugs that inhibit dopamine secretion, estrogens, opiates	Amenorrhea; galactorrhea; depressed libido; osteopenia, hirsutism, acne in women; impotence, oligospermia in men	Pituitary surgery; irradiation; drugs to suppress prolactin (bromocriptine)
Prolactin deficit	Same as GH deficit	Failure of postpartum lactation	
Gonadotropic hormone excess	*Primary* Pituitary tumor *Secondary* Ovarian, adrenal, or testicular failure	Precocious sexual development in children; changes in secondary sex characteristics; hirsutism in women; gynecomastia in men	
Gonadotropic hormone deficit	Suppression of androgens by drugs; e.g., spironolactone, estrogen combined with progesterone, cimetidine	Delayed sexual development in children; in adults: female—amenorrhea, infertility; male—impotence; in both—changes in secondary sex characteristics	Replacement of sex hormones in cyclic pattern

Types of anterior pituitary adenomas

Type	Hormone secreted
Chromophobic	Prolactin (most common), GH, ACTH
Acidophilic	Prolactin, GH
Basophilic	ACTH, TSH (rare)

☐ Neurologic alterations

Tumors larger than 1 cm in diameter (macroadenomas) cause compression of the pituitary and enlargement of the sella turcica; as they expand, they can invade or compress nearby tissue. The major neurologic alteration is caused by pressure on the optic chiasma and optic nerves. Patients experience progressive loss of vision, and if untreated, permanent blindness results. Most adenomas cause midline pressure and damage the fibers subserving vision in the upper temporal fields. This causes loss of vision in one half of the visual field of both eyes (Fig. 29-4).

Other symptoms include headaches that are characteristically bitemporal and bifrontal and result from pressure on the sella turcica.[4] Confusion and impaired memory may occur but are rare. Symptoms of increased intracranial pressure may develop as lesions expand in size.

☐ Endocrine alterations

The clinical picture may be the result of excessive secretion of prolactin, GH, ACTH, or TSH. The signs and symptoms of increased secretion of ACTH and TSH are discussed in the sections of this chapter on adrenal problems and thyroid problems, respectively.

☐ Prolactin excess

Prolactin excess is often caused by pituitary adenomas, usually microadenomas (tumors less than 1 cm in diameter), or hypothalamic dysfunction. Dopamine is the primary hypothalamic inhibitor of prolactin release; interruption of dopamine transmission to the pituitary can result in prolactin excess. Other causes are hypothyroidism, renal failure, and the side effects of drugs. Levels of serum prolactin over 300 µg/ml suggest a prolactinoma.[32] Prolactin excess interferes with normal gonadal function by disturbing the hypothalamic-pituitary-gonadal axis. (See symptoms listed in Table 29-3.) Women usually seek help for endocrine dysfunction before neurologic signs and symptoms from an intrapituitary mass are present. They may complain of amenorrhea or galactorrhea. They often complain of depressed libido. Men frequently seek help for neurologic complaints. They may give a history of depressed libido, infertility, or impotence. Other signs of hypogonadism, such as changes in secondary sex characteristics, may be present.

Growth hormone excess

An excess of GH is almost always caused by a secreting pituitary tumor, although occasionally there is no distinct tumor.[4] Hypersecretion of GH that occurs in children before fusion of the epiphysis results in *gigantism*. Such children reach enormous proportions because of massive growth in both the length and width of bones. Soft tissue enlarges along with the skeleton.

Hypersecretion of GH that occurs after the fusion of the epiphysis results in *acromegaly*. This disorder affects men and women equally and most frequently begins between the second and fourth decades of life. The changes are slow and progressive and frequently go unrecognized for some time. Tables 29-1 and 29-3 present normal functions and structural and functional changes that occur with growth hormone excess. The adult with acromegaly may note an increase in ring, shoe, glove, and hat size. The hands become spadelike in appearance (Fig. 29-6). The enlargement of the mandible causes an under bite and increased spacing of the lower teeth. The forehead and orbital ridges become prominent (Fig. 29-7). Widening of spaces between joints occurs with increased cartilage growth. This leads to osteoarthritis with pain and limitation of joint motion. Changes in the spine may cause nerve root and cord compression.

The following systemic changes can result from excess in growth hormone:

1. Increased metabolic rate
2. Increased sweating and sebaceous gland activity
3. Glucose intolerance (50% of patients) and insulin resistance that can lead to diabetes mellitus

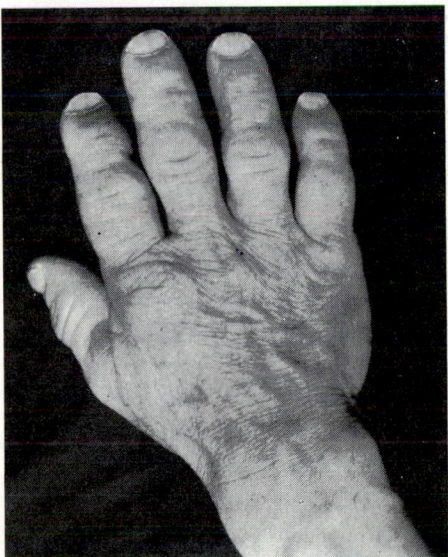

Fig. 29-6 Hand showing characteristics of acromegalic condition. (From Schottelius, BA, and Schottelius, DD: Textbook of physiology, ed 18, St. Louis, 1978, The CV Mosby Co.)

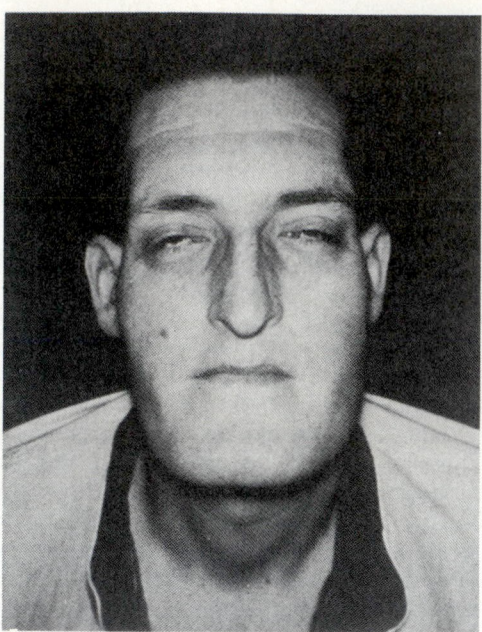

Fig. 29-7 Acromegaly. Note large head, exaggerated forward projection of jaw, and protrusion of frontal bone. (From Rimoin, DL: N Engl J Med 272:923, 1965.)

4. Hypertension (25% of patients) and cardiomegaly can lead to congestive heart failure (CHF)

Many patients with GH excess eventually develop neurologic defects resulting from an expanding lesion. Frequently they do not seek help until then.

☐ Hyposecretion

Hypopituitarism is the hyposecretion of one or more anterior pituitary hormones. In the adult the most frequent cause is a pituitary tumor that compresses normal secretory tissue. In this case, hormonal deficits often occur slowly in a sequential pattern; the order is listed below[32]:

Growth hormone lack
Hypogonadism
Adrenal insufficiency
Hypothyroidism

Because growth hormone deficit in the adult has no striking effects, amenorrhea in premenopausal women or impotence in men may be the first clinical problem. Growth hormone deficit may aggravate hypoglycemia related to other disorders. Later, hypothyroidism and adrenal insufficiency secondary to the lack of TSH or ACTH may develop. These two conditions are discussed later in this chapter.

Panhypopituitarism is present when deficits of all anterior pituitary hormones are present. This can occur as a result of pituitary tumor, injury, or disease, or it can occur iatrogenically (following pituitary ablation).

Table 29-1 lists the characteristic signs and symptoms, etiology, and treatment for hyposecretion of each of the anterior pituitary hormones. The clinical picture may vary

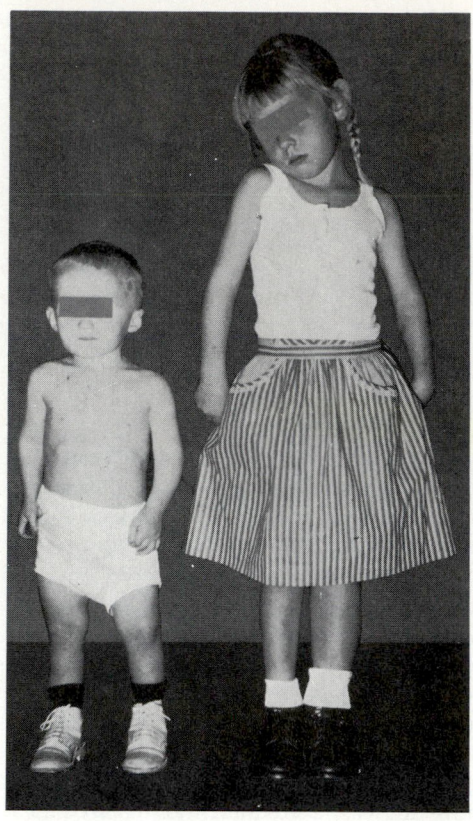

Fig. 29-8 Hypopituitary dwarfism in a 4-year-old boy whose height is 25 inches. Girl is also 4 years old and has a normal height of 39 inches. Dwarf has normal face, as well as head, trunk, and limbs of approximately normal proportions. (From Brashear, HR, and Raney, RB: Shand's handbook of orthopaedic surgery, ed 9, St. Louis, 1978, The CV Mosby Co.)

depending on the hormonal deficit present and the cause of the deficit.

Although deficiency of GH in the adult is usually not significant, congenital deficiency of growth hormone in the child results in short stature (dwarfism). Pituitary dwarfism is a rare disorder and is characterized by short stature that is apparent at about 4 years of age (Fig. 29-8). The child typically appears immature and has increased truncal fat. Bone age and height age are usually approximate, and as the child matures, the body proportions approach those of an adult.

🎛 Assessment

The application of the nursing process to patients with anterior pituitary dysfunction focuses on patients with pituitary surgery and hormonal imbalances related to lack of ACTH and GH. Many of the descriptions of assessment, data analysis, and planning discussed in this section can be applied to later sections in the chapter. The following are some common clinical problems that are seen in several endocrine disorders:

1. Fatigue
2. Nutritional alterations
3. Fluid and electrolyte imbalances
4. Cardiovascular changes
5. Changed body characteristics
6. Intolerance to stress
7. Emotional instability
8. Reproductive alterations

Nursing assessment should include the following:

1. Monitoring for potential complications of the endocrine disorder or its treatment
2. Monitoring for clinical signs and symptoms that indicate the extent of hormonal imbalances
3. Eliciting the patient's and family's perceptions of health problems, their management, and the assistance needed
4. Determining the resources needed by the patient and family to cope with the disorder and to manage it in the hospital and after discharge

Assessment of psychologic and social factors is important for several reasons. The endocrine diagnostic process can be lengthy, frightening, and costly. Stress in the patient with hormonal imbalances should be avoided as much as possible, because stress places an additional burden on the impaired endocrine function. Body image changes and physical problems may influence the person's goals, activities of daily living, and relationships with others. The person's coping abilities may also be diminished because of energy depletion or physiologic crisis. Learning to incorporate a treatment regimen into daily life is often necessary for optimal treatment and, sometimes, necessary to maintain life.

■ SUBJECTIVE DATA

The collecting of information regarding changes in body characteristics is not only important in defining the physiologic problem, but also in identifying potential or present emotional or psychologic problems. Some of the changes that occur with endocrine disorders are irreversible even when the physiologic problem is controlled. Body characteristics are part of the identity of the person, and the patient may have problems dealing with the changes.

The patient's description of the following factors help define the needs for assistance:

1. Fatigue, rest, and sleep patterns
2. Eating patterns (frequency of food intake)
3. Fluid intake and output patterns
4. Cardiovascular history
5. Special hygiene or grooming needs (hirsutism, perspiration, obesity)
6. Discomforts
7. Emotional response
8. Reproductive history
9. Medication usage
10. The endocrine disorder and its treatment

■ OBJECTIVE DATA

Initially, inspection is used to assess the patient's body growth and developmental status and should include the following:

1. Height and weight
2. Body proportions
3. Amount and distribution of muscle mass
4. Fat distribution
5. Skin pigmentation
6. Hair distribution

A great variation exists in these characteristics in the general population and often changes are not obvious. Inspection of family members for like characteristics provides information as to whether the characteristics seen in the patient are caused by heredity or pathophysiologic alterations. The patient's alertness and speech patterns can be assessed when the history is being collected. Physical assessment (Chapter 3) should be thorough in these patients because of the wide spectrum of bodily effects that occur with pituitary dysfunction.

The minimum baseline data should include the following:

Nutritional status: presence or absence of fat pads, truncal obesity, abnormal fat depositions; muscle mass, strength; serum levels of lymphocytes, albumin, glucose

Fluid and electrolyte status: vital signs, urine output, fluid intake; signs of fluid excess (edema, jugular vein distension [JVD], adventitious lung sounds) or deficit (orthostatic blood pressure, poor skin turgor, sunken eyeballs, dry mucous membranes); serum levels of electrolytes, BUN, creatinine

Cardiovascular status: blood pressure level including postural BP; pulses, skin color; signs of hypotension or cardiac failure; serum levels of electrolytes, triglycerides, cholesterol; ECG

■ DIAGNOSTIC TESTS

Usually target organ function is first studied to confirm the presence of a hormonal deficit or excess suggested by the patient's history and clinical findings. Thus measurements of cortisol, T_3 and T_4, and estrogen or testosterone are usually the first tests performed when pituitary disorder is suspected. These are followed by measurements of ACTH, TSH, and FSH and LH. The nontrophic hormones (GH and prolactin) may also be measured.

In comparing the results of these tests, the physician can often learn if the source of the endocrine problems is target gland or hypothalamic pituitary dysfunction. For example, low levels of both trophic and target gland hormones indicate pituitary-hypothalamic hyposecretion, whereas a low level of target gland hormone and a high level of trophic hormone indicates target gland failure.

Further studies may be needed for exact diagnosis. Provocative tests involve the use of a stimulant or suppressant of the hormone and measurements of the effects on hor-

Table 29-5 Tests of anterior pituitary function

Test	Procedure	Interpretation
Hormonal radioimmunoassay TSH, ACTH, prolactin, FSH, LH, GH	Blood sample, no special preparation in most cases Glucose may be administered before blood collection	Used to measure circulating hormonal levels; for hormones secreted in diurnal pattern (ACTH, GH), best obtained in early AM and at intervals throughout day to determine cyclic pattern

Provocative tests
  TSH stimulation
    TRH
	All require basal rate established by pretest assay; stimulant is given and the hormonal levels repeatedly measured	Normal serum TSH begins to rise at 10 min and peaks at 45 min; subnormal values reflect decreased pituitary reserve

ACTH stimulation ACTH, insulin, metyrapone		Normal response of serum cortisol is doubling of normal baseline; subnormal values reflect pituitary or adrenal deficiency
GH stimulation L-dopa, insulin, glucagon, exercise	IV glucose may be given before stimulant	Normal response is a peak in GH levels approximately 60 min after stimulation
Suppression tests ACTH suppression, dexamethasone	Basal rate established by pretest assay; suppressant is given and serum levels of cortisol are measured, as well as urinary excretion of cortisol and its metabolites Collection of 24-hr urine for 17-hydroxycorticosteroids (OHCS)	Dexamethasone normally suppresses ACTH secretion and thus cortisol; less than normal suppression can reflect pituitary, adrenal, or ectopic hypersecretion
GH suppression	75-100 g glucose load Blood sample drawn every 30 minutes for 2 hours	Hyperglycemia normally suppresses GH secretion

monal serum levels. Table 29-5 lists the most common tests of pituitary function. Provocative tests are not used in prolactin excess or deficit because serum levels give confirming data about pituitary function.[32]

Skeletal and skull x-ray examinations are used to assess changes in bone structure and the size of the pituitary gland and sella turcica. Computed tomography (CT) scanning may be used to demonstrate the presence of intrasellar masses and to differentiate a pituitary tumor from an "empty" sella turcica. An enlarged sella turcica may be described as "empty," a condition resulting from herniation of the arachnoid and subarachnoid cistern into the pituitary fossa.[32] The displacement of the pituitary gland is not always clinically significant.

▶ Data analysis: nursing diagnoses

Nursing diagnoses are determined from the assessment of patient data. Possible nursing diagnoses for the person with pituitary dysfunction may include, but are not limited to, the following:

Diagnostic title	Possible etiologies
Activity intolerance	Generalized weakness, immobility
Anxiety	Threat to self-concept, threat of death, change in health status
Body image disturbances	Change in body appearance or function
Fluid volume deficit or excess	Compromised regulatory mechanism; inappropriate sodium and/or water intake; drug side effects; lack of knowledge
Knowledge deficit: hormonal disorder, diagnostic or treatment measures, self-care measures	Lack of exposure, cognitive limitation
Impaired physical mobility	Intolerance to activity: decreased strength, pain, musculoskeletal impairment
Altered nutrition	Compromised regulatory mechanisms; lack of knowledge
Sensory/perceptual alterations: visual	Altered sensory transmission; altered environmental stimuli

Diagnostic title	Possible etiologies
Altered patterns of urinary elimination	Compromised regulatory mechanisms; inappropriate fluid intake; side effects of medications

Planning: expected patient outcomes

Expected patient outcomes for the person in hormonal imbalance may include, but are not limited to, the following:

1. Patient will have restoration of physiologic well-being, as evidenced by:
   a. Stable blood pressure and pulse within optimal limits
   b. Desired weight
   c. Balance of intake and output
   d. Prompt recovery from crisis
2. Patient can independently perform activities of daily living.
3. Patient can explain planned diagnostic, therapeutic, and coping measures.
4. Patient can speak of self in positive terms, listing strengths and ways to deal with deficits.
5. Patient can explain to others the assistance needed because of visual defect, weakness, or immobility.
6. Patient can explain rationale for medications and prescribed modification of food and fluid intake.
7. Patient or significant others will demonstrate requisite knowledge, skill, and resources for self-management of treatment measures:
   a. Describe the hormonal imbalance and relate to signs and symptoms.
   b. Explain the planned treatment measures and effects of treatment.
   c. Explain the prescribed medication program.
      (1) Awareness of the need for lifelong replacement therapy
      (2) Drugs, dosage, and frequency of therapy
      (3) Desired effects and side effects of therapy
      (4) What to do when signs and symptoms of undertreatment or overtreatment occur
   d. Describe the times when extra hormonal therapy is necessary.
   e. Describe need to obtain MedicAlert symbol to wear.
   f. State plans for regular follow-up care

Implementation

ASSISTING WITH ACHIEVEMENT OF THERAPEUTIC GOALS

Pituitary tumor (adenoma) is the most frequent cause of hyperpituitarism, and the most frequent treatment is surgery. If possible, pituitary tissue is not disturbed. Following an adenectomy, hormonal levels are expected to return to normal immediately. External radiation or *yttrium*

(^{39}Y) implantation may also be used for treatment of a hormone-secreting pituitary tumor or pituitary hyperplasia, but hormonal levels are slow to return to normal with these therapies.

Because microadenomas that secrete prolactin are slow growing, treatment may not be recommended if the patient has no annoying symptoms (for instance, galactorrhea) and does not wish to be pregnant.[32] If pregnancy is a desired goal, surgical removal of the adenoma is usually performed because pregnancy induces pituitary enlargement. While suppression of prolactin by bromocriptine mesylate (Parlodel) can restore fertility, this drug is not recommended for use during pregnancy. Other drugs that suppress GH are estrogen, medroxyprogesterone, and chlorpromazine.

Pituitary hypofunction is most often caused by a pituitary tumor, although there are many other causes. Surgery, irradiation, or bromocriptine mesylate are choices of therapy. Irridation and bromocriptine mesylate work by shrinking the tumor.

Sometimes the treatment of hypersecretion of a gland results in a state of hyposecretion. When a total hypophysectomy (removal of the pituitary) is performed, panhypopituitarism results. Even though panhypopituitarism is not expected after a partial hypophysectomy, ^{39}Y implantation, or drug therapy, it can occur as a complication. All patients with these treatments are monitored for hormonal deficiencies.

Radiation therapy or cranial surgery is frightening to most patients and their families, and they need time to share concerns, fears, and questions with the nurse. All questions should be answered as honestly and as completely as possible.

The patient with acromegaly needs to be aware that the surgery or irradiation reduces excess hormone levels. Some of the coarsening features may disappear because soft tissue swelling decreases; glucose intolerance disappears; and visceral enlargement may decrease; but most of the physical changes associated with excessive GH are irreversible.

Surgery
Transsphenoidal surgery

The transsphenoidal approach is most frequently used to resect an adenoma. The sella turcica is entered through the sphenoid sinus, and the tumor is removed with the aid of a surgical microscope (Fig. 29-2). The incision is made between the gums and upper lip. This approach may also be used to implant ^{39}Y. The opening made in the dura mater on entering the sella turcica is frequently patched with a piece of fascia taken from the leg; thus the patient must be prepared for the leg incision. The patch is to prevent a cerebrospinal fluid (CSF) leak. Leaking of CSF may occur for a few days postoperatively but should then stop. The nose may be packed and a gauze sling placed under it to absorb drainage.

Monitoring for the presence of CSF leak is important. The following data should be noted:
1. Complaint of postnasal drip
2. Constant swallowing

**Activities that increase
intracranial pressure**

Coughing
Sneezing
Blowing the nose
Bending over
Straining

**Signs and symptoms of adrenocortical
insufficiency**

Nausea, vomiting
Prolonged lethargy
More fatigue than expected
Slower recovery than expected
Mild hypotension

---

3. Evidence on the nasal sling or gauze pads of a "halo ring" (clear CSF fluid marking around a darker center of serous fluid)
4. Presence of glucose in the nasal drainage

CSF fluid contains glucose, whereas nasal drainage does not. If the glucose test is positive, a specimen should be sent to the laboratory for confirmation.

If a persistent leak occurs, bed rest with the patient's head elevated to place pressure against the patch is prescribed. Most often CSF leaks heal spontaneously, but occasionally surgical repair is necessary. Activities that increase intracranial pressure should be avoided (see the box above).

Headache may be present and is treated with nonnarcotic analgesics or codeine. Persistent headache or nuchal rigidity (neck stiffness) may indicate the presence of meningitis and should be reported immediately. Because of the risk of infection, prophylactic antibiotics may be ordered preoperatively or postoperatively.

Other nursing interventions for the patient with transsphenoidal surgery include the following:

1. Encourage oral fluids and a clear liquid diet as soon as the patient is alert and no longer nauseated from the anesthesia.
2. Increase the diet as tolerated (anorexia may result from a decreased sense of smell).
3. Reassure the patient that the loss of smell is temporary and should improve as soon as the nasal packing or sling is removed.
4. Provide oxygen and humidity as ordered to keep the nasal and oral mucous membranes moist.
5. Provide mouth care:
   a. Avoid toothbrushing to prevent disruption of the suture line.
   b. Use soft cotton swabs to cleanse the teeth.
   c. Offer mouth rinses frequently.

☐ *Transfrontal surgery*

When the pituitary tumor extends beyond the boundaries of the sella turcica (extrasellar), craniotomy is used to obtain adequate surgical exposure. (The care of the patient with a craniotomy is discussed in Chapter 19.) Other intracerebral tumors, disease, or trauma of structures lying near the pituitary may result in temporary or permanent pituitary dysfunction.

■ **CORRECTION OF HORMONAL IMBALANCE**

The patient with panhypopituitarism requires lifelong replacement of cortisol, thyroid, and in most instances, sex hormones, whether the hormonal deficits are caused by disease, trauma, hypophysectomy, or irradiation. The exception to replacement of sex hormones following hypophysectomy is the patient with cancer whose pituitary was removed to eliminate gonadotropic stimulation of tumor growth.

ACTH deficiency and thus glucocorticoid deficiency occurs immediately if the total pituitary has been removed. An intramuscular or intravenous cortisone preparation can be given preoperatively and postoperatively. Oral replacement therapy using cortisone acetate should be started as soon as oral intake is tolerated. Although it occurs rarely after transsphenoidal adenectomy, a temporary ACTH deficiency can result in adrenocortical insufficiency and even *addisonian crisis.* (See the boxes above and below for signs and symptoms.) The patient is treated with replacement therapy as long as necessary. Plasma levels of cortisol will be checked before discharge to make sure that the deficit has been corrected.

To detect adrenocortical deficiency and to determine adequacy of cortisol replacement, frequent monitoring of any patient with potential for adrenocortical insufficiency is necessary. Actions include the following:

1. Taking vital signs every hour after surgery until stable, then every 4 hours
2. Tabulating intake and output every 8 hours
3. Weighing patient daily

Electrolyte studies are ordered at least daily to monitor sodium and potassium levels. Signs of insufficient cortisol

---

Signs of addisonian crisis

Hypotension
Dehydration
Hyponatremia
Hyperkalemia
Hypoglycemia

---

replacement are usually vague and nonspecific. Maintaining the patient's blood pressure at optimal levels is a major clinical guideline that determines the amount of cortisol replacement.

The signs and symptoms listed in the box on p. 956 should be reported and carefully evaluated. Progression of symptoms can be rapid and profound shock can develop. There are five classic signs of adrenocortical deficiency (see the box on p. 956). The treatment of addisonian crisis is discussed on p. 964. The critical treatment measure is the replacement of cortisol.

☐ Diabetes insipidus following pituitary surgery

The removal of the pituitary gland or edema of surrounding tissue can precipitate the sudden onset of *diabetes insipidus*. Disruption of the hypothalamic secretion of ADH can also result in ADH alterations. Diabetes insipidus is usually not permanent, even if all of the pituitary gland has been removed—ADH is produced in the hypothalamus and adequate amounts can be released from there. Monitoring for patients who may develop diabetes insipidus includes the following:

1. Intake and output tabulated every 4 hours
2. Specific gravity determined on each urine specimen (continuously dilute urine with specific gravity of 1.000 to 1.005 is a sign of diabetes insipidus)

Polyuria makes it imperative that fluid intake be maintained to balance the urinary output. When diabetes insipidus occurs, thirst is a frequent complaint. It can usually be managed by providing ice chips and adequate water intake. If fluid deficit is severe, vasopressin (Pitressin) is administered by intravenous route.

☐ Lifelong cortisol replacement

The daily replacement of cortisol in patients with adrenocortical insufficiency is critical; it is necessary to maintain life. Cortisone is the drug of choice, and it is given to correlate with the patient's activity and to mimic the usual diurnal pattern. Because cortisone is ulcerogenic, it should always be given after meals or with milk. Antacids may be prescribed. If an adrenocortical derivative with glucocorticoid properties, such as prednisone, is prescribed, the dosage needs to be equivalent to the antiinflammatory potency of hydrocortisone (Table 29-10).

☐ Thyroid and gonad hormone replacement

Deficiency of TSH and of thyroid hormones usually does not occur on a temporary basis, and it is not seen immediately even after the total pituitary has been removed, since the thyroid stores enough hormone to last for several weeks. If the total pituitary has been removed, the patient will eventually require thyroid replacement.

Gonadotropin deficiency requires lifetime therapy. To maintain libido, secondary sexual characteristics, and well-being, men are given testosterone and women receive estrogen-progesterone preparations. If childbearing is desired, the gonadotropins (LH and FSH) must be replaced.

■ COUNSELING AND TEACHING

Nurses make an important contribution to patients with hypopituitarism when they help them to understand the prescribed regimen for hormonal replacement. The serious nature of adrenocortical insufficiency should be stressed. Specific points to include in the teaching are listed in the box below.

Most adult patients with acromegaly have already learned to deal with their changed appearance and the reaction of others. Nurses can support the patient's adaptive coping mechanisms and be empathetic when choices include socially isolating behaviors. Patients may benefit from suggestions about the following:

1. Minimizing body appearance with make-up and clothes
2. Managing oily skin and hair and perspiration
3. Preventing further limitation in movement by range of motion exercises and physical activity
4. Decreasing discomfort by modifying activities

Teaching for the patient requiring cortisol replacement

1. Never omit a dose of the drug.
2. Notify physician if a dose cannot be taken or not retained.
3. Wear an identification bracelet.
4. Carry information concerning:
   a. Name and dosage of drug to be given in case of an emergency.
   b. Name and phone number of physician to be notified in an emergency.
5. Carry an emergency supply of a rapid-acting cortisone preparation with directions for use (for example, hydrocortisone 100 mg in a sterile syringe).
6. Report to physician any signs and symptoms of adrenocortical insufficiency (p. 956).
7. Avoid stress as much as possible.
8. Notify physician when illness, injury, or emotional crises occur.
9. Maintain regular medical follow-up.

The patient with blindness or visual field defects can be helped to maintain independence while in the hospital and can be referred for visual rehabilitation services (see Chapter 20). Patients treated with bromocriptine alone or as adjunctive therapy must know how to self-administer the drug. For prolactin-secreting tumors, 2.5 to 15 mg of bromocriptine daily usually is effective. Higher doses may be necessary for growth–hormone-secreting tumors. The major side effects are mild nausea, vomiting, and postural hypotension. Repeated hormonal analysis is carried out to monitor the effectiveness of therapy.

■ POSTERIOR PITUITARY DYSFUNCTION

The two hormones of the posterior pituitary are oxytocin and ADH. Refer to obstetrical nursing texts for further information about oxytocin. The two alterations of ADH secretion, ADH excess and deficit, are described in Table 29-6.

■ Pathophysiology

■ HYPOSECRETION OF ADH

The secretion of ADH is an important and normal response to states of stress or hyperosmolality. ADH effects changes in the kidney tubular membrane to increase water absorption to dilute the hyperosmolality and to provide an adequate blood volume during stress. In the presence of ADH, the urine is concentrated. When ADH is absent, water is not reabsorbed in the tubules and a large amount (7 to 11 L/day) of dilute urine is produced.

When the posterior pituitary does not release ADH or the hypothalamus does not secrete ADH in response to a hyperosmolar state, diabetes insipidus results. The potential is great for severe dehydration and vascular collapse if the patient does not replenish fluids lost by the excessive urination. The three classic symptoms that should alert the nurse to diabetes insipidus are *polyuria, dilute urine,* and *polydipsia.*

Often the patient complains of insatiable thirst. Ice water is preferred, although the reason for this is unknown. Voiding may occur so often that there is interference with sleep and the patient complains of tiredness.

■ HYPERSECRETION OF ADH

In the syndrome of inappropriate antidiuretic hormone (SIADH), the patient is unable to excrete dilute urine and therefore retains water. Normally, ADH secretion is self-limiting; in SIADH, there is a continual release of ADH unrelated to plasma osmolality. Hemodilution results in depressed levels of solutes and electrolytes. CNS dysfunction occurs as a result of the hypo-osmolar state in which fluid shifts between intracerebral fluid compartments.

■ Assessment

A history of polydipsia and polyuria should always be explored further. If the patient with diabetes insipidus is able to replenish lost fluids, few other symptoms will be noticed. There can be a severe and sudden onset of dehydration and hyperosmolar fluid imbalance if oral intake is decreased.

Most symptoms of ADH excess (Table 29-6) are nonspecific. Mental status changes can occur with either hyperosmolar or hypo-osmolar fluid imbalances. The patient who is unconscious, such as after intracranial or pituitary

Table 29-6 Alterations in ADH (posterior pituitary) secretion

Alteration	Etiologic factors	Signs and symptoms	Medical therapy
ADH excess: SIADH	Diseased lung and pancreatic tissue (for example, oat cell carcinoma); skull fractures, intracranial lesions, surgery; positive pressure breathing; drugs: chlorpropamide, morphine, thiazides; nephrogenic diseases	*Dilutional hyponatremia:* Serum Na below 130 mEq/L; weakness; lethargy; confusion; convulsions; weight gain; edema	Surgical removal of ADH secreting tissue (pituitary or nonpituitary); water restriction of 800 to 1000 ml/day; hypertonic saline; demeclocycline
ADH deficit: Diabetes insipidus	Head trauma, intracranial surgery or lesion; pituitary disorder; hypophysectomy	Polyuria, polydipsia, dilute urine (specific gravity 1.000 to 1.005); if fluid intake is insufficient: dehydration, vascular collapse; weakness, anorexia	Fluid intake to balance fluid output; vasopressin replacement: Pitressin, lypressin, (deamino-D-arginine vasopressin nasal spray or drops); surgical removal of tumor; drug therapy: thiazide diuretics, chlorpropamide

surgery, cannot relate feelings of discomfort or thirst nor can the nurse assess mental changes. Careful documentation of patterns of fluid intake and output can help alert caregivers to fluid imbalances in these patients.

■ SUBJECTIVE DATA

Subjective data can be obtained from the conscious patient. Data to collect include the following:
1. Fluid intake and output patterns
2. Use of Pitressin: frequency and side effects
3. Presence of thirst

■ OBJECTIVE DATA

The following objective data center around fluid and electrolyte monitoring:
1. Mental status
2. Daily weight
3. Fluid intake and output every 8 hours or more frequently if risk of imbalance is high
4. Urine osmolality, specific gravity, and sodium content
5. Serum sodium and serum osmolality
6. Blood pressure

■ DIAGNOSTIC TESTS

Primary diabetes insipidus is rare, but secondary or iatrogenic diabetes insipidus is seen fairly often. Before diabetes insipidus is conclusively diagnosed, the patient must be shown to have a deficit of ADH, and the patient's kidneys must be able to respond to ADH to rule out nephropathy. (Table 29-7 lists tests of ADH function.)

Another diagnostic problem is the differentiation of ADH deficiency from neurogenic polydipsia (compulsive water drinking). A water deprivation test demonstrates ADH deficiency if urine output continues with no change in urinary osmolality and sodium content when the patient is deprived of water. Close monitoring of vital signs is necessary to detect significant changes before vascular collapse occurs. In neurogenic polydipsia, the water-deprived patient needs continual emotional support to endure the test and may exhibit extreme behavioral responses.

Usually laboratory studies of electrolytes and osmolality confirm the diagnosis of SIADH. A search for an extra-pituitary source of ADH hypersecretion would include x-ray films of the skull, chest, and abdomen.

➡ Data analysis: nursing diagnoses

Nursing diagnoses are determined from the assessment of patient data. Possible nursing diagnoses for the person with imbalances of ADH may include, but are not limited to, the following:

Diagnostic title	Possible etiologies
For the patient with ADH hyposecretion:	
Fluid deficit, potential or actual	Compromised regulation of urinary excretion, inadequate fluid intake, Pitressin underdosage, knowledge deficit
For the patient with ADH excess:	
Fluid excess, potential or actual	Compromised reevaluation of urinary excretion, excessive use of Pitressin, knowledge deficit

See p. 954 for other nursing diagnoses applicable to patients with hormonal imbalance, particularly knowledge deficit.

⌐ Planning: expected patient outcomes

Expected patient outcomes for the person with ADH dysfunction may include, but are not limited to, those for patients with hormonal imbalance listed on p. 955, particularly numbers 1 and 7. The following are specific expected outcomes:
1. Patient with ADH deficit will maintain daily weight and urine volume between 800 and 2000 ml/24 hr.
2. Demonstrate correct use of ADH replacement agent.
3. Patient with SIADH will comply with fluid and, if necessary, sodium restrictions.
4. Suffer no injury during mental status impairment.

Table 29-7 Tests of ADH function

Test	Procedure	Interpretation
Radioimmunoassay of ADH	Blood sample	Clinical findings, sodium content and osmolality of blood and urine more commonly used
Water deprivation test	Water withheld until 2%-5% of body weight is lost; collect urine and serum samples for osmolality and sodium before test and at ordered intervals; measure intake and output every 1-2 hr, weigh every 8 hr	Normal response is an increase in osmolality and sodium content and decrease in urine volume; in diabetes insipidus, no changes occur
Vasopressor stimulation	Baseline urine osmolality obtained before test and after administration of vasopressin	Urine osmolality rises after vasopressin; confirms renal responsiveness to vasopressin and rules out nephrogenic origin of polyuria

⊞ Implementation

■ ASSISTING WITH ACHIEVEMENT OF THERAPEUTIC GOALS

☐ Maintaining fluid balance

Frequent monitoring of these patients and early detection of problems assists in achieving fluid and electrolyte balance. High priority nursing actions that ensure adequate intake for patients with diabetes insipidus include the following:

1. Provide access to and assistance with oral fluid intake, as permitted.
2. Notify physician if fluid intake is inadequate.
3. Maintain ordered flow rates of intravenous infusions.

Water restriction is the key therapeutic measure for SIADH-induced hyponatremia. Fluids may be restricted to as low as 500 ml/24 hr. During changes in electrolyte levels, thirst can be discomforting to the patient. The nurse can enhance the patient's comfort and assist in adherence to fluid restriction by the following:

1. Moistening the patient's mouth frequently by offering ice chips rather than water to allow more frequent intake
2. Offering mouth rinses to the patient
3. Planning with the patient and dietitian the most satisfactory fluid distribution

The use of hypertonic saline solution is usually reserved for patients who have severe hyponatremia, disturbed sensorium, or convulsions. Appropriate safety measures must be provided for the level of mental confusion.

A review of Table 29-6 will indicate other medical treatments that may be necessary.

☐ ADH replacement

The key therapeutic measure for diabetes insipidus is the administration of *Pitressin*. For immediate treatment of a crisis, vasopressin injection is used. Pitressin tannate in oil can provide longer-lasting duration of effect (over 3 days). It is only given intramuscularly; it is often painful and swelling may occur. It is best to warm the vial and to shake it vigorously to disperse the active ingredient.

Most patients use nasal sprays or drops of Pitressin solution to maintain adequate ADH levels. They learn to determine the dosage in response to polyuria and thirst. The patient is cautioned about overdosage and its symptoms. Usually 2 to 3 doses/24 hr are sufficient to maintain a urinary volume under 2000 ml. Overdosage of any Pitressin medication results in symptoms of ADH excess:

1. Weight gain
2. Edema
3. Abdominal cramping
4. Hypertension

Rhinopharyngitis may interfere with the absorption of nasal drops, sprays, or powders. For this reason, patients are taught to report this condition to the physician. Currently, Pitressin "snuff" is not frequently used because of its irritating qualities.

Teaching for the patient with diabetes insipidus

1. Knowledge of medication therapy
   a. Dosage and side effects of prescribed medication
   b. Correct use of prescribed Pitressin nasal spray or drops (Chapter 23)
   c. Signs and symptoms (polyuria, polydipsia) that indicate the need to take prescribed medication
2. Need to report signs of rhinopharyngitis (runny nose and red, painful mucous membranes) to physician
3. Need to seek immediate medical follow-up if symptoms become worse or are not relieved by prescribed medications
4. Need to carry at all times an identification card or a Medic Alert bracelet or necklace indicating the nature of the disorder
5. Probable requirement for lifelong replacement therapy with diabetes insipidus
6. Need for regular medical follow-up care

■ COUNSELING AND TEACHING

A summary of the instruction required for the patient with diabetes insipidus is listed in the box above.

⊞ Evaluation

Evaluation is based on the expected patient outcomes. Key questions are the following:

1. Is fluid and electrolyte balance achieved?
2. Is the patient able to maintain fluid and electrolyte balance by self-care measures?
3. Does the patient understand the prescribed medication plan?

■ ADRENAL GLAND DYSFUNCTION

Dysfunction of the adrenal gland can be manifested as an increased or decreased function of the cortex or an increased function of the medulla (Fig. 29-9). The three major hormones of the adrenal cortex are cortisol, aldosterone, and androgens. The adrenal medulla produces epinephrine and norepinephrine (Table 29-8). The etiology, signs and symptoms, and medical therapy for adrenal gland dysfunctions are listed in Table 29-9.

HYPERFUNCTION (↑)　　　　　　　HYPOFUNCTION (↓)

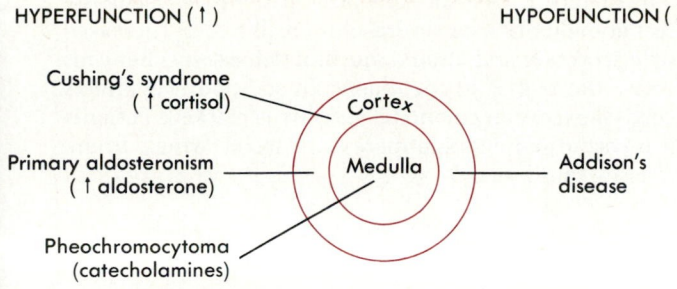

Fig. 29-9 Adrenal gland dysfunctions.

■ Pathophysiology

■ HYPERSECRETION

☐ **Cortisol excess**
☐ *Iatrogenesis*

The most frequent cause of cortisol excess is *iatrogenic,* which means that the cause is induced by therapeutic doses prescribed for a variety of conditions including:

1. Treatment of inflammations, autoimmune diseases, allergies
2. Prevention of rejection in organ transplantation
3. Prevention of excessive fibrosis (scarring) following certain surgeries or diseases
4. Reduction of acute increased intracranial pressure
5. Reduction in size and activity of lymphatic tissue

The term *Cushing's syndrome* is used for all other causes of cortisol excess: adrenocortical tumors, ectopic tissue sources, and exogenous corticosteroid drugs (iatrogenic).

Whether the cause is pathologic or iatrogenic, cortisol excess has widespread effects (Table 29-9). The changes in body appearance may be quite striking:

1. The *adipose deposition* is classic in its distribution to trunk, facies (moon face), and intrascapular areas ("buffalo hump").
2. *Muscle wasting* is most obvious in the legs, thighs, and buttocks.
3. Pale, purplish *striae* result from thinning of skin and weakening of collagenous fibers that expose subcutaneous tissue.
4. Tissue *bruises* easily with ecchymosis formation from lack of collagen support.

Table 29-8　Functions of the adrenal hormones

Gland	Hormones	Functions
Adrenal cortex	Glucocorticoids (cortisol)	Overall effect is to maintain blood glucose level by increasing gluconeogenesis and decreasing rate of glucose use by cells
		Increases protein catabolism
		Promotes lipolysis
		Promotes sodium and water retention
		Antiinflammatory
		Degrades collagen
		Decreases T lymphocyte participation in cellular-mediated immunity by decreasing circulating level of T lymphocytes
		Increases neutrophils by increasing release and decreasing destruction
		Decreases new antibody release
		Decreases eosinophils, basophils, and monocytes
		Decreases scar tissue formation
		Increases RBC formation and possibly increases platelet formation
		Stimulates appetite
		Increases gastric acid and pepsin production
		Maintains emotional stability
	Mineralocorticoids (aldosterone)	Major stimulus is renin-angiotensin system
		Primarily responsible for maintenance of normovolemic state by increasing sodium and water retention in distal tubules
		Causes potassium excretion
		Causes increased excretion of ammonium and magnesium ions
	Androgens	Same functions as gonadal sex hormones
Adrenal medulla	Epinephrine and norepinephrine	Necessary for maintenance of neuroendocrine integrating functions of body
		Elevates blood pressure, increases heart rate, and causes vasoconstriction
		Stimulates conversion of glycogen to glucose for emergency fuel
		Stimulates gluconeogenesis
		Increases lipolysis

Many of the signs and symptoms of cortisol excess are related to its diabetogenic, catabolic, and ketogenic effects:
1. Loss of bone matrix and calcium from bones
2. Decreased glucose intolerance, decreased glucose use, and increased gluconeogenesis
3. Increased ketogenesis and fatty acid mobilization
4. Increased sodium and water retention

The metabolic dysfunctions place patients with cortisol excess at higher risk for several chronic illnesses. Increased gastric secretion and altered mucosal defense mechanisms increase the risk of peptic ulcers. In addition, the effects of cortisol excess on emotional stability is marked. Patients may report insomnia, nightmares, and mood swings. Frank psychoses can develop.

Table 29-9 Adrenal gland dysfunction

Alteration in secretion	Etiology	Signs and symptoms	Medical therapy
Adrenocortical excess	**Primary** Adrenocortical tumor **Secondary** (Cortisol) Adrenocortical hyperplasia because of ACTH stimulation; ectopic cortisol secreting tumor; (aldosterone): increased renin: liver disease, malignant hypertension, congestive heart failure (androgen): ovarian tumors, drug side effects	**Cortisol excess** Body appearance change Hyperglycemia, hypernatremia, hypokalemia Increased susceptibiility to infections Emotional changes Hypertension, edema Weakness, fatigue **Aldosterone excess** Hypertension Hypokalemia Hypernatremia Metabolic alkalosis Headache, edema Severe muscle weakness **Androgen excess** Hirsutism, virilization, amenorrhea in females, precocious sexual development in young boys	Surgery: adrenalectomy (unilateral, bilateral), excision of tumor Irradiation Drugs to suppress cortisol synthesis: mitotane, metyrapone, aminoglutethimide Pituitary ablation Surgery: adrenalectomy, excision of tumor Spironolactone Surgery: adrenalectomy, excision of tumor
Adrenocortical deficiency	**Primary** Addison's disease; infection, hemorrhage; congenital hypoplasia; idiopathic atrophy **Secondary** Adrenal hypoplasia as a result of decreased ACTH **Iatrogenic** Bilateral adrenalectomy; mitotane and cortisol therapy	**Cortisol lack** Weight loss, asthenia Hypoglycemia Intolerance to stress Hyperpigmentation GI complaints: nausea, vomiting, abdominal pain, diarrhea; Addisonian crisis: hypotension, vasomotor collapse, coma, hyperpyrexia **Aldosterone lack** Hypotension, hyponatremia, hyperkalemia **Androgen lack** In males: hypogonadism, impotence, loss of secondary sex characteristics	Replacement therapy: glucocorticoids (cortisone, hydrocortisone); mineralocorticoids (desoxycorticosterone, fludrocortisone); anabolic steroids For addisonian crisis: hydrocortisone phosphate (IV), plasma expanders IV, normal saline solution IV, vasopressors, rest
Adrenal medulla excess	Pheochromocytoma Neuroblastoma	Hypertension, episodic or sustained Headache, episodic Diaphoresis Palpitations, tachycardia Hyperglycemia during attacks	Surgery: excision of tumor Drugs to suppress catecholamines: phentolamine (Regitine); nitroprusside; propranolol; trimethaphan camsylate

---

Conditions for which persons with cortisol excess are at high risk

Hypertension
Diabetes mellitus
Osteoporosis
Peptic ulcer
Psychoses
Infection

Cortisol is immunosuppressive as a result of decreased lymphocyte and antibody production and cell-mediated immunity (Chapter 38). Although the number of neutrophils may be increased, there are decreased fibrin deposits that limit localization of infections and allow systemic spread.

The potency of antiinflammatory action varies among the many preparations; mineralocorticoid activity of most is low (Table 29-10). The metabolic side effects of glucocorticoids place a limit on the dosage employed over time.

Beside the problems caused by corticosteroid therapy (cortisol excess), the patient is also at risk for an episode of *adrenocortical insufficiency* (cortisol deficit) should the medication be stopped suddenly or severe stress occur.

□ Pathogenesis

The most common pathologic cause is excessive stimulation of the adrenal cortex by ACTH, which results in bilateral hyperplasia of the adrenal gland and hypersecretion of cortisol and, often, an excess of androgens. An increase in ACTH release from the pituitary, because of pituitary or hypothalamic dysfunction, is called *pituitary Cushing's syndrome,* or *Cushing's disease.* Very often a pituitary microadema is associated with Cushing's disease.

□ Aldosterone excess

The etiologic factors, symptoms, and medical therapy of aldosterone excess are listed in Table 29-9. Three major effects of aldosterone excess are *hypertension, hypokalemia,* and *hypernatremia.* Hypertension results from the increased blood volume as a result of sodium reabsorption. As the sodium is retained, potassium is excreted and results in hypokalemia. Hypokalemia can result in the following:

1. Changes in excitability of muscle membrane, causing weakness, paresthesia, hypoactive bowel sounds, and deep tendon reflexes
2. Cardiac arrhythmias, changes in ECG patterns, and sensitivity to digitalis preparations
3. Loss of the kidneys' concentrating ability: dilute urine, polyuria, and nocturia
4. Metabolic alkalosis
5. Suppression of renin release and, therefore, aldosterone secretion

Primary aldosteronism is rare and is caused most often by an adrenal adenoma. Secondary aldosteronism can result from pathologic states that increase renin activity secondary to decreased perfusion pressure or volume to the kidneys. Secondary aldosteronism can also result from physiologic responses to reduced sodium intake, increased potassium intake, and an upright position over a long period of time.[32]

□ Androgen excess

Most adrenal adenomas secrete only cortisol, aldosterone, or androgens. When bilateral hyperplasia of the cortex occurs, there is usually an excess of both cortisol and androgens. In contrast, adrenal carcinomas frequently secrete all three hormones in excess. Other causes of androgen excess include primary disease of the ovary and side effects of some medications.

Androgen excess does not produce clinically significant signs in adult men. Two signs of androgen excess in women are *hirsutism* and *virilization*[28]:

1. *Hirsutism:* an increase in coarse, dark hair on the face, abdomen, axillae, and pubes; increased sebaceous gland activity leading to oily skin and acne

---

Table 29-10 Comparison of antiinflammatory and mineralocorticoid potency of derivatives of adrenocorticosteroids

Drug	Antiinflammatory potency*	Mineralocorticoid potency†
Hydrocortisone (Cortef)	1	0.03
Cortisone acetate (Cortone, Cortogen)	0.8	0.03
Prednisone (Deltasone, Meticorten)	4	0.04
Methylprednisolone (Medrol)	6	0.02
Triamcinolone (Aristocort, Kenacort)	5	None
Dexamethasone (Decadron)	30	None
Desoxycorticosterone (DOCA)	None	1
Fludrocortisone (Florinef)	10	4.2

*Potency relative to hydrocortisone, whose potency = 1.
†Potency relative to DOCA, whose potency = 1.

2. *Virilization:* symptoms of amenorrhea or oligomenorrhea, clitoromegaly, frontal balding, deepening voice, and muscle hypertrophy

□ Catecholamine excess

Catecholamines secreted by the adrenal medulla are not essential for life because the sympathetic nervous system also produces these hormones. The functions of epinephrine and norepinephrine are listed in Table 29-8.

Although rare, the most common cause of excess catecholamines in adults is *pheochromocytoma*, a catecholamine-producing tumor of the adrenal medulla (Table 29-9). Similar tumors are sometimes found in the abdomen around the adrenal medulla or anywhere along the sympathetic nervous system trunk.

The prominent sign of catecholamine excess is hypertension, which may be labile, depending on blood levels of the catecholamines, or the blood pressure may stay persistently elevated. Most patients have an elevated blood pressure reading at least 50% of the time.[49] Headache is abrupt, severe, throbbing, and generalized; it usually is of short duration. If hypertension is long standing, the patient may develop hypertensive retinopathy.

Frequently there is a history of paroxysmal attacks that are precipitated by multiple factors. Postural changes (especially flexion or bending of the body), sneezing, abdominal pressure, sexual activity, eating, urination, Valsalva maneuvers, exercise, pain, and changes in environmental or body temperature are some of the major precipitating factors.

In pheochromocytoma, the serum levels of catecholamines and their metabolites in the urine are increased.

■ HYPOSECRETION

The adrenal cortex is essential to life. Without its hormones, cortisol and aldosterone, the body's metabolic processes would respond inadequately to even minimal physical and emotional stressors, such as changes in temperature, exercise, or excitement.

□ Adrenocortical insufficiency

The inability to secrete glucocorticoids, mineralocorticoids, and androgens may occur as a result of atrophy, disease, or destruction of the adrenal gland.

Hypotension, hyponatremia, and hyperkalemia are characteristically seen in patients with primary adrenocortical insufficiency because of a lack of mineralocorticoids. These patients are subject to changes in cardiovascular status because of fluid and electrolyte alterations. A low circulating blood volume and a decreased heart size develop. ECG changes may occur with hyperkalemia.

Conversely, when there is hypoplasia secondary to decreased ACTH secretion, usually only cortisol secretion is decreased. This occurs because ACTH has minimal influence on aldosterone secretion, which is under control of the renin-angiotensin system. However, there may be evidence of hyposecretion of other pituitary hormones.

A review of Table 29-9 explains many of the signs and symptoms that occur with the lack of cortisol because of diminished protein, carbohydrate, and fat metabolism, resulting in:

1. Hypoglycemia
2. Weight loss
3. Weakness, fatigue

Gastrointestinal symptoms (for example, anorexia, nausea and vomiting, or diarrhea) are often the reason that the person initially seeks help. Symptoms of adrenocortical insufficiency most often have a gradual onset and are vague. Asthenia (weakness) is a cardinal complaint, the intensity of which is out of proportion to other overt symptoms. It is usually more severe at times of stress and eventually may require the patient to stay in bed.

The decreased cortisol level is often associated with mental and emotional changes: loss of vigor, depression, irritability, and loss of ability to concentrate. Apathy and generalized weakness contribute to decreased activity.

Hyperpigmentation with a bronzelike discoloration of skin and mucous membranes is a common sign in primary adrenal insufficiency. This is caused by increased levels of melanocyte-stimulating hormone (MSH) in the anterior pituitary. In normal persons, cortisol causes negative feedback inhibition of MSH, one of the precursors of ACTH. This lack of cortisol in adrenal insufficiency allows the MSH level to increase. Persons with secondary insufficiency do not usually have hyperpigmentation because their levels of ACTH and MSH are low.

Iatrogenic adrenocortical insufficiency results from adrenal atrophy induced by corticosteroid therapy. An elevation of serum cortisol levels inhibits the secretion of ACTH and CRH; and thus the stimulation of the cells of the adrenal cortex is decreased. This suppression of the hypothalamic-pituitary-adrenal (HPA) axis may persist for up to 1 year, if corticosteroid therapy is used in large doses or if therapy is prolonged. During the period of HPA axis suppression, stress may precipitate acute adrenocortical insufficiency (adrenal crisis). Measures to reduce the suppression of the HPA axis include administering cortisol in doses that mimic normal secretion of cortisol; for example, cortisol can be given on alternative days in the morning or in a larger dose in the morning and a smaller dose in the early afternoon. Topical administration of corticosteroids causes less suppression than does systemic administration. Gradual tapering of doses before withdrawal of all corticosteroids has been used in the past in the belief that it prevented adrenal crisis; however, it has been shown that HPA suppression is prolonged with this practice.[32] Tapering is used to prevent reactivation or flare-up of the underlying disease and to determine the lowest adequate dosage.

□ Addisonian crisis (adrenal crisis)

Adrenal crisis is a severe and sudden exacerbation of adrenal insufficiency. It can quickly lead to death unless it is treated promptly. It is usually precipitated by stress. Adrenal crisis can occur in any person with adrenal in-

---

Symptoms of adrenal crisis

Hypotension
Shock
Fever
Nausea and vomiting
Confusion

---

sufficiency and is manifested by acute exaggeration of symptoms and vascular collapse. (See the box above.)

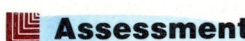 Assessment

■ SUBJECTIVE DATA

Common considerations in assessing patients with pituitary dysfunction (p. 949) are also pertinent for adrenal dysfunction because of the effect of the anterior pituitary on the adrenal glands. The nurse can gain insight into patient needs by considering the following data:

1. Extent of fatigue
2. Patient's perception of body image changes
3. Mood changes
4. Ability to tolerate stress
5. Need for assistance with activities of daily living
6. Sleep patterns
7. Eating patterns
8. Knowledge of the adrenal dysfunction and its treatment
9. Medication regimen
10. Presence of discomforting symptoms

■ OBJECTIVE DATA

Ongoing patient assessment should include the following:

1. Daily weight
2. Temperature and blood pressure every 4 hours
3. Intake and output every 4 hours
4. Skin integrity
5. Activity level
6. Food intake
7. Early signs of infection

The nurse should be alert for clinical findings that indicate excess or deficiency of adrenal hormones, including those of acute crises. Laboratory tests (of serum glucose and electrolyte levels) should be closely monitored.

■ DIAGNOSTIC TESTS

Diagnosis in adrenocortical dysfunction relies heavily on measurements of serum and urinary levels of hormones and metabolites (Table 29-11). There is usually no special preparation needed for tests of blood hormonal values, unless provocative agents are used to test responses of the adrenal gland to a stimulant or depressant. Provocative agents could be medications, diet, or any stimulus that elicits a known response. For example, an upright position or sodium loading can test aldosterone secretion. When such tests are performed, special care must be taken to clarify any questions and avoid the need to reschedule that test. Tests of adrenocortical function are described in Table 29-12.

Special care must be taken if provocative agents are used to test catecholamine secretion in suspected pheochromocytoma; histamine, which depletes catecholamines, may precipitate a hypertensive crisis. Regitine, an adrenergic-blocking agent, may induce severe hypotension. These agents are used infrequently today.

When urinary hormonal levels of metabolites are measured, timed specimens are collected. Important nursing actions include the following:

1. Start and stop the urine collection at the specified times; this is necessary if the pattern of diurnal secretion is to be analyzed correctly.
2. Obtain the specimen container and preservative required by the hospital laboratory; icing the specimen may be necessary.
3. Instruct the patient and involved staff in the procedure recommended by the laboratory.
4. Ensure that all urine voided in the time period is collected.
   a. Just before starting the collection, the patient should void and that urine is discarded.
   b. The last urine collected should be of a voiding at the time the test ends.

Additional tests that the physician may order include the following:

1. Glucose tolerance test
2. Renal function tests (Chapter 32)
3. Roentgenograms of kidney or abdomen
4. Adrenal arteriograms
5. CT scans

➜ Data analysis: nursing diagnoses

Nursing diagnoses are determined from the assessment of patient data. Possible nursing diagnoses for the person with adrenal dysfunction may include those identified on p. 954 (with the exception of sensory/perceptual alterations).

Other nursing diagnoses specific to adrenal hormonal imbalance include the following:

Diagnostic title	Possible etiologies
For the patient with Cushing's disease:	
Potential for infection	Decreased immune response
Altered nutrition: more than body requirements	Excessive intake in relation to metabolic needs; lack of knowledge

Table 29-11 Comparison of laboratory findings in hyposecretion and hypersecretion of adrenal gland

Substance	Hyposecretion	Hypersecretion
Adrenal cortex		
Plasma levels		
Cortisol	Low in all cases of adrenal cortex insufficiency	High in all cases of adrenal cortex hypersecretion
Aldosterone	Low in primary adrenal insufficiency	High in adrenal hyperplasia or aldosterone-secreting tumors
Androgen	Low in primary adrenal insufficiency	High in adrenal hyperplasia or androgen-secreting tumors
ACTH	Low in pituitary hyposecretion of ACTH	High in pituitary hypersecretion of ACTH
	High in primary adrenal deficiency resulting from lack of feedback inhibition by cortisol	Low in primary adrenal hypersecretion because of inhibition of cortisol
MCH	High in primary adrenal insufficiency resulting from lack of feedback inhibition by cortisol	Normal
Urinary		
Cortisol excretion rate	>100 µg/24 hr; >25 µg/24 hr; after dexamethasone is given for 2 days (0.5 mg/6 hr)	
Urinary excretion of cortisol metabolites	All are low in primary adrenocortical hyposecretion	All are high in primary adrenocortical hypersecretion
17-Ketogenic glucocorticoids (17-KGs) 5 to 23 mg/24 hr (m) 5 to 18 mg/24 hr (f)		
17-Hydroxycorticosteroids (17-OHCS) 3-10 mg/24 hr		
17-Ketosteroids (17-KS) (androgens) 5 to 18 mg/24 hr	17-KS may be normal with pituitary lack of ACTH	17-KS may be high in androgen-secreting tumors or enzymatic deficiency
Aldosterone and 18-glucoronide 16 mg/24 hr		Aldosterone elevated in hyperaldosteronism
Adrenal medulla		
Plasma levels		
Epinephrine		
Norepinephrine		
Total catecholamines		All are increased in pheochromocytoma
Urinary excretion		
Total catecholamines		
Epinephrine		All are increased in pheochromocytoma
Norepinephrine		
Metanephrine		Metanephrine is a urinary metabolite of epinephrine
Vanillylmandelic acid (VMA)		VMA is end product of catecholamine metabolism

Diagnostic title	Possible etiologies
For the patient with hypoadrenalism:	
Decreased cardiac output	Reduced fluid and electrolyte intake; inadequate cortisol replacement, noncompliance, lack of knowledge

It is important that there be mutual planning with patients about care needs. The responses to body image changes, the potential of emotional lability, and the fatigue experienced by patients may overwhelm their ability to cope effectively with hospitalization.

Planning: expected patient outcomes

Expected outcomes for the person with adrenal hormonal imbalances include those listed on p. 955. In addition, expected outcomes include, but are not limited to, the following:

1. Patients with *adrenocortical excess* can:
   a. Describe dietary and fluid restrictions.
   b. Explain ways to avoid infections and describe what to do if infections occur.
   c. Describe any therapeutic regimens prescribed for hypertension or diabetes mellitus, if appropriate.

2. Patients with *adrenocortical insufficiency* can perform the following:
   a. Describe ways to increase fluid and sodium intake.
   b. State why medications must be taken daily as prescribed.
   c. Explain the effects of stress on the need for medication.
   d. Identify stressors in own life and ways to control them.
   e. State awareness of the need for additional medication in times of severe stress.

Implementation

ASSISTING WITH ACHIEVEMENT OF THERAPEUTIC GOALS

Certain nursing measures are appropriate regardless of the type of adrenal dysfunction. The *maintenance* of medication regimens is a high priority. Other measures include those that achieve the following:

1. Provision of adequate rest
2. Regulation of blood pressure levels within desired limits
3. Maintenance of fluid and electrolyte balance

Table 29-12 Tests of adrenocortical function

Function test	Procedure and preparation	Interpretation
ACTH stimulation test (various tests available)	Synthetic ACTH given in 500-1000 ml of normal saline at 2 units/24 hr; then 17-OHCS and plasma cortisol levels are measured; alternative is to infuse 25 units of ACTH over an 8 hr period on 2-3 days and measure 17-OCHS and plasma cortisol levels on these days	Normally 17-OHCS excretion increases to 25 mg/24 hr and plasma cortisol increases to 40 μg/100 ml or greater; in patients with secondary adrenal insufficiency, the 17-OHCS rate is 3-20 mg/24 hr and the cortisol level is 10-40 μg/dl
Screening ACTH stimulation test	ACTH, 25 units, is given IM and plasma cortisol level is measured before and at 30 and 60 min intervals	Normally plasma cortisol increases 7 μg/dl
Cortisol suppression test	Twenty-four-hour urine specimen for 17-OCHS is collected for baseline; dexamethasone, 0.5 mg, is given every 6 hr for 2 days; 24 hr urine is also collected for 2 days	Dexamethasone suppresses pituitary secretion of ACTH but does not change steroid excretion; normally by day 2 of dexamethasone, 24-hr urinary level of OHCS should drop more than 50% below baseline, patients with adrenocortical excess (primary) show decrease in 24-hr urine levels; patients with secondary adrenocortical excess have drop, but less than 50%
Screening cortisol suppression test	Dexamethasone 1 mg, given at 12 PM; at 8 AM cortisol level is drawn	Normally cortisol should be less than 5 μg/dl
Mineralocorticoid suppression test (various tests are available)	IV infusion of saline 500 ml/hr for 4 hr	Normally saline infusion depresses plasma aldosterone to <8 μg/dl

Table 29-13 Comparison of clinical problems of Cushing's disease and Addison's disease

Cushing's syndrome	Addison's disease
Hypertension	Hypotension
Hyperglycemia	Hypoglycemia
Hypervolemia	Hypovolemia
Hypokalemia	Hyperkalemia
Immunosuppression	Intolerance to stress
Osteoporosis	

4. Maintenance of adequate nutrition to maintain or achieve desired weight and to keep blood glucose levels within normal limits
5. Provision of an environment that is as restful and as free of stressors as possible

The reasons for the above nursing measures are shown in Table 29-13.

The patient with Cushing's disease/syndrome

Nurses can assist patients with specific therapy directed toward correcting the hormonal imbalance caused by disease. Measures may include one or more of the following:
1. Pituitary surgery or radiation
2. Unilateral or bilateral adrenalectomy
3. Drug therapy to suppress or block synthesis of cortisol (see Table 29-10)
4. Surgery to remove an ectopic source of cortisone

In iatrogenic Cushing's syndrome or when corrective treatment is not feasible, measures include those that control hypertension, hypokalemia, hyperglycemia, hypercalciuria, and hypervolemia.

Nurses can assist patients with the following:
1. Nutrition: calorie and sodium restrictions and potassium supplements
2. Fluid and electrolyte balance: diuretics and potassium supplements; restriction of fluids
3. Blood glucose control: calorie restriction and insulin
4. Blood pressure control: antihypertensive agents and sodium restrictions
5. Safety measures to prevent pathologic fractures when osteoporosis is present

Persons with Cushing's syndrome are at particular risk for *nosocomial infections* because of their immunosuppressed states. Immunosuppression combined with metabolic imbalance and obesity impairs wound healing. Careful handwashing and aseptic technique are essential. Patients must not be exposed to infection, and they should be isolated from other patients with infections. Staff members who have *any* signs or symptoms of infection should not care for these patients.

Adrenal surgery causes considerable hemodynamic and metabolic changes that occur rapidly. A temporary cortisol deficit may occur after unilateral adrenalectomy or resection of an adenoma. The cortisol deficit results from the atrophy of the normal adrenal gland, which is caused by HPA axis suppression by the previously high blood-cortisol levels.

Bilateral adrenalectomy results in a permanent cortisol deficit because surgery changes the hormonal imbalance from cortisol excess to cortisol deficit. After adrenal surgery the patient has iatrogenic adrenal insufficiency and is at risk for adrenal crisis. Hormonal replacement is essential for maintenance of life.

After bilateral adrenalectomy, ACTH levels rise in the absence of the feedback control of cortisol-blood levels. The hypersecretion of ACTH is believed to be responsible for the development of pituitary tumors after bilateral adrenalectomy. In these instances pituitary irradiation is used to prevent pituitary tumor.

Suppressant drug therapy is commonly prescribed preoperatively and may reduce blood levels of (1) cortisone, (2) aldosterone, and (3) androgens (see Table 29-11).

The patient with primary aldosteronism

The treatment of primary aldosteronism is usually surgical resection of the adrenal adenoma or unilateral adrenalectomy. Bilateral hyperplasia is usually treated with sodium restriction, potassium replacement, and the aldosterone antagonist, spironolactone. These same measures may be used preoperatively.

After either surgery or the use of spironolactone, a temporary suppression of renin-induced aldosterone production may be present. If the aldosterone deficit is severe, fludrocortisone may be necessary. If the deficit is mild, treatment of acidosis and hyperkalemia may be achieved with sodium bicarbonate and sodium polystyrene sulfonate (Kayexalate) or furosemide (Lasix). Usually aldosterone production returns to normal within 6 months. Surgery reverses hypertension in a majority of patients.

The patient with pheochromocytoma

The primary treatment of pheochromocytoma is surgical removal of the tumor. The priority in preoperative care is control of hypertension. Medication to control hypertension includes adrenergic blocking agents such as propanolol (Inderal), which is often used to control tachycardia, arrhythmias, sweating, and angina. During a hypertensive crisis, the patient should be admitted to an intensive care unit. Cardiac monitoring and frequent monitoring of vital signs are necessary. When the patient's blood pressure level reaches the desired level, medication can be gradually decreased.

Maintaining blood pressure at a desired level is a major concern during anesthesia, surgery, and the postoperative period. The antihypertensive medication used preoperatively may influence the choice of anesthetic agent; manipulation of the tumor during surgery may release large bursts of hormones causing elevation of the blood pressure. When the tumor is removed sudden hypotention may occur. Hypotension is usually treated with plasma or a plasma substitute. Appropriately administered volume expanders usually control the hypotension, making vasopressors unnecessary.[49]

On the first postoperative day, hypertensive episodes are

common and caused by the response to pain and to hypervolemia caused by the treatment of hypotension following surgery. Currently, the most effective therapy is a rapidly acting diuretic such as furosemide (Lasix).

☐ The patient with Addison's disease

Nursing activities for patients with adrenocortical insufficiency include the following:

1. Administering and teaching hormonal replacement
2. Ensuring frequent and adequate food intake with normal to increased protein content
3. Ensuring normal or increased sodium and fluid intake
4. Treating hypoglycemia
5. Avoiding stressors
6. Ensuring frequent rest periods

The patient's adrenal insufficiency may be partial or complete, thus the doses of hormonal replacement will vary. In mild adrenocortical insufficiency, cortisol may be needed only during periods of stress, and mineralocorticoid insufficiency can be managed with high sodium intake. When cortisol and aldosterone deficit is absolute, as after bilateral adrenalectomy, the usual hormonal replacement is as follows:

1. Cortisone: 37.5 mg daily (25 mg in the early morning and 12.5 mg in the early evening)
2. Fludrocortisone: 0.1 to 0.2 mg daily

Synthetic preparations of cortisol may be used instead of cortisone, but the inability to monitor the blood levels of synthetic preparations is a disadvantage.

☐ Surgery

The patient undergoing adrenal surgery usually has a preoperative state of hormonal excess (cortisol, aldosterone, or catecholamines) that is suddenly reversed by surgery. This rapid change is associated with instability in hemodynamic and metabolic functions and varies according to the hormones involved and the amount of functional adrenal tissue that remains. The patient must be given constant nursing attention until hormonal stability is regained or a maintenance regimen established.

When cortisol deficit is expected after surgery, glucocorticoid replacement is first given by intravenous drip

---

Nursing care of the patient undergoing adrenal surgery

Preoperative

1. Provide supportive care (see p. 967).
2. Assist patient with usual preoperative care.
3. Maintain nutritional status with a high-protein, prescribed calorie diet with adequate minerals and vitamins.
4. Assist with correction of fluid and electrolyte imbalance.
5. Assist with hormonal suppression as prescribed (see Table 29-10).
6. Assist with measures used to prevent or treat crises of adrenal hormonal excess or deficit.
7. Administer prescribed intravenous fluids and glucocorticoid before surgery.

Postoperative

1. Establish monitoring schedule to detect complications of surgery and:
   a. Adrenal crisis
   b. Blood pressure alterations
   c. Blood glucose alterations
   d. Fluid and electrolyte imbalances
2. Because the patient may have unusual activity intolerance, pace postoperative activities with alternate periods of rest and gradual increase in self-care.
3. Provide measures to minimize effects of postural hypotension:
   a. Supply ace bandages or elastic stockings.
   b. Assess effects of posture on blood pressure.
   c. Assist or accompany the patient during ambulation while blood pressure remains labile.

4. Provide measures to decrease risk of infection in the immunosuppressed patient (for instance, strict surgical asepsis, coughing and deep breathing, avoid contact with persons with upper respiratory infections).
5. Administer cortisol replacement as typically prescribed:
   a. Intravenous route for the first 24 hours
   b. Intramuscular route the second day
   c. Oral route when patient is able to tolerate food by mouth
6. Administer mineralocorticosteroid (Fludrohydrocortisone) replacement, if prescribed.
   a. Typically prescribed when cortisol replacement is less than 40 to 50 mg/24 hr in the patient with bilateral adrenalectomy
7. Assist patient and family in learning about required hormonal replacement (see p. 957):
   a. Bilateral adrenalectomy: maintenance dose of cortisol and mineralocorticoids
   b. Unilateral adrenalectomy: doses of cortisol dependent on degree of suppression of HPA axis

throughout the perioperative period and then changed to intramuscular or oral doses. The dosage is adjusted by evaluating measurements of blood pressure, blood glucose, electrolyte, and serum cortisol levels. Monitoring for signs of adrenal insufficiency and adrenal crisis should be frequent. An increase in glucocorticoid medication is often required when blood pressure levels are less than adequate.

Along with hormonal, fluid, and electrolyte replacement, vasopressors may be necessary to maintain adequate blood pressure in the immediate postoperative period. Orthostatic hypotension is not unusual as the patient begins ambulation.

The patient is also observed carefully for signs of hypoglycemia. This condition is most likely to occur if the patient had diabetes mellitus as a symptom, but it can occur in any patient who has adrenal gland surgery. Intravenous solutions containing glucose are usually ordered. If the patient is able to eat, the nurse should check to see that all food on the tray is consumed.

Teaching the patient about adrenocortical insufficiency and the importance of hormonal replacement was discussed previously for the hypophysectomy patient. It is not unheard of for patients to be admitted to the hospital in adrenal crisis because they did not understand the need to take their medication as ordered.

✚ Evaluation

Evaluation is based on the expected patient outcomes. Some questions to consider include the following:

1. Were the patient and his or her family assisted to use resources in order to cope satisfactorily with hospitalization?
2. Were complications minimized and crises detected and treated promptly?
3. Were the following outcomes achieved:
   a. Blood pressure regulation?
   b. Blood glucose regulation?
   c. Weight at desired level?
   d. Fluid and electrolyte balance?
4. Is the patient able to manage self-care regimens?
5. Is the patient aware of the need for hormonal replacement?

■ PARATHYROID DYSFUNCTION

Parathyroid hormone (PTH) is primarily involved with maintenance of calcium and phosphorus levels. See Table 29-14 for the specific effects of PTH on the kidneys, bone, and intestine. PTH and vitamin D are two major regulators of calcium metabolism. PTH excess drives blood calcium levels upward, whereas PTH deficit leads to hypocalcemic states. PTH excess leads to hypophosphatemia, whereas PTH deficit is associated with elevated serum levels of phosphorus.

PTH and vitamin D work together to promote absorption of calcium from the intestine. They both promote bone

Table 29-14 Functions of parathyroid hormone (PTH)

Organ	Effects of PTH
Kidney tubule	Decreases urinary excretion of calcium
	Increases urinary excretion of phosphorus
	Inhibits H$^+$ ion secretion
	Decreases reabsorption of sodium and bicarbonate
	Increases renal threshold for glucose
Gut	Increases calcium and phosphorus absorption from intestinal tract (requires vitamin D)
Bone	Converts osteogenic osteocytes to osteolytic osteocytes
	Decreases the number of osteoblasts
	Decreases bone formation and increases bone breakdown

resorption of calcium. In hypoparathyroidism, PTH deficiency impairs the synthesis of vitamin D to its active form $(1,25\,(OH)_2D)$, and thus vitamin D deficiencies accompany PTH deficits. See Table 29-17 for information about vitamin D synthesis.

Calcitonin, a third regulator of calcium metabolism, has actions antagonistic to PTH and vitamin D. It is not involved in parathyroid disorders; however, it may be used for treatment of severe hypercalcemia. Calcitonin inhibits bone resorption.

■ Pathophysiology

■ PARATHYROID HORMONE (PTH) EXCESS

Primary hyperparathyroidism (Table 29-15) results from increased secretion of PTH, usually by a parathyroid adenoma. Normally, a low serum calcium level stimulates secretion of PTH, whereas a high serum level inhibits its secretion. In primary hyperparathyroidism, PTH does not become suppressed with the elevated serum calcium level (dysfunctional negative feedback system), thus leading to hypercalcemia. In many instances elevated serum calcium is the only sign of parathyroid dysfunction and is detected on routine examination. Mild symptoms of weakness and easy fatigability may be present. In some patients severe effects of hypercalcemia (renal or bone disease) may be evident.

Most of the symptoms are a result of the hypercalcemia. Nausea, vomiting, and anorexia lead to weight loss and fatigue. The effect of increased calcium on the muscles leads to hypotonicity of skeletal muscles, tendon reflexes, and gastrointestinal muscles. Muscle weakness and fatigue are thus common findings. Mental changes may vary from confusion to depression or psychosis. Relatively small elevations of calcium may cause major mental changes, especially in elderly persons.

Table 29-15 Parathyroid dysfunction

Etiology	Signs and symptoms	Medical therapy

PTH hormone excess
 	
Primary
  Adenoma, carcinoma, idiopathic hyperplasia
Secondary
  Renal failure, rickets, PTH-resistant nephropathy, vitamin D intoxication
Ectopic
  PTH-like secreting tumor
	Hypercalcemia and hypophosphatemia:
	Anorexia, nausea, vomiting, fatigue, depression, polyuria, polydipsia, dehydration; bone pain, muscle hypotonia and hyporeflexia; constipation
		Hydration, normal saline infusion
		Furosemide (Lasix)
		Phosphate infusion or oral salts
		Calcitonin — *hypocalcemia*
		Mithramycin
		Dialysis
		Surgical excision of tumor or parathyroidectomy

PTH hormone deficiency
 	
Excision of glands, autoimmune disease, idiopathic
 	
Tetany
	Hypocalcemia:
	  Paresthesia, Chvostek's sign, Trousseau's sign, carpopedal spasm, marked anxiety, seizures, laryngeal stridor, dyspnea, cyanosis, arrhythmias
	Hyperphosphatemia:
	  Soft tissue calcifications; nausea, vomiting, abdominal pain; dry scaling skin, brittle nails; patchy, thin hair
		Calcium salts: give with food but not with dairy products; calcium gluconate, calcium chloride
		Vitamin D supplements: Hytakerol, calciferol
		Dietary calcium and vitamin D
		Antacids (phosphate-binders)

When the serum calcium level rises above 16 to 18 mg/dl, acute hypercalcemic crisis occurs. Severe intractable vomiting leads to dehydration and electrolyte imbalances. Fever, severe mental changes, coma, and cardiac arrhythmias may result, ending in death if untreated.

The hyperplasia and excessive production of PTH may be enough to keep the calcium level normal, but this is at the expense of bone integrity. A variety of bone lesions may develop, bone pain may be severe, and bone fragility can predispose the patient to injury. In contrast to primary hyperparathyroidism, renal failure is characterized by hyperphosphatemia.

Secondary hyperparathyroidism develops from chronic hypocalcemic states, such as renal failure. Hyperplasia of the parathyroid glands develops with an increase in PTH. In some of these patients, the parathyroid glands become autonomous and lose their responsiveness to serum calcium levels (tertiary hyperparathyroidism).

Hyperparathyroidism results in *hypercalcemia* and *hypophosphatemia*. There is increased urinary excretion of both calcium and phosphorus with the following effects:
1. Inability of the kidney to concentrate urine
2. Polyuria
3. Increased risk of renal calculi with subsequent urinary obstruction or infection
4. Calcification of renal tubules

Calcium is lost from bone leading to demineralization of the bone, pathologic fractures, or cystic bone disease causing bone pain.

■ PARATHYROID HORMONE (PTH) LACK

The most common cause of hypoparathyroidism is the surgical removal of the parathyroid glands or an interference with their blood supply. With a diminished level of parathyroid hormone, there is decreased bone resorption, and the serum calcium level falls. Since parathyroid hormone is involved in the renal clearance of phosphate, serum phosphate levels increase. The decreased level of serum calcium results in neuromuscular irritability.

Nerves show decreased thresholds of excitation, repeated responses to a single stimuli, and in severe cases, continuous activity. The neuromuscular irritability is manifested in both peripheral sensory and motor nerves and is responsible for the signs of latent tetany (see the box on p. 972). Convulsions, laryngeal stridor and bronchospasm, and cardiac arrhythmias are possible if treatment is not instituted for the latent tetany.

Acute hypocalcemia (tetany) is life threatening, and the signs of latent tetany should always be promptly reported to the physician.

It is important for the nurse to recognize that the clinical findings of hypocalcemia are more reliable than the total serum calcium level, which measures (1) the ionized (unbound) blood calcium, which is the active metabolic calcium, and (2) the nonionized (bound) calcium, which does not affect neuroactivity. Changes in electroencephalographic (EEG) patterns may be present, and a prolonged

---

Signs of latent tetany

Paresthesia in fingertips and around mouth
Chvostek's sign (facial contraction on tapping facial nerve near jaw angle)
Trousseau's sign (carpal spasm after compression of upper arm with a cuff)
Carpopedal spasm (spasm of wrist and fingers and/or feet and toes)

Q-T interval is frequently seen on the cardiac monitor.

The major problem in hypoparathyroidism is that of hypocalcemia. In prolonged hypoparathyroidism, there may be other problems of calcium imbalance, such as cataract, malabsorption, and decreased growth of skin and nails. Hyperphosphatemia is indicated by calcifications in blood vessels, nerves, and soft tissues.

▣ Assessment

The signs and symptoms of calcium excess and deficit are priority observations when patients are treated for parathyroid dysfunction.

■ SUBJECTIVE DATA

The following subjective data are obtained from the patient:
1. Presence of discomfort (bone pain), fatigue, or paresthesia
2. Elimination patterns (constipation, polyuria)
3. Medication usage
4. Dietary history
5. Knowledge of condition

■ OBJECTIVE DATA

Objective data include the following:
1. Mental status (signs of behavior changes)
2. Intake and output every 8 hours
3. Daily weight
4. Muscle weakness
5. Electrolyte levels (calcium, phosphorus)
6. Condition of skin, hair, and nails

■ DIAGNOSTIC TESTING

Since the maintenance of normal calcium and phosphorus metabolism involves multiple systems besides the parathyroid (skeletal, gastrointestinal, and urinary), when parathyroid function is being assessed, the patient also undergoes diagnostic tests of these other systems. This

Table 29-16   Diagnostic tests for parathyroid function

Test	Procedure	Interpretation
Serum		
Total calcium 4.8-5.2 mEq/L 9.6-10.4 mg/100 ml	Blood sample No preparation	Measures both bound and ionized calcium; increased in primary hyperparathyroidism; decreased in hypoparathyroidism
Phosphorus 1.3-1.75 mEq/L	Blood sample	Decreased with hypercalcemia and elevated in hypocalcemia and in renal failure
Alkaline phosphatase 2-5 Bodansky units	Blood sample	Increased in stages of demineralization, liver disease, and by certain drugs
Parathyroid hormone (PTH) by radioimmunoassay	Blood sample	Elevated in hyperparathyroidism and decreased in hypoparathyroidism
Urine		
Calcium	Collect single specimen	Decreased in hypoparathyroidism
Quantitative	24-hr collection	Elevated in hyperparathyroidism
Phosphorus	24-hr collection	Elevated in renal failure, hypocalcemic states, and PTH excess; decreased with PTH lack
Function tests		
Ellsworth-Howard excretion test (PTH infusion test)	Fasting required; 200 units of PTH extract administered IV; hourly urine collections	Normal response is 5-6 times increased urinary phosphate excretion; an increase of 10 times is found in hypoparathyroidism
Urinary cAMP	Urine sample	High levels of cyclic AMP found in hyperparathyroidism

is necessary to determine whether the problem with calcium and phosphorus metabolism is caused by parathyroid metabolism or other disease states. In addition, ECG, EEG, and sometimes nerve conduction studies may be performed in an effort to detect hypotonicity or neuromuscular irritability.

Tests of parathyroid function are shown in Table 29-16.

Data analysis: nursing diagnoses

Nursing diagnoses are determined from the assessment of patient data. Possible nursing diagnoses for the person with parathyroid disorders include, but are not limited to, those listed on p. 954, and the following:

Diagnostic title	Possible etiologies
For the patient with hypocalcemia:	
Ineffective breathing	Neuromuscular impairment, respiratory obstruction
Decreased cardiac output	Disturbed neurologic mechanisms: arrhythmias
Potential for injury	Sensorimotor deficits during convulsions
For the the patient with hypercalcemia:	
Impaired physical mobility	Pain, neuromuscular impairment

Planning: expected patient outcomes

Expected patient outcomes for the person with parathyroid disorders may include, but are not limited to, those listed on p. 955, particularly numbers 1 and 7. In addition, patients with *hypoparathyroidism* should be able to:
1. Maintain adequate air exchange as shown by adequate blood gases, absence of stridor and dyspnea.
2. Maintain adequate cardiac output; undetected cardiac arrhythmias do not occur.
3. Avoid injury during convulsions.
4. State plans for self-care:
   a. Explain the prescribed drug therapy (calcium, vitamin D).
   b. State reasons for lifelong calcium and vitamin D therapy, if total parathyroid function is lost.
   c. Plan a diet high in vitamin D.
   d. Describe symptoms of tetany or hypercalcemia that require immediate attention.
   e. State plans for ongoing follow-up care.

The patient with *hyperparathyroidism* can:
1. List signs and symptoms of calcium imbalance.
2. Describe symptoms requiring medical follow-up.
3. Explain planned medication regimen, if appropriate.
4. Describe plans for follow-up care.

The patient with *hypercalcemia* should be able to:
1. Maintain optimal mobility by pacing activities and scheduling of analgesics.
2. State ways to maintain optimal health.

Implementation

ASSISTING WITH ACHIEVEMENT OF THERAPEUTIC GOALS

Correction of hyperparathyroidism

Definitive treatment of hyperparathyroidism requires surgical removal of the adenoma or of all but a part of one gland, if hyperplasia is the cause. Treatment varies depending on whether symptoms are present. In mild asymptomatic hypercalcemia when renal function, urinary calcium excretion, and skeletal system x-ray films are normal, surgery may be withheld until abnormalities occur. This patient should be evaluated every 6 to 12 months. Medical treatment of hypercalcemia may be performed preoperatively and in some patients who are not suitable candidates for surgery. Normalization of electrolyte levels reduces the risk of surgery. Hypercalcemia greater than 14 mg/dl requires immediate therapy if cardiac arrhythmias and coma are to be avoided.[32] Several measures can be used. The first step is diuresis; this involves hydration followed by a potent diuretic, such as furosemide (Lasix), for the excretion of several grams of calcium per day. This therapy can only be used in patients with adequate renal function. Intake and output must be monitored closely in all patients receiving this treatment. Replacement of electrolytes other than calcium may be necessary. This may include potassium, phosphorus, and magnesium. Drugs that inhibit bone resorption include calcitonin salmon (Calcimar), mithramycin, and phosphates (Neutra-Phos).

Calcimar may be given in acute hypercalcemia. It has a rapid action and causes an abrupt inhibition of bone resorption. Sensitivity skin testing may be performed with 1 MRC unit applied to the forearm. A rapid fall in the serum calcium level may occur following injection. Mithramycin is a cytotoxic antibiotic that has a potent effect on serum calcium levels; often only one dose is ordered. See Table 29-15 for other agents that are used as adjunctive therapy in selected instances of hypercalcemia.

When serum calcium laboratory results are assessed, the serum protein level must also be assessed. If patients have decreased serum protein content (hypoalbuminemia), less calcium is bound, more is ionized, and thus patients may exhibit signs of hypercalcemia more readily.

Mobilization that provides stress to long bones is known to increase bone formation, whereas immobilization fosters demineralization; thus ambulation should be promoted in these patients. A schedule of progressive activities should be planned with the patient, with attention to his or her level of weakness and pain. Activities should be spaced to lessen fatigue, and pain medication should be given before ambulation. Safety measures to prevent injury from falling are a high priority in these patients, who are weak, may have impaired cognitive function, and often have increased bone fragility.

The patient with hyperparathyroidism may exhibit several problems related to hypercalcemia. Nursing care includes the following:

1. Promoting urinary elimination by ensuring a fluid intake of 3 L/day unless contraindicated
2. Monitoring for signs of renal calculi (Chapter 32)
3. Preventing fecal impaction by careful attention to elimination patterns and use of dietary fiber, fluids, activity, and stool softeners, laxatives, or enemas
4. Providing symptomatic relief and administering prescribed agents for bone pain or gastrointestinal distress
5. Preparing patients for treatments and surgery to decrease anxiety
6. Providing rest periods to minimize fatigue

□ Parathyroid surgery

Partial parathyroidectomy is usually the treatment of choice in primary hyperparathyroidism. The usual surgery involves removing three glands totally and part of the fourth gland. An alternative approach involves removing all four glands and implanting some of the removed tissue into the muscle of the forearm. Implantation avoids vascular failure and death of residual parathyroid tissue left in the neck.[19] If no glandular abnormality is found at the time of surgery, extensive exploration of the neck and surrounding areas for additional glands that could be the source of the symptoms is necessary.

POSTSURGICAL HYPOCALCEMIA. The serum calcium level decreases within 24 hours after successful surgery. The patient must be monitored carefully for signs of tetany. Parathyroid function usually returns to normal in 5 to 7 days following subtotal resection. By this time the remaining parathyroid tissue resumes normal secretion. If mild hypocalcemia occurs, oral calcium is given. If hypocalcemia is severe, calcium gluconate or calcium chloride is given intravenously. Calcium replacement is continued until the serum calcium level returns to normal, usually within a few days. If signs and symptoms of hypocalcemia continue to be present, calcium and/or vitamin D replacement therapy in the same amount as that used to treat hypoparathyroidism will be necessary. While patients are on replacement therapy, they must be monitored carefully for signs and symptoms of hypercalcemia.

If total parathyroidectomy is performed, hypoparathyroidism will develop, and the patient will need the same treatment as any other patient with hypoparathyroidism.

□ Care of the patient with tetany

When the patient has a known risk of tetany, nursing interventions include the following:
1. Frequent assessment of signs of latent tetany (p. 972)
2. Prompt reporting to physician of any signs of hypocalcemia
3. Maintenance of emergency equipment (tracheostomy set and intravenous calcium) at bedside
4. Administering ordered calcium and vitamin D replacement with antacids to patient with hyperphosphatemia
5. Maintaining a quiet, nonstressful environment

The symptoms of hypocalcemia are more severe in patients with alkalosis because alkalosis causes more of the dissolved calcium to bind to serum albumin. If more calcium is bound, less is ionized, and hypocalcemic symptoms occur more readily. Attention to acid-base balance includes the prevention and treatment of causes of alkalosis: hypokalemia and respiratory alkalosis (hyperventilation). Caution should be used with agents that promote alkalosis, such as certain drugs and gastrointestinal intubation.

Providing a nonstressful environment for this patient is a major nursing responsibility. Actions might include the following:
1. Controlled visitation
2. Discussion with family members about avoiding disturbing discussions
3. Explanations of treatments geared to patient's level of understanding and concern
4. Frequent contacts by nursing staff

If tetany develops, the nurse assists as needed in emergency treatment of airway obstruction, cardiac arrhythmia, and seizures. Interventions for these conditions are discussed elsewhere in the text.

□ Management of hypoparathyroidism

The first priority of treatment is the correction of significant hypocalcemia with the measures already discussed. Long-term maintenance of normal serum calcium levels can usually be achieved by daily calcium and vitamin D supplements. Replacement of PTH is not possible.

Large doses of vitamin D_2 or D_3 are required to overcome the lack of PTH on the synthesis of vitamin D. Use of one of the more potent vitamin D preparations such as Calderol or Rocaltrol (Table 29-17) necessitates frequent measurements of serum and urinary calcium.

Dietary intake of calcium may be limited by the necessity for restricting phosphorus intake. When a low phosphorus

Table 29-17 Vitamin D synthesis and synthetic preparations

Metabolic steps	Preparations
Vitamin D_2 (ergocalciferol) skin: photogenesis ingestion	Calciferol (Drisdol, Geltaps)
Vitamin D_3 (cholecalciferol)	Dihydrotachysterol (Hytakerol)
Liver synthesis of vitamin D metabolite, 25 (OH) D (hydroxycholecalciferol)	Calcifediol (Calderol)
Kidney synthesis of vitamin D metabolite, 1, 25 $(OH)_2D$ (dihydroxycholecalciferol) and vitamin 24, 25 $(OH)_2D$	Calcitriol (Rocaltrol)

intake is required, dairy products and egg yolks (good sources of phosphorus and vitamin D) are avoided. Phosphate-binders (such as aluminum-based antacids) may be prescribed to increase excretion of phosphorus. The amounts of elemental calcium contained in calcium preparations varies; for example, a 650 mg calcium lactate tablet contains 87 mg of elemental calcium, whereas an Os-Cal tablet contains 250 mg. Calcium salts may be given as lactate, gluconate, or carbonate; calcium phosphate is contraindicated.

Dosages of vitamin D and calcium are adjusted to maintain a low normal serum calcium and to minimize urinary calcium excretion, to avoid the risk of renal calculi. The lack of PTH results in excessive urinary calcium excretion even in the presence of normal serum calcium levels. Thiazide diuretics and a restricted sodium intake are helpful in decreasing hypercalcinuria.

Medical follow-up with monitoring of laboratory tests of serum and urinary calcium levels is necessary to prevent hypercalcemia, renal colic, and metastatic calcifications. The patient must be well educated for self-management of the illness.

☐ **Counseling and teaching**

Vitamin D appears to be the principal regulator of the level of calcium ions in the body and therefore increases the absorption of calcium. A diet high in vitamin D needs to be followed by the person with hypoparathyroidism. The amount of calcium and vitamin D is gradually adjusted

---

Important information for the patient with hypoparathyroidism

1. Relationship of symptoms of hypocalcemia and hypercalcemia to
   a. Disease
   b. Medication usage
   c. Complications: tetany, hypercalcemia, renal stones
2. Importance of medical care at prescribed intervals and when untoward signs develop
3. Importance of taking prescribed medications daily
4. Importance of informing health care providers of the health problem
5. Consistent dietary inclusion of vitamin D and calcium-rich foods (excepting dairy foods that are high in phosphates)
6. Awareness that dietary intake alone is insufficient to maintain calcium levels in the absence of PTH
7. Need for lifelong management of calcium balance by replacement; the amount necessary is determined by serum calcium levels

---

until the serum calcium level is normal. Recognition of symptoms of hypocalcemia and hypercalcemia is important so that adjustment in dosage can be instituted. Other instructions for patient education are listed in the box below, left.

✚ Evaluation

Questions that the nurse can use to evaluate the nursing care of the patient with parathyroid dysfunction include the following:
1. Were complications prevented in early detection and reporting of signs and symptoms?
2. Is patient prepared to manage treatment measures at home?
3. Is patient aware of need for lifelong replacement therapy, if indicated?

■ THYROID DYSFUNCTION

■ Pathophysiology

Alterations in the thyroid gland may be associated with hyperthyroid, hypothyroid, or euthyroid metabolic states (Table 29-18).

■ GOITER

Any enlargement of the thyroid gland is spoken of as a goiter. A goiter may be caused by various disorders that prevent the synthesis of normal quantities of thyroid hormones. These include the following:
1. Iodide deficiency
2. Congenital metabolic defects preventing synthesis of thyroid hormones
3. Blocking of hormone synthesis by chemical agents (e.g., substances in cabbage, turnips, soybeans)
4. Blocking of hormone synthesis by drugs (for example, thiocarbamides, sulfonylureas, and lithium)

Goiter occurs because of an impairment in hormonal synthesis associated with a reduction of the thyroid hormones T_3 and T_4. It is believed that this reduction prevents the normal feedback inhibition of TSH. The TSH level is increased, which in turn causes an increase in thyroid mass. The thyroid enlargement (Fig. 29-10) may produce hyperplasia and be sufficient enough to allow for adequate hormonal synthesis.

Not all patients with goiter demonstrate an elevated level of TSH. Another hypothesis is that goiter results from the stimulation of the thyroid gland by thyroid growth immunoglobulins.[48] Goiter may be diffuse or nodular; nodules are caused by an adenoma, carcinoma, inflammatory processes, or hemorrhage.

Simple goiter is the term used for thyroid enlargement that is not associated with hyperthyroidism, hypothyroidism, malignancy, or inflammation. It is frequently seen in females, appearing at puberty or during pregnancy.

Table 29-18   Thyroid gland dysfunction

Etiologic factors	Signs and symptoms	Medical therapy
Thyroid hormone deficit **Primary** Congenital, idiopathic; iodine deficiency; chronic thyroiditis; thyrotoxin	Hypothyroidism (early signs): Weight gain, sluggishness, sleepiness, slowed mental process, slurred speech; intolerance to cold; constipation; dry skin, dry sparse hair; infertility, decreased libido; decreased body temperature; menorrhagia in young women	Replacement therapy of thyroid hormones: Thyroid Levothyroxine sodium Liothyronine sodium Thyroglobulin Liotrix
Secondary/tertiary Pituitary or hypothalamic dysfunction	Myxedema: Lethargy, coma; periorbital puffiness; nonpitting edema of feet and hands; large tongue; dull facies; pale, cool, rough, "doughy" skin	
Iatrogenic Radioactive iodine; surgery of thyroid; antithyroid drugs	Decreased urine flow and urine concentration, proteinuria (see text for cardiac, musculoskeletal, and gastrointestinal symptoms)	
Thyroid hormone excess **Primary** Toxic diffuse goiter (Graves' disease) Adenoma Toxic multinodular goiter Thyrotoxicosis Cancer of thyroid	Hyperthyroidism Loss of weight, fatigue Mental status: anxiety, poor concentration, restlessness, emotional lability, irritability, restlessness Nervous system: fine tremors, rapid tendon reflexes, decreased fine coordination Cardiovascular system: tachycardia, increased blood pressure, angina, arrhythmias, cardiac hypertrophy	Reduction of thyroid hormone Antithyroid drugs; sodium iodide, propylthiouracil, methimazole Radioactive iodine Surgery: subtotal or total thyroidectomy
Secondary/tertiary Pituitary or hypothalmic hyperfunction Some ovarian tumors Factitious use use of thyroid medications	Muscle and bone changes: muscle weakness, atrophy, osteoporosis Skin changes: warm, moist skin, intolerance to heat, fine hair Dermopathy: pretibial myxedema, vitiligo, hyperpigmentation Sexual changes: amenorrhea, decreased libido Enlarged thyroid	Thyroid crisis: Antithyroid drugs; oxygen, hypothermia to reduce fever, IV fluids, steroids, sedatives, cardiac drugs as necessary

■ THYROIDITIS

Inflammation of the thyroid gland may be acute, subacute, or chronic and is characterized by painful swelling of the thyroid gland. Acute thyroiditis, infection by a pyogenic organism, and subacute thyroiditis that follows a viral infection are rare.

The most common form of thyroiditis is Hashimoto's thyroiditis, in which the thyroid is infiltrated with lymphocytes and plasma cells. Autoimmunity is considered to be the pathologic basis of this chronic thyroiditis. Early in the disease when functioning thyroid tissue is still present, excessive stored thyroid hormone may be released, resulting in signs and symptoms of transient hyperthyroidism.

As the disease progresses, the thyroid gland may be destroyed, and signs and symptoms of hypothyroidism may develop. Antithyroid antibodies are present in the serum. TSH levels may be elevated in the early stages but serum T_4 and T_3 levels gradually decrease. There is diffuse enlargement of both lobes of the thyroid gland.

■ HYPOTHYROIDISM

Hypothyroidism is a hypometabolic state resulting from a deficiency of thyroid hormone that may occur at any age. Signs of infantile (congenital) hypothyroidism, or *cretinism,* are not usually seen until several months after birth;

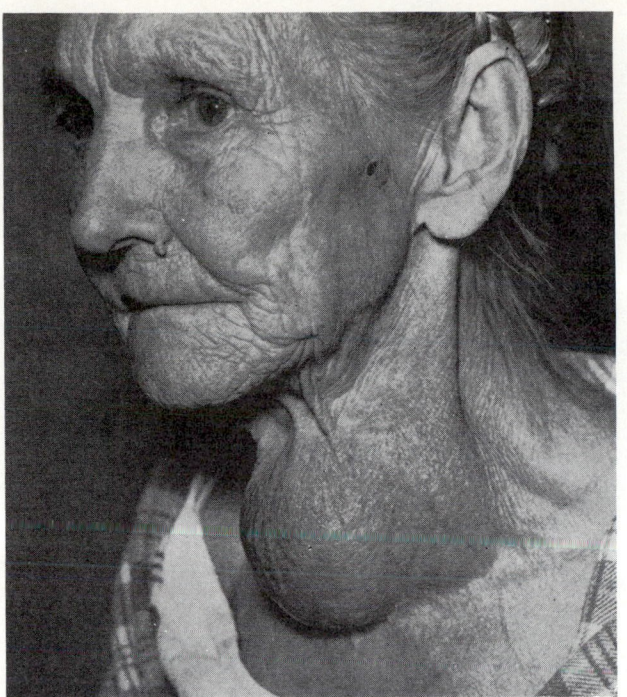

Fig. 29-10 Simple goiter. (From Prior, JA, Silberstein, JS, and Stang, JM: Physical diagnosis: the history and examination of the patient, ed 6, St. Louis, 1981, The CV Mosby Co.)

by then, mental and physical retardation are usually irreversible. Figure 29-11 shows an adult who had untreated infantile hypothyroidism.

In adults the most frequent causes of hypothyroidism are autoimmune thyroiditis, ablative therapy, and idiopathy.[37] It may be secondary to pituitary failure and TSH lack or from hypothalamic disease that causes a deficiency of thyroid-releasing hormone. In hypothyroidism resulting from pituitary or hypothalamic problems, TSH is depressed and no hyperplasia occurs.

The signs and symptoms result from a deficiency of T_3 and T_4, leading to a decrease in the normal metabolic functions that are under the control of these hormones. Usually the pathophysiologic changes develop slowly and early. Symptoms are vague (fatigue, weakness, lethargy, and intolerance to cold). The entire spectrum of signs and symptoms is listed in Table 29-18. *Myxedema* refers to severe hypothyroidism; marked slowing of metabolic functions and fluid accumulation lead to the distinctive features of myxedema.

The characteristics of hypothyroidism vary with the age of onset and the severity of the deficiency. There is an accumulation of hyaluronic acids and alteration of ground substances that results in mucinous edema. This devel-

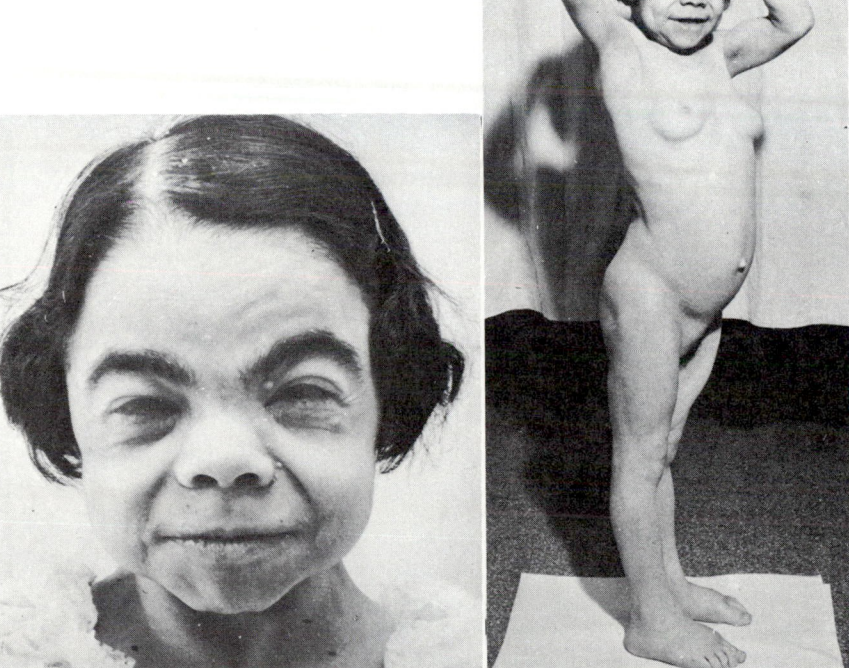

Fig. 29-11 Adult cretin (33 years old, untreated). Note characteristic cretinoid features, dwarfism (height of 44 inches), absent axillary and scant pubic hair, poorly developed breasts, potbelly, and small umbilical hernia. (From Schneeburg, NG: Essentials of clinical endocrinology, St. Louis, 1979, The CV Mosby Co.)

NURSING CARE PLAN

Person with hyperthyroidism

DATA: Mrs. Talbot, a 28-year-old housewife, is admitted for diagnostic evaluation before a thyroidectomy, which is scheduled to be performed in 2 weeks. Graves' disease was diagnosed 2 days ago; hospitalization was delayed until child-care arrangements were made for her 6-year-old step-son. (The marriage occurred 3 months ago.) Initial therapy, started 2 days ago, is Tapazole and Lugol's solution. The ECG report is sinus tachycardia (rate 132).

The nursing history identified the following about the patient:

1. She feels overwhelmed, cries frequently, and fears losing control of temper.
2. She has lost 15 lb in 2 months and is always hungry, although she is eating large amounts of food.
3. She is bothered by heat, others' noisiness, and her own clumsiness.
4. She expects medicine to keep her feeling better and dreads surgery.

The physical examination revealed the following: BP: 140/90; pulse: 136, R: 24. Staring gaze of eyes with proptosis (equal bilaterally); right eye slightly reddened. Skin warm and perspiration present. Increased muscle tone; quick muscle response to sudden noise; fine tremor of both hands. Diffuse enlargement of thyroid visible. *Bruit* present over thyroid.

Collaborative nursing actions include those to prevent further environmental stress that could make the patient more uncomfortable and increase her signs and symptoms.

Nursing actions include monitoring for the following: temperature, pulse, respiration, blood pressure, weight, excessive hunger, and tremulousness.

Nursing diagnosis: Decreased cardiac output: related to environmental stimulation

Expected patient outcomes	Nursing interventions	Rationale
Patient's pulse rate is less than 10 above baseline during first 72 h Pulse rate decreases gradually after 72 h Undetected cardiac arrhythmias do not occur	Assess vital signs, especially heart rate and rhythm at least q4h Instruct patient to report palpitations, chest pain, and dizziness Assess daily weight, daily intake and output; assess for signs of edema, jugular vein distention and pulmonary congestion q8h Decrease known stressors; explain all interventions, and listen to patient Balance periods of activity with rest Administer prescribed drugs and monitor therapeutic response	The early detection of atrial fibrillation or thyroid storm allows prompt treatment and prevents cardiovascular crisis

Nursing diagnosis: Ineffective individual coping: related to personal vulnerability to environmental stimuli

Expected patient outcomes	Nursing interventions	Rationale
Patient explains reason for change in behavior Emotional lability is minimized Patient identifies at least one coping mechanism that will help during periods of nervousness	Discuss reasons for emotional lability Maintain calm, relaxed environment Encourage visitors who are calm and will not upset her Provide privacy (such as a single room) Suggest that others avoid sharing distressing news with her Explain all interventions Avoid stimulants such as coffee, caffeine, and alcohol Help her identify previous coping mechanisms or explore new ones	A supportive environment can reduce environmental stimuli and stressors and assist patient in coping

Person with hyperthyroidism—cont'd

Nursing diagnosis: Altered nutrition: less than body requirements related to increased metabolic needs

Expected patient outcomes	Nursing interventions	Rationale
Patient's normal weight is maintained Patient gains at least 0.5 kg/wk, if weight is below normal	Monitor weight qod to weekly Monitor serum albumin, hemoglobin, and lymphocyte levels Help her plan for high-calorie, high-protein, high-carbohydrate diet with selection from all food groups Suggest six small meals per day or between-meal snacks	Increase nutrient intake to meet increased metabolic demand

Nursing diagnosis: Sensory/perceptual alterations: potential, visual, related to environmental agents

Expected patient outcomes	Nursing interventions	Rationale

Patient's vision does not worsen
Patient can explain measures to protect eyes
	Assess visual acuity, ability to close eyes, and photophobia
	Protect eyes from irritants:
	  Use patches or glasses when in high wind
	  Use artificial tears, if prescribed
	  Elevate head of bed at night
		These measures can prevent corneal injury and minimize risk of loss of vision

Nursing diagnosis: Pain: heat intolerance, diaphoresis related to increased metabolic rate

Expected patient outcomes	Nursing interventions	Rationale
Patient states that she feels more comfortable	Control environmental temperature for comfort (fans may be helpful) Suggest that she take frequent showers Encourage adequate fluid intake and monitor fluid losses	These measures keep her comfortable by increasing heat loss

Nursing diagnosis: Activity intolerance: related to generalized weakness

Expected patient outcomes	Nursing interventions	Rationale
Patient states fatigue is decreased	Assess activity schedule Suggest ways to modify fatiguing activities Identify activities than can be done by others until condition is controlled Schedule rest periods Encourage activities that promote sleep at night	Reduction of energy expenditure is necessary to reduce fatigue in persons with increased metabolism

Continued.

NURSING CARE PLAN

Person with hyperthyroidism—cont'd

Nursing diagnosis: Impaired home maintenance management: related to signs and symptoms

Expected patient outcome	Nursing interventions	Rationale
Patient states plan for home maintenance management	Assist her to identify home maintenance difficulties Assist her to identify persons who can provide temporary help Make referrals as needed, such as to social services Identify persons who can help monitor her compliance with medical regimen	These measures increase resources available to patient and reduce stress from inability to meet expectations of role

Nursing diagnosis: Knowledge deficit: lack of exposure to information

Expected patient outcomes	Nursing interventions	Rationale
Patient explains medical regimen and care needs	Explain how and when to take prescribed medications Describe symptoms of infection to be reported to physician, such as sore throat or fever Describe ways to plan prescribed dietary intake Provide required teaching about care needs (comfort, sleep, and rest)	These measures increase likelihood of compliance with therapy used to achieve euthyroid state and optimal physical status before surgery

---

Thyroid hormone functions

Hormones	Functions
Thyroxine (T_4) Triiodothyronine (T_3)	Regulates protein, fat, and carbohydrate catabolism in all cells Regulates metabolic rate of all cells Regulates body heat production Insulin antagonist Maintains growth hormone secretion, skeletal maturation Affects CNS development Necessary for muscle tone and vigor Maintains cardiac rate, force, and output Maintains secretion of gastrointestinal tract Affects respiratory rate and oxygen utilization Maintains calcium mobilization Affects RBC production Stimulates lipid turnover, free fatty acid release, and cholesterol synthesis
Thyrocalcitonin	Lowers serum calcium and phosphorus levels Decreases calcium and phosphorus absorption in gastrointestinal tract Inhibits bone resorption

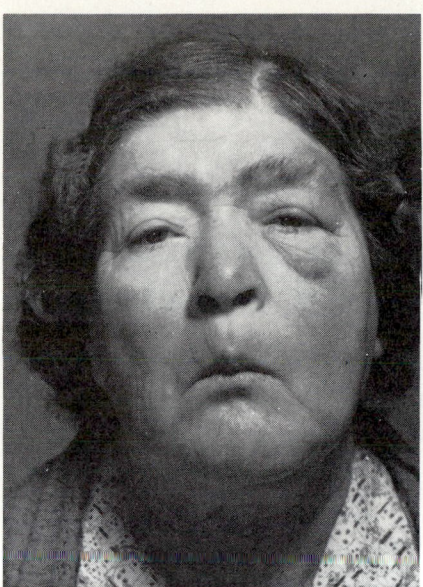

Fig. 29-12   Person with myxedema. (From Schottelius, BA, and Schottelius, DA: Textbook of physiology, ed 18, St. Louis, 1978, The CV Mosby Co.)

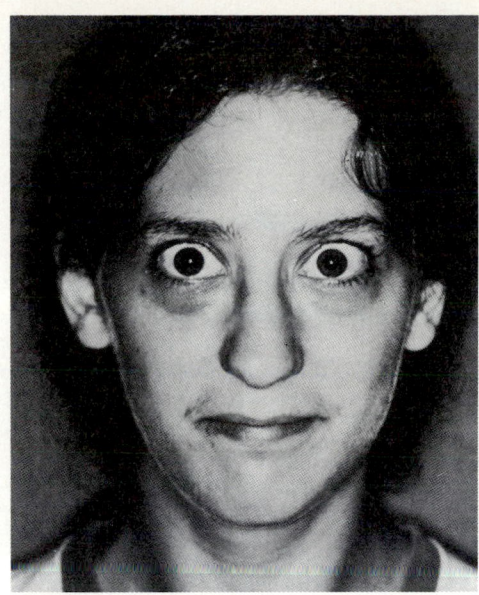

Fig. 29-13   Ophthalmopathy of Graves' disease. (From Kaye, D, and Rose, LF: Fundamentals of internal medicine, St. Louis, 1983, The CV Mosby Co.)

opment is responsible for the thickened tissues of hands, feet, and tongue and around the eyes and for effusions in the pleura, pericardium, and joints.

See Fig. 29-12 for an example of the facies characteristic of myxedema. These patients often have coarse skin that bruises easily (because of increased capillary fragility) and is pale and yellow (because of anemia and hypercarotenemia). Hair becomes sparse, dry, and brittle. Mental processes slow, with loss of initiative, memory deficit, and slurred speech; somnolence, confusion, and even dementia may occur. Muscular and joint stiffness are common. Appetite decreases and decreased peristaltic activity leads to constipation. Despite these marked changes, some individuals do not seem to be aware of the changes in their physical functioning, appearance, or behavior.

Cardiovascular dysfunction is a serious outcome of untreated hypothyroidism. Besides bradycardia, there may be elevation of diastolic blood pressure, cardiomegaly and changes in cardiac output. Hypercholesteremia is often present. Angina or cardiac failure may occur. Diminished heart sounds may represent pericardial effusion. *Pleural effusion* and *ascites* can develop.

Myxedema crises occurs as the myxedema worsens. The patient becomes less responsive and may go into a coma. An infection such as pneumonia, cellulitis, or pyelonephritis may precipitate the coma.

■ HYPERTHYROIDISM

Hyperthyroidism, a hypermetabolic state, is also called thyrotoxicosis. See Table 29-18 for some of the conditions associated with hyperthyroidism.

Hyperthyroidism results from excessive secretion of thyroxine (T_4) or triiodothyronine (T_3). The most common causes are toxic diffuse goiter (Graves' disease) and toxic nodular goiter. In both of these conditions, secretion of T_4 and T_3 becomes autonomous, and the thyroid gland is no longer regulated by TSH.

The cardiovascular system is seriously affected by hyperthyroidism because of the increased metabolic rate and the direct effects of thyroid hormones on the heart.

☐ Graves' disease (toxic diffuse goiter)

Graves' disease, which is characterized by a triad of symptoms—*goiter, hyperthyroidism,* and *exophthalmos* (abnormal protrusion of the eyes, Fig. 29-13)—is thought to be an autoimmune disease and is the result of thyroid-stimulating immunoglobulins (TSI), also called long-acting thyroid stimulator (LATS). The cause of the abnormal development of the immunoglobulins is unknown. Persons with specific haplotypes and monozygotic twins have a higher frequency of Graves' disease.[48]

Retro-orbitally, there is edema with infiltration (fat, mucopolysaccharides, and lymphocytes) that results in proptosis. This process is not closely correlated with the severity of hormonal excess. The forward protrusion intensifies other signs related to the eye that result from increased sympathetic nervous system (for example, stare and lid lag). In severe *exophthalmos,* there may be an inability to close the eye and extraocular muscle weakness.

The amount of thyroid enlargement varies in Graves' disease, but it is diffuse and usually symmetric. An important sign of Graves' disease is a *bruit* heard over the thyroid; this sign reflects increased vascularity.

Sympathetic nervous stimulation is responsible for many of the symptoms of hyperthyroidism listed in Table 29-18. Other symptoms are related to a chronic catabolic state or interactions with other hormones. Atrial fibrillation and congestive heart failure may evolve if hyperthyroidism is not treated.

☐ Toxic multinodular goiter

Milder hyperthyroidism and nodular disease are typical of toxic multinodular goiter. This condition usually occurs after age 50 and is most commonly seen in the elderly. Usually nontoxic nodular disease has been present for many years. In the elderly, signs of increased sympathetic activity (for example, tremors, hyperactivity, and heat intolerance) may not be as marked and can make diagnosis more difficult. Unexplained tachycardia or a decrease in mental status may lead to the diagnosis.

Hyperthyroidism is more common in women than in men, and there is a higher incidence between 20 and 40 years of age. It often appears after episodes of emotional trauma, infection, or increased stress and occurs frequently in persons who have had other endocrine disturbances.

☐ Thyroid storm

Thyroid storm (thyroid crisis) may occur in persons with uncontrolled hyperthyroidism. It is believed that in a thyroid storm, increased amounts of hormones are released into the bloodstream and metabolism is markedly increased. It may be precipitated by infection, stressors, or thyroid surgery undertaken on a patient who was not adequately prepared with antithyroid drugs. The onset often occurs spontaneously. The patient's temperature may rise to 41° C (106° F) as the body becomes unable to release the heat formed with increased metabolism. The pulse will be rapid, and there is marked respiratory distress, apprehension, restlessness, irritability, and prostration. The patient may become delirious and finally comatose, with death resulting from heart failure.

▦ Assessment

■ SUBJECTIVE DATA

Hypersecretion or hyposecretion of the thyroid gland has marked effects on the patient's ability to function, as well as on physiologic processes. The nurse collects data from the patient or a family member about the factors listed below. It is important to ask if there has been a change in any of these factors and when the change was first noted.

Energy level
Mood and mental ability
Ability to carry out activities of daily living
Ability to manage stress
Intolerance to heat or cold
Food intake
Elimination patterns

The interview should help the nurse determine the patient or family's understanding of the disease and its treatment and learn about the care needs of the patient.

■ OBJECTIVE DATA

Initial physical examination should provide the following baseline information about the patient:

Mental status (ability to follow directions)
Nutritional status
Cardiovascular status
Body characteristics
Skin appearance and texture
Hair quality and amount
Eye appearance and extraocular motion
Presence and location of edema
Neck appearance and range of motion
Abdominal girth
Extremities

■ DIAGNOSTIC TESTS

Testing for thyroid function can be made at the hypothalamic, pituitary, thyroid, serum, or peripheral tissue levels. Table 29-19 presents the major test procedures and preparations and their interpretation. The most commonly used tests are serum T_4 and T_3 concentrations and T_3 resin uptake. The T_3 resin uptake test evaluates changes in serum protein concentrations that can alter the binding of T_3 and T_4. T_4 is the more potent hormone. Changes in thyroxine-binding globulins (TBG) and prealbumin may alter free T_4 concentrations and, to a lesser extent, T_3.

An elevated T_4 level often confirms clinical findings of overt hyperthyroidism, whereas T_3 testing is more sensitive in discerning mild hyperthyroidism. TSH radioimmunoassay and stimulation testing can help differentiate primary and secondary hypothyroidism. Investigation of thyroid nodules may require needle biopsy or surgical exploration.

➡ Data analysis: nursing diagnoses

Nursing diagnoses are determined from the assessment of patient data. Possible nursing diagnoses for the person with thyroid hormone imbalance may include, but are not limited to, those identified on p. 954.

Diagnostic title	Possible etiologies
Diagnoses specific to thyroid hormonal imbalances for the patient with hyperthyroidism are the following:	
Ineffective individual or family coping	Inadequate information, temporary role change, crisis
Altered nutrition: less than body requirements	Altered metabolic demands, inability to obtain sufficient food
Sleep pattern disturbance	Anxiety, altered sensory state, environmental change

Table 29-19   Diagnostic tests of thyroid function

Function test	Procedure and preparation	Interpretation
Tests related to serum levels of thyroid hormone		
Serum T_4 concentration	Blood sample, no special preparation	Measures circulating thyroxine that is bound and free; normal, 3-7 $\mu g/100$ ml; can be affected by pregnancy, estrogen, glucocorticoids, and hypoproteinemia.
Serum T_3 concentrations	Radioassay of blood sample; no special preparation	Measures circulating T_3 that is bound; normal values are 100-170 $\mu g/100$ ml
Thyroxine-binding globulin (TBG)	Blood sample, no special preparation	Measures levels of TBG; TBG can be elevated or depressed by other conditions and can alter T_4 and T_3 concentrations
Triiodothyronine (T_3) resin uptake (T_3U)	Blood sample drawn; in laboratory, resin and radioactive T_3 are added to sample of blood; radioactive T_3 will bind to unoccupied sites of thyroxine-binding globulin (TBG); radioactive counts are performed on blood and resins to determine amount of T_3 (radioactive) bound to resin	Measures changes in thyroid-binding protein concentrations Normally 25%-30% of radioactive T_3 will bind to resin If binding sites of protein are saturated by high levels of T_4; higher T_3U levels may indicate hyperthyroidism; low levels may indicate hypothyroidism
Pituitary level test TSH radioimmunoassay	Blood sample, no special preparation	Directly measures TSH levels, measurement aids in differentiating primary and secondary hypothyroidism; values are elevated in primary hypothyroidism because of loss of negative feedback
TSH stimulation test	Baseline level of TSH is measured, 500 ug of TRH is given; 30 min later, TSH again measured	Normally TRH causes a rise in TSH to 15-30 $\mu g/ml$, or an incremental rise of 5 m/u above baseline; a flat response confirms hyperthyroidism; a marked response indicates primary hypothyroidism
Thyroid level test Radioactive iodine uptake (RAIU)	A tracer dose of radioactive iodine (^{131}I) is given by mouth. At 2, 6, and 24 hr following administration, scintillation detector is placed over neck in region of thyroid and amount of accumulated radioactive iodine is measured; excess iodine in any foods, cough medicines, x-ray media, other medications, and enriched iodine foods affect test by giving low readings. Fasting may be required.	Measures level of thyroid activity Normal thyroid will take up 5%-35% of tracer dose; increased uptake occurs in hyperthyroidism; excess tracer dose is excreted in urine and can be measured; urine is collected for 24 hr; decreased amounts in urine indicate hypothyroid state
Thyroid scan	Dose of ^{131}I is given, and scintillation scan is done: a picture of distribution of radioactivity is recorded	Size, shape, and anatomic function of gland assessed; areas of increased or decreased uptake noted; iodine ingestion (in medicines and dyes) before test can modify results
Thyroid ultrasound	No preparation required	Ultrasonography used to find structural abnormalities; cysts, nodules, and other masses

Continued.

Table 29-19 Diagnostic tests of thyroid function—cont'd

Test	Procedure and preparation	Interpretation
Thyroid antibody test	Blood sample	Antibodies to thyroglobulin and microsomes are present in Hashimoto's thyroiditis
Thyroid-stimulating immunoglobulins (TSI)	Blood sample	If TSI antibodies are present: Graves' disease is confirmed
Tests related to peripheral effects of thyroid hormone		
Basal metabolic rate (BMR)	Patient at rest and fasted: amount of oxygen used while at rest is calculated; patient's oxygen use is compared with established norms for people of same sex, age, and size	Normal range is -15% to $+15\%$; in hyperthyroidism patient's BMR will be greater than $+15\%$; in hypothyroidism patient's BMR will be less than -15%; BMR is less accurate than other tests described above but may be used to evaluate therapy
Serum cholesterol level	Blood sample; patient placed on NPO list night before	Normals vary from laboratory to laboratory; high levels found in hypothyroidism and low levels found in hyperthyroidism; data augment other tests

Diagnostic title	Possible etiologies
For the patient with hypothyroidism diagnoses are the following:	
Self-care deficit	Intolerance to activity, cognitive impairment
Constipation	Immobility, inadequate fluid and nutritional intake

Planning: expected patient outcomes

Expected patient outcomes for the person with thyroid disorders may include, but are not limited to those listed on p. 955. Specifically, the patient with *hyperthyroidism* should be able to perform the following:
1. Employ coping measures to decrease anxiety and interpersonal friction.
2. Describe ways to increase caloric and protein intake.
3. State plans for follow-up care:
   a. State symptoms requiring immediate follow-up (signs of remission, thyroid crisis, hypothyroidism).
   b. State plans for regular medical appointments.
4. Describe eye care if exophthalmos is present.

The person with *hypothyroidism* should be able to perform the following:
1. Gradually increase independence in self-care abilities.
2. Employ measures to prevent constipation.
3. State plans for follow-up care:
   a. State symptoms of hypothyroidism or hyperthyroidism requiring immediate follow-up.
   b. State plans for regular medical appointments.
   c. State need for daily replacement therapy.

Implementation

ASSISTING WITH ACHIEVEMENT OF THERAPEUTIC GOALS

Medications

Medications may be used to treat goiter, hyperthyroidism, or hypothyroidism.

The drugs used most commonly to treat *hypothyroidism* are listed in the box on p. 985. It is important that dosages be increased gradually because a sudden increase in metabolic rate can cause cardiac failure.

Thyroid hormone replacement

Unless hypothyroidism is mild and the patient otherwise healthy, levothyroxine therapy is started with doses of 25 to 50 µg. Doses are then increased by increments of 25 to 50 µg until a normal metabolic rate is obtained.[32] Most patients require a dosage of 0.1 to 0.2 mg daily. The daily maintenance dose of thyroid hormones varies widely. The correct dose is determined by clinical status. Diuresis with weight loss and regression of puffiness is an early response. Increased pulse rate, improvement of appetite, and relief of constipation are usually seen next.[48] Most signs of hypothyroidism are eventually reversed.

Adults with hypothyroidism respond quickly to the administration of thyroid hormones. Changes in appearance and physical symptoms occur within 2 to 3 days. Treatment must be continued throughout life. Medication dosage may need periodic adjustments to avoid symptoms of hyperthyroidism or recurrence of hypothyroidism.

Antithyroid drugs

Propylthiouracil or methimazole block thyroid hormone synthesis, thus they reduce the output of thyroid hormone

Replacement therapy for hypothyroidism

Levothyroxine sodium; L-thyroxine (synthetic T₄)
Synthroid
Levothroid

Liothyronine sodium; L-triiodothyronine (synthetic T₃)
Cytomel

Liotrix (synthetic combination of T₄ and T₃)
Euthroid
Thyrolar

Thyroid extract (natural T₃ and T₄ preparation from animal thyroid); potency varies; rarely used today

in hyperthyroidism (see Table 29-20). Usually antithyroid drugs are used before ablation of thyroid tissue by surgery or radioactive iodine.

The patient usually is started on a relatively large dose of an antithyroid drug, and then the dosage is gradually reduced to a level sufficient to maintain the euthyroid state. When antithyroid drugs are used as the primary therapy, they commonly are continued for 6 to 18 months or longer. Some patients stay in remission without further therapy. Others require longer drug therapy, additional therapy, or lifelong therapy.

The patient should see the physician at regular intervals after drugs are discontinued so that early signs of recurrence are noticed. It is important to give the drugs at regularly spaced intervals, since their blood levels are reduced in about 8 hours. Continued use of antithyroid drugs may not be tolerated by some persons. Toxic side effects include agranulocytosis and cholestasis. Skin rashes, joint pains, and diarrhea may also occur.

□ Iodides

Lugol's solution or another iodide solution can rapidly reduce the patient's metabolic rate. It is given for short periods only. Its major use is to decrease thyroid vascularity before surgery. Iodide administration saturates the thyroid gland with iodine and interferes with ablation of the thyroid by ¹³¹I; however, the administration of iodides is contraindicated before ¹³¹I therapy. See Table 29-20 for important interventions for iodide administration.

Iodide may be used in concert with antithyroid therapy preoperatively; it is given after propylthiouracil has reduced the hyperthyroidism.

□ Radioactive iodine

Ablation of the thyroid gland may be achieved by radiation. The most commonly used isotope is ¹³¹I. It is the treatment of choice for older persons. A radioactive isotope of iodine, ¹³¹I is given by mouth, is absorbed rapidly in the stomach, and becomes concentrated in the thyroid. Usually, a single dose is given in a radioactive "cocktail." It takes about 3 weeks for the symptoms of hyperthyroidism to subside, and over 2 months for thyroid function to become normal. Occasionally, remission is not achieved with one dose, and the treatment is repeated after an interval of several months. Hypothyroidism may develop after ¹³¹I therapy, and the onset can occur years after treatment.

Radioactive iodine is not used in pregnant women because iodine readily crosses the placenta and may affect the fetus. Some physicians do not prescribe ¹³¹I for persons in the childbearing years because of the potential for destruction of the gonads.

Patients who receive radioactive iodine for hyperthyroidism need to have the treatment explained to them with special care, and they usually need repeated reassurance that the radioactive properties are quickly dissipated. Because they may be more emotional than other persons, they sometimes think they are experiencing reactions to the

Table 29-20 Antithyroid drugs

Drug	Actions	Interventions
Iodide solutions Compound iodide solution (Lugol's solution) Saturated solution of potassium iodide (SSKI)	Rapid action, block synthesis and release of thyroid hormone; less sustained action; reduce vascularity of the thyroid gland, thus often used in preparation for surgery; saturate thyroid with iodide, thus radioactive iodine studies or treatment of thyroid cannot be done	Explain to patient that compliance with dosage schedule is necessary; give through a straw to avoid staining of teeth; give in milk or fruit juice; teach patient to report toxic symptoms: brassy taste, sore teeth and gums
Propylthiouracil (Propacil) Methimazole (Tapazole)	Block synthesis of thyroid hormone, not the release of stored hormone	Explain to patient that 2-4 weeks are necessary before improvement is noticed; teach patient to report toxic symptoms: fever, sore throat, skin eruptions; leukopenia or pancytopenia may occur

drug long after this is possible. Permanent hypothyroidism is a potential complication of ^{131}I therapy.

□ Surgery

Surgery of the thyroid is the procedure of choice for removal of goiters causing pressure, cancer of the thyroid, and hyperthyroidism in persons under age 40.

Part or all of the thyroid gland may be removed surgically. Total thyroidectomy (complete removal of the thyroid) may be performed for cancer of the thyroid, and the patient must then take thyroid hormones regularly for the re- mainder of his or her life. Hyperthyroidism may be treated surgically by removing approximately five sixths of the gland (subtotal thyroidectomy). In most cases this opera- tion permanently alleviates symptoms, while the remaining thyroid tissue provides enough hormones for normal func- tion. Hypothyroidism, if present, is treated with replace- ment doses of thyroid hormone. The remaining tissue can hypertrophy, however, and hyperthyroidism can recur.

Before thyroid surgery is undertaken, a normal (euthy- roid) state is produced by drug therapy. An ECG is made before surgery to detect evidence of heart damage.

POSTOPERATIVE COMPLICATIONS. The complications following thyroid surgery are extremely serious. Monitor- ing for these complications has the highest priority in post- operative care (see the box at left).

Hemorrhage can result in incisional bleeding or in compression of the trachea and surrounding tissue. Hem- orrhage is most common in the first 12 to 24 hours after surgery.

Although slight hoarseness is normal, the patient is ob- served for any increase in hoarseness and accompanying respiratory difficulty. To recognize early symptoms of la- ryngeal nerve injury, patients are asked to speak as soon as they have reacted from anesthesia and at intervals of 30 to 60 minutes.

Respiratory obstruction can occur for many reasons.

Possible complications following thyroid surgery

Complication

Hemorrhage
Edema about vocal cords and larynx
Laryngeal nerve injury
Tetany

Nursing care of the patient who has undergone thyroid surgery

1. Monitor for postoperative complications.
   a. Laryngeal damage: hoarseness, weak voice, stridor
   b. Hemorrhage or tissue swelling
      (1) Bleeding: check dressing and back of neck by slipping hand gently behind neck and shoulders
      (2) Choking sensation
      (3) Difficulty in swallowing or coughing
      (4) Sensation of dressing being too tight even after it is loosened
   c. Hypocalcemia (tetany)
      (1) Parathesias
      (2) Trousseau's and Chŏstek's signs
      (3) Carpopedal spasm
      (4) Seizure activity
   d. Respiratory distress
2. Maintain equipment at bedside for treatment of laryngeal obstruction (tracheostomy set) and tetany (calcium gluconate).
3. For acute respiratory distress:
   a. Call for immediate medical assistance.
   b. If a physician is not readily available, remove clips or sutures as previously instructed.
4. Encourage high-carbohydrate fluids by mouth and a soft diet as tolerated.
5. Provide comfort.
   a. Use prescribed analgesics.
   b. Local agents (analgesic throat lozenges or gels) ease swallowing; give 30 minutes before meals.
   c. Avoid placing tension on suture line.
   d. After 5 to 7 days, gradual range of motion may be promoted.
6. Teach patient about required drugs (dosage, side effects) and importance of medical follow-up.

These include laryngeal nerve injury, compression of the trachea by hemorrhage, vocal cord edema or spasm, and tetany. Emergency measures for these complications are outlined in the box on postoperative care on p. 986. Injury to the parathyroids is uncommon but may occur. Surgery or inflammaiton may block the normal release of parathyroid hormone and symptoms of tetany caused by calcium deficiency, may appear from 1 to 7 days after surgery. Serum calcium levels are usually monitored, and hypocalcemia is treated by replacement of calcium intravenously. Daily oral doses of calcium are then given until normal function returns.

Postoperative nursing interventions are summarized in the box on p. 986.

ASSISTING WITH COMFORT AND ADL

☐ Hyperthyroidism

Since the advent of antithyroid drugs and ^{131}I therapy, most people with hyperthyroidism can be cared for at home. Although these persons usually are not particularly hyperactive, they are likely to be nervous and irritable. It is important that family and friends understand that extreme sensitivity and irritability are part of the disease; otherwise, they may become upset with the individual and aggravate the situation. It may be necessary to assist these persons with activities requiring fine motor coordination and concentration, although they may appear physically able to perform the activities themselves. They will need an explanation about why they require such assistance.

The following interventions by nurses or caregivers at home are indicated for the person with hyperthyroidism:

1. Maintain a cool, quiet environment.
2. Assist person to obtain sufficient rest.
3. Encourage quiet activities that require gross motor movements (for example, weaving and reading), which the person can do without assistance.
4. Assist person with tasks requiring fine motor coordination (for example sewing and washing dishes).
5. Provide a high-calorie, high-protein diet; snacks between meals may be necessary to maintain weight and meet energy requirements.
6. Discourage the use of caffeinated drinks.
7. If exophthalmos is present:
   a. Encourage use of dark glasses, which afford some protection from wind, sun and dust.
   b. Administer soothing eye drops, such as methylcellulose, 0.5% to 1%, which may prevent drying of the eye and provide comfort.

☐ Hypothyroidism

The patient's slowed mental and physical functioning requires understanding and patience on the part of caregivers. A thorough explanation of the cause of the changes in the patient's physical and mental responses should also be given to family or friends. As thyroid hormone levels return to normal, the patient's physical and mental state will return to normal.

During the time the patient is experiencing hypothyroidism, nursing care includes the following:

1. Minimize environmental stressors, because the patient is less able to respond to them.
2. Administer replacement therapy and monitor patient for effectiveness of therapy and side effects.
3. Provide complete care at first and gradually increase patient's self-care.
4. Prevent constipation and fecal impaction by administrating fluids, fiber, and stool softeners and by encouraging activity.

Evaluation

Evaluation is based on expected patient outcomes. Questions useful in evaluating nursing care of patients with thyroid dysfunction may include the following:

1. Is patient prepared to manage self-care regimen at home?
2. Were complications prevented or promptly identified and treated?
3. Is patient able to achieve desired
   a. Weight?
   b. Energy level and activity?
   c. Sleep and rest?

SUMMARY

1. Normal physiology depends on the proper amounts of hormones being available to act on cell receptors of target tissues.
2. Many factors influence secretory patterns and rates of secretion of hormones. Atrophy and hypoplasia of a gland results in hyposecretion, whereas hypertrophy and hyperplasia results in hypersecretion.
3. The hypothalamic-pituitary-target gland axis is a major regulator of hormonal secretion of the adrenal, thyroid, and gonad glands.
4. Parathyroid hormone, vitamin D, and calcitonin are three regulators of calcium and phosphorus balance. The serum level of calcium is the major regulator or parathyroid hormone secretion.
5. *Giantism* in children and *acromegaly* in adults are conditions resulting from growth hormone excess. Tumors or pituitary hyperplasia may be treated with surgery, irradiation, or growth hormone suppressants.
6. The most common pituitary tumor is a prolactinoma that may present with symptoms of galactorrhea or reproductive dysfunction.
7. Pituitary tumors may cause compression of normal tissue, resulting in hyposecretion of anterior pituitary hormones. They may also compress optic nerve tracts and cause visual field defects.
8. Life-long replacement of cortisol is necessary to maintain life after a bilateral adrenalectomy or pituitary ablation or when disease or injury has destroyed the

pituitary or adrenal cortex (for instance, in Addison's disease).

9. Administration of therapeutic doses of glucocorticoid medications produce iatrogenic Cushing's syndrome and place the patient at risk for adrenocortical insufficiency or crisis.

10. Diabetes insipidus results from ADH deficit and is characterized by polyuria and low specific gravity of urine. Overdosage of ADH replacement by nasal sprays or drops (Pitressin) can induce weight gain and reduce urinary volume.

11. Cardiac problems may develop from several hormonal alterations: growth hormone, cortisol, thyroid hormone, and catecholamines. Cardiac arrhythmias may occur in hypoparathyroidism and hyperthyroidism.

12. Fluid and electrolyte imbalances are predominate features of disorders of the posterior pituitary and adrenal cortex.

13. Hypertension may result from adrenal medullary or adrenal cortical hypersecretion.

14. Nutritional problems are common with hormonal disorders. Excesses of growth hormone and cortisol can induce states of catabolism, ketogenesis, and hyperglycemia. Hyperthroidism increases the amounts of nutrients required.

15. Disorders of growth may be a reflection of hormonal alterations; for instance, in *pituitary dwarfism* and *congenital cretinism* (hypothyroidism). Skin, hair, and nails may be changed in appearance in several of the hormonal disturbances.

16. Skeletal abnormalities and loss of bone integrity is a hallmark of parathyroid dysfunction. *Osteoporosis* from excessive bone resorption of calcium may limit the amount of corticosteroid medications given in chronic inflammatory diseases. *Acromegaly* (growth hormone excess) induces bony growth, which alters the patient's appearance and may cause joint problems and compression syndrome.

17. Hypotension is of particular concern in deficits of ADH and mineral corticosteroids (Addison's disease). Vasopressors may be required immediately after adrenal surgery or to treat Addison's crisis. Large doses of cortisol (over 50 mg/24 hr) have mineralocorticoid effects.

18. Both vitamin D and calcium supplements are necessary to maintain serum calcium levels in *hypoparathyroidism* and to prevent *tetany*.

19. Neuromuscular irritability gives rise to the symptoms of latent tetany and to cardiac arrhythmias, laryngeal obstruction, and convulsions. *Trousseau's* sign, *Chovstek's* sign, *carpopedal spasm*, and *paresthesia* should be reported promptly.

20. The first priority in treatment of hyperparathyroidism is reducing severe hypercalcemia (that is, levels greater than 14 mg/dl); cardiac arrhythmias and coma can result if treatment is delayed.

21. Thyroid enlargement (goiter) may be detected by inspection and palpation and described as diffuse or nodular, and the qualities of symmetry and presence of pain or tenderness noted. *Simple goiter* is the term used to describe enlargement without thyroid hormone alteration.

22. *Hyperthyroidism* has many causes; excesses of T_3 and T_4 induce a hypermetabolic state and excessive sympathetic nervous system stimulation.

23. *Graves' disease* is characterized by hyperthyroidism, goiter, and exophthalmos. TSI antibodies confirm the diagnosis.

24. *Hypothyroidism* often has an insidious onset. A decrease in the metabolic functions under the control of T_4 and T_3 gives rise to multiple symptoms. Fluid re-

---

Putting knowledge to practice

■ Where is each of the endocrine glands located? Review the hormones secreted by each gland.
■ Review the functions of the anterior and posterior pituitary, thyroid, and parathyroid glands. For each function, consider the effect on the body of an excess or lack of that gland's secretion.
■ Review the physiology of stress (Chapter 7). What is the role of the adrenal gland in the stress response?
■ In what way does giving a large amount of a hormone (such as cortisone) to a patient who already is producing a normal amount affect production of the hormone? Why does this reaction take place?
■ How would you explain to a patient who has a high basal metabolic rate (such as occurs with hyperthyroidism) that increased amounts of food are needed?
■ Review in your nutrition text foods high and low in calcium and phosphorus. What vitamin is essential for the body to use calcium effectively?
■ Compare the effects on nutrition of hypersecretion and hyposecretion of the adrenal and thyroid glands.
■ What are latent signs of tetany? What complications require immediate interventions?
■ How many potassium imbalances are caused by disorders of the adrenal cortex and pituitary?
■ Describe cardiovascular effects of thyroid dysfunction.

tention results in weight gain, changes in appearance of skin, and effusions.

25. Hypothyroidism in the elderly may not be detected until severe changes in cardiac or mental status occur.

26. Thyroid hormone replacement reverses most signs of hypothyroidism in the adult; synthroid, in doses of 0.1 to 0.2 mg, is a common drug used for maintenance therapy. Smaller doses of 0.25 to 50 mg may be used to initiate therapy.

27. Treatment of Graves' disease, the most common disease associated with hyperthyroidism, may include medications (iodide or thiamides), ^{131}I, or surgery.

28. Complications or thyroid surgery include hemorrhage, tetany, laryngeal nerve injury, and respiratory obstruction.

REFERENCES AND SELECTED READINGS

1. *Arcangelo, VP: Disorders of the thyroid and parathyroid. In Coogan, JM, editor: Diseases: nurses reference library, Springhouse, Pa, 1983, Intermed Communications.
2. Andreoli, TE, and others: Essentials of medicine, Philadelphia, 1986, WB Saunders Co.
3. Bagdale, JD: Endocrine emergencies, Med Clin North Am 70(5):1111-1128, 1986.
4. Bondy, P, and Rosenberg, L: Metabolic control and disease, Philadelphia, 1980, WB Saunders Co.
5. Camunas, C: Pheochromocytoma, Am J Nurs 83:887-891, 1983.
6. Carlson, HE, editor: Endocrinology, New York, 1983, Wiley Medical Publications.
7. Cooper, DS, and Ridgway, EC: Clinical management of patients with hyperthyroidism, Med Clin North Am 69:953-971, 1985.
8. *Evangelisti, JT, and others: Thyroid storm: a nursing crisis, Heart Lung 12:184-194, 1983.
9. Fairchild, RS: Diabetes insipidus: a review, Crit Care Q 2:111-118, 1980.
10. Geola, F, and Chopra, I: Hyperthyroidism and hypothyroidism, Med Times 108:64-69 and 73-74, 1980.
11. *Gotch, PM: Teaching patients about adrenal corticosteroids, Am J Nurs 81:78-85, 1981.
12. Greenspan, FS, and Forsham, PH: Basic and clinical endocrinology, Los Altos, Calif, 1983, Lange Medical Publications.
13. Hahn, AB, Barking, RL, and Oestreich, SJK: Pharmacology in nursing, ed 15, St. Louis, 1982, The CV Mosby Co.
14. Hamburger, S, and Rush, D: Syndrome of inappropriate secretion of antidiuretic hormone, Crit Care Q 2:119-129, 1980.
15. Harris, RB, and Heany, G: Comprehensive nursing care of the patient with pheochromocytoma, Heart Lung 13(1):82-87, 1984.
16. Hellman, R: The evaluation and management of hyperthyroid crisis, Crit Care Q 2:77-92, 1980.
17. Hoffman, JT: Syndromes of ectopic hormone production in cancer, Nurs Clin North Am 15:499-509, 1980.
18. *Hoffman, JT, and Newby, TB: Hypercalcemia in primary hyperparathyroidism, Nurs Clin North Am 15:469-480, 1980.
19. *Honigman, RE: Deciphering diagnostic studies: thyroid function tests, Nurs 82 12(4):68-71, 1982.
20. Hurley, JR: Thyroid disease in the elderly, Med Clin North Am 67(2):497-516, 1983.
21. *Jones, SG: Adrenal patient: proceed with caution, RN 45(2):69-72, 1982.
22. *Jones, SG: Bilateral adrenalectomy: postop dangers to watch for, RN 34(2):66-69, 1982.
23. Jubiz, W: Endocrinology: a logical approach for clinicians, New York, 1985, McGraw-Hill Book Co.
24. Koppers, LE: Pheochromocytoma—critical care, Crit Care Q 2:93-97, 1980.
25. *Larson, CA: The critical path of adrenocortical insufficiency, Nurs 84 14(10):66-69, 1984.
26. Leeper, RD: Thyroid cancer, Med Clin North Am 69:1079-1095, 1985.
27. Lukert, BP: Hypercalcemia, Crit Care Q 2:11-18, 1980.
28. Malasanos, L, and others: Health assessment, ed 3, St. Louis, 1986, The CV Mosby Co.
29. Mannix, H, and others: Hyperparathyroidism in the elderly, Am J Surg 139:581-585, 1980.
30. *Mazzuca, SA: Does patient education in chronic disease have therapeutic value? J Chronic Dis 35:521-529, 1982.
31. *McFadden, EA, Zaloga, GP, and Chernow, B: Hypocalcemia: a medical emergency, Am J Nurs 83:227-230, 1983.
32. Metz, R, and Larson, EB: Blue book of endocrinology, Philadelphia, 1985, WB Saunders Co.
33. Nasr, H: Endocrine disorders in the elderly, Med Clin North Am 67(2):481-485, 1983.
34. *Nemeroff, DR: Transphenoidal hypophysectomy, J Neurosurg Nurs 13:303-312, 1981.
35. Nicoloff, JT: Thyroid storm and mxydema coma, Med Clin North Am 69(5):1005-1017, 1985.
36. *Coogan, JM, editor: Nurse's clinical library: endocrine disorders, Nursing 84 Books, Springhouse, Pa, 1984, Springhouse Corp.
37. *Sawin, CT: Hypothyroidism, Med Clin North Am 69:989-1003, 1985.
38. Sanford, SJ: Dysfunction of the adrenal gland: physiologic considerations and nursing problems, Nurs Clin North Am 15:481-498, 1980.
39. Schimke, RN: Adrenal insufficiency, Crit Care Q 2:10-27, 1980.
40. Schwartz, S: Principles of surgery, ed 4, New York, 1984, McGraw-Hill Book Co.
41. *Smith, J: Nursing management of diabetes insipidus, J Neurosurg Nurs 13:313-317, 1981.
42. *Solomon, BL: The hypothalamus and the pituitary gland: an overview, Nurs Clin North Am 15:435-451, 1980.
43. Sowers, DK, and Sowers, JR: Pituitary emergencies, Crit Care Q 2:45-54, 1980.
44. Stephens, GJ: Pathophysiology for health practitioners, New York, 1980, Macmillan Publishing Company.

References preceded by an asterisk are particularly well suited for student reading.

45. Stillman, MJ: Transphenoidal hypophysectomy for pituitary tumors, J Neurosurg Nurs 13:112-122, 1981.
46. Tilbian, SM, Conover, MB, and Tilkian, AG: Clinical implications of laboratory tests, ed 4, St. Louis, 1987, The CV Mosby Company.
47. Wake, MM, and Brensinger, JF: The nurse's role in hypothyroidism, Nurs Clin North Am 15:453-467, 1980.
48. Wilson, JD, and Foster, DW: Williams' testbook of endocrinology, ed 73, Philadelphia, 1985, WB Saunders Co.
49. Wyngaarden, JB, and Smith, LH: Textbook of medicine, ed 16, Philadelphia, 1985, WB Saunders Co.

Classic

50. Cataland, S: Hypoglycemia: a spectrum of problems, Heart Lung 7:459-462, 1978.
51. *Clancey, J, and Abruzzi, L: Pituitary tumors, growth disease: nursing intervention of patients with pituitary tumor, J Neurosurg Nurs 10:24-28, 1978.
52. *Hallal, J: Thyroid disorders, Am J Nurs 77:418-432, 1977.
53. *Kubo, WM, and Grant, M: The syndrome of inappropriate antidiuretic hormone, Heart Lung 7:469-472, 1978.

30

The Patient with Hepatic, Biliary, and Pancreatic Problems

DOROTHY R. BLEVINS and VIRGINIA L. CASSMEYER

CHAPTER OBJECTIVES

After studying this chapter, the student should be able to:

- Describe preventive measures for hepatitis.

- Differentiate between focal and diffuse hepatocellular disorders, and explain the pathophysiologic basis for common manifestations of diffuse liver disorders.

- Differentiate between toxic and viral hepatitis, acute and chronic hepatitis, and among hepatitis A, B, D, and non-A, non-B.

- Explain the pathophysiologic bases for the symptoms of cirrhosis.

- Describe care of the patient with a diffuse liver disorder including control of gastrointestinal bleeding.

- Describe the nature of cholecystitis, cholelithiasis, and cancer of the biliary system, types of surgery, and care of the patient experiencing biliary surgery.

- Explain the pathophysiologic bases for signs and symptoms of pancreatitis and pancreatic tumors, and explain care of the patient during an acute phase and following surgery.

- Develop patient outcomes and nursing plans for patients exhibiting common signs and symptoms of hepatic dysfunction.

The liver, biliary system, and pancreas are affected by a variety of pathologic processes that may severely affect digestion and normal metabolic processes. Many of the disorders are chronic and require that the patient make changes in life-style to keep the problem under control. These patients need nursing support in adapting to their chronic health problem and in learning the necessary self-management skills.

■ ANATOMY AND PHYSIOLOGY

■ Hepatic system

The hepatic system is a major system involved in regulation of body functions. The liver is one of the largest organs of the body and consists of two lobes located in the right upper quadrant of the abdomen under the diaphragm.

It extends up under the ribs. The gallbladder lies under the inferior surface of the liver (Fig. 30-1).

The liver is made up of small liver lobules (Fig. 30-2) composed of hepatic cellular plates. Each hepatic cellular plate is usually two cells thick, and between these cells run biliary canaliculi. Hepatic sinusoids, capillaries of the liver, which receive blood from both the portal vein and the hepatic artery, lie on the opposite sides of the hepatic cells. After flowing through the hepatic sinusoids, blood is emptied into the central vein and from there flows into the hepatic vein. The hepatic sinusoids are lined with Kupffer's cells, which are reticuloendothelial cells that phagocytize bacteria and other foreign products.

The liver is ideally structured to receive large supplies of blood to carry out its multiple functions, which are summarized in the box on p. 993. Although only 25% of its blood supply is oxygenated, oxygen extraction by the liver is so efficient that there is little variation in oxygen

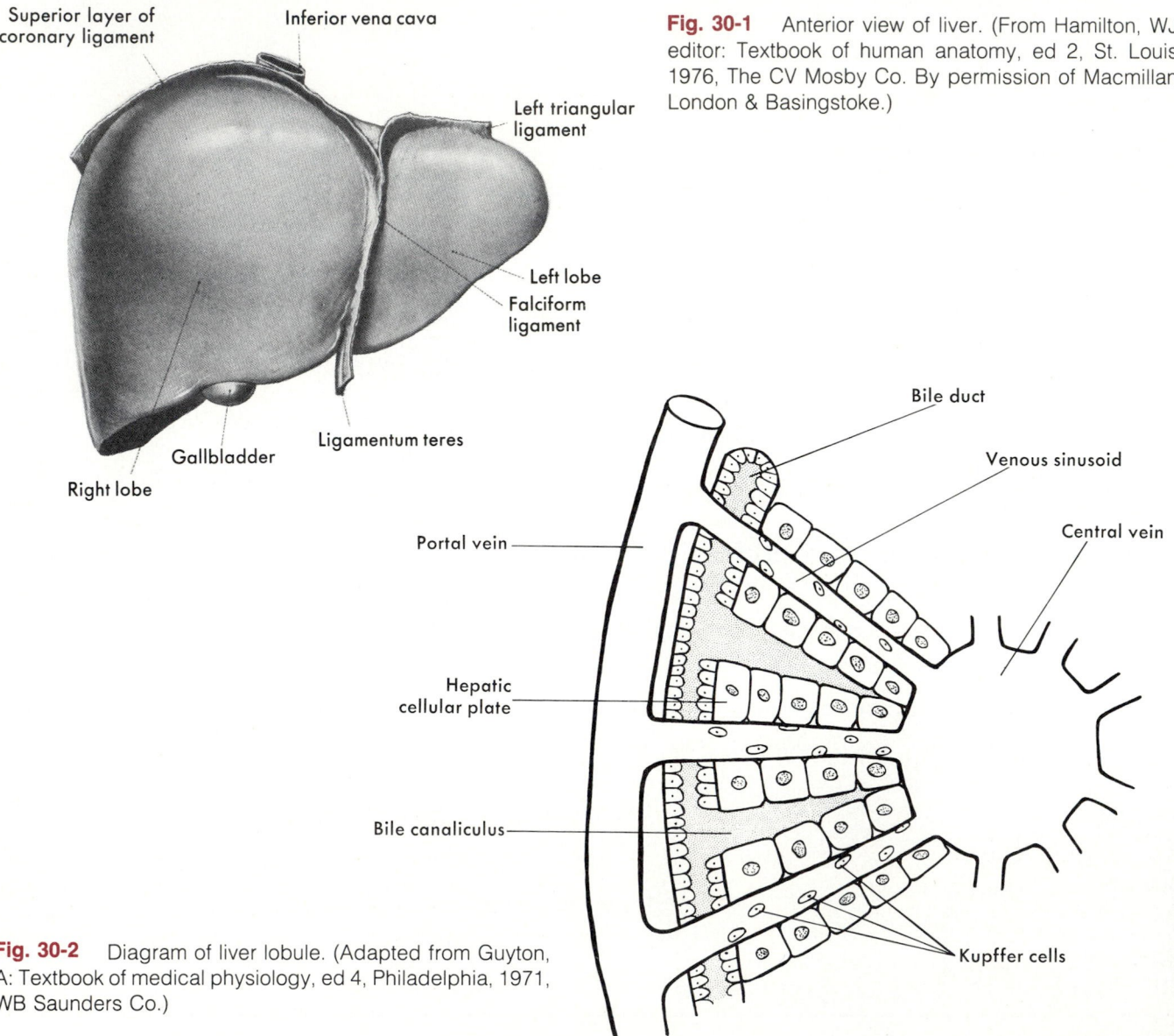

Fig. 30-1 Anterior view of liver. (From Hamilton, WJ, editor: Textbook of human anatomy, ed 2, St. Louis, 1976, The CV Mosby Co. By permission of Macmillan, London & Basingstoke.)

Fig. 30-2 Diagram of liver lobule. (Adapted from Guyton, A: Textbook of medical physiology, ed 4, Philadelphia, 1971, WB Saunders Co.)

Summary of liver functions

1. Carbohydrate, protein, and fat metabolism
   a. Carbohydrate metabolism
      (1) Glycogen formation and storage
      (2) Glucose formation from glycogen (glycogenolysis) and from amino acids, lactic acids, and glycerol (gluconeogenesis)
   b. Protein metabolism
      (1) Protein catabolism
      (2) Protein synthesis
         (a) Albumin
         (b) Globulin
         (c) Clotting factors
         (d) C-reactive protein
         (e) Transferrin
         (f) Enzymes
         (g) Ceruloplasmin, etc.
      (3) Formation of needed amino acids

   c. Fat metabolism
      (1) Oxidation of fatty acids for energy
      (2) Ketone formation
      (3) Synthesis of cholesterol and phospholipids
      (4) Formation of triglycerides from dietary and excessive dietary carbohydrates and proteins
      (5) Formation of lipoproteins
2. Production of bile salts
3. Bilirubin metabolism
4. Detoxification of endogenous and exogenous substances
   a. Ammonium
   b. Steroids
   c. Drugs
5. Storage of minerals and vitamins

---

consumption regardless of the rate of oxygen flow. Receiving 25% of the cardiac output, the liver contains about 15% of the total blood volume. Because it can quickly expel about half of this blood in situations of hemorrhage, the liver is a blood reservoir.

It is helpful to think about the liver as a metabolic factory and a waste disposal facility. For example, the portal vein brings to the liver raw materials absorbed from the small intestine; the liver manufactures finished products, and the hepatic venules and biliary canaliculi distribute these and wastes through blood and bile flow.

CARBOHYDRATE, PROTEIN, AND FAT METABOLISM

The liver plays a major role in the metabolism of the three major food nutrients. Through various enzymatic activities, the liver can oxidize carbohydrates, proteins, and fats for energy or use these nutrients to produce compounds that can be stored for future use or to manufacture needed compounds.

The liver helps to maintain a normal blood glucose level. Immediately after meals, the liver cells extract glucose and other sugars from the sinusoidal blood and utilize them to form glycogen (glycogenesis). Between meals, or in longer fasting states, the liver provides glucose to the blood by breaking down glycogen (glycogenolysis) and forming new glucose from amino acids, glycerol, and lactic acids (gluconeogenesis). The liver provides needed amino acids through the process of deamination. In addition, it is the only source of albumin, which is necessary for the maintenance of osmotic pressure, and of prothrombin (factor II). Normal production of prothrombin is dependent on the following four factors:

1. Ingestion of foods that can undergo synthesis in the intestines
2. Presence of bile in the intestines for production of vitamin K
3. Absorption through the intestinal wall of the vitamin K
4. Use of the vitamin K by the liver in the formation of prothrombin

Other clotting factors are produced by the liver; these include: factor I (fibrinogen), factor V (proacclerin), factor VII (serum prothrombin conversion accelerator), and factor X (Stuart factor). Vitamin K is necessary for factors II, VII, IX, and X.

The waste product of protein deamination, ammonia, is converted to urea by the healthy liver through the Krebs-Henseleit cycle. Urea is then excreted by the kidney.

The liver is involved in multiple aspects of fat metabolism. Fatty acids are released from adipose tissue or derived from food. Triglycerides in the diet are absorbed in chylomicrons and metabolized to fatty acids. Fatty acids may be (1) oxidized, (2) converted to phospholipids, (3) used to form cholesterol esters or (4) reesterified to triglycerides and combined with protein, cholesterol, and phospholipids to form lipoproteins.

BILIRUBIN METABOLISM

Bilirubin is a by-product of the heme portion of red blood cells and is released when red blood cells are destroyed. The bilirubin at this point is not water soluble (unconjugated) and is carried in the blood attached to protein. The liver is responsible for picking up this unconjugated bilirubin, for conjugating it into a water soluble form, and for secreting conjugated bilirubin into the bile. The bilirubin in bile is emptied into the duodenum and is broken down by bacteria into urobilinogen. Some of the urobilinogen is excreted with the feces, giving the stool its brown color. Some urobilinogen is eliminated in the urine, and the remainder returns to the liver and is converted to bilirubin.

■ DETOXIFICATION

The liver has a prime role in detoxification of both exogenous and endogenous substances. It also has a major role in the detoxification of many drugs. All barbiturates (except phenobarbital and barbital) and many other sedatives are inactivated by the liver. The status of the liver plays an important role in the effectiveness or toxicity of these and other drugs. The liver also serves a function in detoxifying corticosterone, aldosterone, estrogen, and testosterone.

■ Biliary system

The biliary system consists of the gallbladder and its associated ductal system (Fig. 30-3). The ductal system provides a pathway for the bile that is formed in the liver to reach the intestine and also functions to regulate bile flow. The liver produces up to 1 L of bile per day. As it is formed, bile is excreted into the hepatic ducts, where it passes into the cystic duct to be stored in the gallbladder.

The capacity of the gallbladder is usually 50 ml but can increase in size under normal conditions. In the gallbladder, bile is concentrated to a solution that is 5 to 10 times as concentrated as that produced in the liver.

Bile contains cholesterol, phospholipids, bile salts, bilirubin, and a very small amount of proteins and electrolytes; 97% of bile is water. Some toxins, drug metabolites, and hormones are excreted in bile. Because bile can be released directly into the duodenum through the common

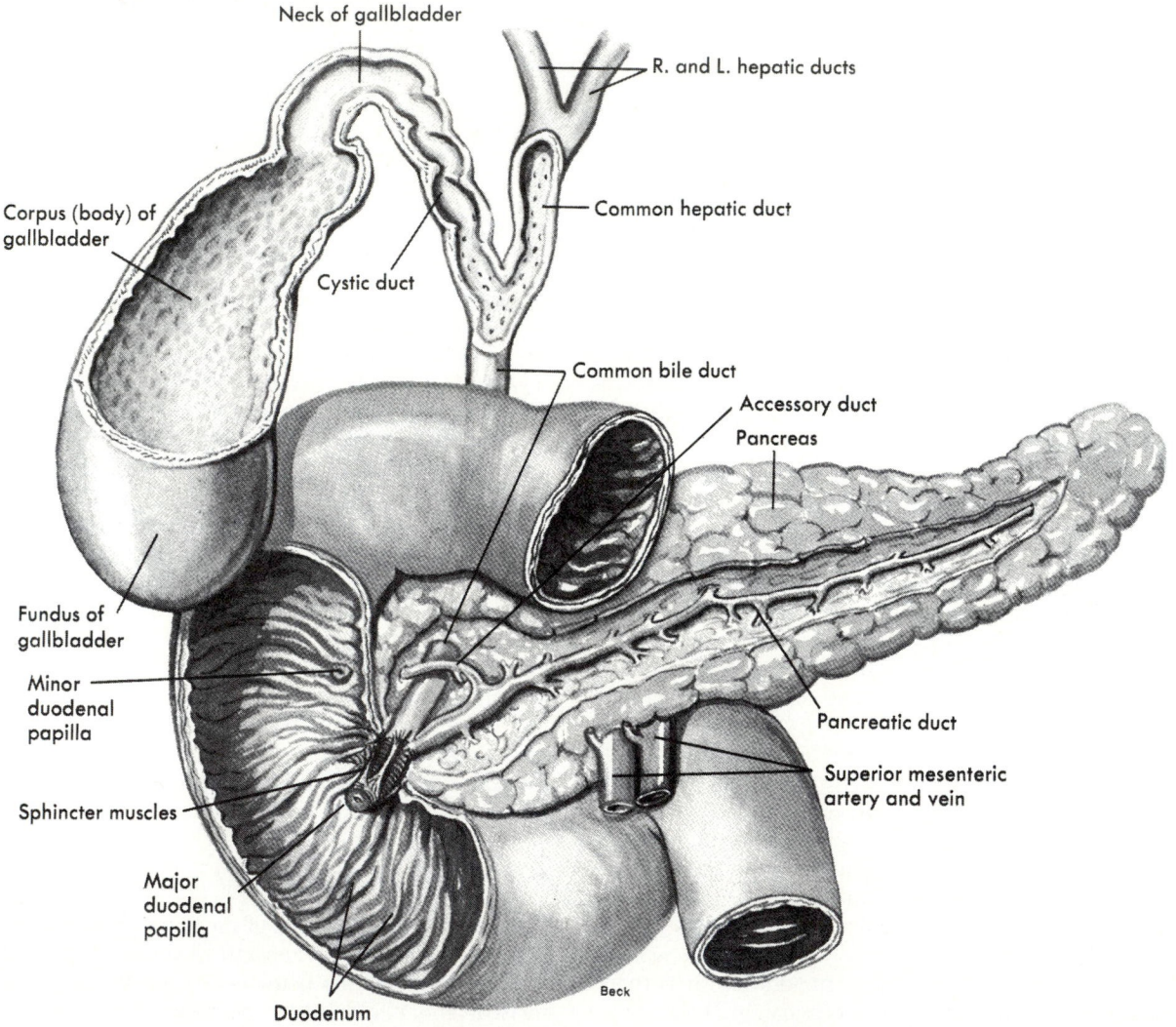

Fig. 30-3 Anatomic schemata of biliary and pancreatic ductal systems. Note head of pancreas surrounds common bile duct. (From Anthony, CP, and Thibodeau, GA: Textbook of anatomy and physiology, ed 12, St. Louis, 1987, The CV Mosby Co.)

bile duct, the removal of the gallbladder has no long-term consequences.

Neural and hormonal mechanisms control the secretion of bile from the gallbladder. Food, particularly lipids in the duodenum, causes the release of cholecystokinin-pancreozymin (CCK) from the mucosa of the duodenum. CCK is released into the blood and travels to the gallbladder. One of its activities is to stimulate the gallbladder musculature to contract. At the same time it causes the muscle of the sphincter of Oddi (at the end of the common bile duct) to relax and permit entry of bile into the duodenum. Gastrin, another gastrointestinal hormone, and vagal stimulation can also cause the gallbladder to contract.

Bile acids are predominantly composed of a cholesterol derivative, and they function in the intestinal metabolism of fats and other substances as follows:

1. Facilitate fat digestion by emulsifying fats for action by intestinal lipases
2. Facilitate absorption of fats, fat-soluble vitamins, iron, and calcium
3. Activate the release of pancreatic and intestinal enzymes

■ Pancreatic system

The pancreatic system includes the exocrine glands of the pancreas (acinar cells) and a ductal system (Fig. 30-3). (The endocrine functions of the pancreas are described in Chapter 29.) Acinar cells release their secretions into ducts that converge to form the main pancreatic duct (duct of Wirsung). Lining the ducts are cells (ductal cells) that secrete a bicarbonate-rich fluid. In most persons, the pancreatic duct merges into the common bile duct at its entry into the duodenum, but in some persons the common bile duct and pancreatic duct do not merge.

The acinar cells of the pancreas secrete multiple digestive enzymes.

1. Proteolytic enzymes: trypsinogen, chymotrypsinogen, and procarboxypeptidase
2. Amylotic enzyme: amylase
3. Lipolytic enzymes: lipases
4. Nucleolytic enzymes: ribonuclease and deoxribonuclease

The pancreatic exocrine secretions are released under the influence of the vagus nerve and secretin, cholecystokinin-pancreozymin (CCK), and gastrin during digestion. Gastrin is released during the gastric phase and stimulates the release of bicarbonate-rich solution. The entry of chyme and acids into the small intestines stimulates the release of secretin and cholecystokinin-pancreozymin. Secretin then stimulates further secretion of the pancreatic bicarbonate-rich solution, and cholecystokinin-pancreozymin stimulates the release of the pancreatic enzyme-rich solution.

■ Physiologic changes with aging

Many of the liver functions do not seem to be affected by aging, even though the weight of the liver lessens and there are identifiable microscopic changes in liver cells.

Most laboratory tests of liver function have the same values in the elderly as in the young with a few exceptions. The exceptions are (1) a decrease in serum albumin levels, (2) an increase in serum globulins, (3) an increase in serum alkaline phosphatase, and (4) an increase in serum cholesterol.[35] Although other factors can be involved, two changes of liver function may prolong or increase the effect of drugs in the elderly: (1) there is less drug binding if hypoalbuminemia exists, and (2) there is diminished biotransformation if the liver enzyme reactions are reduced.[7]

There is an increase of *cholelithiasis* and *cholecystitis* in the aged, however, the reasons for this increase is unknown. The pancreas shows microscopic changes in aged persons and the activity of lipase is said to be decreased, but that of trypsin and amylase remains unchanged. A sufficient volume and concentration of enzymes is secreted from normal digestive functions.[9]

■ PREVENTION AND HEALTH EDUCATION

■ Primary prevention

■ HEPATITIS

An acute inflammation of the liver is termed *hepatitis*; it can be induced by a toxin or a virus.

☐ Toxic hepatitis

Toxic hepatitis can be prevented if the public is informed about precautions in the use of toxic substances. Because cleaning agents, solvents, and related substances sometimes contain substances that are harmful to the liver, the public should read instructions on labels and should follow them explicitly. Dry-cleaning fluids may contain carbon tetrachloride, which can cause liver injury if warnings to avoid inhalation of the fumes and to keep windows open are not heeded. If people must use these agents inside the home, a good practice is to open the windows wide, use the cleaning materials as quickly as possible, and then vacate the premises for several hours, leaving the windows open.

Many solvents used to remove paint and plastic material and to stain and finish woodwork contain injurious substances and should be used outdoors—not in the basement—since dangerous fumes may spread throughout the house. Cleaning agents and finishes for cars should be applied outdoors or in a garage with the door open. Nurses in industry have a responsibility to teach the importance of observing regulations to avoid industrial hazards, such as exposure to nitrobenzene, tetrachloroethane, carbon disulfide, and dinitrotoluol.

Some drugs that are known to cause mild damage to the liver must be used therapeutically. A safe rule to follow is to avoid taking any medication except that specifically prescribed by a physician for a specific ailment.

☐ Viral hepatitis

Viral hepatitis is by far the most important infection attacking the liver. It is a reportable disease in all states.

Statistics from the Centers for Disease Control (CDC) indicate that viral hepatitis is one of the most frequently reported infectious diseases in the United States. It is well accepted that the figures for any given year may be grossly underestimated, because persons with subclinical manifestations are often not reported as having active disease.

Prevention of viral hepatitis is related to knowledge about, (1) the viral agent, (2) routes and modes for transmission, and (3) measures that are effective in controlling transmission. The hepatitis viruses are extremely resistant to such antimicrobial measures as drying, chlorination, disinfectants, heat, ultraviolet light, radiation, and freezing. The viruses are especially refractive to such measures when protected by the presence of serum proteins. At boiling temperatures the viruses can survive for about 20 to 30 minutes. Autoclaving is the best method to ensure destruction of the viruses on contaminated articles. When boiling is the only available way to sterilize needles and other equipment, everything placed in the water sterilizer is *covered completely and boiled for at least 30 minutes*. See Table 30-1 (p. 998) for a comparison of the four types of hepatitis with information about transmission, secretions that may contain the virus, and high-risk groups for each type.

☐ *Hepatitis A*

At a community level of intervention, the risk of hepatitis A is minimized when (1) there are noncontaminated sources of water and food, (2) there is an adequate sewage system to protect water supplies, (3) food handlers receive instruction and supervision in handwashing practices and in the safe care of food, and (4) public education is provided so that all persons decrease person-to-person spread by handwashing.

The spread of hepatitis A is greatest during the 2 weeks before the onset of icterus (jaundice), during the incubation period, and early in the symptomatic phase. Patients are often not diagnosed until the onset of icterus. They should be placed on *enteric precautions* whether at home or in the hospital for 1 week after the onset of icterus. There is no known carrier state for hepatitis A.

Children should be in private rooms, but responsible adults do not require one. The major precaution is good handwashing following elimination. Anyone who must handle feces or potentially contaminated articles (bedpans, diapers, rectal thermometers) should wear gloves and gowns and wash hands thoroughly after completing care. Separate toilet facilities are not necessary if fecal contamination is not a problem. The toilet should be cleaned at least daily.

IMMUNIZATION. Immune serum globulin can be given prophylactically before or after exposure to hepatitis A to provide passive immunity. No vaccine is available to promote active immunity for hepatitis A. Preexposure prophylaxis is recommended for travelers to developing countries who will be eating in settings of poor or uncertain sanitation or visiting extensively with local persons. The recommended dose of immune serum globulin is 0.02 ml/kg for those traveling for less than 2 months and 0.06 ml/kg every

---

Populations at risk for hepatitis B

Certain health care workers
Clients and staff of institutions providing services to mentally retarded persons, to hemodialysis patients, to recipients of frequent blood or blood component transfusions, and to long-term correctional facility inmates
Homosexually active men
Heterosexually active persons with multiple sexual partners
Users of illicit injectable drugs
Household and sexual contacts of HBV carriers
Some American populations (Alaskan Eskimos)
Immigrants and refugees from areas where hepatitis is endemic

---

5 months for those traveling for prolonged periods.

Postexposure use of immune globulin is recommended for selected persons who have had (1) contact with a person who has hepatitis A or (2) exposure to food or water contaminated with hepatitis A virus (HAV). Immune globulin must be given within 2 weeks.

☐ *Hepatitis B*

Table 30-1 lists the routes of transmission of hepatitis B as percutaneous, permucosal, sexual, and through close personal contact. Although concentration of the virus is highest in the blood and serous fluid, the hepatitis B virus (HBV) has been found in many body fluids. The box above lists the populations at risk for hepatitis B; preexposure prophylaxis is recommended for these persons.

Hepatitis B is considered the primary occupational risk for health care workers (see the box below). In 1987 the CDC estimated that there would be 20,000 to 30,000

Health care workers at risk for hepatitis B

Dentists
Medical technologists or staff
Phlebotomists
Intravenous therapy nurses
Surgeons
Pathologists
Oncology and dialysis staff
Dental hygienists
Laboratory and blood bank technicians
Emergency medical technicians
Morticians

HBV infections among health workers in the next year, that 2000 of those who become infected would become carriers, and that about 300 of them would die.[6] Although only 25,000 new cases are reported each year; it is estimated that there are 300,000 new infections in the American population each year. And, there is believed to be a pool of 1,000,000 carriers, half of whom do not know that they are carriers. There is a 6% to 20% chance of getting hepatitis from a needle-stick (in comparison, a 0.3% chance of getting AIDS from a needle-stick) because of the concentration of virus in the blood. Carelessness (or absence) of handwashing after contact with blood, body fluids, or with equipment contaminated with these fluids removes a major barrier against percutaneous or permucosal transmission to health care workers.

All equipment should be treated as if it had been used on an infected person regardless of the patient's diagnosis. There are several reasons for this precaution. Hepatitis B has an insidious onset, often a low-grade intensity of symptoms, and the infected person may not seek medical diagnosis. In addition, about 6% to 10% of persons infected with HBV become carriers and may not be identified as carriers. HBV remains present in blood and body fluids longer than HAV.

The following guidelines are recommended for use with *all* patients to prevent the nurse from contracting hepatitis from persons who are not identified as contagious or who are carriers and to prevent the nurse from transmitting the virus to others.

1. Handwashing before and after patient contact is essential.
2. Disposable needles, syringes, and other equipment in contact with blood are placed in rigid containers that are later incinerated.
3. Needles should not be recapped; instead they should be placed promptly in a puncture proof container.
4. Disposable gloves are suggested for use when handling soiled urinals, catheters, bedpans, or commodes or when the patient or bed linens are soiled by body excreta or secretions.
5. Masks and safety glasses should be worn when splashing of blood or body excretions is expected.
6. Containers for body secretions should be plastic or waterproof.
7. All patients should have their own thermometer if disposable equipment is not used.
8. Good housekeeping practices should be mandatory in bathrooms and in areas where food is prepared or served.

In addition to following these guidelines, the nurse should consult the latest information from the CDC about *blood/body fluid precautions* when a patient is identified as having hepatitis B or as being a carrier of HBV. A carrier state is recognized when the HBsAg test remains positive for 6 months. Isolation is continued throughout hospitalization for hepatitis B. See Chapter 11 for details of blood/body fluid precautions.

Patients with hepatitis B, hepatitis D, or non-A, non-B are instructed how to prevent transmission of the disease to others. Specific instructions for home care include the importance of the following:

1. Handwashing before eating and after use of toilet
2. Separate equipment for hygiene (razor, toothbrush, drinking glass, and so on)
3. Avoiding mucous membrane contact (kissing, sexual contact) until the physician recommends otherwise as based on laboratory results
4. Cleanliness of bathroom and kitchen areas
5. Use of detergents with bleaching agents and hot water cycle for laundry
6. Use of hot water for dishwashing

Special attention to home-going instruction is given when unusual exposure to feces, blood, or secretions is expected (for example, incontinent patients, hemodialysis patients). Disposable gloves should be used by caregivers in these situations. (Although fecal-oral transmission is considered negligible, feces can be contaminated by blood from lower gastrointestinal mucosal sites and the virus can be transmitted through breaks in skin.)

Hepatitis B is rarely transmitted by blood transfusion because screening of blood donors for HBsAg is routinely done. Sharing of syringes and needles by intravenous drug users remains a major mode of transmission of HBV. Providing sterile syringes and needles to drug abusers is a growing trend in some communities because teaching the value of not sharing such equipment seems fruitless unless sterile needles and syringes are available to them.

There is increasing awareness about the lack of regulations (or enforcement) concerning the disposal of infectious material in both hospitals and the community (doctors' offices, clinics, nursing homes, and group homes or institutions). Infectious material should be incinerated prior to transport for deposit in land fills.

IMMUNIZATION. Hepatitis B vaccine, which has been in use since 1982, provides active immunity. It is given as a series of three injections, with the second and third doses given 1 and 6 months after the first injection. The cost is about $110.00. The effect of the vaccine on the developing fetus is not known; however, because the vaccine contains only noninfectious HBsAg particles, pregnancy should not be considered a contraindication to its use, if necessary. In contrast, hepatitis B infection in pregnant women results in a severe infection in the mother and chronic infection in the infant.[1]

Preexposure vaccination is recommended for those in high-risk groups (see the boxes on p. 996). Prevaccination serological screening may be used to identify carriers and previously infected noncarriers who have adequate immunity. The cost of screening must be weighed against the cost of unnecessary, but harmless, vaccination, to identify whether or not vaccination should be done. Hepatitis B vaccine causes no adverse effects or benefits in HBV carriers.[12]

An immune globulin with high amounts of anti-HBs (HBIG) is used in certain postexposure situations: infants exposed perinatally are given HBIG at birth and the HBV series is started at the same time.

Persons who have percutaneous, permucosal, or sexual

Table 30-1 Characteristics of different types of viral hepatitis

	Hepatitis A	Hepatitis B	Non-A, Non-B	Hepatitis D
Age group	Older children and young adults	Young adults because of life-style	All age groups but highest in adults because of more frequent blood transfusions	Same as for hepatitis B
Transmission	Primarily person-to-person through fecal contamination; common source epidemics from contaminated food and water; rare transmission by blood; *not* transmitted by shared utensils and kissing	Percutaneous or permucosal routes through infective blood or body fluids introduced by contaminated needles and sexual contact; spread by personal contact in households and among children; rare transmission by blood transfusion, since screening of blood for presence of HBsAg; *not transmitted* fecal-oral route or by contaminated food or H_2O	Percutaneous through infected blood transfusion and parenteral drug abuse; report of a form of non-A, non-B that is spread by contaminated water and close personal contact in Southeast Asia and North Africa	Routes same as those for hepatitis B
Incubation period	15-50 days; average 28-30 days	45-160 days, average 60-120 days	Variable 14-150 days; 50 days average	Unknown
Secretions that have been found to contain infective agent	Stools of infected persons	Highest in blood and serous fluids; also found in saliva and semen, urine, nasopharyngeal washings, feces and pleural fluid	Blood	Blood
Greatest infectivity	2 weeks before onset of jaundice		Infections occur as either coinfection with hepatitis B or superinfection in hepatitis B carrier	
Clinical onset	Abrupt	Insidious	Insidious	Insidious
Diagnostic serologic tests	Confirmed by IgM-class anti-HAV in serum (found during acute and early convalescent period)	Confirmed by HBsAg, HbeAg, anti-HBe, anti-HBc	None available	Delta antigen in serum during early infection; delta antibodies during or after infection (latter test not yet commercially available)
Indication of protective immunity	IgG-class anti-HAV appears during the convalescent period and indicates immunity	Anti-HBs indicates immunity	No tests available; people have had repeated infections	No test available but can only occur if hepatitis B virus is present
Chronic carriers	None demonstrated	Frequent, 6% to 10% of persons with HBV become carriers	8% of population	Unknown
Mortality	Infrequent (<0.6%)	1%-2%	Unknown	Unknown
Subsequent chronic disease	Virtually absent	About 10% develop chronic disease	High, 20% to 70% develop chronic disease	Frequent in persons who contract a superinfection of hepatitis D

From Advisory Committee on Immunization Practices (ACIP): Recommendations for protection against viral hepatitis, Morbid Mortal Week Rep 34:313-340, 1985.

Table 30-1   Characteristics of different types of viral hepatitis—cont'd

	Hepatitis A	Hepatitis B	Non-A, Non-B	Hepatitis D
High-risk groups	Staff and children at day-care centers where children in diapers are cared for; staff and persons in institutions for custodial care (prisons, institutions for developmentally disabled); international travelers to developing countries	Immigrants/refugees from areas of high HBV endemicity; clients and staff in institutions for mentally retarded; users of illicit parenteral drugs; fetuses of infected mothers; homosexually active men; household and sexual partners of HBV carriers; patients on hemodialysis; male prisoners; health care workers with frequent contact with blood	Persons receiving frequent blood transfusions; international travelers to endemic area	Same as for hepatitis B

exposure to blood or body fluid who are known to be HBsAG-positive and unvaccinated, are treated similarly. Vaccinated persons are checked for anti-HBs and given HBIG immediately, with a booster dose of the vaccine.

☐ **Hepatitis D and non-A, non-B hepatitis**

Review Table 30-1 for information about these most recently discovered types of hepatitis. The transmission routes are similar to those of hepatitis B.

Blood transfusions and parenteral drug abuse are a major source of non-A, non-B hepatitis. A fecal-oral route has been found to exist in Southeast Asia and North Africa for this type of hepatitis. Prophylaxis for non-A, non-B hepatitis is not as effective as it is for hepatitis B. Immune globulin may be given, but its value is uncertain.[1] Preventive health teaching is the best measure for travelers to areas where non-A, non-B hepatitis is endemic. Blood/body fluid precautions used for isolation and health instructions are the same as those for persons with HBV. Hepatitis D requires the presence of hepatitis B virus; thus

Table 30-2   Serologic tests for hepatitis antigens and antibodies

Test*	Hepatitis A virus (HAV)	Hepatitis B virus (HBV)	Hepatitis non-A, non-B
HAV-Ab/IgM	Positive test, develops early in the disease, 4 weeks after infection	Not positive	Not positive
HBsAg	Not positive	Positive test, develops about 3 weeks after infection; it is also positive in chronic infections of HBV and in carrier states	Not positive
HBeAg	Not positive	Develops about 3 weeks before onset of symptoms; usually clears in 1 month	Not positive
HBcAb	Not positive	Develops shortly after core antigens appear; positive in acute and chronic infections; indicated low infectivity	Not positive
HBeAb	Not positive	Develops about 4 weeks before onset of jaundice; may be persistently present in chronic infections	Not positive
HBsAb	Not positive	Develops about 3-4 months after onset of symptoms; reflects clinical recovery and immunity	Not positive

*Ab, antibodies; Ag, antigens; s, surface marker (viral coating); c, core viral material (Dane particle); e, early.

the prophylaxis recommended for hepatitis B should prevent delta hepatitis.[1] Isolation is similar to that for hepatitis B.

Tables 30-1 and 30-2 give information about tests that may be used to detect hepatitis in persons at high risk. HBsAg (formerly called *Australian antigen*) is usually the first test done when symptoms of hepatitis are present. A positive test confirms past or present hepatitis B infection. If the HBsAg test is negative, other tests may be used. Hepatitis A is confirmed by the presence of IgM-class anti-HAV in serum. Hepatitis D may be detected by the presence of hepatitis D antigen in the serum; non-A, non-B hepatitis is detected by a process of exclusion because no serological markers have yet been described. The time at which the various antigens and antibodies appear are well known and guide the physician in selecting the particular test(s) to use.[4]

■ CIRRHOSIS OF THE LIVER

Programs for the prevention of cirrhosis are designed primarily to control the ingestion of alcohol. Prevention of alcohol addiction and early intervention in the disease of alcoholism are two important measures in reducing the incidence and severity of pancreatitis, alcoholic hepatitis and cirrhosis, and selected gastrointestinal disorders.

■ GALLSTONES

It is not possible at this time to prevent gallstones, the most prevalent disorder of the biliary tract. Populations that are at higher risk are people who are obese and those with certain metabolic and hemolytic disorders. Patients who tend to form stones in the ducts are usually advised to be careful of their fat intake and to drink generous amounts of fluids.

■ Secondary prevention: detection of disease

Early detection of disease is always important if treatment is to be most beneficial. This is well illustrated by several disorders to be discussed in this chapter. For example, nonspecific gastrointestinal distress may be noticed by patients long before specific symptoms of tumors of the liver, the pancreas, and bile ducts become apparent. Nurses can encourage persons who complain of vague but persistent symptoms to seek medical evaluation. The use of home remedies or over-the-counter preparations can also delay proper diagnosis of serious illnesses.

■ SPECIFIC HEALTH TEACHING

The nurse can assist in the prevention of toxic hepatitis by teaching the danger of injudicious use of materials known to be toxic (see p. 995).

Further, the nurse should encourage persons who complain of persistent and low-grade symptoms to seek medical diagnosis to aid in early detection of diseases that may be serious or contagious.

All persons should be taught personal responsibility for health practices that decrease the risk of infectious disease: handwashing, hygienic care, and "safe sex." Those who are members of a high-risk group for hepatitis should consult a physician for guidance about serological testing and vaccination. Travelers to areas in which hepatitis is endemic should do so also.

Patients, health care staff, and other caregivers need to be educated about how to prevent the spread of hepatitis; thus they must be given specific instructions about enteric and blood/body precautions.

Major health problems of the liver, biliary system, and pancreas

---

Disorders that are encountered in the liver, the biliary system, and the pancreas include not only those caused by infectious organisms but also abnormalities from changes in structure and function. The more common disorders are outlined below.
1. Disorders of the hepatic system
   a. Focal hepatocellular disorders
      (1) Liver abscess
      (2) Trauma to the liver
      (3) Tumors of the liver
   b. Diffuse hepatocellular disorders
      (1) Hepatitis
      (2) Cirrhosis of the liver
      (3) Hepatic coma
2. Disorders of the biliary system
   a. Cholecystitis
   b. Cholelithiasis
   c. Carcinoma of the biliary system
3. Disorders of the pancreas
   a. Pancreatitis
   b. Tumors of the pancreas

■ DISORDERS OF THE LIVER

A variety of pathologic states can affect the liver. Diseases of the liver may be classified in several ways. In this chapter, disorders secondary to focal damage and disorders secondary to diffuse damage will be discussed.

■ Pathophysiology

■ FOCAL HEPATOCELLULAR DISORDERS

The three most common focal disorders of the liver, their etiologies, signs and symptoms, and medical therapies are listed in Table 30-3. Each disorder will be discussed briefly.

□ **Liver abscess**

Liver abscesses may result from a variety of organisms and are an infectious process. See Table 30-3 for related

Table 30-3 Focal disorders of the liver

Disorder	Etiology	Signs and symptoms	Therapy
Liver abscess	Infection complication of obstructed biliary tract, contiguous viscera, intestinal tract, septicemia; traumatic injury to liver, amebic abscess	Fever, chills Vague abdominal discomfort, tenderness over liver, palpable liver Jaundice, leukocytosis ↑ Serum alkaline phosphatase ↑ SGOT	Surgical incision and drainage and broad spectrum antimicrobial therapy for pyogenic abscess Amebic abscess: emetine hydrochloride, chloroquine, metronidazole (Flagyl)
Trauma to liver	Penetrating stab wounds Blunt wounds (automobile accidents or falls)	Variable signs: pain, shock, abdominal rigidity Blood or bile with peritoneal tap	Drainage Suture and drainage Resection Blood volume management Antimicrobial therapy
Carcinoma of liver	Primary risk factors: hepatitis, cirrhosis, hepatotoxins, trauma Metastasis from any site but commonly from carcinoma of abdominal viscera, breast, lung, kidney, ovary, testes, skin	Weight loss, weakness Jaundice, anemia Ascites, edema Upper right quadrant pain, hepatomegaly Unexplained fever Elevated liver enzymes (SGOT, SGPT) Elevated sedimentation rate	Surgical excision Chemotherapy: methotrexate, 5-fluorouracil, doxorubicin (Adriamycin), mitomycin C; often administered by hepatic artery perfusion Homotransplantation Decompression of biliary tract Palliative radiation

signs and symptoms and some of the tests that may demonstrate altered hepatic function. The mortality rate for untreated liver abscess is 100%. Complications include sepsis, peritonitis from rupture of abscess, and respiratory complications (emboli, infection). Pyogenic abscesses may occur after liver injury, from contiguous extension of infections, or from organisms reaching the liver through blood, lymph, or bile. The most common cause is biliary tract disease (cholangitis, acute cholecystitis).[4]

Entamoeba histolytica is an important worldwide cause of amebic liver abscess and dysentery. In amebic infections the vegetative form of the organism moves from the gut to the small portal canaliculi in the liver, where it becomes activated, releasing enzymes that cause local tissue destruction. Multiple abscesses occur. The clinical manifestations of liver abscess are often nonspecific and are related to the infectious process. Patients present with tenderness of the right upper quadrant, hepatomegaly, and persistent

fever; 20% to 40% show pleural involvement (effusion, pain on breathing, cough, rales).

Biliary peritonitis may follow leakage of bile into the peritoneal cavity. A peritoneal tap or lavage is often done after injury in order to examine the fluid for bile or blood. Signs of peritonitis are shown in the box below, left.

Treatment includes prolonged antibiotic therapy and, often, surgical incision and drainage for pyogenic abscesses and amebicidal therapy for amoebic abscesses. Surgery is rarely done for amoebic abscess.

□ **Trauma to the liver**

Because of its location and size, the liver is frequently subjected to trauma. If the injury is severe, rupture of the liver may occur with severe internal hemorrhage. Injury to the liver may occur with trauma to the chest or abdomen.

Death that occurs shortly after the injury is caused by uncontrollable hepatic hemorrhage. This happens in part because the walls of the hepatic veins are thin, the liver is highly vascular, and the bile mixing with the blood interferes with clotting. Deaths occurring later after injury may be caused by biliary peritonitis, shock, or infections.

Small lacerations or ruptures of the liver, except for temporary peritoneal irritations from blood oozing into the peritoneal cavity, usually heal and leave a subcapsular scar. In some instances a hematoma may become infected, with abscess formation complicating the healing process. Hepatic cysts may also develop. Trauma that causes severe contusions may result in subsequent degeneration of the injured hepatic cells. The prognosis depends on the amount

---

Signs and symptoms of peritonitis

Abdominal tenderness
Rebound tenderness
Muscle rigidity or spasm
Decreased or absent bowel signs
Abdominal distention

of tissue damage, and the final outcome for the patient may not be known for many years after the initial injury.

□ Tumors of the liver

Tumors of the liver may be either malignant or benign. Benign lesions include hemangiomas, cysts, and, rarely, adenomas. These benign tumors occasionally enlarge enough to become symptomatic and present problems in differentiation from a malignant tumor. If the latter occurs, surgical intervention may be required.

Malignant tumors may be metastatic or primary. *Metastatic tumors* are common; they occur 20 times more frequently than primary tumors and rank second to cirrhosis as a cause of fatal liver disease.[28] The liver most commonly receives metastatic cells from tumors in the gastrointestinal tract, the lung, the breast, the kidney, and melanomas of the skin. See Table 30-3 for common signs and symptoms of metastatic lesions of the liver. Metastatic carcinoma of the liver varies from a few small nodules to large nodes. Adjacent nodes may eventually grow together and compress the surrounding liver tissue. Usually different parts of the liver are uniformly involved so that liver biopsy may be a useful diagnostic aid.

Primary hepatic carcinomas may arise within the liver (hepatocellular) or the bile duct cell (cholangiocellular) or may be of mixed origin. Hepatocellular tumors are the most common, but primary liver cancer accounts for only 1% to 2% of malignant tumors found at death in the United States. They are more common in men and usually occur in the fifth and sixth decades of life.

Primary lesions may be multiple or singular, diffuse or nodular, and may spread to only a lobe or to the entire liver. The cancerous cells appear to compress the surrounding normal liver cells and to spread quickly by invading the portal vein branches. Spread may be by direct extension to surrounding tissue. Primary cancers also tend to cause hemorrhage and necrosis. The most common site for metastasis of the primary liver lesion is the lung, but it may metastasize elsewhere. Primary lesions tend to grow rapidly, sometimes without signs or symptoms, and the patient may live only a short time after onset.

Jaundice and ascites are signs that the metastic or primary process is quite far advanced. Extreme weakness is also usually an outstanding symptom. Ascites occurs secondary to compression of the portal vein. Gastrointestinal bleeding may also be present and may confuse the diagnosis. A special blood test that may be used to help diagnose primary liver carcinoma is the high serum concentrations of alpha-fetoprotein (AFP). AFP in concentrations of 500 mg/ml is found in 70% of patients with hepatocellular cancer.[42] (Lower levels may be found in patients with metastatic carcinoma or viral hepatitis.)

■ DIFFUSE HEPATOCELLULAR DISORDERS

Regardless of the specific pathologic condition, disorders secondary to diffuse parenchymal damage present the patient with common problems. These problems will be discussed before the specific disorders of *hepatitis*, acute inflammation of the liver, *cirrhosis*, and chronic fibrotic disease of the liver are discussed.

□ Common manifestation of diffuse hepatocellular disorders
□ *Jaundice*

Jaundice is a symptom complex caused by a disturbance of the physiology of bile pigment and is present in many diseases of the liver, pancreas, and biliary system. There is an excess of bile pigment in the blood, which eventually is distributed to the skin, mucous membranes, and other body fluids and tissues, giving them a yellow discoloration. If the bilirubin has been processed by the liver (extracted, conjugated, and secreted), it is water soluble and can be excreted in urine, which will be dark in color.

The presence of bile pigment in the skin causes *pruritus* (itching) in about 20% to 25% of the patients who have jaundice. Table 30-4 compares the three types of jaundice. Regardless of the type of jaundice, there will be an increase in the *total* serum bilirubin (normal: 0.5 to 1.0 mg/dl). Jaundice can usually be detected when bilirubin concentrations exceed 2.5 mg/dl. The changes in concentrations of conjugated bilirubin (measured by a "direct" laboratory test) and unconjugated bilirubin ("indirect") help in determining the type of jaundice. Serum bilirubin levels must be combined with other laboratory and diagnostic tests and interpreted in view of the history and clinical findings (see p. 993 for differences in bilirubins).

A common reason for *intrahepatic cholestasis* is drug reactions; such as from phenothiazines. Clay-colored stools indicate that bile is not reaching the intestine and suggests *extrahepatic obstruction*. An absence of urobilinogen in the urine supports this inference.

Frequent causes of extrahepatic obstruction are gallstones lodged in the common bile duct, pancreatitis, and carcinoma of the head of the pancreas. Fig. 30-3 shows how pancreatic enlargement can compress the common bile duct.

In hepatocellular damage, there is interference with uptake, conjugation, and excretion of bilirubin into bile. Excretion is the most profoundly affected process and a predominately conjugated hyperbilirubinemia is seen. Jaundice does not imply severity in hepatitis; but in cirrhosis, jaundice suggests a poor prognosis.

□ *Bleeding tendencies and anemia*

Bleeding tendencies and anemia are common complications of liver disease. They may occur in persons with advanced hepatitis, cirrhosis, and biliary duct obstruction. These tendencies are a result of deficiencies in the formation of clotting factors, thrombocytopenia, and a deficiency of erythrocytes. In patients with obstructive jaundice and liver disease, the synthesis of various clotting factors is impaired. If the patient's bile duct is obstructed, absorption of fat and vitamin K (fat-soluble) is reduced. Even if vitamin K is absorbed, severely damaged liver cells cannot synthesize adequate amounts of these factors, especially prothrombin. Other vitamin deficiencies (A, B complex, D) may also result from decreased absorption of fat-soluble vitamins and the inability to store the vitamins.

The patient with liver disease may also develop an en-

Table 30-4 Types of jaundice

Category	Pathology	Possible findings
Obstructive		
Intrahepatic	Suppression of bile flow in canaliculi or small biliary ductiles (chole-stasis)	Direct* bilirubin elevated; alkaline phosphatase elevated; no enlargement of bile ducts seen on scan or ultrasound
Extrahepatic (biliary tract obstruction)	Obstruction of bile flow in large bile ducts	Direct* bilirubin elevated; alkaline phosphatase elevated; enlargement of bile ducts documented by scan, ultrasound; absence of urobilinogen in urine
Hepatocellular	Hepatocyte injury from toxins, viruses (hepatitis) or as part of syndrome of cirrhosis	Transaminases (SGPT, SGOT) elevated 10- to 15-fold; both direct* and indirect† bilirubin may be elevated (direct more than indirect); prolonged prothrombin time
Hemolytic	Excessive amounts of bilirubin are released from RBC's; liver is unable to excrete bilirubin as rapidly as it forms	Usually mild elevation of total bilirubin (indirect more than direct)

*"Direct" measures conjugated bilirubin.
†"Indirect" measures unconjugated bilirubin.

larged spleen as a result of portal hypertension. This is believed to be responsible for the resulting thrombocytopenia and increased red blood cell destruction.

Various other factors contribute to the anemia, including blood loss from gastrointestinal bleeding and decreased red blood cell production secondary to folic acid deficiency and poor protein intake. In addition, alcohol has a direct toxic effect on bone marrow.

☐ **Infection**

The patient with diffuse hepatocellular disease is at risk for infection. Depressed protein synthesis, lymphatic obstruction of the splanchnic organs, impaired Kupffer cells, and depressed bone marrow all play a part. Leukopenia may be present.

☐ **Fluid and electrolyte alterations**

Fluid volume deficit results when body losses exceed body gains and should be considered when the following symptoms are seen:
1. Vomiting
2. Anorexia with decreased intake
3. Hemorrhage
4. Diarrhea
5. Biliary or pancreatic drainage

It is important that nurses understand that patients with *hypoalbuminemia* (serum level below 4.0 g/dl) may have a contracted intravascular volume, *even in the presence of edema and ascites.* This phenomenon is seen most often in cirrhosis and results from the decreased production of albumin and the continued loss of this protein into the peritoneal cavity. As a result, the colloidal osmotic pressure of the blood is decreased (leading to increased fluid filtration through the capillary wall) while the return of fluid to the capillary is impaired. The patient is less able to maintain

adequate perfusion of tissues should blood volume decrease further.

The several factors that lead to *ascites* (accumulation of serous fluid in the peritoneal cavity) are illustrated in Fig. 30-4. The sequence of these mechanisms and how they interact to intensify ascites is not well established. A vicious cycle is established as the albumin lost into the peritoneal cavity further decreases the patient's serum albumin level, resulting in an increase in interstitial fluid. As a result, hydrothorax, ankle, and presacral edema may accompany the ascites. The patient with cirrhosis frequently is unable to excrete normal amounts of urinary sodium. *Hyponatremia* is frequent and reflects the disproportional retention of water in comparison to sodium.

Alterations in renal function may occur because of decreased blood volume, portal hypertension, and increased circulating hormones. Decreased excretion of water, sodium, and metabolic wastes is common. Oliguria, azotemia (nitrogen wastes in the blood), and low urinary sodium (less than 10 mEq/L) may occur abruptly and signal hepatorenal syndrome. Although renal medullary bloodflow is maintained in this condition, there is a marked decrease in renal cortical bloodflow. Precipitants of this condition, which has a mortality rate of nearly 90%, are the following:
1. Diuretic therapy
2. Parecentesis
3. Gastrointestinal hemorrhage

☐ **Hepatitis**

Hepatitis may be defined as any acute inflammatory disease of the liver. Although the term *hepatitis* is most commonly used in conjunction with viral hepatitis, the disease can be caused by toxic injury to the liver, viruses, or bacteria (Table 30-5).

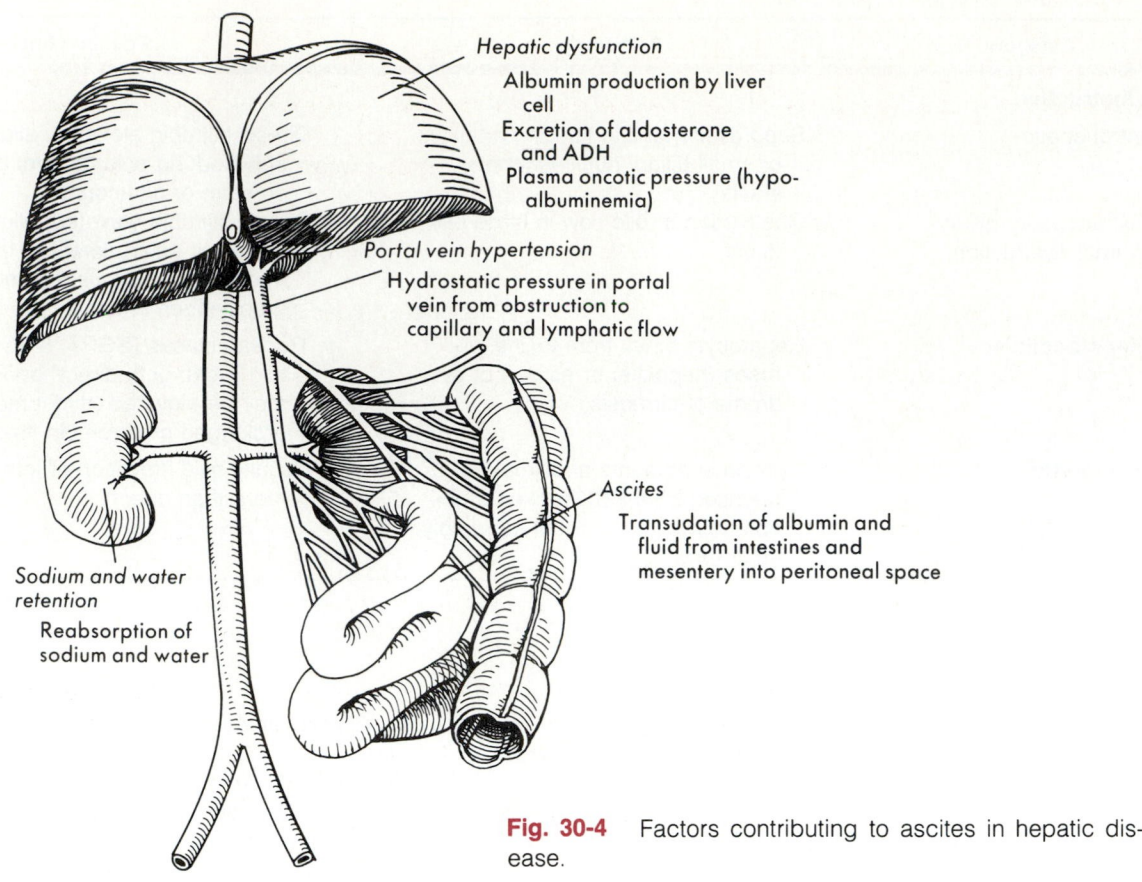

Hepatic dysfunction
Albumin production by liver cell
Excretion of aldosterone and ADH
Plasma oncotic pressure (hypo-albuminemia)

Portal vein hypertension
Hydrostatic pressure in portal vein from obstruction to capillary and lymphatic flow

Ascites
Transudation of albumin and fluid from intestines and mesentery into peritoneal space

Sodium and water retention
Reabsorption of sodium and water

Fig. 30-4 Factors contributing to ascites in hepatic disease.

Table 30-5 Diffuse disorders of the liver

Disorder	Etiology	Signs and symptoms	Medical therapy
Viral hepatitis	Hepatitis virus A, B, non-A, non-B, D (see Table 30-1) Epstein-Barr virus Cytomegalovirus	**Preicteric stage** Anorexia, nausea and vomiting, chills and fever, arthralgia, right upper quadrant tenderness, fatigue	Rest Diet: high calorie, high protein, low fat Avoidance of toxins
		Icteric stage Jaundice (yellow sclera and skin), dark urine, light colored stools	Vitamin K
		Post-icteric stage fatigue	
	Atypical course (see box, p. 1006)	Signs of liver failure similar to those seen in cirrhosis	Treatment based on dysfunction For some: Prednisolone/Imuran; Dialysis; Immunotherapy
Cirrhosis of the liver	Chronic hepatitis Alcohol, malnutrition, hepatotoxins, biliary obstruction, congestive heart failure, metabolic problems, infectious diseases, gastrointestinal diseases	Malaise Gastrointestinal symptoms: anorexia, indigestion, nausea, vomiting, flatulence, altered bowel function	Rest Diet: high calorie, normal to high protein (unless ammonia toxicity is present), low fat, vitamin supplement (A, B, C, D)

Table 30-5   Diffuse disorders of the liver—cont'd

Disorder	Etiology	Signs and symptoms	Medical therapy
Cirrhosis of the liver—cont'd		Malnutrition: muscle wasting, muscle weakness, loss of weight	Bile salts Abstinence from alcohol
		Fluid retention: edema, ascites, abdominal distention, hydrothorax (often on right), weight gain	Sodium and water restriction Furosemide, spironolactone Albumin infusion (salt-poor) Peritoneal-jugular shunt (PJS) Paracentesis
		Jaundice: pruritus, hypoprothrombinemia, steatorrhea, light colored stools, dark urine	Antihistamines, tranquilizer, Vitamin K (Hykinone)
		Hepatomegaly, splenomegaly	
		Hyperestrinism: palmar erythema, gynecomastia, spider angiomas, sparse body hair, testicular atrophy	
		Portal hypertension: caput medusae, hemorrhoids, esophageal varices, edema of lower extremities	Surgical procedures that shunt blood away from liver
		Gastrointestinal bleeding Esophageal varices	Fresh blood transfusion, plasma expanders, normal saline (IV) Esophageal tamponade Iced saline lavage Pitressin (IV) Injection of sclerosing agents Measures to prevent hepatic coma
		Bleeding tendencies, purpura, hematuria, gingival bleeding, epistaxis, melena, hematemesis	Vitamin K Transfusions of whole blood, plasma, platelets
		Anemia: pallor, fatigue, ↓ RBC, hematocrit and hemoglobin	High protein diet with supplements of vitamins and folic acid Splenectomy
Portal system encephalopathy	Precipitating factors: Infection, high protein intake, GI bleeding, blood transfusions, hypokalemia, alkalosis	Impaired attention span, impaired concentration, apathy, insomnia, slurred speech, yawning, asterixis, fetor hepaticus	Protein-free diet Enemas, cathartics Lactulose, neomycin Dialysis, exchange transfusion Corticosteroids
		Coma: muscular rigidity, hyperreflexia, myoclonus seizures	Amino acid (arginine) or levodopa replacement Colon bypass Liver transplant

Common hepatotoxins

Drugs: chlorpromazine, isoniazid, tetracycline, thiazides, thiouracil, acetaminophen
Organic solvents: carbon tetrachloride, methylenedianiline (MDA)
Phosphorus, heavy metals
Plant poisons
Alcohol

☐ Toxic hepatitis

The pathologic changes in the liver will depend on the toxic agent (see the box above). For example, necrosis and fatty infiltrates are present when the causative agent is carbon tetrachloride, whereas cholestasis with portal inflammation is seen when the toxic agent is chlorpromazine.[27]

Two types of chemical hepatotoxicy occur: direct toxic and idiosyncratic. In direct toxic hepatitis, the agent causes toxicity with predictable regularity and is dose dependent. The reactions in idiosyncratic toxic hepatitis are sporadic and not dose dependent, which suggests idiosyncrasy in the host.

☐ Fatty liver and alcoholic hepatitis

The leading cause of liver disease in the United States is alcohol. There are two reversible conditions of alcoholic liver damage: *fatty liver* and *alcoholic hepatitis*. In fatty liver, fatty deposits are seen within hepatocytes and the patient may complain of right quadrant tenderness. Hepatomegaly and elevated levels of transaminases are often present.

Alcohol has at least two effects on fat metabolism that lead to fatty liver:
1. Increased NADPH generation, which promotes fatty acid synthesis and triglyceride formation
2. Inhibition of the release of triglycerides

In addition, acetaldehyde may be directly toxic to the hepatocytes. Factors that may enhance hepatotoxicity of alcohol include malnutrition, genetic susceptibility, and immune processes.[4]

In alcoholic hepatitis, histological examination reveals deposits of hyalin within hepatocytes, leukocytic infiltration and development of connective tissue surrounding hepatocytes and central veins. The clinical presentation is varied; it can be asymptomatic or reflect liver failure. Anorexia, nausea, vomiting, weight loss, and abdominal pain are common.[4]

Cirrhosis, the irreversible condition of alcoholic liver damage, will be discussed later.

☐ Viral hepatitis

ACUTE VIRAL HEPATITIS. Viral hepatitis causes diffuse inflammatory infiltration of hepatic tissue. With typical acute viral hepatitis, there is no collapse of lobules, no loss of lobular architecture, and minimal or no fibrosis. Inflammation, degeneration, and regeneration may occur simultaneously, distorting the normal lobular pattern and possibly creating pressure about the portal vein. Laboratory findings include elevations in serum levels of transaminase (SGOT), prothrombin time, alkaline phophatase, and bilirubin. Symptoms may vary in severity; many patients have very mild symptoms and do not have jaundice. Because the pathologic process is usually distributed evenly throughout the liver, biopsy in most cases is diagnostic for viral hepatitis.

In most instances of nonfatal viral hepatitis, regeneration begins almost with the onset of the disease. The damaged cells are removed by phagocytosis and enzymatic reaction, and the liver returns to normal.

The outcome of viral hepatitis may be affected by such factors as the following:
1. Virulence of the virus
2. Amount of hepatic damage sustained before exposure to the virus
3. Natural barriers to damage and disease of the liver
4. Supportive care patient receives when symptoms appear

The majority of patients recover normal liver function, but the disease may take several courses; different terms describe each of them (see the box below).

The four types of viral hepatitis are described on p. 998. Symptoms of the various types are not clinically distinctive from each other except that acute symptoms may be more severe in hepatitis A. Symptoms usually appear from 4 to 7 days before jaundice is apparent. Anorexia is one of the most frequent symptoms. This preicteric stage lasts for approximately 1 week and then subsides as hepatocellular jaundice occurs.

The icteric stage usually reaches its intensity in 2 weeks and may last from 4 to 6 weeks. The *posticteric* or convalescent stage begins with the disappearance of jaundice and may last from a few weeks to several months. Complete

Atypical courses of hepatitis

Submassive hepatic necrosis	Destruction of substantial group of adjacent cells but without destruction of the greater part of a lobule
Massive hepatic necrosis	Destruction of whole lobule
Fulminant viral hepatitis	Sudden and severe degeneration of the liver
Subacute fatal viral hepatitis	Slower severe degeneration of the liver

recovery is usually expected in 6 months. The disease may relapse during this stage, with recurrence of previous symptoms but to a milder degree.

□ Chronic hepatitis

If hepatitis lasts 6 months, it is classified as chronic hepatitis. Viral hepatitis is only one cause but it is the most common etiology of chronic hepatitis (drugs, toxins, metabolic liver disease, and autoimmune processes are other causes).[4]

□ *Chronic viral hepatitis*

Chronic hepatitis is not seen with hepatitis A. *Chronic active hepatitis* is the most serious form of chronic hepatitis. Twenty percent of cases follow HBV infection.[4] If autoimmunity is determined and there is absence of HBsAg, corticosteroids (prednisolone), and sometimes Imuran may be used. If patients are HBsAg-positive, corticosteroids are seldom used. There is extension of the necrosis with loss of normal structure and function. Very frequently the disease progresses to cirrhosis. If left untreated, most patients will die within 4 to 5 years; about 75% respond well to corticosteroid treatment.

Chronic persistent hepatitis and *chronic lobular hepatitis* are characterized by abnormal liver function tests, fatigue, and hepatomegally for greater than 6 months, but there is no necrosis and no increase in mortality.

□ Cirrhosis of the liver

Cirrhosis of the liver refers to several diseases that are characterized by diffuse inflammation and fibrosis of the liver that result in drastic structural changes and significant loss of liver function. The basic processes leading to cirrhosis are liver cell death with scar tissue formation and regeneration of cell mass that causes distortion of the structure with a resultant change in circulation. Destruction

---

NURSING CARE PLAN

Person with cirrhosis

DATA: Mr. Sartos is a 55-year-old salesman diagnosed with portal hypertension and admitted to the hospital with upper gastrointestinal bleeding. Endoscopy revealed enlarged esophageal and upper gastric veins and a bleeding ulcer. Gastric lavage with iced saline controlled bleeding; 1 U of packed red blood cells was given. Treatment orders included protein and sodium restrictions, fluid restriction, neomycin 1 g every 4 hours, thiamine 1 cc intramuscularly and vitamin K subcutaneously 3 times a day, and spironolactone 25 mg twice a day.

Physical exam revealed: slight jaundice of sclera and skin; ascites and peripheral edema; thin legs and arms and poor musculature; signs of hyperestrinism; mental status—oriented × 3 and coherent; blood pressure was 116/60; pulse was 90; respiration rate was 18.

The nursing history identified the following:
1. Mr. Sartos has participated in Alcoholics Anonymous (AA) for 1 year; he has not been drinking since then.
2. Mr. Sartos had influenza-like symptoms the past 2 weeks but continued with busy schedule. Complains of fatigue, anorexia, and itching.

Collaborative nursing actions include those to prevent further impairment from hemorrhage, ammonia toxicity, and to assist in treatment for ulcer, and for fluid excess. Nursing actions include monitoring for the following:
1. Signs of hemorrhage: hematemesis, decreased blood pressure, tachycardia, restlessness, stools testing positive for guaiac, and cool moist skin.
2. Signs of hepatic encephalopathy: change in mental status, asterixis, change in handwriting, tremors.

Nursing diagnosis: Activity intolerance related to generalized weakness

Expected patient outcomes	Nursing interventions	Rationale
Patient will increase activities gradually.	Encourage bed rest during acute phase. Encourage increasing activity interspersed with rest periods as tolerated. Intervene if patient shows fatigue after prolonged visits by family or friends.	Graduated increase of activity is important so as not to overtax patient who has poor nutritional status and activity intolerance.

Continued.

NURSING CARE PLAN

Person with cirrhosis—cont'd

Nursing diagnosis: Altered nutrition: less than body requirements related to anorexia

Expected patient outcomes	Nursing interventions	Rationale
Patient ingests required nutrients. Signs of muscle wasting decrease.	Assess nutrient intake. Teach patient how to plan and implement a well-balanced, high-carbohydrate, low-protein diet with adequate vitamins. Encourage use of salt substitute or alternative seasonings. Give antiemetics and mouth care if nausea is present. Suggest small frequent meals. Use measures that encourage eating. Support continuation of AA activities while hospitalized.	Food intake within prescribed limitation can influence liver regeneration; nursing measures can influence amount of intake in an anorectic patient. Important that he continue AA participation as he has for past year. AA representatives should be allowed to see patient as condition permits.

Nursing diagnosis: Altered tissue perfusion: related to arterial decreased blood flow and portal vein hypertension

Expected patient outcomes	Nursing interventions	Rationale
Patient's weight and abdominal girth decrease. Edema resolves. Serum sodium and potassium remain normal.	Monitor daily weight and blood pressure; assess edema; measure abdominal girth daily. Monitor intake and output until excess fluid is excreted. Teach patient rationale for sodium restriction. Provide bed rest for ascites. Give prescribed medications (spironolactone and salt-free albumin infusions). Restrict fluids; provide those which are best tolerated and space these fluids throughout 24 hours.	Diuresis in cirrhosis is undertaken slowly because of the contracted, intravascular fluid volume. Diuresis in excess can jeopardize renal perfusion and precipitate hepatic coma.

Nursing diagnosis: Ineffective breathing pattern: related to ascites and immobility

Expected patient outcomes	Nursing interventions	Rationale
Patient's dyspnea is decreased. Breath sounds are clear.	Monitor respirations and breath sounds. Place patient in high-Fowler's position. Encourage patient on bed rest to cough and turn frequently. Encourge deep breathing.	Nursing measures to encourage deep chest excursions are important when ascites and immobility are present.

NURSING CARE PLAN

Person with cirrhosis—cont'd

Nursing diagnosis: Potential impaired skin integrity: related to immobility, poor nutrition, and edema

Expected patient outcomes	Nursing interventions	Rationale
Patient's skin remains intact.	Assess skin daily for signs of possible breakdown. Use measures to prevent skin breakdown. Keep skin clean and moisturized.	Patient has poor nutrition, edema, immobility; all of these are risk factors for decubitus ulcers.

Nursing diagnosis: Pain: itching—jaundice and environmental stimuli

Expected patient outcomes	Nursing interventions	Rationale
Patient states feeling more comfortable.	Avoid heat and heavy clothing and provide a cool environment. Apply antipruritic lotion to skin as needed. Give prescribed antihistamines. Use diversional activities. Keep fingernails cut short. If patient must scratch, provide soft cloth to prevent excoriations.	Measures relieve or avoid environmental stimuli, reduce itching, and promote comfort.

Nursing diagnosis: Potential for infection: related to immunosuppression

Expected patient outcomes	Nursing interventions	Rationale
Patient develops no new infection.	Monitor for signs of infection. Use sterile technique for all intrusive procedures. Encourage pulmonary hygiene. Restrict exposure to persons with infections.	Infection in patient with cirrhosis can be life-threatening and can precipitate hepatic failure with hepatic encephalopathy and septicemia as results. Measures to prevent infection are essential in persons whose immune systems are suppressed

Nursing diagnosis: Ineffective individual coping: related to health crisis

Expected patient outcomes	Nursing interventions	Rationale
Patient will describe at least one coping mechanism.	Assess patient's perception of health and present illness. Identify and support patient's coping strategies. Listen actively if patient expresses feeling of powerlessness, fears, or spiritual distress. Assess and facilitate family support.	Support of patient undergoing health crisis can strengthen use of intrapersonal family resources. One can expect this patient to be discouraged and fearful.

Table 30-6 Types of cirrhosis

Type	Etiology	Description
Laënnec's cirrhosis (nutritional, portal, or alcoholic cirrhosis)	Alcoholism, malnutrition	Massive collagen formation; liver in early fatty stage is large and firm; in late state it is small and nodular
Postnecrotic cirrhosis	Massive necrosis from hepatotoxins, usually viral hepatitis	Liver is decreased in size with nodules and fibrous tissue
Biliary cirrhosis	Biliary obstruction in liver and common bile duct	Chronic impairment of bile drainage; liver is first large then becomes firm and nodular; jaundice is major symptom
Cardiac cirrhosis	Right side congestive heart failure (CHF)	Liver is swollen and changes are reversible if CHF treated effectively; some fibrosis with long-standing CHF
Nonspecific, metabolic cirrhosis	Metabolic problems, infectious diseases, infiltrative diseases, gastrointestinal diseases	Portal and liver fibrosis may develop; liver is enlarged and firm

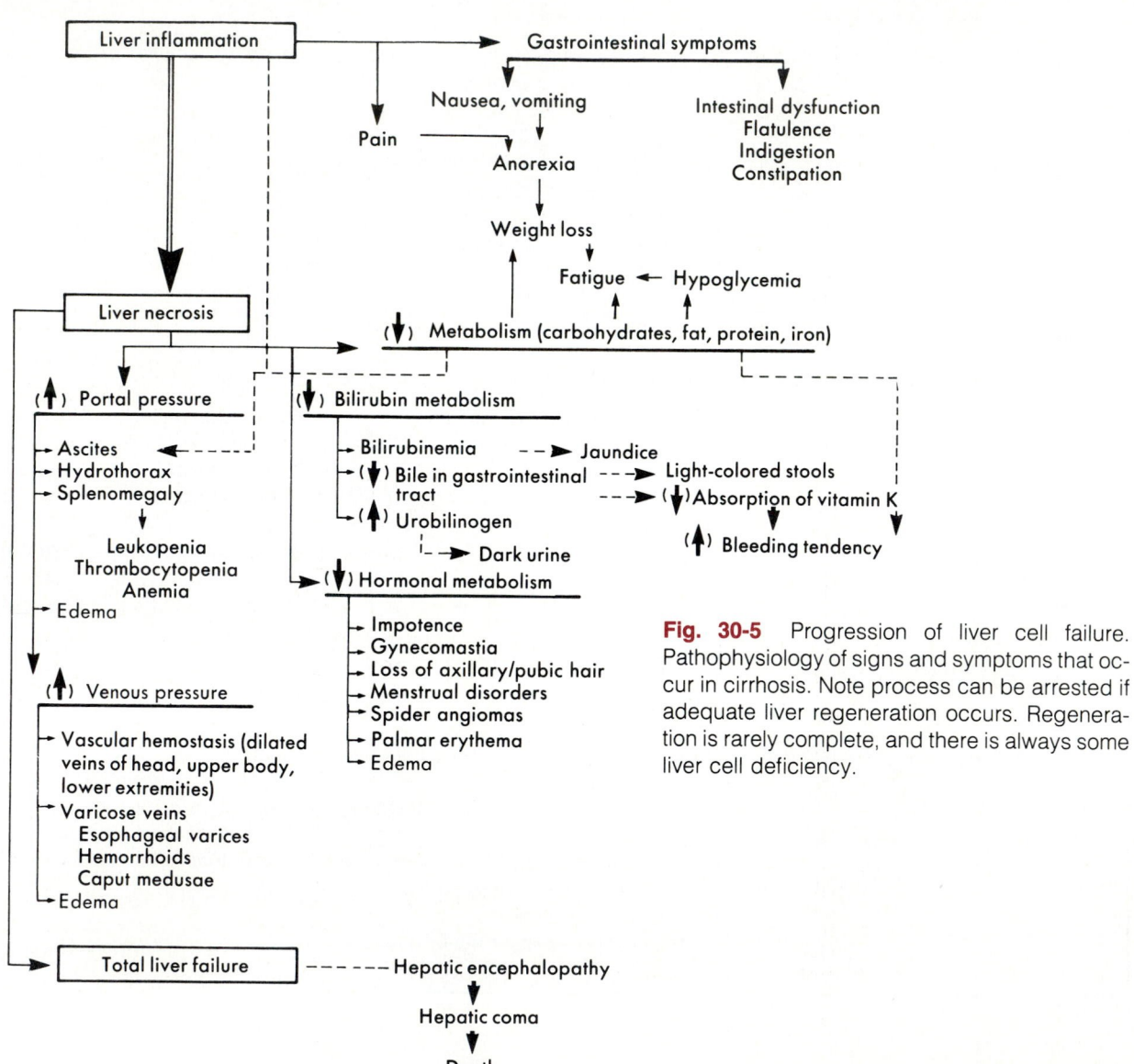

Fig. 30-5 Progression of liver cell failure. Pathophysiology of signs and symptoms that occur in cirrhosis. Note process can be arrested if adequate liver regeneration occurs. Regeneration is rarely complete, and there is always some liver cell deficiency.

of the lymphatic system and the capillary bed (sinusoids) retards the portal vein bloodflow and thereby increases the volume and pressure of blood in the portal vein.

The major types of cirrhosis are described in Table 30-6. Postnecrotic cirrhosis from infectious disease is the most common type on a worldwide basis. More rare nonspecific types account for about 10% of deaths resulting from cirrhosis.

In Laënnec's cirrhosis, the most common type in North America, chronic alcoholism is a frequent cause; it may also be caused by malnutrition associated with other diseases such as pancreatitis, diabetes mellitus, and ulcerative colitis.

The signs and symptoms seen in cirrhosis are similar regardless of the cause and result from the progressive destruction of hepatic cells. Regeneration and proliferation of fibrous tissue cause obstruction of the portal vein. Cirrhosis is manifested clinically by the following alterations, discussed previously: portal hypertension, jaundice, bleeding tendencies and anemia, decreased resistance to infection, ascites, and edema.

Once the disease is established, it usually advances slowly to death. Many people, however, can be helped to live for years if they follow instructions. The liver has remarkable powers of regeneration. Sometimes sufficient collateral circulation can be established and sufficient repair of hepatic tissue can be accomplished so that symptoms subside for long periods. Unfortunately, at other times rapid deterioration occurs. Two crises are often responsible: hepatic coma and bleeding esophageal varices. Fig. 30-5 summarizes the numerous alterations that occur in cirrhosis of the liver.

As the cirrhotic process continues, the patient is prone to develop many life-threatening complications. Death may occur from total liver failure, bleeding esophageal varices,

hepatic coma, or renal failure. Severe ascites and jaundice; neurologic symptoms; and decreased prothrombin, albumin, and sodium levels indicate a poor prognosis.

□ *Portal hypertension*

As circulation in the portal system becomes impaired because of structural changes in the liver, portal hypertension occurs (Fig. 30-6), producing splenomegaly and increasing edema of the lower extremities. As pressure increases in the portal veins, a back flow of blood into the veins emptying into the portal veins occurs. These veins in turn develop collateral channels of circulation. Collateral channels are most likely to occur in paraumbilicus veins, the hemorrhoidal veins, and the veins at the cardia of the stomach that extend into the esophagus. These veins become distended and tortuous because they are not anatomically equipped to handle large volumes of blood. This results in hemorrhoids, esophageal varices, and a ring of varicosities surrounding the umbilicus (caput medusae).

□ *Bleeding esophageal varices*

Bleeding esophageal varices (Fig. 30-7) occur frequently in patients with cirrhosis of the liver. These small vessels

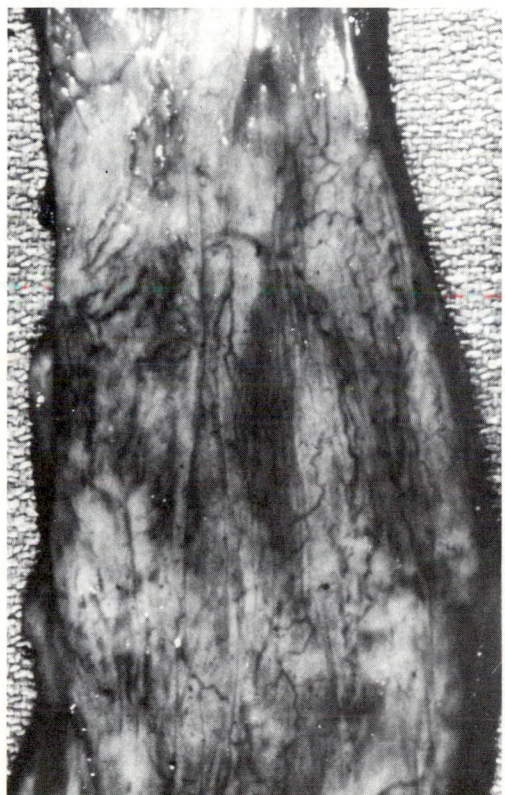

30-7 Esophageal varices. Swollen varices and extensive collateral circulation are evident in segment of esophagus from patient with Laënnec's cirrhosis. (From Groër, ME and Shekleton, ME: Basic pathophysiology: a conceptual approach, ed 2, St. Louis, 1983, The CV Mosby Co. Courtesy department of pathology, University of Tennessee, Knoxville).

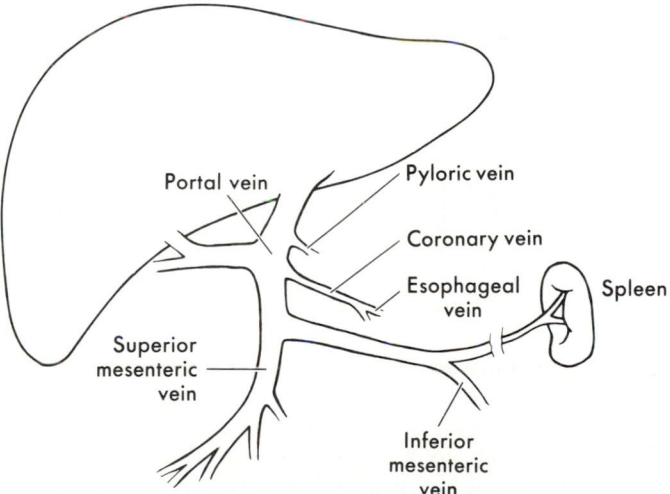

Fig. 30-6 Splanchnic veins. Venous drainage of splanchnic organs. When portal hypertension develops, other vessels can become engorged, leading to stasis and hypoxia of respective organs. (From Groër, MF and Shekleton, ME: Basic pathophysiology: a conceptual approach, ed 2, St. Louis, 1983, The CV Mosby Co.)

Table 30-7 Stages of consciousness, intellectual behavior, and neurologic changes in portal system encephalopathy[3,18]

Stage 1 (Prodromal)	Stage 2 (Impending)	Stage 3 (Stuporous)	Stage 4 (Coma)
Change in sleep pattern	Lethargy	Confused, somnolent	Unconscious
Slow response	Disorientation to time	Stupor but arousable	No intellectual functioning
Shortened attention span	Impaired computation	Disorientation to place	Loss of deep tendon reflexes
Oppressed or euphoric	Decreased inhibition	Anger, rage, paranoia	If response, it is only to deep pain
Irritable	Anxiety or apathy	Increased reflexes	
Tremors	Inappropriate behavior	Clonus	
Some incoordination	Speech slurred	Babinski reflex	
Writing impaired	Decreased reflexes		
	Ataxia		

become tortuous and fragile and may be affected by mechanical trauma from ingestion of coarse food and acid pepsin erosion, which may result in bleeding. Bleeding may also occur as a result of coughing, vomiting, sneezing, straining at stool (Valsalva's maneuver), or any physical exertion that increases abdominal venous pressure. Bleeding is frequently abrupt and without pain. Severe hematemesis and resultant shock may follow, requiring emergency treatment.

□ *Portal system encephalopathy*

Portal system encephalopathy (PSE), formerly called *hepatic coma* or *ammonia toxicity*, is metabolic encephalopathy associated with liver failure. This dysfunction of the central nervous system is thought to be related to several factors. Many patients with hepatic coma have an increase in blood ammonia concentration. Normally, ammonia, which is formed in the intestines from the breakdown of protein by intestinal bacteria, is converted to urea in the liver. When liver failure occurs, ammonia is not converted into urea and ammonia concentration in the circulating blood is increased. In liver failure, ammonia levels may be increased at the same time the detoxification ability of the liver is decreased or when blood is shunted past the liver. There are many factors that can increase blood ammonia levels (see p. 1024).

It has been shown that patients with PSE have increased levels of aromatic or short-chain amino acids (SCAA's) and a decrease in branched-chain amino acids (BCAA's).[3] Normally SCAA's are cleared by the liver. With liver failure they increase and cross the blood-brain barrier. These SCAA's such as phenylalanine, tryptophan, and tyrosine act as weak neurotransmitters and compete with regular neurotransmitters.

Hypokalemia, alkalosis, sedation, and *gastrointestinal bleeding* are common precipitants of PSE. They induce PSE by the following mechanisms:

1. Hypokalemia results in a shift of potassium from the cells to the extracellular fluid in exchange for sodium and hydrogen. The shift of hydrogen ion decreases the H ion concentration in the extracellular fluid and increases that within cells. The change in pH increases the formation of ammonia NH_3 in the extracellular fluids from ammonia NH_4. NH_3 is gaseous and crosses readily into cells where it exerts its toxic effects and where it may become trapped as nondiffusible NH_4.

2. Alkalosis, from any cause, results in an increased formation of NH_3 in extracellular fluids, as described above.

3. In PSE, there is increased sensitivity to depressants, and any hypoxic insult or sedation may precipitate PSE.

4. Blood in the intestines increases the protein content, ammonia formation by bacteria, and ammonia absorption into the portal vein.

When one or more of these conditions exist, the nurse should institute intense monitoring for PSE. Treatment for PSE may be started when the earliest signs are detected. Table 30-7 presents the stages of progression in impaired consciousness, intellectual behavior, and neurologic changes.

Assessment

SUBJECTIVE DATA

The patient's description of complaints or symptoms and course of illness yields useful data for the nurse who is planning care for the patient with liver disease. Among the potential symptoms, the following are explored:

1. Level of fatigue and amount of rest needed
2. Extent of pruritus and measures used to relieve it
3. Severity of anorexia; food intake patterns and likes and dislikes
4. Nausea or vomiting
5. History of ankle edema or ascites
6. Changes noted in mood, alertness, and mental ability
7. Pain: onset, location, measures used to relieve it
8. Episodes of bleeding, lightheadedness, or syncope
9. Known allergies or toxic agents

When viral hepatitis is a potential medical diagnosis, the past history often contributes clues as to the time and type of contact (blood or sera, polluted water, food, shellfish, and so on). The past history is also vital in determining the injurious agent in toxic hepatitis. The patient's de-

Common manifestations of liver disease

Ascites and edema
Bleeding tendencies
Esophageal varices with gastrointestinal bleeding
Malnutrition
Jaundice
Portal system encephalopathy (hepatic coma)

scription of the course of illness in chronic hepatitis or cirrhosis can be helpful in giving the nurse insight into the patient's understanding of the disease, its prognosis, and whether the patient believes there is control over its progress.

When alcohol ingestion is a factor, data from the patient should include the patient's knowledge of the effect of the alcohol and the person's desire to abstain from drinking (see Chapter 13).

■ OBJECTIVE DATA

A thorough physical assessment is required on admission to obtain data for baseline comparisons. There is a possibility that any of the manifestations listed in the box above will be present in a patient with a liver disease; in the patient with cirrhosis, these manifestations will be chronic in nature and subject to progressive worsening.

The patient with liver dysfunction can deteriorate rapidly, and many factors can depress liver function. It is helpful to have the same nurse responsible for documenting changes in mental functioning that can occur as liver dysfunction worsens (see the box below).

Asterixis (liver flap) is a characteristic sign elicited by asking the patient to dorsiflex the wrist while the arm is extended. The patient's hand has a peculiar flapping tremor. *Fetor hepaticus* is a sweet but fetid breath odor. Asterixis, fetor hepaticus, and decreasing consciousness indicate progressing portal system encephalopathy.

Ascites and peripheral edema are monitored by daily

Parameters of mental functioning

Attention span
Ability to concentrate
Irritability
Apathy
Restlessness
Writing patterns
Speech patterns
Level of consciousness

measurements of the abdomen and extremities. All patients with abdominal wounds or bleeding tendencies are monitored for signs of internal hemorrhage (shock).

When caring for the patient with liver disease, the nurse should make ongoing observations about each of the following:

1. Body weight
2. Vital signs
3. Intake and output
4. General appearance: muscle mass, nutritional status, color of skin and sclera
5. Mental status
6. Breath sounds and respiratory effort
7. Abdomen, including abdominal girth
8. Skin: color, presence of spider angiomas, bleeding sites, excoriations, palmar erythema
9. Extremities: edema
10. Color of urine and stools

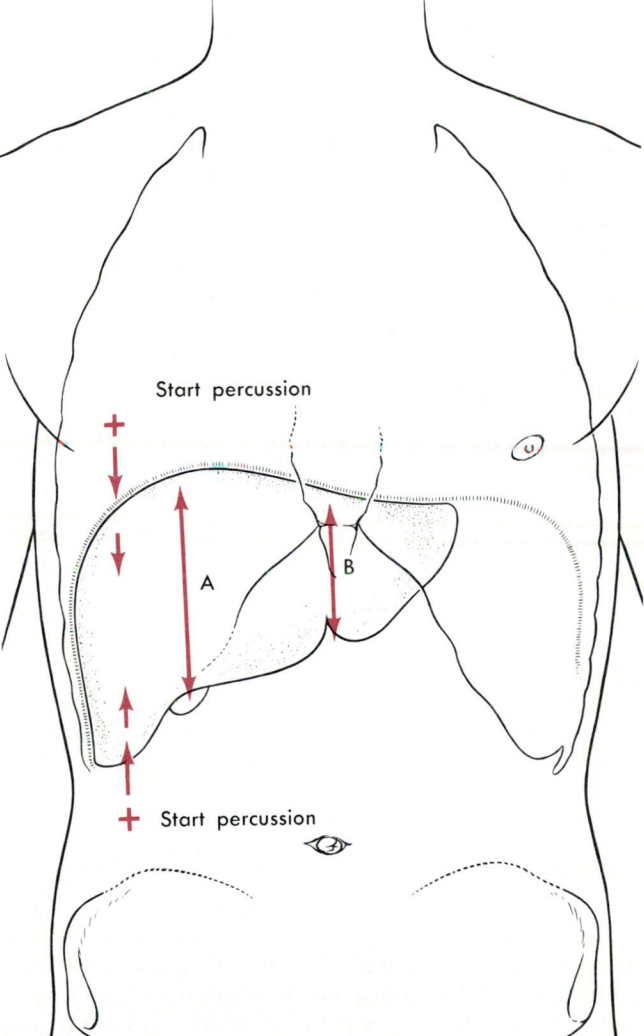

Fig. 30-8 Percussion of liver. Vertical span of liver dullness should measure approximately 6 to 12 cm at midclavicular line, *A*, and 4 to 8 cm at midsternal line, *B*.

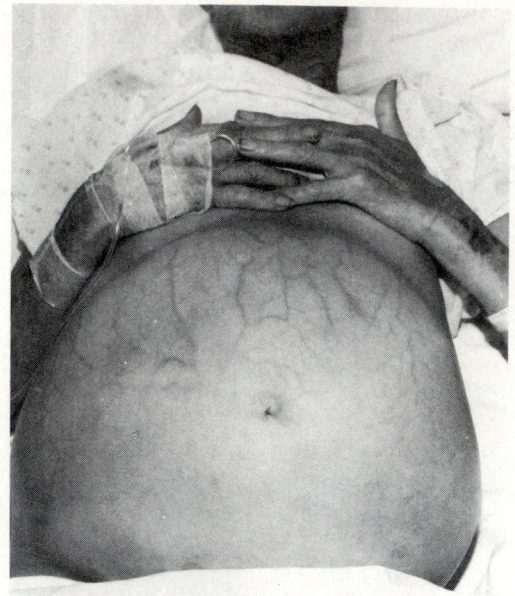

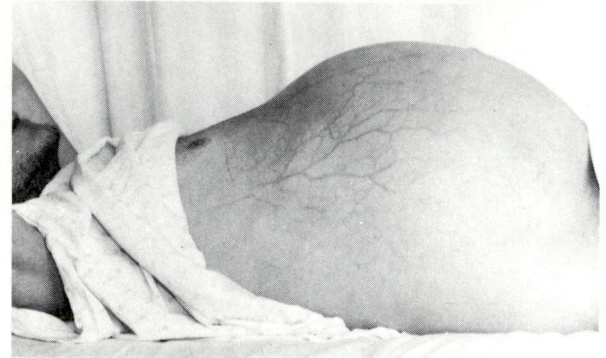

Fig. 30-9 Massive ascites. Note bulging flanks, dilated upper abdominal veins, and everted umbilicus (From Prior, JA, Silberstein, JS, and Stang, JM: Physical diagnosis: the history and examination of the patient, ed 6, St. Louis, 1981, The CV Mosby Co.)

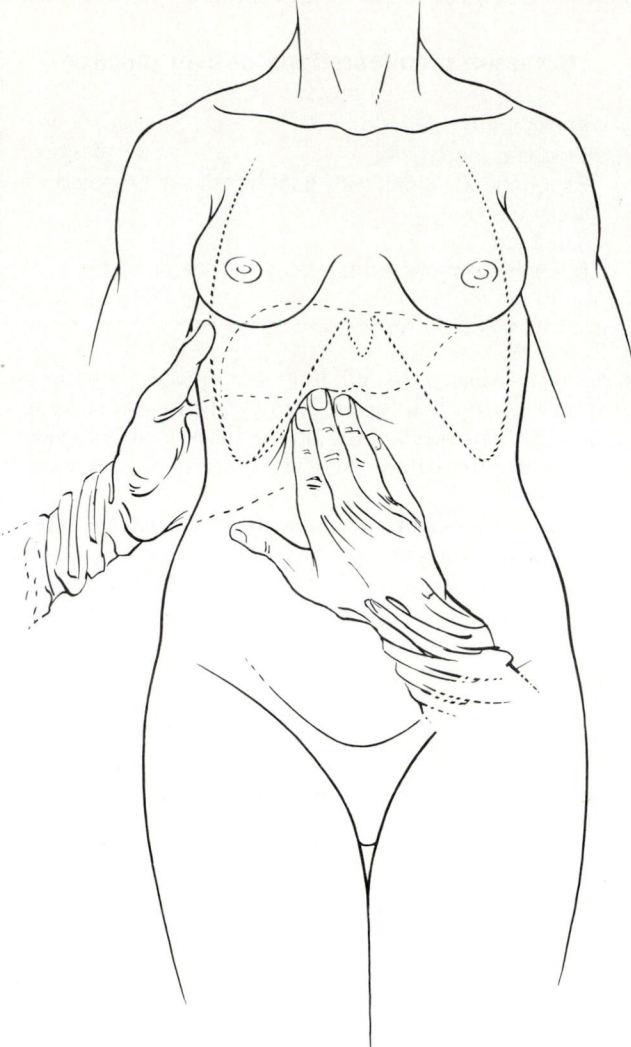

Fig. 30-10 Correct placement of hands for palpating liver.

□ Examination of the liver

The liver may be examined while the abdomen is examined. The abdomen is first observed for the following signs:

1. Striae caused by stretching of skin with ascites
2. Engorged veins caused by obstruction of portal flow
3. Abdominal distention caused by ascites

Auscultation of the abdomen for bowel sounds is done before percussion or palpation. To percuss the liver, start at an area below the umbilicus in the midclavicular line and percuss upward until dullness is heard. Then start at about the fourth intercostal space, midclavicular line, and percuss downward. The vertical span of liver dullness should be approximately 6 to 12 cm in width. If this percussion reveals an enlarged liver, the liver can be percussed in the same manner at the midsternal line. At this point

it normally is 4 to 6 cm in width (Fig. 30-8). Lung consolidation or right pleural effusion can obscure the upper border dullness, while gas in the colon can obscure the lower border dullness.

Percussion is also used to check for the presence of *shifting dullness*. Ascites causes dullness and bulging of flanks when the patient is supine (Fig. 30-9); tympany may be found centrally. If the patient is turned to the side, the bulging and dullness is shifted to the dependent side.

While the patient is lying supine, the abdomen can be examined for presence of a *fluid wave*. In performing this test, the edge of the patient's hand is placed on the midline abdomen to prevent transmission of wave through abdominal wall. One hand of the examiner is placed on the patient's right flank and the opposite hand sharply strikes the left flank. A sharp wave will be felt by the examiner's hand in the presence of a significantly large amount of fluid (ascites).

The liver may also be palpated by deep palpation (Fig. 30-10). The liver edge, if palpable, presents a firm, sharp, regular ridge with a smooth surface. It is considered abnormal when felt more than 1 cm below the costal margin.

■ DIAGNOSTIC TESTS

Multiple tests may be necessary to determine the extent and seriousness of hepatic disease. Some of the laboratory tests are listed in Tables 30-8 and 30-9. Additional studies may include abdominal films, barium swallow and barium enema, and endoscopic examinations. The diagnostic workup will frequently include one or several tests for examination of the biliary tract (p. 1032).

☐ Liver biopsy

Biopsy of the liver presents the risk of hemorrhage because of the vascularity of the liver and the bleeding tendencies that often occur with liver disease. The procedure may be open or closed. The open procedure is done in the operating room, and the usual preoperative procedure is required.

The closed procedure is often done in the patient's bed. This procedure is contraindicated if the patient has an infection of the right lower lobe of the lung, ascites, or a blood dyscrasia, or is unable to cooperate by holding a breath. The procedure consists of inserting a specially designed needle through the chest or abdominal wall into the liver and removing a small piece of tissue for study. Movement by the patient may tear the liver covering. No physical preparation is necessary for a closed procedure but written consent is usually required and food and fluids may be withheld after midnight the night before (see the box on p. 1016).

→ Data analysis: nursing diagnoses

Nursing diagnoses are determined from assessment of patient data. Possible nursing diagnoses for the person with diseases of the liver may include, but are not limited to, the following (see p. 1017):

Table 30-8 Laboratory tests of liver function with possible changes in hepatocellular and biliary disease

Test	Normal	Hepatocellular disease	Biliary disease
Fat metabolism			
Serum total cholesterol	150-250 mg/dl	Decreased	Increased
Cholesterol ester	70%	Decreased	Decreased
Serum phospholipids	150-380 mg/dl	Decreased	Increased
Protein metabolism			
Total serum protein	6-8 g/dl	May be normal	
Albumin	3.2-4.5 g/dl	Decreased	
BUN	10-20 mg/dl	Varies	
Serum prothrombin time	12-15 sec	Increased	Increased
Blood ammonia	< 75 μg/dl	Increased	
Bilirubin metabolism			
Total bilirubin	0.1-1.0 mg/dl	Increased	Increased
Conjugated (direct)	0.1-0.3 mg/dl	Increased	Increased
Unconjugated (indirect)	0.2-0.8 mg/dl	Increased	
Urine bilirubin	None	Increased	Increased
Urine urobilinogen	0.1-1.0 Ehrlich U/dl	Increased	Decreased
Fecal urobilinogen	90-280 mg/day		Decreased
Serum enzymes			
SGOT	5-40 IU/L	Increased (nonspecific)	
Serum glutamic pyruvic transaminase (SGPT)	5-35 IU/L	Increased	
Lactic dehydrogenase (LDH)	90-200 IU/L	Increased (nonspecific)	
Gamma-glutamyl transpeptidase (GGT)	Men: 10-38 IU/L Women: 5-25 IU/L	Increased	
Alkaline phosphatase	30-85 IU/L	Increased (slightly)	Increased
Excretory function			
Bromsulphalein (BSP excretion)	< 5% retained after 45 min	Increased	

Table 30-9 Diagnostic tests used in hepatic diseases

Procedure	Preparation	Interpretation

Radioisotope scanning
  ^{131}I rose bengal
  ^{99}Tc colloidal technetium
  ^{67}Ga gallium citrate
  Risa^{131} radioionated serum albumin
  ^{198}Au colloidal gold
  ^{99}TC-HIDA
	Injection of radioisotope
	A scintillosope detects, amplifies, and records radiation
	No preparation necessary except for ^{67}Ga, for which enema and laxatives will be ordered to prevent absorption by GI tract
		The liver will be outlined by radioisotope scanning techniques to help identify tumors, cysts and abscesses (Fig. 30-11); hepatocellular abscesses and carcinomas show as areas of heavy radioactivity with ^{67}Ga; decreased areas of radioactivity usually are those of nonfunctioning tissue

Ultrasonic hepatography (liver ultrasound)	Preparation includes enema and/or laxatives and sometimes dietary preparation to decrease intestinal gas (low carbohydrate, no carbonated beverages); barium studies should be done after ultrasonic exams or 48 hours before	Use of sound waves to bombard liver and surrounding areas; images caused by differences in sounds reflected by solid tissue, air-filled cavities, and fluid-filled cavities; can help in determining focal or diffuse liver disease
Computerized axial tomography (CAT scan)	No preparation needed; patient must lie still Sometimes dye studies of the biliary system are done at the same time; barium studies should be done after CT scan	Use of CAT scan is becoming more available and provides radiographic visualization of liver and surrounding structures; a computer handles the complex calculations used to analyze the multiple images of serial sections of tissue
Angiography (catheterization of hepatic artery, portal venous system vein)	Preparation includes fasting and obtaining written consent; check for previous reactions to contrast media	The contrast medium provides visualization of the vascular supply of the liver and presence of masses, bleeding, and collateral circulation
Wedged hepatic vein pressure (WHVP) and portal vein pressure	This test may be done with angiography	The degree of portal hypertension can be determined
Percutaneous transhepatic cholangiography	Preparation includes fasting (up to 8 hours); written consent is required; explain that tilting of table will occur and patient must be securely fastened on table; check for previous reactions to contrast media	The contrast medium is directly inserted into biliary ducts and allows visualization of the biliary tree

---

Liver biopsy

1. *Preprocedure*
   a. Explain procedure to patient
   b. Explain need to hold breath during the procedure; help patient practice holding breath and maintaining a sustained exhalation
   c. Report inability of patient to hold breath on command
   d. Give vitamin K as prescribed
2. *Postprocedure*
   a. Maintain bedrest for prescribed period (8 to 24 hours)
   b. Turn patient on *right* side for first few hours with pillow placed under the right side for pressure on liver
   c. Monitor patient
      (1) First hour
         (a) Observe site for hemorrhage every 15 minutes
         (b) Monitor vital signs every 15 minutes
      (2) Up to 24 hours, take vital signs hourly
      (3) Report signs of hemorrhage (increased pulse, decreased blood pressure, cold clammy skin) and peritonitis (increased temperature, pain in lower abdomen)
   d. Provide analgesics as prescribed for mild right upper quadrant or right shoulder pain

Diagnostic title	Possible etiologies
Activity intolerance	Generalized weakness, fatigue
Ineffective breathing pattern	Ascites, neuromuscular impairment, coma
Decreased cardiac output: potential	Potential for hemorrhage and fluid deficit in response to diuretic therapy
Fluid volume excess or deficit	Compromised regulatory mechanisms, inappropriate fluid or sodium intake
Potential for infection	Decreased immune response, pruritis, skin lacerations, intrusive procedures
Potential for injury: falls	Sensory/perceptual deficits, tremors, weakness, impaired cognition
Knowledge deficit: blood/body fluid precautions	Lack of exposure
Altered nutrition: less than body requirements	Anorexia
Pain: pruritis and discomfort	Jaundice, ascites, right upper quadrant distention, improper positioning

⌐ Planning: expected patient outcomes

Expected patient outcomes for the person with hepatic dysfunction may include, but are not limited to, the following:

1. Patient will demonstrate one increase in self-care ability each day.
2. Patient has normal breath sounds and a normal chest x-ray examination.
3. Patient does not develop undetected bleeding and/or hypotension.
4. Patient states that itching is reduced and has no skin lacerations.
5. Patient does not develop undetected oliguria or exceed 1 kg loss of body weight per day.
6. Patient does not develop any new infections and temperature remains at normal level.
7. Patient does not fall or suffer injury.
8. By discharge the patient can give detailed description about ways to manage diuretic therapy, water restriction, and alcohol abstinence.
9. By discharge the patient eats at least 200 g of carbohydrate foods per day.
10. By discharge the patient can explain the disorder and relationships to relevant symptoms and treatment.
11. By discharge the patient is able to describe plans for self-care (activity, rest and sleep, wound care if surgery performed).
12. By discharge the patient can describe signs and symptoms to be reported to physician.
13. If alcoholic, the patient is able to make conscious decision about the use of services such as Alcoholics Anonymous by discharge.

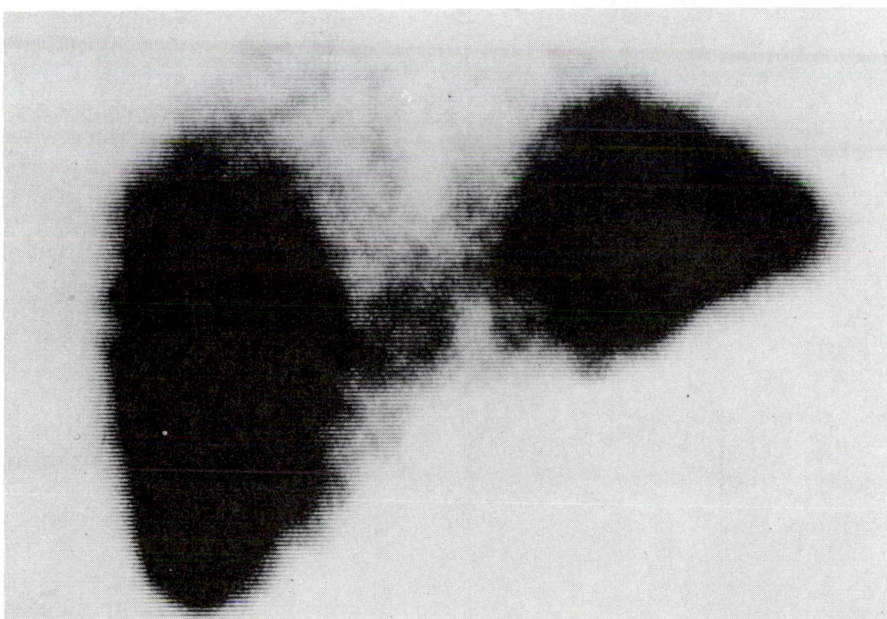

Fig. 30-11 Liver scan showing metastasis to liver (light area on right) of carcinoma of colon. (Courtesy Abbas M Rejali, MD, Department of Radiology, Case Western Reserve University, Cleveland, Ohio.)

▣ Implementation

A wise nurse considers the patient with hepatic disease to have multisystem disorders, to be immunosuppressed, and to be at risk for fluid and electrolyte imbalances, hemorrhage, infections, and coma. Thus, regardless of the specific diagnosis or severity of distress, the nurse should institute a monitoring schedule that ensures early detection of at least those clinical findings listed in the box below.

The frequency of monitoring depends on the current status of the patient, the medical diagnosis, and the estimation of risk. For example, the patient who is actively bleeding from liver trauma or esophageal varices requires continuous monitoring, preferably in an intensive care unit. In contrast, the patient who has bleeding tendencies because of a mild increase in prothrombin time may be monitored by routine vital signs, daily *guaiac* tests for occult blood in the stool, and daily partial prothrombin time and hematocrit.

Institution of new therapeutic agents, a change in therapy (dosage of medication, amount of food, or fluid intake), or the onset of complications necessitates review of the monitoring plan to assess its adequacy.

Priorities in monitoring schedule

Fluid and electrolyte problems

Ascites
Edema
Oliguria
Hypotension

Hemorrhage

Gastrointestinal bleeding
Hypotension
Tachycardia

Infection

Fever
Tachycardia
Abnormal breath sounds
Chills
Malaise
Cloudiness of body fluids

PSE (see Table 30-7)

Mental status impairment
Change in sleep pattern, mood, behavior, perceptual ability
Lethargy
Slurred speech
Incoordination

■ ASSISTING WITH ACHIEVEMENT OF THERAPEUTIC GOALS

Rest, nutrition, and absence of toxin use are principal treatments for patients with liver disorders. Before the nurses' role in implementing these treatments is discussed, this section will discuss other treatments for specific hepatic lesions or dysfunctions.

▢ Medications

The drugs to be described are antimicrobial, chemotherapeutic, immunosuppressive, and antipruritic agents. Diuretics and drugs used to treat bleeding and PSE will be discussed later.

▢ *Antimicrobials*

The nurse will be involved in the administration of antimicrobials to patients with bacterial infections of the liver (liver abscess, wound infections). The specific antibiotic therapy is based on culture and sensitivity studies of material obtained by percutaneous or surgical aspirations of the abscess or on studies of wound drainage. Blood cultures are usually done to determine if septicemia is present. Anaerobic organisms alone or in combination with aerobic organisms account for 50% of liver abscesses; common organisms are *Escherichia coli*, *Klebsiella*, and *Staphylococcus aureus*.[4] Appropriate broad-spectrum antibiotics may be administered for 4 to 6 weeks to a patient with pyogenic liver abscess. Surgical drainage of the abscess is also frequently necessary. See Chapter 11 for details about administration of antibiotics.

Because patients with liver dysfunction may be immunosuppressed, they are subject to a variety of infections including superinfections and nosocomial infections. Therefore, the nurse may be involved in the administration of antibiotics to patients with liver disease who have infections of the urinary tract, pneumonia, peritonitis, or other infections. There is no antimicrobial therapy for hepatitis. The patient with amoebic abscess is treated with amebicidal agents (see Table 30-3). Usually surgery is not done. Medication therapy must be prolonged; for example, metronidazole (Flagyl), 750 mg, might be ordered orally, three times a day for 5 to 10 days followed by diiochohydroxyquin (Diodoquin), 650 mg, three times a day for 20 days. Intravenous administration of metronidazole may also be used. Reconstituted vials of this medication should not be refrigerated and should be used within 96 hours. This drug may cause a reddish-brown color to the urine, gastrointestinal distress (nausea, diarrhea, abdominal cramps, and dizziness). A psychotic episode may be precipitated if metronidazole is combined with alcohol intake or disulfiram.

▢ *Chemotherapy*

Chemotherapy is used to induce regression of primary and metastatic lesions of the liver, it may be part of the overall treatment. Although radiation therapy may be used occasionally to control pain; it is palliative and it does not contribute to survival.[36] Surgical treatment may include

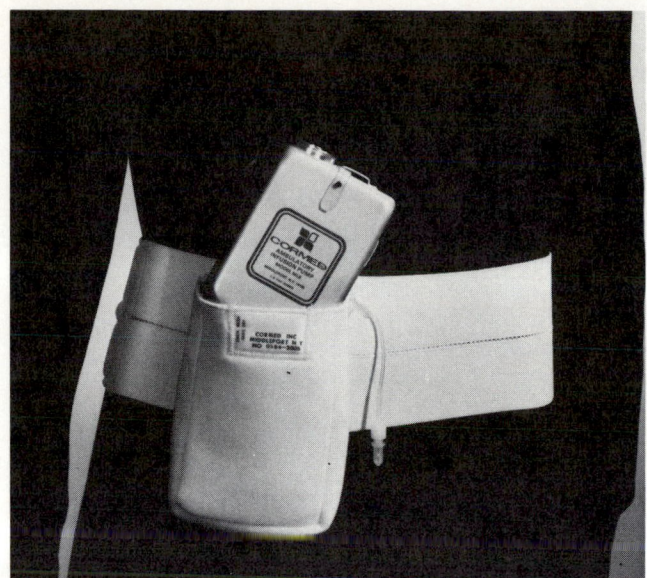

Fig. 30-12 Lightweight, battery-operated infusion pump for ambulatory patient. Flow rate adjustable. Power pack operates for 7 days before needing recharging. (Courtesy CORMED, Inc., Middleport, NY.)

resection (up to 90%), or, in some centers, total removal and transplantation. For many hepatic tumors, the lesion is too far advanced for any treatment other than supportive therapy. Medical interventions are directed toward management of pain, ascites, and other physical problems that arise.

5-Fluorouracil (5-Fu) and doxorubicin (Adriamycin) have been used as single drug therapy. Combination chemotherapy with 5-Fu and 1.3 bis-2 chloroethyl-1-nitrosurea (BCNU), methyl CCNU, or streptozotocin have also been tried.

Chemotherapeutic agents have been given intravenously or by infusion into the hepatic artery by a surgically implanted percutaneous catheter. The catheter can be attached to a pressurized infusion system or an external pump[25] (see Fig. 30-12). Or, the catheter and a continuous drug delivery device are surgically implanted; this method has been more recently developed[41] (see Fig. 30-13). The implantable delivery system allows the patient to be treated at home and is associated with fewer complications than external delivery systems.[24,41] See the box on p. 1020 for characteristics of the Infusaid pump.

There are many care requirements for the patient who is receiving chemotherapy via hepatic artery perfusion. For the patient with an external device, mobility is limited. (Bed rest is mandatory if the femoral artery is the site of catheter insertion.) Catheter care must be meticulous: cleansing and dressing of the insertion site, monitoring for catheter breaks, leaks, dislodgement, clotting and bleeding or infection at the site. All tubing must be securely attached and positioned so as to avoid tension on it. A hemostat should be kept at the bedside to clamp the tubing if it becomes disconnected from the pump or external system. See Chapter 12 for information about the administration of chemotherapeutic agents including precautions for nurses to use in handling them.

□ *Cholestyramine (Questran, Cuemid)*

Cholestyramine may be prescribed because it increases fecal excretion of bile acids and thus reduces pruritus. It is an ion-exchange resin and acts by absorbing intestinal bile salts and combining them to form an insoluble and nonabsorbable complex. The usual dosage is 4 g three times a day before meals and before bedtime. One to three weeks may be needed to develop full antipruritic effect. Diarrhea or constipation may occur.

This medication should not be given with other drugs, since it binds (inactivates) acids. Gastric distress, constipation, skin reactions, and bleeding tendencies have been

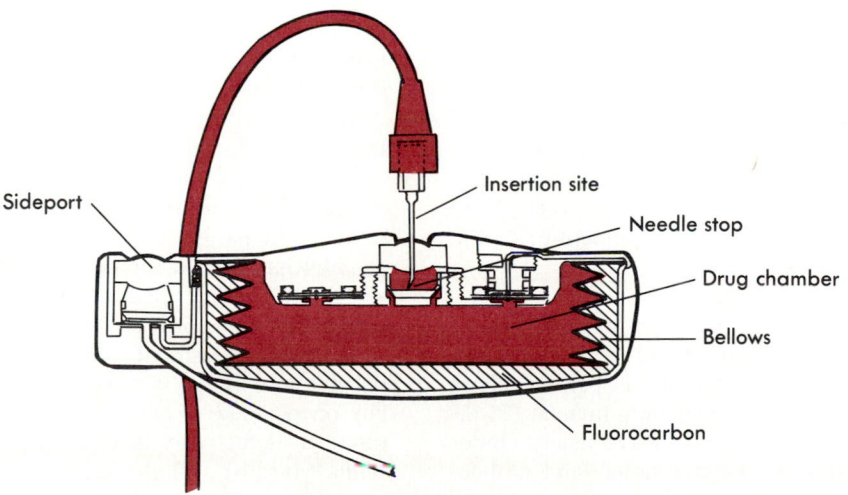

Fig. 30-13 Infusaid pump.

Characteristics of Infusaid pump

1. The pump has two chambers: one for the drug solution and one that contains a fluorocarbon fluid.
2. The two chambers are separated by a flexible metal bellows.
3. The drug reservoir has a capacity of approximately 50 ml (model 400) and is refilled every 2 weeks by percutaneous injection into a special insertion site with the use of a special needle.
4. The fluorocarbon is temperature sensitive and converts from a liquid to vapor at body temperature.
5. The vapor exerts pressure on the bellows, forcing the drug solution from its reservoir into the catheter. This occurs at a constant preset rate, and typically 2 to 3 ml/day of solution is delivered.
6. *Drug dosage* is controlled by manipulating the concentration of the chemotherapeutic agent.
7. The fluorocarbon vapor is reliquefied as the drug chamber is refilled; vaporization again occurs, and the next dosage is delivered.

Instructions regarding self-care for patients with implanted pumps

1. Avoid deep-sea diving, mountain climbing, or long-distance airplane trips. These activities change atmospheric pressure and can change vaporization of the fluorocarbon and thus the delivery rate.
2. Monitor body temperature daily, and report elevations immediately.
3. Avoid long hot baths, saunas, and spas. These can change the flow rate.
4. Avoid contact sports because they can damage the pump.
5. Wear a Medic Alert bracelet or necklace that states that you have an implantable pump and give information such as physician's name.
6. Return for follow-up case as prescribed—usually every 2 weeks.
7. Contact nurse/physician/outpatient department any time questions arise.
8. Other instructions are individualized and concern side effects of the specific chemotherapeutic agents that need to be monitored for and reported.

From Gullatte, M, and Foltz, AT: Hepatic chemotherapy via implantable pump, Am J Nurs 83:1674-1676, 1983.

noted with prolonged treatment. Vitamin K and other fat-soluble vitamins may have to be given intramuscularly for absorption.

☐ *Immune suppressive agents*

Although immune suppression is often present in patients with liver disease, there are at least four instances in which immunosuppressive agents are used:
1. Liver transplantation
2. Reduction of fibrosis in healing process in some conditions
3. Fulminant viral hepatitis
4. In some cases of chronic hepatitis

Agents used are: azathioprine and/or cyclophosphamide, corticosteroids, antilymphocyte globulin (ALG) and cyclosporin A. The combination of prednisone and cyclosporin A has been reported to have shown improvement in patient survival after transplantation.[48]

☐ Reduction of edema and ascites

Edema and ascites are typically found in patients with cirrhosis; however, they may occur in any patient whose liver dysfunction results in (1) hypoalbuminemia; (2) dilutional hyponatremia; and (3) portal hypertension. Under these circumstances, diuresis occurs slowly and is more difficult to accomplish than it would be in a patient with a normal serum colloidal pressure, a normal serum sodium to water ratio, and relatively similar hydrostatic pressures

in portal and systemic venous circulations (see p. 1003).

Sodium restriction and bed rest are usually the first approach to reducing edema. These measures and an adequate diet often result in a spontaneous diuresis that reflects improved hepatic function. The amount of sodium restriction may be based on 24-hour urinary excretion of sodium but is generally not less than 1 g daily. The lack of salt in food makes it less palatable, and the patient may not consume adequate protein and calories. Inadequate intake is reported to the physician and dietitian since adjustments may need to be made in sodium restriction. Salt substitutes may be permitted.

A second intervention that may be used, if hyponatremia is present, is fluid restriction. Fluids may be restricted to as little as 500 ml/day and will usually not exceed 1500 ml/day. The fluid restriction may affect the patient's food intake. The patient is encouraged to assist in planning the distribution of fluid intake. It is not unusual for fluid and sodium to be restricted and bed rest continued when diuretic therapy is ordered.

Nursing assessments to monitor fluid and electrolyte balance in patients with edema or ascites are listed in the box on p. 1021. These assessment measures enable the nurse to detect the onset of hypokalemia, oliguria, azotemia, and PSE (all of which are complications of diuresis in patients with liver dysfunction and are related to excess fluid and potassium losses).

Ascites cannot be mobilized at rates greater than 900

Assessment for patients with edema or ascites

Daily weights
Intake and output
Measurement of abdominal girth
Blood pressure
Mental status

---

mg/day (approximately 2 lb/day of weight loss).[40] Hypovolemia can occur if amounts greater than this are diuresed (unless peripheral edema is contributing the additional fluid). Azotemia and oliguria result from decreased renal perfusion in hypovolemic states. PSE may be precipitated by azotemia, hypovolemia, and hypokalemia.

□ Diuretic therapy

Furosemide (Lasix) alone or with spironolactone (Aldactone) is commonly used to promote diuresis in persons with hepatic dysfunction. Spironolactone provides the benefit of retention of potassium along with the excretion of sodium.

Potassium supplements are often prescribed along with the furosemide and, at times, may be necessary for the patient treated with spironolactone. The nurse should monitor the patient's potassium level and be alert for signs of potassium imbalance (see Chapter 8).

Infusions of salt-poor albumin in 25 g units may be given to promote the effectiveness of diuretic measures. These infusions expand the blood volume, thus, increasing renal blood flow and serum osmotic pressure. They may also decrease the risk of oliguria, azotemia, and encephalopathy. Albumin is administered slowly (4 to 6 hours) daily for brief periods. Its effects are short-term and protein loss into the ascitic fluid continues. Albumin is very viscous and must be infused with a large-bore needle, such as a No. 18. It is often used to improve the patient status during acute crises or to prepare the patient for surgery. The administration of salt-poor albumin may expand the blood volume rapidly. During and following administration, the patient is monitored carefully for signs of pulmonary edema.

□ Paracentesis

A peritoneal tap may be done to obtain fluid for laboratory study but paracentesis places the patient at risk for complications such as shock, hypovolemia, azotemia and encephalopathy. Although once a standard mode of therapy, paracentesis is now used with caution and usually only as a last resort in patients with severe and chronic liver disease.

If the abdomen is taut with fluid and is producing dyspnea and anorexia, paracentesis may be necessary. In general, only small amounts of fluid are removed; this de-creases the risk of rapid fluid shifts and additional protein loss. One liter of ascitic fluid contains as much protein as 200 ml of whole blood. Salt-poor human blood albumin may be administered following this procedure to counteract the shift of fluid and protein into the peritoneal cavity.

□ Peritoneojugular shunt

In chronic and resistant ascites caused by cirrhosis, a LeVeen peritoneojugular shunt (PJS) may be used. The LeVeen PJS allows for the continuous reinfusion of ascitic fluid back into the venous system through a silicone catheter with a one-way pressure sensitive valve. One end of the catheter is implanted in the peritoneal cavity, and the tube is channeled through subcutaneous tissue to the superior vena cava where the other end is implanted. The valve opens when there is a pressure differential greater than 3 mm of water between the abdominal cavity and the thoracic vein, allowing fluid to move from the peritoneal cavity into the superior vena cava.

Persons treated with the LeVeen PJS may also receive furosemide therapy, and the two together have been successful in relieving ascites in some patients. Persons who have a LeVeen PJS may still have severe problems, including disseminated intravascular coagulation, bleeding varices, and congestive failure.[41]

A modification of the PJS, the Denver shunt, is sometimes used when ascites is marked and is the result of malignancy. Malignant ascites may contain a lot of particulate matter that can stop the flow of ascitic fluid through the tubing. The Denver shunt has a subcutaneous pump that can be compressed manually to irrigate the tubing. Increased comfort and improvement of renal and respiratory function have been reported.[31]

When shunts are first implanted and functioning, there can be dramatic changes such as hemodilution of intravascular fluid, decrease in abdominal girth, and increased renal output. As peritoneal fluid is removed, less of a pressure gradient exists between the peritoneal fluid and the jugular vein. To force the valve open, deep breathing is encouraged at regular intervals with the patient in supine position.

□ Control of bleeding

Bleeding tendencies or actual hemorrhage is common in patients with liver disorders. See p. 1002 for the specific factors that may decrease coagulation ability in hepatocellular or biliary tract disease. Also, see p. 1011 for the reason that dilated hemorrhoidal, gastric, and esophageal veins are frequent sites of bleeding when portal hypertension is present.

Gastrointestinal bleeding is not uncommon in patients with jaundice and/or portal hypertension. Patients with cirrhosis or recent alcohol intake may have bleeding from gastritis or peptic ulcers, as well as from hemorrhoidal or esophageal venous rupture.

Bleeding may also be prolonged in tissue injury and in surgical wounds. Assessment measures for bleeding and measures to minimize bleeding are listed in the upper and lower boxes on p. 1022.

Assessment for bleeding

Check the following for bleeding:
  Urine, stool, vomitus, or gastrointestinal drainage
  Mouth
  Wounds
  Skin (for purpura, hematoma, or petechiae)
Monitor vital signs for the following:
  Hypotension
  Postural hypotension
  Tachycardia
Monitor results of the following:
  Prothrombin or partial thromboplastin times
  Platelet count
  Hematocrit level

The nurse assists with specific medical therapies to improve the status of coagulation. A trial of vitamin K (usually daily for 3 days) may be ordered to determine whether the liver is able to manufacture prothrombin when an adequate supply of vitamin K is given. Recall that shunting of blood around the liver or the absence of bile or bacteria in the intestine reduces the supply of vitamin K available to the liver. This will not help if liver cell damage is the cause of reduced prothrombin formation. If this is the case, whole blood or plasma may be given to replace clotting factors at least temporarily. If the patient has a reduced platelet level, platelet transfusion may be given.

Table 30-10 lists the treatment measures used with bleeding esophageal varices. This hemorrhage is often massive and life-threatening; mortality rates are 30% to 60%. Esophagogastric tamponade has been widely used to treat massive hemorrhage; it is accomplished by inserting a special esophagogastric tube (Blakemore-Sengstaken). Esophageal tamponade may be the only specific therapy or

it may be combined with other measures to stop bleeding. These include the following:

1. Intravenous injection of vasopressin (Pitressin), which reduces portal pressure and bloodflow by constricting the splanchnic arterioles and decreasing the blood supply to the liver.
2. Injection of sclerosing solutions into the varices during endoscopy. Sclerosing may be the only treatment used.

Both of these measures have side effects and complications (see the box below), and bleeding may recur after the treatment is completed.

□ *Esophageal tamponade*

The Blakemore-Sengstaken tube is a three-lumen tube with two balloon attachments. One lumen serves as a nasogastric suction tube, the second is used to inflate the gastric balloon, and the third is used to inflate the esophageal balloon (Fig. 30-14). The tube is passed through the

---

Side effects and complications of treatment measures for esophageal bleeding

Vasopressin infusion

Coronary artery vasoconstriction
Abdominal colic
Uterine cramping
Facial pallor
Hypertension

Injection sclerotherapy

Perforated esophagus
Aspiration pneumonia
Pleural effusion
Worsening of ascites
Retrosternal pain

Measures to minimize bleeding

1. Arrange with the laboratory to minimize number of venipunctures.
2. Start IV infusions when blood samples are drawn.
3. Apply pressure for 5 minutes to sites of venipunctures or injections, for 10 minutes to sites of arterial puncture.
4. Suggest patient use a soft toothbrush or cotton swabs for teeth brushing to prevent bleeding gums.
5. Serve the patient with esophageal varices only soft foods (for example, bread rather than toast).
6. Avoid taking temperatures rectally, and use gentle pressure and well-lubricated enema tips if hemorrhoids are present.
7. If injection must be given, use the smallest gauge needle possible.
8. Instruct patient not to strain at stool and to avoid vigorous coughing or blowing of the nose.
9. Avoid clutter in patient's room and give adequate assistance in ambulating to prevent falls.

Fig. 30-14 Blakemore-Sengstaken tube with esophageal and gastric balloons inflated. (Redrawn from Rubber appliances in surgery and therapeutics, Providence RI, Davol, Inc.)

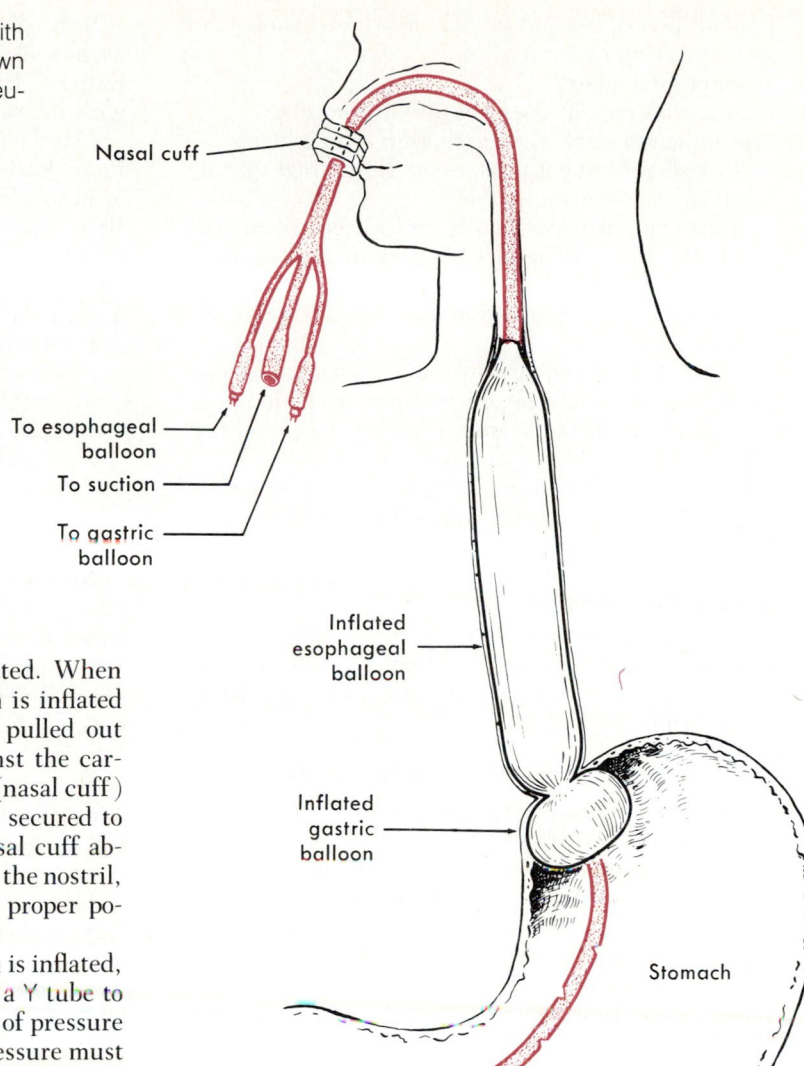

Nasal cuff

To esophageal balloon

To suction

To gastric balloon

Inflated esophageal balloon

Inflated gastric balloon

Stomach

nose into the stomach with the balloons deflated. When the tube is in the stomach, the gastric balloon is inflated and the lumen is clamped; the tube is then pulled out slowly so that the balloon is held tightly against the cardioesophageal junction. A cube of foam rubber (nasal cuff) is placed between the tube and the nares and secured to the face with pressure-sensitive tape. The nasal cuff absorbs excess nasal secretions, reduces trauma to the nostril, and provides traction to maintain the tube in proper position.

If bleeding continues after the gastric balloon is inflated, the esophageal balloon, which is connected by a Y tube to a manometer, is inflated to the desired amount of pressure and then clamped. To stop the bleeding, the pressure must be greater than the patient's portal venous pressure. If bleeding is from esophageal varices, blood will no longer be aspirated from the stomach. If there is still blood present, the stomach may be lavaged with iced saline or a solution of iced alcohol and water may be circulated through the balloon to provide vasoconstriction, as well as pressure.

The nasogastric lumen is usually connected to intermittent gastric suction, which permits easy appraisal of cessation of bleeding and also keeps the stomach empty. It is important to remove all blood from the stomach because the presence of it may precipitate PSE from ammonia produced from the digested blood. Cathartics, antacids, and neomycin or lactulose may be given through the gastric tube with suction temporarily discontinued (20 minutes).

The esophageal balloon can be left inflated up to 48 hours without tissue damage or severe discomfort. The fully inflated gastric balloon with traction exerted on it, however, compresses the stomach wall between the balloon and the diaphragm causing ulceration of the gastric mucosa and severe discomfort. To offset the possibility of necrosis, the physician may release the traction and balloon pressures periodically.

The nurse must stay with the patient while balloons are deflated to secure the tube's position and to detect recurrence of bleeding. Intensive monitoring is also necessary when the balloons are inflated. *Asphyxiation* is a hazard if the inflated esophageal balloon moves into the upper airway. This can happen if the gastric balloon deflates or ruptures and the inflated esophageal balloon moves upward. If this happens, the esophageal balloon is deflated at once and the entire tube is removed.

The nurse will be assisting with therapeutic measures aimed at restoration of blood volume and coagulation factors and the prevention and treatment of PSE.

Nursing care of the patient with esophageal tamponade includes the following:

1. Explain procedure and provide continued support to patient during the procedure.
2. Monitor vital signs.
3. Ensure that patient does not pull at the tube.
4. Provide mouth and nares care every 1 to 2 hours.
   a. Provide patient with tissues, and encourage spitting of saliva into a receptable.
   b. Have patient rinse mouth well to remove any old blood; a Water Pik under low pressure may be used.
   c. Gently suction mouth and throat if patient is weak.
   d. Keep nostrils clean and lubricated with water soluble jelly.
5. Measure and record pressure of esophageal balloon every hour; maintain pressure at prescribed level.
6. Maintain transfusions and infusions at prescribed rate.
7. If iced solutions are used in the balloons, report patient chilling to the physician who may then order a warming blanket.
8. Record intake and output; test gastrointestinal output for occult blood (guaiac).
9. Consult physician concerning permissible patient movement; passive range of motion is usually allowed.
10. Provide comfort measures (for example, rub back, change patient's position).

☐ **Treatment of portal system encephalopathy**

Treatment of PSE centers around finding and treating the precipitating cause (Table 30-5), providing general supportive measures and decreasing ammonia levels (see the box below for common sources of ammonia).

Measures to decrease ammonia levels include the following:
1. Eliminate protein from the diet for several days.
2. Give carbohydrates by mouth or through nasogastric feedings to prevent protein catabolism. At least 200g of carbohydrate should be given in 24 hours.
3. Administer intestinal antibiotics (for example, neomycin) and other agents (such as lactulose) that destroy or alter bacteria in the intestines and subsequently reduce the amount of ammonia absorbed into the blood.
4. Give enemas and cathartics (for example, magnesium sulfate) to empty the bowel and to prevent further ammonia formation.

Sources of ammonia

Exogenous	**Endogenous**
Dietary protein	Azotemia
Whole blood transfusions	Blood in gastrointestinal tract
Ammonium salts	Constipation
Amino acids	Catabolism

Some physicians prefer to rely on cathartics and cation exchange resins to help remove toxins from the bowel rather than to give neomycin or lactulose, which interfere with the manufacture of vitamin K and cause diarrhea.

Many patients with PSE die of renal failure secondary to an inadequate circulating blood volume (hypovolemia) or hepatorenal syndrome (see p. 1003). The treatment of PSE requires careful balancing of fluid administration to maintain adequate perfusion of the kidney without creating an excessive load on the cardiovascular system. Nursing activities include the following:
1. Monitoring desired flow rate very closely.
2. Observing patient for signs of cardiovascular overload (dyspnea, moist respirations, coughing frothy sputum, distended neck veins, restlessness).
3. Monitoring urinary output from indwelling catheter.
4. Monitoring changes in CVP readings that are suggestive of either hypervolemia or hypovolemia.
5. Documenting all fluid losses including diarrhea.

Neomycin (Mycifradin) may be prescribed orally or by rectal instillation. The adult dosage is 4 to 12 g/day. Lactulose is a synthetic disaccharide that is degraded in the lower intestine and acidifies the intestinal lumen.[41] The lowered pH traps ammonia ions (as nondiffusible NH_4), which are then excreted into the stool. The dosage of lactulose syrup (Cephulac) is 30 to 45 ml initially, and as often as hourly until the patient has a bowel movement. Then the dosage is usually lowered to 3 times a day. Lactulose causes a very irritating diarrhea. The skin should be cleansed promptly after each stool.

The patient who has had definite or threatened PSE may be kept indefinitely on a low-protein diet. When protein is added to the diet, it is added gradually and often does not exceed 40 g/day (average intake in the United States is 70 to 80 g/day). In addition, the patient may receive neomycin or lactulose daily. Patients with chronic liver disease may go in and out of PSE; therefore, they are monitored for any change in behavior that would indicate early coma. The patient and family are taught to be alert to subtle changes in the patient's behavior and to seek medical assistance when changes occur.

☐ **Surgery**
☐ *Focal liver disease*

Treatment of liver abscess consists of incision and drainage of the abscess or abscesses and treatment with broad-spectrum antibiotics for pyogenic abscesses. Portal hypertension occurs in rare instances from scarring of the liver as part of the healing process. These patients require close follow-up after discharge from the hospital.

If trauma to the liver has occurred, blood volume replacement is usually required. Emergency surgery may be needed to repair the ruptured liver and local pressure may need to be applied to stop the bleeding. Removal of necrotic tissue may also be indicated, as well as drainage of any bile that may be leaking from the liver surface. The patient may require long-term follow-up to check for signs and symptoms of residual liver damage.

In most instances there is no corrective medical surgical treatment for metastatic or primary carcinoma of the liver because the disease is too far advanced when first diagnosed. Patients are usually alert at this time and will know the prognosis. The patient and family are assisted to live with the prognosis and to do the things they wish to do in the time remaining for the patient (see Chapter 12).

In a few patients with primary tumors, surgery may be possible. If the tumor is limited to a single lobe and there is no evidence of metastases elsewhere, a hepatic lobectomy may be done to remove metastatic as well as primary carcinoma. The remarkable regenerative capacity of the liver permits resection of 70% to 80% of the organ.

Homotransplantation of the liver has been performed in a few medical centers, but the survival rate has been poor. The liver must be transplanted rapidly because of difficulty preserving the organ. Death occurs as a result of rejection or infection secondary to depression of immune response by immunosuppressive therapy. Rapid advances in technology and pharmacologic agents are occurring; however, availability of donor organs and high costs are major limitations.

Hepatic transplantation is done in selected cases of biliary atresia in children and chronic aggressive hepatitis, cirrhosis, and malignancy in adults.[46] Criteria for selection are the following:

1. The person is free of infection.
2. The person is free of coexisting heart disease.
3. Usually, persons selected are no older than 55 years of age.
4. The person is able to meet self-care needs after transplantation.

Organs are obtained from brain-dead donors whose livers are free of disease and who have had adequate maintenance of blood pressure and blood volume. Tissue matching (human lymphocytic antigen) is done; however, transplants have been performed despite the presence in the recipient of cytolytic antibodies against the donor organ and of incompatible blood groups.[46] Both vascular and biliary drainage system reconstruction are necessary.

Complications include rejection, infection, and occlusion of vessels. Measurements of liver function show improvement immediately if a complication does not occur. Immunosuppression is started before surgery and must be continued for life.

□ Portacaval shunts

The only way to achieve permanent lowering of portal pressure is by surgical treatment to reduce bloodflow through the portal system. Fig. 30-15, *A* and *B*, shows two different techniques to decompress the portal vein and one technique, *C,* to decompress the esophageal veins. It must

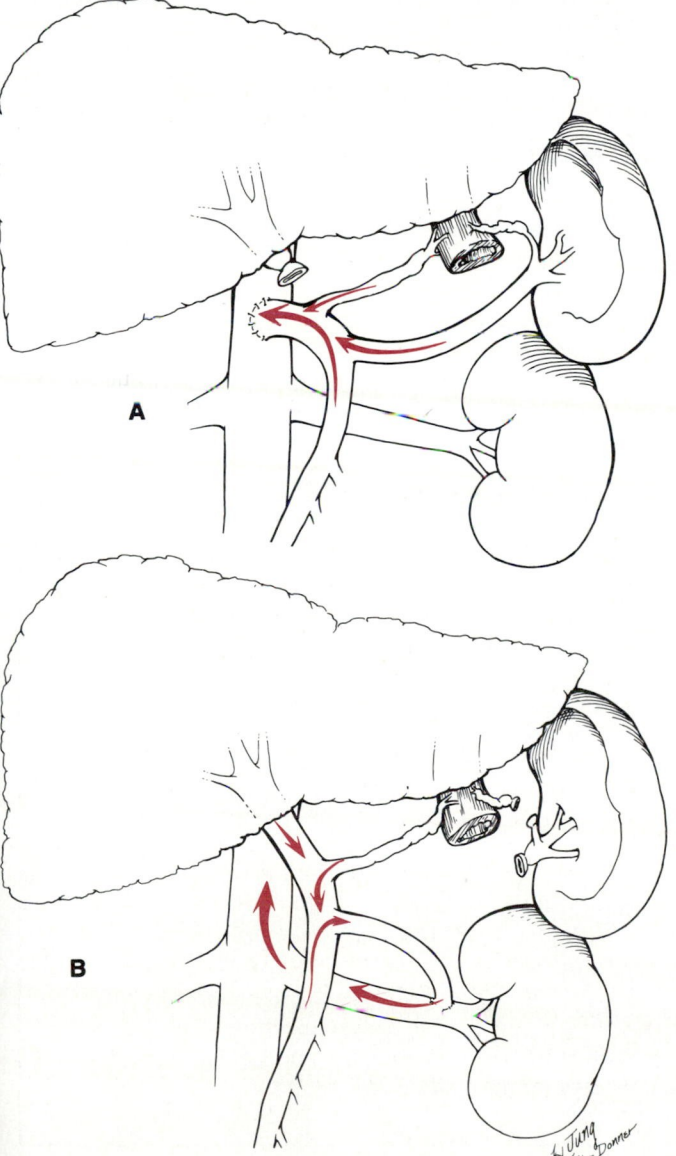
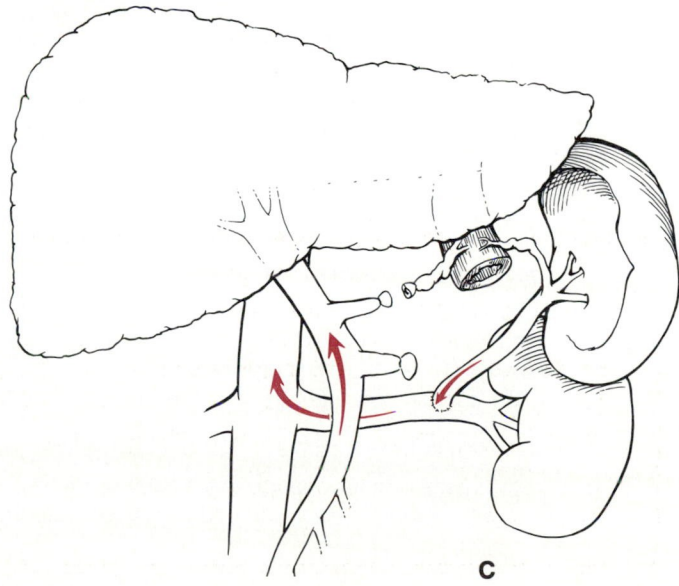

Fig. 30-15 Decompression operations for portal hypertension. **A,** End-to-side portacaval shunt. **B,** Splenorenal shunt. **C,** Distal splenorenal shunt.

be remembered that the patient with liver damage severe enough to cause bleeding esophageal varices is not a good operative risk.

The mortality rate when surgical shunts are used as immediate intervention for bleeding esophageal varices is 50%; it is 10% when performed in well-selected patients with portal hypertension who are not actively bleeding.[9] It is generally believed that a prophylactic shunt is not justified.

Shunts are recommended only when there has been at least one hemorrhage from esophageal varices and all of the following conditions apply:

1. Serum bilirubin level is less than 2 mg/100 ml.
2. Serum albumin is greater than 3.5 g/100 ml.
3. No ascites exist.
4. No neurologic disorder exists.
5. Nutrition is excellent.

The shunts shown in Fig. 30-15 *A* and *B* create a connection between the high-pressure portal system and the low-pressure portal venous system, thereby decompressing the portal system.[46] A major complication is PSE resulting from less venous blood passing through the liver. Nursing care of the patient having liver bypass surgery will be discussed later.

Regional heparization may be employed to prevent thrombosis of the portal vein. A fine polyethylene catheter is inserted into the right gastroepiploic vein during surgery, brought out through the wound, and attached to a continuous drip of heparin and saline solution. The surgeon determines the rate of flow. The catheter must not be obstructed or subjected to tension in any way during the period of insertion, up to 5 to 7 days. If activity is limited during this period, active range of motion of the lower extremities is encouraged.

The nurse assists the patient and family to prepare for surgery of the liver as for any other thoracoabdominal procedure. Special needs are present because of the specific lesion, acuteness of infection or injury, and because of hepatic dysfunction. Surgery, anesthesia, and their resultant changes in hemodynamics or metabolism provide added stress to hepatic function.

The box below summarizes preoperative and postoperative care.

Nursing care of the patient undergoing liver surgery

Preoperative care

1. Assist patients and significant others to cope with anxiety and fear related to trauma or illness, surgery, and unknown outcomes.
2. Institute hemodynamic monitoring as required by severity of shock or hypotension, or risk of these complications (see Chapter 25).
3. Establish baseline data (neurologic, respiratory, renal), and monitor frequently for change in these and for peritonitis.
4. Assist in therapy to improve the patient's physiologic status and to protect the liver from further metabolic insult.
   a. If the prothrombin level is low, vitamin K is given.
   b. If the patient has upper respiratory disease or infection, vigorous respiratory therapy is given; because of the thoracoabdominal approach and postoperative splinting, postoperative atelectasis and pneumonia are frequent complications.
   c. If malnourishment is present, protein hydrolysates are given by total parenteral nutrition (TPN), and blood transfusions and vitamins are given.
   d. Salt-poor albumin may be given to increase blood colloidal pressure and blood volume.
5. Administer antimicrobial (such as neomycin) to rid intestine of bacteria.
6. Avoid sedation and use judicious doses of CNS depressants if hepatic dysfunction is present; chlordiazepoxide (Librium), barbital, or phenobarbital are excreted by the kidney, and thus may be drugs of choice.

If the patient has a **pyogenic abscess**

1. Monitor for signs of rupture of abscess, peritonitis.
2. Control pyrexia by cool sponge baths, antipyretics and cooling blankets.
3. Administer broad spectrum antibiotics as prescribed.
4. Provide comfort measures for chills, fever, and headache.

If the patient has **liver trauma**

1. Monitor intensively for change in hemodynamic, neurologic, and respiratory parameters, and peritonitis.
2. Assist with peritoneal tap, chest tube insertion, and measures used to maintain blood volume

Nursing care of the patient undergoing liver surgery—cont'd

For the patient who has a **portasystemic shunt**

1. Assist in measurement and treatment of edema and ascites and hepatic dysfunction. When hepatic function is poor, coagulation problems, hypoglycemia, hypoalbuminemia, and ammonia excess are common.
2. Assist patient with comfort measures for pruritus and hemorrhoidal pain, and assist with positioning and self-care activities.

Postoperative care

1. Establish schedule for hemodynamic, neurologic, renal, and respiratory monitoring, and for detection of the following:
   a. Hemorrhage, coagulation defects
   b. Hypovolemia, oliguria
   c. Hypoglycemia
   d. Hypoalbuminemia
   e. Infection: wound, subdiaphragmatic
   f. Atelectasis or pneumonia
   g. Fluid and electrolyte imbalance (dilutional hyponatremia, metabolic alkalosis, ascites, edema)
   h. PSE

2. Give prescribed drugs for control of pain observing the same precautions cited under preoperative care.
3. Assist with measures to improve or maintain respiratory function:
   a. Have person cough and deep breathe hourly.
   b. Give respiratory treatments as prescribed.
   c. Change position frequently.
   d. Monitor chest drainage system.
4. Maintain patency and prescribed flow rates of intravenous fluids including blood, plasma, dextran, and parenteral nutrition substances.
5. Maintain patency of gastrointestinal tubes.
6. Nothing by mouth is usually maintained for several days. When food intake is begun, protein intake may be limited and advanced as the patient demonstrates ability to metabolize and excrete protein wastes (BUN, ammonia levels, mental status). Hypoglycemia may occur because of hepatic dysfunction or because of increased insulin capacity from parenteral nutrition.
7. Assist patient with ambulation. This may be slower than after other types of surgery depending on the patient's hemodynamic status. Carefully monitor pulse, blood pressure, and respiratory rate before, during, and after exertion.
8. Maintain asepsis in managing all wounds and insertion sites (cleansing, dressings, and drainage system).
9. Assist patient and family to cope with distress of postoperative period, prolonged and uncertain recovery, and issues related to chronicity, prognosis, and treatment options.
10. Assist with specific therapies, monitoring, and education related to the following:
    a. *Pyogenic abscess*
       (1) Prolonged antimicrobial therapy, recurrence of infection
    b. *Liver trauma*
       (1) Late complications: hemorrhage, cyst and abscess formation, biliary fistulas
    c. *Portasystemic shunts*
       (1) Thrombosis at site of anastomoses: pain, distention, fever, nausea
       (2) Edema in lower extremities: sudden increase in blood flow into vena cava may cause venous congestion
    d. *Peritoneojugular shunt*
       (1) Sudden change from shunting of ascitic fluid into venous system (hemodilution, increased renal output, decrease in abdominal girth)
       (2) Measures to increase shunt's effectiveness
    e. *Transplantation*
       (1) Complications including rejection; infection and need to continue immunosuppressive agents for life

□ Assisting with comfort and ADL

Liver repair and regeneration can be promoted by rest, nutrition, and avoidance of toxins and infection. Rest of the liver can best be provided by decreasing metabolic demands of activity, of infection, of catabolism, and of the stress response.

The physician usually prescribes the desired amounts of rest and activity. In hepatitis, serum enzyme levels may indicate necrosis and may serve as a guide (the higher levels indicate a need for more rest and restricted activity). It is believed that activity and maintaining an upright position decrease hepatic bloodflow, thus preventing optimal circulation to the already compromised liver.[42] Relapses are frequently attributed to premature increases in activity.

Although the physician's prescriptions define whether complete bedrest or some ambulation is allowed, the nurse must use judgment in determining activity levels within these limits. The patient with hepatic dysfunction has overwhelming fatigue and benefits from a paced schedule alternating self-care activities and rest. The schedule should allow rest before meals and before visitation of family. The nurse can use the patient's rating of fatigue and transaminase levels as guide to a graduated increase in activity. As patients recover and acute discomfort recedes, patients may need assistance in finding diversional activities that will dispel boredom, yet not be tiring. Boredom and social isolation are particularly difficult for patients who are placed in isolation. Recurrence of anorexia, enlargement or tenderness of the liver, or lack of progress as indicated by laboratory studies indicate a need to return to bed rest.

There are many sources of discomfort in patients with disorders of the liver. The nurse can promote rest by assisting patients to reduce discomfort by direct physical care measures:

1. Assist patients with ascites to shift position frequently. They often require a high-Fowler's position for ease in breathing. Flotation or air mattresses and a trapeze may be helpful.
2. Provide assistance for acute symptoms of chills, fever, diaphoresis, nausea, vomiting, and diarrhea.
   a. Apply blankets to provide comfort during chills, yet not so many that temperature is increased.
   b. Use tepid sponge baths to lower temperature and apply cool cloths to the forehead.
   c. Change linens or dressings as frequently as necessary.
   d. Provide clean receptacles for emesis and diarrhea and remove them promptly.
   e. Provide quiet, cool, and pleasant environment.
3. Provide measures to decrease pruritus:
   a. Use cool, light, and nonrestrictive clothing and dry, soft bed linens.
   b. Avoid extremes of temperature in baths or compresses.
   c. Avoid stimulating perspiration.
   d. Maintain a cool environment.
   e. Administer prescribed antihistamines or cholostyramine (Cuemid, Questran).
   f. Use distraction to decrease patients' perception of pruritus.

□ Assisting with nutrition

Good nutritional intake is necessary for repair and regeneration of the liver. Rest and nutrition are key treatments for hepatitis, alcoholic lesions of the liver, and cirrhosis. The liver's ability to excrete toxins and to carry on its many other functions may be seriously hampered by inadequate intake of protein and vitamin B. If liver damage has occurred, the organ's ability to store glycogen and vitamins A, B complex, C, and D may also be decreased.

Although fat is a concentrated source of calories, most patients with diffuse liver disorders have some fat intolerance. Oral bile salts may improve the digestion and absorption of fats and fat-soluble vitamins.

A diet high in calories, protein, and vitamins; fairly high in carbohydrates (unless weight reduction is desired); and with moderate amounts of fat is often ordered for patients with liver disease.

A high-protein diet may not be possible if there is potential or actual PSE. In this case, protein restriction becomes necessary. If protein needs to be restricted for some time, the physician may prescribe an enteral or parenteral supplement that has selected BCAAs and a low content of SCAAs. (see p. 1012).

Because alcohol is thought to interfere with hepatic conversion of folic acid to its active metabolites, many persons with cirrhosis have a folic acid deficiency anemia that usually responds well to treatment with oral doses of folic acid. Other nutritional anemias requiring nutritional supplements include vitamin B_{12} and iron deficiency anemias (see Chapter 27).

Anorexia and fatigue interfere with adequate food intake. Although large amounts of food may be prescribed, it is exceedingly difficult for patients to eat these amounts. Foods that are especially high in protein such as meat, fish, poultry, eggs, and dairy products are recommended. The person is often anorexic, and it can become a challenge for the nurse to identify ways to encourage the person to eat the prescribed diet. It is good to remember that the nurse is the health team member who provides this direct assistance to the patient. The following are specific measures to promote nutritional intake:

1. Provide frequent oral hygiene.
2. Provide pleasant atmosphere.
3. Incorporate patient's food preferences.
4. Serve small, frequent feedings.
5. Increase caloric content by adding calories to prepared foods (for example, powdered milk, sauces, butter).
6. Use calorie-rich juices and drinks as fluid allowance, particularly if fluids are restricted.
7. Request use of salt substitutes, herbs, and spices if sodium is restricted.

□ Counseling and teaching

All patients need to be prepared for diagnostic tests, to understand their treatments, and to learn how to imple-

Table 30-10 Teaching content for patients with specific liver disorders

Disorder	Content
Hepatitis	Activity restriction
	Food intake
	Measures to avoid transmission of disease and exposure to toxins
Liver abscess	Long-term compliance with self-administered antimicrobial therapy
	Wound care
	Recurrence of infection; signs to watch for
Liver trauma and surgery	Wound care
Peritoneojugular shunt	Shunt care
	Self-monitoring of abdominal girth and weight
Transplantation	Signs of rejection: fever, tachycardia, enlargement or tenderness of the liver
	Importance of periodic medical tests to detect rejection: serum enzymes, bilirubin, albumin, and clotting times; hepatic perfusion studies (scans)
	Immunosuppression: how to take medication; never to miss a dose; how to monitor for infection or rejection
Cirrhosis	Self monitoring of abdominal girth, ankle edema, body weight, bleeding sites, jaundice
	Compliance and self administration of diuretics: neomycin/lactulose; potassium replacements; fluid, sodium restriction; avoidance of alcohol and other toxins; restriction of activity

ment their therapeutic regimens at home. Patients with chronic hepatic dysfunction need to understand long-term care needs for changes in life-style, diet, fluid intake, and avoidance of toxins, including alcohol. Table 30-10 lists the instructions for patients with various liver disorders. All patients should be taught how to prevent further liver damage from insults of inadequate food, toxins, and infections.

A major focus for many patients is helping them to confront the effect of alcohol on their well-being, and it requires willingness to engage in discussion about alcohol. Denial is a major part of alcoholism and "breaking through" denial is a part of treatment that occurs over time. Discussion of past alcohol intake and its effects on physical health, and social functioning (family, job, involvement with police, and accidents) is a necessary early part of counseling. Confrontation by family members, employers, and friends may be part of intervention (see Chapter 13 for details and for other techniques and support systems to assist persons with alcohol problems).

For patients with alcoholism and cirrhosis, the nurse can assist the patient to develop a more positive self-concept by giving the patient as much control as possible. This could include the following:

1. Involve the patient in goal setting and decision making.
2. Give positive feedback for accomplishments.
3. Support the patient in times of failure.
4. Help the patient recall past accomplishments.
5. Help significant others provide positive feedback.
6. Help the patient find ways to disguise jaundice or ascites.

A different set of issues is the focus of counseling the patient with hepatitis. Often, patients with hepatitis are young adults who find that fatigue and slow recovery interfere with personal and career goals. The nurse can assist the patient and family to cope with these concerns by actively listening and supporting their coping mechanisms. Accurate information about rest requirements and infectiousness, as well as about measures that can be used at home to further recovery should be provided. The patient and family need an opportunity to express their fears and concerns about care requirements, prognosis, and infectiousness.

Evaluation

Evaluation will be based on the identified patient outcomes. For the person with acute liver dysfunction, questions to ask might include the following:

1. Are signs and symptoms returning to normal?
2. Have complications (infection, bleeding, skin breakdown) been avoided?
3. Is the patient getting sufficient rest?

For persons with chronic liver dysfunction, do the patient and family know the following:

1. The nature of the disorder and need for continued medical follow-up?
2. Measures to prevent exacerbations and complications?
3. Signs and symptoms to be reported to the physician?

DISORDERS OF THE BILIARY SYSTEM

Inflammation, stone formation, and carcinoma are the major disorders of the biliary system. The signs and symptoms and medical therapy are listed in Table 30-11.

Pathophysiology

CHOLECYSTITIS

Cholecystitis, inflammation of the gallbladder, may be acute or chronic and is usually associated with gallstones or other obstructions of the bile passage. Cholecystitis is more common in women than in men. Sedentary, obese

Table 30-11 Biliary tract disorders

Disorder	Etiology	Signs and symptoms	Therapy
Cholecystitis	Often associated with cholelithiasis	History of intolerance of fatty foods, gaseous eructations after meals, flatus, diarrhea, abdominal distention Nausea, vomiting Pain: right upper quadrant, referred to right scapula Fever, tachycardia Leukocytosis	Conservative: NPO, nasogastric intubation, IV infusions, meperidine hydrochloride, spasmolytics (papaverine, amyl nitrate), anticholinergics (chronic condition), antibiotics Surgery: cholecystectomy, cholecystostomy
Cholelithiasis Choledocholithiasis	See the box on p. 1031.	As for cholecystitis Biliary colic: intense spasmodic pain with diaphoresis, tachycardia and prostration Jaundice Elevated serum bilirubin Prolonged prothrombin time	Conservative: as for cholecystitis Surgery: choledochostomy, choledocholithotomy, cholecystectomy, ERCP (endoscopy), EPT (endoscopic papillotomy), sphincterotomy, or sphincteroplasty
Choledocholithiasis			Agents to dissolve stones: heparin, Chenodeoxycholic acid (CDC-A), ursodeoxycholic acid (UDC-A)
Carcinoma	High risk in persons with history of cholelithiasis	Jaundice, weight loss, pain, right upper quadrant mass	Surgery: cholesystectomy, choledochoduodenostomy, choledochojejunostomy, cholecystoduodenostomy, biliary drainage

persons are affected more often, and the incidence is highest in the fifth and sixth decades of life.

In acute cholecystitis, the gallbladder is usually very enlarged and resembles a distended sac. Inflammation occurs, and the wall of the gallbladder becomes thickened and edematous. Impaired circulation, edema, and distention produce ischemia, which can proceed to necrosis and gangrene. Perforation of the gallbladder may occur, leading to biliary peritonitis, pancreatitis, and fistula formation. Bacterial invasion can lead to empyema of the gallbladder, ductal cholangitis, abscess formation, and sepsis.

Chronic cholecystitis may produce a variety of structural changes whether or not stones are present. This is not the result of an infectious process but is related to a diseased gallbladder wall with inefficient emptying. It is believed that chronic cholecystitis is caused by chemical or mechanical irritation from stones causing pressure on the mucosa or from biliary stasis. Eventually, because of destruction of the mucosa, outpouchings of the epithelium may form. Bacteria and other irritants may become trapped in these outpouchings, which may maintain a chronic inflammatory process.

The chronic form of the disease is usually preceded by several acute attacks of moderate severity. Persons with chronic disease may not be as ill as those with acute disease

and, therefore, may not seek medical attention until they experience pain from biliary obstruction or develop jaundice (p. 1002).

■ CHOLELITHIASIS

Gallstones in the biliary tract may occur in either sex at any age but are more common in women and the incidence increases with age. Stones may be present for years without symptoms. Sometimes they appear to precede or follow chronic cholecystitis. It is estimated that there are one million new cases of cholelithiasis each year.

It is not completely known why stones form in the biliary tract. Three specific factors contribute to the formation of gallstones: metabolic factors, stasis, and inflammation.

Of patients with gallstones, 20% to 50% are asymptomatic, about 18% will have biliary pain, and 3% will require removal of the gallbladder. The box on p. 1031 lists the factors that lead to precipitation of bile salts, bile pigments, and cholesterol. Most gallstones in Western culture are cholesterol stones (75%); the remaining are bilirubin pigment stones (25%). It appears that a proper relationship between lecithin (a phospholipid), bile salts, and cholesterol is necessary for cholesterol to be soluble in bile. A reduction in the bile salt pool (available in the terminal

Factors increasing the risk of cholelithiasis

Metabolic

Biliary cholesterol saturation
  Estrogens
  Oral contraceptives
  Obesity
  Terminal ileal disease or resection
Increased production of serum bilirubin
  Hemolytic states
  Cirrhosis
Increased serum cholesterol
  Obesity
  Pregnancy
  Diabetes mellitus
  Hypothyroidism
  Hyperlipidemia

Biliary stasis

Biliary tract obstruction
  Fasting
  Parenteral hyperalimentation
Inflammation
  Cholecystitis

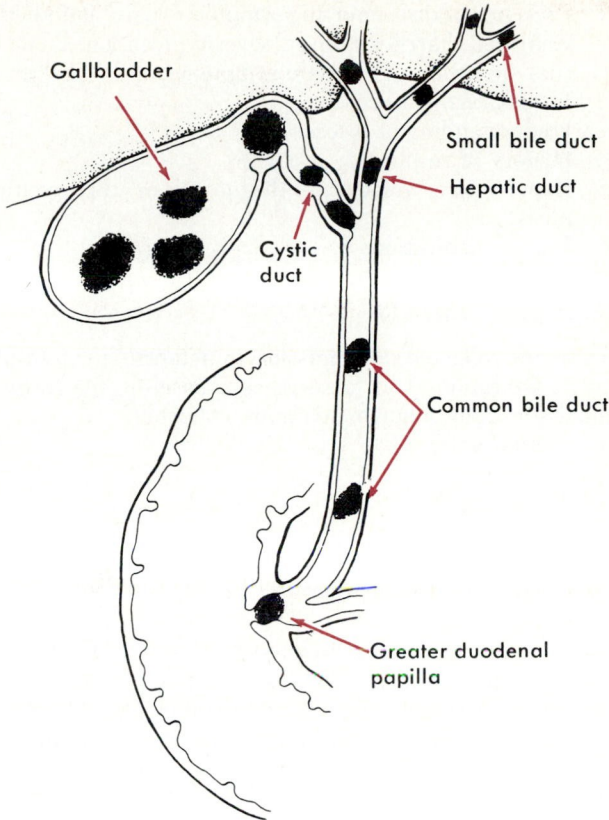

Fig. 30-16 Common sites of gallstones.

ileum for reabsorption) reduces the amount of bile salts in the bile and thereby the solubility of cholesterol. Serum cholesterol levels do not always correlate with the presence of cholesterol gallstones.

Biliary stasis leads to stagnation of bile in the gallbladder and to excessive absorption of water, allowing the salts to precipitate easily. Fasting states reduce the normal stimulation of bile flow from cholecystokinin.

Inflammation of the biliary system causes the bile constituents to become altered. The inflamed gallbladder mucosa absorbs more of the bile acids with a resultant reduction of the solubility of cholesterol.

There may be no signs of cholelithiasis until a stone becomes lodged in a biliary duct, although a history of postprandial indigestion is common. Gaseous eructations occur immediately after a meal, in contrast to several hours later as seen with gastric ulcer. *Biliary colic* can cause one of the most severe pains that can be experienced. The pain, which is caused by spasm of the ducts as they attempt to dislodge the stone, radiates through to the back under the scapula and to the right shoulder.

Stones may lodge anywhere along the biliary tract (Fig. 30-16). If they lodge in the small bile ducts, hepatic duct, or common bile duct, the stones obstruct bile flow and the patient becomes jaundiced. Stones may also cause pressure and subsequent necrosis and infection of the walls of the biliary ducts. Occasionally a stone, because of its location, blocks the entrance of pancreatic fluid and bile into the duodenum. This condition is difficult to differentiate from obstruction caused by malignancy. Complications are similar to those for cholecystitis.

CARCINOMA OF THE BILIARY SYSTEM

Cancer can occur anywhere in the biliary system, and, unfortunately, at present there is no method of early diagnosis. Identification is often made during surgery. Jaundice may be the first sign and indicates that the lesion has developed sufficiently to obstruct bile passage at some point. Spread by direct extension to the liver or peritoneal surface may be the initial manifestation. The prognosis is usually one of rapid deterioration with death ensuing within a few months. Surgery is usually done for palliation. Drainage of the biliary tract or surgical bypass of the area of obstruction can improve the comfort of the patient.

Assessment

SUBJECTIVE DATA

Some patients with biliary tract disease will be admitted for surgery while their disease is quiescent, whereas others will be in an acute stage of the disease. Potential and actual problems may, therefore, be present in individual patients. Minimum data to collect include the following:

1. Presence of discomforting symptoms (pain, jaundice, vomiting, diarrhea): onset, severity, location, factors that aggravate or alleviate symptom
2. Food intake patterns
3. Understanding of disease
4. History of respiratory problems
5. Expectations related to diagnostic or therapeutic measures
6. Use of medications

■ OBJECTIVE DATA

Data are collected on admission to determine extent of present alterations and to serve as a baseline for future comparison. The following data are collected:

1. Mental status
2. Vital signs
3. Body weight
4. Abdominal assessment for distention tenderness or guarding
5. Breath sounds
6. Signs of jaundice

Intake and output measurements are started if patients have any unusual fluid losses or are acutely ill. Urine and stool are examined for color. Dark brown urine, caused by the presence of bilirubin, and a light colored stool, resulting from an absence of bile, may be noted. A dipstick test on urine for bilirubin can be done quickly and easily.

■ DIAGNOSTIC TESTS

It is not unusual for patients with symptoms of biliary tract disease to have numerous diagnostic tests performed on the liver, pancreas, and biliary tract. See Table 30-8 for tests of serum bilirubin, urine bilirubin, urine urobilinogen, and fecal urobilinogen, and Table 30-4 for findings of these tests in obstructive and hepatocellular jaundice. The absence of urinary urobilinogen represents a highly significant finding for suggesting the presence of obstructive jaundice (a history of antibiotic therapy may influence the test results).

Other diagnostic tests are listed in the box on p. 1033. The most frequent test of the biliary tract is an oral cholecystogram. If nonvisualization of the gallbladder is found, the test may be repeated the next day. Barium studies should follow gallbladder studies to prevent a barium-filled colon from obscuring the gallbladder.

Some patients find the oral dye of the oral cholecystogram to be very irritating; diarrhea is not uncommon, and nausea and vomiting can occur. If vomiting soon after ingestion of the tablets is reported, directions are sought about further dosage. Intravenous injection of the dyes may cause allergic reactions in susceptible persons such as dyspnea, chills, diaphoresis, faintness, and tachycardia. Patients are queried about allergies or reactions to x-ray examinations in the past. Some patients report temporary dysuria following the test.

➡ Data analysis: nursing diagnoses

Nursing diagnoses are determined from assessment of patient data. Possible nursing diagnoses for the person with biliary tract disease may include, but are not limited to, the following:

Diagnostic title	Possible etiologies
Ineffective breathing pattern	Pain
Knowledge deficit: dietary requirements, diagnostic and therapeutic measures	Lack of exposure to information
Altered nutrition: more than body requirements	Excessive intake in relation to metabolic needs, lack of knowledge
Pain	Biliary colic and jaundice

Planning: expected patient outcomes

Expected patient outcomes for the patient with biliary tract disease may include, but are not limited to, the following:

1. Patient will not demonstrate behaviors associated with pain.
2. Patient will have normal breath sounds and a normal chest x-ray examination.
3. Patient will describe ways to reduce caloric and fat content in the diet.
4. Patient will describe the purpose of diagnostic and therapeutic measures.

Implementation

■ ASSISTING WITH ACHIEVEMENT OF THERAPEUTIC GOALS

☐ Conservative management

There are a variety of treatment measures used in biliary tract disease (see Table 30-11). Conservative treatment of cholecystitis usually will effect improvement within 1 to 7 days; selective cholecystectomy is performed 4 to 8 weeks after the acute process has subsided.[4] Surgery is usually recommended because recurrent attacks are common.

Food is withheld until acute symptoms subside. If vomiting persists, a nasogastric tube is passed and attached to suction. Meperidine hydrochloride may be given for pain and is preferred because its spasmogenic effect on the biliary tract is less than that which occurs with opiates. The inhalation of amyl nitrite may diminish intestinal and biliary spasms. When food is tolerated, a reducing diet (if appropriate) and careful avoidance of too much fat usually are recommended.

☐ Surgical management

An alternative plan of management includes early cholecystectomy (or cholecystostomy followed by cholecystectomy in 24 to 48 hours).

Radiographic and endoscopic studies for biliary disorders

Cholecystography (gallbladder series)
Explanation

A normal liver removes radiopaque dyes from the bloodstream and concentrates them in the gallbladder. The dye-filled functioning gallbladder shows up as a dense shadow on the x-ray film. Nonvisualization of a dye-filled gallbladder suggests nonfunctioning. If a fatty meal is taken, the normal gallbladder contracts and expels the dye. An x-ray at this time outlines the bile ducts. Stones that are not radiopaque show up as dark patches on the film.

Patient preparation

1. Explain procedure to patient.
2. Check for iodine allergy.
3. If an oral cholecystogram is to be done, administer the Bilopaque or Telepaque tablets as ordered (usual dose is 3 g, but is determined by weight).
4. If an intravenous cholecystogram is to be done, the dye will be administered just before examination in the radiation department.
5. Diet
   a. A low-fat meal is eaten the evening before the test.
   b. No further foods may be taken after the evening meal.
   c. Black coffee, tea, or water may be taken for breakfast.
6. Give prescribed laxatives or enemas.

Cholangiography
Explanation

Visualizes the bile ducts and can demonstrate presence of stones, strictures, or tumors, or the patency of the common bile duct after surgery. In *percutaneous transhepatic cholangiography,* the dye is injected through skin and abdominal wall into a blood vessel or bile duct; in *surgical cholangiography,* the dye is inserted through a needle or catheter into the common bile duct.

Patient preparation

1. Explain procedure to patient.
2. Omit meal before test.
3. Decrease patient's fluid intake.
4. Give laxative, if prescribed.

Endoscopy
Peritonoscopy

Direct visualization of peritoneum and liver, sometimes combined with liver biopsy; air sufflation, which may be painful, may be used.

Endoscopic retrograde cholangiopancreatography (ERCP)

Use of fiberscope to visualize and obtain a biopsy of the biliary and pancreatic tracts; the fiberscope is passed through the oral pharynx to the duodenum and into the biliary and pancreatic ducts. Contrast media may be injected through the endoscope and dilation or sphincterotomy may be used to remove gallstones or enlarge the sphincter.

Patient preparation

1. Written consent is required.
2. Explain procedure to patient.
3. Nothing by mouth is allowed after midnight.
4. Skin is prepared before peritonoscopy.
5. Give sedatives as prescribed.

There is no consensus among physicians as to whether a prophylactic cholecystectomy should be performed for asymptomatic gallstones. Some believe that this should only be done for persons at high risk. However, surgery is performed when there are signs of biliary tract obstruction.

Sometimes after surgery, stones remain in the common bile duct or new stones form. In these instances, attempts may be made to dissolve stones by injecting heparin, CDC-A, or UDC-A through a tube into the duct. Or, an alternative treatment is the removal of stones by sphincterotomy performed during endoscopy.

The terminology used to indicate specific biliary tract surgery is self-explanatory once common terms are understood. *Cholecyst* refers to the gallbladder, *choledocho* refers to the common bile duct, and *lith* refers to a stone (see the box below). Biliary tract anastomoses are palliative operations to provide biliary drainage to the intestine through bypass of an obstructed area.

□ **Biliary drainage**

External biliary drainage is used in empyema, fistula, or when decompression of the biliary tract is required. Drainage is provided by a catheter inserted into the gallbladder (cholecystostomy) or by a T-tube inserted into the common bile duct (choledochostomy) (Fig. 30-17). Usually stab wounds are used to bring these tubes through the skin. The T-tube is inserted to maintain patency of the common bile duct and to ensure drainage of bile out of the body until edema in the common duct has subsided enough for bile to drain into the duodenum normally. (For some patients with extensive ductal disease, the T-tube may be used for long periods of time.) Cholangiograms (op-grams) are commonly performed in the operating room to ensure patency of the common bile duct; radiopaque dye is inserted through the T-tube. Preoperative and postoperative care is summarized in the box on p. 1035.

At first the entire output of bile (normally 500 to 1000 ml/day) may flow through the T-tube, but within 10 days most of the bile will be flowing into the duodenum. If bile is not flowing out the tube or through into the duodenum, it can be assumed that drainage is obstructed and that bile is being forced back into the common bile duct into the

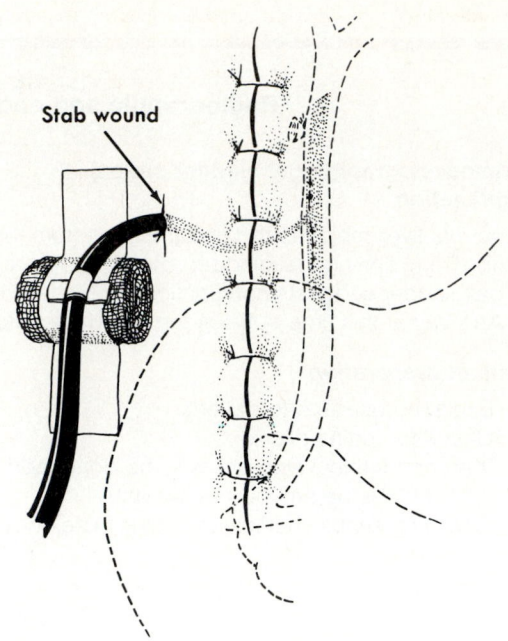

Fig. 30-17 Section of T tube emerging from stab wound may be placed over roll of gauze anchored to skin with adhesive tape to prevent its lumen from being occluded by pressure.

liver. The patient is observed closely for jaundice, particularly in the sclerae.

Occasionally with prolonged external biliary drainage, feeding of bile will be used to improve digestion. This is generally done through a feeding tube. Opaque containers should be used; tomato or grape juice can change its appearance.

Before the T-tube is removed, the patency of the common bile duct must be assessed. The tube is clamped for variable intervals and the patient monitored for signs of distress. If distress occurs, the tube is unclamped immediately and the physician is informed. A cholangiogram is usually performed to confirm patency of the duct before the tube is removed. Following the removal of the T-tube, the patient

---

Surgeries of the biliary tract

Cholecystectomy	Removal of gallbladder
Cholecystostomy	Creation of an opening into gallbladder for drainage
Choledochotomy	Incision into common bile duct
Choledocholithotomy	Incision into common bile duct to remove a stone
Choledochoduodenostomy	Anastomosis of common bile duct with duodenum
Choledochojejunostomy	Anastomosis of common bile duct with jejunum
Cholecystogastrostomy	Anastomosis of gallbladder with stomach

---

Nursing care of the patient undergoing surgery of the biliary tract

Preoperative

1. Carry out actions used in preparing any patient with abdominal surgery (see Chapter 31).
   a. Pay particular attention to improving respiratory function, because the high incision and right upper quadrant (RUQ) pain predispose the patient to *right lower lobe pneumonia* and *atelectasis*.
   b. Explain the types of biliary drainage tubes that are anticipated.
2. Provide care required because of the severity of acute symptoms or the presence of jaundice.
   a. Administer intravenous fluids and antibiotics at prescribed rate.
   b. Administer analgesics (usually meperidine) as prescribed and required.
   c. Provide comfort measures for pruritus, nausea and vomiting, and pain.
   d. Administer vitamin K as prescribed.

Postoperative

1. Place patient in low-Fowler's position, assist to change position frequently.
2. Urge patient to cough and deep breathe at regular intervals (every 1 to 2 hours) until ambulating well.
3. Monitor frequently for signs of hemorrhage (shock) the first few hours preoperatively (hemorrhage is rare, but may occur when the inflamed gallbladder was adherent to the liver and difficult to remove).
4. Give analgesics fairly liberally the first 2 to 3 days.
5. Maintain a dry, intact dressing; usually a drain is inserted near the stump of the cystic duct; some serous fluid drainage is normal initially.
6. Encourage progressive ambulation when permitted.
7. When food is permitted, gradually increase diet to regular with low fat content or fat content as tolerated (appetite and fat tolerance may be diminished if there is external biliary drainage).

Biliary drainage

1. Connect any biliary drainage tubes to closed gravity drainage.
2. Attach sufficient tubing so the patient can move without restriction.
3. Explain to patient the importance of avoiding kinks, clamping, or pulling of the tube.
4. Monitor the amount and color of drainage frequently; measure and record drainage at least every shift.
5. Report any signs of peritonitis (abdominal pain or rigidity, fever) to the physician immediately.
6. Monitor color of urine and stools; stools will be a light color if bile is flowing out a drainage tube but the normal color should gradually reappear as drainage diminishes and disappears.

---

may have chills and fever caused by edema and a local reaction to the bile; these symptoms usually subside within 24 hours.

■ ASSISTING WITH COMFORT AND ADL

Analgesia should be freely administered after biliary surgery in order to control pain and, thereby, increase the patients' willingness to deep breathe, cough, and ambulate. Medication should be scheduled prior to wound care, self-care activities, and ambulation.

Dressings that are moist with drainage are uncomfortable and increase the risk of infection. Great care should be taken to avoid tension on biliary drainage tubes, another source of discomfort.

□ Counseling and teaching

The time available for preoperative teaching is often limited because patients may be acutely ill and undergoing multiple diagnostic procedures and treatments to prepare them for surgery within a short time. Or, conversely, the patient scheduled for elective surgery may come to the hospital the morning of surgery, 1 to 2 hours before surgery. The nurse must be prepared to give essential information in the brief period that is available, as well as to address the patient's expressed concerns. Priority should be given to demonstrating deep breathing and coughing.

It is important after surgery to carefully assess the patient's understanding of postoperative care measures. Instruction is best done when the patient is free of pain.

Persons with prolonged illness, as with biliary tract fistula or metastatic carcinoma, will need supportive care and instructions related to specific symptoms.

The essential points to include in teaching the person with a biliary system disorder are listed in the box on p. 1036. Nursing actions for the problems listed in the box on p. 1036 were discussed on p. 1002.

Patients with complicated biliary tract disease (fistulas,

Teaching for the patient with a biliary system disorder

Postoperative

1. The patient to be sent home with dressings or drainage tube should be informed of the following:
   a. Expected amount of biliary drainage
   b. Frequency of dressing change or emptying of drainage bag
   c. Need to keep dressings dry and skin clean (soap and water is sufficient by time of discharge); a daily shower may be permitted
   d. Technique of dressing change and availability of supplies
   e. Signs to report to physician: excessive drainage, leakage, obstruction (jaundice, lighter colored stools)
2. Resuming normal activities in about 1 month and sexual activities when desired; avoidance of heavy lifting for 6 weeks

Long-term care for chronic condition

1. Dietary restrictions
   a. Low-fat diet if fat is poorly tolerated
   b. Low calorie diet if weight reduction is necessary
2. Drug therapy, if appropriate
   a. Importance of medication in preventing recurrence of symptoms
   b. When and how to use medications such as anticholinergics or antispasmodics
3. Follow-up care
   a. Signs and symptoms to be reported to health care provider (pain, fever, jaundice, dark urine, pale stools, pruritus, tube dislodgement)
   b. Plans for follow-up care

Common problems of patients with biliary disorders

Infection
Malnutrition
Fluid and electrolyte imbalance
Jaundice
Pain

---

structure, abscesses) or malignancy will have decreased energy and progress slowly in ADL. Alternating rest and activity periods and graduated ambulation is necessary.

⊞ Evaluation

Evaluation is based on expected patient outcomes. Questions to ask may include the following:
1. Is patient comfortable?
2. Did the patient remain free of pneumonia or atelectasis in the right lower lobe?
3. Is jaundice decreased?
4. Is the wound healing?
5. Can the patient explain how to reduce calorie and fat intake?

6. Does patient know how to care for self at home, for example, as to medications, care of any drainage systems or dressings
7. Does patient know when and what to report to the physician?

■ DISORDERS OF THE PANCREAS

■ Pathophysiology

Nonendocrine disorders of the pancreas consist primarily of inflammation (pancreatitis) and tumors. The endocrine pancreatic disorder of diabetes mellitus is discussed in Chapter 28.

■ PANCREATITIS

Pancreatitis, an inflammatory disorder, may be acute or chronic. Table 30-12 lists the etiology, signs and symptoms, and medical therapy for these conditions.

☐ Acute pancreatitis

Acute pancreatitis may occur in a single episode or there may be recurrent attacks (relapsing acute pancreatitis). It is an inflammatory process with multiple etiologies (see Table 30-12). Infection may occur secondarily, but it is not a part of the initial disease process. Several mechanisms

Table 30-12 Disorders of the pancreas

Disorder	Etiology	Signs and symptoms	Medical therapy
Pancreatitis	Biliary obstruction Drug toxicity (chlorpromazine, chlorothiazide, isoniazid, corticosteroids)	*Acute pancreatitis:* Epigastric pain, abdominal tenderness Nausea, vomiting Shock, dehydration Fever, tachycardia Jaundice Abdominal rigidity Hyperglycemia Hypocalcemia Serum amylase greater than 300 Somogyi units	Fluid deficit: hydrating fluids, albumin, blood or plasma, electrolyte replacement Inhibition of pancreatic activity: NPO, propantheline (Pro-Banthine) or methantheline (Banthine), nasogastric suction, antacids Pain: meperidine hydrochloride, sympahetic nerve blocks, epidural anesthesia Paralytic ileus: Miller Abbot intubation
Chronic pancreatitis	Alcoholism in adults, cystic fibrosis in children, malnutrition	*Chronic pancreatitis:* Recurring episodes of acute pancreatitis diarrhea, steatorrhea, weight loss, malnutrition, diabetes mellitus, jaundice	Antacids Diet: high calorie, high protein, low fat Pancreatic enzyme replacement: pancreatin, (Viokase), pancrelipase (Cotazym, Pancrease) Fiberoscopy with cannulization and sphincterotomy of spincter of Oddi Pancreatic surgery
Tumors	Adenocarcinomas Ductal cell (90%) Islet cell Acinar cell Insulinoma Cystadenoma	Anorexia, nausea and vomiting, weight loss Pain Jaundice Hyperglycemia Peptic ulcer, diarrhea, steatorrhea	Surgery: pancreatic-duodenal resection (Whipple), cholecystojejunostomy or other bypass operation Chemotherapy Pancreatic resection Pancreatic resection and gastrectomy, cimetidine

may explain the relationship between alcohol and pancreatitis. These include the following:

1. Direct toxic effect of alcohol on acinar cells
2. Spasms of the sphincter of Oddi or pancreatic duct, permitting reflux of duodenal contents
3. Dietary deficiencies
4. Deposits of proteinaceous material in the small ducts

Regardless of specific etiology, pathologic changes appear to be caused by *autodigestion* of pancreatic tissue. It is believed that this is produced by premature activation of proteolytic enzymes that are normally activated only in the duodenum. Activation of the enzymes may result from the following:

1. Specific factors such as endotoxins, exotoxins, or ischemia
2. Reflux of duodenal contents through the pancreatic duct
3. Failure of enzyme inhibition

The activated enzymes digest pancreatic and surrounding tissues. Regardless of the pathogenic mechanism, severe destruction of the pancreas may result.

Acute pancreatitis may be divided into three stages, edematous or interstitial, hemorrhagic, and necrotizing. The mortality rate increases with each succeeding stage.

Pain may result from distention of the pancreatic capsule, from obstruction of bile flow caused by compression of the common bile duct, and from peritoneal irritation. The pain may radiate to the back, flanks, and substernal area and may be more intense when the person is lying supine. Difficulty in breathing may accompany the severe pain. Ascites and ileus distend the abdomen and lead to hypoventilation. Vomiting at first relieves pain, but continued vomiting worsens it. The patient often assumes a flexed posture to relieve pain.

Fluid and electrolyte abnormalities result from vomiting, local edema, ascites, or calcium precipitation into the inflamed pancreas. Hypovolemic shock may ensue if there is severe fluid loss. Shallow respirations may reflect metabolic alkalosis (induced by loss of gastric contents), limited diaphragmatic excursion, or ascites. Decreased breath sounds may be the result of atelectasis or pleural effusion. Rales may be present.

☐ Chronic pancreatitis

In chronic pancreatitis there is permanent damage to the exocrine and endocrine cells and ducts. Normal tissue is replaced by scar tissue; cells atrophy; and protein precipitates obstruct the ductal system. Calcification of the pancreatic tissue continues. The following result:

1. Diminished secretion of enzymes and pancreatic hormones
2. Obstruction, stasis of flow, and secondary infection of pancreatic ducts
3. Malnourishment from poor absorption
4. Steatorrhea, weight loss
5. Hyperglycemia

Pain may be very severe during acute flare-ups of chronic pancreatitis, and for some patients, pain may be chronic. For other patients, between acute attacks the pain may disappear or may be only a vague discomfort.

Distention and distortion of the ductal system may lead to the development of pseudocysts (collections of liquefied necrotic tissue). These cysts may contain digestive enzymes. Large pseudocysts are a serious complication of pancreatitis because of the possibility of rupture, bleeding, and erosion into nearby tissue or into the peritoneal cavity. Infection, abscess formation, and fistula formation may occur. Although small pseudocysts may resolve over time, large ones are surgically removed.

Table 30-13 Diagnostic tests for pancreatic disease

Laboratory tests	Normal	Interpretation
Blood tests		
Amylase, serum	60 to 150 Somogyi units	Serum and urinary enzyme levels are increased when there is cellular injury. (There are other causes of increased serum enzymes, however.) Lower levels may be seen in advanced chronic state of pancreatitis.
Lipase	0 to 1.5 U/ml	
Calcium	4.5 to 5.75 mEq/L 9 to 11 mg/dl	Serum calcium levels are lowered as calcium is deposited into inflamed and necrotic soft tissue.
Bilirubin (direct conjugated)	0.1 to 0.3 mg/dl	Bilirubin levels are elevated when biliary obstruction exists.
Glucose	90 to 120 mg/dl	A transient hyperglycemia may occur in acute pancreatitis; permanent carbohydrate intolerance may occur if beta cells are destroyed in chronic pancreatitis.
Urine tests		
Amylase (urine, 24 hour specimen)	35 to 260 Somogyi U/hour	Increased levels are found in acute pancreatitis.
Radiographic tests		
Flat plate of abdomen	No calcification of pancreas visualized	See serum calcium above.
CAT; ultrasonography	Normal structures visualized	These tests are used to detect calcification, masses, and ductal distention.
Other scans	See p. 1033	These tests are used to detect ductal obstruction and pseudocysts.
Endoscopic retrograde chalangio-pancreatography	See p. 1033	See p. 1033
Other tests		
Pancreatic secretion test (secretin given IV; analysis of duodenal contents)	Volume 117-392 ml/80 min HCO₃ 16-33 mEq/80 min Amylase 439-1921 U/80 min	Decreased release of bicarbonate and/or enzymes are found in chronic pancreatitis. Increased acid secretion is found in Zollinger-Ellison syndrome.
D-xylose test (25 g D-xylose given orally)	5-8 g excreted in urine/5 hours 25-40 mg serum levels in 2 hours	Lowered blood or urinary level indicate malabsorption conditions.
Quantitative fecal fat	7 g/24 hours	Elevated levels show steatorrhea.

TUMORS OF THE PANCREAS

Tumors of the pancreas may be malignant or benign. Benign tumors are usually adenomas or cystadenomas and are relatively rare. Malignant tumors occur more frequently and are most often found in the head of the pancreas. Men are affected far more often than women, usually after middle age. Cancer of the pancreas is the fourth most common cause of cancer mortality in men.

Most malignant tumors of the pancreas appear to begin in the ductal areas, causing eventual blockage and resulting in chronic pancreatitis. Direct extension of the lesion may cause its spread to the posterior wall of the stomach, duodenum, colon, and common bile duct. The tumor may be diffusely spread over the entire gland, or it may be a well-defined growth. It usually grows rapidly, is highly invasive, and metastasizes frequently. Many patients live only 3 to 6 months after diagnosis is confirmed. Symptoms usually occur late in the course of the disease. Pain occurs in about 85% of patients. Jaundice occurs from common bile duct obstruction but is seldom a primary sign.

Islet cell tumors give rise to particular syndromes (see Table 30-13) that are important in the differential diagnosis of hypoglycemia and peptic ulcer. These tumors may be benign or malignant. *Beta-cell pancreatic adenoma (insulinoma)* results in hyperinsulinism and episodes of hypoglycemia. Attacks are precipitated by fasting or exercise, and symptoms are relieved by glucose ingestion or infusion. *Non–beta-cell tumors* result in peptic ulceration of the duodenum or jejunum. Hypersecretion of gastric acid is extremely severe in this Zollinger-Ellison syndrome (see Chapter 31). The patient often gives a history of severe diarrhea and steatorrhea.

Assessment

SUBJECTIVE DATA

The nursing history should be thorough and should carefully document the course of symptoms, particularly pain and vomiting. The use of any medications, alcohol, and home remedies are explored. When alcohol use is a factor in pancreatitis, data are collected about the person's present perception of drinking as a problem for which help is needed (see Chapter 13). Baseline data about food intake patterns and likes and dislikes can help the nurse and dietitian plan for patients with malnutrition or anorexia.

OBJECTIVE DATA

The physical examination should be complete. Special attention is directed to the abdomen to elicit signs of ascites, guarding, or tenderness. Dehydration is usually found in acute pancreatitis. Although unusual, hypocalcemia may occur, therefore, the patient is monitored for the presence of Chvostek's sign and Trousseau's sign. Baseline abdominal girth can help determine further abdominal distention. A brief listing of important data includes the following:

General appearance and posture
Mental status
Body weight
Vital signs
Breath sounds
Abdomen: girth, tenderness, guarding
Chvostek's and Trousseau's signs
Urinalysis for sugar and acetone
Urinary intake and output

DIAGNOSTIC TESTS

Of the greatest value in establishing a diagnosis of acute pancreatitis are measurements of enzyme levels (Table 30-13). With pancreatic trauma, a peritoneal tap may reveal an increased amylase level in the peritoneal fluid. When elevations of SGOT, alkaline phosphatase, and bilirubin occur, obstruction of the common bile duct or liver disease is usually present. Laboratory findings consistent with acute inflammation (leukocytosis) and dehydration may be present.

Radiography, scans, and ERCP are used to diagnose chronic pancreatitis and complications of acute pancreatitis.

Data analysis: nursing diagnoses

Nursing diagnoses are determined from assessment of patient data. Possible nursing diagnoses for the person with pancreatic disorders may include, but are not limited to, the following:

Diagnostic title	Possible etiologies
Activity intolerance	Generalized weakness
Altered health maintenance	Substance abuse, perceptual/cognitive impairment, lack of knowledge
Hopelessness	Long-term stress, failing physical condition, abandonment
Altered nutrition: less than body requirements	Anorexia, inability to obtain food, noncompliance with enzyme replacement
Pain	Pathophysiologic: inflammation; diagnostic tests, improper positioning

Planning: expected patient outcomes

Expected patient outcomes for the person with pancreatic disorders may include, but are not limited to, the following:

1. Patient will gradually increase participation in self-care activities.
2. Patient will state comfort level is increased.
3. Patient will state goal and methods of treating substance abuse.
4. Patient will express less apathy and identify one example of improvement in situation.
5. Patient will take replacement enzymes with bland food.

6. Patient will explain how to implement medical regimen on discharge.
7. Patient/family have access to supportive services for long-term alcoholism control or hospice services when prognosis for pancreatic carcinoma is poor.

▓ Implementation

■ ASSISTANCE WITH ACHIEVEMENT OF THERAPEUTIC GOALS

☐ Acute pancreatitis

Medical treatment is directed toward (1) decreasing secretions of the pancreas, (2) resting the pancreas, and (3) preventing and treating complications (see the box below), and (4) controlling pain.

Rest of the pancreas during the acute phase is achieved by measures that reduce stimulation of the exocrine secretions such as the following:
1. Nothing-by-mouth status
2. Nasogastric suction
3. Anticholinergic drugs or cimetidine
4. Antacids

These measures decrease stimulation of the vagus nerve, and thus of hydrochloric acid, and decrease secretion of the enzymes stimulated by secretin, gastrin, and pancreoenzyme (CCK). Antibiotics are not usually administered in the edematous stage or in the absence of complications. Atropine-like drugs are contraindicated in the presence of paralytic ileus and shock. There is some question of their efficacy in treating pancreatitis, and they are not always used.

Pain relief is usually achieved with meperidine hydrochloride rather than morphine or codeine, since it is less spasmogenic on the sphincter of Oddi. Some patients find that the pain is decreased if they assume a sitting position with the trunk flexed or with their knees drawn up to the abdomen in a side-lying position.

The following nursing interventions are used depending on the presence or extent of dehydration and the presence of complications of acute pancreatitis:
1. Maintain intravenous fluid replacement (blood, albumin, plasma, fluids) and electrolytes as ordered.
2. Monitor vital signs and central venous pressure.

Signs of complications of acute pancreatitis

Paralytic ileus
Shock (hypovolemic, toxic)
Pulmonary complications
Hypocalcemia
Hyperglycemia
Jaundice

---

3. Monitor intake and output every 1 to 4 hours.
4. Administer vasopressors and other measures for shock.
5. Maintain patency of the gastrointestinal tube.
6. Monitor for glucosuria, ketonuria, Chvostek's and Trousseau's signs, and increasing abdominal girth.
7. Encourage deep breathing and coughing.
8. Administer as prescribed for complications: insulin, calcium, antibiotics, vitamin K.

As soon as the acute attack passes, oral fluids and foods are started. Patients are placed on a low-fat bland diet distributed over five to six small feedings per day. When eating starts, the patient is observed carefully for pain, nausea, and vomiting, which indicate continuing inflammation and the need to return to a nothing-by-mouth status.

☐ Chronic pancreatitis

Therapy for the acute attack of chronic pancreatitis includes the therapies discussed above (NPO, suction, antacids, and IV fluids). In addition, as the acute attack subsides, medical attention will turn to confirming the diagnosis, to treating the malabsorption, and, in some instances, to surgery. Pancreatic enzyme replacement drugs contain amylase, lipase, and trypsin. They are taken at mealtimes to aid digestion and to facilitate the absorption of nutrients and fat-soluble vitamins. The patient should observe stools for steatorrhea, which occurs when fat intake is lowered and enzymes improve absorption.

☐ *Surgery*

An exploratory laparotomy may be performed in acute pancreatitis when a diagnosis cannot be established and the possibility of general peritonitis, perforation of an organ, or a bowel obstruction cannot be excluded. If biliary obstruction is present, a surgical or endoscopic procedure may be done to divert or increase bile flow at the sphincter of Oddi and thereby reduce regurgitation of bile into the pancreatic duct.

For the treatment of pseudocysts the surgeon may employ external drainage, construct anastomoses between the pancreas and gastrointestinal tract (for example, pancreatojejunostomy), or resect part or all of the pancreas.

Exploratory surgery is often necessary to diagnose pancreatic tumors. Various techniques may be used when pancreatic tumors are present or to relieve pancreatic duct obstruction. Procedures to relieve obstructive jaundice are sometimes helpful in providing comfort (cholecystostomy, choledochojejunostomy). Often malignant tumors of the pancreas are inoperable by the time diagnosis is made.

Pancreatoduodenal resection is sometimes done when the carcinoma is localized with no evidence of metastasis. Whipple's procedure involves resection of the antrum of the stomach, duodenum, varying amounts of pancreas, and often the gallbladder. Anastomoses are constructed between the stomach, common bile duct and pancreatic ducts, and the jejunum. Malabsorption syndrome follows total pancreatectomy (protein, fat, iron, calcium, phosphate, vitamin B_{12}), as does carbohydrate intolerance.

The patient with extensive pancreatic surgery or disease may have a prolonged postoperative course. Malnourishment, postoperative complications (hemorrhage, fistulas, anastomotic leak, infection) and metabolic derangements may occur. Hemorrhagic and hypovolemic shock can lead to renal failure. Wound care must be meticulous. Drains are usually employed, and dressings should be inspected frequently and changed as often as necessary to maintain dryness. If a pancreatic fistula develops, there can be severe tissue breakdown from digestion of skin and underlying tissues by the pancreatic enzymes. Measurement of biliary or pancreatic drainage is carefully recorded.

■ COUNSELING AND TEACHING

The patient requires teaching directed toward self-care (see the box below), as well as counseling directed toward acceptance of chronic disease or malignancy. Not all patients with pancreatitis have alcoholism as a contributing factor, but those who do are encouraged to seek appropriate services (see Chapter 13).

Patients with chronic pancreatitis and their families require much support. Long-term illness, physical deterioration, and chronic pain combined with alcohol, and, sometimes, narcotic addiction often result in apathy and hopelessness. These factors and the patient's affect or behavior may evoke the same feelings of apathy and hopelessness in health care providers.

The treatment of pain and the offering of support under these circumstances is difficult. Pain control in an acute attack or following surgery will require the use of narcotics. It is best not to address addiction until the patient is physiologically stable and sources of pain are thought to be minimal.

The box below lists measures used to reduce pain from pancreatitis. As the nurse works with the patient to achieve pain control, the patient's hope that efforts will be successful is supported. Pointing out subtle changes that show improvement, as well as the decreased use of narcotics, helps the patient maintain hope.

The nurse who has developed self-awareness about perceptions of patients with chemical dependency and the responses evoked by apathetic patients may be more able to exhibit hopefulness in patient interactions. Patients can be helped to maintain hope by nurses who do the following:

1. Promote self-esteem.
2. Make referrals for treatment of substance abuse.
3. Reinforce the notion that the patient can control pain by prescribed measures.

♯ Evaluation

The expected patient outcomes serve as the basis for evaluating the extent to which patient status was improved. Questions to ask may include the following:

Teaching for the patient with pancreatic disorders

1. After pancreatic surgery
   a. Self-care as to dressings, tubes, medications
   b. Need for low-fat, high-calorie diet, as appropriate
   c. Need for continued medical follow-up care
2. After pancreatitis
   a. Prevention of further attacks (avoidance of alcohol, narcotics, and abdominal injury; medical care when ill)
   b. Reporting symptoms indicating relapse or complications
      1. Pain
      2. Nausea and vomiting
      3. Abdominal distention
      4. Steatorrhea
      5. Polyuria, polydipsia, polyphagia
      6. Weight loss
      7. Fever
   c. Maintaining low-fat, bland diet with several small feedings per day and vitamin supplements
   d. Avoiding rich foods to keep pancreatic secretions at a minimum
   e. Continuing medication therapy (pancreatic enzymes, bile salts, oral hypoglycemic agents, or insulin)—scheduling, rationale, dose, side effects
   f. Need for continued medical follow-up care
3. Pain management
   a. Avoidance of stimulants of pain
   b. Timing of food and enzyme replacements
   c. Use of antacids, cimetidine (Tagamet)

1. Were symptoms relieved?
2. Did serum amylase return to normal?
3. Was there prompt detection and treatment of complications?
4. Was patient adequately prepared to manage the treatment regimen at home?
5. Were patient and family referred to appropriate supportive services?

■ SUMMARY

1. The anatomical structure of the liver has several specialized characteristics: the organization of cellular plates; the portal vein and hepatic arterial blood supply into the sinusoids; the biliary canaliculi emptying into the larger biliary ductules, ducts and common bile duct; and Kupffer's cells lining the blood vessels.
2. The liver is important for proper metabolism of fat, protein, and carbohydrate, for production of plasma proteins, for bile production, and for detoxification.
3. The gallbladder can store and concentrate bile; it can release bile under neural (vagal) and hormonal stimulation (cholecystokinin, gastrin).
4. The secretions of the pancreas are necessary for absorption of nutrients and neutralization of acid chyme. Acinar cells secrete several kinds of enzymes and ductal cells secrete a bicarbonate-rich fluid into the pancreatic ducts.
5. Physiologic changes that occur in aging are shown by some differences in laboratory measurements of albumin, globulins, serum alkaline phosphatase, and cholesterol.
6. In the elderly, prolonged action of drugs and untoward effects may occur because of hypoalbuminemia and diminished biotransformation.
7. The incidence of toxic hepatitis could be reduced by decreased use or proper use of toxins such as petroleum distillates.
8. In America the problem of alcohol addiction contributes to the complexity of preventing hepatitis, cirrhosis, and pancreatitis.
9. There are four known types of viral hepatitis. Measures to control hepatitis A are directed toward handwashing and interrupting the fecal-oral route of transmission. The other three types are spread through blood and body fluid routes.
10. Preexposure and postexposure prophylaxis for hepatitis include immune globulin and HBIG (passive immunity) and hepatitis B vaccine (active immunity).
11. The CDC in Atlanta is the national authority for information about the prevention of infectious diseases.
12. There are many tests that use serological markers (antigens, antibodies) for differentiating the type of hepatitis: HBsAg is one test for hepatitis B. Hepatitis A is detected by absence of hepatitis B markers and the presence of IgM-class anti-HAV.
13. The CDC considers hepatitis B to be the greatest occupational hazard for health workers. Measures to decrease risk include hepatitis B vaccination, handwashing, and blood/body fluid precautions used with all patients.
14. Liver abscesses may be pyogenic and treated with broad-spectrum antibiotics and surgery, or they may be amoebic and treated with amebicidal drugs.
15. Metastatic tumors of the liver are 20 times more prevalent than primary tumors of the liver. Symptoms occur late; jaundice, ascites, and weakness are common.
16. All types of jaundice have increased serum levels of bilirubin; hemolytic jaundice is a problem of excessive red blood cell breakdown; obstructive jaundice is associated with an elevation of conjugated bilirubin (direct) and an absence of urinary urobilinogen, and hepatocellular jaundice is often associated with elevated serum transaminases.
17. A decreased prothrombin time may be associated with hepatocellular inability to form prothrombin or a biliary tract problem that interferes with the absorption of vitamin K.
18. Common problems of hepatocellular disease are jaundice, bleeding tendencies and anemia, infection, and fluid and electrolyte imbalances.
19. Increasingly severe histologic changes in liver cells are seen in alcoholic fatty liver, alcoholic hepatitis and Laënnec's cirrhosis; the latter condition is not reversible.
20. Anorexia and influenza-like symptoms are often more acute in hepatitis A but these symptoms occur in all types of hepatitis. They occur before icterus (jaundice) appears.
21. Most persons with viral hepatitis recover within 6 months and have no residual liver damage. Hepatitis B and non-A, non-B hepatitis may lead to a carrier state, atypical course of illness, chronic hepatitis, or cirrhosis.
22. In the United States, cirrhosis is most commonly a result of chronic alcoholism and is characterized by multiple liver dysfunctions. Portal hypertension and bleeding esophageal varices are two problems that threaten life.
23. Portal system encephalopathy (PSE) is associated with elevations of serum ammonia. Central nervous system dysfunction is manifested in a sequential pattern leading to coma. Asterixis is an early sign.
24. Common precipitants of PSE are hypokalemia, alkalosis, sedation, and gastrointestinal bleeding.
25. Assessment techniques of value in persons with liver diseases include percussion and palpation of the liver, inspection, auscultation, and percussion of the abdomen. Palpating for fluid wave is helpful when ascites is present.
26. In liver biopsy, aseptic technique and assisting the patient to hold his or her breath during the procedure reduce risks of infection and hemorrhage.
27. Rest, nutrition, and abstinence from toxins are three major treatments of liver disorders.
28. Malignant lesions of the liver are treated by resection, palliative use of radiation, and chemotherapy by systemic routes or portal arterial infusion.
29. Diuresis of ascitic fluid is slow and liable to induce

Putting knowledge to practice

- Review the functions of the liver, pancreas, and gallbladder.
- Explain symptoms that indicate impaired function: such as problems in metabolism, digestion and absorption, coagulation, detoxification, and urea formation; and hypoalbuminemia and fluid and electrolyte imbalances.
- List some agents that are toxic to the liver.
- Explain PSE and list observations used to detect it.
- Collect data from a patient with cirrhosis. How can that patient improve or maintain current health status?
- Compare precautions used in enteric and blood/body fluid isolation.
- Interview nurses about approaches they use with patients with alcoholism.
- Compare the nature of pain in biliary tract obstruction, pancreatitis, and malignancy of the pancreas or biliary tract.

complications: hypokalemia, oliguria, azotemia and PSE. 1/Kg of loss of body weight/per day is the maximum safe amount of ascitic fluid loss.

30. Measures to control bleeding in esophageal varices include use of the Blakemore-Sengstaken tube, pitressin infusion, and injection sclerosis. Measures to prevent PSE are also started when there is gastrointestinal bleeding.

31. After one esophageal hemorrhage, elective surgical decompression of the portal vein is done by creating a connection between portal and systemic venous circulation (liver bypass or shunting procedures).

32. Portal system encephalopathy may be treated by neomycin, lactulose and no protein diet. These measures may be used as prophylaxis when there is gastrointestinal bleeding.

33. Review the summary of preoperative and postoperative care on p. 1026.

34. In diffuse liver disorders the nurse assists the patient to recover by promoting rest and nutritional intake.

35. See pp. 1029, 1036, and 1041 for summaries of patient education.

36. Cholecystitis (often associated with cholelithiasis) can be an acute or chronic inflammatory process.

37. Cholecystography is the most common test of gallbladder filling, concentration, and emptying. Not all stones are visualized by this test.

38. In cholecystitis conservative treatment (NPO, pain control, intravenous fluids) may allow later elective surgery.

39. Biliary tract surgery is the treatment of choice when obstructive jaundice is present.

40. Nursing priorities for patients with biliary surgery include measures to prevent RLL complications, to control pain, and to promote wound healing and biliary tube drainage.

41. Acute pancreatitis is often associated with alcoholism and involves autodigestion of pancreatic tissue. Treatment includes measures to reduce pancreatic secretions (nothing by mouth, nasogastric drainage, cimetidine, antacids).

42. Acute attacks of pancreatitis may be seen in relapsing acute or in chronic pancreatitis.

43. Chronic pancreatitis is characterized by permanent structure changes, diminished exocrine and endocrine secretions, malnourishment, and the development of pseudocysts.

44. Pancreatic surgery may be used in patients with pseudocysts and other complications of pancreatitis and in patients with pancreatic tumors or biliary obstruction.

45. Pain control is very complex in chronic pancreatitis. The nurse can promote hope by supporting measures of pain relief, making referrals to resources for chemical addiction, and affirming the patient's self-esteem.

REFERENCES AND SELECTED READINGS
Contemporary

1. *Advisory Committee Immunization Practices (ACIP): Recommendations for protection against viral hepatitis, MMWR 34:313-340, 1985.

2. Altemeier, WA: Pyogenic liver abscess. In Schiff, L, and Schiff, ER, editors: Diseases of the liver, ed 5, Philadelphia, 1982, JB Lippincott Co.

3. *Anderson, FD: Portal-systemic encephalopathy in the chronic alcoholic, Crit Care Q 8(4):40-52, 1986.

4. Andreoli, TE, and others: Cecil essentials of medicine, Philadelphia, 1986, WB Saunders Co.

5. Bodenheimer, HC, Fulton, JP, and Kramer, P: Acceptance of hepatitis B vaccine among hospital workers, Am J Public Health 76:252-255, 1986.

6. Calabreese, L: In Health and Science, The Cleveland Plain Dealer, Aug 11, 1987, 5B.

7. Carnevali, DL, and Patrick, M (editors): Nursing management for the elderly, ed 2, Philadelphia, 1986, JB Lippincott Co.

8. *Cunningham, SM: When a transplant team comes to your operating room, AORN J 39:50-54, 1984.

9. Cutler, BS, and others: Manual of clinical problems in surgery, Boston, 1984, Little, Brown & Co.

10. Deitzen, DC: Surgery of the pancreas, Soc Gastrointest Assist J 5(4):5-6, 1983.

*References preceded by an asterisk are particularly well suited for student reading.

11. Dienslag, JL, and others: Hepatitis B vaccine administered to chronic carriers of hepatitis B surface antigen, Ann Intern Med 96:575-579, 1982.

12. *Dodd, RP: Ascites: when the liver can't cope, RN 47(10):26-30, 1984.

13. *Dougherty, WM: Serum bilirubin, Nurs '82 (11):138-139, 1982.

14. *Fredette, SL: When the liver fails, Am J Nurs 84:64-67, 1984.

15. *Gannon, RB, and Pickett, K: Jaundice, Am J Nurs 83:404-407, 1983.

16. *Garvey, EC, and Manganano, E: Nursing implications of hepatic artery infusion, Can Nurse 5:51-55, 1982.

17. Gillham, MB, Southworth, K, and Dollahite, J: Nutritional treatment for the alcoholic patient, Crit Care Q 8(4):20-28, 1986.

18. Given, BA, and Simmons, SJ: Gastroenterology in clinical nursing, ed 4, St. Louis, 1984, The CV Mosby Co.

19. Goldenberg, DA: Management of bleeding esophageal varices, Crit Care Q 5(2):33-46, 1982.

20. Greenberger, NJ: Chronic pancreatitis and exocrine insufficiency, Hosp Pract 20(1A):33-38, 40-45, 1985.

21. Greenberger, NJ: Gastrointestinal disorders: a pathophysiologic approach, ed 2, Chicago, 1981, Year Book Medical Publishers, Inc.

22. Gruber, M, and Nuwer, N: Treating esophageal varices with injection sclerotherapy, Am J Nurs 82:1214-1216, 1982.

23. Guenter, P, and Slocum, B: Hepatic disease: nutritional implications, Nurs Clin North Am 18(1):71-80, 1983.

24. Gullatte, MM, and Foltz, AT: Hepatic chemotherapy via implantable pump, Am J Nurs 83:1674-1676, 1983.

25. Gurerich, I: Viral hepatitis, Am J Nurs 83:571-586, 1983.

26. Isselbacher, K, and others: Harrison's principles of internal medicine, ed 9, New York, 1980, McGraw-Hill Book Co.

27. Kelber, MB: Pancreatic enzymes: deciphering diagnostic studies, Nurs '82 12(12):65-67, 1982.

28. *King, DE: How to give your portal hypertension patient a fighting chance, RN 46(7):31-37, 1983.

29. Kirkman-Liff, BL, and Dandoy, S: Hepatitis B: what price exposure? Am J Nurs 84:988-990, 1984.

30. Klopp, A: Shunting malignant ascites, Am J Nurs 84:212-213, 1984.

31. Kosel, K, and others: Total pancreatectomy and islet cell autotransplantation, Am J Nurs 82:568-571, 1982.

32. Malasanos, L, and others: Health assessment, ed 3, St. Louis, 1986, The CV Mosby Co.

33. Maloney, JP: Surgical intervention in the alcoholic patient with portal hypertension, Crit Care Q 8(4)63-73, 1986.

34. *Mar, DD: Drug-induced hepatotoxicity, Am J Nurs 82:124-126, 1982.

35. Moertel, CG: Medical management of liver cancer, In Schiff, L, and Schiff, ER, editors: Diseases of the liver, ed 5, Philadelphia, 1982, JB Lippincott Co.

36. *Newell, J: Portal systemic encephalopathy, Nurs Pract 9:26-37, 1984.

37. *Nurses Clinical Library: Gastrointestinal disorders, Springhouse, Pa, Nursing '85 Books, 1985, Springhouse Corp.

38. Quinless, F: Portal hypertension: physiology, signs and symptoms, Nurs '84 14(1):52-53, 1984.

39. Resnick, RH: Cirrhosis. In Conn, HR, and others, editors: Current therapy 1984, Philadelphia, 1984, WB Saunders Co.

40. Roemeling, RV, and others: Chemotherapy via implanted infusion pump: new perspectives for delivery of long-term continuous treatment, Oncol Nurs Forum 13(2):17-24, 1986.

41. Schiff, L, and Schiff, ER, editors: Diseases of the liver, ed 5, Philadelphia, 1982, JB Lippincott Co.

42. Schumann, D: Correction of ascites with peritoneovenous shunting: a study of clinical management, Heart Lung 12:248-257, 1983.

43. Schwartz, SI, and others: Principles of surgery, ed 4, New York, 1984, McGraw-Hill Book Co.

44. Seybert, P, Gardon, KM, and Jackson, BS: The Leveen shunt: new hope for ascites patients, Nurs '79 9(1):24-31, 1979.

45. Smith, GS: Evaluation of patients with portal hypertension, In Rutherford, RB, editor: Vascular surgery, Philadelphia, 1984, WB Saunders.

46. Starzel, TE, and Iwatsuki, S: Transplantation of the liver. In Schiff, L, and Schiff, ER, editors: Diseases of the liver, ed 5, Philadelphia, 1982, JB Lippincott Co.

47. Taylor, DL: Gallstones: physiology, signs and symptoms, Nurs '83 13(6):44-45, 1983.

48. Taylor, DL: Jaundice: physiology, signs and symptoms, Nurs '83 13(8):52-54, 1983.

49. *Thompson, MA: Managing the patient with liver dysfunction, Nurs '81 11(11):100-107, 1981.

50. *Thorpe, C, and Caprini, R: Gallbladder disease: current trends and treatment, Am J Nurs 80:2181-2185, 1980.

51. Tilkian, SM, Conover, MB, and Tilkian, AG: Clinical implications of laboratory tests, ed 4, St. Louis, 1987, The CV Mosby Co.

52. Toskes, PP: Diagnosis of chronic pancreatitis and exocrine insufficiency, Hosp Pract 20(10):97-100, 102-103, 107-108, 1985.

53. Toskes, PP: Recurrent acute pancreatitis, Hosp Pract 20(7):85-88, 90-92, 1985.

54. US Public Health Service, Centers for Disease Control: Isolation techniques for use in hospitals, ed 3, Washington, DC, 1983, US Public Health Service.

55. Williams, SR: Essentials of nutrition and diet therapy, ed 3, St. Louis, 1982, The CV Mosby Co.

56. *Wimpsett, J: Trace your patient's liver dysfunction, Nurs '84 14(8):56-57, 1984.

Classic

57. *Bates, B: A guide to physical examination, ed 3, Philadelphia, 1983, JB Lippincott Co.

58. *Boyer, CA, and Oehlberg, SM: Interpretation and clinical relevance of liver function tests, Nurs Clin North Am 12:275-290, 1977.

59. Simmons, S, and Givens, B: Acute pancreatitis, Am J Nurs 71:934-939, 1971.

UNIT VIII
Problems of Digestion or Elimination

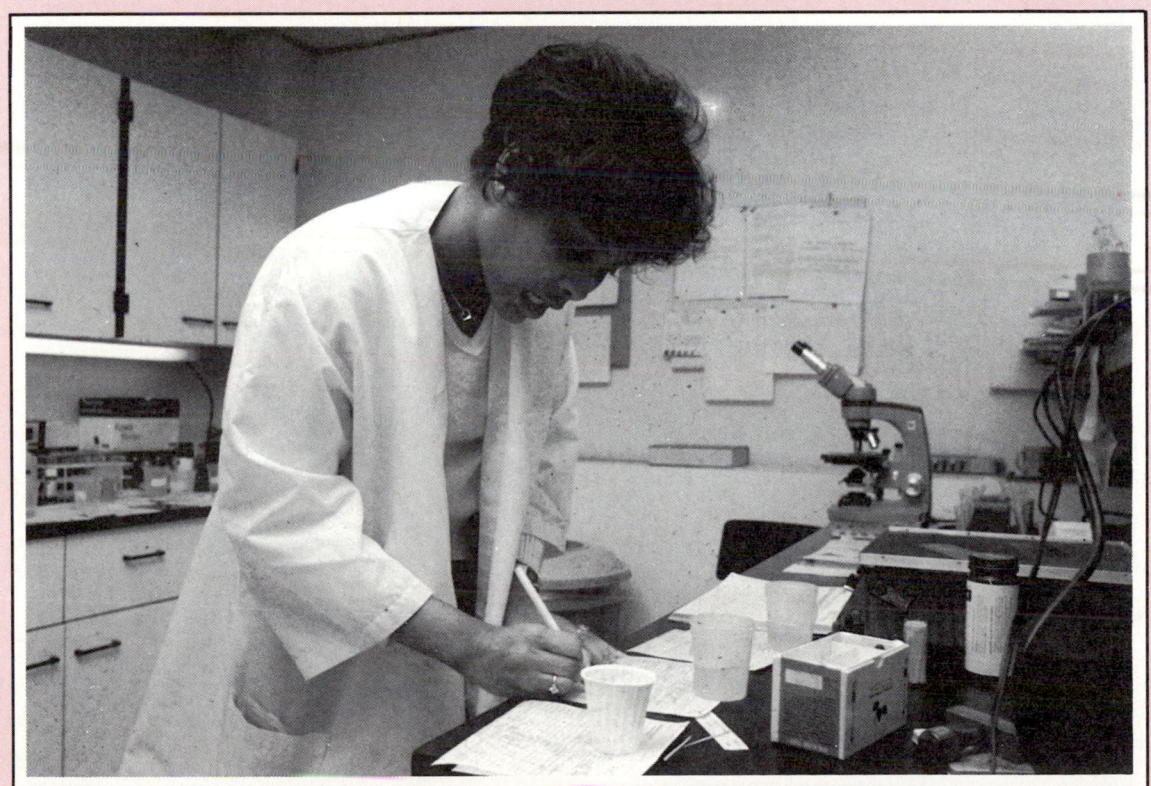

31

The Patient with Gastrointestinal Problems

BARBARA C. LONG and REBECCA ROBERTS

CHAPTER OBJECTIVES

After studying this chapter, the student should be able to:

- Describe measures for prevention and early detection of gastrointestinal (GI) disorders.

- Describe the nature of and nursing interventions for common inflammatory disorders of the mouth (stomatitis), stomach (gastritis), intestines (enteritis), and appendix (appendicitis).

- Describe the causes of dysphagia and heartburn and related therapeutic interventions.

- Differentiate gastric and duodenal ulcers and describe therapeutic modalities and patient teaching for peptic ulcer.

- Explain malabsorption syndrome and nursing interventions.

- Differentiate ulcerative colitis, Crohn's disease, and diverticular disease, and the care required for each.

- Describe the nature and care of the patient with intestinal obstruction, including hernias.

- Describe therapeutic modalities for patients with cancer of the mouth, stomach, and bowel, especially surgery.

- Describe the care of the person with a stoma for fecal diversion.

- Differentiate anorectal lesions and postoperative nursing care for rectal surgery.

■ ANATOMY AND PHYSIOLOGY

Maintenance of adequate nutrition and elimination requires an intact and functioning gastrointestinal tract. Normally, food and fluids are placed in the mouth, chewed (if solid), pushed to the pharynx by the tongue, and swallowed by automatic reflex activity down the esophagus into the stomach. Digestion starts in the mouth and ends in the small intestine, although fluids continue to be reabsorbed in the colon. The anatomical structures of the gastrointestinal tract are illustrated in Fig. 31-1. The liver, gallbladder, and pancreas, which are also involved with digestion, are discussed in Chapter 30.

■ Mouth and esophagus

■ SALIVATION

The cortical thought of food initiates saliva production from the salivary glands. The salivary secretions are made up of *serous secretion,* containing ptyalin for starch digestion, and *mucous* secretion for lubrication. These two secretions account for one half of the upper gastrointestinal tract secretions.

■ MASTICATION

The teeth serve the function of initial food breakdown. No other part of the gastrointestinal tract can perform this function if the teeth are missing. Enzymes can act only on the exposed surfaces of the food particles. Very fine particulation prevents excoriation of the lining of the tract, and the rate of digestion is dependent on the total surface area of food particle exposed. General health teaching for children and adults should stress the reason behind thorough mastication of all food substances that are ingested.

■ SWALLOWING

Swallowing must be accomplished without compromising respiration. The tongue forces the bolus of food into the pharynx, from which point the food moves to the upper esophagus and then down into the stomach. Food is prevented from passing into the trachea by the closing of the epiglottis over the trachea and the opening of the esophagus.

The esophagus is a hollow tube. The upper one third is composed of skeletal muscle and the remainder of smooth muscle. It is lined with mucous membrane, which secretes a mucoid substance for protection. The bolus of food arrives at the cardiac sphincter of the stomach usually within 5 to 10 seconds of ingestion.

The cardiac sphincter prevents reflux of stomach contents into the lower esophagus. This area is heavily layered with mucoid glands. The secretions adhere to the food particles and prevent actual contact with the wall mucosa. The coated particles adhere to each other, forming a bolus for digestion. These secretions act as a protective mechanism for the sphincter zone, since they themselves are strongly resistant to digestion.

■ Stomach

The food bolus enters the stomach, the largest dilated portion of the tract. There is relatively little muscular tone, allowing for increased distension. Movement of food through the stomach and intestines is by *peristalsis,* the alternate contraction and relaxation of the muscle fibers that propel the substance in a wavelike motion.

The mucous membrane lining the stomach is arranged in thick folds known as *rugae* that provide an increased surface area for exposure and contain the openings of the gastric glands. The gastric secretions are clear and colorless and contain water, salts, enzymes, and hydrochloric acid. The amount of enzymes produced is in direct proportion to the amount needed, and the actual food substance stimulates the release of a particular enzyme. The gastric mucosa releases gastrin, which stimulates the production of *pepsinogen* (the precursor of pepsin), *rennin,* and *lipase.* Pepsin and rennin digest protein, and lipase splits fats. The production of hydrochloric acid (HCl) does not appear to depend on the presence of any particular food.

As the food moves toward the pyloric sphincter at the distal end of the stomach, peristaltic waves increase in force and intensity. The fluid bolus now becomes a substance known as *chyme.* Chyme is pumped through the pyloric sphincter into the duodenum. Emptying of stomach contents is regulated by two factors: consistency of the fluid chyme and receptiveness of the duodenum. The average length of time food remains in the stomach after a meal is 2 to 6 hours.

■ Intestines

The small intestine has three parts: the *duodenum,* which connects to the stomach, the *jejunum* or middle portion, and the *ileum.* The large intestine also has three parts: the *cecum,* which connects to the small intestine, the *colon,* and the *rectum.* The primary function of the intestines is to receive the chyme from the stomach and move the chyme forward to facilitate proper absorption of water, nutrients, electrolytes, and bile salts (Fig. 31-2). Secondary functions include secreting mucus and serving as a storage area before waste discharge.

■ MOVEMENT

Contents of the small intestine are propelled toward the anus by peristaltic movements that mix the intestinal contents. Chyme moves slowly and normally takes 3 to 10 hours to move from the stomach to the ileocecal valve (see Fig. 31-1). In the colon, the fecal contents are pushed forward by mass movements that occur only a few times each day. These mass movements are stimulated by gastrocolic reflexes initiated when food enters the duodenum from the stomach, especially after the first meal of the day. This is therefore the most frequent time of the day for defecation to occur.

The defecation reflex occurs when feces enter the rectum. Afferent impulses are transmitted to the sacral segments of the spinal cord, from which reflex impulses are

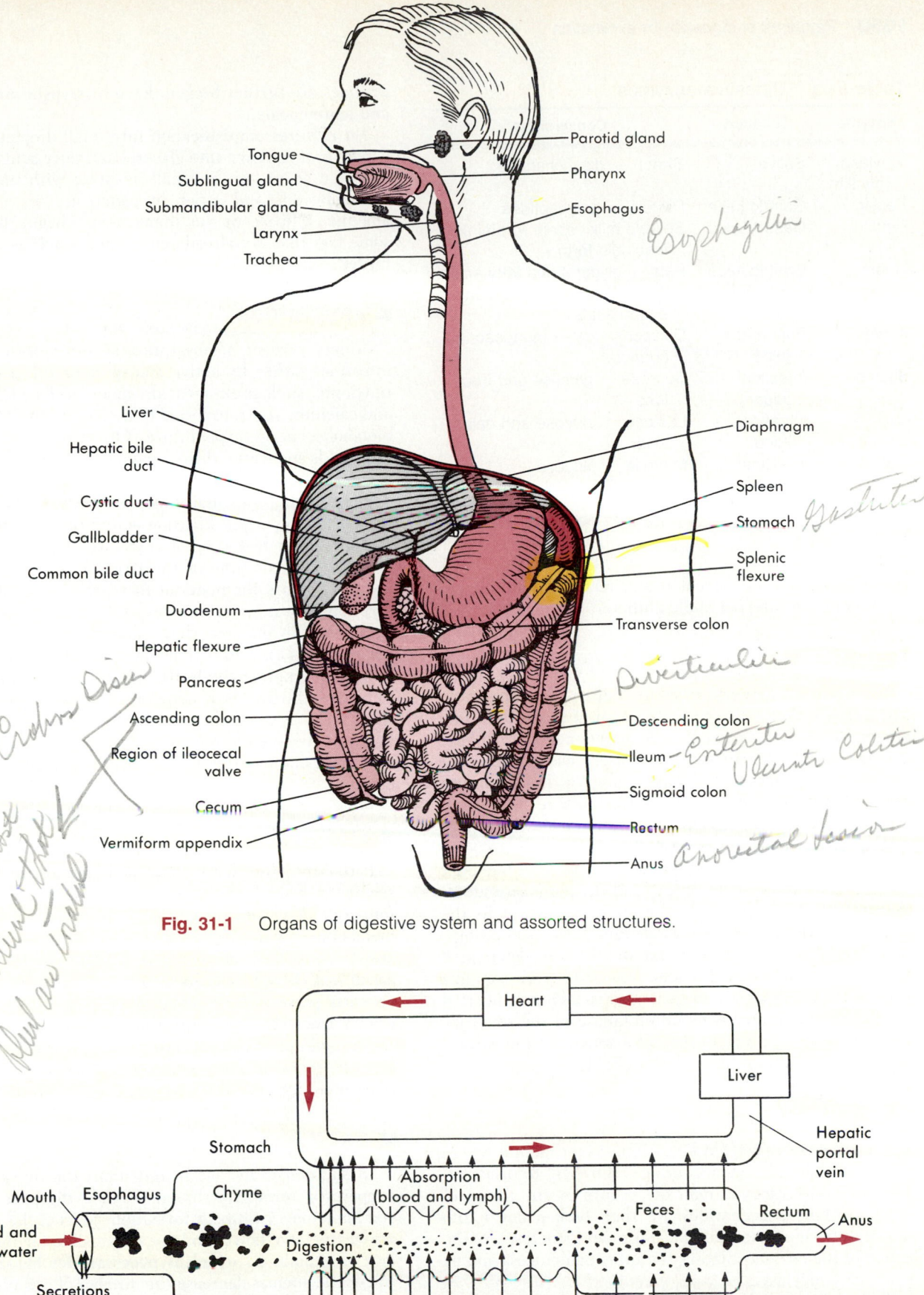

Esophagitis

Gastritis

Diverticulitis

Enteritis

Ulcer Colitis

Anorectal lesion

Crohn's Disease

Whenever
intestinal tract
filled or inflamed

Fig. 31-1 Organs of digestive system and assorted structures.

Fig. 31-2 Summary of gastrointestinal activity involving motility, secretion, digestion, and absorption. (From Vander, AJ, and others: Human physiology, ed 3. Copyright © 1980 by McGraw-Hill Book Co., New York. Used with the permission of McGraw-Hill Book Co.)

Table 31-1 Digestive enzymes

Enzyme	Location	Conversions
Amylase (ptyalin)	Saliva	Starch → disaccharides
Pepsin	Gastric juice	Protein → polypeptides
Renin	Gastric juice	Soluble milk casein (protein) → insoluble form
Lipase	Gastric juice	Fats → glycerol and fatty acids
Trypsin	Pancreatic juice	Polypeptides → peptides and amino acids
Amylase	Pancreatic juice	Disaccharides → monosaccharides
Sucrase	Intestinal juice	Sucrose → glucose and fructose
Lactase	Intestinal juice	Lactose → glucose and galactose
Maltase	Intestinal juice	Maltose → glucose

transmitted back to the colon and rectum, initiating relaxation of the internal anal sphincter.

■ SECRETION

Secretions of the small intestine, biliary, and pancreatic systems provide for the final digestion of food. As chyme enters the small intestine, gastric secretion of hydrochloric acid is slowed. Mucous secretion throughout the tract increases food adhesion, prevents contact of the food with the wall of the mucosa, enhances free passage of the food, neutralizes the small amounts of acid or alkali, and makes some particles more resistant to digestion.

Emptying into the duodenum are the common bile duct (from the liver and gallbladder) and the pancreatic duct. *Bile,* which is produced in the liver and stored in the gallbladder, drains into the duodenum to assist in absorption of fats by emulsifying the fat and breaking down large fat droplets into small droplets. *Pancreatic juice* contains three digestive enzymes, trypsinogen (which is converted into trypsin by the enzyme enterokinase in the small intestines), amylase, and lipase. The actions of the various digestive enzymes are described in Table 31-1.

■ DIGESTION

The digestion of *carbohydrate* begins in the mouth, where the breakdown of polysaccharides (starches) to disaccharides (sucrose, lactose, maltose) occurs by the action of amylase. The disaccharides are then broken down into monosaccharides (glucose, galactose, and fructose) by the action of the enzymes within the intestinal mucosa and by pancreatic amylase.

Protein digestion begins in the stomach with the breakdown of proteins into polypeptides (an intermediate step) by the action of pepsin. In the small intestine, the poly-

peptides are further broken down by trypsin into peptides and amino acids.

Fat requires emulsification into small droplets before it can be broken down into glycerol and fatty acids. Most fat digestion occurs in the small intestine with the emulsification by bile and action of pancreatic lipase. A small amount of lipase in the stomach may begin digestion of some fats that are already emulsified, such as cream and butter.

■ ABSORPTION

Ninety percent of absorption occurs within the small intestine, either by active transport or diffusion. Many nutrients, such as amino acids, monosaccharides, sodium, and calcium, are transported by active transport, requiring metabolic energy expenditure. Other nutrients, such as fatty acids and water, diffuse passively across the cell membrane. Pancreatic lipase and conjugated bile salts must be present in the intestinal lumen for hydrolysis of fats into fatty acids to permit diffusion across the cell membrane.

Approximately 450 ml of chyme reaches the cecum per day. The transit time in the large bowel is slow, taking about 12 hours for material to reach the rectum. Reabsorption of water, electrolytes, and bile salts occurs predominantly in the ascending colon. The colon has the capacity to absorb 6 to 8 times more fluid than is delivered to it daily. Approximately 100 ml of fluid contents remains to be mixed with the residue of feces. Normally, this residue (feces) is evacuated on a fairly regular schedule. The evacuation schedule differs for each individual and may vary from one to three times per day to once every 3 to 4 days.

■ FLUID AND ELECTROLYTE BALANCE

Pathologic alterations occur with the loss of particular segments of small or large bowel or when reabsorption is impaired. The loss of small bowel contents precipitates metabolic acidosis and hypokalemia from the loss of bicarbonate and potassium. This problem may occur with drainage of small bowel contents through a suction tube or fistula or with persistent vomiting of the intestinal contents. Losses from the large intestine comprise mainly loss of water, sodium, and to a lesser extent chloride, resulting in dehydration and hyponatremia. This occurs in conditions in which the rate of peristalsis is increased.

■ BACTERIA

In addition to its role in nutrition, the intestinal tract supports bacterial growth that enhances digestive processes and has a role in antibody formation. Most of the organisms are in the large bowel and are responsible for the production of vitamin K, which is necessary for blood clotting. Antibiotic enemas decrease the number of organisms, thus interfering with vitamin K synthesis. Conditions that inhibit intestinal motility may lead to bacterial overgrowth in the intestines.

■ Physiologic changes with aging

Changes in the gastrointestinal tract structure and function may occur with aging but vary among individuals and may or may not cause altered functioning.

In the mouth, aging teeth become darker and may loosen from loss of supporting bone and gums. Teeth may become uneven or develop fractures, and circulation of the gums is reduced. Gum changes affect the fit of dentures. Salivary gland output decreases, leading to increased dryness of mucous membranes and making them more susceptible to breakdown. Dryness of the mouth may also interfere with chewing.

Changes in the ability to digest and absorb foods are related to decreased secretion of most digestive enzymes and bile production. Absorption of fats and fat-soluble vitamins becomes impaired. The increased residue resulting from decreased digestion and absorption may lead to increased flatulence. Gas-forming foods may be less well tolerated than when the person was younger.

Decreased intestinal motility may result from decreased peristalsis, decreased muscular tone of the intestinal wall, and decreased abdominal muscle strength. Decreased anal sphincter tone may also be present. These changes con-

tribute to the increased occurrence of constipation in the older person.

■ PREVENTION AND HEALTH EDUCATION

Disorders of the digestive system are among the most commonly encountered health problems. Symptoms produced by digestive disorders are numerous and often lead to decreased employment productivity. Gastrointestinal symptoms, such as nausea and vomiting or diarrhea, often result from disorders of other body systems. Interference with functioning of the gastrointestinal system leads to temporary or long-term nutritional imbalances.

■ Primary prevention: prevention of disease

Because the cause of many gastrointestinal disorders is unknown, prevention may not be possible. Some health practices that are either known to be or are thought to be helpful in preventing disorders include good oral hygiene

---

Prevention of gastrointestinal problems: health teaching

Oral hygiene

1. Brush teeth after meals with fluoridated toothpaste.
2. Use denture floss between teeth.
3. Rinse mouth after eating sweets.
4. Have regular dental checkups.
5. Replace misfitting or broken dentures.
6. Strengthen gums under dentures by rubbing with fingers or rinsing with alternating warm and cold liquid.

Nutrition

1. Plan meals based on basic four food groups (Chapter 6).
2. Substitute high-vitamin fruits for sweets, especially at end of meal (for example, apples, apricots, peaches, pears).
3. Avoid *excessive* amounts of foods that are found to irritate the oral mucosa (for example, raw tomatoes, hot peppers).
4. Avoid foods found to irritate one's stomach, such as highly seasoned foods, large amounts of alcohol, or coffee.
5. Include high-fiber foods (vegetables, fruits, whole-grain cereals) in the diet.
6. Avoid foods that may cause food poisoning: unrefrigerated mayonnaise; cream-filled foods; inadequately cooked eggs, poultry, or meat (especially pork); improperly canned foods.

Tobacco use

1. Avoid constant exposure of lips to hot pipe.
2. Avoid chewing tobacco.
3. Discontinue cigarette smoking, if possible.

Stress

1. Identify and remove cause of stress, if possible.
2. Use measures to reduce stress response when stress occurs; for example, relaxation exercises (see Chapter 7).
3. Get adequate sleep on a regular basis.

Early detection of major gastrointestinal disorders

1. *Signs requiring immediate medical follow-up*
   a. *Mouth*
      1. A sore that bleeds easily and does not heal
      2. A lump or thickening
      3. A persistent red or whitish patch
      4. Difficulty chewing, swallowing, or moving tongue or jaws
   b. *Abdomen*
      1. Persistent heartburn, indigestion
      2. Abdominal pain, especially if accompanied by nausea and vomiting
   c. *Elimination*
      1. Change in bowel habits
      2. Blood in the stool
2. *American Cancer Society recommendations for screening for cancer of colon and rectum*
   a. Digital rectal examination by physician every year after age 40
   b. Stool guaiac test done by patient at home every year after age 50
   c. Proctoscopic examination every 3 to 5 years after age 50; following two initial negative tests, 1 year apart.

---

and nutrition, and avoidance of tobacco use and stress (see the box on p. 1051).

■ Secondary prevention: early detection

Early detection of major gastrointestinal health problems can prevent serious complications, such as a ruptured appendix with peritonitis. Persons at high risk for cancer of the colon (p. 1105) need careful screening to detect early signs of cancer because the cancer may be in an advanced stage before any symptoms occur. Guidelines for early detection are listed in the box above.

Major health problems of the gastrointestinal system

Gastrointestinal disorders may be classified according to their overall effect on gastrointestinal function or according to the function of specific areas.

■ CLASSIFICATION BY GENERAL FUNCTION

Disorders of the gastrointestinal (GI) tract may interfere with function in one of three ways: interference with motility and control, with digestion and absorption, and with mechanical passage of food, chyme, and feces.

■ Disorders of motility

Interference with GI motility may occur in any part of the GI tract. Esophageal disorders interfere with swallowing and movement of food to the stomach. Vomiting is reverse peristalsis and may result from delayed gastric emptying. Surgical removal of part of the stomach leads to rapid emptying (dumping syndrome). Intestinal hypermotility produces diarrhea. Fecal incontinence results from loss of control. Decreased intestinal motility may lead to flatulence and constipation. Paralytic ileus is failure of intestinal peristalsis.

■ Disorders of digestion and absorption

Disorders that interfere with the digestion and absorption of food include inflammatory disorders, ulcerations, or malabsorptions. *Inflammatory* disorders may occur in any part of the GI tract (Fig. 31-3) and may be acute or chronic. Acute inflammations are painful and produce swelling of the mucosa that may interfere with absorption. Chronic inflammations create changes in the muscular walls, as well as in the mucosa. *Ulcerations* may also extend through the mucosa into the muscular wall and cause pain. *Malabsorption* disorders may alter digestion when nutrients are not broken down into a form that can be transported across cell membranes, or they may alter absorption of the nutrients across the cell membranes and into the lymphatic or circulatory system.

■ Obstructive disorders

The GI tract may become obstructed at any point from the portal of entry (mouth) to the exit (rectum). Obstruction may occur from mechanical causes that physically impede passage of intestinal contents or from paralytic causes, in which the passageway is open but peristalsis ceases. Mechanical obstructive disorders include tumors, hernias, adhesions, twisting or telescoping of the intestines, and interferences with the vascular supply.

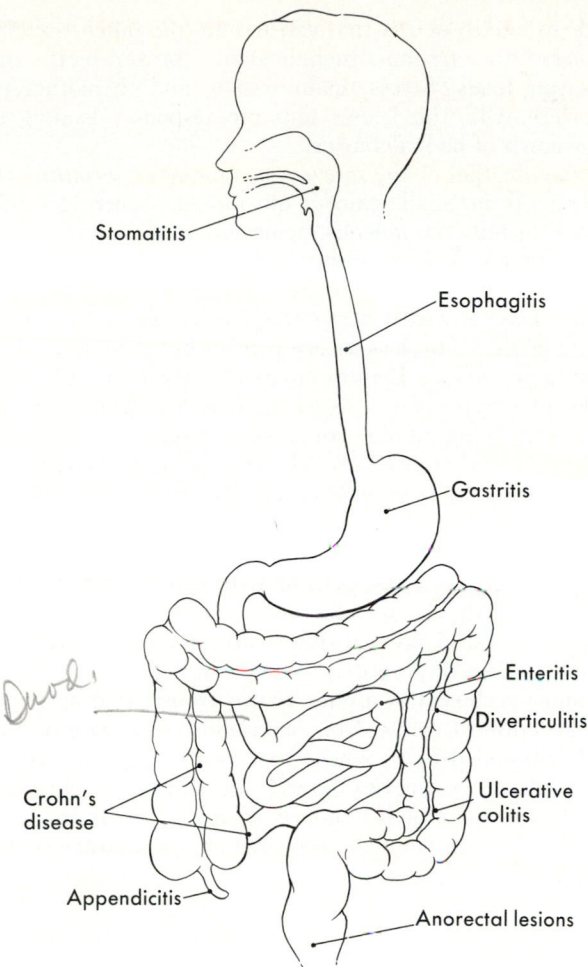

Fig. 31-3 Inflammatory conditions of GI system.

■ CLASSIFICATION BY SPECIFIC FUNCTION

GI disorders can also be grouped by functions of specific areas: ingestion via the mouth and esophagus, digestion in the stomach and duodenum, and elimination via the intestines. Common GI disorder classifications are:

1. Ingestive disorders
   a. Inflammations of the mouth
   b. Esophageal disorders
   c. Cancer of the mouth and esophagus
2. Digestive disorders
   a. Gastritis
   b. Ulcerations of stomach and duodenum
   c. Cancer of the stomach
   d. Malabsorption syndromes
3. Elimination disorders
   a. Acute inflammatory intestinal disorders
   b. Chronic inflammatory intestinal disorders
   c. Ileus: paralytic, intestinal obstruction
   d. Hernias
   e. Anorectal lesions
   f. Colorectal cancer

■ INGESTIVE DISORDERS

■ Vomiting

Although vomiting is a symptom rather than a disorder per se, it is a common disruption of motility of the upper GI tract and therefore is discussed here.

■ PATHOPHYSIOLOGY

Vomiting is often preceded by nausea but may occur alone. It may be a symptom of a disease process (such as infection or uremia) or a response to drugs, visceral injury, pain, psychic trauma, radiation, or motion. Vomiting is initiated by the vomiting center in the brain. It is reverse peristalsis. Vomiting can be defined as forceful ejection of stomach contents. If the pyloric end of the stomach is obstructed, the vomitus will project away from the person (projectile vomiting).

Prolonged and severe vomiting will interfere with nutrition and cause fluid and electrolyte imbalance, specifically dehydration and metabolic alkalosis with loss of potassium, chloride, and hydrogen ions. The act of vomiting produces a strain on the abdominal muscles, and in some postoperative patients it may cause wound dehiscence or bleeding. Vomiting is especially dangerous for anesthetized patients, persons in coma, and infants because they are likely to aspirate the vomitus into the lungs. Aspiration may block oxygen intake (asphyxia) or lead to inflammation of the lung (atelectasis, pneumonitis), especially in an elderly person whose nasopharyngeal reflexes are less acute than those of a younger person.

▦ ASSESSMENT

Subjective data: onset of vomiting, patient's perception of cause
Objective data: examination of vomitus
1. Greenish yellow: bile
2. Bright red: overt bleeding of recent origin
3. Brownish "coffee-ground": blood has been in the stomach for a period of time and is partly digested
4. Fecal odor: intestinal contents from an intestinal obstruction
Vomiting of blood is termed *hematemesis*. It is important to ascertain whether the content expelled from the mouth has been vomited from the stomach or coughed up from the lungs. Bloody sputum usually has a more frothy appearance than hematemesis. "Dry" emesis or retching may occur when the stomach is empty.

▦ IMPLEMENTATION

1. Assisting with achievement of therapeutic goals
   a. If vomiting is anticipated (such as with radiation or motion), give prescribed antiemetic 30 minutes before the event.
   b. If vomiting is present, give prescribed antiemetic by suppository or *deep* intramuscular injection.

2. <mark>Assisting with comfort</mark>
   a. Provide a calm environment to decrease anxiety.
   b. Suggest deep breaths through the mouth if nausea or gagging occurs.
   c. Remove vomitus as soon as possible and provide oral hygiene.
   d. Provide fluids in small amounts after vomiting subsides; ginger ale and other effervescent drinks are usually well tolerated.
   e. Provide solid foods (after vomiting subsides) that are well tolerated, such as crackers, baked potato, or apple.

Inflammatory disorders of the mouth

The mouth is an excellent barometer of general health, reflecting general disease and debility as well as good health. Specific diseases of the mouth most often occur when general nutrition and oral hygiene are poor, when people neglect their teeth, and when smoking is excessive.

In the mouth, inflammation may occur on the mucous membranes, gum, or tongue. Medical treatment depends on the site and causative factor (Table 31-2).

PATHOPHYSIOLOGY

Several factors contribute to the development of oral inflammatory disorders: (1) poor oral hygiene, (2) stress, (3) nutritional deficiencies, (4) debilitating diseases, (5) heavy smoking, and (6) chemotherapy. Poor oral hygiene leads to mouth debris that can irritate the mucous membranes. Other irritants include smoke, broken teeth, and irritating foods. Stress, malnutrition, and chemotherapy interfere with the body's immune response, leading to breakdown of body defenses.

Inflammation of the mucous membranes (*stomatitis*) often results in small, painful ulcerations. Scarring rarely occurs, as only the mucous membrane is usually involved. Inflammation of the gums may cause teeth to loosen. Causative organisms include bacteria, viruses, or funguses.

Aphthous stomatitis occur frequently, especially among young adults. The lesions are painful but usually heal in about 1 to 3 weeks. *Herpetic* stomatitis may occur only once or be recurrent. There is an increased susceptibility in people receiving immunosuppressive drugs.

Thrush is frequently seen when antibiotics are given over a period of time to control other infections. It is thought that the elimination of bacteria permits growth of the existing fungus, causing thrush. Persons at higher risk include denture wearers, persons with debilitating or acute illnesses, or those with impaired immune response.[42]

The parotid gland that drains into the mouth may also become inflamed (parotitis). Acute communicable parotitis (mumps) is caused by a virus that is transmitted by direct contact with the saliva. Noncommunicable parotitis occurs in debilitated persons whose oral hygiene is poor, whose mouths have been permitted to become dry, and who have not chewed solid foods regularly. Elderly persons are more susceptible than younger ones. Usually the *staphylococcus* organism is not present.

Table 31-2 Inflammatory disorders of mouth

Disease	Etiology	Signs and symptoms	Medical therapy
Aphthous stomatitis (canker sores)	Unclear	Ulcer on mucous membranes becomes covered with opaque material; pain	Triamcinolone acetonide in emollient dental paste (Kenalog in Orabase)
Herpetic stomatitis (cold sore, fever blister)	Herpesvirus type 1	Initial burning sensation, vesicle formation on junction of lips to mucosa, secondary infection, crusting	Symptomatic treatment: 70% alcohol initially for drying; petrolatum after vesicular stage; rest; avoidance of stress
Vincent's angina (ulceromembranous stomatitis)	Fusiform bacillus and a spirochete	Malaise, acute painful bleeding gums, fetid breath, ulceration on margins of gums, dysphagia	Gentle debridement by dentist; mouthwashes with warm normal saline or 3% hydrogen peroxide; rest; antibiotics if severe
Thrush (candidiasis)	*Candida albicans* (fungus)	White patches (like milk curds) over inflamed membranes	Nystatin oral suspension Clotrimazole troches (Mycelex) Ketoconazole tablets (Nizoral)
Gingivitis (gums)	Bacterial plaque, malocclusion, food impaction, vitamin deficiency	Red inflamed gums, bleeding with minimal injury, swelling of interdental spaces	Good oral hygiene and dental care
Periodontitis (loss of bone supporting teeth)	Same as for gingivitis	Same as for gingivitis, loose teeth, recession of gums, possible abcess formation	Dental care, dental surgery

⊞ ASSESSMENT

In patients at high risk of developing infections, the mouth is assessed daily for developing or healing inflammations.

☐ Subjective data

The patient is questioned about the presence and extent of the following symptoms: (1) pain in the mouth, (2) loss of appetite, (3) nausea, (4) foul taste in the mouth, and (5) increase or decrease of salivation. The pain is caused by the inflammatory response, and it restricts ability or desire to keep the teeth and mouth clean. This leads to the foul taste and loss of appetite. Swallowing of inflammatory debris may produce nausea.

☐ Objective data

1. Mouth inspection
   a. Cleanliness
   b. Condition of teeth (caries, loose teeth, debris)
   c. Signs of inflammation (redness, edema, ulceration, or white curdlike patches of thrush)
   d. Bleeding of mucous membranes or gums
2. Ability of patient to carry out oral hygiene
   a. Mental status (decreased consciousness or confusion)
   b. Ability to open mouth (pain may limit mouth movement)
   c. Cleanliness of mouth after oral hygiene
3. Ability to ingest and swallow food

➡ DATA ANALYSIS: NURSING DIAGNOSES

Nursing diagnoses are determined from assessment of patient data. Possible nursing diagnoses for the person with a mouth infection may include, but are not limited, to the following:

Diagnostic title	Possible etiologies
Potential fluid volume deficit	Foul taste, mouth discomfort
Altered nutrition: less than body requirements	Difficulty chewing, foul taste, mouth discomfort
Altered oral mucous membrane	Poor oral hygiene, inflammation
Pain: mouth	Inflammation of mouth

⊞ PLANNING: EXPECTED PATIENT OUTCOMES

Expected patient outcomes for the person with a mouth infection may include, but are not limited to the following:
1. The patient's mouth is clean; mucosa pink and moist.
2. Fluid intake is greater than 1500 ml/day; skin turgor is good.
3. Weight remains stable; patient eats a balanced diet.
4. Patient says mouth feels comfortable.
5. Patient can describe risk factors to be avoided to prevent recurrence of oral inflammations.

⊞ IMPLEMENTATION

☐ Assisting with achievement of therapeutic goals
☐ *Medications*

If antibiotics are ordered, they are given on time on a regular schedule to maintain blood levels. If the patient has difficulty swallowing tablets, they are crushed, if possible, or the antibiotics may be given intramuscularly or intravenously. If nystatin is prescribed for oral thrush, the suspension should be held and swished through the mouth for as long as possible before being swallowed.

☐ *Mouth care*

Thorough and frequent mouth care is a must.
1. Frequency
   a. Mild stomatitis: at least every 4 hours
   b. Severe stomatitis: at least every 2 hours
2. Types of solutions
   a. Alkaline mouthwashes, such as sodium bicarbonate or sodium perborate
   b. Hydrogen peroxide diluted 1:4 with normal saline (mix just before use to prevent decomposition)
   c. Lidocaine rinses may be prescribed for stomatitis resulting from chemotherapeutic drugs
3. Removal of dentures if causing pain
4. If the toothbrush causes pain, gently wipe gum and teeth with moistened gauze wrapped around a tongue blade; rinse with solution followed by water

☐ Assisting with comfort and activities of daily living
☐ *Relief of pain*

Pain may be partially relieved by good oral hygiene. Smoking is contraindicated. Cold drinks or sucking on frozen Popsicles may be soothing. Analgesic drugs may be necessary, and lidocaine may be applied to provide topical anesthesia.

☐ *Facilitating eating*

If the mouth is very sore and painful, eating may be difficult, and the patient may need considerable encouragement. Soft foods, including strained meats and fish, pureed vegetables and fruits (except citrus), cooked cereals, soups, flavored gelatin, and ice cream, are best tolerated. Hot spicy foods are to be avoided; cold drinks may be soothing. High-protein, high-calorie drinks such as eggnog serve both nutritional and fluid needs.

☐ *Teaching*

Persons at high risk for developing recurrent oral infections need to know about contributing factors that may be controlled, such as poor oral hygiene, poor nutrition, irritating foods, heavy smoking, and stress (see preventive measures, p. 1051).

⊞ EVALUATION

Evaluation is based on the expected patient outcomes. Interventions may have to be modified based on the severity of the oral infection. The mouth is assessed daily for cleanliness and extent of healing and comfort.

■ Cancer of the mouth

Cancer of the mouth (Table 31-3) accounts for about 4% of all cancers. Men are affected twice as often as women, and occurrences are more frequent after age 40; the average patient age is about 65.[42] Although any part of the mouth may be affected, the lips and the anterior tongue and floor of the mouth are the most common sites.

■ PATHOPHYSIOLOGY

Most oral cancers are squamous cell carcinomas; occasionally the tumor may be a basal cell carcinoma that starts on the skin and spreads to the lips. Risk factors include smoking and alcohol; the combination causes an apparent breakdown in the immune system.[53]

Oral cancers can be classified according to four stages. In stages I and II, there is no lymph node spread or metastasis; tumor size varies from less than 2 cm (I) up to 4 cm (II). In stage III, the tumor size is greater than 4 cm, and there may be a palpable node on one side. In stage IV, the tumor is invasive, and there may be metastasis to the liver or lungs. Either surgery or radiation may be used to treat stage I cancers, and both therapies are used for stages II and III. Stage IV therapy is usually palliative.

Premalignant lesions (that may or may not become malignant) include *leukoplakia* (white patches), *erythroplasia* (red granular patches), and *erythroplakia* (white plaques within red patches). The red patches have a higher potential for malignancy than leukoplakia.[53]

The cure rate for cancer of the *lips* is high because the lesion is easily apparent to the patient and to others. Metastasis to regional lymph nodes has occurred in 10% of people when the case is diagnosed. In some instances a lesion may spread rapidly and involve the mandible and the floor of the mouth by direct extension.

Cancer of the *anterior tongue* and *floor of the mouth* may seem to occur together because their spread to adjacent tissues is so rapid. Metastasis to the neck has already occurred in more than 60% of people when the diagnosis is made because of the tongue's abundant vascular and lymphatic drainage. The mortality is high. Lesions about the base of the tongue may go unnoticed by the patient and may be far advanced when treatment is started.

■ PREVENTION

Preventive measures include the following:
1. Avoid excess exposure to sun and wind on lips.
2. Eliminate smoking or chewing tobacco or betel leaf.
3. Maintain good oral hygiene and dental care.
4. Consult physician for a mouth lesion that does not heal within 2 to 3 weeks.

■ ASSESSMENT

Condition of mouth: the intactness of the mucous membranes is threatened by chemotherapy or radiation

Eating patterns: changes may occur in the ability to cope with certain types of foods, especially solids, and with the ability to swallow. Patients may also have difficulty with choking and aspiration and with nasal returns and drooling when swallowing.

Verbal communication: the ability to speak will vary from some limitation to complete inability to speak, depending on the amount of tissue resected or destroyed.

Concerns: the person's facial appearance will also change depending on the extent of tissue removed or destroyed. Even with reconstructive changes, noticeable changes will be present.

Table 31-3 Cancer of mouth and esophagus

Place	Incidence	Contributing factors	Signs and symptoms	Medical therapy
Mouth				
Lips	4300	Smoking, alcohol	Fissure or painless indurated ulcer	Excision, jaw reconstruction if extensive
Anterior tongue and floor of mouth	17,400	Smoking, alcohol	Ulcer or growth	Local tissue perfusion with antimetabolites, Partial or total excision of tongue Radical neck dissection if extensive Radiation therapy instead of or following surgery
Esophagus	9700	Alcohol, heavy smoking	Dysphagia, regurgitation, aspiration of fluids, foul breath odor	Upper one third: radiation Middle one third: esophagogastrostomy Lower one third: esophagogastrectomy

DATA ANALYSIS: NURSING DIAGNOSES

Nursing diagnoses are determined from assessment of patient data. Possible nursing diagnoses for the person receiving therapy for cancer of the mouth may include, but are not limited to, the following:

Diagnostic title	Possible etiologies
Body image disturbance	Actual/threat of facial/head disfigurement, foul breath
Impaired verbal communication	Resection of oral tissue
Altered nutrition: less than body requirements	Chewing or swallowing difficulties, anorexia
Altered oral mucous membrane	Oral cavity radiation, decreased salivation, mouth dryness

PLANNING: EXPECTED PATIENT OUTCOMES

Expected patient outcomes for the person receiving therapy for cancer of the mouth may include, but are not limited to, the following:

1. Incisions heal without infection.
2. Patient feeds self through appropriate means and consumes a nutritionally balanced fluid or soft diet.
3. Patient has a means of communication and is working to improve speech.
4. Patient interacts with others and states plans for gradual resumption of activities involving others.

IMPLEMENTATION

Surgery

The tongue may be partially excised (hemiglossectomy) or totally excised (glossectomy). If the lymph nodes are involved, a radical neck dissection (Chapter 23) may be performed.

Antibiotics may be given *preoperatively* to decrease the number of bacteria present in the mouth. Prostheses of the palate and jaw may be designed to replace portions of tissue that have been resected. If a prosthesis is to be made, impressions will be taken during the preoperative period; the prosthesis will be fitted when healing has occurred postoperatively. If a composite resection including a radical neck dissection is to be performed, reconstructive surgery will be done, if possible, during the initial procedure; it may also be performed at a later date.

Postoperative care of the patient is focused on promoting an adequate airway, mouth drainage, oral hygiene, comfort, nutrition, and speech (see the box on p. 1058). Good mouth care is essential for comfort, prevention of infection, and promotion of healing. Teeth brushing is usually contraindicated because of discomfort and potential trauma. Sterile equipment is used to prevent introduction of exogenous organisms. Patients are encouraged to assist in their oral hygiene as soon as possible.

Most patients can suction and feed themselves a few days after mouth surgery and are happier doing so. Chewing is difficult without the tongue, and the person has a problem getting the food to the posterior pharynx. Sensation in the mouth is decreased, and the patient has difficulty locating the position of the food in the oral cavity. One method of eating is for the person to use the forefinger to push the food to the posterior pharynx.

The ability to speak is commonly lost for short or long periods after surgery, but if the vocal chords are intact, speech will eventually return. A magic slate may be used for communication; however, many patients have difficulty using this because of visual impairments. Conversation can be carried out so that the patient's responses can be limited to affirmative or negative gestures. Loud noises are disturbing to the patient since the oral tissue loss may create a channel that amplifies sound; therefore the patient should be addressed in a soft, clear voice. Speech retraining may be necessary, and a tape recorder may be useful for the patient to hear his or her own voice to work on improvements.

Radiation

Tumors of the mouth may be treated by radiation in various forms. Needles containing radium, radioactive cobalt, or other radioactive substances may be inserted and left in place for a prescribed time. Seeds containing emanations from radium or radioactive cobalt may be used and left in place indefinitely or else removed. External radiation treatment using x-rays or other radioactive substances may be prescribed.

Radiation therapy produces secondary effects in the mouth that include mucositis, dryness, dental decay, and tightening of the jaw muscle. Some of the changes may be permanent. The initial reaction is an inflammation of the mucous membrane. Sloughing of the tissues may occur and cause a fetid odor. Dentures are not tolerated for some time thereafter because of the sensitivity of the tissues. Dryness of the mouth begins 1 to 2 weeks after radiation is started and may persist throughout life. The dryness makes the mouth feel uncomfortable and gives an unpleasant taste.

Decreased salivary secretion and altered pH of the saliva contribute to rapid dental decay, especially at the gingival margins. An active dental control program is started before radiation therapy is initiated. Fluoride treatments to the teeth may be given and a conscientious toothbrushing regimen is instituted.

The general care of the patient receiving radiation therapy is discussed in Chapter 12. Specific considerations for the patient receiving radiation of the mouth include the following:

1. Provide good oral hygiene.
2. Remove dentures at night; check dentures for fitness.
3. Encourage fluid intake of at least 2500 ml/day unless contraindicated.
4. Encourage chewing sugar-free gum or lozenges to stimulate salivation.

Nursing care of the patient undergoing mouth surgery for cancer

Preoperative care

1. Clarify patient's knowledge of expected changes after surgery.
2. Explain expected postoperative measures (including suctioning, nasogastric tube).
3. Provide openings for patient to begin to express feelings about changes in body image.

Postoperative care

1. Monitoring
   a. Assess facial movement for facial nerve damage (if parotid gland excised): ask patient to raise eyebrows, frown, smile, show teeth, pucker lips.
   b. Assess degree and character of drainage.
      (1) Amount of drainage and presence of blood should be minimal.
      (2) Hemorrhage may occur with wide resection of tongue.
2. Maintaining adequate airway/promoting drainage
   a. Have patient use side-lying position initially.
   b. Have patient use Fowler's position when fully alert.
   c. Suction mouth (except for lip surgery).
   d. Gauze wick may be used to direct saliva into an emesis basin.
   e. Maintain patency of drainage tubes, if used.
3. Promoting oral hygiene and comfort
   a. Clean involved areas of mouth with cotton applicator moistened with hydrogen peroxide and saline.
   b. Mouth irrigations
      (1) Use sterile equipment.
      (2) Use solution of sterile water, diluted hydrogen peroxide, normal saline, or sodium bicarbonate (avoid commercial mouthwashes).
      (3) Protect any dressings from getting wet.
      (4) A catheter may be inserted along the side of cheek and the solution injected with gentle pressure; a spray may also be used.
      (5) Give analgesics as indicated (pain is usually mild).
4. Promoting nutrition
   a. Tube feedings will be used initially with hemiglossectomy.
   b. Oral fluids: place in back of throat with Asepto syringe or feeding cup with attached tubing.
   c. Eating soft foods
      (1) Encourage patient to feed self when possible.
      (2) Teach patient to follow all meals with clear water to cleanse mouth.
      (3) Avoid using fork, which may traumatize new tissue.
   d. Foods
      (1) Avoid long-term use of commercial preparations such as instant breakfast drinks (may cause diarrhea or constipation).
      (2) Fruit-flavored yogurt preparations are less irritating than gelatin preparations and easier to swallow.
      (3) Avoid very hot or cold foods (hot foods irritate new tissue; cold foods may cause facial pain or paralyze oral functions).
5. Promoting speech
   a. Limit patient responses initially to yes-no questions that can be answered by gestures.
   b. Encourage patient when speech returns to speak slowly.
   c. Listen carefully and validate communication before initiating action on requests.
   d. Speak in a soft clear voice.
   e. Refer patient to speech therapist if necessary.
6. Encourage socialization with others.

5. Provide humidity in air for added moisture and comfort.
6. Avoid very hot or cold food, dry bulky foods, or smoking to decrease irritation of sensitive mucous membranes.

□ Counseling

The person with cancer of the mouth faces two threats: threat to life and possible disfigurement. Because the face and neck are readily visible to others, one of the major problems that the person will have to cope with and adapt to is the change in body image. The impact of the loss may be slightly minimized when the grieving process begins early. The full emotional impact of the loss, however, occurs after therapy.

Withdrawal because of not wanting to be viewed by others or because of foul breath odor is often observed in these patients. The patient needs to experience acceptance by health professionals. The family members may need help in understanding patient behavior and in coping with their own feelings concerning the patient's appearance. Patients are encouraged to identify their feelings and are provided with support and explanations as appropriate. Patients are encouraged to mingle with others as soon as clues indicating readiness are observed.

□ Palliative care

Tissue necrosis and severe pain occur in advanced cancer of the mouth, either from failure of treatment or from death of tissue as a result of radiation. The patient usually experiences difficulty in swallowing, fear of choking, and the constant accumulation of foul-smelling secretions.

Good mouth care is extremely important. The danger of severe and even fatal hemorrhage must always be considered. It is very difficult to induce these patients to take sufficient nourishing fluids. A gastrostomy (p. 1063) may be done to permit direct introduction of food into the stomach. Family members caring for the person at home need considerable support from hospice or other community health nurses.

■ Common esophageal disorders

A number of esophageal disorders delay motility in the esophagus. Some of these disorders are described in Table 31-4.

■ PATHOPHYSIOLOGY

Esophageal motility may be impaired by physiologic dysfunction or lack of peristalsis (achalasia), by a narrowed tract (stricture), by lack of structural integrity (diverticulum), or by irritation of the esophageal lining, particularly at the gastroesophageal junction (gastroesophageal reflux, hiatal hernia).

Various degrees of *achalasia* can exist. In addition to the absent peristalsis, the lower esophageal sphincter does not relax with swallowing. In severe conditions the portion of the esophagus above the achalasia dilates, and the person may have difficulty swallowing food and fluids past that point (Fig. 31-4). Chest pain results from esophageal spasms. Increased hydrostatic pressure (such as with the Valsalva maneuver) helps to overcome the increased lower esophageal pressure. Nitrates and calcium channel

Table 31-4   Esophageal disorders

Disease	Etiology	Signs and symptoms	Medical therapy
Achalasia (aperistalsis of esophagus)	Unknown	Dysphagia for liquids and solids, weight loss, substernal chest pain Later: regurgitation	Forceful dilation of lower esophageal sphincter with pneumostatic or mechanical dilators Isosorbide dinitrate, nifedipine
Esophageal strictures	Swallowing of caustic substances Secondary to inflammatory lesions	Dysphagia	Esophageal dilation, resection of stricture
Esophageal diverticulum (pouch in mucosa)	Weakened esophageal wall	Dysphagia, fetid breath	Surgery for severe symptoms (excision of herniated sac)
Gastroesophageal reflux	Incompetent lower esophageal sphincter	Heartburn	Antacids; histamine-2 blockers (cimetidine [Tagamet], ranitidine [Zantac]); bethanechol chloride (Urecholine); metoclopramide (Reglan)
Hiatal hernia (diaphragmatic hernia)	Contributing factors: obesity, trauma, aging	50% asymptomatic, heartburn, dysphagia	No treatment for asymptomatic Heartburn: high-protein, low-fat diet; antacids Surgery for incarcerated hernias through thorax or abdomen

blockers may reduce the lower esophageal sphincter pressure.[42]

Strictures may be corrosive or benign. Corrosive strictures occur from ingestion of a strong alkali (such as Drano) or strong acid (such as toilet bowl cleaner) leading to severe esophageal burns. Benign strictures develop following inflammatory lesions (such as those occurring with gastroesophageal reflux), acute viral or bacterial diseases, or mucosal injury from prolonged presence of indwelling nasogastric tubes.[42] Narrowing of the esophagus makes swallowing difficult.

An *esophageal diverticulum* is a bulging of the esophageal mucosa and submucosa through a weakened portion of the esophageal muscle (Fig. 31-5). As food is ingested, some of it may collect in the pouch formed by the weakened area. After a sufficient amount of food has collected in the pouch, it overflows into the esophagus and is regurgitated.

There is always danger that some of the regurgitated food may be aspirated in the trachea during sleep.

Gastroesophageal reflux occurs when the lower esophageal sphincter (LES), at the junction of the esophagus and stomach, becomes incompetent and permits reflux of gastric material into the esophagus. The acidity of the gastric juice irritates the esophageal mucosa, creating a muscle spasm. Chronic reflux may lead to stricture of the LES (as a result of fibrosis from the inflammatory process), delaying passage of food into the stomach. An incompetent LES may be idiopathic (no known cause) or may be exacerbated by anticholinergic drugs, caffeine, theobromine (chocolate), ethyl alcohol, or smoking. Gastroesophageal reflux may also occur with *hiatus hernia,* a protrusion of part of the stomach through the diaphragm into the thoracic cavity (Fig. 31-6). Obesity and aging are contributing factors to the development of hiatal hernias.

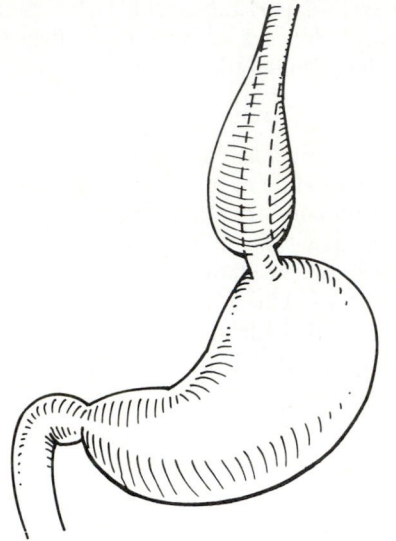

Fig. 31-4   Achalasia.

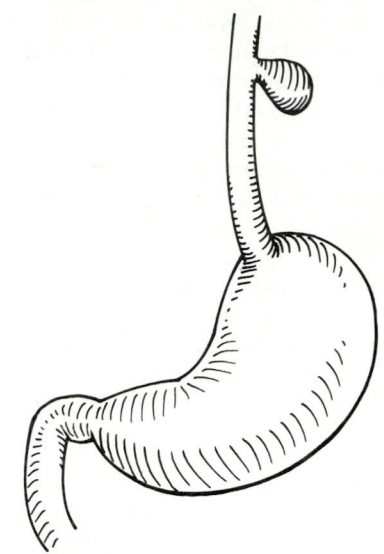

Fig. 31-5   Esophageal diverticulum.

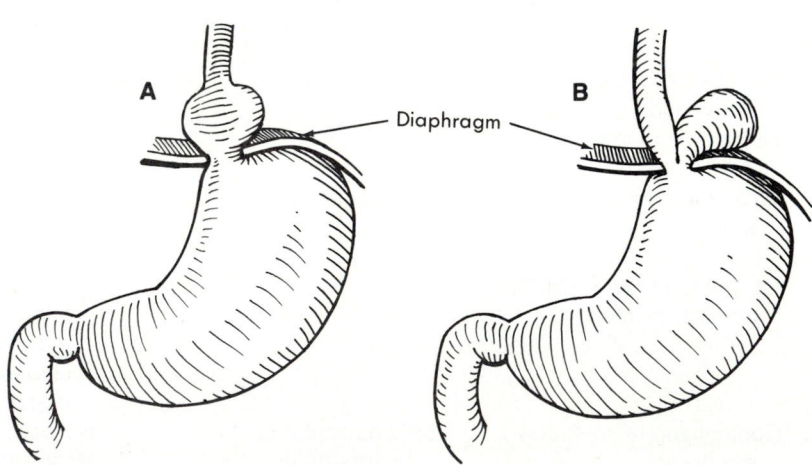

Fig. 31-6   Hiatal hernia, **A,** Sliding hernia. **B,** Paraesophageal hernia.

ASSESSMENT

Subjective data

Dysphagia is a primary symptom of esophageal disorders. Esophageal dysphagia of motor origin characteristically produces dysphagia for both solids and liquids. This differs from dysphagia that results from paralysis of neurologic origin (difficulty swallowing liquids) or dysphagia caused by obstruction of the esophageal lumen (difficulty swallowing solids). If the patient has had dysphagia for a period of time, it is helpful to know what approaches to eating the person has found most useful.

The patient who experiences *regurgitation* is asked if this occurs at night (staining of the pillow may have been observed), and if there is a foul odor of the regurgitated material (seen with esophageal diverticulum).

Heartburn is a substernal "burning" sensation resulting from gastroesophageal reflux. The pain may be referred to the neck or back if severe. It is frequently accompanied by a sour regurgitation of gastric contents but is not accompanied by nausea.

Objective data

The ability to swallow is assessed by placing three fingers over the thyroid cartilage of the larynx (Adam's apple) and asking the person to swallow or by observing the movement of the larynx. If movement is limited, the gag reflex can be elicited by touching the posterior tongue or pharynx lightly with a tongue blade. A further assessment can be made, if necessary, by placing 1 to 2 ml of water in the oropharynx and asking the patient to swallow.

Diagnostic tests

The diagnosis of esophageal disorders is facilitated by x-ray films of the esophagus taken after barium swallow. The patient may be placed in Trendelenburg's position during the x-ray examination or fluoroscopy to identify gastroesophageal reflux.

A water siphon test is a fluoroscopic examination in which barium is swallowed followed by plain water. If the LES is incompetent, the barium will be seen to reflux into the esophagus. Overnight pH recordings measured from swallowed glass electrodes will demonstrate periods of increased gastric reflux.

DATA ANALYSIS: NURSING DIAGNOSES

Nursing diagnoses are determined from assessment of patient data. Possible nursing diagnoses for the person with a common esophageal disorder may include, but are not limited to, the following:

Diagnostic title	Possible etiologies
Potential for aspiration	Impaired swallowing
Pain: heartburn	Reflux of acid gastric contents
Altered nutrition: less than body requirements	Dysphagia
Knowledge deficit	Lack of exposure/recall

PLANNING: EXPECTED PATIENT OUTCOMES

Expected patient outcomes for the person with a common esophageal disorder may include, but are not limited to, the following:
1. Aspiration does not occur.
2. Patient has a nutritionally balanced intake.
3. Patient describes any recommended dietary changes.
4. Patient states he or she is feeling comfortable.
5. Patient describes body position and activity requirements.

IMPLEMENTATION

Assisting with comfort and activities of daily living

People with esophageal disorders who experience *dysphagia* have difficulty swallowing both solids and liquids. Frequent small feedings are suggested. Some patients drink large amounts of fluid while swallowing solids to increase esophageal pressure, thus pushing the food into the stomach. The Valsalva maneuver can also be used to help push the food past the sphincter. Eating with the head elevated encourages movement of food through the esophagus by gravity. Regurgitation of food may occur several hours after eating, especially at night when the body is horizontal (therefore eating is avoided for at least 2 hours before bedtime). People are encouraged to sleep with the upper body elevated; wooden blocks may be used to raise the head of the bed.

Discomfort from heartburn can be decreased by administration of 30 ml of a liquid antacid 1 hour after meals, at bedtime, and whenever heartburn occurs. Gaviscon, which is a mixture of antacids with alginic acid, has been found to be effective in alleviating heartburn. Two to four tablets, when *chewed* thoroughly and then swallowed, produce a viscous antacid foam that coats the esophagus and floats on the gastric contents. If antacids are not effective, medications that increase LES contraction may be prescribed; these include bethanechol chloride (Urecholine) or metoclopramide (Reglan) to be taken 30 minutes before meals and at bedtime. Anticholinergic medications are avoided, because they decrease gastric emptying. Histamine-2 blockers (Tagamet, Zantac) suppress gastric secretions, thus preventing night reflux.

Patient teaching

Prevention is the best approach to treatment of heartburn. Key points for patient teaching are listed in the box on p. 1062. A high-protein, low-fat diet is encouraged. Protein stimulates gastrin release that increases LES pressure. Fats, however, stimulate release of the hormone cholecystokinin that decreases LES pressure. Other foods that decrease LES pressure include caffeine products, chocolate, peppermint and spearmint oils, and alcohol; therefore, these foods should be avoided.

Teaching for the patient with heartburn

1. Eat a high-protein, low-fat diet to prevent esophageal regurgitation.
2. Avoid foods containing caffeine (coffee, tea, colas), chocolate, and alcohol.
3. Eat small frequent feedings to prevent gastric distention and increased gastric acid secretion.
4. Avoid smoking.
5. Avoid lying down or bending over for 2 hours after eating to prevent regurgitation.
6. Avoid lifting or wearing tight belts or girdles after eating to prevent abdominal pressure.
7. Sleep with upper body elevated (bed blocks can be used to elevate the head of the bed).

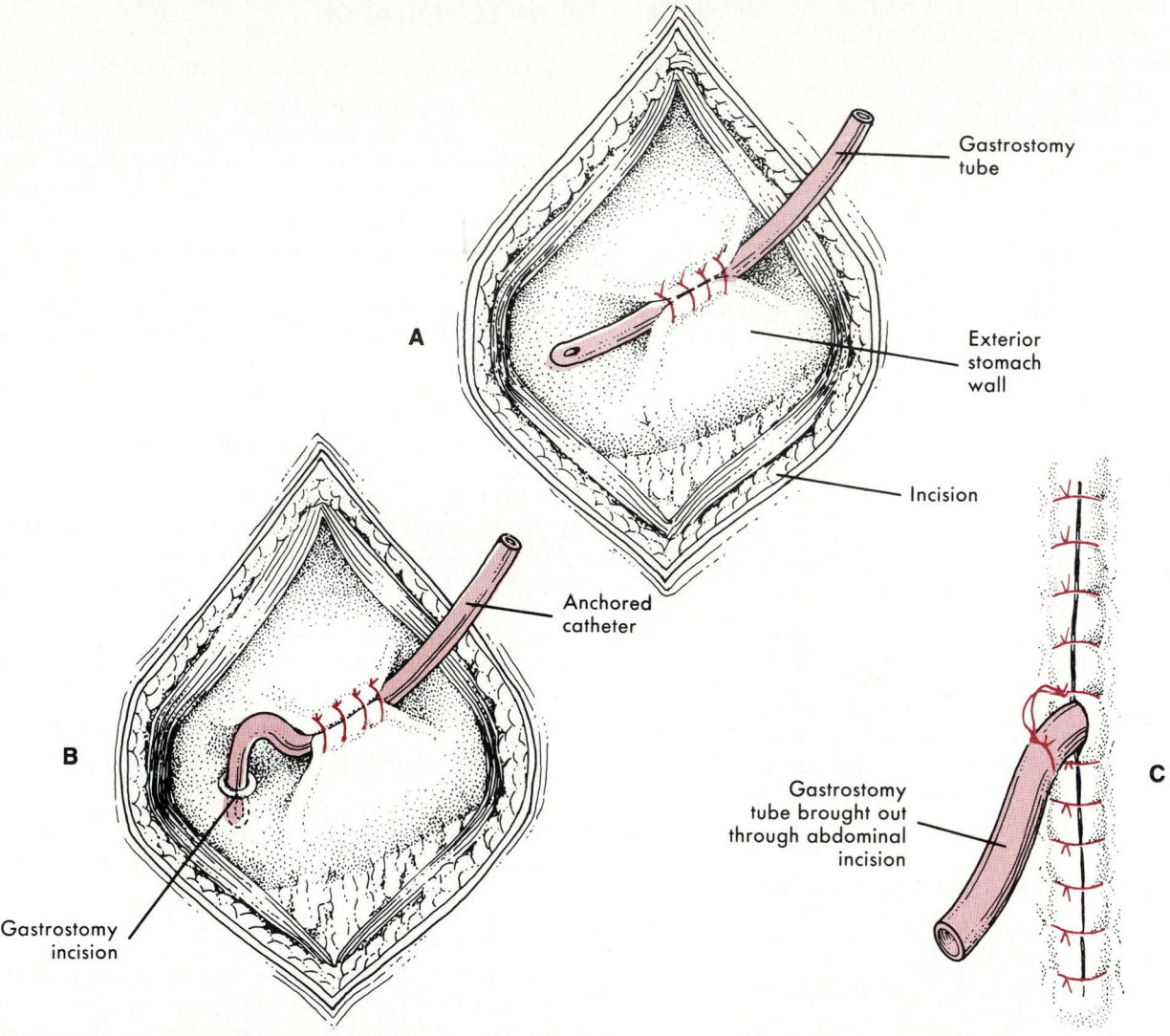

Fig. 31-7 Gastrostomy with tube. **A,** Catheter is laid on greater curvature of exterior stomach wall and sutured to secure it in place. **B,** Anchored catheter is then inserted into stomach. **C,** Abdomen is closed, and gastrostomy tube is sutured in place. A separate stab wound may be made for tube rather than bringing it out through incision line. (From Broadwell, DC, and Jackson, BL: Principles of ostomy care, St. Louis, 1982, The CV Mosby Co.)

■ ESOPHAGEAL DILATION

The physician may dilate the esophagus by the use of dilators (bougies) or inflatable bags for achalasia or esophageal strictures. The procedures may be performed under fluoroscopy to prevent damage to the mucosa. Postoperatively the patient is monitored for *chest pain*, indicating esophageal perforation. Fluids and soft foods are indicated when swallowing produces pain. Most patients will require pain medication in the early postoperative period.

■ GASTROSTOMY

If the person is unable to swallow for a long period of time, he or she may be fed by nasogastric tube feedings (see Chapter 6) or by gastrostomy in which a tube is inserted into the stomach through the abdominal wall.

□ Method

The standard method involves making an incision through the abdominal wall into the stomach and inserting the tube (Fig. 31-7). Either local or general anesthesia may be used for this method. A second method that does not require incision into the abdominal cavity, the *percutaneous endoscopic gastrostomy* (PEG), consists of using an endoscope to push a cannula from the stomach out the abdominal wall (a small skin incision facilitates passage). A string is pulled back up the cannula and attached to a specially prepared catheter that is then pulled through the esophagus and stomach and out the abdominal wall. Internal and external dams hold the catheter in place.

□ Food and fluids

After surgery the gastrostomy tube may be attached to low intermittent suction for 24 hours or fluids may be started the first day. The initial meal consists of a small amount of tap water or glucose in water and is followed by fluids every 4 hours. If there is no leakage of fluid around the tube and if the patient appears to tolerate the clear fluids, blended foods may be added until a full diet is eventually given through the tube. The meal is warmed to room or body temperature before it is given and is diluted if too thick. Directions for giving the feedings are noted in the box on p. 1064.

The psychologic trauma of not being able to eat normally is usually severe. The patient may become depressed and may need a great deal of encouragement. However, as most patients become proficient in feeding themselves, they gradually accept this method of obtaining nourishment as inevitable and adjust remarkably well.

□ Skin care

Irritation of the gastrostomy by the tube and leakage of gastric contents may lead to skin breakdown around the tube exit point. The skin is inspected daily, and signs of inflammation are reported to the physician. The skin around the tube is cleansed daily and a protective ointment applied if leakage occurs (see the box on p. 1064).

□ Continent tubeless gastrostomy

A different type of gastrostomy does not require a tube and therefore lessens the chance of complications from tube irritation or obstruction. A small tube is surgically formed from the stomach wall and then pushed in to form an intussusception valve. The "valve" is brought out flush with the skin surface to form a flat stoma. The valve prevents leakage of stomach contents; therefore, no skin care or dressings are needed. A feeding tube is inserted through the stoma for feedings. The stoma can be closed at a later date.

■ Cancer of the esophagus

Carcinoma is the most common condition causing obstruction of the esophagus and accounts for about 2% of all deaths from cancer in the United States. The incidence is more than twice as high in men as women but is increasing among women. Smokers, alcoholics, and persons with achalasia are at high risk.

The only possible hope for successful treatment lies in very early diagnosis and treatment. Any person who has difficulty in swallowing, no matter how trivial it may seem, should be urged to seek medical advice at once. This applies particularly to people over 40 years of age because cancer of the esophagus occurs more often in middle and later life than at younger ages.

■ PATHOPHYSIOLOGY

Cancer may develop in any portion of the esophagus but is most common in the middle and lower thirds. The tumor may be a squamous cell carcinoma originating in the esophagus or an adenocarcinoma that spreads upward from the stomach. The cancer may spread to adjoining areas by local invasion or by lymphatic spread. Symptoms depend on the area and extent of metastasis. Unfortunately, by the time symptoms are noted (Table 31-3), the disease is often already well established; therefore, the prognosis is generally poor.

■ IMPLEMENTATION

The treatment for cancer of the esophagus is either radiation for the upper third of the esophagus or surgery for the lower two thirds. An *esophagogastrostomy* is a resection of a portion of the esophagus with anastomosis to the stomach. An *esophagogastrectomy* is resection of a lower esophageal section together with a proximal portion of the stomach, followed by anastomosis of the remaining portions of esophagus and stomach.

Considerable psychologic support is usually required as the patient and family begin to cope with the diagnosis, prognosis, and physical debility of the patient. The patient is taught to avoid others with upper respiratory infections and to seek medical help for even minor illnesses. Palliative and supportive care, as described in Chapter 12, are given as indicated.

Nursing care of the patient with a gastrostomy

Promoting skin integrity

1. Inspect skin around gastrostomy for leakage.
2. Wash skin around catheter daily with soap and water. Dry well.
3. Apply a protective ointment (zinc oxide, karaya paste, Stomahesive) around tube opening if irritation or leakage is present.
4. Cover skin around tube.

Promoting gastric function

1. Attach tube after surgery to low intermittent suction.
2. Monitor tubing for patency (free of kinks, draining).
3. Check tube length every 8 hours. Report changes to physician.
4. Measure and record gastrostomy drainage every 8 hours.
5. Monitor for return of peristalsis (bowel sounds, flatus).
6. Monitor for decreased gastric function (nausea, vomiting, feelings of abdominal fullness, abdominal distention) when tube is clamped by order of physician.

Promoting nutrition

1. Giving the feeding
   a. Before each feeding, unclamp tube and aspirate gastric contents. Delay giving feeding if a residual of 75 ml or more is present. Report findings to physician.
   b. Give feeding with patient in high Fowler's or sitting position to prevent esophageal regurgitation.
   c. Warm feeding to room temperature.
   d. Dilute feeding with water if too thick.
   e. Use feeding tube to introduce the liquid into the catheter.
   f. Give 50 ml of water before feeding.
   g. Let prescribed feeding (usually 200 to 500 ml) flow in by gravity over a 10 to 15 minute period.
   h. Flush tube with 50 ml of water after feeding to maintain patency of tube.
   i. Clamp tube when feeding is completed.
   j. Keep patient's head elevated for 30 minutes after the feeding.
2. Monitor intake and output until gastrostomy feedings are well tolerated.
3. Weigh patient daily until weight becomes stable.
4. Monitor for signs of dehydration (dry mucous membranes, thirst, decreased skin turgor).

Promoting comfort

1. Provide mouth care.
2. Encourage patient to express feelings regarding not being able to eat normally.
3. Encourage patient to participate in giving the feeding.

Patient teaching

1. Preparation of food (blenderized food, special formula)
2. Positioning for eating
3. Method of giving the feeding
4. Washing equipment well after feeding; storing equipment in a clean place
5. Maintenance of skin integrity
6. Making plans for returning to usual activities
7. Need for medical follow-up
8. Symptoms requiring immediate medical attention (tube dislodgement, tube occlusion, bleeding, infection, leakage of fluid around opening)

Nursing care of the patient undergoing esophageal surgery

Preoperative care

1. Encourage improved nutritional status.
   a. Encourage high-protein, high-calorie diet if oral diet is possible.
   b. Total parenteral nutrition (TPN) may be necessary for severe dysphagia or obstruction.
2. Provide good mouth care (p. 1055); vary the solution used.
3. Give preoperative preparation appropriate for thoracic surgery (Chapter 24).
4. Give prescribed antibiotics before esophageal resection or bypass.

Postoperative care

1. Promote good pulmonary ventilation.
2. Maintain chest drainage system as prescribed.
3. Maintain gastric drainage system (p. 1070).
4. Maintain nutrition.
   a. Start clear fluids at frequent intervals when oral intake is permitted.
   b. Introduce soft foods gradually with several small meals of bland foods.
   c. Have patient keep head elevated for 2 hours after eating and while sleeping if heartburn occurs.

■ ESOPHAGEAL SURGERY

□ Preoperative care

The care of the person undergoing surgery of the esophagus is described in the box above. Improving the nutritional status is particularly important before surgery because the person is usually malnourished because of dysphagia and anorexia from the foul taste. Total parenteral nutrition is often prescribed, although a temporary gastrostomy may be performed to supply food in the preoperative or early postoperative period.

Good mouth care is essential, especially when the patient is spitting up decomposed food, blood, or pus. Mouthwashes are useful in making the mouth feel fresher and are offered to the patient before eating. The mouthwashes are varied from time to time unless the patient has a preference, because sometimes the flavor of the solution may be identified with the unpleasant throat secretions and becomes almost as distasteful as the secretions.

Preoperative patient teaching includes the care of the patient experiencing chest surgery (Chapter 24) if this is appropriate. A nasogastric tube will be in place after surgery.

□ Postoperative care

The immediate postoperative care centers on prevention of respiratory complications and maintenance of chest and gastric drainage systems. Postoperatively the nasogastric tube is usually left in place until complete healing of the esophageal anastomosis has occurred because esophageal tissue is very friable and because the anastomosis may be under tension. The nasogastric tube is not disturbed to prevent traction on the suture line. Small amounts of bright red blood may drain from the nasogastric tube for 6 to 12 hours after surgery. The color of the drainage then changes to greenish yellow.

When oral intake is permitted, clear fluids are given first until well tolerated; then the diet progresses to soft foods (see the box above). If part of the stomach has been pulled up into the thoracic cavity, the patient may complain of a feeling of fullness in the chest or difficulty in breathing after eating. Smaller, more frequent meals may alleviate this problem. Heartburn (p. 1061) may result from gastric reflux if the esophageal sphincter has been removed or made incompetent.

☰ EVALUATION

The care of specific patients with esophageal disorders is evaluated on the basis of the expected patient outcomes. General questions to be asked are: Is the patient receiving a balanced nutritional input? Is the patient comfortable? Does the patient know (1) how to achieve comfort and a nutritional intake when at home, (2) medication dosage schedule and side effects, and (3) what signs and symptoms need to be reported to the physician?

■ DIGESTIVE DISORDERS

Most digestion takes place in the stomach, duodenum, and jejunum. Gastritis, peptic ulcer, cancer of the stomach, and malabsorption syndrome are the major digestive disorders (Table 31-5).

■ Gastritis

Gastritis (inflammation of the stomach) is a common disorder characterized by anorexia, epigastric fullness and discomfort, and nausea and vomiting. The cause is often undetermined, but gastritis commonly results from stress,

Table 31-5 Digestive disorders

Disorder	Etiology	Signs and symptoms	Medical therapy
Gastritis	Chronic irritants (e.g., alcohol, drugs), bacteria, viruses, stress Corrosive substances	Anorexia, epigastric fullness, nausea/vomiting, epigastric discomfort, hematemesis, or melena Shock and esophageal strictures	Mild: antacid, rest Severe: correction of fluid/electrolyte imbalances, sedatives, antacids, H$_2$ blockers
Peptic ulcer	Contributing factors include smoking, drugs, stress, genetic tendency	Epigastric pain relieved by food or antacids	Antacids; H$_2$ blockers (cimetidine, ranitidine); sucralfate; surgery for intractable ulcers or complications
Gastric cancer	Cause unknown; high incidence with achlorhydria, atrophic gastritis, pernicious anemia	Few early symptoms: anorexia, weight loss, anemia Late symptom: palpable abdominal mass	Subtotal gastrectomy, chemotherapy, radiation
Malabsorption syndrome	Altered digestion, mucosal cell transport, or lymph/blood transport (see Table 31-15)	Steatorrhea, flatulence, abdominal distention, anorexia, weight loss, signs of vitamin and protein deficiencies	Elimination of foods that cannot be tolerated; TPN when necessary; packed RBC for severe anemia

alcohol, or drugs (especially salicylates, indomethacin, sulfonamide, steroids). The disorder may also occur with bacterial or viral infections, from irritation by backflow of bile or pancreatic secretions, with radiation, or from corrosive substances.

■ PATHOPHYSIOLOGY

Drugs, alcohol, bile salts, or pancreatic enzymes may damage the gastric mucosa (erosive gastritis), disrupting the gastric mucosal barrier and allowing a back-diffusion of acid and pepsin into the gastric tissue, causing inflammation. The gastric mucosa responds to most irritating agents by regeneration of the mucosa; therefore the disorders are often self-limiting. With continued irritation, the tissue becomes inflamed and bleeding may occur.

Ingestion of corrosive acids or alkalies can result in inflammation and necrosis of the stomach wall (corrosive gastritis). The necrosis may lead to perforation of the stomach wall with subsequent hemorrhage and peritonitis.

Chronic gastritis may be associated with atrophy of gastric glands and the appearance of patches of thin, gray, or greenish-gray mucosa (atrophic gastritis). The loss of gastric mucosa will result in eventual diminution of gastric secretion and the development of pernicious anemia. Atrophic gastritis may be a precursor to gastric carcinoma. Chronic gastritis may also be associated with peptic ulcer disease or may occur following gastrojejunostomy.[40]

▦ ASSESSMENT

Subjective data include presence of anorexia and nausea and the extent of abdominal discomfort. Objective data include (1) emesis (frequency, amount, presence of blood) and (2) signs of fluid and electrolyte imbalance (thirst, decreased skin turgor, dry mucous membranes, oliguria, muscle weakness).

▶ DATA ANALYSIS: NURSING DIAGNOSES

Nursing diagnoses are determined from assessment of patient data. Possible nursing diagnoses for the person with gastritis may include, but are not limited to, the following:

Diagnostic title	Possible etiologies
Fluid volume deficit: potential	Vomiting
Pain: epigastric	Gastric irritation

▤ PLANNING: EXPECTED PATIENT OUTCOMES

Expected patient outcomes for the person with gastritis may include, but are not limited to, the following:
1. Patient describes feeling more comfortable.
2. Signs of fluid deficit and electrolyte imbalance do not occur.

▤ IMPLEMENTATION

☐ Assisting with achievement of therapeutic goals

Mild gastritis is treated with antacids and rest. With severe gastritis, intravenous fluids and electrolytes are given to maintain fluid balance until symptoms subside. Tea, broth, and ginger ale are then given orally at frequent intervals. Bland feedings of custard, gelatin, and cream soups are usually tolerated after 12 to 24 hours, and then other foods are added gradually. People with chronic superficial gastritis will usually respond to a diet that avoids highly seasoned or greasy foods. Carbonated liquids are well tolerated.

Histamine H_2 blockers (cimetidine, ranitidine, p. 1075) may be prescribed to inhibit gastric acid formation and thus decrease gastric irritation. Sucralfate (p. 1076) may also be prescribed to protect the gastric mucosa by coating it to prevent back diffusion of acid and pepsin that causes irritation.

□ **Assisting with comfort**

Antacids usually help to decrease epigastic discomfort. Good mouth care is indicated if vomiting is present. Rest and a calm environment help to decrease the effects of stress.

■ Stress erosions/stress ulcers

Stress erosions or ulcers are a form of gastritis that may occur with stressful disorders such as shock, severe trauma, major surgery, sepsis, or severe burns. The lesions are usually superficial. The gastric mucosa becomes eroded or superficially ulcerated in multiple sites. Possible causative factors have been identified as mucosal ischemia or mucus deficiency. Stress erosions that are associated with the central nervous system, such as with brain tumors or injury or with cerebrovascular accidents, are termed *Cushing's ulcers* and are characterized by gastric hyperactivity. However, stress erosions from other causes do not demonstrate hyperacidity, and they may result from increased acid back-diffusion (similar to gastric ulcers, p. 1071).

Stress erosions develop within 24 to 48 hours of the stressful episode[40] and signs of upper gastrointestinal bleeding (hematemesis, melena) are noted. Pain is not a prominent symptom.

Stress erosions can be prevented in high-risk persons, such as those in intensive care units, by administration of antacids and H_2 blockers or sucralfate. If bleeding is severe, blood transfusions may be given.

▦ EVALUATION

The patient with gastritis is questioned regarding degree of comfort and thirst. Skin turgor, urinary output, and muscle strength are monitored for severe gastritis with vomiting.

■ GASTROINTESTINAL INTUBATION

GI intubation consists of inserting a tube through the nose into the stomach (nasogastric) or beyond the stomach into the intestines (intestinal). Common uses of GI intubation include the following:
1. Nasogastric
   a. Decompression of stomach
   b. Tube feedings
   c. Removal of gastric contents (gastric hemorrhage or perforation)
   d. After esophageal or gastric surgery to permit healing of suture line
   e. Tests of gastric analysis
2. Intestinal: intestinal decompression

The following section discusses the use of GI intubation for decompression and drainage and the care of persons with a GI tube. Tube feedings are described in Chapter 6.

■ TYPES OF TUBES

Different types of tubes are used depending on the purpose and site (Table 31-6). A *Levin* tube (Fig. 31-8) is most commonly used for gastric intubation; however, because it is a single-lumen tube, damage to the mucosa may result even with intermittent suction. A less traumatic approach is the use of the double-lumen Salem *sump tube*. The larger lumen of the sump tube drains the area, while the smaller lumen provides a continuous flow of air at atmospheric pressure, thus maintaining the suction at a lower level and preventing adherence of the tube against the tissue wall. The air vent should never be clamped off or connected to suction.

The tubes most often used for intestinal decompression are the Miller-Abbott tube and the Cantor tube. The length of these tubes permits their passage through the entire intestinal tract. A small balloon on the tip of each tube acts like a bolus of food when inflated with air or injected with water or mercury. This balloon stimulates peristalsis, which advances the tube along the intestinal tract. If peristalsis is absent, the weight of the mercury in the balloon will usually carry it forward. When a Miller-Abbott tube is used, the mercury is inserted into the balloon of the tube after the tube is passed.

The choice of tube depends on the physician's preference. The Miller-Abbott tube is a double-lumen tube. One lumen leads to the balloon, and the other has openings along its course, permitting drainage of intestinal contents and irrigation. The external end of the tube contains two openings, one for drainage of secretions and the other for inflating the balloon (Fig. 31-9). In irrigating this tube, the nurse must be careful that the correct opening is used—the one marked "suction." The other opening is for inflating or deflating the balloon. It should be clamped off and labeled "do not touch."

The Cantor tube, which is used less often, is a single-lumen tube with only one opening used for drainage. Before the tube is inserted, the balloon is injected with mercury with a needle and syringe. The needle opening is so small that the globules of mercury cannot escape through it. The mercury can be pushed about so that the balloon is elongated for easy insertion.

■ INSERTION OF TUBES

Nasogastric tubes may be inserted by either the nurse or the physician (see the box on p. 1069). *Intestinal* tubes are more difficult to insert because of the addition of the balloon. The intestinal tube can be mechanically inserted only into the stomach. Its passage along the remainder of the GI tract is dependent on gravity and peristalsis. The weight of the mercury in the balloon helps propel the tube through the intestines.

Table 31-6 Nasogastric and intestinal tubes

Tube	Purpose	Characteristic	Use
Nasogastric			
Levin	Removes fluid and gas from stomach (decompression); may also be used to give tube feedings; most commonly used nasogastric tube	Single-lumen; easy to maintain; may cause trauma to stomach wall	Use intermittent suction at low pressure setting
Salem sump	Same purpose as Levin tube; often used for stomach surgery to prevent pulling on the sutures	Double lumen, one for drainage and one to provide an air vent to prevent tube adherence to stomach wall	Use low (30 mm Hg) *constant* suction (preferred) or high *intermittent* suction; attach the larger lumen of tube only to suction
Entron	Tube feedings for gastric feedings only	No. 6 Fr (small bore); has a stylet for easier insertion but no weighted end	Clamp off when not in use; do not attach to suction (collapses)
Dobbhoff enteric	Tube feedings for gastric or intestinal feedings	No. 8 Fr (small bore); has a stylet for easier insertion and a weighted end to pass into intestines	Same as for the Entron tube
Intestinal			
Miller-Abbott	Removes fluid and gas from intestines (decompression); most commonly used intestinal tube	Double lumen, one for balloon inflation and one for drainage	Use low pressure intermittent suction; clamp off balloon tube and attach drainage tube only to suction
Cantor	Same purposes as Miller-Abbott tube	Single lumen; mercury is injected into balloon with needle and syringe prior to insertion	Use low pressure intermittent suction

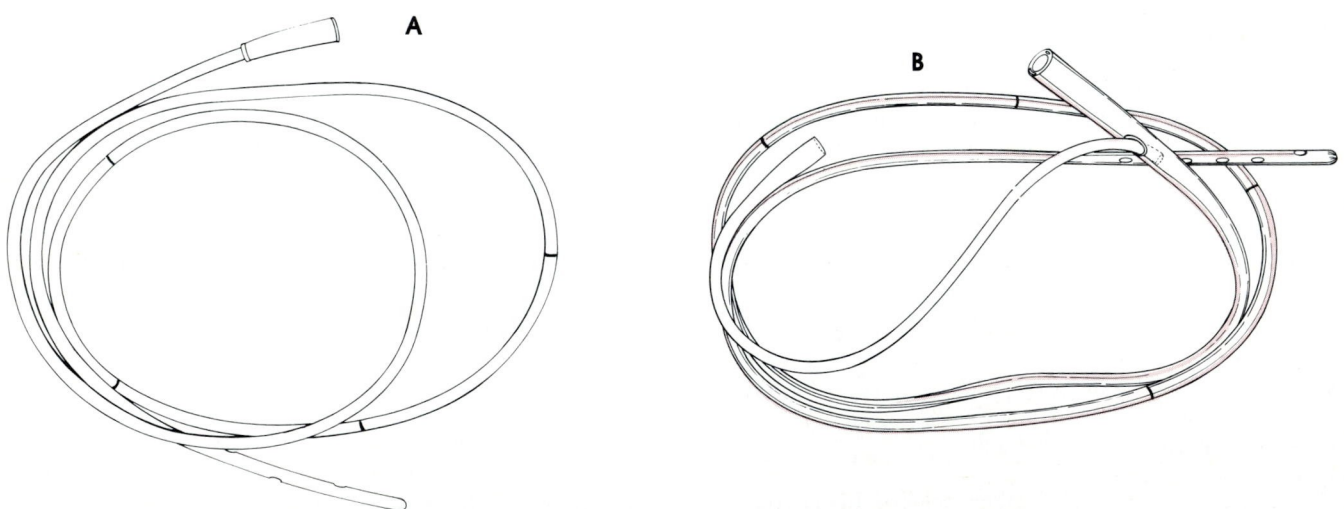

Fig. 31-8 Nasogastric tubes. **A,** Levin tube. **B,** Salem sump tube.

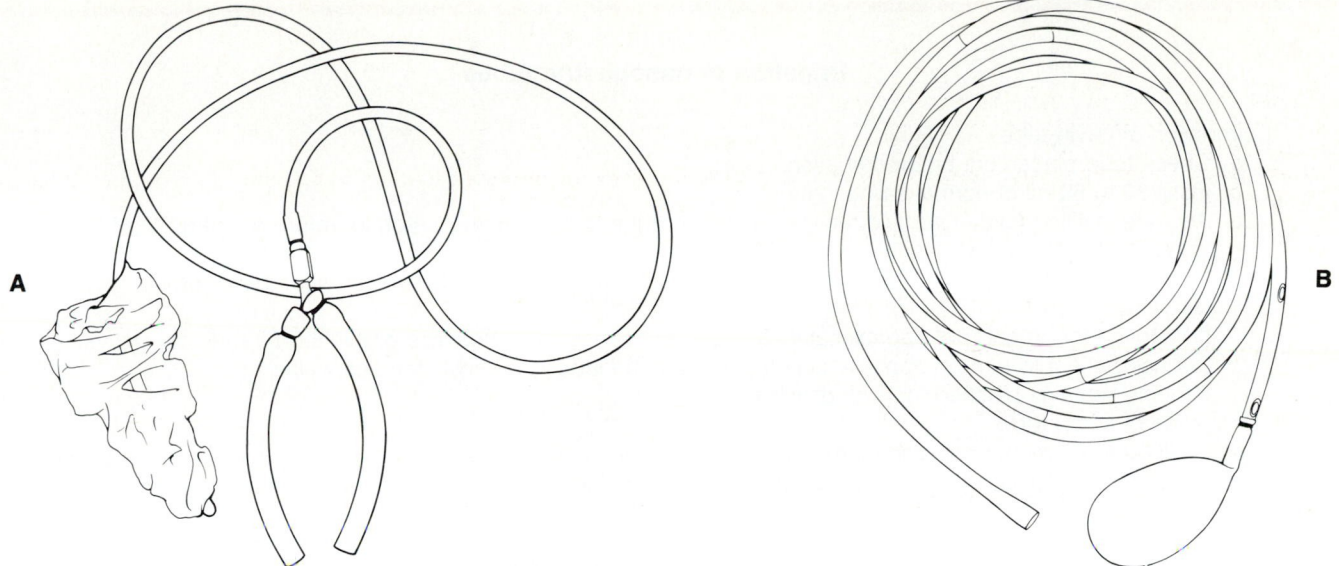

Fig. 31-9   Intestinal tubes. **A,** Miller-Abbott tube. **B,** Cantor tube.

Insertion of nasogastric tube

1. Measure tube to mark desired length of insertion: distance from ear lobe to bridge of nose to xiphoid process. (NEX measurement) or distance of 50 cm + ½ (NEX −50). Mark tube with adhesive tape.
2. Place patient in sitting position with head slightly flexed. Protect clothing and provide patient with tissues
3. Lubricate tip of tube with water-soluble lubricant
4. Insert tube slowly and steadily through nose into pharynx; ask patient to swallow repeatedly while tube is advanced to marked site on tube
5. Ascertain location of tube in stomach by one of the following methods.
    a. Aspirate gastric contents; test with litmus paper for acidity
    b. Instill 20 ml of air into tube while listening to abdomen with a stethoscope; a roar will be heard if tube is correctly placed in stomach
6. Secure tube to nose with adhesive tape (Fig. 31-10)
7. Connect tube to suction:
    a. Levin tube to intermittent suction set at "low" pressure
    b. Sump tube to intermittent suction at "high" pressure or continuous suction at "low" pressure

---

Methods of assessing functioning of gastrointestinal tubes

1. Check the suction machine.
    a. Light is blinking off and on.
    b. Machine is plugged in and turned on.
    c. Tubing connections are tight.
2. Check tubing to identify kinks in the tubing or tubing clamped off by pressure of patient's body.
3. Insert 20 ml of air through tubing while listening with stethoscope for roar sound at abdomen.
4. Irrigate tube with 30 to 60 ml normal saline; a free flow of fluid into the tube and return of fluid mixed with gastric or intestinal contents indicates a patent tube.

Irrigation of nasogastric tubes

1. Irrigation of Levin tubes
   a. Check tube placement before irrigation.
   b. Instill 30 to 60 ml of normal saline in tube.
   c. Aspirate instilled fluid; if no fluid returns, reconnect tube to suction and watch for return drainage; add to fluid intake sheet.
   d. If fluid does not flow easily into tube or return by aspiration or suction, try one or all of the following:
      (1) Rotate tube.
      (2) Move tube in and out approximately 2 to 3 cm (1 to 1½ inches) unless prohibited by medical orders.
      (3) Ask patient to turn on opposite side (tubing may be lodged against stomach wall).
   e. If tubing remains blocked, consult physician.
2. Irrigation of sump tube
   a. Instill 30 to 60 ml normal saline through drainage lumen or smaller vent lumen (without interrupting suction).
   b. When irrigation is completed, inject air through the vent lumen during suction to ensure air patency.

The intestinal tube is passed in the same manner as the nasogastric tube. After the intestinal tube reaches the stomach its passage through the pylorus into the duodenum is facilitated by positioning and activity.

1. Encourage the following patient positions;
   a. Right side for 2 hours, then
   b. Lying on back with head elevated for 2 hours, then
   c. Left side for 2 hours
2. Encourage patient ambulation following passage of tube into the pylorus (often assessed by x-ray film)
3. Advance the tube 2 to 10 cm (1 to 4 inches) at specified intervals to provide slack for peristaltic action
4. Secure tube to face when desired point has been reached; coil extra tubing on bed or pin to clothing

The intestinal tube is usually monitored daily by x-ray film for signs of coiling or telescoping of the tube. Telescoping is movement of bowel along with the tube resulting in intussusception (p. 1101), a serious complication.

■ FACILITATING DRAINAGE

Because the gastric or intestinal fluid must move against gravity to be removed, suction is required. *Intermittent suction* is used for single-lumen tubes; constant suction could damage the mucosal wall if a section of the wall were to be pulled continually against the drainage holes of the tube. Intermittent suction permits the wall to drop away from the tube when suction is not occurring. The Gomco machine which has a high and a low pressure setting is commonly used for intermittent suction. A *low* pressure is used for the Levin and the intestinal tubes; high pressure is used only with the sump tube. Constant suction is usually preferred for the sump tube.

If no visible drainage is occurring or if the patient has nausea, vomiting, or abdominal discomfort, check functioning of the suction apparatus (see the box on p. 1069).

Normal saline is used to irrigate the tube because a hypotonic solution such as water would increase electrolyte loss. Guidelines for *nasogastric* tube irrigation are listed in the box above. It is difficult to aspirate irrigating solution from *intestinal* tubes because of the tubes' length. If no return flow can be obtained, only a small amount of fluid is used and the amount instilled is recorded.

■ PREVENTING INJURY

Pressure of the tube against the nares may lead to irritation and tissue breakdown. The oropharyngeal mucosa or the parotid glands may become inflamed as a result of dry mucous membranes from oral breathing (nares plugged) or from GI bacteria that travels up the tube by capillary action. Discomfort at the jaw angle may indicate a parotitis. Methods to prevent injury from gastric intubation include the following:

1. Tape tube securely to nostril so that it does not press against nostril (Fig. 31-10)
2. Pin tube loosely to clothing to support weight of tube and permit free head movement
3. Prevent oral inflammations
   a. Keep oral mucous membranes moist
   b. Give frequent mouth care
   c. Use ice chips sparingly (ingestion of large amounts of hypotonic water from the melted ice may produce electrolyte loss through suction)
   d. Provide hard candy (sour balls) for sucking to stimulate flow of saliva

■ PROMOTING COMFORT

The presence of the tube in the nasopharynx causes local discomfort, and the person may complain of a lump in the throat, difficulty in swallowing, sore throat, hoarseness, earache, or irritation of the nostril. Methods to promote comfort include the following:

1. Remove excess secretions around nares.
2. Apply *water-soluble* lubricant (K-Y jelly) to tube at nostril to prevent secretion build-up.
3. Provide for relief of sore throat through the use of:
   a. Warm saline gargles
   b. Ice bag to neck
   c. Prescribed throat lozenges
   d. Frequent position changes to relieve pressure of tube on throat
4. Use low- or mid-Fowler's position (unless contraindicated) to prevent esophageal reflux (heartburn).

■ MONITORING FOR COMPLICATIONS

In addition to inflammations of the mouth and parotid glands, the person with GI intubation may experience fluid and electrolyte and pulmonary complications. *Fluid and electrolyte imbalances* result from loss of GI secretions and include dehydration, hyponatremia, and hypokalemia. Loss

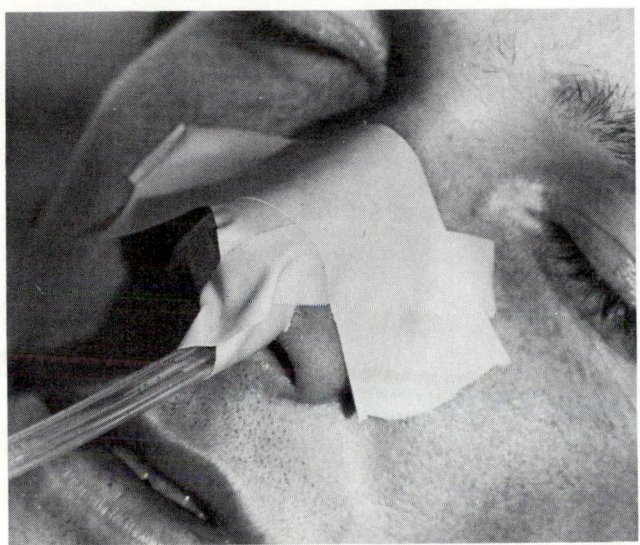

Fig. 31-10 Nasogastric tube secured by crossing tape over patient's nose and applying a second piece of tape over the bridge of the nose. (From Hirsch, J and Hannock, L, editors: Mosby's manual of clinical nursing procedures, St. Louis, 1981, The CV Mosby Co.)

of acid *gastric* contents may lead to metabolic *alkalosis*, whereas loss of alkaline *intestinal* contents may produce metabolic *acidosis* (Chapter 8). The person is monitored for signs and symptoms of these imbalances, and the amount and character of drainage from the tubes is carefully recorded every 8 hours.

Aspiration pneumonia may result from regurgitation of the stomach contents or placement of fluids in an incorrectly positioned tube. The breath sounds are monitored, and the person is encouraged to breathe deeply and cough on a regular basis. Positioning of nasogastric tubes in the stomach is ascertained before fluids are introduced.

■ Peptic ulcer

A peptic ulcer is an ulceration of the mucosa and deeper structures of the upper GI tract (Table 31-7). Ulcers may be acute or chronic. An *acute peptic ulcer* is usually superficial, involving only the mucosal layer. In most cases it heals within a relatively short time, but it may bleed, perforate, or become chronic. A *chronic peptic ulcer* is a deep crater with sharp edges and a "clean" base. It involves both the mucosa and the submucosa. If the ulcer penetrates the stomach wall and becomes adherent to an adjacent organ such as the pancreas, the organ may become the base of the ulcer.

Ulcers in the duodenum occur more frequently than gastric ulcers and have a greater incidence in persons 25 to 50 years of age. Gastric ulcers occur more frequently in persons over 50 years of age.

■ PATHOPHYSIOLOGY

Ulceration of the stomach and duodenum occur through different mechanisms. Persons with *gastric* ulcers have a normal gastric secretion and a normal emptying rate of the stomach but an increased diffusion of gastric acid *back* into the tissue (Fig. 31-11, A). Free acid that has been secreted into the stomach normally diffuses back slowly into the tissue. Rapid diffusion causes an inflammatory reaction in the tissue leading to tissue breakdown and bleeding. Bile acids, alcohol, and salicylates can break down the natural barriers that slow the back diffusion. Cigarette smoking has been shown to increase bile reflux from the duodenum into the stomach.[71]

Table 31-7 Types of peptic ulcers

Type of ulcer	Location	Comment
Esophageal	Lower third of esophagus	Usually result from gastroesophageal reflux
Gastric	Usually on antrum or lesser curvature of stomach	Larger and deeper than duodenal ulcers; gastric malignancy must be ruled out
Duodenal	Usually in first part of duodenum	More common than gastric ulcers, not as well defined
Marginal	Jejunum near site of gastrojejunal anastomosis	Difficult to heal

Persons with *duodenal* ulcers have a normal back diffusion of gastric acid but an increased gastric acid secretory rate and a markedly increased rate of gastric emptying (Fig. 31-11, *B*). Thus there is an increase in the amount of gastric acid in the gastric lumen, and if not buffered with a food such as protein or an antacid, the acid is propelled rapidly into the duodenum. The increased amount of acid in the duodenum irritates the duodenal mucosa, leading to tissue breakdown.

Zollinger-Ellison syndrome refers to peptic ulceration associated with a non–insulin-producing islet cell tumor of the pancreas. The syndrome is characterized by one or more peptic ulcerations in the lower end of the esophagus, stomach, duodenum, and jejunum and by enormous gastric hypersecretion and acidity.

A number of environmental, psychologic, and genetic factors may contribute to the development or delay of healing of peptic ulcers (see the box below). There is a common belief that persons exhibiting certain traits, such as tenseness or a striving for perfection or success, are more likely to develop peptic ulcers, but conclusive evidence to support this belief is lacking. Diet does not appear to be a predisposing factor, although caffeine-containing foods such as coffee or cola may exacerbate an ulcer.

▦ ASSESSMENT

☐ Subjective data

Pain, which is the major symptom of peptic ulcer, has the following characteristics:
1. Usually described as gnawing, aching, or burning
2. Usually confined to a small area of the upper abdomen near the midline
3. May radiate around the costal area to the back
4. Starts 1 to 2 hours after eating when the stomach begins to empty
5. May disappear with ingestion of food or an antacid
6. Frequently occurs at night when the stomach is empty

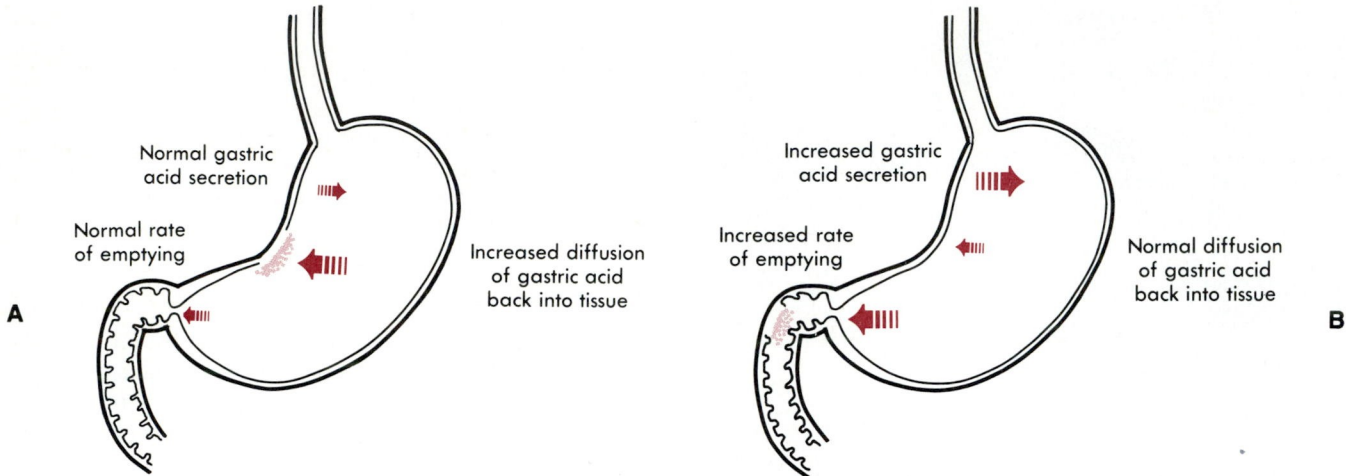

Fig. 31-11 Pathophysiology of peptic ulcer. **A,** Gastric. **B,** Duodenal. Note that the major alteration with gastric ulcers is increased back-diffusion of gastric acid whereas with duodenal ulcers it is increased acid secretion and stomach emptying.

Factors contributing to development of peptic ulcers	
Smoking	Cigarette smokers have increased incidence of peptic ulcers and delayed healing of gastric ulcers.
Drugs	Prolonged aspirin intake may lead to peptic disease. Corticosteroids, salicylates, indomethacin, and phenylbutazone in massive doses may cause acute ulcers or exacerbate an already existing chronic peptic ulcer.
Emotional tension	No direct relationship has been demonstrated between personality and peptic ulcer, but emotional tension can alter gastric functioning. Stress may lead to a stress ulcer.
Genetic factors	A tendency for gastric or duodenal ulcers may be inherited.
Blood group	Duodenal ulcers occur more frequently in persons with type O blood.

Gastrointestinal series (upper GI x-rays)

Purpose

Visualization of the structure and motility of the stomach and intestinal tract by means of ingestion of radiopaque barium

Preparation of patient

1. Diet: No food or fluids 6 to 8 hours before examination (test is postponed if stomach is not empty)
2. Patient teaching
   a. Explain procedure
   b. Time: aproximately 45 minutes
   c. Fluid to drink may taste chalky; patient will need to drink all of fluid

Procedure

1. Patient drinks approximately 250 ml (8 ounces) of barium while standing in front of a fluoroscopy tube
2. Several successive radiographs will be taken
3. The patient will be asked to assume different positions on the x-ray table to outline the stomach and small intestines

After procedure

1. Provide food and fluids
2. Administer laxative, if ordered, to speed elimination of the barium and prevent a fecal impaction
3. Observe stool to determine complete elimination of barium; stool should be brown (barium is white) and of normal consistency

Gastric analysis

Purpose

Aspiration of gastric contents to assess gastric acidity in the fasting and stimulated state

Preparation of patient

1. Diet: no food or fluids 6 to 8 hours before the test
2. No anticholinergic drugs 24 hours before the test (inhibits stimulation of acid secretion)
3. Patient teaching
   a. Explain the procedure
   b. Explain the reason for not smoking for 8 hours before test (smoking stimulates acid secretion)

Procedure

1. Nasogastric tube is inserted (p. 1069).
2. Encourage patient to relax after tube is inserted.
3. Instruct patient to expectorate saliva rather than swallowing (saliva may act as a buffer).
4. Gastric contents are aspirated.
5. Betazole hydrochloride (Histalog) or histamine is given subcutaneously. (Histamine is *not* given to a person with a history of allergies.)
6. Monitor patient for side effects of medication.
   a. Take pulse and blood pressure immediately (a slight increase in pulse and decrease in blood pressure may be noted).
   b. Side effects include flushing, feeling of warmth, slight headache, itching.
   c. Signs of adverse reaction include: shock, intense headache, vomiting, diarrhea.
7. Have epinephrine available to counteract effect of histamine if sensitivity reaction occurs.
8. After histamine preparation is given, stomach contents are aspirated every 10 to 20 minutes until desired number (usually three) of specimens obtained.
9. Tube is then clamped and withdrawn.

After procedure

1. Provide patient with tissues to wipe eyes and nose.
2. Offer mouth care.
3. Food and fluids may be resumed.

Gastroscopy

Purpose

Direct visualization of stomach by means of insertion of a fiberoptic gastroscope (Fig. 31-12)

Preparation of patient

1. Diet: Food and fluids withheld 6 to 8 hours before examination
2. Eyeglasses and dentures removed to prevent their damage
3. Ask patient to void before examination
4. Patient teaching
   a. Explain procedure
   b. Speaking will not be possible when scope is in position
   c. Time: approximately 15 minutes
   d. Sensation: feelings of pressure but no pain
   e. Hoarseness and sore throat may be present for several days after examination

Procedure

1. Topical anesthesia (spray or gargle) applied to throat
2. Valium given parenterally to relax patient
3. Gastroscope inserted through mouth with patient sitting or lying down
4. Air insufflated through scope to visualize mucosa
5. Biopsy may be obtained
6. Scope is removed; patient is asked to sit up immediately and to deep breathe, cough, and expectorate

After procedure

1. No food or fluids until gag reflex returns (2 to 4 hours)
2. Monitor vital signs every 30 minutes for 2 hours
3. Monitor for dyspnea, dysphagia, abdominal pain, fever, bleeding
4. Maintain safety precautions until effect of sedative wears off

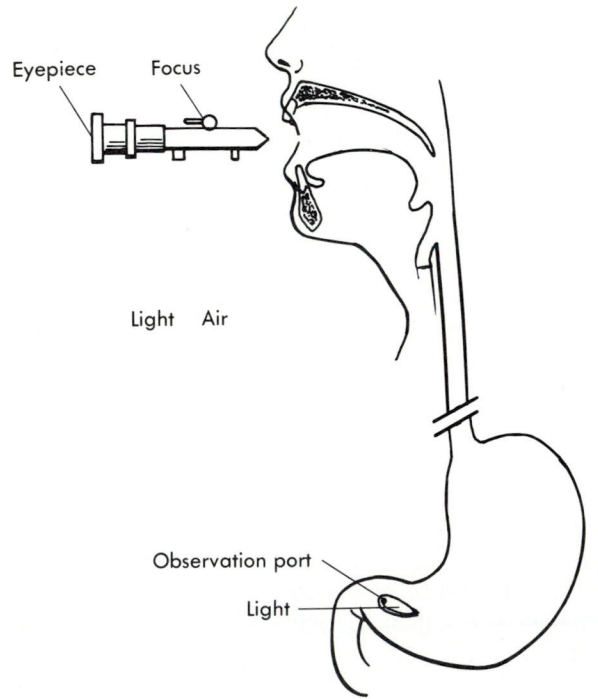

Eyepiece   Focus

Light   Air

Observation port

Light

Fig. 31-12   Stomach may be visualized by means of a fiberscope.

The patient with a peptic ulcer is therefore assessed for the presence, location, and character of pain as well as time of occurrence in relation to food and effectiveness of antacids. Some persons never experience pain, and the peptic ulcer may be discovered accidentally by x-ray or postmortem examination.

☐ Objective data

The patient is monitored for signs of hemorrhage (hematemesis, tarry stools), perforation (severe abdominal pain, abdominal rigidity), or pyloric obstruction (weight loss, projectile vomiting).

☐ Diagnostic tests

The diagnosis of peptic ulcer is made from the patient's history, a gastrointestinal series, gastric analysis, and stool examinations for occult (hidden) blood (p. 1094). Direct visualization of the ulcer by gastroscopy differentiates gastric ulcer from gastric carcinoma. These procedures are described in the boxes on pp. 1073-1074.

Selective *angiography* is becoming useful in the diagnosis and evaluation of treatment of gastric hemorrhage when angiography is combined with endoscopy. With angiography a contrast medium is injected through an arterial cath-

Table 31-8 Drug therapy for peptic ulcer

Drug	Action	Comments
Antacids	Neutralize gastric acid	Generally heal ulcers in 4 to 6 weeks Side effects limited to diarrhea or constipation Lack of adherence to regimen by many patients
Histamine H_2 receptor antagonists (cimetidine, ranitidine)	Inhibit acid secretion	Generally heal ulcers in 4 to 6 weeks Side effects may interfere with administration
Sucralfate (Carafate)	Coats ulcer, prevents action of acid and pepsin on ulcer	Generally heals ulcers in 4 to 6 weeks Longer time span before recurrence Large capsule; may be difficult to swallow
Anticholinergics	Decrease gastric secretions, delay gastric emptying	Less effective than other drugs; now rarely used Side effects usually occur with therapeutic doses

eter for better visualization of bleeding areas and for differentiation between normal and tumor vessels. Following the procedure, the femoral insertion site is observed for signs of bleeding, and vital signs are taken at frequent intervals.

DATA ANALYSIS: NURSING DIAGNOSES

Nursing diagnoses are determined from assessment of patient data. Possible nursing diagnoses for the person with a peptic ulcer may include, but are not limited to, the following:

Diagnostic title	Possible etiologies
Ineffective individual coping	Situational stressors
Knowledge deficit	Lack of exposure/recall, information misinterpretation
Pain: epigastric	Peptic ulceration

PLANNING: EXPECTED PATIENT OUTCOMES

Expected patient outcomes for the person with a peptic ulcer may include, but are not limited to, the following:
1. Pain is decreased, minimal, or absent.
2. Life stressors are identified, and stress management techniques are used.
3. Health-risking behaviors (smoking, alcohol ingestion) are modified, if pertinent.
4. The patient can
   a. Describe factors that contribute to healing.
   b. Describe medication plan to be followed.
   c. Describe plans for follow-up care.

IMPLEMENTATION

Assisting with comfort and healing

The pain of peptic ulcer is directly related to periods of the day when gastric acidity is high, particularly several hours after meals and at bedtime when acid secretion is high and the stomach is empty. Measures to decrease ulcer pain and promote healing include drug therapy (antacids,

histamine H_2 blockers, sucralfate) (Table 31-8) and food to buffer the gastric acidity.

Antacids

Antacids are the most effective therapy for relief of peptic ulcer pain; they act by decreasing gastric acidity. Antacids of choice are the nonsystemic antacids (Table 31-9), which are poorly absorbed from the stomach and therefore do not alter the pH of the blood or interfere with normal acid-base balance. Sodium bicarbonate is readily absorbed and therefore should be avoided as an antacid for relief of ulcer pain. Also, the reaction of sodium bicarbonate and hydrochloric acid forms carbon dioxide, which may cause distention.

Antacids may be administered frequently, and if symptoms are severe, it may be necessary to give them as often as every 30 to 60 minutes. When antacids are given to a person in a fasting state, the buffering power is usually transitory. For maximal effectiveness, antacids should be given 1 and 3 hours *after* meals; this produces a buffering effect that lasts approximately 3 to 4 hours. Aluminum hydroxide becomes less reactive over time and should not be given with anticholinergic drugs or with tetracycline because it interferes with absorption of these drugs. Liquids are more effective than tablets; if tablets are used, they are chewed slowly to permit complete pulverization.

Histamine H_2 receptor antagonists

One of the major stimulants of hydrochloric acid secretion in the stomach is histamine (in addition to gastrin and acetylcholine). In the body, histamine has two types of receptors, H_1 receptors, which mediate histamine action in the smooth muscle (and are blocked by antihistamines), and H_2 receptors, which mediate secretion of hydrochloric acid in the stomach. Histamine H_2 receptor antagonists, therefore, are drugs that block histamine's stimulation of gastric acid, either in the fasting state or the stimulated state.

There are two H_2 receptor antagonists in use for peptic ulcer therapy, cimetidine and ranitidine. *Cimetidine* (Tagamet) may be given orally or intramuscularly; the oral dose may be 300 mg four times a day or 600 mg twice a day before meals and at bedtime. Antacids may interfere

Table 31-9 Commonly used antacids

Drug type	Trade name	Comments
Mixtures		
Magnesium and aluminum hydroxide	Maalox	Preferred antacids
	Mylanta	Minimize possibility of constipation and diarrhea,
	Gelusil	but diarrhea may occur if taken frequently
Magnesium and aluminum hydroxide, calcium carbonate	Camalox	Moderate antacid action
Magaldrate	Riopan	
Magnesium preparations		
Magnesium (Mg) hydroxide, Mg carbonate, and Mg trisilicate	Milk of Magnesia	Laxative effect
		About 10% of the Mg is absorbed; may cause hypermagnesemia
		The hydroxide is fast-acting; the carbonate moderate-acting, and the trisilicate slow-acting
Aluminum (Al) preparations		
Aluminum hydroxide	Alternagel	Constipating
	Amphojel	Only small amounts of Al are absorbed
Aluminum carbonate	Basaljel	Slow-acting
		Prolonged ingestion may cause hypophosphatemia and osteoporosis
Calcium preparations		
Calcium carbonate	Tums	Constipating
	Alka-2	About 10% of the calcium is absorbed; may cause hypercalcemia
		Fast-acting
		May cause acid rebound

with absorption of cimetidine; therefore, the antacids are given at least 1 hour before or after cimetidine. Prophylactic cimetidine (400 mg at bedtime) has been given for periods up to 1 year to prevent recurrences. *Ranitidine* (Zantac) is more potent than cimetidine; it has a greater reduction of acid secretion and a longer duration. It is only given orally, 150 mg twice a day or 300 mg at bedtime. Antacids do *not* interfere with absorption of ranitidine, and ranitidine has fewer side effects than with cimetidine.

□ *Sucralfate*

Sucralfate (Carafate) helps to heal ulcers and decrease pain by coating the ulcer, thus preventing irritation by gastric acid and pepsin (Table 31-8). Sucralfate decreases the absorption of tetracycline and phenytoin; therefore, administration of these drugs should be spaced at least 2 hours apart from sucralfate administration. Antacids should be given at least 30 minutes before or after sucralfate.

□ *Anticholinergic drugs*

Anticholinergic drugs have theoretic value because they decrease gastric acid secretion and delay gastric emptying. Because they are usually prescribed in dosages that produce side effects and are less effective than the other drugs, they are now seldom used except for relief of refractory pain. A newer anticholinergic drug, pirenzepine, appears to accelerate healing of gastric ulcers and enhance the effect of cimetidine.

□ *Food*

Although modifying the diet has not been shown to accelerate healing of an uncomplicated ulcer, regulation of food may promote comfort. Food in the stomach, especially protein, buffers gastric acid; however, food is also a stimulant for gastric acid secretion, which may irritate the ulcer and cause pain. Controversy exists concerning whether ulcer pain is better relieved by three regular meals or six small meals a day. The person with the pain can best judge which approach provides the maximum comfort. The following eating suggestions can be given:

1. Eat meals slowly to prevent overdistention and gastric acid reflux.
2. Eat snacks if pain occurs between meals.
3. Restrict foods that stimulate gastric acid secretion (coffee, tea, cola).
4. If alcohol is consumed (stimulating gastric acid secretion), it should be taken in moderate amounts or less and not on an empty stomach.

Teaching for the patient with a peptic ulcer

Medications

1. Know dosage, administration, action, and side effects.
2. Continue drug for prescribed time, even when symptoms abate.
3. Keep antacids available at all times.
4. Anticipate increased need for antacid during periods of stress.
5. Avoid self-medication with systemic antacids (bicarbonate of soda) that alter acid-base balance.
6. Avoid ulcerogenic drugs such as salicylates, ibuprofen, corticosteroids.
7. Use acetaminophen (Tylenol) or buffered aspirin (if tolerated) for relief of pain.

Smoking

1. Stop smoking if possible.
2. If stopping smoking causes increased discomfort from stress, try to decrease amount smoked.

Eating

1. Eat three balanced meals a day.
2. Eat between meal snacks if this helps to relieve pain.
3. Avoid any foods that increase discomfort.
4. If alcohol is taken, drink in moderation and not on an empty stomach.
5. Avoid stress at mealtimes and plan for a quiet time after eating.

Relaxation and reduction of stress

1. Participate in recreation and hobbies that promote relaxation.
2. Provide for a good night's sleep on a regular basis.
3. Use relaxation techniques to decrease effects of stress.
4. Participate in a reasonable exercise program for promotion of well-being.
5. Structure home and work environment to keep stressors at a reasonable level.
6. Avoid factors found to increase symptoms, if possible.

---

5. Restrict bedtime snacks that may increase nocturnal pain.
6. Avoid any foods that increase discomfort.

☐ **Counseling and teaching**

Ulcer pain typically appears in a cyclic manner, with periods of days to weeks of pain interspersed with periods of little or no pain. Patients therefore need to know what to do at home to prevent or modify the pain. A summary of patient teaching is given in the box above.

In addition to knowing measures for relief of pain, the person with a peptic ulcer needs to understand about factors that contribute to healing and to prevention of ulcer recurrence. These factors include prevention of stress, avoidance of irritating substances that are poorly tolerated, avoidance of ulcerogenic drugs, avoidance of smoking, and maintenance of the medical regimen.

Stress plays a role in the pathogenesis of peptic ulcers, probably by means of the increased acid secretion from vagal stimulation.[52] Thus actions that avoid stressful situations or minimize the effect of stress can be beneficial for healing or for prevention of a recurrence. If removal from stressful environmental influences is impossible, the person must learn to cope with the stressful situations without reactivating the ulcer. (Measures to decrease stress are described in Chapter 7.) Occasionally the person is advised to obtain psychologic counseling for better understanding of the problems and for development of more effective coping behaviors.

Since there seems to be a relationship between *smoking* and irritation of a peptic ulcer, most physicians believe that the person who has a peptic ulcer should give up smoking permanently. To do so is sometimes very difficult, since often the person's life and work situations as well as personality are such that a change of this sort is a major one. Those few persons whose ulcers are reactivated when they attempt to give up smoking are urged at least to moderate the habit.

If every consideration is given to adjusting the prescribed regimen to fit the appropriate physical, economic, and social pattern, the person with an ulcer will be better able to follow the medical treatment.

⊞ EVALUATION

Questions to consider for the person with a peptic ulcer include the following:

1. Has epigastric pain been relieved or minimized?
2. Does the person know measures to relieve the effects of stress in daily living?
3. Has the person made plans to avoid or modify activities that delay healing?
4. Can the person describe
   a. Correct administration of prescribed medications?
   b. Specific actions to take to promote healing of the ulcer and decrease recurrence?
   c. Plans for follow-up care?

Table 31-10 Comparison of different types of vagotomy procedures for peptic ulcer

Type of surgery	Advantages	Disadvantages
Truncal vagotomy with pyloroplasty	Low operative mortality and morbidity	High recurrence rate
Selective vagotomy with pyloroplasty	Preservation of vagal innervation of viscus; fewer side effects than truncal vagotomy	More difficult to perform than truncal vagotomy
Proximal vagotomy	Preserves gastric emptying; low recurrence rate; fewer side effects; no intrusion of GI tract	Newer procedure; requires experienced surgeon
Vagotomy with antrectomy	Lower recurrence rate than for vagotomy with pyloroplasty	Higher operative mortality Greater side effects

Table 31-11 Comparison of subtotal gastrectomy procedures

	Gastroduodenostomy	Gastrojejunostomy
Common term	Billroth I	Billroth II
Procedure	Removal of lower part of stomach (antrectomy) with anastomosis to remaining segment of duodenum (Fig. 31-13, *A*)	Removal of lower part of stomach (antrectomy) with anastomosis to side of the proximal jejunum (Fig. 31-13, *B*)
Common use	Gastric ulcer	Duodenal ulcer
Side effects	Decreased gastric capacity, rapid emptying with decreased effect of pancreatic enzymes (malabsorption)	Same as Billroth I; stasis with subsequent infection in the blind duodenal loop

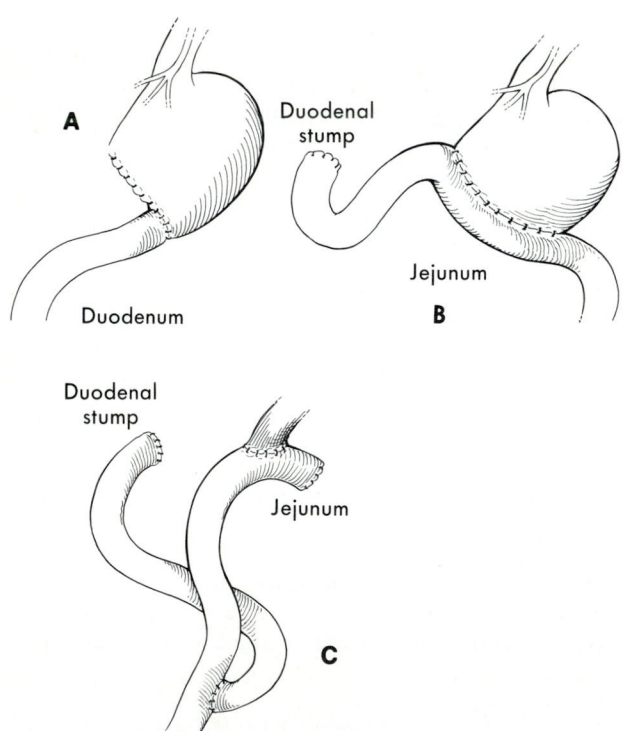

Fig. 31-13 Types of gastric resections with anastomoses. **A,** Billroth I. **B,** Billroth II. **C,** Total gastrectomy.

■ SURGERY FOR PEPTIC ULCER

Emergency surgery is necessary when a peptic ulcer perforates and causes peritonitis or erodes a blood vessel, causing severe hemorrhage. Elective surgery may be performed if the ulcer does not respond to the medical regimen and continues to produce symptoms, if it causes pyloric obstruction, or if a chronic recurring gastric ulcer is thought to be precancerous. The basic surgical procedures for treatment of peptic ulcers are subtotal gastrectomy, vagotomy, and pyloroplasty. Subtotal gastrectomy is now rarely performed alone but is usually combined with a form of vagotomy. Pyloroplasty is also combined with a vagotomy. The several common surgical combinations are listed in Table 31-10.

Subtotal gastrectomies are described in Table 31-11. The Billroth II (Fig. 31-13, *B*) is usually preferred for duodenal ulcers because of decreased duodenal recurrence. The duodenal stump is preserved to permit bile flow into the jejunum to mix with the food, but may develop infection from stasis.

Part of the vagus nerve innervating the stomach is severed in a *vagotomy* for the purpose of decreasing gastric acidity. There are three types of vagotomies currently in use: truncal, selective, and proximal (Fig. 31-14). With both *truncal* and *selective* vagotomies, gastric emptying is inhibited; thus a pyloroplasty or antrectomy (removal of antrum or lower portion of stomach) must be performed to prevent gastric stasis by enlarging the pyloric opening.

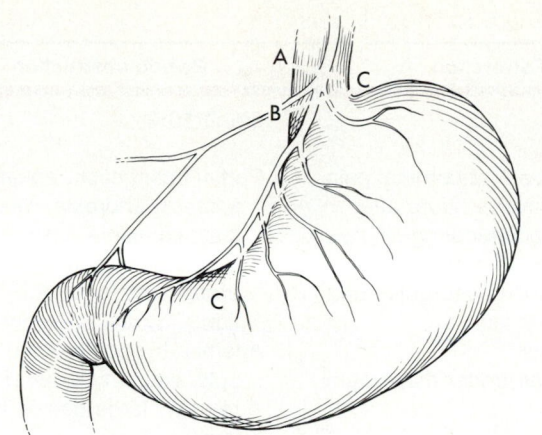

Fig. 31-14 Types of vagotomies: A, Truncal; B, Selective; C, Proximal or parietal cell.

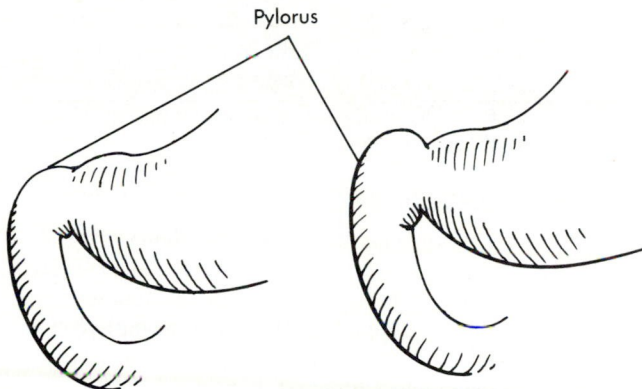

Fig. 31-15 Heineke-Mikulicz pyloroplasty. Longitudinal incision across pylorus is pulled apart and closed in transverse position to widen pyloric outlet.

The *proximal* vagotomy severs only the branches of the gastric portion of the vagal nerve that innervate the upper two thirds of the stomach, thus maintaining effective gastric emptying. Because a pyloroplasty or antrectomy is unnecessary with a proximal vagotomy, there is no intrusion into the gastric lumen and side effects, especially diarrhea, are reduced.

A *pyloroplasty* or drainage procedure widens the pyloric outlet. It is performed with a truncal or selective vagotomy to prevent gastric stasis. One type of pyloroplasty is the Heineke-Mikulicz procedure (Fig. 31-15).

Care of the patient experiencing gastric surgery is described on p. 1082.

■ **COMPLICATIONS OF PEPTIC ULCER**

A peptic ulcer may perforate a major blood vessel and cause hemorrhage, perforate the stomach or duodenal wall, or cause an obstruction at the pyloric end of the stomach.

☐ **Hemorrhage**

Peptic ulcer is the most common cause of massive upper gastrointestinal bleeding. Duodenal ulcers have a higher incidence of bleeding than gastric ulcers. In some cases bleeding is slight, and the only symptoms are tarry stools and a developing iron deficiency. When a major blood vessel erodes, bleeding is massive.

The medical management of hemorrhage is summarized in Table 31-12. Surgery is indicated for uncontrolled bleeding or for recurrence of hemorrhage. Vagotomy with pyloroplasty is preferred to gastrectomy. The drainage from the nasogastric tube is usually dark red for 6 to 12 hours after surgery but should turn greenish yellow within 24 hours. The patient may continue to pass tarry stools for several days postoperatively, but this is usually because the blood from the hemorrhage before surgery has not yet completely passed through the gastrointestinal tract. Stools may be guaiac positive for several days after bleeding stops.

If gastric lavage is indicated, saline is usually used to minimize loss of electrolytes. No evidence supports the use of iced solutions.[11,53]

Nursing interventions during the phase of *severe gastric bleeding* include the following actions:

1. Assisting with achievement of therapeutic goals
   a. Monitor vital signs and urinary output for response to shock therapy.
   b. Monitor nasogastric drainage, emesis, and stools for amount of blood loss (stools may be red or tarry depending on the length of time required for passage).
   c. Test stools daily for occult blood (guaiac) until bleeding has clearly stopped.
   d. Assist with medical treatments (blood transfusions, saline gastric lavage) and monitor patient's response.
   e. Prepare patient for surgery if indicated.
2. Assisting with patient comfort
   a. Provide special mouth care after vomiting (a weak solution of hydrogen peroxide will help remove blood from the oral mucosa).
   b. Administer prescribed sedative/narcotic regularly to decrease apprehension.
   c. Remove all evidence of bleeding as quickly as possible.
   d. Tell patient rationale for blood transfusion.
   e. Tell patient that rest and quiet will help stop the bleeding.
   f. Maintain a calm approach.
   g. Restrict activities only to those deemed necessary until massive bleeding has slowed down or stopped.

☐ **Perforation**

Perforation is an erosion of a peptic ulcer through the muscular wall, providing an opening from the gastrointestinal tract into the peritoneal cavity. Most perforated ulcers are located on the anterior duodenal wall. Immediately on perforation a chemical peritonitis results from contact with the gastrointestinal contents, and bacterial peritonitis results within 12 hours. Symptoms and medical management are listed in Table 31-12. Persons taking corticosteroids

Table 31-12 Complications of peptic ulcer

	Hemorrhage	Perforation	Pyloric obstruction
Occurrence with peptic ulcer	15% to 20%	10%	5% to 10%
Clinical picture	Hematemesis, tarry stools, shock	Sudden severe abdominal pain, usually several hours after eating; abdominal rigidity; decreased abdominal sounds; increased pulse and respiratory rate	Partial obstruction: epigastric fullness, anorexia, weight loss; complete obstruction: projectile vomiting of undigested food, dehydration
Diagnostic findings	Blood in vomitus and stool	Leukocytosis X-ray film: air under diaphragm	Anemia, hypochloremia, hypokalemia, hyponatremia X-ray film: large gastric fluid level
Medical treatment	Bed rest, sedation, blood transfusions, gastric lavage, treatment for shock, cimetidine After bleeding stops: antacids hourly or by continuous drip	Gastric decompression, parenteral fluids, antibiotics, surgery	Gastric decompression, correction of metabolic alkalosis and dehydration Antacids and liquids after 72 hours if obstruction decreased Surgery if obstruction persists

may develop a peptic ulcer and perforation without exhibiting any of the usual symptoms.

Some perforations are minor and close within a short time or wall themselves off. However, most perforations require surgery and should be closed surgically as soon as possible. Surgery may consist of simple laparotomy with closure (oversewing) of the perforation and aspiration from the peritoneum of all escaped GI fluid. A large majority of people who have had a perforated ulcer, however, continue to have recurrences of ulcer symptoms; therefore, most surgeons now perform definitive ulcer surgery, such as vagotomy with gastric resection or pyloroplasty, if the patient's condition permits. A pelvic abscess may require incision and drainage.

Nursing interventions for the person with a *perforated ulcer* include the following activities:
1. Assisting with achievement of therapeutic goals
   a. Connect the nasogastric tube initially to continuous suction until stomach is empty, then maintain at intermittent suction.
   b. Place patient in low Fowler's position to collect escaped fluids in pelvic cavity.
   c. Prepare patient for surgery, if indicated.
   d. Monitor postoperatively for continuing peritonitis and abscess formation (fever, respiratory distress, increased abdominal pain, distention, hyperactive or absent bowel sounds, inability to pass flatus or stool).
2. Assisting with patient comfort
   a. Give analgesic medications at regular intervals for pain control during acute phase.
   b. To decrease apprehension, explain what is being done.

☐ **Pyloric obstruction**

Pyloric obstruction may be caused by edema of tissues around an ulcer or by scar tissue from a healed ulcer located near the pylorus. It may be only a partial obstruction and cause dilation of the stomach, or it may be complete. Obstruction caused by edema and spasm generally responds to medical management (Table 31-12).

At the end of a 72-hour period of gastric decompression, a *saline load test* is performed to assess the degree of gastric emptying: 700 ml of normal saline at room temperature is introduced through the nasogastric tube over a 3- to 5-minute period, and the tube is then clamped. After 30 minutes the stomach is aspirated. A residual volume of more than 350 ml indicates continued pyloric obstruction, and surgery consisting of either a vagotomy with pyloroplasty or gastrectomy is considered. If the saline load test demonstrates improved gastric emptying, oral liquids and antacids are introduced with continued assessment of gastric emptying for several days.

Nursing interventions for the person with a *pyloric obstruction* include the following activities:
1. Monitor for signs of increasing severe abdominal pain and decreased abdominal sounds.
2. Assist with achievement of therapeutic goals.
   a. Assist with gastric lavage and maintain gastric decompression.
   b. Explain saline load test, when pertinent.
   c. Prepare patient for surgery as necessary.

■ **Cancer of the stomach**

Almost all gastric tumors are malignant. The incidence of cancer of the stomach has decreased in recent years;

NURSING CARE PLAN

Person with peptic ulcer

DATA: Mr. Jones is a 42-year-old single computer operator with a history of duodenal ulcer (4 years ago). He has had periods of epigastric distress for the past month with partial relief from Maalox. He was admitted 2 days ago with hematemesis, tarry stools, faintness, and a blood pressure of 96/54 (usual 124/84). Intravenous fluids were initiated. Endoscopy revealed a bleeding duodenal ulcer. A nasogastric tube was inserted and antacids prescribed hourly per tube. Cimetidine was started by intravenous push. His blood pressure is now stable and the nasogastric tube was removed early today. He is taking oral fluids and has been started on a soft diet. The cimetidine has been changed to 300 mg with meals and at bedtime and Maalox 30 ml 1 and 3 hours after meals.

The nursing history identified the following:

1. He is vague about the nature of peptic ulcer or possible complications.
2. He takes aspirin for headaches "from computer eyestrain."
3. He smokes 1½ packs per day; he has tried several times unsuccessfully, to quit.
4. He spends two to three evenings a week at a local bar and "puts down quite a few beers."

Collaborative nursing actions include those to prevent further injury from hemorrhage or perforation. Immediate reporting of and treatment of early signs may prevent serious effects (loss of blood, peritonitis, or death). Nursing actions include *monitoring* for the following:

1. Signs of hemorrhage: hematemesis, decreased blood pressure, restlessness, cool moist skin, stools that test positive for guaiac
2. Signs of perforation: severe, sudden, sharp abdominal pain

Nursing diagnosis: Pain: epigastric related to irritation of gastric acid on duodenal ulcer

Expected patient outcomes	Nursing interventions	Rationale
Patient states epigastric pain is decreased	Give prescribed cimetidine with meals and at bedtime (8:00, 12:00, 5:00, and 9:00)	Cimetidine encourages healing by decreasing gastric acid secretion; give with meals to inhibit food-stimulated HCl secretion
	Give prescribed antacid 1 and 3 hours after meals (9:00, 11:00, 1:00, 3:00, 6:00 and 8:00)	Antacids neutralize HCl; they interfere with absorption of cimetidine if given concurrently
	Teach relaxation measures as appropriate	Relaxation facilitates rest to promote healing

Nursing diagnosis: Altered health maintenance: related to lack of knowledge

Expected patient outcomes	Nursing interventions	Rationale
Patient states plans to decrease smoking and drinking and to avoid aspirin	Teach effects of aspirin, smoking, and alcohol on ulcer formation	If patient knows the direct effects of taking aspirin, smoking, and drinking alcohol, the likelihood of changing these behaviors is increased
	Discuss previous efforts at discontinuing smoking; explore additional ways, especially group programs, such as those provided by the American Cancer Society, American Lung Association, and American Heart Association	Programs that include group support are often more successful than trying to quit smoking by oneself
	Explore with patient reasons for frequent visits to bars, then explore other ways of meeting his needs (such as nonalcoholic drinks or substituting other social activities)	Assisting the person to think about reasons and alternate approaches will increase the potential for a behavioral change
	Suggest patient get his eyes examined (if appropriate); describe analgesics that do not contain aspirin (such as Tylenol and Anacin)	Headaches may be caused by strain from decreased vision; fewer headaches will decrease need for analgesics

Continued.

NURSING CARE PLAN

Person with peptic ulcer—cont'd

Nursing diagnosis: Knowledge deficit: related to lack of recall or exposure

Expected patient outcomes	Nursing interventions	Rationale
Patient describes nature of and therapy for peptic ulcer	Review nature of peptic ulcer and possible recurrence; review factors that contribute to healing (see Table 31-8, p. 1075); review methods of pain relief, including administration and side effects of cimetidine and antacids; review need to report symptoms of bleeding, perforation, or pyloric obstruction to physician immediately	Reinforcement of earlier teaching will help promote retention

nevertheless, gastric cancer is the seventh most common cause of cancer-related deaths.[5] It occurs more frequently in men than women and in blacks and orientals than whites. It rarely occurs in people under the age of 40 and is most frequent between the ages of 50 and 70. Contributing factors, symptoms, and usual medical therapy are summarized in Table 31-5 (p. 1066).

■ PATHOPHYSIOLOGY

Cancer may develop in any part of the stomach but is found most often in the distal third. Most gastric cancers are adenocarcinomas and occur in polypoid, ulcerative, or infiltrative forms. The ulcerative form is the most common and may produce peptic ulcer–type symptoms that, unfortunately, tend to delay diagnosis and encourage self-treatment. Growths located at the entrance or exit of the stomach may lead to signs of esophageal or pyloric obstruction (heartburn or early satiety). In general, however, early signs of gastric cancer are absent.

Gastric cancer may spread directly through the stomach wall into adjacent tissues, to the lymphatics, to the regional lymph nodes of the stomach, to other abdominal organs, or through the bloodstream to the lungs or bones. Involvement of the regional lymph nodes occurs early, followed by involvement of the more distal nodes. There is a tendency toward intraperitoneal seeding, particularly to the peritoneal cul-de-sac. Prognosis depends on the depth of invasion and extent of metastasis.

■ MEDICAL THERAPY

Surgery is the primary therapy for gastric cancer. If the tumor has not spread beyond the stomach, a subtotal gas-

trectomy (gastroduodenostomy or gastrojejunostomy) is usually performed. Tumors high in the cardia of the stomach may require a total gastrectomy (esophagojejunostomy).[40] Palliative subtotal gastrectomy may be performed when hemorrhage or obstruction occurs.

Chemotherapy and radiotherapy may be given for metastatic disease to decrease symptoms and prolong survival. Only about 5% to 10% of persons with gastric cancer have a 5-year survival.

■ Surgery of the stomach

A number of different surgical procedures may be performed on the stomach (Table 31-13). The word form -ostomy means "an opening into," thus gastrostomy refers to an opening into the stomach. If only one prefix precedes the term -ostomy, then the surgical opening is made from the exterior, such as gastrostomy. When two prefixes precede -ostomy, the surgery consists of an opening made between two organs (anastomosis); for example, a gastroenterostomy is an anastomosis of a portion of the stomach (gastro-) with a portion of the small intestine (entero-). The surgical procedures more commonly used for cancer of the stomach are gastroduodenostomy (Billroth I) and gastrojejunostomy (Billroth II) (see Fig. 31-11).

■ PREOPERATIVE CARE

If the nutritional status of the patient is poor, an attempt is made preoperatively to improve nutrition. Total parenteral nutrition (Chapter 6) or a temporary gastrostomy (p. 1063) may be necessary. If the patient is to have surgery for an ulcer, any special dietary prescriptions are continued through the preoperative period.

Table 31-13 Surgeries of the stomach

Name	Description	Comments
Esophagogastrostomy	Anastomosis of esophagus and stomach	Usually involves removal of lower one third of esophagus; tissue graft may be used
Esophagojejunostomy	Removal of stomach (total gastrectomy) and anastomosis of esophagus to jejunum	Two portions of jejunum meeting esophagus are sometimes joined to form a reservoir for food
Gastrectomy	Removal of part (subtotal) or all (total) of stomach	Remaining portions are anastomosed to small intestine
Gastrostomy	Insertion of tube through abdominal wall into stomach	Permits esophageal bypass allowing for nutritional feedings into GI tract
Gastroduodenostomy	Formation of new opening between stomach and duodenum	In Billroth I surgery (Fig. 31-13, *A*) part of stomach is removed and remaining portion is anastomosed to duodenum
Gastrojejunostomy	Anastomosis of stomach with jejunum	In Billroth II surgery (Fig. 31-13, *B*) duodenal stump is closed after excision of lower part of stomach
Antrectomy	Removal of entire antrum (lower portion) of stomach	Usually followed by gastroduodenostomy
Pyloroplasty	Repair of pyloric opening of stomach	To enlarge opening and facilitate stomach emptying
Gastric partitioning	Stapling of stomach to reduce size	Staples applied in two rows partially across stomach for control of massive obesity (see Fig. 6-1)

The major focus of nursing care is teaching the patient. Since the incision for gastric surgery is high in the abdomen, special emphasis is placed on teaching the patient breathing exercises preoperatively (see Chapter 16). The patient should know that a nasogastric tube may be in place for several days postoperatively because of decreased peristalsis from manipulation of the gastrointestinal tract organs during surgery and to prevent trauma or pressure on suture lines.

■ POSTOPERATIVE CARE

The care of the patient after gastric surgery centers on promoting pulmonary ventilation, nutrition, and comfort and teaching the patient. Specific nursing care is listed on p. 1084. Care of the patient with a nasogastric tube is described on p. 1070.

☐ Pulmonary ventilation

Patients with high abdominal incisions are at high risk of developing postoperative pulmonary complications because they are inclined to lie still and breathe shallowly to limit incisional pain. Measures to encourage movement and deep breathing take high priority.

☐ Gastric drainage

Drainage from the nasogastric tube after surgery usually contains some blood for the first 6 to 12 hours, but bright red blood, large amounts of blood, or excessive bloody drainage is reported to the surgeon immediately (Table 31-14). If the nasogastric tube stops draining, the surgeon is also notified, since a buildup of gas or fluid can cause pressure on the suture line resulting in rupture or dislodgement of the sutures. It is the responsibility of the surgeon to adjust the placement of the nasogastric tube so that inadvertent dislodgement of the sutures is prevented. Signs of return of GI functioning (auscultation of bowel sounds, passage of flatus) are reported to the surgeon.

☐ Nutrition

Until the nasogastric tube is removed and the patient is able to drink enough nutritious fluids, fluids are given parenterally. The average patient is given about 3500 ml of fluids intravenously each day (2500 ml for normal body needs plus enough to replace fluids lost through the gastric drainage and vomitus).

Fluids by mouth are restricted for about 12 to 24 hours after the nasogastric tube is removed. Fluids are then introduced slowly until well tolerated. Small amounts of bland food may be added until the patient is able to eat six small meals a day and to drink 120 ml of fluid every hour between meals. The dietary regimen must be adapted to the individual, since some persons tolerate increasing amounts of food and fluids better than others. Vitamins are usually prescribed until the patient is eating a full, well-balanced diet.

Early satiety and regurgitation after meals are common problems after gastric surgery. Eating less food more slowly and chewing thoroughly is usually effective. Persistent early satiety or regurgitation may be caused by edema of the suture line. A nasogastric tube may need to be reinserted until the edema subsides.

☐ Dumping syndrome

After a gastric resection, the dumping syndrome sometimes occurs. It may also occur in patients who had a vagotomy, antrectomy, or gastroenterostomy. The onset may occur during the meal or from 5 to 30 minutes after

Table 31-14 Postgastrectomy complications

Complications	Symptoms	Therapy
Bleeding at anastomotic suture line	Large quantity of blood in nasogastric tube drainage during day 1; may also occur on days 4 to 7	Treatment for upper GI hemorrhage (p. 1079)
Duodenal stump leakage	Severe upper abdominal pain that may radiate to shoulder, fever, leukocytosis; usually occurs on days 2 to 6	Surgery
Gastric retention	Abdominal fullness, nausea, and vomiting after nasogastric tube is removed	Nasogastric suction for 48 hours then feedings resumed slowly; surgery if no improvement
Dumping syndrome	Weakness, faintness, tachycardia, diaphoresis during eating or from 5 to 30 minutes later	Small frequent feedings (low carbohydrate, high fat and protein); fluids only between meals
Blind loop syndrome (stasis in blind loop with bacterial proliferation)	Abdominal pain 15 to 30 minutes after eating; steatorrhea, diarrhea, weight loss	Antibiotics; surgery to change a Billroth II to a Billroth I may be necessary

the meal. The attack may last 20 to 60 minutes. The patient complains of weakness, faintness, tachycardia, and diaphoresis. Other symptoms include a feeling of fullness, discomfort, nausea, and diarrhea.

The symptoms are thought to be caused by the entrance of food directly into the jejunum without undergoing usual changes and dilution in the stomach. The food mixture, more hyperosmolar than the jejunal secretions, causes fluid to be drawn from the bloodstream to the jejunum. The reaction appears to be greater after the ingestion of sugar, since sugar is the most osmotically active food. The symptoms are also attributed to the sudden rise in blood sugar (hyperglycemia), with the entrance of glucose into the bloodstream and the subsequent fall in the blood sugar level. The rapid gastric emptying and the propulsion of chyme into the small intestine are felt to initiate an intensive gastrocolic reflex and cause diarrhea and a feeling of fullness and discomfort.

Teaching for the patient who experiences dumping syndrome includes the following:

1. Eat a low-carbohydrate, high-fat, high-protein diet
2. Drink fluids only between meals
3. Avoid eating large amounts of food at one time
4. Rest after meals (recumbent position for 30 minutes)
5. Take anticholinergic drugs before meals as prescribed

■ TOTAL GASTRECTOMY

Total gastrectomies are now rarely performed. The nursing care of the patient who has had a total gastrectomy (esophagojejunostomy) differs in some ways from that of patients undergoing other types of gastric surgery. A thoracic approach is used, and the nursing care will be the same as that for the patient who has had chest surgery. Drains are usually inserted from the site of the anastomosis, and there may be serosanguineous drainage. There is little or no drainage from the nasogastric tube because there is no longer any reservoir in which secretions may collect, and there is no stomach mucosa left to secrete.

Following a total gastrectomy the maintenance of good nutrition is difficult because the patient can no longer eat regular meals and because the food that is taken is poorly digested and therefore poorly absorbed from the intestines. Since the patient also becomes anemic, ferrous sulfate, folate, and vitamin B_{12} are often prescribed. These patients rarely regain normal strength. Most of them are semiinvalids as long as they live.

■ Malabsorption syndrome

Malabsorption syndrome is a group of signs and symptoms resulting from inadequate absorption of fat in the small intestine. Because fat-soluble vitamins (A, D, E, and K) require fat for absorption, decreasing absorption of these vitamins usually accompanies fat malabsorption. In addition, fat malabsorption often is accompanied by decreased absorption of protein, carbohydrate, and minerals. Different signs and symptoms specific to various nutrients result from malabsorption of nutrients other than fat.

Adult lactase deficiency is a common disorder found among most populations of the world with the exception of northern European Caucasians and their descendants. In North America, Blacks, Jews, Orientals, American Indians, Eskimos, and Mexicans are frequently affected. Lactase deficiency is usually a congenital disorder, although symptoms may not occur immediately. It also occurs occasionally after a subtotal gastrectomy.

Some adults have an intolerance to gluten found in grains (wheat, rye, barley, oats). The disorder may be termed *adult celiac disease, celiac sprue,* or *gluten enteropathy*. These persons often have a history of childhood celiac disease or evidence of disease in relatives. Tropical sprue is different than celiac sprue and is endemic to the Caribbean, Southeast Asia, and India.

■ PATHOPHYSIOLOGY

Malabsorption results when there are (1) alterations of digestion so that nutrients are not broken down into a form that can be transported across the cell membranes of the villi; (2) alterations in the transportation of nutrients across the cell membranes of the villi so that nutrients cannot be absorbed; and (3) alterations in the transport of nutrients, particularly fat, from the villi through the lymphatic or circulatory systems (Table 31-15).

Lactase deficiency results from a lack of the enzyme lactase, which hydrolyzes lactose (a disaccharide found in milk) into glucose and galactose for absorption. The undigested lactose acts as an osmotic agent drawing water into the intestinal lumen and a substrate for bacterial fermentation, producing abdominal distention and discomfort.

Intolerance to gluten found in grains leads to atrophy of the intestinal villi and microvilli. The proximal jejunum is the area most affected. This disorder is thought to be a hypersensitivity response. Tropical sprue has both a nutritional and infectious basis, responding to treatment with antibiotics, as well as to diet therapy.

▨ ASSESSMENT

The stool is assessed for presence of a light, greasy, bulky, mushy appearance and a foul odor. This is a sign of *steatorrhea* (excess fat in the stool). The stools float because of their low specific gravity and because of gas produced by action of intestinal bacteria on the undigested fat. Stools may be limited to one bulky stool a day or may be frequent. If the malabsorption is caused by a lactase deficiency, the patient will have a watery fermentive diarrhea. Malabsorption causes flatulence and abdominal distention. Decreased fat absorption leads to weight loss, weakness, fatigue, and anorexia.

If malabsorption is severe, the person will have signs of *vitamin deficiency* (bleeding, bone pain and fractures, hypocalcemia, anemia, inflammation of the tongue, muscle tenderness, peripheral neuritis, and dermatitis). *Protein deficiency* will be evidenced by edema, hypoalbuminemia and loss of muscle mass. The skin will be dry and scaly and may be hyperpigmented.

Table 31-15 Causes of intestinal malabsorption

Factors affecting absorption	Mechanism	Examples
Altered digestion (intraluminal phase)	Decreased gastric function	Subtotal gastrectomy
	Decreased pancreatic lipase	Pancreatic insufficiency: pancreatitis, cancer of pancreas, cystic fibrosis, Zollinger-Ellison syndrome
	Decreased conjugated bile salts	Liver disease, biliary tract obstruction, enteric fistulas
		Drugs that precipitate bile salts (neomycin, cholestyramine)
Altered mucosal cell transport (mucosal phase)	Genetic abnormalities	Lactase deficiency
	Small bowel disease	Crohn's disease, celiac disease, tropical sprue, Whipple's disease, infectious or allergic enteritis, parasitic infections, small bowel ischemia
	Inadequate surface	Intestinal resection or bypass
	Drugs	Para-aminosalicylic acid, colchicine, irritant laxatives, neomycin
	Radiation	Radiation enteritis
Altered lymph/blood transport (transit phase)	Lymphatic obstruction	Lymphoma
	Altered blood supply	Superior mesenteric thrombosis

If acute generalized malabsorption is present, the patient is monitored for signs of *bleeding* (ecchymosis, hematuria), tetany, and skin breakdown.

→ DATA ANALYSIS: NURSING DIAGNOSES

Nursing diagnoses are determined from assessment of patient data. Possible nursing diagnoses for the person with a malabsorption syndrome may include, but are not limited to, the following:

Diagnostic title	Possible etiologies
Diarrhea	Malabsorption
Knowledge deficit	Lack of exposure/recall
Altered nutrition: less than body requirements	Malabsorption
Pain: abdominal, bone, muscle, dry mucous membranes	Malabsorption

PLANNING: EXPECTED PATIENT OUTCOMES

Expected patient outcomes for the person with a malabsorption syndrome may include, but are not limited to, the following:
1. Diarrhea and steatorrhea are decreased
2. Patient states feeling comfortable
3. Patient describes diet to be followed and signs indicating need for dietary reevaluation
4. Patient consumes nutrients that can be tolerated

IMPLEMENTATION

□ **Assisting with achievement of therapeutic goals**
□ *Promoting nutrition*

If intolerance to a specific substance is present, that substance is omitted from the diet. Thus, in adult *lactase deficiency,* all foods containing milk products or added lactose are avoided. Milk substitutes (such as Ensure Plus, Isocal) are available, and vegetable oils are used instead of butter. Some persons can tolerate some cheeses and yogurt. Calcium substitutes are required.

If *gluten intolerance* is present, all cereal grains and their products (except for rice) are excluded. This is a difficult diet to follow because many commercial foods, including some instant coffees, contain some wheat filler. Corn, soybean, and gluten-free flour are available for cooking.

If *generalized acute malabsorption* is present, the patient may require total parenteral nutrition (Chapter 6) or intravenous albumin, calcium, magnesium, and potassium. Packed red blood cells may be necessary if anemia is severe.

□ **Providing comfort**
□ *Mouth care*

Dry mucous membranes and enlarged tongue (if present) lead to oral discomfort. Good mouth care every 4 hours to maintain hydration will ease discomfort.

□ *Bone and muscle pain*

Analgesics may be prescribed for bone or muscle pain. Aspirin may be contraindicated because of the bleeding tendency from vitamin deficiencies. Gentle handling of the extremities is indicated to prevent further discomfort and possible pathologic fractures.

Foods containing lactose or gluten

Foods containing lactose

Dairy products
Baked foods containing milk, butter, cheese
Commercial foods processed with lactose
Instant coffee
Chocolates
Cold cuts, hot dogs

Foods containing gluten

Foods containing wheat, rye, barley, oats
Commercial baked goods and pastas
Commercial salad dressings
Ice cream, candies
Beer, ale
Instant coffees using wheat flour as a filler

☐ Anal care

The rectal area may become irritated if diarrhea is present. Provide for gentle personal hygiene after *each* loose stool.

☐ Counseling and teaching

Because there is no "cure" for malabsorption syndrome, persons with these problems must learn to adjust their diets for life. Teaching the person includes the following:

1. Avoid all foods containing that which is not tolerated (see the box above).
2. Read carefully the labels of prepared foods.
3. Follow the appropriate diet (lactose-free or gluten-free for life).
4. Reevaluate diet if symptoms reoccur.

⊞ EVALUATION

Evaluation of the care of the person with malabsorption syndrome is based on the expected patient outcomes. Questions to consider are: Does the patient know the types of food to be avoided? Have fatty stools and diarrhea decreased? Is the person comfortable?

■ ELIMINATION DISORDERS

The major disorders of the intestines are inflammatory disorders (acute and chronic) that may interfere with absorption and disorders that interfere with passage of the chyme and fecal matter (paralytic ileus, intestinal obstruction, hernias, and masses). Anorectal lesions, which may be inflammatory or vascular (hemorrhoids), may interfere with passage of feces because of the discomfort produced.

■ Common bowel dysfunctions

Changes in intestinal movement may create flatulence or constipation if movement is inhibited or diarrhea if movement is accelerated. Loss of control leads to fecal incontinence. Nursing actions include preventing the dysfunctions when possible and promoting comfort when the dysfunctions occur.

■ FLATULENCE

☐ Pathophysiology

Gas collects in the GI tract as a result of swallowed air, as gas formed by the action of intestinal bacteria, and as carbon dioxide formed by the action of bicarbonate with hydrochloric acid or fatty acids. Normally the gas is either reabsorbed or is expelled. When gastrointestinal motility is decreased, the gas collects in the stomach or intestines, causing abdominal distention and pain.

▦ Assessment

"Gas pains" can cause severe abdominal discomfort. The abdomen is distended over the entire area (as differentiated from lower abdominal distention occurring from a full bladder). The abdomen has a drumlike sound if tapped.

▦ Implementation

Some of the following interventions may help to decrease the intestinal gas volume when a pathologic condition is not present:

1. Avoid activities that increase repetitive swallowing of air.
2. Maintain an erect position after meals to facilitate gas rising to the fundus of the stomach and being expelled.
3. Eat a low-fat diet to decrease carbon dioxide production.
4. Take antacids containing hydroxide and simethicone (Maalox Plus, Mylanta) 1 hour after meals to neutralize acid and reduce flatus.
5. Avoid gas-forming carbohydrates that produce more discomfort (for example, selected vegetables, fruit, or bran).
6. Ambulate to increase peristalsis to move the gas through the intestinal tract, if discomfort is present.

■ CONSTIPATION

☐ Pathophysiology

Constipation may result from decreased motility of the colon or from retention of feces in the lower colon or rectum. In either case, since water is reabsorbed in the colon, the longer the feces remain in the colon the greater the reabsorption of water, and the dryer the stool becomes. The stool is then more difficult to expel from the anus.

Occasional constipation is not detrimental to health, although it can cause a feeling of general discomfort or abdominal fullness, anorexia, and anxiety in some persons.

Habitual constipation leads to decreased intestinal muscle tone, increased use of Valsalva maneuver (bearing down using a closed glottis) as the person attempts to pass the hardened stool, and increased incidence of hemorrhoids.

Assessment

Constipation is identified by defecation of a hard, formed stool or a frequency considerably less than the person's usual pattern. The person may also report feelings of rectal pressure or fullness and may experience straining at stool. If the stool is permitted to remain in the colon until it becomes exceedingly hard, a *fecal impaction* occurs. Digital examination by means of inserting a gloved finger in the rectum may identify a fecal impaction. Hardened stool may be palpated in the lower left abdominal quadrant. Some persons are at high risk for developing constipation and fecal impaction; high-risk factors include the following:

Nutritional depletion

Dehydration

Radiographic examinations using barium

Prolonged bedrest or inactivity

Prolonged use of constipating medications (aluminum-based antacids, anticholinergics, antihistamines, antidepressants, narcotics, phenothiazines, salts of bismuth, calcium, iron)

Implementation

1. Assisting with achievement of therapeutic goals
    a. Encourage a diet containing adequate high-fiber foods (raw or cooked vegetables and fruits, whole-grain cereal products).
    b. Encourage a fluid intake of at least 2000 to 2400 ml/day (8 to 10 glasses) unless contraindicated.
    c. Encourage all hospitalized patients to be as active as possible within the limits of their activity prescription.
    d. Facilitate change of a constipating antacid with one that has a more laxative effect in high-risk persons (see Table 31-9, p. 1076).
    e. Use suppositories to initiate defecation in persons who lack innervation of rectum (paraplegics).
    f. Encourage use of prescribed laxatives after extensive barium studies.
2. Teach the patient
    a. Effect of diet, fluids, and activity in preventing constipation.
    b. Planning of daily schedules to permit time for defecation after breakfast and dinner.
    c. Avoiding use of laxatives on a regular basis (decrease muscle tone and mucus production; may lead to water and electrolyte imbalances).

■ DIARRHEA

□ Pathophysiology

The definition of diarrhea is based on the consistency of the stool and not on the number expelled per day. Diarrhea results primarily from pathologic disorders that increase the fluid content of the stool or that increase intestinal transit time. The end result is a watery stool. Common causes of diarrhea include the following:

1. Increased fluid content of stool
    a. Intestinal infections
    b. Chronic bowel disorders
    c. Malabsorption disorders
    d. Biliary tract disorders
    e. Postgastrectomy syndrome
    f. Saline laxatives
    g. Antacids (magnesium based)
    h. Caffeine
2. Increased motility
    a. Stress
    b. Gastric or intestinal resection
    c. Surgical intestinal bypass
    d. Antibiotics

Severe diarrhea can lead to excessive losses of water, sodium, potassium, and bicarbonate, leading to dehydration, hyponatremia, hypokalemia, and metabolic acidosis (see Chapter 8). Distention of the intestines and frequent contractions from the rapid motility lead to abdominal cramping, although discomfort may be absent (such as with diarrhea caused by stress). Increased peristalsis may produce high-pitched bowel sounds occurring at frequent intervals (borborygmi).

Assessment

The stool is monitored for consistency (soft to liquid) and amount. Abdominal cramping may occur only immediately before and during defecation, or it may occur irrespective of time and situation. Perineal irritation may result from the frequent defecation.

Implementation

1. Assisting with achievement of therapeutic goals
    a. Facilitate rest of the bowel
        (1) Administer medications as prescribed (see Table 31-16). If diarrhea occurs primarily after meals, give antidiarrheal medications 30 to 60 minutes before meals for maximum effectiveness.
        (2) Diet: control food intake to decrease intestinal stimulation and to prevent irritation of inflamed mucosa
            (a) Give only fluids for 24 to 48 hours for severe diarrhea
            (b) Give the patient a high-protein, high-calorie, low–dietary fat diet when foods are permitted
    b. Assist with fluid and electrolyte replacement
        (1) Monitor for signs of fluid and electrolyte imbalance (thirst, dry mucous membranes, decreased skin turgor, headache, muscle weakness, fatigue, abdominal cramps, distention)
        (2) Monitor and facilitate parenteral fluids and electrolytes as prescribed for severe diarrhea
        (3) Give oral fluids for moderate diarrhea; fluids high in sodium and potassium, such as fruit juices and bouillon, are recommended.

Table 31-16 Drugs that are commonly prescribed for diarrhea

Drug	Action
Systemic effect	
Diphenoxylate (Lomotil, Colonil)	Decrease intestinal motility; side effects; constipation, sedation
Camphorated tincture of opium (paregoric)	
Loperamide (Imodium)	
Local effect	
Bismuth salts (for example, Pepto-Bismol)	Binds with bacterial toxin; side effect: black stool
Kaolin with pectin	Limited value; may protect the irritated, inflamed intestinal wall

2. Assisting with comfort
   a. Provide for personal hygiene after *each* loose stool
   b. Provide rest periods if fatigue is present

■ FECAL INCONTINENCE

□ Pathophysiology

Voluntary emptying of the rectum occurs when the external anal sphincter (under cortical control) relaxes and the abdominal and pelvic muscles contract. Conditions that interrupt transmission of messages to and from the brain (cortical lesions, spinal cord lesions), cause injury to the sphincter (trauma, fistulas, abscess), or cause perineal muscle relaxation (childbirth, perineal surgery, aging) may lead to fecal incontinence.

Assessment

Fecal incontinence is characterized by involuntary passage of stool. Data to be collected include the following:
1. Frequency of defecations
2. Nature of the stool
3. Awareness of need to defecate
4. Ability to contract abdominal and perineal muscles
5. Willingness of person to participate in exercise or bowel control program.

Implementation

1. Assisting with achievement of therapeutic goals
   a. Provide a high-fiber diet to facilitate a formed stool.
   b. Provide a fluid intake of about 3000 ml/day to promote a soft stool.
   c. Administer a stool softener daily, if necessary, to keep the stool soft.

Bowel training program

1. Include patient and family/friend in the planning.
2. Determine when bowel evacuation usually occurs (most frequent times are after breakfast or dinner).
3. Determine whether a morning or evening program is more suitable for patient.
4. Insert glycerine or bisocodyl (Dulcolax) *suppository* 30 minutes before expected time of defecation; give suppository at *same time every day*.
5. Have patient sit on toilet if possible for defecation.
6. If necessary, massage abdomen toward the sigmoid area (left lower quadrant) to encourage defecation; digital rectal stimulation may also stimulate defecation.

---

   d. Plan a bowel training program to prevent incontinence if control is not feasible. Within a few days the patient will probably defecate only once a day when stimulated. If the stool remains soft, the program may be changed to every other day. Consistency in carrying out the plan is important for success (see the box above).
   e. If fecal incontinence is uncontrollable, identify the defecation pattern. Place the patient on the toilet or commode at the time that defecation is anticipated. Protective disposable pants are available to provide the person with a sense of security and dignity.
2. Assisting with comfort
   Assist the person to cleanse the anal and perineal areas as soon as possible after fecal incontinence to eliminate odor and prevent skin breakdown.
3. Counseling and teaching
   a. Provide empathic communication. The person may have feelings of regression, inadequacy, or uncleanliness as a result of the loss of control. The person needs to feel accepted as an adult and accept the condition as a situational physical condition and not personal inadequacy.
   b. Encourage patients to participate in all or some of their own management to the extent that is possible, thus providing them with a sense of control.
   c. Teach perineal exercises for weak perineal muscles (Chapter 32).

■ Acute inflammatory intestinal disorders

Inflammation of the intestines (enteritis) is a common occurrence and may occur alone or in combination with gastritis (p. 1065). Gastroenteritis is often of viral origin.

Table 31-17 Acute inflammatory intestinal disorders

Disease	Etiology	Signs and symptoms	Medical therapy
Gastroenteritis	Virus	Abdominal cramps, nausea and vomiting, diarrhea, headache	Nothing by mouth until nausea and vomiting subside, then fluids and bland diet; rest
Food poisoning	*Staphylococcus aureus:* enterotoxin in fish, meats, unrefrigerated mayonnaise or cream-filled foods; skin and respiratory tract of food handlers	Nausea and vomiting, abdominal pain, decreased temperature; diarrhea is variable	Bed rest, fluids
	Salmonella: inadequately cooked pork, poultry, eggs	Nausea and vomiting, abdominal pain, chills, fever, weakness	Bed rest, fluids
	Clostridium botulinum: improperly canned or smoked foods	Nausea and vomiting, double vision, flaccid paralysis of face and throat, dryness of skin and mucous membranes	Botulinum antitoxin, maintenance of ventilation and oxygen, parenteral fluids
Appendicitis	Appendiceal kinking or occlusion, obstruction by fecalith, infection by colon bacilli or streptococcus	Sudden onset, pain in mid-epigastrium becomes localized in right lower quadrant, nausea and vomiting, low grade fever, leukocytosis	Appendectomy when diagnosis confirmed
Amebiasis	Parasite found in tropical climates where sanitation is poor	Early: abdominal cramps, intermittent diarrhea/constipation, flatulence Late: frequent liquid stools containing blood, mucus; fever, colicky abdominal pain	Amebicidal drugs
Trichinosis	Roundworms transmitted by inadequately cooked food, especially pork	Edema of eyelids, muscle stiffness, weakness, fever, pain on eye motion, dyspnea	Symptomatic: bed rest, analgesics, steroids, thiabendazole

Some foods may cause irritation of the intestinal mucosa leading to mild symptoms of belching, abdominal discomfort, and diarrhea. Bacteria and parasities may also cause intestinal inflammations (Table 31-17). The appendix may become inflamed (appendicitis); appendicitis is most common in males aged 10 to 30.

■ PATHOPHYSIOLOGY

□ Enteritis

Acute enteritis can be caused by direct bacterial or viral infection or by the effect of neurotoxins produced by bacteria. This produces either an increased secretion of water and salt into the gut lumen or an increase in motility, causing large amounts of undigested food and fluid to be excreted. In the latter case, large amounts of gas and foul smelling stool result. With profuse diarrhea, large amounts of fluid and electrolytes may be lost, leading to dehydration, hyponatremia, and hypokalemia (see Chapter 8).

□ Parasitic infections

The most common parasitic infections are amebiasis and trichinosis (Table 31-17). *Amebiasis* is caused by the pro-

tozoan parasite that primarily invades the large intestine and secondarily the liver. The active motile form of the protozoa, the trophozoite, is not infectious and, if ingested, is easily destroyed by digestive enzymes. However, the inactive form (cyst) is highly resistant to extremes in temperature, most chemicals, and the digestive juices. When the cyst is swallowed in *fecally contaminated food or water,* it easily passes into the intestines, where the active trophozoite is released and enters the intestinal wall. Here it feeds on the mucosal cells, causing ulceration of the intestinal mucosa. Although the disease exists chiefly in tropical countries, it also prevails wherever sanitation is poor. The cyst can survive for long periods outside the body.

Trichinosis is caused by the larvae of a species of roundworm, which become encysted in the striated muscles of humans, hogs, and other animals (rodents) that eat infected pork in garbage. Trichinosis has a worldwide distribution with the highest incidence occurring in Europe and the United States. It occurs more often in hogs that have been fed garbage than in those fed on grain. The larvae do not form cysts in pork; therefore, they are not visible to the naked eye and cannot be seen by food inspectors.

Trichinosis is transmitted through inadequately cooked food. *Pork* is the most common source of infection. When infected food is eaten, live encysted larvae develop within the intestine of the host; they mate and produce eggs that hatch in the uterus of the female worm. The larvae are discharged in huge numbers into the lymphatics and lacteals of the host's small intestine at the rate of about two every hour for about 6 weeks. They pass to the muscles of the host, where they become encysted by the reaction of the host's body and may remain for many years.

The trichinosis parasite can be killed by cooking at a temperature of 60° C (140° F) for 30 minutes per pound of meat or by freezing at a temperature of −18° C (0° F) for 24 hours. They are not killed by smoking, pickling, or other methods of processing. Sausage and other infected pork products carelessly prepared are a common source of infection in humans.

☐ Appendicitis

Appendicitis is an inflammation of the vermiform appendix, located near the ileocecal valve. The inflammation may be initiated by obstruction from a fecalith (a stonelike mass formed from feces) or bacterial infection. A small part of the appendix may be edematous or necrotic, or the entire appendix may be involved. Pressure within the appendix builds up rapidly leading to early necrosis of the appendiceal walls with subsequent perforation. Heat and external pressure (such as that resulting from enemas) increases the appendiceal pressure facilitating rupture of the appendix.

Although the typical symptoms of acute appendicitis (anorexia, nausea, and vomiting combined with abdominal pain that becomes located at McBurney's point halfway between the umbilicus and right ileal crest) are common findings, many variations of these symptoms may occur. The pain may be located in other parts of the abdomen as a result of the stretching of the appendix or the location retrocecally or adjacent to the ureter.

☐ Peritonitis

If peritonitis (inflammation of the peritoneum) results from a perforated appendix, adhesions form quickly in an attempt to wall off the infection, and the omentum helps to enclose areas of inflammation, forming an abscess. As healing occurs, fibrous adhesions may form, leading to intestinal obstruction at a later date. At other times the fibrous adhesions may disappear completely. Local reactions of the peritoneum include redness, edema, and the production of large amounts of fluid containing electrolytes and proteins. Hypovolemia, electrolyte imbalance, dehydration, and finally shock develop if the infection is not contained. Intestinal peristalsis is halted by a severe peritoneal infection.

⬛ ASSESSMENT

Subjective data to be collected for the person with an acute inflammatory disorder of the intestines include anorexia, nausea, and presence and extent of abdominal discomfort. If food poisoning is suspected, the person is questioned concerning possible sources of food contamination. Abdominal pain is usually diffuse except if acute appendicitis is present. With appendicitis, there is often rebound tenderness over McBurney's point if pressure is applied lightly, then released suddenly.

Objective data to be collected include the following:
1. Emesis: frequency, amount, presence of blood
2. Stools: frequency, character, amount if liquid, presence of foul odor
3. Flatulence
4. Signs of fluid and electrolyte imbalance (thirst, dry mucous membranes, hemoconcentration, oliguria, muscle weakness)

➡ DATA ANALYSIS: NURSING DIAGNOSES

Nursing diagnoses are determined from assessment of patient data. Possible nursing diagnoses for the person with an acute inflammatory disorder of the intestines may include, but are not limited to, the following:

Diagnostic title	Possible etiologies
Diarrhea	Intestinal inflammation
Fluid volume deficit	Diarrhea
Pain: abdominal	Intestinal inflammation

⬛ PLANNING: EXPECTED PATIENT OUTCOMES

Expected patient outcomes for the person with an acute inflammatory disorder of the intestines may include, but are not limited to, the following:
1. Stools decrease in number and are of normal consistency.
2. Patient states feeling more comfortable.
3. Patient is hydrated (moist skin and mucous membranes, good skin turgor).

⬛ IMPLEMENTATION

☐ Assisting with achievement of therapeutic goals
☐ *Initial care for appendicitis*

When appendicitis is suspected, the patient usually is hospitalized at once and placed on bed rest for observation and the necessary diagnostic procedures (serum WBC, urinalysis, flatplate abdominal x-ray film) that must be performed. Because an operation may be performed shortly after admission, the patient is not given anything by mouth while reports of the blood count are awaited. Parenteral fluids may be given during this time. Narcotics are not given until the cause of the pain has been determined because they would mask signs or symptoms. Sometimes an ice bag to the abdomen is ordered to help relieve pain. *Heat and enemas are contraindicated.* A rectal examination is performed by the physician to help establish the diagnosis, and the patient is given an explanation of why the procedure is necessary. Surgery consists of an appendectomy (removal of the appendix).

☐ *Maintaining hydration*

When nausea and vomiting are present, the person is given nothing by mouth until symptoms subside. With severe vomiting, fluids and electrolytes will be replaced intravenously and a sedative such as sodium phenobarbital or an antiemetic such as prochlorperazine (Compazine) or trimethobenzamide (Tigan) will be given parenterally or by suppository. When vomiting subsides, tea, broth, and ginger ale are given orally every hour. Bland feedings of custard, gelatin, and cream soups are usually tolerated after 2 to 24 hours. Intake and output are carefully measured and recorded.

☐ Assisting with comfort

Abdominal cramping from diarrhea may be relieved by constipating agents containing an opiate, such as paregoric, or diphenoxylate (Lomotil), which is chemically related to meperidine (Demerol) (see Table 31-16). Belching and defecation also often relieve the discomfort. If appendicitis is ruled out, heat to the abdomen may offer some relief.

☐ Environmental control

If a parasite is identified as the cause of the inflammation (such as in amebiasis), excretion precautions may be observed. Cleanliness is stressed, and patients should know that it is important to wash their hands well after bowel movements and before meals to prevent spread of infection.

■ Chronic inflammatory bowel disorders

Ulcerative colitis and Crohn's disease (regional enteritis) are chronic nonspecific inflammatory disorders of the bowel. These disorders are often confused with each other but are different entities (Table 31-18). Both disorders may become exacerbated by stress. Many theories have been suggested about the possible causes of these two disorders; more recent studies are exploring the immunologic mechanisms as possible etiologic factors.

Diverticulitis is a focal bowel disorder involving inflammation of diverticula (outpouchings in the colon wall), especially the sigmoid colon (Fig. 31-16). Diverticula occur more commonly in elderly people.

The etiologies, signs and symptoms, and usual medical therapies of chronic bowel inflammatory disorders are listed in Table 31-19.

■ PATHOPHYSIOLOGY

Ulcerative colitis and *Crohn's disease* differ in terms of location and type of lesions. Ulcerative colitis starts in the rectosigmoid colon and spreads upward. Crohn's disease can affect both the small and large intestines, and the areas of inflamed tissue are often separated by normal tissue. The lesions of ulcerative colitis are mucosal ulcerations that bleed easily. As the lesions advance, the bowel mucosa becomes edematous and thickened with scar formation. The colon may lose its elasticity and absorptive capability. The lesions of Crohn's disease are granulomatous ulcers that may involve deeper structures. The ulcers may perforate and form fistulas (Fig. 31-17). Scar tissue may lead to intestinal obstruction.

The loss of absorptive capability in both ulcerative colitis and Crohn's disease leads to anorexia, weight loss, malaise, and diarrhea. Severe diarrhea leads to dehydration from fluid loss, hypokalemia from loss of potassium-rich intestinal secretions, and hypoproteinemia from loss of protein through the damaged intestinal epithelium.[71]

Diverticula are formed when weakened areas of the colon are pushed outward into pouches by increased pressure within the colon. The cause is thought to be a low intake of dietary fiber, often found in the diet of persons living

Table 31-18 Comparison of Crohn's disease and ulcerative colitis

	Crohn's disease	Ulcerative colitis
General appearance	Usually normal	May feel and look ill
Age	Bimodal: 20 to 30 years and 40 to 50 years	Mostly young adults
Area affected	Mainly terminal ileum, cecum, and ascending colon (right side)	Colon only, primarily the descending colon (left side)
Extent of involvement	Segmental areas of involvement	Continuous, diffuse areas of involvement
Inflammation	Mostly submucosal	Mostly mucosal
Mucosal appearance	Cobblestone effect; granulomas	Ulcerations
Cancer potential	Normal incidence	Increased incidence
Character of stools	No blood; may have some fat; three to four semisoft per day	Blood present; no fat; frequent liquid stools
Reasons for surgery	Fistulas; intestinal obstruction	Poor response to medical therapy; hemorrhage; perforation
Complications	Fistulas; perianal disease; strictures; vitamin and iron deficiencies; fistulas to other organs	Pseudopolyps; hemorrhage; toxic megacolon; cachexia; perforation less often, causes peritonitis

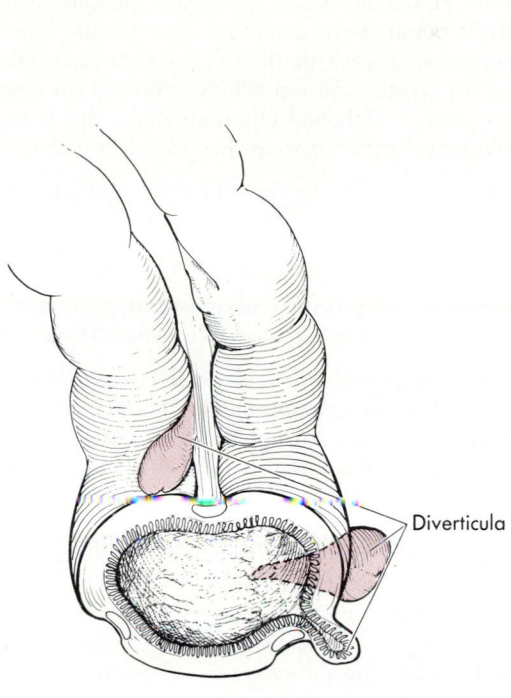

Fig. 31-16 Diverticuli of colon.

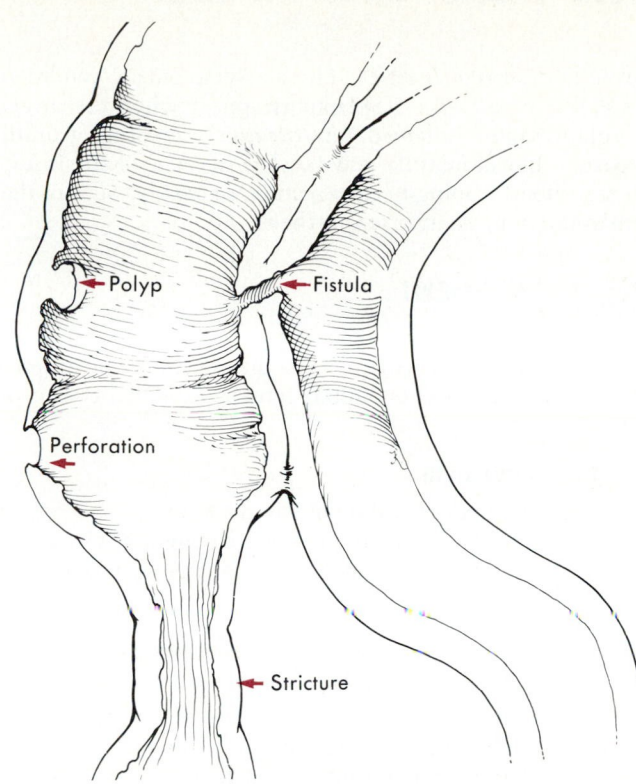

Fig. 31-17 Selected complications of chronic inflammatory bowel disorders.

Table 31-19 Chronic inflammatory bowel disorders

Disease	Etiology	Signs and symptoms	Medical therapy
Crohn's disease	Unknown	Periods of exacerbation and remission Acute: colicky or steady right lower quadrant pain, malaise, moderate fever, mild diarrhea, mucus or pus in stool Chronic: weight loss, anemia, fistula formation, intestinal obstruction	Diet: high-calorie, high-protein, high-vitamin Sulfonamides, azathioprine (Imuran) Surgery for fistulas or intestinal obstruction (colectomy or colostomy)
Ulcerative colitis	Unknown	Periods of exacerbation and remission Severe diarrhea (15 to 20 stools/day containing blood, mucus, pus); anorexia; weight loss; anemia; low grade fever Severe: weakness, debility, cachexia, dehydration, hypokalemia, hypoproteinemia	Diet: high-calorie, high-protein, high-vitamin (avoid milk) Sulfonamides, adrenocorticosteroids Surgery for refractory disease or complications (total colectomy with permanent ileostomy)
Diverticulitis of colon (inflamed mucosal pouches)	Older age, low intake of dietary fiber	May be asymptomatic Intermittent lower left quadrant pain aggravated by emotional tension or eating Constipation alternating with diarrhea	Diet: high in vegetable fiber, unprocessed bran Bulk stool additives; analgesics (pentazocine [Talwin]), anticholinergics (dicyclomine [Bentyl], propantheline [Pro-Banthine]) Bed rest, sedation, and parenteral or oral fluids for severe episode Surgery for complications of perforation or obstruction (colectomy, temporary colostomy)

in industrialized societies. The nonsymptomatic condition is called *diverticulosis*. Symptoms appear when the diverticula become inflamed (*diverticulitis*), creating painful spasms. Bowel motility may be slow because of the insufficient fiber, leading to constipation, or fast because of the inflammation, leading to diarrhea.

ASSESSMENT

Both subjective and objective data are collected about the patient's knowledge of the disorder, the nutritional status, pattern of elimination, comfort, and ability to cope with stress.

□ Subjective data

1. Patient's understanding of the disorder
2. Patterns of bowel elimination: frequency, character, amount; presence of blood, fat, mucus, or pus
3. Pain: location, character, frequency, relief with passage of stools, relief measures taken
4. Nutritional status
   a. Intolerance to certain foods
   b. Intake of caffeinated drinks, alcohol
   c. Appetite, presence of nausea
   d. Usual weight, recent weight loss
   e. Weakness, fatigue
5. Sleep: interference because of diarrhea or pain
6. Stress
   a. Perceived sources of stress in daily life
   b. Occupation: nature, hours of work, job satisfaction
   c. Usual coping methods and present effectiveness
7. Social relationships
   a. Extent of social activities and interferences as a result of illness
   b. Availability and perceived support of significant others
8. Sexual: effect of illness on sexual relationships
9. Medications taken at home: type, dosage, effect

□ Objective data

1. Weight
2. Temperature
3. Observable eating patterns
4. Signs of dehydration with severe ulcerative colitis (decreased skin turgor, dry mucous membranes)
5. Stool: number, character, amount, presence of blood (overt, positive guaiac test), pus, mucus
6. Condition of perianal skin with severe diarrhea
7. Behavior: signs indicating stress or anxiety (for example, restlessness, pacing, twisting hands, verbal comments indicating concerns)

Information about the patient's understanding of the nature and precipitating factors are helpful for planning necessary teaching. The diet of the person with ulcerative colitis or Crohn's disease is analyzed in terms of nutritional adequacy. The person's usual daily intake can be compared to the basic four food groups to determine quality of nutrient intake. Anorexia and intolerance to milk products are characteristic of ulcerative colitis. With severe ulcer-

ative colitis or Crohn's disease, there is weakness from loss of weight because of the decreased nutrient intake and decreased absorption. Cachexia may result. The diet of the person with diverticulitis is assessed for intake of dietary fiber (fruits and vegetables, whole grain cereals).

The pattern of bowel elimination for the person with chronic bowel inflammation may vary as follows:

Ulcerative colitis	Severe diarrhea (15 to 20 stools/day) stool may contain blood, pus, mucus
Crohn's disease	Mild diarrhea; stool may contain mucus, fat or pus; no blood
Diverticulitis	Constipation or constipation alternating with diarrhea; stool may contain blood

With ulcerative colitis, abdominal cramps may occur with or without bowel movements. The colicky right lower quadrant abdominal pain of Crohn's disease and the left lower quadrant abdominal pain of diverticulitis are often relieved by a bowel movement. The pain of diverticulitis may be aggravated by eating.

Symptoms of chronic inflammatory bowel disorders may be exacerbated by stress or tension. Knowledge of the patient's perception of the effect of stress on the onset of symptoms and of the patient's usual coping patterns are useful for planning measures to relieve or reduce effects of stress.

□ Diagnostic tests

Chronic inflammatory bowel disease is diagnosed by means of radiographs, sigmoidoscopy or colonoscopy, and biopsy. Laboratory tests are conducted for the presence of anemia and for blood in the stools.

□ *Radiographs*

The *barium enema* (see the box on p. 1095), also called a lower GI series, helps to identify the lesions of chronic inflammatory bowel disorders, as well as complications such as fistulas, strictures, polyps, megacolon, or perforation (Fig. 31-17).

□ *Endoscopy*

The lower portion of the colon may be visualized by a 30 to 65 cm flexible fiberoptic sigmoidoscope (Fig. 31-18). The upper portion of the colon requires a 105 to 185 cm fiberoptic colonoscope, and is a more exacting procedure. Sigmoidoscopy and colonoscopy are described in the boxes on p. 1096.

□ *Stool examination for occult blood*

Occult blood may be identified by one of three tests: guaiac (Hemoccult), benzidine, or orthotoluidine (Occultest). The *guaiac* test is the least sensitive but does not require special preparation. With the *benzidine* or *orthotoluidine* tests, false readings may be obtained by the ingestion of meat (false positive) or vitamin C in quantities greater than 500 mg/day (false negative). Patients are questioned about taking these substances before the benzidine or orthotoluidine tests are performed.

Barium enema

Purpose

Visualization of the structure of the colon by means of insertion by enema of radioopaque barium

Preparation of patient

1. Diet: nothing by mouth after midnight
2. Cleansing of colon: enemas, laxatives and/or rectal suppository (colon must be free of fecal matter for better visualization)
3. Patient teaching
   a. Explain procedure
   b. Time: approximately 30 to 45 minutes
   c. Sensation: similar to tap water enema
   d. May be tiring

Procedure

1. Instillation of barium in rectum (a rectal tube with a balloon may be used to help patient retain the barium)
2. Fluoroscopy then films to observe and record the barium flow and filling
3. Air insufflation to outline lesions when ulcerative colitis or polyps are suspected
4. Films also taken when barium is expelled to check for barium retention

After procedure

1. Provide food and fluids after test is completed
2. Observe stools for expulsion of barium
3. Assess patient for possible fecal impaction (absence of stools, hard mass in rectum, small amount of thick, liquid stool)
4. Give prescribed laxative or enema to remove residual barium
5. Plan a rest period for debilitated or elderly patient

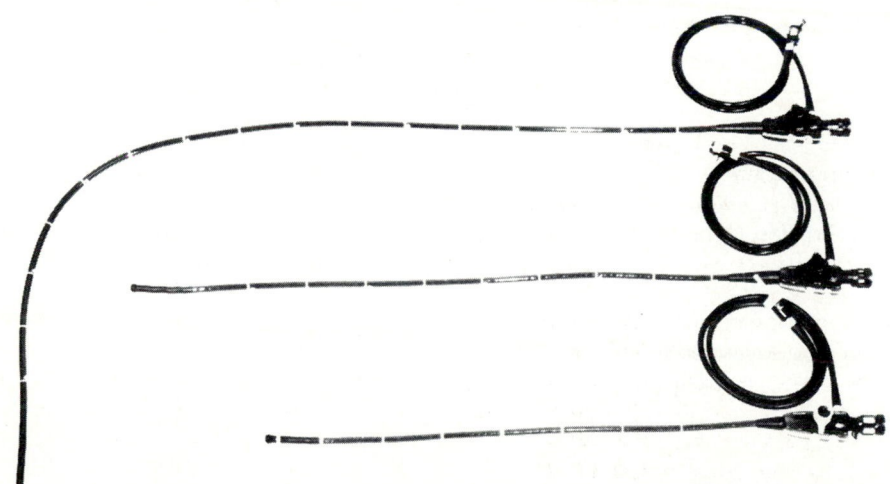

Fig. 31-18   Flexible colon fiberscopes. (From Given, BA, and Simmons, SJ: Gastroenterology in clinical nursing, ed 3, St. Louis, 1979, The CV Mosby Co.)

Sigmoidoscopy

Purpose

Visualization of sigmoid colon

Patient preparation

1. Diet: light supper, light breakfast
2. Bowel preparation: enemas or rectal suppositories (omitted for ulcerative colitis or Crohn's disease)
3. Patient teaching
   a. Explanation of procedure
   b. Time: approximately 10 to 15 minutes
   c. Sensation: urge to defecate and some light abdominal cramping may be experienced

Procedure

1. Position: knee-chest (side-lying for elderly or debilitated persons)
2. Scope inserted and advanced to sigmoid flexure
3. Air insufflation for better visualization
4. Swabbing or suctioning of retained feces

After procedure

1. Clean anus of lubrication
2. Allow rest period
3. Monitor patient for sudden severe abdominal pain (bowel perforation is a rare complication)

Colonoscopy

Purpose

Direct visualization of entire colon

Patient preparation

1. Diet: clear liquid for 3 days, nothing by mouth for 8 hours before examination
2. Bowel preparation: laxatives 1 to 3 days before examination, enemas until clear the night before
3. Consent form signed
4. Patient teaching
   a. Explanation of procedure
   b. Time: ½ to 2 hours
   c. Sensations: discomfort is minimal with analgesic medication; feelings of pressure may be experienced

Procedure

1. Premedication: IV infusion of diazepam (Valium) and meperidine (Demerol)
2. Scope is inserted and advanced to cecum
3. Air insufflation for better visualization
4. Biopsy taken if indicated

After procedure

1. Observe stools for gross blood (hemorrhage)
2. Monitor for abdominal pain (perforation)
3. Monitor vital signs for 4 to 6 hours
4. Plan a rest period

DATA ANALYSIS: NURSING DIAGNOSES

Nursing diagnoses are determined from assessment of patient data. Possible nursing diagnoses for the person with chronic inflammatory bowel disease may include, but are not limited to, the following:

Diagnostic title	Possible etiologies
Constipation	Diverticulosis
Ineffective individual or family coping	Chronicity of disorder, situational crises
Diarrhea	Chronic bowel disease
Potential fluid volume deficit	Diarrhea
Knowledge deficit	Lack of information or recall, information misinterpretation
Altered nutrition: less than body requirements	Loss of nutrients in diarrhea, anorexia
Pain: abdominal, anal irritation	Bowel disease, diarrhea
Sexual dysfunction	Malnutrition, diarrhea
Potential impaired skin integrity	Malnutrition
Sleep pattern disturbance	Pain, diarrhea

PLANNING: EXPECTED PATIENT OUTCOMES

Expected patient outcomes for the person with a chronic inflammatory bowel disorder may include, but are not limited to, the following:

1. Frequency of stools decreases (if diarrhea was present) or increases (if constipation was present) to approximately 3 to 7 per week.
2. Patient states feeling more comfortable.
3. Patient is hydrated (moist skin and mucous membranes, good skin turgor).
4. Patient eats a high-protein, high-calorie, high-vitamin, well-balanced diet.
5. Skin of elbows, sacrum, rectal area is intact.
6. Patient sleeps for longer periods.
7. Family/friends can describe
   a. Approaches to promote patient independence and control of own daily activities
   b. Approaches to cope with own feelings regarding patient's illness
8. The person can describe
   a. Nature of illness and prescribed therapy
   b. Diet to be followed
   c. Measures to decrease bowel motility
   d. Measures to promote relaxation and rest
   e. Plans to participate in social activities
   f. Alternative coping measures, if appropriate
   g. Health maintenance
      (1) Plans for following prescribed medical regimen
      (2) Symptoms requiring medical attention (changes in nature of diarrhea or abdominal pain, persistent anorexia or nausea, skin inflammations)
      (3) Plans for regular follow-up care

IMPLEMENTATION

☐ **Assisting with achievement of therapeutic goals**
☐ *Promoting nutrition*

For *ulcerative colitis or Crohn's disease,* total parenteral nutrition (TPN) is commonly used for the acutely ill person or for the one with severe disease and marked weight loss. It is followed by an elemental diet similar to that given in tube feedings to allow rapid absorption in the upper GI tract and minimal load on the colon. These approaches are described in Chapter 6. Palatability is a problem with the oral intake of elemental diets. Serving fluids chilled and offering a variety of flavors increases patient acceptance. A low-residue, high-protein, high-calorie diet is then gradually introduced.

Milk is poorly tolerated by some persons with ulcerative colitis. Foods known to exacerbate symptoms should be avoided; these foods may include alcohol, caffeine, high-fat foods, and raw vegetables and fruits. Vitamin supplements are usually needed, especially vitamin B_{12}. When anemia is present, iron dextran (Imferon) is given by Z-track injection, because oral intake of iron is ineffective as a result of the intestinal ulceration.

With acute *diverticulitis,* intravenous fluids or a clear liquid diet may be prescribed to allow the bowel to rest. When the person is asymptomatic, a diet high in vegetable fiber (fruits and vegetables, whole grain cereals) is encouraged. Unprocessed wheat bran may be added to foods but should be started in small amounts and increased slowly over a 4- to 6-week period to 10 to 25 g/day.[4] Bran initially causes abdominal distention and excess flatus. The purpose of the high-fiber diet is to increase stool bulk and bowel transit time, thus increasing the diameter of the colon and leading to decreased intraluminal pressure.

☐ *Medications*

Medications for *ulcerative colitis* and *Crohn's disease* include corticosteroids and sulfasalazine. *Corticosteroids* are given in high doses for a limited period for severe disease. Dosages are then decreased and given on an alternate-day schedule; the drug is discontinued when remission can be maintained by sulfasalazine.

Sulfasalazine is given to decrease inflammation and the frequency of recurrent attacks.[42] Because it is given for maintenance as well as therapeutic purposes, instructions to the patient include the following:

1. Take sulfasalazine in equally divided doses with a full glass (240 ml) of water.
2. If gastric upset occurs, take medication after meals or food.
3. Maintain a fluid intake adequate to provide a urinary output of at least 1500 ml/day.

4. Report side effects such as continuous headache, photosensitivity, rash or peeling of skin, aching of joints, unusual bleeding or bruising, jaundice, continuous nausea and vomiting.
5. Male infertility may occur.

Bulk additives such as psyllium seed (Metamucil) and stool softeners such as docusate sodium (Colace) may be prescribed for persons with *diverticular disease*. Anticholinergic drugs may be given to slow peristalsis and to decrease spasms in the sigmoid colon.[42]

☐ Assisting with comfort and ADL

Bed rest may be prescribed for the acutely ill patient, and care must be taken for thin people that bony prominences are protected by pressure-reducing devices, such as an alternating-pressure mattress, foam pad, or sheepskin.

The commode or bedpan is emptied as often as it is used, even when the bowel movement is small. Room deodorizers may be used to dispel unpleasant odors. The commode or bedpan may be padded if the patient spends much time sitting on it.

The perineal area is washed as necessary, at least several times a day when profuse diarrhea is present. An analgesic ointment, such as dibucaine (Nupercaine) or zinc oxide may be applied to the anus to relieve discomfort. Medicated wipes (such as Tucks) may be more comfortable than toilet tissue. Sitz baths three times a day are beneficial to the skin and circulation and to provide rectal comfort.

☐ Counseling and teaching
☐ *Psychologic aspects*

Ulcerative colitis and Crohn's disease are lifelong illnesses with periods of exacerbation and remission that can disrupt the person's life. Emotions and stress have been noted to play a role in exacerbations. If the disease is of long duration, the patient is usually thin, nervous, and apprehensive, and is inclined to be preoccupied with physical symptoms. Insecurity, dependency, and depressed or hostile behavior may be present. Family and friends may take over control of the person's life, adding to the person's feelings of loss of self-control.

The caregiver may also experience feelings of frustration and dissatisfaction. Empathic communication over time is usually needed to establish a helping relationship. It may be necessary to plan to spend time with the person and with the family on a regular basis.

The person with chronic inflammatory bowel disease can be helped to identify possible sources of life stressors and to examine ways to possibly reduce or modify the stress. The person's usual coping mechanisms can be assessed for effectiveness, and alternate coping strategies can be discussed as appropriate (see Chapter 7). Knowledge about the illness, diagnostic tests, and therapy may help to decrease anxiety. Patients need to be included in planning of activities to gain some control over their lives. During periods of remission, the person may need to be encouraged to participate in social activities.

☐ *Promoting sexuality*

Sexual response may be decreased by chronic inflammatory bowel disease and may interfere with sexual relationships. Malnutrition and frequent diarrhea lead to decreased libido. The person is given an opportunity to discuss any sexual concerns, and the nurse assists the person to communicate these concerns with the involved party. Alternate ways of meeting sexuality needs can be explored (see Chapter 33).

☐ *Patient teaching*

Patient teaching is important on an ongoing basis to help the person learn effective self-care. Main points to be included in teaching are listed in the box on p. 1099. Pamphlets about inflammatory bowel disease to be used in patient teaching can be obtained from the National Foundation for Ileitis and Colitis.*

■ SURGERY

Ulcerative colitis can be treated by surgery. The trend is toward earlier surgical intervention for the acutely ill person and for persons experiencing frequent exacerbations. Surgery is clearly indicated when complications are present, including massive hemorrhage, perforation of the colon, strictures, and medically unresponsive toxic megacolon (dilation and hypertrophy of the colon).

Different types of surgery may be performed. The most common procedure is removal of the diseased colon and rectum, with the end of the ileum being brought out through the abdominal wall (*ileostomy*). If the rectum is only mildly diseased, an ileorectal anastomosis may be performed with preservation of rectal function.

A different type of surgical approach is the *continent ileostomy* or Kock's pouch (Fig. 31-19). An intraabdominal reservoir with a nipple valve is formed from the distal ileum to provide continence. The capacity of the pouch increases slowly over months until it can hold approximately 500 ml. Contents of the pouch are removed several times a day by catheterization. Difficulties have occurred with valve failure and in keeping the ileal contents from becoming too thick and plugging up the stoma.

An *ileoproctostomy* consists of resection of the colon, removal of the rectal *mucosa*, leaving the rectal muscle intact, and anastomosis of the *ileum* with the *anal sphincter* (Fig. 31-20). This type of surgery permits elimination through the anus, but because the feces will be highly liquid, bowel incontinence may occur.

Crohn's disease does not respond well to surgery and has a high recurrence rate. Surgery is indicated when complications occur (bowel obstruction, fistulas, abscesses). Types of surgery include (1) segmental *resection* of the diseased bowel with anastomosis (preferred method) or (2) bowel *bypass* by anastomosing the ileum to the disease-free colon, leaving the diseased bowel intact.

---

*National Foundation for Ileitis and Colitis, 295 Madison Ave, New York, NY 10017.

Teaching for the patient with a chronic bowel disorder

1. Diet
   a. Ulcerative colitis or Crohn's disease: eat a high-protein, high-calorie, high-vitamin diet (avoid milk products with ulcerative colitis).
   b. Diverticulitis
      (1) Eat high-fiber foods (fruits and vegetables, whole grain cereals).
      (2) Add unprocessed wheat bran slowly over a 4- to 6-week period.
2. Elimination
   a. Take medications as prescribed.
   b. Drink at least 8 glasses fluid daily.
   c. Keep rectal area clean; use analgesic rectal ointment or take sitz bath for anal discomfort.
3. Promotion of rest
   a. Use relaxation measures (such as breathing exercises) when emotional tension is present.
   b. Identify a source for an ongoing supportive relationship.
   c. Maintain a regular sleep schedule.
   d. Schedule daily activities to avoid fatigue; take rest periods as necessary.
4. Health maintenance program
   a. List signs indicating possible exacerbation or complications (abdominal pain, increasing diarrhea or constipation, presence of blood or pus in the stool, fever, progressive weight loss).
   b. Plan for regular follow-up care.

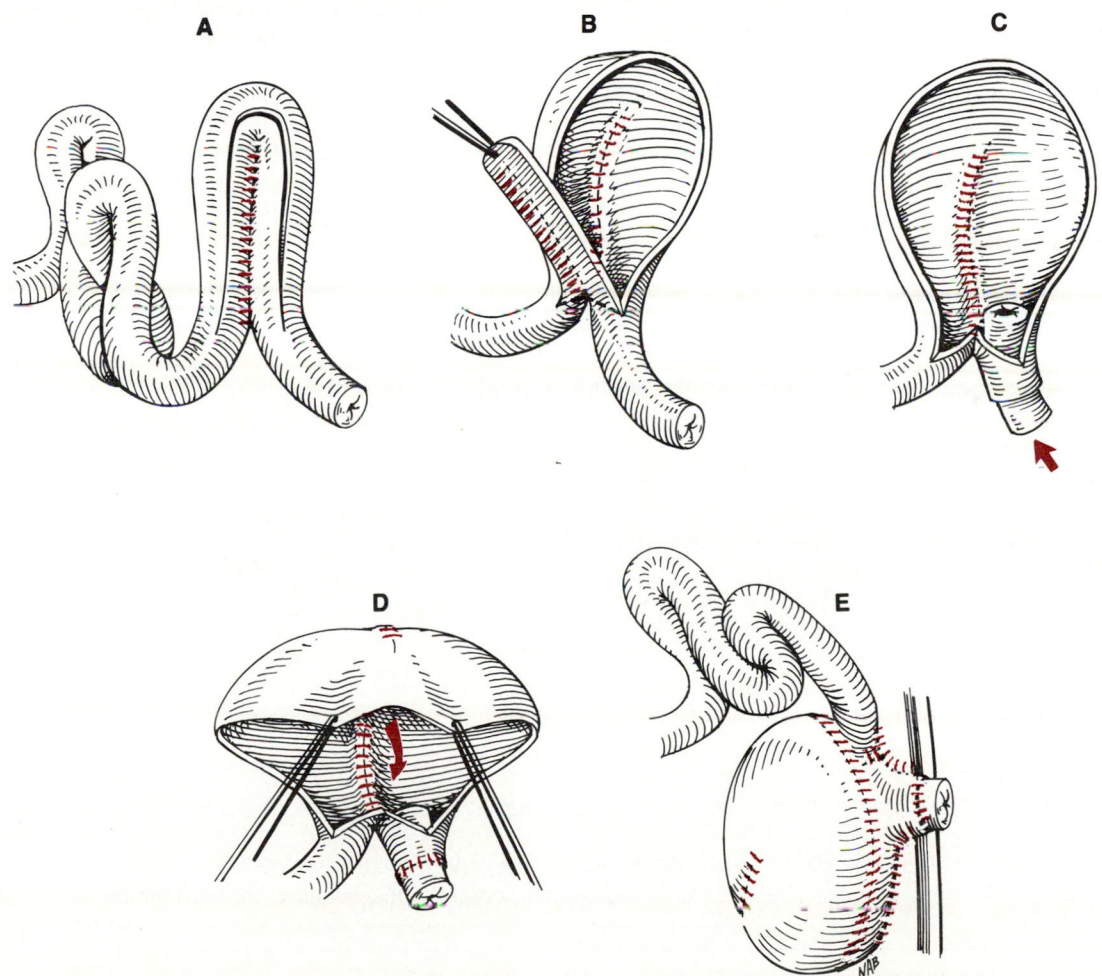

Fig. 31-19   Continent ileostomy. **A,** Loop of bowel sewn together. **B,** Removal of anterior portion. **C,** Nipple valve made by pushing bowel back on itself. **D,** Pouch formation. **E,** End brought through stoma.

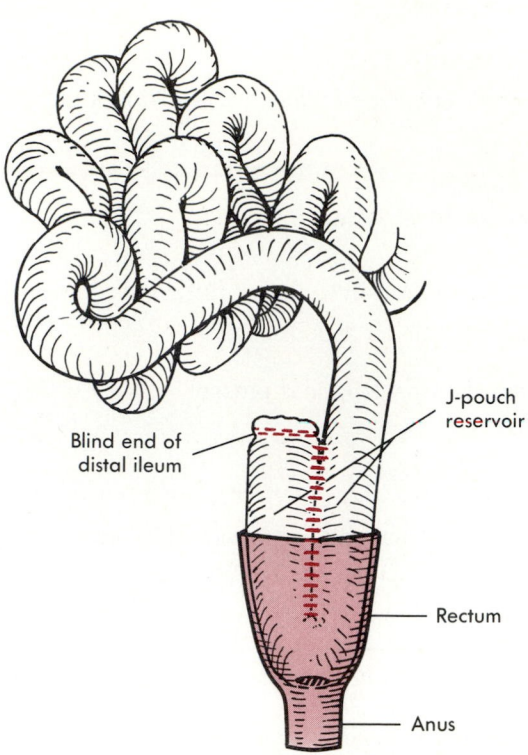

Fig. 31-20 Ileoanal anastomosis with a valveless ileal reservoir. Side-to-side anastomosis of a **J**-loop of terminal ileum is incised at apex and anastomosed to anal sphincter; remaining rectal mucosa provides support. Defecation occurs through anus.

For *diverticular disease* surgery is restricted to people experiencing recurrent episodes of diverticulitis. The involved portion of the colon is resected with an end-to-end anatomosis. The nursing care for persons experiencing bowel surgery is discussed on p. 1106.

■ ILEOSTOMY CARE

The general care of the patient with an ileostomy is similar to that of the patient with a colostomy (p. 1113).

Fecal drainage from the ileostomy stoma begins within 72 hours. It is liquid and may be constant. Commonly, patients will have approximately 1500 ml/day of drainage, although it may go slightly higher. Within 10 to 15 days, the ileostomy output will be a soft, slightly formed stool. The terminal ileum adapts to the loss of the colon and begins to reabsorb water. Patients with ileostomies have "toothpaste" consistency stools within 3 to 6 months after the adaptation of the ileum. Drainage usually occurs 2 to 4 hours after a meal, although there may be a small amount of output intermittently throughout the day.

Exceptions to this pattern of ileostomy elimination are seen in patients who have had previous bowel resections or resections of the ileum for Crohn's disease. The more small intestine that is lost, the greater the chance of a high volume of very liquid output with resultant dehydration.

□ Maintaining fluid and electrolyte balance

An excessive loss of fluid through the stoma may occur during the initial period after surgery, as a result of unabsorbed medications, or with diarrhea. Diarrhea for a

---

Teaching for the patient with an ileostomy

1. Promoting fluid and electrolyte balance
   a. Look for signs of dehydration (dry skin and mucous membranes, thirst).
   b. Increase fluid intake if stool output markedly increases or signs of dehydration occur. Drink fluids containing electrolytes (for example, Gatorade, bouillon).
   c. Avoid routine laxatives.
   d. Monitor closely for increased fecal output when taking antibiotics.
   e. When traveling, drink bottled water and avoid uncooked fruits and vegetables.
2. Promoting nutrition and absorption
   a. Start with bland low-residue foods.
   b. Introduce new foods (especially high-fiber foods) slowly.
   c. Avoid several high-fiber foods at one meal to prevent blockage.
   d. Chew foods thoroughly.
   e. Avoid foods that cause problems such as gas or obstruction (these may include coconut, corn, celery, Chinese foods).
   f. Avoid foods that cause odors (these may include onions, cabbage, fish, spicy foods).
   g. Use liquid or chewable medications rather than enteric coated, time-released, or hard tablets, if possible.

person with an ileostomy is defined as very "hot" liquid output, in which the pouch must be emptied hourly or more frequently.[13] During these periods the person is monitored for signs of fluid and electrolyte imbalance. The patient is taught how to promote fluid and electrolyte balance (see the box on p. 1100).

□ Promoting nutrition

The patient may be kept on a low-residue diet for 6 weeks to decrease the amount of bulky and undigested foods as the intestinal tract recovers from the surgical intervention. As the person begins to add foods, it is recommended that only one high-fiber food be added at a time and that the person chew the food well. Foods should not be eliminated from the diet unless the person is unable to tolerate them after two or three trials.

Food blockage (a large mass of undigested food, especially high-fiber foods) may occur with an ileostomy. The food becomes lodged at a kink, or narrowing, in the bowel and blocks the lumen. The result is a mechanical bowel obstruction. Blockage most commonly occurs when a person eats several high-fiber foods in one meal or does not chew the foods properly.

If the ileostomy becomes blocked, the person should get into a knee-chest position and gently massage the area below the stoma. Stomal edema will develop with a food blockage, and the pouch should be changed to accommodate the swelling. Diarrhea usually follows the removal of the obstruction, and the patient will need fluid replacement. Abdominal pain in the peristomal area is generally present for 3 to 5 days after obstruction. If the obstruction is not passed following the use of the knee-chest position, the patient should notify the physician.

☐ EVALUATION

Evaluation is based on expected patient outcomes. Data is collected concerning the patient's comfort and knowledge about diet, elimination, rest and sleep, and need for medical follow-up.

■ Intestinal obstruction

Intestinal obstruction (ileus) occurs when there is impedance to the normal flow of intestinal contents, either because of inhibition to neural stimulation for peristalsis (paralytic ileus) or because of blockage (mechanical/organic ileus). *Paralytic ileus* results mainly from handling of the bowel during abdominal surgery, from peritonitis, or from pain of thoracolumbar origin (see the box below). *Mechanical obstructions* of the small intestines are primarily adhesions, whereas in the large bowel, neoplasms are the major cause. A *volvulus* is a twisting of the bowel (Fig. 31-21). *Intussusception* is a telescoping of a segment of the bowel within itself. Hernias may cause bowel obstruction when a loop of bowel becomes strangulated in the defect (p. 1104). The clinical manifestations and medical therapy of intestinal obstruction are outlined in Table 31-20.

■ PATHOPHYSIOLOGY

When peristalsis ceases, the involved intestinal area becomes distended by gas and fluid. Approximately 8 L of fluid are secreted into the stomach and small intestines per day; most of this fluid is normally reabsorbed in the colon. When peristalsis ceases, however, much of the fluid remains in the stomach and small intestine. The retained

---

Causes of intestinal obstruction

Paralytic ileus

Manipulation of abdominal viscera during abdominal surgery
Peritoneal irritation (peritonitis)
Pain of thoracolumbar origin
  Rib or spinal fractures
  Myocardial infarction
  Pneumonia
  Pyelonephritis
  Ureteral or biliary calculi
  Retroperitoneal hemorrhage
Sepsis
Hypokalemia causing decreased muscle tone of bowel
Intestinal ischemia

Mechanical intestinal obstruction

Adhesions
Hernias
Neoplasms
Inflammatory bowel disease
Foreign bodies, gallstones
Fecal impaction
Strictures: congenital, radiation
Intussusception

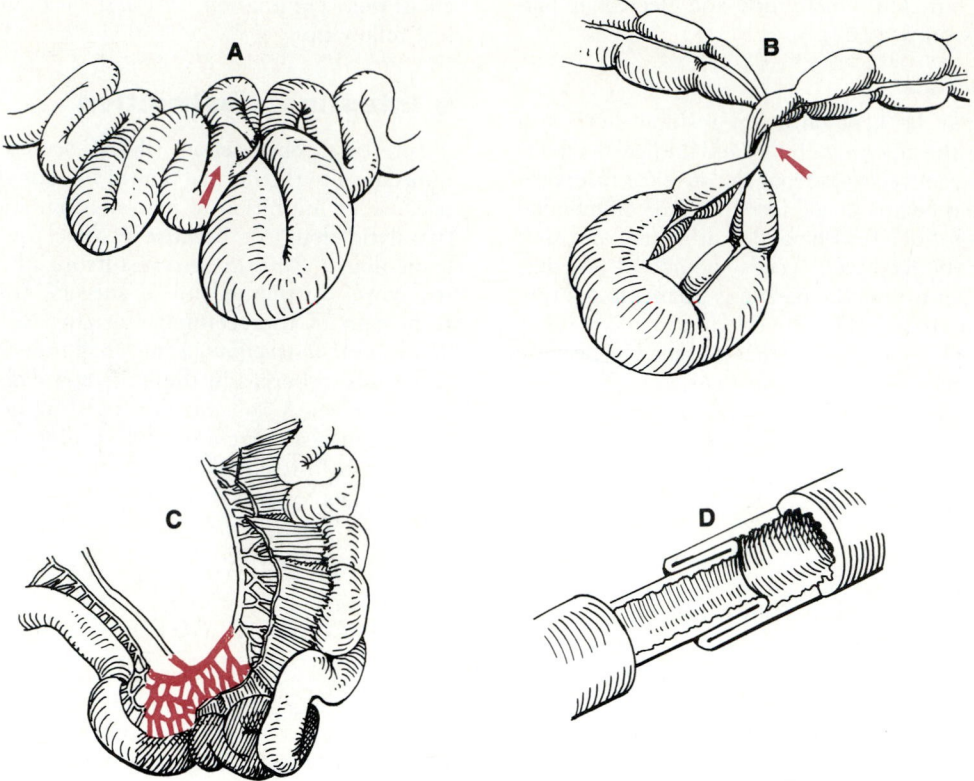

Fig. 31-21   Some causes of intestinal obstruction. **A,** Constriction by adhesions. **B,** Volvulus. **C,** Mesenteric thrombosis. **D,** Intussusception.

Table 31-20   Obstructive disorders of the intestinal tract

Disorder	Obstruction	Signs and symptoms	Therapy
Paralytic ileus	Disturbance of neural stimulation of bowel	Continuous abdominal pain, distention, vomiting, obstipation, decreased or absent bowel sounds	Restricted oral intake, IV fluids, GI suction
Mechanical intestinal obstruction	Physical impedance to flow of bowel contents	Colicky abdominal pain, vomiting, constipation, high-pitched bowel sounds	Same as above; surgery
Hernia	Strangulation of bowel in weakened ring or incision	Lump in weakened area, especially with straining; pain with incarceration	Herniorrhaphy
Cancer of the bowel	Growth narrows lumen of bowel	Blood in stool, changes in bowel patterns	Resection of bowel, with or without a stoma

fluid increases pressure on the mucosal wall and, if not removed, results in ischemia, necrosis, bacterial invasion, and eventually peritonitis. Loss of the fluids leads to hypovolemia (shock) and dehydration. Loss of sodium and chloride ions causes a shift of potassium from the cells, leading to hypokalemic alkalosis.

When mechanical obstruction occurs, peristaltic waves proximal to the affected area increase in an effort to move the intestinal contents past the obstruction. These peristaltic movements create a high-pitched abdominal sound.

As the abdomen distends from the distended gut, pulmonary ventilation may become impaired from pressure on the diaphragm. Pressure on the bladder may cause urinary retention. Constipation occurs with mechanical obstruction because some feces usually pass around the obstruction. When peristalsis ceases completely, as with paralytic ileus or complete organic obstruction, no bowel movement occurs (obstipation).

ASSESSMENT

The following parameters need to be monitored in the patient who is thought to be developing an intestinal obstruction:
1. Bowel sounds: presence and character
   a. Loud, frequent, high-pitched sounds are heard as obstruction is developing.
   b. Bowel sounds are not heard when peristalsis ceases.
   c. Weak bowel sounds and passage of flatus occur as peristalsis returns (flatus is a more significant sign).
2. Vomiting: assess type and frequency
   a. Profuse, nonfecal vomiting is seen with obstruction of the proximal small bowel.
   b. Occasional fecal-type vomitus is seen with obstruction of the distal bowel.
3. Abdominal pain: location and character
   a. Cramping pain occurs as obstruction develops.
   b. Pain becomes more constant and diffuse with distention.
4. Abdominal distention: use a tape measure to determine change in size; always measure at the same site (usually across the umbilicus).
5. Urinary output: amount
   a. Monitor total output (decrease seen with dehydration).
   b. Monitor amount of urine at each voiding for signs of urinary retention.
6. Vital signs
   a. Fever, tachycardia, and hypotension are seen with dehydration.
   b. Fever may also indicate more obstruction or peritonitis.

□ Diagnostic tests

X-ray films of the abdomen (flat plate and upright) are taken to identify air- and fluid-filled areas of obstruction. Serum blood tests will indicate alterations from normal (hemoconcentration) when dehydration occurs. There will be a decrease in sodium and potassium and an increase in hematocrit, plasma bicarbonate, serum pH, and blood urea nitrogen (BUN).

DATA ANALYSIS: NURSING DIAGNOSES

Nursing diagnoses are determined from assessment of patient data. Possible nursing diagnoses for the person with an intestinal obstruction may include, but are not limited to, the following:

Diagnostic title	Possible etiologies
Ineffective breathing pattern	Abdominal distention
Fluid volume deficit	Abnormal loss of GI fluids
Pain: abdominal	Abdominal distention
Urinary retention	Abdominal distention

PLANNING: EXPECTED PATIENT OUTCOMES

Expected patient outcomes for the person with an intestinal obstruction may include, but are not limited to, the following:
1. Patient is hydrated (moist skin and mucous membranes, good skin turgor).
2. Patient states feeling more comfortable.
3. Patient voids at regular intervals; output equals fluid intake.
4. Breath sounds are clear; respirations are easy and regular.

IMPLEMENTATION

□ Assisting with achievement of therapeutic goals

Conservative medical therapy consists of oral intake restrictions, parenteral fluids and electrolytes, and gastric or intestinal suctioning until bowel function returns.

□ *Promoting hydration*

Fluids containing electrolytes are given parenterally in large quantities (3000 to 4000 ml/day) to prevent dehydration. The physician determines the amount to be given based on the amount of gastric drainage from nasogastric or intestinal intubation; thus it is important that accurate measurement of gastric drainage be made. Flow sheets are helpful for careful monitoring of intake and output. The patient is monitored for signs of fluid overload (bounding pulse, neck vein distention, cough). Central venous pressure (Chapter 9) may be monitored in high-risk patients (elderly, cardiac disease).

□ *Promoting pulmonary ventilation*

Abdominal distention creates pressure on the diaphragm, inhibiting chest expansion. Nursing measures to promote aeration of the alveoli include the following:
1. Fowler's position to release pressure on diaphragm
2. Deep breathing exercises
3. Encouraging patient to breathe through the nose and not swallow air to prevent further distention

☐ Promoting comfort

Pain and vomiting often leave the patient physically and emotionally exhausted. Assistance in simple activities such as turning in bed may be necessary. Comfort measures associated with nasogastric intubation (p. 1070) are helpful. The patient may need encouragement that the decompression will ease the discomfort from the distention.

Since oral fluids are usually restricted, mouth care is important for prevention of infection in addition to comfort. If the patient is poorly nourished, measures to keep the skin soft and intact and free from pressure are indicated.

☐ Surgery

Surgery is usually performed for relief of mechanical and vascular obstruction. The operative procedure varies with the cause and the location of the obstruction and the general condition of the patient. If constricting bands or adhesions are found, they are cut, and it may be necessary to resect the occluded bowel and anastomose the remaining segments.

Care of the patient undergoing intestinal surgery is described on p. 1106.

✚ EVALUATION

Evaluation is based on expected patient outcomes. Questions to consider are: Is the patient hydrated? Has fluid overload been avoided? Have pulmonary and urinary complications been avoided? Is the patient relatively comfortable?

■ Hernias

Hernias account for a large number of intestinal obstructions. A hernia is a protrusion of an organ or structure from its normal cavity through a congenital or acquired defect. In addition to a loop of bowel, a hernia may contain peritoneal fat, a section of bladder, or a portion of the stomach, depending on its location.

If the protruding structure of the organ can be returned by manipulation to its own cavity, it is called a *reducible* hernia. If it cannot, it is called an *irreducible* or *incarcerated* hernia. When the blood supply to the structure within the hernia becomes occluded, the hernia is said to be *strangulated*. Some types of hernias are described below.

Types of hernias

Inguinal
    Indirect   Loop of intestine passes through abdominal ring and follows course of spermatic cord into inguinal canal

    Direct   Loop of intestine passes through posterior inguinal wall

Femoral   Loop of intestine passes through femoral ring down into femoral canal

Umbilical   Loop of intestine passes through umbilical ring

Incisional   Loop of intestine or other organ protrudes through weakened scar

A hernia that is not incarcerated can very often be reduced by the person lying down with the feet elevated or by lying in a tub of warm water and pushing the mass gently back toward the abdominal cavity.

Surgery is frequently performed for large hernias or when there is a high risk of incarceration. A *herniorrhaphy* consists of suturing the defect in the fascia. In the postoperative period following repair of an *umbilical* or large *incisional* hernia, a nasogastric tube may be used to prevent postoperative vomiting and distention with subsequent strain on the suture line.

Because of postoperative inflammation, edema, and hemorrhage, *swelling of the scrotum* often occurs after repair of an indirect inguinal hernia. This complication is extremely painful, and any movement of the patient causes discomfort. Ice bags help to relieve pain. The scrotum is usually supported with a suspensory or is elevated on a rolled towel. Urinary retention may occur because of the discomfort in movement producing hesitancy in urination. Ecchymosis of the lower abdominal wall or upper thigh may occur after extensive manipulation during surgery. The ecchymosis fades in a few days. Sexual functioning is not affected.

The patient who has had elective surgery for a hernia is restricted from driving for at least 2 weeks. Physical activities should not include any heavy lifting, pulling, or pushing for at least 6 weeks.

■ Cancer of the bowel

Malignant tumors of the colon and rectum are among the most commonly occurring malignancies in the United States, third following cancer of the lung and prostate in men, and second following cancer of the breast in women.[5] The incidence of bowel cancer is significantly higher in developed countries whose inhabitants are of Northern European descent, and it is lower in Japan, India, Africa, and some Latin-American countries. The incidence of bowel cancer also increases with age and reaches a peak in people in their late 70s. Clinical manifestations and types of surgery are outlined in Table 31-21.

■ ETIOLOGY

Although the cause of cancer of the bowel remains unknown, environmental and genetic factors and preexisting disease appear to be influential (see the box on p. 1105). The high incidence of colorectal cancer in industrial countries relates to a diet high in animal fat, protein, and refined carbohydrates that are low in dietary fiber. A direct causative relationship has not been established. Low-fiber diets decrease colonic transit time and potentially increase contact of endogenous or exogenous carcinogens with the bowel mucosa. Popular literature often suggests that certain foods are carcinogenic; however, research has not yet identified specific foods as carcinogenic for bowel cancer. Genetically, some "cancer families" have been identified in which cancers of certain body areas, including the bowel, are transmitted as dominant traits.

Table 31-21 Cancer of the colon

Location	Signs and symptoms	Surgery
Ascending	Occult blood in stool, anemia, nausea/vomiting, right upper quadrant pain, palpable mass	Right colectomy with anastomosis
Descending colon	Gross blood in stool, progressive constipation with increased frequency, pencil-shaped stools	Left colectomy with anastomosis
Sigmoid colon and rectum	Rectal bleeding, constipation and increased frequency, sensation of incomplete bowel evacuation	Sigmoid: left colectomy with anastomosis Upper rectum: resection with anastomosis Lower rectum: abdominoperineal resection with colostomy

---

Risk factors for colorectal cancer

Age: over 40
Past history
    Colon polyps (adenomas)
    Cancer: colorectal, breast, genital
    Ulcerative colitis
    Polyposis syndromes
    Immunodeficiency disease
Family history: colorectal cancer, polyposis syndromes

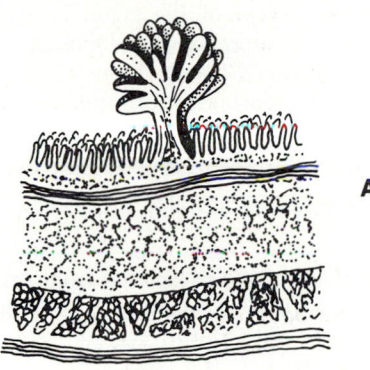

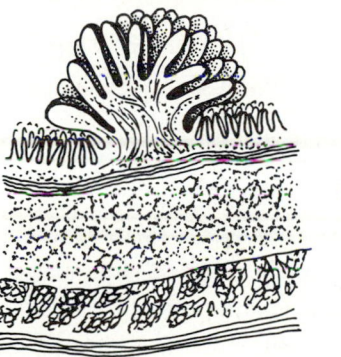

Fig. 31-22 Colon polyps. **A,** Tubular adenoma (note pedicle). **B,** Villous adenoma.

■ PREVENTION

No primary prevention measures are known to be effective for colorectal cancer. High-fiber low-fat diets cannot be considered preventive measures because of the lack of a causal relationship.

Secondary prevention involves early detection. Anyone who develops a change in bowel patterns, a change in the shape of the stool, or the passing of blood should consult a physician. The American Cancer Society's recommended guidelines for screening of people over age 40 include:

1. Digital rectal examination yearly after age 40.
2. Occult blood stool test yearly after age 50.
3. Proctosigmoidoscopy every 3 to 5 years after age 50, following two negative yearly examinations.

■ PATHOPHYSIOLOGY

Polyps are *benign* growths (adenomas) on the colonic mucosa; they are considered to be premalignant. The two major types of polyps are the more common *tubular adenoma* that is a globelike structure attached to the bowel wall by a "stem" (peduncle), and the *villous adenoma,* a large soft polyp that has several fingerlike projections but no peduncle (Fig. 31-22). Villous adenomas are more likely to become malignant.

Cancer of the colon may develop in one of two ways. In the cecum and *ascending* colon, the lesions tend to develop as polyps that grow as cauliflower-like masses protruding into the lumen of the colon. These lesions may ulcerate, but obstruction of the colon is uncommon. Eventually, the lesions penetrate the colon wall and extend into surrounding tissue.

In the *descending* colon, especially the rectosigmoid portion, an annular lesion is more common. The early lesion is a small polypoid mass that becomes plaquelike. The plaque grows circumferentially, encircling the colon wall, and then contracts, causing narrowing of the lumen. Obstruction may result from formed stool on the left side that is unable to pass through the narrowed lumen. These lesions also eventually penetrate the colon wall and extend into adjacent tissue.

Cancer of the colon may spread by direct extension or through the lymphatic or circulatory systems, seeding at distant points in the peritoneum or at distant points in the colon. The liver is the major organ of metastasis because the colonic blood vessels empty into the portal vein leading to the liver.

■ DIAGNOSTIC TESTS

Diagnosis of cancer of the colon is made by physical examination, sigmoidoscopy, colonoscopy, and barium enema examination. Cancer of the rectum can be accurately diagnosed by pathologic examination of a biopsy specimen taken during a proctoscopic examination. Stools are examined for occult blood (p. 1094).

□ Carcinoembryonic antigen monitoring

Carcinoembryonic antigen (CEA) is an antigen seen in fetal life. It was originally isolated from patients with colonic cancer, but it is also seen in persons with ulcerative colitis, cirrhosis, and other forms of cancer and in chronic cigarette smokers.

The CEA test is not useful as a screening test for colonic cancer; however, it is useful as an indicator of the effects of therapy. For example, a drop in CEA level would suggest the effectiveness of the therapy. A continued high level or rise in level would suggest recurrence or spread of the tumor.

■ MEDICAL THERAPY

□ Surgery

Treatment of cancer of the colon is always surgical and the tumor, surrounding colon, and lymph nodes are resected. The amount of bowel resected is based on removal of all tissue supplied by the blood vessel of the diseased tissue. Surgery is performed in one of the following ways: (1) the diseased portion of the bowel is removed (resected), and the remaining ends are joined together in an end-to-end anastomosis (EEA); or (2) the diseased portion of the bowel is removed, and the functioning end is brought out onto the abdominal surface forming a "stoma" (p. 1111).

Resection with anastomosis can be performed for cancer of the ascending, descending, or sigmoid colon and upper rectum (Fig. 31-23 *A*, *B*, and *C*). These surgeries are performed through abdominal incisions, and natural defecation is maintained. The anastomosis may be done by suturing or stapling techniques. A greater amount of rectal tissue can be removed by the use of the stapling technique for anastomosis.

Growths in the lower rectum require removal of the entire rectum and sigmoid colon by means of an abdomi-

noperineal resection (p. 1108); this surgery requires formation of a stoma. Care of the person experiencing bowel surgery is described below.

Obstruction or perforation of the colon usually requires a temporary colostomy, followed later by closure of the colostomy. Prognosis after surgery depends on the stage and location of growth. Low-lying colorectal stage C cancers have a lower survival rate than high-lying colonic cancers.[71] Duke's stages of colorectal cancer are listed below:

Stage A: Confined to bowel mucosa
Stage B: Invading muscle wall
Stage C: Lymph node involvement
Stage D: Metastases or locally unresectable tumor

□ Other therapies

Radiation therapy is generally ineffective in the treatment of colorectal cancer. It may be used preoperatively in large, locally extensive growths to retard growth; this prevents cells that may accidentally be dislodged during surgery from seeding themselves at other locations.

Chemotherapy is used for metastatic disease and for persons with a high risk of recurrence.[71] It is most effective for liver metastasis. The chemotherapeutic agent of choice is 5-fluorouracil (5-FU), either alone or in combination with other agents.

■ Bowel surgery

Surgery of the bowel may be performed for different reasons, including bowel obstruction, ulcerative colitis, and bowel cancer. The major concern with any type of bowel surgery is contamination by fecal contents. Preoperative preparations are directed toward minimizing this problem. Many of the people experiencing bowel surgery are elderly, because the largest number of bowel surgeries are performed for bowel cancer. Elderly persons have a higher risk for postoperative pulmonary embolism and fluid imbalances.

■ PREOPERATIVE CARE

Preoperative care consists primarily of preparing the bowel so that it will be free of stool, and of decreasing the intestinal bacteria. This is accomplished by (1) a low-residue diet for several days followed by clear liquids the day before surgery, (2) bowel cleansing by means of enemas and laxatives for several days before surgery, and (3) oral antibiotic therapy. Neomycin is usually the chosen antibiotic because it is not absorbed through the intestinal tract, has low toxicity, and has broad-spectrum activity against colonic bacteria. Erythromycin may also be prescribed. Vigorous mechanical cleansing or purging may be poorly tolerated by some persons, such as the acutely ill or elderly; therefore, these approaches may be modified.

Patient teaching includes preparing the patient for postoperative procedures, such as nasogastric intubation and the need for parenteral fluids for several days until peristalsis returns. Ventilatory measures, as well as leg exer-

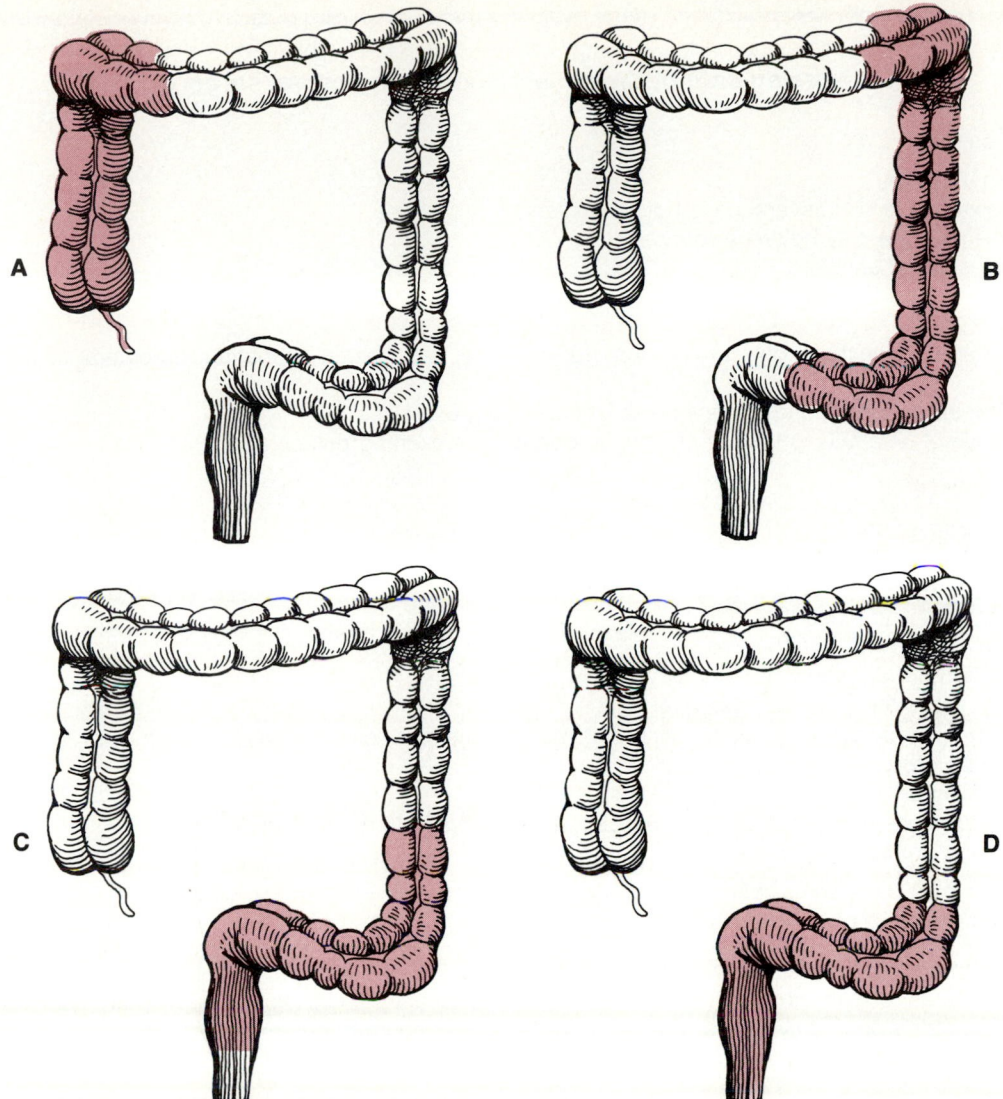

Fig. 31-23   Bowel resection. **A,** Right hemicolectomy. **B,** Left hemicolectomy. **C,** Anterior rectosigmoid resection. **D,** Abdominoperineal resection.

cises (Chapter 16), will also be important postoperatively, especially for the elderly patient.

■ POSTOPERATIVE CARE

Extensive handling of the GI organs during surgery causes a marked inhibition of peristalsis. Care during the early postoperative period is directed at (1) preventing a buildup of fluid and gas by the use of nasogastric intubation, (2) preventing pulmonary complications, (3) maintaining fluid and electrolyte balance, (4) promoting elimination, and (5) promoting comfort.

Atelectasis and pulmonary embolism may result from decreased respiration and circulation. Incisional pain may limit chest expansion and the patient may require much encouragement to move, ambulate, and breathe deeply.

There is a high risk of pulmonary embolism after perineal resection. Venous congestion in the pelvic veins leads to stasis of circulation; platelets adhere to the vessel walls, especially at bifurcation of pelvic blood vessels, leading to formation of blood clots with possible embolism.

The length of time required for peristalsis to return depends on the extent of bowel manipulation. Presence of bowel sounds and passage of gas signals the return of function. It is not unusual after a resection of the bowel for diarrhea to occur after peristalsis returns. Usually it is temporary and soon disappears. When the stool becomes normal, the patient is advised to avoid becoming constipated, because a hard stool and straining to expel it could possibly injure the anastomosis, depending on its location.

The care of the patient experiencing bowel surgery is summarized in the box on p. 1108.

Nursing care of the patient undergoing bowel surgery

Preoperative care

1. Preventing infection
   a. Give low-residue diet several days before surgery.
   b. Give clear liquids day before surgery.
   c. Give prescribed antibiotic.
   d. Give prescribed enemas and laxatives.
2. Teaching
   a. Explain special postoperative procedures (for example, nasogastric intubation, parenteral fluids for several days).
   b. Teach deep breathing and coughing exercises and leg exercises.
   c. Teach use of side rails to facilitate turning in bed without exerting pull on abdomen.

Postoperative care

1. Promoting oxygenation
   a. Encourage turning and deep breathing exercises.
   b. Encourage patient to be active.
2. Maintaining fluid and electrolyte balance
   a. Maintain patency of GI tube.
   b. Record amount of drainage accurately.
   c. Maintain prescribed flow of parenteral fluids.
   d. Monitor for signs of fluid loss (dry skin and mucous membranes, decreased skin turgor) or overhydration, especially in the elderly.
3. Promoting elimination
   a. Monitor for signs of returning peristalsis (passage of flatus, return of bowel sounds).
   b. Encourage increasing ambulation.
   c. Monitor character of initial stools.
4. Promoting comfort
   a. Give good oral hygiene until oral fluids are taken freely.
   b. Lubricate nares with water-soluble lubricant.
   c. Use measures to maintain moisture of oral mucous membranes (rinse mouth, chew gum, suck hard candy).
   d. Give analgesics on a fairly regular basis during the first 48 hours to prevent severe pain.
5. Teaching
   a. Drink at least 2000 ml of fluid daily to avoid constipation.
   b. Avoid use of laxatives without medical approval; stool softeners or Metamucil may be used.
   c. Avoid heavy lifting for at least 6 weeks after surgery.

■ ABDOMINOPERINEAL RESECTION

Malignant growths in the lower two thirds of the rectum are removed by means of an abdominoperineal resection (Fig. 31-23, *D*). The operation is performed through two incisions: a low midline incision of the abdomen and a wide elliptic incision about the anus. Through the abdominal incision, the sigmoid colon is divided and the lower portion is freed from its attachments and temporarily left beneath the peritoneum of the pelvic floor. The proximal end of the sigmoid is then brought out through a small stab wound on the abdominal wall and becomes the permanent colostomy. Through the perineal incision, the anus, rectum and distal portion of sigmoid are removed. The perineal wound may be closed around Penrose drains, or it may be left wide open to heal slowly from the inside outward (Fig. 31-24). The open perineal wound will take longer to heal than a usual incision. Care of the patient with an abdominoperineal resection is summarized in the box on p. 1110.

Many patients complain of *phantom rectal sensations* and of feeling the necessity to defecate. An explanation of cortical perception and transmission of nerve impulses often helps the patient cope with these sensations.

Urinary retention is a common occurrence following rectal excision. Factors that influence urinary retention include loss of pelvic support, chronic urinary tract infection, enlarged prostate, or nerve injury. Loss of pelvic support increases problems with micturition when the patient is supine; thus micturition may improve with ambulation. If nerve injury is present, problems with urinary retention

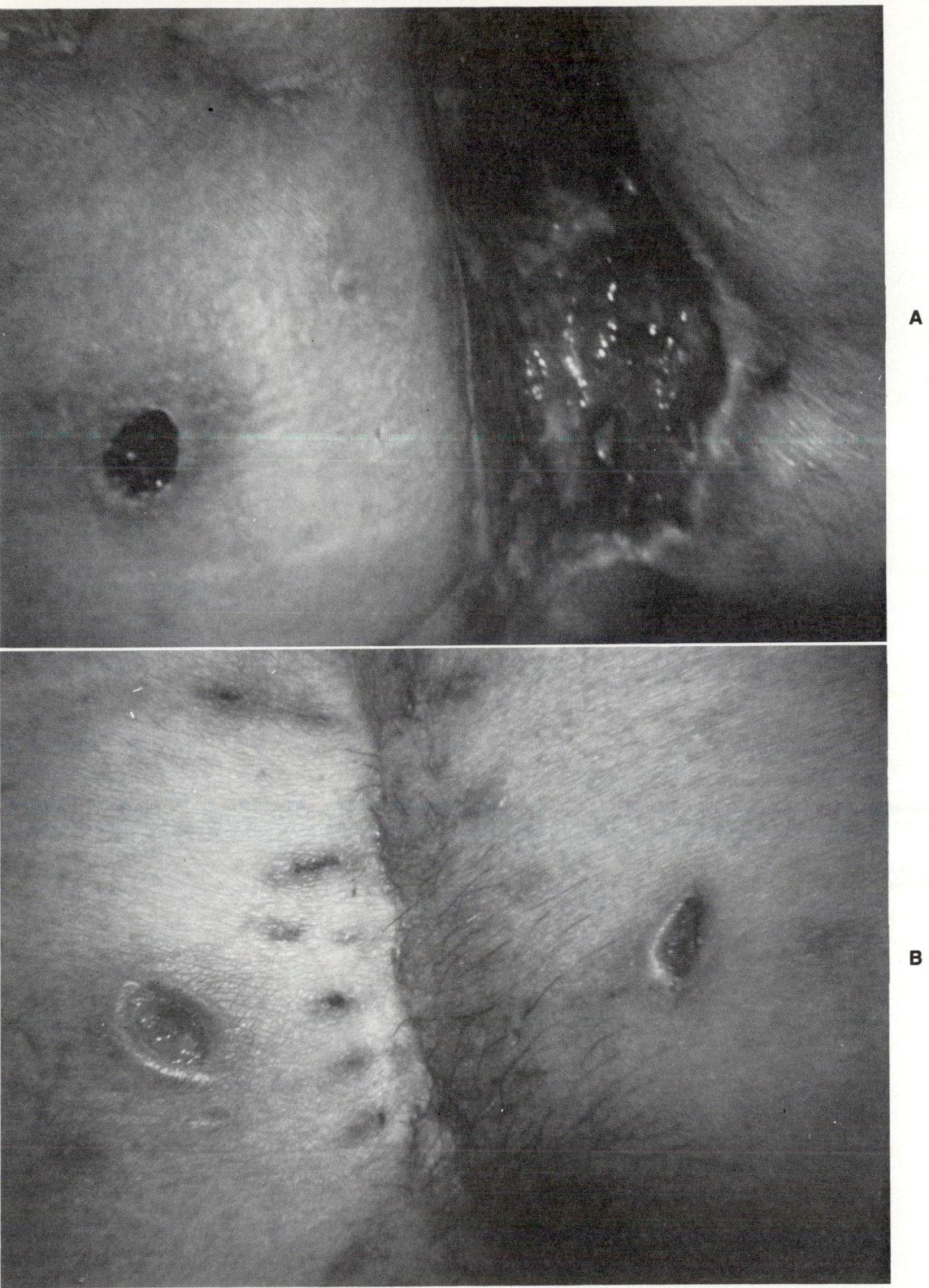

Fig. 31-24 Perineal wound following an anteroposterior resection for cancer in rectum.
A, Postsurgical wound; note site of sump drain to left of wound. **B,** Following healing;
perineum is completely closed; shape of buttocks looks normal.

Nursing care of the patient with an abdominoperineal resection

Preoperative care

1. Prepare patient as for other bowel surgery.
2. Prepare patient for a stoma (p. 1112).
3. Prepare patient for a perineal incision: wound may be open and, if so, will take longer to heal.

Postoperative care

1. Provide care as for other bowel surgery.
2. Preventing complications
   a. Shock: monitor for early signs and institute shock measures.
   b. Hemorrhage
      (1) Check perineal dressing frequently: initial drainage is profuse and serosanguineous.
      (2) Reinforce initial dressings as necessary.
      (3) Report excessive bleeding to physician.
   c. Thrombophlebitis/pulmonary embolism
      (1) Encourage leg exercises (Chapter 16) until patient is ambulatory.
      (2) Encourage use of elastic stockings with elderly patients or those with poor leg circulation.
      (3) Encourage ambulation when permitted.
3. Promoting healing
   a. Maintain low continuous suction of sump catheters, if present.
   b. Change perineal dressing as frequently as needed after first 24 hours.
      (1) Record precise directions for dressing change on nursing care plan.
      (2) Irrigate wound with normal saline solution by use of catheter, hand-held shower massage, or Water Pik.
      (3) Cover with dry dressings and hold in place with a T-binder (the T "top" is wrapped around the waist and the T strap is brought up between the legs).
   c. Substitute sitz baths for irrigation when patient is ambulatory; maintain free flow of water on perineal wound in sitz tub (rubber ring may be helpful).
   d. Provide stoma care (p. 1113).
4. Promoting urinary elimination
   a. Maintain patency of indwelling catheter.
   b. Monitor for residual urine when catheter is removed.
      (1) Keep accurate intake and output records.
      (2) Monitor for lower abdominal distention, patient discomfort, restlessness.
   c. Use measures to encourage voiding if patient has inability to initiate stream.
5. Promoting comfort
   a. Assist patient to find a comfortable position in bed: side-lying is usually preferred.
   b. Assist patient to turn frequently.
   c. Try a foam pad under buttocks for supine position.
   d. Give narcotics at regular intervals until severe pain decreases (about 3 days postoperatively).

---

and urinary tract infections may persist for several months with partial resolution of retention but with urinary incontinence experienced at night.

Sexual difficulties may occur in about 40% of males following abdominoperineal resection. Difficulty with ejaculation is more commonly seen than impotence (difficulty with erection), but they may occur together.

Convalescence after an abdominoperineal resection is prolonged and may require many months. During this time the individual should remain under close supervision.

■ Fecal diversion: stomas

Diversion of the fecal stream may be performed for GI diseases or for trauma. Common reasons for ostomy surgery include the following:

Type	Reason
Ileostomy	Ulcerative colitis, familial polyposis
Temporary colostomy	Trauma: gunshot wounds, stab wounds
	Complications of diverticulitis, volvulus, bowel ischemia, perforation
Permanent colostomy	Cancer of colon and rectum

Table 31-22 Comparison of ileostomy and colostomies

	Ileostomy	Ascending colostomy	Transverse colostomy	Sigmoid colostomy
Location	Ileum	Ascending colon	Transverse colon	Sigmoid colon
Type of drainage	Liquid-to-paste consistency	Liquid-to-soft	Soft	Soft-to-formed
Bowel regulation	No	No	No	Only with irrigations
Fluid imbalance	Monitor for dehydration if high output diarrhea	Same	May occur with bouts of diarrhea	Usually not a problem unless there were previous resections
Skin irritation	Occurs easily because of digestive enzymes	Same	Can occur from exposure to stool	Same as transverse colostomy
Other complications	Food blockage Prolapse of stoma Stricture	Prolapse Stricture	Prolapse Stricture	Prolapse Stricture Constipation

Diversion of the fecal stream may be temporary or permanent. In a *temporary diversion* the fecal stream is rerouted to allow the GI tract an opportunity to heal or to provide an outlet for the stool when an obstruction is present. A *permanent diversion* implies that the intestine cannot or will not be reconnected; thus, a return to a normal elimination mode will not occur.

■ SURGICAL SITES

When the small bowel (ileum) is the site of diversion, the ostomy is called an *ileostomy.* The surgical diversion of the large colon will result in a *colostomy.* The anatomic location of the colostomy will determine the name, that is, *ascending colostomy, transverse colostomy,* or *sigmoid colostomy.* The effects are different for each type of ostomy (Table 31-22).

The two main types of functioning stomas are the end stoma and the loop stoma. A nonfunctional end stoma is referred to as a *mucous fistula.*

When an *end stoma* is created surgically, the proximal bowel is brought out through an incision in the abdominal wall, folded over on itself (forming a cuff) and sutured. The stomal surface is the mucosal lining or inner layer of the intestinal wall (Fig. 31-25). The remaining *distal* bowel may be surgically removed, oversewn to form a Hartmann's pouch (Fig. 31-26), or brought to the skin surface to form another stoma, the mucous fistula (Fig. 31-27). If the proximal and distal stomas are adjacent (Fig. 31-28), they are referred to as a *double-barreled ostomy.*

The *loop stoma* is created by bringing the bowel through an abdominal incision, sliding a support under the bowel, and opening the upper wall of the bowel (Fig. 31-29). The posterior wall remains intact. There is one stoma, but there are two openings: proximal and distal. The loop ostomy is generally a temporary procedure.

Patients who do not receive adequate bowel preparation before a loop or double-barreled procedure may have a

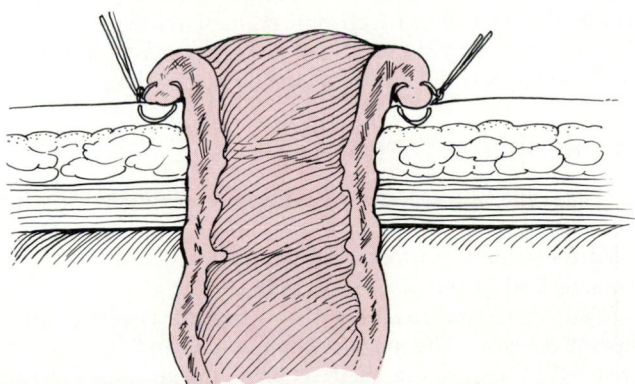

Fig. 31-25 Formation of an end stoma.

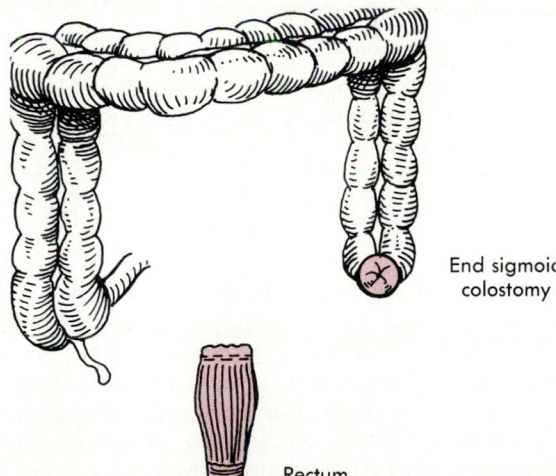

End sigmoid colostomy

Rectum

Fig. 31-26 End sigmoid colostomy with an oversewn rectum left intact (Hartmann's pouch).

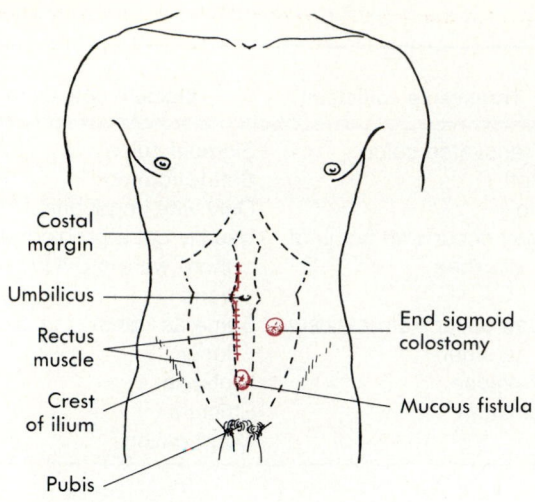

Fig. 31-27 End sigmoid colostomy and mucous fistula.

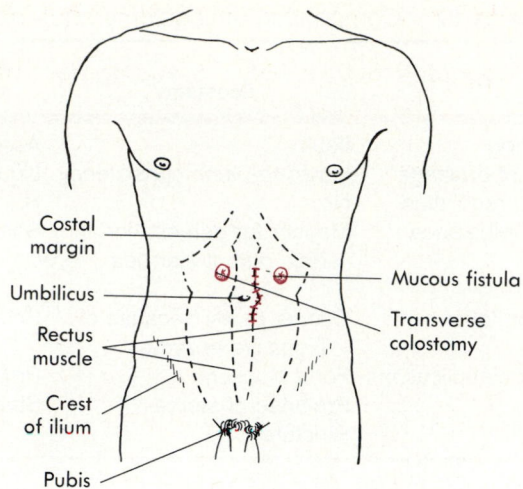

Fig. 31-28 Transverse colostomy with adjacent mucous fistula.

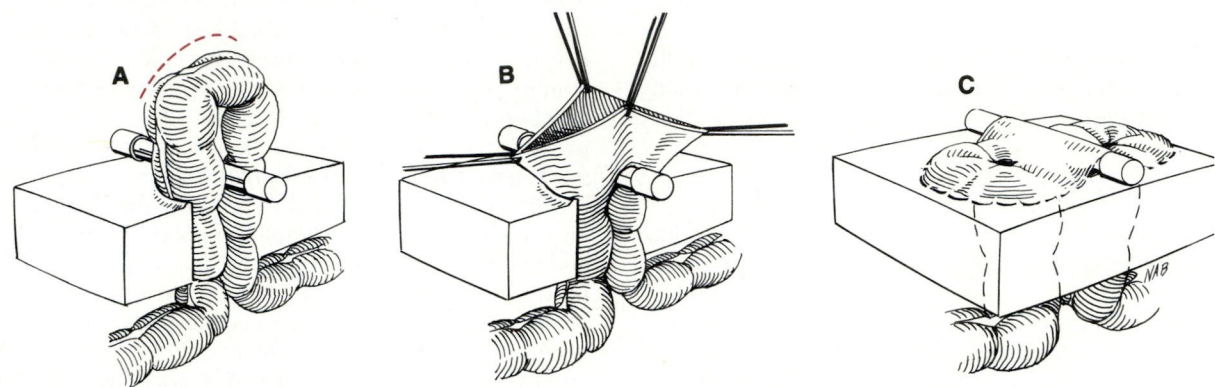

Fig. 31-29 Loop colostomy. **A,** Bowel brought through incision and supported with rod. **B,** Incision in anterior wall. **C,** Edges are folded over to make two openings in one stoma.

bowel evacuation through the rectum. Patients should be told this may occur. Mucus may continue to be passed through the rectum.

■ PSYCHOLOGIC RESPONSE TO OSTOMY SURGERY

When the physician first tells the person of the probable need for an ostomy, the immediate reaction is likely to be shock and disbelief. Whether the ostomy is to be temporary or permanent, it is difficult for most people to accept. It is not unusual for the person to be sad, withdrawn, and depressed after learning of the need for ostomy surgery.

Removal of any part of the body involves a sense of loss. Thus, the person facing ostomy surgery may experience grief and mourning over the lost part, which includes shock, denial, anger, and depression. (See Chapter 15 for a discussion of these reactions.) The change in body image may result in feelings of guilt, shame, or disgust. Usually

the formation of the stoma is viewed as mutilating surgery, but for some individuals the surgery may be a relief or release from coping with chronic pain, diarrhea, or debility. No matter what reaction is expressed, patients need time and the support of others to work through their feelings.

■ PREOPERATIVE CARE

The general preoperative and postoperative care for bowel surgery (p. 1108) is followed for the person scheduled for ostomy surgery. Guidelines for ostomy care are summarized in the box on p. 1113.

Counseling and teaching are important aspects of preoperative care. The patient and family and friends are assisted in identifying their feelings and reactions to the proposed surgery. The patient's knowledge of the surgery, as well as responsiveness to information, is assessed. Some people are very upset by the impending surgery and want little information. However, it is important for each person

Suggested preoperative teaching for the patient requiring a stoma

1. Simple explanation with drawings of anatomy of the GI tract
2. Explanation of surgery
   a. Areas to be removed
   b. Effect on bowel function
3. Definition of terms: colostomy (or ileostomy), stoma, pouch
4. Explanation of appearance/sensation of stoma and basic management
5. Availability of nurse/enterostomal therapist after surgery to teach patient the care of the stoma
6. Availability of Ostomy Visitor (p. 1117)

Nursing care of the patient with a colostomy or ileostomy

1. Prepare the person for surgery by describing the ostomy, answering questions, and dispelling misconceptions.
2. Monitor the stoma postoperatively for swelling, color, function, and intactness of mucocutaneous suture line.
3. Assess the readiness of the person to view the stoma and to begin learning about care of the ostomy.
4. Promote acceptance of the change in the body through own facial expressions and empathic interactions.
5. Instruct the person in the care of the ostomy through use of a detailed and individualized care plan.
6. Provide the person with written instructions and supplies.
7. Provide necessary follow-up care.

to know, at least, what is meant by ostomy surgery and the type of management it will require. Many people have misconceptions about the ostomy that add to the preoperative anxiety. Dispelling these myths and giving correct information can lessen the fears of an ostomy. Some suggested information is listed in the box above.

■ POSTOPERATIVE CARE

☐ Stoma drainage

The stoma is assessed regularly for color and to ensure intactness of the stoma-skin suture line. A red color denotes viability. A stoma that has impaired circulation will appear dark, dusky, or black.

The stoma secretes mucus immediately following surgery and will continue to do so. During the first 24 to 48 hours, the stomal drainage is mucoid and serosanguineous. As intestinal function returns, flatus will be produced. Fecal drainage is initially liquid for all ostomies. Drainage from a colostomy may then change quickly depending on its location (Table 31-22).

☐ Protecting the skin

Fecal drainage from the stoma can be very irritating to the skin surrounding the stoma; therefore, the skin needs protection. *Skin barriers* are substances that are applied to protect the skin. The most commonly used barriers are 4 × 4 inch squares or pectin-based *wafers* that are cut to fit snugly around the stoma. *Pastes* are useful to fill in creases or folds in poor locations and to supplement wafers for a longer seal. Powders must be covered with a *sealant* (spray, liquid, gel, wipe) before a pouch can be applied.

Peristomal skin infections may be bacterial or fungal. The most common is a yeast infection from *Candida albicans*. The skin becomes bright red with papular lesions in an irregular area; secondary skin changes occur as the process continues, and dry, scaling areas develop. Treatment involves the use of nystatin (Mycostatin) powder sealed with a skin sealant.

☐ Changing the pouch

Products for ostomy care are available in a variety of styles, shapes, and sizes. Pouches are available in clear and opaque plastics, and covers are designed to make the wearing of a pouch more comfortable (Fig. 31-30).

An effective pouching system protects the skin, contains the stool, molds to the body contour, allows comfortable bending and movement, and is inconspicuous and odorproof. Selection of an effective pouching system is crucial to the rehabilitation process.

Preparing the patient to care for the stoma facilitates incorporation of the body changes into the new body image. Most persons do not wish to look at the stoma immediately. They are not pushed to look at the stoma but are gently

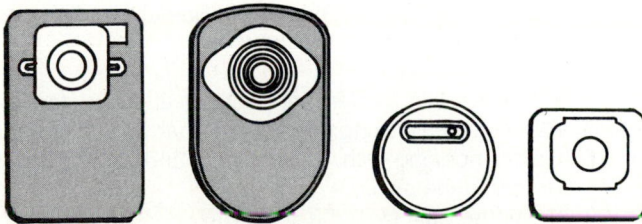

Fig. 31-30 Closed end pouches and patches for regulated colostomies.

encouraged to look at it as they evince interest in doing so.

A patient who is unable (or refuses) to participate in self-care creates a management problem. The patient, family member or friend, nurse, and physician need to discuss the problem openly. Someone must be prepared to care for the stoma after the patient is discharged from the hospital. If the patient is unwilling to assume an active role, an early consultation with a psychiatric nurse clinician may be helpful.

The patient is taught the steps of changing the pouch (see the box below) and is given written instructions prior to discharge. A minimum of three lessons are generally needed. Lessons should begin when the patient is receptive to instruction.

During the first lesson, the patient observes the steps of the procedure. The nurse informs the patient that the stoma has no touch sensation, and the red color means the stoma has healthy blood supply. Questions and concerns are addressed. During the second lesson, the patient assists with preparing the pouch, cleansing the skin and stoma, and centering the pouch around the stoma. The patient changes the pouch with supervision as needed for the third lesson. Some persons need more practice, and additional sessions are scheduled. A visiting nurse referral may be needed for assessment of the patient's ability to adapt to the ostomy in the home environment.

Before discharge, the patient needs a temporary supply of pouches and skin barriers, a list of what supplies to order, and the names of local suppliers. A prescription for ostomy supplies may be needed for insurance reimbursement.

☐ **Promoting regular elimination: colostomy irrigation**

Irrigation may be ordered after a sigmoid colostomy. There is controversy about the long-term effects of irrigations. The purpose of regular colostomy irrigations is to stimulate emptying of the colon at a convenient and regular time.

Pouch appliance procedure

Pattern

1. The pattern should be ⅛ inch larger than the stoma.
2. A paper towel may be used to trace a pattern.
3. Always label the pattern for "top" or "skin" side.

Skin barrier (Stomahesive, Hollihesive, Reliaseal, Colly-Seel)

1. Use either a fourth, a half, or a full wafer, depending on the size of the stoma and the abdomen.
2. Round the corners to conform to the shape of the adhesive on the pouch.
3. Trace the pattern on the paper side.
4. Cut hole on pattern line.
5. Smooth sides of the opening with your finger.

Pouch

1. Pouch opening should be slightly larger than the opening of the skin barrier (paper can cut the stoma).
2. Trace pattern on the paper side of the pouch (use the opening from the skin barrier that has already been cut off).
3. Cut the hole larger than the line of the pattern (cut outside of the line).
4. Smooth edges around the opening.
5. Remove paper backing from the pouch, center the openings, and apply the shiny side of the skin barrier to the pouch.

Applying the system

1. Remove the old pouch and skin barrier carefully.
2. Cleanse the skin with warm water.
3. Pat the skin dry.
4. Warm the skin barrier (the pouch is already attached).
5. Remove the backing; save this paper, it can be used as a pattern in the future.
6. Center opening with stoma; press and seal to the skin; hold your hand against the pouch to help seal the skin barrier to the skin.
7. Close the bottom of the pouch.

From Broadhurst, BB, and Broadwell, DC: Ostomy care for children, Unpublished material, 1981.

A patient who is free of stool between irrigations can wear a closed-end pouch with a gas-relief valve or stoma "cap," a small square pouch with an absorbent dressing. The stoma will continue to secrete mucus and expel flatus between irrigations, so an ostomy covering with a gas filter is desirable (Fig. 31-30). Some persons are unable to regulate the colostomy with irrigations and decide to wear drainable pouches instead of irrigating.

Persons who have irrigated their colostomies successfully for years may develop irregular results with irrigation secondary to aging. As one ages, there is a decrease in mucus production and peristalsis. This is often frustrating for patients who may feel they have failed, because the elimination pattern is unpredictable.

Various types of commercial irrigation sets are available, and they all require similar supplies: an irrigation sleeve that fits over the stoma and is long enough to drain into the toilet, a cone tip for the insertion of water into the stoma (Fig. 31-31), an enema bag to contain the solution, and clips to close the top and bottom of the sleeve.

When ordered, irrigations are begun after the bowel has begun to function and the stool is beginning to become soft, usually between the fifth and seventh postoperative day. The procedure for irrigation is outlined in the box at right.

The irrigation procedure is usually performed in the bathroom. The patient may wish to sit on a chair with a pillow and face the commode until the perineal wound heals. Subsequently the patient sits on the toilet (Fig. 31-32). Cramping during an irrigation may be caused by inserting the water too rapidly or from water that is too cold. Rate of flow varies with the pressure (height of the bag) and caliber of the tube.

☐ Promoting nutrition

Anyone with an ostomy should eat balanced meals at regular intervals, and chew foods slowly and thoroughly. Patients need to be informed that certain foods such as seeds, kernels, and other undigested residue will be visible in the stool.

Persons with a *colostomy* do not need a restricted diet, although many persons develop their own food preferences.

They should be informed which foods tend to cause gas in order to avoid these foods as desired. Most pouches are odor-proof, and some are available with gas-relief valves that make gas less of a problem.

Persons with an *ileostomy* need to avoid high-fiber or high-residue foods for 4 to 6 weeks after surgery. High-fiber foods can then be added one at a time in small amounts. If the person is unable to tolerate the food after two or three trials, the food can be eliminated from the diet.

Colostomy irrigation

1. Remove old pouch.
2. Clean skin and stoma with water.
3. Apply irrigating sleeve and belt.
4. Fill bag with desired amount of warm water (250 to 1000 ml).
5. Hang bag so bottom of bag is at shoulder height.
6. Remove air from tubing.
7. Gently insert irrigating cone snugly into stoma, holding it parallel to floor.
8. Let water run in slowly until patient identifies need to expel stool.
9. Remove cone and allow solution to drain into container.
10. When most of stool is expelled (about 15 minutes) rinse sleeve with water and close up bottom end.
11. Encourage activity to complete bowel emptying (about 30 to 45 minutes).
12. Remove sleeve and apply clean pouch.

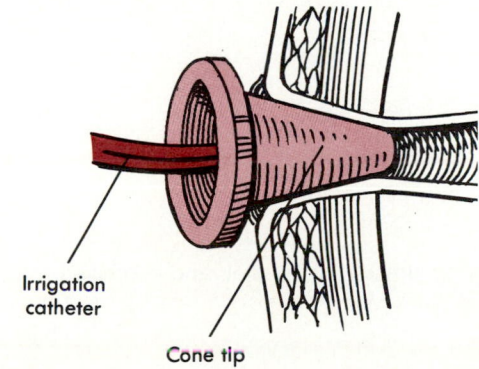

Fig. 31-31   Cone irrigating tip inserted in stoma.

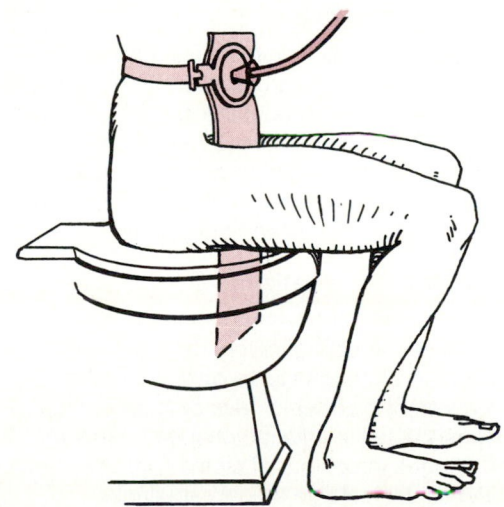

Fig. 31-32   Colostomy irrigation with person sitting on toilet; irrigating sleeve drains into toilet.

□ **Promoting return to normal activity**

For most persons whose condition warrants it, optimal recovery is achieved within 3 months, and they can return to their normal activities, including work. Questions about activities need to be discussed before the patient goes home. Traveling is possible for the ostomate. Preparations to be considered are listed in the box below. With careful planning the person with an ostomy can participate in activities enjoyed before the surgery.

□ **Promoting sexuality**

The opportunity for the patient and significant other to ask questions regarding the return to normal sexual functioning needs to be provided. It is most often the nurse who hears cues such as, "I guess I'll never be able . . . ,"

or, "I wonder what my spouse . . . ." The nurse takes this opportunity to clarify this concern with the person. Arrangements can be made, if desired by the patient, for the significant other to be present when a frank discussion of sexual functioning is carried out by the nurse or physician. Many persons will not verbalize their concerns about sexuality so that a deliberate meeting must be planned to facilitate expression of these concerns. The patient and sexual partner can be assisted to consider sexual positions that may be more facilitating and less problematic if a bag is worn.[58]

About 15% of men with ostomies have decreased sexual activity that may be related either to nerve injury or to psychologic reasons. The successful return to sexual activity depends on psychosexual functioning before surgery

---

Teaching for the patient with a stoma

Promoting nutrition and elimination

1. Eat a balanced diet. Avoid foods that cause diarrhea or constipation.
2. Drink at least 2500 ml of fluids daily (6 glasses).
3. Avoid foods that cause flatus, as desired.

Promoting return to normal activities

1. Participate in activities enjoyed before surgery.
2. Avoid direct contact sports such as football. Activities such as swimming, tennis, and planned exercise programs are all possible.
3. When traveling:
   a Wear seat belt above or below stoma.
   b. Hand-carry regular ostomy supplies to facilitate care if baggage is misplaced.
   c. Use disposable bags.
   d. Carry plastic bags for disposal of used supplies.
   e. Take extra supplies for unexpected events requiring extra days.
   f. Eat moderately. Use restraint when eating new foods.
   g. Use caution about water intake in areas where "traveler's diarrhea" is a high risk.

Promoting sexuality

1. Allow time to ease into sexual relations.
2. Resume sleeping in bed with partner if this was habit before surgery.
3. Talk with partner about the stoma.
4. Empty the pouch before intercourse.
5. Use an attractive cover over the pouch.
6. Tape pouch to abdomen or groin.
7. Experiment with different positions.

Preventing complications

Report the following symptoms to physician or nurse enterostomal therapist:
1. Changes in configuration, color, consistency, or odor of stool
2. Bleeding through stoma or rectum
3. Persistent diarrhea or lack of stool evacuation despite medications, treatment, fluids, diet, and exercise program
4. Persistent skin irritation despite treatment
5. Changes in contour of stoma (prolapse, inversion)
6. Persistent leakage around appliance
7. Signs of dehydration and electrolyte imbalance

and adaptation and coping following surgery. Counseling may be helpful if nerve injury is not present and sexual difficulties are being experienced. Women have a decreased incidence of nerve injury because of the larger pelvis. Ostomy surgery does not interfere with contraception, pregnancy, or delivery. A pamphlet entitled *Sex and the Ostomate* is available from the United Ostomy Association.*

☐ Community resources

During and after hospitalization, the patient and significant others have additional resources available to assist in adapting and coping with the ostomy. A representative from the local chapter of the United Ostomy Association can be requested to visit the patient either preoperatively or postoperatively. This visitor can share how he or she has learned to live well with the ostomy. The patient may wish to become a member of the Association and through meetings learn how others in the community are effectively dealing with the ostomy.

The enterostomal therapist, a nurse with additional education in providing ostomy care, should be consulted (if available) to assist or coordinate instruction. The social worker, clinical nurse specialist, dietitian, and clergy are consulted as needed.

The American Cancer Society in certain locations will assist with providing ostomy supplies to persons with financial need. They also can provide assistance with information about home supplies, medications, and transportation.

■ CLOSURE OF COLOSTOMY

If the colostomy was performed to relieve obstruction or to divert the fecal stream to permit healing of a portion of the bowel, the person will be readmitted to the hospital at a later date for a further examination and for possible resection of any diseased portion of the bowel. The ostomy subsequently may be closed.

In preparation for a resection of the bowel and closure of the colostomy, the physician may order irrigation of the colostomy and probably both openings of a loop colostomy. The irrigation fluid, usually normal saline solution, is instilled into each opening as ordered. For irrigation of the distal stoma, the patient should sit on the bedpan or the toilet. Unless the distal bowel is obstructed, the solution instilled into the distal loop will be expelled through the rectum. The returns are inspected before being discarded.

■ REQUIREMENTS BEFORE DISCHARGE

The following instructions are given to the patient before discharge from the hospital:
1. Written information about the ostomy
2. Written instructions for application of the pouch
3. A list of supplies to order
4. A temporary supply of items needed for pouch changes

---

* United Ostomy Association, 36 Executive Park, Irvine, CA 92714.

5. A measuring guide and instructions for determining the size of pouches to order
6. List of surgical supply stores in the area
7. Information about the United Ostomy Association and the local chapter
8. Phone numbers of the primary nurse, the enterostomal therapist, the physician, and the visiting nurse service

■ Anorectal lesions

■ PATHOPHYSIOLOGY

The anorectal area may develop fissures, abscesses, or fistulas (Table 31-23). A *fissure* is usually the result of trauma caused by passage of hard-formed stool that overstretches the anal lining. It does not heal readily. An *anal abscess* may develop in an anal fissure, and if the sinus tract draining the abscess does not close, a chronic draining *fistula* may develop.

Hemorrhoids occur frequently as a result of congestion in the veins of the hemorrhoidal plexus. Heredity, occupations requiring long periods of standing or sitting, the erect posture assumed by human beings, structural absence of valves in the hemorrhoidal veins, increase of intraabdominal pressure caused by constipation, straining at defecation, and pregnancy are factors that predispose to development of hemorrhoids. Hemorrhoids may be internal (above the internal sphincter) or external (outside the anal sphincter). Many persons have both internal and external hemorrhoids.

▦ ASSESSMENT

Pain and bleeding are the two major symptoms of hemorrhoids. Data to be collected include the following:
1. Pain
   a. Onset: with defecation, sitting, or walking
   b. Character: constant or episodic; sharp or throbbing
2. Bleeding: presence, amount, color (bright or dull red)
3. Stool: consistency (hardness), streaked with blood or pus

Bleeding is usually bright red because of the close proximity of the bleeding site. Internal hemorrhoids often bleed with defecation, whereas external hemorrhoids rarely bleed. Rectal bleeding must not be confused with menstrual bleeding in women.

▶ DATA ANALYSIS: NURSING DIAGNOSES

Nursing diagnoses are determined from assessment of patient data. Possible nursing diagnoses for the person with an anorectal lesion may include, but are not limited to, the following:

Diagnostic title	Possible etiologies
Constipation	Anal discomfort
Pain: rectal	Anal disorder

Table 31-23 Common anal lesions

Lesion	Description	Symptoms	Treatment
Anal fissure	Slitlike ulceration in epithelium of anal canal	Pain with defecation; bleeding; constipation	Stool softeners; analgesic ointments; sitz baths; surgical removal of fissure if medical therapy ineffective
Anal abscess	Abscess in tissue around anus	Persistent throbbing anal pain with walking, sitting, defecation; systemic signs of infection	Incision and drainage of abscess
Anal fistula	Hollow track leading through anal tissue from anorectal canal through skin near anus	Purulent discharge near anus	Fistulectomy or fistulotomy
Hemorrhoids	Varicosities of lower rectum and anus	Bleeding with defecation; pain if thrombosed	Analgesic ointments for mild discomfort; injection, ligation, or hemorrhoidectomy for severe discomfort

Table 31-24 Treatment of hemorrhoids

Procedure	Description	Comments
Incision	Drainage of blood from thrombosed hemorrhoid	Dry dressing for 12 to 24 hours
Injection	Sclerosing solution injected into submucosal area	Bleeding stops in 24 to 48 hours
Ligation	Constriction of hemorrhoids by rubber bands	Destroyed tissue sloughs off within 1 week
Hemorrhoidectomy	Excision of hemorrhoids	Preoperative: stool softener Postoperative: dressings may be omitted; stool softeners; first defecation is painful; monitor for excessive bleeding.

PLANNING: EXPECTED PATIENT OUTCOMES

Expected patient outcomes for the person with an anorectal lesion may include, but are not limited to, the following:

1. Stool is soft and formed.
2. Patient states feeling more comfortable.

IMPLEMENTATION

□ Assisting with achievement of therapeutic goals
□ *Promoting normal stools*

Chronic constipation may precipitate anal lesions. Once the lesion is present, defecation may initiate rectal spasms such that the person may delay defecation. This leads to formation of a hard stool as water is reabsorbed in the colon, causing further discomfort. Measures are therefore instituted to promote passage of a soft stool, including activity, adequate fluids (at least 2000 ml/day), and dietary fiber. A stool softener may be prescribed.

□ *Promoting healing*

Abscesses are incised and drained. Dressing containing purulent drainage must be changed frequently to protect the skin. Hemorrhoids may be incised, injected, ligated, or excised (see Table 31-24).

□ **Anorectal surgery**
□ *Preoperative care*

The patient may be given a laxative and is encouraged to eat a full, normal diet until a few hours before a local anesthetic is given. Stool softeners are often given to facilitate passage of the stool through the rectum postoperatively, and a bulk laxative such as psyllium (Metamucil) may be given to increase the bulk of the stool. An enema may be prescribed 1 to 2 hours before surgery.

□ *Postoperative care*

Because the operations are often considered minor, there may be a tendency to minimize anorectal surgery. In reality,

---

Nursing care of the patient after anorectal surgery

1. Assessment
   a. Monitor vital signs every 4 hours for 24 hours.
   b. Monitor for signs of restlessness, thirst.
   c. Inspect rectal area or dressing every 2 to 3 hours for 24 hours.
   d. Monitor urinary output.
2. Promotion of comfort
   a. Assist patient to a position of comfort; side-lying is often preferred.
   b. Use floatation pad under buttocks for sitting.
   c. Give analgesic medications as prescribed during first 24 hours.
   d. Use moist heat after first 12 hours: rectal compresses or sitz baths 3 to 4 times/day.
3. Promotion of elimination
   a. Give stool softener as prescribed.
   b. Give an analgesic shortly before first bowel movement, if possible.
   c. If an enema is prescribed, use a well-lubricated catheter or small rectal tube.
4. Patient teaching
   a. Take a sitz bath after each bowel movement for at least 1 to 2 weeks after surgery.
   b. Eat adequate dietary fiber; drink at least 2000 ml of fluids/day, and exercise moderately.
   c. A stool softener may be desired every day or every other day until healing is completed.
   d. Report the following symptoms to physician: rectal bleeding, continued pain on defecation, suppurative drainage.

---

the surgery may cause as much discomfort as many major surgeries. The pain, which results from rectal spasms, may inhibit urination and defecation. Patients worry considerably about passing the first stool, which can be uncomfortable. Pain can be minimized by the use of analgesics, sitz baths, and stool softeners.

During the first 12 hours after surgery, hemorrhage is a possibility. Blood may collect in the anal canal and not be expelled; therefore, other signs of hemorrhage are monitored (vital signs, restlessness, thirst). Moist heat (sitz baths) are avoided during this period, as moist heat will encourage further bleeding by dilating the blood vessels. The postoperative care of the patient experiencing anorectal surgery is summarized in the box above.

⊞ EVALUATION

Evaluation is based on the expected patient outcomes. Questions to be asked are: Is the patient comfortable? Does the patient know what to do after he/she goes home?

■ SUMMARY

1. GI signs requiring immediate medical follow-up include (1) a sore that bleeds easily and does not heal, a lump or thickening or a persistent red or whitish patch in the mouth, (2) persistent heartburn or indigestion, (3) abdominal pain accompanied by nausea and vomiting, and (4) a change in bowel habits or the presence of blood in the stool.
2. Factors placing the person at high risk for inflammatory mouth disorders include poor oral hygiene, stress, nutritional deficiencies, debilitating diseases, heavy smoking, and chemotherapy.
3. Common inflammatory disorders of the mouth include aphthous or herpetic stomatitis, Vincent's angina, thrush, gingivitis, and periodontitis.
4. Parotitis may be of the communicable type (mumps) or noncommunicable; the latter is often seen in debilitated persons with poor oral hygiene.
5. Good mouth care involves frequent care (at least every 2 to 4 hours), cleaning of the teeth, and rinsing the mouth with a solution such as alkaline mouthwash, hydrogen peroxide diluted 1:4 with saline, or a lidocaine rinse.
6. Contributing factors to cancer of the mouth and esophagus include alcohol and heavy smoking or chewing tobacco.
7. Premalignant (higher potential for becoming malignant) lesions of the mouth include white or red patches.
8. Following surgery of the mouth or esophagus for cancer, tube feedings may be necessary for several days.
9. Swallowing is impaired by common esophageal disorders including achalasia (aperistalsis of esophagus), esophageal stricture, esophageal diverticulum, or gastroesophageal reflux.

Putting knowledge to practice

■ Examine written instructions given at your hospital to patients scheduled for diagnostic GI tests and x-ray examinations. How could you use these tools most effectively?

■ Practice testing a stool sample for occult blood (guaiac test).

■ Compare drug content and costs of antacids in your local drugstore.

■ Examine the different types of nasogastric and intestinal tubes; which part of each tube is connected to suction and where would you place fluids for irrigation?

■ Explain why loss of large amounts of gastric secretion may lead to metabolic alkalosis, whereas loss of large amounts of intestinal secretions may lead to metabolic acidosis.

■ Develop a 1-day meal plan for a person with adult lactase deficiency.

■ Write a care plan for a 23-year-old male, height 6 feet, weight 130 pounds, admitted to the hospital with an exacerbation of ulcerative colitis.

■ Examine different types of products available for stoma care. Where in your community can the person obtain these products? What would be the average monthly cost?

■ What resources are available in your community for people with ostomies?

---

10. Esophageal disorders of motor origin produce dysphagia for both solids and liquids; with paralysis of neurologic origin, the dysphagia is mainly for liquids, and with obstruction, there is dysphagia for solids.

11. A hiatal hernia consists of herniation of the upper part of the stomach through the diaphragm, causing heartburn.

12. Heartburn is relieved by taking antacids; eating a high-protein, low-fat diet in small frequent feedings; avoiding smoking; avoiding lifting, bending, or lying down immediately after eating; and sleeping with upper body elevated.

13. A gastrostomy is insertion of a feeding tube directly through the abdominal wall into the stomach; feedings consist of blenderized foods or special formulas.

14. Acute gastritis is a common occurrence; stress erosions (or ulcers) are a form of gastritis resulting from stress; chronic gastritis may lead to pernicious anemia or gastric cancer.

15. Gastric ulcers result from increased back diffusion of gastric acid into the tissues; gastric acid and emptying rate are normal. Duodenal ulcers result from increased gastric acid emptied more rapidly into the duodenum.

16. The major therapy for peptic ulcers is drug therapy, primarily antacids, histamine H_2 antagonists, and sucralfate.

17. Antacids are given 1 and 3 hours after meals for maximal effect; they should not be given within 1 hour of cimetidine.

18. Teaching the person with a peptic ulcer includes information about medications, suggestions for eating, and avoidance of smoking and stress, if possible.

19. Surgery for peptic ulcer may include a Billroth II (gastrojejunostomy, the most common), Billroth I (gastroduodenostomy), or vagotomy (with or without pyloroplasty).

20. Complications of peptic ulcer include hemorrhage, perforation, or pyloric obstruction.

21. Dumping syndrome occurs from entrance of a hyperosmolar mixture directly into the jejunum after gastric surgery.

22. Malabsorption syndrome is a group of disorders resulting from inadequate absorption of fat in the small intestine; common malabsorption syndromes include lactase deficiency and celiac sprue.

23. Inflammation of the intestines (enteritis) may result from viruses, bacteria, or parasites. Common parasitic infections include amebiasis (from fecally contaminated food or water) or trichinosis (from improperly cooked pork).

24. Although symptoms of appendicitis may be atypical, a common site of abdominal pain is McBurney's point (halfway between the umbilicus and right iliac crest).

25. If appendicitis is suspected, heat is avoided (increases pressure within appendix leading to rupture); enemas are also avoided (increased intraluminal pressure may also lead to a ruptured appendix).

26. Ulcerative colitis affects primarily the left colon with a continuous area of mucosal involvement; the liquid stools contain blood, but not fat. Crohn's disease affects segmental areas of the ileum, cecum, and right colon, involving submucosal layers; the frequent semisoft stools contain fat but not blood. Surgery may be useful for ulcerative colitis but not for Crohn's disease.

27. Diverticular disease involves outpouching of the colon wall; diverticulitis is the inflammatory condition, diverticulosis the quiescent phase. A high-fiber diet is encouraged to increase bowel transit time and stool bulk.

28. Care of the person with ulcerative colitis or Crohn's disease includes a low-residue, high-protein, high-calorie diet, medications (corticosteroids, sulfasal-

azine), comfort measures following diarrhea and to protect skin, and promotion of sexuality.

29. Intestinal obstruction may result from inhibition of peristalsis (paralytic ileus) or from mechanical obstruction, such as by adhesions, volvulus, intussusception, hernias, or cancer. Therapy consists of inserting a nasogastric tube, restricting oral intake, and removing the source of obstruction, if possible.

30. Hernias may occur in the inguinal, femoral, or umbilical areas from mural defects or in weakened scars from previous abdominal surgeries. Of concern is the possible entrapment (incarceration) of a loop of bowel. The treatment is surgical.

31. Risk factors for bowel cancer (the second most common form of cancer) are being older than 40 years of age, past history of colon polyps, colon cancer, cancer of the reproductive organs, ulcerative colitis, or polyposis disorders, or a family history of colorectal cancer or polyposis syndromes.

32. Recommendations for early detection of colorectal cancer include a digital rectal examination yearly after age 40; occult blood stool test yearly after age 50; and proctosigmoidoscopy every 3 to 5 years after age 50, following two negative yearly examinations.

33. Colon polyps (adenomas) are benign growths that are premalignant; the villous adenomas are more likely to become malignant than the pedunculated tubular adenomas.

34. Cancers of the ascending colon are of the cauliflowerlike mass type, and because the chyme is liquid, there is less probability of obstruction. Cancer of the descending colon is usually an annular lesion that may narrow the lumen and obstruct the more solid feces.

35. Surgery for cancer of the colon and upper rectum usually consists of resection with anastomosis; surgery for the lower rectum consists of an abdominoperineal resection with a colostomy.

36. Types of stomas include an end stoma (end of bowel brought out abdominal wall to form a single stoma), loop stoma (loop of bowel brought out abdominal wall and opened, creating one stoma with two openings), and double-barreled ostomy (ends of both proximal and distal ends of resected colon brought out to form two stomas).

37. Stoma care includes cleaning the skin to prevent skin breakdown, early treatment of excoriated skin, and application of pouches to prevent leakage.

38. Persons with a sigmoid colostomy may be able to regulate elimination by colostomy irrigations.

39. Teaching the person with a colostomy includes promoting nutrition and elimination, promoting return to normal activities and sexuality, and preventing complications.

40. Inflammatory anorectal lesions include anal fissures, anal abscesses, and anal fistulas, hemorrhoids are varicose veins of the rectum.

41. Relief of discomfort from anal lesions may include measures to prevent constipation (which irritates the lesions) and sitz baths.

REFERENCES AND SELECTED READINGS
Contemporary

1. Abrams, JS: Abdominal stomas, Littleton, Mass., 1984, Wright-PSG.
2. *Alterescu, V: Colostomy, Nurs Clin North Am 22:281-290, 1987.
3. *Alterescu, V: The ostomy: what do you teach the patient? Am J Nurs 85:1250-1253, 1985.
4. Altman, DF: Gastrointestinal diseases in the elderly, Med Clin North Am 67(2):1250-1253, 1985.
5. American Cancer Society, 1987 Cancer facts and figures, New York, 1987, The Society.
6. American College of Surgeons: Manual of preoperative and postoperative care, ed. 3, Philadelphia, 1983, WB Saunders Co.
7. *Backer, CL, and LoCicero, J: Surgical management of esophageal disorders, CCQ 9(3):12-19, 1986.
8. *Beber, CR: Freedom for the incontinent, Am J Nurs 80:483-484, 1980.
9. *Beck, ML: Two intestinal tests: one oral, one anal, Nursing '81 11(7):20-25, 1981.
10. *Beck, ML: Three common GI tests and how to help your patient through each, Nursing '81 11(4):34-35, 1981.
11. Berk, JE (editor): Bockus' gastroenterology, ed 4, Philadelphia, 1985, WB Saunders Co.
12. *Broadwell, D: Peristomal skin integrity, Nurs Clin North Am 22:321-332, 1987.
13. Broadwell, DC, and Jackson, BS: Principles of ostomy care, St. Louis, 1982, The CV Mosby Co.
14. *Burkhart, C: Upper GI hemorrhage: the clinical picture, Am J Nurs 81:1817-1820, 1981.
15. Burkitt, DP: Etiology and prevention of colorectal cancer, Hosp Pract 19(2):67-77, 1984.
16. *Bustin, MP, and Iber, FL: Management of common nonmalignant GI problems in the elderly, Geriatrics 38(3):69-75, 1983.
17. Clark, JB, Queener, SF, and Karb, VB: Pharmacological basis of nursing practice, ed 2, St. Louis, 1986, The CV Mosby Co.
18. Clinical news: Comparing Moi-Stir to lemon-glycerin swabs, Am J Nurs 87:422-424, 1987.
19. Crohn, BB, Ginzburg, L, and Oppenheimer, GD: Regional ileitis: a pathologic and clinical entity, JAMA 251:73-79, 1984.
20. Crooms, JW and Kovalcik, PJ: Obstructing left-sided colon carcinoma, Am Surg 50:15-19, 1984.
21. *Didich, JM: How to gauge abdominal girth accurately, Nursing '81 11(7):32-33, 1981.
22. *Dobkin, KA, and Broadwell, DC: Nursing considerations for the patient undergoing colostomy surgery, Sem Oncol Nurs 2:249-255, 1986.
23. *Doering, KJ, and LaMountain, P: Flow charts to facilitate caring for ostomy patients. I. Preoperative assessment, Nursing '84 14(9):47-49, 1984.

*References preceded by an asterisk are particularly well suited for student reading.

24. *Doering, KJ, and LaMountain, P: Flow charts to facilitate caring for ostomy patients. II. Immediate postoperative care, Nursing '84 14(10):47-49, 1984.

25. *Doering, KJ, and LaMountain, P: Flow charts to facilitate caring for ostomy patients. III. Recuperative care, Nursing '84 14(11):54-57, 1984.

26. *Doering, KJ, and LaMountain, P: Flow charts to facilitate caring for ostomy patients. IV. Discharge outcome assessment, Nursing '84 14(12):47-49, 1984.

27. *Doughty, DB: Colorectal cancer: etiology and pathophysiology, Sem Oncol Nurs 2:235-241, 1986.

28. Eastwood, GL: GI problems in the elderly, Cancer 39(5):59-82, 1984.

29. Englert, DM, and Guillory, JA: For want of lactase . . . , Am J Nurs 86:902-906, 1986.

30. *Erickson, P: Ostomies: the art of pouching, Nurs Clin North Am 22:311-320, 1987.

31. *Feickert, DM: Gastric surgery: your crucial pre- and postop role, RN 50(1):24-35, 1987.

32. Ferguson, E, Jr.: Operations of choice of cancers of the colon and rectum, Am Surg 50:121-127, 1984.

33. Given, B, and Simmons, S: Gastroenterology in clinical nursing, ed 4, St. Louis, 1984, The CV Mosby Co.

34. Goligher, JC: Procedures conserving continence in the surgical management of ulcerative colitis, Surg Clin North Am 63(1):49-59, 1983.

35. *Greitzu, S: Close up on cancer care: colorectal cancer, when a polyp is more than a polyp, RN 49(9):22-30, 1986.

36. Groer, MW, and Shekleton, ME: Basic pathophysiology: a conceptual approach, ed 2, St. Louis, 1983, The CV Mosby Co.

37. *Huffman, J: Living with limitations, Geriatr Nurs 4:107-108, 1983.

38. *Joachim, G: An update on inflammatory bowel disease, AAOHN 34(4):171-173, 1986.

39. *Johnson, S: A safer gastrostomy for the high-risk patient: percutaneous endoscopic gastrostomy, RN 49(3):29-32, 1986.

40. Kaye, D, and Rose, LF: Fundamentals of internal medicine, St. Louis, 1983, The CV Mosby Co.

41. *Khan, AH: Colorectal carcinoma: risk factors, screening, early detection, Geriatrics 39:42-47, 1984.

42. Krupp, MA, Schroeder, SA, and Tierney, LM, Jr: Current medical diagnosis and treatment 1987, Norwalk, Conn, 1987, Appleton & Lange.

43. *Lamphier, TA, and Lamphier, RA: Upper GI hemorrhage: emergency evaluation and management, Am J Nurs 81:1814-1817, 1981.

44. *Lewicki, LJ, and Leeson, MJ: The multisystem impact on physiologic processes of inflammatory bowel disease, Nurs Clin North Am 19(1):71-79, 1984.

45. Maklebust, J: United Ostomy Association visits and adjustment following ostomy surgery, J Enterost Ther 12:84-92, 1985.

46. *McNamara, JP: Esophageal cancer, Nursing '82, 12(3):64-65, 1982.

47. *Messner, R, Gardner, SS, and Lewis, S: Crohn's disease: more than a chronic illness, Occup Health Nurs 33(12):604-609, 1985.

48. *Messner, RL, Gardner, SS, and Webb, DD: Early detection: the priority of colorectal cancer, Cancer Nurs 9(1):8-14, 1986.

49. Metheny, NM: Fluid and electrolyte balance: nursing considerations, Philadelphia, 1987, JB Lippincott, Co.

50. *Myer, SA: Overview of inflammatory bowel disease, Nurs Clin North Am 19(1):3-10, 1984.

51. *Podiasky, P, and Rudzinski, HM: Percutaneous endoscopic gastrostomy, AORN J 45:1403-1411, 1987.

52. Price, SA, and Wilson, LM: Pathophysiology: clinical concepts of disease processes, ed 2, New York, 1982, McGraw-Hill Book Co.

53. Rakel, RE (editor): 1987 Conn's current therapy, Philadelphia, 1987, WB Saunders Co.

54. *Ramos, LY: Oral hygiene for the elderly, Am J Nurs 81:1468-1469, 1981.

55. *Rubin, DM: New hope for colitis patients, AORN J 38:783-793, 1983.

56. *Schulmeister, L: Join the fight against oral cancer, Nursing '87 17(5):66-67, 1987.

57. *Shipes, E: Psychosocial issues: the person with an ostomy, Nurs Clin North Am 22:291-302, 1987.

58. Simmons, KN: Sexuality and the female ostomate, Am J Nurs 82:409-411, 1983.

59. Sleisinger, M: and Fordtran, JS: Gastrointestinal disease: pathophysiology, diagnosis, and management, ed 3, Philadelphia, 1983, WB Saunders Co.

60. *Smith, DB: Clinical rounds: colostomy irrigations, so simple? J Enterost Ther 10:22-23, 1983.

61. *Smith, DB: The ostomy: how is it managed? Am J Nurs 85:1246-1249, 1985.

61a. *Starkey, JF, Jefferson, PA, and Kirby, DF: Taking care of a percutaneous endoscopic gastrostomy, Am J Nurs 88:42-45, 1988.

62. Steiner, R, Banks, PA, and Present, DH: People, not patients: a source book for living with inflammatory bowel disease, New York, 1985, National Foundation for Ileitis and Colitis, Inc.

63. *Stotts, NA, Fitzgerald, KA, and Williams, KR: Care of the patient critically ill with inflammatory bowel disease, Nurs Clin North Am 19(1):61-70, 1984.

64. United Ostomy Association, Inc: Sex, courtship, and the single ostomate, Los Angeles, 1981, The Association.

65. United Ostomy Association, Inc: Sex and the male ostomate, Los Angeles, 1982, The Association.

66. *Watson, PG: Meeting the needs of patients undergoing ostomy surgery, J Enterost Ther 12:121-124, 1985.

67. *Watts, RC: The ostomy: how is it created? Am J Nurs 85:1242-1243, 1985.

68. Way, LW: Current surgical diagnosis and treatment, ed 6, Los Altos, Calif 1983, Lange Medical Publications.

69. *Wicks, LJ: Treatment modalities for colorectal cancer, Sem Oncol Nurs 2:242-248, 1986.

70. *Wilson, C: The diagnostic work-up for the patient with inflammatory bowel disease, Nurs Clin North Am 19(1):51-60, 1984.

71. Wyngaarden, JB, and Smith, LH: Cecil textbook of medicine, ed 17, Philadelphia, 1985, WB Saunders Co.

32

The Patient with Urinary Problems

H. FRED FARLEY

CHAPTER OBJECTIVES

After studying this chapter, the student should be able to:

- Describe interventions for urinary retention and urinary incontinence.

- Describe the causes and methods of prevention of urinary tract infections (UTI). Differentiate between upper and lower UTI.

- Describe pathophysiologic differences among, signs and symptoms of, and therapeutic modalities and nursing interventions for glomerular disorders.

- Describe the pathophysiology of obstructive urinary disorders.

- Describe the pathophysiology and interventions for renal calculi.

- Compare different approaches to prostatectomy and describe the related nursing interventions.

- Describe the care of the person undergoing surgery of the urinary tract.

- Differentiate between acute and chronic renal failure, including pathophysiology, signs and symptoms, medical therapy, and nursing interventions.

- Explain the physiologic principles of dialysis and describe the types of dialysis and related care.

- Describe the care of the person with a kidney transplant.

Maintaining homeostasis, or the state of dynamic equilibrium, of the internal environment is essential for life. The body must have a means for eliminating wastes that are produced by metabolism. Furthermore, the body must regulate fluid volume, electrolyte composition, and acid-base balance. The kidneys and other structures of the urinary system play major roles in the regulation of the internal environment. Some of the urinary disorders discussed in this chapter may lead to destruction of renal tissue, with subsequent alterations in fluid and electrolyte balance, excretion of body wastes, and regulation of body processes.

This chapter begins with a brief review of the major concepts relating to anatomy and physiology of the urinary system. (For a more intensive review, the reader is referred to a physiology text.) The next part of the chapter describes major urinary disorders, some of which may lead to renal failure. The last part of the chapter discusses renal failure, both acute and chronic, and includes the treatment modalities of dialysis and kidney transplantation.

■ ANATOMY AND PHYSIOLOGY

The urinary system consists primarily of the kidneys, ureters, bladder, and urethra (Fig. 32-1). Although the prostate gland is primarily a male reproductive organ, it is discussed in this chapter because enlargement or infection of the prostate impinges on the urinary tract.

■ Kidneys
■ ANATOMY

The kidneys are two bean-shaped organs that lie behind the parietal peritoneum at the costovertebral angle. The *nephron* is the functional unit of the kidney, and each kidney contains approximately 1 million of these units. The structures of the nephron involved in the process of urine formation include the glomerulus within the Bowman's capsule, the proximal convoluted tubule, the loop of Henle, the distal convoluted tubule, and the collecting tubule (Fig. 32-2). Bowman's capsule and both convoluted tubules lie within the cortex of the kidney, whereas the loop of Henle and the collecting tubules are in the medulla (Fig. 32-3). Urine from many collecting tubules drains into larger tubules that form the pyramids in the medulla; urine then drains into the kidney pelvis.

■ RENAL PHYSIOLOGY

The functions of the kidney are summarized in the box on p. 1126. These functions, accomplished during the formation of urine, are described in the succeeding paragraphs.

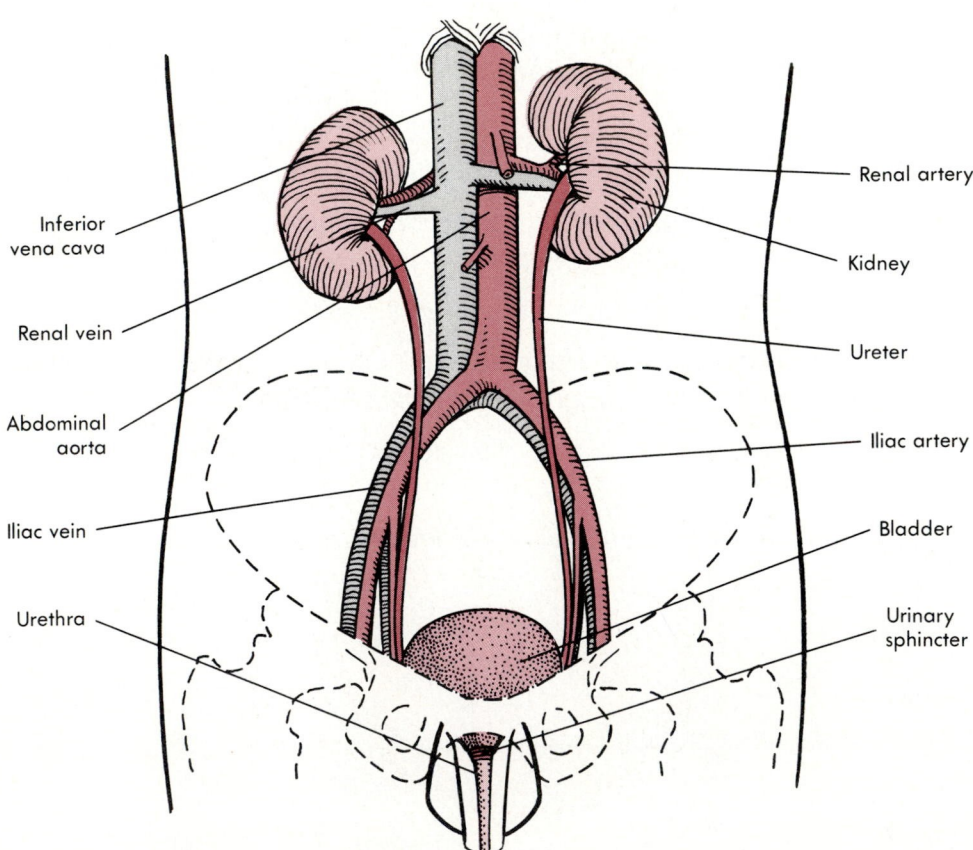

Inferior vena cava

Renal vein

Abdominal aorta

Iliac vein

Urethra

Renal artery

Kidney

Ureter

Iliac artery

Bladder

Urinary sphincter

Fig. 32-1 Kidneys and other structures of urinary system.

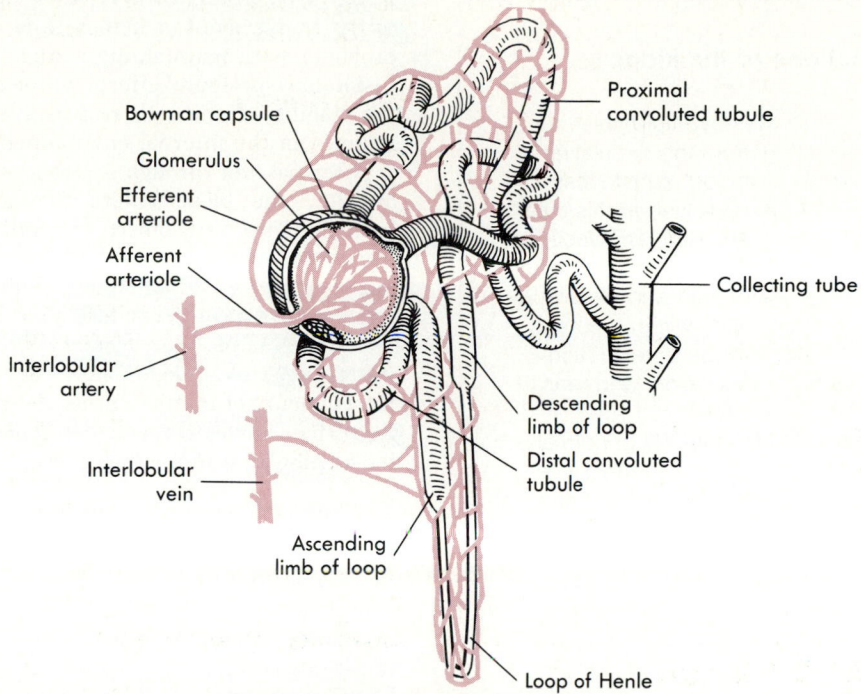

Bowman capsule

Glomerulus

Efferent
arteriole

Afferent
arteriole

Interlobular
artery

Interlobular
vein

Ascending
limb of loop

Proximal
convoluted tubule

Collecting tube

Descending
limb of loop

Distal convoluted
tubule

Loop of Henle

Fig. 32-2 Nephron.

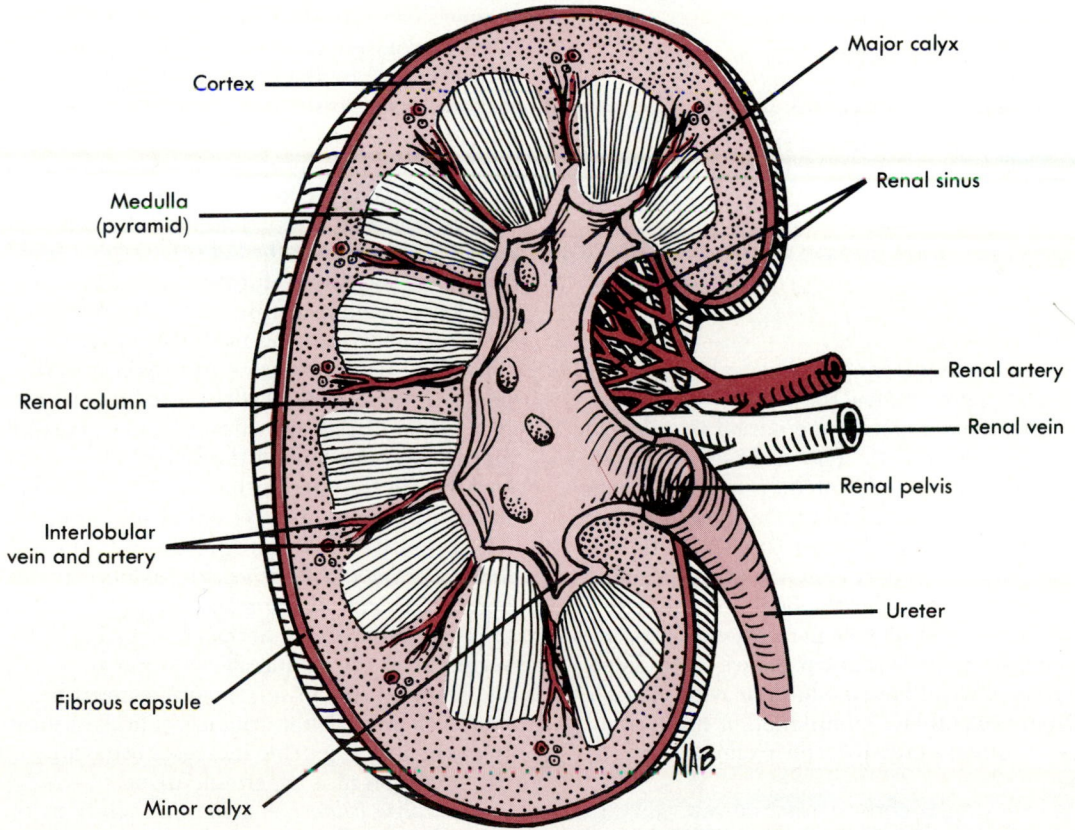

Cortex

Medulla
(pyramid)

Renal column

Interlobular
vein and artery

Fibrous capsule

Minor calyx

Major calyx

Renal sinus

Renal artery

Renal vein

Renal pelvis

Ureter

Fig. 32-3 Frontal section of kidney.

Major functions of the kidneys

Ultrafiltration	Remove fluid volume from the circulating blood; substances dissolved in this fluid are also removed
Fluid and elect- rolyte control	Maintain correct balance of fluid and electro- lytes within a normal range by excretion, secretion, and reab- sorption
Acid-base balance	Maintain pH at normal range by directly ex- creting H⁺ ions and forming bicarbonate for buffering
Excretion of waste products	Direct removal of meta- bolic waste products contained in the glo- merular filtrate
Blood pressure regu- lation	Regulate blood pressure by controlling circulat- ing volume and renin secretion
RBC production	Erythropoietin secreted by kidneys stimulates bone marrow to pro- duce RBCs
Regulation of calcium- phosphate metabo- lism	Vitamin D activation reg- ulated by kidneys

☐ **Ultrafiltration**

The ultrafiltrate arising from the glomerular capillaries (*glomerular filtrate*) approximates 180 L/day. The amount of glomerular filtrate in a given time period is called the *glomerular filtration rate* (GFR). The GFR in an average-sized man is approximately 125 ml/minute (7.5 L/hour) or the equal in 1 day of about 60 times the plasma volume. The average GFR in a woman is about 10% less. The same forces that affect fluid transport between vascular and interstitial spaces in other parts of the body (see Chapter 8) also affect filtration in the glomerular capsule. The GFR is affected by changes in hydrostatic pressure (for example, with decreased renal blood flow in shock or with arteriolar constriction from sympathetic stimulation or medications) or by changes in osmotic pressure (for example, with hypoproteinemia).

The kidneys receive 25% of the cardiac output, and renal blood flow approximates 600 ml/minute. This blood supply to the kidneys is basic to the formation of glomerular fil-

trate, or beginning urine, and to the nutrition and respiration requirement of kidney cells. Severe and prolonged problems with maintaining cardiac output and renal perfusion have profound effects on the formation of urine and the viability of the cells responsible for maintaining consistency in the internal environment.

After passing through a series of progressively smaller arteries, the blood enters the afferent arteriole that branches into the glomerular capillaries. The *glomerulus*, located in Bowman's capsule, is the first functional portion of the nephron. When blood enters the glomerular capillaries at a pressure not less than 60 to 70 mm Hg, an ultrafiltrate of plasma is formed. This *ultrafiltrate* (primitive urine) contains approximately the same concentration of the elements of plasma minus the proteins. This ultrafiltrate then passes through the remainder of the nephron for modification into actual urine.

☐ **Fluid and electrolyte control**

Were it not for some conserving mechanism in the kidneys, a person would be depleted of fluid and salts within 3 to 4 minutes. The *proximal convoluted tubule* reabsorbs up to 85% to 90% of water in the ultrafiltrate; up to 80% of filtered sodium; and the majority of filtered potassium, bicarbonate, chloride, phosphate, glucose, and protein.

Dehydration would still occur if the body did not have an additional mechanism within the kidneys to conserve filtered water. This mechanism allows urine to be concentrated to less than 1% of the daily filtered volume. The kidneys can vary the amount of fluid excreted so precisely that intake over that required for normal fluid balance is excreted and intake under that required for normal fluid balance leads to further concentration of the urine. The mechanisms responsible for this increased urine concentrating ability and precision in excreting appropriate urine volume exist in the loop of Henle and the distal convoluted and collecting tubules. The *loop of Henle* reaches into the medullary portion of the kidney, which is highly hypertonic in comparison to the filtrate. In the *descending* portion of the loop, sodium diffuses into the filtrate as the tubule passes deeper into the medullary area, and water moves out of the primitive urine in response to the high sodium concentration. The result is a reduction in volume of the glomerular filtrate and a dramatic increase in its osmolality. In the *ascending* limb of the loop of Henle, sodium is reabsorbed into the interstitium, but the loop is impermeable to the movement of water either into or out of the tubule. The primitive urine now presented to the *distal convoluted* and *collecting tubules* is greatly reduced in volume but hypotonic because of the reabsorption of sodium. The influence of antidiuretic hormone (ADH) on these last two segments of the tubule allows water to be reabsorbed into the interstitium in an amount compatible with maintenance of proper fluid balance. The reabsorption of water from the forming urine increases osmolality and results in the excretion of a hypertonic urine.

Electrolyte balance is achieved mainly in the distal convoluted and collecting tubule portions of the nephron. As with fluid, the major conservation site for electrolytes is

Table 32-1 Fluid and electrolyte control by kidney

Site	Function	Effect	Physiologic basis
Glomerulus	Filtration of water and electrolytes	Beginning of urine formation	Hydrostatic pressure
Proximal convoluted tubules	Reabsorption of large amounts of water, sodium, potassium, bicarbonate, chloride, phosphate	Conservation of fluid and electrolytes	Reabsorption by acitve and passive transport Bicarbonate reabsorption controlled by acid-base imbalance

Loop of Henle
  Descending limb
  Ascending limb
	Diffusion of sodium into tubule
	Reabsorption of water
	Reabsorption of sodium
		Reduction in urine volume; urine is hypertonic
		Urine becomes hypotonic
			Medulla of kidney is hypertonic
			Water remains in loop because membrane is impermeable to water

Distal convoluted tubule and collecting tubule	Reabsorption of water Secretion of potassium, hydrogen and ammonia ions as needed Reabsorption of sodium	Fluid and electrolyte control depending on body needs	Water is reabsorbed as needed by effect of ADH Extra potassium is secreted Hydrogen and ammonia ions are secreted, depending on acid-base imbalances Sodium is reabsorbed by effect of aldosterone

the *proximal convoluted tubule* where the vast majority of all filtered electrolytes are reabsorbed, thus preventing rapid depletion of these substances. The precise regulation of body electrolyte composition occurs in the distal tubular segments. Depending on the concentrations of electrolytes presented to the tubular cells in the primitive urine and the concentrations of these substances in the interstitium, tubular cells secrete or further reabsorb electrolytes into the urine (Table 32-1).

Regulation of *acid-base balance* is achieved by the kidney through regeneration or excretion of bicarbonate ions in the proximal tubule. During acidosis, either metabolic (when kidney function is not impaired) or respiratory, the kidney excretes hydrogen ions and conserves bicarbonate ions. During alkalosis the opposite effect occurs, that is, conservation of hydrogen ions and excretion of bicarbonate ions (see Chapter 8).

☐ Excretion of waste products

Metabolic wastes are excreted in the glomerular filtrate. Creatinine is little modified in its passage through the nephron; creatinine contained in the glomerular filtrate is excreted unchanged in the urine. Other wastes, such as urea, are excreted unchanged in the glomerular filtrate but undergo reabsorption during passage through the nephron. The amount of waste material excreted in urine in such an instance is only a fraction of that originally contained in the glomerular filtrate.

Excretion of drugs by the kidneys occurs through both filtration at the glomerular level and secretion into the urine by distal tubular cells. Penicillin is an example of a drug secreted by tubular cells.

☐ Blood pressure regulation

Renal regulation of blood pressure is controlled by the renin-angiotensin-aldosterone system. *Renin* is a hormone released by the juxtaglomerular apparatus (adjoining the glomerulus) in response to sodium depletion, renal artery hypoperfusion, or stimulation of the renal nerves through the sympathetic pathway. *Angiotensinogen,* which is produced in the liver, is activated to *angiotensin I* in the presence of renin. An enzyme in the lungs converts angiotensin I to the active form, *angiotensin II.* Angiotensin II is a powerful *vasoconstrictor* that also stimulates the release of aldosterone by the adrenals. *Aldosterone* increases sodium reabsorption by the kidney; water follows the sodium, leading to an increase in blood volume (see Fig. 26-18). A low GFR, seen with numerous kidney diseases (such as glomerulonephritis, nephrotic syndrome, polycystic disease, renal trauma, renal failure) usually leads to hypertension by activation of the renin-angiotensin-aldosterone system (See Chapter 26 for a discussion of hypertension.)

☐ Stimulation of red blood cell production

Red blood cell (RBC) production is controlled by the kidneys. *Erythropoietin* is a hormone that is secreted by the kidneys. Erythropoietin stimulates bone marrow to produce RBCs. Persons with chronic renal failure often have serum hematocrit values of 18% to 30% (normal values are 42% to 47%). This decrease in hematocrit values is the result of decreased secretion of erythropoietin from the diseased kidneys compounded by bone marrow toxicity, decreased life span of RBCs and increased bleeding, all of which are associated with the altered metabolic state present in chronic renal failure.

☐ Regulation of calcium-phosphate metabolism

Calcium-phosphate metabolism is also controlled by the kidneys. Vitamin D prohormone is converted to its active form by the kidneys. Active vitamin D regulates not only GI absorption of calcium but also its deposition within the bone matrix, as well as the metabolism of calcium and phosphorus.

A constellation of signs and symptoms that cannot as yet be explained arises in patients with chronic renal failure. This suggests that there may be some functions of the kidneys that we are not yet aware of. Because of this, nephrology remains an area rich with research questions.

■ Lower urinary tract

■ ANATOMY

The *ureters* arise as extensions of the kidney pelves and empty into the bladder in an area called the *trigone* (Fig. 32-4). These small tubes are composed of smooth muscle; their function is to propel urine from the kidney into the bladder. Spasm and severe colic-type pain result from obstruction of the ureters. The *bladder,* situated behind the symphysis pubis, is a collecting bag for the urine. The mucous membrane is arranged in folds called rugae that, together with the elasticity of the muscular walls, can distend the bladder considerably to hold large amounts of urine. A layer of skeletal muscle encircles the base of the bladder, forming the *external urinary sphincter.* The bladder is innervated by both the sympathetic and parasympathetic

nervous system, whereas the ureters receive fibers only from the sympathetic nervous system.

The *urethra* transports urine from the bladder to the external meatus. Male and female urethras differ in length and accessibility of reproductive organs. The female urethra is short (about 4 cm long), exits anterior to the vagina (see Fig. 34-1), and is separate from the reproductive organs. The male urethra (see Fig. 34-3) is 18 to 20 cm long and transports semen as well as urine. The urethra is innervated by both the sympathetic and parasympathetic nervous systems.

The *prostate gland* is a male reproductive gland about the size of a walnut that encircles the upper portion of the male urethra (Fig. 32-4). It is shaped like a doughnut with the urethra passing through the "hole." When the prostate is enlarged, the urethra is squeezed, causing obstruction of urinary flow. Numerous prostatic ducts empty into the urethra. Bacteria from urinary tract infections may travel up these ducts, causing prostatic infection.

■ MICTURITION

Urine flows out the kidney pelves and is propelled through the ureters by peristaltic action. About 200 to 300 ml of urine can collect in the bladder before the urge to void is initiated. Baroreceptors in the bladder wall are triggered by the stretching of the bladder walls, which causes reflex stimulation of parasympathetic nerves to the bladder, resulting in bladder contractions. When the motor nerves to the external urinary sphincter are inhibited, the

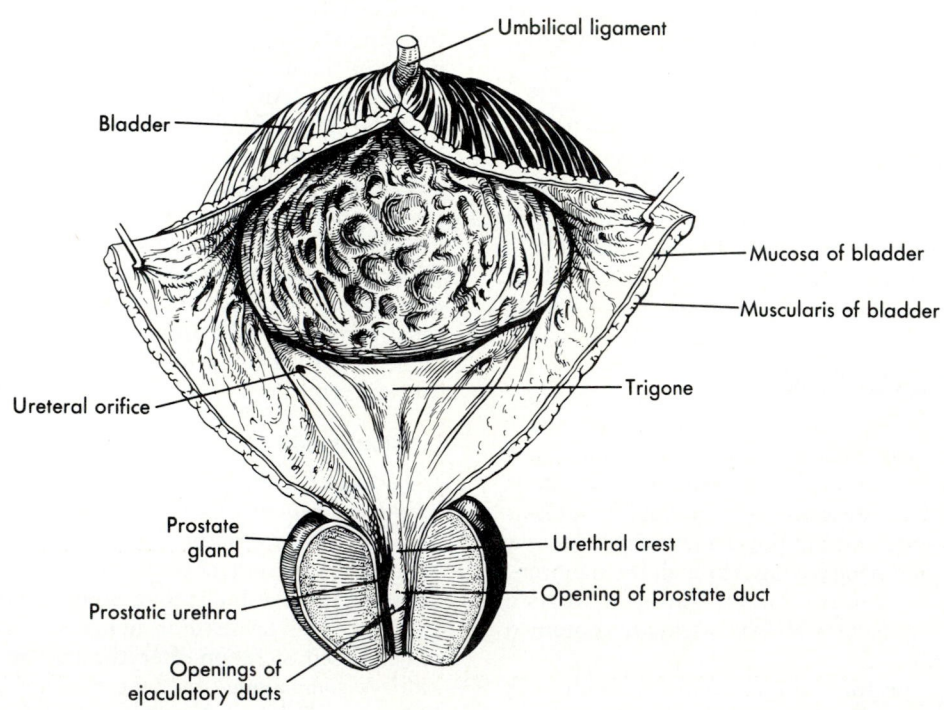

Fig. 32-4 Interior of urinary bladder and some associated structures. (From McClintic, JR: Human anatomy, St. Louis, 1983, The CV Mosby Co.)

muscle relaxes, opening the sphincter and permitting urine to be expelled. Stimulation of the sphincter muscles can keep the sphincter contracted against strong bladder contractions. Voluntary control over micturition can be exerted by stimuli transmitted over descending spinal pathways from the brainstem.

Use of a large balloon (30 ml) indwelling catheter (such as after a transurethral resection of the prostate) can stimulate the parasympathetic nerves, causing uncomfortable bladder contractions. Pressure on the sphincter by the balloon can also create an urge to void, although the bladder has been emptied by the catheter.

■ Physiologic changes with aging

A direct relationship exists between blood supply to the kidneys and renal function. The rate of blood flow to the kidneys is about 5 to 10 times greater than that to the heart, liver, and brain. Glomerular capillary pressure, which is the force that promotes ultrafiltration, is controlled by blood flow to the kidneys. Therefore, physiologic alterations in the vascular bed can lead to changes in renal function.

Arteriosclerotic changes in renal arteries are the most common form of renal vascular pathology.[17] Arteriosclerotic changes occur to some extent in most normal individuals with aging. The degree of morphologic change experienced depends on the specific arteries affected and the extent of involvement.

Aging is also known to cause predictable increases in both systolic and diastolic blood pressure.[27] This slow increase in blood pressure begins at birth and continues through adulthood. Untreated hypertension further accelerates the development of atherosclerosis, which can lead to renal failure.

Changes also occur in kidney structure and function with aging. About 40% of glomeruli are lost by age 70. The glomerular and and tubular basement membranes thicken, leading to a 46% decrease in GFR from age 20 to 90.[9] If heart failure is also present with compensatory vasodilation, renal ischemia is increased further and the risk of renal failure is increased.

The ability to concentrate urine and sensitivity to ADH stimulation also decreases with age. Elderly persons have greater difficulty eliminating heavy solute loads and are slower to conserve fluids with fluid restriction.[19] Electrolyte imbalance may occur more readily from a decreased ability to conserve sodium, excrete potassium, and form and excrete ammonia.

Urinary incontinence may occur in acutely ill elderly persons who lack energy for voluntary control or who may be confused or disoriented. Stress incontinence may be noted in women with relaxed perineal muscles or in males following prostatectomy. Benign prostatic hypertrophy (p. 1167) occurs in more than half of all men over age 50 and 75% of men over age 70; the enlarged prostate presses on the urethra, resulting in urinary symptoms.

■ PREVENTION AND HEALTH EDUCATION

Two measures can be effective in reducing the incidence of renal failure: (1) identification of individuals at risk and (2) identification and control of environmental factors that can result in renal failure. The box below summarizes conditions and substances that can result in injury to the kidneys.

Renal dysfunction can be somewhat elusive. Renal function can be described as being on a continuum (Fig. 32-

---

Conditions and substances that can result in kidney damage

Inadequate perfusion

1. Hypovolemia
2. Blood loss (surgery, trauma)
3. Plasma loss (burns, surgery, acute pancreatitis)
4. Sodium and water loss (prolonged diarrhea or vomiting, gastrointestinal tract drainage, sustained high fever)
5. Cardiac failure
6. Myocardial infarction
7. Cardiac arrhythmias
8. Congestive heart failure
9. Septic shock

Toxic substances

1. Solvents (carbon tetrachloride, methanol, ethylene glycol)
2. Heavy metals (lead, arsenic, mercury)
3. Antibiotics (kanamycin, gentamicin, polymyxin B, amphotericin B, colistin, neomycin, phenazopyridine)
4. Pesticides
5. Poisonous mushrooms

| Normal renal functioning | Diminished | Renal insufficiency | Renal failure |

Fig. 32-5   Continuum of renal function.

Factors contributing to the development of hypertension

High sodium intake
Family history of hypertension
Advanced age
Race (Black)
Obesity
Stress
Drugs, such as amphetamines, alcohol, nicotine

---

5)—at one end of the continuum is normal renal function, while at the other end is renal failure. It is when persons near the point of renal failure that they begin to exhibit signs and symptoms. Two other points on this continuum are decreased renal reserve and renal insufficiency. *Decreased renal reserve* exists when renal function has diminished to the point at which additional physiologic stress results in signs and symptoms. This stress could result from intercurrent illness, infection, or dietary overindulgence. Signs and symptoms of decreased renal reserve usually resolve once the stress is removed. *Renal insufficiency* is defined as the reduced capacity of the kidney to perform its functions. Renal insufficiency is generally experienced when the GFR is 20% to 40% of normal. The person with renal insufficiency typically requires symptomatic management by the physician. It is important to follow these two points on the renal function continuum, because proper management can prevent the loss of more renal functioning and eliminate the need for more aggressive therapy. Regular physical examination, including serum

---

Urinary tract infections

Prevention

1. Cleanse perineal area properly; a shower is more desirable than a bath.
2. Drink adequate volume of fluid, 3 to 4 L/day.
3. Void frequently during waking hours, every 2 to 3 hours during day.

Treatment

1. Seek prompt medical attention for symptoms.
2. Continue with drug therapy even though symptoms abate.
3. Follow steps 1 through 3 listed above.
4. Follow-up care with repeated urine cultures are essential.

---

chemistry evaluation, can aid in the detection of changing renal status.

Hypertension remains a major cause of renal disease. Early detection and treatment of hypertension can prevent or arrest renal complications. Persons at high risk for hypertension should be screened regularly. Factors contributing to the development of hypertension are listed in the box at left.

Urinary tract infections (UTI) are a significant source of morbidity in the United States. These infections contribute to illness during the active stage but also can lead to the development of chronic renal failure. Although the vast majority of UTIs clear spontaneously, there remains a portion significant enough to warrant consideration as a health problem. Early detection and treatment of a UTI decrease the probability of renal complications. The box below, left summarizes health care practices helpful in prevention and treatment of a UTI.

Major health problems of the urinary system

The major health problems of the urinary system can be categorized in a number of ways. The following common disorders will be discussed in this chapter.

1. Urinary dysfunction
   a. Urinary retention
   b. Urinary incontinence
2. Urinary tract infections
   a. Pyelonephritis
   b. Lower urinary tract infection
3. Glomerular disorders
   a. Glomerulonephritis: acute, chronic
   b. Nephrotic syndrome
4. Obstructive disorders
   a. Urinary calculi
   b. Benign prostatic hypertrophy
   c. Urethral strictures
   d. Neoplasms: renal, bladder, prostate
5. Other urinary disorders
   a. Cystic disease
   b. Vascular disorders
   c. Toxic nephropathy
   d. Trauma

Another major health problem of the urinary system is congenital disorders. Congenital disorders include structural malformation, lack of or poor development of one or both kidneys, dysplasia, and polycystic disease. Any of these conditions can result in morbidity in adults. (For more information about congenital disorders the reader is referred to a pediatric nursing text.)

Any of the preceding disorders can lead to loss of renal function resulting in what is called renal failure. Renal failure is classified as (1) acute or (2) chronic. Acute and chronic renal failure will be discussed at the end of this chapter.

■ URINARY DYSFUNCTION

■ Urinary retention

Under normal conditions a person who is consuming an adequate diet, including adequate fluid intake, will have a urinary output approximately equal to fluid intake. Inadequate urinary output may occur either when the kidneys are not producing urine or when the flow of urine is blocked between the kidneys and the urethral opening. This blockage is called *urinary retention*.

■ PATHOPHYSIOLOGY

Causes of urinary retention can be categorized as either mechanical or functional. A mechanical obstruction exists when there is a blockage of urine flow. This blockage can exist anywhere within the urinary system from the collecting ducts to the urinary meatus. Some mechanical obstructions are congenital; however, most obstructions observed in the adult are acquired. A functional obstruction exists when there is an obstruction that cannot be attributed to a mechanical problem. The major causes of urinary retention are summarized in the box at right.

▨ ASSESSMENT

☐ Subjective data

The patient is asked questions to provide data on the following:
1. Understanding of the disorder
2. Voiding patterns, including dysuria, frequency, urgency, hesitancy (see Table 32-2)
3. Dietary habits, including fluid intake
4. Presence of suprapubic pain
5. History of urinary problems

☐ Objective data

Objective data should include intake and output, assessment of level of hydration, palpation for bladder distention, and visual inspection of urine for color, clarity, sedimentation, and odor.

Major causes of urinary retention

Type of retention	Cause
Mechanical obstruction	
Congenital	Urethral stricture
	Urinary tract malformation
	Spinal cord malformation
Acquired	Calculus
	Inflammation
	Trauma
	Tumor
	Hyperplasia
	Pregnancy
Functional obstruction	Neurogenic bladder dysfunction
	Ureterovesical reflux
	Decreased peristaltic activity of the ureter
	Detrusor muscle atrophy
	Anxiety, such as fear of pain after surgery
	Medications, for example anesthetics, narcotics, sedatives, and antihistamines

☐ Diagnostic tests

Diagnostic tests include urinalysis. This test yields information about probable locations and causes of urinary disease and some information as to the extent of the illness. Urinalysis is a test that assists in establishing tentative diagnoses and predicting additional tests and observations required to make precise diagnoses. Urinalysis also indicates abnormalities of nonrenal and nonurologic origin (for example, diabetes mellitus). Table 32-3 indicates possible normal and abnormal findings.

A urine culture should be performed to determine the presence of infection that could be leading to the urinary dysfunction (p. 1149). Urine chemistry assessments may also be ordered. Serum creatinine and blood urea nitrogen

Table 32-2 Possible causes of urinary symptoms

Symptom	Definition	Possible causes
Dysuria	Painful urination	Urinary tract infection (UTI)
Frequency	Voiding at frequent intervals	UTI, retention with overflow, excess fluid intake
Urgency	Need to void immediately	Bladder irritation from inflammation, trauma, tumor
Hesitancy	Difficulty initiating voiding	Partial urethral obstruction

Table 32-3 Urinalysis

Test	Normal	Abnormal
Color	Amber-yellow	Red indicates hematuria (possible urinary obstruction, renal calculi, tumor, renal failure)
Clarity	Clear	Cloudy: debris, bacterial sediment (urinary infection)
pH	4.6-8.0 (average 6.0)	Alkaline on standing or with UTI
		Increased acidity with renal tubular acidosis
Specific gravity	1.003-1.035	Usually reflects fluid intake; the less the fluid intake, the higher the specific gravity
		If specific gravity remains low (1.010-1.014), renal disease is suspected
Protein	0-8 mg/dl	Proteinuria may occur with high-protein diet and exercise (particularly prolonged)
		Seen in renal disease
Sugar	0	Glycosuria occurs after a high intake of sugar or with diabetes mellitus
Ketones	0	Ketonuria occurs with starvation and diabetic ketoacidosis
Red blood cells	0-4	Injury to kidney tissue (see hematuria)
White blood cells	0-5	Urinary tract infection (UTI)
Casts	0	UTI, renal disease

(BUN) are important diagnostic tests to ascertain the level of renal function. Creatinine clearance tests may also be performed. These urinary system tests are summarized in Table 32-4.

DATA ANALYSIS: NURSING DIAGNOSES

Nursing diagnoses are determined from assessment of patient data. Possible nursing diagnoses for the person with urinary retention may include, but are not limited to, the following:

Diagnostic title	Possible etiologies
Anxiety	Threat to self-concept, threat to and/ or change in health status
Fluid volume deficit	Decreased fluid intake
Pain	Pathophysiologic: visceral disorders, distention
Urinary retention	Obstruction, position for voiding, immobility, inability to initiate stream, stress, fear, effect of medications (narcotics, anesthetics, sedatives, antihistamines)

PLANNING: EXPECTED PATIENT OUTCOMES

Expected patient outcomes for the person with urinary retention may include, but are not limited to, the following:
1. Patient or significant other can verbalize signs and symptoms of retention.
2. Bladder is not palpable after voiding.
3. Patient voids 200 to 400 ml at each voiding.
4. Patient maintains fluid intake of at least 2400 ml each day.

IMPLEMENTATION

Assisting with achievement of therapeutic goals

Interventions for urinary retention are aimed at reestablishing urine flow. Some mechanical obstructions must be corrected by surgical intervention; others, such as that caused by an enlarged prostate, may require temporary urethral catheter drainage.

Promotion of micturition

If the person is having difficulty eliminating urine from the bladder in the absence of mechanical obstruction, measures that encourage voiding are attempted before catheterization is instituted. These measures may include ensuring a position that facilitates voiding (positional stimuli), running water or blowing bubbles in water (auditory stimuli), or pouring water over the perineum or placing the hands in water (tactile stimuli). Having the person sit in lukewarn water may help relax the urinary sphincters. Bethanechol chloride (Urecholine) may be given to initiate voiding by stimulation of the bladder detrusor muscle. Persons with long-term problems may be taught to carry out intermittent catheterizations (p. 1136) rather than maintaining an indwelling catheter.

Catheter usage and types

Assisted urinary drainage is used in a variety of clinical situations in both acute and chronic care. Major reasons for catheter drainage include the following:
1. Relieve temporary anatomic or physiologic urinary obstruction.
2. Permit healing of various parts of the urinary system postoperatively.
3. Permit accurate measurement of urinary output in severely ill patients.

Table 32-4   Selected renal function tests

Test	Normal results	Purpose/significance	Nursing implications
Specific gravity of urine	1.010-1.026	Measures ability of kidneys to concentrate urine	First morning void is usually in the high normal range in healthy individual False high is caused by presence of radiographic dyes
Osmolality of urine	400-600 mOsm/kg	Excellent indication of renal function Osmolality is total concentration of particles in solution	No special preparation
Urine chemistries	Sodium: 130 to 220 mEq/L Potassium: 39 to 90 mg/24 hrs Calcium: 100 to 300 mg/24 hrs	Urine electrolytes reflect ability of kidney to excrete and reabsorb electrolytes	Abnormal results may be caused by disease processes other than renal disorders, for example, elevated urine calcium in hyperparathyroidism or prolonged immobilization
Creatinine clearance	Men: 100 to 150 ml/min Women: 85 to 125 ml/min	Clearance is rate at which a substance is excreted in terms of plasma concentration Because diet and metabolic state have little influence on it, serum creatinine is excellent for determining glomerular filtration rate.	Procedure 1. Patient empties bladder and time is noted 2. *All* urine is saved for 24 hours 3. Exactly 24 hours after start of procedure the patient voids and specimen is saved 4. Total urine volume and urine creatinine is measured 5. Serum creatinine is determined at end of 24 hour period 6. Creatinine clearance is then calculated by formula: $$\text{Clearance: } \frac{UV^*}{P^*}$$ $^*U$ = Urine creatinine concentration $^*V$ = Urine volume $^*P$ = Plasma creatinine concentration
Serum creatinine	Men: 0.85 to 1.5 mg/dl Women: 0.70 to 1.25 mg/dl	Indicates ability of kidneys to excrete nitrogenous wastes	No specific preparation for test Diet and metabolic rate have little effect on serum creatinine
BUN	5-20 mg/dl	Indicates ability of kidneys to excrete nitrogenous wastes BUN gives a rough estimate of GFR	BUN can be affected by high-protein diet, blood in GI tract, catabolic state (injury, infection)

4. Relieve inability to void.
5. Achieve continence.
6. Prevent retention of urine in certain types of persons with neurogenic bladder dysfunction.
7. Permit irrigation to prevent obstruction of urine flow.

Reestablishment of the flow of urine is an immediate treatment goal. The type of catheter used to provide drainage in the presence of obstruction depends on the location of the blockage.

Straight catheters (Fig. 32-6) are used for single catheterizations. The various catheters have different usages:
1. Robinson—intermittent catheterization (ease of insertion)
2. Coudé—prostatic hypertrophy (avoid trauma to gland)
3. Whistle-tip—presence of hematuria and blood clots (less chance of blockage)
4. Filiform (thin, stiff catheter)—urethral stricture

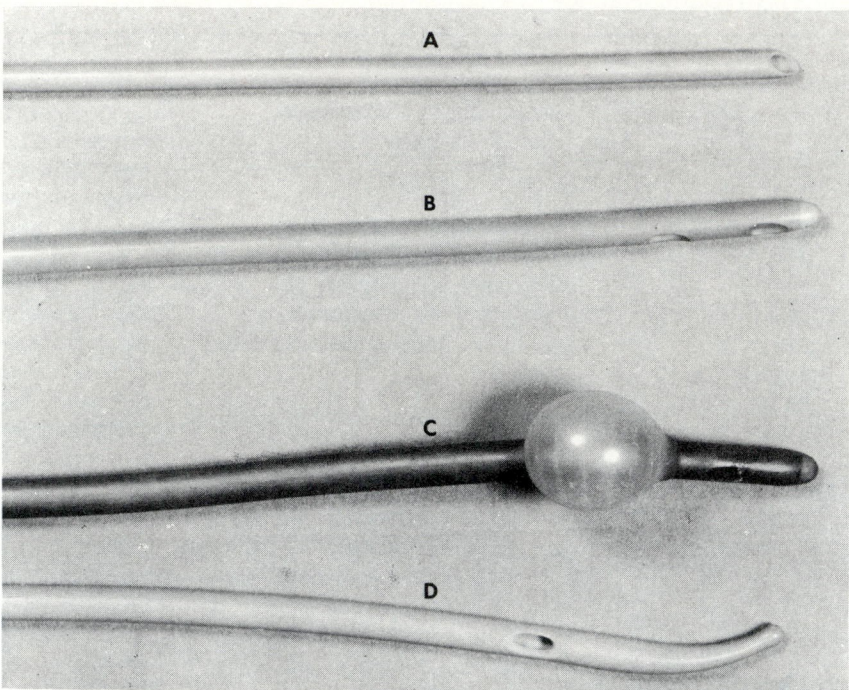

Fig. 32-6 Urethral catheters. **A,** Whistle-tip catheter. **B,** Many-eyed Robinson catheter. **C,** Foley catheter. **D,** Coudé catheter.

The *Foley catheter* is the most frequently used self-retaining catheter; it is used when continuous drainage is required. The Foley catheter has a double lumen with an inflatable balloon at the distal end. The balloon is inflated with either normal saline or sterile water after it has been placed well within the bladder (Fig. 32-7). Indwelling urethral catheters must be securely anchored to prevent

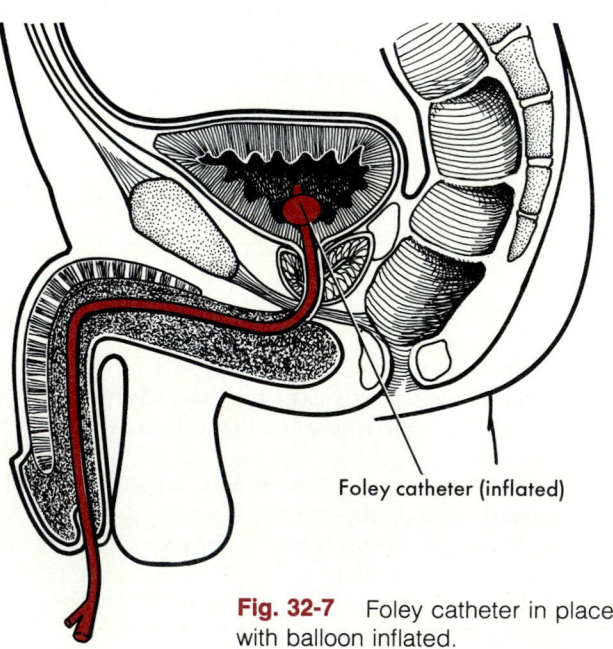

Foley catheter (inflated)

Fig. 32-7 Foley catheter in place with balloon inflated.

accidental dislodging of the catheter (Fig. 32-8). Proper anchoring will prevent accidental traction (possible injury to the bladder or urethra) and yet keep the catheter from moving in and out of the urethra (possible irritation and infection). Guidelines for maintenance of an indwelling urinary drainage system are listed in the box on p. 1135.

□ *Difficulties following catheter removal*

It is normal to note some dribbling of urine for a few hours after an indwelling urethral catheter has been removed because of dilation of the sphincter muscles by the catheter. Dribbling of urine that persists longer than a few hours is reported to the physician; this symptom may indicate damage to the sphincters. Stress incontinence may persist for several months if the catheter has been in place for more than a few days.

Inability to initiate voiding may occur when the catheter is removed. The person is encouraged to drink fluids to stimulate the sphincters and is assessed for distention. Measures to promote voiding are encouraged. Persons should not go longer than 8 hours without voiding unless fluid intake has been restricted.

Cystitis (inflammation of the bladder) may develop after catheter removal because of incomplete emptying of the bladder as muscle tone is reestablished. Any abnormalities in color, odor, or sediment in the urine are reported.

□ *Home care for persons with indwelling catheters*

It is not uncommon for persons to be discharged to home requiring catheter drainage on a temporary or permanent

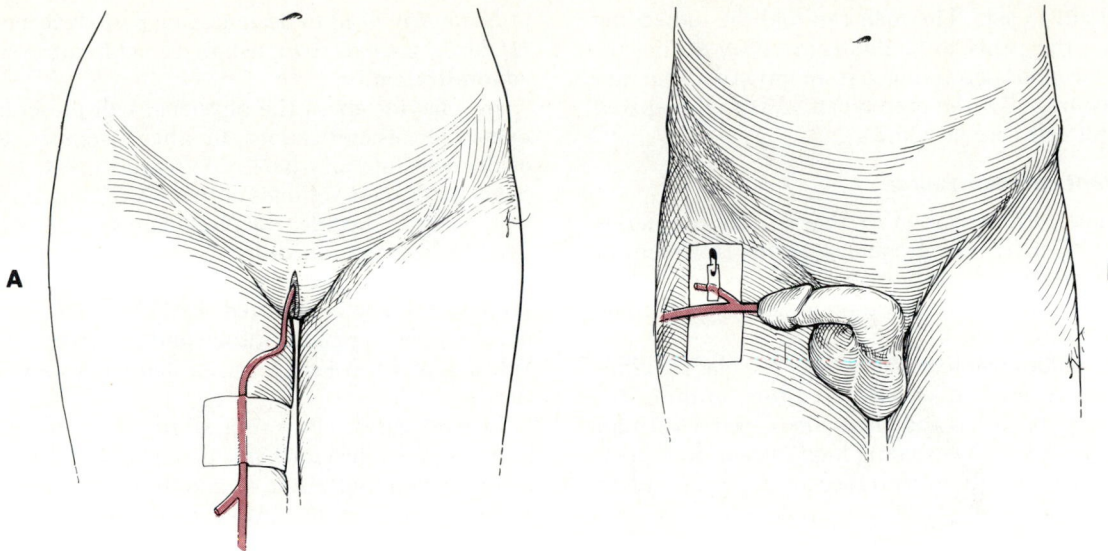

Fig. 32-8   Anchoring of Foley catheter. **A,** In female patient. **B,** In male patient. Proper anchoring prevents accidental traction that could result in injury to bladder or urethra and yet keeps catheter from moving in and out of urethra.

basis. Ideally, frequent disconnection of the catheter and drainage tubing should be avoided. However, persons at home must disconnect the tubing at night to change from a leg bag to the overnight drainage bag and reverse the procedure in the morning. To lessen the risk of contamination, the person should wash the hands and then wipe the catheter and tubing with 70% alcohol before disconnection and reconnection. The disconnected ends of the

drainage bags are protected with a connector cap or with a sterile gauze secured in place with a rubber band.

A shower or tub bath with a catheter in place is generally permitted unless there is an unhealed surgical incision. The adhesive tape holding the catheter in place will need to be replaced after bathing.

There is no need for men or women to remove an indwelling catheter before intercourse, a question persons

---

Maintenance of drainage system

Action	Rationale
Never disconnect the catheter except to irrigate	Prevent introduction of bacteria
Collect urine samples by inserting a small-bore needle into the drainage port that has been cleansed with alcohol or povidone-iodine.	Maintain closed system and prevent introduction of bacteria
Never elevate drainage bag above level of the patient's bladder or cavity being drained; suspend bag from the bed frame when the patient is recumbent and from below the knee when the patient is ambulatory.	Prevent reflux of urine back into bladder; drainage bags are available with antireflux valves
Drainage bags and tubing should never be allowed to rest on the floor.	Prevent contamination of system
Observe tubing for kinks and loops.	Obstructions will result in reflux of urine
Empty drainage bag into a measuring container that is used only for that particular patient; cleanse measuring container regularly.	Prevent cross-contamination of drainage system
Cultures of urine are usually ordered at regular intervals when a patient has an indwelling catheter.	Provides data on changing numbers and types of organism present in urine before symptoms appear
Observe collecting system daily for sedimentation and leaks.	Replace when sediment or leaks are present

may be hesitant to ask. The man can fold the indwelling catheter over the penis to facilitate insertion during intercourse. Questions pertaining to resumption of usual lifestyle are encouraged so the person can be as well prepared as possible for self-care at home.

□ *Intermittent catheterization*

Intermittent catheterization of the urinary bladder is being used with increasing frequency in the treatment of neurogenic bladder dysfunction secondary to spinal cord trauma, birth defects, urinary retention, and some chronic diseases.

Because periodic complete emptying of the bladder eliminates residual urine (an excellent culture medium for multiplication of bacteria) and maintains a good blood supply to the bladder wall by avoiding high intrabladder pressures, infections are often decreased, even when only a clean technique is used.

The goals of intermittent catheterization may vary from patient to patient but are generally to prevent urinary retention and its sequelae (UTI and renal damage) and to achieve continence. The patient should know exactly what is expected of the treatment plan to elicit full cooperation.

The hospitalized patient with intermittent catheter drainage of the bladder may be one for whom the treatment is temporary (as in the early phases of spinal cord trauma), one who is learning the technique for home use, or one who has been using intermittent catheterization before hospital admission. Even though the clean technique is suitable for home use, sterile technique is necessary during hospitalization to decrease the possibility of hospital-acquired infection when the catheterization is performed by hospital personnel. When hospitilized, the patient who customarily performs self-catheterization may continue to use clean technique if this method is used at home, but preferably a sterile catheter will be used each time or special precautions will be taken to store the reusable catheter in a closed container. Specimens for culture must be obtained by the usual sterile catheterization technique to avoid contamination of the specimen. The patient is informed about the reasons why sterile precautions are necessary in the hospital setting.

A No. 14 Fr Robinson catheter is generally used for an adult. The volume of urine obtained with each catheterization is recorded to ensure that schedule adjustments can be made if necessary. The adult bladder should not be permitted to hold more than 300 ml at any time, since greater amounts lead to overdistention of the bladder with greater susceptibility to infection. The frequency of catheterization is determined by the amount of residual urine (more than 200 ml means that more frequent catheterization is necessary). Usually such individuals will need catheterization every 4 to 6 hours. A small amount of residual urine (less than 200 ml) after voiding means that the person will only need to do self-catheterization every 8 to 12 hours. Some persons eventually will be able to manage with once-a-day catheterization. Some individuals may also have to catheterize themselves at night if they have a large output of urine at night. It is important to realize that the person who normally does not perform self-catheteriation at night

at home may need to do so during periods where the fluid intake is greater than usual, as with intravenous fluid administration.

In some instances the physician will prescribe the frequency of catheterizations; in other instances, adjustment of the schedule may be a nursing judgment. If the nurse notes that excess volumes of urine are being obtained with a prescribed schedule, the physician is consulted about the need to alter the schedule.

Color, clarity, and odor of the urine are noted; and any symptoms of a UTI reported. Periodic urine specimens are obtained and sent for culture and sensitivity. Some individuals are given long-term antibiotic therapy prophylactically.

In most cases, clean (not sterile) catheterization technique is prescribed for home use. Hand washing is advised before each catheterization, and the meatal area is cleansed with soap and water. After inserting the catheter and draining the bladder, the catheter is removed and washed with soap and water before being stored in a clean, closed container for the next use. The catheter is reused until it becomes either too soft or too hard to be directed properly.

Most individuals require much support during the actual teaching but very quickly become comfortable with the procedure. Initially, a mirror is used to teach women where to place the catheter. The woman should learn to catheterize while sitting on the commode, using palpation to locate the urethral meatus. Men may sit or stand to catheterize themselves. It is important that men use generous amounts of lubricant to avoid urethral irritation; women generally do not require lubrication of the catheter.

If sterile catheterization technique is needed for home use, more time and practice will be required to learn good sterile technique. Careful explanation of sterilization of equipment must be provided, and planning for adapting sterile intermittent self-catheterization to the individual's usual life-style must be worked out with the person.

If teaching of self-catheterization is performed on an outpatient basis or if hospitalization is short, follow-up for adjustment of schedule and other concerns of adaptation to home routine should be provided. This may be done by the primary nurse, by the physician, or by referral to a home health care nurse. Ongoing urologic care with periodic urine cultures is essential.

□ **Counseling and teaching**

Specific patient teaching depends on the underlying cause of urinary retention and need for indwelling catheter or intermittent catheterization.

1. Rationale for the type of care required
2. Maintenance of adequate fluid intake
3. Use of Credé method of emptying bladder
4. Intermittent catheterization: techniques, frequency, adaptation of catheterization routine to life-style, procurement of supplies, need for ongoing care
5. Indwelling urethral catheter: maintenance of catheter patency, caring for the equipment, dealing with catheter problems, procurement of supplies, need for ongoing care
6. Signs of retention to be reported to physician

✄ EVALUATION

Questions to ask in evaluation of the person with urinary retention may include the following:

1. Is the person experiencing any bladder discomfort?
2. Is the person drinking at least 3 L of fluid per day?
3. Is urinary output comparable to fluid intake?
4. Is the person emptying bladder with each voiding?
5. Does the person going home with an indwelling catheter or with intermittent catheterization know the required care?

■ Urinary incontinence

Urinary incontinence, the involuntary expulsion of urine, may be encountered in a number of temporary and permanent conditions. Inability to control urination is a problem that frequently leads to emotional distress and can seriously impair an individual's socialization patterns if not managed either by the person or by others in a way that makes the person feel physically and emotionally comfortable and socially acceptable. Several types of incontinence have been identified (Table 32-5).

■ PATHOPHYSIOLOGY

Persons with urinary incontinence often present baffling management problems. Solutions require that the nurse understand the physiologic basis of incontinence.

Bladder and sphincter control is necessary to have urinary continence. Such control requires normal voluntary and involuntary muscle action coordinated by a normal urethrobladder reflex. Understanding this coordinated sequence of nerve stimuli and muscle action will help the nurse understand how continence is maintained.

As bladder filling occurs, the pressure within the bladder gradually increases. The detrusor muscle (the three-layered bladder wall) responds by relaxing to accommodate the greater volume. When a certain point of filling is reached, usually 150 to 200 ml of urine, the parasympathetic stretch receptors located in the bladder wall are stimulated. The stimuli are transmitted through afferent fibers of the reflex arc to the reflex center for micturition. Impulses are then carried through the efferent fibers of the reflex arc to the bladder, causing reflex contraction of the detrusor muscle. The internal sphincter, which is normally closed, reciprocally opens, and the urine enters the posterior urethra. Relaxation of the external sphincter and perineal muscles follows, and the bladder content is released. Completion of this reflex act can be interrupted and voiding postponed through release of inhibitory impulses from the cortical center, which results in voluntary contraction of the external sphincter. If any part of this complex function is upset, there is apt to be urinary incontinence.

The five major causes of urinary incontinence and the nature of the incontinence they cause are outlined in Table 32-6.

Cerebral clouding is most common in the aged. In many instances the elderly person is incontinent because of a lack of awareness of the need to empty the bladder. This type of incontinence is often not associated with any definite pathologic problem at the cerebral level. Cerebral clouding also occurs in acutely ill persons, who may be so ill that cerebration is dulled. They may not be able to think or may not have the energy to exercise voluntary control. Likewise a person who is comatose is incontinent because of loss of the ability to control voluntarily the opening of the external sphincter. As soon as urine is released into the posterior urethra, the bladder contracts and empties. This is the reason why voiding sometimes occurs under anesthesia.

Infection anywhere in the urinary tract may lead to incontinence because bacteria in the urine cause irritation of the mucosa of the bladder and stimulate the urethrobladder reflex abnormally.

Table 32-5 Types of incontinence

Type	Definition	Related factors
Stress	Involuntary loss of <50 ml urine with increased abdominal pressure	Relaxed pelvic muscles associated with age, obesity, incompetent bladder outlet
Reflex	Involuntary loss of urine when a specific volume is reached, occurring at somewhat predictable intervals	Neurologic impairment such as spinal cord lesion
Urge	Involuntary loss of urine occurring soon after a strong sense of urgency to void	Decreased bladder capacity, bladder infection, increased fluid intake, increased urine concentration, overdistention of bladder
Functional	Involuntary unpredictable loss of urine	Sensory, cognitive, or mobility deficits
Total	Continuous and unpredicable loss of urine	Neurologic dysfunction; independent contractions of detrusor muscle as a result of surgery, trauma, or disease affecting spinal cord nerves; fistulas

Modified from North American Nursing Diagnosis Association; McLane, AM, editor: Classification of nursing diagnoses: proceedings of the seventh conference, St. Louis, 1987, The CV Mosby Co.

Table 32-6 Major causes of urinary incontinence

Cause of urinary incontinence	Factors involved				
	Awareness of need to void	Cortical ability to inhibit voiding	Reflex arc	Bladder response to filling	Result
Cerebral clouding	Impaired	Impaired	Intact	Normal	Uncontrolled voiding because of reflex response
Infection	Intact	Intact, but overcome by strong reflex response	Abnormally stimulated	Heightened	Voiding because of strong reflex response (urgency)
Disturbance of CNS pathways (cortical lesions)	Diminished	Impaired	Intact	Heightened	Voiding because of reflex response
Disturbance of urethrobladder reflex					
Upper motor neuron lesion	Destroyed	Destroyed	Intact but deranged	Heightened	Voiding because of reflex response
Lower motor neuron lesion	Destroyed	Destroyed	Destroyed or impaired	Diminished to absent	Distention or incomplete emptying
Tissue damage	Intact	Intact, but not functional because of poor muscle response	Intact	Normal	Loss of control of voiding because of muscular impairment

Disturbance of the central nervous system pathways may occur in diseases such as cerebral embolus, cerebral hemorrhage, brain tumor, meningitis, or traumatic injury of the brain. Adequate voluntary (cortical or cerebral) control of bladder function is prevented in these situations. Urgency incontinence may be present as a result of the inability to inhibit completion of the urethrobladder reflex by the higher centers.

Disturbance of the urethrobladder reflex may result from lesions of the spinal cord or damage to peripheral nerves of the bladder. This form of incontinence may be seen in persons with spinal cord malformations, injuries, or tumors, and those with compression of the cord caused by fractures of the vertebae, herniated disk, metastatic tumor, or postoperative edema of the spinal cord. This type of difficulty can result in two types of responses known as *neurogenic bladder*. The person with a neurogenic bladder has no way of knowing when voiding is occurring.

Lesions above the S2 level of the spinal cord or impairment of the cerebrocortical centers do not destroy the reflex arc for voiding, although they may derange it. Such lesions destroy the potential for cortical control to inhibit the reflex. The result is an "upper motor neuron" or "automatic" bladder. The bladder is hypertonic and has a small capacity (less than 150 ml). The increased detrusor tone and increased sensitivity to small amounts of urine present in the bladder result in precipitous reflex voiding and the potential for vesicoureteral reflux.

Damage to nerves in the cauda equina or sacral segments of the spinal cord may cause destruction of the reflex arc by interruption of its afferent, efferent, or central components. The result is a "lower motor neuron" or "flaccid" bladder. The bladder is hypotonic with capacities of 500 ml or more. Overflow incontinence, retention of residual urine, and the potential for vesicoureteral reflux are problems imposed by a hypotonic bladder.

Overflow incontinence is considered to be caused by pressure exerted on the distended bladder by the abdominal muscles. Residual urine, urine remaining in the bladder after incomplete emptying, provides a medium for the growth of bacteria, and a UTI is common.

Tissue damage to the sphincters of the bladder from instrumentation, surgery, or accidents, scarring following urethral infections, lesions involving the sphincter, or relaxation of the perineal structures may cause urinary incontinence. The latter cause of incontinence is seen occasionally following childbirth. The problem is local in nature and does not involve the nervous system.

ASSESSMENT

□ Subjective data

The following questions are asked when assessing incontinence:

1. Is there a total inability to control urination?
2. What is the frequency of incontinence?
3. Can anything be associated with precipitating incontinence (stress, fear, laughing, exercise)?
4. Is pain or burning present with incontinence?
5. Is there a state of awareness to void before incontinence?
6. Does dribbling occur?

□ Objective data

Important objective data to obtain include the following:

1. Volume of urine output
2. Characteristics of urine
3. Palpation of bladder to identify residual urine
4. Patient's level of consciousness to determine ability to cooperate
5. Patient's ability to follow directions
6. Is there a physiologic reason for incontinence (for example, spinal cord injury)

□ Diagnostic tests

Diagnostic tests should include an evaluation of renal functions. This is done by obtaining urinalyses, urine cultures, urine electrolytes, blood urea nitrogen, serum creatinine, and creatinine clearance.

Normally the bladder contains little or no urine after voiding; however, certain disease states inhibit the bladder from emptying completely. Some common conditions in which incomplete emptying of the bladder occurs are benign prostatic hypertrophy, urethral strictures, and interruptions in bladder innervation. Urine left in the bladder after voiding is called *residual urine.*

One way to determine the amount of residual urine is to *catheterize* the person immediately after voiding. This may be ordered by the physician on a one-time or on a repeated basis. Before catheterizing the person, the physician is consulted regarding the plan for establishing urinary drainage. If a large amount of residual urine is suspected, the physician may wish the catheter to be left in place in the bladder. *Residual urine volumes of 50 ml or less indicate near normal or returning bladder function.*

To avoid passing a catheter to measure residual urine volumes, x-ray examination of retained urine may be performed. In this procedure a radiopaque substance excreted by the kidneys is injected intravenously. As the dye is excreted in the urine, it passes into the bladder. A sufficient amount of urine containing the radiopaque material is allowed to accumulate in the bladder before the person is instructed to void. Immediately after voiding an x-ray film is taken. Any urine retained in the bladder will be visualized on the radiograph. This means of determining residual urine is used in conjunction with other studies requiring visualization of the urinary tract.

Cystometric examination is performed to evaluate bladder tone. In general, the examination is indicated when incontinence is present or when there is evidence of neurologic dysfunction of the bladder. A Foley catheter is inserted before the examination. After the person assumes a supine position, a liter bottle of normal saline or sterile distilled water and a cystometer are connected to the catheter. Fluid is instilled at a constant and specified rate; measurements of the pressure exerted on the fluid by the bladder musculature are recorded after the instillation of every 50 ml of fluid. The person is asked to report feelings of fullness, the need to void, and any urgency or discomfort. Fluid is instilled until urgency occurs or it is determined that the sensation is absent. During cystometric examination, bethanechol chloride (Urecholine) may be administered to determine its effect on enhancing the tone of a flaccid bladder, or an anticholingeric medication may be given to assess relaxation in a hyperactive bladder. There is no specific care required after cystometric examination.

Electromyography may be used to evaluate sphincter tone and intactness of nerve pathways.

DATA ANALYSIS: NURSING DIAGNOSES

Nursing diagnoses are determined from assessment of patient data. Possible nursing diagnoses for the person with urinary incontinence may include, but are not limited to, the following:

Diagnostic title	Possible etiologies
Bathing/hygiene, toileting self-care deficit	Cognitive impairment, depression
Body image disturbance	Loss of body functions, change in life-style, change in social involvement
Ineffective individual coping	Situational crisis, maturational crisis
Impaired home maintenance management	Unavailable support system, lack of knowledge
Functional incontinence	Altered environment, sensory deficit
Reflex incontinence	Neurologic impairment
Stress incontinence	Relaxed pelvic muscles, overdistention
Total incontinence	Neurologic impairment
Urge incontinence	Decreased bladder capacity, bladder infection, overdistention of bladder
Potential impaired skin integrity	Irritation
Altered patterns of urinary elimination	Sensorimotor impairment

PLANNING: EXPECTED PATIENT OUTCOMES

Expected patient outcomes for the person with urinary incontinence may include, but are not limited to, the following:

1. The person is free of perineal skin excoriation.
2. The person is free of urinary odor.

3. The person or significant others can describe or state the following:
   a. The relationship of adequate hygiene to the maintenance of skin integrity
   b. The relationship of adequate fluid intake to facilitate bladder training
   c. The bladder training plan
   d. How to care for minor skin problems if they occur
   e. How to obtain professional and community resources
      (1) Agencies that are available when necessary
      (2) How to obtain and maintain any needed supplies and equipment (drainage systems, commodes, protective padding, special beds)
      (3) Where and when to seek assistance if problems are encountered
   f. Plans for follow-up care

■ IMPLEMENTATION

□ Assisting with achievement of therapeutic goals

□ *Control of urinary incontinence*

No problem of bladder retraining or management of uncontrolled incontinence is likely to be successful without the cooperation of the individual involved. The probable outcomes of the management program should be included in planning for implementation of the program.

Control of urinary incontinence is largely dependent on its cause. Measures include treatment of associated conditions, programs of bladder retraining, surgical procedures, or the use of internal or external drainage devices. Both the person and nurse need to know that rehabilitation may take weeks or months to accomplish. The person often becomes discouraged by recurring accidental voiding and needs a great deal of encouragement. It is often helpful to teach the physiology of voiding so that there is better understanding of the problem. Consistency in carrying out any plan for bladder control is often the key to success.

□ *Sphincter dysfunction*

Repair of a sphincter that has been cut is almost impossible. When the *external sphincter* has been damaged, the person will be incontinent on urgency. A voiding schedule can be planned so that voiding occurs before the bladder is full enough to exert sufficient pressure to open the internal sphincter involuntarily. When the *internal sphincter* is damaged, there may be no acute feeling of the need to void. Here the problem is not one of incontinence but of retention. To assure regular emptying of the bladder, a regular voiding schedule is necessary. If both sphincters are damaged, there will be total incontinence.

□ *Stress incontinence*

Urinary incontinence that occurs during coughing, straining, or heavy lifting is termed *stress incontinence*. It is seen primarily in women who have relaxed pelvic musculature, but it may also occur in men following prostatectomy. When bladder pressure is suddenly increased, urine enters the proximal third of the urethra then returns to the bladder when the pressure is decreased after ex-

ertion. Some of the urine escapes through the urethra. Usually the person is continent at night because bladder pressure is decreased in the recumbent position.

CONSERVATIVE THERAPY. *Perineal exercises* are helpful in controlling mild stress incontinence. The exercises consist of tightening and relaxing perineal and gluteal muscles and can be performed in a number of ways. Much of the problem of incontinence caused by a relaxed perineum in women can be prevented if perineal exercises are taught before and following childbirth. These exercises also may be included as part of the health teaching of any woman. Following are different methods for performing perineal exercises.

1. Tighten the perineal muscles as if to prevent voiding. Hold for a count of 10, then relax (Kegel exercises, see Chapter 34).
2. Inhale through pursed lips while tightening perineal muscles.
3. Bear down as if to have a bowel movement. Relax then tighten perineal muscles.
4. Hold a pencil in the fold between the buttock and thigh.
5. Sit on toilet with knees held wide apart. Start and stop the urinary stream.

SURGERY. Surgery may be indicated for severe stress incontinence. A *vesicourethropexy* (Marshall-Marchetti-Krantz operation) consists of fixation of the urethra to the fascia of the rectus muscle of the abdomen with support given to the neck of the bladder. A suprapubic incision is usually made, but a transvaginal repair may be carried out if there is scar tissue around the urethra from vaginal surgery. A urethral catheter is inserted postoperatively and maintained for 5 to 6 days. The urine may be pink, but the urethral catherer is not irrigated as a rule. It is not uncommon for difficulty in voiding to be experienced immediately after the indwelling catheter is removed. The woman is observed for signs of vaginal bleeding. Straining and use of Valsalva's maneuver should be avoided until healing has occurred, and mild laxatives may be given to prevent straining from constipation. Surgeons differ in the amount of activity permitted in the early postoperative period.

A newer surgical procedure that is less invasive is the *Stamey* procedure, a suspension of the bladder neck by sutures passed adjacent to the ureterovesical junctions.[10] A small incision is made above and lateral to the symphysis pubis. The needles are introduced suprapubically and the positions are checked by cystoscopy (a bulge can be noted at the junction wall) before suturing. The procedure is then repeated on the opposite side. A percutaneous suprapubic catheter is inserted following the suturing; the catheter is removed when spontaneous voiding occurs, which may take several days. There is minimal postoperative discomfort. Antibiotics are given for 2 weeks postoperatively. The patient should refrain from sexual activity until permitted (usually 1 to 2 months).

□ *Urge incontinence*

Incontinence caused by urinary tract infection (UTI) is generally temporary, responding to treatment of the infection by systemic antibiotics. Specific causes of infection such as obstruction must be identified and corrected when possible. Provision must be made for adequate fluid intake of 3000 ml or more per day unless contraindicated by the person's medical condition. Because of heightened bladder sensitivity to even small amounts of urine, urgency to void demands rapid response by the nurse to the request for help to void.

The person who has a brain tumor, meningitis, or traumatic injury to the brain that prevents adequate voluntary control of bladder function and causes urgency incontinence by inhibiting cortical control over the urethrobladder reflex may also respond to a bladder retraining program. If the person's condition or response prohibits such a program, an internal or external drainage device should be used.

□ Neurogenic bladder dysfunction

Persons with injuries of the spinal cord experience a transitory period of "spinal shock" in which urinary retention occurs. This is treated with continuous or intermittent catheter drainage that aims to prevent a UTI and overdistention of the bladder. Following this acute stage, further management depends on the exact nature of any residual neurogenic bladder dysfunction. Persons with a lesion above the sacral segments and who have an intact urethrobladder reflex may initiate voiding by pinching or stroking trigger areas of the thighs or suprapublic area. In persons with a lower motor neuron lesion, the use of the *Credé method,* which consists of exerting manual pressure over the bladder, may be ordered to provide for more complete bladder emptying. The appropriateness of this technique must be determined by the physician as based on the person's complete urologic status. An increasing number of persons with neurogenic bladder dysfunction are being taught intermittent self-catheterization using clean technique to prevent infection and manage incontinence. Maintenance of a regular schedule is stressed, and the frequency of catheterization is determined on an individual basis.

Certain medications are sometimes used alone or in conjunction with an intermittent catheterization program in the management of incontinence related to neurogenic bladder dysfunction. Alpha adrenergic drugs such as ephedrine sulfate are used to increase urethral resistance. Anticholinergic drugs such as propantheline (Pro-Banthine) are prescribed to control the reflex bladder activity.

□ Urinary drainage for incontinence

Occasionally there are justifications for the use of an indwelling catheter for the incontinent patient. Such reasons include the need to protect a surgical incision or to permit healing of a decubitus ulcer in the area. Indwelling catheterization, however, presents many potential dangers, such as UTI, urethritis, epididymitis, and urethral fistulas. All other means to manage incontinence should be tried before resorting to catheterization. Proper catheter management is essential.

In males, *external drainage* can be easily accomplished by

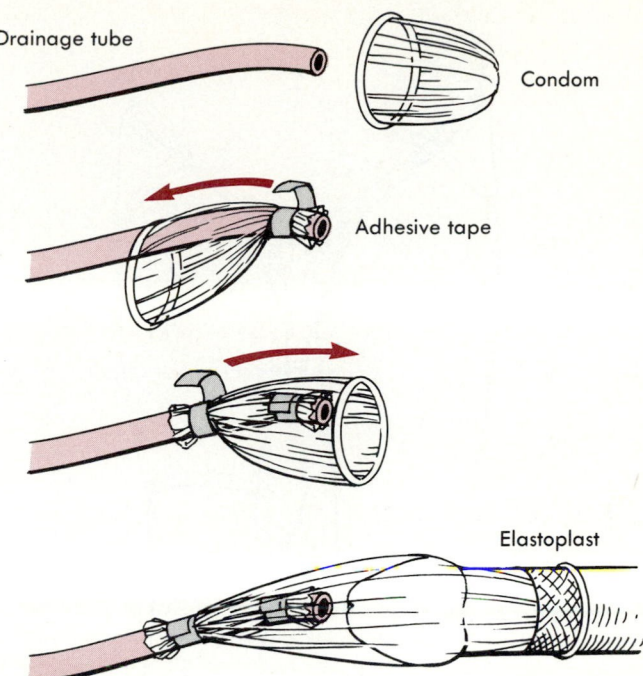

Fig. 32-9 One method of making external drainage apparatus.

applying a watertight apparatus to the penis. The following is one method. Select a condom of the correct size. Puncture a hole in the closed end of the condom with an applicator stick. Attach the punctured end of the condom to a firm rubber or plastic drainage tube with either a 3 mm (⅛-inch) piece of rubber tubing or a strip of adhesive tape (Fig. 32-9). Before applying the condom, clean and dry the penis thoroughly and check it for edema, skin breaks, or discoloration. Invert the condom and roll it onto the penis. There should be no roll at the top that could cause constriction. At least 2.5 cm (1 inch) of the condom should remain between the meatus and drainage tube to allow for penile erection. There should not be so much slack as to cause twisting and subsequent interference with drainage. Elastoplast is then applied over the condom and around the penis (never touching the skin). *Under no circumstances should adhesive tape be used.* The Elastoplast must not be constricting.

The external catheter should be removed daily, and the skin washed and checked. Frequent checking is necessary to determine whether edema or irritation is present and to ensure proper drainage. This is especially important in men with loss of sensation. The external device is attached to straight drainage or to a leg bag.

For persons who need external catheter drainage indefinitely, a rubber urinary appliance (sometimes called an incontinence urinal) may be used (Fig. 32-10). There are several models available, and the one best suited to the person's needs is selected. Two appliances are recommended to allow for cleaning and drying. They should be washed in mild soap, turned inside out, and thoroughly dried before using.

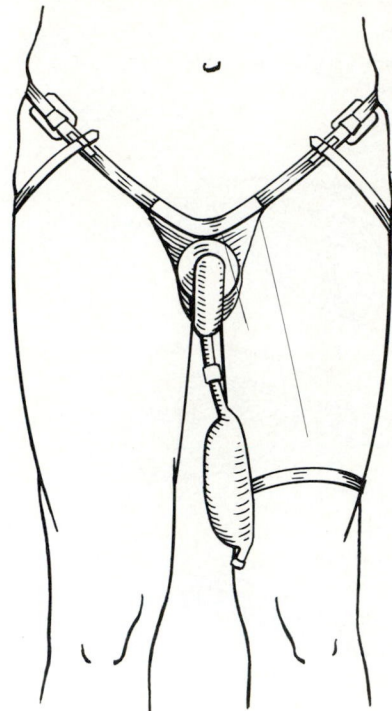

Fig. 32-10 Rubber urinary appliance. Bag is emptied by drain valve at bottom of bag.

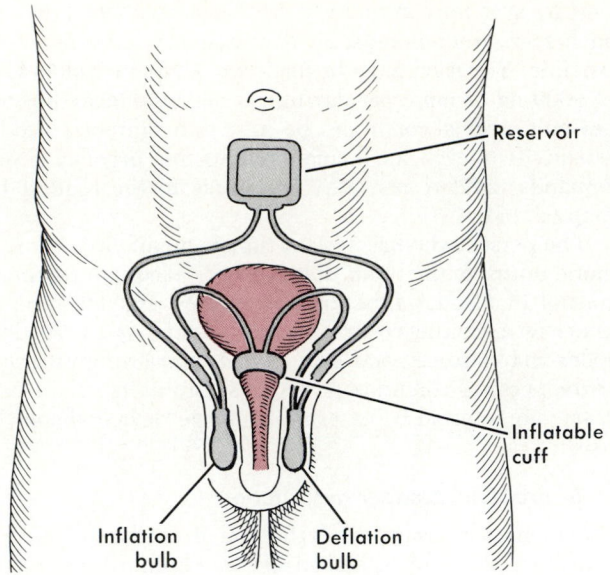

Fig. 32-11 Artificial bladder sphincter. Compression and release of inflation pump bulb inflates cuff surrounding urethra stopping urine flow. Compression and release of deflation pump bulb deflates inflatable cuff, returning fluid to storage reservoir. This releases urethral constriction, permitting urine to flow.

Most persons prefer to manage their own incontinence if they are at all able to do so. The nurse supports and encourages this, offering assistance as necessary and instruction in basic principles of skin care, equipment selection, and maintenance. The choice of management method should take into account the person's ability to manage as independently as is possible.

Implantation of an *artificial urinary sphincter* can be used to achieve continence when other methods have failed. In this procedure a hydraulically activated sphincter mechanism is placed around the urethra or bladder neck. The sphincter is made to open and close at will by squeezing one of two bulbs implanted under the skin of the labia or scrotum (Fig. 32-11). Postoperative nursing care of the person with such an implant includes observation for and reporting of fever or pain on inflation of the device, swelling of the genitalia, and recurrence of incontinence. Complications of the procedure include erosion of the urethra, abscess, cellulitis, and mechanical malfunctions in the system. Men have had more success with the artificial sphincter than have women.

In some instances none of the above measures are appropriate or successful. Therefore, nursing goals of assisting the person to remain clean, free of odor, and free of decubiti may require external urinary protection; the type varies with the sex, functional status, and physical status of the person. Interventions that nurses can carry out independently include the following:

1. Encourage fluids to the limits of any prescribed restriction.

2. Use aseptic techniques when handling the urinary drainage system.
3. Evaluate patient for participation in a bladder retraining program.
4. Encourage activity to prevent stasis of urine.
5. Give meticulous skin care to prevent breakdown (essential).
6. Encourage self-care of incontinence, whenever possible.
7. Be supportive to patient by providing a relaxed atmosphere when providing care for incontinence.

□ **Assisting with comfort and ADL**

Because the person who experiences incontinence may at times have bladder control, the nurse should respond immediately when assistance to toilet is requested. Offer assistance to toilet shortly after each meal. The person should also be encouraged to limit intake of fluids for 2 to 3 hours before bedtime.

Meticulous skin care is absolutely essential when caring for the person with urinary incontinence. Without proper cleansing, the person will be subject to skin breakdown, which, as a result of continued incontinence, is extremely difficult to heal. When a person who is incontinent also has a diminished level of consciousness, the person should be assessed frequently to ensure dryness. A person who has been incontinent must be cleaned and dried immediately.

Low airflow beds (Flexicare) are showing promise in control of skin breakdown in immobile patients. This therapy offers some hope in the care of the bedridden incontinent person. The protective cover of the bed provides a one-way barrier that draws water away from the patient and assists in keeping the patient dry. The airflow also aids in drying the skin.

□ Counseling and teaching

The individual with urinary incontinence often experiences alterations in body image. The person must receive adequate counseling to deal with this problem. Counsel the person about available resource and support groups that exist in the community. The person should also be encouraged to resume an active life-style whenever possible. Teaching must include the following:

1. Care of any drainage systems that may be used
2. Perineal exercises for control of stress incontinence
3. Measures to maintain skin integrity
4. Signs and symptoms of urinary tract infection (frequency, dysuria)

□ *Bladder retraining*

When incontinence is caused by dulled cerebration in the elderly, by confusion, or by acute illness, control can usually be established if a persistent retraining schedule is carried out (see the box below). A voiding schedule is developed and must be strictly adhered to until the person gradually relearns to recognize and react appropriately to the feeling of having to void. A successful program of this type, leading to complete rehabilitation, or continence, requires mental competence of the individual. Otherwise someone else must always remind the person to follow the schedule. However, with proper support, bladder retraining is possible even when the incontinent person is not fully mentally competent.

People ordinarily void on awakening, before retiring, and before or after meals. If a diuretic such as coffee has been taken, it is usually necessary to void about 30 minutes later. Using this knowledge, the nurse can begin to set up a schedule for placing the person on a bedpan or taking the person to the toilet. Then if a record is kept for a few days of the times the person voids involuntarily, it is usually

possible to determine the normal voiding pattern. If the schedule based on the pattern of incontinence is not successful, toileting every 1 to 2 hours should be carried out on a 24-hour basis.

During the retraining program, *mobilization* of the individual, attention to the *position* assumed for voiding, and adequate *fluid intake* contribute to reduction of the possibility of infection. Complete emptying of the bladder eliminates the possibility of residual urine acting as a medium for bacterial growth, while a high fluid intake provides for internal bladder irrigation.

Elderly persons isolated from their families and familiar surroundings, confused by institutionalization, or suffering feelings of loss of self-esteem frequently respond well to mobilization in bladder retraining programs. Their circulation is enhanced by the imposed mobility, their awareness is increased, and they respond to the attention given them. In instances in which nurses believe that it is easier to change bed linen than it is to establish an appropriate bladder retraining program, a disservice is done to the individual and more work is actually created for the nurse. The person becomes subject to UTI and skin breakdown, and feelings of worthlessness are increased. For those who can be continent, incontinence is an indignity.

When it is possible, toileting should be carried out in surroundings that will remind the person of the voiding function; that is, the person should be taken to the bathroom where the toilet can be used. If this is not possible, a bedside commode can be an adequate substitute. Many men can void into a urinal more easily if allowed to stand at the bedside. The use of a bedpan is unfamiliar and distasteful to most persons, but in instances where women must remain in bed, voiding into a bedpan can be facilitated if the head of the bed is rolled up as high as allowed. This kind of positioning is more consistent with the position normally assumed for voiding and facilitates complete emptying of the bladder. Few persons can void adequately in the supine position.

Providing adequate amounts of fluids, a minimum of 3000 ml per day, is necessary to ensure that there will be adequate amounts of urine produced and present in the bladder to stimulate the voiding reflex at the proper times. Fluids may be given at scheduled times, the largest portion being given during the day before 4:00 PM to decrease the frequency of voiding through the night. Persons on fluid restriction because of medical problems should, of course, receive no more fluids than the amount prescribed.

⊞ EVALUATION

Questions to ask for evaluation include the following:
1. Is adequate urinary drainage being maintained?
2. Is the patient aware of professional and community resources available?
3. Can the patient state maintenance of necessary equipment?
4. Is the patient's skin free of excoriation?
5. Can the patient state plans for follow-up care?
6. Can the patient describe bladder training program?

Bladder retraining

1. Establish patient's usual voiding patterns.
2. Plan toileting based on the patient's usual pattern; assist patient as necessary.
3. If no voiding pattern can be determined, plan toileting for every 1 to 2 hours.
4. Encourage patient to use normal toileting position.
5. Encourage patient to empty bladder completely.
6. Provide for a fluid intake of 3000 ml/day for adequate urine volume.
7. Schedule most fluids to be taken before 4 PM.

■ URINARY TRACT INFECTIONS

UTI is a significant source of morbidity in the United States and also is significant in the development of chronic renal failure. Infection occurs in both acute and chronic stages in all portions of the urinary tract.

Table 32-7 summarizes factors contributing to infection of the urinary tract. Although the great majority of non-complicated urinary infections are asymptomatic and clear spontaneously, there remains a portion significant enough to warrant consideration as a health problem. There is no controversy among those practicing preventive health care regarding the question of the need for screening of asymptomatic infections; however, there exists difficulty in identifying the specific risk groups in which the detection and treatment of these infections yield significant improvement in the person's health. As the health care of our population becomes more oriented toward prevention of health problems, specific target populations will be better defined and the number of screening programs for asymptomatic UTI will increase.

Females seem more predisposed to UTI than males. Factors postulated in their higher infection rates include a shorter urethra close to the rectum and the lack of prostatic fluid protection present in the male. Infection rates for females approximate 1% of school-aged girls and 4% of women through the childbearing years.[11] Incidence of infection in females increases directly with sexual activity and with aging. Pregnancy does not seem to increase infection rates, although spontaneous clearing of infections is decreased during pregnancy, and there is a higher incidence of acute kidney infections progressing upward from the lower urinary tract.

Structural and functional abnormalities of the urinary

Table 32-7 Risk factors associated with development of UTI

Risk factor	Common examples
Female	Short urethra
Structural abnormality	Strictures
	Incompetent ureterovesical junction anomalies
Obstruction	Tumors
	Prostatic hypertrophy
	Calculi
	Iatrogenic causes
Impaired bladder innervation	Congenital spinal cord malformation
	Spinal cord injury
	Multiple sclerosis
Chronic disease	Gout
	Diabetes mellitus
	Hypertension
	Sickle cell disease
	Chronic renal disease
Instrumentation	Catheterization
	Diagnostic procedures

tract, obstruction of the flow of urine, and impaired bladder innervation promote infection of the urinary tract. Mechanisms involved include stasis of urine, which provides a culture medium for bacteria; reflux of infected urine higher into the urinary tract; and increasing hydrostatic pressure.

Certain chronic health problems predispose persons to UTI by changing the metabolism of tissues, creating extrarenal obstructions, and altering the function and structure of kidney tissue. Common among these health problems are diabetes mellitus, gout, hypertension, polycystic kidney disease, multiple myeloma, and glomerulonephritis.

Instrumentation of the urinary tract is associated with high rates of infection. Catheterization, even when performed without breaks in asepsis, results in significant infection of the bladder. *Nosocomial infections* account for a sizeable percentage of all UTIs. Drug-resistant strains of *Staphylococcus* and *Pseudomonas*, along with various other organisms commonly found in hospitals, are frequently those involved in nosocomial UTIs. Prevention and control of all urinary tract infections can be most significantly influenced through a lowering of this nosocomial infection rate.

Urinary tract infections may occur in the upper portion of the urinary tract (pyelonephritis) or in the lower urinary tract (cystitis, urethritis). The etiology, signs and symptoms, and usual medical treatment of these conditions are described in Table 32-8.

■ Pyelonephritis

Pyelonephritis refers to bacterial infection of kidney tissue. This infection usually begins in the lower urinary tract and ascends into the kidneys. The lower UTI may be asymptomatic, and kidney involvement may be the first indication of infection in the lower tract. Often the diagnostic workup of a person with pyelonephritis reveals previously unknown urinary tract obstruction or the presence of other chronic kidney disease. *Escherichia coli* is the most common organism identified with pyelonephritis, and resistance to antibiotic therapy rarely results. Pyelonephritis is most commonly associated with (1) pregnancy; (2) obstruction, instrumentation, or trauma of the urinary tract; and (3) chronic health problems including diabetes, analgesic abuse, polycystic kidney disease, and hypertensive kidney disease.

The most significant efforts in preventing pyelonephritis are through early detection and adequate treatment of lower UTI. Anyone with symptoms of dysuria, cloudy urine, or frequent small voidings should be examined for UTI and appropriately treated. Persons complaining of fever and costovertebral tenderness should be encouraged to seek medical attention.

■ PATHOPHYSIOLOGY

Pyelonephritis is among the most common diseases of the kidney and occurs in both acute and chronic forms. Acute pyelonephritis is caused by bacterial infection. Bacterial infection can be a result of bacteria ascending the urinary tract to the kidneys. It may also develop as a result

Table 32-8 Urinary tract infections

Disorder	Etiology	Signs and symptoms	Medical therapy
Pyelonephritis	Bacteria from ascending route Hematogenous Lymphatic spread	Sudden fever Chills Costovertebral tenderness Leukocytosis WBCs in urine	Antibiotics Bed rest for acute episode Hydration
Cystitis/urethritis (lower UTI)	Bacteria from ascending route	Urgency Frequency Dysuria Suprapubic discomfort Cloudy urine with WBCs	Antibiotics Hydration
Prostatitis	Bacteria from ascending route Reflux of infected urine from bladder Introduction of rectal bacteria through direct, lymphatic, or hematogenous spread	Fever Chills Low back pain Perineal pain Urgency Frequency Dysuria Tender prostate Urethral discharge	Antibiotics Bed rest for acute episodes Sexual abstention Analgesics Stool softeners Sitz baths

of seeding of bacteria from the blood stream. Although acute pyelonephritis may temporarily affect renal function, rarely does it progress to the level of renal failure.

Chronic pyelonephritis also results from a bacterial infection, however, other factors such as urinary reflux and urinary tract obstruction also play a part. Chronic pyelonephritis destroys renal tissue permanently through repeated inflammation and scarring. The process of developing chronic renal failure from repeated kidney infections occurs over a number of years or after several extensive and fulminant infections. It is estimated that pyelonephritis represents the original diagnosis in one third of all persons with chronic renal failure.

ASSESSMENT

□ Subjective data

When pyelonephritis is suspected, it is important to obtain the following subjective data:
1. Presence of fever or chills
2. Nausea or vomiting
3. Presence of flank pain
4. Has the person experienced frequency or urgency
5. Has the person complained of fatigue
6. Is anorexia present

□ Objective data

Whenever pyelonephritis is suspected a urine specimen is obtained. The urine is examined for color, clarity, sedimentation, concentration, and odor. It is important that the person's temperature be taken at least every 6 hours because bacteremia may occur. The nurse should also assess for tenderness over the kidneys or flank areas on palpation.

□ Diagnostic tests

Diagnostic tests include urinalysis to assist in determining the level of functioning of the kidneys. A urine culture and sensitivity should also be obtained (p. 1149). Blood cultures may also be necessary to identify the source of infection. Renal biopsy (p. 1152) may be required in chronic pyelonephritis to make the differential diagnosis.

A number of radiologic examinations may be necessary to evaluate the patient with suspected pyelonephritis, particularly in the chronic form. These examinations and their nursing implications are listed in Table 32-9.

□ *Maintaining hydration*

Large amounts of free-flowing urine help to wash away ascending bacteria in the urinary tract and to promote complete emptying of the bladder (urinary stasis provides a medium for bacterial growth). If urinary function is decreased, however, fluid overload may occur. Interventions, therefore, include the following:
1. Encourage fluid intake of more than 3000 ml/day unless contraindicated by oliguria or other symptoms of renal failure.
2. Assess intake and output every 8 hours.
3. Assess for signs of fluid overload (changes in mentation, moist breath sounds, peripheral edema, sudden weight gain).

□ *Medications*

The course of antibiotic therapy may extend over weeks, and the person may need to be reminded of the necessity to continue taking medication even when symptoms disappear. The urine is recultured 2 weeks after drug therapy has been discontinued and every month thereafter for the next several months. Should infection become chronic,

Table 32-9 Common radiologic examinations of the urinary tract

Test	Purpose	Procedure	Nursing implications
Retrograde pyelography	Visualization of urinary tract	1. Ureteral catheterization required 2. Radiopaque material (Hypaque, Renografin) gently injected 3. Radiographs are taken of the renal collecting structures	Patient may experience discomfort in region of kidneys as dye is injected Pain may be experienced if too large a volume of dye is injected and renal pelvis becomes distended
Intravenous pyelography (IVP)	Determine size and location of kidneys Demonstrate presence of cysts or tumors Outline filling of renal pelvis Outline ureters and bladder	1. Radiograph of abdomen (KUB) is taken to identify size and position of kidneys 2. Radiopaque dye is given intravenously 3. Radiographs of the kidneys are taken at 3-, 5-, 10-, and 20-minute intervals	Bowel cleansing required Fluids are often withheld for up to 8 hours to produce slight dehydration The patient is informed that a feeling of warmth, flushing of the face, and a salty taste in the mouth may occur as the dye is injected The patient is observed for signs and symptoms of a reaction to the dye including respiratory distress, diaphoresis, urticaria, instability of vital signs, or unusual sensations. Cardiopulmonary resuscitation equipment and emergency medications should always be available for immediate use.
Kidney, ureters, and bladder (KUB) radiograph	Gross visualization of kidneys, ureters, and bladder Calcifications and stones can be located	Radiograph of abdominal region obtained	Bowel cleansing may or may not be ordered
Urethrography	Visualization of urethral size and shape	Radiography of urethra taken after instilling 20 ml of radiopaque water-soluble lubricant	No special preparation
Computed tomography (CT)	Visualization of kidneys and renal circulation	Whole body CT scanner segments kidneys Can be done with IV contrast dye	If dye is used same implications apply as listed for IVP
Renal angiography	Visualization of renal circulation Particularly useful in evaluating renal artery stenosis	Procedure is similar to IVP, however, the contrast dye is often injected directly into the femoral artery by passing a catheter through the artery to the level of the renal arteries	Nursing implications are the same as in IVP Patient must be observed for bleeding at arterial puncture site, especially within first 4 hours; the pressure dressing is checked for fresh bleeding; the puncture site is checked for tenderness or swelling; vital signs and distal pulses must be assessed frequently (q 15 min × 4 hours); bed rest should be maintained for 8 hours after the procedure

Table 32-9 Common radiologic examinations of the urinary tract—cont'd

Test	Purpose	Procedure	Nursing implications
Renography	Visualization of urinary tract Measures renal bloodflow Measures renal tubular and excretory function	Involves scintillation scanning or photography Radioactive isotope such as iodo-hippurate sodium tagged with I^{131} or I^{125} is injected intravenously Scintillating probes placed over the kidneys record the photographs	Because only trace doses of bound isotopes are used, no special precautions are necessary
Ultrasound	Used to distinguish between abnormal fluid collections and solid masses. Used to identify obstructions and detect abscesses. Often used to diagnose abscesses, ureteral leaks, and obstructions in renal transplant recipients	Sound waves are used to outline internal body structures. The procedure is accomplished by computer interpretation of tissue densities	Procedure is painless and noninvasive. A full bladder assists in outlining structures

drug therapy may continue indefinitely; the goal is to reduce and control the bacterial population of the urinary tract to prevent renal damage.

➡ DATA ANALYSIS: NURSING DIAGNOSES

Nursing diagnoses are determined from assessment of patient data. Possible nursing diagnoses for the patient with pyelonephritis may include, but are not limited to, the following:

Diagnostic title	Possible etiologies
Fluid volume excess	Renal failure, compromised regulatory mechanism, excess fluid intake
Potential for infection	Renal failure, lack of knowledge, decreased nutrition
Altered nutrition: less than body requirements	Anorexia
Pain	Inflammation
Altered patterns of urinary elimination	Anatomical obstruction, urinary infection

⊡ PLANNING: EXPECTED PATIENT OUTCOMES

Expected patient outcomes for the person with pyelonephritis may include, but are not limited to, the following:
1. Person is comfortable.
2. Person does not appear malnourished.
3. Person or significant other can state or explain the following:
   a. Name, dosage, frequency, and side effects of medications

   b. Rationale for continued antibiotic therapy even when symptoms are no longer present
   c. Rationale and method for maintaining adequate fluid intake
   d. Signs and symptoms of kidney infection and the need to seek health care when symptoms occur
   e. Plan for follow-up urine cultures and health care

⊞ IMPLEMENTATION

☐ Assisting with achievement of therapeutic goals

Interventions include maintaining hydration, promoting nutrition if anorexia is present (see Chapter 31), and administering antibiotic therapy.

☐ Assisting with comfort

Medicate as prescribed for flank pain. Back massages often provide short-term relief of discomfort. Encourage rest during the acute phase to conserve energy for healing.

☐ Teaching

Points to be considered in teaching the person with pyelonephritis include the following:
1. Take the antibiotics for the prescribed period even after symptoms abate; infection may still be present even if asymptomatic.
2. Monitor urinary output and report decreased output (may indicate decreased renal function).
3. Monitor weight daily until therapy is discontinued by physician; a sudden increase in weight indicates fluid retention.
4. Report signs of recurrence to physician (flank pain, fever, chills).

5. Report for ongoing medical follow-up as instructed; repeated urinary cultures will be needed to identify recurrence.

✠ EVALUATION

Evaluation of the person with pyelonephritis is based on nursing diagnoses and goals. Questions to ask in this evaluation process include the following:

1. Is the person comfortable?
2. Is the person maintaining an adequate fluid and nutritional intake?
3. Can the patient state the need to maintain antibiotic therapy after symptoms subside?
4. Does the patient know the signs and symptoms that should be reported immediately to the physician?

■ Lower urinary tract infections

Infections of the lower urinary tract involve the urinary bladder (cystitis) and the urethra (urethritis). The etiologic factors and general preventive and management principles are the same as for infections of the upper urinary tract. For further discussion on prostatitis see Chapter 34.

Three considerations are important in preventing infection of the lower urinary tract: (1) preventing or minimizing morbidity, which can accompany these infections; (2) preventing recurrence of the infection; and (3) preventing renal damage from untreated or inadequately treated ascending infection. Because individuals with a lower UTI seek medical attention as a result of symptoms or are identified through routine urinalysis or screening of populations at high risk, both education and the public and community health case findings assist in decreasing UTI and its complications.

The symptoms that bring the person to medical attention typically include urgency, burning on urination (dysuria), and slight to gross hematuria. Most persons, however, are asymptomatic or minimally symptomatic, the infection being identified only on routine examination of the urine. Bacteriuria and positive urine cultures serve as the basis for diagnosing a lower UTI. Growth of a single pathogen in excess of 1×10^5 organisms/ml of urine in a properly obtained and stored midstream specimen indicates infection.

■ PATHOPHYSIOLOGY

Most infections of the lower urinary tract result from gram-negative organisms, such as *Escherichia coli, Klebsiella, Proteus, Enterobacter,* or *Pseudomonas,* that originate in the person's own intestinal tract and ascend through the urethra to the bladder. During micturition, urine may flow back up the ureters (*vesicoureteral reflux*) and carry bacteria present in the bladder up through the ureters to the kidney pelvis. Whenever stasis of urine occurs, such as with incomplete emptying of the bladder, renal calculi, or genitourinary obstructions, the bacteria have a greater opportunity to grow and a more alkaline media, which favors their growth and multiplication.

A UTI will occur primarily when host resistance is impaired. The major factors in preventing a UTI are tissue integrity and blood supply.[47] A break in the surface of the mucous membrane lining permits the bacteria to invade the tissue and cause infection. Breaks in tissue integrity result from erosions caused by tips of indwelling catheters or rough-edged renal stones, from neoplasms, or from invasion of the tissue by parasites such as *Schistosoma*. In the bladder, blood supply to the tissues can be compromised when the pressure within the bladder is markedly increased, as may occur with overdistention of the bladder, contracture of the bladder neck, or obstruction of the urethra by an enlarged prostate, metastatic growth, or urethral stricture.

▦ ASSESSMENT

☐ Subjective data

Specific questions are directed at eliciting the presence of abnormal findings. *Dysuria* (painful urination) is usually described as "burning with urination" and is usually associated with frequency and urgency when a UTI is present. *Frequency* of urination is voiding at frequent intervals, either in small or large amounts; therefore, the approximate amount must be ascertained when the symptom is present. Small amounts may be caused by infection. Large amounts may be the result of an increased fluid intake or the effect of a diuretic. If frequency is associated with suprapubic discomfort and sense of fullness but not with dysuria, the cause may be retention of urine in the bladder with frequent overflow of the excess amounts. *Urgency* refers to the need to void immediately. It commonly accompanies frequency in persons with a UTI. A person with *nocturia* awakens at night with the need to urinate. Additional data include the number of times this occurs per night, the amount of fluid intake over 24 hours, and whether this is a change in the usual pattern.

Pain resulting from urinary disorders is located in different areas depending on the organ involved. Pain from the kidney is usually experienced over the kidney site in the back between the twelfth rib and the iliac crest (costovertebral angle). Pain from the ureters may begin over the kidney are but then radiate to the front along the course of the ureter and down into the groin. Pain from the bladder is usually suprapubic. Any discomfort from prostatic disease is usually felt in the perineum.

☐ Objective data

Objective data includes assessment of body temperature for fever and inspection of urine specimens for color, clarity, and odor (indicating presence of bacteria).

☐ Diagnostic tests

The most common diagnostic tests for UTI include urinalysis and urine culture with sensitivity testing. A clean-catch specimen is usually obtained for these tests.

☐ *Urinalysis*

Ideally, the urine specimen is collected from the first voiding of the day. This sample is preferable because it is concentrated and abnormal constituents are more likely to be present. The person is given a clean container in which to catch urine. Cleansing the meatus before collecting the specimen decreases likelihood of external contamination; mild soap followed by water or a special antiseptic solution may be used. At least 50 to 100 ml of urine is collected for the test to ensure a sufficient amount to determine specific gravity in addition to microscopic analysis. If analysis of the urine cannot be performed immediately, the specimen must be refrigerated to retard bacterial growth.

The urine is inspected for gross changes. Normal urine color varies from pale to deep yellow depending on the specific gravity. A very dark shade suggests that the urine may be concentrated (high specific gravity) or that there may be an increased excretion of bilirubin. Certain medications and foods may change the color of urine.

Hematuria, blood in the urine, may be detected overtly or may be present microscopically without visual signs. If blood is observed in the urine of a women having her menstrual period, the vaginal orifice can be blocked with cotton balls and an additional specimen obtained to ascertain the source of the blood. Hematuria without pain is usually caused by disease of the kidney, bladder, or prostate. Hematuria with pain may be the result of calculi, a clot from renal bleeding, or bladder infection.

Cloudy urine may result from precipitation of phosphate salts in an alkaline urine or from bacterial growth. A urinary or vaginal discharge may also give the urine a cloudy appearance.

☐ *Urine culture*

Urine cultures are used to confirm suspected infections, to identify causative organisms, and to determine appropriate antimicrobial therapy. Cultures are also obtained for periodic screening of urine when the threat of UTI persists.

Urine in a properly collected and stored sample is considered to be normal if it contains 10,000 or fewer organisms per milliliter. Organisms of this magnitude are the result of normal urethral flora and do not signify UTI. A UTI is diagnosed when bacterial counts in a properly collected and stored sample reach 100,000 or more organisms per milliliter and the organisms are of one or very largely one bacterial type.[56] Contamination of the urine specimen during collection is most likely when bacterial counts include predominant colonies of *Staphylococcus, Streptococcus,* and diphtheroids, when two or more organisms contribute significantly to the total bacterial count, or when repeated cultures yield differing results. All of these results are indicative of a need to repeat the culture, paying particular attention to the collection of the specimen and to its handling.

Specimens for urine culture may be obtained either by catheterization or by midstream voiding (see the box below). It should be made clear, however, that *urethral catheterization should never be used routinely in collecting urine for culture because of the risk of introducing additional bacteria into the bladder.* Catheterization may be necessary to obtain a sterile urine specimen when the person is unable to void after being adequately hydrated or if the person is incontinent of urine. When a catheter is passed, meticulous attention is given to nontraumatic aseptic technique. After urine flow from the catheter is established, 5 to 10 ml of urine should be collected directly into a sterile specimen container. Care must be taken to ensure that the rim and the inside of the container are not touched by the catheter or by the hands. If a culture tube with a cotton plug is used as specimen container, care must be taken to keep the tube upright to prevent moistening the cotton and thereby contaminating the specimen. Cultures may also be ordered on the urine taken from the renal pelvis during

---

Directions for collecting a midstream urine specimen

Equipment needed
Sterile container for the urine
Three sponges (cotton or gauze) saturated with cleansing solution

General directions
Only outside of collecting container is touched
Urine is collected in container well after urinary stream is started

Special directions
Female

Labia are kept separated throughout procedure
Meatus is cleansed with one front-to-back motion with each of the three cleansing sponges

Male

Foreskin is retracted if man is uncircumcised
Glans is cleansed with each of the three cleansing sponges

ureteral catheterization or when ureterostomy or nephrostomy tubes are in place.

In collecting a voided specimen for culture, the nurse must decide if the patient is capable of independently obtaining the specimen or if nursing or medical personnel will need to collect a midstream specimen. Most persons who are ambulatory and are given precise and unhurried direction will be able to collect their own midstream urine specimen.

The first voided specimen of the day should be used whenever possible because bacteria will be more numerous. If the specimen is not cultured immediately, refrigeration is mandatory to prevent growth of organisms in the specimen.

▶ DATA ANALYSIS: NURSING DIAGNOSES

Nursing diagnoses are determined from assessment of patient data. Possible nursing diagnoses for the person with lower UTI include, but are not limited to, the following:

Diagnostic title	Possible etiologies
Pain	Inflammation
Altered patterns of urinary elimination	Urinary infection

▦ PLANNING: EXPECTED PATIENT OUTCOMES

Expected patient outcomes for the person with lower UTI may include, but are not limited to, the following:
1. The person will have relief of symptoms.
2. The person will have sterile urine or bacterial urine count of less than 1×10^4 to 1×10^5.
3. The person will have identified or corrected any disease or abnormality that would contribute to reinfection or relapse.
4. The person or significant other can state or explain the following:
   a. Signs and symptoms of lower UTI
   b. When and how to take prescribed medication
   c. Plan for follow-up care including urine cultures
   d. Rationale and means of increasing fluid intake to 3 to 4 L/day

▦ IMPLEMENTATION

☐ Assisting with achievement of therapeutic goals

Treatment goals for a lower UTI include sterilizing the urine and identifying any illness or urinary tract abnormality that may be contributing to the infection. After culture and sensitivity studies a 10- to 14-day course of antibiotic therapy is instituted. It is crucial that urine culture be obtained before initiating drug therapy to ensure appropriateness of antimicrobial medication and to decrease the development of resistant strains of organisms. The urine should be recultured every few months during the following year to reconfirm urine sterility.

A more extensive urologic workup including IVP and voiding cystogram may be performed for men and young children after a repeated or even first, UTI or when infection does not abate. This workup is performed on women when infection occurs repeatedly or cannot be cleared up with treatment. The rationale for this extensive workup is that a UTI is not common in men and children and that a significant portion of infections in these populations, and in women with persistent infection, involves abnormality of the urinary tract.

Medications commonly used in the treatment of a UTI include urinary antiseptics such as sulfisoxazole (Gantrisin) or nitrofurantoin (Furadantin) and systemic antibiotics. Sulfonamides are widely used; they are usually effective against the organisms causing a large percentage of UTIs, are safe, and are less likely than most systemic antibiotics to contribute to growth of resistant organisms. Prescribed antibiotics must be given on time on a regular schedule to maintain adequate blood levels.

Additional interventions include increasing fluid intake to 3000 ml/day unless contraindicated. Increased fluids dilute the urine, which lessens irritations and burning, and provides a continual flow of urine to discourage stasis and multiplication of bacteria in the urinary tract. Sitz baths may provide comfort for persons with urethritis.

☐ Assisting with comfort and ADL

The person with a lower UTI may experience pain or itching in the perineum. Sitz baths may provide relief of these symptoms.

☐ Counseling and teaching

Patient education concerning the problem, the requirements for antibiotic therapy, and follow-up care should facilitate completion of drug regimens for eradication of bacteria. By educating the person about the causes, proper hygiene, and recognition of early symptoms, recurrences can be eliminated or treated early. This will reduce morbidity in the long run. Females should be instructed in good perineal hygiene.

✚ EVALUATION

The nurse's success in dealing with the person with lower UTI can best be evaluated by eradication of infection in the individual. The care of specific patients with lower UTI is evaluated on the basis of expected patient outcomes. General questions to ask include the following:
1. Is the person free of fever?
2. Is the person free of pain and itching?
3. Can the person describe the antibiotic regime?
4. Can the person describe signs and symptoms of UTI?
5. Can the person state follow-up plan for health care?

■ GLOMERULAR DISORDERS

Glomerular disorders, which are a group of diseases that result from injury to the glomeruli, are termed *glomerulonephritis*. The glomerulus plays an essential role in the

Classification of glomerular diseases

Primary glomerulonephritis

Acute diffuse proliferative glomerulonephritis
Rapidly progressive glomerulonephritis
Membranous glomerulonephritis
Minimal change disease
Membranoproliferative glomerulonephritis
Chronic glomerulonephritis

Secondary to systemic diseases

Systemic lupus erythematosus
Goodpasture's disease
Wegener's granulomatosis
Bacterial endocarditis
Diabetes mellitus

functioning of the kidneys; therefore, any injury to the glomerulus is likely to result in some change in renal functioning.

There are several different diseases of the glomerulus resulting in a number of classification systems to assist in defining glomerulonephritis[17] (see the box above). For purposes of discussion, in this chapter glomerulonephritis is discussed as either acute or chronic; the nephrotic syndrome is described as a component of glomerulonephritis. Table 32-10 provides a summary of the major glomerular disorders, including etiology, signs and symptoms, and medical therapy.

Acute glomerulonephritis

Glomerulonephritis is a disease that affects the glomeruli of both kidneys. Etiologic factors are many and varied; they include immunologic reactions (lupus erythematosus, streptoccal infection), vascular injury (hypertension), metabolic disease (diabetes mellitus), and disseminated intravascular coagulation (DIC). Glomerulonephritis exists in acute, latent, and chronic forms. The most common form of *acute glomerulonephritis* occurs 2 to 3 weeks after a streptococcal infection. Common sites of infection include the throat (tonsillitis, strep throat) and the skin (impetigo).

Children of preschool and grade-school age are most likely to develop the illness. Of all individuals developing acute poststreptococcal glomerulonephritis, approximately 1% to 2% will develop end-stage renal failure in which dialysis or transplantation is required to prevent death. Approximately 90% of children and 50% of adults with acute glomerulonephritis attain full recovery from illness, although recovery may require up to 2 years.[23] Little can be inferred from the severity of the acute episode regarding prognosis. Persons with mild illness may develop chronic disease, and those with severe illness may completely recover and have no recurrence of the illness.

Prevention of acute poststreptococcal glomerulonephritis involves prompt medical treatment of sore throats and upper respiratory tract infections. Cultures should be obtained, and when indicated appropriate antibiotics prescribed.

PATHOPHYSIOLOGY

Normal glomerular membranes consist of three types of cells: epithelium, basement membrane, and endothelium.

Table 32-10 Glomerular disorders

Disorder	Etiology	Signs and symptoms	Urine	Medical therapy
Acute glomerulo-nephritis	Poststreptococcal infection, systemic lupus erythematosus, hypertension, DM, disseminated intravascular coagulation	Headache, malaise, facial edema, mild fever, flank pain, oliguria, shortness of breath, elevated BUN and creatinine	Protein 1-3+, casts, blood	No specific therapy; antibiotics for residual streptococcus, bed rest, dietary protein and sodium restriction as needed
Chronic glomerulo-nephritis	May follow acute glomerulonephritis; often no history of infection	Usually asymptomatic initially, hypertension; may progress to renal failure	Albumin, casts, blood	No specific therapy; treatment for exacerbation of acute episodes
Nephrotic syndrome	Associated with allergic reaction, herpes zoster, diabetes mellitus, sickle cell disease, severe congestive heart failure, pregnancy	Massive edema with anorexia, fatigue, shortness of breath, hypoalbuminemia, hyperlipidemia	Large amount of protein, casts	No specific therapy; bed rest and corticosteroids for severe edema

Any or all three of these cells may be affected by glomerulonephritis. Acute glomerulonephritis is the result of an antigen-antibody reaction with glomerular tissue that produces swelling and death to capillary cells. The antigen-antibody reaction activates the complement pathway, resulting in chemotaxis of polymorphonuclear (PMN) leukocytes with release of lysosomal enzymes that attack the glomerular basement membrane (GBM). The response in the GBM is an increase in the three types of glomerular cells. The various disease entities tend to attack specific cells, therefore, differential diagnoses is usually made by renal biopsy. The ability to make a differential diagnosis has been greatly aided by the tremendous increase in knowledge about the immune system (Chapter 37).

Signs and symptoms reflect damage to the glomeruli with leaking into urine by protein (proteinuria) and red cells (hematuria). As the disease process continues, scarring occurs leading to decreased glomerular filtration producing oliguria and retention of water, sodium, and nitrogenous wastes. This results in fluid overloading, edema, and azotemia as noted by shortness of breath, dependent edema, headache, weakness, and anorexia.

ASSESSMENT

□ Subjective data

The person with acute glomerulonephritis is likely to present with some signs and symptoms of renal failure, and the person is assessed for changes in voiding patterns and presence of headaches and flank pain. Because glomerulonephritis frequently occurs after a streptococcal infection, the person may complain of recent flulike symptoms.

□ Objective data

Objective data include evaluation of the extent of fluid retention and characteristics of the urine, as a baseline for ongoing assessment and evaluation:
1. Breath sounds, for signs of rales (crackles)
2. Pitting edema of dependent body parts (legs, sacrum)
3. Body weight: weigh daily for increase
4. Blood pressure, for elevations
5. Urine, for signs of increased blood, cloudiness, casts, increased specific gravity

□ Diagnostic tests

The most important immediate diagnostic test is urinalysis to determine presence of proteinuria, hematuria, and cellular debris. BUN and serum creatinine are obtained to determine renal function. Immunologic tests such as antigen-antibody titers and immunoelectrophoresis may be obtained.

A composite urine for creatinine clearance and protein can also provide important information. Instructions for obtaining a composite urine specimen are provided in the box below.

□ *Renal biopsy*

The differential diagnosis for glomerulonephritis can often be difficult to establish. A renal biopsy may be necessary to assist in diagnosis and establishing a definitive treatment plan. The biopsy can be performed either through a skin puncture (closed biopsy) or through an incision (open biopsy). The use of a fluoroscopic guided needle biopsy now allows for most renal biopsies to be obtained by the closed method.

Inherent in taking a biopsy specimen of this vascular tissue is a potential threat of hemorrhage. Throughout the procedure, care is given to prevent and to detect early loss of blood. Before biopsy is performed, a thorough medical evaluation with particular attention to detection of any abnormality in bleeding or coagulation time is carried out. The patient's blood is usually typed and cross-matched with 2 units of blood; the blood is held for the patient until any threat of bleeding has passed.

An open biopsy carries less risk of hemorrhage and provides better visualization of the kidney; however, the risk of infection is increased, and a longer period of recovery is required.

PREPROCEDURE CARE. Preparation before biopsy includes discussing the procedure with the patient. Topics covered include the necessity for the examination, the procedure itself, the care to be anticipated, and any questions of concern to the patient. The preparation of the patient

---

Instructions for composite urine specimen

1. The bladder is emptied and the urine *discarded* at the appointed time to start the test.
2. Urine from *all* subsequent voidings is saved.
3. Specific directions for storing the urine should be given. Some specimens need to be kept cold during the collection period; some need preservatives added; some need no special care.
4. The person should void into a separate receptacle before defecation to prevent contamination of the specimen.
5. The bladder is emptied and the urine *added* to the collection at the appointed time to end the test.
6. The designated amount (properly labeled) is sent to the labortory.
7. If an aliquot (5 to 10 ml sample of the total specimen) is the designated amount, the total amount collected is (1) measured and recorded on the specimen requisition and (2) mixed well before the aliquot is selected.

is shared by the physician and nurse. In most institutions it is necessary to have the patient sign a special permit before having the biopsy performed. The biopsy may be carried out in the patient's room, in the radiology department, or in the operating room.

PROCEDURE. The procedure for *percutaneous (closed) biopsy* is as follows: Before the biopsy, the patient is taken to the radiology department for localization of the kidney. This is accomplished with a plain film, a dye contrast film, or fluoroscopic location. The position of the kidney in relation to body landmarks is marked on the skin in ink. The lower pole of the kidney is located, this being the site for biopsy, since it contains the fewest number of large vessels. The patient is then transported to the area where the biopsy will be performed. Sedation is usually not required except for children or adults who are restless and unable to relax sufficiently to follow necessary instructions during the test. The patient is placed prone over a sandbag or firm pillow and an additional soft pillow. The body should be bent at the level of the diaphragm, with the shoulders on the bed and the spine in straight alignment. Blood pressure and pulse rate are determined at this point and are recorded. Cleansing of the skin is carried out to remove as many surface contaminants as possible. The physician identifies the location for biopsy, and a local anesthetic agent is injected. As the biopsy is being taken, the patient is instructed to hold his or her breath. Pain may be felt in the kidney region as the tissue sample is taken. The needle is withdrawn immediately, and direct pressure is applied to the site for 20 minutes. A pressure bandage is then applied.

POSTPROCEDURE CARE. After the procedure the patient is turned supine and is kept flat and motionless for the next 4 hours. One small pillow may be used under the head. Coughing and other activity that increases abdominal venous pressure is to be avoided during this time. Blood pressure and pulse should be taken each 15 minutes for 1 hour, every 30 minutes during the next hour, and every hour for an additional 2 to 3 hours to assess for hemorrhage. The patient should remain in bed for at least 24 hours following the procedure. All urine is observed for hematuria, and bed rest is maintained until the urine is clear. Initially, the urine is likely to demonstrate blood, but rarely continues after a 24-hour period. Caution the person against any heavy lifting for a period of 10 days.

DATA ANALYSIS: NURSING DIAGNOSES

Nursing diagnoses are determined from assessment of patient data. Possible nursing diagnoses for the person with acute glomerulonephritis may include, but are not limited to, the following:

Diagnostic title	Possible etiologies
Activity intolerance	Generalized weakness, electrolyte imbalance
Fluid volume excess	Renal failure, compromised regulatory mechanism, excess fluid intake, excess sodium intake

Diagnostic title	Possible etiologies
Potential for infection	Increased susceptibility
Altered nutrition: less than body requirements	Anorexia
Altered patterns of urinary elimination	Renal failure

PLANNING: EXPECTED PATIENT OUTCOMES

Expected patient outcomes for the person with acute glomerulonephritis may include, but are not limited to, the following:

1. Person does not display signs or symptoms of fluid volume excess.
2. Person maintains adequate nutritional intake.
3. Person remains free of signs and symptoms of infection.
4. The person or significant other can explain the following:
   a. The rationale for therapy (prolonged bed rest, maintenance of fluid balance)
   b. Dietary changes (decreased sodium intake, adequate caloric intake, controlled protein intake)
   c. Medication program to be followed at home
   d. Plans for a health maintenance program to include:
      (1) Measures to prevent further infection
      (2) Signs and symptoms that require immediate medical attention
      (3) Plans for follow-up health care

IMPLEMENTATION

Assisting with achievement of therapeutic goals

The care of the person with acute glomerulonephritis can be complex because of the overall ramifications of the disease. The following section emphasizes some of the aspects of this care.

Control of infection

Persistent infection is treated promptly to help further decrease antigen-antibody complex formation. Persons with poststreptococcal glomerulonephritis are given a prophylactic antibiotic; the drug of choice is penicillin. Rationale for this therapy is based on preventing further infections that could reactivate the nephritis. Prophylactic therapy may be continued for months after the acute phase of illness. Exposure to any infection must be avoided, because even mild infections may reactivate nephritis.

Activity

Bed rest is instituted until clinical signs disappear; this may involve a period of several months. Ambulation is allowed when blood sedimentation rates and blood pressure are normal and edema abates. If ambulation causes an increase in proteinuria or hematuria, bed rest is reinstituted. Because the period of bed rest may be long and the person usually does not feel ill, the nurse may need to continue reinforcing the importance of bed rest and assist in planning diversionary activities and the constructive use of time. For small children this can present no small problem. When bed rest is reinstituted after periods of ambulation, the person may become depressed. Helping the person to express concerns and feelings can serve as a basis for helping to make realistic plans about the illness and its sequelae.

☐ *Maintenance of fluid balance*

Edema and fluid overloading are anticipated and treated initially with dietary sodium restrictions. The amount of restriction depends on the severity of fluid retention, and it is maintained until dependent edema and circulatory overload are no longer a problem. Diuretics are generally reserved for managing severe fluid overload and pulmonary edema. The nurse is constantly alert for signs of fluid overload. Blood pressure elevation is treated with antihypertensive drugs only after fluid control has proved unsuccessful in controlling hypertension. Dietary protein is reduced only when BUN and creatinine levels are elevated. The diet should contain sufficient carbohydrate to prevent protein being used for energy. This helps maintain nitrogen balance.

☐ **Assisting with comfort and ADL**

Because of the need for bed rest during the acute phase of this disease, the person may need to have assistance with most ADL. As the condition progresses, the nurse closely assesses the person's ability to carry out ADL. Activity, as tolerated, is encouraged during all phases of recovery. Pain medication is administered, as prescribed, for flank pain.

☐ **Counseling and teaching**

Because of the long-term nature of glomerulonephritis, patient teaching is important. The person generally shows little to no change from normal in renal function, but proteinuria, hematuria, and cellular debris may exist microscopically. Although fatigue may be present, these persons usually feel well, therefore, they often must be convinced of the need to continue prescribed treatment and to return to routine follow-up care. Teaching includes the following:

1. Nature of the illness
2. Effect of diet and fluids on fluid and electrolyte balance
3. Medication regimen (dose, frequency, side effects)
4. Need to pace activities and rest when fatigue is noted
5. Avoidance of trauma and infection (may exacerbate the illness)
6. Signs and symptoms indicating need for medical attention (hematuria, headache, edema, hypertension)
7. Importance of follow-up health care

✚ EVALUATION

Questions to ask for evaluation may include the following:
1. Are signs of fluid retention decreased?
2. Is the person eating a balanced diet according to prescribed guidelines (low salt, sufficient carbohydrate)?
3. Are signs of infection absent?

4. Can the person tolerate activity without undue fatigue?
5. Can the person describe the nature of the disease and self-care activities?

■ Chronic glomerulonephritis

Although chronic glomerulonephritis (CGN) may follow the acute disease, the majority of persons give no history of the disease. In most instances no evidence of predisposing infection can be found. The course of chronic glomerulonephritis is extremely varied. Some persons with minimal impairment in renal function continue to feel well and show little progression of disease. With other individuals the progression of renal deterioration may be slow but steady and end in renal failure. In still other individuals the progression of disease is rapid.

■ PATHOPHYSIOLOGY

CGN is characterized by slow progressive destruction (sclerosis) of glomeruli and gradual loss of renal function. The glomeruli have varying degrees of hypercellularity and become sclerosed (hardened) as the disease progresses. This results in decreased renal function and increased presentation of signs and symptoms of renal failure. The kidneys decrease in size; eventually there is tubular atrophy, chronic interstitial inflammation, and arteriosclerosis[47] (Fig. 32-12). The underlying pathophysiologic

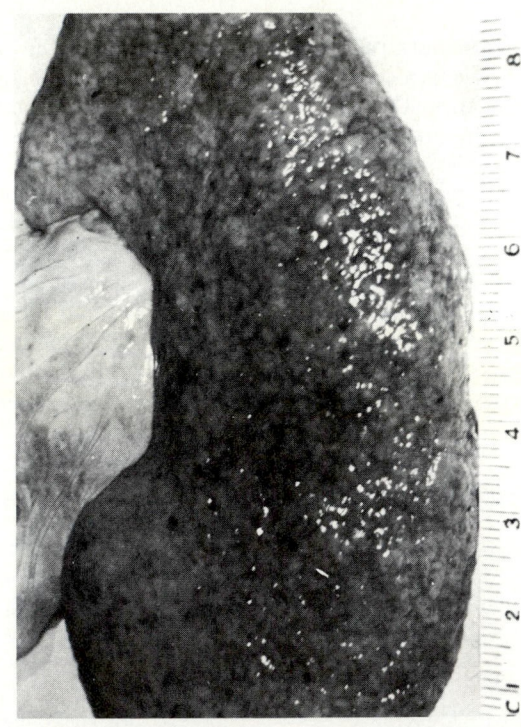

Fig. 32-12 End-stage chronic glomerulonephritis. Note pebbly surface corresponding to surviving hypertrophied nephrons amid atrophy. (From Anderson, WAD, and Kissane, JM: Pathology, ed 7, St. Louis, 1977, The CV Mosby Co.)

changes are the immune responses described for acute glomerulonephritis.

Various symptoms of failing renal function, none of which may seem severe, may lead the person to seek health care. There may be a slow onset of recurrent dependent edema, or there may be mild headache, especially in the morning. Dyspnea on exertion or difficulty sleeping in a flat position may be noted. Blurring of vision may lead the person to an ophthalmologist, who may be the first to suspect chronic renal disease based on ocular vascular changes. Occasionally, chronic nephritis is discovered during routine physical examination or may be discovered by a school nurse who observes marked visual changes and lassitude in a student. Early in the disease urinalysis shows the presence of albumin, casts, and blood. At this point renal function tests may be normal. The ability of the kidneys to regulate the internal environment will begin to decrease as more and more glomeruli become scarred and the amount of functional renal tissue is reduced. Finally, when few intact nephrons remain, hematuria and proteinuria decrease, the specific gravity of the urine becomes fixed, and the nonprotein nitrogen level in the blood increases.

ASSESSMENT

☐ Subjective data

General questions to ask include: (1) Have you experienced shortness of breath, headaches, weakness, or anorexia? (2) Have you noticed any change in your pattern of urination, either frequency or volume? and (3) Do you recall a recent infection of symptoms of a virus? It is also important to determine if there is a history of renal problems in the past.

☐ Objective data

It is important to establish baseline vital signs including temperature, pulse, respirations, and blood pressure. Vital signs are assessed frequently, at least every 6 hours, until stable. The person is assessed daily for edema. Daily weighing is one of the best means of assessing the person's fluid status. Intake and output should be assessed at least every 8 hours until stable. The urine is assessed for color, clarity, specific gravity, and odor.

☐ Diagnostic tests

Urinalysis is essential to determine the presence of proteinuria, hematuria, and cellular debris. BUN and serum creatinine are obtained to determine renal function. Immunologic tests such as antigen-antibody titers and immunoelectrophoresis may also be obtained. A composite urine for creatinine clearance and total protein can also provide important data about renal function. Renal biopsy (p. 1152) may be necessary to make the differential diagnosis.

DATA ANALYSIS: NURSING DIAGNOSES

Nursing diagnoses are determined from assessment of patient data. Possible nursing diagnoses for the person with

chronic glomerulonephritis may include, but are not limited to, the following:

Diagnostic title	Possible etiologies
Activity intolerance	Generalized weakness, electrolyte imbalance
Ineffective individual coping	Changes in body integrity, altered affect caused by changes in body chemistry
Fluid volume excess	Renal failure, compromised regulatory mechanism, excess fluid intake, excess sodium intake
Altered health maintenance	Lack of knowledge
Potential for infection	Altered immune response
Knowledge deficit	Lack of exposure, and/or recall
Altered nutrition: less than body requirements	Anorexia
Altered patterns of urinary elimination	Renal failure

PLANNING: EXPECTED PATIENT OUTCOMES

Expected patient outcomes for the person with chronic glomerulonephritis may include, but are not limited to, the following:

1. Signs and symptoms of infection are absent.
2. Blood pressure is under control.
3. Person maintains adequate nutritional intake within the prescribed dietary limitations.
4. Person states feeling comfortable and knows how to control pain after discharge.
5. The person or significant other can explain the following:
   a. The rationale for therapy (prolonged bed rest, maintenance of fluid balance)
   b. Dietary changes (decreased sodium intake, adequate caloric intake, controlled protein intake)
   c. Medication program to be followed at home
   d. Plans for a health maintenance program to include the following:
      (1) Measures to prevent further infection
      (2) Signs and symptoms that require immediate medical attention
      (3) Plans for follow-up health care

IMPLEMENTATION

☐ Assisting with achievement of therapeutic goals

No specific therapy exists to arrest or reverse the disease process. With some forms of CGN, steroid therapy may be attempted, although results of this therapy in arresting disease are not well documented. Treatment of renal failure begins when the illness destroys so much kidney tissue that the individual's kidneys are no longer able to independently control the internal environment.

With any exacerbation of hematuria, hypertension, and edema, the person is put to bed and treatment similar to that for acute glomerulonephritis is instituted. Signs of pulmonary edema and congestive failure are monitored. Treatment is symptomatic and supportive.

☐ Assisting with comfort and ADL

During periods of exacerbation, the person may need assistance with ADL. The dependency that the person experiences may lead to frustration and depression, which are common problems in persons with a chronic illness. Whenever the condition permits, the person is encouraged to be independent in ADL.

☐ Counseling and teaching

The teaching for the person with chronic glomerulonephritis is the same as for acute glomerulonephritis (p. 1154). Care involves teaching the person to live healthfully, to avoid infections, to eat a balanced diet with moderate sodium intake if prescribed, to appropriately administer medication, and to maintain follow-up health care visits and report to the physician any exacerbations in signs and symptoms.

Women with CGN who become pregnant appear to be susceptible to toxemia and to spontaneous abortion. The woman who has had nephritis of any nature should be urged to see a physician if she plans on pregnancy. When pregnancy does occur, she should remain under close health supervision.

The person also needs to know what resources are available in the community to assist with chronic renal disease. The National Kidney Foundation is organized at the local level to assist in locating resources.

✠ EVALUATION

The evaluation of the person with chronic glomerulonephritis is dependent on identified nursing diagnoses. Attention is given to assessing the person's attainment of the specific patient outcomes. General questions include the following:

1. Can the person state the signs and symptoms that require immediate medical follow-up?
2. Is the person able to maintain an adequate diet within prescribed restrictions?
3. Is the person free of pain?
4. Can the person state the signs and symptoms of infection?
5. Can the person state the medication regimen including doses, frequency, and side effects?

■ Nephrotic syndrome

Nephrotic syndrome is not a single disease entity but is a constellation of symptoms. In nephrotic syndrome there is damage to the glomeruli and quantities of protein are lost in the urine. This condition has been associated with allergic reactions (insect bites, pollen, acute glomerulonephritis), infections (herpes zoster), systemic disease (diabetes mellitus, sickle cell disease), circulatory problems (severe congestive heart failure, chronic constrictive peri-

carditis), and pregnancy. Known glomerular disease is the most common precipitating event in adults; in children the syndrome appears frequently with no evidence of a causative factor. In approximately 25% of children and 50% to 75% of adults who develop nephrosis the disease progresses to renal failure within 5 years.[44] In other individuals (particularly children) there may be remissions or nephrosis may exist in a chronic form. Other than treating the underlying illness, little can be done to prevent a recurrence of nephrosis.

■ PATHOPHYSIOLOGY

The initial change in nephrotic syndrome is a derangement of cells in the glomerular basement membrane, resulting in increased membrane porosity with loss of large amounts of protein into the urine (proteinuria). As protein continues to be excreted, serum albumin is decreased (hypoalbuminemia), thus decreasing the serum osmotic pressure. The capillary hydrostatic fluid (push) pressure in all body tissues becomes greater than the capillary osmotic (pull) pressure, and generalized edema results (Fig. 32-13). As fluid is lost into the tissues, the plasma volume

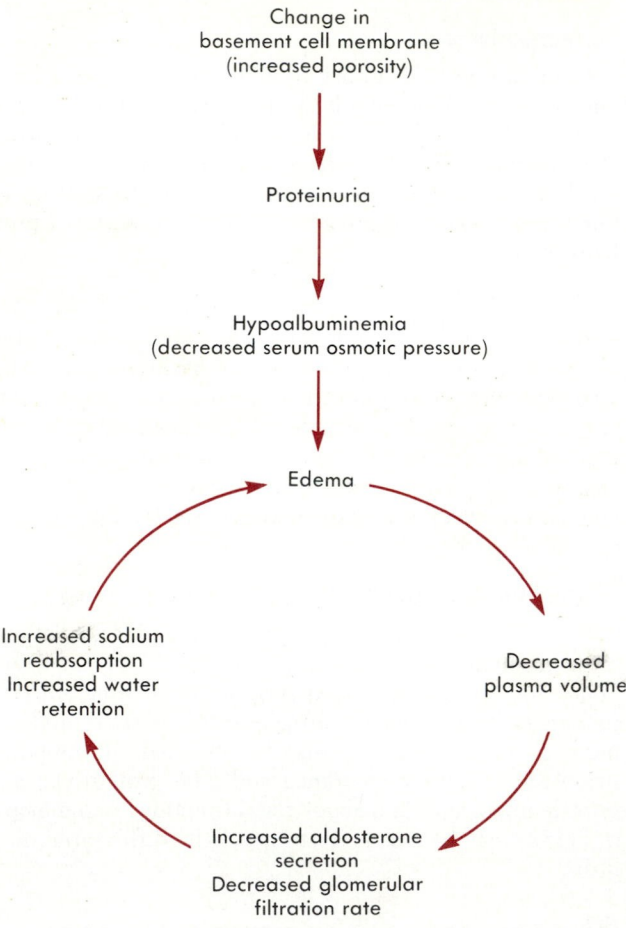

Fig. 32-13 Pathophysiologic changes in nephrotic syndrome.

decreases, stimulating secretion of aldosterone to retain more sodium and water and decreasing the glomerular filtration rate to retain water. This additional fluid also passes out of the capillaries into the tissue, leading to even greater edema. Altered renal function and development of symptoms of renal failure occur as a result of progressing glomerulonephritis. Loss of appetite and fatigue are common. Women usually have amenorrhea or other disturbances in their reproductive cycle.

ASSESSMENT

Subjective data

The person with nephrotic syndrome displays signs and symptoms as described with acute glomerulonephritis (p. 1152). General questions for the person with nephrotic syndrome include the following:

1. Have there been changes in voiding patterns?
2. Is the person experiencing headaches or nausea?
3. Has appetite changed? Any anorexia?
4. Is fatigue present?

Objective data

The person with nephrotic syndrome is assessed for signs of fluid retention and infection:

1. Edema: amount, location, degree of pitting
2. Intake and output: monitored every 8 hours until stable
3. Daily weights and abdominal girths
4. Condition of skin: assess frequently as severe edema may lead to skin breakdown
5. Respiratory status: monitored at least each shift (as renal failure progresses, pulmonary edema may develop)
6. Signs and symptoms of infection

Diagnostic tests

The diagnosis of nephrotic syndrome is made on the basis of proteinuria, hypoalbuminemia, and hyperlipidemia. It is essential that serum albumin, cholesterol, and triglycerides be obtained. Urinalyses and a composite urine specimen (p. 1152) for total protein are collected. A renal biopsy is sometimes used as a means of definitive diagnosis.

DATA ANALYSIS: NURSING DIAGNOSES

Nursing diagnoses are determined from assessment of patient data. Possible nursing diagnoses for the person with nephrotic syndrome may include, but are not limited to, the following:

Diagnostic title	Possible etiologies
Activity intolerance	Bed rest, immobility, generalized weakness, imbalance between oxygen supply and demand
Ineffective breathing pattern	Pulmonary edema, fatigue
Ineffective individual coping	Situational crisis
Fluid volume excess	Renal failure, decreased cardiac output

Diagnostic title	Possible etiologies
Altered health maintenance	Lack of knowledge, situational crisis
Potential for infection	Decreased nutrition, immobility
Altered nutrition: less than body requirements	Anorexia
Pain	Renal failure, immobility
Altered patterns of urinary elimination	Renal failure, sensorimotor impairment

PLANNING: EXPECTED PATIENT OUTCOMES

Expected patient outcomes for the person with nephrotic syndrome may include, but are not limited to, the following:

1. Independence in ADL is maintained.
2. The person remains free of infection.
3. Edema and blood pressure are controlled; pulmonary edema and congestive heart failure do not occur.
4. The person or significant other can describe the following:
   a. Measures to prevent infection
   b. Name, dosage, frequency, and side effects of prescribed medications
   c. Dietary prescriptions and appropriate meal plans
   d. Signs and symptoms requiring immediate attention
   e. Plans for follow-up care

IMPLEMENTATION

Assisting with achievement of therapeutic goals

Treatment of nephrotic syndrome is directed toward reducing albuminuria, controlling edema, and promoting general health. Corticosteroids may be useful in controlling the illness, but the response to them will vary from remission of nephrosis to no response. Prednisone is the steroid preparation most frequently prescribed. The diet should contain normal to increased amounts of protein (1 g/kg body weight per day) and be high in calories. Periodic determination of proteinuria and measures of renal function enable the physician to monitor response to treatment and level of kidney function.

To control edema, sodium intake is reduced and diuretics are employed to increase excretion of fluid. When diuretics are administered over prolonged periods, hypokalemia usually results. Potassium may be supplemented through dietary intake; medication supplements should be initiated only after attempts to increase serum potassium through dietary means have failed. Bed rest is usually ordered when edema is severe; however, immobility is contraindicated for prolonged periods.

Persons with nephrosis need to direct particular attention toward preventing infection, since body defenses are impaired by urinary protein losses and edematous tissues are particularly susceptible to injury. When infection is suspected, it is important to give immediate attention to the problem. Culture and sensitivity studies are done and appropriate antibiotics are prescribed. The person is informed of the importance of prescribed medication and diet therapy and of the need for follow-up health care.

The nephrotic syndrome is usually complicated by periods of marked edema. During this time meticulous skin care is essential to prevent breakdown. Close monitoring of oral and parenteral fluid is necessary.

Usually a sodium and protein restricted diet is prescribed. This often results in a diet that is not appetizing to the patient. Appetite may also be diminished as a result of fluid overload. This all results in the potential for inadequate nutrition.

☐ Assisting with comfort and ADL

The patient may tire easily and therefore require assistance with ADL. The patient should be encouraged to be independent but not be allowed to overdo.

As edema increases, the patient becomes increasingly uncomfortable. Careful positioning and frequent changes in position may increase comfort while also protecting the skin. Males may develop edema in the scrotum, which can be particularly uncomfortable. A sling to support the scrotum will not only provide comfort but will also aid in reducing swelling (see Chapter 34).

☐ Teaching

As the patient begins to convalesce the teaching plan should include the following:
1. Medication teaching
2. Nutrition teaching
3. Self assessment of fluid status including edema and weight gain
4. Signs and symptoms requiring immediate attention (increase in edema, fatigue, headache, infection)
5. Need for follow-up care

▦ EVALUATION

The care of specific patients with nephrotic syndrome is evaluated on the basis of expected patient outcomes. General questions to ask include the following:
1. Is the person's blood pressure under control?
2. Can the person state the signs and symptoms of fluid retention?
3. Can the person state the names, dosages, time and side effects of prescribed medications?
4. Is the person comfortable?

■ OBSTRUCTIVE DISORDERS

Obstructive disorders are a significant source of morbidity. Obstruction of the urinary tract can occur in any portion of the urinary tract from the urinary calyces to the meatus. The signs and symptoms that a person displays are usually characteristic of the location and extent of the obstruction. The box above summarizes the locations and major causes of the common urinary tract obstructions.

Location and causes of urinary tract obstruction

Location	Major causes
Kidney	Calculi
	Ptosis
	Polycystic disease
Ureteral obstruction	Calculi
	Trauma
	Nephroptosis ("floating" or dropped" kidney)
	Enlarged lymph nodes
	Lymphosarcoma
	Reticulum cell sarcoma
	Hodgkin's disease
Lower urinary tract	Bladder neoplasm
	Urethral strictures
	Trauma
	Chronic inflammation
	Calculi
	Tumors
	Benign prostatic hypertrophy (BPH)

Obstruction of the urinary tract produces pathophysiologic changes leading to symptoms of obstruction. Therapy consists of reestablishing drainage and relieving the acute discomfort. In the following pages, the pathophysiology of and therapy for urinary obstruction will be discussed. Several major causes of urinary obstruction are then described in more detail; these topics include the following:
1. Urinary calculi
2. Benign prostatic hypertrophy
3. Urethral strictures
4. Neoplasms: renal, bladder, prostate

■ Pathophysiology of urinary obstruction

Obstruction of any part of the urinary system from the kidney to the urethra will generate pressure that may cause functional and anatomic damage to the renal parenchyma (Fig. 32-14). When any part of the urinary tract is obstructed, urine collects behind the obstruction producing a dilation of the structure. Muscles of the affected areas contract in an effort to push the urine around the obstruction. Partial obstruction may produce slow dilation of structures above the obstruction without functional impairment. As the obstruction increases, however, pressure builds up in the tubular system behind the obstruction causing a backflow of urine and dilation of the ureter (*hydroureter*). The urine backup eventually reaches the kidney causing dilation of the kidney pelvis (*hydronephrosis*). Pres-

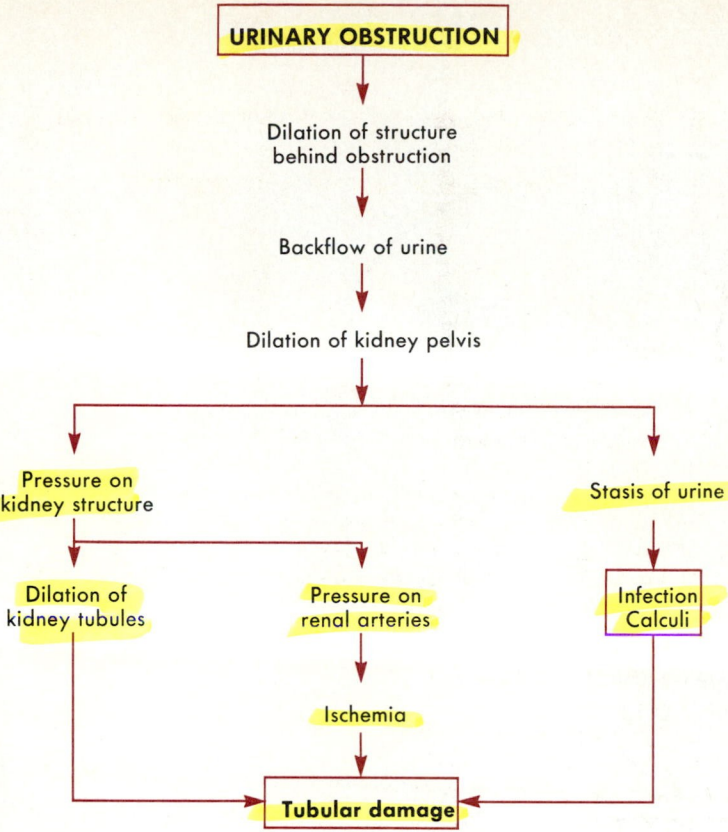

Fig. 32-14 Pathophysiology of uncorrected urinary obstruction.

sure buildup in the renal pelvis leads to destruction of kidney tissue and eventual renal failure.

With obstruction urine flow is decreased even to the point of stagnation. This stagnant urine provides a good culture medium for bacterial growth, and rarely is obstruction seen without some infection. The specific effects that occur with obstruction depend on the location of the obstruction, the extent of obstruction (partial or complete), and the duration. Obstruction in the *lower* urinary tract causes bladder distention. If this is prolonged, muscle fibers become hypertrophied and *diverticuli* (herniated sacs of bladder mucosa) develop between the hypertrophied muscle bands. Because the diverticulum holds stagnant urine, infection often occurs, and bladder stones may form.

Obstruction of the *upper* urinary tract leads even more quickly to hydronephrosis because of the small size of the ureters and kidney pelvis. Increased pressure causes partial ischemia of arteries between the renal cortex and medulla and dilation of the renal tubules leading to tubular damage. Stasis of urine in the dilated pelvis predisposes to infection and calculi, which add to the renal damage. Some urine can flow back up the renal tubule into the veins and lymphatics as a compensatory mechanism to prevent kidney damage. The unaffected kidney then takes on increased elimination of waste products. With prolonged obstruction the unaffected kidney hypertrophies and may function as effectively alone as both kidneys did before the obstruction. Obstruction of both kidneys leads to renal failure.

Hydronephrosis can occur without any symptoms as long as kidney function is adequate and urine can drain. An acute upper urinary tract obstruction will cause pain, nausea, vomiting, local tenderness, spasm of the abdominal muscles, and a mass in the kidney region. The pain is caused by the stretching of the tissues and by hyperperistalsis. Because the amount of pain is proportional to the rate of stretching, a slowly developing hydronephrosis may cause only a dull flank pain, whereas a sudden blockage of the ureter such as may occur from a stone causes a severe stabbing (colicky) pain in the flank or abdomen. The pain may radiate to the genitalia and thigh and is caused by the increased peristaltic action of the smooth muscle of the ureter in an effort to dislodge the obstruction and force urine past it.

The nausea and vomiting frequently associated with acute ureteral obstruction are caused by a reflex reaction to the pain and will usually be relieved as soon as pain is relieved. A markedly dilated kidney, however, may press on the stomach causing continued GI symptoms. If the renal function has been seriously impaired, nausea and vomiting may be symptoms of impending uremia.

When the bladder is distended from lower urinary tract obstruction, the person will experience lower abdominal discomfort and a feeling of the need to void although voiding may not be possible. The bladder may be palpated above the symphysis pubis. With partial obstruction such as by benign prostatic hypertrophy the man first complains of increasing urinary frequency because the bladder fails to empty completely at each voiding and therefore refills more quickly to the amount that causes the urge to void (usually 250 to 500 ml). Nocturia may also be present.

■ Therapy for urinary obstruction

The person with a sudden obstruction is usually acutely ill and may have severe colic but will not be able to remain in bed until the pain has been relieved. It is not unusual to see a person with acute renal colic walking the floor doubled up and vomiting. Narcotics such as morphine and meperidine and antispasmodic drugs such as propantheline bromide (Pro-Banthine) and belladonna preparations are usually necessary to relieve severe colicky pain. After narcotics have been given, the patient will be dizzy and must be protected from injury. As the pain eases, the patient can usually be made relatively comfortable in bed. As soon as the nausea subsides large amounts of fluids are urged.

If a *ureter* becomes obstructed, a catheter must be placed directly into the renal pelvis. This prevents renal damage that otherwise would occur as pressure in the kidney increases because of continued urine formation. When there is complete obstruction of a ureter, a *nephrostomy* or *pyelostomy* tube may be inserted surgically into the renal pelvis. The surgical incision is located laterally and posteriorly in the kidney region. Catheters used as nephrostomy or pyelostomy tubes are usually of the Pezzer (mushroom) or Malecot (batwing) types (Fig. 32-15). An alternate form of drainage for a ureteral obstruction is the surgical placement of a ureterostomy tube (a whistle-tip

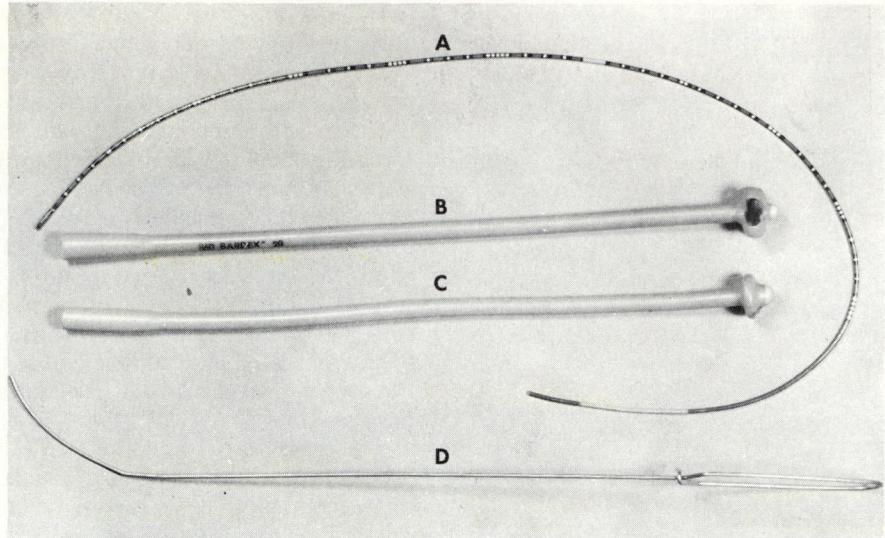

Fig. 32-15 **A** to **C,** Catheters used to drain renal pelvis. **A,** ureteral catheter. **B,** Malecote (batwing) catheter. **C,** Pezzer (mushroom) catheter. **D,** Stylet used to insert urethral catheter into male patient.

or many-eyed Robinson catheter, No. 6 or 8 Fr) that is passed through an incision in the upper outer quadrant of the abdomen into the ureter above the obstruction. The catheter is then passed through the ureter to the renal pelvis.

If the ureter is unobstructed or partially obstructed, the *renal pelvis* may be drained by a ureteral catheter, which is passed up the ureter to the renal pelvis by a cystoscope (p. 1167). Ureteral catheterization is performed before

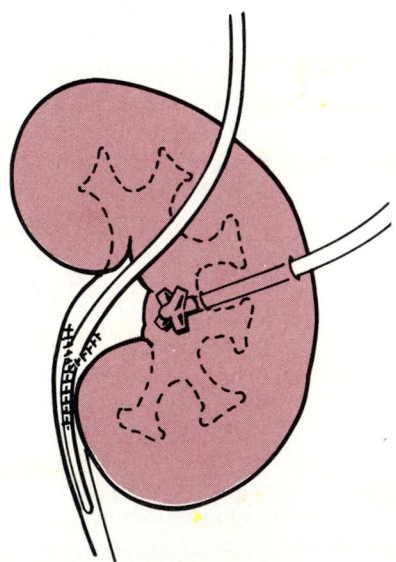

Fig. 32-16 Placement of splinting catheter after repair of ureteropelvic stricture. Note use of nephrostomy tube for drainage of urine during healing of anastomosis.

gynecologic and lower abdominal surgery when there is danger of not recognizing and accidentally injuring the ureter during the operation. Ureteral catheterization is also used after surgery involving the ureters to prevent stricture as the ureter heals. When used for this purpose, the catheter is referred to as a *splinting catheter* (Fig. 32-16). Whether it is expected to drain urine will depend on its relation to other catheters used.

Adequate anchorage of nephrostomy catheters must be provided to prevent accidental dislodgement and trauma to the tissues in which they lie. The openings made for these tubes are essentially fistulas that rapidly decrease in size on removal of the catheter. Even 30 minutes after removal of this type of catheter it is often impossible to reinsert a similar-sized tube. When a catheter is inserted during surgery, it is usually sutured in place. In this case, additional anchorage consists of affixing the tube to the skin with adhesive tape after the skin has been cleansed. When the tube is not sutured in place, it should be anchored to the skin at *two points* using adhesive—with some slack in the tubing between the anchor points.

Free drainage of catheters leading to the renal pelvis is of the utmost importance. Because the normal renal pelvis has only a 5 to 8 ml capacity, great pressure can be exerted on renal structures even when these catheters are obstructed for only a few minutes. Care must be taken to prevent kinking of the tubes while the patient is in the side-lying position in bed.

In some cases nephrostomy tubes may be left in place for several months, with the patient returning to the hospital later for their removal. Occasionally, the nephrostomy tube serves as a form of urinary diversion for long-term use. The person at home with a catheter draining the kidney pelvis must know how to obtain medical assistance quickly should the catheter obstruct or become dislodged.

When obstruction occurs below the *bladder,* constant drainage must be provided to prevent renal damage, which may occur because of inadequate emptying of the lower urinary system. One means of providing drainage is by the use of a *cystostomy* tube (usually a Foley, Malecot, or Pezzer catheter), which is placed directly into the bladder through a suprapubic incision. This method is usually used when the urethra is completely obstructed or when the prolonged use of a urethral catheter is to be avoided in a male patient. During some operative procedures both a cystostomy tube and a small urethral catheter will be inserted to drain the

bladder. Both catheters must be monitored for patency. If patency is assured, it is not necessary to record the output from each catheter separately, since both tubes drain the bladder. The catheters will not necessarily drain equal amounts of urine. As is true with nephrostomy and ureteral catheters, secure anchorage of these catherers is also necessary.

■ Urinary calculi

Urinary stones (*urolithiasis*) may develop at any level in the urinary system (kidney, ureters, bladder) but are most commonly found within the kidney (nephrolithiasis). Fig. 32-17 illustrates the most common locations of calculi formation. At least 1% of the people in the United States will develop urolithiasis. About one-third of the individuals who have recurrent upper urinary tract calculi will eventually have the affected kidney removed.

No demonstrable cause can be found for over half of the urinary stones that occur (idiopathic). A major predisposition is urinary tract infection. Chronic hypercalciuria and hyperphosphaturia, as seen with hyperparathyroidism, hypervitaminosis D, and excess calcium and alkali intake, may lead to precipitation of calcium salts in the urine. Other predisposing factors can be noted in the box below.

■ PREVENTION

Measures can be taken to decrease the potential for renal stones in persons at high risk. Adequate hydration (intake of 2500 ml/day or more unless contraindicated) will help to prevent urinary stasis that can lead not only to stone formation but also to a UTI. Persons restricted to bed

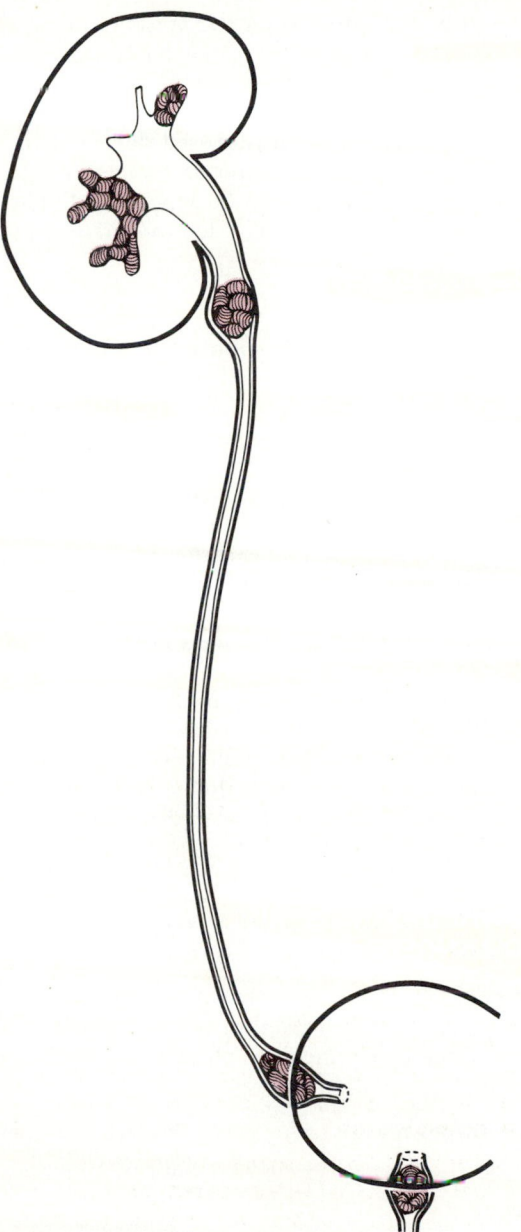

Fig. 32-17 Most common locations of renal calculus formation.

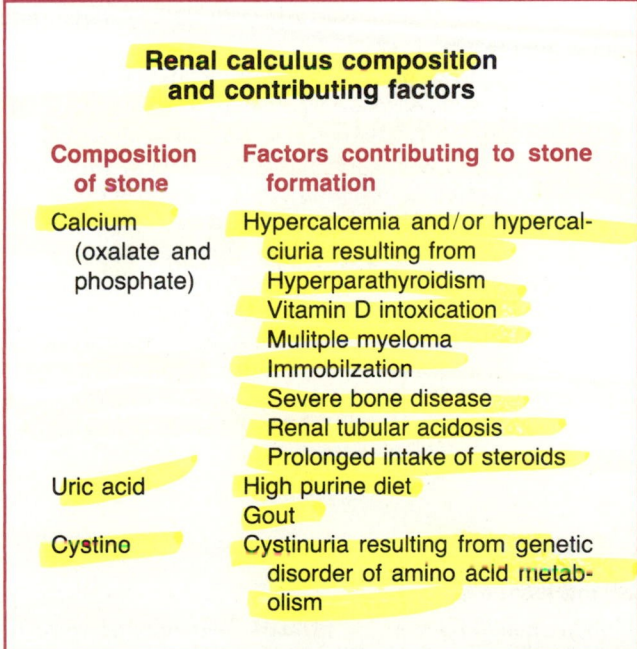

Renal calculus composition and contributing factors

Composition of stone	Factors contributing to stone formation
Calcium (oxalate and phosphate)	Hypercalcemia and/or hypercalciuria resulting from Hyperparathyroidism Vitamin D intoxication Mulitple myeloma Immobilzation Severe bone disease Renal tubular acidosis Prolonged intake of steroids
Uric acid	High purine diet Gout
Cystine	Cystinuria resulting from genetic disorder of amino acid metabolism

Table 32-11 Acid and alkaline ash food groups

Acid ash	Alkaline ash	Neutral
Meat	Milk	Sugars
Whole grains	Vegetables	Fats
Eggs	Fruit (except cran-	Beverages (coffee,
Cheese	berries, prunes,	tea)
Cranberries	plums)	
Prunes		
Plums		

From Williams, SR: Nutrition and diet therapy, ed 6, St. Louis, 1989, The CV Mosby Co.

should be encouraged to turn and move frequently, exercising their arms if the legs are immobilized. Changing the body position of a bedfast patient by means of a Circ-Olectric bed or tilt table or by sitting up in a wheelchair (if permitted) can help to prevent urinary stasis. Even with exercises and the use of a wheelchair, however, paraplegics and quadriplegics often develop renal calculi. *Persons with indwelling catheters need scrupulous aseptic technique in catheter care to prevent infection and require adequate hydration and good catheter drainage to wash away minerals that can be deposited at the tip of the catheter.*

Persons at risk for developing calcium oxalate or phosphate or magnesium ammonium phosphate stones may be placed on an acid ash diet (Table 32-11) to promote excretion of an acid urine.

■ PATHOPHYSIOLOGY

Urinary calculi result in obstruction of the urinary tract; the obstruction may be partial or complete. Complete obstruction leads to hydronephrosis with its associated signs and symptoms.

The pathophysiologic processes associated with urinary stones tend to be mechanical in nature. Urinary calculi (stones) are crystallizations of minerals around an organic matrix such as pus, blood, devitalized tissue, tumors, or urates. The mineral composition of renal calculi varies. About three-fourths of stones are calcium and oxalates; others stones are calcium phosphate, uric acid, and cystine. Increased concentration of urine solutes, resulting from low fluid intake, as well as increased organic matter from urinary tract infections or urinary stasis, may provide the nidus for stone formation. In addition, infection increases the alkalinity of the urine (by the production of ammonia), resulting in precipitation of calcium phosphate and magnesium ammonium phosphate.

▦ ASSESSMENT

☐ Subjective data

Pain (*renal colic*) is the primary symptom in an acute episode of renal calculi. The location of the pain depends on the location of the stone. If the stone is in the pelvis

of the kidney, the pain is caused by hydronephrosis and is more dull and constant in character, occurring primarily in the costovertebral angle. As the stone moves along the ureter, the pain can be excruciating and is intermittent in character. It is caused by spasm of the ureter and anoxia of the wall of the ureter from the pressure of the stone. Pain follows the anterior course of the ureter down to the suprapubic area and radiates to the external genitalia. Often a stone is "silent" causing no symptoms for years; this is especially true of very large renal stones. Extremely small smooth stones may be passed without the person's awareness. Nausea and vomiting often accompany renal colic.

☐ Objective data

The urine is monitored for the presence of blood. *Gross hematuria* may occur if the stone has rough edges, and microhematuria is usually present. Whenever a stone is suspected, all urine is strained to determine the presence of stones that are frequently passed during voiding. Patterns of urination are also noted because frequency or voiding in small amounts may be experienced. The acidity or alkalinity of the urine can be determined with pH paper.

☐ Diagnostic tests

Urinalysis, to determine the presence of casts, crystals, and blood cells, and urine culture, to identify UTI, are performed. A 24-hour urine collection is made to measure calcium oxalate, phosphorus, and uric acid levels. A nitroprusside urine test may be performed to check the presence of cystine.

BUN and serum creatinine tests are important to determine the level of renal function. Because urinary stones are frequently composed of calcium, phosphorus and uric acid, these serum levels are usually obtained.

Calcium stones are radiopaque and can be noted with a KUB (kidney, ureter, bladder) x-ray examination; uric acid stones usually cannot be seen in radiographic studies. An intravenous pyelogram (IVP) (p. 1146) may also be obtained. IVP may demonstrate dilation of the ureter above an obstructing stone. Very small stones, however, may be washed away during radiographic studies. Ultrasound of the kidneys may also be ordered to detect hydronephrosis.

➡ DATA ANALYSIS: NURSING DIAGNOSES

Nursing diagnoses are determined from assessment of patient data. Possible nursing diagnoses for the person with urinary calculi may include, but are not limited to, the following:

Diagnostic title	Possible etiologies
Fear	Surgery, treatment, pain
Fluid volume excess	Compromised regulatory mechanism
Potential for infection	Urinary stasis
Knowledge deficit	Lack of exposure/recall

Diagnostic title	Possible etiologies
Pain	Visceral inflammation
Altered patterns of urinary elimination	Anatomical obstruction
Urinary retention	Obstruction

PLANNING: EXPECTED PATIENT OUTCOMES

Expected patient outcomes for the person with urinary calculi may include, but are not limited to, the following:
1. Person remain comfortable.
2. Signs or symptoms of fluid volume excess are absent.
3. Signs or symptoms of urinary retention are absent.
4. Hematuria is decreased or absent.
5. Person or significant other can state the following:
   a. A plan to achieve a daily fluid intake of 4 to 5 L, sufficient to maintain a dilute urine
   b. The need to be as active as possible and prevent long periods of immobilization
   c. Menus to include any dietary restrictions
   d. Name, dosage, desired action, and side effects of medications prescribed to acidify or alkalinize the urine
   e. Plans for follow-up care, including signs and symptoms requiring immediate medical attention.

IMPLEMENTATION

Assisting with achievement of therapeutic goals

About 90% of urinary calculi are passed spontaneously. Therefore, *the urine of all patients with relatively small stones should be strained.* Urine can be strained easily by placing two opened 4-inch × 8-inch gauze sponges over a funnel. The urine from each voiding is strained, and one needs to watch closely for the stone because it may be no bigger than the head of a pin and the patient may not realize that it has been passed.

Stones smaller than 5 mm have a good chance of being passed. If there is no infection or obstruction, the stone may be left in the ureter for several months. The person is observed closely but permitted to carry out usual activities. A person who is up and about is more likely to pass a stone than one who is in bed. Fluids should be taken freely (3000 ml/day or more) to promote passage of the stone and prevent infection.

Patients frequently have two or three attacks of acute renal colic before the stone passes. This is probably because the stone gets lodged at a narrow point in the ureter causing temporary obstruction. The ureters are normally narrower at the ureteropelvic and ureterovesical junctions and at the point where they pass over the iliac crest into the pelvis. If the stone is to pass along the ureter by peristaltic action, the patient will have some pain. The patient is involved in determining when pain medication is needed.

If the stone fails to pass, one or two ureteral catheters may be passed through a cystoscope up the ureter and left in place for 24 hours. The catheters dilate the ureter, and when they are removed the stone may pass into the bladder.

If there are *signs of infection,* an attempt is made to pass a ureteral catheter past the stone into the renal pelvis. If such an attempt is successful, the catheter is left as a drain, because pyelonephritis will quickly follow if adequate urinary drainage is not reestablished. When there is a catheter in each ureter, each catheter is labeled and should drain into a separate drainage bag. The catheters must be checked frequently to see that they are draining. Patients with ureteral catheters are usually confined to bed to prevent possible dislodgement of the catheters.

If the stone has passed to the lower third of the ureter, it can sometimes be removed by *manipulation.* Special catheters with corkscrew tips, expanding baskets, and loops are passed through the cystoscope, and an attempt is made to "snare" the stone. This procedure is performed with the patient under anesthesia. The aftercare of a patient on whom manipulation has been carried out is the same as that following cystoscopy. Any signs suggestive of peritonitis or a decreased urinary output are carefully watched for, since the ureter occasionally is perforated during manipulation.

Surgical interventions for renal calculi

Surgical intervention is often indicated when a large stone (greater than 1 cm) is producing pain, obstruction, or infection. The operation for removal of a stone from the ureter is a *ureterolithotomy* (Fig. 32-18, C). A radiograph is taken immediately preceding surgery, since the stone may have moved, and it is desirable to make the incision

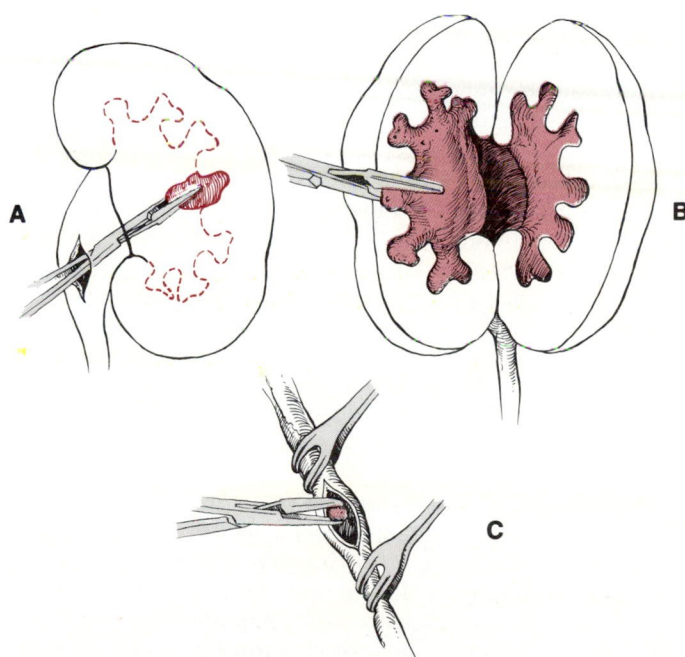

Fig. 32-18 Location and methods of removing renal calculi from upper urinary tract. **A,** Pyelolithotomy, removal of stone through renal pelvis. **B,** Nephrolithotomy, removal of staghorn calculus from renal parenchyma (kidney split). **C,** Ureterolithotomy, removal of stone from ureter.

into the ureter directly over the stone. If the stone is in the lower third of the ureter, a rectus incision is made. If it is in the upper two thirds, a flank approach is used. If the patient has a ureteral stricture that causes stones to form, plastic surgery to relieve the stricture may be carried out as part of the operation.

Removal of the stone through or from the renal pelvis is known as a *pyelolithotomy* (Fig. 32-18, *A*). Removal of a stone through the parenchyma is a *nephrolithotomy* (Fig. 32-18, *B*). Occasionally, the kidney may have to be split from end to end (a kidney split) to remove the stone. Patients in whom such a split is done may have severe hemorrhage following surgery.

Bladder stones may be removed through a suprapubic incision, or they may be crushed with a lithotrite (stone crusher) that is passed transurethrally. This procedure is known as a *litholapaxy*. Following bladder stone removal, the bladder may be irrigated (intermittently or constantly) with an acid solution such as magnesium and sodium citrate (G solution) or Renacidin to counteract the alkalinity caused by the infection and to help wash out the remaining particles of stone. If there has been a suprapubic incision, the care of the incision is similar to that following a suprapubic prostatectomy (p. 1170). Nursing care of the person undergoing kidney surgery is discussed on p. 1165.

☐ *Lithotripsy*

Until the early 1980s, surgery was frequently required to remove a urinary stone. *Percutaneous lithotripsy* is now a common method for the removal of urinary stones.[24] This technique is accomplished by creating a percutaneous nephrostomy tract through an incision 1/4 to 1/2 inch over the region of the kidney. An endoscope is then passed through the tract and a snare basket is used to retrieve the calculi. If the calculi cannot be removed, ultrasonic lithotripsy is used to disintegrate the stone. Complications of percutaneous lithotripsy are rare; however, hemorrhage, urinoma, sepsis, and abscess may develop. The person may also experience pain similar to renal colic postoperatively. Pain is managed by administering meperidine hydrochloride. The person may also experience copious drainage from the nephrostomy tract opening. This drainage consists of serous drainage, as well as urine. Dressings should be changed frequently to prevent infection and aid in patient comfort. Urinary drainage from the incision may be experienced for 3 to 4 days following the procedure. Patients are usually prescribed a 2-week course of antibiotic therapy after the surgery.

Transcutaneous shock wave lithotripsy is another recent development in the treatment of urinary stones.[13] This technique was developed in Germany and has been used at a growing number of facilities in the United States since 1985. Shock wave lithotripsy is accomplished by submerging the patient in a large tub of warm water and aiming ultrasonic waves over the area of the urinary calculi. Fluoroscopy is used to locate the stones. The water bath is necessary to allow for the passage of the shock waves into the body. Repeated firing of the ultrasonic waves results in the disintegration of the calculi. It may require 1500 or more shock waves to break up a large stone. The patient is usually sedated with diazepam (Valium) during the procedure. Pain of moderate intensity may be experienced during the passage of each sound wave; therefore, epidural or general anesthesia may be used. Aiming of the sound waves is best accomplished when the patient is able to control both breathing and movement while in the water bath. Therefore, local anesthesia is preferred for this procedure.

Following lithotripsy the patient is observed for signs of bleeding. Blood pressure is monitored frequently for the first several hours following the procedure. Urinary output is also closely monitored for both quantity and quality. Blood initially may turn the urine cherry red to pink for the first several hours. The urine should then clear. Immediately following the procedure the patient may experience redness or bruising on the skin at the site of the lithotripsy. Pain may also be experienced in this region from the force of the ultrasonic shock waves. Pain is usually localized to the skin as a result of the shock waves entering the body.

The patient may also experience pain similar to renal colic following lithotripsy, usually as a result of the passage of fragments of the pulverized urinary stone through the lower urinary tract. Renal colic is usually controlled by the use of narcotic analgesics. The patient can be discharged within a few days following the procedure if complications, which are rare, are not experienced. Because renal colic pain often occurs 3 or more days after lithotripsy, the person should be made aware of this potential side effect. The person is also informed about the use of pain medications and signs and symptoms that require immediate reporting to the physician.

Occasionally urinary obstruction may occur as a result of stone fragments blocking the flow of urine. The patient is instructed to observe the volume of urine output for several days following discharge. The patient is also weighed daily for several days following lithotripsy in order to detect urinary retention. Flank pain may indicate urinary obstruction. When these symptoms are present, the patient should contact the physician immediately.

☐ Assisting with comfort and ADL

When the person is experiencing renal colic, it can be very difficult to eliminate pain. Every effort should be made to medicate the person before pain has reached intense levels. Narcotic analgesics are usually prescribed and should be administered liberally. Because of the nature of the pain, the person may not tolerate activity. Assistance with ADL is given as required. When the person is comfortable, activity is encouraged.

☐ Counseling and teaching

The person who has had urinary calculi must be instructed in methods to prevent development of future stones. Patient teaching should include the following:
1. Methods to prevent urinary tract infection
   a. Drink at least 2500 ml fluids each day.
   b. Avoid situations that lead to urinary stasis whenever possible (such as long periods of inactivity).
   c. Practice good hygiene.

2. Dietary prescriptions, including a variety of menus that include necessary dietary restrictions (acid or alkaline ash diets)
3. Names, dosages, and side effects of medications
4. Need to report signs and symptoms of recurrence of calculi to physician

□ Long-term care

Persons who have recurrent renal calculi benefit from ongoing prophylactic therapy, which is determined by the type of stone being produced. *All persons with recurrent renal stones should drink fluids in sufficient quantity to produce very dilute urine and nocturia.* This may amount to a daily intake of up to 4 to 5 L of fluid.[55] The purpose of the increased fluid intake is to rinse away any precipitates that can serve as a nidus for stone formation.

Any underlying identifiable cause of calciuria is treated to prevent recurrence of calcium stones. Hydrochlorothiazide (HCTZ) in doses of 50 mg twice a day may be prescribed for persons with hypercalciuria to decrease urinary excretion of calcium. Persons receiving HCTZ therapy must be monitored carefully for signs of electrolyte imbalances especially hypokalemia.

As previously stated, more than 50% of calcium stones are idiopathic. Foods high in calcium are sometimes restricted, but a very low-calcium diet is usually unsatisfactory because it is unpalatable. The solubility of oxalate salts is not pH dependent; therefore manipulation of pH is not useful. Sodium or potassium phosphate, 1.5 to 2.0 g/day, may be prescribed to decrease levels of urinary calcium.

Phosphatic calculi develop in alkaline urine; thus their prevention depends on keeping the urine acid and preventing a UTI. Medications such as ascorbic acid or ammonium chloride may be given for a time to increase urine acidity.

The Shorr regimen has given beneficial results in the prevention of phosphatic calculi. A diet containing only 1300 mg of phosphorus daily is prescribed, and 40 ml of aluminum hydroxide gel is taken after meals and at bedtime. The aluminum combines with the excess phosphorus, causing it to be excreted through the bowel instead of through the kidney, thus decreasing the possibility of stone formation. Constipation frequently results from this regimen.

Prophylaxis for *uric acid* stones consists of alkalinizing the urine by the administration of sodium bicarbonate and acetazolamide (Diamox) sufficient to maintain a urine pH of 6.0 to 6.5. Allopurinol (Zyloprim) usually is prescribed to inhibit synthesis of uric acid.

⊞ EVALUATION

The care of specific patients with urinary calculi is evaluated on the basis of expected patient outcomes. General questions to ask include the following:

1. Does the patient have signs or symptoms of pain?
2. Is the patient maintaining normal urination patterns?
3. Can the patient state the necessity for surgical intervention?

Table 32-12 Types of urologic surgery

Site	Surgery	Description
Kidney	Nephrectomy	Removal of a kidney
	Partial nephrectomy	Removal of part of a kidney
	Pyelolithotomy	Incision into renal pelvis for removal of calculi
	Nephrolithotomy	Incision into kidney parenchyma for removal of calculi
	Nephropexy	Fixation of a floating kidney
	Pyeloplasty	Plastic repair of ureteropelvic junction
Ureters	Ureterolithotomy	Incision into ureters for removal of calculi
	Ureterectomy	Excision of a ureter
	Ureterostomy	Creation of a new outlet for a ureter
Bladder	Cystectomy	Removal of the bladder
	Segmental bladder resection	Partial removal of the bladder

4. Can the patient state signs and symptoms requiring immediate medical attention?

■ Urologic surgery

Surgery of the urinary tract may be performed for various reasons, such as renal calculi, tumors, multiple cysts, trauma, congenital defects, "floating" kidney (nephroptosis), or renal hypertension. The types of surgeries are described in Table 32-12.

■ PREOPERATIVE CARE

General preoperative preparation for surgery (Chapter 16) is appropriate for the urologic patient. Patient concerns may be focused not only on the diagnosis but also on possible changes in urinary elimination. For many patients, interruption in urinary elimination is temporary. If one kidney is removed, adequate waste removal can be maintained by the remaining kidney or by even less than half of one kidney remaining functional. The remaining kidney may grow to handle the extra load. If an entire kidney is removed, a drain may be placed to remove serous fluid from the space previously occupied by the kidney. In this situation there will be no urinary drainage. Urinary drainage will occur with partial nephrectomy.

Partial removal of the bladder will decrease capacity of the bladder to about 60 ml immediately postoperatively, but the elastic tissue of the bladder will regenerate so that the person is able to retain from 200 to 400 ml of urine within several months. If the entire bladder is removed, diversion of the urinary tract is necessary.

Instructions in deep breathing and coughing exercises are crucial with kidney surgery because of the high flank incision interfering with ventilation.

■ POSTOPERATIVE CARE

The basic needs of the patient requiring urologic surgery are the same as those of any other surgical patient. Special emphasis is placed on promotion of ventilation and adequate urinary output, prevention of distention and hemorrhage, and attention to drainage tubes and dressing (see the box at right).

☐ Ventilation

Surgery of the kidney or upper ureters usually involves a flank incision that can influence respiratory status. Because the incision is directly below the diaphragm, deep breathing is painful and the patient is reluctant to take deep breaths or to move about. Splinting of the chest is common, and therefore atelectasis or other respiratory complications must be guarded against. In addition, because of the placement of the incision there is a greater incisional pull every time the person moves, as compared with an abdominal incision. The patient is often reluctant to turn in bed or to get up to ambulate. Most patients will be more comfortable turning themselves if they are given time, side rails to hold onto, and encouragement. Incisional pain usually requires a narcotic every 3 to 4 hours for 24 to 48 hours after surgery, and turning, ambulation, and deep breathing exercises can be planned so that these activities occur at the time the analgesic has the greatest effect. Patients may lie on the affected side unless a nephrostomy tube is in place. Even then they can be tilted to the affected side with pillows placed at the back for support. It must be ascertained that the tube is not kinked and that there is no traction on it.

☐ Urinary output

The urinary output is monitored carefully for several days postoperatively to ascertain adequate renal functioning and drainage. The output should be at least 50 ml/hour, preferably greater, to prevent urinary stasis and subsequent infection. A urinary output of 20 to 30 ml/hour in a patient with satisfactory fluid intake (at least 1200 ml/day) and in the absence of signs of urinary retention is reported immediately to the physician. Urinary output includes drainage from nephrostomy or cystostomy tubes, urethral or ureteral catheters, and an estimate from urine-soaked dressings. Daily weights are compared with the preoperative weight and with each other to identify fluid retention.

☐ Distention

Following kidney surgery most patients have some abdominal distention that may result in part from pressure on the stomach and intestinal tract during surgery. Patients who have had renal colic before surgery frequently develop paralytic ileus postoperatively. This condition may be related to the reflex GI tract symptoms caused by postoperative pain. Because of the problem of abdominal disten-

---

Nursing care following urologic surgery

1. Promote ventilation:
   a. Encourage breathing exercises.
   b. Encourage frequent self-turning in bed.
   c. Encourage ambulation.
2. Monitor output and maintain patency of urinary catheters.
3. Prevent complications:
   a. Change wet dressings to protect skin.
   b. Restrict food and oral fluids if paralytic ileus is present.
   c. Encourage fluids to 3000 or more ml/day when permitted.
   d. Monitor for bright red blood on dressing or in urine.

---

tion following renal surgery, food and fluids by mouth are often restricted 24 to 48 hours postoperatively. By the fourth postoperative day most patients tolerate a regular diet. Fluids are then usually forced to 3000 ml/day.

☐ Hemorrhage

Hemorrhage may follow such operative procedures as prostatectomy, nephrolithotomy or nephrectomy. It occurs most often when the highly vascular parenchyma of the kidney has been incised. The bleeding may occur on the day of surgery, or it may occur 8 to 12 days postoperatively, during the period when tissue sloughing normally occurs with healing. The presence of bright red blood on the dressing or in the urine is reported immediately to the physician. The patient is observed for signs of shock. Because many patients with urologic disease have hypertension, the blood pressure may be relatively high but still represent a marked drop for the individual. Comparisons should therefore be made with baseline data.

If hemorrhage occurs, a pressure dressing is applied over the incision while the physician's arrival is awaited. Measures to prevent shock are instituted. Several liters of sterile physiologic saline solution for irrigation should be available.

☐ Dressings

There may be large amounts of urinary drainage following urologic surgery, except after nephrectomy. The drainage may be pink or dark red but should not be bright red. If the surgery involves a flank incision, drainage is usually the heaviest on the posterior edge of the dressing because of gravity flow. It is important therefore to turn the patient on the side opposite the surgery to examine the posterior edge of the dressing. When a suprapubic incision is present, drainage is heaviest on the side and in the inguinal region.

The dressings are usually held in place by Montgomery straps and must be changed frequently. Urinary drainage irritates the skin, has an unpleasant odor, and leads to discomfort. If a drain is present, the end of the drain should be placed over dressings, then covered with additional dressions to absorb the drainage. If a drainage tube is present, presence of large amounts of drainage on the dressing with little drainage coming from the tube indicates blockage of the tube. If a large amount of drainage is present, a disposable drainage bag used for urinary stomas may be applied over the drainage site.

□ Drainage tubes

A catheter is usually inserted during surgery to drain urine from the operative area and permit healing to occur. Different types of drainage tubes may be inserted, and each tube is connected to a separate drainage system. It is important to know the purpose of the catheter and the area to be drained.

■ Benign prostatic hypertrophy

Benign prostatic hypertrophy (BPH) is an adenomatous enlargement of the prostate gland. More than half of all men over 50 years of age and 75% of men over 70 have some symptoms of prostatic enlargement. The cause is not known but appears to be related to changing hormone levels that are experienced during the aging process.

■ PATHOPHYSIOLOGY

The prostate is an encapsulated gland, weighing about 20 g, that encircles the male urethra below the bladder neck. The signs and symptoms associated with BPH are the result of the enlargement of the prostate causing a partial or complete obstruction of the lower urinary tract.

One of the early symptoms of benign prostatic hypertrophy is nocturia (awakening at night to void) and urinary frequency in general. The man notices that the urinary stream is smaller and more difficult to start (hesitancy). The bladder muscle must contract more forcibly to push the urine past the partial obstruction, and the overworked muscles hypertrophy. Stagnant urine is held in trabeculae, or cellules, formed by sagging of the atonic mucous membranes between hypertrophied muscle bands. The bladder will not empty completely at each voiding (residual urine); this urine becomes alkaline from stasis and is a fertile medium for bacterial growth. The man will then complain of symptoms of cystitis (frequency, urgency), and bladder stones may occur. Some men develop hematuria from rupture of blood vessels that have become overstretched. Destruction of renal function can eventually occur from back pressure up the ureter to the kidney. Acute urinary retention is not uncommon.

■ ASSESSMENT

□ Subjective data

The most frequent and disturbing symptoms of BPH include dysuria and nocturia. The man is asked about urinary patterns, including the presence of frequency, hesitancy, dribbling, number of times he must get up at night to void, and the force of the urinary stream. *Hesitancy* refers to difficulty in initiating voiding that is often accompanied by a decrease in the force and flow of the urinary stream. The man is asked if he has to strain to start or maintain the urinary flow.

Because urinary tract infection may occur as a result of stasis of urine, the man is assessed for chills and pain or burning on urination.

□ Objective data

Patterns and amounts of urination are noted. The abdomen above the symphysis pubis is palpated to assess urinary retention.

□ Diagnostic tests

Urinalysis is performed to determine the presence of casts, crystals, and blood cells, and a urine culture is obtained to assess for infection. BUN and serum creatinine are important to determine the level of renal function. An IVP (p. 1146) is usually obtained to evaluate the functions and structure of the kidneys and urinary tract.

Enlargement of the lateral lobes of the prostate gland may be palpated by digital rectal examination. Enlargement of the middle lobe is diagnosed by signs of partial obstruction of the urethra, and the obstruction and bladder trabeculae are visualized by cystoscopy.

□ *Cystoscopy*

Cystoscopy is the direct examination of the bladder using an instrument called a *cystoscope* (Fig. 32-19). The cystoscope relies on a flexible optic fiber to provide illumination into the urinary tract. The instrument is attached to the illuminating source then slowly passed through the urinary tract, thus enabling direct visualization of the urethra, ureteral orifices, and bladder.

PREPROCEDURE CARE. Fluids are forced for several hours before the procedure. This ensures a continuous flow of urine, in the event that specimens need to be collected, and aids in preventing multiplication of bacteria

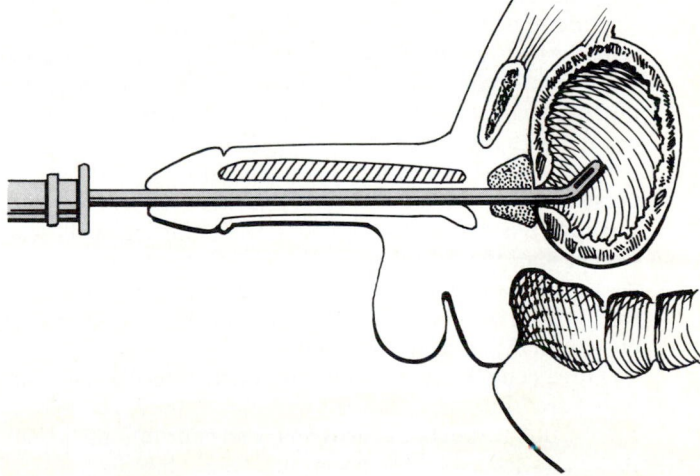

Fig. 32-19 Cystoscope inserted for examination of bladder.

that may be introduced during the procedure. If radiographs are to be taken during the procedure, bowel preparation may be ordered.

METHOD. If the patient is relatively comfortable and relaxed, the cystoscope can be passed with little discomfort, provided there is no obstruction in the urethra. A local anesthetic such as procaine may be instilled into the urethra before insertion of the cystoscope. Any discomfort felt during this procedure is the result of contraction or spasm of the bladder sphincters; this can be decreased through deep-breathing exercises and general relaxation on the part of the patient. A sedative such as diazepam may be given to the anxious person. General anesthesia is required when the person is overly apprehensive or when much manipulation is anticipated. In these instances, anesthesia reduces the possibility of trauma to the urethra or perforation of the bladder caused by sudden vigorous movement of the patient during the examination.

When the patient is awake, passing the instrument will be followed immediately by a strong desire to void. This occurs as a result of the pressure the instrument exerts against the internal sphincter. During the examination the bladder is distended with distilled water to make visualization more effective. As the bladder becomes increasingly distended, the urge to void increases.

During cystoscopy a number of tests may be performed on the urinary system. *Cystography* involves the injection of a radiopaque dye such as methiodal (Skiodan) or air as a contrast medium to visualize the bladder and determine its size, shape, and any irregularities. Bladder capacity may be measured through instillation of distilled water. A *voiding cystourethrogram* can reveal reflux of urine into the ureters on voiding, a bladder malfunction that can lead to pyelonephritis.

Ureteral catheterization (with a nylon, radiopaque, No. 4 to 6 Fr catheter) can be performed through the cystoscope. The catheter is inserted into the ureteral opening in the bladder, into the ureter, and into the renal pelvis (Fig. 32-20). This procedure may involve one or both ureters. It is performed (1) when culture and analysis of urine from individual kidneys is required; (2) when tests of renal function are to be performed on the kidneys separately; and (3) when visualization of the urinary tract is desired and intravenous pyelogram visualization has been inadequate, obstruction is present, or sensitivity to intravenous radiopaque material is noted.

POSTPROCEDURE CARE. Care should be taken that the person does not stand or walk alone immediately after cystoscopy. Blood that has drained from the leg while the person is in the lithotomy position will flow back into the vessels of the feet and legs as the person stands. Accidents caused by dizziness and fainting can occur from the sudden change in distribution of blood.

Three complications of cystoscopy that need to be monitored are bleeding, perforation of the bladder, and spread of infection throughout the urinary tract or into the bloodstream (sepsis). Observation for frank bleeding (pink-tinged urine is normal) is necessary. Urinary output and voiding pattern are monitored to detect obstruction, and

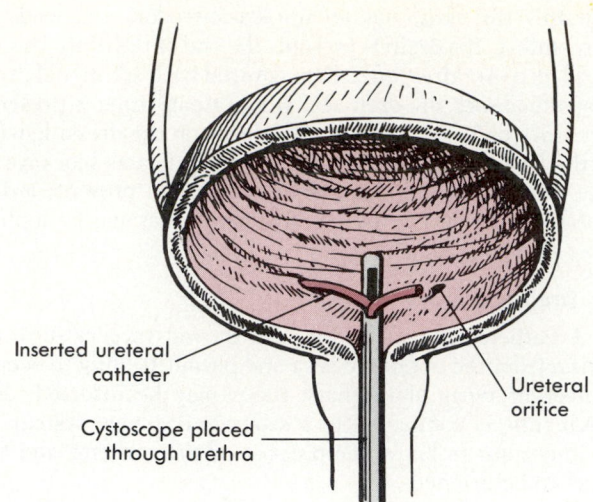

Fig. 32-20 Ureteral catheterization through cystoscope. Note ureteral catheter inserted into left orifice. Right ureteral catheter is ready to be inserted.

fluid intake is increased to prevent stasis. Mild analgesics are given for discomfort, and warmth is provided if the patient complains of being chilly. Vital signs are monitored as necessary.

➡ DATA ANALYSIS: NURSING DIAGNOSES

Nursing diagnoses are determined from assessment of patient data. Possible nursing diagnoses for the person with BPH may include, but are not limited to, the following:

Diagnostic title	Possible etiologies
Fluid volume excess	Compromised regulatory mechanism
Potential for infection	Urinary statis
Pain	Bladder spasms, retention
Potential impaired skin integrity	Irritation from dribbling of urine
Social isolation	Loss of urinary function
Altered patterns of urinary elimination	Anatomical obstruction, dribbling, urgency, frequency
Urinary retention	Obstruction

▦ PLANNING: EXPECTED PATIENT OUTCOMES

Expected patient outcomes for the person with BPH may include, but are not limited to the following:
1. The man remains comfortable.
2. The man does not display signs or symptoms of urinary retention.
3. The man's skin remains intact.
4. The man verbalizes the need for necessary diagnostic procedures.

◼ IMPLEMENTATION

□ Assisting with achievement of therapeutic goals

If urinary retention is present, an indwelling urinary catheter is usually inserted to relieve the retention and is maintained if the degree of obstruction is severe. Urinary tract infection is treated with antibiotics. Surgery is the primary treatment for BPH (see below).

□ Assisting with comfort

Pain from bladder spasms (either before or after surgery) is controlled with prescribed analgesics or antispasmodics such as belladonna preparations. The man is encouraged to void at the initial urge and to empty the bladder completely with each voiding.

□ Surgery

During surgery the capsule of the prostate gland is left intact, and the adenomatous soft tissue is removed by one of four surgical routes: transurethral, suprapubic, retropubic, or perineal (Table 32-13).

□ *Transurethral prostatectomy*

Transurethral prostatic resection (TURP) is performed when the major enlargement exists in the medial lobe that directly surrounds the urethra. There must be a relatively small amount of tissue requiring resection so that excessive bleeding will not occur and the time required to complete the surgery will not be prolonged. A resectoscope (an instrument similar to a cystoscope but equipped with a cutting and cauterization loop attached to electric current) is passed through the urethra. The bladder is irrigated continuously during the procedure. The patient is grounded against electric shocks by a lubricated metal plate placed under his hips. Tiny pieces of tissue are cut away, and the bleeding points are sealed by cauterization (Fig. 32-21). A transurethral prostatectomy may be performed with the patient under general or spinal anesthesia.

Following a TURP, a large (No. 24 Fr) three-way Foley catheter with a 30 ml balloon is usually inserted into the urethra. After the retention balloon of the catheter is inflated, the catheter is pulled down so that the bag rests in the prostatic fossa and provides hemostasis. Traction may be applied to the Foley catheter to increase pressure on the operative area to control bleeding. The large size catheter (No. 24 Fr) is used to facilitate removal of clots from the bladder. Because the catheter retention balloon exerts pressure on the internal sphincter of the bladder, the patient continually feels the urge to void. If the catheter is draining properly, the strongest of these sensations usually passes momentarily. Attempting to void around the catheter causes the bladder muscles to contract and results in a painful "bladder spasm."

Discuss the physiology of the "need to void" with the patient preoperatively so that spasms will be seen as an expected event and not an abnormal complication. Teach the patient that the catheter produces the sensation of fullness and that *not* straining to pass urine around the

---

Table 32-13   Comparison of types of prostatic surgery

	Transurethral resection	Suprapubic resection	Retropubic resection	Perineal resection	Radical perineal resection
Reason for surgery	Enlargement of medial lobe surrounding urethra	Extremely large mass of obstructing tissue	Large mass located high in pelvic area	Large mass located low in pelvic area	Cancer of prostate gland
Location of incision	No incision; removal by way of urethra	Low midline abdominal incision through bladder to prostate gland	Low midline abdominal incision into prostate gland (bladder not incised)	Incision between scrotum and rectum	Large perineal incision between scrotum and rectum
Drainage tubes	Three-way Foley catheter with 30 ml bag in urethra, constant irrigation for 24 hr	Cystotomy tube or drain through incision; Foley catheter with 30 ml bag in urethra	Foley catheter with 30 ml bag in urethra, constant irrigation for 24 hr	Foley catheter with 30 ml bag in urethra	Foley catheter with 30 ml bag in urethra; drain in incision
Bladder spasms	Yes	Yes	Few	Few	Few
Dressing	None	Abdominal dressing easily soaked with urinary drainage	Abdominal dressing; no urinary drainage	Perineal dressing; no urinary drainage	Perineal dressing; urinary drainage
Complications	Hemorrhage; water intoxication; incontinence	Hemorrhage; wound infection	Hemorrhage; wound infection	Hemorrhage; wound infection	Urinary incontinence; wound infection; impotence; sterility

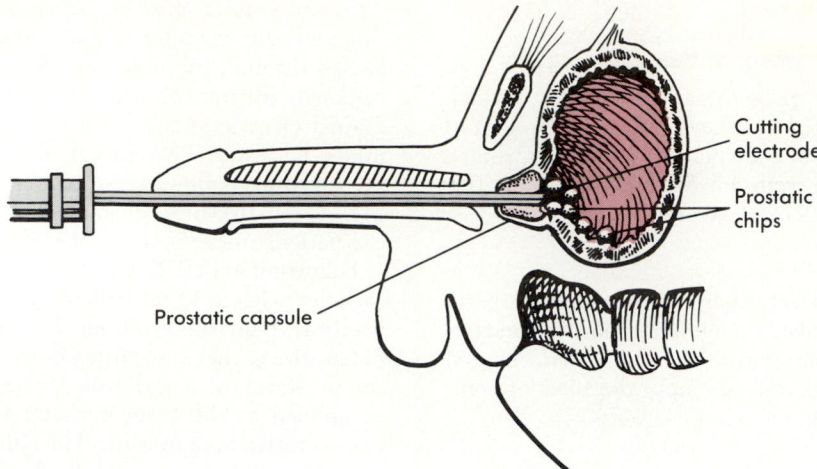

Cutting
electrode

Prostatic
chips

Prostatic capsule

Fig. 32-21 Transuretheral resection of prostate gland by means of resectoscope. Note enlarged prostate gland surrounding urethra and tiny pieces of prostatic tissue that have been cut away.

catheter and drinking large amounts of fluids will reduce irritation and spasm. Narcotics are given to lessen the pain sensation; belladonna and opium suppositories are prescribed to relieve bladder spasms. As the nerve endings become fatigued, the frequency and severity of spasms decrease. This usually occurs by the end of 24 to 48 hours.

The bladder is constantly irrigated by a three-way drip apparatus with normal saline or another solution prescribed by the surgeon. The purpose of constant irrigation is to keep the bladder free of clots that would block the drainage of urine.

A full bladder increases pressure on the outside of the prostatic fossa "milking" the bleeding vessels. Straining to have a bowel movement may also cause prostatic hemorrhage as can enemas, rectal tubes, and rectal thermometers, all of which are avoided for about a week postoperatively.

Persistent bladder discomfort, bladder spasms, or failure of a catheter to drain properly usually signifies one of the following serious complications, which require immediate medical attention: (1) hemorrhage and clot retention, (2) displacement of the catheter, or (3) unsuspected perforation of the bladder during surgery.

Sometimes patients develop *water intoxication,* formerly known as transurethral resection (TUR) syndrome, as a result of excessive irrigating solution being absorbed into the venous sinusoids during surgery. Cerebral edema may result. Confusion and agitation on the part of the patient may be the first signs of this condition.

Constant bladder irrigation is usually discontinued after 24 hours if no clots are draining from the bladder. The catheter may then be manually irrigated every 4 hours until removed, usually 3 to 5 days after surgery.

Following removal of the catheter, the patient should measure and record the time and amount of each voiding. The patient may not be able to void after removal of the catheter because of urethral edema. When this occurs, the

catheter may need to be reinserted. Continence should also be assessed since the internal and external sphincters lie above and below the prostate gland, close to the operative area, and may have been disturbed during surgery.

About 2 weeks after TURP, when desiccated tissue is sloughed out, there may be a secondary hemorrhage. The patient, who probably is home at this time, must contact the physician immediately should there be any bleeding.

□ *Suprapubic prostatectomy*

The alternate methods of prostatectomy are open operations. In the *suprapubic resection* the prostate gland is removed from the urethra by way of the bladder; this type of resection is performed when a large mass of tissue must be resected. The usual method of draining urine following surgery is illustrated in Fig. 32-22, *A.* There will be some type of hemostatic agent placed in the prostatic fossa and urine will be drained by Foley catheter or cystotomy tube or both.

Hemorrhage is a possible complication, and the precautions are the same as those taken following TURP. Because there is some oozing of blood from the prostatic fossa, continuous bladder irrigations are usually ordered for the first 24 hours.

Cystotomy tubes are usually removed 3 to 4 days postoperatively; urethral catheters generally remain until the suprapubic wound is healed. After the urethral catheter has been removed, the nursing care of the patient is similar to that for the patient undergoing transurethral resection. If the suprapubic wound should reopen and drain, a urethral catheter is usually reinserted.

□ *Retropubic prostatectomy*

In a retropubic prostatectomy a low abdominal incision similar to that used for suprapubic prostatectomy is made, but the bladder is not opened. Rather, it is retracted and the adenomatous prostatic tissue is removed through an incision in the anterior prostatic capsule (Fig. 32-22, *B*).

Sphincter muscles are seldom damaged by retropubic prostatectomy, and there is no urine fistula. A large Foley catheter is inserted postoperatively, but bladder spasms are not usually a problem. When the Foley catheter is removed, the patient seldom has difficulty voiding. Hemorrhage from the prostatic fossa and wound infection may complicate the surgery; therefore, precautions to prevent bleeding as discussed under TURP are taken. There should be no urinary drainage on the abdominal dressing. If urinary drainage on the abdominal dressing, purulent drainage, fever, or increased pain with ambulation occurs, the phy-

sician should be notified because these symptoms may indicate deep wound infection or pelvic abscess. Hospitalization generally is required for about 1 week after a retropubic prostatectomy.

□ *Perineal prostatectomy*

The perineal approach is used primarily for confirmed or suspected cancer of the prostate (Fig. 32-22, *C*). The incision is made between the scrotum and rectum. In addition to removal of the adenomatous prostate tissue, adjacent tissue may be excised when cancer is confirmed. Preoperative and postoperative care is similar to that given a patient having radical perineal surgery.

□ **Counseling and teaching**

Common to all patients undergoing prostatectomy are concerns regarding sexual functioning and the ability to be continent of urine. The nurse may need to provide an opportunity during interactions with the patient to promote expressions of these concerns by the patient. Impotence occurs physiologically when the perineal nerves are cut during a radical perineal prostatectomy and not with the other types of prostatectomies. If the man believes that the surgery will or may produce impotence, however, this may occur because of psychologic influences. Urinary incontinence frequently follows transurethral or suprapubic prostatectomy. Most men have some difficulty with continence after any type of prostatectomy. The patient should understand that this is normal for a period after surgery, and he should be taught perineal exercises to hasten recovery of control over voiding.

The following points should be included in preparing the patient for discharge from the hospital: (1) Vigorous exercises, heavy lifting, and sexual intercourse should be

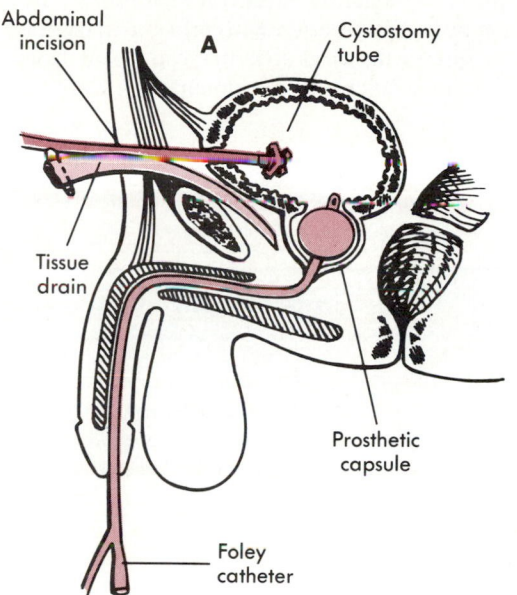

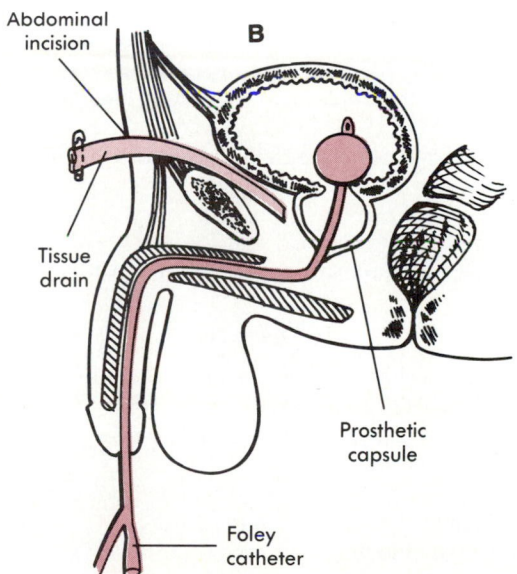

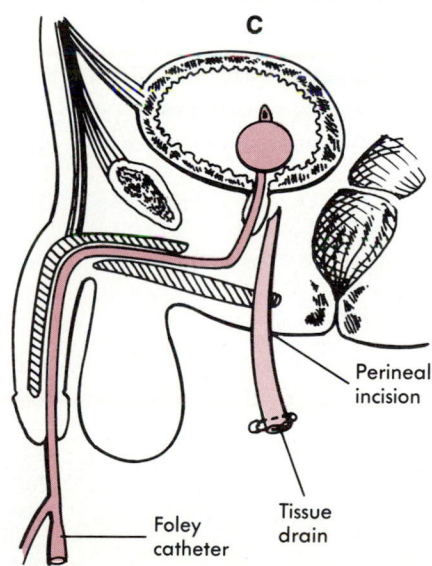

Fig. 32-22 Three types of prostatectomies. **A,** Suprapubic; note placement of inflated Foley catheter in prostatic fossa. **B,** Retropubic. **C,** Radical perineal; note tissue drain placed in incision between scrotum and rectum.

avoided for about 3 weeks after returning home. (2) Driving during this period is also not advised. (3) Straining with defecation should be avoided; stool softeners or mild cathartics may be prescribed as home-going medication. (4) Fluids are encouraged to prevent stasis and infection and to keep stools soft. (5) The patient is instructed to notify his physician should his urinary stream diminish. The urinary stream also will be checked on the patient's postoperative visit to the physician. This is important because urethral mucosa in the prostatic area is destroyed during surgery and strictures may form with healing.

⊞ EVALUATION

The care of specific patients with BPH is evaluated on the basis of expected patient outcomes. General questions to ask include the following:

1. Does the person appear to be comfortable?
2. Is the person maintaining a normal urination pattern?
3. Can the person state the necessity for any surgical interventions?
4. Can the person demonstrate exercises to regain urinary sphincter muscle function?
5. Can the person explain the rationale for potential sexual dysfunction following surgery?

■ Urethral strictures

A urethral stricture is a narrowing or constriction of the lumen of the urethra. Urethral strictures can be congenital or acquired. Congenital urethral strictures can occur in isolation or in combination with other urinary tract anomalies. Acquired urethral stricture can result from trauma secondary to accident or instrumentation, infection, mus-

---

NURSING CARE PLAN

Person with transurethral resection prostatectomy for benign prostatic hypertrophy

DATA: Mr. Smith is a 72-year-old retired automobile mechanic. He had been in his usual state of good health until about 4 months ago when he started to develop nocturia. Several weeks later he noted difficulty initiating voiding. He also noted mild dribbling after voiding. On physical examination his physician noted moderate enlargement of his prostate. He is being admitted for cystoscopy and possible TURP. His vital signs are stable. He is married and states that his wife provides him support at home. He lives in a two-story, single-family home.

The nursing history obtained on admission identified the following:
1. He has not been hospitalized before.
2. He does not take any medications.
3. He enjoys outdoor activities and exercises daily by walking 2 to 3 miles.
4. His expectations are that he will have the procedure and return to his normal life-style within a few days.
5. His wife is in constant attendance and tends to answer any questions that are asked of the patient.

Collaborative nursing actions include those to monitor for postoperative complications, including bleeding and dysuria. Specific nursing actions include monitoring the following:
1. Signs and symptoms of hemorrhage: hematuria; increased pulse; decreased blood pressure; restlessness; cool, moist skin
2. Inability to void once urinary catheter is removed

Nursing diagnosis: Altered patterns of urinary retention: related to obstruction secondary to TURP

Expected patient outcomes	Nursing interventions	Rationale
Retention of urine does not occur	Monitor urinary output and characteristics	Detect retention early
	Maintain constant bladder irrigation as prescribed during first 24 hours	Prevent clots from obstructing urine flow
	Maintain patency of indwelling urinary catheter by irrigating	Prevent clots from obstruction catheter
	Encourage high fluid intake (2500 to 3000 ml/day)	Promote urinary flow
	After catheter is removed, continue to monitor for signs of retention	Detect retention early

NURSING CARE PLAN

Person with transurethral resection prostatectomy for benign prostatic hypertrophy

Nursing diagnosis: Pain: related to bladder spasm

Expected patient outcomes	Nursing interventions	Rationale
Patient states feeling more comfortable	Teach patient not to try to void around catheter	Reduce likelihood of spasm
	Monitor patient at regular intervals for 48 hours to identify early signs of bladder spasm	Identify presence of spasms so that medication may be administered
	Give prescribed medications (analgesics, antispasmodics)	Relieve symptoms
	Tell patient spasms will decrease in intensity and frequency within 24 to 48 hours	Encourage patient that discomfort is temporary

Nursing diagnosis: Fluid volume excess: potential, related to absorption of bladder irrigation solution

Expected patient outcomes	Nursing interventions	Rationale
Early signs of water intoxication are identified	Monitor patient for signs of water intoxication during first 24 hours: confusion, agitation, warm moist skin, anorexia, nausea and vomiting	Early detection can lead to early treatment

Nursing diagnosis: Potential for injury: hemorrhage or infection related to surgery

Expected patient outcomes	Nursing interventions	Rationale
Infection does not occur	Monitor vital signs, report signs of shock or fever	Prevent shock before it occurs
Bleeding is minimized	Monitor appearance of urine for persistent bright red color rather than expected dark red beyond first few hours postoperatively	Urine should change from cherry pink to amber in the first 2 to 3 postoperative days
	Teach patient to avoid Valsalva maneuver	May initiate prostatic bleeding during initial postoperative period because of pressure
	Avoid use of rectal thermometers, rectal examinations, or enemas for at least 1 week	May initiate prostatic bleeding
	Maintain strict asepsis of urinary drainage system, irrigate only when necessary	Minimize potential of introducing organisms that could cause infection
	Encourage high fluid intake	Increase urinary output that will reduce potential of infection

Nursing diagnosis: Incontinence, stress or urge: related to catheter removal following surgery

Expected patient outcomes	Nursing interventions	Rationale
Patient achieves urinary control	Assess patient for dribbling after catheter is removed	Detect incontinence
	If dribbling occurs:	
	a. Tell patient this is common occurrence and continence will return	Patient needs to be reassured this is normal
	b. Teach perineal exercises	Assist in bladder control

Continued.

NURSING CARE PLAN

Person with transurethral resection prostatectomy for benign prostatic hypertrophy— cont'd

Nursing diagnosis: Sexual dysfunction: potential, related to TURP

Expected patient outcomes	Nursing interventions	Rationale
Sexual functioning is maintained	Give patient opportunity to discuss feelings about effects of prostatectomy on sexual intercourse	This is a difficult subject for many patients to raise
	Provide information as necessary	Lack of knowledge may create anxiety and lead to sexual dysfunction
	a. Probable return of previous level of functioning	
	b. Occurrence of retrograde ejaculation (urine may have a milky appearance)	
	Avoid sexual intercourse for 3 to 4 weeks after surgery	Bleeding and discomfort may occur

Nursing diagnosis: Knowledge deficit: related to TURP

Expected patient outcomes	Nursing interventions	Rationale
Patient describes activity restrictions and need for medical follow-up	Teach patient:	May initiate bleeding
	a. Avoidance of heavy activites for 3 to 4 weeks (check with physician regarding resumption of long walks)	
	b. Avoidance of straining at stool for 4 to 6 weeks; use of stool softeners or laxatives as necessary	Straining may initiate bleeding; stool softeners will reduce the need to strain at stool
	c. Fluid maintenance of at least 2500 ml to 3000 ml/day	Will reduce potential of infection and clot formation
	d. Instructions for medical follow-up	Follow-up is essential to ensure no complications have developed

cular spasm, or pressure from the outside, by adjacent structures, or by growing tumors. Urethral strictures occur more often in men than women, primarily because of the length of the urethra. A common cause of strictures in the past was the instillation of silver nitrate in the male urethra for the treatment of gonorrhea.

Strictures may be corrected by dilation of the urethra; this is accomplished by inserting splinting catheters into the urethra past the area of stricture. The size of the splinting catheter can be increased, causing a gradual dilation of the urethra. The procedure may be accomplished during a single visit or over a period of time. The person may experience pain during the procedure, therefore, a local or spinal anesthetic may be used. Complications are infrequent but may include hematuria.

Urethral strictures may also be repaired by transurethral

visual urethrotomy or by urethroplasty with end-to-end anastomosis or with an inlay graft. Care of the person after transurethal visual urethrotomy is similar to that after a TURP (p. 1169). The urethroplasty is open surgical repair through a lower abdominal approach; the care of the patient is similar to that following other urologic surgeries (p. 1166).

■ Neoplasms

Neoplasms of the urinary system are a significant source of morbidity. The major neoplasms are found in the kidney and bladder. Cancer of the prostate causes urinary problems by pressure on the urethra, leading to obstruction (Table 32-14). Tumors growing anywhere within the abdominal cavity can result in renal involvement through

Table 32-14   Tumors of the urinary tract

Site	Incidence	Signs and symptoms	Medical therapy
Kidney	2%	Hematuria Dull flank pain Flank mass Unexplained weight loss Fever Polycythemia	Nephrectomy Radiation
Bladder	5%	Intermittent hematuria Anemia Cystitis Suprapubic pain RBCs, WBCs and bacteria in urine	Transurethral fulguration or excision of small papillomas Segmental or total cystectomy Intravesicular chemotherapy if the bladder is not removed Palliative chemotherapy
Prostate	20%	Urethral obstruction Low-back pain Hematuria Anemia	Radical resection of prostate Radiation Hormonal therapy

metastasis or invasion, or by pressure of the tumor creating urinary obstruction. Urinary diversion (p. 1177) may be required in treating urinary neoplasms.

■ RENAL NEOPLASMS

Malignant renal tumors, primarily adenocarcinomas, account for 2% of all cancers. Small benign renal tumors (adenomas) may occur without causing significant damage or symptoms. Renal cell carcinomas rarely occur before the age of 40 years, are more commonly seen in the 50- to 70-year age range, and occur twice as often in men as in women.

Hematuria is the most frequent symptom of renal cell carcinoma. Unfortunately, the hematuria is often intermittent, lessening the person's concern and causing procrastination in seeking medical care. Any person with hematuria should have a complete urologic examination, because it is only by immediate investigation of the first signs of hematuria that there is any hope of cure. Other symptoms may include dull flank pain, flank mass, weight loss, fever, and polycythemia. Hypertension may result from stimulation of the renin-angiotensin system.

An IVP may show a distortion of renal outline suggesting a kidney tumor. Small tumors in the parenchyma may not be apparent on a routine pyelogram but may be identified by CT scan. A CT scan is also useful in differentiating between renal cell carcinoma and renal cyst. Angiography may also be performed to differentiate a cyst from a tumor.

Unless the person is a poor surgical risk or has extensive metastases, the diseased kidney is removed (*nephrectomy*) through a transabdominal, thoracoabdominal, or retroperitoneal approach. The first two approaches are preferred to secure the renal artery and vein and prevent any spread of malignant cells. (See p. 1165 for care of the person requiring urologic surgery.)

Following surgery for a malignant tumor that is radio-sensitive, the patient is usually given a course of x-ray therapy. Hospitalization is not always necessary during this time. Radiation may also be used over the metastatic sites as palliative treatment for the person with an inoperable tumor. Chemotherapy has not yet proved of value in the treatment of renal cell carcinomas. The survival rate after therapy depends on the extent of metastasis. The 10-year survival rate is very low, especially since many persons do not seek initial treatment until the disease is far advanced.

■ TUMORS OF THE BLADDER

The most common site of cancer in the urinary tract is the bladder. Cancer of the bladder occurs 3 times more often in males than in females and multiple tumors are common, with about 25% of patients having more than one lesion at the time of diagnosis. This figure increases to about 50% in patients with papilloma, grade I carcinoma, over a 5-year period. Approximately 40% of the tumors involve the trigone, and an additional 45% involve the posterior and lateral bladder walls.

In the past 25 years, the incidence of bladder cancer in men has increased over 20% while the incidence in women has decreased over 25%. Known factors predisposing to bladder cancer are exposure to the chemicals beta-naphthylamine and xenylamine, infestation with *Schistosoma haematobium*, and cigarette smoking.

□ Pathophysiology

Tumors of the bladder range from small benign papillomas to large invasive carcinomas. Most of the neoplasms are of the transitional cell type since the urinary tract is covered with transitional epithelium. These neoplasms begin as papillomas; therefore, all papillomas of the bladder are considered premalignant and are removed when identified. Squamous cell carcinoma occurs less frequently and has a poorer prognosis. Other neoplasias include adenocarcinoma (which is often inoperable) and rhabdomyosarcoma (seen in infants).

Grades I (well differentiated) and II (medially differentiated) bladder tumors are usually superficial, while grades III (poorly differentiated) and IV (anaplastic) tumors are usually invasive. Bladder cancers are *staged* according to the depth of invasiveness:

Stage O:	Mucosa
State A:	Submucosa
Stage B:	Muscle
State C:	Perivesical fat
State D:	Lymph nodes

Painless *hematuria* is the first symptom in the majority of bladder tumors. It is usually intermittent, and the individual may fail to seek treatment. Painless hematuria occurs also in nonmalignant urinary tract disease and in cancer of the kidney; therefore, any hematuria should be investigated. Cystitis may be the first symptom of a bladder tumor because the tumor may act as a foreign body in the bladder. Renal failure from obstruction of the ureters sometimes is the reason given for seeking medical care. Vesicovaginal fistulas may occur before other symptoms develop. The last two conditions indicate a poor prognosis because usually the tumor has infiltrated widely.

□ Diagnostic tests

Cytologic examination of the urine may identify malignant cells before the lesion can be visualized by cystoscopy. The diagnosis is established by cystoscopic visualization of the bladder with biopsy. Clinical determination of the invasiveness of the tumor is important in establishing a therapeutic regimen and in predicting the prognosis. Any person who has had a papilloma removed should have a cystoscopic examination every 3 months for 2 years and then at less frequent intervals if there is no evidence of a new lesion. The necessity for frequent examination should be fully explained by the urologist, and the explanation should be reinforced by the nurse. Emphasis should be placed on the necessity for repeated cystoscopies, since papillomas tend to recur without symptoms until they are far advanced tumors.

□ Surgery

Small tumors with minimal tissue layer involvement may be adequately treated with *transurethral fulguration or excision*. A Foley catheter may or may not be inserted after surgery. The urine may be pink tinged, but gross bleeding is unusual. Burning on urination may be relieved by forcing fluids and applying heat over the bladder region by means of a heating pad or a sitz bath. The patient is discharged within a few days after surgery.

If the tumor involves the dome of the bladder, a *segmental resection* of the bladder (p. 1165) may be carried out. Over half of the bladder may be resected. A *cystectomy*, or complete removal of the bladder, usually is performed only when the disease appears curable. Complete removal of the bladder requires permanent urinary diversion (p. 1177).

□ Radiation

External cobalt radiation of large invasive tumors is often given before surgery to retard tumor growth. Supervoltage irradiation can be given when the patient physically cannot tolerate surgery. Radiation is not curative and has little value in patient management if the tumor is deemed inoperable. Internal radiation (radioisotopes or radon seeds) are rarely used since the introduction of better methods of external radiation.

□ Chemotherapy

Chemotherapy is primarily palliative. 5-Fluorouracil (5-FU) and doxorubicin (Adriamycin) are the most commonly used agents. Thiotepa may be instilled into the bladder as a topical treatment. The patient is dehydrated 8 to 12 hours before thiotepa treatment, and the drug remains in the bladder for 2 hours.

■ CANCER OF THE PROSTATE

The prostate gland is the second most common site of cancer among men. There is a familial tendency for the disease. Prostate cancer is responsible for 10% of all deaths from cancer in men. It rarely occurs before age 50 and the incidence increases with age. The younger the man at the age of onset, the more lethal is the disease. Although cancer may start anywhere within the prostate gland and may be multifocal in origin, it usually arises in the peripheral lobes resulting in a palpable nodule. Early detection of nodules on palpation can lead to early treatment and improve the prognosis significantly. For this reason all men over age 40 should have an annual rectal examination.

Prostate cancer usually begins with changes in voiding patterns, including frequency, urgency, and nocturia because of the increase in gland size impinging on the urethra. Complete urethral obstruction can develop. Hematuria can occur resulting in anemia. Treatment is primarily surgical.

□ Radical prostatic resection

In patients in whom a diagnosis of prostatic cancer is made before local extension of the cancer or distant metastasis, a radical resection of the prostate gland usually is curative. The entire prostate gland, including the capsule and the adjacent tissue, is removed. The remaining urethra is then anastomosed to the bladder neck.

Because the internal and external sphincters of the bladder lie in close approximation to the prostate gland, it is not unusual for the patient to have urinary incontinence after this type of surgery. The perineal approach is most used, but the procedure may be accomplished by the retropubic route (see p. 1171).

□ *Preoperative care*

If the surgery is to be done via a perineal approach, the patient is given a bowel preparation (enemas, cathartics, antibiotics) and only clear fluids the day before surgery to prevent fecal contamination of the operative site. Postoperatively, when food is permitted, a low-residue diet may be given until wound healing is well advanced.

Radical prostatectomy results in physiologic sexual dysfunction from disruption of genital innervation. Ninety percent of patients lose emission, ejaculation, and erectile potency. Ten percent do have satisfactory erections, possibly because some nerves escape damage during surgery. Both the man and his sexual partner are made aware of this sexual dysfunction before surgery. The information is given by the physician, but the involved persons need opportunities to share their concerns about the proposed surgery.

□ *Postoperative care*

URINARY DRAINAGE. The patient returns from surgery with an indwelling urethral catheter. A large amount of urinary drainage on the dressing for a number of hours is not unusual. This can be managed by use of an ostomy bag around the dressing. Urinary drainage should decrease rapidly. There should not be the amount of bleeding that follows other prostatic surgery.

Because the catheter is not being used for hemostasis, the patient usually has little bladder spasm. The catheter is used both for urinary drainage and as a splint for the urethral anastomosis; therefore, care is taken that it does not become dislodged or blocked. The risk of blockage is greatest during the first hour. The catheter may be irrigated intermittently or continuously as ordered by the physician. The catheter is usually left in the bladder for 2 to 3 weeks.

FECAL CONTROL. Fecal incontinence may occur after surgery as a result of relaxation of the perineal musculature. Control of the rectal sphincter usually returns readily. Return of function can be facilitated by perineal exercises (p. 1140) started within a day or two after surgery and continued after rectal sphincter control returns, to strengthen bladder sphincters (unless the bladder sphincters have been permanently damaged).

PSYCHOLOGIC SUPPORT. The patient with cancer of the prostate gland is often very depressed after radical prostatectomy because he suddenly realizes the implications of being impotent and perhaps permanently incontinent. At times the man may have difficulty talking to his sexual partner about his concerns and the effect of his impotence on their relationship. The nurse can encourage each person to share his and her feelings separately, then gently encourage and facilitate mutual sharing by the partners.

■ Urinary diversion

Urinary diversion procedures are surgical procedures that divert the urinary flow from its normal flow patterns to a newly created opening, usually on the abdominal wall. Although urinary neoplasms are one of the major reasons for urinary diversions, these procedures may also be performed for neurogenic bladder dysfunction, chronic progressive pyelonephritis, urinary birth defects, or irreparable urinary tract trauma.

■ URINARY DIVERSION PROCEDURES

The most common urinary diversion procedures include ureterostomy, ileal conduit, and colonic (sigmoid) conduit (discussed below). These procedures require the placement of an external stoma; the urine is then collected in an ostomy pouch. Newer procedures being studied include a continent ileal conduit, continent vesicostomy, and carbon conduit. These procedures offer hope of control over the flow of urine without the use of an external stoma and ostomy pouch.

A *cutaneous ureterostomy* is used when the physical condition of the person prohibits more extensive surgery. This is usually temporary therapy followed by more extensive treatment. One or both ureters are excised from the bladder and diverted through the abdominal wall to form a small stoma. If both ureters are diverted, each is diverted separately, resulting in two stomas. Initially the ureterostomy stoma will appear pink, but it will turn pale in several weeks. Complications of ureterostomy include stricture of the ureter at the stoma. This stricture is treated by dilation. Untreated strictures can result in hydronephrosis; UTI is also a common complication.

The *ureteroileocutaneous anastomosis* (commonly called *ileal conduit* or *ileal loop*) is the most common permanent urinary diversion. A 15 to 20 cm section of the ileum is resected with the mesentery and blood supply intact, and the ileum itself is then anastomosed (Fig. 32-23). The ureters are excised from the bladder and anastomosed to one end of the resected ileal portion; that end is then sutured closed to form a pouch. The open end of the resected ileal portion is then brought through the abdominal

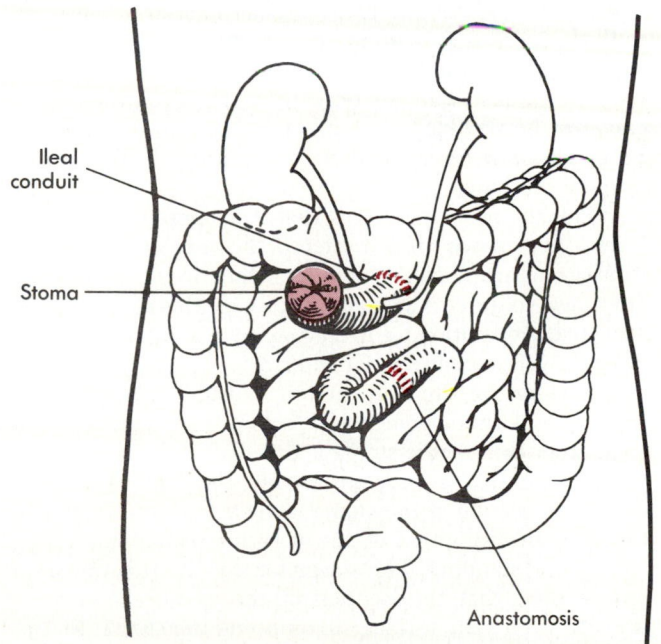

Ileal conduit

Stoma

Anastomosis

Fig. 32-23   Ileal conduit or ileal loop.

wall to the skin surface to create a stoma. The urinary bladder may be left intact or resected, depending on the reason for the diversion.

The *colonic conduit or loop* is similar to the ileal conduit, however, a segment of the colon is resected to serve as a conduit. Any section of colon can be resected. The colonic conduit is preferred by some surgeons because it has been shown to reduce the incidence of urinary reflux in some people.[4]

In both the ileal and colonic conduit, the stoma should be bright red in color. Complications of conduit surgery include hemorrhage, infection, separation of the anastomosis, and paralytic ileus. Procedural complications include leakage at the ureter anastomosis, obstruction of the ureter, mucocutaneous separation, and stoma necrosis.

■ PREOPERATIVE CARE

Changes in body image can be a significant effect of any procedure that leads to the formation of a stoma, therefore, it is important to prepare the patient appropriately for the surgery. Individuals who have been well informed about the surgery do better both in the immediate postoperative period and in the long term. The person's questions must be answered honestly and completely. The goals for preoperative teaching must reflect the individual patient's needs. Not every person will want to see a stoma model or urinary pouches before surgery; however, certain basic information must be conveyed. The person should be able to describe the surgical procedure and expected outcomes.

The person is instructed concerning the appearance of the stoma. Anatomical charts, models, and simple drawings are ways of explaining the placement of the stoma. It is stressed that work, hobbies, physical activities, diet, and clothing should not change significantly after surgery.

If the person is willing, he or she may be given an opportunity to handle a urostomy appliance to dispel any misconceptions. The person can be reassured that stoma care will be provided immediately after surgery and that he or she will be assisted in mastering self-care before hospital discharge.

When the nurse perceives that it is appropriate, a visit from a person who has mastered the care of a urostomy can be reassuring to the patient. Many local cancer societies have volunteers available to provide this support. Preoperative preparation for ureterostomy is similar to that for other bowel procedures (Chapter 31).

The stoma for the ileal conduit is usually placed on the right side of the abdomen just below the waist, whereas location of the colonic stoma is determined by the portion of the bowel that is resected. Ideally, the determination of the exact location of the stoma is made before surgery and includes an evaluation of the person's body when lying, sitting, and standing. The reason for this careful evaluation is to ensure that the location of the stoma allows for a smooth, even skin surface surrounding the stoma, for optimal adherence of the appliance.

■ POSTOPERATIVE CARE

□ Immediate care

Following a *cutaneous ureterostomy*, the patient generally returns from surgery with catheters inserted through the ureters to maintain drainage of the renal pelves. The catheters are usually left in place for 7 to 14 days. Patency of the catheters must be maintained to prevent hydronephrosis.

Following a *conduit procedure*, splinting catheters may be in place through the stoma; these catheters are usually removed on the second or third postoperative day. A nasogastric tube with suction is also used for 2 to 3 days postoperatively to allow for the return of effective intestinal peristalsis and healing of the intestinal anastomosis. Nothing is permitted by mouth until the return of bowel sounds or passing of gas; the diet is then gradually advanced from small amounts of fluids to a normal diet.

During the immediate postoperative period, urinary output is monitored closely; decreased urinary output could signal obstruction of urinary drainage or complications such as dehydration or renal failure. Urine is tested for presence of blood. Blood in the urine is expected in the immediate postoperative period; however, it should clear within the first few postoperative days.

The abdominal incision is assessed daily for healing and signs and symptoms of infection. Care of the abdominal incision is sometimes complicated by the leakage of urine into it; this complication is minimized by using appropriate drainage bags postoperatively.

□ Stoma care

Adequate skin care is essential postoperatively in any type of urinary diversion procedure. Care must be taken to prevent the leakage of urine onto the skin surrounding the stoma. When catheters are in place during the immediate postoperative period, urine drainage is usually not a problem. However, when no catheters are present, it is essential that a properly fitting stoma pouch or temporary postoperative drainage bag be applied. An appropriate appliance has an opening cut so that the hole fits around the stoma with no more than 3 mm ($\frac{1}{8}$ inch) of skin exposed.

Several commercially available adhesives are available to apply the pouch to the stoma. These products, such as United's Skin-Prep or Hollister's Skin-Gel, provide for good adhesion and skin protection. Some skin sealant products contain alcohol that can cause irritation and drying of skin. Tincture of benzoin should be avoided because it can result in severe skin reactions. A skin barrier product such as Stomahesive or Hollihesive may be used during the postoperative period to prevent skin excoriation or to protect already excoriated skin.

The stoma pouch is changed to observe the stoma, to assess the mucocutaneous suture line postoperatively, and to allow for patient teaching of stoma care. The box on p. 1179 summarizes the procedure for changing the stoma pouch. After the patient has mastered stoma care and the

---

Changing a urinary pouch

1. Assemble needed supplies before starting.
2. Empty the pouch and gently remove the appliance from the skin.
3. Cleanse the skin surrounding the stoma with mild soap and water. Rinse completely. Pat dry. Any mucous secretions should be washed from the stoma gently.
4. Place a rolled piece of gauze or cotton ball over the stoma opening to absorb draining urine until the pouch is reapplied.
5. Measure the diameter of the stoma and cut a corresponding opening in the skin barrier (if used) and the pouch or select the corresponding size of precut pouch.
6. Apply skin sealant around the stoma if desired. Allow the area to dry completely.
7. Attach the pouch to the skin barrier. The pouch and skin barrier may be applied to the skin separately or together. In the early postoperative period it is easier to attach the pouch to the skin barrier and then to apply the system in one piece to the skin.
8. Apply the pouch and skin barrier around the stoma, keeping the adhesive area free of wrinkles or creases. Press gently but firmly into place and hold for approximately 30 seconds.
9. The valve at the bottom of the pouch must be closed or attached to a drainage collection bag.

---

stoma is healing well, the pouch should only be changed when a leak develops. The patient is instructed to assess the stoma for color and bleeding and to assess the surrounding skin each time the pouch is changed. The physician is contacted for changes in the color of the stoma or bleeding from the stoma.

☐ Permanent appliance

Approximately 7 days after surgery, the patient can be measured for a permanent appliance. The stoma is measured using a commercially available measurement card. These cards have several holes, labeled for size, that are placed over the stoma. The correct size allows for approximately 1.5 to 3 mm of skin to show between the card and the stoma. Another method is to measure the diameter of the stoma and add 3 to 6 mm to that measurement. Because the stoma may continue to shrink for 6 to 8 weeks after surgery, the patient is taught to measure the stoma so that the individual can continue to adjust the size of the appliance during healing.

Several types of appliances are available (Fig. 32-24 and 32-25). Appliances all have two things in common, a pouch to collect urine and a valve at the bottom to drain urine. There are three basic types of bags:

1. Permanent—can be washed and reused
2. Semidisposable—fit over a permanent disk attached to the skin
3. One-piece disposable—discarded after each use

All pouches adhere to the body with some type of adhesive to form a watertight seal. The type of pouch used depends largely on individual preference, body build, and physical or visual impairments. The person is encouraged to examine different types; however, guidance may be necessary in making a final selection. An enterostomal therapist may be helpful in assisting with the selection. Before discharge, the person must be instructed on how to manage the care of the pouch.

If a reusable pouch is selected, the patient is instructed to place 10 ml of full- or half-strength vinegar into the pouch twice a day. The vinegar decreases urinary odor and disinfects the pouch. A pouch with an antireflux valve is recommended to prevent urinary tract infection from the pouch.

Odor is not a problem in persons with urinary diversion. The presence of an unpleasant odor usually is a sign of UTI, alkaline urine, or inadequate cleaning techniques. Alkaline urine is associated with crystals, recurrent UTI, stoma and loop stenosis, and hyperkeratosis of the skin. Alkaline urine can be treated by acidification of urine by diet (p. 1162).

In summary, a teaching plan for the person with a urinary diversion includes the following:

1. Nature of the urinary diversion
2. Assessment of stoma appearance and changes that require medical attention
3. Method for measuring correct size of stoma appliance
4. Methods to protect the skin and to treat skin excoriations
5. Correct pouch application
6. Care of permanent appliances
7. Signs and symptoms of UTI
8. Need for follow-up care

■ OTHER URINARY DISORDERS

Several disorders of the urinary tract do not fit into the classifications discussed thus far. These disorders, polycystic disease, vascular disorders, toxic nephropathy, and trauma, will be discussed in this section.

■ Polycystic disease

Polycystic disease is an inherited defect that involves the kidneys bilaterally. The kidneys are usually enlarged and filled with cysts. Polycystic disease is categorized into two groups, infantile and adult. Infantile polycystic disease is an autosomal recessive trait. The infant usually develops

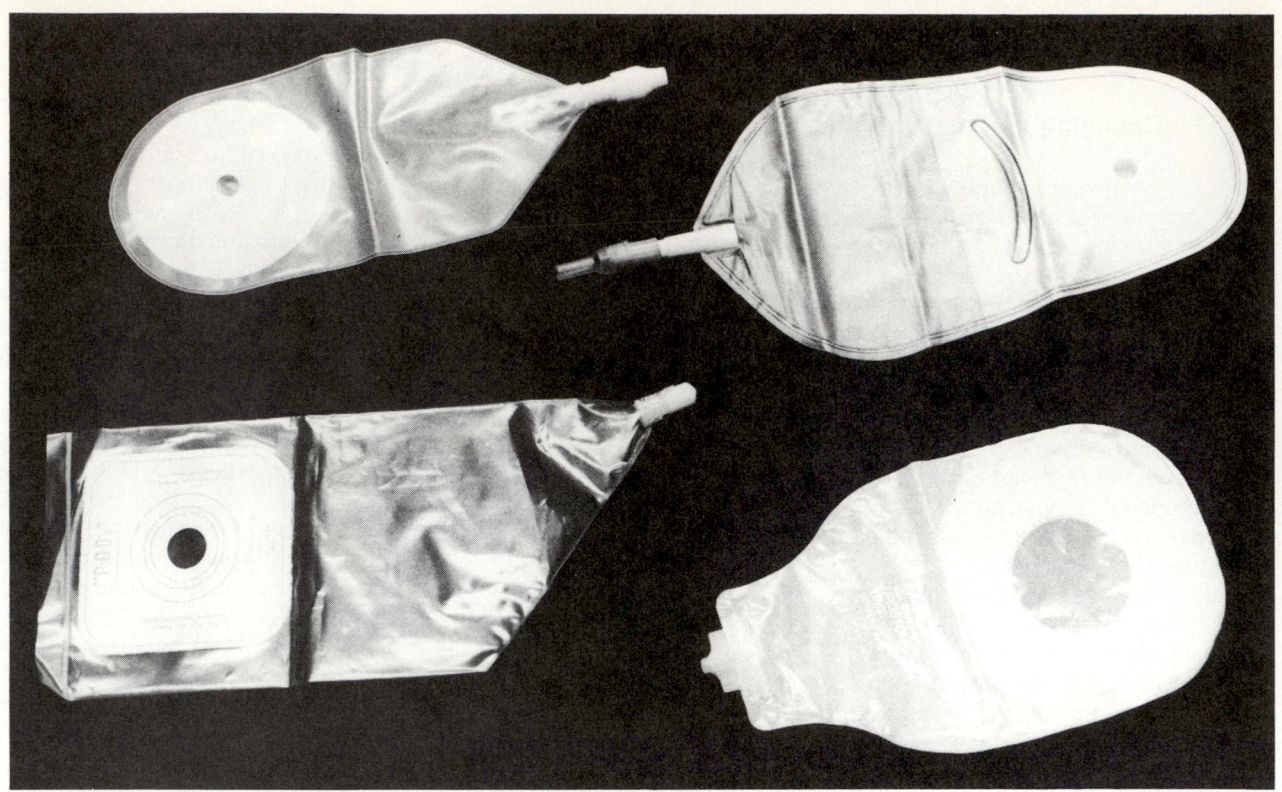

Fig. 32-24   Examples of postoperative drainage bags for urinary stoma.

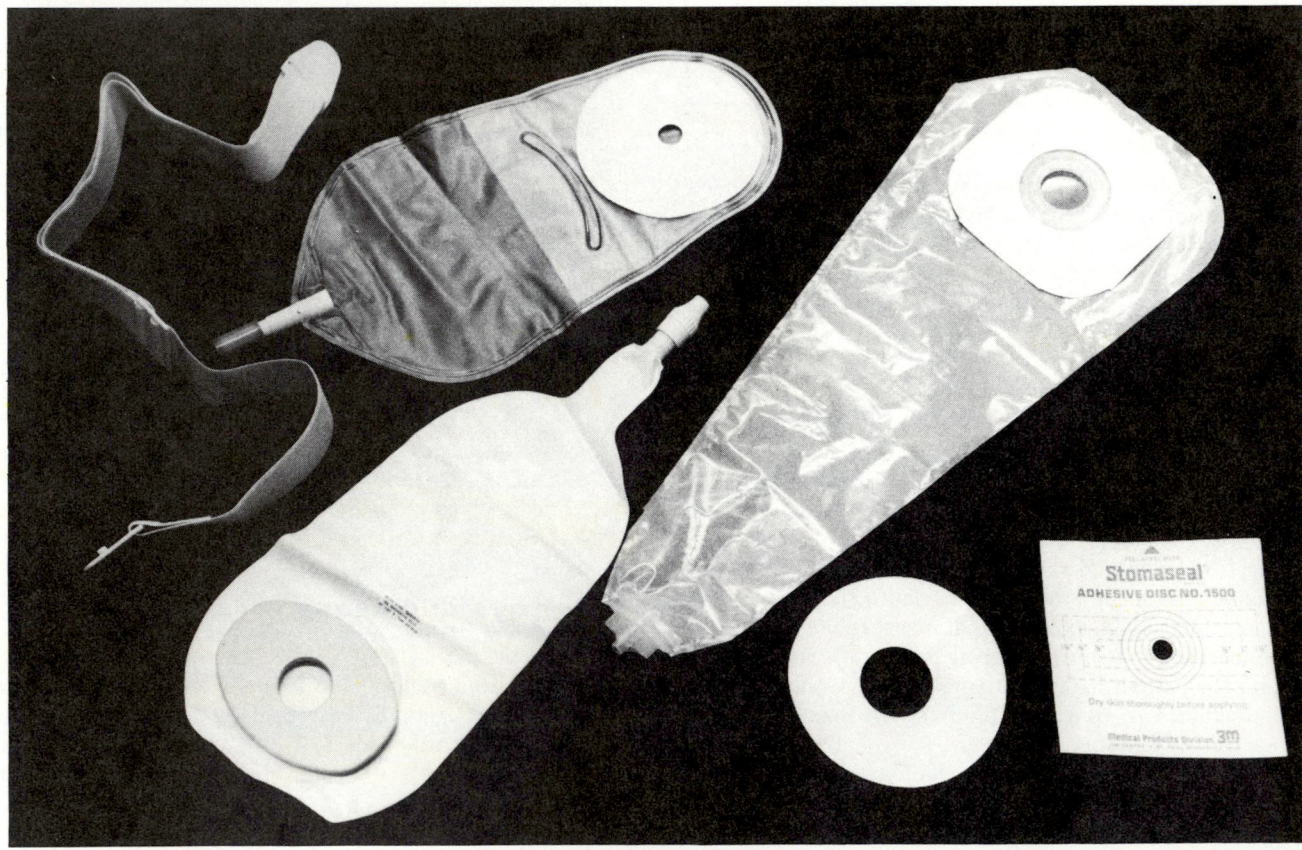

Fig. 32-25   Some examples of urinary appliances used by persons for long-term management of urinary tract diversion. Adhesive tape disks and belt are also shown.

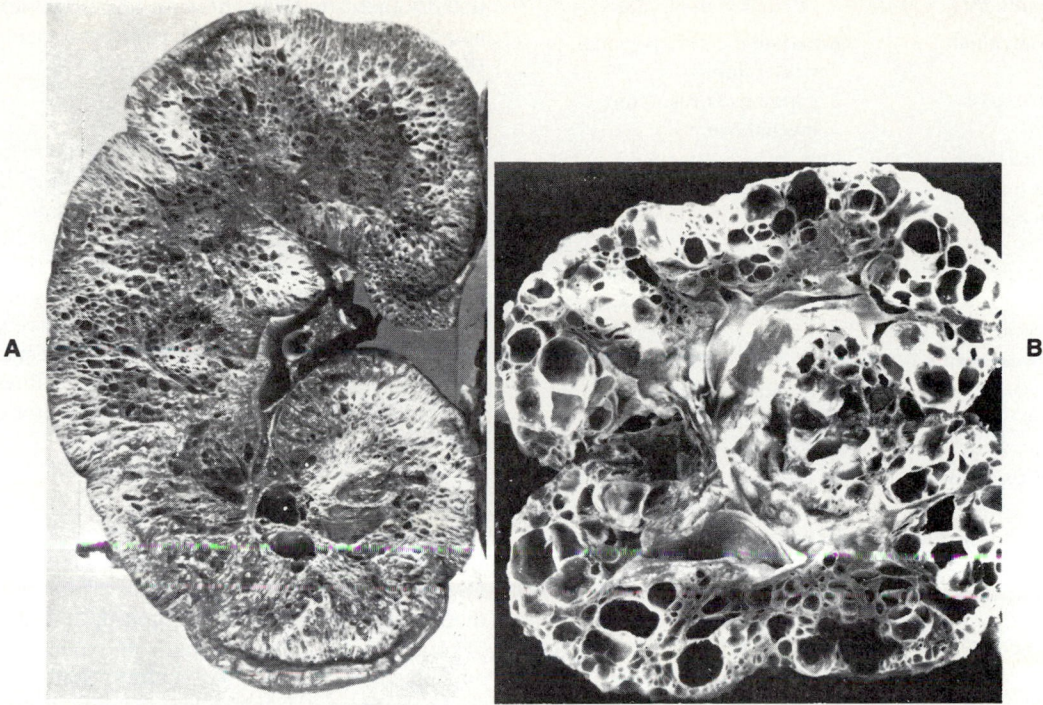

Fig. 32-26   Polycystic disease of kidney. **A,** Newborn infant. **B,** Adult. (From Anderson, WAD, and Kissane, JM: Pathology, ed 7, St. Louis, 1977, The CV Mosby Co.)

symptoms and dies within a few months after birth. Adult polycystic disease is an autosomal dominant trait affecting about 1 in 500 persons. Adults with this disorder generally develop symptoms in the third to fourth decade of life. End-stage renal disease is usually reached 10 to 15 years after symptoms arise.

There is no preventive care for polycystic disease. However, early detection and medical care can prevent and control infection of the diseased kidneys and retard the development of end-stage renal failure.

■ PATHOPHYSIOLOGY

As polycystic disease progresses, cysts in the kidneys enlarge and rupture (Fig. 32-26). The ruptured cysts become infected and scar tissue develops, thus decreasing the number of functioning nephrons. The size of the cysts also increases gradually, creating pressure on the surrounding parenchyma and causing ischemic atrophy.

▓ ASSESSMENT

☐ Subjective data

The patient is questioned about the presence and extent of discomfort and pain in the flank. Colicky pain may be experienced when clots are passed down the ureter. Symptoms of uremia may be present when renal function has deteriorated to the point of end-stage renal disease. Fever, chills, and general malaise may be experienced by the patient.

☐ Objective data

Hematuria and hypertension are each (independently) present in approximately 50% of all cases of polycystic disease. It is common for both hematuria and hypertension to be present in the same individual. On physical examination, the enlarged kidneys appear as large palpable abdominal masses. Serum and urine electrolytes and creatine clearance tests provide accurate data about renal function. A urine culture is obtained to determine the presence of UTI.

☐ Diagnostic tests

While a retrograde pyelograph and KUB can give valuable data about the size of the kidneys, the IVP is most often used to confirm the diagnosis of polycystic disease.

➡ DATA ANALYSIS: NURSING DIAGNOSES

Nursing diagnoses are determined from assessment of patient data. Possible nursing diagnoses for the person with polycystic disease may include, but are not limited to, the following:

Diagnostic title	Possible etiologies
Impaired adjustment	Disability requiring change in life-style, incomplete grieving, loss of body function
Anxiety	Threat to self-concept, change in health status

Diagnostic title	Possible etiologies
Ineffective individual coping	Situational crisis, personal vulnerability
Fluid volume excess	Compromised regulatory mechanism
Anticipatory grieving	Loss of body function
Impaired home maintenance management	Chronic debilitating disease, change in support mechanisms
Hopelessness	Failing physical condition, long-term stress
Altered nutrition: less than body requirements	Anorexia
Pain	Renal inflammation
Powerlessness	Illness-related regimen, life-style of helplessness
Altered renal tissue perfusion	Decreased blood flow to kidneys
Altered patterns of urinary elimination	Urinary infection, anuria

PLANNING: EXPECTED PATIENT OUTCOMES

Expected patient outcomes for the person with polycystic disease may include, but are not limited to, the following:
1. Person states feeling comfortable.
2. Person does not display signs or symptoms of fluid volume excess.
3. Person eats a balanced diet.
4. The person or significant other can state or describe the following:
   a. Signs and symptoms of infection and blood loss requiring immediate medical attention
   b. Plans for follow-up health care
   c. Appropriate health screening and follow-up care for children
   d. Dosages, reason for taking, and side effects of prescribed medication

IMPLEMENTATION

□ Assisting with achievement of therapeutic goals

Interventions for the patient with polycystic disease centers largely on preventing infection and bleeding. Infection is difficult to eradicate in persons with polycystic kidneys, and when infection is uncontrolled it leads to further destruction of kidney tissue. Frequent culture of the urine is performed and instrumentation and catheterization of the urinary tract are avoided whenever possible. Antibiotic therapy is often instituted. When antibiotics are ordered, they should be given on time and on a regular schedule to ensure adequate blood levels. The patient's urinary output must be closely monitored.

□ Assisting with comfort and ADL

Analgesic drugs may be necessary in control of flank pain associated with enlarged kidneys.

When bleeding from ruptured cysts becomes severe enough to turn the urine from pink to red, bed rest is usually instituted. At these times the patient will require assistance with ADL. Otherwise independence in ADL should be encouraged.

□ Counseling and teaching

The patient will need to be instructed to be alert to signs and symptoms of infection and bleeding. The emotional overtones of this illness can be severe for both the individual and the family. Challenges exist in helping the person deal with an illness on an individual basis when relatives have died of the same disease and children have not yet developed symptoms. Counseling regarding family health care and the individual's role in passing on a potentially fatal disease to children will, at times, be required. The patient should be instructed to monitor urinary output and report changes to the physician.

EVALUATION

The evaluation of nursing care of patients with polycystic disease is made on the basis of the identified nursing diagnoses. General questions to ask include the following: (1) Can the patient state signs and symptoms of infection and bleeding? (2) Can the patient state plans for follow-up health care? (3) Is the patient dehydrated or fluid overloaded? (4) Is the patient receiving a balanced nutritional input? and (5) Is the patient comfortable?

■ Vascular disorders

Renal diseases resulting from vascular disorders are caused by one of two processes: *renal artery stenosis,* which is a narrowing of the main renal artery, or *nephrosclerosis,* which is sclerosis of renal arterioles. *Diabetic nephropathy* is also a vascular disorder that occurs as diabetes progresses.

■ RENAL ARTERY STENOSIS

Renal artery stenosis causes approximately 5% of all hypertension.[48] Stenosis of the renal arteries is usually classified as either arteriosclerosis or fibromuscular dysplasia. In either case, the end result is a narrowing of the lumen of the arteries supplying the kidneys. Obstruction of the renal arteries can also be caused by aneurysms, thromboses, and emboli.

□ Pathophysiology

Renal stenosis results in a major reduction in circulation to the kidneys.[34] This change in perfusion causes increased secretion of renin and activation of the renin-angiotensin-aldosterone system (Chapter 26). The end result is accelerated hypertension, which left untreated leads to further pathologic changes in the kidneys. These changes include nephrosclerosis.

The signs of renal artery stenosis follow:
1. Hypertension
2. Disparity in size of kidneys
3. Delayed appearance of contrast medium in renal arteriograph

4. Hyperconcentration of contrast medium in calyceal system on IVP
5. Lesion evidenced on renal arteriograph

☐ Medical therapy

Medical treatment will include vigorous antihypertensive therapy to control blood pressure. Prolonged hypertension will ultimately result in further renal involvement. When a well-defined lesion exists in the renal artery, vascular surgery may be performed to remove the affected area.

■ NEPHROSCLEROSIS

Renal artery stenosis results in hypertension, and hypertension can cause nephrosclerosis. Hypertension is a major precipitating factor of renal disease. It is estimated that approximately 10% of individuals with essential hypertension develop severe renal damage, and approximately 1% will develop end-stage renal disease and die unless supportive care is provided.[23]

Preventive care includes greater screening efforts to detect persons with elevated blood pressure early in the disease process. Adequate treatment and follow-up must be provided for those with hypertension. Another important measure is the education of persons regarding the nature of hypertension, the diet and medication regimen and the importance of periodic follow-up care. Yearly blood pressure monitoring of all persons with elevated blood pressure is a minimal preventive care measure.

☐ Pathophysiology

Peripheral vasculature is subject to adverse changes when hypertension is present. The kidney and brain circulation are most frequently affected.

Regardless of the origin (essential or renal), hypertension that is untreated over a period of time leads to the sclerosing of renal arterioles. The blood supply to glomeruli, tubules, and interstitium gradually decreases. Scarring and death of renal tissue occur, and signs of renal insufficiency develop when damage to the kidneys has become extensive. This destructive process is called *nephrosclerosis*.

By the time signs and symptoms indicating kidney involvement develop, the disease has progressed to an extreme point. Deterioration in renal function progresses gradually unless an acute or malignant phase of hypertension occurs to accelerate the process. Signs and symptoms are those of chronic renal failure.

☐ Medical therapy

Treatment of nephrosclerosis is directed toward early detection and treatment of hypertension. Causative factors are sought, and treatment to lower blood pressure is begun. When significant renal damage exists, stabilizing the person's current level of renal function or slowing deterioration of renal tissue is the treatment goal. Control of hypertension is continued, and management of end-stage disease and uremic symptoms provides for comfort and increased independence in daily living, although renal function may not improve.

■ DIABETIC NEPHROPATHY

Persons with diabetes develop vascular changes at a more accelerated rate than nondiabetic persons. These changes, which are a normal part of the aging process, result in chronic renal failure. This process of accelerated vascular change is most evident in persons with Type I diabetes, which develops in childhood. In controlling the carbohydrate intake of the person with diabetes, abnormal metabolism of fats occurs, resulting in elevated serum cholesterol levels. Immunofluorescent and electron microscopic studies of the renal vasculature suggest that large quantities of lipids leak into these blood vessels and precipitate on the vessel walls. The vascular changes caused by diabetes result in two distinct processes: glomerulosclerosis and nephrosclerosis. As described earlier, nephrosclerosis develops from the sclerosing of the renal arterioles.[44] Glomerulosclerosis is the scarring of the loops in the glomerulus. Pathologic changes occur in the basement membranes of the kidney. The first indication of renal involvement in the person with diabetes is usually proteinuria.

▥ ASSESSMENT

The nursing assessment for persons with vascular disorders of the kidney is the same as that outlined for chronic renal failure (p. 1194).

▤ IMPLEMENTATION

The nursing implementation for persons with vascular disorders of the kidney is the same as that outlined for chronic renal failure (pp. 1199-1202).

If the person undergoes surgery for revascularization of the renal artery, the implementation is the same as that outlined for general renal surgery (p. 1165).

■ Toxic nephropathy

Toxic nephropathy or chemical-induced nephritis is an idiosyncratic reaction resulting in damage to the tubules and interstitium of the kidneys. This disease process was first noted in patients who were sensitive to sulfonamide drugs. Many substances are now associated with chemical-induced nephritis. A list of the most common of these substances appears in Table 32-15.

■ PATHOPHYSIOLOGY

Toxic nephropathy usually begins within 15 days of exposure to the chemical. The inflammatory process disrupts the ability of the glomeruli to filter. Furthermore, the capillary membrane is altered to the extent that it becomes permeable to plasma proteins and blood cells resulting in proteinuria and hematuria. Loss of protein in the urine produces decreased serum proteins, leading to edema. Fever and eosinophilia are additional signs of inflammation. A rash may also occur. Oliguria, or a urine output of 400 ml or less in a 24-hour period, occurs in approximately 50% of all cases.

Table 32-15 Substances associated with chemical-induced nephritis

Category	Substance
Solvents	Carbon tetrachloride
	Methanol
	Ethylene glycol
Heavy metals	Lead
	Arsenic
	Mercury
Antibiotics	Kanamycin
	Gentamicin
	Amphotericin B
	Colistin
	Neomycin
Analgesic, urinary	Phenazopyridine
Pesticides	
Poisonous mushrooms	

ASSESSMENT

Subjective data

Data to obtain from the person with toxic nephropathy include the following:
1. Recent exposure to a toxic substance that may affect kidney function
2. Changes in voiding patterns and decreased urinary volume
3. Presence of flulike symptoms (fever, chills, rash)
4. Unexplained weight gain

Objective data

Data to be collected related to urinary output and fluid retention include the following:
1. Urine output (decreased amount)
2. Color, characteristics, and specific gravity of the urine
3. Breath sounds for rales (crackles) and moist cough, indicating pulmonary edema
4. Presence of peripheral edema
5. Blood pressure elevations

Diagnostic tests

Tests usually performed to diagnose chemical-induced nephritis usually include urinalysis (for proteinuria and hematuria), serum creatinine and BUN to assess renal function, and KUB x-ray examinations. A renal biopsy may be performed to confirm the diagnosis.

DATA ANALYSIS: NURSING DIAGNOSES

Nursing diagnoses are determined from assessment of patient data. Possible nursing diagnoses for the person with toxic nephropathy may include, but are not limited to, the following:

Diagnostic title	Possible etiologies
Activity intolerance	Bed rest, generalized weakness
Anxiety	Change in health status
Fluid volume excess	Compromised regulatory process
Altered nutrition: less than body requirements	Anorexia

PLANNING: EXPECTED PATIENT OUTCOMES

Expected patient outcomes for the person with toxic nephropathy may include, but are not limited to, the following:
1. The person rests comfortably.
2. Signs of fluid overload are not present.
3. The person eats a well-balanced diet based on dietary prescriptions.
4. The person or significant other can explain the following:
   a. Rationale for removing environmental factors
   b. Prescribed dietary changes
   c. Medication regimen including dosages, effects, and side effects of all prescribed medications
   d. Need for follow-up medical care

IMPLEMENTATION

Assisting with achievement of therapeutic goals

A detailed description of the implementation of care for the person with acute renal failure is found on p. 1191 This should be reviewed because the person with toxic nephritis will often be treated for acute renal failure.

The medical management of the person with toxic nephritis includes the immediate withdrawal of the suspected chemical.[17] Conservative medical management includes treating any symptoms, bed rest, and control of diet to limit the workload on the kidneys and to reduce symptoms. A sodium-restricted diet may be necessary to maintain fluid balance. Proteins may be restricted if renal function is severely compromised. Hemodialysis may be instituted to facilitate the removal of nephrotoxins from the blood. Steroids may be administered for their antiinflammatory response.

Nursing care includes continuous assessment of the person's fluid status, including the presence of edema, adventitious breath sounds, and blood pressure changes. The person's weight should be obtained daily. When edema is present, meticulous skin care is required to prevent breakdown.

Control of environment

Prevention of chemical-induced nephritis is best managed by identifying causative agents and removing them from the environment. Many people are exposed to these agents as a result of their medical regimen. It is therefore imperative that the health care professional be aware of these agents, as well as the signs and symptoms associated with chemical-induced nephritis. Early detection and removal of the causative agent improves the prognosis.

□ **Counseling and teaching**

The person must be instructed about the environmental factors that lead to toxic nephropathy, including the measures to be taken to eliminate the hazards. The rationale for fluid balance and dietary restrictions must also be emphasized.

✚ EVALUATION

The care of the specific patient with toxic nephropathy is evaluated on the basis of expected patient outcomes. General questions to ask include the following: Is the person resting comfortably? Has fluid overload been prevented? Is the person maintaining adequate caloric intake? Can the person state plans for follow-up care?

■ Trauma to the urinary tract

Assessing intactness of the urinary tract structures must be a part of the evaluation of any person with traumatic injury to the lower trunk. Injuries particularly conducive to urinary tract damage include fractures of the pelvis and sharp blows to the abdomen or flanks.

■ TRAUMA OF THE LOWER URINARY TRACT

Pelvic fractures may result in *bladder perforation* and *ureteral* and *urethral tearing*. After bladder perforation or ureteral or urethral injury, urinary output may be scant or absent, the urine may be bloody, and symptoms of peritonitis may appear. Treatment is directed toward stabilizing the patient and surgically repairing the perforation or laceration. After stabilizing the patient, a cystotomy may be performed to provide urinary drainage when the injury involves the bladder or urethra. When the ureters are involved, splinting catheters may be required. When injury is extreme, urinary diversion may be required (p. 1177). The immediate treatment goal is to provide for adequate urinary drainage to prevent damage to the kidneys.

■ KIDNEY TRAUMA

A sharp blow to the body, particularly to the lower back or flanks, may result in contusion, tearing, or rupture of a kidney (Fig. 32-27). Signs and symptoms of trauma to the kidneys include frank bleeding from the urinary meatus, hematuria, pain, and tenderness of the upper abdominal quadrant and flank on the involved side. Signs of shock may be present if hemorrhage was extensive. Treatment includes controlling bleeding, preventing shock, and promoting drainage of the urinary tract. Vital signs, fluid balance, and hematocrit levels are monitored to assess hemostasis. Complaints of pain may indicate development of ureteral colic, signifying obstruction of the ureter by a clot. Surgical intervention is required to control severe hemorrhage; spontaneous healing of the kidney is otherwise permitted. Nephrostomy with catheter placement may be required to permit adequate urinary drainage. Bed rest is maintained until gross hematuria clears; thereafter, activity is progressed according to continued absence of hematuria. In the presence of extensive damage a nephrectomy may be required.

A kidney may become loosened and "float" or become displaced (*nephroptosis*). If symptoms of obstruction occur in the presence of nephroptosis, the kidney may be sutured to its anatomic site (*nephropexy*) to eliminate kinking of the ureter. Postoperatively, the patient is positioned with the hips elevated to prevent tension on the suture line.

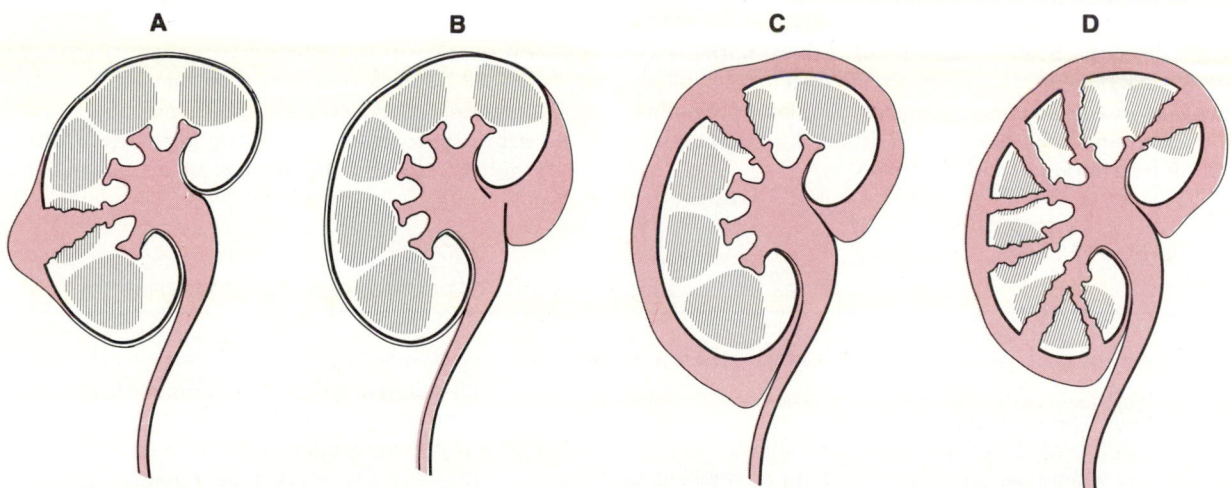

A   B   C   D

Fig. 32-27 Four degrees of renal trauma. **A,** Urine is extravasating from split in renal parenchyma but confined under renal capsule. **B,** Urine is extravasating through tear in renal pelvis. **C,** Urine is extravasating through rent in kidney and capsule and surrounds kidney and renal pelvis. **D,** Kidney is shattered and urine is extravasating in all areas. (From Winter, CC, and Morel, A: Nursing care of patients with urologic diseases, ed 4, St. Louis, 1977, The CV Mosby Co.)

■ RENAL FAILURE

Renal failure is the inability of the kidneys to function. *It is a state of total or nearly total loss of the kidneys' ability to excrete waste products, to maintain fluid and electrolyte balance (including acid-base balance), and to control blood pressure.* The person in renal failure cannot independently sustain life.

Renal failure may be acute in onset or may develop slowly and progressively over a course of several years. When renal failure occurs suddenly, such as, within a few days, biochemical changes are often dramatic and the person has little time to adjust to these changes. The person becomes very ill and usually requires care in a hospital critical care unit.

When renal failure occurs as the end result of a chronic kidney illness in which kidney tissue is destroyed progressively over the course of several months or years, control of symptoms and preservation of functional abilities are achieveable goals. Dietary adjustment, medications, and attention to preventing additional illnesses compensate for loss of kidney function in early stages of progressing renal failure. As renal function continues to deteriorate, dialysis or transplantation becomes necessary to support life.

■ Acute renal failure

■ EPIDEMIOLOGY

Acute renal failure generally follows an identifiable trauma of either toxic or ischemic nature.[29] The health of the individual before the insult is usually good to adequate. The major causes of ischemic and toxic injuries to the kidney are listed in Table 32-16. Other conditions that can precipitate acute renal failure are (1) acute glomerular disease, (2) acute severe infection of kidney tissue, (3) bilateral occlusion of the renal arteries, (4) mechanical obstructions in the urinary tract, and (5) hemoglobinemia and myoglobinemia. All of these conditions lead to massive and rapid destruction of kidney tissue.

■ PATHOPHYSIOLOGY AND CLINICAL SIGNS

Renal ischemia occurs when blood flow to the kidneys is reduced. The response of the normal kidney is *vasoconstriction*, which compounds the problem of reduced renal blood flow and increases renal ischemia. Perfusion problems affect both kidneys. When ischemia is prolonged, renal tubular tissue dies and frank renal failure develops.

Substances that are toxic to the cells of the renal tubules affect the kidneys bilaterally. The kidney with its large blood flow and ability to concentrate fluid in the medullary portion (where the tubules are located) creates conditions in which exposure of tubular cells to toxins is maximized. Damage to the cells leads to decreased glomerular permeability and tubular obstruction.

The course of acute renal failure is usually characterized by an initial oliguric phase followed in a number of days to a few weeks by a diuretic period. Major problems during the *oliguric* phase include inability to excrete fluid loads, to regulate electrolytes, and to excrete metabolic waste materials (Table 32-17). During the *diuretic* phase large amounts of fluid and electrolytes are lost.

□ Oliguric phase
□ *Inability to excrete fluid loads*

Because of the decreased kidney function, fluids are retained in the body, resulting in fluid overload and edema (Chapter 8). When fluid overload is excessive, congestive heart failure and pulmonary edema may occur. Hypertension accompanies acute renal failure when the person is hypervolemic, although this is usually not a finding when fluid balance is controlled.

Inability to excrete fluid loads leads to decreased urinary output. Either *oliguria* (urinary output below 400 ml/day) or *anuria* (urinary output below 100 ml/day) may be present, although oliguria is more common. Classically, the patient in acute renal failure shows a fall in urinary output within 1 to 2 days to between 50 and 400 ml/day. The urine *specific gravity is low* (1.010), and the osmolality of the urine approaches that of the person's serum (280 to 320 mOsm). Specific gravity and urine osmolality remain

---

Table 32-16 Conditions and substances that produce ischemic or nephrotoxic injury to the kidney

Ischemic conditions*	Toxic substances†
Hypovolemia	Solvents (carbon tetrachloride, methanol, ethylene glycol)
Blood loss (surgery, trauma)	
Plasma loss (burns, surgery, acute pancreatitis)	Heavy metals (lead, arsenic, mercury)
Sodium and water loss (prolonged diarrhea or vomiting, GI tract drainage, sustained high fever)	Antibiotics (kanamycin, gentamicin, polymyxin B, amphotericin B, colistin, neomycin, phenazopyridine)
Cardiac failure	
Myocardial infarction	Pesticides
Cardiac arrhythmias	Mushrooms
Congestive heart failure	
Septic shock	

*Inadequate perfusion of the kidney.
†Injury to the kidney cells.

Table 32-17   Symptoms caused by physiologic changes in acute renal failure

Symptoms	Physiologic effects	Findings
Oliguric phase		
Nausea, vomiting, drowsiness, confusion, coma, GI bleeding, asterixis, pericarditis	Inability to excrete metabolic wastes	Increased BUN and creatinine levels
Nausea, vomiting, cardiac arrhythmias, Kussmaul's breathing, drowsiness, confusion, coma	Inability to regulate electrolytes	Hyperkalemia, hyponatremia, acidosis
Edema; congestive heart failure; pulmonary edema; hypertension	Inability to excrete fluid loads	Fluid overload, hypervolemia
Diuretic phase		
Urinary output of up to 4 to 5 L/day, postural hypotension, tachycardia	Increased production of urine	Hypovolemia, loss of sodium and potassium in urine
Increasing mental alertness and activity	Slowly increasing excretion of metabolic wastes	Initially, high BUN (fluid loss greater than solute loss), gradual return of BUN to normal

within this fixed range and reflect tubular damage with loss of concentrating ability.

□ Electrolyte imbalances

The three major electrolyte problems are retention of potassium, excretion of sodium, and acidosis.

POTASSIUM IMBALANCE. In the normal individual the potassium ion is exchanged in the distal convoluted tubule of the nephron for either sodium or hydrogen ions; for the healthy person there is no mechanism in the body to conserve the potassium ion. However, in the individual with acute renal failure in whom a large number of tubular cells are no longer functional, no mechanism exists to remove potassium from the body. *Hyperkalemia* is said to exist when the serum concentration of this ion reaches a level of 5.5 mEq/L or higher. Serum concentrations of 7 to 10 mEq/L can be quickly reached in acute renal failure and are incompatible with normal cardiac function and life.

In monitoring for signs of potassium toxicity, electrocardiography and laboratory determinations of serum potassium are the most reliable indicators. Rarely does the patient become symptomatic, and pulse changes must not be relied on to indicate the degree of rise of potassium in the patient's system.

SODIUM IMBALANCE. *Hyponatremia* in acute renal failure most commonly develops with overhydration of the patient. The oliguric patient cannot excrete large volumes of urine; when the administration of sodium-free or low-sodium intravenous or oral fluids continues in such an individual, the serum is diluted and the serum concentration of sodium falls.

In this situation hyponatremia is accompanied or caused by hypervolemia. In the very acutely ill, the situation commonly occurs when the patient receives numerous drugs and fluids in an attempt to treat coexisting life-threatening problems. When the volume of drugs and fluids cannot be reduced to a safe level, dialysis is required to remove the excess fluid and restore sodium balance.

Signs and symptoms of hyponatremia include warm, moist, flushed skin; muscle weakness, muscle twitching; and behavioral changes involving confusion, delirium, coma, and convulsions. Serum sodium concentrations will be below 130 mEq/L. The hematocrit and hemoglobin values suddenly fall without evidence of bleeding; this is caused by hemodilution.

Increases in total body content of sodium also occur in acute renal failure. Commonly, this occurs when the patient is receiving medications high in sodium content and excess sodium in the diet. Edema and increasing blood pressure indicate retention of sodium and fluids even though the serum sodium concentration is normal or below normal.

METABOLIC ACIDOSIS. Acidosis develops when hydrogen ion secretion and bicarbonate ion production diminish in the tubular cells. The pH of the blood decreases, the carbon dioxide content decreases, and central nervous system symptoms of drowsiness progressing to stupor and coma may appear. Although the lungs are unable to compensate totally for the increasing acid load, they help determine the rate at which acidosis develops and the frequency or need for dialysis. In compensating for increased metabolic acid loads, the lungs attempt to excrete more carbon dioxide. Kussmaul's breathing is noted.

□ Inability to excrete metabolic wastes

Decreased kidney function alters the body's ability to get rid of metabolic waste materials, producing typical signs and symptoms referred to as *uremia*. BUN and serum creatinine values rise sharply. In the person who has already sustained illness and trauma, BUN values may increase at a rate of 30 mg/100 ml/day. Signs and symptoms include neurologic manifestations such as confusion, convulsions, coma, and asterixis. GI bleeding may result from uremic gastritis or colitis. Decreased cellular immunity causes an increased tendency for infections to develop. Bruising and bleeding result from changes in blood coagulation factors. Pericarditis (Chapter 25) is thought to develop as a result of pericardial irritation from accumulated metabolic wastes.

☐ Diuretic phase

After a period of oliguria or anuria that may last a few days to 2 weeks, patients recovering renal function pass into another distinct phase of illness characterized by increased urinary output. Increased output indicates that the damaged nephrons are healing and are able to begin excreting urine. At first daily urine volume increases slowly, although within 1 to 2 days diuresis up to or exceeding 4 to 5 L/day may occur. Although fluid can be excreted, the kidneys are not yet healed. Often there is inability to excrete proportional amounts of waste materials, and BUN may rise or remain elevated as urine volume increases. At times excessive excretion of sodium and potassium occurs during diuresis. Complete recovery of renal function is slow and requires anywhere from days to several months. Return of the renal function to normal or near normal levels is evidenced when the kidney can both conserve and dilute urine and when serum electrolytes and nonprotein nitrogen levels become normal.

■ PROGNOSIS

Recovery from an episode of acute renal failure depends on the underlying illness, the condition of the patient, and the careful, supportive management given during the period of kidney shutdown. Mortality associated with acute tubular necrosis approaches 40%; these statistics largely reflect the deaths of severely ill persons in whom renal failure is a sequela to extensive underlying illness. Owing to the more widespread availability of dialysis, mortality directly attributable to decreased renal function from potassium intoxication, fluid overload, and acidosis has been reduced. The potential for recovery of renal function for those who survive the acute episode of tubular insufficiency is good. Although recovery statistics indicate that kidney tissue may regenerate more completely after toxic injury than it does after ischemic injury, follow-up studies of persons years after episodes of acute tubular insufficiency show normal to near normal renal function.[23]

For those in whom acute renal failure has been caused by glomerular disease or severe infection of kidney tissue, the prognosis may not be as favorable. Return of renal function is determined by the extent of scarring and obliteration of functional renal tissue that has occurred during the acute episode of kidney failure. A significant number of adults who develop acute glomerulonephritis show some decrease in renal function, which may remain at a level at which biochemical abnormalities are not produced or may progress to a chronic form of renal failure.

■ PREVENTION OF ACUTE RENAL FAILURE

The incidence of acute renal failure can be reduced through identification and observation of populations at risk and identification and control of environmental risk factors. The greatest incidence of acute renal failure occurs in persons who have undergone major trauma, extensive burns, aortic surgery, massive blood loss, or severe myocardial infarction with or without associated arrhythmia. Acute renal failure also frequently occurs in patients with sepsis and in those having abnormal intravascular coagulation, such as DIC, because these acutely ill persons are prime candidates for inadequate kidney perfusion. Frequent monitoring of urinary output and detection of excessive losses of body fluid will help to identify instances of inadequate renal perfusion before development of renal failure.

Significant factors in preventive care for the general population include control of nephrotoxic drugs, increased medical supervision of persons with sore throats and upper respiratory tract infections, and increased case finding and treatment of individuals with bacteriuria and obstructive disease of the urinary system. Attempts to control the distribution and identification of nephrotoxic drugs and chemicals is largely accomplished through the Food and Drug Administration (FDA). Identification of nephrotoxic drugs and chemicals, enforced labeling of these substances, and drug dispensing by prescription only are examples of this agency's attempts to promote public health. Proper labeling and storage of potentially toxic drugs and chemicals in the home can reduce further the number of accidental ingestions of nephrotoxic substances.

▨ ASSESSMENT

☐ Subjective data

Assessment should include questions that ascertain the following:

1. Voiding patterns, including any recent changes
2. Unexplained weight gain
3. Presence of nausea and anorexia
4. Family history of renal disease
5. Recent history of flulike symptoms
6. Presence of nephrotoxins, including those in environment, at work, and in medications

☐ Objective data

Objective data must include the measurement of fluid intake and urine output in a 24-hour period. Daily weights are essential because they provide the best measure of fluid status. Blood pressure, including postural changes, is measured frequently until stable, and the pulse rate and rhythm are also recorded. Fluid status is assessed by observing for skin turgor and peripheral edema and auscultating breath sounds. The person is assessed for the presence of halitosis that can result from acidosis and from ammonia secretion. The person is observed carefully for any changes in mental status.

☐ Diagnostic tests

Diagnostic tests include urinalysis. Creatinine urinary clearance is followed closely to monitor changes in kidney function. Serum creatinine and BUN are also obtained. Serum chemistries must be followed closely to ensure that the person is maintaining homeostasis. Specific tests used to assist in making the diagnosis and identifying the cause of acute renal failure include KUB, IVP, cystoscopy, and renal ultrasound. In some cases a renal biopsy may be performed to provide the differential diagnosis.

When oliguria or rising serum creatinine and BUN values are noted, the physician must determine whether the decreased output and decreased renal function are the results of inadequate renal perfusion or of frank renal failure. This distinction directs treatment. In instances of poor kidney perfusion, restoring circulating volume by adding fluids and otherwise increasing cardiac output prevents death of kidney tissue and subsequent renal failure. In contrast, the treatment of true renal failure is supportive and is based on careful balance of input and output of fluid, electrolytes, and wastes. In addition to the urine sodium concentration as a diagnostic sign, the physician may wish to challenge the patient's ability to excrete fluid. In this instance usually 100 to 500 ml of fluid is given as rapidly as possible intravenously. A poorly perfused but intact kidney should respond with increased urinary output. During this treatment the patient must be closely monitored for signs and symptoms of congestive heart failure and pulmonary edema. The kidney in acute failure will be unable to produce a greater urine flow in response to this fluid challenge. The physician may give furosemide, 40 to 80 mg intravenously, in an attempt to produce a greater flow of urine. The test may be repeated if there is no response to the initial trial, although subsequent attempts to produce urine in this manner are contraindicated.

➡ DATA ANALYSIS: NURSING DIAGNOSES

Nursing diagnoses are determined from assessment of patient data. Possible nursing diagnoses for the person with acute renal failure may include, but are not limited to, the following:

Diagnostic title	Possible etiologies
Activity intolerance	Bed rest, generalized weakness, lethargy
Anxiety	Threat to self-concept, change in health status, situational crisis
Ineffective breathing pattern	Anxiety, fluid volume excess
Fluid volume excess	Compromised regulatory mechanism
Potential for infection	Decreased nutrition, urinary stasis
Altered nutrition: less than body requirements	Anorexia
Pain	Visceral inflammation, diagnostic tests
Altered patterns of urinary elimination	Anatomic obstruction, infection

▣ PLANNING: EXPECTED PATIENT OUTCOMES

Expected patient outcomes for the person with acute renal failure may include, but are not limited to, the following:

In the *oliguric* phase the person demonstrates control of internal environment through the following:
1. Absence of pulmonary edema
2. Absence or control of peripheral edema
3. Control of blood pressure (range between 170/100 and 100/60 mm Hg)
4. Restored or maintained mental alertness
5. Control of electrolyte balance
   a. Sodium range of 125 to 145 mEq/L
   b. Potassium range of 3.0 to 6.0 mEq/L
   c. Bicarbonate above 14 mEq/L
6. Control of protein catabolism
   a. BUN below 100 mg/dl
   b. Creatinine below 12 mg/dl
   c. Absence of skin breakdown
7. Absence of bleeding
8. Resolution or control of intercurrent illness (congestive heart failure, shock)
9. Absence of infection
10. Absence of injury resulting from decreased level of awareness and strength
11. Absence of toxicity from inadequately excreted medication

In the *diuretic* phase the person or significant others can state, identify, or describe the following:
1. Extent of recovery of kidney function
2. Any preventable environmental or health factor involved in generating the illness
3. A diet to maintain positive nitrogen balance and sufficient caloric intake
4. Signs and symptoms of dehydration and sodium and potassium loss
5. Plans for follow-up care

▦ IMPLEMENTATION

☐ Oliguric phase

During the oliguric phase of acute renal failure, development of hyperkalemia, severe acidosis, severe fluid overload and pulmonary edema, infection, convulsions, or pericarditis indicate need for immediate intervention.

Included among these problems are the major causes of death resulting from acute kidney failure.

☐ *Control and excretion of metabolic waste buildup*

Because the patient's ability to excrete metabolic wastes (nonprotein nitrogen products and acids) cannot keep pace with production of these substances, alternative routes of excretion and control over production of these materials must be found. Means available to accomplish this include providing carbohydrate to spare protein stores, preventing additional tissue trauma, and increasing excretion of wastes through the lungs and through renal dialysis. Of these, dialysis is by far the most efficient and is the only true means available for controlling the internal environment of the severely ill hypercatabolic person. Daily laboratory tests will determine blood nonprotein nitrogens and bicarbonate levels, which serve as a guide for determining the frequency of dialysis.

Decreasing the production of metabolic wastes can be

influenced through dietary means. Calories in the form of carbohydrates and fats provide energy and spare body protein stores, thus decreasing nonprotein nitrogen production. The body recycles urea to synthesize amino acids for protein building so that some regeneration of tissues can occur even though protein intake is curtailed.

Preventing infections and tissue breakdown decreases production of metabolic wastes. Aseptic technique should be rigorously pursued in all treatments performed on the patient. Indwelling lines and catheters are a common source of infection and are to be avoided when possible. *The patient should be isolated from anyone with an infection, including other patients, health care personnel, and visitors.* Detecting existent infections early so that treatment can be instituted promptly decreases tissue breakdown. When the patient is extremely weak and immobile, frequent turning and repositioning to prevent decubiti must be performed. Skin care for patients with edematous tissues should include observation and prevention of pressure and trauma; these tissues are particularly prone to breakdown.

In compensating for increased metabolic acid loads, the lungs attempt to excrete more carbon dioxide. To maximize this pathway for acid excretion, pulmonary hygiene should be carried out. Preventing atelectasis and maintaining maximal lung expansion are goals of nursing care.

□ *Control of fluids*

The oliguric or anuric patient is unable to excrete more then minimal amounts of fluid. Nursing care is directed toward three broad objectives: (1) monitoring for signs of fluid overload, (2) maintaining the patient's energy expenditure at a level compatible with the individual's state of health, and (3) controlling or helping the patient to control fluid intake.

All observations regarding the patient's state of hydration need to be recorded so that hour-to-hour and day-to-day comparisons can be made. Any finding indicating retention of fluids is reported to the physician. Edema can first be noted in dependent areas such as the feet and legs, in the presacral area, and around the eyes. The patient is observed carefully for signs of pulmonary edema and congestive heart failure. Central venous or arterial monitoring lines will help to provide data for short-term comparisons in managing the fluid balance of the critically ill person. Accurate recording of intake and output is extremely important as are daily weight records.

The patient in renal failure is unable to excrete fluid loads, and much energy is expended just to maintain current functional status. Positioning and activity are determined daily based on assessment of the energy level and ability to ventilate adequately.

Controlling fluid intake is essential when the ability to excrete fluid is limited. All fluid (parenteral and oral) must total only slightly more than daily output if severe overhydration is to be avoided. When the patient is neither to gain nor lose additional body fluid, the physician will calculate the patient's fluid replacement using the following as a guide: intake will approximate 500 ml/day plus urinary output and adjustments for additional fluid lost through fever, diarrhea, and wound drainage. Fortunately, when sodium intake is controlled, extreme thirst does not develop.

Devices that allow 50 to 150 ml of fluid to be isolated from the main intravenous solution container and drip chambers that allow precise control of fluids through administration of smaller drops of fluid are added safety measures when giving fluids parenterally to anuric or oliguric individuals. Accuracy in fluid balance records is essential. For the patient who is unable to take medications with small amounts of fluid, medications may be given in soft foods such as applesauce.

□ *Interventions for hyperkalemia*

Interventions to control the rise of serum potassium and to prevent cardiac arrest include those that (1) decrease the intake of potassium, (2) decrease the liberation of potassium from body tissues, (3) protect the cardiovascular system, and (4) assist in removal of potassium from the body by nonrenal means.

Decreasing the intake of potassium is achieved by administering intravenous feedings or a diet in which the potassium content is very low or absent. All fluids and drugs that the patient receives intravenously should be checked for potassium content. Some medications (for example, most penicillin preparations) contain large amounts of this ion.

Controlling the breakdown of body tissues is extremely important in preventing a rapid rise in serum potassium.

Protecting the cardiovascular system from high levels of extracellular potassium (K^+) *is essential.* When high K^+ levels occur and the patient is exhibiting cardiovascular effects, renal dialysis is required. Because it takes several hours to get the dialysis treatment underway and for the K^+ to be reduced to safe levels, other therapy is instituted. Hypertonic glucose (25%) may be given with 1 unit of regular insulin per 2 g of glucose. Over a 30-minute period, 200 to 300 ml of fluid is given to promote the movement of K^+ back into the cells. This lowers the serum K^+ level and reduces cardiac instability resulting from the high serum K^+ levels. The K^+ levels will begin to fall in 1 hour and will remain lowered for 4 to 6 hours.[11] In addition to hypertonic glucose, calcium gluconate may be given intravenously to reduce the irritability of cardiac cells caused by the hyperkalemia.

To *promote the excretion of potassium* from the body when the kidneys are nonfunctional, an exchange resin such as sodium polystyrene sulfonate (Kayexalate) may be ordered for the patient as a temporary measure before a dialysis treatment when (1) the serum K^+ level is high and rising rapidly; (2) the serum K^+ level is rising, although at a controlled rate, and other metabolic disturbances do not necessitate dialysis; or (3) control of a rising serum K^+ is required before a patient's transfer to an acute care area where dialysis can be provided. This drug reduces serum potassium by exchanging sodium for potassium ions in the intestinal tract. It can be administered orally, through a nasogastric tube, or by enema. The medication is given orally when the patient's condition permits; oral daily doses range from 15 to 60 g/day. When sodium sulfonate is administered in enema form, the usual dose is 50 g of exchange resin for each enema; it may be repeated daily or as necessary to lower serum potassium. The medication is a powder that when mixed becomes a thick paste within a few seconds; therefore, preparation should take place at the bedside just before administration. Often mannitol is used to mix the powdered sodium sulfonate, because it induces an osmotic shift of fluid into the bowel producing diarrhea, which helps to expel the medication, additional K$^+$, and additional fluid from the GI tract. If spontaneous bowel movements do not occur, a cathartic or cleansing enema can be given to ensure the elimination of potassium from the bowel.

□ **Maintenance of adequate nutrition**

Most persons in acute renal failure are too ill to tolerate oral feedings either initially or for sustained periods of time. Some patients who are able to tolerate fluids orally find that eating food compounds the nausea they experience as a result of an altered biochemical environment and accompanying GI tract irritation. Intravenous hypertonic glucose in amounts of 100 g/day or more provides a temporary source of energy that slows the burning of the body's own

---

Nursing care of the patient in the oliguric phase of acute renal failure

Assisting with achievement of therapeutic goals

1. Fluid and electrolyte imbalance
   a. Assist in maintaining adequate nutrition.
   b. Assist patient in remaining within limitations of diet (protein, sodium, potassium, phosphorus, and fluid limits).
   c. Maintain fluid restrictions.
   d. Keep accurate records of intake and output.
   e. Weigh patient daily.
   f. Monitor vital signs frequently, including postural signs.
   g. Assess fluid status of patient
   h. Administer phosphate binding medications as prescribed.
2. Activity
   a. Maintain strict bed rest in acute phase.
   b. Assist patient with ADL to conserve energy.
   c. Promote early ambulation.
   d. Maintain safe environment for patient.
3. Prevention and treatment of infection
   a. Assess patient for signs and symptoms of infection.
   b. If catheterization is required, maintain strict asepsis during insertion. Meticulous catheter care is essential.
   c. Maintain pulmonary hygiene while patient is on bedrest.
   d. Turn patient frequently.
   e. Administer antibiotics as prescribed.
4. Altered bleeding tendency
   a. Protect patient from injury.
   b. Administer stool softeners as prescribed.
   c. Instruct patient to use soft toothbrush.
   d. Assess patient for signs of bleeding
      (1) Bruising
      (2) Perform guaiac tests on stools, emesis, and NG returns
      (3) Changes in vital signs

5. Altered neurologic status
   a. Assess orientation at least every 8 hours.
   b. Assess level of consciousness at least every 8 hours.
   c. Report any change in mental status to physician immediately.
   d. When patient is ambulatory, assess motor skills at least every 8 hours.

Assisting with comfort and ADL

1. Assist patient with ADL to conserve energy.
2. Instruct patient to deep breath when experiencing nausea
3. Provide fluid in small amounts; ginger ale and other effervescent soft drinks are often tolerated better than other fluids.
4. Administer antiemetics as prescribed.
5. Provide patient with moist cloth to keep lips and mouth moist.
6. Meticulous mouth care is essential to protect teeth and mucous membranes.
7. Meticulous skin care is essential to prevent skin breakdown.
   a. Assess skin for pruritus and rashes.
   b. Bathe patient every day or more often if necessary, using super fat soap.
   c. Administer antipruritics (diphenhydramine [Benadryl], cyproheptadine [Periactin]) as prescribed.

Control of environment

1. Protect patient from chilling.
2. Maintain a calm, supportive environment.
3. Reverse isolation may be instituted.
4. Use humidifier during dry months.

protein stores. For patients who are severely ill or nauseated, maintaining positive nitrogen balance is not feasible. The total caloric intake for the patient on IV therapy will be influenced by the amount of fluids that can be tolerated in a 24-hour period.

If the patient is able to tolerate oral feedings, dietary protein and potassium are avoided unless dialysis has been initiated. In this case modest amounts of protein and potassium are allowed, thus increasing protein available for tissue building and increasing the palatability of the diet. Foods high in carbohydrate and fat content are encouraged. A total intake of 2000 calories per day is desired although often not achieved because of anorexia and nausea. The care of the patient during the oliguric phase of acute renal failure is summarized in the box on p. 1191.

□ Diuretic phase

Medical treatment during the diuretic phase is symptomatic. Electrolyte imbalances are likely to persist and are treated as in the oliguric phase. When polyuria is present, dehydration can become a potential problem and fluid replacement then becomes necessary.

Nursing implementation is directed toward detection of fluid losses and electrolyte imbalances. The care is the same as described in the oliguric phase with the exception of the following:
1. Fluid and electrolyte imbalance
   a. Assess patient for adequate hydration.
   b. Assess for changes in mental status indicative of low serum sodium levels.
   c. Irregular apical pulses are indicative of hypokalemia.
2. Activity
   a. Encourage independence in ADL as tolerated.
   b. Encourage early ambulation as tolerated.
3. Coping with illness
   a. Encourage the development of a nurse-patient relationship that will assist the patient in expressing perceptions of illness.
   b. Promote independence in patient.
   c. Involve significant other in care of patient.

□ Teaching

During the diuretic phase, the patient is usually ready for the start of the education process that is necessary for patients with kidney disease. These teaching plans must include the following elements:
1. Cause of renal failure
2. Identification of preventable environmental or health factors contributing to the illness (for example, hypertension, nephrotoxic drugs)
3. Prescribed medication regimen
4. Prescribed dietary regimen
5. Signs and symptoms of returning renal failure
6. Signs and symptoms of infections
7. Need for on-going follow-up care

■ Chronic renal failure

Chronic renal failure (CRF) exists when the kidneys are no longer capable of maintaining an internal environment consistent with life and when return of function is not anticipated. For the majority of individuals the transition from health to a state of chronic or permanent disease is a slow one extending over a number of years. Recurrent infections and exacerbations of nephritis, obstruction of the urinary tract, and destruction of vessels from diabetes and long-standing hypertension lead to scarring of kidney tissue and progressive loss of renal function. Some individuals, however, develop total irreversible loss of renal function acutely; such loss of renal function usually develops in a matter of a few hours or days and follows a direct traumatic insult to the kidneys.

Chronic renal failure exists as a major health problem in the United States. Approximately 8 million individuals now have chronic kidney disease; approximately 60,000 persons die each year as the result of renal failure.[37]

■ PROGNOSIS

The individual with chronic renal failure can to some extent control and manage the symptoms of the disease. Although renal function that has been lost as a result of destruction of kidney tissue cannot be recovered, the life of the person can be maintained by limiting the intake of substances that require renal excretion and by providing alternative routes of excretion for waste products and electrolytes. By adhering to a prescribed management routine, albeit quite strict and demanding, life may be sustained. For some individuals medication and diet therapy alone may control uremic symptoms; other individuals may require dialysis or transplantation to control the symptoms of their disease.

■ PREVENTION

Obstruction and infection of the urinary tract and hypertensive disease are common and often asymptomatic causes of renal damage and renal failure. A significant reduction in the incidence of renal failure can be affected through increasing attention to general health promotion. Yearly physical examinations in which blood pressure is determined, urinalysis is performed, and the person is questioned about dysuria or pain in the urinary tract assist in early detection of diseases that may lead to renal failure.

General health maintenance can reduce the number of individuals progressing from renal insufficiency into frank renal failure. Care is aimed toward adequately treating medical problems and closely supervising the person's health status in times of stress (infection, pregnancy).

■ PATHOPHYSIOLOGY AND CLINICAL MANIFESTATIONS

During chronic renal failure, some of the nephrons (including the glomerulus and tubules) are thought to remain intact while others are destroyed (intact nephron hypothesis). The intact nephrons hypertrophy and produce an increased volume of filtrate with increased tubular reabsorption in spite of a decreased GFR. This adaptive method permits the kidney to function until about three-fourths

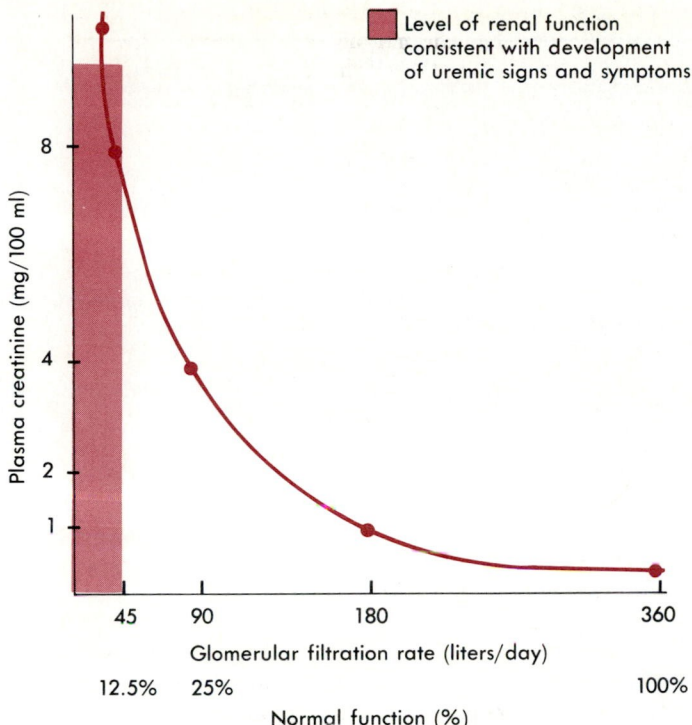

Level of renal function consistent with development of uremic signs and symptoms

Fig. 32-28 Glomerular filtration and plasma creatinine levels.

of the nephrons become destroyed. The solute load then becomes greater than can be reabsorbed, producing an osmotic diuresis with polyuria and thirst. Eventually, as more nephrons are damaged, oliguria occurs with retention of waste products.

The point at which the patient becomes obviously symptomatic and displays signs of typical renal failure occurs when approximately 80% to 90% of renal function has been lost (Fig. 32-28). At this level of renal function, creatinine clearance values will fall to 15 ml/minute or less.

The symptoms of uremia usually develop so slowly that the patient and family often do not recall the time of onset of the illness. Common symptoms include the following:

1. Early symptoms—lethargy, headaches, physical and mental fatigue, weight loss, irritability, depression.
2. Later symptoms—anorexia, persistent nausea and vomiting, shortness of breath on either mild or no exertion, and pitting edema; pruritus may be absent, mild, or severe

□ Biochemical changes

Although the clinical course of chronic renal disease varies, there are common features of the illness. Signs and symptoms result from disordered fluid and electrolyte balance, alterations in regulatory functions of the body, and retention of solutes. Common findings include the following:

1. Azotemia (excess serum nitrogenous products)
2. Metabolic acidosis

3. Hyperkalemia
4. Fluid and sodium imbalances
5. Hyperuricemia
6. Hyperphosphatemia, low or normal serum calcium levels
7. Hyperpigmentation of skin
8. Neuromuscular signs (muscle twitching, numbness in feet and legs)

The mechanisms for azotemia, metabolic acidosis, and hyperkalemia are the same as for acute renal failure. Fluid and sodium imbalances may include either abnormal retention or excretion of sodium and water; thus urinary volume can be decreased, normal, or increased.

The varied serum levels of uric acid seem to have no definite relationship to the exact level of kidney function.[51] Increased serum phosphate levels result from decreased renal excretions of phosphate and simultaneous reduction in ionized serum calcium. Through increased production of parathormone, the body may reestablish a normal serum calcium level, although this is accomplished at the expense of the person's bone matrix. Excess serum calcium phosphate may precipitate out into the kidney parenchyma, leading to further nephron damage.

Anemia universally accompanies chronic renal disease. Hematocrit values of 16% to 22% are not abnormal for these individuals. Anemia results from both a decreased production of RBCs and a decrease in longevity of the cells in circulation.

Hypertension is usually present. Elevated blood pressure appears to be the result of increased total body water, a renally released vasopressor, or an inadequately secreted vasodepressor.[44]

Glucose intolerance may be seen, although usually not of sufficient severity to warrant treatment. The rising blood sugar level appears to result from an altered biochemical environment produced by the failing kidneys and does not signify the development of diabetes mellitus.

□ Organ system involvement

The effects of chronic renal failure on organ systems are summarized in Table 32-18. Note that there can be involvement of any or all of the body systems.

□ Alterations in fertility

As end-stage renal failure develops, most women note changes in their menstrual cycle. Bleeding may occur at more widely spaced intervals, may be heavier or lighter in flow than normal, or may cease all together. This obvious change in reproductive cycle is usually accompanied by changes in fertility. Ovulation may occur normally or may occur only a few times a year. Pregnancy in uremic women is of much lower incidence than in the normal population. In men impotence may occur as chronic renal failure progresses toward end-stage disease. Dialysis or more vigorous treatment of uremia is indicated to return or maximize reproductive function. It should be stressed that sexual activity of some persons with chronic renal failure may remain quite normal even though changes in reproductive ability are present.

Table 32-18 Summary of organ system involvement in patients with chronic renal failure

System	Manifestation	Cause
Integumentary		
Skin	Pallor	Anemia
	Gray/bronze pigmentation	Pigment retained
	Dry and scaly	Decreased size of sweat glands
		Decreased activity of oil glands
	Pruritus	Dry skin; phosphate deposits
Nails	Thin, brittle	Protein wasting
Hair	Dry	Decreased activity of oil glands
	Brittle	Protein wasting
Gastrointestinal		
Oral cavity	Halitosis (fetor uremicus)	Urea converted to ammonia by saliva
	Bleeding of gums	Change in platelet activity
Stomach	Nausea, vomiting, anorexia	Serum uremic toxins
	Gastritis, ulceration	Serum uremic toxins
Lower bowel	Constipation	Aluminum hydroxide given as phosphate binders
Cardiovascular	Hypertension	Fluid overload
		Renin-angiotensin mechanism
	Congestive heart failure	Fluid overload, anemia
	Arteriosclerotic heart disease	Chronic hypertension
		Calcification of soft tissues
	Pericarditis	Uremic toxins in pericardial fluid
		Fibrin formation on epicardium
Pulmonary	Uremic "lung" or pneumonitis	Uremic toxins in pleural space and lung tissue
Neurologic	Fatigue, headache, sleep disturbance	Uremic toxins
	Muscle irritability	Electrolye imbalances
	Seizures	Cerebral swelling resulting from fluid shifting
Hematologic	Anemia	Suppression of RBC production
		Decreased survival time of RBCs
		Loss of blood through bleeding
		Loss of blood during dialysis
	Bleeding	Mild thrombocytopenia
		Decreased activity of platelets
Metabolic	Carbohydrate intolerance	Decreased sensitivity to insulin in peripheral tissues
		Delayed production of insulin by pancreas
		Increased survival time of insulin
	Hyperlipidemia	Increased production of serum triglycerides
		Increased output of glycerides by liver as a result of elevated insulin levels
Endocrine	Hyperparathyroidism	Elevated serum phosphate results in decreased serum calcium, which stimulates parathyroid
	Infertility	Mechanism unknown
	Sexual dysfunction	Mechanism unknown

ASSESSMENT

The nursing assessment of the person in chronic renal failure is extremely complex, particularly because of the multisystem involvement and chronicity of the disorder. The assessment must include physical, psychologic, and social parameters. The initial nursing history and physical assessment must elicit adequate information to generate the appropriate nursing diagnoses. Fig. 32-29 provides an example of the subjective data to be collected for the person in chronic renal failure, and Fig. 32-30 includes the objective data to be obtained.

Once an initial data base is obtained, it must be continuously updated. All subsequent assessments are determined by the medical regimen and nursing interventions for each patient. Some areas of ongoing assessment are listed in the box on p. 1199.

□ Diagnostic tests

A wide variety of diagnostic tests are required of the person in chronic renal failure once the diagnosis has been made. Many tests will be required to confirm the initial

Text continued on p. 1199.

HEMODIALYSIS NURSING NOTES
ADMISSION HISTORY

41   (Inpatient)/Patient Notes (Outpatient)

DATE	HOUR	I. **Perception of Illness**
		Why, initially, did you come to the hospital?
		What does the doctor plan for you while you are here?
		What do you expect is going to happen to you when you start dialysis?
		II. **History of Past Illness (Include dates and hospitalizations).**

		MEDICATIONS	DOSE	FREQUENCY	LAST DOSE TAKEN	REASON FOR TAKING

		Do you receive any special treatments or exercises?
		III. **Activity**
		Do you have difficulty walking or getting in and out of a chair?
		Can you climb stairs?
		Are you employed?
		What are your usual daytime activities?
		What are your recreational interests?

Fig. 32-29   Hemodialysis nursing notes: admission history.

DATE	HOUR	IV.	**Nutrition**
			Are you on a special diet?
			Do you have difficulty following diet?
			How many meals do you eat a day?
		V.	**Sleep Habits**
			Do you sleep through the night at home?
			What helps in getting to sleep at night?
			What are your usual sleeping habits?
		VI.	**Elimination**
			How often do you urinate?
			Do you have any difficulty with urination?
			Frequency Pain on urination
			Urgency Other
			Have you ever had urinary tract infections?
			Twenty four hour urine output cc/24 hrs
			Color of urine?
			What are your usual bowel habits?
			Do you have difficulty with diarrhea or constipation?
			How often do you use enemas or laxatives?
		VII.	**Reproductive System**
			When was your most recent menses?
			Have you recently had a change in menses?
			Have you had any changes in sexual function recently?
			Do you have any concerns about reproductive or sexual functions?
		VIII.	**Social**
			Do you live with anyone?
			Upon whom do you rely when you need help?
			What type of dwelling do you live in?
			Do you have to climb stairs?

Admitting Nurse _____

Fig. 32-29, cont'd.   Hemodialysis nursing notes: admission history.

HEMODIALYSIS NURSING NOTES
ADMISSION ASSESSMENT

41   (Inpatient)/Patient Notes (Outpatient)

DATE	HOUR		
		A) **Vital Signs**	
		Temperature	
		Pulses	Apical
			Radial
			Rhythm
		Weight	
		Height	
		B) **Cardiopulmonary**	
		Vascular Access	
		Peripheral Pulses:	Right Left
		Radial	
		Femoral	
		Popliteal	
		Pedal	
		Peripheral Edema?	
		Periorbital Edema?	
		Friction Rub?	
		Neck Vein Distention?	
		Cough? Sputum? Smoking Habits?	
		Adventitious Breath Sounds?	
		Shortness of Breath?	
		C) **Neuromuscular**	
		Orientation	
		Level of Alertness and Responsiveness?	
		Muscle Tone and Strength, Symmetry?	
		Weakness or Loss of Function of Extremities?	
		Balance	
		Numbness, Tingling or Tremors?	

Fig. 32-30   Hemodialysis nursing notes: admission assessment.

DATE	HOUR	Patient Experiencing Difficulties with:
		Sight
		Speech
		Touch
		Taste / Smell
		D) Skin
		Color
		Turgor
		Temperature
		Lesions
		Condition of Nails
		E) General
		Presence of:
		Nausea
		Vomiting
		Headache
		Blurring of Vision

Admitting Nurse _____

Fig. 32-30, cont'd.   Hemodialysis nursing notes: admission assessment.

Monitoring parameters for the person with chronic renal failure

1. Intake and output every 8 hours
2. Fluid excess: palpating for edema, auscultating breath sounds, checking blood pressure at least every 8 hours, daily weight records
3. Cardiac rhythms every 8 hours
4. Level of consciousness every 8 hours
5. Signs of electrolyte imbalances
6. Presence of fatigue and shortness of breath
7. Signs of GI bleeding (bleeding gums, guaiac positive stools)
8. Presence of pruritus and evidences of skin excoriations
9. Presence of discomfort: muscle cramping, headaches, ocular irritations
10. Insomnia
11. Anorexia, bad taste in mouth, daily dietary intake
12. Signs of infection

diagnosis of chronic renal failure. Refer to the section in this chapter dealing with a specific diagnosis.

As renal failure progresses the person will continue to have serum chemistries monitored, to ensure that adequate treatment is being provided. Serial creatinine clearance and serum creatine, as well as BUN, are monitored. As complications develop, other diagnostic tests will be used to provide necessary data; the specific tests will depend on the body system that is involved.

→ DATA ANALYSIS: NURSING DIAGNOSES

Nursing diagnoses are determined from assessment of patient data. Possible nursing diagnoses for the person with chronic renal failure may include, but are not limited to the following:

Diagnostic title	Possible etiologies
Activity intolerance	Bed rest, immobility, generalized weakness
Adjustment, impaired	Disability requiring change in life style, impaired cognition, assault to self-esteem
Anxiety	Threat to self-concept, threat of death
Constipation, colonic	Change in life-style, immobility, medications
Comfort, altered: pain, itching	Diagnostic tests, treatment, uremia
Coping, ineffective individual	Situational crisis
Fluid volume excess	Compromised regulatory mechanism
Home maintenance management, impaired	Insufficient family resources, impaired functioning
Hopelessness	Failing physical condition
Knowledge deficit	Lack of exposure, cognition limitation
Mobility, impaired physical	Intolerance to activity
Nutrition, altered: less than body requirements	Anorexia
Protective mechanisms, altered	Decreased RBCs, decreased platelet activity
Sexual dysfunction	Physical limitations, medications
Urinary elimination, altered patterns	Anatomical obstruction, urinary infection, anuria

This is not an exhaustive list. As end-stage renal disease progresses, most patients develop numerous complications, expanding the list of nursing diagnoses.

⊔ PLANNING: EXPECTED PATIENT OUTCOMES

Expected patient outcomes for the patient with chronic renal failure may include, but are not limited to, the following:

1. Patient does not develop additional signs of fluid retention.
2. Patient eats a balanced diet within the dietary and fluid prescriptions.
3. Patient participates in activities without increased fatigue.
4. Patient can state feeling comfortable: itching is minimized.
5. Patient sleeps reasonably well during night and awakens refreshed.
6. Patient does not develop infections or additional GI bleeding.
7. Patient does not injure self.
8. Patient describes nature of chronic renal failure.
9. Patient describes menus to include dietary prescriptions.
10. Patient describes need for rest periods and need to pace activities to prevent fatigue.
11. Patient knows the names and can find the telephone numbers of community local support groups.
12. Patient describes symptoms to be reported to physician and need for medical follow-up.

⊔ IMPLEMENTATION

The nurse collaborates with the physician to meet the treatment goals (see the box on p. 1200) through control of fluid balance, regulation of electrolyte balance, and prevention of metabolic waste buildup. Nursing care guidelines are summarized in the box on p. 1202.

Treatment goals for the person with chronic renal failure

1. Stabilization of the internal environment as demonstrated by the following:
   a. Mental alertness, attention span, and appropriate interaction with the environment
   b. Absence or control of peripheral edema, absence of pulmonary edema
   c. Control of electrolyte balance:
      Sodium   125 to 145 mEq/L
      Potassium   3 to 6 mEq/L
      Bicarbonate   >15 mEq/L
      Calcium   9 to 11 mg/dl
      Phosphate   3 to 5 mg/dl
   d. Serum albumin >2 g/dl
   e. Control of protein catabolism and protein breakdown products
      Urea nitrogen <100 mg/dl
      Creatinine   <15 mg/dl
      Uric acid   <12 mg/dl
   f. Absence of joint inflammation and pain
2. Infection and abnormal bleeding are not present.
3. Blood pressure is controlled at less than 160/100 mm Hg sitting and less than 30 mm Hg postural change on standing.
4. Anorexia, nausea, and pruritus are absent or controlled.
5. Intercurrent illness is resolved or controlled (heart failure, infection, dehydration).
6. There is no toxicity from inadequately excreted medication.
7. Nutrient intake is sufficient to maintain positive nitrogen balance.

□ Assisting with achievement of therapeutic goals
□ *Fluids and diet*

It is important to adhere to the fluid prescriptions. Fluid intake must be sufficient to maintain renal function without producing diuresis or fluid retention. The person needs to understand the effects of excessive or inadequate fluid intake and signs indicating fluid retention or dehydration in order to maintain the fluid prescriptions both during hospitalization and at home.

Although severely restricted *sodium* diets are *not* now usually prescribed, most persons with CRF require some salt restrictions. If a no-added salt (NAS) diet is prescribed, a normal diet is followed except that no extra salt is added to prepared foods, and obviously salted foods are omitted. For more restricted diets, the specific amount of sodium permitted is prescribed; the dietitian can be especially helpful to patients in planning meals that meet the sodium

restriction. *Salt substitutes should be avoided* by all persons with CRF because these substitutes contain large amounts of potassium.

Potassium intake may need to be restricted. If severe hyperkalemia is present, measures to remove the excess serum potassium must be taken (p. 1190). If hyperphosphatemia is present, dietary restriction of *phosphates* will be necessary. Food high in phosphorus include meat, poultry, fish, eggs, and legumes.

Protein intake is reduced to decrease azotemia, acidosis, and hyperkalemia, and to relieve distressing GI symptoms. Some protein is needed to help maintain nitrogen balance. The preferred proteins are those that contain more essential amino acids (such as fish, poultry, eggs, milk). A newer approach to protein replacement that promotes positive nitrogen balance is the use of mixtures of essential amino acids and ketoacid analogs. *Carbohydrates* are encouraged to provide energy without placing an undue load on the kidneys.

□ **Medications**

When kidney function is impaired, drugs are not excreted easily, thus their effects may be prolonged. Persons with CRF must therefore be monitored closely for signs of side effects or toxicity. These persons must have the necessary information to monitor themselves at home. Because hypertension commonly occurs with CRF, antihypertensive drugs may be prescribed (Chapter 26).

Measures to decrease high phosphate levels help to protect the kidney from further damage (p. 1193). Antacids containing aluminum hydroxide or carbonate (Amphojel, ALternaGEL, Basaljel) bind phosphorus in the intestinal tract and allow it to be eliminated. These drugs should be taken at meals to bind the phosphates in the food. The drugs should not be taken with other medications because they also bind drugs in the intestinal tract. Aluminum preparations are *constipating,* therefore stool softeners are usually required.

Anemia may be treated with iron supplements if an iron deficit has been shown to exist. Transfusions are generally avoided, unless the person has excessive fatigue and shortness of breath, because transfusions depress the patient's stimulus to red cell production in addition to the usual possible transfusion complications.

Vitamin supplements may be necessary if the diet is severely restricted. Folic acid supplements may be prescribed because dietary sources of folate (folic acid) may be restricted in CRF and because the food preparation may further decrease the amount of folate ingested.

□ *Promotion of safety*

Persons with CRF are at greater *risk for infection*. In addition, significant rises in serum potassium can be averted by preventing tissue breakdown. Potassium is largely an intracellular cation, and extensive tissue damage can liberate a lethal amount of this ion into the system of the person with CRF. Prevention and control of infection is similar to that for acute renal failure (p. 1190). The person is counseled to avoid exposure to individuals with known infections and to avoid extreme fatigue, which lowers body resistance. Persons are encouraged to seek medical attention for early signs of infection.

GI *bleeding* needs to be diminished when possible. Urea is broken down to ammonia by the action of intestinal bacteria. Because ammonia is a mucosal irritant, ulceration and bleeding can occur. Antacids can be administered every 2 to 4 hours to decrease GI irritation. A soft toothbrush is recommended for oral care to decrease gum irritation with bleeding. The person is instructed to observe and report signs of melena.

Neurologic changes occurring with CRF can lead to *injuries*. The buildup of osmotically active particles and fluid in the body occurring in uremia produces changes in the brain cells that may lead to confusion and impairment in decision-making ability. Convulsions and coma may occur. Fluid accumulation and hypertension can produce visual changes. The patient's awareness of the environment needs assessment. At times the person may need to be helped in limiting activities to a level commensurate with mental processes and level of awareness. For instance, blurred vision and delayed reaction time contraindicate driving an automobile. Individuals caring for the patient need to be aware of the possibility of seizure activity and take appropriate precautions. Correction of abnormal body chemistries will help prevent coma or convulsions.

Assisting with comfort and ADL

Rarely does the person with CRF have acute sharp pain; however, these persons are subject to a wide variety of chronic discomforts, including pruritus, cramping, numbness and tingling in the hands and feet, headaches, and irritation of the eyes. These discomforts are decreased through control of uremia and fluid and electrolyte imbalances.

Pruritus

Most persons with end-stage renal disease develop pruritus. Patients relate that itching is of a deep sensation. Factors that appear to exacerbate the itching include increasing levels of serum phosphorus, dry skin, and warm moist heat. Itching is largely symptomatic, and measures that are effective in controlling it vary. Keeping the skin moist and supple through use of lotions and bath oils, controlling the room temperature during sleep to prevent excessive warmth, and bathing with a vinegar solution are measures alone or in combination that may provide some relief from itching. Antipruritic medications may be prescribed. Injury to the skin from vigorous scratching may lead to skin infections. Fingernails can be trimmed closely, and a soft cloth rather than fingernails, should be used to scratch the skin.

Other discomforts

Muscle cramping in the lower extremities and hands may be temporarily relieved by heat and massage for some persons. *Ocular irritation* in chronic renal failure is caused by hyperphosphatemia leading to calcium deposits in the conjunctiva, which cause burning and watering of the eyes.

Methylcellulose (artificial tears) placed in the conjunctival sac every few hours helps to reduce irritation.

Fatigue and insomnia

Insomnia and fatigue are common complaints of persons with CRF, resulting from uremia, pruritus, and recurring occupation with thoughts concerning the disease state and resultant changes in life-style. Treatment for anemia will help decrease fatigue. Plans for daily activities should include provision of rest periods. Naps taken late in the day are avoided to prevent interference with sleep. Measures to promote sleep are appropriate.

Oral hygiene

Decreased salivary flow and ammonia from breakdown of urea can lead to irritation of the oral mucous membranes and produce discomfort and anorexia. Oral hygiene several times a day, especially before meals, is recommended. Lip emollients can help keep lips moist.

Counseling and teaching

The patient with end-stage renal disease presents a unique opportunity for the nurse to promote optimum health through counseling and teaching.

Facilitating coping

Numerous alterations in life-style, group membership, and feelings regarding the self occur for the person with chronic renal failure. The numerous physical changes that occur often make it difficult to carry on activities that were once normally pursued. *Chronic fatigue* may make it impossible for the person to continue to be employed. Because the patient is often tired and not feeling well, it may be difficult to plan in advance for social events. The former roles of the sick member of the family must often be taken on by another. When roles cannot easily be changed or additionally assumed by other members of the family, serious threats to the organization of the family group occur. Physical appearance also changes and is of much concern to most persons. As uremia progresses, the individual often becomes thin and weaker and appears sallow. Thoughts concerning death and the quality of life are common.

Denial often becomes a chief defense mechanism for the patient. With it the individual can periodically forget the constant threat of life. The use of this mental mechanism for the person with chronic renal failure can be quite appropriate as long as it is not manifested by maladaptive or harmful behavior. Inappropriate uses of denial involve continuous dietary indiscretion and failure to take prescribed medications.

Patients with chronic renal failure need the hope and encouragement that with treatment discomfort will be lessened and they will be allowed to pursue what seems most productive and important to them. Hope should not be focused on cure, but on learning to manage a new style of life. In managing the changes that occur as a result of chronic renal failure, the patients should be encouraged to be as independent and as active as possible. Patients should be taught to manage the treatment and should be given the responsibility of doing so. Nursing care should be provided as part of the team approach that assists patients in identifying problems and resources to meet them, and helps patients and their families adjust to the changes in their life-style.

□ *Patient teaching*

To promote self-care, every aspect of health care promotion pertaining to end-stage renal disease must be conveyed to the patient and significant others who may be participating in care (see the box at left). Education about *medications,* concerning prescribed, over-the-counter, and folk medicines, is carried out with the person. The use of popular medications that are sold without prescription must be discouraged. All medications should be prescribed by the physician. Aspirin may be hazardous because it is normally excreted by the kidneys and may rapidly build to toxic levels and prolong bleeding time. Many cold preparations contain large amounts of sodium. Remembering to take prescribed medication can be a problem for the person who may have many pills to take each day, especially if the person is confused. Correlating pill-taking times with major activities of the day or use of mechanical devices to separate out the daily allotment of pills may be helpful. Patient teaching includes the following:

1. Nature of chronic renal failure
2. Diet regimen, including fluid restrictions
3. Medication regimen, including action, dosage, frequency, and side effects
4. Relationships between diet, fluid restriction, medication, and blood chemistries
5. Relationships between symptoms and their causes
6. Need for rest periods, and need to pace activities to prevent fatigue
7. Availability of community resources
8. Symptoms that must be reported to the physician (changes in urinary output, edema, weight gain, dyspnea, infection, behavioral changes)
9. Need for continued medical follow-up

⊞ EVALUATION

General questions to ask in evaluating the care of the person with chronic renal failure include the following:

1. Are there any signs of additional fluid retention?
2. Is the patient following the required fluid and diet prescriptions?
3. Are there signs of excessive fatigue?
4. Is the person scratching excessively?
5. Is the person sleeping reasonably well at night?
6. Have infection, additional GI bleeding, and injuries been prevented?
7. Can the person describe the nature of CRF, rationale for therapy, therapeutic regimen, and symptoms to be reported?

■ Dialysis

Dialysis involves the movement of fluid and particles across a semipermeable membrane. It is a treatment that can help restore normal fluid and electrolyte balance, control acid-base balance, and remove waste and toxic material from the body. It can sustain life successfully in both acute and chronic renal failure where substitution for or augmentation of normal renal function is needed. Specifically, dialysis is used to remove excessive amounts of drugs and

---

Nursing care of the patient with chronic renal failure

Assisting with achievement of therapeutic goals

1. Encourage the person to remain within prescribed fluid restrictions.
2. Encourage a diet high in carbohydrates and within the prescribed limits of sodium, potassium, phosphorus, and protein.
3. Administer phosphate binding agents (aluminum gels) with meals as prescribed.
4. Give prescribed stool softeners when patient is taking aluminum antacids.
5. Administer vitamin and mineral supplements as prescribed.
6. Protect the patient from infection.
7. Assess patient's environment and protect from injury as appropriate.
8. Prevent further GI bleeding through use of soft toothbrush and antacids.

Assisting with comfort and ADL

1. Use measures to decrease itching; give prescribed antipruritics as necessary.
2. Provide heat and massage for muscle cramping of hands and lower extremities.
3. Provide artificial tears for ocular irritations.
4. Encourage rest for fatigue.
5. Use measures to promote sleep, as appropriate.
6. Provide good oral hygiene several times a day, especially before meals.

Counseling and teaching

1. Provide person with opportunities to discuss feelings about chronicity of disease.
2. Provide counseling if denial interferes with therapy.
3. Encourage hope by helping the person learn how to manage the new life-style.
4. Teach the person about the nature of CRF, rationale for therapy, therapeutic regimens, and need for follow-up care (see Patient teaching on this page).

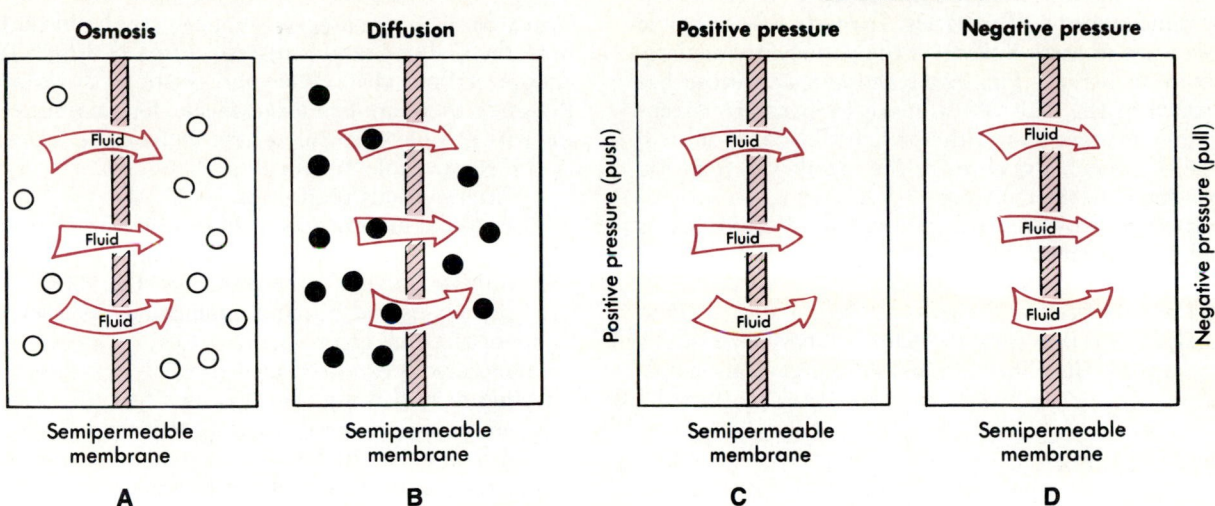

ULTRAFILTRATION

Osmosis | **Diffusion** | **Positive pressure** | **Negative pressure**

Semipermeable membrane (A) | Semipermeable membrane (B) | Semipermeable membrane (C) | Semipermeable membrane (D)

Fig. 32-31 Dialysis is based on principles of **A,** osmosis, and **B,** diffusion and ultrafiltration. Ultrafiltration occurs when either **C,** positive pressure or **D,** negative pressure is placed on system. Ultrafiltration can be maximized by exerting both positive and negative pressure on system simultaneously.

toxins in poisoning of both an intentional and accidental nature, to correct serious electrolyte and acid-base imbalances, to maintain kidney function when renal shutdown occurs as a result of transfusion reactions, to temporarily replace renal function in persons with acute renal failure of various origins, and to permanently substitute for loss of renal function in persons with chronic end-stage renal disease.

■ PHYSIOLOGIC PRINCIPLES OF DIALYSIS

Dialysis is based on three principles: diffusion, osmosis, and ultrafiltration (Fig. 32-31). *Diffusion* involves the movement of *particles* from an area of greater to an area of lesser concentration. In the body this usually occurs across a semipermeable membrane. Diffusion is involved in the clearance of solute from the patient's body in both hemodialysis and peritoneal dialysis. Diffusion results in the movement of urea, creatinine, and uric acid from the patient's blood into the dialysate solution. This solution contains fewer particles to be removed from the bloodstream and higher concentrations of particles to be added to the blood (Fig. 32-32). Because the dialysate contains no protein waste products, the concentration of these substances in the blood will decrease because of random movement of the particles across the semipermeable membrane into the dialysate. The same principle applies to the movement of potassium ions. Although the concentration of red blood cells and protein is high in blood, these molecules are quite large and do not diffuse through the membrane pores; hence they are not lost from the blood.

Osmosis involves the movement of *fluid* across a semi-

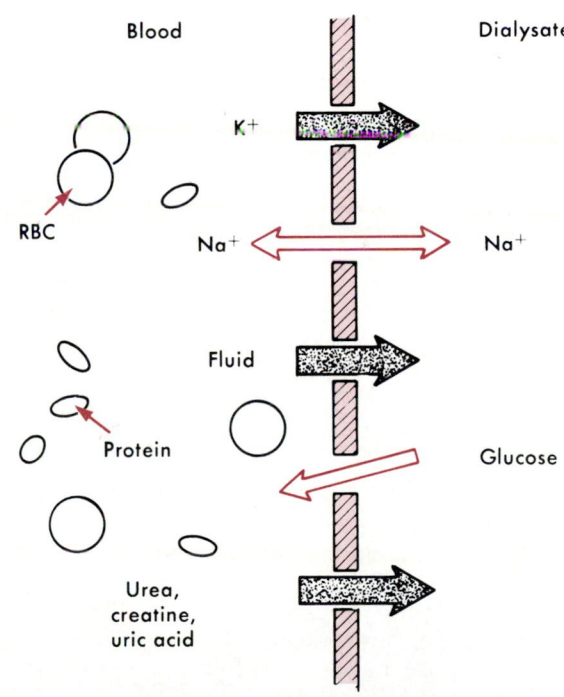

Fig. 32-32 Osmosis and diffusion in dialysis. Net movement of major particles and fluid is illustrated.

permeable membrane from an area of lesser to an area of greater concentration of particles. Osmosis is responsible for movement of extra fluid from the patient, particularly in peritoneal dialysis. Fig. 32-32 shows that glucose has been added to the dialysate to make its particle concentration greater than that of the patient's blood. Fluid will then move through the pores of the membrane from the patient's blood to the dialysate.

Ultrafiltration involves the movement of fluid across a semipermeable membrane as a result of an artificially created pressure gradient. Ultrafiltration is more efficient than osmosis for removal of fluid and is used in hemodialysis for this purpose. During dialysis, osmosis and diffusion or ultrafiltration and diffusion occur simultaneously.

■ HEMODIALYSIS

□ Procedure

Hemodialysis involves shunting the patient's blood from the body through a dialyzer in which diffusion and ultrafiltration occur and back into the patient's circulation.

To perform hemodialysis there must be access to the patient's blood, a mechanism to transport the blood to and from the dialyzer, and a dialyzer (area in which the exchange of fluid electrolytes and waste products occurs). Presently there are five major means for gaining access to the patient's bloodstream. These include the following:
1. Arteriovenous fistula (Fig. 32-33, *A*)
2. Arteriovenous graft (Fig. 32-33, *B*)
3. External arteriovenous shunt (Fig. 32-33, *C*)
4. Femoral vein catheterization (Fig. 32-33, *D*)
5. Subclavian vein catheterization (Fig. 32-33, *E*)
The indications and nursing implications for each access is summarized in Table 32-19.

Many persons expect to leave the dialysis treatment with a feeling of well-being. Few persons feel this way; most experience some minor discomfort that diminishes within several hours after dialysis. The greatest feeling of well-being seems to occur the day after dialysis.

A dialysis treatment lasts from 3 to 5 hours, depending on the type of dialyzer used and the time necessary to correct the fluid, electrolyte, acid-base, and waste problems that are present. Dialysis for an acute problem may

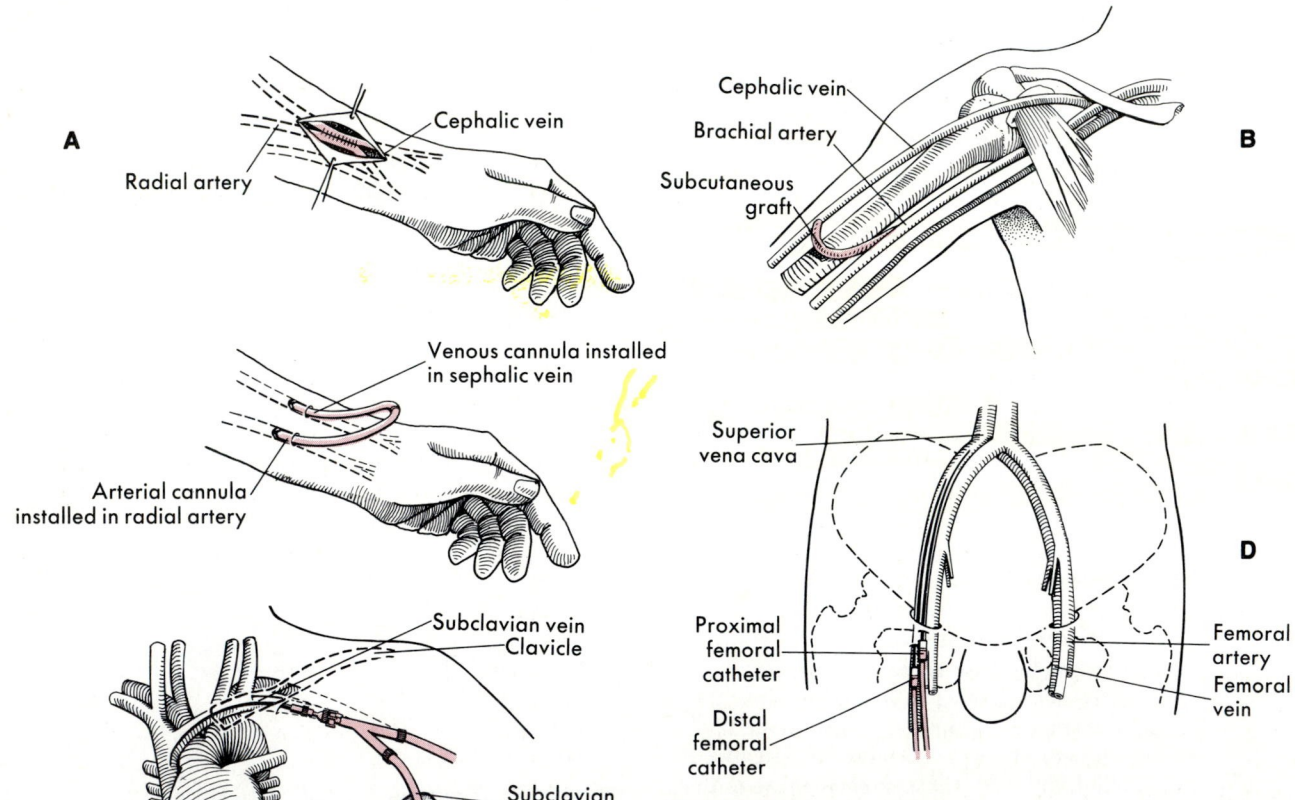

Fig. 32-33 Frequently used means for gaining vascular access for hemodialysis includes **A,** arteriovenous fistula, **B,** arteriovenous graft, **C,** external arteriovenous shunt, **D,** femoral vein catheterization, and **E,** subclavian vein catheterization.

Table 32-19 Indications and nursing implications for the major types of vascular access for hemodialysis

Type	Indications	Advantages	Nursing implications
Femoral vein catheterization	Immediate access Need for access seen as short duration	Ease of access Can be used immediately	Assess patient frequently for bleeding from insertion sites Requires frequent irrigation with heparin solution to maintain patency Sterile technique is essential when working with catheters
External shunt	Long term (weeks to months) needed for vascular access Access required within a few hours	Ease of access Can be used immediately	Assess patient frequently for bleeding at insertion site Assess patency of access frequently by observing continuous flow of blood through shunt Shunt is potential source of infection
Subclavian vein catheterization	Immediate access Short or long duration of vascular access	Does not restrict patient's activity Requires only one catheter	Assess patient frequently for bleeding from insertion site Sterile technique is essential when working with catheter Requires irrigation with heparin solution to ensure patency
Arteriovenous fistula and graft	Permanent access required	Is least likely of all the accesses to develop an infection Once maintained it provides easy access	Assess patency of fistula or graft by palpating or auscultating bruit Instruct patient to avoid compression of fistula by tight clothing or carrying objects with arm bent Patient must be instructed to assess fistula for signs and symptoms of infection including pain, redness, swelling or excessive warmth

be carried out daily or as often as the condition of the patient warrants. Hemodialysis for chronic renal failure is usually performed two or three times a week.

Nursing care of the patient during hemodialysis should center around (1) monitoring the physical status of the patient before and during dialysis for evidence of physiologic imbalance and change, (2) comfort and safety needs of the patient, and (3) helping the patient to understand and adjust to the care and changes in life-style. This latter objective involves educating the person as to the specifics of the treatment program (diet and medications in particular) and how these relate to altered kidney function. The person is encouraged to express concerns and feelings, and attempts must be made to help the individual work through these feelings. If dialysis is performed at home, the patient and back-up person must be able to institute all the care described.

The environment must provide protection from conditions that would promote infection. Because there is the potential for blood spills as a result of the treatment, all equipment must be easily cleaned. Great care must also be taken to dispose properly all soiled articles to prevent cross-contamination between patients.

Because the person spends a great deal of time at the dialysis center, the environment should present an atmosphere that is warm and inviting. Activities should be available to assist the person in using the time on dialysis as fully as possible. Art and music therapy both provide effective and productive diversion.

□ **Predialysis care**

Before the procedure, patients should have an opportunity to become familiar with the dialysis unit. They should be given an explanation of what will happen and what will be expected of them during the treatment. Patients often want to know (1) what types of pain will be experienced during the treatment, (2) how long and how often the dialysis will be, (3) what they should feel like during and after the treatment, (4) what they will be allowed to do during dialysis, and (5) if family members may be present during the therapy. Monitoring activities include the following:

1. Record weight.
2. Obtain baseline vital signs.
3. Assess patient for fluid overload (pedal edema, periorbital edema, neck vein distention, adventitious breath sounds).
4. Assess vascular access for patency and infection.

A blood sample is drawn to determine the level of serum electrolytes and waste products, and the patient's physical status is assessed.

Patients should be told that they may experience some

headache and nausea during the treatment and for a few hours afterward. Headache and nausea result from change in fluid, acid-base, and waste balance during dialysis. The symptoms should never be extreme, and relief should be attained from rest and sleep, mild analgesics, or antiemetics. Postural hypotension may also occur following dialysis; it is transitory in nature and caused by a relative depletion of intravascular volume secondary to fluid removal. The hypotension may produce dizziness and faintness. Relief should be obtained within a few hours with rest. The patient is assured that all of these symptoms will abate and that frequent monitoring during the procedure will help to control the degree of change that occurs during dialysis and the development of these symptoms.

☐ Care during hemodialysis

When the patient has an external shunt, no pain should be experienced during initiation of dialysis. However, pain of a moderate degree may be present when venipuncture is performed in an arteriovenous fistula. A local anesthetic is used in most dialysis centers before insertion of the needles.

Nursing care includes measures to increase the patient's physical comfort. Lying relatively immobile for even a few hours can produce pressure over bony prominences and general restlessness. Changing the patient's position increases tolerance to limited movement. Mouth care is required if the patient is nauseated and vomiting. Because an upper extremity is generally kept immobile during dialysis, the patient may need help with activities requiring the use of both hands.

Activity during dialysis is largely a matter of individual preference. Some persons sleep throughout their treatment; others read or carry on various activities.

Eating during dialysis is largely a matter of individual preference. Some individuals may become quite hungry, while for others the smell of food causes nausea. Patients may ask that they be allowed to eat foods not generally allowed during dialysis. Practice indicates that either allowing or discouraging eating freely during dialysis is a matter of individual unit philosophy. Because of the frequency of nausea, vomiting, and disequilibrium many patients experience during hemodialysis, it may be best to discourage eating to decrease the potential of aspiration.

☐ *Physiologic imbalances*

HYPOVOLEMIA. Most physical problems that occur during dialysis are related to hypotension from removal of fluid and disequilibrium from a rapid reduction in extracellular electrolytes and wastes. Hypovolemia and shock can occur during dialysis as a result of rapid removal of fluid from the intravascular compartment. Because this can occur faster than reequilibration of intracellular and intravascular volume relationships, the person may appear edematous and yet exhibit signs of shock. Signs and symptoms that indicate that the intravascular volume is being rapidly depleted are anxiety, restlessness, dizziness, nausea and vomiting, diaphoresis, tachycardia, and hypotension. Activities to prevent hypovolemia include the following:

1. Check blood pressure and pulse every 30 to 60 minutes (more frequently if signs of shock present); blood pressure should show only a slight increase.
2. Monitor blood flow and dialyzer pressure settings carefully to prevent too rapid blood flow (usual flow rate for adult is 200 to 250 ml of blood per minute).
3. Withhold rapid-acting antihypertensives the morning of dialysis (unless person is severely hypertensive).
4. Evaluate need for withholding medications that predispose to hypovolemia (analgesics, tranquilizers, hypnotics, nitroglycerin).

In treating a patient who shows signs of hypovolemia, initial nursing measures include determining the blood pressure and pulse, placing the head of the bed in a flat position, and raising the patient's feet. Administration of normal saline solution may be necessary to restore blood pressure. Throughout a hypotensive episode vital signs, level of consciousness, and any complaints offered are closely monitored. Vomiting frequently accompanies hypotension. Because an upper extremity must be maintained fairly immobile during the dialysis, it may be awkward for the patient to clear the mouth if vomiting should occur. The patient is helped to a safe position so that aspiration is avoided.

The patient is weighed before and after dialysis to determine amount of fluid loss during treatment. When the weight losses of several dialysis treatments are correlated with the patient's blood pressure, pulse, and other indications of hypovolemia, an individual pattern of the patient's tolerance to fluid removal can be determined. This trend or pattern can be used to help adjust the rate and overall effect of the dialysis in keeping with the patient's physiologic tolerance.

DISEQUILIBRIUM PHENOMENON. A disequilibrium phenomenon occurs for many dialysis patients toward the end of or after dialysis. Disequilibrium results when excess solutes are cleared from the blood more rapidly than they can diffuse from the body's cells (particularly those of the central nervous system) into the vascular compartment. Hence, disequilibrium exists in the concentration of solute inside and outside the cells. Because particle content is greater inside the cells, water is taken in and edema results. Intracellular pH changes are also present. To some degree this process occurs with all patients with each dialysis procedure and helps to explain why patients do not feel their best immediately after treatment. *Severe disequilibrium*, or *disequilibrium phenomenon*, is most likely to be seen in the person whose blood chemistry values are exceptionally high before dialysis. Signs and symptoms of disequilibrium include *headache, restlessness, mental confusion*, and *nausea* and *vomiting*. Severe disequilibrium may result in convulsions, especially in children when BUN levels exceed the concentration of 100 mg/ml.

Treatment includes anticipation of severe disequilibrium. Often when a patient is beginning dialysis treatments, the procedures are kept short and may be spaced more frequently than normal during the first week. This allows solute to be cleared from the body without producing the extremely wide swings in body chemistry that would result in severe disequilibrium. Keeping the patient quiet, reducing environmental discomfort such as temperature extremes and bright lights, and closely supervising the patient to ensure physical safety are nursing care requirements. Mild analgesics may help to relieve headache. If disequilibrium becomes severe and the patient is still on dialysis, the therapy may be discontinued.

BLOOD LOSS. Care of the patient on dialysis should also include preventing blood loss. To prevent the patient's blood from clotting as it flows through the dialyzer, heparin is administered. Protamine sulfate is not generally given to the patient to counteract the effect of heparin. The patient is watched for signs of bleeding anywhere in the body. At the end of the treatment when dialysis needles are removed from the fistula, pressure dressings are applied to the puncture sites. They are observed at frequent intervals to detect hemorrhage. During and shortly after dialysis, treatments that cause tissue trauma should not be performed. These commonly include venipuncture and intramuscular injections. The patient who has had recent surgery, dental extractions, or recent trauma to soft tissues will have clotting times monitored frequently during dialysis to prevent hemorrhage. These patients need to be closely observed for signs of bleeding.

□ Postdialysis care

Following dialysis, the person's weight is again recorded and postural vital signs are assessed.

□ Patient teaching

A sample teaching plan is described below. Major teaching points specific to hemodialysis include the following:

1. The process of dialysis and relationship to the person's own body needs.
2. Care of the vascular access, including monitoring for complications (absent thrill or bruit over artery indicating no blood flow, constriction of fistula, infection, hemorrhage).
3. Where to obtain care if complications occur.

Example of care plan for teaching the patient on hemodialysis

Date	Hour	Teaching/learning needs	RN signature
		Chronic renal failure being treated by hemodialysis	
Start	**Stop**	Plan	
		1. Introduce patient to hemodialysis unit using available printed material and a visit to unit when appropriate.	
		2. Explain normal kidney function.	
		3. Explain kidney failure specific to patient's pathophysiology.	
		a. Types	
		b. Causes	
		4. Explain and reinforce medication regimen.	
		a. Purpose of each prescribed medication	
		b. Common side effects	
		c. Dosage and times of each medication	
		d. Prescription filling procedure	
		5. Reinforce dietary instructions.	
		a. Protein	
		b. Potassium	
		c. Sodium	
		d. Fluids	
		e. Calories	

Continued.

Example of care plan for teaching the patient on hemodialysis—cont'd

		6. Instruct patient in necessity for and care of vascular access.	
		a. Procedure for assessing presence of thrill and bruit; who to notify if thrill or bruit is absent	
		b. Guarding against constriction of fistula, that is sleeping on arm or wearing tight clothing	
		c. Hygiene and removing dressing after dialysis	
		d. Signs and symptoms of infection, that is, redness, swelling or tenderness	
		e. Measures to control hemorrhage should it develop while away from dialysis unit	
		7. Instruct patient about process of hemodialysis.	
		a. Explain principles of dialysis in sufficient detail for learning level of patient.	
		b. Describe hemodialysis in full detail to patient.	
		c. Explain common sights and sounds of dialysis unit to patient.	
		d. Describe common complications of hemodialysis, as well as usual treatments, to patient.	
		(1) Hypotension	
		(2) Nausea	
		(3) Vomiting	
		(4) Cramping	
		8. Instruct patient in interpretation of laboratory data and effects of hemodialysis, diet, and medications on these values.	
		9. Introduce patient to alternative modes of treatment of ESRD.	
		a. Free-standing hemodialysis centers	
		b. Self-dialysis (home)	
		c. Peritoneal dialysis	
		d. Transplantation	
Date		Status of problems at discharge:	
Date		Patient knowledge:	
Date		Follow-up plans:	

RN signature _____

4. Common complications of hemodialysis.
5. Changes in medication schedule required before and after dialysis treatments.
6. Ways to schedule dialysis treatments for minimal interference with life-style.
7. Alternative modes of treatment for end-stage renal disease.

■ PERITONEAL DIALYSIS

In peritoneal dialysis the dialyzing fluid is instilled into the peritoneal cavity and the peritoneum becomes the dialyzing membrane (Fig. 32-34). In comparison with hemodialysis treatments, which last 3 to 6 hours, peritoneal dialysis is maintained continuously for up to 36 hours. The procedure, once instituted, becomes largely a nursing responsibility. Peritoneal dialysis is used in treating acute and chronic renal failure. It can be performed in the hospital or at home.

The major advantages of peritoneal dialysis include the following:

1. The procedure provides a steady state of blood chemistries.
2. Any location can be used, and machinery is not needed.
3. The process can be easily taught to patient or family.
4. Few dietary restrictions are required; because of the loss of protein across the peritoneal membrane into the dialysate, the patient is usually placed on a high-protein diet.
5. The patient has more control over daily life.
6. The procedure can be used for persons who are hemodynamically unstable.

□ Procedure

Access to the peritoneum is gained through introduction of a catheter into the peritoneal space. For acutely ill patients, and those who are chronically ill and require sporadic dialysis, a sterile catheter is inserted for each procedure. For the chronically ill person treated on a routine basis, a special catheter can be placed into the peritoneal space, the catheter remains until it malfunctions or another form of treatment is selected for the patient. These catheters present a continued potential entrance for organisms into the peritoneum.

To insert a peritoneal catheter, the physician cleanses the abdomen and anesthetizes a small area in the midline of the abdomen about 5 cm (2 inches) below the umbilicus. A small incision is made, and the many-eyed nylon catheter is inserted into the peritoneal cavity (Fig. 32-34).

A dressing is placed around the protruding catheter. Dialysis is initiated for the person with a permanent catheter by carefully cleansing the catheter and surrounding skin with a bactericidal agent before the catheter is connected to the dialysate line. Approximately 2 L of sterile dialysate warmed to body temperature is attached by tubing

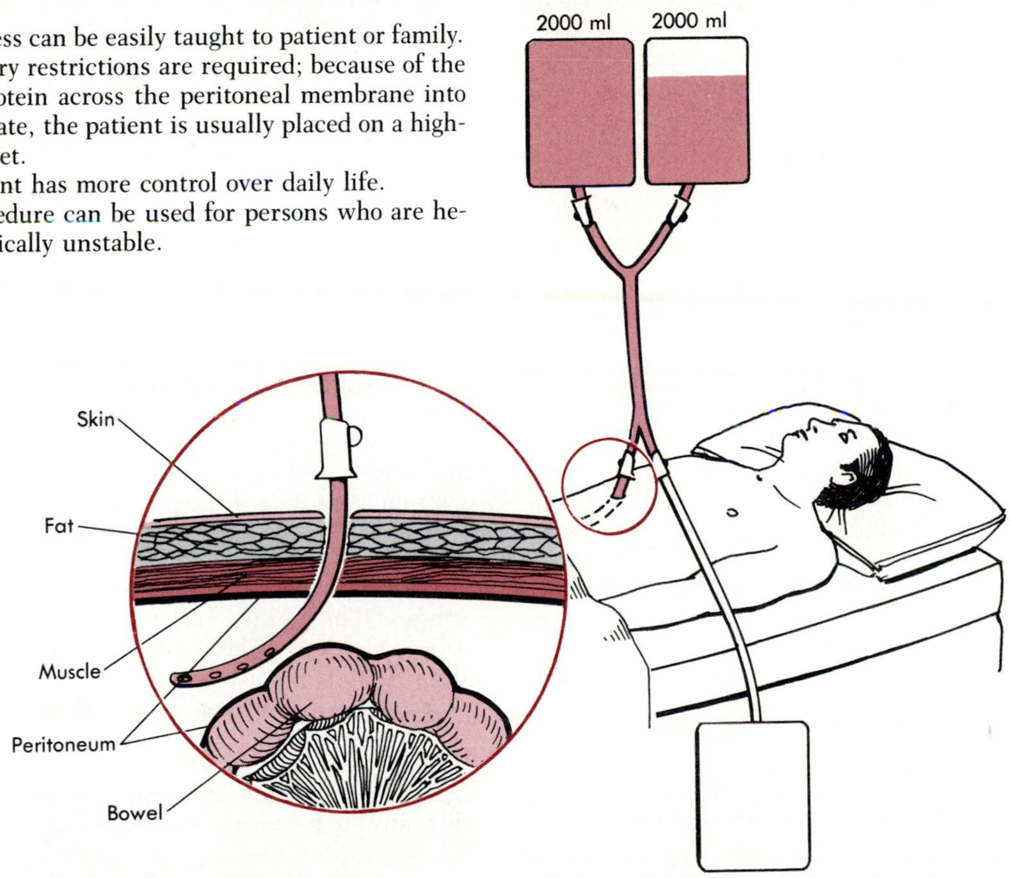

Fig. 32-34 Patient receiving peritoneal dialysis. Dialysis fluid is being inserted into peritoneal cavity.

to the catheter and allowed to run into the peritoneal cavity as rapidly as possible. This usually takes about 10 minutes. The tubing is then clamped, and 10 to 30 minutes are allowed for osmosis of fluid and diffusion of particles into the dialyzing solution. This is called a *dwell time*. At the end of the dwell time the tubing is unclamped and the fluid is allowed to flow by gravity from the abdomen.

Fluid should drain in a steady stream. Drainage time should average about 10 to 15 minutes. The first drainage may be pink tinged as a result of the trauma of catheter insertion; however, this should clear with the second or third drainage. At no time should fluid draining from the abdomen appear grossly bloody. After fluid has drained from the abdomen, another cycle is started immediately. After the dialysis has been completed, the permanent catheter is again cleansed and a sterile cap is applied to the tip; the temporary catheter is removed, and the incision is covered with a dry sterile dressing. The small abdominal wound from the catheter should heal completely in 1 to 2 days.

□ Preprocedure care

Weight, blood pressure, and pulse are recorded before the procedure is initiated. These values serve as baseline information to assess changes in the patient's condition. For persons undergoing insertion of a peritoneal catheter before dialysis, assessment should be made of their knowledge of the procedure and their anxiety level. A mild sedative may help the severely anxious person to better tolerate the insertion of the catheter. It is important that these patients void just before catheter insertion; this decompresses the bladder and prevents accidental puncture during catheter placement.

□ Care during peritoneal dialysis

The person undergoing acute peritoneal dialysis may be confined to bed during the treatment as a result of general fatigue and the constant fluid exchanges that take place. Comfort measures and diversionary activities should be of high priority. During the dialysis, the patient is able to turn from side to side and move about in bed as desired as long as the catheter remains undisturbed. The patient is provided assistance with hygiene care as needed. If peritoneal dialysis is carried out at home, the patient and a backup person need to be able to do all steps of the procedure to ensure that therapy is not interrupted when the patient is too ill to dialyze alone.

Nursing activities during peritoneal dialysis include the following:
1. Maintain strict aseptic technique to prevent infection.
2. Monitor vital signs frequently.
3. Maintain strict intake and output records.
4. Assess catheter site for signs of infection.
5. Assess patient for edema.
6. During cycles maintain accurate record of each cycle, including the following:
   a. Type of dialysate
   b. Amount of dialysate infused
   c. Amount of dialysate recovered
   d. Time dialysate was left indwelling
   e. Characteristics of recovered dialysate

□ Complications of peritoneal dialysis

Complications most commonly associated with peritoneal dialysis include hypotension and hypovolemia, inadequate drainage of fluid from the peritoneal space, pain, atelectasis, respiratory distress, and peritonitis. As with hemodialysis, *hypotension* is most likely to result from rapid removal of fluid from the intravascular space. In addition to checking vital signs and observing the patient's behavior, records of fluid balance are crucial in determining the amount of fluid that has been removed. The net gain or loss of fluid from the abdomen should be determined at the completion of each cycle. To decrease the amount of fluid that is being removed from the vascular space, the physician may decrease the hypertonicity of the dialysate and may increase the rate at which fluid is administered through an intravenous line.

Drainage of fluid from the abdomen can be slow or impossible to start. Generally, this problem results when the tip of the catheter has become lodged against abdominal tissues. It may also result from plugging of the catheter with blood or fibrin that has accumulated as a result of tissue trauma. A small amount of heparin may be added to the dialysate to decrease the chance of a clot forming in the catheter. When the dialysate does not drain freely from the abdomen, the patient should be turned from side to side in an attempt to reposition the catheter in the peritoneal cavity. In addition, firm pressure may be applied to the abdomen with both hands and the head of the bed may be raised. If the flow of the dialysate does not increase, the physician is called to irrigate the catheter or reposition it.

Severe *pain* should not be experienced during peritoneal dialysis. Moderate levels of pain are often experienced as fluid is instilled and withdrawn from the peritoneal cavity. Procaine hydrochloride may be instilled with the dialysate in an attempt to control the patient's discomfort. Mild analgesics may be ordered for administration at 3- to 4-hour intervals during the procedure.

When the patient is markedly overhydrated and shows evidence of congestive failure and pulmonary edema, *respiratory difficulty* may be encountered as the dialyzing fluid infuses. The quality and rate of respiration should be closely observed. The head of the bed can be raised to decrease the pressure of the dialysate on the diaphragm. The amount of dialyzing fluid used for each cycle may be decreased when respiratory distress becomes prolonged and severe. The patient, although encouraged to eat while being dialyzed, may find that this increases respiratory difficulty. To help overcome additional pressure created by a full stomach, frequent small meals may be provided.

Peritonitis is an ever present threat during peritoneal dialysis. Aseptic technique must be rigidly maintained during insertion of the catheter and throughout the procedure. Care should be taken to avoid contaminating the solution or the tubing when dialysate solution is hung. Cultures of the dialysate fluid are performed routinely to ensure continued attention to asepsis and to identify organisms if peritonitis should develop subsequently. The patient should be observed for signs of peritonitis. These include an elevated temperature and tenderness or pain of the abdomen.

☐ Other approaches to peritoneal dialysis

Several advances in the management of patients with chronic end-stage renal disease have led to two variations of peritoneal dialysis. These technologies emphasize home- and self-dialysis.[52,54] *Continuous ambulatory peritoneal dialysis* (CAPD) is one development that is leading to safe self-dialysis that is practical and relatively inexpensive when compared to hemodialysis and that promotes patient independence. Bascially, CAPD involves continuous contact of dialysate with the peritoneal membrane. Approximately 2 L of dialysate are maintained interperitoneally and exchanged by the patient through a permanent peritoneal catheter 4 to 5 times a day.[2] No special equipment is required for the exchanges, and the patient can therefore lead a fairly normal life-style. Exchanges can take place at home or at work by connecting an empty bag to the catheter and opening a clamp to allow drainage. A full dialysate bag is then instilled and the patient has completed an exchange.

The second method is *continuous cyclic peritoneal dialysis* (CCPD). CCPD differs from CAPD in that a machine known as a *cycler* is used to instill and drain dialysate from the patient. The machine has a series of clamps that are controlled by timers. The timers open and close the clamps in sequence to allow for instillation and drainage of dialysate from the patient. The cycle times for patients with chronic renal failure generally allow for the patient to be dialyzed in 6 to 8 hours. A patient can therefore connect up to the cycler at bedtime, set the machine, and be dialyzed while sleeping. A number of alarms are built into the cycler to protect the patient from such malfunctions as dialysate that is too hot or cold, long or short dwell times, improper return of fluid, and changes in catheter pressures. The greatest advantage of CAPD and CCPD over other forms of dialysis is that both offer the patient unprecedented freedom in managing their own care.

☐ Teaching the patient

The teaching requirements for the patient undergoing peritoneal dialysis are consistent with the teaching plan for hemodialysis. However, the patient will need to be instructed in the specifics of the process of peritoneal dialysis. If CAPD is planned, training should be accomplished in a home training center that is equipped to assist the patient in dealing with home care.

■ Kidney transplantation

Kidney transplants are performed to prolong the lives of persons with chronic renal failure. Transplantation is not without problems, however, and persons undergoing kidney transplantation, in essence, exchange the limitations of a program of chronic hemodialysis for the problems of possible rejection. Unless the kidney has been donated by an identical twin, the body senses the graft as a foreign tissue and attempts to reject it. Graft survival has improved in recent years because of better blood typing and leukocyte typing for histocompatibility antigens and because of newer immunosuppressive drugs, such as cyclosporine.

■ DONOR SELECTION

Kidney allografts may be obtained from cadavers, matched family members, or an identical twin. Although more than half of the transplanted kidneys are from cadavers, better results are obtained from related donors. Currently, success rates 1 year after transplantation are 50% to 60% when a cadaveric kidney is used, 70% to 80% when a matched sibling or parent donated the kidney, and 90% when an identical twin is the organ donor.

Cadavers should be free of renal disease, neoplasms (excluding those of the central nervous system and skin), infectious agents such as AIDS, and sepsis. Permission for cadaver donation is given by next of kin or by persons who plan in advance to donate their organs.

The major requirement for the donated kidney is histocompatibility. Rejection occurs from a cell-mediated (type IV hypersensitivity) response or from a humoral (type II cytotoxic hypersensitivity) response (Chapter 38). The important antigens are the human leukocyte antingen (HLA) and the ABO blood groups. For the ABO groups the same rules apply as for blood transfusions.

Graft survival from living related donors is significantly increased by *donor-specific transfusion*.[30] Shortly before transplantation the recipient receives three transfusions of the donor's blood, each 2 weeks apart. After these transfusions, if the recipient and donor blood cross-match is still compatible, transplantation is performed. The purposes of donor-specific transfusion are (1) to identify recipients who would respond unfavorably to the donated organ and (2) to desensitize the recipient to the donor's tissue.

Related donors must be in good health, be highly motivated to be a donor, have good mental health, and not be receiving drugs such as barbiturates, which depress reflexes and electrical brain activity. The donor is given a complete medical evaluation and in some cases may be referred to a psychiatrist for further evaluation.

Viability of the donor kidney must be maintained until the time of transplantation surgery. Preservation times of 24 to 72 hours have been reported with proper technique. Methods include washing out the formed blood elements and perfusing a heparinized electrolyte solution at 2° to 4° C. Use of a pulsatile flow pump and oxygenator helps to preserve the kidney beyond 6 to 12 hours.

■ TRANSPLANT REJECTION

Rejection of a new kidney because of the body's immunologic response to foreign substances leads to tissue

Table 32-20 Common side effects of immunosuppressive therapy and nursing interventions

Side effect	Nursing intervention
Leukopenia	Observe for signs of infection Reverse isolation Antibiotic therapy as prescribed
GI irritation and bleeding	Perform guaiac tests on stool, vomitus, and NG aspirate Administer antacids as prescribed Provide calm, supportive environment Assess postural vital signs
Increased appetite	Reinforce diet teaching Encourage low-sodium diet
Alopecia	Suggest use of wig Encourage patient that hair will grow back Provide emotional support
Acne	Encourage frequent bathing Instruct in use of appropriate soaps
Delayed wound healing	Maintain sterile technique for dressing changes Assess wound each dressing change for signs of infection Encourage adequate protein in diet
Change in mental status (mood swings)	Observe patient for changes in behavior and report to physician Provide calm supportive environment Provide diversional activities

necrosis and a nonfunctioning kidney. Rejection is the leading cause of graft failure. Survival of the graft depends on the suppression of the immune response, usually achieved by immunosuppressive drugs. The most commonly used drugs are the following:

1. Cyclosporin A—drug of choice to prevent rejection; can be nephrotoxic, therefore kidney function is monitored carefully
2. Antimetabolites (azathioprine [Imuran] and cyclophosphamide)—often given together because lower doses of each can be given, thus reducing side effects of both drugs
3. Corticosteroids—high doses required for immunosuppression may create significant risks and side effects
4. Antilymphocytic globulin (ALG)—required high doses may cause an Arthus reaction (Chapter 38); is used mostly as adjunct therapy

Side effects of therapy with immunosuppressive medications and nursing interventions are listed in Table 32-20.

□ Types of rejection

Rejection may occur as a hyperacute event, as an acute event, or as a slow and progressive decline in renal function. *Hyperacute rejection* occurs immediately after surgical implantation. Following arterial anastomosis, circulating cytotoxic antibodies instantly infiltrate and infarct the foreign tissue. The hyperacute rejected kidney is usually removed immediately to prevent further complications. *Acute rejection* typically begins within the first 2 weeks but may

be seen 2 or more years after transplantation. Most transplant patients undergo at least one episode of acute rejection. The delay in the occurrence of the first attack is related to the time it takes for T-lymphocytes to become sensitized. Signs and symptoms indicative of acute rejections are listed in the box below.

Chronic rejection is a slow progressive process. It occurs secondary to cell-mediated and humoral immune responses. The signs and symptoms are similar to those that

---

Signs and symptoms of acute rejection of a transplanted kidney

1. Decrease in urine output
   a. Oliguria
   b. Anuria
2. Fever greater than 37.7° C (100° F); may be masked by steroids
3. Pain or tenderness over grafted kidney
4. Edema
5. Sudden weight gain, 2 to 3 pounds in 24 hours
6. Hypertension
7. General malaise
8. Rise in serum creatinine value
9. Decrease in creatinine clearance

occur in acute rejection; however, they occur more slowly. In most instances the patient will eventually lose all renal function as chronic rejection progresses.

□ Therapy for transplant rejection

Immunosuppressive drugs are usually given to treat, as well as to prevent, tissue rejection. Large doses of methylprednisolone (Solu-Medrol) may be administered intravenously. A newer drug, muromonab-CD3 (OKT3) has been shown to be effective in treating steroid resistant rejections, and it reduces the adverse effects of large doses of steroids. OKT3 reacts with receptors on T-cell surfaces, preventing lysis of cells. Other immunosuppressive drugs that are being given are reduced or discontinued when OKT3 therapy is given. Local graft irradiation may also be used to destroy infiltrating lymphocytes.

■ PREOPERATIVE CARE

Nursing care of the person in the preoperative phase includes physical and emotional preparation for the surgery. The nature of the surgery and location of the transplant, the possible need for postoperative dialysis, the use of immunosuppressive drugs, and the need for infection prevention after surgery are explained to the patient and family. They should also be prepared for the possibility of the kidney not functioning after transplantation. Throughout the period from the patient's acceptance as a transplant candidate to the time of surgery, opportunities are provided for the patient and family to discuss their concerns and anxieties regarding transplantation.

The person must be in optimal physical condition for transplantation. Dialysis may be required before transplantation to ensure optimal fluid and electrolyte balance, acid-base balance, and removal of wastes. The integrity of the vascular access must be maintained. Before surgery the extremity containing the vascular access may be wrapped to draw attention to it and identify it as containing the patient's access for dialysis. This identification will help all individuals caring for the person to avoid using the affected extremity for blood pressure determinations, drawing of blood, or intravenous infusions.

■ SURGERY

During surgery the transplanted kidney is placed in the iliac fossa (Fig. 32-35). Generally, the peritoneal cavity is not entered. The patient's own kidneys are not disturbed unless they are infected or are the cause of significant hypertension, in which case the recipient undergoes bilateral nephrectomy before transplant surgery. The recipient's kidneys are left intact whenever possible to maintain erythropoietin production, blood pressure control, and prostaglandin synthesis and metabolism. The donor ureter is used to the extent that is possible. If long enough, the donor ureter is connected to the bladder in such a way as to prevent reflux of urine. If the ureter is short, a ureteroureterostomy may be performed. A catheter is placed in the wound to promote drainage of accumulating fluid.

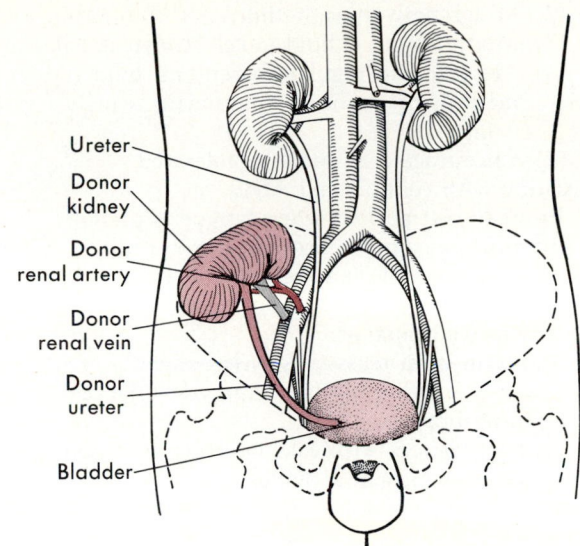

Fig. 32-35 Location of transplanted kidney showing anastomosis of renal artery, renal vein, and ureter.

Labels: Ureter; Donor kidney; Donor renal artery; Donor renal vein; Donor ureter; Bladder

■ POSTOPERATIVE CARE

Fluid and electrolyte balance must be monitored carefully because the patient may have little or no urinary output for a number of hours to weeks after transplantation. Parameters indicating disturbed fluid and electrolyte balance are listed in the discussion of chronic renal failure (p. 1193). Any drainage from the dressing or tubes is carefully calculated into the patient's fluid balance record.

In the operating room an indwelling catheter is inserted into the bladder to promote drainage of urine and to prevent bladder distention and pressure on the newly anastomosed ureter. If gross hematuria or clots are noted in the drainage system, the physician is notified immediately. Urinary drainage is monitored hourly during the early postoperative period.

Additional immediate postoperative care includes protecting the patient from infection, observing for signs and symptoms of rejection or other complications such as hemorrhage or hypovolemia, and identifying the effects of medications that have been administered during the entire postoperative period. The postoperative care is summarized below:

1. Assisting with achievement of therapeutic goals
   a. Immediate postoperative period
      (1) Maintain sterile technique in caring for wound and urinary drainage catheter.
      (2) Encourage early ambulation.
      (3) Administer medications as prescribed.
      (4) Assess patient for signs and symptoms of an infection both at surgical incision and systemically.
   b. Fluid and electrolyte balance
      (1) Maintain accurate intake and output.

(2) Weigh daily at same time.

(3) Monitor signs of fluid and electrolyte imbalance.

(4) Monitor and regulate parenteral fluid replacement as prescribed by physician (usually 1 ml/ 1 ml).

(5) Encourage oral intake as tolerated.

2. Assisting with comfort and ADL
   a. Promote rest periods when fatigue is present.
   b. Administer pain medication as prescribed.
   c. Assist with ADL as necessary but encourage independence.

3. Control of environment
   a. Maintain calm reassuring environment.
   b. Reverse isolation may be required while patient is immunosuppressed.
   c. Restrict visitors with colds or other infections.
   d. Provide diversional activities.

■ TEACHING THE PATIENT

Because of the possibility of delayed rejection following transplantation, the person must know the expected therapy to be followed and signs to be monitored:

1. Actions, dosages, and potential side effects of medications

2. Signs and symptoms of graft rejection and information to report to physician

3. Measures to prevent infection: avoidance of persons with upper respiratory infections; dental prophylaxis, regular medical check-ups, and avoidance of immunization with live-virus vaccines

4. Signs and symptoms of infection and actions to take

5. Accurate monitoring of intake and output

6. Monitoring of daily weights

7. Need to avoid trauma to graft site because it is superficially placed

8. Need to preserve dialysis access

9. Need for medical follow-up

10. Resources for assistance with illness and rehabilitative concerns, and means of contact with the resources

■ SUMMARY

1. The kidneys are essential for the following:
   a. Regulating electrolytes
   b. Eliminating wastes
   c. Regulating fluid volume
   d. Maintaining acid-base balance
   e. Regulating blood pressure
   f. Stimulating production of RBCs
   g. Regulating calcium-phosphate metabolism

2. The kidneys regulate blood pressure by controlling fluid volume as well as mediating the renin-angiotensin-aldosterone system.

3. Hypertension is a leading cause of renal disease that could be minimized by early detection and adequate treatment.

4. Urinary retention can result in hydronephrosis that leads to permanent damage to the kidneys.

5. Control of urinary incontinence is largely dependent on its cause. Accurate diagnosis of the cause of the incontinence is therefore essential before a program to reestablish continence is developed.

6. Females are more likely to develop UTI than are males. Approximately 1% of all school age girls and 4% of all women in their childbearing years are diagnosed as having UTI.

7. If untreated, lower UTIs can migrate to the kidneys resulting in pyelonephritis.

8. Untreated streptoccal infections can lead to the development of acute glomerulonephritis.

9. The clinical manifestations of the nephrotic syndrome include the following:
   a. Severe generalized edema
   b. Pronounced proteinuria
   c. Hyperalbuminemia
   d. Hyperlipidemia
   The presence of these findings defines nephrotic syndrome.

10. Corticosteoids are usually prescribed for the treatment of the nephrotic syndrome because of their antiinflammatory effect.

11. Obstruction of any part of the urinary system from the kidney to the urinary meatus may lead to hydronephrosis and may cause functional and anatomical damage to the renal parenchyma.

12. Lithotripsy is fast becoming the treatment of choice for renal stones because of the noninvasive nature of the treatment and the short recovery period.

13. An alkaline-ash diet is often effective in preventing the recurrence of renal stones.

14. More than 75% of all men over 75 years of age will develop benign prostatic hypertrophy requiring treatment. A transurethral prostatectomy is the treatment of choice but can only be employed if there is a relatively small amount of tissue to be removed; otherwise bleeding can be excessive.

15. An essential component of the preoperative teaching plan for the person about to undergo any urostomy surgery is preparation for the presence of the ostomy and a drainage appliance.

16. Major components of the treatment of a person with polycystic disease are prevention, early detection, and treatment of any infections that develop so that renal function can be preserved.

17. Proteinuria is never considered a normal finding.

18. Because a major cause of toxic nephropathy is antibiotic therapy, the nurse must observe all patients on nephrotoxic antibiotics for signs and symptoms of decreasing renal function.

19. In managing acute renal failure the goal is to decrease the production of metabolic wastes; this can be accomplished by close dietary restriction including limiting intake of proteins.

20. Because of the potential to develop hyperkalemia, severe acidosis, severe fluid overload, infection, and sei-

---

Putting knowledge to practice

- Plan a one-day menu for a person with nephrosis who weighs 60 kg. Use the following daily prescription: 2800 to 3000 calories, 1g/kg protein, and 500 mg sodium.
- Examine the chart of a patient with acute renal failure. Draw a graph of the reported electrolytes, BUN, serum creatinine, and creatinine clearances. Include a line showing the normal values of each finding. How did the patient's laboratory findings compare to the "typical clinical picture."
- Develop a care plan for a person about to undergo surgery for a permanent ileal conduit. Outline the elements of the teaching care plan that must be instituted both before and after surgery.
- What criteria are used for selection of the type of dialysis prescribed for specific patients with renal failure? List the physiologic parameters that must be considered in selecting a mode of dialysis.
- Develop a list of the community resources that are available in your area for persons with end-stage renal disease. It will be helpful to contact the local affiliate of the National Kidney Foundation to assist in obtaining this information.
- Explore the procedure in your community for organ recovery and allocation for renal transplantation. Review the process by which individuals are placed on a recipient list and the length of time that is normally required to get a transplant.

---

zures in the oliguric phase of acute renal failure, prompt medical management of the patient is required. The nurse observes for the signs and symptoms of these life threatening problems.

21. Maintaining adequate caloric intake for the person with chronic renal failure is accomplished by selecting foods high in carbohydrates and fats.

22. Phosphate binding agents such as ALternaGEL and Amphojel must be administered at mealtimes to be effective in binding dietary phosphate.

23. Hemodialysis is not a cure for end-stage renal disease but rather a treatment necessary to sustain life.

24. Antihypertensive medications should be withheld until after the hemodialysis treatment to safeguard against hypotensive episodes during the treatment.

25. Because peritonitis frequently occurs as a result of peritoneal dialysis, great care must be taken to limit all potential causes of infection. This is best managed by observing strict aseptic technique whenever handling the catheter.

26. Acute tubular necrosis frequently follows renal transplantation and often is managed by hemodialysis. Return to dialysis immediately after transplantation may lead to anxiety and depression in the patient.

27. The body will attempt to reject any foreign tissue that is introduced, therefore immunosuppression is instituted to prevent the rejection of the transplanted kidney. Immunosuppression will be required as long as the transplanted kidney remains functional.

REFERENCES AND SELECTED READINGS
Contemporary

1. *Alt, D, Balduf, R, and Thompson, E: When a vascular access site complicates care, RN 49(10):36-39, 1986.
2. *Arenz, R: Do-it-yourself dialysis, RN 44:57-60, 1981.
3. *Barta, M: Correcting electrolyte imbalances, RN 50(2):30-33, 1987.
4. *Brogna, L, and Lakaszawski, ML: The continent urostomy, Am J Nurs 86:160-163, 1986.
5. Chambers, J: Save your diabetes patient from early kidney damage, Nurs 83 13:58-63, 1983.
6. *Chambers, JK: Fluid and electrolyte problems in renal and urologic disorders, Nurs Clin North Am 22:815-826, 1987.
7. Cianci, J, and others: Renal transplantation, Am J Nurs 81:354-355, 1981.
8. *Conti, MT, and Eutropius, L: Preventing UTIs: what works? Am J Nurs 87:307-309, 1987.
9. Cope, R, Coe, R, and Rossman, I: Fundamentals of geriatric medicine, New York, 1983, Raven Press.
10. Fowler, JE, and Crowley, JL: Stress urinary incontinence: endoscopic suspension of the vesical neck, AORN J 45:922-933, 1987.
11. Goldberger, E: A primer of water, electrolyte and acid-base syndromes, ed 7, Philadelphia, 1986, Lea & Febiger.
12. Hadley, E, and others: Bladder training and related therapies for urinary incontinence in older people, Proceedings from the National Institute of Aging workshop, April 26-27, 1983, Bethesda, MD, 1983, National Institute of Aging.
13. *Harwood, C: Pulverizing kidney stones: what you should know about lithotripsy, RN 48(7):32-37, 1985.
14. *Irwin, B: Now—peritoneal dialysis for chronic patients too, RN 44:49 52, 1981.

---

*References preceded by an asterisk are particularly well suited for student reading.

15. *Kadas, N: Reducing fluid overload without dialysis, RN 49(5):27-31, 1986.
16. Lancaster, L: The patient with end-stage renal disease, ed 2, New York, 1984, John Wiley & Sons.
17. Leaf, A, and Cotran, R: Renal pathophysiology, Oxford, 1985, Oxford University Press.
18. Lu, L: Incontinence stress index: measuring psychological impact, J Gerontol Nurs 3(7):18-25, 1987.
19. Matheney, N: Fluid and electrolyte balance: nursing considerations, Philadelphia, 1987, JB Lippincott Co.
20. *McCormick, KA, Scheve, AA, and Leahy, E: Nursing management of urinary incontinence in geriatric inpatients, Nurs Clin North Am 23:231-264, 1988.
21. Ouslander, JG, Kane, R, and Abrass, I: Urinary incontinence in elderly nursing home patients, JAMA 248(1):1194-1198, 1982.
22. *Palmer, MH: Incontinence: the magnitude of the problem, Nurs Clin North Am 23:139-158, 1988.
23. Papper, S: Clinical nephrology, ed 2, Boston, 1981, Little, Brown, and Co, Inc.
24. *Percutaneous lithotripsy for renal calculi, Am J Nurs 85:772-773, 1985.
25. *Petillo, MH: The patient with a urinary stoma: nursing management and patient education, Nurs Clin North Am 22.263-280, 1987.
26. *Plawecki, HM, and others: Chronic renal failure, J Gerontol Nurs 13(12):14-17, 1987.
27. Porth, C: Pathophysiology, ed 2, Philadelphia, 1986, JB Lippincott Co.
28. *Prewit, D: Postoperative complications: an overview, Nephrol Nurse 5:27-32, 1983.
29. *Randolph, G: Bringing them back out of renal shutdown, RN 44:34-39, 108-112, 1981.
30. Robbins, K, Richard, A, and Ronselli, M: Donor specific transfusions as pretreatment for living related donor transplants and nursing implications, Nephrol Nurse 5:4-8, 1983.
31. Rosman, J: Low-protein diet reduces kidney failure, RN 48(6):70-71, 1985.
32. Ruge, CA: Shock (wave) treatment for kidney stones, Am J Nurs 86:400-401, 1986.
33. Salvatiena, O, and others: Deliberate donor specific blood transfusions prior to living-related renal transplantation, Ann Surg 192:543-552, 1980.
34. Schrier, R: Renal and electrolyte disorders, Boston, 1980, Little, Brown and Co., Inc.
35. *Smith, DAJ: Continence restoration in the homebound patient, Nurs Clin North Am 23:207-218, 1988.
36. *Solomon, J: Does renal failure mean sexual failure? RN 49(8):41-43, 1986.
37. *Stark, J, and Hunt, V: Helping your patient with chronic renal failure, Nurs 83 13(9):56-63, 1983.
38. *Stark, J: Acute renal failure, Nurs 82 12:26-33, 1982.
39. Steinhiser, SA, and Plawecki, HM: OKT3 for the treatment of patients with acute renal allograft rejections, ANNA J 14:127-129, 1987.
40. *Strangio, L: Believe it or not: peritoneal dialysis made easy, Nurs 88 18(1):43-46, 1988.
41. *Underwood, MA: Urinary tract infections, Crit Care Q 3:63-70, 1980.
42. Williams, SR: Nutrition and diet therapy, ed 5, St. Louis, 1985, The CV Mosby Co.
43. Younger, S, and others: Psychosocial and ethical implications of organ retrieval, N Engl J Med 313(5):321-323, 1985.

Classic

44. Black, DAK: Renal disease, ed 4, Oxford, England, 1979, Blackwell Scientific Publications, Inc.
45. Fennel, S: Percutaneous renal biopsy, Am J Nurs 75:1292-1294, 1975.
46. *Hartman, M: Intermittent self-catheterization, Nurs 78 8:75-77, 1978.
47. Lapides, J, editor: Fundamentals of urology, Philadelphia, 1976, WB Saunders Co.
48. Maxwell, MH, and others: Comparative study of renovascular hypertension: demographic analysis of the study, JAMA 220:1195, 1972.
49. Mooney, TO, Cole, T, and Chilgren, R: Sexual options for paraplegics and quadriplegics, Boston, 1975, Little, Brown and Co., Inc.
50. Pallay, V: Clinical testing of renal functions, Med Clin North Am 55:231-241, 1971.
51. Papper, S: Renal failure, Med Clin North Am 55:335-357, 1977.
52. Popvitch, RP, and others: Continuous ambulatory peritoneal dialysis, Ann Intern Med 88:449-456, 1978.
53. Report of the Coordination Committee: Research needs in nephrology and urology, vol 5, p 3, National Institute of Arthritis, Metabolism and Digestive Disorders, Public Health Service, DHEW Publication No (NIH) 78-1485, 1978, Washington, DC.
54. Robson, MD, and Oroponlous, DG: Continuous ambulatory peritoneal dialysis: an orientation in the treatment of chronic renal failure, Dialysis Transplant 7:999-1103, 1978.
55. Rous, SN: Urology in primary care, St. Louis, 1976, The CV Mosby Co.
56. Stamm, W: Guidelines for prevention of catheter-associated urinary tract infections, Ann Intern Med 82:386-390, 1975.
57. Stroot, VR, and others: Fluids and electrolytes: a practical approach, ed 2, Philadelphia, 1977, FA Davis Co.
58. US Department of Health, Education and Welfare, Centers for Disease Control: Outline for surveillance and control of nosocomial infections, Atlanta, 1974, The Department.

UNIT IX
Sexual and Reproductive Problems

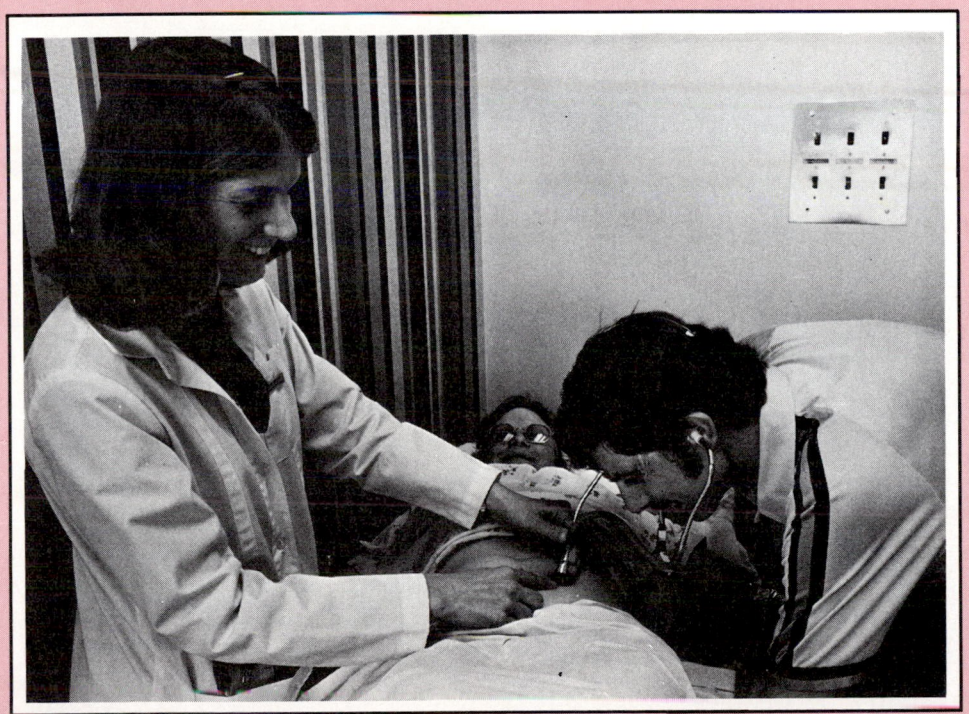

33

Sexuality in Health and Illness

NANCY FUGATE WOODS

CHAPTER OBJECTIVES

After studying this chapter, the student should be able to:

- Describe changes that occur during the phases of human sexual response.
- Describe changes in sexuality that occur with aging.
- Differentiate types of sexual variation.
- Identify ways in which illness and environment affect sexuality.
- Identify types of alterations in sexual health and related nursing interventions.
- Describe methods of prevention of sexual problems.
- State approaches that facilitate assessment of sexual health.
- Describe levels of intervention for persons with alterations of sexual health.

■ SEXUALITY AND HEALTH

Human sexuality is not merely a biologic phenomenon, but one that pervades the total person. A complex interrelationship exists among biologic, psychologic, and sociocultural aspects of our sexuality. The very complexity of human nature makes it difficult to define sexuality, much less sexual health. Nevertheless, the recognition of the importance of sexuality as a component of health has led the World Health Organization to suggest the following definition[68]:

Sexual health is the integration of the somatic, emotional, intellectual, and social aspects of sexual being, in ways that are positively enriching and that enhance personality, communication, and love.

Sexual function, sexual self-concept, and sexual roles and relationships are important dimensions of sexual health. Sexual function refers to the ability of an individual to give and receive sexual pleasure, whereas sexual self-concept refers to the image one has of oneself as a man or a woman and the evaluation of that image as masculine or feminine. Sexual self-concept includes body image and the evaluation of one's body and self within the context of the culture. Sexual relationships are the interpersonal relationships in which one's sexuality is shared with another.

■ Evolution of human sexuality

The evolution of our sexuality illustrates the complexity and interrelationship of the dimensions of our sexuality. From the moment of conception a variety of factors come into play to influence our sexuality, not only as children but also as adults. In early embryonic life the X or Y chromosome from the paternal sperm sets in motion a process analogous to a relay race; that is, each component has control of the process for a time, eventually yielding control to another[65] (Fig. 33-1). The chromosomes tag the undifferentiated fetal gonads as male or female, thus setting in motion another process by which hormonal secretions of the testes in turn affect not only the appearance of the genitals but also pathways in the brain.

The appearance of the infant's genitals at birth initiates another series of events, those primarily dependent on socialization of the child. The behavior of other persons during infancy and early childhood and the appearance of

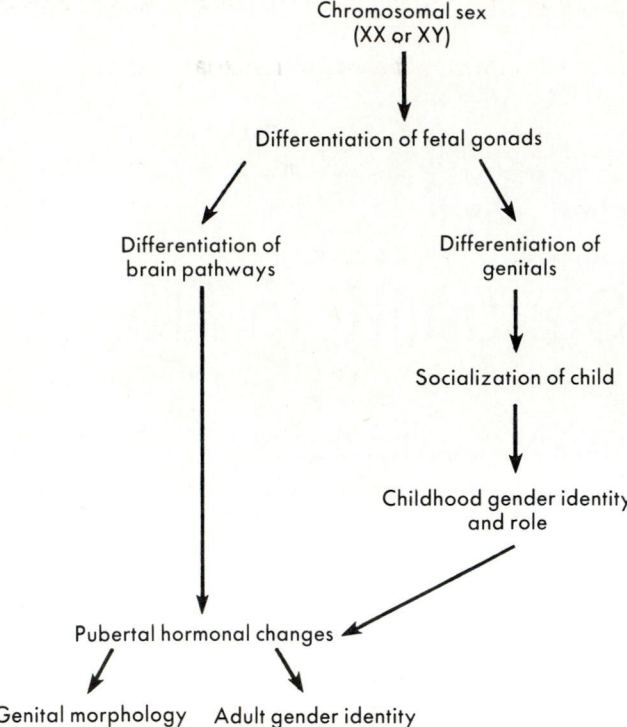

Fig. 33-1 Evolution of sexuality.

the child's external genitals are instrumental in the evolution of childhood gender identity and role. In fact, gender identity seems to be well established by the time a person is 18 months of age. At puberty, biologic influences again come to the fore as hormones influence the genital structure and eroticism.

Thus from conception we are all sexual beings subject to multiple influences throughout life. If the previous processes proceed without interference, the person's biologic sex is congruent with gender identity and gender role.

This complex set of biologic and psychosocial variables begun at conception has a pervasive influence on the remainder of our lives. The biologic component of sexuality (sexual function or expression) constantly interacts with the psychologic components (gender identity, thoughts, and feelings), as well as with social factors (such as sanctioned role and mores and folkways regulating sexual expression). Such complexity mandates a holistic approach to conceptualizing a person's sexual problems and concerns.

■ Physiologic aspects of human sexuality

■ PHASES OF THE HUMAN SEXUAL RESPONSE

Masters and Johnson, pioneers in the scientific study of the physiologic aspects of sexual behavior, demonstrated that sexual response is a cyclic phenomenon consisting of four phases[63] (see the box on p. 1221). The physiologic changes seen during human sexual response (Table 33-1)

Definition of terms

Biologic sex	Female or male
Gender identity	Person sees self as man or woman
Gender role	Outward manifestations of masculinity or femininity

Phases of the human sexual response

Phase	Description
Excitement	Increase in sexual tension evidenced by swelling of genitalia and vaginal lubrication
Plateau	Intensification of sexual tension with more pronounced genital swelling
Orgasm	Involuntary climax and release of sexual tension evidenced by muscle contraction
Resolution	Dissipation of muscle tension and swelling

depend on two main principles: myotonia and vasocongestion. It is through the congestion of pelvic blood vessels and involuntary muscular contractions in the pelvic organs and other parts of the body that changes supportive of orgasmic experience are attained.

☐ Excitement phase

The excitement phase is the initial component of the cycle. It develops from sexually arousing stimuli such as touch. An increase in sexual tension is observed during this phase. Vasocongestive changes are seen in the external genitals and the breast in both women and men. In ad-

dition, a sex flush, which looks like a red, maculopapular rash, appears over the chest in some persons. An increase in both the heart rate and blood pressure is evident, paralleling the level of sexual excitement.

☐ Plateau

The plateau phase is a consolidation period during which sexual tension becomes intensified. Vasocongestion continues. The uterus continues to elevate in the pelvis, which creates a tenting effect in the innermost portion of the vagina. The sex flush continues to spread, sometimes involving the neck, face, and arms. Hyperventilation occurs in both sexes, along with heart rates of 100 to 175 beats per minute. There is elevation of systolic blood pressure (20 to 60 mm Hg for women, 20 to 80 mm Hg for men) and diastolic blood pressure (10 to 20 mm Hg for women, 10 to 40 mm Hg for men).

☐ Orgasm

Orgasm, the involuntary climax of sexual tension, involves only a small portion of the sexual response cycle. The climactic release of sexual tension is evident in contractions throughout the body. Uterine contractions are also noted in women with orgasm, much like those characteristic of labor.

☐ Resolution

During the resolution phase, the changes involving the blood vessels, sexual organs, and muscular tension are reversed. The uterus and testes return to their normal positions. Cardiovascular and respiratory rates quickly return to normal. Occasionally a thin film of perspiration may appear over the entire body. Women may at this time

Table 33-1 Sex organ changes during sexual response

Phase	Changes in female	Changes in male
Excitement	Vaginal lubrication Vagina becomes longer and wider Uterus begins to elevate in pelvis Clitoris becomes longer and wider Labia minora extend outward Nipples enlarge, areolae become engorged, breast size increases	Penis becomes erect Scrotal sac tenses Testes begin to rise toward perineum Nipples enlarge
Plateau	Clitoris retracts Labia and outer part of vagina (orgasmic platform) become congested Uterus continues to rise in pelvis	Diameter of penis continues to increase Testes increase in size 50% and elevate close to perineum
Orgasm	Orgasmic platform contracts rapidly (throbbing sensation) Uterine contractions Rectal sphincter contractions	Expulsive contraction along entire urethra to expel semen Internal bladder sphincter contractions (prevent semen from entering bladder) Rectal sphincter contractions
Resolution	Vasocongestion decreases rapidly from vagina/labia and slowly from clitoris and breasts Uterus descends to usual position	Rapid loss of penis size to 1 to 1.5 times usual size Slower resolution of penis size to usual size Testes descend into scrotum

begin another sexual response cycle immediately; men have an obligatory period during which they cannot be restimulated to higher levels of sexual tension.

■ TRIPHASIC CONCEPT OF HUMAN SEXUAL RESPONSE

Recently Kaplan[57] has suggested a triphasic concept of human sexual response. She delineates three phases—desire, excitement, and organsm—that are related components of sexual response but are governed by separate neurophysiologic systems. This notion is useful for understanding not only the physiology of sexual response, but also the consequences of pathophysiologic conditions, the etiology of sexual dysfunction, and appropriate therapies.

□ Desire phase

The desire phase refers to the experience of a sexual appetite or drive produced by the activation of a neural system in the brain. Sexual desire is experienced as sensations that move the person to seek sexual experiences. It is likely that the sexual centers of the brain have either neural or chemical connections with the pleasure and pain centers of the brain. The pleasure centers are stimulated when we have sex, which accounts for the pleasurable quality of sexual behavior. On the other hand, the pain centers can inhibit the sexual system. Some persons suggest that the pleasure center is stimulated by release of endorphins in sexual behavior. If a sexual object or situation produces pain, then it will cease to evoke desire.

Testosterone is important in mediating sexual desire in both men and women. Luteinizing hormone and the neurotransmitters serotonin and dopamine also may be important in mediating sexual desire. Bonding to another person and love are powerful stimuli to sexual desire. Many stimuli seem to be capable of evoking sexual desire, such as sight, smell, and other sensory cues, and some of these are conditioned by culture. Fear and pain, however, are potent inhibitors.

The connections between the sex center and other parts of the brain also make it possible for people to "turn off" sexual desire when other stimuli are more important or when it is not to the individual's advantage to pursue sexual activity. Hypoactive desire and inhibited sexual desire are common problems of the sexual desire phase.

□ Excitement phase

The excitement phase is similar to the excitement and plateau phases described by Masters and Johnson and is produced by reflex vasodilation of the genital blood vessels. This vasodilation causes the genitalia to swell and changes their shape to adapt to their reproductive function. The vasocongestion is primarily a parasymphathetically mediated response, and an intense sympathetic response such as that produced by fear and anxiety can instantly lead to loss of erection. It is believed that erection is governed by two spinal reflex centers. The thoracolumbar center (psychogenic) appears to respond more to psychic stimuli, whereas the sacral center is stimulated from tactile input to the genitalia. It is believed that the spinal reflex centers and the higher neural connections are analogous in men and women. Disorders of the excitement phase include difficulty in attaining or maintaining erection in men and difficulty with swelling and lubrication in women.

□ Orgasm phase

The orgasm phase corresponds to orgasm as described by Masters and Johnson. It is also a genital reflex governed by spinal neural centers, but it consists of reflex contractions of certain genital muscles. Disorders of the orgasm phase include inadequate ejaculatory control (premature ejaculation) and retarded ejaculation in men and orgasmic dysfunction in women. Other disorders include painful intercourse and sexual phobias.

■ REQUIREMENTS FOR SEXUAL RESPONSE

The requirements for the physiologic sexual response include intact sexual organs, adequate vasculature to support the vasocongestive changes, functional innervation of the genital organs, and the appropriate hormonal milieu.[58] The changes of myotonia and vasocongestion are thought to be mediated by the autonomic nervous system. Perception of the sexual experience at cortical levels requires intact sensory pathways from the genitals and other peripheral structures to the cortex. The capacity to stimulate oneself or a partner sexually depends on the presence of intact motor pathways from higher centers to the effector muscles involved. It should also be noted that thoughts and feelings or visual, auditory, and olfactory-gustatory stimuli alone may result in arousal to orgasmic experience even in the absence of tactile perception.

Adequate hormonal milieu, with appropriate hormonal release, influences both the structure and function of the genitals; for example, the decreased estrogen levels during menopause are believed to be responsible for a decreased amount of vaginal lubrication. Finally, the presence of intact genital structures is usually thought to be a requisite for sexual response, but substitution of prosthetic devices for sexual organs is an option beginning to be explored. Although each of these components is important in sexual response, it is possible for humans to have profound sexual pleasure even when one or more of these is absent.

■ Sexuality and aging

Changes in sexual function become accentuated during middle age (see the box on p. 1223), although their onset is gradual and they probably begin long before they are perceived. Men need more time to attain an erection, and once attained, it is likely to be less full than in earlier years. The testes elevate more slowly with sexual excitement, and vasocongestive changes in the scrotum and testes are less noticeable. With prolongation of the plateau phase, middle-aged men actually achieve much better control over ejaculation than they had as young adults.

Orgasm is perceived as happening more quickly, and feelings of ejaculatory inevitability may disappear entirely.

Factors that influence sexual interest and activity in middle and old age

Women	Men
Marital status: availability of a partner	Past sexual experience
Age	Age
Enjoyment of sex in earlier years	Objective and subjective health ratings
	Social class

Resolution of sexual tension becomes more rapid with age, and the obligatory refractory period (a period during which the man cannot be restimulated to orgasm) becomes longer. With aging, men actually gain better control of ejaculation, and because of reduced ejaculatory demand, they may be satisfied not to ejaculate with each intercourse.

In women, menopausal changes may lead to delay in production of vaginal lubrication and diminished expansion of the vaginal barrel. Changes in external genitals and the breasts are apparent. The woman's orgasmic experience becomes shorter, and resolution occurs more rapidly.

Studies of healthy aging individuals indicate that a decline in overall interest and activity is seen with age. However, men from each age range tend to report greater interest and activity than women in each respective age range. Several factors can influence sexual interest and activity in middle and old age. Level of sexual activity in youth appears to be related to that in older years.[33]

As men age, an interest-activity gap appears; that is, they desire more sexual activity than they are able to experience. This gap grows as men age; however, it remains small for women. Women without a socially acceptable partner may adaptively inhibit their sexual interest. The wider interest-activity gap for men may reflect their socialization to express more interest in sex. Other social factors, such as the role loss associated with children leaving the parents' home and retirement, are likely to influence the older person's sexual interests.

■ Variations in sexual expression

Sexual behavior is a product of society and culture and our biology. Each culture has a set of norms that prescribes which behaviors are sexual and which are acceptable. In cross-cultural comparisons of sexual behavior, a wide variety of sexual expression is found. In Western society, sex is frequently equated with penis-in-vagina intercourse. Yet a wide range of behaviors exists encompassing sexual meaning (for example, talking, sharing thoughts and feelings, or just touching another person). This wide range of behaviors causes us to question what is "normal." Yet normal can refer to prevalence of a behavior, optimal function, a statistical distribution, or fashionable or socially acceptable behavior. Comfort[55] suggests that as professionals we do not restrict our definition of normal to what we, personally, admit to enjoying. Instead he recommends that we consider the following questions:

1. What does the behavior mean to the individual?
2. Does the behavior enrich or impoverish the sexual life of the individual and those persons with whom sexual relations are shared?
3. Is the behavior tolerable to society?

Variation in sexual behavior is bounded only by one's imagination and to some extent by the culture. Different types of sexual expression are described in the box below.

Sexual intercourse may be restricted to marriage or to a similar relationship in some societies. In others, there may be legitimized extramarital rights, and in some, premarital sexual freedom is encouraged. The position for intercourse varies between cultures and within cultures. Usually the position assumed for intercourse reflects other aspects of the culture; for example, in cultures where families sleep in the same quarters, often side-to-side positions are used to afford some privacy from other occupants of the room.

Culture also dictates whether the woman plays an active or passive role in sexual activity and the duration of the act of intercourse. Precopulatory stimulation may be brief or lengthy, and the type used, such as kissing, painful acts, and manipulation of the breasts or genitals, varies with the

---

Sexual variations

Heterosexuality	Choice of adult sexual partner of opposite sex
Homosexuality	Choice of adult sexual partner of same sex
Bisexuality	Choice of adult sexual partners of same and opposite sex
Transvestism	Sexual satisfaction achieved by dressing in clothing of opposite sex
Incest	Sexual relations with close relative, for example, child
Zoophilia	Choice of sexual object is an animal
Fetishism	Sexual object is an inanimate object
Voyeurism	Sexual satisfaction achieved by watching others
Exhibitionism	Sexual satisfaction achieved by exposing genitals
Sadism	Sexual satisfaction achieved by inflicting pain
Masochism	Sexual satisfaction achieved by receiving pain

culture. Sexual frequency may also be governed by norms, and in some cultures is prohibited during menses, lactation, pregnancy, or before hunts or battles.

Heterosexuality is the most prevalent form of sexual expression among adults of known societies, but it is rarely the only type of sexual behavior in which humans engage. Homosexual behavior is found in most species of mammals; in humans it is most common among adolescents and males. Since "normal" sexual response may be determined by cultural norms as well as physiologic, phylogenetic, legal, statistical, moral, and social standards, it is impossible to state a hard and fast definition of what constitutes the "normal state."

■ HOMOSEXUALITY

Homosexuality is the most common sexual variation, yet it is poorly understood by health professionals. It has been viewed as an illness, a criminal offense, and a life-style in Western society. Recently the American Psychiatric Association removed homosexuality from the "illness" classification; however, the social climate remains less liberated. Although the majority of society still seems to subscribe to the definition of homosexuality as an illness, only a minority of homosexuals classify themselves as ill.

Kinsey[59,60] estimated that 13% of women and 37% of men had had at least one homosexual experience leading to orgasm. The extent to which these persons engaged in homosexual behavior varied greatly. Thus Kinsey suggested that a continuum existed on which the two poles represented exclusive heterosexuality (0) and homosexuality (6), and the five remaining categories (1 through 5) represented a combination of the two. Individuals in categories 1 and 5 had predominant heterosexual or homosexual orientations. Those in categories 2 and 4 still had a clear preference for heterosexual or homosexual relations, but retained an active interest in the other form. Category 3 represented persons who had equal heterosexual and homosexual interests.

The Institute for Sex Research[54] conducted a large-scale study of the sexual dimensions of homosexual experience in the San Francisco Bay area. Although the authors of the report are careful to point out that their results may not mirror the entire homosexual population, the study did include men and women, both white and black. Results revealed that homosexuality encompasses more than the person's sexual tendencies. Although there was variability on the homosexual-heterosexual continuum for both male and female homosexuals, there was more heterosexuality in the feelings and behaviors of homosexual women than men.

Most of the homosexual men and women were relatively covert about their homosexuality. The mother and siblings were more likely to be aware of the individual's homosexuality than other family members. Families were more likely to be aware of the person's homosexuality than other members of society. In most cases friends, employers, and colleagues were aware of the person's homosexuality.

Homosexual men or women could not be stereotyped as sexually hyperactive or inactive; instead, the amount of activity varied with each individual. Public cruising (purposive search for a sexual partner) was infrequent among lesbians. Of those homosexuals involved in public cruising, most conducted their sexual activity in their own homes. Gay bars were the most popular cruising locales.

Homosexual men had many more sexual partners than did lesbians. There seemed to be more emphasis placed on sexual activity among males. This may be a function of lesbians' preference for relationships based more on emotions than on sex, or it may merely be a function of the problems male homosexuals have in meeting partners. For both male and female homosexuals, a relatively steady relationship with a love partner was a meaningful event.

The male homosexual subculture seemed to place more emphasis on youth than did women. Social prestige did not seem to be a major determinant in sexual appeal.

A variety of sexual techniques was used. Male homosexuals most frequently employed fellatio, hand-genital stimulation, and anal intercourse. Female homosexuals most frequently engaged in masturbation with their partners and in cunnilingus. Men and women both specified receiving oral-genital sex as a preferred technique.

Sexual problems encountered included difficulty in meeting a suitable sexual partner, maintaining affection for the partner, and meeting the other's sexual request. There was a lower incidence of these problems among lesbians. Whereas almost two thirds of the male homosexuals had at some time contracted a sexually transmitted disease from homosexual sex, only one of the lesbians had done so. More women than men had considered stopping their homosexuality, but only a minority in each case had done so. At interview, more men than women regretted their homosexuality.

About 20% of the homosexual males had been married, and more than 33% of the white lesbians and almost 50% of the black lesbians had been married once. They did not perceive their homosexuality as having a particular affect on their children.

Homosexual men and women seemed to have more friends than their heterosexual counterparts. Their friends included both homosexuals and heterosexuals. Lesbians were more involved in activities outside the home or with others than were homosexual males. Men were more likely than women to have had social difficulties, but few had been arrested because of their homosexuality.

When homosexual respondents were compared with their heterosexual counterparts in terms of adult psychologic adjustment, it appeared that the dysfunctional and asexual homosexuals were less well off than those in the heterosexual group. However, homosexual adults who have come to terms with their homosexuality are no more distressed psychologically than heterosexual men and women.[54] Thus therapists would do well to consider why a person's homosexuality is problematic and examine ways to enhance the person's life rather than direct therapy at changing the person's sexual orientation.

■ SEXUALITY AND ILLNESS

People today seem to be more comfortable in expressing their concerns about their sexual health than has previously been the case. As a result of this increased comfort, nurses are increasingly expected to provide accurate information about sexuality and health, as well as to listen with comfort and understanding to the sexual concerns patients describe. Although many persons can openly describe their problems, others are too embarrassed or lack the vocabulary necessary to do so. For this reason it is important that nurses have a frame of reference to help them identify persons at risk for sexual problems or concerns.

There are many ways in which illness may affect sexuality and sexual function. Illness may influence sexuality through changes in body structure or function, use of certain medications, or alteration in the person's body image.

■ Changes in body structure

Changes in the structure of the nervous system, circulatory system, or genital organs may result in sexual health problems. Many examples of these structural changes and the probable mechanism by which they interfere with sexual health are given in Table 33-2. Anatomic disruptions are probably best exemplified by the spinal cord–injured person who has sustained irreversible damage to neural pathways that interferes with some methods of sexual function (Chapter 19).

■ Changes in body function

Many illnesses alter physiologic processes essential to the sexual response, including nervous transmission, vasocongestion, hormonal metabolism myotonia, and perception of pleasurable sensation. Table 33-3 illustrates some illnesses that have the potential to interfere with sexual

Table 33-2   Changes in body structure and sexual health

System	Probable mechanism of interference
Central and peripheral nervous systems	
Spinal cord injury	Disrupts integrity of peripheral nerves and spinal cord reflexes involved in sexual response (for example, erection)
Spinal cord tumors	
Herniated disk	
Multiple sclerosis	
Spina bifida	
Amyotrophic lateral sclerosis	
Tumors of frontal or temporal lobes	May interfere with function of centers controlling sexual drive
Cerebrovascular accident	
Trauma to frontal or temporal lobes	
Cardiovascular system	
Thrombus formation in vessels of penis	May interfere with blood supply to penis, thus interfering with erection
Leriche's syndrome	
Sickle cell disorders	
Leukemia	
Trauma to vasculature supplying sexual organs	
Reproductive/sexual system	
Prostatectomy, radical perineal	May destroy nerve supply, interfering with sensory and motor aspects of sexual response
Abdominal perineal resection	
Lumbar sympathectomy	May result in disturbed ejaculation
Rhizotomy	May result in impotence, as well as disturbed ejaculation
Absence of penis or penile injury	Precludes or discourages intromission
Penectomy	
Imperforate hymen	
Congenital absence of vagina	
Pelvic exenteration	
Vaginectomy	
Obstetric trauma or poor episiotomy	Leaves gaping vaginal opening or painful scarring, thus discouraging intercourse
Damage to pubococcygeus muscle	

Table 33-3 Influence of changes in body function on sexual health

Physiologic interferences	Hypothesized mechanism of action	Physiologic interferences	Hypothesized mechanism of action
Systemic diseases		Trauma to penis	
Pulmonary disease	Debility, pain, and	Vaginal infections	
Renal disease	depression probably	Senile vaginitis	
Malignancies	interfere with sexual	Vulvitis	
Infections	desire and expression	Leukoplakia	
Degenerative diseases		Bartholin's cyst	
Some cardiovascular diseases		Allergic response to vaginal sprays and deodorants	
Metabolic disruptions		Vaginitis following radiation therapy	
Cirrhosis	Hepatic problems in men	Pelvic inflammatory disease	
Mononucleosis	result in estrogen	Fibroadenomas	
Hepatitis	buildup from inability	Endometriosis	
	of liver to conjugate	Uterine prolapse	
	estrogens; similar pro-	Anal fissures, hemorrhoids	
	cesses occur in	Pelvic masses	Local irritability, damage
	women along with	Ovarian cysts	to genitalia, and con-
	general debility	Prostatitis	sequent interference
Hypothyroidism	By depression of CNS	Urethritis	with reflex mecha-
Addison's disease	function, general debi-		nisms involved in
Hypogonadism	litation, and depres-		erection and ejacula-
Hypopituitarism	sion, libido may be		tion
Acromegaly	decreased, and im-		
Feminizing tumors	paired erectile abilities	**Medical or surgical castration**	
Cushing's disease	in men may result	Orchiectomy	Lowered androgen
Diabetes mellitus		Radiation therapy	levels depress libido
		Oophorectomy, adrenalec-	and lead to impo-
Diseases of the genitalia		tomy	tence, retarded ejacu-
Priapism	Each of these problems		lation, or impaired
Peyronie's disease	involves damage to		sexual responsiveness
Balantitis	genital organs, which		
Phimosis	may result in painful		
Genital herpes	intercourse		

Modified from Kaplan, HS: The new sex therapy, New York, 1974, Quadrangle Press.

response and the hypothesized mechanisms by which they affect sexual response.

In general, it appears that the extent of a physiologic disorder and its chronicity determine relative frequency of sexual problems. Diabetic women have a higher rate of difficulty with lubrication than do nondiabetic women, particularly women who have been diabetic for 6 years or longer and who have neuropathy.[50] This relationship between chronicity and dysfunction is also observed in men with diabetes. A high incidence of problems with erection, however, is found among diabetic men during the first year after diagnosis. It is believed in this instance that the lack of diabetic control (physiologic derangement) is responsible for the sexual dysfunction.[66] For chronic illnesses as a group, it is easy to hypothesize a relationship between perception of health status, degree of fatigue, metabolic derangements, altered roles, fear of dying, and the demands of a chronic illness on the partner and changes in the sexual relationship.

Although some medical-surgical conditions do not interfere directly with sexual functions, their perceived seriousness or the presence of symptoms discourages persons from engaging in their usual sexual practices. One very common example is associated with cardiac disease, more specifically myocardial infarction. Although marital sex probably does not demand a great energy expenditure, many persons are fearful of attempting intercourse after having a heart attack. One study of married men who had had myocardial infarctions demonstrated that heart rates with orgasm were much lower in this group than among the younger group studied by Masters and Johnson.[56] An active physical conditioning program did produce significant improvements in the frequency and quality of sexual activity for men who had had a myocardial infarction. This energy expenditure associated with sex seemed to be better tolerated by those who exercised regularly.

In general, the literature indicates that the postmyocardial infarction patient may return to regular sexual ac-

Table 33-4 Drug effects on human sexual behavior

Drug or drug category	Effect	Probable mechanism of action
Oral contraceptives	Positive	Permits separation of sexual activity from concern about conception
Antihypertensives Guanethidine (Ismelin) Reserpine (Serpasil) Mecamylamine (Inversine) Trimethaphan (Arfonad) Spironolactone (Aldactone)	Negative	Peripheral blockade of nervous innervation of sex glands
Antidepressants Imipramine (Tofranil) Desipramine (Norpramin, Pertofrane) Amitryptyline (Elavil) Nortriptyline (Aventyl) Protriptyline (Vivactil) Phenelzine sulfate (Nardil) Tranylcypromine sulfate (Parnate) Pargyline (Eutonyl)	Negative	Central depression; peripheral blockade of nervous innervation of sex glands
Antihistamines Diphenhydramine (Benadryl) Promethazine (Phenergan) Chlorpheniramine (Chlor-Trimeton)	Negative	Blockade of parasympathetic nervous innervation of sex glands
Antispasmodics Methantheline (Banthine) Glycopyrrolate (Robinul) Hexocyclium (Tral) Poldine (Nacton)	Negative	Ganglionic blockage of nervous innervation of sex glands
Sedatives and tranquilizers Chlorpromazine (Thorazine, Megaphen) Prochlorperazine (Compazine) Thioridazine (Mellaril) Mesoridazine (Serentil) Chlordiazepoxide (Librium) Diazepam (Valium) Benperidol Phenoxybenzamine (Dibenzyline) Chlorprothixene (Taractan)	Negative and positive	Central sedation; blockade of autonomic innervation of sex glands; suppression of hypothalamic and pituitary function Tranquilization and relaxation
Ethyl alcohol	Negative Transiently positive	Central depression; suppression of motor activity; diuresis Release of inhibitions; relaxation
Sex hormone preparations Cyproterone acetate Methandrostenolone (Dianabol) Nandrolone phenpropionate (Durabolin)	Negative	Antiandrogenic effects on sexual function; loss of libido; decreased potency
Potassium nitrate (saltpeter)	Questionable	Diuresis
Cantharis (Spanish fly)	Negative	Irritation and inflammation of genitourinary tract, systemic poisoning
Yohimbine	Questionable	Stimulation of lower spinal nerve centers
Narcotics and psychoactive drugs Morphine Heroin Cocaine Marijuana LSD Amphetamines	Negative Transiently positive	Central depression; decreased libido and impaired potency Release of inhibitions; increased suggestibility; relaxation
L-Dopa and p-chlorophenylalanine	Questionable	Improvement of well-being
Amyl nitrite	Questionable	Vasodilation of genitourinary tract; smooth muscle relaxation
Caffeine	Questionable	CNS stimulant
Vitamin E, selenium	Questionable	Supports fertility in laboratory animals

From Woods, NF: Human sexuality in health and illness, ed 3, St. Louis, 1984, The CV Mosby Co.

tivity provided there are no symptoms of congestive heart failure. However, certain conditions that increase energy expenditure during intercourse are to be avoided. These include having intercourse shortly after a meal or soon after alcohol consumption, since both increase the heart rate and metabolic demands. Extremes in temperatures and anxiety-provoking or secretive situations should also be avoided. The energy expenditure in climbing two flights of stairs appears to produce a greater increase in heart rate than does orgasm.[60]

■ Effects of pharmacologic agents

Pharmacologic agents that have the potential to affect sexual drive, as well as performance, are listed in Table 33-4. The relationship between extent of physiologic problems and degree of sexual dysfunction may be demonstrated by pharmacologically induced changes. For example, alcohol induces transiently positive changes; in small doses it initially promotes relaxation and release of inhibitions, as do other psychoactive drugs. However, in larger doses, alcohol has negative effects on sexual function, leading to central nervous system depression and interference with motor activity.

Several categories of drugs have demonstrably negative effects on sexual function. These include antihypertensives, antidepressants, antihistamines, antispasmodics, sedatives, and tranquilizers, ethyl alcohol, some sex hormone preparations, and some narcotics and psychoactive drugs.

■ Body image changes

The extent to which distortion of body image influences sexuality often depends on the perceptions of two persons: oneself and a significant other. Multiple variables may influence the body image of a woman who has had a mastectomy. Although one might suspect that the extent of surgery and pain in the operative area would be most important, the value she assigned to her breasts, her preoperative body image, and social factors such as the quality of her preoperative sexual relationship are also influential. In one study the quality of the relationship the woman had with her husband before the surgery was the most important determinant of her return to sexual functioning after surgery.[66]

The visibility of a defect plays an important role in sexual adaptation. Visibility of a disability seems to be just as disruptive of marital and family relations as it is of other social relationships.[66]

Finally, the meaning and significance one attaches to the changed body part may interfere with sexual behavior. The amputee who views the loss as castration, the woman who sees her hysterectomy as a neutering surgery, and the person who equates an ostomy with loss of adult control are likely to experience problems with self-image and, in turn, sexual adjustment. Thus both society's perception of the person and the individual's concept of self can interfere with sexual health. Some common health problems

---

> **Some health problems resulting in body image changes that may raise sexual concerns**
>
> **Surgically induced**
>
> Mastectomy
> Ostomy
> Hysterectomy
> Amputation of limb or limbs
>
> **Traumatically induced**
>
> Burns
> Lacerations, scarring
> Amputations
>
> **Others**
>
> Dermatologic disorders
> Obesity
> Congenital anomalies of sexual organs (for example, absence of penis, hypospadias)
> Unusual breast size, including immaturity or hypertrophy

---

resulting in body image change are listed in the box above.

Several authorities believe that the interpersonal components of sexual problems are of primary importance. They advise that both partners be involved in the treatment of sexual problems.

■ Environmental restrictions

Environmental factors such as privacy, competing stimuli, and segregation interfere with sexual expression. Institutionalization rarely affords sufficient privacy for sexual expression. Many institutions segregate persons on the basis of sex. For whatever reason this may be done, the act of segregation may elicit a range of adaptation, including masturbation, homosexual activity, or withdrawal from human warmth.[64] Often these adaptive behaviors are punished, and those who resort to them are stigmatized. In some institutions staff members may assume an in loco parentis stance, treating even aging persons as if they required protection from their sexual desires.

■ SEXUAL CONCERNS, DIFFICULTIES, AND DYSFUNCTIONS

People have a variety of sexual problems ranging from concerns about sexual phenomena to alterations in sexual health. Each type of problem usually is the consequence of antecedents, and each requires somewhat different therapeutic approaches.

■ Sexual concerns

Sexual concerns constitute a source of worry, dissatisfaction, or discomfort but do not produce difficulty in sexual function, profound problems in the sexual relationship, or a greatly altered sexual self-concept. Sexual concerns arise because of misinformation or lack of information, conflicting values, difficulty communicating about sexual issues, and anxiety or guilt about sexual phenomena.

These concerns are usually amenable to sex education strategies, such as permission giving, provision of limited information, values clarification exercises, rehearsal of communication, validation of normalcy, and provision of anticipatory guidance.

■ Sexual difficulties

Sexual difficulties create discomfort in the sexual relationship, may occasionally interfere with sexual function, and sometimes may challenge the person's sexual self-image. Sexual difficulties include the following:

1. Inability to relax
2. Disinterest in sexual activity
3. Sexual dissatisfaction
4. Inability to please or be pleased by a partner
5. Problems in the timing of sexual activities

These difficulties are amenable to counseling approaches, including relaxation training, exploration of alternatives in the sexual repertoire, provision of specific suggestions, and training in communication skills.

■ Alterations in sexual health

Contemporary systems for classification of *sexual dysfunction* include desire phase, arousal phase, and orgasm phase dysfunctions, coital pain, and dissatisfaction with sexual frequency.[43,58] Although this schema addresses the functional dimension of sexual health, it does not address the dimensions of self-concept and relationships. The following paragraphs describe alterations in sexual function, sexual self-concept, and sexual relationships as a basis for a diagnostic taxonomy for nursing practice.

■ ALTERATIONS IN SEXUAL FUNCTION

□ Alterations in sexual desire

Alterations in sexual desire include low sexual desire and sexual aversion. Low sexual desire reflects lack of interest in sex. Low frequency of self-stimulation and activity with a partner and diminished desire for sexual activity, incidence of fantasy, erotic dreams, or seeking erotic stimulation define this alteration. Low sexual desire and aversion are part of a continuum on which aversion includes a clearly negative response to the idea of sex.

Physiologic and psychosocial factors contribute to alterations in sexual desire. Depression, severe stress, certain pharmacologic agents, low androgen levels, and certain illnesses can interfere with sexual desire. Pharmacologic agents such as narcotics, sedatives, and alcohol, centrally acting antihypertensives (such as reserpine and methyldopa), and testosterone antagonists are associated with low sexual desire.

Illness-associated malaise, thought processes, and fear and anger produced by interpersonal conflicts, as well as concerns about intimacy or sexual self-concept, can also inhibit sexual desire. Anxiety and guilt linked to childhood experiences such as sexual abuse, pressure to have sex, and repeated unpleasant experiences may also interfere with sexual desire. Common diagnoses in nursing practice include the following:

Low sexual desire related to chronic pain, medication regimen, partner's poor health and inability to have intercourse, or depression

Sexual aversion related to rape trauma[50,53]

Therapies for low sexual desire and sexual aversion relate to underlying causes when this can be determined. When low sexual desire is related to chronic pain, the strategies may include identification of positions of maximum comfort and alternative stimulation that does not intensify pain. Sexual aversion typically is treated in the context of intensive sex therapy or psychotherapy.[58]

□ Alterations in sexual arousal

Many alterations in sexual arousal exist for men and include decreased subjective arousal, difficulty attaining an erection, difficulty maintaining an erection, and decreased subjective arousal combined with difficulty in some aspect of attaining or maintaining an erection. Alterations in women's sexual arousal include decreased physiologic arousal and decreased physiologic combined with decreased subjective arousal. Diminished vasocongestion is a symptom of diminished physiologic arousal, whereas loss of erotic sensation is a symptom of diminished subjective arousal.[58]

Alterations in sexual arousal typically reflect body-mind-social interaction. Transient episodes of alterations in arousal are common. Pharmacologic agents such as certain antihypertensives, sedatives, and tranquilizers may interfere with physiologic sexual arousal in both men and women. Diseases affecting vascular function, such as diabetes, can impair vasocongestion.[49] As people age, vasocongestive responses to sexual stimuli and vaginal lubrication appear more slowly, and the response may be less intense than in younger years. Anxieties about sexual performance and fear of failure are commonly associated with alterations in sexual arousal.

Alterations in sexual arousal commonly encountered in nursing practice include the following:

Decreased vasocongestion and vaginal lubrication related to diabetic neuropathy

Decreased vaginal lubrication related to anxiety about pain with intercourse

Difficulty attaining an erection related to a medication

Difficulty maintaining an erection related to fear of failure.[50]

Strategies for treating alterations in sexual arousal include reducing anxiety about the problem and correcting or transcending the physiologic problems if possible. Anxiety can be reduced through desensitization exercises in which the person is instructed to use erotic imagery to approximate sexual situations evoking anxiety.

Structuring sexual encounters so they are not demanding is a second strategy. Exercises that emphasize pleasure rather than pressure to perform often begin by refocusing the person's attention on sensual aspects of touch without genital touching for a period of time. After the person has pleasure in sensual experiences without anxiety, sexual activity is gradually reintroduced.

Physiologic problems can sometimes be modified to restore sexual function. Drug regimens can be modified and strategies can be introduced to persons to amplify erotic sensations in parts of their bodies not affected by disease. A penile prosthesis may be implanted in men as a method of treatment for organic erectile dysfunction.

☐ Alterations in orgasm

Alterations in orgasm in men include problems with ejaculation and orgasm and with the perception of pleasure associated with orgasm. Ejaculatory problems include premature ejaculation and inhibited ejaculation. *Premature ejaculation* occurs when men ejaculate too rapidly for their own or a partner's pleasure. Often men with premature ejaculation do not perceive erotic sensations that occur before orgasm and progress rapidly from very low to very high levels of arousal. Anxiety about sex is common, and many men have learned to make their sexual encounters quick. *Inhibited ejaculation,* sometimes referred to as retarded ejaculation, implies the inability to ejaculate during sexual activity or the need for an extended period of time to ejaculate, even with adequate stimulation. Inhibited ejaculation is often associated with anger or lack of trust. Physiologic alterations and medications can interfere with ejaculation.[50,57]

Alterations in orgasm for women include *anorgasmia*, a global inability to have orgasm, and situational anorgasmia, the inability to have orgasm in certain situations. Anorgasmia with intercourse is common. Inadequate stimulation, self-observation, and fear of loss of control over sexual or aggressive impulses often produce these alterations.

Both physiologic and psychosocial mechanisms can produce orgasm phase alterations. Because a person has a physiologic problem does not justify attributing the alteration to the disease; instead, an emotional or congitive process may be involved.

Therapeutic strategies for anorgasmia include structuring situations for sexual activity that reduce anxiety. Distraction from self-observation through the use of fantasy and imagery along with self-pleasuring exercises often reduce anxiety sufficiently to enhance awareness of erotic sensation and orgasm.

Strategies for premature ejaculation include use of the start-stop techniques (p. 1235), in which stimulation is withdrawn intermittently, or the source of stimulation is stopped intermittently to increase awareness of erotic sensations and to increase tolerance of pleasure associated with arousal. Retarded ejaculation is treated with a combination of relaxation and stimulation techniques, and these are sometimes enhanced by the use of imagery.

☐ Pain with coitus

Vaginismus is a relatively rare sexual problem characterized by an involuntary, conditioned spasm of the vaginal outlet, thus causing it to shut tightly. This problem precludes sexual intercourse, but vaginismic women may be orgasmic with alternative methods of sexual stimulation.

Dyspareunia, or painful intercourse, may be attributable to a number of factors ranging from a full lower bowel to feelings of aversion toward sexual intercourse. It is sometimes felt by women with steroid alterations, for example, the postpartum mother and postmenopausal women.

■ ALTERATIONS IN SEXUAL SELF-CONCEPT

An individual's sexual self-concept can be changed dramatically because of developmental transitions or health-related events. In response to surgery or injury that produces changed body image or in response to taking on the identity of a disease, sexual self-concept may change. Moreover, embarrassment and shame associated with bodily changes can produce anxiety about sexual relationships.

Nursing diagnoses commonly associated with alteration in sexual self-concept include the following:

Altered sexual self-concept related to identification with an illness

Anxiety about sexual encounters related to changed body image (for example, after ostomy surgery)

Anxiety about sexual encounters related to feelings of inadequacy as a man or woman

Altered sexual self-concept related to a partner's lack of acceptance of change in one's body

Strategies for enhancing sexual self-concept include those directed at accepting and transcending alterations in body image, transcending the sick role, obtaining support from a partner, and enhancing perception of one's sexual self-concept as positive.

■ ALTERATIONS IN SEXUAL RELATIONSHIPS

Sexual relationships can be changed by developmental transitions and changes in health status. Value conflicts about sexual activity, difficulty communicating about sexual issues, dissatisfaction with sexual frequency, a partner's inability to provide sexual stimulation, inability to please a partner, and conflicts about the timing of sexual activity may all occur as people experience ill health.

Some examples of nursing diagnoses related to alterations in sexual relationships include the following:

Value conflicts related to using alternative forms of sexual expression required by the illness, by partner's inability to reconcile roles as caretaker/lover, by partner's lack of acceptable sexual outlet, or by partner's inability to provide sexual stimulation because of reduced mobility

Adjustment, impaired sexual related to dissatisfaction with decreased sexual frequency

Strategies for promoting healthy sexual relationships include facilitating involvement that is mutually acceptable to both partners. Communicating clearly and comfortably about concerns and problems, negotiating mutually acceptable solutions to conflicts, obtaining adequate information about the consequences of health problems for sexuality, and clarifying sexual values can enhance the quality of sexual relationships.

■ Gender disorders

Although many gender disorders exist, they are encountered less often in nursing practice than the problems discussed earlier. Recently the media have called attention to transsexualism, a gender identity problem that may be encountered in some medical-surgical services.

Transsexualism refers to the condition of people who are convinced that they are "trapped in the body of the wrong sex." These persons believe that they belong to the opposite sex and desire the body, appearance, and social status of the opposite sex. Many actually live in the role of the opposite sex before treatment. Male-to-female transsexuals are usually treated initially with hormonal therapy, and later surgical revision of the genitals is performed. The surgery involves removal of the male genitals and revision of the scrotal and neighboring tissue to resemble the female genitals. Usually the surgery is cosmetically successful, and an artificial but functional vagina can be created. These women are, of course, sterile, since they have neither ovaries nor uterus.

The female-to-male transsexual has a less cosmetically effective and functional surgical transformation. In a series of procedures, the breasts and vulva are revised and a phallus is created. Hormonal therapy is also used to effect the transformation. Often the creation of the penis requires extensive grafting and surgical revision, and the female-to-male transformation is consequently more difficult and usually less satisfactory. After the transformation these men are also sterile.

Both men and women electing transsexual surgery require considerable emotional support. They usually have careful psychologic assessments before and following the surgery. Because of their cultural conditioning, nurses sometimes find it difficult to relate appropriately to the transsexual. Often it is necessary to analyze one's attitudes and values carefully to be accepting of these patients.

Transsexualism should not be confused with *tranvestism*, the act of dressing in the clothing of the opposite sex. Additionally, transsexuals are not homosexuals.

Hermaphroditism is a congenital condition in which the reproductive structures appear ambiguous. Early life experiences seem to have profound impact on our gender

identities. It is important, therefore, that sexual assignment be correctly established early in life to prevent gender confusion later.

┌───┐
│ **Knowledge base prerequisite for sexual** │
│ **counseling** │
│ │
│ Understanding of sexual response │
│ Knowledge of the variety of sexual behaviors that │
│ exist in our society and their prevalence │
│ Understanding of the types of sexual dysfunctions │
│ Awareness of the relationship between age, life │
│ events, pathologic conditions, behavioral prob- │
│ lems, pharmaceutic agents, and sexual function │
└───┘

■ NURSING PRACTICE

■ Prerequisites for intervention

Three prerequisites are important before practitioners can help individuals with their sexual problems:

1. A knowledge base
2. Awareness of own value system
3. Ability to communicate genuinely and therapeutically with patients

■ KNOWLEDGE BASE

The knowledge base that is required is listed in the box above. Without such knowledge the nurse has no basis for discriminating between normal and abnormal responses or the interpretation of patient's concerns and thus no basis for education or counseling.

■ AWARENESS OF OWN VALUE SYSTEM

In addition to an adequate knowledge base, an awareness of one's own value system, including the biases and beliefs about appropriate and inappropriate sexual behavior, is also important. Unless professionals can accept their own sexuality and are comfortable with their own behavior, it is difficult to convey comfort to others. Self-acceptance is seen as prerequisite to the development of a nonjudgmental and tolerant approach. Just as individuals have belief systems related to sexual phenomena, so do professionals. This does not imply that the sex educators or counselors must condone every variety of sexual activity. Rather, it is essential that they be aware of their own feelings and values and attempt to keep them in perspective by acknowledging them. This assists them in maintaining a supportive climate that encourages sharing of feeling by patients and simultaneously permits professionals to acknowledge the validity of their own beliefs.

Furthermore, there are some issues about which the professional has such strong beliefs that these values would interfere with effective intervention. An example encountered in practice is the health professional whose basic conviction is that homosexuality is an illness or deviation rather than a variation in sexual expression or orientation. No matter how extensive the professional's training, knowledge base, and therapy skills, such a strong basic belief is likely to interfere greatly with the ability to relate objectively to a homosexual's sexual problems. Often professionals need to acknowledge their inability to deal with sexual problems because of their own value systems. Topics likely to elicit biases among health professionals include abortion, alternative life-styles, and sexual variations.

THERAPEUTIC COMMUNICATION

Finally, the professional needs to be able to communicate genuinely and therapeutically with patients. Often this involves using the person's own language, which may be different from that of the health professional. Without the ability to interact accurately and empathetically with individuals, the most sophisticated knowledge base and objective attitudes are of little benefit.

Nurses frequently encounter behavioral problems that involve the individual's sexuality. One common problem is the patient who acts out sexually, for example, by making inappropriate sexual gestures, using explicit sexual language, or exposing the sexual organs. Two general principles are helpful in coping with such a situation:

1. Analyze what meaning this behavior might have for the patient.
2. Assert the right as a human being to establish limits that protect the nurse's integrity.

In responding to a patient who has exhibited sexual behavior that is deemed inappropriate, one can analyze why the behavior occurs and share this observation with the patient. Is the patient attempting to gain control in a situation in which he or she has little or no control? Is the patient trying to obtain validation of his masculinity or her feminity? Is the patient unaware that the behavior has sexual overtones or is making the nurse uncomfortable?

Nurses have the right to establish limits with patients to protect their own integrity. Violation of certain body boundaries, for example, touching the breasts or buttocks of the nurse or exposing one's genitals, is not behavior that nurses must tolerate to be "accepting of patients." Nurses' responses, however, can address three important points:

1. The inferred meaning of the behavior can be shared—"I know you feel helpless right now. . ."
2. The boundary can be established—"That's not acceptable behavior."
3. The patient's sexuality can be validated—"You're a good looking guy, but that's just not acceptable behavior."

Some patients cannot respond appropriately to these strategies, and in some instances the nurse may need to believe that not working with this patient is permissible.

Prevention of sexual problems

Nurses may prevent sexual problems among patient populations through three strategies: education of patient groups likely to have sexual concerns, provision of anticipatory guidance throughout the life cycle, and promotion of a milieu conducive to sexual health.

EDUCATION OF PATIENT POPULATIONS

Education of patient populations implies more than mere dissemination of information. Just as nurses are being educated to provide sex education, patients may also need assistance in exploring the attitudes and values that shape their sexual behavior and in developing the ability to communicate comfortably about sexual phenomena. Thus providing accurate knowledge about sex and sexuality is not synonymous with education for a healthy sexuality.

ANTICIPATORY GUIDANCE

Nurses are often in strategic positions to provide anticipatory guidance at sensitive points in the life cycle. Adolescence and middle age are two life periods during which anxiety about sexuality is likely to surface. By informing individuals about the usual changes experienced at these points (for example, nocturnal emissions or concerns about masturbation in adolescents or worry about effects of menopause on the ability to function sexually among middle-aged persons), nurses can assist individuals to cope realistically with major changes in their bodies. Adults with young children can also benefit from anticipatory guidance regarding their children's sexuality.

PROMOTION OF A MILIEU CONDUCIVE TO SEXUAL HEALTH

Some approaches useful in developing a milieu conducive to sexual health include minimizing guilt felt in conjunction with sexual thoughts, feelings, and behavior. This may be accomplished by assisting persons in examining objectively the consequences of their activities within a reality-oriented framework. Reduction of performance anxiety (for example, concern about how well one is able to function) can be facilitated by helping individuals to understand the relationship between being attentive to their own performance at the expense of losing touch with their sexual feelings. "Spectatoring" refers to the habit of watching oneself or a partner perform. Just as in athletics, one cannot be both spectator and a performer without minimizing the effectiveness of the performance.

Often individuals need to be advised to modify their environments to reduce competing stimuli. Use of anxiety-provoking settings or those settings prone to interruption can help establish dysfunctional patterns. (The relationship between anxiety and orgasmic dysfunction and premature ejaculation has been well established.)

Finally, maintenance of good general health facilitates optimum sexual functioning. Fatigue, pain, and malaise are stimuli that compete with sexual pleasure.

■ Assessment

■ THE SEXUAL HISTORY

Many health care providers may not be experienced in eliciting a sexual history and at first may be uneasy. No doubt this uneasiness is conditioned by social prohibitions about discussing intimate matters such as sexual experiences or behavior. However, health professionals are expected to be informed, willing to discuss sexual matters openly with patients, and prepared to educate and counsel them appropriately. Nurses who are hesitant to deal with sexual matters with patients are helped by working through their own feelings about sex and sexual matters. Seeking counsel from other nurses or health professionals who are comfortable with the topic is often helpful. Some nurses may find it helpful to attend a workshop on sexuality for nurses.

Although there is no single approach to taking a sexual history, application of certain principles facilitates both the patient's and the nurse's comfort. Absolute requirements for history taking include the following:

1. Provision of privacy, such as in a closed room
2. An atmosphere of trust between patient and nurse, such as assurance of confidentiality for the patient
3. Comfort on the part of nurses with their own sexuality

Some principles for promoting patient-nurse comfort are listed in the box above, right. The sexual history itself may be therapeutic. Within the context of obtaining the data, the nurse can provide permission for the patient to discuss concerns, provide limited information or suggestions, or validate the normalcy and acceptability of the patient's concerns and practices.

It may be necessary for both patient and nurse to define their terms. Street language may be unfamiliar to the nurse, and highly technical language may be confusing to the patient. The nurse may need to become familiar with some commonly used street language to be sure of what the patient is reporting.

The technique of moving from less sensitive to more sensitive areas paves the way for both the patient and nurse. For example, the nurse may explore a woman's sexual role before discussing her ability to have orgasm, her menstrual history before her experience with sexual variations, and her personal experiences with sex education before her actual sexual experiences. In all of these situations, the decision to pursue the topics depends on the cues presented by the patient that sexual concerns are present.

Principles that facilitate obtaining a sexual history

Action	Effect
1. Obtain sexual history early in nurse-patient relationship	Legitimizes sexuality as part of health; Provides permission for patient to discuss sexual concerns
2. Avoid overreaction or underreaction to patient's comments	Facilitates truthful data gathering
3. Use language patient understands	Facilitates accurate data gathering
4. Move from less sensitive to more sensitive areas	Facilitates patient-nurse comfort
5. Terminate sexual history by inquiring if patient has additional questions or concerns	Conveys a willingness by nurse to further explore sexual matters

■ BRIEF SEXUAL ASSESSMENT

A brief assessment can be incorporated in the nursing history by means of three questions. (See the box below.) The first of these questions deals with the person's role, the next with the affective-cognitive elements of sexuality, and the last with biologic aspects of sexual function. The questions may be modified to deal with illness, hospitalization, life events, or any other relevant entity that may influence or interfere with sexual health.

The questions may also be adapted to elicit the patient's expectations of changes resulting from procedures or hospitalization that he or she is about to experience. These

Brief sexual history

1. Has your (illness, pregnancy, or hospitalization) interfered with your being a (husband, wife, father, mother)?
2. Has your (abortion, heart attack, etc.) changed the way you see yourself as a (woman, man)?
3. Has your (colostomy, hysterectomy, etc.) changed your ability to function sexually (or your sex life)?

brief items invite the patient to explore sexual concerns. Often it is unnecessary for the nurse to ask the second and third questions, since many patients proceed to state their concerns about masculinity, femininity, and sexual functioning without further prompting.

■ Promotion of sexual health

■ PRINCIPLES FOR PROMOTING SEXUAL HEALTH

Mims[33] cites some basic principles involved in the promotion of sexual health. The first of these principles acknowledges that there is no single set of appropriate sexual values in our society. Rather, the professional needs to accept that major conflicts of values exist. A second principle is that education (provision of accurate and adequate information) is more helpful than indoctrination. Although it is often tempting to impose one's own solutions or values on others, growth of the individual is more likely to be fostered by guidance rather than indoctrination. Finally, it is suggested that individuals be assisted in making their own informed choices rather than conforming to guidelines established by a professional or an agency. It is the individual, and not the health professional, who will have to cope with the consequences of the individual's choice.

■ LEVELS OF INTERVENTION

Annon[53] presents an extremely useful distinction between the various levels of intervention possible for persons with sexual concerns or problems. He terms these levels permission, limited information, specific suggestions, and intensive therapy. These are listed in order of sophistication, with permission requiring the most basic preparation and intensive therapy requiring specific educational preparation in sex therapy techniques. Annon's contention is that sexual problems may be resolved on a variety of levels and do not always require counseling or intensive therapy.

□ Permission

Often individuals merely want to know that they are normal, acceptable, and not "perverted." They seek out the health professional for validation of their sexual normalcy. This type of intervention requires minimal preparation on the part of the professional. Permission may be applied to thoughts, fantasies, dreams, and feelings, as well as to overt sexual behaviors. At times nurses will be asked to provide individuals with permission not to engage in certain sexual behaviors if this is their choice. This may relieve individuals from feeling pressured to conform to someone else's standards for sexual behavior that are not necessarily their own.

People with disabling diseases that interfere with their usual forms of sexual expression may seek permission to discuss alternative approaches to sexual pleasure. For example, cord-injured persons may welcome the permission

from staff members to discuss alternatives to penis-vagina intercourse. Women who do not experience orgasm with every act of intercourse may be seeking permission not to do so, even though some of their friends insist that "normal women do." A common concern among young married couples is the normalcy of oral-genital sex. Often these couples merely seek reassurance that this variation is not perverted or, on the contrary, that is it not mandatory to engage in this practice unless both partners are comfortable with it.

□ Limited information

The next level of intervention can also be therapeutic and preventive. It involves providing information to individuals that is directly relevant to their particular problems or concerns. Some common areas of sexual concern that may require only limited information include worry about breast and genital shape, configuration, and size; masturbation; sexual intercourse during menstruation; and oral-genital sex. A woman who is about to have a hysterectomy is often concerned that she will no longer be able to have intercourse or that she will have no more sexual desire. Informing the woman in advance of the surgery that this is not true may remove unnecessary barriers from the resumption of sexual activity. Similar information would be helpful to a man about to undergo a prostatectomy. Even though the man having a transurethral resection is likely to have retrograde ejaculation, he may still have an erection and enjoy intercourse. Having this information before surgery may avert later sexual problems.

□ Specific suggestions

Before giving individuals specific suggestions regarding direct attempts to help change their behavior and reach a designated goal, it is essential to obtain a detailed sexual history including the following:
1. Description of the problem; its onset and course
2. The person's ideas about the cause of the problem and why it persists
3. Past attempts at treatment and their effectiveness
4. The patient's current goal for treatment

Some specific suggestions may relate to the conditions conducive to optimum sexual functioning, specific approaches to use given certain illnesses or surgeries, and directives for coping with some sexual dysfunctions. One specific suggestion often incorporated in sexual counseling is that a couple having difficulties with intercourse abstain from it for a specified period. This admonition is designed to reduce the "pressure to perform" perceived by a member of the dysfunctional couple.

Specific suggestions can be given to *cord-injured persons,* including positions most likely to be comfortable, care of the indwelling catheter before and during intercourse, and techniques available to stimulate the noninjured partner. Use of imagery (fantasy) can also be incorporated as a specific suggestion.

Ostomy patients often have concerns about accidents involving their appliances during intercourse. Specific suggestions might include emptying the appliance before initiating sexual activity, employing cosmetic covers for the stoma bag, or avoiding excess pressure over the stoma site until the ostomy incision is well healed.

Cardiac patients can be counseled to minimize their cardiac work load during sexual activity by avoiding intercourse in very hot or very cold rooms and within 3 hours of eating a big meal or drinking alcoholic beverages and by allowing plenty of time for rest after intercourse. Patients who have had myocardial infarctions are counseled to consult a nurse practitioner or physician if they have chest pain or palpitations during or after intercourse or if they feel extremely tired afterward.

Nurses can offer some rather simple directives for coping with specific sexual dysfunctions. The man whose problem is premature ejaculation can be taught to use the squeeze technique or the partner may learn to apply it. The squeeze technique consists of applying pressure over the coronal ridge of the glans, exerting enough pressure for 3 to 4 seconds to relieve the feeling of ejaculatory inevitability. Women who have inadequate lubrication and have painful intercourse as a consequence of steroid starvation during the postpartum period or menopause may benefit from the use of a water-soluble lubricant such as K-Y jelly.

☐ Intensive sexual therapy

The intensive sexual therapy approach combines techniques and concepts of psychotherapy with special approaches to intervention with individuals or couples having sexual problems. Usually the problems involved are one or more of the sexual dysfunctions discussed earlier. These forms of therapy usually require intensive preparation beyond that provided in most schools of nursing. However, an awareness of the sexual dysfunctions enables nurses to refer persons with complex problems to trained therapists.

■ SUMMARY

1. Human sexuality is a complex set of interrelating biologic and psychosocial variables that begin at conception and continue through life; components include biologic (sexual function or expression), psychologic (gender identity, thoughts, and feelings), and social factors (such as sanctioned role and mores and folkways regulating sexual expression).
2. The physiologic phases of human sexual response may be divided into four categories (excitement, plateau, orgasm, resolution) or three categories (desire, excitement, orgasm).
3. The excitement and plateau phases are characterized by vasocongestion of pelvic blood vessels, leading to swelling of genitalia and by vaginal lubrication, the orgasm phase by myotonia (involuntary muscle contractions in the pelvic organs and other parts of the body), and the resolution phase by muscle relaxation and return of normal blood flow.
4. Although generally a decline in overall interest and sexual activity is seen with age, many persons continue with an active sexual life into old age; the level of activity appears related to the extent of sexual activity during youth.
5. Sexual expression varies and includes heterosexuality, homosexuality, bisexuality, transvestism, incest, zoophilia, fetishism, voyeurism, exhibitionism, sadism, and masochism; social norms influence expected sexual expressions.
6. Illness may affect sexuality and sexual function through changes in body structure, changes in body functions, effects of pharmacologic agents, body image changes, or environmental restrictions (privacy, competing stimuli, partner segregation).
7. Sexual concerns and difficulties generally do not produce profound problems in sexual response although they may temporarily interfere with sexual functioning; sexual concerns and difficulties are usually amenable to sex education and counseling.
8. Alterations in sexual health include alterations in sexual function (desire, arousal, orgasm), in sexual self-concept, and in sexual relationships.
9. Alterations in sexual desire include low sexual desire and sexual aversion. Therapy is directed toward underlying causes; intensive sex therapy or psychotherapy is often required for sexual aversion.
10. Alterations in sexual arousal reflect body-mind-social interaction and may result from drugs, diseases affecting vascular function, age, and anxiety about sexual performance. Transient episodes of alteration in arousal are common. Therapies include anxiety-reducing aproaches and exercises that emphasize pleasure rather than pressure to perform.
11. Alterations in orgasm include ejaculatory problems in men and anorgasmia in women; both physiologic and pyschologic mechanisms can produce orgasm phase alterations. Therapies include anxiety-reducing strategies for anorgasmia and relaxation-stimulation techniques for ejaculatory problems.
12. Alterations in sexual self-concept may result from disease or injury. Therapies include strategies toward accepting and transcending body image changes, transcending the sick role, obtaining partner support, and enhancing a positive self-concept.
13. Alterations in sexual relationships during illness result from value conflicts about sexual activity, problems with communication, or difficulties in sexual functioning. Therapies include promoting communication and providing education to resolve conflicts and promote sexuality.
14. Nursing interventions for persons with sexual concerns, sexual difficulties, and alterations in sexual response include awareness of the nurse's own value system, therapeutic communication, prevention of sexual problems through education, anticipatory guidance, and promotion of a milieu conducive to sexual health.
15. Levels of intervention for persons with sexual problems include giving permission for engaging or not

---

Putting knowledge to practice

- What instances in your own life shaped some of your feelings about yourself as female or male?
- What nursing behaviors would increase your comfort in describing your own sexual history?
- Examine your beliefs about homosexuality. In what ways might your beliefs help or hinder working with homosexual patients who have sexual concerns?
- Examine the list of diseases in Table 34-3 and the list of medications in Table 33-4. Have any of these conditions existed for patients for whom you have provided care recently? How might their sexual response have been affected? Did they express any concerns about their sexuality or sexual response? Discuss the nursing care that could have been offered.

---

engaging in sexual behaviors (inner or overt), providing limited information directly related to the particular problems or concerns, giving specific suggestions, or providing intensive sexual therapy. The type of intervention depends on the level of expertise of the provider.

REFERENCES AND SELECTED READINGS
Contemporary

1. *Allen, M: A holistic view of sexuality and the aged, Holistic Nurs Pract 1(4):76-83, 1987.
2. *Assey, JL, and Herbert, JM: Who is the seductive patient? Am J Nurs 83:530-532, 1983.
3. *Bachers, E: Sexual dysfunction after treatment for genitourinary cancers, Sem Oncol Nurs 1(1):18-24, 1985.
4. *Baggs, J, and others: Sexual counseling of women with coronary heart disease, Heart Lung 16:154-159, 1987.
5. Bell, A, Weinberg, M, and Keifer-Hammersmith, S: Sexual preference: its development in men and women, Bloomington, 1981, Indiana University Press.
6. Bernhard, L: Sexuality expectations and outcomes in women having hysterectomies, Chart 83(10):11-15, 1986.
7. *Bernhard, L, and Dan, A: Redefining sexuality from women's own experiences, Nurs Clin North Am 21:125-136, 1986.
8. *Boyer, G, and Boyer, J: Sexuality and aging, Nurs Clin North Am 17:421-427, 1982.
9. Brink, P: Cultural aspects of sexuality, Holistic Nurs Pract 1(4):12-20, 1987.
10. *Byers, JP: Sexuality and the elderly, Geriatr Nurs 4:293-297, 1983.
11. *Campbell, M: Sexual dysfunction in the COPD patient, DCCN 6(2):70-74, 1987.
12. *Cohen, J: Sexual counseling of the patient following myocardial infarction, Crit Care Nurse 6(6):18-29, 1986.
13. *Cooley, M, and others: Sexual and reproductive issues for women with Hodgkin's disease: overview of issues, CA Nurs 9:188-193, 1986.
14. Donlou, J, and others: Psychosocial aspects of AIDS and AIDS related complex: a pilot study, J Psychosocial Oncol 3(2):39-55, 1985.
15. *Driver, JD: Elders and sexuality, J Nurs Care 15(2):8-11, 1981.
16. Dunn, M: Sexual questions and comments on a spinal cord injury service, Sexuality and Disability 6:126-134, 1983.
17. *Fischman, S, and others: Changes in sexual relationships in postpartum couples, JOGNN 15(1):58-63, 1986.
18. *Frank-Strombert, M: Sexuality and the elderly cancer patient, Sem Oncol Nurs 1(1):49-55, 1985.
19. Friend, R: Sexual identity and human diversity: implications for nursing practice, Holistic Nurs Pract 1(4):21-41, 1987.
20. *Fuentes, RJ, and others: Sexual side effects: what to tell your patients, what not to say . . . commonly prescribed drugs, RN 46(2):34-41, 1983.
21. *Grunbert, K: Sexual rehabilitation of the cancer patient undergoing ostomy surgery, J Enterost Ther 13:148-152, 1986.
22. Halstead, L, and others: Disability SARs and the small group experience: a conceptual framework, Sexuality and Disability 6:183-196, 1983.
23. *Heinrich, K: Effective response to sexual harrasment, Nurs Outl 35(2):70-72, 1987.
24. *Hogan, RM: Human sexuality: a nursing perspective, ed 2, New York, 1984, Appleton-Century-Crofts.
25. *Hogan, RM: Influences of culture on sexuality, Nurs Clin North Am 17:365-376, 1982.
26. *Johnson, CD, and others: Alcohol and sex: alcohol induced problems of sexual function, Heart Lung 12(1):93-97, 1983.
27. *Kus, R: Sex, AIDS, and gay American men, Holistic Nurs Pract 1(4):42-51, 1987.
28. Lion, E: Human sexuality in nursing process, New York, 1982, John Wiley & Sons, Inc.
29. *Lamb, M: Sexual dysfunction in the gynecologic oncology patient, Sem Oncol Nurs 1(1):9-17, 1985.
30. *MacElveen-Hoehn, P: Understanding sexuality in progressive cancer, Sem Oncol Nurs 1(1):56-62, 1985.
31. *Marks, RG: Sexual side effects: how drugs can change fertility, RN 46(3):61-63, 1983.
32. *Mims, FH: Sexual stress: coping and adaptation, Nurs Clin North Am 17:395-405, 1982.

---

*References preceded by an asterisk are particularly well suited for student reading.

33. Mims, FJ, and Swensen, M: Sexuality: a nursing perspective, New York, 1980, McGraw-Hill Book Co.

34. Moses, A, and Hawkins, R: Counseling lesbian women and gay men: a life issues approach, St. Louis, 1982, The CV Mosby Co.

35. *Papadoupolous, C, and others: Sexual activity after coronary bypass surgery, Chest 90:681-685, 1986.

36. Paul, W, and others: Homosexuality: social, psychological and biological issues, Beverly Hills, Calif, 1982, Sage Publications.

37. *Persaud, D: Assessing sexual functions of the adult with traumatic quadriplegia, J Neurosurg Nurs 18(1):11-12, 1986.

38. *Price, J: Promoting sexual wellness in head-injured patients, Rehabil Nurs 10(6):12-13, 1985.

39. *Roberts, N: Advising patients on sex after surgery, AORN J 32:55-61, 1980.

40. Savage, JS: Effect of crisis on female sexual identity, Issues Health Care Women 3:151-160, 1981.

41. *Schain, W: Breast cancer surgeries and psychosexual sequelae: implications for remediation, Sem Oncol Nurs 1:200-205, 1985.

42. *Sex and aging: a game people play, Geriatr Nurs 3:263-264, 1982.

43. Shover, L, and others: Multiaxial problem-oriented systems for sexual dysfunctions, Arch Gen Psychiatry 39:614-619, 1982.

44. Spengler, A: Radical prostatectomy and sexuality, Sexuality and Disability 6:155-166, 1983.

45. Spennrath, S: Understanding the sexual needs of the elder patient, Canad Nurs 78:25-29, 1982.

46. Szasz, G: Sexual incidents in an extended care unit for aged men, J Am Geriatr Soc 31:407-411, 1983.

47. Valentich, M, and others: Facilitating the sexual integration of the head-injured person in the community, Sexuality and Disability 7:28-42, 1984.

48. Waterhouse, J, and others: Development of the sexual adjustment questionnaire: impact of cancer and surgery, Oncol Nurs Forum 13(3):53-59, 1986.

49. Woods, JS: Drug effects on human sexual behavior. In Woods, NF: Human sexuality in health and illness, ed 3, St. Louis, 1984, The CV Mosby Co.

50. *Woods, NF: Human sexuality in health and illness, ed 3, St. Louis, 1984, The CV Mosby Co.

51. *Woods, N: Toward a holistic perspective of human sexuality: alterations in sexual health and nursing diagnoses, Holistic Nurs Pract 1(4):1-11, 1987.

52. Zalar, MK: Role preparation for nurses in human sexual functioning, Nurs Clin North Am 17:351-363, 1982.

Classic

53. Annon, J: The behavioral treatment of sexual problems, Honolulu, 1974, Enabling Systems, Inc.

54. Bell, A, and Weinbereg, M: Homosexualities, New York, 1978, Simon & Schuster, Inc.

55. Comfort, A: The normal in sexual behavior: an ethnological point of view, J Sex Ed Ther 2:1-7, 1975.

56. Hellerstein, H, and Friedman, FH: Sexual activity and the postcoronary patient, Arch Intern Med 125:987-999, 1970.

57. Kaplan, HS: Disorders of sexual desire and other new concepts and techniques in sex therapy, New York, 1979, Simon & Schuster, Inc.

58. Kaplan, HS: The new sex therapy, New York, 1974, Brunner/Mazel, Inc.

59. Kinsey, AC, Pomeroy, WB, and Martin, CW: Sexual behavior in the human male, Philadelphia, 1948, WB Saunders Co.

60. Kinsey, AC, and others: Sexual behavior in the human female, Philadelphia, 1953, WB Saunders Co.

61. Larson, J: Heart rate and blood pressure responses of coronary artery disease patients during sexual activity and a two-flight stair climbing test, Master's thesis, Seattle, 1978, University of Washington.

62. Masters, W, and Johnson, V: Homosexuality in perspective, Boston, 1979, Little, Brown & Co.

63. Masters, W, and Johnson, V: Human sexual response, Boston, 1966, Little, Brown & Co.

64. Masters, W, and Johnson, V: Human sexual inadequacy, Boston, 1970, Little, Brown & Co.

65. Money, J, and Ehrhardt, A: Man and woman, boy and girl, Baltimore, 1972, The Johns Hopkins University Press.

66. Rubin, A, and Babbott, D: Impotence and diabetes mellitus, JAMA 168:498-500, 1958.

67. Woods, NF, and Earp, JA: Women with cured breast cancer: a description of women's experiences four years after mastectomy, Nurs Res 27:279-285, 1978.

68. World Health Organization: Education and treatment in human sexuality: the training of health professionals, Tech Rep Series, No 572, Geneva, 1975, The Organization.

34

The Patient with Reproductive Problems

BARBARA C. LONG and GREER GLAZER

CHAPTER OBJECTIVES

After studying this chapter, the student should be able to:

- Describe measures for prevention of genital infections and early detection of cancer.
- Identify health teaching regarding menstruation and menopause.
- Describe methods and effects of sterilization, and assessment methods and counseling for infertility.
- Describe the types and effects of inflammatory and structural disorders of the reproductive tract in females and males.
- Identify the incidence and different sites of cancer of the reproductive tract in females and males.
- Describe nursing care for persons experiencing surgery of the reproductive tract.

Professionals and lay people have become more enlightened about prevention of problems of the reproductive system. This increased awareness has led many persons to initiate requests for information about or treatment of reproductive system problems. Although men and women are better informed today about matters relating to reproductive health, many neglect preventive measures and ignore signs or symptoms of illness because of embarrassment and the special significance that they attach to the reproductive organs.

In spite of advances in medicine, science, and technology, diseases and disorders of the genital system continue to threaten the lives and the physical and emotional health of men and women, sometimes needlessly. Many of these problems are preventable; many of them can be treated and cured.

■ ANATOMY AND PHYSIOLOGY

■ Female genital system

■ EXTERNAL STRUCTURES

The external genitalia, or vulva, of the female consist primarily of the labia majora, labia minora, and clitoris (Fig. 34-1). Two glands are located in this area: Skene's glands, opening into the urethral orifice, and Bartholin's glands, situated at each side of the vaginal opening near the base of the labia. These glands are common sites of infection.

■ INTERNAL ORGANS

The female internal reproductive organs, consisting of the vagina, uterus, fallopian tubes, and ovaries, are shown in Fig. 34-1. These organs are located within the cavity of the true pelvis unless their size is increased by disease or pregnancy.

□ Vagina

The vagina leads from the external structures to the uterus. The length of the vaginal canal varies, and the posterior wall is longer than the anterior wall. The uterine cervix protrudes into the upper vagina, creating recesses (fornices) around the margins of the cervix.

The vagina is lined with pink mucous membrane arranged in folds called rugae. Physiologic events such as pregnancy and pathologic conditions such as infections often alter the color of the vaginal mucosa because of congestion with blood. The membrane is lubricated by vaginal secretions that are normally acid during the years of ovarian function; neutral or alkaline secretions are normally found in postmenopausal women. An alkaline medium promotes growth of bacteria.

□ Uterus

The uterus consists of three portions: the fundus (upper crest), the main body (corpus), and the neck (cervix). In adult females the position of the uterus may vary. It is usually anteverted (tipped forward) and slightly anteflexed (bent forward at an angle), but it may also be retroverted, retroflexed, or in midposition. During menopause the uterus decreases in size.

The uterus has three functional layers: parametrium or outer layer, myometrium or middle muscular layer, and endometrium or mucous membrane lining. The outer surface of the uterus is covered by the peritoneum. Reflection of the peritoneum posteriorly between the uterus and rectum creates a space known as the cul-de-sac of Douglas. This space is a common entry site for endoscopy or for surgical drainage of the peritoneal cavity.

□ Ovaries

The ovaries are endocrine glands as well as reproductive organs. Their functions are to store follicles, to produce mature ova, and to produce and secrete estrogen, progesterone, and androgens. Ovarian functions are readily disturbed by acute and chronic diseases. The functions can also be altered or interrupted by surgery, radiation, and the ingestion of drugs such as oral contraceptives. After menopause the ovaries undergo rapid regressive changes and decrease in size.

■ ENDOCRINE FUNCTIONS

The major hormones produced by the ovaries are estrogen and progesterone. *Estrogen* is the hormone responsible for the development of secondary sex characteristics at the time of puberty. After puberty the primary function of estrogen is to cause development of the endometrium in preparation for implantation of a fertilized ovum. Estrogen causes the retention of calcium and phosphorus and thus promotes bone growth. After menopause the decline in estrogen levels may account for some of the symptoms that sometimes occur, such as hot flashes, osteoporosis (loss of calcium from bone), and vaginal atrophy. *Progesterone* enhances the action of estrogen on the endometrium. It also prevents muscular contractions of the myometrium as an aid for maintaining pregnancy should the ovum become implanted.

Secretion of ovarian hormones is cyclic, with each cycle requiring an average of 28 days. Unless stimulated by pituitary hormones, however, the ovaries do not fulfill their hormone-secreting and ovum-producing functions.

The phases of the menstrual cycle are illustrated in Fig. 34-2 and described in the box on p. 1241. The secretory (luteal) phase is the least variable part of the menstrual cycle. Irregular menstrual cycles are most frequently related to longer or shorter menstrual or proliferative (follicular) phases.

On the day of ovulation, about 25% of women experience pain in the lower abdomen on the side of ovulation. This pain (mittelschmerz) is probably a result of peritoneal irritation from follicular fluid or blood released from the ovary with the ovum. This sign rarely occurs with every cycle and is therefore an unreliable indicator of ovulation. If the pain occurs on the right side and is severe, it may be mistaken for appendicitis.

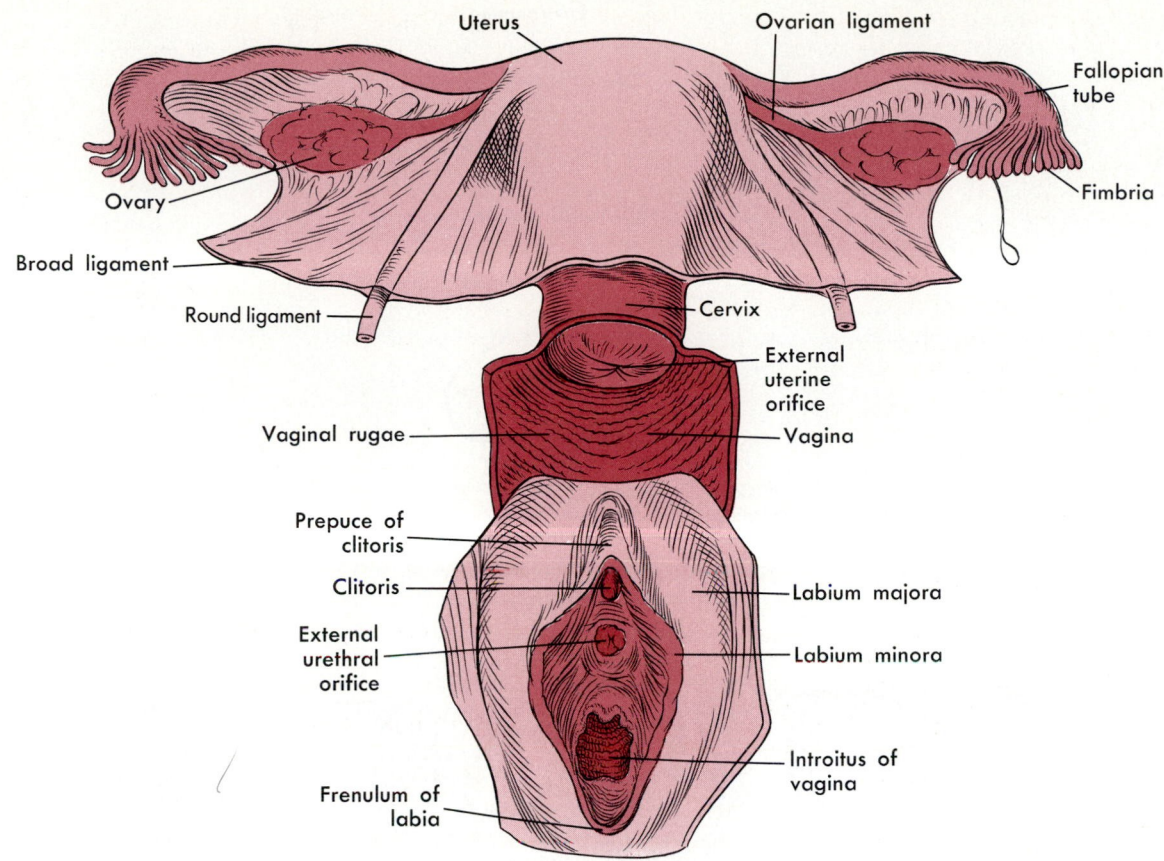

Fig. 34-1 Female internal organs of reproduction. Major ligaments are shown.

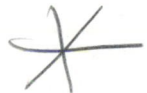

Menstrual cycle

Menstrual phase (menstruation): Day 1 to day 4
  Estrogen and progesterone withdrawn before onset of menstrual flow
  Shedding of endometrial lining
Proliferative (follicular) phase: Day 5 to day 14
  Regrowth of endometrial tissue
  Secretion of follicle-stimulating hormone (FSH) by the pituitary gland
  Development in ovary of a mature graafian follicle containing a mature ovum
  Secretion of increasing amounts of *estrogen* by graafian follicle
  Suppression of FSH when estrogen level becomes high, leading to secretion of luteinizing hormone (LH) by pituitary
    gland
Secretory (luteal) phase: Day 15 to days 25 to 28
  Rupture of graafian follicle releasing ovum (ovulation) starts the secretory phase
  Movement of ovum through fallopian tube to uterus
  Formation of corpus luteum at site of ruptured graafian follicle
  Production of *progesterone* by corpus luteum
  Stimulation by progesterone of endometrial cell growth
  Significant decrease in progesterone level if implantation does not occur; menstrual phase then begins again

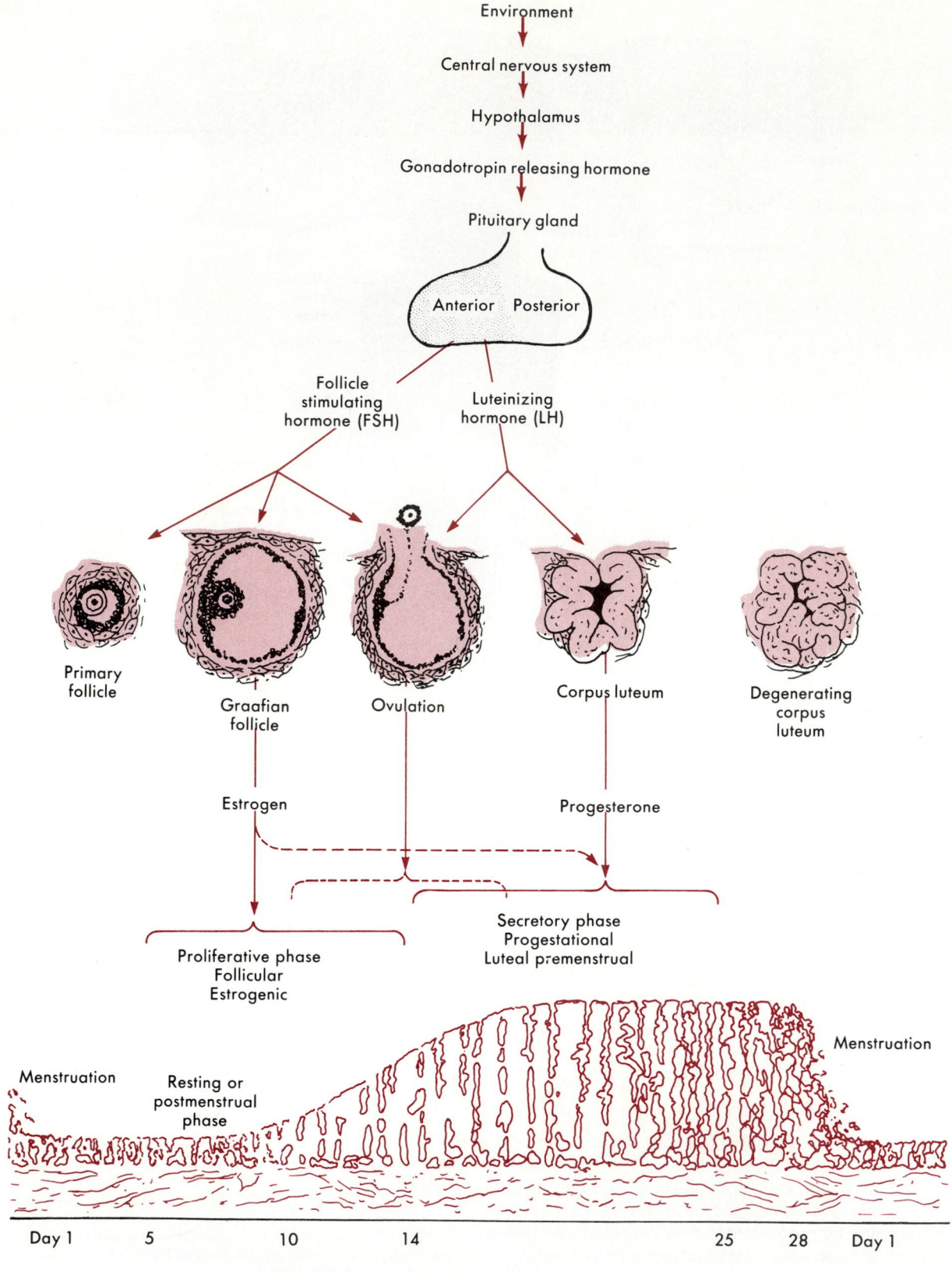

Environment

Central nervous system

Hypothalamus

Gonadotropin releasing hormone

Pituitary gland

Anterior   Posterior

Follicle stimulating hormone (FSH)

Luteinizing hormone (LH)

Primary follicle

Graafian follicle

Ovulation

Corpus luteum

Degenerating corpus luteum

Estrogen

Progesterone

Proliferative phase
Follicular
Estrogenic

Secretory phase
Progestational
Luteal premenstrual

Menstruation

Resting or postmenstrual phase

Menstruation

Day 1   5   10   14   25   28   Day 1

Fig. 34-2   Hormone control of menstrual cycle.

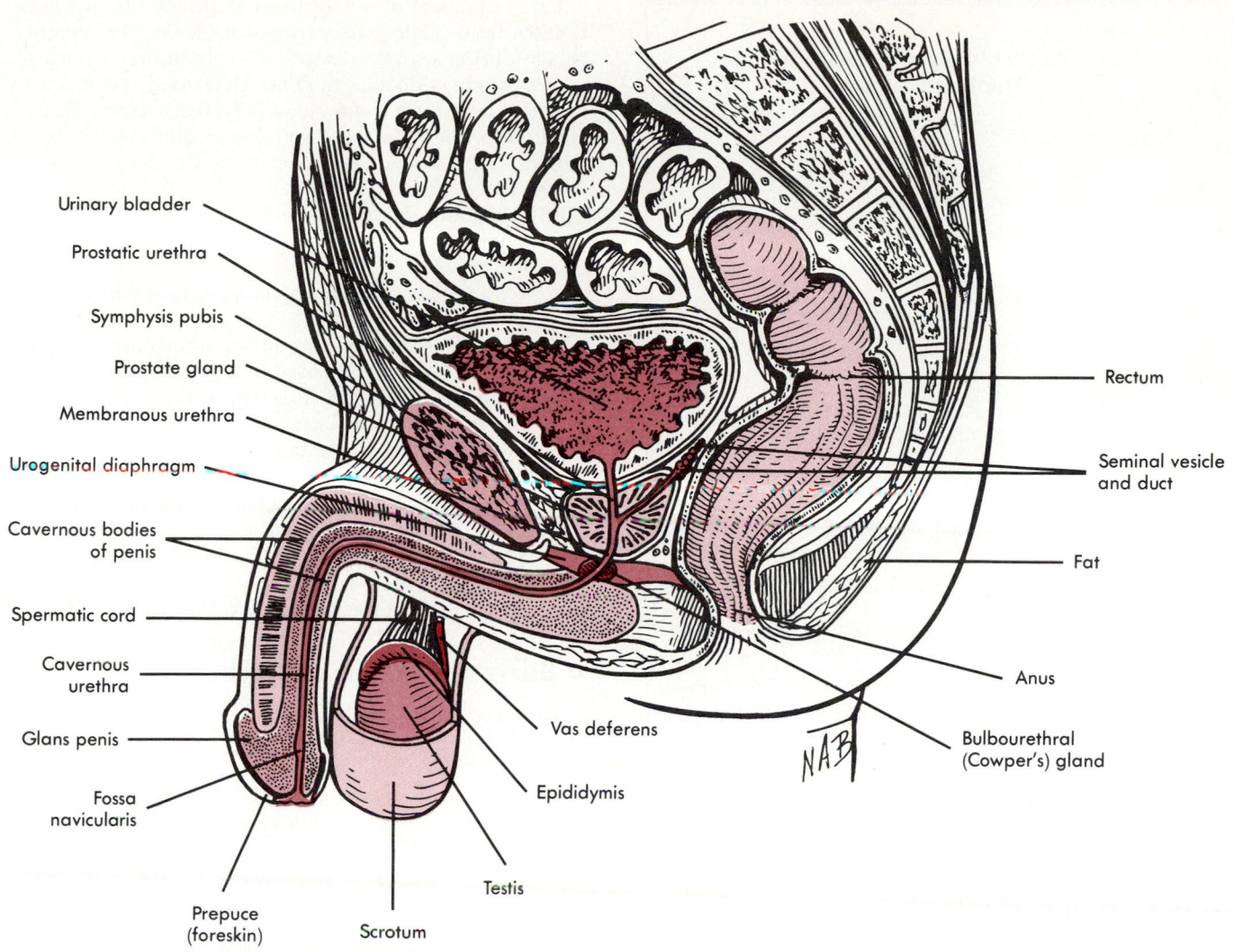

Urinary bladder

Prostatic urethra

Symphysis pubis

Prostate gland

Membranous urethra

Urogenital diaphragm

Cavernous bodies
of penis

Spermatic cord

Cavernous
urethra

Glans penis

Fossa
navicularis

Prepuce
(foreskin)

Scrotum

Testis

Epididymis

Vas deferens

Rectum

Seminal vesicle
and duct

Fat

Anus

Bulbourethral
(Cowper's) gland

Fig. 34-3   Male organs of reproduction.

■ Male genital system

The male reproductive organs and associated structures are shown in Fig. 34-3. The male reproductive organs produce sperm, suspend the sperm in a liquid, and deliver the sperm into the vagina to fertilize an ovum. Another important function is secretion of male hormones, the androgens. Sperm are produced in the testes and are conveyed through the vas (ductus) deferens to the urethra. Semen consists of sperm with fluids from the seminal vesicles and the prostate gland. The prostate gland is important clinically because of its affinity for congestive, inflammatory, hyperplastic, and malignant disease. Because the prostate gland encircles the urethra, even benign enlargement (hypertrophy) may lead to obstruction of the urethra.

The male hormone *testosterone* is produced by the interstitial cells of the testes and is responsible for development of the genitalia during puberty and for maintaining the genitalia in a functional state during life. Androgenic hormones are also responsible for the development of sec-

ondary sex characteristics including growth of body hair and thickening of the vocal cords. Testosterone secretion is closely related to pituitary gland function, and the rate of secretion is determined by levels of luteinizing hormone (LH) in the blood. Secretion of testosterone decreases slowly with age.

■ Physiologic changes with aging

Menopause, which occurs in the middle-aged woman, results in physiologic changes from the hormonal decrease (see the box on p. 1244). When ovulation ceases, no progesterone is produced and estrogen diminishes. In the male, androgen production decreases steadily during adulthood to about age 60 years, then levels off.

The physiologic changes do not diminish the elderly person's ability to engage in sexual intercourse (see Chapter 33) but may lead to discomfort or complications. The vaginal dryness and narrowed introitus may cause dyspa-

---

Physiologic changes in reproductive tract with aging

Female

Uterus	Decreased size
Ovaries	Atrophy, with decreased size
Vagina	Decreased width and length
	Vaginal entrance (introitus) narrowed
	Vaginal secretions decrease and become more alkaline

Male

Testes	Decreased size and firmness
Seminal fluid	Decreased amount and viscosity
Prostate gland	Hypertrophy (enlargement)
Penile erection	Slower, decreased frequency of involuntary morning erections

---

reunia (painful intercourse). Vaginal infections occur more readily in the alkaline medium. Muscle weakness may lead to cystocele, rectocele, or uterine prolapse.

PREVENTION AND HEALTH EDUCATION

Prevention of infection

Vaginal infections may result from the presence of large numbers of invading organisms or from decreased resistance to infection. Those women in whom the natural barriers to infection are at a minimum (low estrogen levels, thinness of the vaginal epithelium, or reduced acidity of the vagina) are at greatest risk (see the box below).

Risk factors for vaginal infections

Aging
Diabetes
Pregnancy
Malnutrition
Inadequate perineal hygiene
Excessive douching
Use of vaginal inserts
Oral contraceptives
Broad-spectrum antibiotics
Intercourse with infected partner

Large numbers of organisms may invade the vagina or urethra from inadequate personal hygiene, from another person during sexual intercourse, or from use of unclean articles such as douche nozzles. Decreased resistance to infection may result from vaginal secretions becoming more alkaline, providing a more suitable medium for bacterial growth. Vaginal yeast infections may be a side effect of drugs such as the tetracyclines or oral contraceptives. Preventive measures include the following:

1. Wiping from front to back (female) after bowel movements
2. Voiding shortly after intercourse to wash away organisms
3. Using a condom (male) during intercourse if either partner has been exposed to a genital infection
4. Recognizing signs of infection in the sexual partner and urging medical attention
5. Abstaining from intercourse if one partner has a genital infection
6. Avoiding douching (which may alter vaginal pH) unless advised by a physician for treatment
7. Seeking immediate medical attention for early signs of vaginal infection (abnormal vaginal discharge, vaginal itching), especially in persons at high risk.

Early detection of cancer

Dramatically decreased rates of death from cancer are associated with early detection and treatment. Persons at high risk for cancer of the cervix include women who were sexually active at an early age and those with multiple sex partners. High-risk factors for endometrial cancer include early problems with menstruation or ovulation or late menopause, lack of progestin with prolonged estrogen therapy, and obesity.[2] (See the box below.)

The decline in deaths from cervical cancer is primarily the result of increased use of the Papanicolaou (Pap) smear for mass screening, combined with more frequent and more thorough gynecologic examinations. Cancer of the cervix

---

Risk factors for uterine cancer

Cancer of the cervix

First sexual intercourse at early age
Multiple sexual partners

Cancer of the endometrium

History of infertility
Failure of ovulation
Prolonged estrogen therapy without added progestin
Late menopause
Combination of diabetes, high blood pressure, and obesity

Examinations for prevention of uterine cancer as recommended by the American Cancer Society

1. Pap test once every 3 years after two initial negative tests 1 year apart
2. More frequent Pap tests for persons at high risk
3. Endometrial tissue sample at menopause for persons at high risk for endometrial cancer

is easier to detect through the Pap smear than is cancer of the endometrium.

Health teaching for prevention of uterine cancer includes regular pelvic examinations that include a Pap smear. Recommendations of the American Cancer Society to detect cancer early are listed in the box above.

■ Health teaching related to menstruation and menopause

■ MENSTRUATION

Menstruation occurs on an average of every 28 days; the normal range is 26 to 34 days. The menstrual flow usually lasts for 3 to 7 days (average 4 days). Normally 30 to 180 ml (average 50 ml) of menstrual fluid is lost during the period. One half to three fourths of the fluid is blood, and the remainder is mucus, fragments of endometrial cells, and desquamated vaginal epithelium.

Normally menstrual fluid does not clot unless it is re-

tained in the uterus or vagina for a prolonged time. It is believed that the endometrium produces an anticoagulant that prevents clotting of blood in the uterus. An occasional very small clot may occur during the first 24 hours, and this is probably a particle of endometrial tissue. Large clots or pus in the menstrual flow are never normal.

During pregnancy menstruation ceases, and then returns within 6 to 8 weeks after delivery, although lactation suppresses the menses for varying periods of time. Unless disease occurs, the menstrual periods recur during adult life until menopause.

Menstruation is a manifestation of normal body function and should be treated as such. The "period" and "monthly period" are accurate terms to use if the woman does not wish to say "menstruating." Terms such as "being sick," "on the rag," or "having the curse" are to be avoided because of their negative connotation. Suggestions for health teaching related to menstruation are listed in the box below.

To become knowledgeable about the patterns of their menstrual cycles, women are encouraged to keep a written record. Establishing this habit makes it possible to predict the onset of the next menstrual period and to determine the range of cycles and duration of flow. Should it be necessary to seek the attention of a health professional for any reason, the date of onset of the last menstrual period (LMP) is known.

■ PREMENSTRUAL SYNDROME

Premenstrual syndrome (PMS), which occurs in more than 25% of all menstruating women, is the presence of symptoms in the premenstruum or early menstruation with the absence of postmenstrual symptoms. Identical symptoms must occur in three consecutive cycles to confirm a diagnosis of PMS. Symptoms vary considerably among

Health teaching for menstruation

1. Knowledge of the physiologic process
2. Factors that may alter the menstrual cycle: stress, fatigue, exercise, acute and chronic illness, changes in climate or working hours, pregnancy
3. Personal hygiene
   a. Wear pads during early period of heavy flow
   b. Change tampons frequently to decrease risk of toxic shock syndrome
   c. Consult a physician if tampons cause discomfort
   d. Take a daily bath for comfort (warm bath may relieve slight pelvic discomfort)
4. Exercise
   a. Exercise is not contraindicated and may help prevent discomfort
   b. Modify exercise if fatigue occurs
5. Diet
   a. Restrict salt intake if fluid retention is present
   b. Consult physician if fluid retention persists after menstruation
6. Discomfort (dysmenorrhea)
   a. For mild discomfort take aspirin or acetaminophen, apply warmth, rest
   b. For prolonged severe discomfort, consult physician.

Table 34-1 Activities to modify PMS discomforts

PMS symptoms	Activity
Behavioral changes	Increase intake of foods rich in vitamin B_6 (yeast, wheat germ, whole-grain cereals, liver, legumes); decrease dairy products intake; increase outdoor exercise
Water and sodium retention	Restrict salt intake; restrict intake of coffee, tea, cola, chocolate; increase intake of foods rich in vitamin B_6 (see above)
Increased appetite, (especially for sweets), headache, fatigue	Restrict free sugar, sodium, and animal fat intake; substitute complex carbohydrates for simple sugars
Depression	Increase intake of green leafy vegetables, legumes, and whole-grain cereals (high in B vitamins)

Adapted from Abraham, G: Nutritional factors in the etiology of the premenstrual tension syndrome, J Reprod Med 28:446-464, 1983.

women and may include behavioral changes (tension, irritability, mood swings, anxiety, crying, depression, insomnia), fatigue, signs of water and sodium retention (edema, weight gain, breast enlargement and tenderness, and abdominal bloating), palpitations, increased appetite, headache, and backache.[1] The symptoms result from changes in hormone levels and altered glucose tolerance.

The nurse can assist women with PMS by acknowledging the existence of the syndrome and its attendant symptoms, which may be severe for some women. Because some women have been made to feel that the symptoms are nonexistent or exaggerated, the nurse can encourage them to keep a menstrual-symptom calendar to document the cyclic nature of the symptoms.[48]

Different activities can be suggested to modify the discomforts (Table 34-1). Women can also be encouraged to plan activities during the symptom-free part of their cycles. Because fatigue may exaggerate PMS symptoms, adequate rest, sleep and relaxation are helpful. Women can seek detailed guidance and information from one of several centers specifically studying PMS (see the box top, right).

■ DYSMENORRHEA

Although menstruation is a normal physiologic process, some women experience varying degrees of discomfort (menstrual cramps). Dysmenorrhea is the greatest single cause of absenteeism by women from school or work. Dysmenorrhea may result from various causes (see the box at right). Primary dysmenorrhea often disappears after pregnancy or by age 25 years.

Premenstrual tension centers

National Center for PMS and Menstrual Distress
15 Smith Road
Bedford, NH 03102

The National PMS Society
Box 11467
Durham, NC 27703

PMS Action, Inc.
P.O. Box 9326
Madison, WI 53715

Rocky Mountain PMS Society
P.O. Box 16453
Salt Lake City, UT 84116

From Wilson, MA, and others: JOGN Nurs. 13(2)suppl:15s, 1984.

Women who are consistently unable to engage in usual activities because of pain associated with menstruation should be urged to seek health care for diagnosis and treatment of any existing secondary dysmenorrhea.

Treatment of secondary dysmenorrhea is aimed at the organic cause. Surgical and pharmacologic interventions may be appropriate depending on the severity and type of pathology. If the uterus is found to be in an abnormal position and can be manually returned to a normal position, a pessary may be inserted for a trial period to learn whether malposition is the cause of dysmenorrhea. Dilation of the cervical canal is done when a cervical stricture is found and thought to be the cause of dysmenorrhea.

If no organic cause of dysmenorrhea can be found, the woman is advised to try rest, moderate exercise, and avoidance of constipation. Local application of heat and mild analgesics are usually prescribed. Aspirin is a prostaglandin antagonist. Heat causes vasodilation of blood vessels, thereby increasing the blood flow and relieving ischemia, increasing elimination of the menstrual flow, and decreasing muscle hypertonus.

Causes of dysmenorrhea

Primary dysmenorrhea

High concentration of uterine prostaglandins

Secondary dysmenorrhea

Pelvic inflammatory disease
Endometriosis

Medications that usually give the best relief of discomfort are the prostaglandin synthetase inhibitors (PGSIs), including ibuprofen (Motrin, Rufen), mefenamic acid (Ponstel), and naproxen (Naprosyn, Anaprox). These drugs are effective when started at the onset of bleeding. The medication may be given with milk or with meals if gastric irritation occurs. Oral contraceptives have also been used to suppress ovulation by inhibiting prostaglandin levels.

Other measures that may be explored include systematic relaxation, exercise, muscle toning, massage, effleurage, breathing techniques, manual pressure on the abdomen, and orgasm. Biofeedback and autogenic training have also been used. Positive attitudes toward menstruation and alternative interventions from which to select the most useful are helpful for the woman experiencing dysmenorrhea.

■ MENOPAUSE

Menopause, or the *climacteric*, is the transitional phase between reproductive and nonreproductive ability. Menopause is said to have occurred when there has been no menstrual flow for 1 year (although some women have periods even after 1 year of amenorrhea). During the climacteric, which usually lasts for 12 to 18 months, there is a gradual decline in ovarian function. The ovaries gradually cease to produce ova and estrogen, and as a result the menses become scanty, irregular, and farther apart, until they stop altogether.

Natural menopause may occur between 35 and 60 years of age (average age 51 years). Early menopause may be caused by a number of factors (see the box below).

Menopause may be artificially induced by such procedures as irradiation of the ovaries, surgical removal of both ovaries, or hysterectomy. Each of these has one common consequence, namely, cessation of menstruation. However, surgical removal or irradiation of the ovaries results in menopause with all its physiologic changes, whereas ovaries left intact after hysterectomy will continue to function provided the age of climacteric has not yet been reached.

Physiologic changes in the genital organs as a result of loss of hormonal functioning are listed on p. 1243. Women can still enjoy sexual activity after menopause. There may be changes in the skeletal system; about 30% of women develop osteoporosis from the effect of lack of estrogen on calcium balance.

Factors associated with early menopause

Excessive exposure to radiation
Poor general health
Inadequate spacing between pregnancies
Hypothyroidism with severe obesity

□ Counseling and teaching

Most women have heard of the "change of life." The negative image of menopause is reinforced by the media, books, health professionals, and the general public. Depending on the climate in which they were reared and on their own changes in attitude toward normal functions of the reproductive organs, women may feel more or less free to discuss menopause and their feelings and concerns during this period of life. Because many problems related to the reproductive organs occur in this age group, and because it is important for mental health that women be helped to make menopause as comfortable as possible, it is important for nurses to identify women who can profit from interventions.

Education regarding menopause should precede its onset (see the box on p. 1248). Women approaching menopause, regardless of whether it is an event of normal aging or is artificially induced, need to know what menopause is, why it occurs, the effects menopause has on reproductive and sexual ability, what can be done to make menopause more comfortable, and those symptoms that require medical attention.

Many women go through the climacteric with little awareness of its occurrence. Some women, however, experience hot flashes (flushes), which are felt as waves of warmth accompanied by flushing of the skin, especially the face, neck, and arms, and perspiration. The hot flash is the perception of the spread of heat from an anatomic point of origin on the body to other areas of the body. Hot flashes may be so mild that they are hardly noticed or so severe that they produce distress. Estrogen may be prescribed by the physician for severe discomfort. During estrogen therapy women should be seen at least every 6 months for examination and for review of menopausal symptoms. The examination should include the breasts and reproductive organs, Pap smear, and blood pressure.

Feelings of depression and uselessness may occur, particularly among women who have been highly invested in the maternal role. Peer support groups may be very helpful in these situations.

Publications that may help the woman during the climacteric include *Our Bodies Ourselves**, *The Menopause: A Positive Approach†*, and *Menstruation and Menopause‡*.

■ INTERFERENCES WITH REPRODUCTION

The ability to have children may be modified either to prevent conception or to terminate a pregnancy (see the box on p. 1248). Some persons are unable to procreate. The topics of contraception and abortion are covered in maternity nursing texts and are not repeated here.

---

*Boston Women's Health Book Collective: New York, 1980, Simon & Schuster, Inc.
†Reitz, R.: Philadelphia, 1979, Chilton Book Co.
‡Weideger, P.: New York, 1976, Alfred A. Knopf, Inc.

Health teaching for menopause

1. Knowledge about menopause
   a. Cessation of ovarian function with cessation of menstruation over 12 to 18 months
   b. Changes in reproductive ability
      (1) Conception still possible during the period of change
         (a) Contraception should be used for 1 year after last menstrual period
         (b) Rhythm method unreliable contraceptive method during this period
      (2) Ability to conceive ceases when menopause completed
   c. Sexual ability still present
   d. Physical symptoms vary from mild to severe; estrogen therapy may be given to relieve severe symptoms
2. Promotion of health and physical appearance
   a. Moderate exercise to maintain muscle tone and help prevent osteoporosis
   b. Dietary control to prevent weight gain
   c. Activities that encourage self-esteem and interest outside of self
   d. Peer support groups during menopause, if necessary
   e. Medical attention required for recurrence of bleeding or other vaginal discharge
3. Prevention of discomfort
   a. Prevention of dyspareunia: local application of lubricant or vaginal cream
   b. Relief of vaginal itching: vitamin E or estrogen therapy
   c. Relief of vasomotor reactions (hot flashes)
      (1) Moderation of factors identified by the person as exacerbating hot flashes (excitement, alcoholic beverages heavy eating, excessive clothing, impairment of heat loss in hot weather)
      (2) Vitamin E or B complex vitamins

Interferences with reproduction

Contraception Process of temporary prevention of impregnation or conception

Sterilization Process of making an individual incapable of reproducing, either permanently or until the process is reversed

Abortion Termination of a pregnancy before the fetus is viable

Infertility Inability to achieve a pregnancy within a stipulated time (at least 1 year) of unprotected sexual intercourse

---

■ Sterilization

Voluntary sterilization has become increasingly acceptable to both men and women as a method of preventing pregnancy. It is the most commonly used method of fertility control for married couples older than 30 years. Sterilization may also be performed in selected instances where pregnancy would create risks to the health or life of the woman or infant (for example, heart disease, severe diabetes, probable genetic defects in the infant).

Because sterilization may be a permanent method of contraception, it is absolutely necessary to obtain voluntary, informed consent. Patients receiving federal funds for sterilization must be at least 21 years old and mentally competent.

■ METHODS OF STERILIZATION

Methods of sterilization are described in Table 34-2. The abdominal approaches are favored by some physicians because they are familiar with the female pelvic anatomy as viewed from the abdomen and because the fallopian tubes are free and suspended in this position, which makes them easy to see, manipulate, and ligate or cauterize. The vaginal approach is favored by some physicians and women because of the absence of a visible scar, ease of peritoneal entry, and rapid postoperative recovery; however, because of its higher complication rate, it is less frequently used today.

Successful sterilization (conception prevented) is dependent on the technique used, the surgeon's experience in performing the procedure, and the length of the tube removed. The main causes of failure in the female are recanalization of the fallopian tube, erroneous ligation, and pregnancy resulting from tuboperitoneal fistula. In the male spontaneous recanalization (reanastomosis) may occur; the cause is unknown but duplication of the vas deferens has occasionally been noted.

Table 34-2   Methods of sterilization

Method	Description	Comments
Female		
Tubal sterilization		
ABDOMINAL		
Minilaparotomy	Ligation or cutting of fallopian tubes under direct vision through small abdominal incision	Local or general anesthesia Complications: wound infection, hematoma, bladder injury Advantages: good chance for sterility reversal
Laparoscopy	Electrocoagulation of segment of fallopian tubes by laparoscopy through small abdominal incision	Local or general anesthesia Advantages: minimal discomfort, short procedure
VAGINAL		
Culpotomy	Ligation or cutting of fallopian tube through small incision in cul-de-sac of Douglas	Local, spinal, or general anesthesia Higher complication rate than laparoscopy (infection, hemorrhage)
Culdoscopy	Electrocoagulation of segment of fallopian tubes by culdoscope through small incision in cul-de-sac of Douglas	Local anesthesia Higher complication rate than laparoscopy
Male		
Vasectomy	Removal of a segment of vas deferens through small incision in scrotum	Local anesthesia Complications rare Bruising, mild edema, and mild discomfort common

■ EFFECTS OF STERILIZATION

□ Physiologic effects

Although tubal sterilization usually terminates a woman's ability to bear children, ovarian hormones and menstrual functioning are not altered and artificial menopause is not induced. Ability to derive satisfaction from sexual intercourse should not be impaired, and some women may experience greater enjoyment from intercourse free from fear of pregnancy.

Because vasectomy interrupts the continuity of the vas deferens, sperm are prevented from being ejaculated with other components of the semen. However, sperm are still produced and the ejaculate is not noticeably diminished in amount. Residual fertility lasting for a variable period is present because of sperm in the semen beyond the point of occlusion of the vas. Sperm *gradually* disappear from the ejaculate; thus conception is possible in the immediate postoperative period. Semen analysis will determine when sperm have finally disappeared.

□ Psychologic effects

Men and women who elect sterilization seem to have little or no regret after the surgery if they understand what to expect during and after the procedure and are able to express their feelings and have questions answered before the procedure. Persons with preexisting emotional problems have reported depression, loss of self-esteem, guilt, and difficulty in sexual adjustment after surgery.

■ PREOPERATIVE CARE

Preoperative counseling is indicated to identify men and women before surgery who may later have strong regrets and emotional problems. One aim of counseling before surgery is to confirm that the decision for sterilization is made as objectively as possible. Previous experience with other methods of contraception can be explored and reasons for dissatisfaction with the methods determined. It may be that there is lack of knowledge about contraceptive methods, and with adequate information the couple might choose a means other than sterilization. Young persons and those who are unhappy about pregnancies or who have marital problems are poor candidates for sterilization. They may want to change their minds at a later date. The discussion of sterilization methods should be based on the federal government's informed consent guidelines (see the box on p. 1250).

■ POSTOPERATIVE CARE

Many of the sterilization procedures are performed on an outpatient basis, and the patient can be discharged when

---

Informed consent guidelines (federal) relating to sterilization

1. Choice is made by patient, without pressures (for example, loss of welfare benefits, wrath of health care provider).
2. Benefits and risks of sterilization are described:
   a. Benefits: permanent, no further costs or decision making.
   b. Risks: usual surgical risks, possibility of future pregnancy (not 100% effective).
3. Alternative contraceptive methods are described.
4. Patient is encouraged to ask questions.
5. Explanations are given about the entire sterilization procedure, costs, and possible side effects (effects on hormones, weight changes, menstrual changes, sexual response).
6. Written instruction and risk factors are explained to patient.
7. Written consent to the procedure is signed by patient and witnessed.

---

the effects of general anesthesia have worn off and vital signs are stable. If the patient expresses feelings of guilt or regret about having been sterilized, a review of the reasons for sterilization and positive effect on sexual relationships may need to be repeated. Teaching guidelines following a sterilization procedure are described in the box below.

■ STERILIZATION REVERSAL

Requests for reversal of previous sterilization may be made because of divorce and remarriage, death of children, or change in economic status, as well as for other reasons. The chances of reversing the effects of sterilization are improving as a result of refinement of microsurgical techniques.

Reconstruction of the fallopian tubes involves an end-to-end anastomosis of the ligated or dissected tubes with or without insertion of plastic lumen. Success of restoration of tubal function is partly dependent on the original surgery performed, especially regarding the length of the tubal portion excised. Ligation of the tubes produces adhesions that must be dissected away to the point of tubal patency; this reduces the amount of remaining tubal structure. Also the length of the fallopian tube remaining after reconstruction may play a role in permitting adequate time for the fertilized ovum to undergo maturational changes in preparation for implantation.

In the male, reconstruction consists in attempting to rejoin the severed ends of the vas deferens. Success is measured by the presence of sperm in the semen after

---

Teaching for the patient who has had a sterilization procedure

Woman

1. Rest for 24 to 48 hours after procedure
2. No heavy lifting or strenuous exercise for 1 week
3. Abstain from sexual intercourse
   a. Abdominal method: until wound is healed and no discomfort is present
   b. Vaginal method: 1 week
4. Report to physician signs of fever, persistent abdominal pain, or bleeding from incision

Man

1. Apply ice to scrotum, take sitz baths for minor discomfort and swelling
2. Wear scrotal support for 48 hours
3. Rest for 48 hours after procedure
4. No heavy lifting or strenuous exercise for 1 week
5. Abstain from sexual intercourse for 3 days
6. Use an alternate method of contraception until physician reports semen no longer contains sperm
7. Report to physician signs of fever, persistent scrotal pain, or profuse incisional bleeding

reconstruction. A notable point is that although sperm reappear in the semen, the pregnancy rate after reconstruction is low; the reason for this is unknown.

■ Infertility

It has been estimated that 10% to 15% of all couples in the United States are unwillingly childless. Approximately 50% of couples who undergo assessment and treatment for infertility are likely to conceive. Although infertility is most often attributed to women, in about 40% of infertile marriages the man is infertile.[44]

The fertility of a couple is affected by coital frequency and the age of the man and the woman. Increased coital frequency enhances fertility. Frequent ejaculation improves sperm motility unless ejaculation is excessive, resulting in depletion of available sperm. Fertility peaks at age 24 years in women and age 25 years in men.

■ CAUSE AND PREVENTION

There are many causes of infertility in men and women (see the box below). Some are preventable or correctable, others are not. There is no known cause in 10% to 20% of infertility problems.

One of the most common preventable causes of infertility in women is infection of the pelvic organs, especially as a result of gonorrhea, which causes obstruction of the fallopian tubes. Such serious consequences are preventable through prophylactic use of penicillin for women exposed to gonorrhea and through early diagnosis and treatment of all vaginal and cervical infections. Gonococcal cultures should be obtained every 6 months for women with multiple partners. If infection is present and the woman has an IUD, the device should be removed.

Many of the ovarian and hormonal problems that cause infertility produce symptoms such as menstrual irregularities and ill health before a problem with conception is ever recognized. Many of these problems can be managed with hormone therapy, provided women seek help at an early age or as soon as deviations are noticed. Birth control pills should be avoided by women who have not established normal menses.

In males, bilateral undescended testes (cryptorchidism) should be corrected surgically before puberty. In later life cryptorchidism may produce sterility because of failure of the testes to develop their sperm-producing function, even if the condition is surgically corrected. Destruction of testicular tissue by infectious processes can be prevented through prompt treatment when symptoms first appear.

▥ ASSESSMENT

It is important that couples who wish to have children seek medical advice if they are unsuccessful after about a year of trying to achieve pregnancy. Infertility evaluation often requires a long time.

Attempts to correct infertility are based on data obtained through a detailed history and physical examination as well as from laboratory tests and clinical studies. A sexual history is taken and sexual practices are reviewed. Suggestions about sexual intercourse are given if this seems to be the problem. The couple should attempt to attend the first interview together because they share responsibility for infertility, information is needed by both partners, and this may be their first opportunity to confront their feelings about being infertile.

☐ Examination of the man

Many physicians prefer to carry out examination of the man first, because it is more easily accomplished and less time consuming. Stricture and varicoceles (dilated veins of the spermatic cords) may be corrected by surgery.

If sperm count and motility of sperm are low, thyroid extract and vitamins may be prescribed along with a well-balanced diet, rest, and moderate exercise. A lack of vi-

---

Causes of infertility

Disorder	Effect
Female	
Obstructions of fallopian tubes	Interfere with transport of ovum
Diseases of body or cervix of uterus	Inhibit passage of active sperm
Hormonal deficiencies	Inhibit release of ovum
	Inhibit development of endometrium for implantation
Male	
Obstruction of vas deferens	Interfere with transport of sperm
Diseases of testes, undescended testes, hormonal deficiencies	Inhibit development of sperm
Sperm-bound immunoglobulins	Inhibit sperm penetration of ovum

---

Examination for infertility

Tests	Data obtained
Male	
Multiple semen examination	Determine presence, number, and motility of sperm
Testicular biopsy if sperm count low or absent	Presence of sperm indicates obstruction of vas deferens
Female	
Basal body temperature chart	Determines that ovulation is occurring
Postcoital test of cervical secretions	Measure ability of sperm to penetrate cervical mucus and remain active, and quality of the mucus
Endometrial biopsy, serum progesterone and estradiol levels, laparoscopic inspection of ovaries	Determine whether ovulation is occurring (if in question)
Rubin test (uterotubal insufflation)	Determine patency of fallopian tubes
Hysterosalpingography (x-ray after insertion of contrast media)	Determine patency of uterus and fallopian tubes
Hormonal tests for males and females	Determine whether the problem is hormonal

---

tamins A and E in the diet may cause some atrophy of the sperm-producing structures. The couple are advised to have intercourse every other day during the fertile period (usually 12 to 16 days before the beginning of the next menstrual period). When the man is completely aspermatic, conception is impossible, and the couple should be counseled regarding the alternatives open to them.

□ Examination of the woman

If the man is found to be fertile, examination of the woman is carried out (see the box above). If sperm are being destroyed by vaginal and cervical secretions, smears from these sites are studied. If the secretions are too acid or too alkaline, medicated douches may be prescribed. A douche with sodium bicarbonate taken just before intercourse has been found to increase the motility of sperm in many cases. Tubal strictures or obstructions are sometimes repaired by plastic surgery, but the rate of success in restoring tubal function is very low. Underlying metabolic diseases are corrected if possible.

■ COPING WITH INFERTILITY

Couples who wish to have children but find themselves unable to do so experience immeasurable emotional distress. Feelings of inadequacy are common, as are anger and guilt. The infertile couple must confront feelings about lack of control, self-image, self-esteem, and sexuality. Couples who are informed that they will never be able to have children experience a life crisis with all of its ramifications, and they have a strong need to grieve. For those who are told they are a normal, fertile couple, but for whom pregnancy does not result despite months or years of tests, studies, examinations, and advice, feelings of frustration alternating with hope are common.

All of these couples require emotional support, including encouragement to grieve, to express their anger and other feelings in order to regain objectivity and to avoid premature decisions and actions about alternatives. The urgent need for such support is reflected in the emergence of support groups organized by infertile individuals and couples.

■ ALTERNATIVE INFERTILITY APPROACHES

Among the alternatives available to infertile couples are adoption, remaining childless, artificial insemination, in vitro fertilization, and surrogate motherhood.

Artificial insemination is the placement of a few drops of donor semen in the cervicovaginal, intracervical, or intrauterine (more painful) area. It is simple, safe, inexpensive, and highly successful. The major indication for artificial insemination is male infertility. Previous loss of children because of Rh or ABO incompatibility or severe hereditary defects transmitted by the man are other indications. Therefore, artificial insemination is not reserved exclusively for infertile couples.

Artificial insemination is homologous (AIH) when the partner's semen is used and heterologous (AID) when donor semen is used. Criteria for donor selection is based on semen analysis as well as on a complete history and physical examination. Donor candidates with venereal disease, diabetes, hepatitis, blood diseases, prostatic infection, AIDS, and a family history of hereditary disorders are excluded. Fertility of donors must be proved by semen analysis.

In vitro fertilization (IVF) involves recovering one or more of the woman's ova from her ovarian follicles through laparoscopy and fertilizing the ova with the partner's sperm in a petri dish. If fertilization and cleavage occur, the resulting embryos are transferred into the woman's uterus about 48 hours after the ova retrieval has taken place. This procedure is indicated for women with complete blockage of the fallopian tubes, for oligospermia of the male, and for cases of unexplained infertility. The chance of a successful pregnancy is at best about 20% per IVF attempt, so the odds are very much against any one couple achieving a pregnancy.[29]

Surrogate mothers are women who contract to conceive by artificial insemination and give the baby to the semen donor after delivery. There are many social, moral, psychologic, and legal implications surrounding this approach.

Major health problems of the reproductive system

The major problems of the reproductive system include inflammation, structural disorders, tumors, and sexually transmitted diseases. The first three types of disorders are discussed separately for women and men because of the inherent anatomic differences. Sexually transmitted diseases (see Chapter 35) are discussed as a separate topic because the problems are common to both women and men. The various disorders that fall within the cited categories are as follows:

1. Female disorders
   a. Inflammatory disorders: vaginitis, cervicitis, pelvic inflammatory disease, toxic shock syndrome
   b. Structural disorders: relaxed vaginal outlet, uterine displacement, prolapse of uterus, fistulas
   c. Tumors: ovarian tumors and cysts, endometriosis, uterine fibroid tumors, cervical polyps, and cancer of the cervix, endometrium, and ovary
2. Male disorders
   a. Inflammatory disorders: urethritis, prostatitis, epididymitis, orchitis
   b. Structural disorders: hydrocele, spermatocele, varicocele, torsion of spermatic cord
   c. Tumors: cancer of the testes, prostate gland, penis

■ DISORDERS IN WOMEN

■ Inflammatory disorders

■ TYPES OF INFLAMMATORY DISORDERS

Inflammations of the female reproductive tract are seen most commonly in the vagina, cervix, or fallopian tubes and adjacent areas (Table 34-3). Many of these infections can be prevented (p. 1244).

Table 34-3 Inflammatory disorders of the female reproductive tract

Disorder	Etiology	Signs and symptoms	Medical therapy
Vulvitis/vaginitis	*Candida, Trichomonas, Gardnerella,* coliform bacteria, *Gonococcus,* herpes simplex	Itching of vulva or vagina, vaginal discharge, dyspareunia	Antifungal agents, antibiotics (oral, topical, douches), sitz baths
Cervicitis	*Gonococcus, Streptococcus, Staphylococcus,* herpes virus, *Chlamydia*	Mucopurulent discharge, erosion of cervix	Cauterization of cervix, antibiotics
Pelvic inflammatory disease (salpingitis)	*Gonococcus, Chlamydia,* coliform bacteria, *Streptococcus, Mycoplasm,* anaerobic bacteria	Severe abdominal pain, lower abdominal cramps, intermenstrual spotting, dyspareunia, fever and chills, malaise, nausea and vomiting, foul-smelling purulent vaginal discharge	Penicillin, tetracycline, amoxicillin, rest; heat to abdomen, analgesics, oral contraceptives, therapy for 3 months, sexual abstinence until recovery
Toxic shock syndrome	Toxin from *Staphylococcus aureus*	High fever, vomiting, watery diarrhea, sore throat, myalgia, erythematous rash with desquamation; if severe, impaired renal, hepatic, cardiopulmonary function	Antibiotics, rapid hydration, supportive therapy for septic shock

■ PATHOPHYSIOLOGY

□ Vulva and vagina

Normally the vagina is protected from infection by its pH and the presence of *Döderlein's bacilli*. If the vaginal pH is altered, if the invading organisms are numerous, or if the woman's resistance is decreased by aging, malnutrition, stress, disease, or the use of drugs, the risk of infection is increased. Yeast organisms grow best in an acid pH <4.7, whereas *Trichomonas* and organisms causing nonspecific vaginitis thrive in a pH >5 (more alkaline).

Organisms causing infection of the vulva and vagina are most often introduced from outside sources such as clothing, hands, douche nozzles, or other contaminated articles or during intercourse. In sexually active women reinfection may occur after treatment unless their sexual partners are also successfully treated.

Women of menopausal and postmenopausal age often develop vaginitis (sometimes referred to as atrophic or senile vaginitis). Increased alkalinity of the vaginal secretions is a contributing cause, and the pyogenic bacterial invasion of the thin vaginal mucosa produces symptoms of burning, pruritus, and *leukorrhea* (whitish-yellow vaginal discharge).

Inflammation may also occur in Bartholin's glands or less frequently in Skene's glands. The infection is usually unilateral but may be bilateral. With infection the duct from the gland becomes partially or completely obstructed, resulting in severe redness, enlargement of the gland, and edema of the surrounding tissues. The area becomes tender, and walking may become painful. The usual result of the infectious process is an abscess. Occasionally, acute bartholinitis subsides, leaving fibrotic or scar tissue. When this occurs, a Bartholin's cyst develops. The cyst may vary in size, from a few centimeters in diameter to the size of a hen's egg, is mobile, and nontender.

□ Cervix

Cervicitis, infection of the cervix, is the most common gynecologic disorder, affecting more than half of all women. There are two forms of cervicitis, acute and chronic, of which the chronic is the most frequent. Cervicitis usually progresses from the acute to the chronic form if not treated, and it may go undetected for a long time. In fact, the cervix may heal and appear quite healthy after the disease has spread upward. This condition presents few symptoms, and those symptoms that occur do not ordinarily lead women to seek medical attention. If the vaginal discharge is slight, the woman may not become concerned.

Cervicitis may follow childbirth or abortion or it may be caused by infection of a cervical laceration or erosion. In untreated cervicitis the tissues are constantly irritated, and there is some evidence that this irritation predisposes to cancer.

□ Fallopian tubes

Inflammation of the fallopian tubes, *salpingitis,* may be local or more often may spread to the ovaries, pelvic peri-

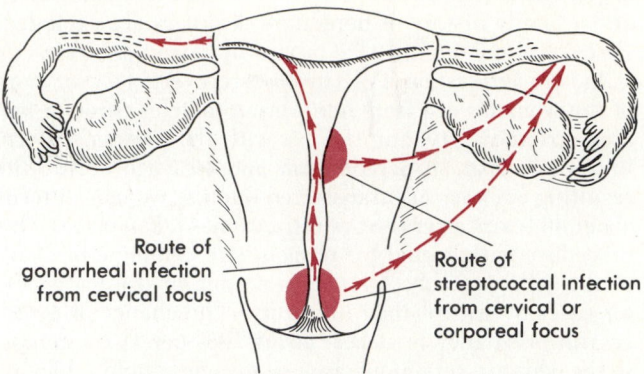

Fig. 34-4 Two chief routes of pelvic infection. (From Novak, ER, Jones, GJ, and Jones, HW, Jr: Novak's textbook of gynecology, ed 9, Baltimore, 1975, The Williams & Wilkins Co.)

toneum, pelvic veins, or pelvic connective tissue. This widespread inflammation is termed *pelvic inflammatory disease (PID)*. The pathogens may invade the pelvic organs during sexual intercourse, childbirth or the postpartum period or after abortion. PID is reported to occur five times more often among women using intrauterine devices (IUDs) for birth control than among women using other methods.

Pathogenic organisms are usually introduced from outside the body and pass up the cervical canal into the uterus. They seem to cause little trouble in the uterus but pass into the pelvis by way of the fallopian tubes, through thrombosed uterine veins, or through the lymphatics of the uterus (Fig. 34-4). The invaded structures become host to an acute or chronic inflammatory process.

Many of the pathogens causing PID lodge in the fallopian tubes. Purulent material collects in the tubes, adhesions form, strictures may occur, and sterility is a frequent result. Adhesions resulting from inflammation may cause such distress that complete removal of the uterus, fallopian tubes, and ovaries is necessary. Although generalized peritonitis can occur, the infection usually remains confined to the lower abdomen and pelvis. A severe inflammatory process may lead to dehydration, electrolyte imbalances, and prostration.

□ Toxic shock syndrome

Toxic shock syndrome, although not exclusively a reproductive disorder, occurs most commonly in menstruating females, especially among those using superabsorbent tampons. The syndrome has been associated with toxins produced by *Staphylococcus aureus*. It is suggested that the organism gains entry to the circulation through lesions in the vagina produced by tampons. Superabsorbent tampons provide a milieu favorable to bacterial growth because they can contain a large amount of menstrual blood and may be left in place several hours. Sepsis results from the effect of the toxins.

⬛ ASSESSMENT

☐ Subjective data
☐ *Itching*

Itching is a major symptom of vulvular or vaginal infection. The itching may result from irritation from the vaginal discharge or from end products of the inflammatory response. The degree of itching experienced is monitored for signs of decreasing intensity as the inflammation subsides. Itching is most intense with *Trichomonas* infections.

Causes of vulvar or vaginal itching other than infection include epithelial changes seen with menopause, high urinary sugar content as in diabetes mellitus, pediculosis pubis, scabies, allergies, pinworms, or cancer of the vulva. With severe pruritus there are usually excoriations of the skin caused by scratching, and secondary infection may result. Dysuria may occur as a consequence of local irritation of the urinary meatus.

☐ *Pain*

Pain is primarily a symptom of PID. In *acute* PID there is usually severe cramping lower abdominal pain; in *chronic* PID the pain is typically dull and aching and may be located in the lower back as well as the lower abdomen. Occasionally women have been thought neurotic because of ongoing reports of the diffuse pain, only to have chronic PID diagnosed later.

☐ Objective data
☐ *Vaginal discharge*

Vaginal discharge is a major finding in most inflammations of the female genital tract. The *character* and *amount* of the discharge are monitored because these differ depending on the type and severity of the disorder (see the box below). Normally, many women have a scant, thin, whitish vaginal discharge, primarily at the time of ovulation.

Types of vaginal discharges with inflammation

Inflammation	Discharge
Vaginitis	
Candida	White, curdlike, cheesy, sweetish odor
Trichomonas	Yellow to green, frothy, foul odor, copious
Gardnerella	Grayish white, fishy or foul odor, scanty
Cervicitis	Whitish yellow (mucopurulent), amount varies

➡ DATA ANALYSIS: NURSING DIAGNOSES

Nursing diagnoses are determined from assessment of patient data. Possible nursing diagnoses for the woman with a gynecologic inflammation may include, but are not limited to, the following:

Diagnostic title	Possible etiologies
Knowledge deficit	Lack of exposure/recall, information misinterpretation
Pain: itching	Inflammation, vaginal discharge
Sexual dysfunction: dyspareunia	Vaginal inflammation, discomfort from PID

⬛ PLANNING: EXPECTED PATIENT OUTCOMES

Expected patient outcomes for the woman with a gynecologic inflammation may include, but are not limited to, the following:
1. Patient states feeling more comfortable.
2. Patient can describe how infections of the reproductive organs occur and spread.
3. Patient can describe potentially undesirable effects of infections of the reproductive tract.
4. Patient can state signs that indicate improvement or lack of response to therapy.
5. Patient can describe methods to prevent infection of sexual partner.
6. Patient can describe plans for sexual abstinence until inflammation subsides.

⬛ IMPLEMENTATION

Usual methods for medical therapy are given in Table 34-3. Some alternative therapies developed by women are included in Table 34-4.

☐ Assisting with achievement of therapeutic goals
☐ *Medications*

The major types of prescribed medications are antibiotic, antifungal, or amebicidal agents (see the box on p. 1256). The medications should be used by the patient for the prescribed number of days. They may be prescribed to be taken orally, used topically, or as a suppository (to be placed in the vagina) or douche. Douching is also used to apply heat to promote healing by increasing circulation and for comfort. If both heat and topical medications are prescribed, the topical medication is applied after the douche.

☐ *Supportive therapy*

Patients with severe PID are usually hospitalized for intensive therapy. They are usually placed on bed rest in mid-Fowler's position to provide dependent drainage so that abscesses will not form high in the abdomen where they might rupture and cause generalized peritonitis. Fluids are given intravenously to correct dehydration and acidosis.

Table 34-4 Alternative therapies for vaginitis

Infection	Intervention	Dosage	Administration
Monilia	Gentian violet	Few drops/qt water 0.25% to 2% (over-the-counter drug)	Douche or local application
	Vinegar (white)	1 Tbsp/1 pt water	Douche every day for 5 to 7 days; twice daily for 2 days
	Acidophilus culture	2 Tbsp/1 pt water	Douche twice daily
	Acidophilus yogurt	1 application to labia hourly	
	Plain yogurt	and as needed for symptom relief	
Trichomonas	1 handful chapparel chamomile	Steep in 1 qt water for 20 min	Douche 2 to 3 times/wk for 2 wk
Nonspecific vaginitis	Vinegar douche	5 Tbsp/2 qt water	Every other day for 1 wk
	Salt (sea)	1 Tbsp/1 qt water	Every other day for 1 wk
	1 tsp goldenseal and 1 clove minced garlic	Steep in 1 qt boiling water	Douche every day for 1 wk
	1 tsp goldenseal	Steep in 1 pt water; strain through cloth	Douche every day for 1 wk
	Povidone-iodine (Betadine) gel		Twice daily for 1 wk

From Fogel, CI, and Woods, NF: Health care of women: a nursing perspective, St. Louis, 1981, The CV Mosby Co.

Drugs commonly prescribed for inflammations of the female reproductive tract

Drugs	Route
Antibiotic	
Ampicillin	Oral
Procaine penicillin G	Oral
Tetracylcline	Oral
Antifungal	
Clotrimazole (Gyne-Lotrimin)	Vaginal, topical
Micronazole (Monistat)	Vaginal, topical
Nystantin (Mycostatin, Nilstat)	Vaginal, topical, oral
Amebicidal	
Metronidazole (Flagyl)	Oral

☐ *Surgical procedures*

Surgical intervention may be necessary in selected instances as described below.

INCISION AND DRAINAGE OF ABSCESS. An abscess of a Bartholin's gland may need to be incised and drained (I & D). After I&D a small amount of purulent drainage tinged with blood is expected, but any active, bright red bleeding should be reported to the physician. Relief from pain occurs almost immediately after I&D. The woman may experience soreness or mild pain for about a day. Peritoneal irrigations or sitz baths serve the purpose of cleansing and giving comfort. Warm water can be used to cleanse the involved area after each voiding or bowel movement.

CAUTERIZATION OF CERVIX. When cervical lacerations or erosions are present, the area is usually cauterized. Silver nitrate sticks may be used to remove very small lesions. For larger areas requiring cauterization, an electric cautery unit is used. The woman is informed that a small, lubricated sheet of lead will be placed against the skin under the lumbar areas as a safety device for grounding electrical charges and that there will be slight bleeding, which will be controlled by a tampon or packing inserted by the physician. The odor of burning tissue when cautery is used is distressing to some patients. They are told to expect an odor but that the odor is insignificant and that the procedure is over quickly. Slight discomfort may be experienced.

Instructions for follow-up care vary, but usually include the following:

1. Leave the tampon or packing in place as long as the physician advises (usually 8 to 24 hours).
2. Report to the hospital or physician's office if bleeding is excessive (more than occurs during a normal menses).
3. Do not douche or have sexual relations until the next visit to the physician unless specific instructions have been given for resumption of intercourse.
4. An unpleasant discharge caused by sloughing of destroyed cells may appear 4 to 5 days after cauterization; frequent warm baths will help this condition.

REMOVAL OF REPRODUCTIVE ORGANS. If a tubal abscess develops with PID, a salpingectomy (removal of the fallopian tubes) may be necessary. In severe chronic PID

Teaching for the woman with an inflammation of the reproductive tract

1. Knowledge of spread of infection and its effects
2. Application of vaginal medication
   a. Wash hands before and after procedure
   b. Lie down after insertion to facilitate distribution of medication in vagina
   c. Do not douche after insertion of medication
   d. Wear a minipad
3. Sexual intercourse
   a. Abstain, if possible, to prevent discomfort and spread of infection to partner
   b. If abstention not feasible, advise male to use a condom
4. If repeated infections have occurred:
   a. Use an alternative brand of birth control pill or alternative method of control
   b. Use only clean equipment if douches are used
   c. Restrict sexual intercourse
   d. Encourage sexual partner(s) to seek medical attention
5. Report signs of further infection (increased vaginal discharge, bleeding, pain, fever).

---

more reproductive organs may also need to be removed. Surgery of the reproductive tract is discussed on p. 1262.

☐ Assisting with comfort

Itching is the primary discomfort with inflammations of the vulva and vagina. Frequent bathing and sitz baths may be helpful. Soothing lotions may be prescribed. Vinegar douches that decrease the alkalinity of the vagina may also relieve the pruritus.

Pain is the primary discomfort with PID. Heat (hot water bottle or electric heating pad) applied to the abdomen may promote circulation and ease the discomfort. Analgesics are often necessary to relieve the pain.

Dyspareunia (discomfort with intercourse) may be present as a result of inflammation. Abstinence is advised until the inflammation subsides.

☐ Counseling and teaching

Women with PID are usually of childbearing age. If severe or chronic PID is present, infertility may result from adhesions in the fallopian tubes or from removal of reproductive organs. The woman needs opportunities to identify her feelings regarding potential or actual infertility. Many women with inflammations of the reproductive tract can be treated on an ambulatory basis. Women who are hospitalized will require further therapy at home (see the box above).

■ Structural disorders

■ TYPES OF STRUCTURAL DISORDERS

Women may experience problems with relaxation of the vaginal outlet, displacement or prolapse of the uterus, or fistulas that may develop between the bladder or rectum and the vagina (Table 34-5).

■ PATHOPHYSIOLOGY

Most of the structural problems of the reproductive tract experienced by women result primarily from stretching and weakening of the ligaments supporting the uterus or of the muscles of the perineum. When the pelvic supporting tissues are relaxed, the urinary bladder may sag below the uterus and press against the vaginal wall (*cystocele*) (Fig. 34-5). This leads to stress incontinence (see Chapter 32). Similarly the posterior vaginal wall may weaken and the rectum may herniate into the vagina (*rectocele*). The weakened rectal wall predisposes to constipation and hemorrhoids.

The uterus itself may be displaced, either flexed forward (anteflexion) or backward (retroflexion) or tilted backward (retroversion) (Fig. 34-6). In addition the uterus may lose its support and descend (*prolapse*) into the vaginal canal. With complete uterine prolapse, the cervix protrudes beyond the vaginal orifice. Cystoceles, rectoceles, and uterine prolapse are more commonly seen in older women.

Fistulas are abnormal passageways between two organs. *Vesicovaginal fistulas* are openings between the bladder and vagina and lead to leakage of urine through the vagina. Because the vagina does not have a sphincter, urinary incontinence results. *Rectovaginal fistulas*, which are less common, are passageways between the rectum and vagina. These lead to fecal incontinence and uncontrollable flatus expulsion. Both types of fistulas may close spontaneously but frequently need to be repaired surgically. If so, 3 to 4 months are required for the inflammation to subside before surgery can be attempted.

■ ASSESSMENT

Women with structural disorders of the reproductive tract often experience low-grade discomfort in the pelvic

Table 34-5   Structural problems of the female reproductive tract

Disorder	Etiology	Signs and symptoms	Medical therapy
Relaxed vaginal outlet	Unrepaired childbirth lacerations, loss of pelvic muscle tone from repeated pregnancies or congenital weakness	Dragging pain in back of pelvis, stress incontinence, constipation, hemorrhoids	Plastic surgery
Uterine displacement	Congenital, PID, endometriosis, pregnancy, pelvic tumors, trauma	May be asymptomatic; dysmenorrhea, backache	Postural exercises, vaginal pessary
Uterine prolapse	Childbirth injuries, muscle relaxation due to age	Bearing down sensation, backache	Vaginal pessary, hysterectomy
Fistulas	Radiation of cervix, gynecologic surgery, trauma during childbirth	Vaginal leakage of urine, gas, or feces	Surgical removal of fistula (fistulectomy)

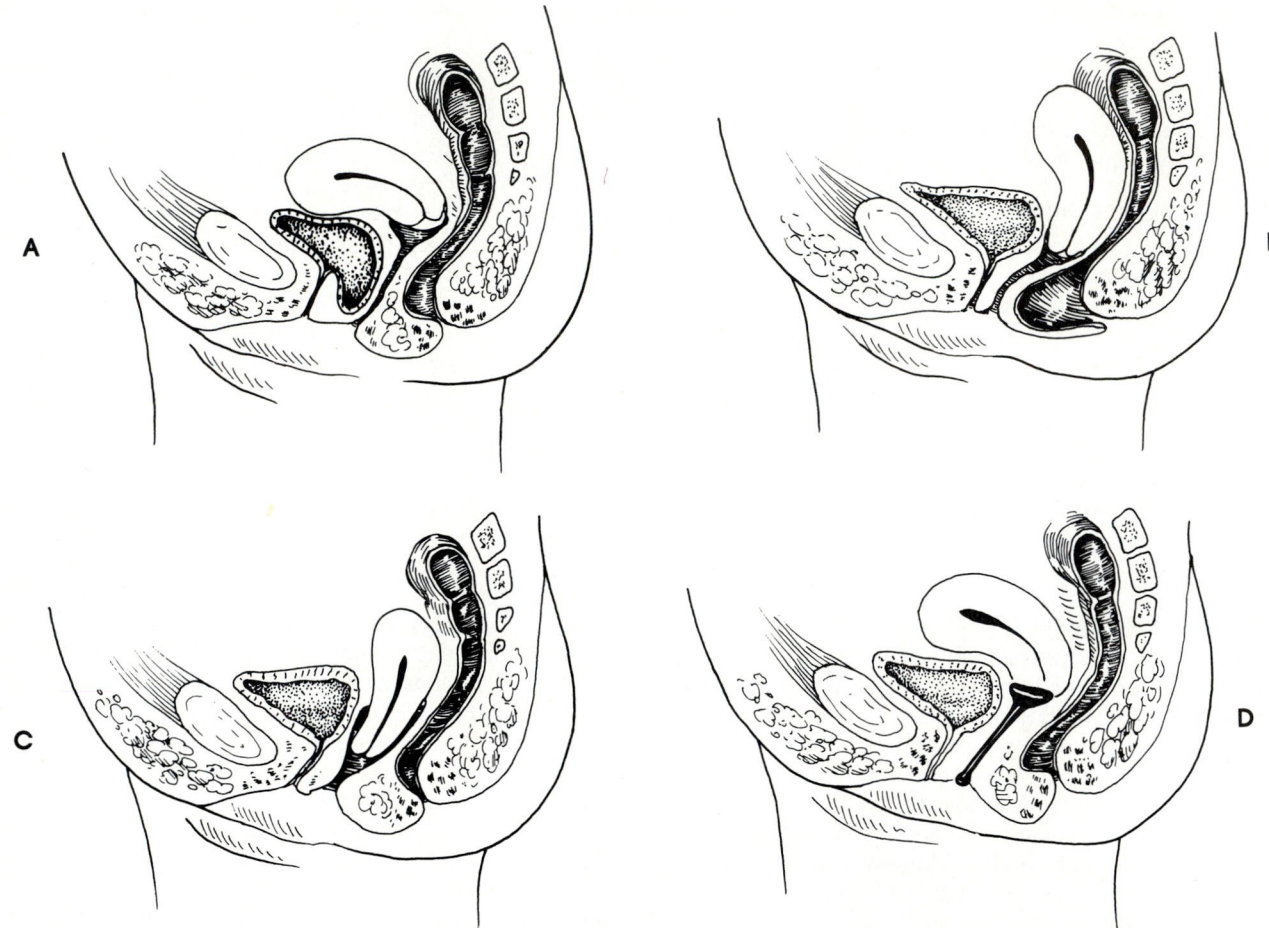

Fig. 34-5   Abnormalities of vagina. **A,** Cystocele: downward displacement of bladder toward vaginal orifice. **B,** Rectocele: pouching of rectum into posterior wall of vagina. **C,** Prolapse of uterus into vaginal canal. **D,** Stem pessary in place to maintain normal anatomic position of uterus.

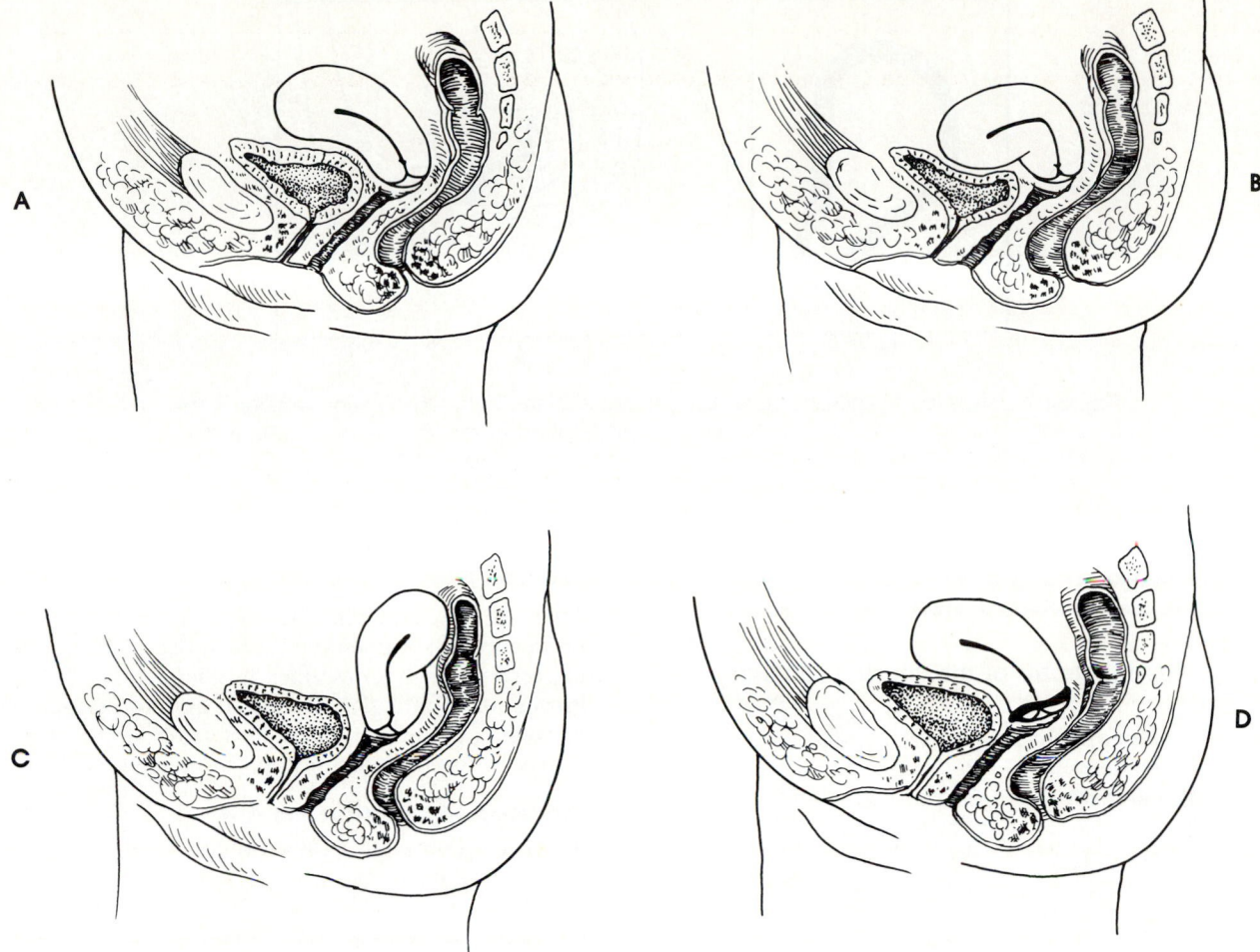

Fig. 34-6 Normal and abnormal positions of uterus. **A,** Normal anatomic position of uterus in relation to adjacent structures. **B,** Anterior displacement of uterus. **C,** Retroversion, or backward displacement, of uterus. **D,** Normal anatomic position of uterus maintained by use of rubber S-shaped pessary.

area and back. In addition, problems with urinary or fecal control may be present. Data to be collected if incontinence is present include the following:

1. Extent of incontinence
2. Pattern of incontinence: incontinence from a cystocele is intermittent, occurring mostly during stress (such as laughing or crying); incontinence from fistulas is continual seeping
3. Usual methods of coping (for example, use of pads, plastic pants, avoidance of fluids before social occasions)
4. Feelings regarding incontinence

➡ DATA ANALYSIS: NURSING DIAGNOSES

Nursing diagnoses are determined from assessment of patient data. Possible nursing diagnoses for the woman with a gynecologic structural disorder may include, but are not limited to, the following:

Diagnostic title	Possible etiologies
Stress incontinence	Relaxed pelvic muscles
Pain: backache	Vaginal or uterine structural disorders

◱ PLANNING: EXPECTED PATIENT OUTCOMES

Expected patient outcomes for the woman with a gynecologic structural disorder may include, but are not limited to, the following:

1. Woman states feeling comfortable.
2. Woman performs self-care measures to manage the condition.
3. Woman seeks help from a health professional when appropriate.

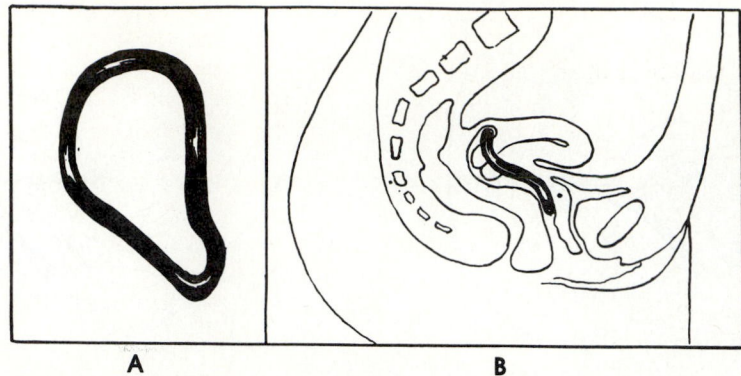

Fig. 34-7 **A,** Albert Smith pessary. **B,** Pessary in place to hold posterior vaginal fornix, and with it attached cervix, well backward and upward in pelvis. (From Beacham, DW, and Beacham, WD: Synopsis of gynecology, ed 10, St. Louis, 1982, The CV Mosby Co.)

Surgeries for repair of structural problems

Anterior colporrhaphy	Repair of cystocele
Posterior colporrhaphy	Repair of rectocele
Marshall-Marchetti	Suspension of bladder in correct position
Fistulectomy	Removal of fistula
Stami procedure	Small incision made through cystoscope to elevate urethra

---

 IMPLEMENTATION

□ Assisting with achievement of therapeutic goals

If symptoms are severe enough to interfere with the woman's ability to function effectively, the primary medical therapies are the use of a *pessary* (plastic ring inserted to support the uterus [Fig. 34-7]) or *surgery* to repair weakened muscles and walls or fistulas (see the box above).

□ *Preoperative care*

If the rectum is involved, preoperative laxatives and enemas are usually given to reduce bowel contents. Clear liquids are given 24 hours before surgery.

□ *Postoperative care*

Repair may be accomplished vaginally or through a suprapubic incision. In the latter method, a suprapubic tube may be inserted and maintained for several days to permit healing (see Chapter 32). An indwelling urethral catheter is inserted after anterior colporrhaphy to keep the bladder empty and to allow edema to subside to prevent pressure on the incison.

After surgery involving the rectum, laxatives may be given to prevent strain on the incision. Care of the patient after rectal surgery is described in Chapter 31.

Prevention of infection is effected by good perineal care after voiding or defecation. A heat lamp at the perineal area may be used for comfort and to promote healing.

□ **Assisting with comfort and ADL**

Pain from structural disorders is usually low grade. Aspirin and acetaminophen usually suffice as analgesics, if required.

Psychologic discomfort related to incontinence is usually more of a problem. The woman can be helped to explore her feelings about the incontinence and possible effects on sexual functioning. Before surgery is planned, alternative methods of keeping dry can be explored. For a vesicovaginal fistula, a menstrual rubber cap (Tassette) may be attached to a catheter and leg bag urinal. For stress incontinence, menstrual pads or padded plastic pants may be helpful.

Dribbling of fecal matter into the vagina from a rectovaginal fistula is particularly distressing and may be temporarily lessened by a high enema; this is useful prior to social situations. Constipating diets to decrease fecal leakage are not useful because they eventually cause pressure that may aggravate the condition and increase the size of the fistula.

□ **Counseling and teaching**

Kegel exercises can be learned by women to help prevent stress incontinence and prolapse of the uterus, bladder or rectum. The Kegel muscle is a major support muscle for the pelvic floor. The muscle surrounds the urethra, vagina, and rectum; it may be felt by placing a finger along the upper vaginal wall while tightening the perineum. Because the muscle may lose tone if not exercised, women are encouraged to do Kegel exercises 100 times a day for life. Kegel exercises consist of tightening the Kegel muscle and holding the contraction for a count of 10, then relaxing; it is repeated 100 times.[20]

Preoperative and postoperative teaching include the following:

1. Preoperative
   a. Do Kegel exercises as instructed.
   b. Do pelvic exercises to assist in repositioning of uterus:
      (1) Knee-chest position for 5 minutes three times a day
      (2) Lie on abdomen 2 hours a day
   c. Seek medical consultation for symptoms of lower abdominal pain or incontinence.
2. Postoperative
   a. Use douches or mild laxatives as prescribed (gently inserting douche nozzle).
   b. Avoid heavy lifting, prolonged standing or sexual intercourse until permitted (usually about 6 weeks).
   c. Expect loss of vaginal sensation for several months (normal response).
   d. Avoid enemas after rectal surgery until healing is complete.
   e. Report signs of infection or pain to physician.

■ Tumors

■ BENIGN TUMORS

Many different types of benign neoplasms affect the female reproductive tract. The more common sites for these tumors are the ovaries or myometrium of the uterus (Table 34-6).

□ Ovarian tumors

Most ovarian tumors are benign and are often asymptomatic. There are numerous types depending on the site and tissue involved. Ovarian cysts occur frequently. Simple cysts are thin-walled structures containing serous fluid and are often seen during menopause. Corpus luteum cysts result from an exaggeration of the process of formation and resorption of the corpus luteum. Follicle cysts arise during the evolution or involution of the graafian follicle. Cysts do not become malignant. Severe pain may result if a cyst becomes twisted on its pedicle, and the symptoms may resemble appendicitis.

Polycystic ovarian disease (Stein-Levanthal) is characterized by enlargement of the ovaries, with numerous cystic follicles encased in a fibrotic capsule. Effects of these tumors are often not noted unless there is compresson of a neighboring organ or blood supply, a menstrual disorder, or infertility.

□ Endometriosis

Endometriosis is a condition in which endometrial cells that normally line the uterus are seeded throughout the pelvis and occasionally extend to as distant a location as the umbilicus (Fig. 34-8). With each menstrual period the endometrial cells are stimulated by the ovarian hormones and bleed into the surrounding areas, causing an inflammation. Subsequent adhesions may be so severe that pelvic organs become fused together, occasionally causing a stricture of the bowel or interference with bladder function. Encased blood may lead to palpable tumor masses, which often occur on the ovary and are known as *chocolate cysts.* Occasionally these cysts rupture and spread endometrial cells still farther throughout the pelvis.

Usually endometriosis progresses gradually and does not produce symptoms until the age of 30 to 40 years. Occasionally, however, symptoms appear when the woman is in her teens. Approximately half of the women with endometriosis are infertile, and endometriosis is sometimes first detected when a woman complains of inability to conceive.

If the woman is young and wants children, the treatment for endometriosis is usually as conservative as possible. Pregnancy is beneficial, because menstruation ceases during this time. If a young woman has endometriosis, she and her husband usually are advised to have their family

Table 34-6 Benign tumors of the female reproductive tract

Type	Signs and symptoms	Medical therapy
Ovarian tumors and cysts	Increased abdominal size; fatigue; sense of pelvic fullness	Oral contraceptives for suspected cysts Ovarian cystectomy Oophorectomy
Endometriosis	Pain that increases in severity during menstruation, dyspareunia, irregular menstrual cycles	Antiovulation drugs (oral contraceptives, danazol), analgesics Surgery: younger than 35 years, resection of lesions; older than 35 years, total hysterectomy, salpingectomy, oophorectomy
Uterine fibroid tumors	Menorrhagia, low back pain, dysmenorrhea, constipation, irregular enlarged uterus	Small tumors: no treatment Severe symptoms or rapidly growing tumors: myomectomy or hysterectomy
Cervical polyps	Leukorrhea, abnormal vaginal bleeding	Surgical removal (polypectomy)

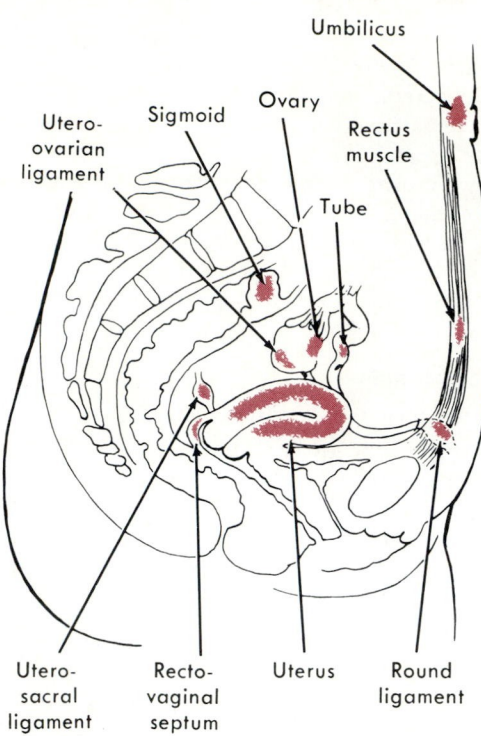

Fig. 34-8 Sites of endometrial implants.

early, because the fertility rate is low, sterility caused by adhesions may occur, and a hysterectomy may have to be done within a reasonable period of time. Nursing the infant is also recommended because it delays the onset of menstruation after delivery. Menopause stops the progress of this condition.

☐ Uterine fibroid tumors

Fibroid tumors are the most common tumors of the female genital tract. They are discrete benign tumors of the uterine muscle and connective tissue. The sizes of myomas are variable. Most are found in the body of the uterus (corporeal) but some occur in the cervix or may involve the broad ligament. Submucous tumors may impinge on the blood vessels of the endometrium and produce bleeding. As they grow larger they may impinge on the opposite uterine wall and distort the cavity of the uterus. In some instances submucous tumors develop pedicles and may protrude through the vagina or cervix, resulting in infection or ulcerations.

Fibroid tumors of the uterus tend to disappear spontaneously with menopause. They rarely become malignant. Infertility may result from a myoma that obstructs or distorts the uterus or fallopian tubes. Myoma in the body of the uterus may cause spontaneous abortions, and those near the cervical opening may make the delivery of a baby difficult and may contribute to hemorrhage postpartally. Myomectomy is the procedure of choice during childbearing years.

☐ Cervical polyps

Cervical polyps form when an area of the mucosa proliferates. These growths are usually visible at the cervical os as bright red, vascular, fragile areas. They are most often pedunculated and appear to protrude from the cervical canal. Polyps may occur singly or in clusters.

Because of the vascularity of the polyp, bleeding is a common symptom. The bleeding is small in amount and occurs between menstrual periods and closely resembles that of early cancer of the cervix. Especially characteristic is the contact bleeding produced by coitus, by douching, or by vaginal examination.

The pedicle by which the polyp is attached is usually quite small, and the polyp can easily be removed by twisting the pedicle at its base or by biopsy. Tissue examination of removed polyps is essential because epidermoid cancer arises from cervical polyps in a small percentage of cases.

■ SURGERY OF THE REPRODUCTIVE TRACT

☐ Types of surgery

Minor surgical procedures are performed primarily for diagnostic purposes. Major surgery involves removal of one or more reproductive organs (see the box on p. 1263).

☐ *Minor procedures*

PREOPERATIVE CARE. Dilation and curettage (D and C) is the standard procedure for investigating any irregular bleeding. In addition it may be performed to correct a cervical stricture or to treat dysmenorrhea. Cervical biopsy and conization of the cervix are done to test for the presence of malignancy. All of these procedures may be performed on an outpatient basis. Cervical biopsy does not require anesthesia, whereas local or general anesthesia may be used for D and C or conization. The usual preoperative preparation is given; shaving is rarely required.

POSTOPERATIVE CARE
VAGINAL BLEEDING

Bleeding is monitored every 15 minutes for 2 hours and then as necessary thereafter. The blood loss is best recorded in estimated milliliters. A blood loss of at least 60 ml is required to saturate a perineal pad. It is important to record each pad change as well as blood loss. Any excessive bleeding is reported to the physician. More blood is lost by conization of the cervix than with the other procedures, and oozing may be controlled by packing inserted at the time of surgery.

DISCOMFORT

Mild abdominal cramping may be experienced postoperatively. Mild analgesics such as codeine sulfate and acetylsalicylic acid are usually ordered to relieve pain. Abdominal pain after D and C that is continuous, sharp, and not relieved by analgesics should be reported immediately to the surgeon; this type of pain may indicate perforation of the uterus.

Surgeries of the female reproductive tract

Procedure	Description
Minor procedures	
Dilation and curettage (D and C)	Dilation of the cervix and scraping of uterine walls
Cervical biopsy	Punch biopsy of the cervix
Conization of cervix	Removal of cone-shaped portion of cervix
Major procedures	
Oophorectomy	Removal of ovaries
Salpingectomy	Removal of fallopian tubes
Hysterectomy (vaginal, abdominal)	Removal of uterus, either through the vagina or abdomen
Radical hysterectomy	Removal of uterus, upper vagina, and parametrium
Pelvic exenteration	Removal of pelvic viscera (bladder, rectosigmoid) and all reproductive organs

---

TEACHING

1. Rest more than usual for first 24 hours postoperatively.
2. Avoid heavy lifting or marked exertion for 4 weeks.
3. Leave tampon or packing in place as advised (usually 8 to 24 hours).
4. Report to physician bleeding that is more than usually experienced during normal menses.
5. No douches or sexual intercourse until advised by physician.

□ Major procedures

PREOPERATIVE CARE. Preparation of the patient for gynecologic surgery is similar to that for major abdominal surgery. Functioning of other systems within the pelvis (urinary, intestinal) is evaluated, particularly if there are any symptoms of dysfunction.

PSYCHOLOGIC PREPARATION

Removal of reproductive organs can significantly affect the woman emotionally, and time may be needed to help her adjust to the proposed changes. The reproductive organs are a major component of "womanhood," and loss of these organs creates a change in body image. Women see menstrual functioning as a symbol of femininity; therefore, with sudden cessation of menstruation some women state feelings of being "less of a woman."

Feelings of sexuality in terms of sexual relations are also threatened. Some women worry that sexual relations may be hindered or be less satisfactory. In actuality, many women find after hysterectomy that sexual relations are enhanced because fear of pregnancy has been removed. Except in rare instances of pelvic exenteration, sexual intercourse is possible after healing has occurred.

Women who experience some difficulties in adjusting may be those of childbearing age and those at menopause.

The latter are still adjusting to life's changes and may be at a crisis period in their life. The nurse's role is to help the woman explore her feelings and to correct myths or misunderstandings before surgery to facilitate an easier recovery.

PHYSIOLOGIC PREPARATION

Close proximity of the urinary tract and bowel to the reproductive organs requires measures to prevent infection. Preoperative measures are also taken to prevent postoperative thromboembolism:

1. Antibiotics to treat or prevent infection
2. Bowel preparation if bowel will be involved
   a. Mechanical cleansing (laxatives, enemas)
   b. Liquid diet for 24 hours
3. Medicated douches if there is high risk of infection
4. Persons at high risk for thrombophlebitis (varicose veins, obesity, diabetes mellitus)
   a. Low-dose heparin
   b. Support stockings
   c. Discontinuation of oral contraceptives 3 to 4 weeks preoperatively.

POSTOPERATIVE CARE. General care of the patient after major gynecologic surgery is essentially the same as that after abdominal surgery. Measures to prevent respiratory complications are important. Fluid and electrolyte balance is monitored carefully.

PREVENTION OF THROMBOEMBOLISM

Thrombophlebitis and pulmonary embolism are major postoperative complications after pelvic surgery as a result of venous stasis in the major pelvic veins. Symptoms may be absent until signs of pulmonary embolism occur (chest pain, hemoptysis) 1 week later. Because the involved veins are usually deep in the thigh, the only local symptoms may be pain and swelling in the thigh and a positive Homan's sign (pain with dorsiflexion of foot). Preventive activities are described in the box below.

URINARY COMPLICATIONS

Urinary *retention* is a common occurrence after gynecologic surgery as a result of handling of the bladder during surgery. An indwelling urinary catheter is usually inserted for 3 to 5 days postoperatively until muscle function returns. Suprapubic drainage by means of a small polyethylene catheter introduced into the bladder by means of a large-bore needle or trocar may be used in place of the standard urethral catheter. Urinary *infection* (a common postoperative occurrence) is minimized with use of suprapubic drainage.

Urinary *fistula* may result despite careful surgical technique. It is identified by leakage of urine through the vagina. Many such fistulas close spontaneously. The woman may be placed on her stomach and gentle intermittent suction applied to the indwelling catheter to encourage healing of the fistula.[3]

Nursing care of a woman undergoing major gynecologic surgery

Preoperative care

1. Identify patient's understanding of planned surgical procedure and correct misunderstandings
2. Encourage and support self-exploration of feelings related to proposed surgery
3. Provide support stockings for persons at high risk for thromboembolism
4. Teach breathing and leg exercises

Postoperative care

1. Monitor
   a. Fluid and electrolyte balance
   b. Breath sounds and respiratory excursion
   c. Abdominal distention
   d. Pain in abdomen
   e. Pain in thighs
   f. Dressing
   g. Signs of urinary tract infection
2. Encourage breathing exercises every 2 to 4 hours until patient becomes active
3. Urinary drainage
   a. Maintain patency of indwelling urinary catheter
   b. When catheter removed, monitor for leakage of urine in vagina (signs of urinary fistula)
4. Provide pain medication through third postoperative day on a fairly regular schedule, then as needed thereafter
5. For gas pains, apply heat (hot water bottle, electric heating pad) to abdomen, encourage ambulation, try a rectal tube
6. Prevent thrombophlebitis
   a. Teach patient to avoid sharp flexion of knee or thighs; no pillows under knees
   b. Continue support stockings for patients at high risk
   c. Encourage leg exercises every hour while awake until ambulating freely
   d. Lower head of bed to flat position for a short time every 2 hours for 24 hours, then every 4 hours until ambulating freely
   e. Encourage walking, increasing distance
7. Continue providing emotional support
8. Teach patient
   a. Resume home activities gradually
   b. Car riding permitted after first week at home, but no driving for 3 to 4 weeks, especially with standard shift car
   c. Avoid heavy lifting, riding over rough roads, walking swiftly, jogging, or dancing (activities that tend to cause pelvic blood congestion) for 6 to 8 weeks
   d. Resume preoperative sexual activities such as cuddling or closeness immediately
   e. Resume sexual intercourse in 4 to 6 weeks
   f. Report immediately to physician any signs of thromboembolism
   g. Return for postoperative medical evaluations as instructed

GASTROINTESTINAL PROBLEMS

Gastrointestinal function usually returns 24 to 72 hours after surgery, depending on the extent of handling of the intestines. Persistent nausea and vomiting with severe abdominal distention may indicate ileus, and all oral intake is stopped and a nasogastric tube inserted. Most patients, however, have return of function. Abdominal distention with abdominal cramping may result from collection of gas in the sluggish bowel. Ambulation and heat encourage expulsion of the gas (see Chapter 31).

PSYCHOLOGIC SUPPORT

Postoperatively, almost all patients feel depressed for several days. The patient often is unable to explain why she is depressed and crying. Grieflike responses to loss of a body part may appear as they do after loss of other body parts. Feelings of guilt, shame, and remorse are common. Encouraging the woman to continue activities associated with being feminine, such as using makeup, arranging her hair, and wearing her own clothing, often helps the woman to regain her feminine perspective. During this time she needs understanding and empathic care. Families may need to be helped to accept these responses calmly, and a husband may need help in understanding her need for reassurance of his continued love and affection.

■ Cancer

Malignancies in the female reproductive tract occur primarily in the uterus (cervix and endometrium) and in the ovaries (Table 34-7); they may also occur, although less frequently, in the vagina or vulva. Cancer of the reproductive tract now ranks third to cancer of the breast and colorectum in females.[2]

The death rate from cancer of the *cervix* has fallen steadily over the past 40 years. This decline has been attributed to early detection through annual examinations (including a Papanicolau smear) and improved surgical and radiotherapeutic techniques. Cancer of the cervix identified and treated early at the preinvasive stage is 100% curable, thus *early detection* (p. 1244) *is vitally important.*

The incidence of *endometrial* cancer is not decreasing significantly partly because it is primarily a disease of postmenopausal women and women are living longer.

Cancer of the *ovary* has had a steady slow *increase* in incidence but appears to be leveling off.[2] Because it is asymptomatic in the early stages, it is often far advanced before diagnosis is made. The only effective means of assuring early diagnosis is a pelvic examination every 6 months, including careful ovarian palpation, and surgical exploration of any questionable ovarian growth. The Pap test does *not* reveal ovarian cancer.

■ PATHOPHYSIOLOGY

□ Cancer of the cervix

Most cervical cancers are squamous carcinomas that arise in the intraepithelial layers (preinvasive stage or carcinoma in situ). It usually takes 2 to 10 years for squamous cell carcinoma to become invasive beyond the basement membrane. Spread usually occurs by direct extension or by means of the lymph system. Therapy depends on the stage (extent of spread) (Table 34-8).

□ Cancer of the endometrium

Cancer of the endometrium is primarily a slow-growing adenocarcinoma. Because it occurs mostly in postmenopausal women, estrogen stimulation unopposed by progesterone is thought to be implicated. Prolonged use of estrogen without addded progestin during menopause increases the risk of endometrial cancer. Cancer of the endometrium is usually diagnosed when the postmenopausal woman seeks medical care for vaginal bleeding. Although the incidence is twice that for cancer of the cervix, the death rate is lower.

Table 34-7   Cancer of the female reproductive tract

Site	Incidence	Usual age (yr)	Signs and symptoms	Medical therapy
Cervix	2.5%	30 to 50	Early: may be asymptomatic, vaginal discharge, spotting between menses Late: dark, foul vaginal discharge, pain	Conization of cervix for cancer in situ in young women; hysterectomy, radiation (internal, external)
Endometrium	8%	50 to 70	Early: postmenopausal bleeding Late: uterine enlargement, pain	Hysterectomy and bilateral salpingo-oophorectomy, radiation (internal, external), progestin for metastases
Ovary	4%	All ages	Early: asymptomatic Late: ascities, edema of legs, pain	Salpingo-oophorectomy; hysterectomy may also be necessary; chemotherapy, radiation

Table 34-8 Stages of cancer of female reproductive tract

Stage	Cervix	Endometrium	Ovary
0	Confined to epithelium	Confined to epithelium	–
I	Confined to cervix	Confined to corpus	Confined to ovary
II	Extends outside cervix but does not involve pelvic wall or lower third of vagina	Involves corpus and cervix	Involves ovaries with pelvic extension
III	Involves pelvic wall and lower third of vagina	Involves pelvic and vaginal wall (but not bladder or rectum)	Intraperitoneal metastases
IV	Involves bladder, rectum, or metastatic spread	Involves bladder, rectum, or metastatic spread	Involves metastatic spread

Cancer of the ovary

Ovarian cancer causes more deaths than cancer of the uterus. The pathophysiology of ovarian cancer is complex, and there are a great variety of tumors. The ovaries may be a site of metastasis from the gastrointestinal tract, breast, pancreas, or kidneys. The risk for ovarian cancer increases with age, with the highest rates for women aged 65 to 84.[2]

DIAGNOSTIC TESTS

Pelvic examinations

Pelvic examinations are useful for visualization of changes in the vulva, vagina, and cervix; for palpation of internal organs, especially the ovaries and surface of the uterus; and for obtaining Pap smears.

Women are advised to avoid douching and applying any vaginal preparation (medicinal or deodorant) for at least 24 hours before examination. They should void immediately before the examination, because an empty bladder makes palpation of the pelvic organs easier, decreases patient discomfort, and eliminates possible distortion of the position of pelvic organs caused by a full bladder. The technique for performing pelvic examinations is described in most physical examination texts.

After the pelvic examination a woman may need assistance in removing her legs from the stirrups and getting down from the table. Elderly women merit careful assistance after the pelvic examination because unnatural positions, such as the knee-chest and lithotomy positions, may alter the normal circulation of blood sufficiently to cause faintness.

Papanicolaou (Pap) test

The Pap test is a cytologic test that makes it possible to detect abnormal cells, not all of which are cancerous. However, the Pap test has made it possible through routine use to detect precancerous conditions and cancer of the cervix early enough to make treatment of these conditions almost 100% successful. For detection of atypical cells, the Pap test is 95% accurate. False negative reports are most frequently the result of an inadequate sample or improperly fixed slide (see the box at right).

The Pap test involves microscopic examination of cells collected from the vaginal pool, exocervix, and endocervical canal. Samples of cells are obtained by using a vaginal pipette with a rubber tip and a specially designed wooden spatula. Secretions containing exfoliated cells are preferably obtained from the cervix or external os.

Glass slides should be labeled and ready for use. A solution of 95% alcohol and ether in a wide-mouthed jar is used because rapid fixation of the smear is essential. The secretions are collected, smeared on the glass slide, and immediately placed back to back in the fixative solution to prevent drying out and cell distortion.

Do-it-yourself Pap tests are available. These can be used by women who are reluctant or unable to visit a physician for examination.

Obtaining endometrial cells for study

The Pap test is not ideal for detecting endometrial cancer, although samples may be obtained by cervical aspiration when performing a Pap test. Less than half of women with uterine cancer have an abnormal Pap test result at the time of routine Pap test screening. Probably the main reason the Pap test is inadequate is that cells rarely ex-

---

Guidelines for Pap tests

1. Ideal time for a Pap test is 5 to 6 days after menstrual termination.
2. Avoid tub bath or douche for 48 hours before the test.
3. Delay a Pap test for at least 1 month after use of *topical* antibiotics (produce rapid, heavy shedding of cells).
4. Slight vaginal bleeding (spotting) after the test may occur; excessive bleeding should be reported to the physician.
5. Medications such as tetracycline or digitalis may alter the results.[13]

Endoscopic procedures for visualization of pelvic organs

Colposcopy   Visualization of vagina and cervix under low-power magnification
Culdoscopy   Insertion of a culdoscope through posterior vaginal vault into cul-de-sac of Douglas for visualization of fallopian tubes and ovaries
Hysteroscopy   Insertion of a hysteroscope through the cervix for visualization of inside of the uterus
Laparoscopy   Insertion of a laparoscope (under local anesthesia) through small incision in abdominal wall (inferior margin of umbilicus), which is insufflated with carbon dioxide; permits visualization of all pelvic organs (Fig. 34-9)

---

foliate from the endometrium in the early stages of uterine cancer.

One method of obtaining endometrial cells for study is by *vacuum curettage*. The procedure and apparatus used for vacuum curettage are similar to those used in suction curettage for performing an abortion, except that the curette is much thinner. With the patient under general anesthesia, the cervix is dilated and the suction tip is inserted through the cervix into the uterus. Suction is applied and the entire uterine cavity is suctioned to secure specimens. Vacuum curettage is considered to be at least as good as conventional endometrial biopsy for diagnosing endometrial cancer.

An *endometrial biopsy* is performed by presenting a small curette into the uterus and obtaining several strips of endometrial tissue. The specimens are taken from several sites of the uterine cavity to increase the chances of ob-

taining malignant cells. For diagnosis of endometrial cancer, the biopsy method is considered to be about 90% accurate.

☐ Ultrasound

Ultrasound has become a useful diagnostic tool for gynecologic problems. It can be used to locate pelvic masses, displaced IUDs, ectopic pregnancies, and prostatic neoplasms.

☐ Endoscopy

The pelvic organs and surrounding tissues can be directly visualized by endoscopy. Endoscopic procedures include colposcopy, culdoscopy, peritoneoscopy (laparoscopy), and hysteroscopy (see the box above). The most common procedure is the laparoscopy (Fig. 34-9). De-

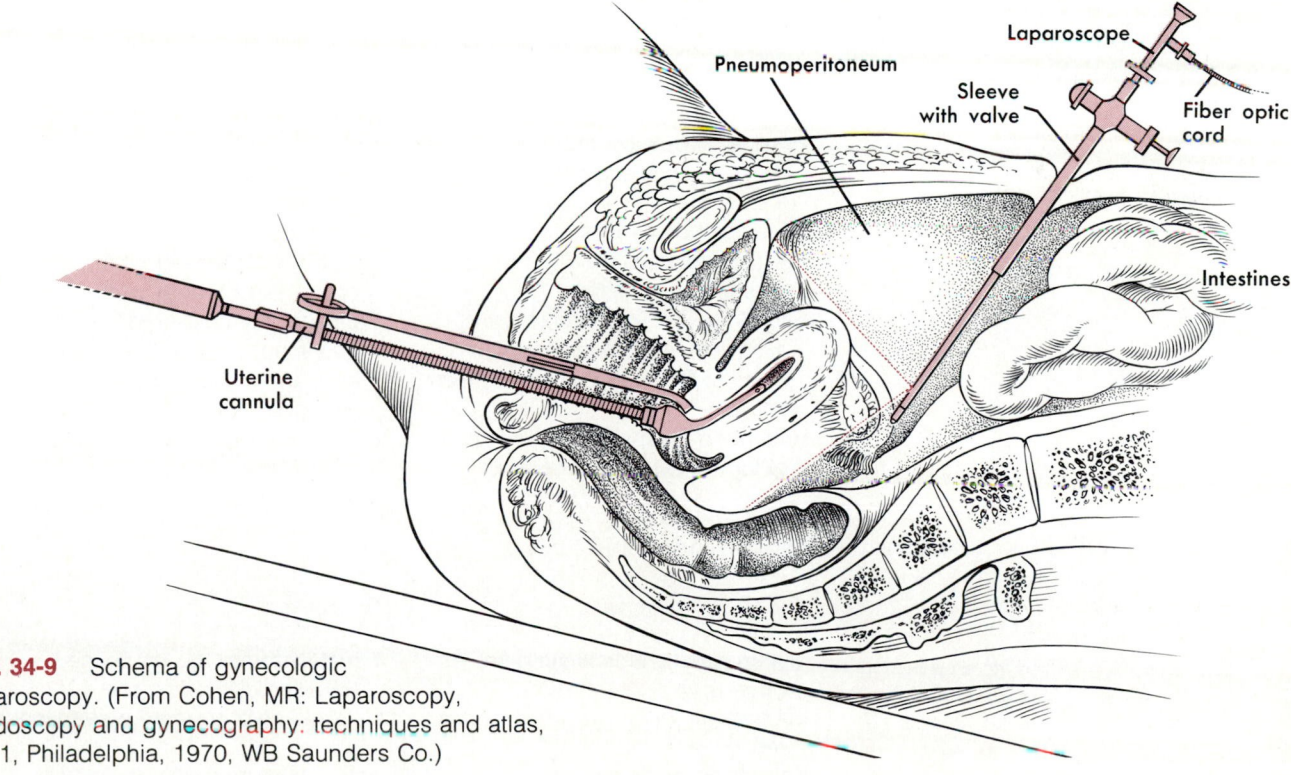

Fig. 34-9   Schema of gynecologic laparoscopy. (From Cohen, MR: Laparoscopy, culdoscopy and gynecography: techniques and atlas, vol 1, Philadelphia, 1970, WB Saunders Co.)

Care of the woman after hysterectomy for cervical cancer

DATA: Mrs. Conn, age 42, saw her gynecologist 2 weeks ago because of bleeding between periods and occasional postcoital bleeding. The result of her Pap smear 5 years previously had been negative. The Pap smear this time was positive and a cervical biopsy confirmed cancer of the cervix, stage I. She was admitted yesterday for a total hysterectomy.

Admission notes indicate that Mrs. Conn is married and has two teenagers, a boy and a girl. Her husband accompanied her to the hospital and appeared to be supportive. Mrs. Conn is a bank teller and likes to read, knit, and watch TV. She has varicose veins but states these do not bother her. Her preoperative concerns centered mainly on the cancer: "I hope they get it all." She also stated, "Well, at least I hadn't planned any more children. My boy joked and said, 'You're going to be neutered like our cat was!' I wonder how it feels to be so-called neutered. I hope it won't affect my sex life." The nurse explored Mrs. Conn's knowledge of the surgery and explained that the surgery would not physically affect sexual relationships.

Mrs. Conn returned from the recovery room alert with an IV running and stable vital signs. The dressing was dry. She had an order for morphine sulfate (MS) 0.010 q3h prn and received a half-dose in the recovery room. Monitoring activities included checking vital signs, breath sounds, urinary output, fluid intake, and dressing checks.

Nursing diagnosis: abdominal, related to abdominal incision

Expected patient outcomes	Nursing interventions	Rationale
Patient states feeling more comfortable	Give analgesic on a regular basis for first 24 h, then as necessary	Giving the analgesic regularly will prevent severe pain and thus be more effective; morphine sulfate (MS) also reduces anxiety
	Encourage frequent changes of position in bed and early ambulation	Activity decreases pain by increasing circulation and reducing muscle tension; ambulation will also encourage peristalsis, decreasing possibility of gas pains

Nursing diagnosis: Body image disturbance: potential, related to loss of uterus

Expected patient outcomes	Nursing interventions	Rationale
Patient verbalizes concerns about loss of uterus	Provide patient opportunities to express feelings and concerns about loss of uterus	Patient may feel freer to talk about her feelings if opportunities are provided
	Be empathetic about patient's feelings, which may include grief, guilt, shame, or remorse	Feelings associated with grief may also be expressed when grieving over loss of a body part
	Encourage her to continue activities associated with femininity, such as fixing hair, makeup, wearing own apparel	Feelings of femininity will emphasize "feminine" rather than "neuter," and that she herself has not changed
	Help her make plans for resumption of former activities	If life pattern is not changed, her thoughts about her body changes may diminish

Nursing diagnosis: Constipation: potential, related to pelvic surgery

Expected patient outcomes	Nursing interventions	Rationale
Stool is soft and formed	Monitor stool characteristics and frequency	Peristalsis may be decreased from handling of pelvic viscera
	Encourage oral fluids when permitted	Hydration will promote a soft stool
	Encourage ambulation	Ambulation promotes peristalsis

Care of the woman after hysterectomy for cervical cancer—cont'd

Nursing diagnosis: Altered patterns of urinary elimination: related to pelvic surgery

Expected patient outcomes	Nursing interventions	Rationale
Patient voids in sufficient quantities	Monitor urinary output until she voids sufficiently Monitor for distention above symphysis pubis and for lower abdominal discomfort other than incisional pain	Handling of bladder during pelvic surgery may decrease bladder muscle tone, leading to urinary retention (Mrs. Conn did not have an indwelling catheter)

Nursing diagnosis: Altered peripheral tissue perfusion: potential, related to pelvic venous stasis from surgery

Expected patient outcomes	Nursing interventions	Rationale
No leg or thigh pain occurs	Monitor for discomfort in legs/thighs	Early detection will ensure early treatment of thrombophlebitis
	Encourage leg exercises and frequent turning in bed until ambulating well	Exercises promote venous return (muscle pumps)
	Avoid use of knee gatch or pillows under knees; encourage patient to keep knees flat when in bed	Pressure on popliteal veins or sharp knee flexion may increase venous stasis
	Encourage patient to lie completely flat in bed for short periods q2h for 24 h, then q4h until ambulating well	Lying flat for periods of time will help blood return from the pelvic veins
	Encourage ambulation	Ambulation promotes venous return (muscle pumps)
	Provide antiembolic stockings	Mrs. Conn is at higher risk for thrombophlebitis because of varicose veins (sluggish circulation) and sedentary life pattern

Nursing diagnosis: Knowledge deficit: related to surgery

Expected patient outcomes	Nursing interventions	Rationale
Patient describes self-care	Teach patient: When activities can be resumed (see text)	Activities are resumed gradually to permit healing; heavy activities are avoided for 6-8 weeks
	Signs of thrombophlebitis to be monitored and reported	Thrombophlebitis may occur 7-10 days postoperatively, after patient goes home
	Signs of vaginal bleeding to be reported	Bleeding could indicate impaired healing
	Need for medical follow-up	To ensure that metastasis has not occurred
	Reinforce the preoperative explanations of the surgery and effect on sexual relationships	Preoperative anxiety may have decreased her awareness; hysterectomy does not interfere with satisfactory sexual relationships
	Find out what she has told her daughter about regular Pap smears	Regular Pap smears enhance early detection of cervical cancer
	Suggest she use support hose in her job as a bank teller	Preventive measure for thrombophlebitis because of her varicose veins

pending on the organs and structures inspected, these methods are valuable for determining the cause of abnormal bleeding, in evaluating the stage of malignancies, and for inspecting organs for size, shape, and position.

Most of the procedures used for visualizing the pelvic organs can be performed on an outpatient basis; this allows the physician to schedule the procedure at the appropriate time of the menstrual cycle.

Maintaining asepsis throughout any of the endoscopic procedures is important in preventing infection. Air may enter the abdominal cavity during the procedures and cause discomfort; a prone position with a pillow under the abdomen may increase comfort. Douching and intercourse should be avoided for about 1 week following a culdoscopy. Complications such as hemorrhage and infection are rare,

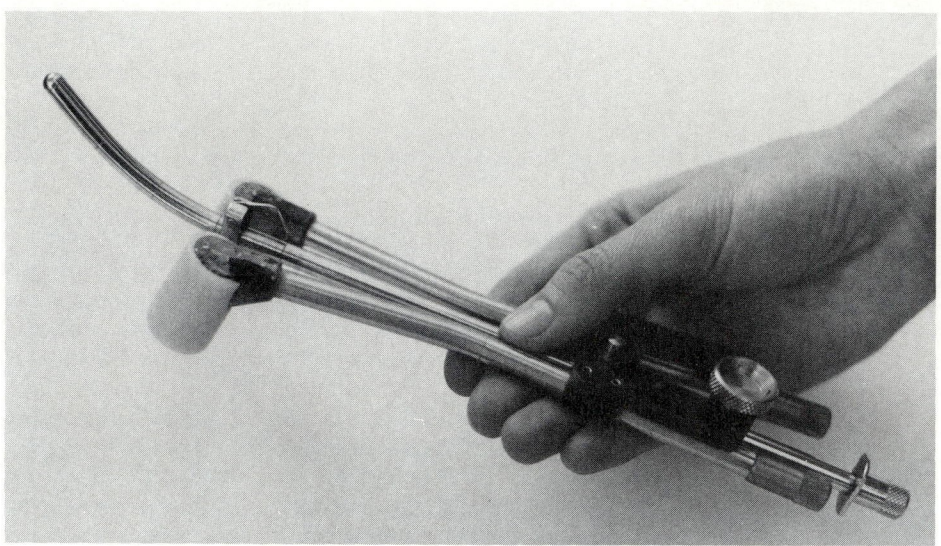

Fig. 34-10 Assembled configuration of tandem and colpostat before placement.

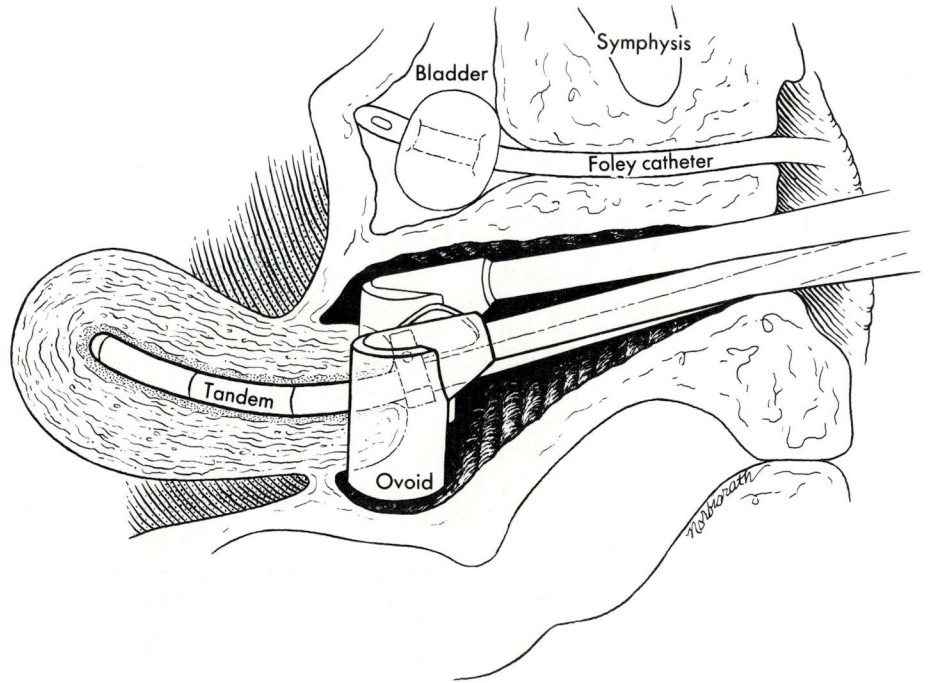

Fig. 34-11 Placement of tandem and colpostats before vaginal packing.

but women should be cautioned to report fever or pain in the lower abdomen.

■ TREATMENT MODALITIES

□ Surgery

Total abdominal hysterectomy (TAH) with or without bilateral salpingo-oophorectomy (BSO) is the most common treatment for gynecologic cancer (Table 34-7). Care of the patient experiencing gynecologic surgery is described on p. 1262. The woman with cancer not only experiences the same feelings associated with loss of reproductive organs as other women but is at the same time facing the concerns related to cancer (see Chapter 12). This is therefore a period of high anxiety for the woman, and she requires considerable empathy and emotional support as she works through her feelings.

□ Radiotherapy

Intracervical, intrauterine, or external whole pelvic irradiation may be given preoperatively to shrink the tumor to facilitate safety of the operation. Radiation may also be used as adjunct therapy postoperatively. Guidelines for radiation therapy are described in Chapter 12. Premenopausal women who receive pelvic irradiation will lose their ovarian function.

Radiation of the pelvic organs may create problems in sexual functioning. Patients have reported lack of libido, marked pain or discomfort with intercourse, and feelings of a narrow or shortened vagina.[13] These problems may add to the woman's feelings of sexual inadequacy from interferences with reproductive function.

□ *Intracavitary implant*

Radium or cesium may be inserted through a tandem placed in the uterine cavity (Figs. 34-10 and 34-11). During an intracavitary implant, it is important that all normal tissues remain in their natural position and that the radioactive substance is not placed nearer than is anticipated and provided for by the protective materials used. Gauze packing is usually inserted into the vagina to push both the rectum and the bladder away from the area being irradiated. A urinary catheter is inserted before therapy to prevent bladder distention. Low-residue diet and cleansing enemas are given before therapy, and the enema is repeated after therapy to prevent bowel distention.

Nursing care consists of the following guidelines:
1. Keep patient flat in bed; may turn side to side
2. Provide analgesics for severe uterine contractions from dilation of cervix
3. Provide good perineal care; there will be foul-smelling vaginal discharge from cell destruction; a deodorant is helpful
4. Encourage fluids to 3000 ml/day to maintain urinary adequacy
5. Follow general guidelines for internal radiation
6. Plan care that includes measures to decrease social isolation.

Radiation sickness may result as a systemic reaction to the breakdown and reabsorption of cell proteins. Local reaction may include cystitis and proctitis. Vaginal discharge will continue for some time after termination of therapy, and the patient may need to take douches for as long as the odor and vaginal discharge persist. Some vaginal bleeding may occur for 1 to 3 months after irradiation of the cervix. The woman who is at home should report persistent rectal irritation to the physician. The patient is usually discharged from the hospital within a day or two after the applicators are removed, but may return for another course of radiation.

Complications to watch for after radiation of the uterus are vesicovaginal fistulas, ureterovaginal fistulas, cystitis, phlebitis, and hemorrhage. Each is caused by the radiation or by extension of the disease process. The patient is urged to report even minor symptoms to her physician.

□ Chemotherapy

Chemotherapy has not significantly improved cancer of the uterus and therefore is rarely used in this situation. Chemotherapy is used more often for cancer of the ovaries. Combinations of drugs such as cisplatin, doxorubicin, and cyclophosphamide may be given. The drugs are not curative, but some long-term remissions may result.[47]

■ DISORDERS IN MEN

■ Inflammatory disorders

Nonspecific pyogenic organisms as well as specific organisms such as the gonococci and tubercle bacilli may cause stubborn infections of the male reproductive system. Urethritis, prostatitis, epididymitis, and orchitis are the most common infections (Table 34-9). Infecting organisms may reach the genital tract by direct spread through the urethra, or they may be borne by blood or lymph.

■ PATHOPHYSIOLOGY

□ Prostatitis

Prostatitis is commonly associated with urethritis. It may be acute or chronic; recurrent episodes of acute prostatitis may cause fibrotic tissue to form. The fibrosis causes a hardening of the prostate gland that may initially be confused with carcinoma. In the granulomatous form of prostatitis, the enlargement may take 3 to 6 months to resolve.

□ Epididymitis

Epididymitis is one of the most common inflammations of the male reproductive system. It is frequently a complication of gonorrhea or the first indication of tuberculosis of the genitourinary tract. It may follow instrumentation or prostatectomy.

Traumatic or chemical epididymitis is a sterile inflammation caused by direct injury or reflux of urine down the

Table 34-9 Inflammatory disorders of the male reproductive tract

Disorder	Etiology	Signs and symptoms	Medical therapy
Urethritis	*Chlamydia trachomatis*, urea-plasma, urealyticum	Urgency, frequency, and burning with urination, purulent urethral discharge	Antibiotics
Prostatitis	*Chlamydia trachomatis, Neisseria gonorrhoeae*	Perineal pain, fever, dysuria, urethral discharge	Antibiotics, rest, hydration, analgesics, stool softener, sitz baths
Epididymitis	Same as for prostatitis	Sudden scrotal pain, scrotal edema	Antibiotics, injection of procaine around spermatic cord, bed rest with scrotal elevation, analgesics
Orchitis	Pyogenic bacteria, gonoccoci; may follow mumps or tuberculosis; may result from trauma or surgical manipulation	Same as for epididymitis; nausea and vomiting, pain radiating to inguinal canal	Same as for epididymitis

vas deferens. The chemical form is frequently seen in military recruits during basic training as a result of straining with a full bladder, which causes urinary reflux.

Bilateral epididymitis usually causes sterility. Untreated epididymitis leads rather rapidly to necrosis of testicular tissue and septicemia, which can be fatal.

□ **Orchitis**

When mumps are contracted after puberty, approximately 18% of the cases are complicated by orchitis (inflammation of the testes). Orchitis may also be caused by bacteria or it may follow septicemia. Usually both testes are involved, and if it is bilateral, sterility often results. Sterility does not occur with unilateral involvement.

■ **PREVENTION**

Because urethral infection spreads so readily to the genital organs, men should not be catheterized unless it is absolutely necessary. Some trauma to the urethral mucosa is likely to accompany catheterization or the passage of instruments, such as a cystoscope, because of the length and curvature of the male urethra. The distal part of the urethra is not sterile, and trauma makes the urethra susceptible to attack from bacteria. Fluids should be given liberally after passage of instruments through the urethra.

Any postpubertal male who is exposed to mumps usually is given gamma globulin immediately unless he has already had the disease. If there is any doubt, globulin usually is given. Although gamma globulin may not prevent mumps, the disease is likely to be less severe, with less likelihood of orchitis developing and subsequent sterility.

■ **DIAGNOSTIC TESTS**

The site of the infection will influence treatment. The physician may obtain segmented bacteriologic localization

cultures to make the determination. Four sterile culture tubes are used for collection. The patient must be well hydrated, have a full bladder, and be able to cooperate.

1. The first 5 to 10 ml of a voiding is collected.
2. After approximately 200 ml have been voided, a 5 to 10 ml midstream specimen is collected.
3. The patient is asked to stop voiding, and the prostate gland is massaged rectally until prostatic secretions are collected.
4. The next 5 to 10 ml of urine are collected, and the bladder is then emptied.
5. The specimens are refrigerated and taken to the laboratory for culture within 4 hours.

■ **INTERVENTION**

□ **Assisting with comfort**

Mild to moderate discomfort may be experienced by the man with an inflammation of the genital tract. *Heat* may be applied for prostatitis by means of sitz baths, but is *contraindicated for epididymitis or orchitis* because of possible destruction of sperm cells. *Cold* is applied in the latter cases for relief of swelling and discomfort. If an ice cap is used, it should be placed under the scrotum and should be removed for short intervals every hour to prevent ice burns. A plastic glove may be filled with crushed ice; with the palm of the glove placed under the scrotum, the fingers provide cold to the sides.

Swelling and discomfort of the scrotum can also be relieved by elevation of the scrotum, either on a folded towel or with adhesive strapping known as a Bellevue bridge (Fig. 34-12).

□ **Counseling and teaching**

The female nurse must be particularly sensitive to the reactions and feelings of male patients who have diseases of the reproductive system. The patient may feel more comfortable discussing his problems with a male nurse. However, it is incumbent on all nurses to provide a comfortable environment in which these patients can verbalize their concerns and feelings.

Patient comments with subtle sexual connotations may reveal concerns the patient has regarding his sexuality, and he often must be given permission to discuss these concerns. The patient may "try out" his sexuality on a female nurse. Rejections from her may be perceived by the patient as less threatening than rejection by a loved one would be.

Certain reproductive disorders in the male are accompanied by a high incidence of sexual dysfunction. The patient may be worrying needlessly about possible sterility (inability to conceive a child) or impotence (inability to have an erection). If the patient does have a condition in which the incidence of sexual dysfunction is high, the nurse needs to know the specific patient situation, because these dysfunctions do not always occur in each disorder (see the box below, left).

Teaching includes the need to continue antibiotic therapy for the prescribed length of time (which may be lengthy in chronic prostatitis).

■ Structural disorders

Structural disorders of the testes and scrotum may occur in some men (see the box at the bottom of the page).

Immediate medical attention should be sought for any swelling of the scrotum or the testes within it. Any acute swelling of sudden onset must be considered twisting (torsion) of the spermatic cord until proved otherwise.

Hydrocele is treated by aspiration of the fluid. Usually no therapy is needed for *spermatocele*, although aspiration or surgical excision may be done. *Varicocele* is often seen in men with low fertility. Ligation of the spermatic vein has been shown to improve semen quality.

Torsion of the spermatic cord interrupts the blood supply, leading to ischemia and severe pain that is not relieved and may be aggravated by scrotal elevation. Absence of pain indicates infarction and necrosis; gangrene may be a serious sequela. Unless the testis is gangrenous it is not excised, because it may still produce hormones even if spermatogenesis is destroyed. The testis is fixed surgically to the scrotal wall (orchiopexy). The contralateral testis is usually fixed prophylactically at the same time.

Body image disturbances may include fears of castration, loss of masculinity, sterility, and impotence. The possibility of these fears being justified depends on the degree of insult to the testis and the functioning of the remaining testicle.

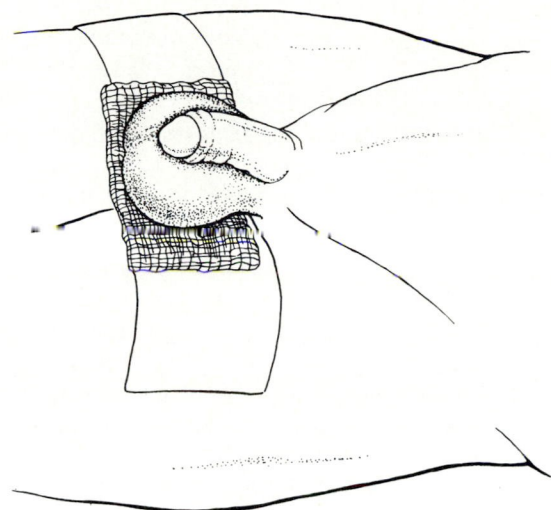

Fig. 34-12 Bellevue bridge.

Male reproductive disorders that may affect sexual functioning

Sterility	Impotence
Bilateral epididymitis	Radical prostatectomy
Severe bilateral orchitis	External radiation of pelvic floor
Torsion of testes	Total penectomy

Structural disorders of testes and scrotum

Hydrocele	Benign nontender collection of clear amber fluid within the outer covering of the testes, leading to scrotal swelling
Spermatocele	Benign nontender cystic mass attached to epididymis containing milky fluid and sperm
Varicocele	Dilation of spermatic vein, primarily on left side (because of longer left spermatic vein)
Torsion of spermatic cord	Kinking and twisting of spermatic cord and artery

Table 34-10 Cancer of the male reproductive tract

Site	Incidence	Usual age (yr)	Signs and symptoms	Medical therapy
Testes	0.1%	18 to 35	Painless enlarged testis, gynecomastia	Surgery: orchiectomy; radiation, chemotherapy
Prostate gland	20%	>60	Urethral obstruction, low back pain, anemia	Surgery: radical resection of prostate gland, radiation, hormonal therapy
Penis	0.01%	50 to 70	Nodular growth on foreskin, fatigue, weight loss	Surgery: partial or total penectomy

■ Tumors

Tumors of the male reproductive tract are usually malignant. The more common tumors involve the testes, prostate gland, and penis (Table 34-10).

■ PATHOPHYSIOLOGY

□ Cancer of the testes

Cancer of the testes is the second most common malignancy in men between the ages of 18 and 35 years and is the second most common cause of death from cancer in this age group. The most common type of testicular cancers is seminomas, which usually spread slowly through the lymphatics. Embryonal tumors invade the spermatic cord and metastasize early to the lungs.[24]

Removal of the testis, with examination of the nodes, is indicated for testicular cancers. *Biopsy of the testis is contraindicated* because of the highly metastatic character of testicular carcinoma. Seminomas respond to radiotherapy whereas embryomas do not. Combination chemotherapy may be given for metastatic disease; cisplatin, vinblastine, and bleomycin are commonly used. The prognosis following treatment of seminomas is a 5-year cure rate of 90%; however, the prognosis for other types of testicular cancer is poor.

□ Cancer of the prostate gland

The prostate gland is the second most common site of cancer among men; it is responsible for 10% of all deaths from cancer in men. It rarely occurs before the age of 60 years, incidence increases with age, and there is an increased familial risk. (Prostatic cancer is discussed in Chapter 32.)

□ Cancer of the penis

The incidence of penile cancer is highly dependent on hygienic standards as well as cultural and religious practices. It almost never occurs in a male who was circumcised at birth. Circumcision after puberty does not decrease the risk of cancer when compared with the incidence among uncircumcised males. Circumcision removes the prepuce, or foreskin, which provides a haven for bacteria. The bacteria act on desquamated cells producing smegma, which is irritating to the tissue of the glans penis and the prepuce. This chronic irritation is considered to be carcinogenic. Trauma and sexually transmitted diseases are felt to be coincidental to penile cancer rather than causative.

■ PREVENTION

Regular testicular self-examination (TSE) is recommended to detect cancer of the testes in its early stages when it is most likely to be localized and most curable. *All young men should be taught testicular self-examination.* (See the box below.) By performing TSE routinely, each man can get to know what is normal for him and more readily identify any lumps or abnormalities. Any swelling that is not normal should be examined by a physician. Nine of ten testicular cancers are detected by the patient or his sexual partner.

■ DIAGNOSTIC TESTS

Because prostatic tissue is rich in acid phosphatase, there is usually an increase in serum acid phosphatase with cancer of the prostate. Diagnosis of cancer of the prostate gland is confirmed by *prostatic biopsy*. If the transrectal route is used for biopsy, no bowel preparation is required. Vital signs are monitored for possible hemorrhage because of the high vascularity of the gland. Bleeding may be from

---

Testicular self-examination (TSE)

1. Perform TSE after a bath or shower when scrotum is warm and most relaxed
2. Grasp testis with both hands and palpate gently between thumb and fingers (Fig. 34-13):
   a. The testis should feel smooth, egg-shaped, and firm to touch
   b. The epididymis, found behind the testis, should feel like a soft tube

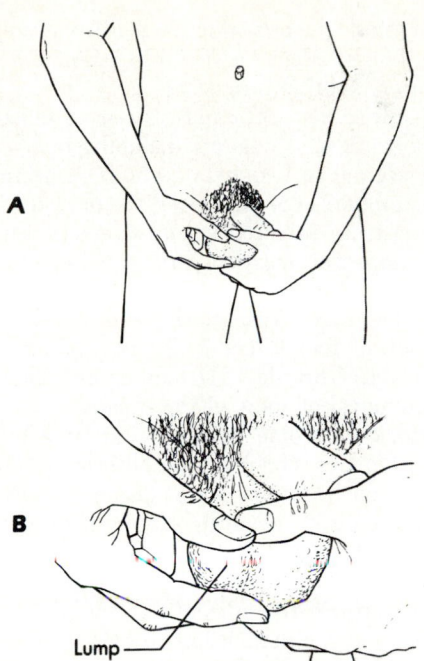

Fig. 34-13 Testicular self-examination. **A,** Grasp testis with both hands; palpate gently between thumb and fingers. **B,** Abnormal lumps or irregularities are reported to physician. (Adapted from Fred Hutchinson Cancer Research Center, Cancer Control Program: Self breast and testicular exam [grant no 2 R18-Ca 16404], Seattle 1980, Cancer Control Program.)

the urethra or the bladder and may be internal. The patient is observed for fever, acute urinary retention, rectal bleeding, pain or swelling of the scrotum.

■ SURGERY

□ Surgery of the testicle

Orchiectomy consists of en bloc excision of the spermatic cord, the contents of the inguinal canal, and the testis with the tunica attached. The adjacent area is explored for metastases.

□ *Preoperative care*

In addition to usual preoperative care, psychologic preparation for surgery is important. The man will usually be concerned about the effects of castration. *Unilateral* removal of a testis will *not* demasculinize him or cause sterility. Prostheses are available to replace the removed testis.

□ *Postoperative care*

ACTIVITY. Bed rest may be instituted for 24 to 48 hours after extensive removal of tissue, but ambulation usually is begun within 12 hours after surgery. Leg exercises are important if bed rest is to be maintained. The scrotum is elevated on a rolled towel, or the man may wear an athletic supporter while in bed. An athletic supporter or tight undershorts should be worn for support when the patient is ambulating.

POSTOPERATIVE COMPLICATIONS. The two major problems after scrotal surgery are edema and intrascrotal hemorrhage. *Edema* may be controlled by ice bags for the first 12 hours and a compression dressing for 3 to 5 days.[3] Ice is best applied by filling a rubber glove with crushed ice. Signs of hemorrhage or complaints of increasing discomfort are reported to the physician.

TEACHING
1. Avoid prolonged standing, which increases scrotal edema.
2. Wear athletic supporter or tight undershorts until healing is complete.
3. Take 20-minute tub baths three times per day for 1 week after discharge.
4. Avoid heavy lifting for 4 to 6 weeks.

□ Penile surgery

If the cancer is confined to the prepuce, circumcision may be adequate. If the lesion is on the glans, partial penectomy or amputation of the penis is required. If the shaft of the penis is involved, total amputation may be necessary. The decision is based on the amount of penis remaining after excision with an adequate tumor-free margin. The remaining penis must be long enough for the patient to void standing, direct the stream, and not void on himself. If this is possible, the sexual function will probably be retained. If total amputation is required, a perineal urethrostomy is performed in which the urethra is redirected to an opening between the scrotum and the anus. With spread of the cancer to the scrotal contents, radical removal is required, either hemipelvectomy or hemicorporectomy.

Sexual counseling is indicated for the patient with a total penectomy. Some patients with urethrostomy have experienced orgasm and ejaculation following stimulation of the perineal, scrotal and testicular regions.

■ RADIATION

Although the normal testis is shielded during external radiation of an involved testis, it does receive radiation scattered from the abdomen and thighs. A period of 70 days is required to determine whether spermatogenesis has been affected. Spermatogenesis may be decreased for 7 months to 5 years or more. Although genetic defects are possible after irradiation, there is currently no evidence to cause serious concern. Genetic counseling may be helpful for those couples desiring children.

Radiation for prostatic cancer may be delivered by external beam or by implant. The testes are shielded during external radiation. Erectile dysfunction may occur.

Iodine-125 retropubic prostatic implantation may be used initially or after failure of external radiation therapy. Complications of iodine-125 implantation include blood loss from multiple needle punctures during implantation, deep vein thrombosis, pulmonary emboli, hematomas, and abscesses. Potency is retained. Risk of incontinence and serious rectal complications such as rectourethral fistulas increases with the size of the gland and the intensity of the implant seed.

■ HORMONE THERAPY

Estrogen therapy may be used for advanced prostatic cancer when metastasis has occurred, especially to the bone. Bilateral orchiectomy to eliminate androgen may be combined with estrogen therapy. In males, estrogen frequently causes gynecomastia (enlargement of the breasts), loss of libido, arrest of spermatogenesis, and testicular atrophy.

Estrogen helps to decrease pain and reduce tumor size. The use of hormone therapy provides a longer symptom-free period but makes palliation more difficult when symptoms recur. If endocrine is delayed, symptoms recur earlier but longer palliation is possible.

■ SUMMARY

1. Premenstrual syndrome (PMS) consists of behavioral changes, fluid retention, fatigue, headach, backache, or increased appetite, which occurs repeatedly in many women before and during menstruation.
2. Dysmenorrhea is a common cause of absenteeism from work or school. Interventions include prostaglandin inhibitors, rest, heat applications, and moderate exercise.
3. Methods of sterilization include tubal ligation in the female and vasectomy in the male; although sterilization may be reversed in some cases, it is not always successful.
4. Infertility may result from obstructed fallopian tubes or vas deferens, from uterine or testicular disorders, or from hormonal deficiencies. Couples who are assessed as infertile need support in coping with the infertility and in examining alternative strategies (remain childless, adopt, artificial insemination, in vitro fertilization, mother surrogate).
5. Genital infections occur most often in females with low estrogen levels, who are malnourished, who have alkaline vaginal secretions, or who have been exposed to large numbers of organisms. Good personal hygiene, protection from infected sexual partners, and avoidance of unprescribed douching can help to prevent genital infections.
6. Pelvic inflammatory disease (PID) is a widespread inflammation of female pelvic organs; spread is up the genital tract. Chronic PID may cause adhesions requiring removal of some of the organs.
7. Toxic shock syndrome, which occurs mostly in menstruating females who use superabsorbent tampons, is associated with toxins from *Staphylococcus aureus*. Treatment consists of antibiotics and supportive care similar to that given septic shock.
8. In the male, the common genital inflammatory disorders are urethritis, prostatitis, epididymitis (most common), and orchitis. Bilateral epididymitis usually causes sterility.
9. Common structural disorders in the female are a relaxed vaginal outlet leading to stress incontinence, displacement or prolapse of the uterus, or fistulas; the treatment is primarily surgical. Perineal (Kegel) exercises may help prevent stress incontinence by strengthening the Kegel muscle.
10. Common structural disorders in the male are hydrocele, spermatocele, varicocele, or torsion of the spermatic cord.
11. Common *benign* genital tumors in the female include ovarian cysts and tumors, uterine fibroid tumors, cervical polyps, and endometriosis (seeding of endometrial cells in the pelvis). Cervical polyps are removed for biopsy. Uterine fibroid tumors are removed only when growth is rapid or when size is causing other difficulties.
12. Removal of the uterus (hysterectomy) ends menstruation but does not lead to menopausal symptoms if the ovaries are left intact.

Putting knowledge to practice

■ Compare and contrast the experiences of several women who are postmenopausal. How do their experiences compare with the discussion in the text?

■ Review the procedure for douches. What are the main purposes? What solutions are used most often? Why is the practice of frequent unprescribed douching not recommended?

■ Examine the chart of a woman who has had a hysterectomy. What was her psychologic response to the removal of the uterus? How would you respond to a woman in this situation who was crying and saying that she felt "less than a woman"?

■ Check the lastest issue of *Cancer Facts and Figures* published by the American Cancer Society for the latest data on estimated new cases and deaths for genital cancers and compare with the data cited in the text.

13. The most common genital cancer in females is cancer of the endometrium, occurring primarily in postmenopausal women. However, ovarian cancer causes more deaths than uterine cancer. The incidence of cancer of the cervix has decreased because of better screening by means of Pap smears.

14. Women should have a Pap test at least every 3 years after two initial negative tests 1 year apart. Persons at high risk for cervical cancer (early sexual activity, multiple sex partners) should have more frequent Pap tests.

15. Most genital cancers in males are prostatic cancers occurring primarily in men over age 60. Young men have a higher incidence of cancer of the testes, that can be detected early by testes self-examination (TSE).

REFERENCES AND SELECTED READINGS

1. Abraham, G: Nutritional factors in the etiology of the premenstrual tension syndrome, J Reprod Med 28:446-464, 1983.
2. American Cancer Society: 1987 cancer facts and figures, New York, 1987, The Society.
3. American College of Surgeons, Committee on Pre- and Postoperative Care: Manual of preoperative and postoperative care, ed 3, Philadelphia, 1983, WB Saunders Co.
4. Babaryan, R: When to refer: evaluation of scrotal masses, Hosp Pract 20(3):51-53, 1985.
5. Bachmann, G: Optimizing the postmenopausal years, Contemp OB/GYN 24:127-136, 1984.
6. Berkus, M, and Daly, J: Cone biopsy: an outpatient procedure, Am J Obstet Gynecol 137:953-958, 1980.
7. *Boarini, JH, Bryant, RA, and Ingang, SF: Fistula management, Sem Oncol Nurs 2:287-292, 1986.
8. *Brown, L: Toxic shock syndrome, MCN 6:57-59, 1981.
9. *Brown, MA: Primary dysmenorrhea, Nurs Clin North Am 17(1):145-173, 1982.
9a. Cashavelly, BJ: Cervical dysplasia: an overview of current concepts in epidemiology, diagnosis, and treatment, Cancer Nurs 10:199-206, 1987.
10. Cosper, B, Fuller, S, and Robinson, G: Characteristics of posthospitalization recovery following hysterectomy, JOGNN 10:7-11, 1981.
11. Crawford, E: Diagnosis and treatment of prostatitis, Hosp Pract 20(9):77-80, 1985.
12. Crosson, K: A patient teaching aid for the pelvic exenteration patient, Oncol Nurs Forum 8:53-56, 1981.
13. *Edlund, BJ: The needs of women with gynecologic malignancies, Nurs Clin North Am 17(1):155-163, 1982.
14. Federation of Feminist Women's Health Centers: A new view of a woman's body, New York, 1981, Simon & Schuster.
15. *Fogel, CI, and Woods, NF: Health care of women: a nursing perspective, St. Louis, 1981, The CV Mosby Co.
16. *Frank, EP: What are nurses doing to help PMS patients? Am J Nurs 86:136-140, 1986.
17. *Galt, PL: Taking your part in the fight against testicular cancer, Nurs 81 11(5):45-50, 1981.
18. *Googe, MCS: The inflatable penile prosthesis: new developments, Am J Nurs 83:1044-1047, 1983.
19. *Hampton, BG: Nursing management of a patient following pelvic exenteration, Sem Oncol Nurs 2:275-286, 1986.
20. *Henderson, JS, and Taylor, KH: Age as a variable in an exercise program for the treatment of simple urinary stress incontinence, JOGNN 13:266-272, 1987.
21. Hogan, R: Human sexuality: a nursing perspective, ed 2, New York, 1984, Appleton-Century-Crofts.
22. Houghton, B: Vasectomies affect women, too, Am J Nurs 81:821-825, 1981.
23. Jusenius, K: A teaching aid for the radical hysterectomy patient, Oncol Nurs Forum 10(2):71-75, 1983.
24. Krupp, MA, Schroeder, SA, and Tierney, LM: Current medical diagnosis and treatment 1987, Norwalk, Conn, 1987, Appleton & Lange.
25. Kuczynski, H: Pros and cons of douching: the nurse's role in counseling, JOGNN 9:90-93, 1980.
26. Lamb, M: Ovarian cancer: patient information booklet, Oncol Nurs Forum 12(5):83-86, 1985.
27. Lamb, M: Sexual dysfunction in the gynecologic oncology patient, Sem Oncol Nurs 1(1):9-17, 1985.
28. Managing the patient with testicular cancer: Nursing Grand Rounds, Nurs 86 16(8):42-45, 1986.
29. *Marrs, R: In vitro fertilization's future looks bright, Contemp OB/GYN 20:135-141, 1982.
30. *Menning, BE: The psychosocial impact of infertility, Nurs Clin North Am 17(1):155-163, 1982.
31. Mims, F, and Swenson, M: Sexuality: a nursing perspective, New York, 1980, McGraw-Hill Book Co.
32. *Nachtigall, L, and Nachtigall, R: Evaluating newly menopausal women, Contemp OB/GYN 25:65-91, 1985.
33. Novak, ER, Jones, GS, and Jones, HW, Jr: Novak's textbook of gynecology, ed 10, Baltimore, 1980, The Williams & Wilkins Co.
34. *O'Laughlin, KM: Changes in bladder function in the woman undergoing radical hysterectomy for cervical cancer, JOGNN 15:380-385, 1986.
35. *Papanier, M, and Villano, K: Total abdominal hysterectomy: perioperative patient care, AORN J 42:368-373, 1985.
36. *Robertson, C: Treatment modalities for gynecologic cancers, Sem Oncol Nurs 2:275-280, 1986.
37. *Rosenthal, M: Grappling with the emotional aspects of infertility, Contemp OB/GYN 27:97-106, 1985.
38. *Rubin, D: Gynecologic cancer: cervical, vulvular and vaginal malignancies, RN 50(5):56-63, 1987.
39. *Rubin, D: Gynecologic cancer: uterine and ovarian malignancies, RN 50(6):52-57, 1987.
40. Sandelowski, M: Women, health and choice, Englewood Cliffs, NJ, 1981, Prentice-Hall, Inc.
41. Sargis, N: Detecting ovarian cancer: a challenge for nursing assessment, Oncol Nurs Forum 10(2):48-53, 1983.
42. Scrinivas, V, and others: Penile carcinoma, Hosp Pract 20(1):154-159, 1985.
43. *Smith, DB: Gynecologic cancers: etiology and pathophysiology, Sem Oncol Nurs 2:270-274, 1986.

*References preceded by an asterisk are particularly well suited for student reading.

44. Speroff, L, Glass, RH, and Kase, N: Clinical gynecologic endocrinology and infertility, ed 3, Baltimore, 1983, The Williams & Wilkins Co.

45. Studva, K, and White, L: Cancer prevention and detection: cervical cancer, Ca Nurs 7(4):335-345, 1984.

46. *Torrington, J: Pelvic inflammatory disease, JOGNN 14(suppl):21-31, 1985.

47. Way, LW: Current surgical diagnosis and treatment, ed 6, Los Altos, Calif, 1983, Lange Medical Publications.

48. *Wilson, MA: Menstrual disorders: premenstrual syndrome, amenorrhea, JOGNN 13(suppl):11s-19s, 1984.

49. Woods, NF: Human sexuality in health and illness, ed 3, St. Louis, 1984, The CV Mosby Co.

50. Woods, NF, Most, A, and Dery, GK: Prevalence of perimenstrual symptoms, Am J Pub Health 72:1257-1264, 1982.

35

Sexually Transmitted Diseases

WILMA J. PHIPPS and ELLEN F. OLSHANSKY

CHAPTER OBJECTIVES

After studying this chapter, the student should be able to:

- Define sexually transmitted diseases (STDs).

- Describe the transmission, prevention, and control of STDs.

- List the causative agent, incubation period, signs and symptoms, medical therapy, and long-term effects of gonorrhea, syphilis, herpes genitalis and chlamydia infection.

- Describe the subjective and objective data to be collected from a person suspected of having an STD.

- Write a teaching plan for a unit on the prevention of STDs for a sex education course for adolescents.

■ Epidemiology and etiology

Sexually transmitted diseases (STDs) are diseases that are *usually* or *can* be transmitted from one person to another with heterosexual or homosexual intercourse or intimate contact with the genitalia, mouth, or rectum. In addition to the five classic venereal diseases (syphilis, gonorrhea, chancroid, lymphogranuloma venereum, and granuloma inguinale), the STD category includes genital herpes infection, *chlamydia trachomatis* nonspecific urethritis, trichomoniasis, candidiasis, pediculosis, pubis (crabs), scabies, genital or venereal warts, hepatitis B infections, molluscum contagiosum, and G. *vaginalis* (previously referred to as *Cornybacterium vaginalis* or *Haemophilus vaginalis*) vaginitis. The diseases classified as STDs and their causative organisms are listed in the box below.)

These latter STDs might be considered the "new generation" of STDs, although they have probably existed since antiquity. Because of improved laboratory and epidemiologic methods, their prevalence, modes of transmission, and clinical consequences are better understood than in earlier decades. In addition, many of the newly recognized STDs have become epidemic or hyperendemic as a consequence of changing sexual behavioral patterns. Not only has the incidence of many STDs increased, but for agents with multiple modes of transmission (for example, hepatitis B virus, enteric pathogens), the proportion of infections that are transmitted sexually has also increased. In addition to the immediate consequences of STDs there are newly recognized effects on maternal and infant morbidity as well as on human reproduction and fertility.

All states require that each case of syphilis and gonorrhea be reported to the state or local health officer. Chancroid, granuloma inguinale, and lymphogranuloma venereum are also reportable in most states. Herpes genitalis, trichomoniasis, and candidiasis are not reportable in any state. The true incidence of STDs is *not* known because of variable reporting requirements and also because many cases are not reported by the clinicians who treat them.

In explaining the trends of reported cases of STDs in the United States, *three changes* occurring in recent years are often referred to in the literature. The *first* of these concerns use of antibiotics and changes in the antibiotic susceptibility of pathogenic organisms. The widespread, perhaps indiscriminate, use of penicillin and other antibiotics between the late 1940s and early 1950s parallels the decline in both syphilis and gonorrhea. It is said that the organisms developed a greater resistance to antibiotics over time and that antibiotics have therefore become less effective than previously. There is no firm evidence to indicate a decrease in effectiveness of penicillin against syphilis. However, the gonococcus tends to develop resistance to antibiotics.

A *second* explanation for the rise in incidence of STDs is that they are more likely to occur if a social system is permissive. During times of war and other catastrophes, it is easier for agencies to control interpersonal behavior, whereas in times of peace and absence of national crisis, civil liberties tend to flourish. The incidence curve of syphilis and gonorrhea after the years of World War II seems to support this thesis.

The *third* explanation centers around sexual behavior patterns and includes permissiveness. Concern has been expressed particularly about the prevalence of gonorrhea among adolescents and young adults who are considered to be promiscuous. In fact, rates for gonorrhea show young adults of 20 to 24 years of age accounted for 40% of reported cases of gonorrhea, while persons 15 to 19 years of age accounted for 25% of cases. The highest morbidity for males was in the 20- to 24-year age group; for females it was in the 15- to 19-year age group.[27]

The above discussion makes an assumption of sexual promiscuity, and in doing so, requires acknowledgement of advances in contraceptive technology, especially "the pill." These social changes are often termed the three *P*s (permissiveness, promiscuity, and the pill).[38] The underlying idea is that, with the advent of antibiotics and the pill, people began to lose fear of untreated venereal disease and pregnancy and that sexual promiscuity increased significantly, leading to increased exposure to infection.

If the definition of promiscuity is that sexual relations are not restricted to one partner, studies show that patients diagnosed in clinics as having STD are not promiscuous. In one study 66.4% of patients having an STD named only one sexual contact.[38] It must be realized, however, that persons may hesitate to admit to having more than one sex partner for any number of reasons.

In the past, prostitution has been considered a major

Sexually transmitted diseases

Type of organism	Disease
Bacteria	Gonorrhea, chancroid, granuloma inguinale, *Gardnerella vaginalis*
Spirochete	Syphilis
Chlamydia	Nongonococcal urethritis, epididymitis, cervicitis, PID, lymphogranuloma venereum
Virus	Herpes genitalis, hepatitis B, cytomegalovirus, AIDS, genital warts
Protozoa	Trichomoniasis
Yeast	Candidiasis
Parasites	Pediculosis pubis, scabies

force in the transmission of STDs. Before World War II it was estimated that approximately 75% of all STDs could be traced to prostitutes and that at least 10% of all prostitutes had contracted an STD at least once. Today less than 5% of patients with syphilis can be classed as prostitutes. Also, most persons with gonorrhea are single and under 25 years of age, and most clients of prostitutes are usually older, married men. *Chlamydia trachomatis* and herpes are two STDs that are very common in middle-class America.

Before 1960, homosexuals were rarely mentioned in the literature as carriers of STDs. Since the early 1970s much more attention has been given to the risk of STDs among homosexual and bisexual men. Homosexual men carry pathogens in the rectum and colon, including gonococcus, *Giardia,* ameba, *Shigella,* and *Camphylobacter.* Although lesbians are at low risk for contracting STDs and gay males are at higher risk, it is important to note that sexual orientation does not prescribe individual forms of sexual behavior.

The condom was the main method of contraception used before the advent of antibiotics and oral contraceptives. The use of the condom may have prevented the spread of the STDs by providing a mechanical barrier to the organisms. The pill revolutionized contraception practices, and it is known that neutralization of the vaginal and cervical environment by estrogenic substances predisposes to infection. It would appear that individual characteristics of persons engaging in sexual activity need to be more closely studied before any conclusions about permissiveness, promiscuity, and use of the pill can be made.

SEXUAL TRANSMISSION

The STDs are contagious diseases spread almost exclusively by contact during sexual intercourse; that is, when mucous membrane surfaces come in contact during genital, oral, or anal sexual activity. Because the causative organisms survive only very briefly outside a warm, moist environment, there is almost no way to contract STDs from toilet seats, towels, or bed linens. Although STDs are not usually transmitted in public restrooms, conditions caused by fungi, bacteria, and lice can be transmitted from water in unclean toilet bowls. Women using a conventional toilet expose the vaginal and anal area to pathogens that can be introduced by the back splash of contaminated toilet water.

There are some notable exceptions to sexual transmission. During pregnancy the fetus may become infected in utero by placental transmission, and the infant may acquire congenital syphilis or be stillborn. Infants of mothers with gonorrhea may contract infections of the eyes (ophthalmia neonatorum) during birth, and unless treated, this can lead to permanent blindness.

Prevention and health education

Prevention and control measures for STDs include three levels of prevention. *Primary prevention* is directed at preventing the disease. This includes educating uninfected persons so that they can avoid contact with an infected person, identification and treatment of exposed persons who are asymptomatic, interviewing persons with infection for identification of contacts, examination and preventive treatment of contacts, educational programs for the public, and active involvement of professionals in programs of control. The goal of these efforts includes eradication of the reservoir of disease in the population. *Secondary prevention* is directed toward prevention of complications, and *tertiary prevention* focuses on decreasing the effects of complications.

CONTACT INVESTIGATION

In the prevention and control of STDs especially gonorrhea, emphasis was once placed on interviewing for information regarding sexual contacts. The named contacts were sought out for examination and treatment. Lay people knowledgeable about the required reporting to the local health department of some of the diseases were very hesitant to name their sexual contacts. Young people often feared that their parents and the parents of the sexual partner would find out about their infection. Minors need to know that they can probably obtain treatment without parental consent. Presently most states permit physicians to treat minors for STD without obtaining parental consent, and several states are proposing changes in existing legislation restricting treatment of minors. People also may perceive reporting of STDs as a threat from an official agency and may hesitate to name their contacts out of a sense of protection if they do not know that no punishment is involved.

Interviewing the patient for contacts is done at the time of the initial visit in the event that the patient does not return for follow-up. This interview is probably best done after the patient is examined, the type of infection is determined, and treatment is prescribed. If assessment is accompanied by information giving, the person should be better informed about STDs and how they are treated, and be more willing and able to give information about sexual contacts.

Interviewing for contacts involves two aspects. The patient is first asked to name sexual contacts. Second, the patient is interviewed for "cluster suspects," who are friends or acquaintances who may have been exposed to the same contacts, or who have symptoms of an STD. Since one focus of STD control is on increasing self-referrals, the patient is asked to advise known contacts and cluster suspects to present themselves for examination and preventive treatment. Confidentiality is stressed. There is reason to believe that patients do not name all their contacts at the time of the first interview and that a reinterview will usually result in additional names of contacts. Because of the understandable reluctance of many people to name their sexual contacts, the patient may be given the responsibility of informing the contacts and advising them of their need for treatment. (The contacts are not named, but instead cards that permit both examination and treatment without identification are given to the contact by the patient.) The local health departments cooperate in locating, examining, and treating these contacts as necessary.

Whenever possible, the contacts of the infected person are located and advised to have an examination and tests as soon as possible. If the sexual contacts do not have symptoms of infection at the time of the first examination, treatment is instituted to abort infection. Giving preventive treatment to named contacts who have no clinical evidence of infection has gained popularity and acceptance in the United States, and there are indications that this same approach is being used more often in management of patients having the "minor" STDs.

CURRENT AND FUTURE NEEDS

The epidemic nature of some STDs makes it evident that measures for control of spread need to be even more vigorously applied and that new measures may be necessary to check the spread of infection. Efforts to implement mass education and screening programs need to be continued. Program efforts are directed toward creating public awareness of the problem of STDs and their control methods and informing the public of the possible serious consequences of these diseases. There also is a need to expand screening, contact treatment, and diagnostic and treatment programs.

Little is known about some of the STDs. Surveillance over some of them is inadequate, so that even the true incidence of several sexually transmitted infections is not known. Treatment of several of these diseases is poorly understood because knowledge of the natural history of the causative organisms is inadequate. Such knowledge is necessary to understand the epidemiology of these diseases so that treatment and prevention can be better directed than is now possible. Diagnostic methods need to be improved so that they are more reliable and inexpensive for large numbers of people. Alternative therapies for prophylaxis require the development of agents to be used specifically and with discretion for treatment of exposed individuals, for the treatment of persons allergic to specific drugs, and for the management of pregnant women.

In order to better understand the modes of transmission and circumstances surrounding spread of the STDs, knowledge of human behavior is required. There has been considerable research in recent years regarding sexual behavior patterns, contraceptive practices, and permissiveness. Although this has been helpful, there is little consensus about whether these variables influence the incidence and spread of STDs. Further study will add to the pool of knowledge, which can be applied in programs of detection, treatment, and prevention.

Signs and symptoms

Vaginitis, cervicitis, lower abdominal pain, urethritis, epididymitis, pharyngitis, proctitis, and skin or mucous membrane lesions are common in persons with STDs (see Table 35-1). Some people may be asymptomatic.

Table 35-1   Selected sexually transmitted diseases

Disease	Incubation period	Signs and symptoms	Medical therapy
Gonorrhea	Men: 3 to 30 days Women: 3 days to an indefinite period	Men: purulent urethral discharge, dysuria, epididymitis, prostatitis Women: asymptomatic in early stages; cervicitis with purulent discharge, bartholinitis, salpingitis	Amoxicillin 3.0 g or ampicillin 3.5 g orally or aqueous procaine; penicillin G 4.8 million units IM or ceftriaxone 250 mg IM; Probenemid 1.0 g orally along with amoxicillin, ampicillin, or penicillin
Syphilis	3 weeks (9 days to 3 months)	Positive serologic tests, chancre in stage I	Benzathine penicillin G 2.4 million units IM
Herpes genitalis	3 to 14 days	Vesicles that rupture and form ulcerations, pain, inguinal lymph node enlargement, dysuria, flulike symptoms	Symptomatic; topical acyclovir
Chlamydia	5 to 10 days or longer	Women: painful or difficult urination, abnormal vaginal discharge or bleeding, pain or bleeding with coitus, irregular menses. One third are asymptomatic. Men: testicular pain, nonspecific urethritis or epididymitis	Tetracycline 500 mg 4 times daily for 7 days or erythromycin 500 mg daily for 7 days for persons unable to take tetracycline; usually also treated with penicillin because high percentage also have gonorrhea
Condylomata acuminata (genital warts)	1 to 6 months	Horny papules on vulva, vagina, cervix, perineum, anal canal, urethra, glans penis	Cryotherapy

■ Medical therapy

Treatment depends on the causative organisms identified through the history, physical examination, and laboratory tests and is discussed in detail in the following pages. It is not unusual for an individual to harbor two or more organisms simultaneously.

▣ Assessment

■ SUBJECTIVE DATA

The following information is collected from the person suspected of having an STD:

1. Exposure to STD contact
2. Prior STD history, treatment
3. Sexual orientation: "Have you been having sex with men, women, or both?"
4. Timing of last sexual activity
5. Number of sexual partners in the past 2 months
6. Women are questioned about:
   a. Vaginal discharge
   b. Vulvar itching
   c. Dysuria
   d. Urinary urgency
   e. Lower abdominal pain
   f. Rectal symptoms
   g. Sore throat
   h. Genital lesions
   i. Skin rashes or itching
   j. Menstrual periods
7. Heterosexual men are questioned about:
   a. Urethral discharge
   b. Dysuria
   c. Genital lesions
   d. Skin rashes
   e. Itching
   f. Testicular pain
   g. Sore throat
8. Gay or bisexual men are asked the same questions as heterosexual men plus the following:
   a. Rectal symptoms such as pain, bleeding, discharge, and diarrhea
9. If hepatitis is also suspected, the person is questioned about:
   a. Dark-colored urine
   b. Clay-colored stools
   c. Fatigue
   d. Jaundice

■ OBJECTIVE DATA

Objective data include the following:

1. Inspection and palpation of the integumentary system, reproductive system, and anorectal area.
2. Examination for women includes the following:
   a. Inspection of skin of lower abdomen, inguinal area, hands, palms, and forearms
   b. Inspection of pubic hair for lice and mites
   c. Inspection and palpation of external genitals, including perineum and anus
   d. Speculum examination of vagina and cervix
   e. Bimanual pelvic examination
   f. Palpation for inguinal and femoral lymphadenopathy
   g. Inspection of mouth and throat, including tonsils
3. Examination of heterosexual men includes the following:
   a. Inspection of the skin and pubic hair
   b. Inspection of the penis, including the meatus, with retraction of the foreskin and "milking" of the urethra
   c. Palpation of the scrotum
4. Examination of homosexual or bisexual men is the same as for heterosexual men plus the following:
   a. Inspection of the mouth, throat including the tonsils, and anorectal area
   b. Anoscopic examination if there are rectal symptoms

■ DIAGNOSTIC TESTS

Specific diagnostic tests are used to establish the diagnosis of each of these diseases. Diagnostic tests will be discussed under the specific disease later in this chapter.

➡ Data analysis: nursing diagnoses

Nursing diagnoses are determined from assessment of patient data. Possible nursing diagnoses for the person with a sexually transmitted disease, may include but are not limited to, the following:

Diagnostic title	Possible etiologies
Altered health maintenance	Lack of knowledge, cultural practices, lack of material resources
Knowledge deficit	Lack of exposure/recall, information misinterpretation, lack of familiarity with information sources

▣ Planning: expected patient outcomes

Expected patient outcomes for the person with a sexually transmitted disease may include, but are not limited to, the following:

1. Person and/or partner can explain the etiology and factors contributing to the STD.
2. Person and/or partner can state the name, dosage, and schedule of administration of drug therapy, as well as its possible side effects.
3. Person and/or partner can explain the need for adherence to the entire treatment regimen.
4. Person and/or partner can state the implications for sexual activity during the infectious stages of the STD.
5. Person and/or partner can state effects of the STD on the reproductive system of oneself and one's partner.
6. Person and/or partner can state indications for seeking immediate health care.

Recommendations from the CDC for the use of condoms

The following recommendations for proper use of condoms to reduce the transmission of STD are based on current information:

1. Latex condoms should be used because they offer greater protection against viral STD than natural membrane condoms.
2. Condoms should be stored in a cool, dry place out of direct sunlight.
3. Condoms in damaged packages or those that show obvious signs of age (e.g., those that are brittle, sticky, or discolored) should not be used. They cannot be relied upon to prevent infection.
4. Condoms should be handled with care to prevent puncture.
5. The condom should be put on before any genital contact to prevent exposure to fluids that may contain infectious agents. Hold the tip of the condom and unroll it onto the erect penis, leaving space at the tip to collect semen, yet assuring that no air is trapped in the tip of the condom.
6. Adequate lubrication should be used. If exogenous lubrication is needed, only water-based lubricants should be used. Petroleum- or oil-based lubricants such as petroleum jelly, cooking oils, shortening, and lotions) should not be used since they weaken the latex.
7. Use of condoms containing spermicides may provide some additional protection against STD. However, vaginal use of spermicides along with condoms is likely to provide greater protection.
8. If a condom breaks, it should be replaced immediately. If ejaculation occurs after condom breakage, the immediate use of spermicide has been suggested. However, the protective value of postejaculation application of spermicide in reducing the risk of STD transmission is unknown.
9. After ejaculation, care should be taken so that the condom does not slip off the penis before withdrawal; the base of the condom should be held while withdrawing. The penis should be withdrawn while still erect.
10. Condoms should never be reused.

From US Department of Health and Human Services, Public Health Service; Condoms for the prevention of sexually transmitted disease, MMWR 37(9):133-137, 1988.

7. Person and/or partner can explain necessity for treatment of sexual partner or partners.
8. Person and/or partner can accept the occurrence of the STD.
9. Person and/or partner can explain how to prevent the transmission of STD's by using "safe sex" practices including the type of condom to use, when and how to apply it, and how to remove it. Recommendations on the proper use of condoms to prevent transmission of STDs can be found in the box above.

Implementation

COUNSELING AND TEACHING

The nurse's first responsibility in STD control is to educate patients who may develop or have a sexually transmitted infection. Nurses must be knowledgeable about the diseases most prevalent, the signs and symptoms, methods used in diagnosis, treatments used, and where individuals can obtain help and information. They also can influence the knowledge and attitudes of their colleagues and peers toward STD and its control. Nurses can exert influence in the community by taking an active role in programs of education. Perhaps the best way to reduce the risk of STD is for a person to know his or her sexual partner. Sexual activity with different partners increases the risk of infection.

Preventive measures such as washing or showering with soap and water and using a condom are recommended but are no guarantee against STD. Good laundry and personal hygiene practices also may help reduce risk.

Before nurses can be effective in working with patients who have STDs, they must confront their own feelings and attitudes about STDs. The patient is often young, fearful of pain, and unaccustomed to surroundings in a clinic or physician's office. Young patients especially fear that their families and friends may learn they have an STD.

Once the diagnosis, tentative or conclusive, is made, focus should first be placed on obtaining a cure and preventing complications and reinfection. Many lay people know that the treatment for syphilis and gonorrhea is penicillin, but they may not be fully informed about this and other aspects of treatment. Because some of the diseases respond to penicillin or other antibiotics, many people believe that all genital infections can be cured easily, and this is not so. Some people believe that antibiotics not only cure an infection but that they produce immunity against reinfection as well. Persons receiving an antibiotic or other medications for STDs must be informed of the action of the drug, its duration of effectiveness, side effects, chances of cure, and the need for follow-up. They need to be advised that treatment failures do occur and that reinfection rates are high. Return visits should be encouraged whenever possible, because adequacy of treatment of all of the STDs is evaluated best by laboratory analysis for the specific organism.

■ PROVIDING SOCIAL AND EMOTIONAL SUPPORT

Many patients focus on how the diseases are spread rather than on the consequences of having an infection. For single persons, contracting an STD and securing help means they must admit to sexual activity, and some of them may feel guilty. Patients with an STD have not only a physical but a social, emotional, and perhaps economic problem as well. They need constructive and comprehensive help. The nurse who is successful in working with persons having an STD is one who can create an atmosphere of trust in which the person feels free to discuss all aspects of the problem.

Persons who seek help recognize they have a problem; they want to get better and stay well. Because of this they are highly motivated to do what is necessary, and receptive to information and advice, and are attentive when advice is given. Nurses can take advantage of the patient's readiness to learn and motivation to improve and maintain health.

■ PROMOTING SELF-CARE

Persons treated for sexually transmitted infections need information about self-care. To understand their therapy and to responsibly engage in self-care, they must be informed about the sexual nature of the infection, how it is transmitted, and the possibility of reinfection and infection of their sexual partner or partners. The patient needs to know that it is important for sexual partners to be checked for signs of infection, to be advised of what the signs are, and have a culture done for asymptomatic infection. Patients should be advised to abstain from intercourse until cured. It also should be stressed that condoms should be used to prevent infection or reinfection, if persons do engage in intercourse even when advised not to.

Teaching about hygiene and personal health practices is beneficial in reducing the chances of secondary infection, recurrence, and infections of various types in the future. Frequent bathing and hand washing are indicated. It is known that many of the organisms causing STDs are destroyed by soap and water. For women, *douching* is contraindicated unless it is prescribed for the purpose of applying heat or applying medication. All women should be informed that, for personal cleanliness, frequent douching at any time is *not* advisable, because this may disturb the vaginal and cervical environments and predispose the woman to infection. If douching is prescribed by the physician, the patient should be instructed in the procedure.

If the lesions are present on body surfaces, the patient should be instructed in their care. Unless contraindicated, a hot bath is taken two to three times a day; and lesions are kept as dry as possible between baths. Both men and women should be advised to wear cotton underwear, and women should be advised to avoid wearing pantyhose, because they tend to trap moisture and prevent circulation of air to the genitalia. Unless they are specifically prescribed as local medications, the patient should not apply any lotion, cream, or ointment to any of the lesions associated with STDs.

Self-examination is important for sexually active people, especially those with more than one partner. Inspecting skin, mouth, genitals, and perianal areas for lesions and discharges is recommended. In addition, people can learn to casually inspect their partners during the initial period of lovemaking to identify any signs of STDs. Urinating after sexual activity can be helpful in cleansing the urethra of organisms.

■ PROMOTING HEALTHY SEXUAL ATTITUDES

Opportunities for promoting healthy attitudes about sexual activity and STDs frequently arise. These topics are approached tactfully and with consideration of the patient's feelings. Adolescents especially require an approach that indicates understanding balanced with the ability to help them set limits. Developmental tasks of adolescence require that young people find means of sexual gratification within the context of meaningful sexual relationships. In their search, adolescents need to be reassured that mutually rewarding relationships involving sexual gratification can be fulfilling. However, within this context, adolescents need to recognize that consequences of their behavior may include unwanted pregnancy and STD.

Development of prophylactic vaccines, especially for gonorrhea and syphilis, needs to be given high priority. To accomplish this, techniques for growing the organisms need to be developed, and this in turn requires knowledge of the natural history and evolution of specific organisms, including viruses.

History has revealed that treatment alone has never conquered any of the major communicable diseases, but that programs through which the public becomes better informed and demands services, as well as the development of protective vaccines, have almost always been universally successful in preventing disease.

⊞ Evaluation

Evaluation is based on the expected patient outcomes. Questions to be asked include the person's and/or partner's ability to do the following:

1. State the factors that contributed to the present infection with STD (multiple sexual partners; not practicing safe sex).
2. State the drug therapy to be followed including name of drug, dosage, schedule of administration, and side effects.
3. Explain why the therapy must be taken without inter-

ruption (to prevent resistant strains of organisms from developing).

4. State why he or she should not engage in sexual activity while the STD is infectious.
5. State effects of STDs that may develop in the reproductive system of either partner.
6. State signs and symptoms (fever, pain, discharge) that indicate need for immediate health care.
7. Explain what is meant by practicing "safe sex" including what type of condom to use, when and how to apply it, and how to remove it.
8. Verbalize that she or he has an STD and identify ways to prevent further STD infections.

■ GONORRHEA

■ Epidemiology, etiology, and pathophysiology

There is no clinical difference in the infections caused by resistant strains of *N. gonorrhoeae* and those caused by sensitive strains. When there are a high number of resistant strains in a community, there is more likely to be an increase in sequelae of acute gonococcal infections such as pelvic inflammatory disease (PID), gonoccocal ophthalmia, and disseminated gonococcal infection (DGI).[30]

The costs of patient management in communities with a high rate of resistant strains of *N. gonorrhoeae* are increased because of (1) additional laboratory tests, (2) added

drug costs, (3) extra clinic visits, and (4) more extensive disease intervention.

Not all laboratories are prepared to test for all three forms of resistant strains. Therefore, emphasis is placed on identification of plasma-mediated resistance to penicillin by having all isolates of *N. gonorrhoeae* tested for beta-lactamase production.[30]

The incidence of gonorrhea in the United States from 1970 through 1986 is shown in Fig. 35-1. Although the rate decreased slightly from a peak in 1974, it is still the most commonly reported communicable disease in the country. The incidence of gonorrhea is accepted to be much higher than shown because it is known that the cases of many patients treated by private physicians are never reported to public health authorities and therefore are not reflected in the statistics. It is generally accepted that only 25% to 50% of cases treated by private physicians are reported. In addition, women have few, if any, signs or symptoms of gonorrhea and thus are often not diagnosed. For this reason, it is commonly believed that the actual number of cases per year in the United States is probably more than 2 million.

Compounding the problem is the rapid increase of cases of gonorrhea caused by resistant strains of *N. gonorrhoeae* (Fig. 35-2). The number of resistant strains has been increasing rapidly with a 98% increase reported in 1985, and an additional 90% increase in 1986.[31] Clinically significant resistance to the three widely used classes of drugs—the penicillins, the tetracyclines, and the aminoglycosides—has been reported.[30] Plasma-mediated resis-

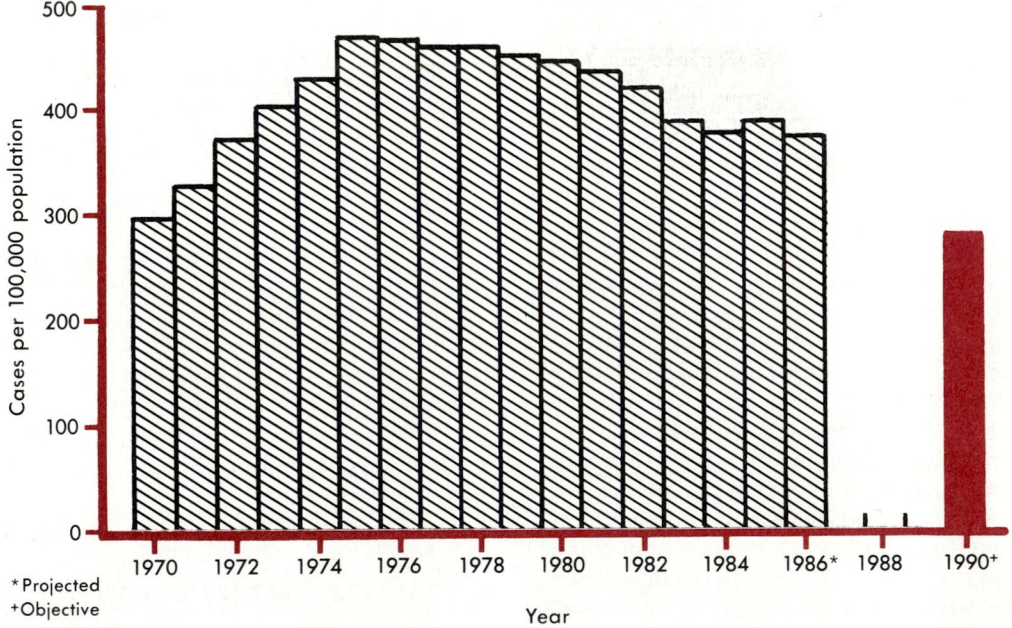

Fig. 35-1 Incidence of gonorrhea in the United States by year, 1970 to 1990. The 1990 rate is the desired goal of 280 cases per 100,000 population. (From Centers for Disease Control: Progress toward achieving the national 1990 objectives for sexually transmitted diseases, MMWR 36(12):173-176, 1987.)

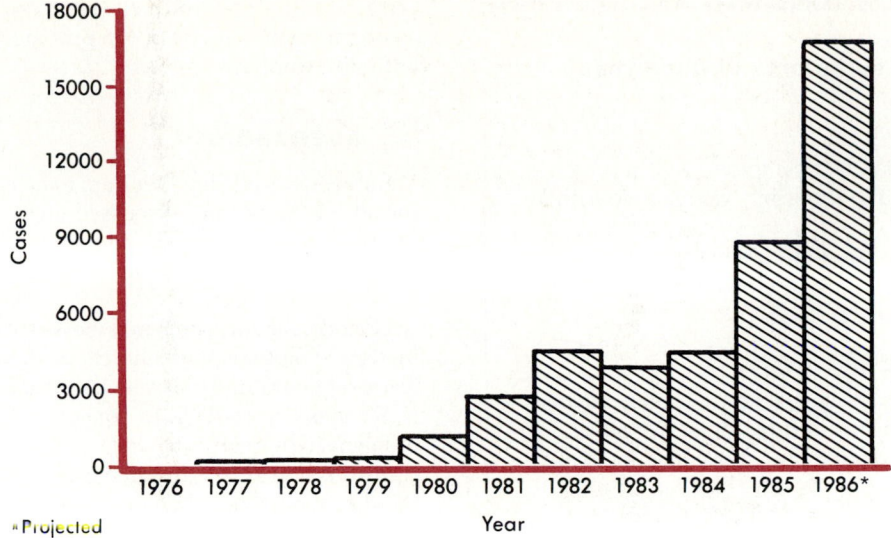

*Projected

Year

Fig. 35-2 Cases of gonorrhea caused by resistant strains in the United States, 1976 to 1988. (From Centers for Disease Control: Progress toward achieving the national 1990 objectives for sexually transmitted diseases, MMWR 36(12):173-176, 1987.)

tance to penicillin (penicillinase-producing N. *gonorrhoeae*) first emerged in 1976.

Resistant strains of the gonococcus can be *plasma-mediated, chromosomally mediated,* or *both* and many varieties have been identified. The three most important in terms of the public health are (1) plasma-mediated resistance to penicillin (PPNG); (2) chromosomally mediated resistance to penicillin (CMRNG); and (3) plasma-mediated, high-level tetracycline resistance (TRNG).[30]

Young adults 20 to 24 years of age are at highest risk of acquiring gonorrhea, with the next highest rates found among teenagers 15 to 19 years of age. In fact, 1 of every 30 teenagers in this age group will acquire gonorrhea each year.

It is estimated that the total cost of gonorrhea to the United States is at least $1 billion yearly. Women and their offspring suffer the major physical, emotional, and economic burden. Pelvic inflammatory disease occurs in 10% to 20% of women with gonorrhea; and even when treated, these women are likely to suffer from recurrent salpingitis, ectopic pregnancy, infertility, and menstrual abnormalities and may face surgical removal of the pelvic organs, as well as fetal loss.

Asymptomatic persons or those with few symptoms are an important reservoir for infection, because they usually remain untreated. As many as 10% to 40% of gonorrheal infections in men are asymptomatic, and in women as many as 80% of infections are asymptomatic. Homosexual men can harbor reservoirs of anorectal and pharyngeal infections.

Gonorrhea, often referred to as "GC" or "the clap" by lay people, is caused by N. *gonorrhoeae.* Gonorrhea is of great concern because of its epidemic rise, high reinfection

rate, and seriousness of residual effects. The incubation period is 3 to 30 days in men and 3 days to an indefinite period in women.

■ Prevention and health education

Prevention of gonorrhea and its complications can be achieved in three stages. The first and most crucial stage is prevention of the disease. The second stage involves prevention of complications of the disease such as pelvic inflammatory disease. The third stage is reversal of the damage caused by the disease, such as by tubal reconstruction.

Early treatment of infected persons is currently the most effective measure to prevent new infection of sexual partners. Mechanical methods such as condoms appear to be effective when used. Education to acquaint people with the symptoms of gonorrhea, the efficacy of condoms, and the availability of diagnostic and treatment resources is also important. Early detection through contact tracing and screening can reduce the serious complications of gonorrhea. Experiments are currently in progress to develop and test an effective vaccine for gonorrhea. See p. 1281 for discussions of contact investigation, which is necessary for all STDs.

■ Signs and symptoms

The most common signs and symptoms are listed in the box on p. 1288. In *men,* the gonococcus is introduced into the anterior urethra during sexual activity. Because most men are diagnosed and treated early, complications and residual effects of gonorrhea are uncommon among men.

Signs and symptoms of gonorrhea

Heterosexual men

1. Urethritis—often first symptom
2. Severe dysuria—especially with first voiding in morning
3. Purulent discharge from urethra
4. Swelling of the penis and balanitis—rare symptoms

Homosexual and bisexual men

1. Rectal gonorrhea is common—usually asymptomatic and discovered by rectal culture
2. Pharyngeal gonorrhea—usually asymptomatic

Women

Women rarely have early, distressing symptoms such as men have. When symptoms are present, they include the following:
1. Slight purulent vaginal discharge
2. Vague feeling of fullness in pelvis
3. Discomfort or aching in abdomen
4. If bladder is involved—burning, frequency, and urgency, which usually cause the person to seek medical attention

The first three symptoms are so slight that they may be ignored.

Sterility from orchitis or epididymitis can occur as a residual effect, but this is rare.

The incidence of *asymptomatic* gonorrhea in men is believed to be low; however, there is an increasing awareness of the importance of men with asymptomatic infection in the transmission of gonorrhea. Some men have been found to have no symptoms of infection despite positive tests for gonorrhea 2 weeks after exposure.

Gonorrhea in women most often begins as *asymptomatic* cervicitis, and the infection can be present for extended periods without causing noticeable signs. Hence there are a high number of infected, *asymptomatic* women. These women do not receive treatment unless gonorrhea is diagnosed through screening or unless the woman is identified by the sexual partner and presents herself for treatment. Frequently, complications are the first indicators of gonorrhea in women. Salpingitis is the most common complication, with 10% to 20% of women presenting themselves with symptoms of *salpingitis* as the first sign of infection. During the course of treatment for salpingitis, many women are surgically sterilized. In cases of untreated gonorrhea, the residual effects of chronic pelvic inflammatory disease, infertility, and ectopic pregnancy are well known.

Other complications of untreated gonorrhea in both men and women include dermatitis, carditis, meningitis, and arthritis. The incidence of these complications is higher among women because of the prolonged period of infection without symptoms.

Assessment

Subjective and objective data to be collected are the same for all STDs and are discussed on p. 1283.

DIAGNOSTIC TESTS

Gonorrheal infection may be suspected on the basis of history, symptoms, and clinical evidence obtained by physical examination. However, identification of the organism is necessary to confirm the diagnosis and to rule out other problems. In men the diagnosis is confirmed by gram-stained smear of the discharge from the penis. Culture of the discharge from the penis is usually reserved for those whose smears are negative in the presence of strong clinical evidence.

Gram-stained cervical smears are inadequate for diagnosing gonorrhea in women. These smears are negative in about 50% of women having gonorrhea and are falsely positive in some cases. Therefore, cultures from the cervix, urethra, throat, and anus are usually taken. Because of the great length of time required to obtain reports of cultures for gonorrhea, treatment is usually instituted on a presumptive basis.

Data analysis: nursing diagnoses

The nursing diagnoses are the same for all STDs and are discussed on p. 1283.

Planning: expected patient outcomes

See p. 1283 for a discussion of the patient outcomes for any of the STDs.

Implementation

ASSISTING WITH ACHIEVEMENT OF THERAPEUTIC GOALS

☐ **Medications**

Therapy for gonorrhea presents a greater problem than for syphilis, because the gonococcus tends to develop resistance to antibiotics. It also is believed that inadequate therapy is common in the United States. Several drug regimens are in use, with emphasis on single-dose treatment to avoid problems with follow-up and patient cooperation.

The treatment regimen recommended by the CDC[32] is as follows:
1. Amoxicillin 3.0 g or ampicillin 3.5 g by mouth or aqueous procaine; penicillin G (APPG) 4.8 million units IM or ceftriaxone 250 mg IM; probenecid 1.0 g by mouth is given along with amoxicillin, ampicillin, or penicillin

2. In addition to the above, tetracycline HCL 500 mg by mouth 4 times daily for 7 days or doxycycline 100 mg by mouth twice daily for 7 days

3. In persons in whom tetracyclines are contraindicated (pregnant women, children under 8 years) or not tolerated, erythromycin base or stearate 500 mg by mouth 4 times daily for 7 days or erythromycin ethyl-succinate 800 mg by mouth 4 times daily for 7 days

Tetracycline is effective against nongonococcal organisms such as *chlamydia,* which are frequently present in persons with gonorrhea. Disadvantages to the recommended regimen includes multiple-dose, multiple-day therapy, which some persons may not comply with. When compliance is poor, resistant strains of *C. trachomatis* may develop.[32]

In areas of the country where antibiotic resistant strains of *N. gonorrhoeae* are endemic or hyperendemic (those areas in which more than 3% of the gonorrhea cases reported in a 2-month period are caused by penicillinase-producing *N. gonorrhoeae*) the following therapy is recommended:

1. Ceftriaxone 250 mg IM

2. Plus, doxycycline 100 mg by mouth, twice daily for 7 days or tetracycline HCL 500 mg by mouth 4 times a day for 7 days

3. If tetracyclines are contraindicated or not tolerated, erythromycin in the amounts recommended above is given

□ Counseling and teaching

Counseling and teaching is the same for all types of STDs and is discussed in detail on p. 1284.

□ Providing social and emotional support

See p. 1285 for discussion about social and emotional support.

□ Promoting self-care

See p. 1285 for discussion of ways to promote self-care.

□ Promoting healthy sexual attitudes

Promoting healthy sexual attitudes is discussed on p. 1285.

⊞ Evaluation

Evaluation is the same for all STDs and is discussed on p. 1285.

■ SYPHILIS

■ Epidemiology, etiology, and pathophysiology

Syphilis is the third most frequently reported communicable disease in the United States, exceeded only by chickenpox and gonorrhea.[27]

Reported cases of syphilis reached an all-time high during World War II, with 575,593 cases being reported in 1943.

The number of cases dropped sharply in the 1950s and began to rise again in the 1960s. There was a steady yearly increase in the number of cases until 1977, when the total

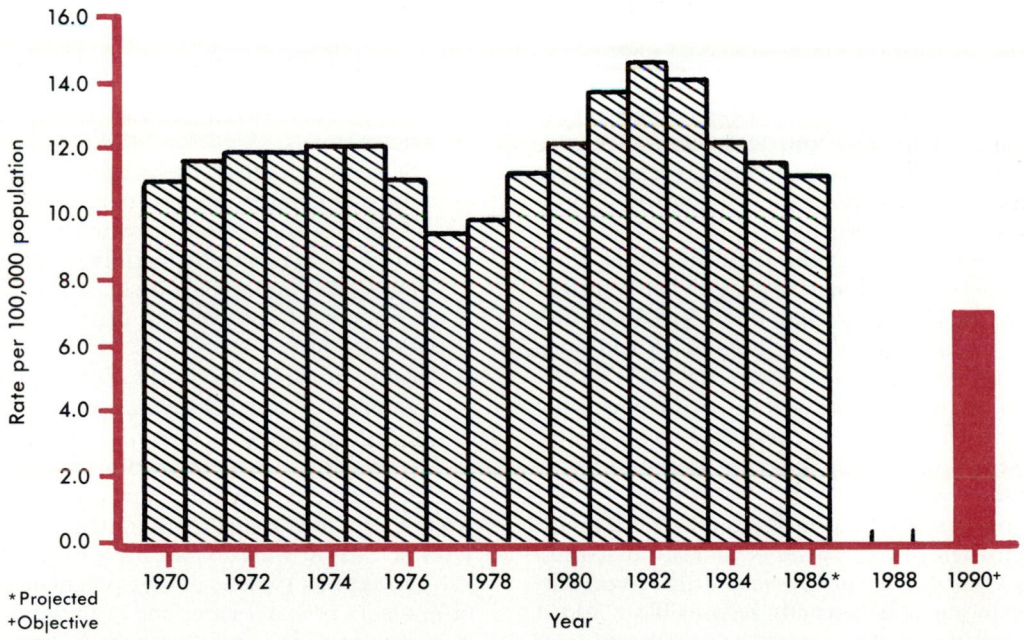

Fig. 35-3 Incidence of primary and secondary syphilis in the United States, 1970 to 1990. The 1990 rate is the desired goal of 7 cases per 100,000 population. (From Centers for Disease Control: Progress toward achieving the national 1990 objectives for sexually transmitted diseases, MMWR 36(12):173-176, 1987.)

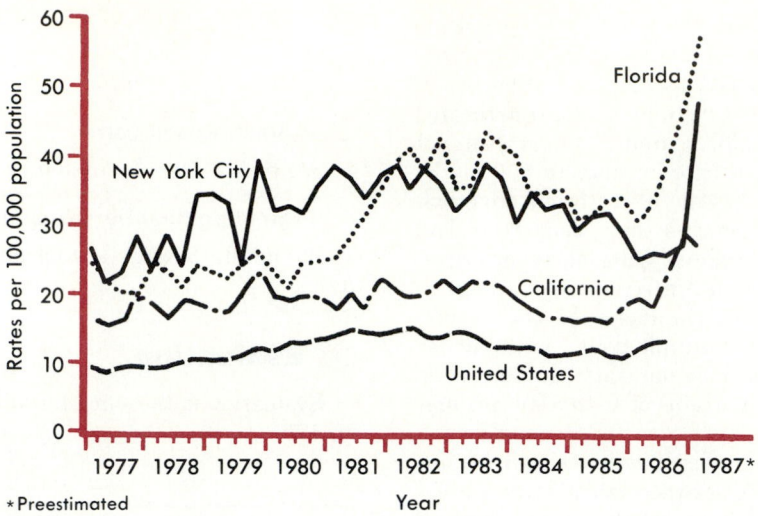

Fig. 35-4 Incidence rates of primary and secondary syphilis, by quarter in the United States and selected areas 1977 to 1988. (From Centers for Disease Control: Increases in primary and secondary syphilis, United States, MMWR 36(25):393-396, 1987.)

number of cases of infectious syphilis (both primary and secondary) decreased. This decrease has persisted each year through 1986 (Fig. 35-3).

Recently there has been a marked increase in the number of cases of infectious syphilis (primary and secondary) reported to the CDC. In the first 46 weeks of 1987,[31] 323 cases of syphilis were reported. This number exceeded the total number of cases reported in 1986 by 32%.[35] The CDC projected annual incidence of syphilis for 1987 would be the highest rate since 1950. The greatest increases were reported in Florida, New York City, and California (see Fig. 35-4). Fifty-six percent of all cases and 83% of the increase occurred in these three areas. In addition, 11 other states reported increases in the incidence of syphilis. In these 14 areas (13 states and New York City) the relative increases were greatest for females and heterosexual males of all racial and ethnic backgrounds.[35] The greatest absolute increases were among blacks.

The figures also reveal that the incidence went down among homosexual/bisexual men, especially white males. This decrease in incidence is believed to result from safer sexual practices by this population because of education about how to prevent AIDS.

The cause of the increase in syphilis is unknown, but suggests a shift in epidemiology of the disease in the United States. Possible reasons for this increase identified by the CDC include the following:

1. Anecdotal reports from persons interviewing syphilis patients and their sexual partners indicate that prostitution that involves *nonintravenous* drugs (especially "crack" cocaine) may be partially responsible.

2. Routine use of spectinomycin to treat gonorrhea in areas where resistant strains of *N. gonorrhoeae* are common may have contributed to the increase in syphilis because spectinomycin does not appear to cure incubating syphilis. This is supported by data from New York City,

Florida, and Los Angeles where spectinomycin was used. However, it does not explain the nationwide increase in syphilis.

3. In some of the high-incidence areas there had been a decrease in the amount of money allocated to syphilis control prgrams and fewer interviewers were available in six of the high-incidence areas. However, the relationship between the number of interviewers and the increase in the incidence of syphilis was *not* statistically significant.

The increases in infectious syphilis among females and heterosexuals are causing concern for three reasons.

1. An increase in syphilis in females will probably be followed by increased incidence and deaths from congenital syphilis.

2. The marked increase in syphilis among inner-city, heterosexual minority groups indicates that high-risk sexual activity is *increasing* despite the risk of HIV infection. This is especially alarming because among these groups risks are already increased because of the high prevalence of intravenous drug abuse in their communities.

3. Studies in Africa and in the United States suggest that genital ulcer diseases such as primary syphilis increase the risk of HIV transmission.[35]

The trends for early congenital syphilis (CS) have paralleled the trends for primary and secondary syphilis among women. Factors thought to contribute to the sustained level of early CS are (1) an increase in the incidence of early infectious syphilis among pregnant women, (2) lack of available prenatal care, and (3) failure of the prenatal system to provide timely serologic testing and prompt follow-up.

In addition, it is believed that the greatest percentage of cases of syphilis go unreported and thus the incidence is much greater than the figures indicate.

Syphilis is caused by a spirochete, *Treponema pallidum*, that gains entry into the body through either the mucous membrane or skin during intercourse. The organism is readily destroyed by physical and chemical agents, including heat, drying, and mild disinfectants such as soap and water.

The incubation period for syphilis is usually 3 weeks. However, symptoms can appear as early as 9 days or as long as 3 months after exposure, which is the case for rectal infections in homosexual men.

■ Prevention and health education

As with gonorrhea, three levels of prevention are important. The first is prevention of the initial infection by finding and treating those with the disease so that they cannot spread it to others. Secondary prevention is directed at early treatment of cases to prevent late syphilis or congenital syphilis. Finally, efforts can be made to treat the complications of syphilis when they occur. Contact investigation, which is necessary for all STDs, is discussed on p. 1281.

■ Signs and symptoms

The signs and symptoms of the four stages of syphilis are listed in Table 35-2. If syphilis is adequately diagnosed and treated during the primary stage, the other stages can be prevented.

⧉ Assessment

The subjective and objective data to be collected from a person suspected of having any STD are discussed on p. 1283.

■ DIAGNOSTIC TESTS

Syphilis is most often diagnosed by standard serologic tests. Massive screening programs in the past made serologic diagnosis of syphilis very common. Mass screening with the VDRL test is no longer practiced except on high-risk populations, pregnant women, sexually active women, and couples who are applying for a marriage license. Dark-field microscopic examination of tissue scrapings from lesions or material obtained by aspiration of regional lymph nodes also reveals the presence of the spirochete, especially during the primary and secondary stages. A presumptive diagnosis is made on the basis of suspicious lesions, positive serologic tests, known exposure to infection, and involvement of regional lymph nodes. False-positive VDRL reactions are common among persons previously treated for syphilis, but fluorescent treponemal antibody (FTA) and absorption (ABS) tests are more specific (Table 35-3). Also, once a VDRL test is positive, it remains so and is not useful for identifying reinfection. Infectious mononucleosis, hepatitis, pregnancy, viral pneumonia, malaria, chickenpox, measles and smallpox vaccination, narcotic

Table 35-2   Stages of syphilis

	Primary	Secondary	Latent	Late
Duration	2-8 weeks	Appears 2-4 weeks after chancre appears; extends over 2-4 years	5-20 years	Terminal if not treated
Signs and symptoms	Hard sore or pimple on vulva or penis that breaks and forms painless, draining chancre; may be a single chancre or groups of more than one; may be present also on lips, tongue, hands, rectum, or nipples; chancre heals leaving almost invisible scar	Depends on site; low-grade fever, headache, anorexia, weight loss, anemia, sore throat, hoarseness, reddened and sore eyes, jaundice with or without hepatitis, aching of joints, muscles, long bones; sores on body or generalized fine rash; condylomata accuminata (venereal warts) on rectum or genitalia	No clinical signs	Tumorlike mass, gumma, on any area of body; damage to heart valves and blood vessels; meningitis; paralysis; lack of coordination; paresis; insomnia; confusion; delusions; impaired judgment; slurred speech
Communicability	Exudates from lesions and chancre are highly contagious	Exudates from lesions highly contagious; blood contains organisms	Contagious for about 2 years; not contagious to others after that; blood contains organisms; may be transmitted placentally to fetus	Noncontagious; spinal fluid may contain organisms

Table 35-3 Serologic tests for syphilis (STSs)

Type	Description	Examples	Comments
Flocculation	Antibody-antigen reaction produces a precipitation (flocculation)	VDRL RPR	Used primarily for screening; performed in standard laboratories
Complement fixation	Complement is used up in antigen-antibody reaction (fixed); hemolysis occurs	Reiter (Wasserman outdated)	Nonspecific; used less frequently; performed in standard laboratories
Fluorescent antibody	Antigen of killed *Treponema pallidum* is labeled with a fluorescent dye	FTA FTA-ABS	More specific than flocculation or complement-fixation test; differentiates false-positive from true syphilis positive results; performed in special laboratories
T. pallidum immobilization	Serum is mixed with live *T. pallidum;* presence of antibody decreases organism mobility	TPI	Most sensitive test; performed only at CDC laboratory in Atlanta

addiction, and terminal malignancy have also been associated with false-positive VDRL results.

▦ Implementation

■ ASSISTING WITH ACHIEVEMENT OF THERAPEUTIC GOALS

☐ Medications

Syphilis can be successfully treated at any stage of the disease, although treatment may have to be more prolonged in latent and late syphilis. Although syphilis can be cured in late stages, the damage to the body is much less easily managed.

Because penicillin continues to be effective in the treatment of syphilis, it remains the drug of choice. All types of penicillin are effective, but penicillin G benzathine is preferred because it is long-acting and can be given in a limited number of injections.

Patients with primary, secondary, and latent syphilis (and their contacts) are usually given 2.4 million units of penicillin intramuscularly. Patients with late syphilis are generally given 2.4 million units intramuscularly at 7-day intervals until a total of 7.2 to 9.6 million units has been given. When the use of penicillin is contraindicated because of drug sensitivity, tetracycline HCL 500 mg orally 4 times daily for 15 days is given. Persons with latent syphilis (more than 1 year's duration) are treated with tetracycline HCL 500 mg orally 4 times daily for 30 days. Compliance with this regimen may be especially difficult, and the patient will need follow-up reminders to take the drug daily.

In addition, although tetracycline is believed to be effective in treating syphilis, it has been evaluated less extensively than penicillin. The most effective therapeutic results have been achieved in cases in which a single dose of medication such as benzathine penicillin IM was given. Compliance with any oral medication regimen can be difficult especially when the person is a chronic drug abuser and engages in other high-risk behaviors.

☐ Counseling and teaching

Counseling and teaching for all types of STDs is the same. It is discussed on p. 1284.

☐ Providing social and emotional support

Social and emotional support for the patient with an STD is discussed on p. 1285.

☐ Promoting self-care

The ways in which self-care can be promoted can be found on p. 1285.

☐ Promoting healthy sexual attitudes

The promotion of healthy sexual attitudes is the same for all persons with an STD (see p. 1285).

▦ Evaluation

The outcomes to be evaluated in the person with syphilis are the same as those for a patient with any STD and are discussed on p. 1285.

Pregnant women with penicillin sensitivity pose problems for treatment. In the large dosage required to treat syphilis, tetracycline produces mottling and staining of fetal teeth and possible abnormal bone formation. If given the usual adult dose, inadequate placental transfer of tetracycline is likely, and congenital syphilis would probably develop. Erythromycin in a dose of 30 g over a period of 15 days seems to be the best alternative treatment for pregnant women with syphilis. Neurosyphilis is treated with intravenous penicillin. Contacts are treated with 2.4 million units of penicillin G benzathine.

■ ACQUIRED IMMUNODEFICIENCY SYNDROME (AIDS)

Although AIDS is a sexually transmitted disease, its most profound effect is on the immune system and for that reason it is discussed in Chapter 38.

■ HERPES GENITALIS

■ Epidemiology, etiology, and pathophysiology

Herpes genitalis (genital herpes, HVH-2) is caused by infection with *Herpesvirus hominis* type 2 (HVH-2). Herpes genitalis was the most important STD of the 1970s. Its chronicity, frequent recurrences, and difficult treatment and prevention distinguish it from other STDs. It is estimated that about 400,000 to 600,000 new cases occur annually.[26] Conservative estimates are that 15% to 20% of Americans now suffer from genital herpes, and it is believed that because of poor control measures the number of cases is increasing dramatically. Its peak incidence parallels the young age groups affected by other STDs. Once acquired, herpes genitalis is a lifelong disease and carries with it not only intense and recurrent discomfort, but also anxieties about future childbearing, malignancy, and sexual and marital function. In early pregnancy women infected with herpes have an increased chance of miscarriage. Because genital herpetic lesions endanger the fetus during delivery, caesarean delivery is often necessary. Genital herpes has also been associated with cervical cancer. It is now generally accepted that HVH-2 is spread by sexual contact.

The incubation period is 3 to 7 days. The primary lesion appears as a vesicle on the external genitalia in men; often on the rectum in homosexual men; and on the vagina, cervix, or external genitalia in women. These lesions often ulcerate, especially when located on moist surfaces. Following primary herpes, the virus persists in a *latent or unrecognized* form in most patients. It is believed that latent infections are localized in the ganglia of sensory nerves to the genitalia. When the host factors favor it, the *latent infection* becomes clinically apparent as *recurrent herpes*.

■ Prevention and health education

Primary prevention of herpes depends on limiting sexual contact between infected individuals and uninfected partners. There is preliminary evidence that the herpes virus may survive on towels for up to 20 minutes; therefore it is important to use separate linens. Refraining from sexual intercourse while lesions are present and for 10 days after they heal is essential. Sexually active young persons should be taught to look at themselves and prospective partners for such lesions. In some communities there are groups of individuals with herpes who have chosen to restrict themselves to sexual contact only with others who already have been exposed to herpes. Condoms may be helpful. Transmission to the fetus may be prevented by caesarean section. Infected neonates may develop subsequent mental retardation or die. If drug therapy for HVH-2 is effective, it will help limit new infections by eradicating at least some of the reservoir of infected individuals by preventing reactivation of HVH-2.

Secondary prevention is aimed at reducing or eliminating complications such as cervical cancer. A yearly Pap smear is recommended. Another important complication of the disease is its ability to create great psychologic pain and anxiety, to disrupt normal social and sexual relationships, and to stigmatize its victims. In the event that secondary prevention is not possible, efforts to detect and treat cervical cancer in its early stages are essential.

▨ Assessment

The subjective and objective data to be collected from any person suspected of having a sexually transmitted disease is discussed on p. 1283.

■ SIGNS AND SYMPTOMS

The common signs and symptoms of primary infection are the following:
1. Local inflammation
2. Pain
3. Enlargement of inguinal lymph nodes
4. Generalized signs of infection
   a. Photophobia
   b. Headache
   c. Flulike symptoms

Primary infections are associated with local inflammation, pain, enlargement of the inguinal lymph nodes, and generalized signs of infection such as photophobia, headaches, and flulike symptoms. Although primary herpetic lesions begin as single or multiple reddish papules that then develop into clear, fluid-filled vesicles, once they rupture they form ulcerations that may fuse with other lesions to form large ulcerated areas. The disease tends to be more extensive in women than in men. In some women cervical infection accompanies the external lesions, and in certain cases it may be the only infected site. Cervical involvement may be mild or severe with extensive ulceration and pus. Genital lesions often worsen during the first 10 to 15 days but usually heal within 3 to 4 weeks. These symptoms will usually lead the individual to seek medical attention.

Vaginal discharge is common among women, and discharge from the urethra is usual in men having primary infections. Urinary tract involvement may occur and is reflected in symptoms of dysuria or urinary retention. The lesions can cause severe pain, requiring hospitalization for parenteral analgesia. Subclinical infections in which patients are unaware of any problem occur in only about 10% of the cases of genital herpes. Unfortunately, about 75% of all patients have at least one recurrence. Fortunately, recurrent infections are usually milder and of shorter duration than primary infections and usually produce local rather than systemic reaction. The patient experiencing a recurrent infection often has prodromal signs of paresthesia and burning at the site where the lesion will erupt. Factors known to predispose to recurrent infection include fever, emotional upsets, premenstrual states, and overexposure to heat and sunshine. Although the mode of recurrent infection is not clear, it has been theorized that during primary infection the virus ascends sensory nerve sheaths, localizing in corresponding nerve ganglia, and that when the environment becomes favorable, the virus is reactivated. Recurrent herpes usually begins with abnormal sensation or itching of a localized genital area. Lesions of recurrent infections usually occur in the site of primary infection. Herpes encephalitis may also occur.

■ DIAGNOSTIC TESTS

Diagnosis of herpes genitalis is made by isolation of the virus from specimens obtained from lesions. Pap smears or fluid from the vesicles collected in transport medium demonstrates cellular characteristics of viruses.

Implementation

■ ASSISTING WITH ACHIEVEMENT OF THERAPEUTIC GOALS

□ Symptomatic therapy

Treatment for genital herpes has most often been symptomatic, because there is no known cure for the disease. Acyclovir appears capable of inhibiting the replication of herpetic viruses in vitro; and in clinical trials with patients who had antibodies against herpes simplex viruses, acyclovir prevented active herpes infections.[81] Acyclovir ointment, 5%, is recommended for genital herpes. The ointment is applied to cover all lesions every 3 hours, six times a day for 7 days. The acyclovir treatment reduces viral shedding and the duration of the disease in patients with primary initial infections who are treated within 6 days of the onset of symptoms. *It does not prevent recurrences.* There is no effective treatment to prevent recurrences or to shorten their duration.

Symptomatic treatment consists of using Burow's solution or hydrogen peroxide and soap and water to cleanse the lesions. The involved areas are blown dry with a hair dryer, and the skin is then dusted with cornstarch. Women are advised to use a mirror to examine the vulva, vagina, and cervix for hidden lesions.

■ COUNSELING AND TEACHING

Persons with herpes should abstain from sexual contact while the lesions are present and for 10 days after the lesions heal. Risk of transmission during asymptomatic periods is unknown. Some advise using condoms to prevent transmission of the disease.

■ PROVIDING SOCIAL AND EMOTIONAL SUPPORT

Because herpes genitalis is a recurrent disease with no cure, patients infected with the virus require considerable support. Some infected persons tend to withdraw from an active social life rather than face the possibility of making a commitment that will require them to share knowledge of their disease with another person. For this reason, in some communities support groups have been formed for persons who have herpes genitalis.

■ CHLAMYDIAL INFECTION

■ Epidemiology, etiology, and pathophysiology

Chlamydia trachomatis infections are recognized as the most prevalent of the STDs in the United States. Because it is not a reportable disease, the actual number of cases is unknown. It is estimated, however, that each year 3 to 4 million Americans suffer from epidemic chlamydial infections. In England and Wales, where nongonococcal urethritis (about half the cases of which are caused by *C. trachomatis*) is a reportable disease, the incidence has nearly doubled in the last decade.[24]

Chlamydial infections are responsible for about 20% of diagnosed pelvic inflammatory disease cases, and it is estimated that about 11,000 women each year become involuntarily sterilized and 3600 suffer ectopic pregnancies as a result of this organism.[25] Chlamydial infections can be transmitted to infants during delivery, causing conjunctivitis and pneumonia in many. Table 35-4 shows how the infection can be transmitted between male and female sexual partners and from females to infants. It also lists the various ways the disease is manifested in males, females, and infants.

■ Prevention and health education

Primary prevention of chlamydial infections consists of limiting sexual contact with infected partners. Secondary prevention requires early diagnosis and treatment.

Risk assessment factors require special attention. Age, number of sex partners, socioeconomic status, and sexual preference are predictors of infection with C. *trachomatis*.[28] These factors include the following:

1. Age—Infection rates are 2 to 3 times higher in sexually active women under age 20 than in those over age 20. The rates for women between 20 and 29 years of age are considerably higher than for women over age 30. The rates of urethral infection are higher for teenage males than for adult men.

2. Number of sex partners—Persons with several sex partners are at higher risk of infection.

3. Socioeconomic status—Some studies have shown that persons of lower socioeconomic status are at increased risk for infection with C. *trachomatis*.

4. Sexual preference—The prevalence of urethral chlamydial infection among homosexual men is one-third that among heterosexual men. However, 4% to 8% of homosexual men seen in STD clinics have rectal chlamydia infection.

Assessment

■ SIGNS AND SYMPTOMS

Chlamydial infections are usually diagnosed on the basis of history and pelvic examination. Women notice painful or difficult urination, abnormal vaginal discharge or bleed-

Table 35-4 Chlamydia trachomatis infections

Males	Females	Infants
Transmission		
Males ⇌ Females ⟶ Infants		
Infections		
Urethritis	Cervicitis	Conjunctivitis
Postgonococcal urethritis	Urethritis	Pneumonia
Proctitis	Proctitis	Asymptomatic pharyngeal carriage
Conjunctivitis	Conjunctivitis	Asymptomatic gastrointestinal carriage
Pharyngitis	Pharyngitis	
Subclinical lymphogranuloma venereum	Subclinical lymphogranuloma venereum	
Complications		
Epididymitis	Salpingitis	
Prostatitis	Endometritis	
Reiter's syndrome	Perihepatitis	
Sterility	Ectopic pregnancy	
Rectal strictures*	Infertility	
	Vulvar/rectal carcinoma*	
	Rectal stricture*	

From Centers for Disease Control, Chlamydia Trachomatis Infections, Policy Guidelines for Prevention and Control, MMWR Suppl. 35:54, 1985.
*Associated with lymphogranuloma venereum.

ing, and possibly dyspareunia or other pelvic pain. Other women, however, are asymptomatic. Men usually have nonspecific urethritis or may seek treatment for epididymitis.

■ DIAGNOSTIC TESTS

There are several tests used to confirm the presence of *C. trachomatis* infection. These include (1) cell culture, (2) identification of organism by immunologic techniques, and (3) measurement of serum antibody response to the organism. The cell culture is considered the best test but it is not available in all laboratories, it is quite costly ($15 to $40), and it takes 4 days to obtain the results.

In areas of high incidence of chlamydial infections or in patients who have gonorrhea, the patient usually is treated for a chlamydial infection whether it has been confirmed by a laboratory test or not.[15] The reason for this is that

chlamydial infection is found fairly often in persons diagnosed with gonorrhea.

▦ Implementation

■ ASSISTING WITH ACHIEVEMENT OF THERAPEUTIC GOALS

☐ Medications

Tetracycline HCL, 500 mg orally four times daily for 7 days is given for chlamydial infections. Erythromycin 500 mg orally 4 times daily for 7 days may be used for patients unable to take tetracyclines for reasons cited previously (Table 35-1). Doxycycline, minocycline, or sulfamethoxazole may be prescribed but are less commonly used. As mentioned above patients are usually treated with penicillin simultaneously because so many of them also have gonorrhea. Penicillin alone is not effective in treating *C. trachomatis*.

☐ Counseling and teaching

It is important that the patient encourage their sexual partner(s) to seek care as soon as possible to avoid reinfection of the patient and complications in the partner.[15] Patients who are sexually active should be advised to wear condoms or use spermicides to reduce reinfection.

☐ Providing social and emotional support

Social and emotional support of these patients is as important as it is with any person with an STD (p. 1285).

■ LYMPHOGRANULOMA VENEREUM

■ Epidemiology and etiology

Lymphogranuloma venereum (LGV) is a systemic, sexually transmitted disease caused by *Chlamydia* organisms. Other species of *Chlamydia* are the causative organisms of trachoma and psittacosis. The disease is contracted by vaginal, anal, or oral intercourse; and primary inoculation with the organism may occur at any site involved in close contact. The incubation period is 7 to 12 days. Lymphadenitis of regional lymph nodes draining the site of primary infection occurs, and the disease spreads by way of the lymphatic system.

LGV is most prevalent in the tropics. In the United States it is found most often in the southern states, but epidemiologic studies are needed to determine its true incidence. Reports of the incidence of LGV indicate less than 500 cases annually. The symptoms of LGV resemble those of other sexually transmitted diseases, and its reported incidence may be influenced by this.

■ Pathophysiology

There are three clinical phases of infection in LGV: (1) inoculation and appearance of the primary lesions, (2) lymphatic spread and generalized symptoms, and (3) late complications. In individual cases any one of the phases may be absent or go unnoticed.

The primary lesion, which is transient, appears as a papule, small erosion, or vesicle. The most common sites of the primary lesion are the prepuce and glans in men and the vagina and cervix in women. Because it is painless, the primary lesion may go unnoticed, especially in women. Localized edema may be present. If the rectum is infected, there is a bloody discharge followed by a mucopurulent discharge, diarrhea, and cramping.

Involvement of the lymphatics occurs 1 to 4 weeks after the appearance of the primary lesion. If the primary lesion is on the penis, anal margin, clitoris, or upper vulva, the superficial inguinal lymph nodes are involved. Infection of the vagina or cervix as the primary site produces involvement of the deep iliac and anorectal lymph nodes. The large lymph nodes, or buboes that appear are firm and lobular. The skin over the superficial nodes is bluish red and adheres to the nodes.

Assessment

SIGNS AND SYMPTOMS

The first indication of infection in most patients is a feeling of stiffness and aching in the groin followed by swelling in the inguinal area. Symptoms of nongonococcal urethritis may be present. Constitutional symptoms of infection may or may not appear at this time. The involved lymph nodes may suppurate, causing extensive scarring. Obstruction of the lymphatics may result, leading to chronic edema and ulceration. Lymphatic spread of the infection is accompanied by generalized symptoms. Mild to severe fever, malaise, nausea, and vomiting may occur. Abdominal pain, symptoms of cystitis, and urinary retention are common when pelvic lymph nodes are involved. Acute proctocolitis is common in homosexual men.

Among the most severe complications of LGV are development of perianal abscesses, rectovaginal or rectovesical fistulas, and rectal strictures. In the last clinical phase, generalized infection is indicated by blood values showing anemia, leukocytosis, and an elevated sedimentation rate.

DIAGNOSTIC TESTS

LGV is isolated from aspirate from an affected lymph node. The LGV complement-fixation test (LGV-CFT) is a test for antibodies. A positive LGV-CFT test along with a careful history and physical examination affords the best chances for diagnosing LGV.

Implementation

ASSISTING WITH ACHIEVEMENT OF THERAPEUTIC GOALS

☐ Medications

Early antibiotic therapy is essential for controlling and reducing morbidity from LGV, and it is generally agreed that treatment should not be delayed until diagnostic test results are obtained. Tetracycline in a dosage of 500 mg four times a day for at least 2 weeks is the treatment of choice. If drug sensitivity or pregnancy precludes use of tetracycline, erythromycin, 500 mg four times daily for 2 to 6 weeks, is used.

If cost is not a factor, doxycycline, 100 mg two times daily for 2 weeks, is preferred because it is better tolerated than tetracycline. Other drugs that are effective in treating LGV are chloramphenicol, minocycline, and rifampin. Sexual partners should receive the same therapy. If lymphadenopathy does not respond to therapy in 1 to 2 weeks, an alternate drug may be required. In some patients therapy must be continued for as long as 6 weeks. Sexual partners should also receive the therapy for the same period of time.

☐ Other therapy

Fluctuant lymph nodes may be aspirated to prevent scarring and destruction of lymphatic channels. This is done only in conjunction with antibiotic therapy. Surgical removal of the lymph nodes is not advised, because this may increase lymphedema and elephantiasis.

If rectal stricture supervenes, rectal dilation at 2-week intervals may be attempted. Development of fistulas is especially distressing and requires that surgical repair be accomplished. LGV is a disease characterized by remissions and exacerbations, and thorough surveillance is important. Antibiotic therapy should be reinstituted as soon as symptoms of reactivation occur. Biopsy of lesions and lymph nodes is advised in chronic cases of LGV, because cancer may develop in the ulcerative lesions and may be overlooked as a result of similarity in appearance.

☐ Counseling and teaching

See p. 1284 for discussion of points to be covered.

☐ Providing social and emotional support

The social and emotional support for patients with LGV is the same as for patients with any STD. See p. 1285 for further discussion.

CHANCROID

Epidemiology, etiology, and pathophysiology

Chancroid is a sexually transmitted disease caused by a gram-negative bacillus, *Haemophilus ducreyi*. Although chancroid is less common in the United States, with only about 2,000 cases reported annually, there is a need for surveillance to determine any increase in incidence.

Since the early 1980s epidemics have occurred in Boston, New York City, Dallas, Florida, and Orange County, California, and the disease has become endemic in these U.S. areas.

Although it is found worldwide, chancroid is most prevalent in tropical and semitropical areas in the Orient, the

West Indies, and North Africa. The disease occurs more often in men than in women and more often among non-white than white people. It is possible that returning military personnel may have introduced the disease into areas where it did not previously exist.

The incubation period varies from 1 to 14 days and averages 4 to 5 days. The primary lesion appears as an inflamed macule that rapidly progresses to vesicle and pustule stages. By the time the patient seeks medical care, the lesions have usually become ulcerated. Multiple lesions in various stages of progression may be seen and are caused by rupture of vesicles and pustules and autoinoculation. There may be single or multiple ulcers that are nonindurated and painful. Inguinal lymphadenopathy may or may not be present.

Assessment

SIGNS AND SYMPTOMS

In women, the lesions of chancroid are most often found on the labia, anus, clitoris, vagina, and cervix. A few women do not have any lesions but may have signs of mild vaginitis. In men the lesions appear on the prepuce, glans, or shaft of the penis.

The ulcers found in chancroid are typically ragged and irregular. They are highly infectious and autoimmunity may occur, resulting in multiple lesions. The ulcers appear excavated, have a granulating, purulent surface, and are painful. Often, edema of the surrounding tissues is present. Involvement of the inguinal lymph nodes occurs in about 50% of all cases of chancroid within 2 weeks after appearance of the primary lesion. The buboes are most often unilateral, painful, and spherical in shape. The skin over the buboes is inflamed. The buboes tend to become softer as abscesses form. These abscesses in turn may suppurate and rupture, further spreading the infection. Generalized symptoms of infection usually appear when inguinal abscesses form.

DIAGNOSTIC TESTS

Diagnosis of chancroid depends on growth of the organism on special media. A specimen is collected by aspiration of a vesicle, pustule, or lymph node, or from the margin of an ulcer.

Implementation

ASSISTING WITH ACHIEVEMENT OF THERAPEUTIC GOALS

Medications

The treatment of choice is erythromycin, 500 mg orally four times daily for 7 days, or ceftriaxone 250 mg IM once. Other antimicrobial therapies are available but are not considered to be as effective.

Other therapy

Fluctuant inguinal nodes should be aspirated to prevent pain and spontaneous rupture.

DONOVANOSIS

Epidemiology and etiology

Donovanosis, commonly called granuloma inguinale or granuloma venereum, is believed to be most often transmitted by sexual contact. The infection is caused by a gram-negative bacillus, *Calymmatobacterium (Donovania) granulomatis*, widely referred to as Donovan bacillus. The incubation period is unknown but is about 8 to 12 weeks.

Donovanosis is common in tropical and subtropical areas and rarely occurs in the United States. It is very common in New Guinea, India, and the Caribbean. The disease is mildly contagious and probably requires repeated exposures for spread of infection. Predisposing factors are poorly understood. The disease is more common in men than women and is especially common among homosexual men.

Assessment

SIGNS AND SYMPTOMS

In donovanosis, lesions appear on the genitalia and in the perianal area. The most common sites of lesions are the prepuce and glans in men and the vagina and labia in women. The infection first appears with development of subcutaneous nodules. These elevated areas eventually ulcerate, producing sharply defined, painless lesions. The ulcers enlarge slowly and bleed on contact. With ulceration, the infection tends to spread along the pubic region. Involvement of the lymph nodes is uncommon but can occur and produce occlusion of the lymphatics, resulting in elephantiasis.

DIAGNOSTIC TESTS

Smears of exudates taken from the lesions do not always demonstrate the causative organism, even when donovanosis is present. Therefore, a sample of tissue is taken from the lesion, is crushed between two slides, and is stained. The specimen is examined for the presence of Donovan bodies, which represent the intracellular stage of the causative organism. Examination of a tissue sample also makes it possible to differentiate between donovanosis and cancer.

Implementation

ASSISTING WITH ACHIEVEMENT OF THERAPEUTIC GOALS

Medications

Tetracycline, streptomycin, and gentamycin are antibiotics used to treat the infection.

■ TRICHOMONIASIS

■ Epidemiology, etiology, and pathophysiology

A protozoan, *Trichomonas vaginalis,* is the causative organism of trichomoniasis. Evidence suggests that the incubation period ranges between 4 and 28 days.[38] Trichomoniasis may well be the most frequently acquired STD in the United States, with an estimated incidence of 3 million cases occurring annually. *T. vaginalis* organisms are found in 3% to 15% of women under the care of private physicians, 13% to 23% of women attending gynecologic clinics,[38] and 50% of women who have gonorrhea. There is no documentation of the rate at which asymptomatic carriers become symptomatic. Older women who experience changes in vaginal pH often exhibit the disease in the absence of new sexual contact.

Trichomoniasis is frequently viewed as an innocuous infection, yet there are serious implications for health. During the postpartum period in women who have trichomoniasis, the rate of persistent fever, prolonged vaginal discharge, and endometritis is twice as high as in women who do not harbor the organism. About 90% of patients with trichomoniasis have cervical erosions and leukorrhea, and it has been suggested that chronic irritation may predispose to cervical cancer. Interpretation of cervical cytology, as in the Pap test, is unreliable in the presence of trichomoniasis, because the infection produces atypical cervical cells. Unless repeated cervical smears are taken, cancer of the cervix may be missed. Trichomoniasis results in urethritis; it also causes prostatitis in men 40% of the time; and, finally, reversible sterility can occur as a result of inhibition of sperm motility by toxins produced by the organism.

■ Assessment

■ SIGNS AND SYMPTOMS

Only 25% of women harboring the organism are asymptomatic. Pruritus of the vulva and vagina is the predominant symptom among women. The itching may be so severe as to awaken the patient, and excoriation from scratching is common. Secondary infection of the broken skin may result.

Classically, the symptoms of trichomoniasis in women are a copious, frothy, green or greenish-yellow vaginal discharge, inflammation of the labia minora and lower vagina, and a red-speckled appearance of the vaginal canal and cervix. A small number of patients present this classic picture that is usually described in texts. Most patients have a vaginal discharge, but it is small in amount and yellow, and there is some inflammation of the labia and vagina. Itching is almost universally present, however; and dyspareunia, dysuria, and urinary frequency may also occur.

In men, urethritis and its symptoms of purulent discharge, itching, burning, and inflammation are the signs of trichomoniasis most often seen. Prostatitis, epididymitis,

and urethral stricture may occur as complications among men. However, these consequences of trichomoniasis have not been extensively studied and are not well documented.

■ DIAGNOSTIC TESTS

Diagnosis of trichomoniasis is most often made by preparing a hanging drop slide containing a specimen of the discharge and observing the motile organism under the microscope. Serologic and skin tests are currently being investigated but lack reliability so far. Because of the high incidence of coexisting gonorrhea, smears or cultures for gonococci should also be taken.

■ Implementation

■ ASSISTING WITH ACHIEVEMENT OF THERAPEUTIC GOALS

☐ Medications

The recommended treatment is metronidazole (Flagyl) 2.0 g by mouth in a single dose. An alternative regimen would be metronidazole 250 mg orally three times daily for 7 days.

Both partners should be treated simultaneously to prevent reinfection by the untreated partner at a later date. Vaginal inserts of metronidazole are less effective. The drug is known to cross the placental barrier. For this reason, it is not given to pregnant women until after the first trimester.

■ CANDIDIASIS

■ Epidemiology, etiology, and pathophysiology

Candidiasis, commonly called monilial infection or monilial vaginitis, is an infection caused by a yeast form, *Candida albicans.* The overall incidence of candidiasis in the United States is unknown. There is disagreement about whether yeast infections such as candidiasis should be classed as sexually transmitted. The organism is commonly found on mucous membrane surfaces in women who have no symptoms of infection. The greatest incidence of candidiasis occurs during the ages of maximal sexual activity. The causative organism is frequently cultured from the urethra of regular male sexual partners, and urethritis and balanitis (inflammation of the glans penis) occur in up to 10% of men who engage in sexual activity with infected women. Women who respond to therapy and become reinfected are usually married women having one sex partner.

C. albicans is found in the mouth, gastrointestinal tract, and vagina of 25% to 50% of women. Differentiation between colonization and true infection may be difficult in some cases. Colonization rate and the chance of true infection increase in diabetic persons, during pregnancy, and with diseases or therapies that impair body defenses (use of broad-spectrum antibiotics, corticosteroids, and oral contraceptives).

Assessment

SIGNS AND SYMPTOMS

Women having symptoms of candidiasis most often complain of pruritus of the vulva. A vaginal discharge that is thick, white, and curdlike is characteristic. The vulva appears inflamed and edematous, and excoriations from scratching are often present. White patches that appear to adhere to the mucosal surfaces are often seen in the vagina. Similar white, curdlike patches appear on the mucous membrane surfaces and tongue in newborn infants infected by the organism, causing a condition known as thrush.

Little is known about candidiasis occurring among men. Symptoms of balanitis may be present; especially in uncircumcised men. Asymptomatic urethritis occurs in up to 10% of infected men.

DIAGNOSTIC TESTS

Diagnosis may be suspected from the patient's history of predisposing factors and symptoms, but it is usually made by microscopic examination of a smear of the discharge.

Implementation

ASSISTING WITH ACHIEVEMENT OF THERAPEUTIC GOALS

☐ **Medications and other therapy**

Therapy consists of treatment with fungicidal creams, ointments, or tablets. The commonly used fungicides are miconazole, nystatin, and candicidin. Relief from itching may be obtained from tepid sodium bicarbonate baths and clothing that allows adequate ventilation. Application of talcum powder or cornstarch is also helpful.

GARDNERALLA VAGINALIS

Etiology

G. vaginalis (previously known as *Cornyebacterium vaginalis* or *Haemophilus vaginalis*) can be cultured from 23% to 96% of women with vaginitis and is recovered from up to 50% of asymptomatic women.

Assessment

SIGNS AND SYMPTOMS

G. vaginalis infection is characterized by a small amount of homogeneous gray or grayish white discharge. The discharge usually has a disagreeable odor, and because it is less irritating than discharges caused by other organisms, pruritus is mild or absent. On inspection, the vaginal walls are slightly reddened, and the discharge appears to adhere to the mucosal lining. Some women are asymptomatic despite positive cultures.

DIAGNOSTIC TESTS

Diagnosis is confirmed by microscopic examination of a smear or culture of the vaginal discharge.

Implementation

ASSISTING WITH ACHIEVEMENT OF THERAPEUTIC GOALS

☐ **Medications**

Treatment of *G. vaginalis* consists of oral ampicillin given four times a day for 5 days; cephalosporin, 500 mg four times a day for 7 to 10 days; tetracycline, 500 mg four times a day for 14 days; or oral metronidazole, 250 mg three times a day for 7 days. Many physicians recommend treating the patient's sexual partner at the same time.

CONDYLOMATA ACCUMUNATA (GENITAL WARTS)

Epidemiology, etiology, and pathophysiology

Genital warts caused by the human papilloma virus (HPV) are the third most common STD. There are between 500,000 and 1 million cases per year in the United States. Genital warts occur in or around the vulva, vagina, cervix, perineum, anal canal, urethra, and glans penis. They enlarge during pregnancy and may cause hemorrhage or obstruction during delivery. The disease is most common in adolescent girls and young women. The HPV can remain dormant for decades before recurrences appear.

Diagnosis

Diagnosis is made by clinical appearance or histologic examination.

Implementation

ASSISTING WITH THE ACHIEVEMENT OF THERAPEUTIC GOALS

☐ **Cryotherapy**

Recently the Centers for Disease Control recommended cryotherapy as the treatment of choice. Podophyllum, which was previously recommended, is less effective and is toxic if applied to a wide area at one time. It still may be used in a 25% solution in benzoin to treat one or two lesions. Neither treatment cures the disease.

☐ **Counseling and teaching**

Because genital warts sometimes undergo malignant change, the patient is advised to have regular medical care. Malignant changes, especially in the cervix, may not be apparent for 5 to 40 years.

■ OTHER SEXUALLY TRANSMITTED DISEASES

In addition to those diseases already enumerated, hepatitis B infection, pediculosis pubis, and scabies are also considered to be STDs.

Viral hepatitis (see Chapter 30), including A, B, and non-A, non-B, is more prevalent among homosexuals and prostitutes than the rest of the population, and is believed to be transmitted by sexual contact.

Pediculosis pubis, also known as "crabs," is caused by pubic lice. Although lice can be transmitted by bedding or clothing, they are often transmitted during sexual contact. They produce erythematous, itchy papules. The lice adhere to hair around the pubic area, anus, abdomen, and thighs. Diagnosis is made by observation of lice or microscopic observation of nits at the base of hair. Recommended treatment is 1% Kwell lotion or shampoo. One treatment per episode is necessary, but itching may persist.

Scabies, caused by mites known as *Sarcoptes scabiei*, is transmitted by close body contact, bedding, and clothing. Diagnosis is made from linear burrows, often characterized by a reddened papule containing the mite. Common sites are finger webs, wrists, elbows, ankles, and the penis. Nocturnal itching is common. A one-time use of 1% Kwell shampoo is recommended. Family, household, and sexual contacts should also be treated.

■ SUMMARY

1. The term *sexually transmitted diseases* refers to diseases that are usually transmitted by heterosexual or homosexual intercourse.
2. The five classic venereal diseases are gonorrhea, syphilis, chancroid, lymphogranuloma venereum, and granuloma inguinale.
3. Three changes have affected the incidence of STDs in the United States since World War II: (1) antibiotics and antibiotic resistance, (2) social permissiveness, and (3) sexual behavior patterns.
4. The highest incidence of STDs is in young adults and adolescents. This is believed to be because of permissiveness, promiscuity, and "the pill."
5. Contact investigation is important to identifying persons who may have been exposed to an STD and in trying to identify the source of the infection.
6. Condoms are recommended to prevent the transmission of STDs. Latex condoms are recommended because they provide greater protection against viral STDs than natural membrane condoms.
7. Gonorrhea is considered to be of epidemic proportions in the United States and 1 of every 30 teenagers between 15 and 19 years of age are infected with it each year.
8. A major concern in the treatment of gonorrhea is the increased resistance of the organism to penicillin and other antibiotics.
9. Gonorrhea in women is often asymptomatic and is only diagnosed when complications such as salpingitis occur.
10. In 1987 there was a marked increase in the number of cases of infectious syphilis reported to the CDC. The cause of this increase is not known but may be related to the use of spectinomycin to treat gonorrhea.
11. The greatest increase in syphilis has been among inner-city heterosexuals who engage in high-risk sexual activity.
12. The drug of choice in the treatment of syphilis is penicillin G benzathine 2.4 million units IM.
13. Herpes genitalis is a lifelong disease with no cure. It can be transmitted to the fetus during delivery and thus caesarean delivery is often recommended.
14. Treatment for herpes genitalis is symptomatic, and acyclovir ointment applied to the lesions reduces viral shedding and the duration of disease. It does not prevent recurrences.
15. *Chlamydia trachomatis* infections are recognized as the most prevalent STD in the United States.
16. *C. trachomatis* can be spread between sexual partners during intercourse and from mothers to infants.
17. Chlamydial infections are most common in women under the age of 20. They are also more common in persons with several sex partners.
18. The treatment of choice for chlamydial infections is tetracycline, 500 mg four times daily for 7 days.
19. Condylomata accumunata (genital warts) is caused by the papilloma virus; it is most common in adolescent girls and young women.
20. Genital warts are of particular concern because they can undergo malignant changes after a latent period of 5 to 40 years.

Putting knowledge to practice

- What is the incidence of STDs in your community?
- How does the incidence in your community compare with the incidence in other parts of the country?
- What services are available for detection and treatment of STD?
- Are human sexuality and prevention of STDs taught in your local schools?
- Are similar teaching programs available for adults in the community in which you reside?

REFERENCES AND SELECTED READINGS
Contemporary

1. Brown, ZA, and others: Effects on infants of a first episode of genital herpes during pregnancy, N Engl J Med 317:1246-1251, 1987.
2. Campbell, C, and Herten, R: VD to STD: redefining venereal disease, Am J Nurs. 81:1629-1634, 1981.
3. Darrow, W: The gay report on sexually transmitted diseases, Am J Public Health 71:1004-1011, 1981.
4. DeMaria, T: Sexually transmitted diseases. In Woods, N (editor): Human sexuality in health and illness, ed 3, St. Louis, 1984, The CV Mosby Co.
5. Dirubbo, NE: The condom barrier, Am J Nurs 87:1306-1309, 1987.
6. DiSaia, PJ, and Creasman, WT: Clinical gynecologic oncology, St. Louis, 1981, The CV Mosby Co.
7. Dodson, MG, and Faro, S: The polymicrobial etiology of acute pelvic inflammatory disease and treatment regimens, Rev Infect Dis., 4(suppl):5696-5702, 1985.
8. Eschenbach, D: Recognizing chlamydial infections, Contemp Obstet Gynecol 16:15-30, 1980.
9. Feldblum, PJ, and Fortney, JA: Condoms, spermicides and the transmission of human immunodeficiency virus: a review of literature, Am J Public Health 78:52-54, 1988.
10. Graduate education, gonorrhea: CDC recommended treatment schedules, 1979, Obstet Gynecol 55:255-258, 1980.
11. Hacker, S, and others: Factors influencing the success of a community VD program held in a university facility, Public Health Rep 95:247-252, 1980.
12. Herpes on delivery, Emerg Med 12:105-108, 1980.
13. Lafferty, WE, and others: Recurrences after oral and genital herpes simplex virus infection, N Engl J Med 316:1444-1449, 1987.
14. Landrum, S, and others: Racial trends in syphilis among men with same-sex partners in Atlanta, Georgia, Am J Public Health 78:66-67, 1988.
15.* Loucks, A: Chlamydia an unheralded epidemic, Am J Nurs 87:920-922, 1987.
16.* Lutz, R: Stopping the spread of sexuality transmitted diseases, Nurs 16:47-50, March 1986.
16a. McElhouse, P: The "other" STDs as dangerous as ever, RN 52-58, June 1988.
17. Miles, P: Sexually transmissible diseases: fourteen sexually transmissible diseases currently recognized by the Centers for Disease Control, Atlanta, Georgia, JEN 6(3):6-12, 1980.
18. Oill, P: Herpesvirus type 2 infection of the genital tract, JEN 6(3):13-16, 1980.
19. Rees, E: The treatment of pelvic inflammatory disease, Am J Obstet Gynecol 138:1042-1047, 1980.
20. Ridenour, N: Chlamydia, Nurse Pract 5(5):45-48, 1980.
21. *Romanowski, B, and Harris, J: Sexually transmitted diseases, Clin Symp 36(1):2-32, 1985.
22. *Smith, LS: Ethnic differences in knowledge of sexually transmitted diseases in North American Black and Mexican-American migrant farmworkers, Res Nurs Health 11:51-58, 1988.
23. Strauss, R, and Glimp, T: Sexually transmitted diseases, Top Emerg Med 7(2):73-84, 1985.
24. Thompson, SE, and Washington, AE: Epidemiology of sexually transmitted Chlamydia trachomatis infections, Epidemiol Rev 5:96-123, 1983.
25. US Department of Health and Human Services, Public Health Service: STD fact sheet, ed 35, HHS pub no (CDC) 81-8195, Atlanta, 1981, Centers for Disease Control.
26. US Department of Health and Human Services: Sexually transmitted diseases: treatment guidelines: morbidity and mortality, MMWR no. 31S-62S, 1982.
27. US Department of Health and Human Services, Public Health Services: Annual Summary 1983, reported morbidity and mortality in the United States, 32(54):Atlanta, 1984, Centers for Disease Control.
28. US Department of Health and Human Services, Public Health Services: Chlamydia trachomatis infections, policy guidelines for prevention and control, MMWR 34(3S):54S-73S, 1985.
29. US Department of Health and Human Services, Public Health Service: 1985 STD treatment guidelines MMWR (suppl) 34(4S):76S-108S, 1985.
30. US Department of Health and Human Services, Public Health Service: Antibiotic-resistant strains of Neisseria gonorrhoeae: policy guidelines MMWR 36(5S):1S-18S, 1987.
31. US Department of Health and Human Services, Public Health Service: Progress toward achieving the 1990 objectives for sexual diseases, MMWR 36(12):173-176, 1987.
32. US Department of Health and Human Services, Public Health Service: Self-reported changes in sexual behaviors among homosexual and bisexual men from the San Francisco City Clinic Cohort, 36(12):187-189, 1987.
33. US Department of Health and Human Services, Public Health Service: Increases in primary and secondary syphilis—United States, MMWR 36(25):393-396, 1987.
34. US Department of Health and Human Services, Public Health Service: Sentinel surveillance system for antimicrobial resistance in clinical isolates of Neisseria gonorrhoeae, MMWR 36(35):585-593, 1987.
35. US Department of Health and Human Services, Public Health Service: Continuing increase in infectious syphilis—United States, MMWR 37(3):35-38, 1988.
36. US Department of Health and Human Services, Public Health Service: Condoms for the prevention of sexually transmitted diseases, MMWR 37(9):133-137, 1988.
37. Wilcox, R: Sexual behavior and sexually transmitted disease patterns in male homosexuals, Br J Vener Dis 57:167-169, 1981.

Classic

38. Darrow, WW: Changes in sexual behavior and venereal disease, Clin Obstet Gynecol 18:255-267, 1975.
39. Rein, MF, and Chapel, TA: Trichomoniasis, candidiasis, and the other minor venereal diseases, Clin Obstet Gynecol 18:73-88, 1975.

---

*References preceded by an asterisk are particularly well suited for student reading.

36

The Patient with Problems of the Breast

BARBARA C. LONG

The breasts are associated functionally with the reproductive system as an organ for milk production in the postpartum woman. The female sex hormones influence the development of the breasts and the production of milk.

The breasts are also associated with feelings of sexuality and are an integral component of sexual behavior. The development of the breasts in the female adolescent indicates her approaching womanhood and emphasizes her femininity. The breast, especially the nipples which are erectile tissue, are erogenous areas in sexual activity. The advertising media emphasize the desirability of the female breast; femininity is typified by a fashion model's breasts, whereas masculinity is typified by the flat, expansive chest of the lifeguard. Diseases of the breast, therefore, evoke varied feelings and cause fears and concerns that influence the practice of breast self-examination or the seeking of diagnostic and therapeutic care.

The most common diseases of the breast are dysplasia (fibrocystic disease), fibroadenoma, cancer, and infections. Although these diseases occur primarily in women, *they can also occur in men.* Cancer requires the most extensive nursing care and is discussed in more detail.

■ PREVENTION AND HEALTH EDUCATION

■ Avoidance of common breast problems

■ PREMENSTRUAL BREAST DISCOMFORT

Tenderness, discomfort, and swelling of the breasts before menstruation are normal functional changes in the breasts that respond to monthly cyclical changes in estrogen and progesterone. Water retention contributes to the swelling. Women who experience some of these problems can be taught to reduce dietary salt intake during the immediate premenstrual period. Increased physical activity during this time will improve cardiovascular dynamics and help reduce the tight, puffy feeling.

■ BREAST DISCOMFORT DURING PHYSICAL ACTIVITY

Bras provide support for the breasts and help prevent sagging and pulling on the underlying muscles. All but small-breasted women may find physical activity uncomfortable unless a bra is worn. A *jogbra,* which does not contain metal clips or fasteners and which has seams on the outside of the fabric away from the skin, may provide greater comfort for physical activity.

■ Early detection of malignancy

■ EXAMINATIONS OF THE BREAST

Mortality from breast cancer can be prevented in many instances through early diagnosis and treatment. The American Cancer Society recommends examinations of the breast as listed on p. 1305.

Guidelines for breast self-examination

1. Perform BSE regularly each month
   a. Premenopausal women: 7 to 8 days after conclusion of the menstrual period
   b. Postmenopausal women: at a set time each month (such as the first day of the month)
2. Use a systematic approach (one of the three listed here)
   a. Palpate in concentric circles beginning at outer rim of breast tissue and move toward nipple
   b. Divide breast into quadrants and examine area in each quadrant from outer perimeter toward nipple
   c. Palpate inner half then outer half of breast
3. Examine the entire breast tissue, including the tail (Fig. 36-1) and the nipple
4. Carry out examination in both the horizontal and vertical body positions (Fig. 36-2)
5. Use the flat parts of the fingers for palpation

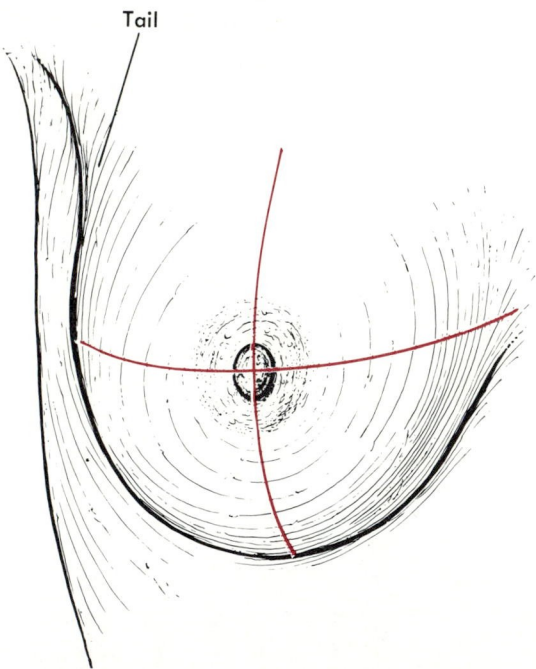

Fig. 36-1 Breast mass includes "tail" that extends from upper, outer quadrant toward axilla. (From Malasanos, L, and others: Health assessment, ed 3, St. Louis, 1986, The CV Mosby Co.)

1. Monthly breast self-examination by *all* women over 20 years of age
2. Women at high risk before age 50: mammography yearly; breast examination by physician every 2 years
3. Women 20 to 40
   a. One baseline mammogram between ages 35 to 40
   b. Breast examination by physician every 3 years
4. Women 40 to 49: breast examination by physician and mammography every 1 to 2 years
5. Women over 50: breast examination by physician and mammography yearly

Studies have shown that the groups of women who are least likely to have regular breast examinations by a physician are elderly, poorly educated, low-income, and black. Some of the reasons are as follows:

Lack of knowledge
Low priority set on preventive measures
Lack of income
Fear of finding a tumor
Concern over possibility of breast removal
Fear of death
Possible life changes if breast cancer is found
Embarrassment
Examination is considered too trivial for a busy physician

Most breast cancers (about 90%) are discovered by self-examination. Breast cancer is usually curable when discovered early and treated immediately. All women, beginning at high school age, should know how to carry out breast self-examination.

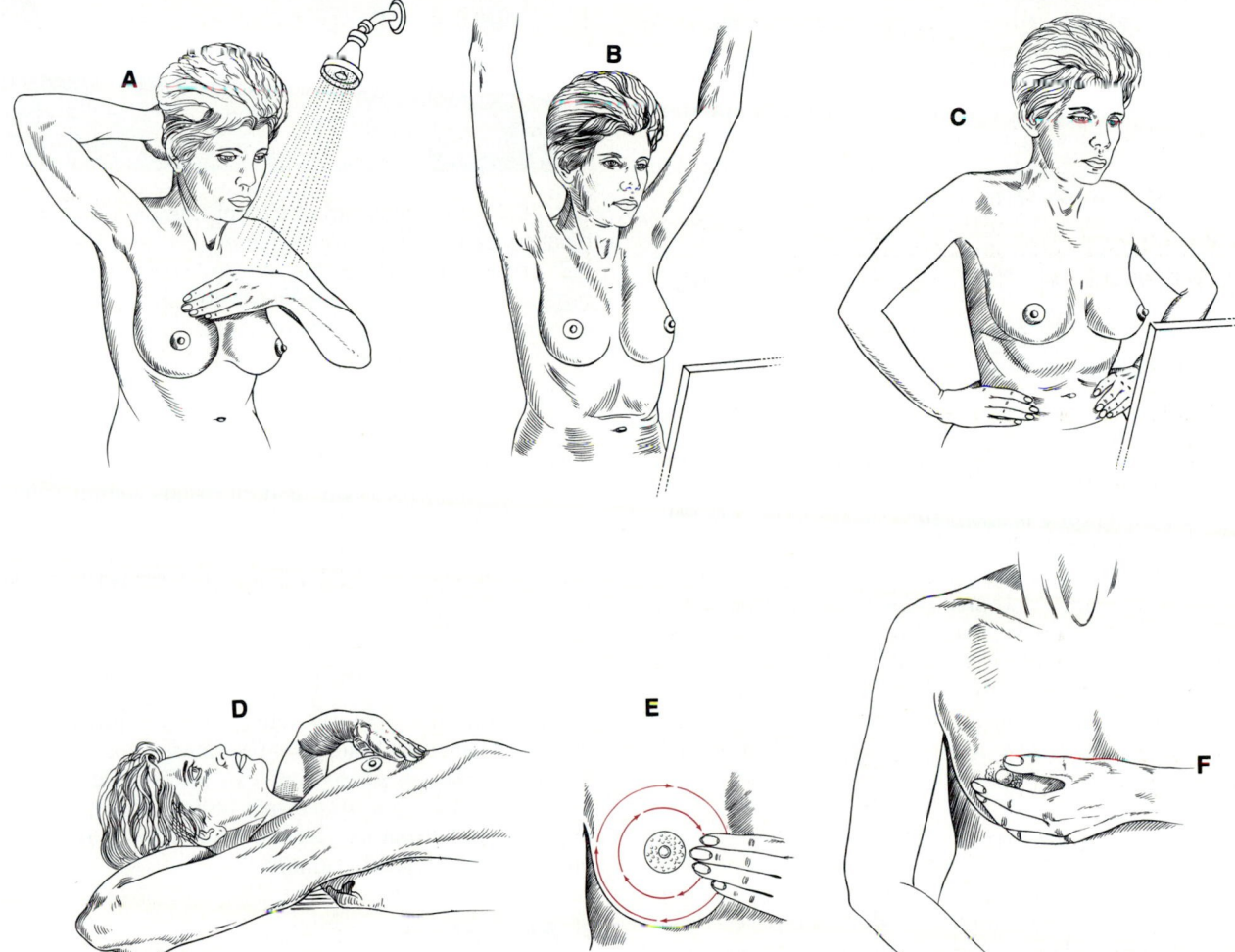

Fig. 36-2 Breast self-examination. **A,** Examine breasts during bath or shower, since flat fingers glide easily over wet skin. Use right hand to examine left breast and vice versa. **B,** Sit or stand before a mirror. Inspect breasts with hands at sides, then raised overhead. Look for changes in contour or dimpling of skin. **C,** Place hands on hips and press down firmly to flex chest muscles. **D,** Lie down with one hand under head and pillow or folded towel under that scapula. **E,** Palpate that breast with other hand using concentric circle method. It usually takes three circles to cover all breast tissue. Include the tail of the breast and the axilla. Repeat with other breast. **F,** End in a sitting position. Palpate the areola areas of both breasts, and inspect and squeeze nipples to check for discharge.

■ BREAST SELF-EXAMINATION (BSE)

Nurses working in the hospital or community settings have the responsibility of teaching women how to examine their breasts and of explaining why it is necessary. Patients can be asked during the admission history if they practice BSE, and necessary instructions can be given when feasible.

Women need to have opportunities to *practice* doing BSE while receiving feedback from the nurse on correct technique and interpretation of any palpable findings. Practice makes women feel more confident about doing BSE, and they are then more apt to practice BSE on a regular basis.

When working with groups of women, arrangements can be made with the American Cancer Society or the local health department for showing movies developed for the general public describing the traditional method of self-examination. Models of breasts are available for women to practice palpation of lumps.

Some women have engorgement of the breast premenstrually, and the breasts normally may have a lumpy consistency at this time. The condition usually disappears a few days after the onset of menstruation. Guidelines for BSE are listed in box on p. 1304.

■ DIAGNOSTIC TESTS FOR BREAST EVALUATION

■ Radiographs
■ MAMMOGRAPHY

Mammography is an x-ray examination of the breast used to detect early lesions before they are palpable (Fig. 36-3). Mammography is about 90% accurate in detecting early breast cancer. It does have limitations, particularly in the penetration of dense breasts as in adolescents, young nulliparous women, or women with large breasts. A low energy x-ray beam is used to delineate the breast structures; this radiation dose is acceptable for use in frequent reexaminations. During the examination the breast is pressed firmly against the film holder, causing momentary mild discomfort, and several films are taken of each breast.

■ XERORADIOGRAPHY

Xeroradiography is similar to mammography except that an aluminum plate with an electrically charged selenium layer is used in place of the familiar black and white mammogram x-ray film. The resulting film is blue and white (Fig. 36-4). Xeroradiography is thought to provide sharper contrast of blood vessel patterns and tissue densities.

■ THERMOGRAPHY

Increased metabolism and increased blood supply to a malignant lesion increase the skin temperature and vas-

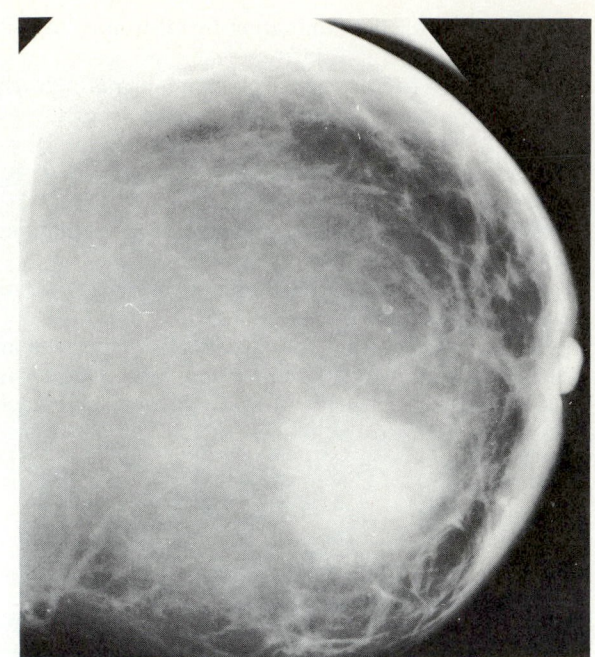

Fig. 36-3 Mammogram of patient with area of density indicating carcinoma. (From Cramer, LN, and Lapayowker, MS: Applied anatomy of the female breast: surgical radiographic and thermographic. In Masters, FW, and Lewis, JR, Jr, editors: Symposium on aesthetic surgery of the face, eyelid, and breast, vol 4, St. Louis, 1972, The CV Mosby Co.)

cularity of the breast. Thermography is a technique that measures and records the heat emissions coming from the breast. Thermography is used less frequently because of a high number of false-positive results. Its use is primarily as a screening device with follow-up of any positive results by mammography.

■ ULTRASONOGRAPHY

Ultrasound is currently being evaluated for its possible value in detecting lesions in the dense breasts of young women. Although ultrasound can differentiate the presence of a cystic mass, it does not indicate calcium deposits or tissue configurations, facts considered important in the diagnosis of malignant tumors.

■ Aspiration

Aspiration of an identified soft breast mass may be performed if a cyst is suspected. A large-bore needle is inserted into the mass and the contents withdrawn and sent to the laboratory for cytologic studies. Cysts usually contain a brownish-greenish fluid. The only discomfort is associated with insertion of the needle. If cytologic tests are positive, a biopsy is performed. If the tests are negative and there are characteristics of cystic disease, no further tests are performed. If there are some doubts, despite the neg-

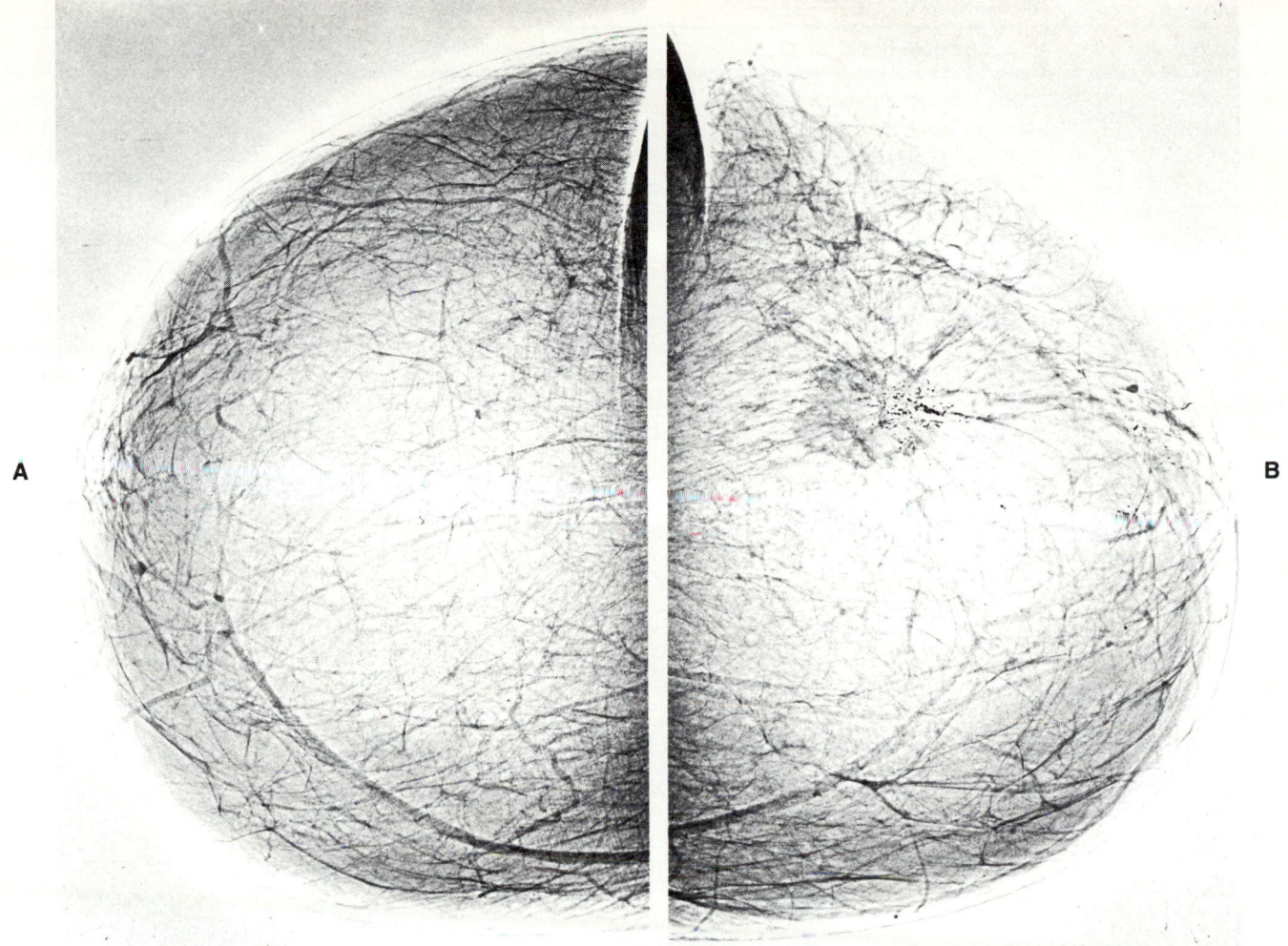

A   B

Fig. 36-4   Xeroradiographs. **A,** Normal left breast. **B,** Right breast shows mass with spiculated margins characteristic of neoplasm. (Courtesy University Hospitals of Cleveland, Ohio.)

ative results, further radiographic studies may be performed.

■ Breast biopsy

Biopsy is the only way to determine conclusively whether a tumor is benign or malignant. Most lesions (80%) are found to be benign.

The procedure is usually performed with a patient under local or general anesthesia in an ambulatory surgical suite. An incision is made and a portion of the mass (or the entire mass if it is very small) is removed and sent to the laboratory for examination. Following the procedure the patient may experience mild discomfort. Results will be available immediately if a frozen section is done, or within 48 to 72 hours.

Sometimes the small lesion size makes location of the lesion difficult or uncertain when biopsy is attempted. Therefore, to locate areas for surgical biopsy, a small meth-

ylene blue dye mark is made within the area of the breast using a syringe and needle during mammographic monitoring. This is done in the X-ray department a few hours before the surgical biopsy, and the mark is made while the patient is under local anesthesia. No color disfiguration is apparent on the breast surface as a result of this procedure, but the mark ensures that the biopsy tissue corresponds to the site identified by mammogram. This procedure requires preinstruction to the patient and support in the X-ray department.

■ BENIGN BREAST DISORDERS

The major benign breast disorders are fibrocystic in nature (dysplasia), benign tumors (fibroadenomas), or infections (mastitis, with or without breast abscess) (Table 36-1).

Table 36-1   Benign breast disorders

Disorder	Characteristics	Signs and symptoms	Medical therapy
Dysplasia (fibrocystic disease)	Refers to several cystic nodular disorders of the breast that become painful during menstruation; seen mostly in women age 30 to 50; estrogen hormone a causative factor	Painful, often multiple and bilateral soft masses in breast; may increase in size or remain the same	Aspiration of probable cyst; biopsy of doubtful cyst to confirm diagnosis; yearly mammograms; intermittent diuretics for premenstrual breast engorgement; symptomatic pain relief
Fibro-adenoma	Fibroplastic tumors commonly seen in young women under age 25	Firm, round, freely movable, nontender mass in breast	Surgical excision with patient under local anesthesia on outpatient basis
Mastitis	Inflammation of breast, usually from cracked or infected nipples	Pain, redness, swelling of breast, fever	Systemic antibiotics; incision and drainage if an abscess forms; symptomatic pain relief

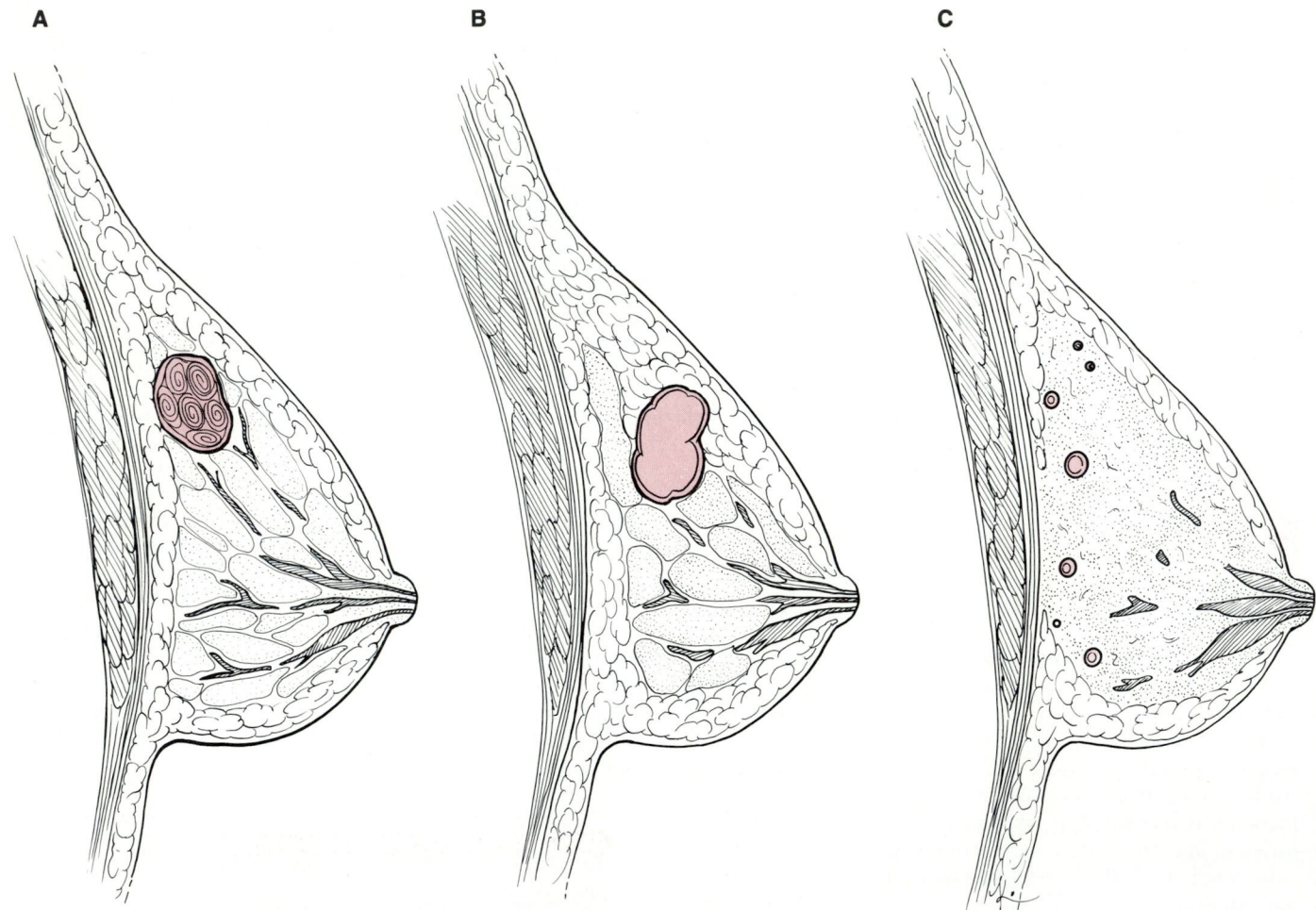

A   **B**   **C**

Fig. 36-5   Benign breast disorders. **A,** Fibroadenoma. **B,** Cyst. **C,** Adenosis (fibrocystic disease).

■ Pathophysiology

Benign breast disorders are usually characterized by one or more movable breast masses, often seen bilaterally (Fig. 36-5). The nodularity may be discrete or diffuse. If tenderness is present, it usually occurs or is increased premenstrually. Any nipple discharge, which may be clear, green, or brownish (but not bloody), is usually spontaneous, especially just before menstruation. Women who take oral contraceptives may experience some nipple discharge that ceases when the pill is discontinued.

Males may have overdevelopment of breast tissue (gynecomastia) as a result of estrogen production during puberty or older age, adrenal or gonadal tumors, or certain drugs, for example, amphetamines, antidepressants (tricyclic), antihypertensive agents, antineoplastic agents, cimetidine, diazepam, digitalis, estrogen, human chorionic gonadotropin, isoniazid, and phenothiazines.

▦ Assessment

Data are collected concerning the person's feelings and knowledge about the disorder, including the following:
1. Concerns about the mass
2. Knowledge of benign versus malignant tumors
3. Knowledge regarding breast self-examination
4. Presence of discomfort

➡ Data analysis: nursing diagnoses

Nursing diagnoses are determined by assessing patient data. Possible nursing diagnoses for the person with a benign breast disorder may include, but are not limited to, the following:

Diagnostic title	Possible etiologies
Anxiety	Fear of cancer
Knowledge deficit	Lack of information/recall, information misinterpretation
Pain	Breast disorder

▦ Planning: expected patient outcomes

Expected patient outcomes for the person with a benign breast disorder may include, but are not limited to, the following:
1. Signs of anxiety are decreased.
2. The woman reports breasts feel more comfortable.
3. The woman demonstrates correct technique for BSE.
4. The woman describes
   a. Difference between benign and malignant breast disease
   b. Plans to do monthly BSE
   c. Plans for yearly medical follow-up

▦ Implementation

■ ASSISTING WITH COMFORT

Breast discomfort may be decreased by mild analgesics (such as aspirin or acetaminophen), by application of heat or cold, or by breast support. Heat may be applied by application of a warm damp washcloth covered by a dry towel and heating pad or hot water bottle. Some people experience relief from an ice bag or a washcloth wrung out in cold water.

Wearing a firm brassiere both day and night may also help to relieve breast discomfort. The brassiere should fit well and give good support, especially for the upper outer breast quadrant.[44]

■ COUNSELING AND TEACHING

☐ Reducing anxiety

Most women who identify a breast mass immediately think of cancer and are, therefore, usually very anxious before the diagnosis is verified. Even after being told that the condition is benign, some women continue to have some anxiety. *Mild* anxiety is useful as this acts as a stimulus for continuing medical follow-up.

The woman who is moderately or severely anxious needs an opportunity to express her concerns to an empathic listener. As the anxiety decreases, the woman is better able to deal with any discomfort and continue her usual activities.

☐ Teaching

The risk of breast cancer in women with mammary dysplasia is twice that for women in general. It is *very important*, therefore, that these women know how to perform accurate breast self-examination and how to recognize masses that differ from the masses of their dysplasia (Table 36-2). More frequent medical follow-up than that specified for asymptomatic people is indicated.

The role of methylxanthines in the reduction of symptoms in benign breast disorders is controversial. Omission of coffee, tea, and chocolate from the diet may help some people and is worth a try.

■ Evaluation

Evaluation is based on expected patient outcomes. Questions to ask may include the following:
1. Is breast discomfort lessened?
2. Does the person know:
   a. The difference between benign and malignant disease?
   b. The method and frequency of breast self-examination?
   c. The frequency of medical follow-up?

■ CANCER OF THE BREAST

The breast is the leading site for cancer in women but is now second to lung cancer in the number of deaths from cancer in women. It is estimated that 1 out of 10 women in the United States will develop cancer of the breast, and this probability increases with age.[1]

Table 36-2 Differences between benign and malignant breast masses

Benign	Malignant
Usually bilateral; may be unilateral	Unilateral
Found often in outer quadrants but may occur anywhere	Found most often in upper outer quadrant and tail or in central nipple portion
Single or multiple	Usually single
Well-circumscribed	Irregular
Soft or firm	Firm
Movable	Nonmovable
Usually have cyclic tenderness; may be nontender	Nontender
No skin changes	Later findings: skin thickened; dimpling
	Very late: ulceration
No palpable lymph nodes	Palpable lymph nodes except in early period
No nipple retraction; discharge usually bilateral, serous, or greenish	Nipple retraction; discharge usually unilateral and may be bloody

■ Pathophysiology

Breast cancer is not one disease but many, depending on the tissue of the breast involved, its estrogen dependency, and the age of onset. Premenopausal breast malignancy is different from postmenopausal malignancy. Treatment response and prognoses differ with various malignancies.

Some tumors are termed *estrogen dependent;* they contain receptors that bind estradiol, a type of estrogen, and their growth is stimulated by estrogen. These receptors are not present in normal breast tissue or in tissue with dysplasia. Presence of estrogen-dependent tumors is identified by an estrogen receptor assay test (ERA) that is performed on biopsied tissue. Postmenopausal women have a higher incidence of hormone-dependent breast cancers. These cancers respond to hormone treatment (endocrine chemotherapy, oophorectomy, or adrenalectomy).

Malignant breast tumors differ from benign tumors (Table 36-2). They are usually solitary, irregularly shaped, firm, nontender, nonmobile masses with a tendency to adhere to the pectoral muscles and to the skin, causing retraction or dimpling of the skin. The skin may become thickened, giving it an "orange peel" effect. Involvement of the lymph nodes is present in about two thirds of the women at the time of diagnosis. Favored sites for metastasis are the lungs, bone, liver, brain, adrenal glands, and ovaries.

Breast cancers are classified using the TNM classification (described in Chapter 12). *T* refers to tumor size, *N* to nodal involvement, and *M* to metastasis. The classification of breast cancer (Table 36-3) serves as a basis for prognosis and direction for treatment.

■ Prevention

■ PERSONS AT RISK

Cancer of the breast cannot be prevented, but cure is more likely if cancer is identified early and treatment started immediately. Most tumors are located by the woman herself; therefore, all women should practice breast self-examination (p. 1304). Persons who are at high risk should know of their risk (see the box on p. 1311, top) and are urged to have careful follow-up. A major factor that places the woman at risk is a long, uninterrupted time period of cyclic hormone changes, that is, early menarche, late menopause, and no pregnancy.

■ Medical therapy

■ SURGERY

Different types of surgery may be performed to remove breast tumors with or without removal of the breast and underlying tissue (see the box on p. 1311, bottom). The type of surgery depends on the extent of the growth and degree of spread. The current recommendations for sur-

Table 36-3 TNM classification of breast cancers

Stage	Tumor size	Nodal involvement	Metastasis
I	Less than 2 cm (T1)	None (N0)	None (M0)
II	Less than 5 cm (T1 or T2)	Movable axillary nodes (N1)	None (M0)
III	Greater than 5 cm with invasion of skin or attached to chest wall	Movable or fixed axillary nodes (N1 or N2)	None (M0)
IV	Any size (any T)	Any nodes (any N)	Yes (M1)

High-risk factors associated with breast cancer

Sex	Female (99% in women)
Age	Over age 50 (80% over age 35)
Familial history	Mother/sister, especially with premenopausal or bilateral breast cancer
Menstrual history	Menarche before age 11; menopause after age 50
Pregnancy	First live birth after age 30; or nullipara
Medical history	Primary breast cancer (risk increased 7 times for a second primary breast cancer); uterine endometrial cancer; mammary dysplasia

---

gery for most patients with potentially curable breast cancer are either partial mastectomy with axillary dissection and radiation therapy or *modified* radical mastectomy.[21] A radical mastectomy (the most deforming procedure) may be necessary in selected cases in which the tumor has invaded the muscle.

■ RADIATION THERAPY

Radiation therapy is being used more extensively following a partial mastectomy. It may also be effective in combination with surgery and chemotherapy for women with large or stage III breast cancers.[21]

☐ External beam therapy

External beam treatments are usually given daily for approximately 5 weeks. The woman will have an extended period of fatigue and depression from the catabolism and loss of tissue. She may also experience nausea, heartburn from transient esophagitis, and cough from transient pneumonitis. Lymphedema may occur.

☐ Interstitial therapy

Iridium (^{192}Ir) needles may be implanted in the breast with the patient under general anesthetic. The patient is placed in a single room and experiences little discomfort after the implantation. Ambulation is permitted within the room. Radiation precautions of internal therapy (Chapter 12) are followed. The needles are removed by the physician after three days, and the patient is discharged. The patient's needs are similar to those of patients receiving other internal radiation therapy.

■ CHEMOTHERAPY

Hormonal therapy with tamoxifen citrate (Nolvadex) has been found useful as an adjuvant treatment for *postmenopausal* women who have estrogen receptor–positive tumors. The drug may be given alone or in combination with other chemotherapeutic drugs.

A CMF *chemotherapeutic* regimen (cyclophosphamide, methotrexate, fluorouracil) appears to be more effective for *premenopausal* women.[21] The drugs are indicated when nodes are positive.

▦ Assessment

If a malignant breast tumor is suspected or diagnosed as such, the following subjective data are obtained as a baseline for planning:

Types of surgery for removal of breast tumors

Lumpectomy	Simple removal of the tumor mass
Partial mastectomy	Removal of tumor mass and 2.5 to 7.5 cm (1 to 3 inches) of surrounding tissue
Subcutaneous mastectomy	Removal of all underlying breast tissue, leaving skin, areola, and nipple intact
Simple mastectomy	Removal of entire breast but not axillary nodes
Modified radical mastectomy	Complete removal of breast (with or without pectoralis minor) and removal of some axillary lymph nodes
Radical mastectomy	Complete removal of breast, axillary lymph nodes, pectoralis muscle (major and minor), and adjacent fat and fascia

---

1. Concerns about the diagnosis and forthcoming therapy
2. Feelings and thoughts about sexuality and the relationship of the breast to these feelings
3. Thoughts about feelings of the sex partner (if appropriate) concerning the forthcoming potential therapy options
4. Future goals, life expectancies, zest for living, and actual or perceived responsibility to others
5. Usual coping mechanisms
6. Family relationships and the existence and availability of support persons
7. Knowledge about BSE (for examination of other breast)

If possible, data are obtained from the sex partner (if appropriate) regarding attitudes about the forthcoming therapy. This identifies possible conflicts in perceptions, the degree of support that can be anticipated from the sex partner, and the potential effects of the partner's feelings on the woman's adaptation and relationships.

Objective data include observations about the woman's behavior and vital signs, which might indicate signs of high anxiety.

Data analysis: nursing diagnoses

Nursing diagnoses are determined by assessing patient data. Possible nursing diagnoses for the person with cancer of the breast may include, but are not limited to, the following:

Diagnostic title	Possible etiologies
Activity intolerance	Fatigue
Anxiety	Fear of surgery, cancer, removal of breast, change in family relationships
Body image or self-esteem disturbance	Loss of breast, difficulty making decisions
Knowledge deficit	Lack of information/recall, information misinterpretation
Impaired physical mobility	Restricted shoulder movement
Pain	Mastectomy
Altered sexual patterns	Loss of breast

Planning: expected patient outcomes

Expected patient outcomes for the person with cancer of the breast may include, but are not limited to, the following:

1. Signs of anxiety are decreased.
2. Patient participates in decision-making, as appropriate.
3. Patient participates in arm exercises with planned rest periods.
4. Patient describes
   a. Breast prostheses and reconstruction possibilities
   b. Plans for continued exercises at home and rest periods as needed

c. Types of clothing to be worn
d. Activities to prevent lymphedema
e. Symptoms to be reported to surgeon
f. Plans for regular BSE of remaining breast
g. Plans for resumption of previous sexual activity
h. Resources for support during early rehabilitation period
i. Community resources (American Cancer Society, Reach to Recovery)

Implementation

PREOPERATIVE CARE

Assisting with coping with preoperative anxiety

Because much emphasis is placed on the breast as a symbol of attractiveness, the thought of losing a breast becomes almost intolerable to many women. This is particularly true of those who depend largely on physical attractiveness to hold the esteem of others and to secure gratification of their emotional needs. Psychologists have pointed out that there is a symbolic connection between the breasts and motherhood that is severely threatened when a breast must be removed. In addition, cancer of the breast often occurs at menopause or soon after when some women feel that they have lost much of their sexual attractiveness. Surgical removal of the breast may save a woman's life, but it also may make her feel less feminine.

Although she may try to conceal fear, any woman who is hospitalized for removal of a breast tumor is anxious, and some may be in a state of near panic. Most fears are related to sexual acceptance, social isolation, disfigurement, recurrence, and death. Many of these women have been unable to discuss their worries and feelings with those close to them, including their spouse. The nurse can help the patient express feelings and understand what breast surgery means to her as a person. The woman who is having breast surgery has a special need to feel understood and accepted by all persons who are providing care.

Simple explanations with repetition may decrease the patient's fears of the unknown. If the patient does not fully comprehend the physician's explanation, the nurse can repeat the explanation and report this to the physician, who in turn can talk with the patient again and clarify any misconceptions, alleviating needless anxiety. Since attention span, memory, and perception are limited when anxiety levels are high, it is helpful if the nurse can be present when information is given to the patient. The nurse can then repeat, reinforce, or clarify given information.

Assisting with decision making

When the diagnostic work is completed and the classification of the tumor has been made, the physician, often with the consultation of the hospital tumor board members (medical, surgical, and radiation oncologists), discusses and proposes the treatment protocol by which the tumor would be most successfully destroyed and which offers the best prognosis for the patient. The patient and family are often involved at this point in this treatment decision plan.

If the patient is not involved, she should ask to be told the findings of the diagnostic measures and the reasons for the therapy plan being described to her.

There are currently many treatments for breast malignancy; the primary therapies are surgery and radiation. If the malignancy is small, nonaggressive, and present in a young woman, she may have several options for therapy that offer her a comparable prognosis with the knowledge available at this time. Every woman should realize, however, that the latest therapy found in magazines may or may not be *best* for her. Nurses have an advantage in assisting a patient in understanding factors involved in decision making from the expertise of the medical professional while taking into consideration the subjective hesitations of the woman.

In some instances, such as an inflammatory carcinoma that rapidly invades the mammary lymphatics, there may be only one treatment plan (immediate radiation). In this situation a nursing diagnosis of *powerlessness* may be identified from collected data because the woman has no alternatives from which to choose. Letting the patient make decisions about other aspects of her life and activities of daily living, whenever possible, helps the patient hold onto a sense of control of her life.

The physician's explanation of breast reconstruction (p. 1319) is important; this information often helps decrease the anxiety of the woman who fears deformity from loss of a breast, and may facilitate the decision making regarding therapy.

The American Cancer Society sponsors a volunteer program, Reach to Recovery, in which the patient has an opportunity to visit with a carefully selected and trained volunteer who has had a mastectomy. This assures the patient that she will receive practical help from someone who has made a satisfactory adjustment to the same operation. Although most of the patient visits by the volunteer from Reach to Recovery occur during the postoperative period, preoperative visits can be requested and may be very helpful to some women.

□ Preoperative teaching

Preoperative teaching includes the following information if a mastectomy is planned:

1. A catheter attached to suction may be used to drain the incision.
2. The arm on the affected side will be elevated.
3. Sitting up and turning in bed should be done by *pushing* up on the unaffected side rather than pulling.
4. Postoperative exercises will be started early.

■ POSTOPERATIVE CARE

□ Wound care

Following the completion of the mastectomy and closure, a stab wound may be made and a catheter inserted and attached immediately to a low, constant suction, such as that provided by a Hemovac or other low suction systems. The purpose of the catheter is to remove blood and serum that may collect under the skin flaps and that would pre-vent healing and predispose the tissue to infection. There is usually no drainage from around the incision when a catheter is draining properly. The catheter may be clamped for short periods of ambulation and is usually removed within 3 to 5 days or when the amount of drainage is less than 5 to 10 ml in 24 hours.

The dressing is checked often for the first few hours to detect hemorrhage or excessive serous oozing. The bedclothes under the patient must be examined for blood that may flow down from the operated region. Any evidence of bleeding is reported to the surgeon. Dressings may be removed in 24 hours, or they may not require changing for several days after the operation. The skin sutures are often removed on the sixth to eighth postoperative day. Usually this is after the patient's discharge from the hospital.

□ Postmastectomy activity and exercise

When the patient returns from surgery, she is placed in a semi-Fowler's position to decrease venous oozing. The arm is elevated to enhance circulation and prevent edema. The pillows are arranged so that the hand is higher than the arm and the arm is above the level of the right atrium. *No blood pressure readings, injections, or blood testing* should be done on the *affected* arm because of potential circulatory impairment or infection (to prevent lymphedema). A sign or tape should be placed on this side of the bed with this message.

Exercises are essential to prevent shortening of muscles, stiffness, and contracture of the shoulder girdle, and to preserve muscle tone so that the affected arm can be used without limitations. To prevent additional deformities, exercises should be bilateral ones with the patient using both arms simultaneously. The time to start specific postoperative exercises depends on the extent of the operation and whether skin grafting has been necessary (as with radical mastectomy).

Slings are to be avoided. Gentle exercises started early in the postoperative course help decrease muscle tension as well as regain muscle function more quickly.

Early exercises for postmastectomy patient

Surgical day	Flex and extend fingers; pronate and supinate forearm
First postoperative day	Squeeze rubber ball
As soon as tolerated	Brush teeth and hair

The patient must know what motion is intended in each exercise. For example, the patient may brush her hair with the arm on the affected side, but she may lower her head and hunch her shoulders in such a way that she does not get normal use of the shoulder girdle. The whole intent of the exercise may, therefore, be lost.

The patient is encouraged under close supervision to exercise each day more and more to the limits of incisional pulling and pain. A specific exercise schedule planned by nurse and patient together is imperative. It is an important aspect of nursing care for the patient.

Continuing exercises are as recommended by the American Cancer Society (see the box on p. 1316). Exercises are begun with 5 repetitions, working up to a maximum

NURSING CARE PLAN

Patient following mastectomy for cancer

DATA: Mrs. Litton, age 35, discovered a lump in her right breast quite accidentally while bathing. She is not familiar with breast self-examination. Mammography and a breast biopsy confirmed the diagnosis of cancer. In a conference with the surgeon and plastic surgeon, Mrs. Litton elected to have a modified radical mastectomy with consideration of breast reconstruction in 6 months.

Mrs. Litton was very quiet during the admission procedure. The primary nurse talked with her the evening before surgery, and Mrs. Litton stated that her major concern was "whether they would get it all." She is glad to know that breast reconstruction can be done in the near future because she doesn't think she wants to go through life with a deformed chest. She also said her husband had supported the surgery, and they both feel it will not affect their relationship. Mr. Litton accompanied his wife to the hospital for admission and spent the evening with her. Her mother is caring for their 3- and 6-year-old daughters while Mrs. Litton is hospitalized.

After surgery, Mrs. Litton returned to the division with intravenous fluids and a wound catheter attached to a Hemovac suction. Vital signs were stable.

Collaborative nursing actions included monitoring the dressing and catheter for wound drainage and observing the arm for signs of enlargement (lymphedema). Medical orders included keeping her right arm elevated on pillows to prevent lymphedema. A sign was placed on her door reminding others to avoid blood pressure readings and injections, or taking blood samples from Mrs. Litton's right arm.

Nursing diagnosis: Pain: related to surgical incision

Expected patient outcomes	Nursing interventions	Rationale
Patient states feeling more comfortable	Give prescribed narcotic on a regular basis for first 24 hr; then re-evaluate	Expected incisional pain is better controlled if not allowed to become severe; patient will participate in exercises earlier if comfortable
	Encourage deep breathing and coughing (DB & C) every 2-4 hr	Narcotic will ease discomfort from DB & C; these exercises will prevent lung problems that would increase her discomfort

Nursing diagnosis: Impaired physical mobility: related to shoulder immobility

Expected patient outcomes	Nursing interventions	Rationale
Patient participates early with arm exercises	Demonstrate early exercises (keep instructions simple) Visit her every 2 hours to provide encouragement	Because of discomfort and narcotic, she may have difficulty concentrating
	Explain rationale of exercises to husband so he can encourage wife	Exercises will help prevent stiffness and contractures of shoulder from disuse

Nursing diagnosis: Body image disturbance: related to loss of breast

Expected patient outcomes	Nursing interventions	Rationale
Patient begins to look at incision and to talk about loss of breast	Spend planned time talking with her	She may need to deny her feelings initially
	Give her opportunities to talk about her feelings	As she begins to think about her surgery, she may need reassurance that the nurse is interested and willing to listen to her concerns
	Don't push her but listen to what she says	
	Observe for signs of touching her dressing and use this as an opening to discuss her thoughts about her surgery	
	Check with her surgeon about a Reach to Recovery volunteer visitor and then explain the program	Interacting with someone who has been through the experience is often helpful in adjustment
	Encourage her to put on makeup and wear her own clothes as soon as possible	She may need reassurance of her femininity

Nursing diagnosis: Knowledge deficit: related to lack of information

Expected patient outcomes	Nursing interventions	Rationale
Patient states: Plans to do BSE regularly on other breast and to teach her daughters when older	Teach BSE: demonstration with return demonstration	Women who have a chance to practice BSE under supervision are more confident about doing BSE
	Explain high risk of daughters for breast cancer and need for continued monitoring	Mother's breast cancer is a high-risk factor for daughter
Plans to continue exercises until full shoulder ROM returns	Demonstrate exercises to be done later; give her booklet from American Cancer Society with instructions	Seeing a demonstration and having written material for reference will promote follow-up of the activity
Plans for rest periods at home	Explain reason for expected fatigue after surgery and help her to plan her day to include rest periods	Care of young children is tiring and she still needs additional energy for healing; rest will give her additional energy for coping
Where to obtain breast prostheses, if needed	Encourage visit by Reach to Recovery volunteer; if not, discuss types of prostheses and where to obtain them	She may postpone reconstructive surgery or may want to use a soft prosthesis before surgery
Symptoms to be reported to physician	Instruct her to report signs of arm edema, redness or infection of incision, or any mass in other breast	Lymphedema and incisional breakdown are better treated if identified early; she is at high risk for cancer in other breast

---

Postmastectomy arm exercises

Exercise: climbing the wall

1. Stand facing wall with toes 6-12 inches from wall.
2. Bend elbows and place palms of hands against wall at shoulder level.
3. Move both hands parallel to each other up the wall as far as possible until incisional pull or pain occurs.
4. Move both hands down to starting position.
5. Goal is complete extension with elbow straight.
6. Activities that use the same action: reaching top shelves, hanging out clothes, washing windows, hanging curtains, setting hair.

Exercise: elbow pull-in

1. Extend arms sideways to shoulder level.
2. Clasp hands behind neck.
3. Pull elbows forward until they touch.
4. Return to position 2.
5. Unclasp hands and extend arms sideways at shoulder level.
6. Lower arms to side.

Exercise: back scratch

1. Place hand of unoperated side on hip for balance.
2. Bend elbow of affected arm, placing back of hand on small of back.
3. Work hand up the back slowly until fingers reach opposite shoulder blade.
4. Lower arm and straighten both arms.

Exercise: rope pull

1. Attach a rope over a shower rod, hook, or over top of an open door.
2. Sit on a chair (with door between legs if using a door) and grasp each end of rope.
3. Alternately pull on each end, raising affected arm to a point of incisional pull or pain.
4. The goal is to raise the affected arm almost directly overhead.

---

of 20 repetitions unless otherwise specified. The woman is instructed to move slowly and rest when pain occurs. With exercise, full range of motion will return; that is, both arms can be extended equally high above the head. This will not be achieved before 2 to 3 months; therefore, the patient must learn and be motivated in the hospital so she will continue exercises at home on a regular basis. Following radical mastectomy, full muscle power for horizontal adduction may be less.

☐ Promoting comfort

Pain in the operated area may be referred to the affected arm or shoulder. Sensations of numbness and tingling over the chest that are painful may cause the patient to take short, shallow breaths in the early postoperative period. She is kept comfortable with analgesics, and a deep breathing and coughing routine is started. Each chest excursion may painfully discourage compliance, and the patient may need considerable encouragement.

Phantom symptoms of the missing breast occur in those women who had painful breasts or nipples before the surgery. This can be very disconcerting to the woman, and reassurance may be needed that these sensations will eventually disappear.

The body requires increased energy for healing and for coping with the grief of the loss of the breast. *Fatigue* occurs not only in the early postoperative period but often for up to 6 weeks after surgery. The woman needs to know that this is a normal reaction and that she should plan for rest periods.

☐ Providing psychologic support

After surgery, denial of the changes in body image may take the form of the woman speaking about "the cancer" and "the mastectomy" but never dealing with her loss or her fears on an emotional level. Denial here is a conservation of energy. If she is to express herself on an emotional level, she must have someone who is capable and responsible to support her according to *her* need. If she does not receive this professional assistance, the impact of her loss occurs at a later date when support systems may not be available.

Avoidance of looking at the dressing or incision can be expected initially. The incision is large, and the feeling experienced by most women is that of mutilation. Postponing looking at the incision delays the impact of the realization that the breast is indeed gone. Preparing the woman in advance concerning the size of the incision is helpful, but she still needs considerable support when viewing the incision and her new image. She is usually physically capable when she feels stronger and begins to socially respond to others. She is encouraged to look at the incision several times before discharge from the hospital while health professionals are available for support.

Feelings of anger and resentment may occur and if present frequently are projected onto female staff or friends. Families may also express anger or anxiety and may complain without cause about the care the patient is receiving. Feelings of decreased self-worth and self-esteem on the part of the patient plus increased dependency needs often produce depression.

The feeling of being isolated and alone during this experience can be helped by interaction with others who have had the same experience such as visitors from the Reach to Recovery program. The Reach to Recovery volunteers hold the potential of motivating the patient, extending hope, and providing visible evidence that femininity, personality, and activity can be retained. They can be good resource people as the patient moves from hospital to community. Often whether or not the patient has the opportunity to use this resource depends on a nurse's initiating the contact.

After the patient is discharged, she may experience periods of depression if she perceives that her recovery is slow or if she tries to reenter her previous activities and responsibilities before her energy reserves return. She may have difficulty sleeping or concentrating if she is still acutely grieving with little recognition or little support. Although she will be aware of this, she usually will be unable to express her needs; significant others can be told of her continuing need for support and patience and can help to extend the kind of support needed.

☐ **Sexual adaptation**

Woods[48] has identified a number of factors that can influence sexual adaptation following mastectomy (Fig. 36-6) Women with very small or very large breasts may have long-unresolved feelings about breast size and may also experience more difficulty in obtaining a satisfactory breast prosthesis. They may perceive the surgery as mutilating, and withdraw from the sexual relationship, fearing rejection from their partner. Women who felt sexually inade-

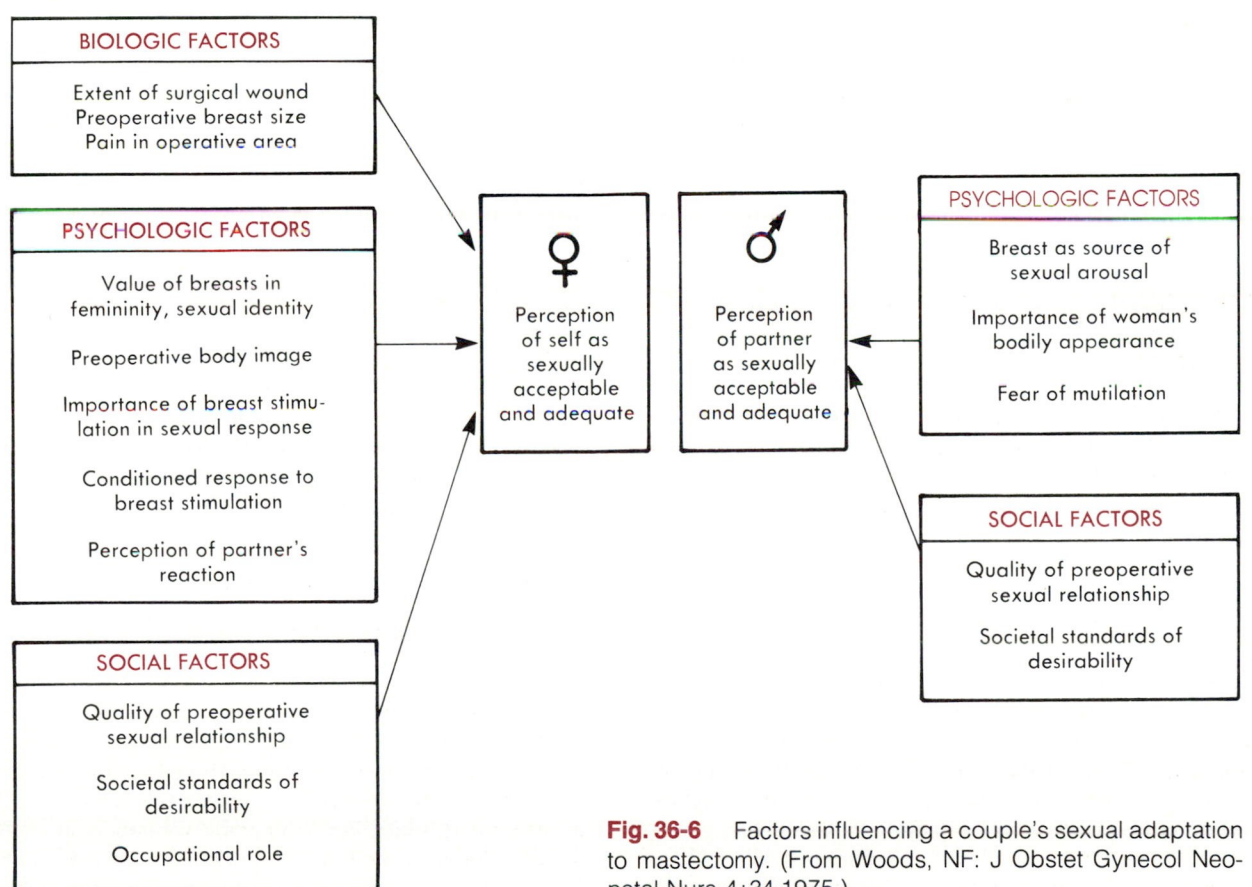

Fig. 36-6 Factors influencing a couple's sexual adaptation to mastectomy. (From Woods, NF: J Obstet Gynecol Neonatal Nurs 4:34,1975.)

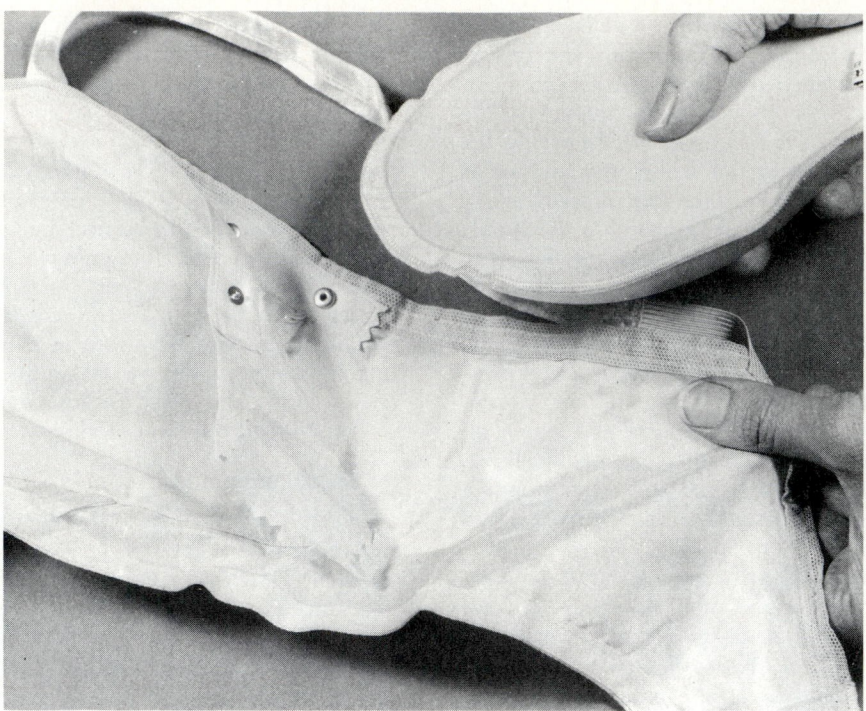

Fig. 36-7 Inner pocket that will hold padding or prosthesis securely can be made in patient's own brassiere. Note snaps that simplify removal of padding.

quate before surgery may find these feelings enhanced postoperatively and use the surgery as a reason for withdrawing from sexual relationships.

The nurse can initiate a discussion with the patient concerning her thoughts and feelings about return to sexual activity (if appropriate) and can encourage the patient to talk about her concerns with her sexual partner. Sexual and marital counseling is helpful for couples who are unable to communicate their feelings openly with each other.

□ Breast prostheses and clothing

Unless a breast reconstruction has been done immediately following breast removal, information about breast prostheses is given to the patient whenever she asks about them or appears interested. The Reach to Recovery volunteer is a good resource person for current information and suggestions concerning prostheses and clothing. She may accompany the patient as she shops for her first prosthesis, serving as a support person. Breast prostheses are not fitted until at least 6 weeks postoperatively or until the incision is healed and is no longer tender.

Until the incision is well healed, the woman is advised to wear one of her own brassieres, which can be lightly padded with a soft, fluffy filling (Fig. 36-7) or a temporary soft prosthesis, available from Reach to Recovery, that will not shift and embarrass her. Opaque, loose-hanging gowns are usually most acceptable to the patient. All clothing should have wide armholes to prevent constriction of the underarm, leading to lymphedema.

Breast prostheses vary in price, type, and weight (Figs. 36-8 and 36-9). Women want prostheses to make them look symmetric and *feel* bilaterally weighted. Even small-breasted women will change posture if weighting is not balanced. Firm, molded prostheses have a disadvantage of remaining elevated when the woman is lying supine, whereas fluid types have a more natural look.

□ Lymphedema

Many patients develop a slight edema of the upper arm that disappears within a week. A few patients, however, develop a severe edema that persists, that may become permanent, and that is caused by surgical interruption of lymph channels and nodes. The incidence is greater in persons who are obese, develop infections, or are subjected to irradiation. Some surgeons order an elastic sleeve that gives additional support to the vessels in the arm; this should extend from the wrist to the shoulder. It is similar to an elastic support stocking and usually may be removed when the patient is in bed. A diuretic such as chlorothiazide (Diuril) may be ordered to help relieve the edema.

□ Teaching

In addition to teaching points stressed earlier, the patient is taught to report symptoms indicating infection or poor healing of the incision. Since the woman is at high risk for developing cancer in the other breast, she needs to carry out monthly breast self-examinations for early identification of another lesion. The points to be stressed in teaching are included in the summary of the care of the patient with a mastectomy listed in the box on p. 1320.

■ Breast reconstruction

Recent improvements in plastic surgery techniques have made surgical breast reconstruction a viable alternative to breast prosthesis for many women. For some women, however, breast reconstruction is not essential to their positive self-image and esteem, femininity, or sexual experience. Some do not want the added surgery and accompanying anesthesia, the cost of time and money, or the pain. They are comfortable and active and successful without the added surgery. Other women consider it important for their self-esteem and continuing relationships with others. Breast reconstruction is contraindicated when there is an aggressive tumor, a probability that metastasis has occurred, or a concern about adequate healing.

The benefits of breast reconstruction include avoidance of an external prosthesis that has the potential for slipping out of place, greater choice of clothing (including lower neck lines), and loss of self-consciousness about appearance. Some women say they feel better about themselves.

Breast reconstruction can be performed immediately after surgery, in 6 months or more after surgery, or 1 to 2 months following chemotherapy or radiation therapy. Women who allow time after the initial surgery to cope with the loss of the breast may be more satisfied with breast reconstruction. The decision for reconstruction should be made in combination with the surgeon, plastic surgeon, and patient. The goal of reconstruction is a breast mound and nipple-areola complex that is similar to the remaining breast. The new breast will not have the exact contours of the natural breast; it is generally a little rounder and flatter and will not sag. However, the breasts will be similarly proportioned and positioned symmetrically.[5]

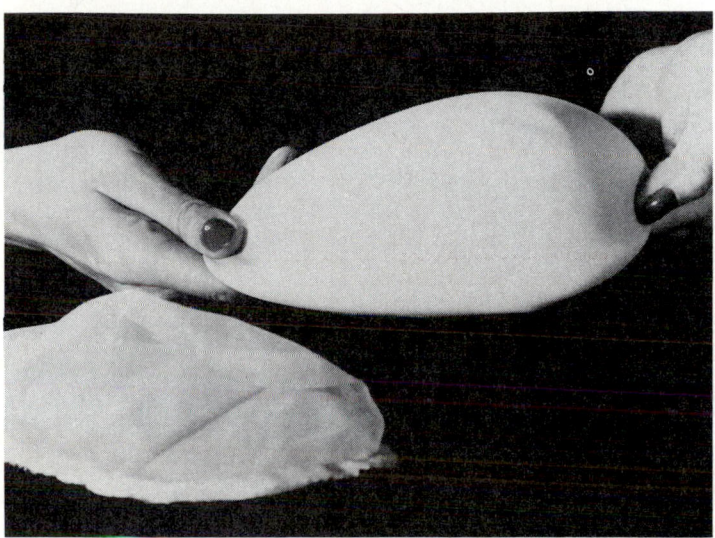

Fig. 36-8   Foam-covered, liquid-filled breast prosthesis. (Courtesy Camp International, Jackson, Mich.)

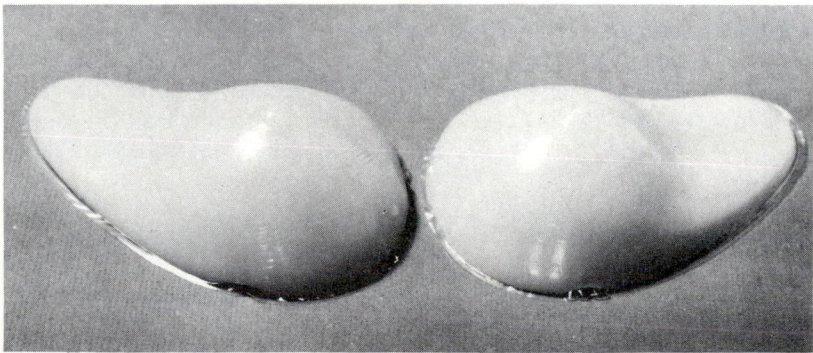

Fig. 36-9   Silicone-filled breast prostheses. (Courtesy Camp International, Jackson, Mich.)

Nursing care of the patient who has had a mastectomy

Preoperative care

1. Help patient explore feelings about loss of breast and fears related to cancer
2. Provide simple explanations; repeat as necessary
3. Teach patient:
   a. Expectation of catheter to drain wound
   b. Need for postoperative exercises

Postoperative care

1. Give immediate care
   a. Place patient in semi-Fowler's position
   b. Wound care:
      (1) Attach catheter to suction drainage
      (2) If Hemovac suction is used, empty when half-full to maintain suction
      (3) Check dressing and bed for signs of drainage
   c. Elevate arm on pillow
   d. Monitor circulation of arm on affected side; report signs of swelling and numbness of lower arm or inability to move fingers
   e. Avoid blood pressure readings, blood testing, or injections in affected arm
   f. Teach patient to sit up in bed by *pushing* up on elbow of *unaffected* side, rather than pulling up with arm
   g. Encourage deep breathing and coughing
   h. Give analgesics for comfort
2. Encourage postmastectomy arm exercises
   a. Start gentle exercises early (see p. 1313)
   b. Start special mastectomy exercises (see p. 1316) when prescribed
3. Encourage rest periods; monitor for fatigue
4. Provide emotional support
   a. Continue to help patient explore feelings
   b. Prepare patient in advance concerning size of incision and be with her, if possible, when she looks at incision
   c. Encourage patient to identify feelings about resuming sexual activities (if appropriate) and to discuss these feelings with sexual partner
5. Teach patient
   a. Wear a brassiere padded with a soft fluffy filling or temporary soft prosthesis until incision is healed
   b. Substitute a regular breast prosthesis later
   c. Avoid clothing that constricts the underarm
   d. Avoid injections and blood pressure measurements in affected arm
   e. Report symptoms indicating need for immediate medical attention:
      (1) Edema of affected arm
      (2) Redness or infection of scar
      (3) Breakdown of scar tissue
      (4) Mass in other breast or axillae
   f. Plan to do monthly breast self-examination on remaining breast

---

Table 36-4 Types of reconstruction breast surgery

Surgery	Description	Comments
Implants		
Silicone implant	Implant inserted into a pocket beneath the pectoralis major muscle	Simplest procedure Ambulatory surgery or overnight hospital stay Requires ample residual skin Result is less symmetric than in other surgeries No ptosis
Tissue expansion	Temporary or permanent expandable bag inserted in submuscular pocket; bag is expanded slowly over time by saline injections in subcutaneous port	Common procedure Ambulatory surgery or overnight hospital stay Useful following modified radical mastectomy if enough tissue present Requires frequent office visits
Flap grafts		
Abdominothoracic	Flap graft advanced from area below breast	Three-day hospital stay Provides better breast detailing than implants More prominent abdominal scar
Latissimus dorsi	Flap graft advanced from latissimus dorsi muscle (lateral upper back)	Five-day hospital stay Useful following radical surgery when tissue lacking Implants may be needed Horizontal back scar
Transabdominal	Flap graft using rectus abdominus muscle tunneled from lower abdomen to breast area	Seven-day hospital stay Useful following radical surgery when tissue lacking Horizontal scar on lower abdomen Removes some abdominal fat (lipectomy)

The two major approaches to breast reconstruction are the submuscular insertion of an implant to provide breast form or the muscle flap grafts from the upper or lower abdomen or from the back (Table 36-4). (Flap grafts are discussed in Chapter 39.) The tissue expansion method of implant surgery has become one of the more commonly used procedures when enough tissue is present. For the woman who lacks sufficient tissue following radical mastectomy, or in some cases a more extensive modified radical mastectomy, the transabdominal flap graft is being used with increasing frequency, although the latissimus dorsi flap graft is also commonly used.

■ SILASTIC IMPLANT

When the skin covering the areas of removed breast tissue is not too tight and the pectoralis muscle is intact, a Silastic or silicone gel implant may be inserted (Fig. 36-10). It is soft and flexible, better approximating breast tissue than the older-model silicone implants. Other types of implants include the temporary saline bag and the three permanent types: the combination saline/silicone gel, the all-silicone gel or Silastic, and the urethane-foam–covered implants.

The skin covering the chest where the implant is to be inserted can be "stretched" (like stretching of the abdomen during pregnancy) by gradually expanding the area below the skin. An all-saline sac or a combination saline/silicone gel sac is implanted under the muscle; the sac is then slowly expanded over a 3-month period by adding saline by injection into a receiving port placed subcutaneously below the axilla. When the desired volume has been achieved, the temporary sac is surgically removed and the permanent silastic implant is inserted into the enlarged space, or the injection port is removed from the permanent implant. The woman will experience minimal discomfort with this procedure.

The woman is asked not to smoke for at least 1 week before surgery because complications occur more frequently among smokers.[10] Possible complications of breast implant surgery may include hematoma/seroma or infection in the early postoperative period, rupture of the implant, capsular contraction following hematoma or infection, and asymmetry or malposition.[40] Postoperative teaching includes the following:

1. Report signs of drainage, fever or other signs of infection.
2. Wear a bra continuously until healing occurs to maintain the implant position and alignment.
3. Avoid raising arms (such as to wash hair or reach cupboards) for 1 to 3 weeks, as instructed.
4. Avoid hard pushing movements, for one to three weeks in order to avoid separation of the pectoralis muscle where the implant has been inserted and to avoid pulling out the sutures.
5. Avoid heavy lifting for 6 weeks.

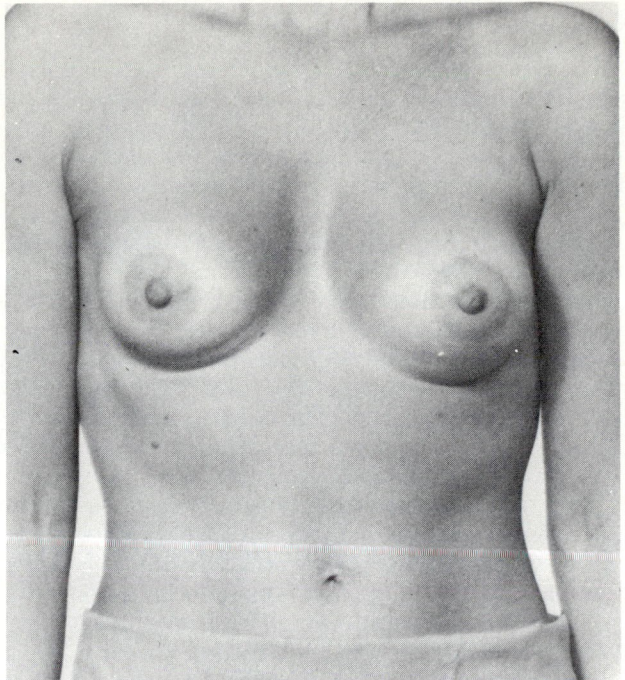

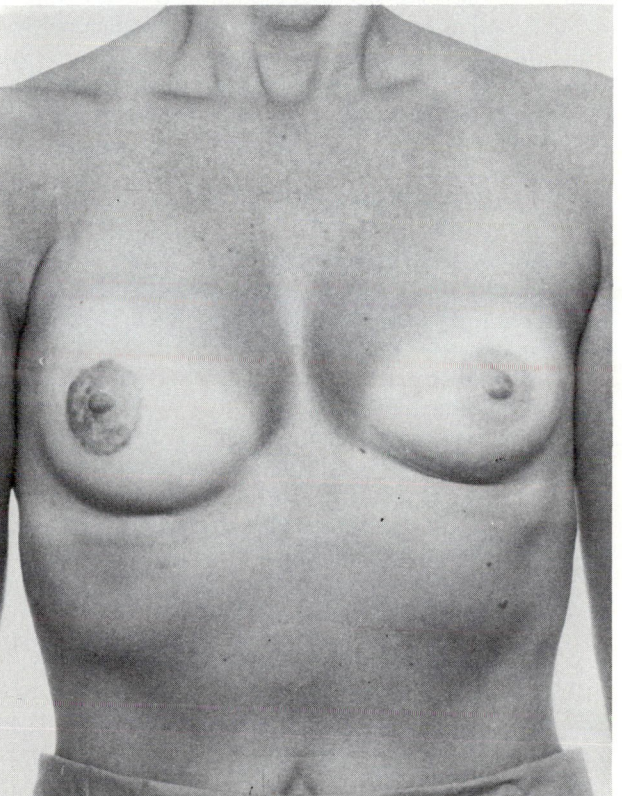

Fig. 36-10   Removal of early intraductal carcinoma in right upper quadrant with implant at time of surgery. **A,** Preoperative view. **B,** Two years after surgery.

■ TRANSABDOMINAL ISLAND FLAP

The transabdominal island flap (TAIF) method creates a breast that better approximates breast tissue than the Silastic implant. TAIF surgery involves transferring a section of abdominal skin and fat and part of the rectus abdominis muscle to the breast area by tunneling under the skin. The tissue is then shaped as a new breast.

The *original* nipple is no longer "saved" because there is always a question about the possible spread of cancer cells into the nipple. Creation of a new areola and nipple is performed as ambulatory surgery at a later date. The areola is formed by free grafting of tissue, either from part of the other areola (if it is large) or from skin of the upper thigh just below the pubic hair. The nipple is more difficult to fashion; the more common approach is to create folds of tissue with local skin and fat flap grafts.

TAIF involves more extensive surgery than the implant procedure and usually requires a week-long hospital stay. Following surgery, the patient will experience abdominal discomfort, tightness, and paresthesia. The abdomen will be flatter but the waistline may be temporarily larger.[19] Possible complications after TAIF surgery include hematoma/seroma, infection, or flap necrosis in the early postoperative period. Fat necrosis is identified by the appearance of a local indurated area. Hernias and abdominal-wall weakness may occur later.

Preoperatively, a liquid diet is prescribed for 24 hours to aid bowel decompression, which is necessary for a relaxed abdominal wall. Postoperative care includes the following[19]:

1. To prevent pull on abdominal incisions, position patient with head elevated and knees flexed.
2. Monitor and empty suction drains from breast and abdomen every 30 minutes for 24 hours; notify physician if drainage is >50 ml/hr.
3. Monitor color and temperature of new breast tissue (it should be paler and cooler than surrounding tissue but not mottled or cold).
4. To aid flap oxygenation, give prescribed isoxsuprine (Vasodilan) and oxygen by nasal cannula.
5. If nausea is present, give prescribed antiemetic to prevent pull on abdominal incision from vomiting.
6. To prevent infection, clean umbilicus and tape over incision with cotton swab saturated with hydrogen peroxide.
7. To ease pull on abdominal incisions, suggest patient ambulate during first week by leaning slightly forward with knees flexed.
8. Teach patient to do the following:
   a. Avoid raising arms above shoulder level for 4 weeks.
   b. Avoid heavy lifting for 6 weeks.

The Reach to Recovery program of the American Cancer Society has a program of volunteers who have had breast reconstruction because of cancer. This is an additional resource for patients and professionals.

⊞ Evaluation

Questions to be considered in evaluating care of women who have had therapy for cancer of the breast may include the following:

1. Has she had an opportunity to discuss her feelings and begin dealing with her change in body image?
2. Has she identified people to turn to for support when she feels depressed or needs help?
3. Has she been exercising during her hospital stay and does she know the home exercises?
4. Is she aware of the possibilities of breast reconstruction?
5. Is she aware that she will fatigue easily for at least six weeks after therapy is completed and needs to plan rest periods?
6. Does she know where to obtain a breast prosthesis?
7. Can she perform breast self-examinations and does she plan to carry them out monthly?
8. Is she aware of the need for yearly follow-up by a physician?

■ METASTATIC DISEASE

The progress of breast malignancy is from the primary mass foci (often more than one) through intramammary lymphatics to regional nodes and then to systemic dissemination, or from primary mass to extension of local structures (skin, rib) and then to systemic disseminated disease. The most usual metastases of breast malignancy are to bone, lung, liver, and brain.

Therapy for disseminated breast cancer is specific to the area involved. If the tumor was estrogen dependent, hormonal therapy, adrenalectomy, ablation of the ovaries (by surgery or radiation), or hypophysectomy may be performed. The sequelae of these therapy interventions require further physiologic and psychologic adaptations.

The care of the patient with advanced metastatic disease is discussed in Chapter 12.

■ SUMMARY

1. A baseline mammogram should be obtained by a woman between 35 and 40 years of age, then repeated every 2 years until age 49, and yearly thereafter.
2. Most breast cancers are discovered by BSE; therefore, BSE should be performed by all women over age 20.
3. Lumps from benign breast disorders are usually seen bilaterally and are discrete, tender, and freely movable. Lumps from malignant tumors are usually solitary, irregularly shaped, nontender, and nonmobile.
4. Common benign breast disorders include fibrocystic disease, fibroadenomas, and mastitis.
5. Breast discomfort from benign breast lesions may be decreased by mild analgesics, heat or cold, or by breast support.

Putting knowledge to practice

- Consider how you would feel if you discovered a lump in your breast.
- Practice doing breast self-examination (or teaching someone else); consider the consequences of having breast cancer but not finding it early because of not doing monthly BSE. (Mark your calendar *now* to remind you to do BSE until it becomes one of your regular routines.)
- Talk with volunteers from Reach to Recovery; ask them for suggestions of how you can most help anyone facing surgery for breast cancer.
- Check some of the clothing stores in your community for available breast prostheses. Compare types and prices.
- Practice teaching postmastectomy exercises to someone else.
- What resources are available to women in your community to help detect breast cancer and facilitate assistance if it is detected? Visit a breast clinic, if one is available, and identify the services provided.

---

6. Radiologic tests for breast cancer include mammography, xeroradiography, and thermography. The only way to determine conclusively whether a tumor is malignant is by breast biopsy.

7. High-risk factors for breast cancer are having a mother or sister with breast cancer (especially premenopausal), menarche before age 11, menopause after age 50, or first live birth after age 30.

8. The most common surgical procedures for breast cancer are partial mastectomy with axillary dissection and radiation therapy, and modified radical mastectomy.

9. Chemotherapeutic regimens are more effective for premenopausal women, whereas hormonal therapy for estrogen receptor–positive tumors is more effective in postmenopausal women.

10. Loss of a breast is a traumatic experience for many women and may lead to feelings of decreased femininity and self-worth. Women need considerable support during this time.

11. Reach to Recovery, sponsored by the American Cancer Society, consists of specially trained volunteers who can provide support and information to women having mastectomies.

12. Shoulder exercises following a mastectomy are started early and continued until the shoulder regains full movement.

13. Breast prostheses of various types may be purchased to wear in a bra after the incision has healed.

14. Lymphedema (swelling of the upper arm) may result after mastectomy because of interference with lymphatic drainage. Elevating the arm after surgery and starting exercises early can help to prevent lymphedema.

15. New advances in breast reconstruction have made this an option for many women who are not satisfied with a breast prosthesis. Types of breast reconstruction include a Silastic implant and a transabdominal island flap.

REFERENCES AND SELECTED READINGS

Contemporary

1. American Cancer Society: Cancer facts and figures 1987, New York, 1986, The Society.

2. American Cancer Society, Reach to Recovery: Exercises after mastectomy, patient guide, New York, 1983, The Society.

3. Argenta, LC: Reconstruction of the breast by tissue expansion, Clin Plast Surg 11:257-264, 1984.

4. *Black Americans' attitudes toward cancer and cancer tests: highlights of a study, Cancer 31:4, 1981.

5. Breast reconstruction following mastectomy, New York, 1982, American Cancer Society and American Society of Plastic and Reconstructive Surgeons.

6. Cancer treatment: an annotated bibliography of patient education materials, NIH Pub No 81-2152, Bethesda, Md, 1981, National Institutes of Health, Office of Cancer Communications.

7. *Chavez, A: Conservation surgery with radiotherapy: an alternative in breast cancer, Sem Oncol Nurs 1:195-199, 1985.

8. *Choices: realistic alternatives in cancer treatment, New York, 1980, Avon Books.

9. Cohen, BE, and Cronin, ED: Breast reconstruction with latissimus dorsi musculocutaneous flap, Clin Plast Surg 11:287-302, 1984.

10. Cohen, IK, and Turner, D: Immediate breast reconstruction with tissue expanders, Clin Plast Surg 14:491-498, 1987.

11. Deffebach, RR, and others: Lumpectomy and irradiation in the treatment of early carcinoma of the breast, West J Med 4:136-139, 1982.

12. *Dinner, M, and Coleman, C: Breast reconstruction: use of autogenous tissue, AORN J 42:490-496, 1985.

12a. Edeiken S: Mammography and palpable cancer of the breast, Cancer 61:263-265, 1988.

13. *Eich, SJ: Promising early breast cancer treatment without mastectomy, Cancer Nurs 8:51-58, 1985.

---

*References preceded by an asterisk are particularly well-suited for student reading.

13a. *Feather, BL, and Lanigan, C: Looking good after your mastectomy, Am J Nurs 87:1048-1049, 1987.

14. *Frank, DI: You don't have to be an expert to give sexual counseling to a mastectomy patient, Nurs 81 11(1):64-67, 1981.

15. Gant, TD, and Vasconez, LO: Post-mastectomy reconstruction, Baltimore, 1981: The Williams & Wilkins Co.

16. *Greitzu, S.: Breast cancer: the risks and options, RN 49(10):26-32, 1986.

17. Hellman, S, and others: Cancer of the breast. In DeVita, V: Cancer: principles and practices of oncology, ed 2, Philadelphia, 1985, JB Lippincott Co.

18. Hery, M, and others: Conservative treatment (chemotherapy/radiotherapy) of locally advanced breast cancer, Cancer 57:1744-1749, 1986.

19. Hutcheson, HA: TAIF: new option for breast reconstruction, Nurs 86 16(2):52-53, 1986.

19a. *Hutcheson, HA: Breast reconstruction using abdominal tissues: a nursing diagnosis approach, Plast Surg Nurs 7(1):11-16, 1987.

20. *Knobf, MKT: Primary breast cancer: physical consequences and rehabilitation, Sem Oncol Nurs 1:214-224, 1985.

21. Krupp, MA, Schroeder, SF, and Tierney, LM, Jr, editors: Current medical diagnosis and treatment 1987, Norwalk, Conn, 1987, Appleton & Lange.

22. *Jussak, PF: Male breast cancer, Innovations in Oncol Nurs 2(1):1-5, 1986.

23. Leffall, LD: Breast cancer in black women, Cancer 31:4-6, 1987.

24. Levitt, SH: Primary treatment of early breast cancer with conservation surgery and radiation therapy, Cancer 55:2140-2148, 1985.

25. *Lewis, RM, Ellison, ES, and Woods, NF: The impact of breast cancer on the family, Sem Oncol Nurs 1:206-213, 1985.

26. Little, JW: Nipple-areola reconstruction, Clin Plast Surg 11:351-363, 1984.

27. *Marszalek, EJ, and Solomon, JS: A breast counseling service, Am J Nurs 81:1658-1659, 1981.

28. Maxwell, GP: Selection of secondary breast reconstruction procedures, Clin Plast Surg 11:253-256, 1984.

29. *McKann, CF: The changing role of surgery in the treatment of breast cancer, Sem Oncol Nurs 1:176-180, 1985.

30. *Morra, ME: Breast self-examination today: an overview of its use and its value, Sem Oncol Nurs 1:170-175, 1985.

31. *Nash, JA: Breast cancer: screening detection and diagnosis, Semin Oncol Nurs 1:163-169, 1985.

32. Radiation therapy and you: a guide to self-help during treatment, pub no 80-2227, Washington, DC 1985, National Institutes of Health.

33. Reich, D: Estrogen receptors and advanced breast cancer, CA Nurs 4(3):247-248, 1981.

34. Rozin, RR, and Skornich, YG: Contemporary options in the operative treatment of breast cancer, Clin Plast Surg 11:231-235, 1984.

35. Saltzstein, SL: Potential limits of physical examination and breast self-examination in detecting small cancers of the breast, Cancer 54:1443-1446, 1984.

36. *Sawyer, PF: Breast self-examination: hospital-based nurses aren't assessing their clients, Oncol Nurs Forum 13(5):44-48, 1986.

37. *Schain, WS: Breast cancer surgeries and psychosexual sequelae: implications for remediation, Sem Oncol Nurs 1:200-205, 1985.

38. Schain, WS, Jacobs, E, and Wellische, DF: Psychosocial issues in breast reconstruction: intrapsychic, interpersonal, and practical concerns, Clin Plast Surg 11:237-252, 1984.

39. Scheflan, M: Building a breast without a prosthesis: the transverse abdominal island flap, Clin Plast Surg 11:303-315, 1984.

40. Scheflan, M, and Kalisman, M: Complications of breast reconstruction, Clin Plast Surg 11:343-350, 1984.

41. *Solomon, J: The good news about breast reconstruction, RN 49(11):47-48, 1986.

42. *Stromberg, M: Screening for early detection, Am J Nurs 81:1652-1657, 1981.

43. *Vogel, CL: Systemic therapy for breast cancer, Sem Oncol Nurs 1:188-194, 1985.

44. *Wilcox, PM: Benign breast disorders, Am J Nurs 81:1644-1651, 1981.

45. *Wiley, KR: Postbiopsy care, Am J Nurs 81:1600-1662, 1981.

46. *Wellisch, DK: The psychologic impact of breast cancer on relationships, Sem Oncol Nurs 1:195-199, 1985.

Classic

47. *Winkler, WA: Choosing the prosthesis and clothing, Am J Nurs 77:1433-1436, 1977.

48. Woods, NF: Influences on sexual adaptation to mastectomy, JOGN Nurs 4:33-37, 1975.

UNIT X
Problems of Physiologic Defense Mechanisms

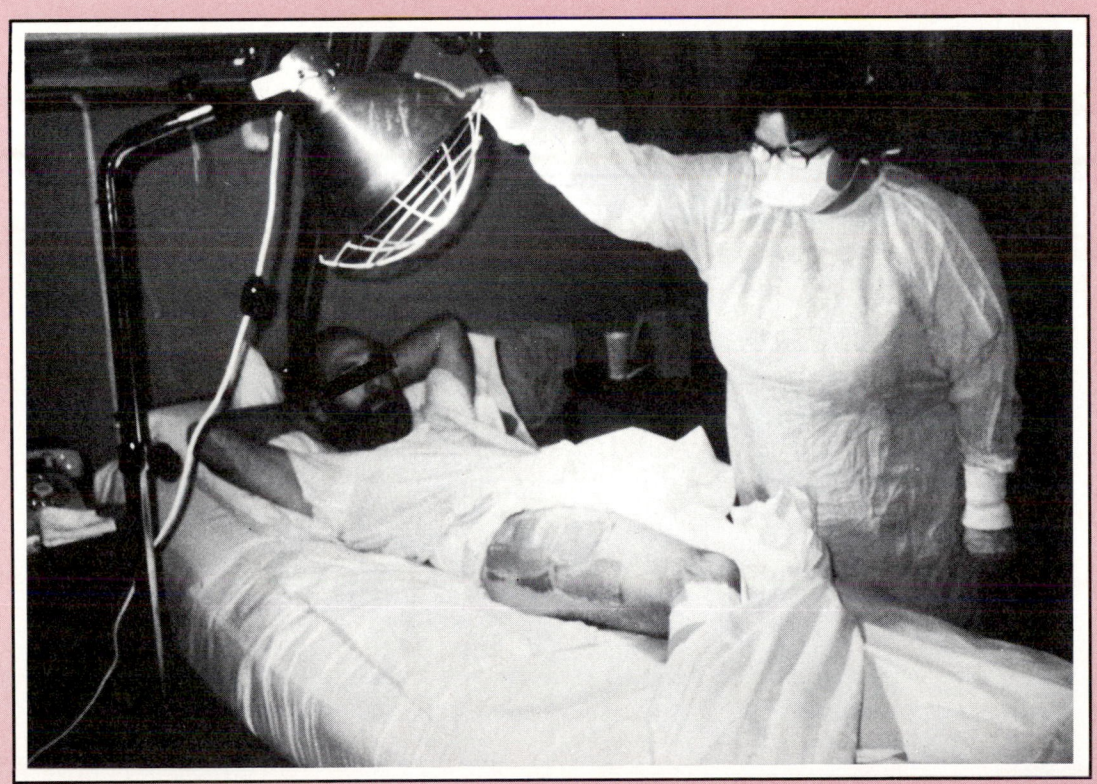

37

Biologic Defense Mechanisms of the Human Body

E. RONALD WRIGHT

CHAPTER OBJECTIVES

After studying this chapter, the student should be able to:

- Differentiate between the concepts of self and nonself.

- Identify the external and internal nonspecific biologic defense mechanisms.

- Define the steps of the inflammatory process, containment of infection, and resolution of inflammation.

- Explain the bases for the five cardinal signs of inflammation.

- Define antigens and antibodies and describe the antigen-antibody interactions.

- Differentiate between B cells and T cells and describe the humoral and cell-mediated responses to antigens.

- Explain the immunologic bases for passive and active immunizations, cancer, AIDS, and tissue transplantation.

■ CONCEPT AND SCOPE OF BIOLOGIC DEFENSE

The human body has developed a wide variety of mechanisms designed to protect itself from the encroachment of antagonistic agents in its environment. Those agents can be *exogenous* (from outside the body), for example, foreign animal cells, parasites, microorganisms, drugs, toxins, or inorganic substances; or they may be *endogenous* (from within the body), for example, damaged or worn-out tissues and cells, obstructive agents, or neoplasms. Life as we know it could not exist without the ability to withstand and deal with these extrinsic and intrinsic onslaughts. In this chapter the array of interactive biologic mechanisms designed to provide this protection are described and the consequences of their failure or inappropriate functioning briefly discussed.

The significance for medical-surgical nursing practice of an understanding of how these mechanisms function cannot be overemphasized. Much of preventative, compensatory, and restorative nursing practice is built on the maintenance and restoration of the systems and mechanisms of these biologic functions. Knowledge of these basic structures and mechanisms helps in the understanding of the following:

1. Resistance and immunity to infectious diseases
2. Diagnosis of diseases and physiologic functions
3. Rejection of tissue transplants and reactions to transfusions

---

Biologic defense mechanisms

Structural	Skin, mucous membranes
Chemical	pH, blood proteins
Cellular	White blood cells, phagocytes
Special proteins	Interferon, immunoglobulins
Tissue	Lymph nodes, thymus gland

---

4. Adaptations of the aging process
5. Development of allergic and hypersensitivity reactions
6. Immunization against infectious diseases
7. Expression of autoimmune diseases and immunodeficiencies
8. Signs and symptoms of local and systemic inflammations
9. Development and treatment of neoplastic disease

■ Concept of self versus nonself

Every human being can be regarded as a "one of a kind" collection of tissues, cells, and molecules that comprises a biologic unit of *self*. The exact nature of this unit is determined by a combination of genes inherited from one's parents, which encode for a unique array of structures and proteins that is not repeated exactly in any other individual. The only exception to this occurs in the case of identical twins. Therefore, every other individual or cell or biologic product can be considered to be *nonself*. It is the function of the biologic defense mechanism of the body to recognize and protect against encroachment by nonself agents, while maintaining, monitoring, and supporting all that is self.

These defense mechanisms are composed of structural, chemical, cellular, special protein, and tissue elements that form an interrelated system of protection throughout the entire body (see the box at left). The mechanisms serve to protect self from both external and internal destructive agents by the following:

1. *Exclusion* of harmful agents from the body
2. *Recognition* of harmful agents within the body
3. *Response* designed to rid the body of the harmful agents that do gain access (Fig. 37-1)

The sources of these harmful nonself materials are generally external and include nonliving materials of the environment such as potentially harmful inorganic chemicals and compounds produced by other living organisms. The most serious external threats to biologic integrity, however, come from the living organisms that constantly surround the body. Some of these organisms pose no real threat because the mechanical, biochemical, and metabolic pro-

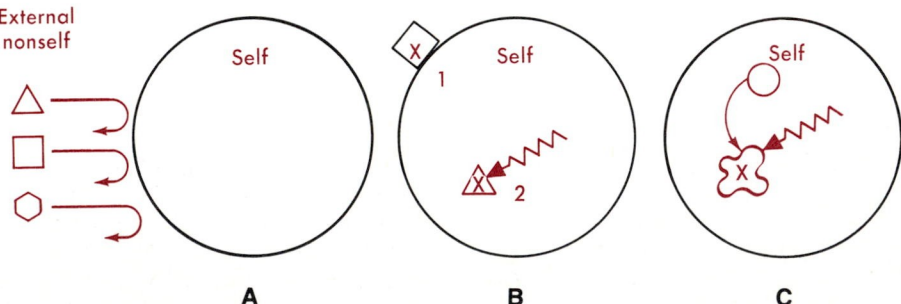

Fig. 37-1 Mechanisms of biologic defense in human body. **A,** Exclusion of external nonself. **B,** Destruction of external nonself by (1) nonspecific external mechanisms and (2) nonspecific or specific internal mechanisms. **C,** Destruction of altered self. X indicates nonspecific mechanisms; ⤳ indicates specific mechanisms.

cesses of the human body will not support them or offer them shelter. There are a myriad of living forms, on the other hand, for which the human body would be an ideal haven for growth and survival. Most of these organisms, if allowed to penetrate the body, would wreak havoc on the normal functionings of the body. The living forms that come to mind in this regard are the organisms classified as pathogenic (disease causing). Although it is true that the progress of these organisms in the body can be altered by external agents such as antibiotics, the eradication of the offending organism from the body must be accomplished by the host's own adaptive mechanisms.

In addition to protection against external agents, the defense mechanisms also protect against the accumulation of damaged or dysfunctional self material. If it were not for these processes that carry out the systematic, specific removal of damaged or worn-out cellular material, the body would become clogged with debris. Still another general function of these systems is recognition of the alteration of self to a potentially dangerous state. When this defense function falters, cancer results.

The overall importance of this system has recently been illustrated by the problems that develop when one part of the defense mechanisms is compromised by the infection of the human body with human immunodeficiency virus (HIV). Infection with HIV leads to the progressive destruction of one group of cells of this system, the helper T cells (see p. 1340). Without the protection afforded by these cells, the body becomes susceptible to the following: (1) infection by a variety of microorganisms that normally do not cause symptomatic infections (such as yeasts, herpes zoster, atypical mycobacteria); (2) infection by normally noninfective parasites (such as *Pneumocystis carinii*, *Toxoplasma*, *Cryptosporidium*); and (3) development and spread of cancers that are normally halted by the immune system (such as Kaposi's sarcoma, lymphomas).

On the other hand, if the immune response system incorrectly identifies self as nonself, it would bring to bear its destructive mechanisms against healthy cells or tissues. The result of such an inappropriate action against self produces cell and tissue damage referred to as autoimmune disease. Among the diseases caused by this failure in distinguishing self from nonself are rheumatoid arthritis, autoimmune thyroiditis, and systemic lupus erythematosis.

◼ Recognition of self from nonself

It follows from the above discussion that a critical feature of the protective mechanisms of the immune response system of the human body is the ability to discriminate between self and nonself materials. This is accomplished by the presence of certain specific protein molecules that are embedded in the cell membrane of all human body cells (Fig. 37-2). The recognition process then occurs at the cell membrane surface. Immunoresponsive cells (lymphocytes) have specific protein molecules embedded in their membranes that recognize foreign (nonself) proteins. A person's own immunoresponsive cells recognize nonself proteins on cells that are genetically different, and this

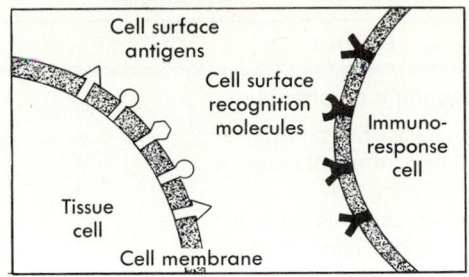

A. CELL SURFACE MARKERS

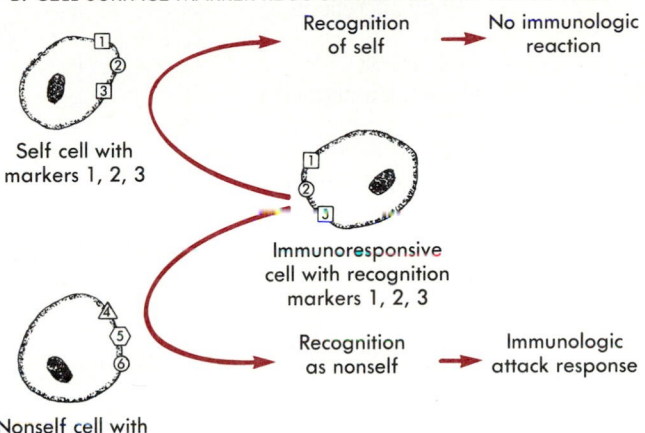

B. CELL SURFACE MARKER RECOGNITION OF SELF vs. NONSELF

Fig. 37-2   Cell surface markers for recognition of self versus nonself.

triggers a sequence of cellular reactions within the immune response system. This sequence of cellular reactions leads to the elaboration of materials and cells that attack the nonself materials. Contact with self proteins (markers) does not produce an immune attack. This explains why cells from different species or genetically dissimilar members of the same species cannot be transplanted from one host to another without triggering an immunologic attack and rejection of the tissue.

◼ Scope of defense mechanisms

The array of defense mechanisms that have been adapted to protect the normal human body is formidable and complex. For the sake of orderly presentation they may be divided into *nonspecific* and *specific* mechanisms (Table 37-1). The specific and nonspecific mechanisms can be further divided on the basis of where the lines of defense are formed, that is, *external* for the mechanisms of mechanical exclusion, biochemical destruction, and microbial competition and *internal* for the physiologic reactions. The nonspecific mechanisms are nonselectively directed against *any* foreign substance. The specific mechanisms are specifically elicited by *unique* substances to which the body has *acquired* the ability to respond.

Table 37-1 Biologic defense mechanisms

External	Internal
Nonspecific mechanisms	
Mechanical exclusion	Reticuloendothelial system
Physical structures	Blood
Skin	Cellular components
Mucous membranes	Fluid components
Specialized structures	Opsonins
Physical actions	Complement
Biochemical factors	C-reactive protein
Body secretions	Phagocytosis
pH	Inflammatory response
Lysozyme	Interferon
Microbial antagonism	
Specific mechanisms	
Immunoglobulin A	Antigen processing by macrophages
In mucosal secretions	Primary immune response
In mucosal cells	Humoral immune response
	Synthesis of circulating antibodies by B cells
	Interaction of antibodies with antigen
	Cell-mediated immune response
	Sensitization of T cells
	Lymphokines
	Combined immune response
	Secondary immune response

■ Concept of immunity

The objective of the biologic defense mechanisms is to provide the host with protection. The ultimate protection would be total resistance to encroachment or damage by an organism or agent; this is usually termed *absolute immunity*. Absence of such protective barriers is called *susceptibility*. Although generally applied to immunity from infectious organisms, these terms can be used to describe the relative susceptibility to encroachment by any external agent. *Nonspecific immunity* (or *innate immunity*) is provided when the external and internal nonspecific defense mechanisms serve as the barrier excluding or destroying the invading agent. *Specific immunity* protects against a single unique agent through the development of specific antibodies or responsive cells in the body. It is *acquired* from prior contact with that agent (antigen) or through the introduction of specifically protective antibodies or cells into the body.

The acquisition of specific immunity may result from *natural* encounter or *artificial* introduction. Immunity acquired naturally means under natural conditions, such as recovery from a disease. Immunity acquired artificially means that the antigen or protective antibodies were purposely introduced into the body (for example, by vaccination). The immunity may be *active* or *passive*. When the antibodies are produced within the body, the immunity is active. When the protective antibodies are received from some other source, the immunity is passive. Thus when antibodies are transferred from the mother across the placenta, the child is said to have a natural passive immunity; when a vaccine is given, so that antibodies are produced within the body, the immunized individual is characterized as having an artificial active immunity. Table 37-2 summarizes the different types of specific acquired immunities.

Specific or nonspecific immunity to harmful agents is a relative state. The effects of different dosages of an infectious organism or the toxic products of such organisms in experimental studies clearly demonstrate that administration of sufficiently large numbers of an organism or high dosages of a toxin can overwhelm even the most highly immunized animal. Further, when the normal mechanisms of defense are breached, even in the highly resistant host, disease can result. Thus acquired immunity to infection is not always an absolute condition but depends on a large number of complex variables. These include not only the defense mechanisms of the host but also the dosage, route of contact, and virulence of the harmful agent.

Table 37-2 Types of acquired specific immunity

Type of immunity	Acquisition of immunity	Development	Duration	Protection	Example
Active Antibodies synthesized by body in response to antigenic stimulation	*Natural* Natural contact with antigen through clinical or subclinical case	Develops slowly; protective levels reached in a few weeks	Long term; often lifetime	Specific to antigen contacted	Recovery from childhood diseases (for example, chickenpox, measles, mumps)
	Artificial Immunization with antigen	Develops slowly; protective levels reached in a few weeks	Several years; extended protection with "booster" doses	Specific to antigen immunized against	Immunization with live or killed vaccines; toxoid immunization
Passive Antibodies produced in one individual are transferred to another	*Natural* Transplacental and colostral transfer from mother to child	Immediate	Temporary, to several months	All antigens to which mother has immunity	Maternal immunoglobulins in neonate
	Artificial Injection of serum from immune human or animal	Immediate	Temporary, to several weeks	All antigens to which source has immunity	Injection of pooled human gamma globulin; injection of animal hyperimmune sera

■ EXTERNAL NONSPECIFIC DEFENSE MECHANISMS

■ Anatomic structures and mechanical actions

■ SKIN AND MUCOUS MEMBRANES

The first line of defense against penetration by foreign materials, including pathogenic microorganisms, is the skin and mucous membranes. The intact skin is an extremely efficient physical barrier to harmful agents and environmental forces, such as heat, cold, and trauma. This protection is afforded by the keratinized surface cells, which provide a tough, dense, waterproof covering. Beneath this outermost layer is a dense layer of highly vascularized connective tissue (see Fig. 39-1).

Even though some of the fatty acids derived from sebaceous gland secretions have antimicrobial activity, the environment provided by the skin does allow the growth of microorganisms on its upper layers and within hair follicles and sweat glands. For the most part these resident microorganisms are nonpathogenic; however, when these organisms gain entrance to the tissue of a host exhibiting reduced resistance, they may cause significant problems. Because even thorough scrubbing with soap and water removes only the surface organisms, the skin can never be considered sterile.

Any time the physical integrity of the skin is broken, such as in surgery, indwelling venous catheterization, or physical irritation or trauma, the risk of microorganisms gaining entrance to the body is significant. The skin must be kept relatively dry because the continued presence of moisture tends to cause maceration of the skin. Further, when essential oils are lost from the skin surface, they should be supplemented by lotions to maintain the resilience and unbroken texture of the surface cells. Adequate care of the skin of the hospitalized patient is not just a luxury but a necessity for the provision of an extremely important aspect of biologic defense.

Mucous membranes protect the eye and line all body tracts that have external openings. When intact, the mucous membranes, like the skin, are basically impervious to foreign materials and microorganisms. The surfaces are covered by a viscous secretion that tends to trap and inactivate microorganisms. The mucous membrane of the respiratory tract is further protected by the surface activity of the ciliated epithelial cells, which sweep foreign material out of the tract. The mucous membranes are highly vascularized so that the internal defense mechanisms are readily available to attack any microorganisms that do gain access to the surface of these cells.

Also found in the mucosal secretions and in high concentration within the secretory mucosal cells of the respiratory and intestinal tracts are a specific class of immunoglobulins (antibodies) known as immunoglobulin A (IgA). These specific antibodies are secreted from the mucosal cells and have antibacterial, antiviral, and antitoxic properties. These antibodies serve to prevent microbial adherence and colonization of these tracts by pathogens.

■ SPECIALIZED STRUCTURES AND MECHANICAL FUNCTIONS

Other structures and functions of the human body that are generally taken for granted actually serve extremely important roles in defense. The filtration action of the nasal hairs serves to trap particles and microorganisms. The flushing action of saliva and urine prevents the buildup of organisms. The eyes are protected from entrance of dirt particles and organisms by the lids and lashes. Foreign material that does gain entrance to the eye tends to be washed out by tears. The constant movement of foods through the stomach and intestines prevents the buildup of organisms or toxic waste products. Even the action of vomiting and the watery stools of diarrhea are active mechanisms of removal of harmful products from the gastrointestinal tract. Dysfunction or blockage of any of these processes means that special measures must be taken to protect against the establishment of pathogenic organisms and the buildup of toxic materials.

■ Biochemical factors

Many areas of the body are protected not only by mechanical barriers but also by the presence of specific antimicrobial chemicals that provide added protection.

■ SKIN

The acetic acid and salt concentration of perspiration is toxic to many pathogenic microorganisms. Some of the fatty acids released to the skin surface by the sebaceous glands also serve to inhibit the growth of some microorganisms.

■ GASTROINTESTINAL TRACT

In the stomach the acidity (approximate pH 2) of the gastric juice kills many organisms and detoxifies certain potentially toxic substances. For this reason, when gastric acidity is low, special precautions must be taken to avoid introduction of organisms through the nose and mouth. Low gastric acidity is characteristic in neonates; therefore, special care should be taken in feeding and handling babies to prevent exposure to pathogens by the oral route. The upper intestine is generally freed of organisms by the action of bile and other proteolytic enzymes.

■ VAGINA

Vaginal secretions allow certain harmless acid-producing bacteria to colonize the vagina and create an acidic environment. This reduces the chance of the colonization of the vagina by pathogens. When either the amount or the acidity of the vaginal secretions is decreased, there is a much greater chance that the vaginal infection will develop. Because vaginal secretions are not present before puberty and are greatly decreased after menopause, young girls and older women are more prone to vaginitis. Birth control pills may cause a shift in the composition of pH of the vaginal secretions, which increases the possibility of colonization of the vagina, especially by the causative agent of gonorrhea, *Neisseria gonorrhoeae.*

■ LYSOZYME

The most ubiquitous antimicrobial factor in the body is the enzyme lysozyme. It is capable of lysing (splitting) the bacterial cell wall of many gram-positive organisms, causing their destruction. Lysozyme is present in mucus, tears, saliva, and skin secretions and is also found in many of the internal fluids and cells of the body. Within the body it tends to work in combination with complement and other blood factors to destroy bacteria directly.

■ Microbial antagonism

The skin and mucosal surfaces offer varying nutritional and environmental conditions for the growth and multiplication of certain microbial cells. Although the surfaces of the body are constantly exposed to temporary contamination by organisms from the environment, most of these organisms, known as *transient flora*, do not find conditions suitable for the colonization of the body; however, many microorganisms, known as *normal microbic flora*, do colonize the skin and mucosal surfaces. Although this normal flora varies from site to site within the body and may vary in response to environmental, hygienic, and physiologic changes, it is capable of reestablishment and reflects a fairly predictable pattern. Table 37-3 provides an overview of the body areas normally colonized and shows which organisms most often make up the normal flora of the various areas.

The maintenance of this balanced microbic flora serves to make it difficult for pathogenic organisms to establish themselves on the body surfaces. Because the normal flora have a selective advantage in their environmental niche, they compete for nutrients and space. Some release antimicrobial substances to retard the growth of transient organisms seeking to occupy the same site. Such microbial interference is called *microbial antagonism*.

Most of the normal microbic flora are basically nonpathogenic; however, some overtly pathogenic organisms, such as *Staphylococcus aureus* and *Streptococcus pyogenes*, can be part of the normal flora. The individual who harbors such organisms without demonstrating any symptoms of disease is known as a *carrier*. This carrier state is of significance because the carrier may be unknowingly shedding organisms into the environment and infecting others.

The protective effects of the normal microbic flora become most apparent when something upsets the microbic balance within the body. The use of broad-spectrum antibiotics sometimes creates such an effect. The imbalance

Table 37-3 Distribution of normal microbic flora

Region of body	Sterile areas	Nonsterile areas	Microorganisms
Skin	None	All skin	*Staphylococcus, Bacillus, Coryne-bacterium, Mycobacterium, Streptococcus,* transient environmental organisms
Respiratory tract	Larynx, trachea, bronchi, bronchioles, alveoli, sinuses	Nose, throat, mouth	*Staphylococcus, Candida, Streptococcus, Neisseria, Pneumococcus,* oral organisms
Gastrointestinal tract	Esophagus, stomach, upper small intestine	Esophagus and stomach (transiently), large intestine	Gram-negative rods, *Streptococcus, Bacteroides, Proteus, Clostridium, Lactobacillus*
Genitourinary tract	Cervix, uterus, fallopian tubes, ovaries, prostate gland, epididymis, testes, bladder, kidney	External genitalia, anterior urethra, vagina	Skin organisms, *Lactobacillus, Bacteroides*
Body fluids and cavities	Blood, pleural fluid, synovial fluid, spinal fluid, lymph, etc.	None	

may allow a segment of the normal flora to gain ascendency, causing adverse reactions. An example of this phenomenon is seen when certain orally administered antibiotics induce marked shifts in the normal intestinal flora, allowing organisms that are generally suppressed by the growth of competitors to thrive to an unusual degree. This imbalance may induce uncomfortable gastrointestinal tract problems or even allow gastroenteritis to develop.

■ INTERNAL NONSPECIFIC DEFENSE MECHANISMS

Once a foreign agent (living or nonliving) penetrates the external resistance barriers, it is met by an even more complex array of defense mechanisms, which provides for the recognition, capture, and disposal of the foreign material. The key to this process is the specific recognition and vigorous action taken against the foreign material while at the same time protecting the host tissues from extensive damage. The physiologic reactions that serve to contain and inactivate the foreign agent are carried out through interactions of cells and molecules of the blood, reticuloendothelial system, vascular system, and body tissues.

■ Reticuloendothelial system

The reticuloendothelial system (RES) is a widespread system of phagocytic (devouring) cells scattered throughout various body tissues (Fig. 37-3). The role of these cells is to ingest foreign particulate matter and damaged host tissues. Some of the phagocytic cells are *fixed* in a variety of tissues, such as lymphoid tissue, liver, spleen, bone marrow, lungs, and blood vessels. Within the different tissues

these anchored cells have been given unique names (Table 37-4). It is the function of the fixed cells to capture and destroy foreign materials found in the fluids of their environment.

Other cells making up the reticuloendothelial network are not stationary and are called *wandering macrophages*. Depending on where they are found, they may be known as monocytes (in the bloodstream) or histiocytes (in loose connective tissues). The wandering macrophages carry out the important role of final cleanup of a damaged site in preparation for repair. The cells have the capacity to engulf and destroy virtually any type of foreign material or debris within the body. The macrophages also play an important role in the specific response mechanisms.

■ Blood

Blood is one of the primary sources of elements designed to provide protection against injurious agents. The blood transports these active factors to the site of an injury or intrusion and through specific vascular changes concentrates these materials at the site. Both the fluid and cellular constituents of blood contain these factors.

■ CELLULAR COMPONENTS

The cellular components of blood that are of importance in this nonspecific response include granulocytes, lymphocytes, monocytes, and thrombocytes (platelets). The granulocytes, also referred to as polymorphonuclear leukocytes (PMNs), and the monocytes are the most important because of their phagocytic activity.

One of the key methods of nonspecific defense is the ingestion of microorganisms and other particulate matter by the phagocytic white blood cells. The phagocytes carry

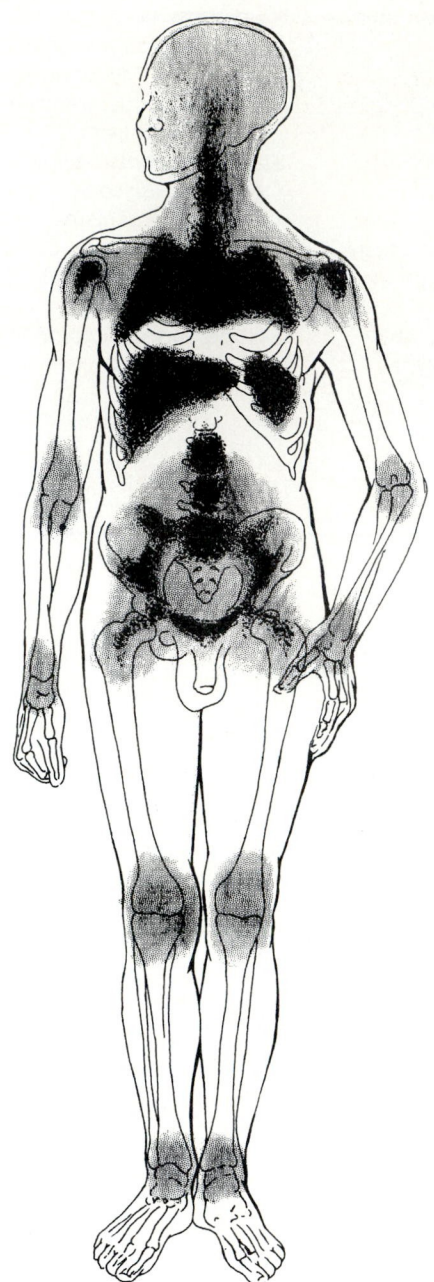

Fig. 37-3 Reticuloendothelial system. Note anatomic distribution of maximal activity in system, as indicated by black areas over body. To produce such an image certain radioactive colloidal particles are given to subject, and radiation detection techniques delineate tissue uptake. Note definition of liver, spleen, and active bone marrow in axial skeleton and proximal parts of long bones. (From Smith, AL: Microbiology and pathology, ed 12, St. Louis, 1980, The CV Mosby Co.)

Table 37-4 Distribution and names of macrophages in various tissue sites

Tissue	Macrophage
Peripheral blood	Monocyte
Loose connective tissue	Histiocyte
Liver	Kupffer's cells
Spleen and reticuloendothelial system	Wandering or fixed macrophage
Lung	Alveolar macrophage or dust cell
Granulomatous tissue	Epithelioid and giant cells
Peritoneal cavity, pleural cavity, and bone	Macrophages

out the process of *phagocytosis* in several discrete steps (Fig. 37-4). Most infecting microbes are quickly and efficiently destroyed by phagocytosis; however, some pathogens exhibit methods of escape from this destruction. Some bacteria, such as strains of the streptococci and staphylococci and *Bacillus anthracis* (anthrax), actually produce factors that will kill the phagocyte. Other organisms resist ingestion or digestion. Some organisms may survive within the phagocytes or reticuloendothelial cells and multiply there. This may lead to the transport of the organism to other sites in the body or serve as a chronic focus of continued infection.

The granulocytes can be divided on the basis of their structure and function into neutrophils, eosinophils, and basophils. The "granules" found within these cells represent discrete packets of degradative enzymes used to digest the ingested materials. The neutrophils are the most numerous in circulation and are the most efficient and responsive phagocytic cells involved in the inflammatory process. Where there is adequate blood supply to a region, the phagocytes are constantly available to move from the blood vessels to the site of injury or infection. The neutrophils and monocytes are actually attracted to the scene by chemicals released during infection or injury. This cellular response to chemical attraction is known as *chemotaxis*, and the substances released are called *chemotactic substances*.

■ FLUID FACTORS

The fluid portion of uncoagulated blood is called *plasma*. Some of the components of plasma provide important constituents for the internal defense mechanisms. Plasma transports the *circulating antibodies* produced in specific response to antigenic stimulation. These antibodies, when bound to their specific antigens, enhance the ability of white blood cells to engulf the clumped and sticky antigens. The antibodies of the blood that create this coating effect are known as *opsonins*. Another plasma constituent, *fibrin*, may create a meshwork around the injured area, causing the sealing off of the area. Microorganisms may also become

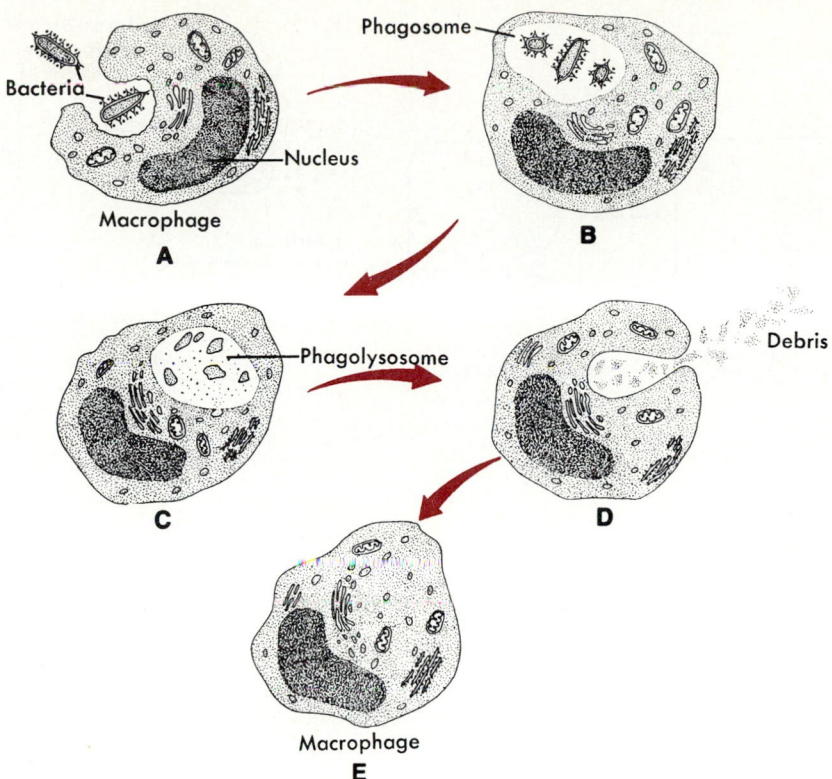

Fig. 37-4   Phagocytosis sketched in macrophage. **A,** Opsonized bacteria engulfed by phagocyte (macrophage). **B,** Phagosome formed. **C,** Phagosome becomes phagolysosome; bacteria digested. (To this point process of phagocytosis is comparable to either macrophage or neutrophil, not shown.) **D,** Debris is egested. (Neutrophil would succumb here.) **E,** Macrophage returns to resting state. (From Smith, AL: Microbiology and pathology, ed 12, St. Louis, 1980, The CV Mosby Co.)

trapped within this meshwork, where they are more easily captured by the phagocytic cells.

One of the most important constituents of plasma is a complex series of 11 proteins known by the singular name of *complement*. The primary role of complement is to provide specific lysis (rupturing) of cell membranes. The initiation of the "complement cascade" is most often triggered by the binding of the first complement protein to complement-binding antibodies that have already bound to their antigens. Thus complement serves to accentuate or complete the action of an antibody. The antibody by itself cannot produce cell lysis, but with the recruitment of complement to join in the reaction, the cell may be ruptured. However, other nonimmune substances can also activate complement. Complement is considered a nonspecific component of the plasma because it is not increased by immunization. In addition to its cytolytic effects, complement is involved in leukocyte chemotaxis, release of histamines, enhancement of phagocytosis by PMNs, viral neutralization, and bactericidal activity.

C-reactive protein is a beta globulin found in the serum of individuals with any type of severe inflammatory process.

Both infectious and noninfectious inflammations elicit the formation of this protein in the plasma. The protein forms a precipitate with a constituent of the cell wall of *Streptococcus pneumoniae* known as the C polysaccharide; hence its name. The amount of C-reactive protein found in the serum is roughly proportional to the severity of the inflammation; therefore, a test for this protein is useful in the diagnosis and management of hard-to-differentiate diseases that have a hidden inflammatory aspect, such as bacterial endocarditis, cryptic abscesses, rheumatic fever, and certain types of cancer.

■ Interferon

Interferons are a group of low molecular weight proteins produced by certain virally infected cells. The protein is released into the extracellular environment, and when taken up by uninfected cells it can protect those cells from viral multiplication. This antiviral action is exerted before the specific antibody levels can reach protective levels. The interferons are synthesized by the cells of many different animal species, but they are species specific; that is, bovine

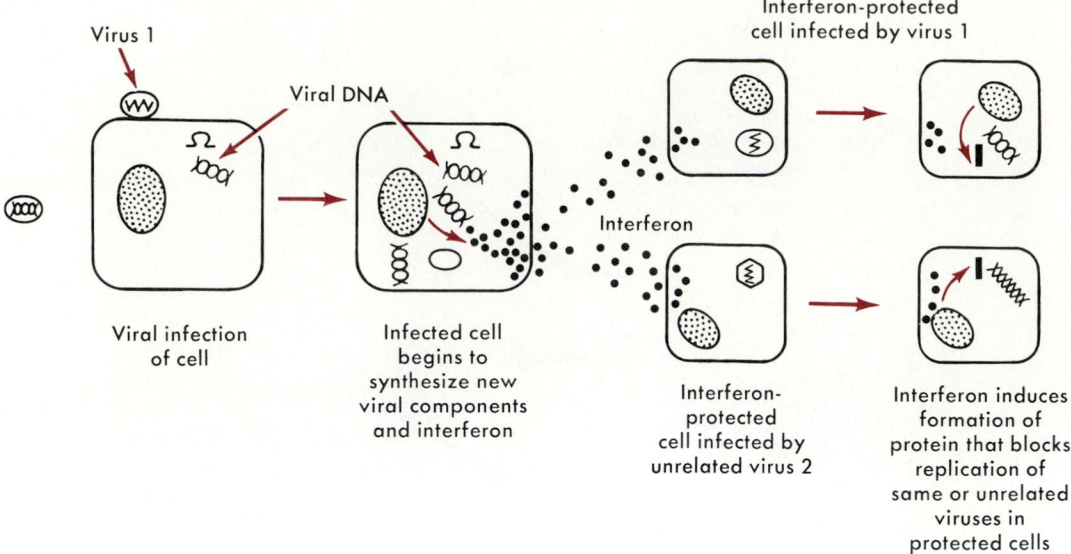

Virus 1

Viral DNA

Viral infection of cell

Infected cell begins to synthesize new viral components and interferon

Interferon

Interferon-protected cell infected by virus 1

Interferon-protected cell infected by unrelated virus 2

Interferon induces formation of protein that blocks replication of same or unrelated viruses in protected cells

Fig. 37-5 Mechanism of interferon action.

interferon will not adequately protect human cells. In general, the product of a viral infection is the same regardless of the viral agent that initiated its formation. Therefore, interferons can be described as being host specific but viral nonspecific.

Interferons are produced by cells infected with infectious viral particles, inactivated viruses, or even laboratory synthesized double-stranded polynucleotides. Virtually all tissue cells are capable of producing interferons when properly stimulated, but the lymphocytes are the primary source of interferon in the plasma. The stimulation seems to be tied to the recognition of the "foreign" nucleic acid, which signals the infected cells to synthesize and liberate interferon for a few hours (up to about 24 hours). The interferon acts on the uninfected cells, causing them to synthesize another protein that remains within the protected cell. This protein inhibits the synthesis of the viral particle without blocking normal cell synthetic functions (Fig. 37-5). Interferon itself has no direct effect on the viral particles, nor does it interfere with the entry of the viral particle into the interferon-protected cell. This interferon-mediated protection lasts only about 24 hours.

That interferon plays a significant role in the recovery from viral infections seems inescapable; however, it has never been shown conclusively that interferon is a necessary part of defense against viral infection. Because naturally occurring deficiencies have never been demonstrated, and there is no mechanism for selective inhibition in experimental animals, it is not possible to specifically evaluate the role of interferon as a defense mechanism.

Interferon has great potential as an antiviral agent because of its protective effects against a wide range of viruses and its low toxicity in the body. There are certain significant limitations to its therapeutic use, however:

1. Species specificity, which until recently meant it had to be produced in human tissue culture, which is both difficult and expensive
2. Difficulty in purification, which makes recovery of large quantities impractical
3. Lack of any effect on viral synthesis already in progress
4. Inability to deliver protective doses to susceptible host cells
5. Short duration of activity

Recent breakthroughs in genetic engineering have made it possible to produce and isolate interferon from bacteria cultures, which greatly reduces the expense and increases the availability of interferon.

Interferon has been shown to be effective in two other clinically important situations: (1) protection of patients whose immunity has been suppressed because of cancer chemotherapy, immunodeficiency disease, or organ transplant and (2) treatment of certain cancers. Interferon has been experimentally successful in protecting immunosuppressed or immunodeficient patients from viral infections by herpesvirus, cytomegalovirus, and influenza virus. Interferon, in addition to its antiviral activity, has been shown to have antitumor activity. Clinical trials with certain human cancers (osteogenic sarcomas and breast cancer) have demonstrated tumor regression after interferon therapy. Interferon may become another chemotherapeutic agent that can be used in cancer therapy.

■ Inflammatory response

When injury occurs in the body, all of the nonspecific and, to some degree, the specific defense mechanisms are directed toward localizing the effects of the injury, protecting against microbial invasion at the site, and preparing the site for repair. This process is called *inflammation*. When inflammation occurs at a particular site in the body, the suffix *-itis* is added to the site designation to indicate the pathologic state; for example, an inflammatory response on the pericardium is termed pericarditis, and of the bladder, cystitis.

The inflammatory response can be initiated by any type of injury, for example, heat, cold, irradiation, chemicals, trauma, infection, immunologic injury, or neoplasm. Whatever the stimulus, the response of the body is the same, but the extent of the involvement of the various facets of the nonspecific response system depends on the extent and severity of the injury.

■ STEPS OF THE INFLAMMATORY RESPONSE

Three major physiologic responses occur in the inflammatory process: vascular response, fluid exudation, and cellular exudation (Table 37-5). The *vascular response* consists of a transitory vasoconstriction (stress response) followed immediately by vasodilation. This occurs as a result of chemical substances such as histamine or kinins released at the site of injury or invasion. The amount of blood flow to the area is thus increased *(hyperemia)*, causing redness and heat. Blood flow slows as the capillaries dilate. Permeability of the capillary walls is increased, facilitating fluid and cellular exudation. *Fluid exudation* from the capillaries into the interstitial spaces begins immediately and is most active during the first 24 hours after injury or invasion. Initially, the fluid exudate is primarily serous, but as the capillary wall becomes more permeable, protein (albumin) is lost into the interstitial spaces. This increases the colloid osmotic pressure in the interstitial spaces,

which encourages more fluid exudation. The swelling of tissue from the fluid in the interstitial spaces is called *edema* (Chapter 8). *Cellular exudation* refers to the migration of white blood cells (leukocytes) through the capillary walls into the affected tissue. An increased number of white blood cells are attracted to the vessels in the affected area as a result of chemotactic substances being released from the tissues by cell injury and complement activation. The white blood cells adhere to the capillary wall and then pass ameboid fashion through the widened endothelial junctions of the capillary wall. Neutrophils (PMNs), which make up about 60% of the circulating white blood cells, are the first leukocytes to respond, usually within the first few hours. The neutrophils ingest the bacteria and dead tissue cells *(phagocytosis);* then they die, releasing proteolytic enzymes that liquefy the dead neutrophils, dead bacteria, and other dead cells (pus). Monocytes and lymphocytes appear later. The macrophages continue the phagocytosis, and the lymphocytes play a role in the antigen-antibody response at the site.

The five cardinal symptoms of inflammation, identified many centuries ago, are redness *(rubor)* and heat *(calor)* caused by the hyperemia, swelling *(tumor)* caused by the fluid exudate, pain *(dolor)* caused by the pressure of the fluid exudate and by chemical (bradykinin) irritation of the nerve endings, and *loss of function* of the affected part caused by the swelling and pain.

■ CONTAINMENT OR SPREAD OF INFECTION

The inflammatory response serves to prepare the tissue for healing and to contain the spread of bacterial invasion. To prevent the spread of bacteria, fibroblasts are attracted to the area and secrete fibrin, a threadlike substance that

Table 37-5   Steps of the inflammatory response

Steps	Mediators	Outcome
1. Injury	Physical, chemical, biologic, immunologic stimulus	Cell and tissue injury
2. Vascular response		
a. Vascular dilation	Histamine, plasmin, serotonin, kinins, prostaglandins released or activated by injury	Dilation of vessels causing stasis of blood and margination of leukocytes
b. Fibrin clot formation	Activation of clotting mechanism	Containment of irritants
3. Fluid exudation	Histamine, kinins, prostaglandins cause opening of venule—endothelial cell junction	Fluid exudation into tissues
4. Cellular exudation		
a. Leukocyte exudation	Chemotactic substances released by complement activation, clot formation, and injured cells	Passage of leukocytes from blood to site of injury and accumulation there
b. Attack and engulfment of foreign materials	Neutrophils and macrophages	Removal and digestion of bacteria, foreign particles, and damaged tissues
5. Healing	Fibroblasts produce collagen fibers and tissue regeneration	Resolution of inflammation and formation of scar tissue

encircles the affected area to wall it off from healthy tissue. If there is interference with this walling-off process, bacteria can spread into the surrounding tissue. This explains why an abscess should not be incised and drained until it has "come to a head," or until the walling-off process is completed.

Bacteria may fail to be contained locally and spread to other parts of the body by means of the lymph system or bloodstream (see the box below). If picked up by the lymph stream, the bacteria will be carried to the nearest lymph node. These nodes are located along the course of all lymph channels, and here too bacteria can be ingested and destroyed. If the bacteria are virulent enough to resist the action in the lymph nodes, leukocytes are brought in by the bloodsteam to attack and engulf the bacteria in the node. The node then becomes swollen and tender because of the accumulation of phagocytes, bacteria, and destroyed lymphoid tissue. This is known as *lymphadenitis*. Swollen lymph nodes can be palpated primarily in the neck, axilla, and groin.

Moderate to severe inflammatory responses can produce generalized systemic effects. Products from the breakdown of bacteria and white blood cells can affect the temperature-regulating center in the hypothalamus and produce fever. A severe infection without accompanying fever may suggest a poor prognosis. Loss of appetite (anorexia) and fatigue may by caused by conservation of body energy needed to resist the infection. The body increases the production of white blood cells to help fight the infection, and *leukocytosis* (serum white blood cell levels >10,000/mm³) may occur. With infection blood sedimentation rate is also increased, that is, when an anticoagulant is added to the blood in the laboratory, the red blood cells settle to the bottom of a test tube more rapidly than normal. This in-

crease in the sedimentation rate is believed to be caused by an increase in fibrinogen (a blood protein essential to the healing process). The sedimentation rate is elevated during the acute inflammatory stage of infection. Its elevation is an indication that the body's defense mechanism for the repair of damaged tissue is operating. Because the sedimentation rate gradually returns to normal as tissues heal, it also is used to determine when physical activity can be safely resumed after an acute infection.

No healing will occur until inflammation has subsided and pus and dead tissue have been removed. Pus is a local accumulation of dead phagocytes, dead bacteria, and dead tissue. The bacteria most commonly causing this reaction are the staphylococci, streptococci, *Neisseria,* and *P. aeruginosa (pyocyanea)*.

Inflammations can be classified as either acute or chronic. *Acute* inflammations are those characterized by a sudden onset and an increase in the fluid exudative response. *Chronic* inflammations have a slower, more insidious onset, and they are characterized by increased cellular exudation.

■ RESOLUTION AND HEALING

After the infected area is clean, new cells are produced to fill in the space left by the injury. They may be the normal structural cells, or they may be fibrotic tissue cells known as *scar tissue*. If they are fibrotic cells, they will not function as formerly but only serve to fill in the injured area. Some body cells readily regenerate; for instance, after the bowel has healed it is almost impossible to find the injured area. The respiratory tract also regenerates its tissues readily. Liver tissue has the capacity to regenerate its tissue, but over a longer period of time. Some nerve cells are always replaced with fibrous tissue. If a large amount of tissue is destroyed, structural cells may not be replaced, regardless of the type of tissue. (See Chapter 18 for discussion of wound healing.)

■ SPECIFIC DEFENSE MECHANISMS

■ Concept of specific immunity

Nonspecific response mechanisms are often inadequate to cope with foreign agents. This is especially true when the agent is capable of multiplication and invasion of host tissues, as is the case with infectious disease microorganisms (viruses, bacteria, fungi). The body responds by activation of the specific immune response system.

The fundamental nature of the specific immune response is characterized by diversity, specificity, recognition, memory, and action. Among the most intriguing aspects of immune response is its *diversity of ability to respond* while at the same time responding with *specificity of action*. Almost any conceivable organic molecular array on the surface of a molecule has been shown to be able to induce a series of cellular events culminating in the production of *antibodies*. These antibodies combine with the inducing

---

Some types of inflammations

Cellulitis	Inflammation involving cellular and connective tissue
Lymphadenitis	Inflammation of lymph nodes
Lymphangitis	Inflammation of lymphatic vessel
Bacteremia	Presence of bacteria in blood
Septicemia	Systemic disease associated with pathogenic microorganisms and their toxins in the blood
Abscess	Collection of pus localized by a zone of inflamed tissue
Sinus	Suppurating channel from an abscess to the surface or into a body cavity
Peritonitis	Inflammation of the peritoneum
Pleuritis	Inflammation of the pleura
Empyema	Collection of pus in a body cavity, especially the pleural cavity

antigen by virtue of combining sites on the antibody molecule, which exhibit an extremely narrow specificity. The remainder of the antibody molecule is chemically and structurally quite similar to all other antibody molecules with distinctly different combining site specificities. *Recognition* and *memory* are two other aspects of this system that make it unique. The normal organism recognizes its own antigenic makeup and will not produce antibodies against its own antigens. This is known as *recognition of self*. At the same time, this intricate system of self-recognition must be able to recognize extremely subtle changes in its own cells when incipient tumors that differ only slightly in antigenic constitution are forming. Further, once the immune system has responded to an antigen, subsequent encounters with that antigen will produce an even more vigorous and rapid response. This response includes a wide variety of mechanisms designed to take *action* against the offending agent. Many of these actions are among the most potent biochemical and cellular reactions that the body is capable of producing, yet they are focused so discretely that the foreign agent is rapidly destroyed with a minimum of damage to the host.

Antigens and antibodies

ANTIGENS (IMMUNOGENS)

An antigen is defined as a substance that, when introduced into an animal, elicits the formation of antibodies, or specifically sensitized cells. The antigen must be recognized as "nonself" or "foreign" material within the body. Although most antigens are naturally occurring proteins of at least 10,000 molecular weight, other substances such as polysaccharides, nucleoproteins, lipoproteins, and glycoproteins may also serve as antigens. The bulk of the antigen consists of subsurface molecular structures that do not elicit an immune response but do serve as carrier for the multiple *antigenic determinants* on the surface. Most antigens have multiple antigenic determinants and are termed *multivalent antigens;* however, some molecules may be monovalent.

Certain molecules, because of their small size, cannot by themselves induce the synthesis of antibodies; however, when they are coupled with a high molecular weight carrier, they can serve as antigenic determinants. These molecules are known as *incomplete antigens*, or *haptens*. These molecules take on special significance in the consideration of hypersensitivities (allergies to low molecular weight compounds such as certain drugs and antibiotics) (Chapter 38).

ANTIBODIES (IMMUNOGLOBULINS)

The body's response to the introduction of an antigenic substance is the production of a specific, soluble *antibody* or a sensitized (antigen reactive) lymphocyte population. The type of antigen introduced will determine the immune response: antibody synthesis, antigen-reactive lymphocyte, or a combination of both.

The circulating antibodies represent modified (that is, antigen specific) globulin proteins found in blood serum. The serum contains several distinct protein fractions, which are separable on the basis of their net electrical charge, molecular size, and molecular conformation into several fractions: albumin, alpha globulins, beta globulins, and gamma globulins (Fig. 37-6). The antibody activity of the serum is characteristically associated with the gamma globulin fraction. Those gamma globulins with the ability to bind antigens are called *immunoglobulins*.

Five different classes of immunoglobulins are actually produced within the body. Each immunoglobulin class varies in structure, distribution in the body, and in protective function. Some of these variations in function have significant clinical implications, for example, only one class of immunoglobulins, IgG, can cross the normal placenta; immunoglobulin E(IgE) binds to receptors on the membranes of mast cells and basophils to mediate one type of

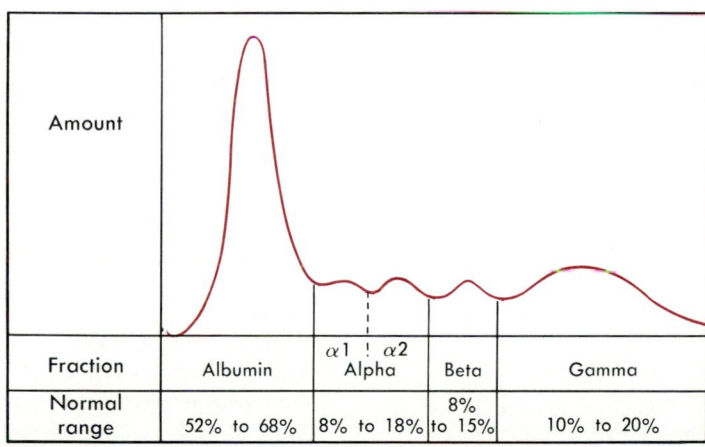

Amount				
Fraction	Albumin	$\alpha 1$ ¦ $\alpha 2$ Alpha	Beta	Gamma
Normal range	52% to 68%	8% to 18%	8% to 15%	10% to 20%

Fig. 37-6   Electrophoretic separation of major serum proteins. Majority of antibody activity lies within gamma globulin fraction. Gamma globulin fraction will rise with active synthesis of antibodies in response to antigenic stimulation.

Table 37-6 Characteristics of immunoglobulin classes

Immunoglobulin class	Function	Body distribution	Activate complement	Cross placenta
IgA	Protects mucosal surfaces from bacteria, viruses, and toxins	Mucosal and exocrine secretions	No	No
IgD	Does not have antibody function but may play a role in signaling B cell differentiation	Membrane of circulating B cells	No	No
IgE	Protects against parasitic infections and responsible for Type I hypersensitivity	Membrane of mast cells and basophils	No	No
IgG	Protects against microorganisms and toxins in blood and body fluids	Major immunoglobulin in serum and other body fluids	Yes	Yes
IgM	Protects against microorganisms in blood	Confined to vascular system	Yes	No

allergic reaction. Table 37-6 summarizes the characteristics of the different immunoglobulin classes.

ANTIGEN-ANTIBODY INTERACTIONS

When an immunoglobulin comes in contact with its specific antigen, a physical interaction occurs between the two, causing a reversible binding of the antibody to the antigen. The affinity that the antibody has for the antigen and the avidity, or tightness, of the binding depend on the location and spatial arrangement of the antigenic determinants on the surface of the antigen and how well the antigen-combining site on the antibody molecule "fits" the antigenic determinant. Because the antigen is usually multivalent and the antibody is generally at least bivalent, the antigen molecules may be cross bound and clumped (agglutinated, precipitated) by antibody molecules (Fig. 37-7).

Within the body the binding of antibody to the antigen can be direct beneficial effects, such as detoxification of toxins, inactivation of viruses, or, coupled with complement, the direct lysis of cells. However, in most cases the antigen-antibody combination initiates and facilitates the

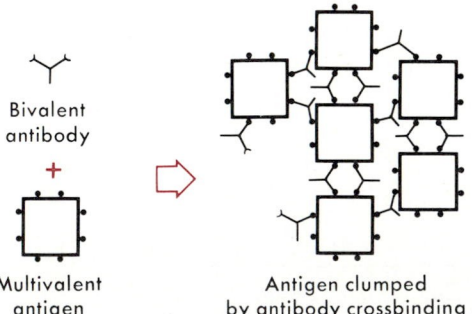

Bivalent antibody

+

Multivalent antigen

Antigen clumped by antibody crossbinding

Fig. 37-7 Clumping of multivalent antigen by its specific antibody.

nonspecific defense mechanisms (phagocytosis, complement, inflammatory response, and so forth).

■ Immune response system

■ CELLS INVOLVED

The cells in the specific immune response are all derived from the original undifferentiated stem cells of the bone marrow. The stem cell has the possibility of developing into any of the blood cells of the body depending on various signals and influences. The primary cells of the immune response system develop from the lymphocytic cell population (Fig. 37-8).

One population of lymphocytic cells undergoes differentiation under the influence of the thymus gland. These cells are known as *thymus-dependent lymphocytes* or *T cells*. They are primarily responsible for providing activated cells that directly attack foreign materials in the body. This arm of the specific immune response system is known as *cell-mediated immunity* (CMI). This division of the immune response system provides primary protection against chronic bacterial infection (tuberculosis, leprosy), fungal infections (thrush, athlete's foot), protozoan infections (pneumocystis, toxoplasmosis), intracellular virus infections (measles, herpes), and foreign tissues (tissue transplants) (Table 37-7). The T cells also produce cells that exercise control of immunologic response. *T helper cells* (designated as T_H or T_4 cells) enhance immunoglobulin production by B cells and amplify cell-mediated immune response. *T suppressor cells* (designated T_S or T_8 cells) inhibit immunoglobulin synthesis and T cell cytotoxic activity.

Another population of lymphocytes undergoes differentiation independent of thymic control and is referred to as *thymus-independent lymphocytes* or *B cells*. The designation, "B cell," comes from the fact that in the chicken, where these cells were first detected, they are differentiated in a single organ, the *bursa of Fabricius*. No such single organ site has been found in humans, so the site in

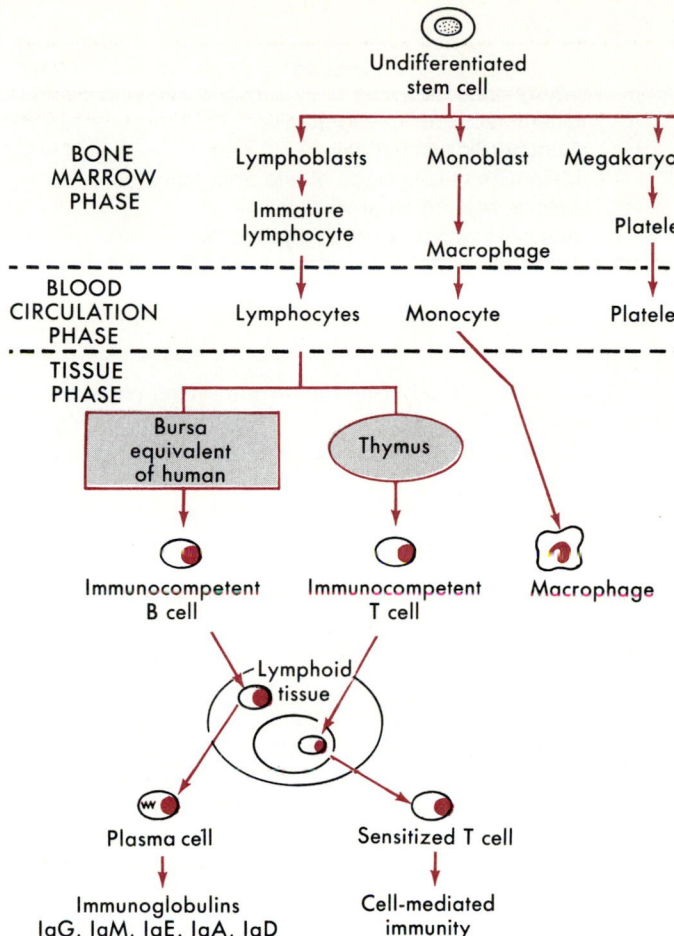

Fig. 37-8   Development of B and T cell lymphocytes.

the human is simply referred to as the *bursa-equivalent*. The process of commitment to the B cell lineage probably occurs in the bone marrow during cell maturation. The B cells produce immunoglobulins that appear in blood, lymph, mucus, and virtually all body fluids. This division of immune response provides the body's primary protection against acute bacterial infections (staphylococcal or streptococcal infections), biologic toxins (diphtheria or tetanus toxin), and certain viral infections (common cold, rabies, polio).

The proteins (markers) on the membranes of immune response cells vary according to the type of immune response cell it is. B cell lymphocytes have immunoglobulins present on their surface that are missing from T cell lymphocytes. All T cells have a marker called T_1; helper T cells have a unique marker known as T_4; and suppressor T cells have a marker known as T_8. It is possible then to identify each of these cell types by their unique surface markers.

The role of the lymphocytes (B or T cells) is to recognize the presence of an antigen and to initiate specific mechanisms of disposal. Just as important, the lymphocyte must recognize a component of host tissues as self and protect that tissue from immunologic reactions.

Table 37-7   Protection provided by humorally mediated and cell-mediated immune response systems

Characteristic	Specific immune response system	
	Humorally mediated system	Cell-mediated system
Lymphocytes	B cells	T cells
Immunologically active effector	Plasma cells producing circulating immunoglobulins	Antigen-specific activated T cell producing lymphokines, cytotoxic T cells
Memory cells	B memory cells	T memory cells
Control cells	—	T helper cells (T_4)
		T suppressor cells (T_8)
Primary protection against	Acute bacterial infections	Chronic bacterial infections
	Biologic toxins	Fungal infections
	Extracellular virus infections	Protozoan infections
		Intracellular virus infections
		Foreign tissues

Table 37-8 Lymphokines liberated by activated T cell lymphocytes

Lymphokine	Function
Lymphocyte-derived chemotactic factors	Chemotactic for macrophages
Lymphocytotoxins	Nonspecific lysis of cells
Macrophage inhibition-activation factors	Maintains macrophage at site and activates it
Interferon	Inhibits replication of viruses
Lymphocyte-activating factors (interleukins)	Activates nonsensitized lymphocytes

The *macrophage* appears to act nonspecifically, but its role in the immune response is critical. First, the macrophage seems to be responsible for initially capturing, processing, and presenting the antigen to the lymphocytes. Capture of the antigen occurs by phagocytosis as described earlier in this chapter. The processing of the antigen is poorly understood, but there is evidence that the macrophage digests and concentrates the antigen. This processed signal is transferred to the surface of the macrophage for presentation to lymphocytes. An antigen presented to lymphocytes in this manner triggers the series of events within the lymphocytes that leads to full immunologic response. An antigen that escapes this processing will stimulate only a weak immune response or none at all.

At the other end of the immune response the macrophage is activated to its maximum of phagocytic efficiency by the release of stimulatory, soluble substances, known as *lymphokines,* by activated lymphocytes (Table 37-8). In this way the macrophage is stimulated at the site of an immune reaction. Other of the soluble lymphokines serve to attract the macrophages to the site by chemotaxis.

■ ORGANS AND TISSUES INVOLVED

The organs and tissues of the specific immune response system include the central organs (bone marrow and thymus) and the peripheral organs (lymph nodes, spleen, and lymphatic vessels). Within the central organs the immune response cells are synthesized and matured, whereas within the peripheral organs the mature cells are concentrated.

The *thymus* serves as the control organ of the immune system. It is the site of differentiation of the T cell lymphocytic populations and through certain soluble thymic hormones serves to regulate the overall immune system. The activity of the thymus reaches its peak in childhood, and the organ begins to shrink in size after puberty. If the thymus is removed (thymectomy) very early in the life of an animal, a severe state of immunodeficiency is induced and T cell–mediated immunity never develops. After thymectomy, a wasting disease develops, characterized by stunted growth, diarrhea, and death from massive infection by intestinal or respiratory tract normal flora. The B cell function is also reduced, pointing to the cooperative effect between the two basic systems. In the adult animal the loss of the thymus creates less severe reactions, probably

because of an already functional, long-lived population of T cells.

The *lymph nodes* and *spleen* serve as the primary sites of localization of the immune response cells. The lymph node serves to filter the lymph drained from a region of tissue. The structure of the lymph node (Fig. 37-9) consists of an inner medullary and paracortical region primarily populated with T cells and an outer cortex composed of clusters, or germinal centers, of B cells known as follicles. The spleen is structured on somewhat the same pattern, with diffusely packed T cell areas and germinal centers of tightly packed B cells. In certain types of antigenic stimulation, either the T cell areas or the B cell areas will show tissue proliferation, whereas the other area remains quiescent. By the same principle, if there is a basic primary immunodeficiency of one system, the corresponding area of lymph nodes and spleen may degenerate.

During the course of the immune response reaction, within the lymph nodes there is significant proliferation of specific cells or migration of phagocytic cells to the site, which may lead to lymph node enlargement. Enlargement of the lymph nodes in a region may be the result of infection, immune disease, intrinsic neoplasm of the lymph node, or metastatic spread of malignant cells to the node. The presence of an enlarged spleen or enlarged lymph nodes is virtually always an important clinical finding.

■ Immune response

■ PRIMARY IMMUNE RESPONSE

□ Antigenic challenge

When an antigen is introduced into the body, it can trigger a wide or narrow spectrum of response mechanisms. The specific pattern of response depends on the amount of antigen introduced, the site of introduction, and the type of antigen introduced.

Small amounts of a noninvasive, large, particulate antigen introduced at a single body site are quickly and efficiently handled at a local site with little or no systemic involvement beyond the local lymph node. Because the inflammatory response and local lymph node can localize the spread of the antigen, the immune response may go completely unnoticed by the host organism. Larger, particulate antigens are readily cleared, but small, soluble antigens are more difficult to clear from the circulation.

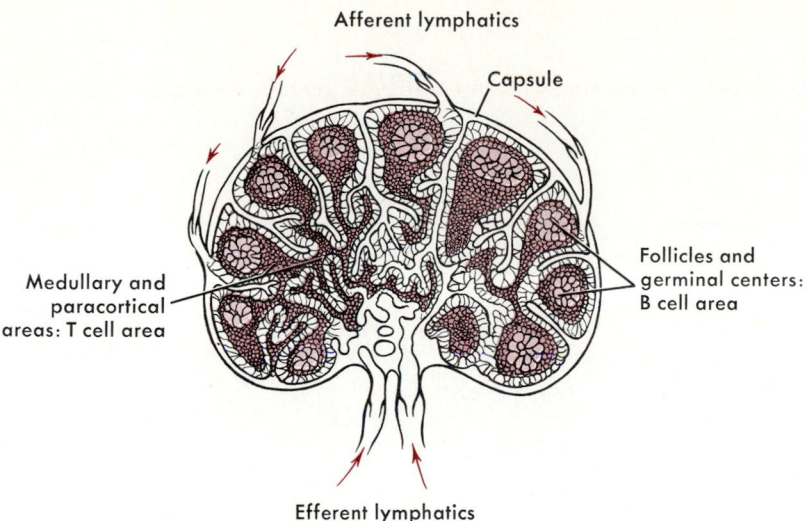

Afferent lymphatics

Capsule

Follicles and germinal centers: B cell area

Medullary and paracortical areas: T cell area

Efferent lymphatics

Fig. 37-9   B and T cell areas of lymph node.

Large amounts of an antigen may allow the antigen to escape from the local site by simply overwhelming the local defense mechanisms. Even though the lymph nodes and reticuloendothelial organs can clear 80% to 90% of an antigen on a single pass, if the amount of the antigen is extremely large, some antigen may escape the local site.

Highly invasive antigens (for example, bacteria such as *Staphylococcus aureus* or *Streptococcus pyogenes*) or those introduced directly into the bloodstream by blood transfusion, intravenous catheterization, or injection can immediately establish a systemic type of immune response. This is why extreme care must be exercised in the use of any type of medical procedure that could allow the introduction of organisms into the general circulation. The localization action of the immune response is critical to efficient functioning of the response.

☐ **Humoral response**

When the antigen is introduced for the first time, one of three basic mechanisms of response will be elicited: a response mediated primarily by B cells, the humoral response; a response in which the T cells are primarily involved, the cell-mediated response; or a combined type of response.

If the antigen is of the type that triggers a humoral response, the first time the body is exposed to the antigen the B cell system responds with the synthesis of circulating immunoglobulins (Fig. 37-10). The encroaching antigen is phagocytosed by a lymph node macrophage or tissue-active macrophage. The macrophage processes the antigen and presents the antigenic stimulus to a B cell, which has been preprogrammed to respond to the introduced antigen. These antigen-specific B cells bear receptors on their surface, which allow them to recognize their antigenic stimulant. Only a few lymphocytes within a lymph node have the ability to respond to the antigen. The stimulated B cell

then begins a process of proliferation (increase in number) and differentiation (change in structure and function). The progeny of the stimulated cell increase in number within the lymph node, forming *clones* of specifically adapted lymphocytes. With each generation of new cells within the clone, the lymphocytes become more differentiated toward a cell population ideally suited for the synthesis and release of immunoglobulin. These cells are known as *plasma cells*. With the development of this cell population in the lymph node (several days after the introduction of the antigen), antibodies can be detected in the lymph node. However, it is not until about 1 to 2 weeks after the antigenic challenge that detectable levels of specific antibodies appear in the serum. The plasma cell population of the lymph node and the levels of antibody in the blood continue to increase for another 2 to 3 weeks, and then both begin to retreat.

Two types of immunoglobulins are produced and released into the circulation. *Immunoglobulin M* (IgM or macroglobulin) is especially effective at attaching to particulate antigens such as bacterial cells and with the activation of the complement system in the serum, causes the lysis of those cells. Because IgM antibodies are so large, they cannot leave the blood vessels, so they are restricted to a role in the bloodstream.

Immunoglobulin G (IgG) makes up about 85% of the antibodies found in the serum. This immunoglobulin is smaller and can move from the blood and lymph into virtually all body fluids and can also cross the placenta from maternal circulation into fetal circulation. This class of immunoglobulin provides most of our protection against bacterial, viral, and toxic agents in the body. Usually when the term *antibody* is used, this is the type of immunoglobulin that is meant.

Some of the lymphocytes of the activated clone may become "memory cells," which are much more responsive,

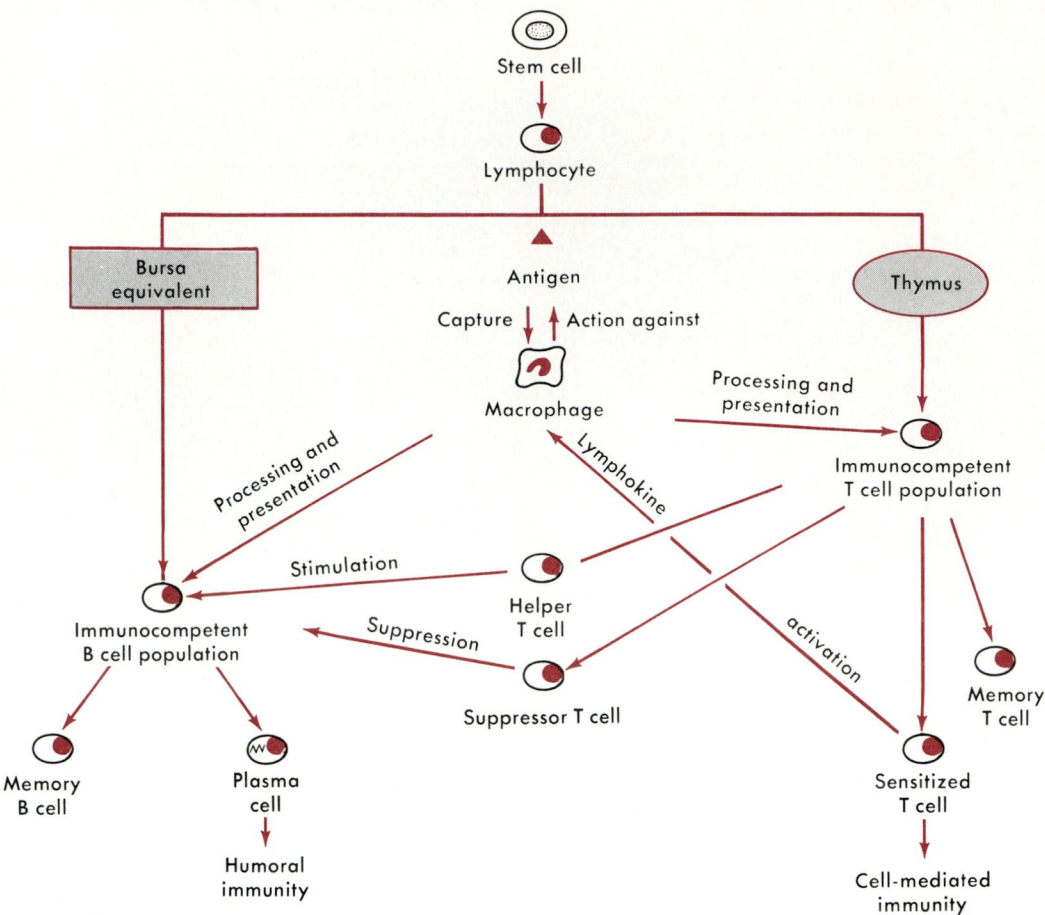

Fig. 37-10   Combined response of B and T cell systems.

both in time of reaction and efficiency of antibody synthesis, to subsequent contact with the antigen.

The humoral response serves to protect the body from such agents as microbial toxins, bacteria within the extravascular spaces in the blood and on mucosal surfaces, and viruses that must pass through the circulatory system to reach their site of infection (for example, poliomyelitis virus).

☐ **Cell-mediated response**

Certain antigens trigger a response mediated by T cell proliferation and reaction. A T cell that has received its antigenic stimulus is referred to as a *sensitized T cell lymphocyte* (Fig. 37-10).

The initial steps of the cell-mediated response, those involving the antigen processing by the macrophage, seem to be the same as in the humoral response. Following presentation of the antigenic stimulus of lymph node T cells, there is proliferation in the T cell domain. Circulatory antibodies are not released; rather, activated lymphocytes are released into the circulation. These cells migrate to the site of the entrance of the antigen into the body, where

the invading agent or residual antigen is found. These activated lymphocytes, along with macrophages, infiltrate the regions of the tissue and begin a direct attack on the antigen or tissue cells labeled with the antigen. The T cells participating in this direct attack are known as *killer T cells.*

To amplify the site reaction further, the sensitized lymphocytes activate the nonspecific phagocytotic cells (macrophages, PMNs, and noncommitted lymphocytes) in the region of the antigen. This is accomplished through the release of the soluble lymphokines (Table 37-8), which recruit additional cells to attack the antigenic materials.

The cell-mediated response is especially effective in protection against diseases that grow and do their damage intracellularly where the circulating immunoglobulins cannot reach them. Diseases of this type include viral and rickettsial diseases and those produced by certain chronic types of infective agents, fungal pathogens and tubercle bacillus being the most outstanding examples. One other important function of this system is the provision of *cancer cell surveillance.*

☐ Combined immune response

Most antigens do not cause a purely humoral or purely cell-mediated response; rather, both types of response are evoked. Likewise, our protection against most harmful antigens is the result of both of these specific response systems being brought to bear on the antigen involved. In the *combined type of response,* an initial perturbation occurs within the T cell areas of the lymph node. This becomes obvious within about 2 days after the introduction of the antigen. About 3 to 5 days later, the B cell areas begin to proliferate.

To mount a maximal immune response, the cooperative action of the three central cell types is necessary. The macrophage serves to capture, process, and present the antigen to immunocompetent cells of both T and B cell ancestry. The T cells aid in the direct cell-mediated response, but a population of T cells also serves to interact with the B cell and a T cell population controls the development of an effective immune response. A *helper T cell* population cooperates with the B cells to enhance the activation and proliferation of the immunoglobulin synthesizing cells. The existence of the helper T cell explains the observation noted earlier in this chapter that the removal of the thymus from the neonate not only compromises the cell-mediated immune response but also significantly reduces the host's ability to mount a humoral immune response. T helper cells also mediate the normal expression of the cell-mediated immune response; therefore, the reduction or loss of this population of cells as occurs in acquired immunodeficiency syndrome would lead to progressive loss of immune response protection.

Another group of T cells also exerts an effect on the synthesis of circulating antibodies. Cells known as *suppressor T cells* may provide a negative control function over B cell clones and other T cell clones, preventing the expression of an immunologic response.

■ SECONDARY IMMUNE RESPONSE

As emphasized at the outset of this section, one of the touchstone characteristics of the specific response system is the ability of the system to remember prior contact with an antigen and to provide a more complete protective reaction on subsequent contact. The first contact between the immune response system and an antigen leads to the *primary response,* the events of which have been laid out in the preceding paragraphs. When antibody synthesis is measured in a primary response, there is a significant lag time to the appearance of antibodies in the circulation (Figs. 37-11 and 37-12). Immunoglobulins of the IgM class are the first to appear, but they maintain protective levels for only a short period. Specific IgG antibodies follow and reach protective levels within 12 to 14 days, but they too fall off fairly quickly with only this initial exposure.

When the "primed" immune response system encounters the antigen again, a *secondary response* ensues, which is more rapid, of greater intensity, and longer lasting than the primary response. This secondary response is also termed an *anamnestic response.* This "remembered" response is a characteristic of both the B and T cell systems. The prior contact with the antigen is stored in special memory cells of both cell lines. As illustrated in Fig. 37-11, the memory cells respond immediately to the antigenic signal, so that the lag time between exposure to the antigen and production of protective antibody levels is greatly reduced. This phenomenon provides the basis for active immunization and "booster" doses to maintain the protective levels of immunity. In an immunized individual the memory cells elicit the rapid response in time for the immune system to overwhelm the pathogen or toxin before it can produce its damage.

■ DEVELOPMENTAL ASPECTS OF THE IMMUNE RESPONSE

Lymphoid cells first appear in the fetus as stem cells in the fetal liver at about the end of the first trimester. The lymphoid tissues of the thymus also develop fairly early in

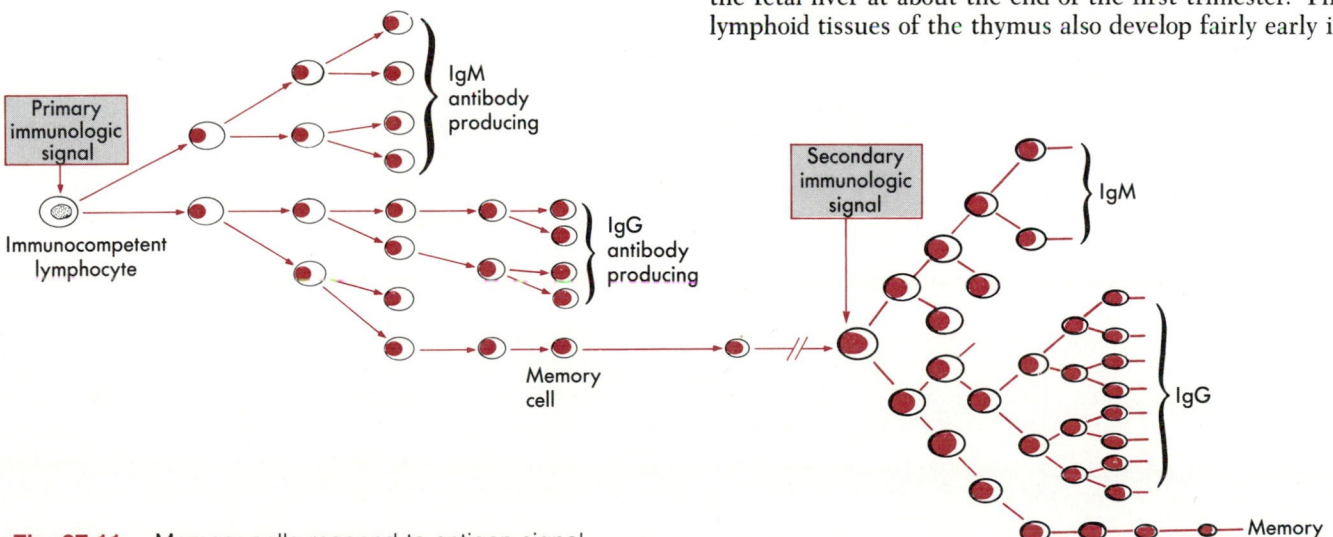

Fig. 37-11   Memory cells respond to antigen signal.

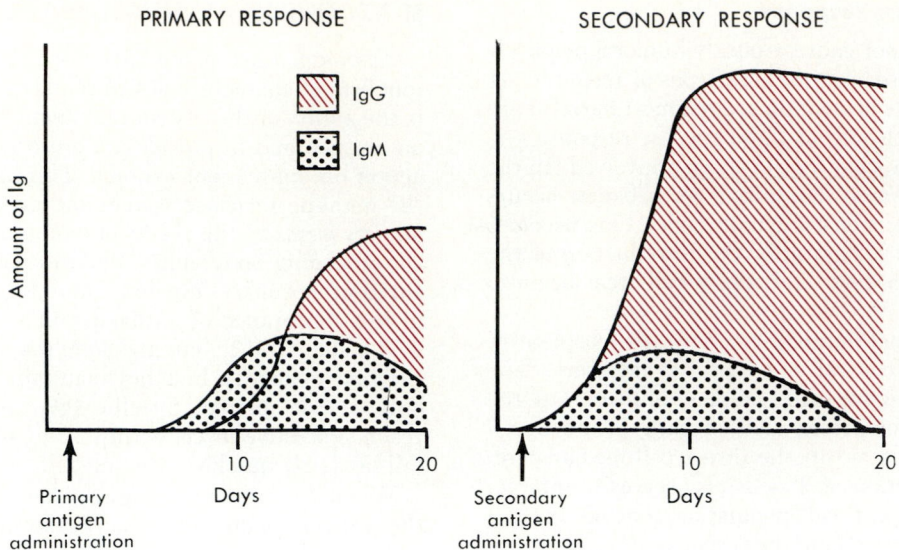

Fig. 37-12 Primary and secondary humoral responses.

the fetus. At birth, however, the lymph nodes and spleen are still underdeveloped, but T and B cell responsiveness is fully functional. The fetus is capable of some immune response if challenged by an in utero (within the uterus) infection, such as in the case of congenital syphilis or rubella. Unless the fetus has been exposed to a congenital infection, at birth the neonate-synthesized immunoglobulin levels are low (Fig. 37-13). The child does have high levels of transplacentally acquired maternal IgG antibodies. These maternal antibodies have a half-life of about 30 days in the child, and this coupled with the increase in blood volume in the growing infant leads to a drop in the IgG levels of the blood over the first 3 months. Thereafter the rate of the child's own synthesis of IgG provides for a steady

increase in the immunoglobulin concentration within the serum. IgM levels reach adult concentrations by about the age of 9 months.

Numerous studies in both animals and humans have shown that during the aging process there is a progressive loss of immunologic vigor. The prime immunologic age probably is achieved during the late teens, when virtually the full complement of immunities has been developed and the responsiveness of the system peaks. The middle years are characterized by a plateau and slowly falling curve until the later years of life, when a sharp decline in both the cell-mediated and humoral response systems becomes evident. This loss in immunologic sensitivity is associated with an increasingly less effective and more misdirected

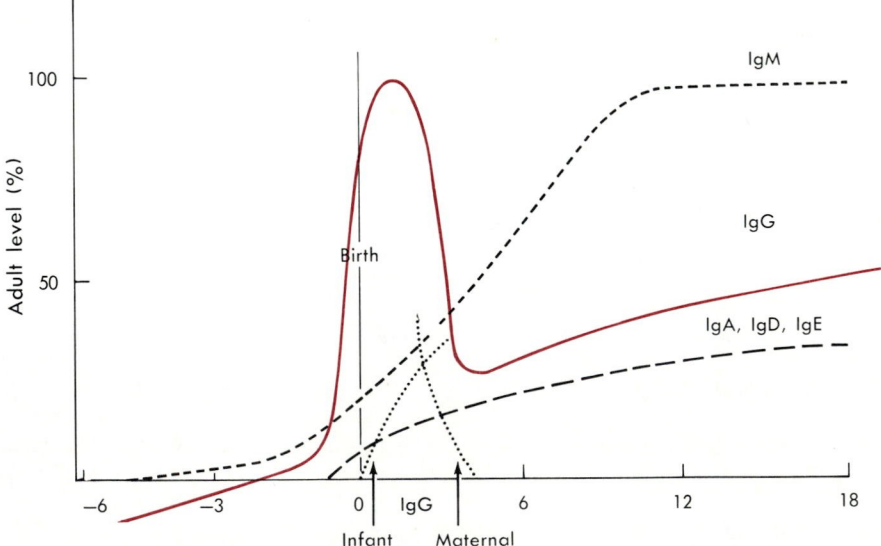

Fig. 37-13 Immunoglobulin levels in fetus and neonate.

immune response. There is an increasing frequency of autoimmune disease, susceptibility to pathogenic and opportunistic microorganisms, and incidence of cancer.

■ DEVELOPMENT OF IMMUNE TOLERANCE

Immune tolerance is defined as the state of immunologic nonresponsiveness. By some mechanisms the body becomes tolerant to self while maintaining responsiveness to foreign materials. Evidence establishes that self-tolerance is acquired during embryonic development; however, the exact mechanisms by which it develops remain an issue. During fetal development the immune system is presented with antigens from the developing tissues; these become identified as self-antigens, so that when exposed to these antigens postnatally the individual is tolerant of them.

One proposed mechanism by which this state could be induced is known as the *clonal selection theory*. This theory states that when potentially responsive clones of B or T cells come into contact with an antigen prenatally, the responsive cell line is killed, thus eliminating the responsiveness of that antigen from the body. This produces a state of *natural tolerance*. This theory is supported by experimental data that show that by exposing experimental animals to foreign antigens in utero a tolerance to that antigen is developed; however, some antigens introduced in this manner are found to be more *tolerogenic* (capable of inducing tolerance) than others. Further, the clonal selection theory does not explain how it is possible to break tolerance in adults, as indicated in certain experimental studies or as in the case of certain of the autoimmune diseases (see Chapter 38). In many cases tolerance is not the result of the total elimination of specifically reactive cells but of the blocking of expression or temporary inactivation of the responsive cells. The action of suppressor T cells or the failure of mobilization by helper T cells plays a significant role in maintaining the state of self-tolerance.

■ APPLICATIONS AND IMPLICATIONS OF IMMUNE RESPONSE

■ Immunization

Long before the mechanisms of immune response were worked out, it was recognized that recovery from certain diseases conferred protection against subsequent exposure. Dating from the days of Jenner's vaccination with cowpox exudate to protect against smallpox (1798), through the success of Pasteur with anthrax and rabies (1880s), to the present, the specific protective mechanisms of the immune system have been used to protect against serious infectious diseases.

■ PASSIVE IMMUNIZATION

Temporary protection, usually measured in days or at most weeks, is afforded by the acquisition of preformed antibody from another host. As the acquired antibodies are used up through binding with antigen or by being catabolized, the protection is lost.

Transplacental passive immunization occurs through the transfer of IgG antibodies from the maternal circulation across the placenta to the fetal blood. Some immunoglobulins are acquired through the colostrum of the mother's milk.

Artificial passive immunization may be necessary if the individual to be immunized has suffered exposure to a serious infectious agent to which he has no immunity or if the individual's own immune system is impaired or deficient. The sources of these preformed antibodies are pooled human adult gamma globulin or heterologous (from another species) globulin fractions. Pooled human gamma globulin has been used to modify the effects of measles, particularly in premature infants, in children with primary immunodeficiencies, and in patients undergoing immunosuppressive therapies. Persons who have contact with persons with hepatitis and smallpox may also be protected by this method. It should be noted, however, that isolated gamma globulin preparations tend to form small protein aggregates, and these, if injected intravenously, could lead to severe anaphylactic reactions. For this reason the material is always administered *intramuscularly*.

The most commonly used heterologous antibody fractions are antitetanus and antidiphtheria antisera derived from horse globulins. Because these are foreign proteins, they can lead to the development of serum sickness (Chapter 38). Serum sickness is more likely to occur in individuals already primed by previous contact with horse globulin; thus multiple use of heterologous sera is to be avoided.

■ ACTIVE IMMUNIZATION

The objective of active immunization is to provide effective long-term immunity by establishing within the individual's body the capacity to produce effective levels of immune response and to establish a population of sensitive cells that can respond to a subsequent antigenic contact.

Immunizing agents ideally should be noninjurious to the individual being immunized. To accomplish this, the pathogenic effects must be modified while at the same time maintaining the antigenicity of the agent. Bacteria exotoxins such as those produced by the diphtheria and tetanus bacteria can be successfully detoxified by formaldehyde treatment without destroying the major antigenic determinants on the protein molecule. Such detoxified antigenic materials are called *toxoids*. The use of *killed vaccines* of viruses and bacteria can also provide a safe antigen for immunization. Killed vaccines include those for pertussis (whooping cough), typhoid, and cholera and the Salk poliomyelitis vaccine. The protection conferred by these vaccines is generally inferior to that produced by live vaccines. A number of the most successful vaccines consist of living organisms that have been modified so that they are nonvirulent. The *attenuated live vaccines* provide excellent protection, but there is some risk in their use because of the slight risk of reversion to the virulent form of the organism or the possibility that the individual being immunized has some degree of immunodeficiency in which case the attenuated organism might produce pathologic effects. Live vaccines that are of importance include those for measles, mumps, and tuberculosis (BCG) and the Sabin poliomyelitis vaccine.

The provision of protective levels of residual immunity depends on the inducement of the right type of response (that is, cell mediated or humoral), in sufficient amounts, at the right place (that is, where the immune response can contact the antigen), and against the right antigenic determinants (that is, the antibodies formed produce an inactivating effect). Simply the induction of an immune response is not sufficient to provide protection. For example, the early killed virus measles vaccines elicited a splendid production of circulating antibodies against the measles virus, but protection against measles is most effectively mediated by cellular immune responses. The humoral protection did not prevent infection.

Another problem of immunization for which provision must be made is the *interference* that one antigen may have with another if the two are given simultaneously. The live virus vaccines occasionally interfere with each other; they each interfere with the development of immunity by the other. This is probably the result of interferon production. Some live virus vaccines contain more than one strain of the virus, and these can cross-inhibit. In the case of the Sabin oral polio vaccine, three separate doses are required because there are three strains within the same vaccine. With the initial dose, immunity to only one strain may develop if the strain interferes with the other two.

■ COMPLICATIONS OF IMMUNIZATION

Although immunization is the most successful approach to the control of many infectious diseases, there are small but still real risks involved. The development of postvaccination encephalitis or other neural autoimmune complications is a serious risk with vaccines such as those for smallpox or rabies. Children with immunodeficiencies may be overwhelmed by vaccination with live vaccine. With viral vaccines, which are produced in monkey kidney of human cell culture, there is a slight risk of the introduction of oncogenic (cancer causing) viruses. A fetus may be significantly at risk if the mother receives a live virus vaccine during pregnancy. Vaccines such as live influenza should never be administered to a pregnant woman. It is still unclear whether the rubella virus harms the fetus, so it too should be avoided. Besides these rather serious risks, general discomfort is to be expected from some forms of immunization. The typhoid vaccine, for instance, is composed of large numbers of killed salmonella bacteria; because the endotoxic cell wall materials of these cells is a pyrogenic (fever producing) substance, fever and malaise are not uncommon sequelae. The influenza vaccines often produce febrile reactions in children.

■ Cancer immunology

One of the functions of the cell-mediated immune response system is the recognition and destruction of cancer cells within the body. It is postulated that, by the same mechanisms that are operative in allograft rejection, the immune system continually protects against the establishment of certain types of tumor growths. The recognition of these cells as nonself is based on the appearance of "new" surface antigens that allow identification. A growing body of evidence supports the view that this is a vital function of the immune system. Patients in whom the cellular immune system is impaired (immunosuppressed) or defective (immunodeficient) for significant periods are at especially high risk of certain neoplastic diseases. To these data is coupled the observation that cancers are most prone to appear early in life before the immune system is fully functional or in later life as the system becomes less effective.

Cancers may become established in the body by escaping the surveillance mechanisms or by growing so rapidly that they outdistance the immune system's ability to respond. Experimentally, if a few thousand tumor cells are transferred from a cancerous animal to a noncancerous animal, the latter is capable of responding and destroying the tumor; however, if the tumor cell load is increased to several billion cells, the tumor may become established. The humoral immune system may actually serve to protect the developing cancer by producing noncytotoxic antibodies (*enhancing antibodies*) that coat the tumor cell surfaces and mask the surface from recognition by sensitized lymphocytes. As a tumor grows, it is capable of both specific and nonspecific suppression of the immune system. This further reduces the effectiveness of a response.

Some of the new surface antigens, (known as *tumor-specific transplantation antigens* [TSTA]) appearing on the cancerous cell are shed into the circulation and can be immunologically detected there. Some of these antigens, such as carcinoembryonic antigen (CEA) and alpha fetoprotein (α-FP), are present during fetal development but are not expressed in the adult. Their reappearance lends support to the theory that cancer represents a dedifferentiation to a more primitive cell caused by the introduction of oncogenes (Chapter 12). These antigens, termed *oncofetal antigens* (OFA), are of some significance in early detection, diagnostic confirmation, and determination of malignant disease progress.

Some very early progress has been made in stimulating, both specifically and nonspecifically, the body's immunologic response to cancers in the hope of preventing further growth of the tumors. With further knowledge of both the cancer process and the immune response mechanisms, the possibility of using immunotherapy, immunoprophylaxis, and immunodiagnosis as specific tools against malignancies seems quite realistic.

■ Immunologic disorders

As expected in such an interrelated, complex system as is operative in the mechanisms providing biologic defense, there are innumerable points at which the system may malfunction. The immunologic disorders that have been characterized may result from the following:

1. Nonresponsiveness
2. Blocked responsiveness
3. Limited responsiveness
4. Misdirected responsiveness
5. Overresponsiveness

The underlying causes of the disorders may be attributed to developmental defect, infection, malignancy, trauma, metabolic state, or pharmacologic intervention. The severity of the disorders ranges from creation of a minor nuisance (for example, mild hayfever) to a life-threatening situation (for example, anaphylactic shock). The disorders may be classified into the following general categories:

1. Immunodeficiencies: deficiencies in the proper expression of the immune response system, parts of the system, or individual cell types within the system
2. Gammopathies: abnormal production of immunoglobulins
3. Hypersensitivities: exaggerated or inappropriate response to specific antigens
4. Autoimmunities: immunologic attack on self-antigens

Each of these immunologic disorders is discussed in Chapter 38.

HIV infection and acquired immunodeficiency syndrome

In Chapter 38 *acquired immunodeficiency syndrome* (AIDS) will be discussed in detail, but an understanding of the syndrome is based on the recognition of the underlying pathologic process.

AIDS is caused by the *human immunodeficiency virus* (HIV), which is classified as a *retrovirus*. A retrovirus is a virus whose genetic information is coded in the form of RNA rather than DNA. When the virus enters a host cell, it converts its RNA code into a DNA message that the host cell can read. This DNA viral message is transported to the host cell nucleus where it becomes associated with the host cell's normal genetic information. The viral message that has been incorporated into the host cell DNA is then replicated along with the host cell DNA each time the host cell divides. In addition, the viral message redirects the host cell metabolism to ignore normal function and give its attention to reproducing viruses that are released from the infected cell. Obviously such a subverted cell cannot carry out its normal functions nor meet its own needs; therefore, dysfunction and death of the cell follow.

Viruses get into cells by recognizing and binding the receptors on the cell membrane. You will remember that earlier in this chapter it was pointed out that the T cells of the immune response system can be classified into T helper (T_H or T_4) or T suppressor (T_S or T_8) cells based on the presence of certain cell membrane markers: T_4 marker identifies T helper cells; T_8 marker identifies T suppressor cells. It so happens that the receptor for HIV is the T_4 surface markers; this explains why HIV causes the loss in T helper cells in the body. With the progressive infection and destruction of T helper cells the ability of the body to mount a normal immune response to infectious agents or cancer cells becomes less efficient.

Tissue transplants

The transfer of healthy tissues and organs from one individual to replace damaged or diseased tissues in another has been surgically possible for many years. Early attempts failed because of the rejection of the foreign cells and tissues by the body. With the growing knowledge of the immune response, the mechanisms of this rejection process become more apparent, and it is now possible to make judgments and predictions concerning the likelihood of success of transplantation. It has now become possible to control the course of the graft transfer process to favor the acceptance of the transplanted tissue.

The antigenic determinants of the tissues that lead to graft rejection are primarily found on the surface of the cells within the transplanted tissues. These antigens are known as *histocompatibility antigens* and are controlled by independently segregating genes within the chromosomal structure of the animal. They are also called *human leukocyte (HLA) antigens*. Some of the histocompatibility antigens are more antigenic than are others; thus some antigens are referred to as major and others as minor. The major transplantation antigens are those of the ABO and Rh blood groups and the HLA antigens (Chapter 38).

Graft rejection can be minimized by the use of chemical (drug) or physical (radiation) agents that nonspecifically or specifically interfere with the development of an immune response reaction against the foreign tissue. Clinically, four types of chemical immunosuppressive agents are effective in providing the transitional protection needed to promote the graft establishment (Table 37-9).

Glucocorticoids, especially prednisone, are significantly antiinflammatory and impair lymphocyte (B and T cell) activation and function. Prednisone exerts a wide spectrum of activity against all immune response and inflammatory response mechanisms. Although it suppresses the cell-mediated system to a greater degree than the humoral system, the continued high dosage needed to maintain cell-mediated suppression creates significant risks in reducing the responsiveness of the humoral system. Often lower dosages of prednisone and azathioprine are used together because they seem to act synergistically.

Antimetabolites and alkylating agents, such as azathioprine and cyclophosphamide, act nonspecifically against rapidly dividing cells within the body, and for this reason they are also used for cancer chemotherapy. They interfere with DNA synthesis and with the B and T cell systems.

A more specific immunosuppression of the T cell system is achieved with the use of *antilymphocytic serum* (ALS). ALS blocks the action of the sensitized cells in circulation while leaving the lymph node B cell system only slightly suppressed. This leaves the host with protection against the humorally protected infectious agents while providing protection against the most active rejection system.

The newest of the immunosuppressive therapeutic

Table 37-9 Effect of selected drugs on the immune system

Drug	Immune system impairment	Indications for immunosuppressive therapy
Corticosteroids	Impairment of T cell function Catabolism of immunoglobulins (decreased IgG) Lymphocytopenia Type 1 hypersensitivity: vasoconstriction, eosinopenia Type 3 hypersensitivity: decreased vascular permeability Type 4 hypersensitivity: decreased macrophage function	Diseases where immune disorder is unknown Tissue and organ transplantation Autoimmune diseases
Antimetabolites (azathioprine)	Interference with RNA, DNA, and protein synthesis Depression of bone marrow and antibody reproduction Decreased primary immune response	Autoimmune diseases Tissue transplantation Dermatologic disease (pemphigus, psoriasis) Neoplasia
Alkylating agents (cyclophosphamide)	Interference with DNA, RNA, and protein synthesis Lymphocytolytic effect Suppression of primary immune response	Autoimmune diseases Tissue transplantation Inflammatory disease of unknown cause
Antilymphocytic serum (ALS, ALG)	Inhibition of lymphocyte stimulation by specific antigens Inhibition of lymphocyte mobility Agglutination and lysis of lymphocytes in the presence of complement	Renal transplantation Bone marrow transplantation Autoimmune diseases
Antibiotics (actinomycin D, chloramphenicol, tetracycline, cyclosporine)	Interference with DNA-directed RNA synthesis Suppression of primary immune response Inhibition of protein synthesis	None, except for cyclosporine (tissue transplantation)

agents is *cyclosporine* (previously called cyclosporin A), an antibiotic derived from fungi that exerts its action on the T lymphocytes. Recent success with this drug has greatly improved the prognosis after transplantation.

■ SUMMARY

1. The concept of "self" refers to the collection of tissues, cells, and molecules that is unique to each human being. Every other individual, cell, or biologic product is therefore considered as "nonself." The body has mechanisms to recognize and protect against encroachment by nonself agents.

2. Biologic defense mechanisms may be structural (skin and mucous membranes), chemical (pH, blood proteins), cellular (WBC, phagocytes), special proteins (interferon, immunoglobulins), or tissue (lymph nodes, thymus gland). These mechanisms may be external or internal and specific or nonspecific.

3. External nonspecific biologic defense mechanisms include the skin and mucous membranes (first line of defense), nasal hairs, tears, peristalsis, antimicrobial chemicals (acidity, lysozyme), and the microbial antagonism of normal skin flora.

4. Internal nonspecific defense mechanisms are carried out by the phagocytes in the reticuloendothelial system and the blood, other blood components, interferon, and the inflammatory response.

5. Interferons enhance synthesis in uninfected cells of a protein that inhibits entry of any viral particles into the interferon-protected cell for about 24 hours.

6. The inflammatory response consists of an immediate vascular dilation to facilitate margination of leukocytes on the vessel walls before exudation. This is followed by exudation first of fluid to the injured area, then of phagocytes to remove and digest foreign substances.

7. The five cardinal symptoms of inflammation and their causes are redness and heat (vascular dilation), edema (fluid exudate), pain (pressure on the fluid exudate and chemical irritation of the nerve endings), and loss of function (swelling and pain).

8. Infection is contained by fibroblasts walling off the affected area; interference with this process may lead to spread of the infection.

9. The immune response is a biologic defense mechanism consisting of specific responses to specific antigens.

10. Antigens are substances that elicit the formation of antibodies when introduced into the body; there are

---

Putting knowledge to practice

- Examine an infected wound; describe your findings in terms of the underlying biologic response mechanisms.
- Prepare a short presentation for a group of new mothers on the need for and basis of immunizations.
- What would you say to a person with a kidney transplant who asks why immunosuppressive drugs must be taken for life?
- In what way do interferons differ from immunoglobulins?

---

five different types of immunoglobulins (antibodies), each with different structures and functions.

11. The two types of cells involved in the immune response are T cells that attack foreign material directly in the body (cell-mediated immunity) and B cells that produce immunoglobulins (humoral immunity). T helper cells enhance immunoglobulin synthesis and T cell cytotoxic activity, whereas T suppressor cells inhibit these actions.

12. Lymphokines are soluble substances released by activated T cells; their functions include attracting and activating macrophages for phagocytosis, nonspecific lysis of cells, inhibiting replication of viruses (interferons), and activating nonsensitized lymphocytes (interleukins).

13. Three basic mechanisms of response may be elicited when an antigen is first introduced (primary immune response): humoral response (primarily B cells), cell-mediated response (primarily T cells), or combined B cell–T cell immune response.

14. An important characteristic of the specific response system is the ability of the system to remember prior contact with an antigen (during the primary immune response) and to provide a more complete protective reaction on subsequent contact (secondary immune response). The secondary response is more rapid, of greater intensity, and longer lasting than the primary response.

15. Immunity, or nonsusceptibility to specific antigens, may be natural or acquired artificially through immunization. Passive immunization is the receipt of antibodies either transplacentally (infant) or by injection (gamma globulin and antitetanus or antidiphtheria antisera). With active immunization, persons develop their own antibodies from injection of killed vaccines or toxoids. Passive immunization is temporary protection, whereas active immunization provides long-term immunity.

16. Persons who are immunosuppressed or immunodeficient have a higher risk for certain neoplastic diseases because the body does not recognize the cancer cells as nonself. Tumors may also suppress specific and nonspecific immune responses, thus reducing effectiveness of the responses.

17. The receptor for the AIDS retrovirus (HIV) is the surface marker of the T helper cells, leading to dysfunction and death of these cells; this makes the individual with AIDS more susceptible to infections.

18. The body recognizes tissue transplants as foreign (nonself) and evokes the immune response to destroy the new tissue; graft rejection can be minimized by suppression of the immune response with drugs or radiation.

REFERENCES AND SELECTED READINGS

1. Baradana, EJ: A conceptual approach to immunodeficiency, Med Clin North Am 65:959-962, 1983.
2. Barrett, JT: Textbook of immunology, ed 5, St. Louis, 1987, The CV Mosby Co.
3. Bellanti, JA: Immunology III, Philadelphia, 1985, WB Saunders Co.
4. Beverly, PC: Antibodies and cancer therapy, Nature 297:358-359, 1982.
5. Bloom, BR: Natural killer cells to rescue immune surveillance? Nature 300:214-217, 1982.
6. Bornstein, DL: Leukocytic pyrogen: a major mediator of the acute phase reaction, Ann NY Acad Sci 389:323-326, 1982.
7. Boyd, RF: General microbiology, St. Louis, 1984, The CV Mosby Co.
8. *Durham, JD, and Cohen, FL: The person with AIDS: nursing perspective, New York, 1987, Springer Publishing Co.
9. *Fauci, AS: Activation and regulation of human immune responses and implications in normal and disease states (NIH Conference), Ann Intern Med 99:61-65, 1983.
10. Friedland, GH, and Klein, RS: Transmission of the human immunodeficiency virus, N Eng J Med 317:1125-1135, 1987.
11. Gewurz, HJ, and others: C-reactive protein and the acute phase response, Am Intern Med 27:345-348, 1982.
12. Goodwin, JS: Searles, RP, and Tung, SK: Immunological responses of a healthy elderly population, Clin Exp Immunol 48:403-407, 1982.
13. *Griffin, JP: Hematology and immunology: concepts for nursing, Norwalk, Conn, 1986, Appleton-Century-Crofts.

---

*References preceded by an asterisk are particularly well suited for student reading.

14. *Gurevich, I: The competent internal immune system, Nurs Clin North Am 20(1):151-161, 1985.

15. Hall, NR, and Goldstein, AL: Thinking well: the chemical links between emotions and health, NY Acad Sci 34:40-45, 1986.

16. *Hastings Center Report: AIDS, the emerging ethical dilemmas, Hastings-on-Hudson, NY, 1985, Hastings Center.

17. Herberman, RB: Natural killer cells, Hosp Pract 17:93-97, 1982.

18. Honjo, T: Immunoglobulin genes, Ann Rev Immunol 1:499-503, 1983.

19. *Hood, LE: Interferon: getting in the way of viruses and tumors, Am J Nurs 87:459-465, 1987.

19a. Horoszewkz, JS, and others: Interferon: a review of its development and potential clinical applications, Hosp Formul 22:776-779, 1987.

20. *Jett, MR, and Lancaster, LE: The inflammatory-immune response: the body's defense against invasion, Crit Care Nurs 5:64-66, 1983.

21. *Lind, M: The immunologic assessment: a nursing focus, Heart Lung 9:658-660, 1980.

22. LoBugho, AF (editor): Clinical immunotherapy, New York, 1980, Marcel Dekker, Inc.

23. Male, D: Immunology: an illustrated outline, St. Louis, 1986. The CV Mosby Co.

24. *Matje, D.: Stress and cancer: a review of the literature, Cancer Nurs 9:339-401, 1984.

25. McMichael, AJ, and Fabre, JW (editors): Monoclonal antibodies of clinical medicine, New York, 1982, Academic Press, Inc.

26. *Merigan, TC: Human interferon as a therapeutic agent: current status, Science 308:1530-1535, 1983.

27. Mims, CA, and White, DW: Viral pathogenesis and immunology, Oxford, 1984, Blackwell Scientific Publications, Ltd.

28. *National Institute's of Health: Understanding the immune system, No. 84-529, Washington, DC, 1983, US Dept of Health and Human Services.

29. Panam, S: The emergent importance of lymphokines, JAMA 249:166-167, 1983.

30. Playfair, JHL: Immunology at a glance, ed 2, Oxford, 1984, Blackwell Scientific Publications, Ltd.

31. *Porth, CM: Pathophysiology, ed 2, Philadelphia, 1986, JB Lippincott Co.

32. Riley, V.: Psychoneuroendocrine influences on immunocompetence and neoplasia, Science 212:1100-1103, 1981.

33. *Roitt, I, Brostoff, J, and Male, D: Immunology, St. Louis, 1985, The CV Mosby Co.

34. Schaller, JG, and Hansen, JA: HLA relationships to disease, Hosp Pract 16:41-45, 1981.

35. Slamon, DJ, and others: Expression of cellular oncogenes in human malignancies, Science 224:256-260, 1984.

36. Stites, DP, Stobo, JD, Fudenberg, HH, and Wells, JV (editors): Basic and clinical immunology, ed 6, Norwalk, Conn, 1987, Appleton & Lange.

37. Unane, ER: Antigen-presenting function of the macrophage, Ann Rev Immunol 2:395-397, 1984.

38. *Weksler, ME: The senescence of the immune response, Hosp Pract 16:55-58, 1981.

38

The Patient with Immunologic Problems

BARBARA C. LONG and E. RONALD WRIGHT

CHAPTER OBJECTIVES

After studying this chapter, the student should be able to:

- Identify the immune response in immunodeficiencies, gammopathies, hypersensitivities, and autoimmunities and give examples.
- Describe methods of immunosuppression and the care of the immunodeficient person.
- Describe the nature of AIDS and related care.
- Compare and contrast the four types of hypersensitivities.
- Describe the pathophysiologic bases of type I hypersensitivities and related interventions.
- Describe blood transfusion and tissue transplant reactions.

Immunologic alterations occur in a wide variety of diseases. In some disorders the immunologic basis is clear-cut, such as in allergic disorders and immunodeficiency diseases. In some instances, as in systemic lupus erythematosus (SLE), immunologic response is known to have a role, but the relative significance of the immunologic factors is not clear. In still other disorders, such as neoplasias, the role of the immunologic response as the causative agent is even less well documented.

The structure and function of the immune response is discussed in the preceding chapter (37). These concepts are basic to understanding the pathophysiology of immunologic problems.

Because immunologic factors are operative in such a wide variety of disorders, much of the information about the disorders is found elsewhere in the text. This chapter describes the various categories of immune disorders and discusses in more detail those disorders not described elsewhere.

■ PHYSIOLOGIC CHANGES WITH AGING

The extent of immunologic changes with aging varies among individuals depending on multiple factors, such as genetics, nutritional status, and presence of disorders that deplete the immune system. In general, however, the immune response is decreased with aging, primarily in the following:

1. Increased frequency and severity of infections, with slower recovery and less probability of developing immunity after an infection[4]
2. Increased potential for cancer because of decreased immune surveillance (see Chapter 37)

The decreased immune response results primarily from atrophy of the thymus gland and development of fewer killer T cells. The balance of regulating T cells and antibody percentages changes, although the total number of lymphocytes is usually unchanged. Lymphocytes are also redistributed, with fewer seen in the germinal centers of the lymph nodes and more in the bone marrow. Autoantibodies increase in number, but the effect is unclear be-

cause autoimmune diseases do not increase.[35] Elderly persons may demonstrate a decreased response to skin tests because of the decreased response to foreign antigens.

Major health problems of the immune system

Immunologic disorders occur when the immune response malfunctions. The disorders may be a result of immune deficiencies, abnormal production of immunoglobulins, excessive response to specific antigens, or immune response to self-antigens (Table 38-1). Each of these major categories will be discussed in this chapter. The majority of immunologic problems (other than the great variety of autoimmune diseases discussed throughout the text) are hypersensitivity disorders, so these disorders will be discussed in more detail.

■ IMMUNODEFICIENCIES

The following discussion of immunodeficiencies is divided into general immunodeficiencies and AIDS because of the pandemic nature of AIDS.

■ General immunodeficiencies

■ PATHOPHYSIOLOGY

Protection of the host depends on an intact immune system. Interference with development of cells and tissues of the immune response leads to immunodeficient disorders. Because the cells and tissues of the immune response system develop sequentially, if a defect in that development appears, the severity of the resulting deficiency reflects the stage of development at which the abnormality arose (Fig. 38-1). Deficiencies may exist in immunoglobulin synthesis (B cell deficiency), cellular immune functions (T cell deficiency), or phagocyte defects.

Immunodeficiencies may be primary or secondary. Pri-

Table 38-1 Classification of immunologic disorders

Category	Immune response	Examples
Immunodeficiencies	Deficiencies in the proper expression of immune response system, part of the system, or specific cells	Primary deficiencies, deficiencies associated with other diseases, acquired immunodeficiency syndrome (AIDS)
Gammopathies	Abnormal production of immunoglobulins	Multiple myeloma, hypergammaglobinemia
Hypersensitivities	Exaggerated or inappropriate response to specific antigen	Anaphylaxis, allergies, transfusion reactions, graft rejections
Autoimmunities	Immunologic attack on self-antigens	Rheumatoid arthritis, SLE, glomerulonephritis

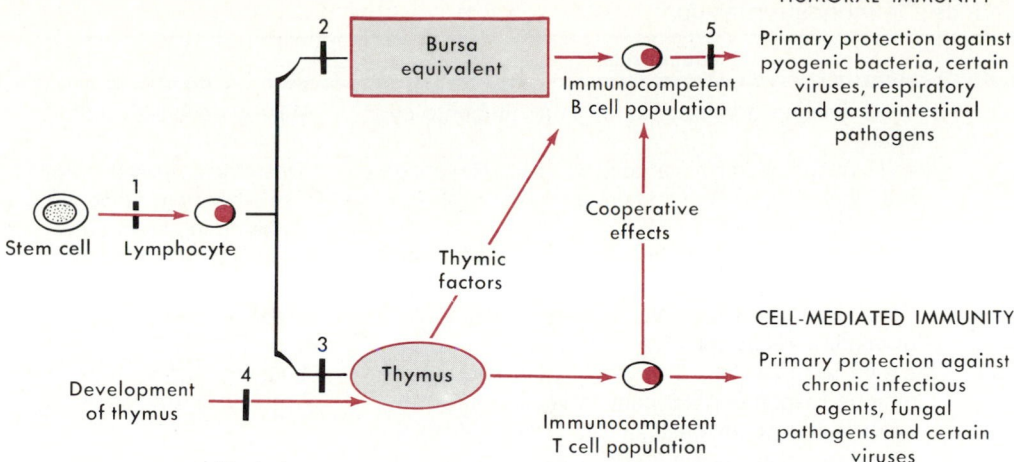

Fig. 38-1 Causes of immunodeficiencies. Abnormalities at *1* result in combined humoral and cell-mediated immunodeficiency. Blockage at *2* produces agammaglobulinemia. Blockage at *3* or *4* results in drastic reduction of T cell–mediated function and, because of cooperative effects on B cell system, some reduction in humoral response. Abnormalities in synthesis of specific immunoglobulin classes are reflected by blockage at *5*. Some blockages result in complete deficiency, whereas others show up as reduction in response.

mary immunodeficiencies, those resulting from improper fetal development, are genetic disorders in children. Some primary immunoglobulin deficiencies may not become evident until the person is an adult, and these are termed *common variable immunodeficiencies* (CVI). Persons with CVI develop recurrent virulent infections and display a high incidence of malignancies, hematologic disorders, and autoimmune diseases.

Secondary immunodeficiencies are a nonspecific depression of the immune response as a result of some interference with the immune system. These deficiencies are present to one degree or another in most of the major disease conditions experienced by persons in addition to the normal response to aging. Thus when caring for a person beyond the age of 60 years or with any acute disease condition, the concepts of immunodeficiency must be considered. Sit-

uations in which immunodeficiency plays a major role are listed in the box below, left.

Major stress of any type may affect immune response as a result of increased corticosteroid production and alterations in protein metabolism. A form of immunodeficiency, immunosuppression, may result from or be deliberately created by the use of radiation, drugs, or antigens and antibodies (Table 38-2).

■ ASSESSMENT

□ Subjective data

Subjective data to obtain from the person with immunodeficiency include the following:
1. Knowledge of the immunodeficiency
2. Knowledge of prevention of infection
3. Occurrence of recurrent infections (type)
4. Concerns related to the immunodeficiency

Recurrent viral or fungal infections are suggestive of T cell–mediated deficiencies, whereas recurrent bacterial infections may have an underlying B cell (immunoglobulin) deficiency.

□ Objective data

Objective data include monitoring for early signs of infection (fever, pain, nasal discharge, cough, and enlarged nodes). The skin is inspected daily for lesions.

□ Diagnostic tests
□ *T cell (cellular) deficiency tests*

T cell function can be screened by delayed hypersensitivity skin testing to common antigens. Specific antigens,

---

**Disorders influenced
by immunodeficiencies**

Protein-calorie malnutrition
Alcoholism
Infections (especially viral)
Cancer
Autoimmune diseases
Lymphomas (including Hodgkin's disease)
Allergies
Trauma
Transplantation

Table 38-2 Induced immunosuppression

Method	Comments	Use
Antigen administration	Specific antigen administered in small amounts over time	Allergy desensitization
Antibody administration	Specific antibody administered to combine with antigen and block contact with immunocompetent cell	Obstetrics: prevent sensitive Rh-negative mother from responding to Rh-positive fetus during pregnancy
Antilymphocytic serum (ALS)	Prepared from serum of horse immunized with human lymphocytic tissue; when administered to humans produces lymphocytopenia, thus fewer cells available for immune response	Restricted use as a result of side effects (serum sickness, anaphylactic shock, nephritis)
Irradiation	Destroys lymphocytes, thus fewer cells available for immune response; total body irradiation affects hematopoietic system, gastrointestinal (GI) system, and central nervous system (CNS)	Local irradiation: renal allografts Total body irradiation: organ transplantation
Drugs	Corticosteroids impair T cell function and cause catabolism of immunoglobulins and lymphocytopenia Cytotoxic drugs destroy rapidly dividing immunologically stimulated cells	Diseases where immune disorder is unknown (for example, autoimmunities); tissue and organ transplantation
	Cyclosporine (Sandimmune) acts against T helper cells and facilitates development of T suppressor cells	Organ transplantation
	Muromonab-CD3 (OKT3), a monoclonal antibody, reacts with receptors on T cell surface preventing lysis of cells	Organ transplantation

including purified protein derivative (PPD), *Candida* organisms, mumps antigen, streptokinase, and streptodornase, are injected intradermally. Reactions are read after 24 to 48 hours to determine hypersensitivity. The test is to determine the hypersensitivity, not the presence of disease. A person who does not react to any of these antigens is said to be *anergic*.

Sensitization with dinitrochlorobenzene (DNCB) is an additional test for suspected anergic patients. DNCB is a chemical to which natural sensitivity does not occur. Following application of DNCB to the skin, contact sensitivity can be elicited after 1 to 2 weeks if T cell function is present.

□ *B cell (humoral) deficiency tests*

ELECTROPHORESIS. The movement of colloid (protein) particles in an electrical field is called electrophoresis. In an applied electrical field, different proteins migrate at different rates because of their different sizes and shapes, and this property can be used to analyze plasma protein content. The plasma proteins consist of albumin and globulins, which can be further divided into alpha globulins, beta globulins, and gamma globulins (immunoglobulins). The serum proteins are subjected to electrophoresis in a medium that stabilizes the migration so that the proteins can be stained and examined.

QUANTITATIVE IMMUNOGLOBULIN TEST. Three of the immunoglobulins—IgG, IgA, and IgM—can be measured quantitatively, whereas IgD and IgE are present in amounts too small to measure. Venous blood is collected; no special preparation is required.

⇨ DATA ANALYSIS: NURSING DIAGNOSES

Nursing diagnoses are determined from assessment of patient data. Possible nursing diagnoses for the person with an immunodeficiency may include, but are not limited to, the following:

Diagnostic title	Possible etiologies
Knowledge deficit	Lack of exposure/recall, information misinterpretation
Potential for infection	Decreased immune response, lack of information

PLANNING: EXPECTED PATIENT OUTCOMES

Expected patient outcomes for the person with an immunodeficiency may include, but are not limited to, the following:
1. Signs of infection do not occur.
2. The person can describe measures to avoid infection.
3. The person can describe signs dictating immediate medical attention.
4. The person can explain the need for continued medical follow-up.

IMPLEMENTATION

□ Replacement therapy

Specific replacement therapy may be given for primary immunodeficiencies. When B cell deficiency is present, gamma globulin or fresh frozen plasma free of HB$_s$Ag (hepatitis B surface antigen) may be given at monthly intervals. Gamma globulin is a purified concentrated solution of antibodies, mostly IgG, found in normal plasma.

When giving gamma globulin intramuscularly, a large-bore (18 to 20-gauge) needle is recommended, and the solution is injected slowly. Large amounts need to be divided and given at separate sites. Plasma therapy is better tolerated by the individual than large doses of gamma globulin, and all five immunoglobulins are included in the plasma. Homologous serum hepatitis and transfusion reactions, however, are potential risks with plasma therapy.

Replacement therapy for T cell–mediated immune deficiencies is more complex. Transfer factor (extracted from lymphocytes of humans who have demonstrated delayed hypersensitivity reactions), thymosin (a thymic hormone), and bone marrow transplants have been used.

☐ **Prevention of infection**

The most important factor in the care of the immunodeficient or immunosuppressed person is protection from infection. Care differs depending on whether the degree of immunosuppression is minimal, moderate, or severe:
1. Care for minimal immunosuppression
   a. Use good medical asepsis.
   b. Avoid persons with infections.
   c. Give meticulous cleaning and protect even minor skin breaks.
   d. Avoid injections as much as possible.
   e. Maintain nutrition at optimal level.
   f. Maintain adequate fluid hydration (intake of more than 1500 ml/day).
2. Care for moderate immunosuppression
   a. If severe leukopenia is present, place person in a single room to decrease infection potential.
   b. If person is acutely ill, give mouth care, perineal care, and pulmonary hygiene to prevent infection.
   c. Use same protective measures as for minimal immunosuppression.

---

3. Care for severe immunosuppression
   a. Use protective isolation by laminar air flow units (Chapter 12).
   b. Use same protective measures as for moderate immunosuppression.

☐ **Teaching**

People who are immunosuppressed, as well as their families, need to know the nature of immunosuppression and how to avoid infection (see the box below, left).

⊞ EVALUATION

Questions to ask may include the following:
1. Has infection been prevented during hospitalization?
2. Does the person know
   a. The nature of immunodeficiency?
   b. How to prevent and identify infection?
   c. The need for continued medical follow-up?

■ Acquired immunodeficiency syndrome (AIDS)

AIDS is a secondary immunodeficiency disorder, first seen in the United States in 1978. The disease originated in Central Africa, then spread to other parts of Africa, the United Kingdom, and Haiti from where it then spread to the United States. It is currently found in 100 countries and in all 50 states. The incidence of AIDS is increasing in all major U.S. cities. It is expected that by 1991 over a quarter of a million persons in the United States will be diagnosed with AIDS and that more people will be dying of AIDS than from auto accidents.

■ ETIOLOGY

The cause of AIDS is a retrovirus (HIV) that has been isolated in most body fluids of infected persons including blood, semen, vaginal secretions, saliva, tears, breast milk, CSF, amniotic fluid, and urine. Epidemiologic evidence, however, has implicated only blood, semen, vaginal secretions, and breast milk in HIV transmission.[16]

The mode of transmission is similar to that of hepatitis B, through sharing of blood or body fluids primarily by sexual contact, needle injection, or mother to fetus (see the box on p. 1358). Persons at highest risk are homosexual or bisexual males with multiple sex partners and intravenous drug users. The incidence of AIDS is increasing with heterosexual contacts, which are the leading route of HIV infection in Third World countries. The male-female ratio is 1:1 in Africa and 13:1 in the United States.[26]

Transmission of AIDS through multiple blood transfusions remains steady at 2%.[16,26] Donated blood is now screened for HIV antibodies and not used if found positive. False negative results do occasionally occur, however. The HIV virus can be transmitted by whole blood, blood cellular components, plasma, and clotting factors but not by other products prepared from blood (such as immunoglobulins or albumin). Clotting factor concentrates are now treated

---

┌─────────────────────────────────────┐
**Teaching for the patient
with immunodeficiency**

1. Explain immunodeficiency, that is, the inability of the body to fight infection.
2. Take measures to prevent infection
   a. Avoid persons with infections (especially colds).
   b. Avoid bumping or breaking the skin.
   c. Inspect skin daily for lesions.
   d. Eat a balanced diet (Chapter 6).
   e. Drink at least 6 glasses of fluid per day.
   f. Avoid becoming fatigued.
   g. Get a regular amount of sleep each night.
3. Report signs of infection to physician immediately.
4. See physician on a regular basis as instructed.
└─────────────────────────────────────┘

Modes of HIV (AIDS retrovirus) transmission

Known routes (high risk)

Sexual
    Homosexual or bisexual men (major route)
    Heterosexual (men to women or vice versa)
Blood
    Transfusion of blood and blood components
    Needle sharing
    Needle sticking (low risk)[26]
Perinatal
    Intraplacental
    Breast-feeding

Undemonstrated routes (unlikely infection)

Personal contacts
Toilet seats
Insects

---

by heat to inactivate HIV, thus providing an additional safety factor for hemophiliacs. HIV cannot be transmitted to blood *donors*.

■ SOCIETAL RESPONSES TO AIDS

Society's fear of AIDS is disproportionate to the actual threat. It is primarily a disease of young adults who are sexually promiscuous or who are drug users sharing needles. Some people's fears are based on *inadequate information or information interpreted incorrectly* to reflect the person's innate fear of AIDS. Underlying this morbid fear may be the present lack of a cure for AIDS. Some high-risk persons such as homosexuals have met with discrimination such as loss of employment or insurance. Children with AIDS have been prevented from attending school, despite the fact that AIDS has not been shown to be trans-mitted by personal contact or toilet seats. A positive result has been a change in behavior noted among homosexual and bisexual men, more of whom are engaging in healthy rather than unsafe sexual practices.

■ PATHOPHYSIOLOGY AND CLINICAL MANIFESTATIONS

The immunologic basis of AIDS is the destruction of T_4 cell (helper T cells) by the human immunodeficiency virus (HIV). The virus attaches to markers on a T_4 cell and enters the cell. The DNA viral message that moves to the T_4 nucleus redirects the T_4 metabolism to ignore normal function (leading to T_4 cell death) and to replicate HIVs. The new HIV components then attach to new T_4 cells and repeat the action (Fig. 38-2). (For further information on T helper cells and HIV, see Chapter 37.) Loss of T helper cells thus places the person at high risk for infection.

Development of AIDS occurs through phases (Fig. 38-3). Persons may become infected with HIV and develop HIV antibodies *but not develop AIDS*. The percentage who do develop AIDS is not known at this time. These persons can *transmit the virus* by sexual or blood-borne transmission in the absence of symptoms.

The CDC classification of HIV infection includes four groups (see the box on p. 1359). The initial acute HIV infection (Group I) is a mononucleosis-like syndrome associated with a positive serum test for HIV antibodies. Group II includes the persons who test positively for HIV antibodies but have no symptoms.

One sign that develops early is *persistent generalized lymphadenopathy* (PGL) that lasts for more than 3 months and involves at least two extrainguinal nodes in the absence of any other illness or drug known to cause lymphadenopathy (Group III). About 20% of persons with PGL develop AIDS.

HIV disease (Group IV) includes several subcategories. Subgroup A (*constitutional disease*) includes one or more symptoms in the absence of concurrent illness or infection. In addition to PGL, the symptoms may include fever, night sweats, fatigue and diarrhea lasting more than 1 month, and severe weight loss greater than 10% of total body weight. These symptoms are noted in the nonacute period

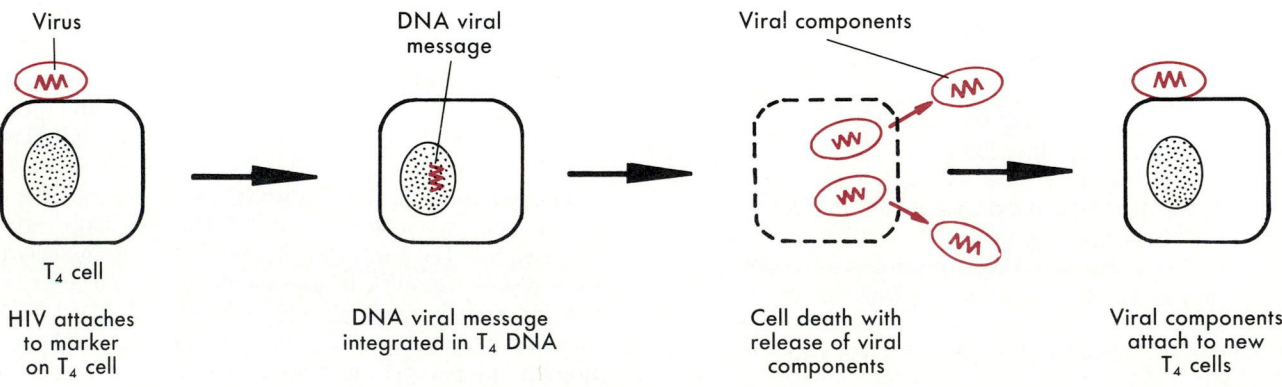

Fig. 38-2   Mechanism of HIV action.

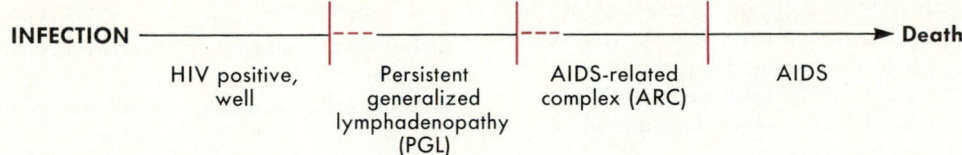

Fig. 38-3   Development of AIDS. However, only some persons proceed from infection to AIDS and death.

of AIDS between periods of acute illnesses. If at least two of these symptoms occur in the absence of any of the AIDS-related diseases, together with at least two laboratory abnormalities (such as decreased T_4 cell count, increased serum globulins, or decreased reaction to skin tests), the condition is termed *AIDS related complex* (ARC).

Persons with *AIDS* are those that are reliably diagnosed as having diseases indicative of underlying cellular immune deficiency. These diseases are illustrated in subgroups B, C, D, and E of Group IV that include neurologic disease (see Chapter 19), opportunistic infections, secondary cancers, and other HIV infections that occur with AIDS.

Opportunistic infections are those that have an opportunity to thrive as a result of the defect in the immune system. The most common opportunistic infection is pneumonia caused by the *Pneumocystis carinii* protozoa that only causes disease in immunodeficient hosts. The disease (PCP) can occur insidiously or can progress rapidly to death. Symp-

toms include dyspnea, dry nonproductive cough, fever, and hypoxemia (see Chapter 24). Bilateral lung consolidation requires intubation and assisted ventilation. Even with therapy (trimethoprim-sulfamethoxazole, pentamidine, or zidothymidine [Retrovir]), PCP is a frequent cause of death in the person with AIDS.

Kaposi's sarcoma (a type of skin cancer) is discussed in Chapter 39. It occurs in about 15% of persons with AIDS and has been noted more commonly in homosexual and bisexual men, although the incidence in this group is decreasing. If Kaposi's sarcoma is the only concurrent disorder in the person with AIDS, survival is longer than when opportunistic infections are present.

The clinical course of AIDS does not follow each classification group in order. Periods of acute opportunistic infections that may or may not respond to treatment may occur. Symptoms (that may develop slowly or suddenly) are exacerbated, followed by partial resolution to a chronic

---

CDC classification of HIV infection

*Group I: acute infection

Mononucleosis-type syndrome

*Group II: asymptomatic infection

No symptoms other than the seroconversion (HIV antibody positive)

*Group III: persistent generalized lymphadenopathy (PGL)

PGL > 3 months; no concurrent illness or infections

*Group IV: other HIV disease

Subgroup A: constitutional disease

Presence of generalized symptoms (fever and diarrhea >1 month, weight loss >10% of baseline); no concurrent illness or infection

Subgroup B: Neurologic disease

Dementia, myelopathy, encephalitis, or peripheral neuropathy; no concurrent illness or infection

Subgroup C: opportunistic infections

Parasite: *P. carinii* pneumonia, cryptosporidiosis (enterocolitis), toxoplasmosis (CNS disseminated disease), isosporiasis (coccidiosis)

Bacterial: mycobacterial infection (disseminated), Salmonella bacteremia, tuberculosis

Viral: cytomegalovirus (liver, retina, lungs, colon), herpes simplex, herpes zoster, progressive multifocal leukoencephalopathy, oral hairy leukoplakia

Fungal: candidiasis (oral, esophagus, intestines), cryptococcosis (meninges, lungs, disseminated), histoplasmosis (disseminated), toxoplasmosis

Subgroup D: secondary cancers

Kaposi's sarcoma, non-Hodgkins' lymphoma, primary lymphoma of the brain

Subgroup E: other disorders

Disorders not listed above, such as secondary infections, or other neoplasms

*All groups include a positive test for HIV antibodies.

From Centers for Disease Control: Classification system of human T-lymphocyte virus type III/lymphoadenopathy-associated virus infections, MMWR 35:331-337, 1986.

condition, often with residual damage. The person at this point may be independent in self-care or may need some partial home care. Once the Group IV conditions start, however, there is a wasting away until eventually the person is totally disabled. Death ensues because of overwhelming disseminated infection.

ASSESSMENT

☐ Subjective data

Because AIDS is an immunodeficiency disease, the same parameters of assessment (p. 1355) are pertinent for AIDS. Additional data are gathered because of the presence of opportunistic infections and probable short life span.
1. Knowledge of AIDS
2. Nutritional data, such as likes and dislikes, problems with eating, weight loss
3. Dyspnea: occurrence, actions found helpful
4. Discomfort: location, character, extent, and actions found helpful
5. Availability of supportive others
6. Feelings and concerns about condition

☐ Objective data

Types of observations to be made depend on the concurrent disorders and may include the following:
1. Skin: specific lesions, lack of integrity
2. Breath sounds
3. Condition of mouth and anus
4. Stools: frequency and character
5. Signs of anxiety

☐ Diagnostic tests

The *ELISA* test (Enzyme Linked Immuno-Sorbent Assay) is a simple test designed to screen blood or plasma for the presence of *antibodies* of HIV. The test indicates previous infection with HIV; it does *not* diagnose AIDS. Antibodies develop after 6 to 12 weeks of infection. The test is repeated if found positive.

The *Western blot* test is used if the ELISA test is positive. The test is more complicated than the ELISA but separates the viral particles by electrophoresis and is more reliable. This test is also repeated if found positive to rule out an occasional false positive result.

DATA ANALYSIS: NURSING DIAGNOSES

Nursing diagnoses are determined from assessment of patient data. Because of the varied diseases that accompany AIDS, the identified nursing diagnoses will vary greatly among persons with AIDS. Possible nursing diagnoses may include, but are not limited to, the following:

Diagnostic title	Possible etiologies
Anxiety	Threat to self-concept, threat of death, change in health status/socioeconomic status/role functioning, interpersonal transmission, unmet needs
Ineffective breathing pattern	Decreased energy, fatigue
Impaired gas exchange	Ventilation/perfusion imbalance
Anticipatory grieving	Probable death
Potential for infection	Decreased immune response
Knowledge deficit	Lack of information/recall, information misinterpretation
Altered nutrition: less than body requirements	Chewing/swallowing difficulties, anorexia, fatigue
Altered oral mucous membranes	Infection, malnutrition
Pain	Skin, oral and anal lesions
Impaired skin integrity	Mechanical forces (pressure, shearing)
Social isolation	Alteration in physical appearance, altered state of wellness, fear of contagion, unacceptable life-style

PLANNING: EXPECTED PATIENT OUTCOMES

Expected patient outcomes for the person with AIDS may include, but are not limited to, the following:
1. Nosocomial infection does not occur.
2. Breathing is easy.
3. Skin integrity remains intact.
4. Patient eats nutritionally balanced meals.
5. Patient states feeling more comfortable and rested.
6. Patient has had opportunities to explore feelings and concerns.
7. Patient has opportunities to interact with supportive others.
8. Patient can describe maintenance of optimal nutrition.
9. Patient can describe methods to protect self and others from infection.
10. Patient can describe optimal sexual practices.
11. Patient can describe maintenance of social contacts.
12. Supportive others can describe maintenance of patient support.
13. Supportive others can describe methods of protecting selves from infections.

IMPLEMENTATION

☐ Prevention of infection

Prevention of infection for the person with AIDS requires additional measures to those of other immunodeficient persons. A private room is not required for the hospitalized patient if the patient is cooperative and not coughing. The other patient in the room should not be immunosuppressed nor have an infectious disease that is not similar to that of the AIDS patient. CDC recommends blood and body fluid precautions (see Chapter 11) to prevent health care worker exposure to potentially contaminated blood or body fluids. Precautions include the following:

1. Wash hands before and after patient contact.
2. Use gloves when touching blood or body fluids; wash hands after removing gloves.
3. Use gown if soiling of clothing with blood or body fluids is likely.
4. Use masks or eye coverings if the potential exists for spraying of the face by body fluids.
5. Place used needles in a prominently labeled puncture-resistant container designated specifically for disposal; do not bend or recap needles.
6. Double-bag and label articles contaminated with blood or body fluids and send for decontamination or processing.
7. Clean up spilled blood promptly with a solution of 5.25% sodium hypochlorite (bleach) diluted 1:10 with water.
8. Avoid direct patient care or handling patient-care equipment if weeping dermatitis of skin lesions is present in health care worker.

□ Promoting nutrition

Encouraging adequate nutrition can be a challenge when the person is acutely ill. The person may not want to eat because of fatigue, difficulty with swallowing, oral lesions, or anorexia. Useful measures are those that conserve energy, provide oral comfort, or provide desirable foods that are easy to swallow. In some instances TPN may be necessary; however, it does not reverse the wasting effects of the disease and is therefore generally palliative.[52]

□ Providing physiologic supportive care

The type of physiologic care required by the person with AIDS depends on the type of opportunistic infections or tumors present. Persons with *respiratory* conditions need ventilatory measures such as deep breathing and coughing exercises and possibly postural drainage or mechanical ventilation.[45] Oxygen may also be required. Persons with severe *diarrhea* need special care as described in Chapter 31. Activity and self-care are encouraged to the extent possible, depending on the patient's condition.

□ Promoting comfort

Actions taken to promote comfort depend on the source and extent of the discomfort. Skin lesions may need protection and padding. Mouth care is given for oral lesions and special anal care (washing, soothing ointments) for anal discomfort.

□ Counseling and teaching

The person with AIDS, at present, faces the prospect of high probability of death within 3 years from the time of symptom occurrence. During this time the person can expect to be ill with more than one opportunistic infection or tumor and to face the possibility of being shunned by others because of the fears and stigma that presently accompany this disorder. At a time when the person most needs the support of family and friends, some will draw away. Providing the person and significant others opportunities to explore their feelings and to deal with the anxieties is a nursing responsibility (see Chapter 7). Support groups and networks may be additional sources of support (see reference 49).

Social isolation may be imposed on the patient by others who are afraid of disease transmission or by the patient who does not want to pass AIDS on to others. Teaching about the nature of AIDS and methods of transmission may help decrease the social isolation. Alerting the involved others to the effect on the patient of the social isolation may facilitate more social interaction. During the patient's hospitalization, nurses also need to include measures to promote social interaction in the care plan, such as planning time to talk with the patient and supporting and reinforcing interactions of the patient with others.

Anticipatory grieving also needs to be considered for both patient and significant other. Every person will respond differently while working through feelings about the patient's decreased life span. The concepts and ideas pertaining to dying (see Chapter 15) need to be considered when working with the person with AIDS.

Teaching also includes methods of preventing infection, including measures appropriate to immunodeficiencies (see the box on p. 1357) and measures specific for AIDS (see the box below). Patients are urged to eliminate sexual contacts or at least to restrict the number of sex partners. If sexual contacts are continued, anal intercourse should be eliminated and condoms used. Persons with AIDS require continued medical attention.

□ Home care

The bulk of care provided persons with AIDS takes place outside the hospital, and home care needs vary from home-

---

Teaching for the patient with HIV-positive antibodies

1. Do not donate blood or organs.
2. Avoid intimate kissing.
3. Restrict sexual contacts; if continued, avoid anal intercourse and oral-genital sex, use a condom, and avoid exchange of body fluids or contact of body fluids with mucous membranes.
4. Avoid sharing articles that may become contaminated with blood (such as toothbrushes, razors, needles).
5. Clean any surfaces contaminated with blood using bleach freshly diluted 1:10 with water. (Clean the surface first with a disinfectant-detergent because organic material may neutralize the bleach.)
6. Inform health care professionals of the positive antibody status when receiving health care.

maker assistance to intensive physical care.[49] Therefore, nursing care varies from helping a person maintain independence to assisting, providing, or supervising direct care. Financial resources may be severely strained. Good support persons who provide care often need support themselves.

✠ EVALUATION

Evaluation is based on expected patient outcomes. Questions to ask may include the following:
1. Are there any signs of additional infections?
2. Has skin breakdown in the bedfast person been prevented? (Additional skin lesions may be caused by concurrent skin disorders that are not preventable.)
3. Is the person eating a nutritious diet?
4. Is the patient resting more comfortably?
5. Have signs of anxiety decreased and has patient been given opportunities to talk about concerns?
6. Is the patient interacting with supportive others and with other persons in the environment?
7. Can the person and supportive others describe methods of AIDS transmission and plans for prevention of transmission?

■ GAMMOPATHIES

■ Pathophysiology

Gammopathies, better termed *hypergammaglobulinemias,* are elevated levels of gamma globulin in the serum. The normal synthesis of an immunoglobulin is the result of the proliferation of plasma cell differentiation of a single clone of B cells in response to an antigenic signal. In gammopathies a single clone or multiple clones of plasma cells begin to overproduce immunoglobulin product in response to inappropriate antigenic stimulation.

Monoclonal (M-type) *gammopathies* involve a single B cell clone and are commonly referred to as plasma cell dyscrasias. A common monoclonal gammopathy is multiple myeloma.

Polyclonal gammopathies involve the overproduction of virtually all classes of immunoglobulins. The major causes are infectious diseases (especially chronic bacterial infections such as lung abscess and osteomyelitis), connective tissue diseases (such as SLE and rheumatoid arthritis), and chronic active liver disease. IgG and IgM are the most commonly involved immunoglobulins, and the degree of immunoglobulin level reflects the severity of the disease. The development of high levels of dysfunctional gamma globulins depresses the synthesis of normal immunoglobulins, which renders the person susceptible to infection.

■ Multiple myeloma
■ PATHOPHYSIOLOGY

Multiple myeloma is a monoclonal plasma cell malignancy seen in both men and women, occurring in middle and old age. It is characterized by widespread bone destruction, anemia, hypercalcemia, and hyperuricemia.

These symptoms are traced to the proliferation of plasma cell tumors from the bone marrow into the hard bone tissue, causing an erosion of the bone. Frequent recurrent infections (especially of the respiratory tract) and spontaneous pathologic fractures occur because of the production of ineffective immunoglobulins, which, in turn, depress the production of normal antibodies. Renal failure may result from precipitation of urate and calcium crystals. (For additional information, see Chapter 27.)

■ MEDICAL INTERVENTION

Radiation therapy may be given for palliative treatment of localized bone pain and pathologic fractures. Chemotherapy is the major treatment. Alkylating agents, specifically melphalan, are given in combination with adrenocorticosteroids. Several weeks may elapse between the initiation of therapy and signs of improvement. The average survival time is 3 years, but survival may be prolonged with periods of exacerbation and remission.

■ SUPPORTIVE NURSING CARE

Ambulation and adequate hydration are vitally important to prevent renal complications from the increased amounts of urates and calcium being excreted in the urine. Fluid intake should be sufficient to ensure a urinary output of a minimum of 1500 ml/24 hr. Ambulation may be difficult because of the skeletal pain and the possibility of fractures. A lightweight spinal brace and analgesics may facilitate ambulation.

Measures to prevent infection are instituted; they include avoidance of persons with upper respiratory tract infections. Medical attention should be sought for any signs of infection, and antibiotics are often given, since infections are usually caused by gram-positive organisms. Rest periods are planned if fatigue from anemia is present.

■ HYPERSENSITIVITY REACTIONS

■ Pathophysiology

The immune response system that has been previously sensitized is designed to provide an immediate, effective, protective reaction to subsequent encounters with the sensitizing antigen. This of course is a positive factor in the provision of immunity; however, under a given set of conditions or because of an idiotypic reactivity to a particular antigen, the response of the immune system may produce detrimental effects. This inappropriate response is usually manifested as a tissue-damaging overreaction to the antigen; thus it is termed *hypersensitivity* or *allergy.* The antigenic stimulants invoking the reactions are referred to as *allergens.* Hypersensitivities, then, are classic expressions of the immune system, but they take place in inappropriate sites, in excessive amounts, or with inappropriate involvement of nonspecific tissues. Whether an allergic response occurs and to what degree depend on a combination of interrelated factors (see the box on p. 1363).

Table 38-3   Summary of hypersensitivity reactions

| | Hypersensitivity type | | | |
| Property | Immediate (humoral) | | | Delayed (cellular) |
	I Anaphylactic	II Cytotoxic	III Immune complex	IV Cell mediated
Immune system mediators	IgE (IgG) bound to mast cells	IgG or IgM (+ complement)	IgG or IgM + complement	T cells, macrophages
Allergens	Exogenous antigens	Foreign cells or alteration of cell surface antigens	Soluble antigens	Infectious agent, contact allergens, foreign tissues, cancer cells
Response to intradermal skin test	Wheal and flare within 30 min, edema	Not done	Erythema and edema within 3 to 8 hr	Erythema and induration within 24 to 48 hr
Pathophysiologic effects	Release of histamines, kinins, SRS-A from mast cells, which affect smooth muscle shock organs	Direct cytotoxic destruction of cells	Acute inflammatory reaction; primarily polymorphonuclear neutrophil leukocytes	Tissue destruction, primarily lymphocytes and macrophages
Examples	Systemic anaphylaxis, atopic allergies, hay fever, insect sting reactions	Hemolytic disease of the newborn (Rh), transfusion reactions	Serum sickness, Arthus reaction, glomerulonephritis	Tuberculin reaction, skin graft rejection, poison ivy

---

Factors influencing hypersensitivity responses

Increased responsiveness of the host
Increased amount of allergen
Nature of allergen
Entrance of allergen through appropriate site
Short time period between contacts

Hypersensitivities can be broadly divided into two categories based on the components of the immune system involved in mediating the hypersensitivity reaction: humoral or immediate response (B cell mediated) and cellular or delayed response (T cell mediated). The humoral response can be further subdivided into type I anaphylactic, type II cytotoxic, and type III immune complex (Table 38-3). Since type I, II, and III hypersensitivities are the result of interactions involving circulating antibodies, these reactions can be transferred from a sensitized host to a nonsensitized host by serum transfer. Type IV cell-mediated sensitivities can be transferred only by lymphocyte exchange.

■ Type I hypersensitivities (anaphylactic)

The type I hypersensitivities may take different forms depending on the type and amount of allergen and the degree of sensitization (Table 38-4). Anaphylactic shock is the most serious, life-threatening form and requires immediate medical intervention.

The less severe and more common forms of type I hypersensitivities are the atopic allergies, seen in about 15% of the population. *Atopic* refers to an inherited hypersensitivity. It is the tendency to become hypersensitive that is inherited, not the allergy to a specific substance. What persons become hypersensitive to is determined by the allergens to which they are exposed.

■ PATHOPHYSIOLOGY

Type I hypersensitivities are associated with the reactions mediated by the IgE class of immunoglobulins. The IgE immunoglobulins attach to the surface of mast cells and basophils, providing a site for allergens to bind to the cells. This causes the cell to release vasoactive substances, including histamine (Fig. 38-4).

Thus in type I reactions the detrimental symptoms are not at the site of the antigen-antibody reaction but at the site of the organs or tissues where the histamine and other mediators exert their action. If those mediators remain confined to a local area, the tissue reactions remain localized and are referred to as *local anaphylaxis*. The local hypersensitivity that most people demonstrate to a mosquito bite, the wheal-flare type of reaction, is the classic example of this type of reaction. The reaction may also become localized in the nose and eyes (hay fever), in the bronchial passages (allergic asthma), or in the skin (atopic dermatitis). If, however, the mediators become released systemically, the response is known as *systemic anaphylaxis*, which can produce *anaphylactic shock* (Chapter 9).

Histamine's three main effects are the following:

Table 38-4 Type I hypersensitivities (allergies)

Disorder	Etiology	Signs and symptoms	Medical therapy
Anaphylactic shock	Penicillin, heterologous antiserum, insect stings, pollen, x-ray contrast media, food	Initial itching and sneezing, apprehension Edema of face, hands, and other body parts; dyspnea, wheezing, shock	Epinephrine subcutaneously; Benadryl intramuscularly; aminophylline to relax bronchial spasm; tracheal intubation for tracheal edema; control of shock
Urticaria (hives)	Foods, especially eggs, fish, and nuts; drugs such as penicillin Chronic: stress, exposure to heat and cold	Skin lesions: pale pink elevated edge on an erythematous background (wheal) Pruritus	Self-limiting; epinephrine or antihistamines may be given
Atopic			
Allergic rhinitis (hay fever)	Pollens and spores of molds	Sneezing, itching, and watery eyes, running nose	Antihistamines; corticosteroids on a temporary basis for severe cases; desensitization (Chapter 23)
Allergic asthma	External antigens	Wheezing, coughing, dyspnea	Epinephrine, bronchodilators (for example, aminophylline) (Chapter 24)
Atopic dermatitis	Fibers in wool, furs, and nylon; detergents, soaps, perfumes, and cosmetics; changes in temperature; stress	Pruritus; vesicles; oozing and crusting lesions; scaling	Wet dressings, topical steroids (Chapter 39)

1. Constricts smooth muscle such as in the bronchi, resulting in bronchial spasm
2. Increases vascular permeability, resulting in urticaria (hives) or tissue edema
3. Increases mucous secretions, as occurs in hay fever and asthma

The symptoms will be determined by the organ affected. Different etiologic factors cause different symptoms (Fig. 38-5).

For type I reactions to occur, the hypersensitive individual must initially come into contact with the allergen that triggers the synthesis of the specific antiallergenic IgE antibodies. This primary contact is known as a *sensitizing dose*. On subsequent contact with the allergen (termed the *shocking or challenging dose*), the individual exhibits the symptoms of type I sensitivity.

ASSESSMENT

All patients should be questioned about allergies and sensitivities to drugs before drug therapy is initiated. If there is any positive history, the physician is consulted before a new drug is given, and if it is given, the patient is watched closely for allergic responses.

It is usually possible to determine specific allergens to which a person is hypersensitive by taking a history that includes the following:

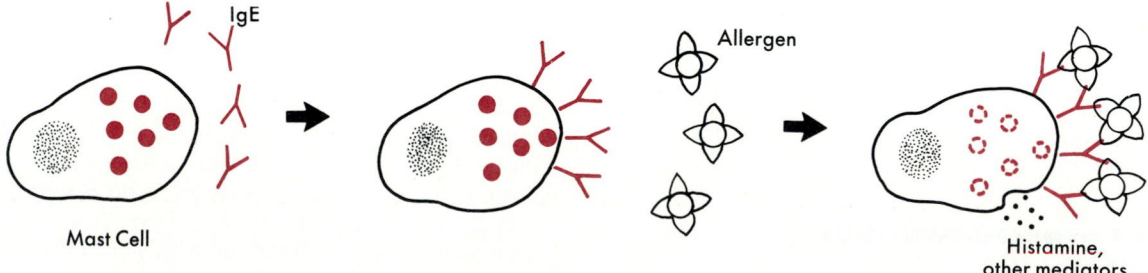

Fig. 38-4 Type I hypersensitivity. IgE binds to mast cell; allergen then binds to IgE, causing degranulation of mast cell with release of histamine and other mediators.

ALLERGY

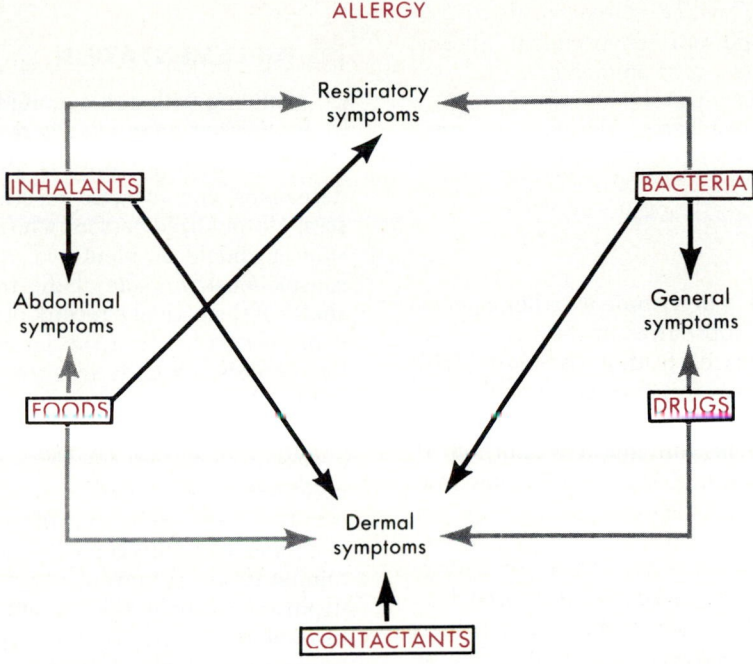

Fig. 38-5   Causes of allergic responses and symptoms produced.

Table 38-5   Allergy skin tests

Test	Method	Time of reading	Positive signs	Use
Intradermal	Allergens are injected intradermally at spaced intervals on forearm or intrascapular area; control tests with diluent alone done concurrently	15 to 30 min	Wheal with surrounding erythema	Allergies to pollen, feathers, animal dander, dust
Scratch	Skin cleaned with alcohol and allowed to dry; skin scratched superficially (1 to 4 mm long), and extract applied to scratch	30 min	Erythema	Same as for intradermal
Patch	Sensitizing substance applied to small (1-inch) gauze square and covered with tape	48 hr	+Erythema only ++Erythema and papules +++Erythema, papules, and vesicles ++++All of above and bullae or ulceration	Allergies to clothing, detergents, perfumes, cosmetics

1. History of allergic reactions in the past (type, frequency, perceived cause)
2. Familial history of allergies
3. Recent exposure to sensitizing substances
4. Changes in living, working, or environmental conditions
5. Characteristics of present environment (house, clothing, plants and trees, or animals)
6. Increased stress in recent past
7. Types of symptoms: respiratory, dermal, or general
8. Alleviating factors, either prescribed by a physician or self-prescribed

□ Diagnostic tests
□ *Skin testing*

Skin tests are often used to determine whether a person has a sensitivity to certain substances in the external environment. Several methods of testing are used (Table 38-5). Occasionally 1 drop of a test extract is instilled into the eye to test for sensitivity (conjunctival test). Redness of the conjunctiva and tearing will appear within 5 to 15 minutes in an allergic person. Tests for allergenic substances are usually done in a series.

□ *Use test*

A person with a food allergy is asked to keep a food diary for at least a week. On the basis of this diary, suspect foods such as milk, wheat products, and eggs may be removed from the diet (elimination diet) until symptoms subside and then added one at a time in an attempt to identify the offending foods. Reaction to the use test may be immediate or over a period of time. Some persons become discouraged during the testing and may need encouragement to adhere to the testing schedule.

➡ DATA ANALYSIS: NURSING DIAGNOSES

Nursing diagnoses are determined from assessment of patient data. Possible nursing diagnoses for the person with an allergy may include, but are not limited to, the following:

Diagnostic title	Possible etiologies
Knowledge deficit	Lack of exposure/recall, information misinterpretation
Health maintenance, altered	Environmental changes, lack of knowledge

▉ PLANNING: EXPECTED PATIENT OUTCOMES

Expected patient outcomes for the person with an allergy may include, but are not limited to, the following:
1. Patient demonstrates a decrease in symptoms.
2. Person describes plans to alter habits or environment.
3. Person can describe substances that are allergenic and approaches for avoidance.
4. Person can describe rationale for immunotherapy and need to continue regular injections (if pertinent).

5. Person can describe need for constant availability of an anaphylaxis emergency kit for self-treatment (if anaphylaxis is a possibility).
6. Person can describe drug therapy to relieve symptoms.

▉ IMPLEMENTATION

□ **Assisting with achievement of therapeutic goals**
□ *Preventing anaphylactic reaction*

Persons with a history of allergies are at high risk for developing anaphylactic reactions from drugs or animal sera. Hospitalized persons who are sensitive to certain substances should be identified, and the information posted conspicuously outside of the room, on the medical order sheets of the patient's record, or in both places. In addition, many hospitals use a special color identification bracelet for the person who is sensitive to certain substances.

If immunization is necessary, animal sera should be avoided and another type given, if possible. When it is necessary to use animal serum, the individual should first be tested for sensitivity to the substance. An intradermal skin test preceded by a scratch or eye test is recommended. If animal sera, allergenic extracts, or contrast media containing iodide are given, a syringe containing 1:1000 epinephrine hydrochloride, an antihistamine such as diphenhydramine (Benadryl), and isoproterenol (Isuprel) should be readily available. The patient is kept under surveillance for at least 20 minutes. Any reaction that occurs within a few minutes forewarns of an impending emergency.

□ *Therapy for anaphylaxis*

At the first signs of anaphylaxis, epinephrine hydrochloride (1:1000) 0.3 to 0.5 ml (less for children), is given subcutaneously. A tourniquet may be applied proximal to the injection site, and epinephrine may be injected into the site. Diphenhydramine (Benadryl) 50 to 100 mg is injected intramuscularly. Aminophylline may be given to relax bronchial spasm, and tracheal intubation may be necessary to maintain an airway if tracheal edema results. Oxygen is given to offset inadequate oxygenation from hypovolemia and bronchial spasms (Chapter 9).

□ *Desensitization (immunotherapy)*

An attempt may be made to slowly desensitize a person by injecting small but increasingly larger doses of the allergen at regular intervals (usually 1 to 4 weeks) over a long period. This treatment may take up to 5 years. It is about 80% effective against pollens causing hay fever but is less effective against asthma or dermatitis. It is essential that the person understand that desensitization is of little value until the environment is controlled; otherwise the constant exposure to allergens will only increase antibody response.

□ Control of environment

Persons whose allergies are caused by environmental inhalants will need a room free of house dust, animal

Table 38-6 Methods of decreasing environmental inhalant antigens

Area	Method
Floors	No wool carpets or felt rug pads; washable throw rugs over wood or tiled floors may be used
Furniture	No kapok stuffing; foam-stuffed furniture is preferable
Clothing	No wool; place closet garments in plastic bags
Bedding	
Pillows	No feathers; use foam or Dacron-filled
Mattress	Use foam mattress over a covered box spring; allergy-free covers
Blankets	Washable cotton
Pets	No fur-bearing pets
Cleaning	Daily damp dusting; no shaking of articles
Air	Air conditioning, if possible; electrostatic filters
Plants	Avoid dried plants
Furnace	Change filters monthly

dander, fungus spores, and other allergens. Because 90% of the airborne particles in the house (for example, house dust) are 5 μm or less in size, an electrostatic filter will be necessary. An electrostatic filter attracts particles by means of highly charged metal plates, which can be removed for cleaning. These filters come in portable models for room use or can be attached to the central heating system. Methods of decreasing environmental inhalant antigens are listed in Table 38-6.

□ **Teaching**

Several facts concerning allergens are helpful to understand:
1. Persons who believe they have "rose fever" are really allergic to pollenating grasses; persons who believe they are allergic to goldenrod are really allergic to ragweed; both roses and goldenrod are insect pollenated.
2. Persons may be allergic to the pollen of one tree and not another; therefore, knowing which tree is pollenating at the time symptoms appear is necessary.
3. Persons who are allergic to pollenating grasses will have the same symptoms no matter which grass is pollenating. If they move from one geographic area to another, they will become sensitized to whatever grasses are present in that area.

Teaching for the patient with allergies

1. Avoid allergens when possible
   a. Seasonal inhalants
      (1) Air-condition the house, if possible
      (2) Use electrostatic window filter if house is not air-conditioned
      (3) Plan vacations outside the ragweed area during the peak of pollenating season, if possible
   b. Environmental inhalants (Table 38-6)
   c. Drugs
      (1) Remind physician of allergy when new medication is prescribed
      (2) Read all labels of nonprescription drugs before taking new drug
      (3) Wear a MedicAlert bracelet indicating the known drug allergy
   d. Food
      (1) Examine labels of new prepared food for presence of allergen
      (2) Avoid eating unknown foods when traveling
   e. Contact allergens
      (1) Use a nonallergenic soap or detergent and cosmetics and take these when traveling
      (2) Use Ivory soap if allergic to most soaps and detergents
2. If sensitive to insect stings
   a. Keep a sting emergency medical kit readily available
   b. If sting occurs:
      (1) Swallow uncoated antihistamine tablet
      (2) Place isoproterenol tablet under tongue
      (3) Inject 1:1000 epinephrine hydrochloride (A family member should also know how to do this)
      (4) Seek medical help immediately
3. Continue medical follow-up if medications are required

Table 38-7   Types of blood components

Blood component	Description	Usage	Comments
Red blood cells (RBC)			
Packed RBC (PRBC)	RBC separated from plasma and platelets	Anemia Moderate blood loss	Decreased risk of fluid overload as compared to whole blood
Washed RBC	RBC washed with sterile isotonic saline before transfusion	Previous allergic reactions to transfusions	Increased removal of immunoglobulins and protein
Frozen RBC	RBC frozen in a glycerol solution; cells are washed after thawing to remove the glycerol	Storage of rare type blood Storage of autologous blood for future use	Relatively free of leukocytes and microemboli Expensive
Leukocyte-poor RBC	RBC from which most leukocytes have been removed	Previous sensitivity to leukocyte antigens from prior transfusions or from pregnancy	Fewer RBC than packed RBC Washed leukocyte-poor RBC units have more RBC than nonwashed
Neocytes	RBC units with high number of reticulocytes (young RBC)	Transfusion-dependent anemias	Fewer problems with iron overload Expensive
Other cellular components			
Platelets: Random donor packs	Platelets separated from RBC by centrifuge; given in 50 ml of plasma	Thrombocytopenia DIC	Plasma base is rich in coagulation factors Platelets preparations can also be packed, washed, or made leukocyte-poor
Pheresis packs	Platelets from an HLA-matched donor, separated by pheresis	Allosensitized persons with thrombocytopenia	Requires specialized techniques
Granulocytes	Granular leukocytes separated by pheresis	Granulocytopenia from malignancy or chemotherapy	Allergen sensitization may occur with chills and fever
Plasma components			
Fresh frozen plasma (FFP)	Freezing of plasma within 4 hr of collection	Clotting deficiencies Liver disease Hemophilia Defibrination	Preserves factors V, VII, VIII, IX, X and prothrombin Minimizes hepatitis risk Administered through a filter
Factor concentrates VIII and IX	Prepared from large donor pools	VIII: Hemophilia A IX: Hemophilia B	Increased risk of hepatitis (VIII, IX) and thromboembolism (IX) Given in small volumes
Cryoprecipitate	Precipitated material obtained from FFP when thawed	Hemophilia A Infection of burns Hypofibrinogenemia Uremic bleeding	Contains factors VIII, XIII and fibrinogen

Serum albumin:
  Normal serum albumin (NSA)
  Plasma protein fraction (PPF)
	Albumin chemically processed from pooled plasma	Hypovolemic shock
		Hypoalbuminemia
		Burns
		Hemorrhagic shock
			No risk of hepatitis
			Does not require ABO compatibility
			Lacks clotting factors
			Hypotension may occur if PPF is given faster than 10 ml/min[46a]

Immune serum globulin	Obtained from plasma of preselected donors with specific antibodies	Hypogammaglobulinemia Prophylaxis for hepatitis A	Given intramuscularly

4. Persons may be allergic to spores of molds and not realize it. Molds are most likely to be found inside the house in warm, damp basements or in crawl spaces under the house. They are also found outside the house in leaves of certain trees, wheat, and corn.
5. For pollens and spores, the highest counts (amounts in the air) occur between 12 midnight and 8 AM.

Prevention of exacerbations requires knowledge of ways to avoid the allergens and when to seek medical assistance. Important points in the teaching of patients with allergies are summarized in the box on p. 1367.

✚ EVALUATION

Evaluation is based on expected patient outcomes. Questions to consider include the following:
1. Does the person know how to avoid the specific allergens?
2. Have plans been made to decrease contact with the allergen?
3. Does the person know when to seek medical help?

■ Type II hypersensitivities (cytotoxic)

■ PATHOPHYSIOLOGY

The underlying mechanisms of type II hypersensitivities involve the direct binding of *IgG* or *IgM* immunoglobulins to an antigen on the *surface of a cell* (see Fig. 37-7). This antibody labeling then triggers the destruction of the cell by phagocytic attack, nonspecific lymphocytic attack, or cell lysis.

■ BLOOD TRANSFUSION REACTIONS

The type II hypersensitivity is classically illustrated by the reactions that occur in mismatched blood transfusion reactions. Blood replacement therapy is used when there has been excessive blood loss (whole blood or blood components) or in treatment of diseases of the hematopoietic system. Replacement therapy may be whole blood or one or more of the blood components (Table 38-7). Blood transfusions are not without dangers to the recipient; therefore, the transfusion of 1 unit (500 ml) of blood for minor therapy is not recommended.

□ Pathophysiology

Many antigens are found on the surface of red blood cells, but in terms of potential immunologic reaction the major clinically significant systems are the ABO and Rh systems.

□ ABO system

The four major human blood groups are listed in the box above. Since type AB contains both antigens, persons with type AB may receive blood from any type (Fig. 38-6). Persons with type O may donate blood to other types, but since both antigens are absent in type O, they may not receive another type without having a reaction.

Major blood groups	
A	Antigen A is present
B	Antigen B is present
AB	Both antigens A and B are present
O	Neither antigen A nor B is present

Within the serum, individuals possess naturally occurring antibodies to the red blood cell (RBC) surface antigens of the ABO blood groups that are not present on their own RBCs. Thus a person with type A blood will possess anti-B antibodies within the serum. These antibodies, called *isohemagglutinins,* are usually of the IgM class. The antibodies are capable of cross-reacting with the A or B antigens on the surface of the "foreign" ABO types. On transfusion, mismatched blood will be immediately coated by the isohemagglutinins, causing agglutination of the introduced cells and the rapid lysis (breakdown) of the cells. The products released by the lysed cells are then dumped into the bloodstream.

□ Rh system

The Rh system is more complex because at least 27 different antigens are in this system. The most immunogenic is the D antigen. When the term *Rh positive* is used, the presence of antigen Rh-D is implied; *Rh negative* indicates the absence of antigen D. Approximately 85% of the population have Rh-positive blood.

When the person with Rh-negative blood is first exposed to Rh-positive blood, Rh antibodies are formed. On subsequent exposures to Rh-positive blood, the Rh antibody binds to its corresponding antigen on the surface of the RBCs containing the Rh antigen. The Rh-antigen RBCs are then rapidly broken down by macrophages in the spleen with conversion of hemoglobin to bilirubin resulting in jaundice.

□ HLA system

Human leukocyte antigens (HLA) are found on many types of tissue cells and on blood leukocytes and platelets. The system is more complex than the RBC antigen sys-

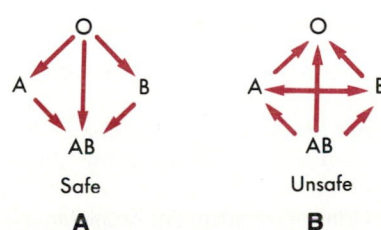

Fig. 38-6 Blood groups and the groups each can receive blood from and give blood to. **A,** Safe. **B,** Unsafe.

tems, and literally thousands of combinations of the antigens can occur. Sensitization may occur through pregnancy or through exposure to platelets and white blood cells (WBCs) during transfusions. Repeated transfusions of blood cells may lead to transfusion reactions.

□ Prevention of transfusion reactions

Prescreening of potential blood donors is essential. Blood received from volunteer donors through the American Red Cross Blood Service or hospital blood banks is preferable to that of paid donors, who may be less likely to report past or present diseases that may affect the recipient.

After the blood has been collected, the blood group and subgroups including Rh typing are identified, and the blood is tested for syphilis, hepatitis, and HIV antibodies. The blood must be cross-matched with blood from the recipient to determine compatibility and prevent an acute hemolytic reaction. Cross-matching consists of mixing samples of the donor's blood and the recipient's blood and examining for cell clumping or hemolysis.

Most of the serious reactions that now occur during transfusions are the result of human error. Safeguards include the following:

1. Blood must be kept cold until ready to use (warm blood is a good medium for bacterial growth).
2. Blood that has remained at room temperature for more than 30 minutes should not be returned to refrigeration for reissue.
3. Blood should be administered within a 4-hour period.
4. The unit of blood must be labeled with the patient's name, and the label must be checked against the patient's wristband before the blood is given.
5. All blood products should be administered through filters to prevent embolism from clots.
6. If blood must be warmed (such as during rapid massive blood replacement), use a temperature-controlled device only (no water bath, incubator, or microwave oven) to prevent RBC hemolysis from temperatures over 37° C (98.6° F).
7. The patient must be monitored throughout the blood administration.

□ Complications of blood transfusions
□ *Immunologic transfusion reactions*

Immunologic reactions that can occur with blood transfusions include acute hemolytic, delayed hemolytic, allergic, febrile, graft versus host disease, and noncardiac pulmonary edema (Table 38-8). The most serious reaction is the acute hemolytic reaction that occurs during administration of the first 50 ml of blood transfused. Several hours after a hemolytic reaction, the urine becomes red (port-wine urine) and the urinary output is diminished. The urine contains RBCs and albumin. This reaction is thought to be caused by the release of a toxic substance from the hemolyzed blood that causes a temporary vascular spasm in the kidneys, resulting in renal damage, and blockage of the renal tubules by the hemoglobin precipitated out in the acid urine (hemoglobinuria). If the patient receives more than 100 ml of incompatible blood, irreversible shock

with complete renal failure may occur, and death may follow.

As blood cells disintegrate (lyse), large amounts of potassium are released into the bloodstream; if renal function is impaired, hyperkalemia will develop. If this occurs, the patient may be treated with renal dialysis. Because fever is a sign of both acute hemolytic reaction and the less serious pyrogenic reaction, the transfusion is stopped until the diagnosis is made.

□ *Nonimmunologic reactions*

Complications other than those of immunologic origin include the following:
1. Fluid overload
   a. Occurs mostly in elderly persons and those with congestive heart failure or severe anemia (hemoglobin less than 5 g/dl)
   b. Can be prevented by use of packed cells
   c. If it occurs, slow down or stop infusion (depending on severity of symptoms)
2. Air embolism
   a. Results when blood is administered under air pressure following severe blood loss
   b. If occurs, place patient in left side-lying Trendelenburg position (diverts air away from pulmonary artery)
3. Complications of massive blood replacement (exchange of one blood volume in 24 hours)
   a. Thrombocytopenia with abnormal bleeding (from platelet deterioration)
   b. Cardiac arrhythmias (from cold blood)
   c. Electrolyte level imbalances
      (1) *Hyperkalemia* (potassium released as RBCs break down)
      (2) *Hypocalcemia* (binding of sodium citrate from donor blood with recipient's serum calcium ions)
4. Transmission of disease
   a. Hepatitis: occurs in 7% to 10% of blood transfusions; blood is screened for hepatitis A and B, but no screening test is available for non-A, non-B hepatitis
   b. AIDS: a rare complication; donated blood is tested but test is not 100% accurate; the number of new infections among blood product recipients has decreased; HIV is now inactivated in blood products by heat treatment
   c. Syphilis and malaria: incidence is rare
   d. Cytomegalovirus: symptoms occur in about 40 days (fever, malaise, splenomegaly); the condition is benign and treatment is symptomatic
5. Transfusion hemosiderosis
   a. Defined as an iron overload from chronic transfusions for hematopoietic disorders
   b. If it occurs, RBC or neocytes are given for future transfusions to decrease number of transfusions required

□ Autologous blood transfusions

One method of preventing immunologic blood transfusion reactions and disease transmission is by using the

Table 38-8   Immunologic reactions to blood transfusions

Reaction	Cause	Mechanism	Symptoms	Occurrence	Action
Acute hemolytic	Recipient antibody incompatible with transfused red cells	RBCs agglutinate, rapid hemolysis Capillary plugging (type II hypersensitivity)	Lumbar pain Constriction of chest Pain in vein Fever, chills Hemoglobinuria Signs of shock	Shortly after initiation of transfusion	Stop transfusion Continue IV saline Blood unit and blood sample from patient sent to lab for immediate testing Treat for shock and renal failure
Delayed hemolytic	Anamnestic immune response	Slow hemolysis	Jaundice Anemia	Days to weeks after transfusion	Monitor adequacy of urinary output and degree of anemia
Allergic	Transfer of an antigen or a reaginic antibody from donor to recipient	Immune sensitivity to foreign serum protein (type I hypersensitivity)	Urticaria Anaphylaxis (wheezing, dyspnea, shock)	Within 30 minutes after initiation of transfusion	Mild: give antihistamine, continue transfusion Severe: stop transfusion; give aqueous epinephrine (0.5 ml of 1:1000 solution)
Febrile	Reaction of antigen on WBC or platelets Bacterial contamination	Leukocyte agglutination Bacterial pyrogens	Fever, chills	Within 30-90 min after initiation of transfusion	Stop transfusion Continue IV saline Antipyretics after ruling out hemolytic reaction Transfuse with leukocyte-poor blood or washed RBC
Graft versus host disease	Immunodeficient person receives lymphocytes	Engraftment of donor lymphocytes, which are then "rejected"	Dermatitis Stomatitis Diarrhea Liver dysfunction	Delayed	Steroids Azathioprine Symptomatic therapy
Noncardiac pulmonary edema	Donor antibodies react with recipient HLA antigen	Infiltration of pulmonary bed by microaggregates, which block blood flow	Fever, chills Urticaria Cough Orthopnea Cyanosis Shock	During transfusion or shortly thereafter	Stop transfusion Continue IV saline Give oxygen as needed Steroids Furosemide

person's own blood for replacement. There are two approaches for using autologous blood, planned collection and autotransfusion. In *planned autologous transfusion*, blood is collected at regular intervals before the time when usage is anticipated, such as before surgery. The blood is then stored or frozen until needed. This method is especially useful for persons with rare blood types, for those whose religious beliefs preclude receiving donor blood, or for those with planned surgeries for which blood transfusions are expected.

Autotransfusion consists of collecting, filtering, and immediately reinfusing the person's own blood, such as in the emergency room or during selected surgical procedures involving large blood loss. The blood is suctioned into a bag and passed through a filter to remove aggregates of fibrin, RBCs, platelets, and other microaggregates.[9] Anticoagulant is added through a volume control system. When the bag is full, it is disconnected from the system, and the blood is transfused into the patient with an administration set and a standard or a microembolic filter. Blood that has been contaminated by gastrointestinal contents or that is close to a malignant tumor is not autotransfused.

Autotransfusion is safe and cost effective, uses warm blood, and contains more RBCs than stored blood, but platelet, fibrinogen, and clotting factors are decreased. The potential exists for nephrotoxic effect from RBC damage with release of hemoglobin.

■ Type III hypersensitivities (immune complex)

■ PATHOPHYSIOLOGY

The type III hypersensitivities result from the union of soluble antigens with immunoglobulins of the IgM and IgG classes. The complexes that are formed are too small for phagocytosis, so rather than being removed by the reticuloendothelial system (RES), they are deposited in body tissues. This causes an inflammatory response, usually intravascular. Immune complexes are a common factor of connective tissue (collagen) disorders, especially lupus erythematosus and rheumatoid arthritis. Complexes may also be trapped in glomeruli, which results in glomerulonephritis.

■ SERUM SICKNESS

A type III hypersensitivity of clinical significance is serum sickness, which can develop from 1 to 3 weeks after the administration of a large amount of "foreign" serum (for example, horse serum). It may also occur with the administration of certain drugs, particularly antimicrobials such as penicillin.

Itching and discomfort at the injection site are usually the first symptoms noted. These are followed by lymphadenopathy, fever, urticaria or erythematous rash, facial edema, and joint pain. Objective signs of arthritis may be present.

Serum sickness is a self-limiting disease. Mild symptoms respond well to antihistamines and salicylates. More severe symptoms are treated with a steroid such as prednisone, with relief of symptoms often obtained within hours. Epinephrine is given if an anaphylactic reaction occurs.

■ Type IV hypersensitivities (cell mediated)

■ PATHOPHYSIOLOGY

Type IV hypersensitivities are cell mediated (delayed type) involving T cells. Antigens identified as foreign to the body can cause a reaction in two ways, by direct or by indirect action. The T lymphocyte can destroy the antigen directly by attaching itself to the antigen cell wall, breaking down the cell membrane, and causing lysis and death of the cell. This direct action approach appears to be a major factor in transplant rejections. The indirect approach consists of activating nonspecific phagocytic cells (macrophages and polymorphonuclear leukocytes) through release of lymphokines by the sensitized T lymphocytes.

Clinical examples of type IV hypersensitivities are microbial hypersensitivity reaction, allergic contact dermatitis (Chapter 39), and tissue transplant rejection.

■ MICROBIAL HYPERSENSITIVITY REACTION

An example of microbial hypersensitivity is the body's reaction to the tubercle bacillus. The body does not react initially when the bacillus invades a nonsensitized host.

However, as the cell-mediated response is activated, tissue destruction (cavitation) and general toxemia result. After the initial sensitization, subsequent contact with the tubercle bacillus will elicit a hypersensitivity reaction. This is the basis of the tuberculin skin test.

■ TISSUE TRANSPLANT REJECTION

The rejection of foreign cells and tissues by the body is a beneficial function of the immune system primarily mediated by a type IV hypersensitivity. If it were not for this mechanism, the human body would be a haven for the inappropriate establishment of growth of any animal cell that penetrated the external defense mechanisms; however, this process is regarded as a disservice when it operates to prevent the positive aspects of the exchange of tissues between hosts.

□ Pathophysiology

The antigenic determinants of the tissues that lead to graft rejection are primarily found on the surface of the cells within the transplanted tissues. These antigens are known as *histocompatibility antigens* and are controlled by independently segregated genes within the chromosomal structure of the animal. They are also called human leukocyte antigens (HLA) (p. 1369).

□ Tissue typing

In preparation for a tissue transplant from another person (allograft), the closest match of donor-recipient transplantation antigens is sought. This is done by tissue typing for the major antigenic determinants (ABO, Rh, and HLA). The recipient's serum is then cross-matched with donor lymphocytes for compatibility.

□ Tissue response

When nonmatched skin is transferred to the new host, a first-set rejection occurs (see the box below). If another skin graft is taken from the same donor and is transplanted to a different site on the same recipient, the graft rejection is more rapid. This accelerated reaction or second-set rejection is so rapid that the graft may never be vascularized before it is sloughed. Graft rejection can be minimized by induced immunosuppression (see Table 38-2).

First-set rejection of nonmatched allograft

1 to 3 days	Skin becomes vascularized
6 to 10 days	Sensitized lymphocytes appear in regional lymph nodes; lymph nodes enlarge
12 to 14 days	Vascular bed begins to deteriorate; graft becomes necrotic and is sloughed off

Table 38-9   Some diseases with autoimmune aspects

Disease	Autoantigen	Comments
Pernicious anemia	Intrinsic factors of parietal cells	Specific autoantibodies detectable
Autoimmune hemolytic anemia	Antigens on the surface of RBC	RBC surface antigens may be altered by drugs
Systemic lupus erythematosus	Nucleoproteins, DNA, many other antigens	Multiple autoimmune responses
Guillain-Barré syndrome	Myelin	
Glomerulonephritis	Cross-reactive streptococcal antigens	May also result from direct attack of glomerular basement membrane
Rheumatic fever	Cross-reactive streptococcal antigens Immunoglobulin G	
Rheumatoid arthritis	Antibodies to gamma globulin	Rheumatoid factor is IgM that reacts with IgG
Ulcerative colitis	Colon cells	
Myasthenia gravis	Skeletal and heart muscle	Thymectomy improves
Male infertility	Sperm cell	Agglutinins formed against sperm cells
Multiple sclerosis	Brain cells	Not proved to be autoimmune
Sympathetic uveitis	Uveal tissues	Release of sequestered uveal antigen
Autoimmune thyroiditis	Thyroid hormones and tissues	Autoantibodies and sensitized lymphocytes

Some allografts circumvent immunorejection because of their site in the body. Corneal and cartilage grafts survive without the need for immunosuppression because these sites are avascular. By some (as yet unknown) mechanism, the fetus developing within the uterus enjoys this same privileged status.

■ AUTOIMMUNE DISEASES

Individuals sometimes respond immunologically to some of their own antigens. The chance that the control mechanisms will be lost increases with the age of the person. The symptoms of such a self-attack are referred to as *autoimmune disease* or *autohypersensitivity*. For the most part, these self-reactions are not immunologically initiated; the causative agent lies outside the immune system, but the immune response serves as the pathogenic mechanism. The incidence of autoimmune disease is higher in young women and in persons with a familial history of autoimmune disease.

Self-reactive immunoglobulins are often associated with certain pathologic states in the body but many times can also be isolated from the serum of "normal" individuals as well, especially in older persons. Autoantibodies have been demonstrated against nuclear material in systemic lupus erythematosus, against gamma globulins in rheumatoid arthritis, against gastric parietal cells in pernicious anemia, and against platelets in autoimmune thrombocytopenia. Sensitized lymphocytes have been demonstrated in the Guillain-Barré-Strohl syndrome and autoimmune thyroiditis.

Many diseases for which no etiologic agent could be identified had been classified as autoimmune, only to be removed from that category when some cryptic, latent, or slow-growing agent was identified within the cells or tissue

under attack. Some of the diseases listed as autoimmune-associated diseases in Table 38-9 will probably be removed from that list as the initiating factor or microorganism is identified. The care of persons having these diseases is discussed elsewhere in this text.

■ SUMMARY

1. Major health problems of the immune system may be categorized as immunodeficiencies, gammopathies, hypersensitivities, and autoimmunities.
2. Immunodeficiencies may result from deficiencies in B cells or T cells or from both cells combined. Most primary immunodeficiencies are genetic; the major secondary immunodeficiencies encountered in general practice are immunosuppression and acquired immunodeficiency syndrome (AIDS).
3. Immunosuppression may be induced by administration of antigen, antibodies, or antilymphocytic serum, by radiation, or by drugs (corticosteroids, cytotoxic drugs, cyclosporine, or OKT3).
4. The major interventions for immunodeficiencies are replacement therapy and prevention of infection.
5. AIDS is caused by a retrovirus (HIV). Some persons test positive for HIV antibodies from an initial infection but may never develop AIDS; others may show some persistent generalized lymphadenopathy (PGL) without developing AIDS. Persons who develop AIDS related complex (ARC) usually develop AIDS, which ends in death.
6. The AIDS virus is transmitted by sexual contact, blood (especially by use of shared needles), or from mother to child prenatally or by breast-feeding; AIDS is not transmitted by personal contact, toilet seats, or insects.

Putting knowledge to practice

■ Write down some concerns you might have if assigned to provide care for a person with AIDS; examine each concern in terms of its basis (fact, fear, values). Then think about ways to deal with these concerns.
■ Think about the following questions and raise the issues in group discussions: What is society's role in providing the expensive health care required for persons with AIDS? Should children who are HIV positive be allowed to attend school? Should persons who are HIV positive be allowed to teach school or give patient care? If persons are HIV positive, who should have access to this information? What are the rights of the person with AIDS versus those of society? For example, what actions should be taken with an HIV positive person who does not take the recommended actions to prevent transmission?
■ Ask a nurse who has had experience giving care to persons with AIDS to discuss her or his experience related to meeting patients' needs.
■ Examine the chart of a patient who has received a blood transfusion. What safeguards were taken to prevent transfusion reaction? If a reaction was noted, what actions were taken?

---

7. Because AIDS is an immunodeficiency disease, the person is highly susceptible to infections, especially opportunistic infections such as *Pneumocystis carinii* pneumonia.

8. Gammopathies are excessive production of immunoglobulins; the most common gammopathy is multiple myeloma (an excess of plasma cells).

9. Hypersensitivity reactions are exaggerated or inappropriate responses to specific antigens (allergens).

10. Type I hypersensitivities are associated with reactions mediated by IgE immunoglobulins that are attached to mast cells; when the allergen binds to the IgE, histamine is released, producing a systemic (anaphylaxic shock) or a local allergic reaction.

11. Therapy for anaphylaxis includes epinephrine to constrict blood vessels and dilate the bronchioles, counteracting the effect of histamine; allergies are treated with desensitization and control of environment to decrease allergens.

12. Type II hypersensitivities are cytotoxic reactions from the direct binding of IgG or IgM immunoglobulins to the surface of foreign cells to trigger cell destruction; an example is blood transfusion reactions.

13. The major antigens on RBCs are the AB antigens, Rh antigens, and HLA antigens. AB blood group indicates presence of both A and B antigens; O blood group indicates absence of either antigen. Absence of an antigen produces antibodies (isohemagglutins) that will cause agglutination of donor RBCs containing the missing antigen. Therefore, people with type O blood may donate blood to other types but may not receive another type without having a hemolytic reaction.

14. Immunologic reactions to blood transfusions include hemolytic (most serious), allergic, febrile, graft-versus host disease, and noncardiac pulmonary edema. Diseases that may be transmitted by blood transfusions include hepatitis, AIDS, syphilis, malaria, and cytomegalovirus.

15. Autologous blood transfusions consist of using the person's own blood for replacement, either by stored blood previously collected or by autotransfusion of blood from excessive bleeding.

16. Type III hypersensitivities are characterized by immune complexes formed by the union of IgM or IgG immunoglobulins with soluble antigens; the small complexes get trapped in body tissues causing an inflammatory response. An example is serum sickness that occurs after administration of a large amount of foreign serum.

17. Type IV hypersensitivities are cell-mediated (T cell) reactions, differing from the other three types, which are humoral (B cell) reactions. T cells destroy foreign antigens directly (as in transplant rejections) or they may release lymphokines to activate macrophages.

18. Rejection of transplanted tissue is more rapid if previous sensitization has already occurred by an earlier reaction; immunosuppressive drugs are given to prevent tissue rejection.

19. Autoimmune diseases are the result of an immune response to one's own antigens, usually as a result of an agent from outside the immune system.

REFERENCES AND SELECTED READINGS

1. *Allen, J, and Mellin, G: The new epidemic: immune deficiency, opportunistic infections, and Kaposi's sarcoma, Am J Nurs 82:1718-1722, 1982.

2. *Anderson, D: AIDS: an update on what we know now, RN 49(3):49-53, 1986.

3. *Baker, GAB: Administering blood safely, AORN J 37:1102-1112, 1983.

4. *Baron, M, and Tafuro, P: The extremes of age; the newborn and the elderly at increased risk for the development of infection, Nurs Clin North Am 20(1):181-190, 1985.

---

*References preceded by an asterisk are particularly well suited for student reading.

5. *Bennett, JA: AIDS: epidemiology and update, Am J Nurs 85:968-972, 1985.

6. *Bennett, JA: AIDS: what precautions do you take in the hospital? Am J Nurs 86:952-953, 1986.

7. *Bennett, JA: Nurses talk about the challenge of AIDS, Am J Nurs 87:1150-1155, 1987.

8. *Bennett, JA: What we know about AIDS, Am J Nurs 86:1015-1020, 1986.

9. *Benson, ML, and Benson, DM: Autotransfusion is here: are you ready? Nurs 85 (15(3):46-60, 1985.

10. *Birdsall, C: How do you avoid transfusion complications? Am J Nurs 85:312, 1985.

10a. *Birdsell, C, Carpenter, K, and Considine, R: How is autotransfusion done? Am J Nurs 88:108-111, 1988.

11. Brown, ML: AIDS and ethics: concerns and considerations, Oncol Nurs Forum 14(1):69-73, 1987.

12. Bryant, JK: Home care of the client with AIDS, J Commun Health Nurs 3(2):69-74, 1986.

13. CDC guidelines: recommendations for preventing transmission of AIDS, AORN J 43:528-532, 1986.

14. Centers for Disease Control: Public Health Service guidelines for counseling and antibody testing to prevent HIV infection and AIDS, MMWR 36:509-515, 1987.

15. Centers for Disease Control: Classification system of human T-lymphocyte virus type III/lymphadenopathy-associated virus infections, MMWR 35:331-337, 1986.

15a. Centers for Disease Control: Human immunodeficiency virus infection in the United States: a review of current knowledge, MMWR 36(suppl 5-6):1-48, 1987.

16. Centers for Disease Control: Recommendations for prevention of HIV transmission in health-care settings, MMWR 36(2S):3S-17S, 1987.

17. *Cecchi, R: Living with AIDS: when the system fails, Am J Nurs 86:46-47, 1986.

17a. Chung, CL, and others: Ethical implications: screening for and treatment of AIDS, Health Educ 18(4):4-7, 1987.

18. *Cianci, J, and Lamb, J: Organ transplantation: matching donors and recipients, Am J Nurs 81:544-545, 1981.

19. *Coleman, DA: How to care for an AIDS patient, RN 49(7):16-21, 1986.

20. *Committee on Transfusion Practices, American Association of Blood Banks: The latest protocols for blood transfusions, Nurs 86 16(10):34-41, 1986.

21. Croman, LC: The relationship between nutrition, infection, and immunity, Med Clin North Am 69(3):519-531, 1985.

22. *Dhundale, K, and Hubbard, PM: Home care for the AIDS patient: safety first, Nurs 86 16(9):34-36, 1986.

22a. Durham, JD, and Cohen, FL: The person with AIDS: nursing perspectives, New York, 1987, Springer Publishing Co.

23. Espersen, S: Nursing support of host defenses, CC Nurs Q 9(1):51-56, 1986.

24. Farrell, B: AIDS patients: values in conflict, CC Nurs Q 10(2):74-85, 1987.

25. Farthing, CF, and others: A colour atlas of AIDS, London, 1986, Wolfe Medical Publications Ltd.

26. Friedland, GH, and Klein, RS: Transmission of the human immunodeficiency virus, New Engl J Med 317:1125-1135, 1987.

27. *Fruth, R: Anaphylaxis and drug reactions: guidelines for detection and care, Heart Lung 9:662-664, 1980.

28. *Fuller, BF: Organ graft rejection: the biological process, AORN J 41:738-745, 1985.

29. *Gaunder, BN: Insect bites and stings: managing allergic reactions, Nurs Pract 11(3):16-20, 1986.

30. Goedert, JJ: What is safe sex? New Engl J Med 316:1339-1342, 1987.

31. *Griffin, JP: Nursing care of the critically ill immunocompromised patient, CC Nurs Q 9(1):25-34, 1986.

32. Gurevich, I, and Tafuro, P: Nursing measures for the prevention of infection in the compromised host, Nurs Clin North Am 20(1):257-266, 1985.

33. *Hood, LE: Interferon, Am J Nurs 87:459-464, 1987.

34. *Jassak, PF, and Spiewak, PL: Interleukin-2, Am J Nurs 87:464-467, 1987.

35. Kaye, D, and Rose, LF: Fundamentals of internal medicine, St. Louis, 1983, The CV Mosby Co.

36. Krupp, MA, Schroeder, SA, and Tierney, LM, Jr: Current medical diagnosis and treatment, Norwalk, Conn, 1987, Appleton & Lange.

37. *Kuhn, R: Organ transplantation: issues and actions, Heart Lung 15(2):21A-24A, 1986.

38. *LaCamera, DJ, Masur, H, and Henderson, DK: The acquired immunodeficiency syndrome, Nurs Clin North Am 20(1):241-256, 1985.

39. *Lewis, HR, and Lewis, ME: What you and your patients need to know about safer sex, RN 50(9):53-58, 1987.

40. *Lind, M: The immunologic assessment: a nursing focus, Heart Lung 9:658-661, 1980.

40a. McCloskey, JE: AIDS: risks from casual contacts discounted, Ohio Nurs Rev 63(3):14, 1988.

41. Mennies, JH, and others: An overview of adult allergic disorders, Nurs Pract 10(6):16-23, 1985.

42. *Mitchell, C, and Smith, L: Dilemmas in practice: if it's AIDS, please don't tell, Am J Nurs 87:911-914, 1987.

43. *Peabody, B: Living with AIDS: a mother's perspective, Am J Nurs 86:45-46, 1986.

44. *Phillips, A: Are blood transfusions really safe? Nurs 87 17(6):63-65, 1987.

45. *Price, DM, and Scimeca, AM: The epidemic of the 80s, Cancer Nurs 7:283-290, 1984.

46. *Querin, JJ, and Stahl, LD: 12 simple sensible steps for successful blood transfusions, Nurs 83 13(11):34-43, 1983.

46a. Rakel, RE: Conn's current therapy, Philadelphia, 1988, WB Saunders Co.

47. *Randall, BJ: Reacting to anaphylaxis, Nurs 86 16(3):34-39, 1986.

48. *Rieger, PT: Monoclonal antibodies, Am J Nurs 87:469-473, 1987.

49. *Schietinger, H: A home care plan for AIDS, Am J Nurs 86:1021-1028, 1986.

50. Selwyn, P: AIDS, what is now known: history and immunology, Hosp Pract 21(5):67-76, 1986.

51. Selwyn, P: AIDS, what is now known: epidemiology, Hosp Pract 21(6):127-164, 1986.

52. Selwyn, P: AIDS, what is now known: clinical aspects, Hosp Pract 21(9):119-139, 1986.

53. Selwyn, P: AIDS, what is now known: psychosocial aspects, treatment prospects, Hosp Pract 21(10):125-164, 1986.

54. *Smith, L: Reactions to blood transfusions, Am J Nurs 84:1096-1101, 1984.

55. *Smith, SL: Immunosuppressive drugs used in clinical practice, CC Nurs Q 9(1):19-24, 1986.

56. Steinhiser, SA, and others: OKT3 for the treatment of patients with acute renal allograft rejection, ANNA J 14(2):127-129, 1987.

57. Sticklin, LA: Interleukin-2 and killer T cells, Am J Nurs 87:468-469, 1987.

58. Van Devanter, NL, and others: Counseling HIV-antibody positive blood donors, Am J Nurs 87:1026-1030, 1987.

59. Wyngaarden, JB, and Smith, LH: Cecil textbook of medicine, ed 17, Philadelphia, 1985, WB Saunders Co.

39

The Patient with Dermatologic Problems

BARBARA C. LONG

CHAPTER OBJECTIVES

After studying this chapter, the student should be able to:

- Describe the psychologic effect of skin disorders.
- Differentiate skin inflammations resulting from bacteria, viruses, fungi, and parasites and describe appropriate therapy.
- Describe methods of applying medications to the skin.
- Describe measures for relief of pruritus.
- Differentiate between contact and atopic dermatitis and methods of prevention.
- Describe the pathophysiology of psoriasis and therapeutic measures.
- Describe the different types of skin tumors and surgical interventions.
- Describe the different types of grafts and measures to promote healing.
- Identify different types of cosmetic surgeries.

The skin is the largest organ of the body. It is exposed to the external environment and provides the first line of defense of the body; yet at the same time it is affected by changes in the internal environment. General health maintenance requires maintenance of healthy skin. Skin changes may result from environmental changes (such as heat and cold, sunlight, and lack of moisture), from systemic disorders, and from disorders of the skin itself. In this chapter the major health problems of the skin of adults and surgical correction of impairments of the skin and underlying tissue (plastic surgery) are discussed. General assessment of the skin is discussed in Chapter 3.

■ ANATOMY AND PHYSIOLOGY

■ Anatomy

The skin is composed of two main layers, the epidermis and the dermis. The *epidermis* is composed of two parts, a thin layer of closely packed dead squamous cells covering a second layer of cells containing melanin, which gives skin its color. The dead cells are constantly being shed and replaced by deeper cells. Blood vessels do not reach into the epidermis (Fig. 39-1).

The second main layer, the *dermis*, is composed of bundles of collagen fibers that act to support the epidermis. It is well supplied with nerves and blood vessels and contains the sweat glands, sebaceous glands, and hair follicles.

Below the dermis is the subcutaneous tissue, consisting of loose connective tissue and fat. It is loosely attached to underlying structures in most body areas.

■ Physiology

The skin has numerous functions (see the box on p. 1379). Fat-soluble substances can penetrate the skin by passing through the hair follicles and sebaceous glands. Atrophic or senile skin contains fewer hair follicles; thus permeability of fat-soluble substances through the skin is decreased in the elderly.

The epidermis can be weakened by scraping or stripping the surface, such as by dry razors or by removal of tape. Once the barrier has weakened, permeability to substances such as bacteria or drugs is increased. Large amounts of drugs can be absorbed by extensive denuded skin areas. Epidermis that becomes overdry may crack and lead to breaks in the surface. If it remains wet for long periods, it becomes macerated and the moisture provides a medium for bacterial growth.

Blood vessels of the skin assist in control of body temperature by constriction in cold environments to promote

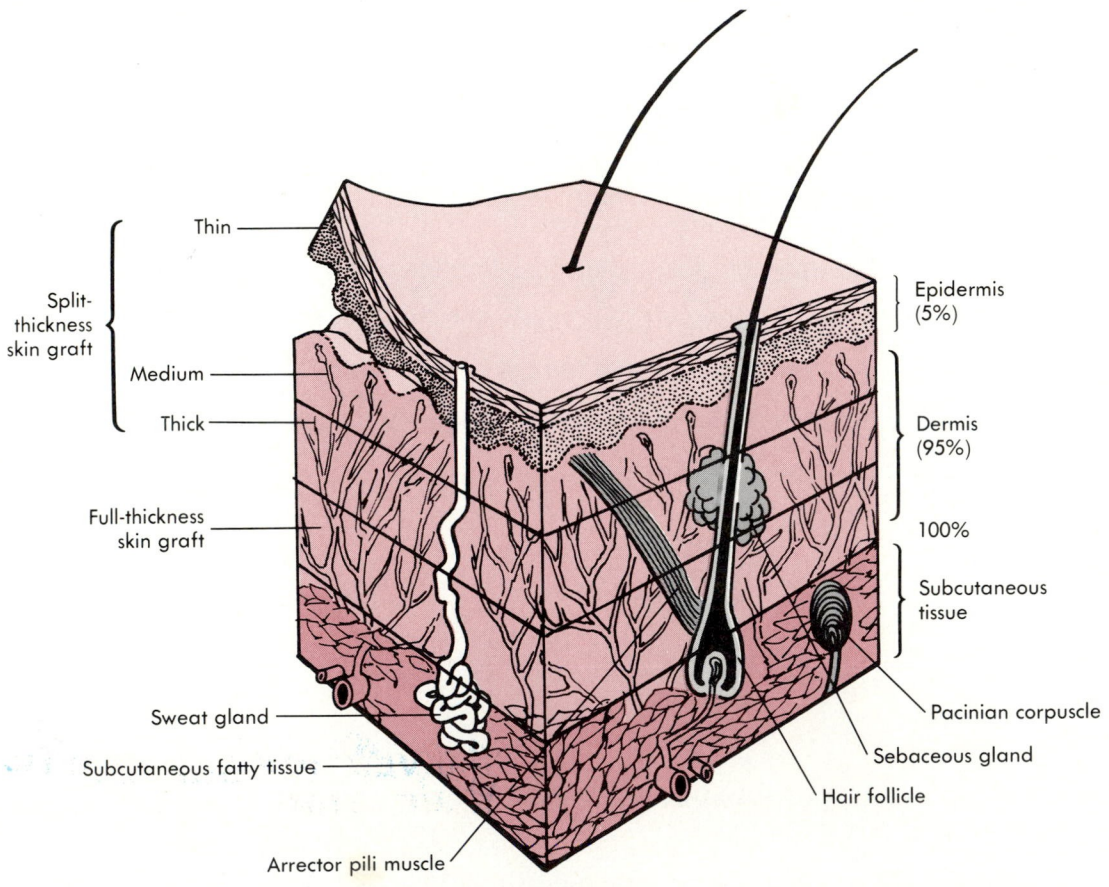

Fig. 39-1   Structures of the skin and skin layers.

Functions of the skin

Protection from environment; pathogenic organisms, foreign substances, heat, rays
Heat regulation
  Conduction: transfer of heat by direct contact to other objects or air
  Convection: removal of heat by air currents on skin
  Evaporation: removal of heat by water loss from skin surface
Sensory perception: sensory receptors in skin
Excretion: removal of water and electrolytes
Production of vitamin D: effect of sunlight

Table 39-1 Normal skin and hair changes seen in elderly persons

Assessment parameters	Changes caused by aging
Skin	
Color	Hyperpigmentation in exposed areas
	Hypopigmented areas
Moisture	Dry skin (sometimes scaly)
Elasticity, turgor	Decreased elasticity
	Loose folds
	Decreased turgor
Texture	Some rough areas
	Thinner, more transparent skin
Lesions	Skin tags on face and neck
	Seborrheic keratoses
	Senile angiomas
	Stasis dermatitis
	Bruises (capillary fragility)
Hair	
Consistency	Thinner on head and body
	More bristly on face, in nose
Distribution	Loss of hair on head and body
	Increased hair on face

conservation of heat and by dilation in warm environments to promote loss of heat by radiation. These mechanisms help maintain a constant internal body temperature.

Skin changes with aging

As people grow older changes occur in the skin and hair (Table 39-1) that make differentiating normal from abnormal changes more difficult. The changes result primarily from loss of subcutaneous tissue, degeneration of collagen and elastic fibers, loss of melanocytes, increased capillary fragility, decreased secretion of sweat glands, hormonal changes, and overexposure to environmental elements. The skin wrinkles and becomes looser, and spotty pigmentation develops on sun-exposed areas.

The elderly person is also more likely to have one or more chronic diseases and to be taking medications that can cause skin changes. Dry skin may cause itching and may lead to skin breakdown if scratched. Toenails become thicker and difficult to trim; fingernails become more brittle and develop longitudinal ridges. Body hair changes in consistency and distribution.

■ PSYCHOLOGIC EFFECTS OF DERMATOLOGIC PROBLEMS

There is a certain degree of "beauty orientation" in Western culture. Cosmetics to enhance good looks are extensively used by men and women. It is no wonder that skin diseases or physical defects that detract from "good looks" produce psychologic reactions.

Emotional reactions to a deformity or defect must not be underestimated. Pride in oneself, the ability to think well of oneself and to regard oneself favorably in comparison with others are essential to the development and maintenance of a well-integrated personality. Every person with a defect or handicap, particularly if it is conspicuous to others, suffers some threat to emotional security. The ex-

tent of the emotional reaction and the amount of maladjustment that follow depend on the individual's makeup and ability to cope with emotional insults. It is not unusual for the individual to withdraw from a society that is unkind. The defect may be used to justify failure to assume responsibility or to justify striking out against an unkind society.

Skin diseases that produce marked disfigurement of visible body surfaces can therefore result in alterations in body image. Feelings of decreased worth by persons with large draining lesions or with severe disfigurement are reinforced during interactions with others. Some people are repelled by the sight of severe skin diseases, or may experience a threat to their own body integrity and physically withdraw to avoid interaction. Some persons may experience nonverbal messages of disgust when others view their disfigurement for the first time. This is markedly poignant when those nonverbal messages are sent by significant others or by health professionals.

In working with the person with severe skin disease the nurse first examines his or her own feelings that could be expressed nonverbally in a negative manner. The patient and family are assisted to cope with their feelings.

■ PREVENTION AND HEALTH EDUCATION

Prevention of dermatologic conditions not only relieves the patient of discomfort but is cost effective because many skin conditions are chronic. In addition, maintenance of

---

Prevention of skin disorders

Maintenance of healthy skin

1. Avoid strong or harsh soaps or detergents.
2. Keep skin well hydrated; apply lubricating lotion or cream to dry areas after bathing.
3. Avoid scraping or stripping skin surface by dry razors or removal of tape.
4. Dry damp areas (such as between toes) well to prevent maceration of skin.
5. Wear loose clothing on hot days to permit loss of heat by evaporation.

Avoidance of causative agents

1. Avoid agents that cause skin disorders in most persons, for example, poison ivy, excessive sunlight.
2. Avoid specific agents known to cause a skin disorder in self.
3. Use protective skin lotions when exposed to excessive sunlight.

Observation of skin changes

1. Note and report changes in size, color, or general appearance of pigmented skin areas, particularly moles.
2. Note and report changes in size and appearance of existing skin lesions.

Avoidance of self-treatment

1. Do not use previously prescribed prescriptions on new and different skin lesions.
2. Seek medical advice when skin conditions develop.

---

intact healthy skin has a positive effect on one's well-being. Prevention of dermatologic conditions includes maintenance of healthy skin, avoidance of causative agents (when possible), observations of skin changes, and avoidance of self-treatment (see the box above).

Major health problems of the skin

There are numerous types of skin conditions, many of which only rarely occur. Some of the more common skin conditions discussed include the following:

1. Inflammatory skin conditions
   a. Bacterial infections: folliculitis, furuncles, and carbuncles
   b. Viral inflammations: herpes simplex, herpes zoster, warts
   c. Fungal inflammations: candidiasis, dermatophytoses
   d. Parasitic infestations: pediculosis, scabies
2. Acne
3. Dermatitis: contact, atopic, or stasis
4. Scaling papular disorders: psoriasis, pityriasis rosea, lichen planus
5. Tumors of the skin: keratoses, hemangiomas, premalignant lesions, malignant lesions
6. Skin disorders in blacks

■ INFLAMMATORY SKIN DISORDERS

■ Types of inflammatory skin disorders

The skin may become inflamed from bacteria, viruses, or funguses or by parasitic infestation.

■ BACTERIAL SKIN INFECTIONS

Most bacteria that normally inhabit the skin are nonpathogenic. Pathogenic bacteria that penetrate the outer skin layer may cause a superficial skin infection or superficial folliculitis or they may penetrate deeper, causing a deep folliculitis or a furuncle (Table 39-2).

Superficial folliculitis occurs most often with uncleanliness, maceration, exposure to oils and solvents, traction on the hair from tar therapy, or occlusion therapy. Furuncles and carbuncles occur most often in obese, poorly nourished, fatigued, or otherwise susceptible persons with poor hygiene, in debilitated elderly people, and in persons with inadequately treated diabetes mellitus.

■ VIRAL SKIN INFLAMMATIONS

Viruses may cause either simple or more serious skin inflammations (Table 39-3). One of the most common viruses found in humans is the *herpes simplex* virus (HSV). It occurs as two similar yet serologically different strands, type 1 and type 2. The type 1 virus is found primarily in lesions of the face and mouth (fever blister, cold sore), eye (keratitis), and brain (encephalitis). Type 2 is associated with lesions of the genitalia that can be transmitted by sexual contact (see Chapter 35). Factors that may precipitate recurrence of herpes simplex lesions include fever, upper respiratory tract infection, exhaustion, and stress. Lesions are also more common during the menses or after direct exposure to the sun's rays.

Herpes zoster (see Plate 1) is caused by the same virus (varicella zoster, V-Z) that causes varicella (chicken pox). Varicella is believed to be the primary infection in a nonimmune host, whereas herpes zoster is thought to be the response in a partially immune host. Although herpes zoster is far less communicable than chicken pox, persons who have not had chicken pox may develop it after exposure to the vesicular lesions of persons with herpes zoster. For this reason, susceptible persons should not care for patients with herpes zoster.

Table 39-2 Bacterial skin infections

Type	Description	Signs and symptoms	Medical therapy
Folliculitis	Infections of the hair follicles, primarily by *Staphylococcus;* occurs frequently after tar or occlusive therapy	Itching of hairy areas, pustules in hair follicles; abscess may develop	Saline or Burow's solution soaks; topical antibiotics
Furuncles (boil)	Deep folliculitis or nodule around hair follicle	Local swelling and redness; severe local pain; core turns yellow and "points" in 3 to 5 days; may rupture spontaneously	Systemic antibiotics; hot moist compresses (discontinued when drainage starts); incision and drainage (I & D); topical antibiotics after I & D
Carbuncle	Cluster of furuncles		
Cellulitis	Diffuse spreading infection of skin and subcutaneous tissue, usually resulting from cocci	Area is red, warm, swollen, painful with poorly defined borders; fever, malaise, leukocytosis	Hot moist dressings; systemic antibiotics; rest

Table 39-3 Viral skin inflammations

Type	Description	Signs and symptoms	Medical therapy
Herpes simplex (fever blister, cold sore)	Infection by herpes simplex virus; may occur anywhere but seen primarily on lips, mouth, genitalia	Initial burning and itching; appearance of painful, small, grouped vesicles; crust forms, healing within 10 to 14 days	Primarily symptomatic; early application of 70% alcohol or moistened styptic pencil may help; analgesics
Herpes zoster (shingles)	Acute vesicular eruption by the V-Z virus along a nerve pathway	Cluster of skin vesicles along course of peripheral sensory nerves; usually one side, primarily on thorax or face; crust develops and drops off in 10 to 14 days; pain, malaise, fever, itching; neuralgic pain may persist	Primarily symptomatic; relief of pain, rest; calamine lotion for itching; steroids to decrease incidence of neuralgia Postherpetic neuralgia: tranquilizers, vitamin E
Herpetic whitlow	HSV infection of finger seen most often in health care professionals	Vesicles on finger preceded by intense itching/pain; fever, chills, and malaise may occur	Primarily symptomatic; elevation and immobilization of finger; analgesics
Warts (verruca)	Benign growths from a viral infection; plantar warts on soles of feet grow inward; anogenital warts have a cauliflower appearance	Small, circumscribed, painless, hyperkeratotic papules, usually on hands, may disappear spontaneously; pain with plantar warts; itching with anogenital warts	Removal by electrodesiccation or cryosurgery

Herpes zoster can be serious in any adult and may even lead to death from exhaustion in elderly debilitated persons. It is one of the most drawn out and exasperating conditions found in elderly patients and leads to discouragement and demoralization. Contrary to popular thought, one episode of herpes zoster does *not* provide immunity, and the disease may recur.[46] Herpes zoster often occurs in persons with Hodgkin's disease and in those with lymphoid and some bone cancers, because of reduced cell-mediated immunity.

■ FUNGAL INFLAMMATIONS

Fungi are larger and more complex than bacteria. They may be unicellular, such as yeast, or multicellular, such as molds. Fungi may cause common skin disorders (Table 39-4).

Yeasts thrive in warm, moist environments such as the mouth and vagina. Problems occur when there is an overgrowth, commonly occurring with pregnancy, use of oral contraceptives, poor nutrition, antibiotic therapy, diabetes

Table 39-4 Fungal skin inflammations

Type	Description	Signs and symptoms	Medical therapy
Candidiasis (moniliasis)	Overgrowth of yeastlike fungus, primarily in mouth and vagina	Mouth: white spots like milk curd Vagina: cheesy discharge, itching	Ketoconazole (Nizoral) orally, nystatin (Mycostatin) orally or vaginally, clotrimazole (Mycelex) troches or vaginal cream
Dermatophytoses			
Tinea capitis	Fungal infection of scalp (ringworm of scalp)	Round lesion with erythema, slight scaling and some pustules around edge; temporary alopecia	Antifungal medication by shampoo or topical application
Tinea corporis	Fungal infection of nonhairy parts of body (ringworm of body)	Flat lesions with clear centers and red borders	Oral griseofulvin and topical application of antifungal medication
Tinea cruris	Fungal infection of groin (jock itch)	Brown to red lesion extending outward from groin, itching	Same as for tinea corporis
Tinea pedis (athlete's foot)	Fungal infection between and under toes	Cracks between toes, maceration, vesicular lesions; toenails may become thickened and discolored	Oral griseofulvin for weeks or months, antifungal topical medication

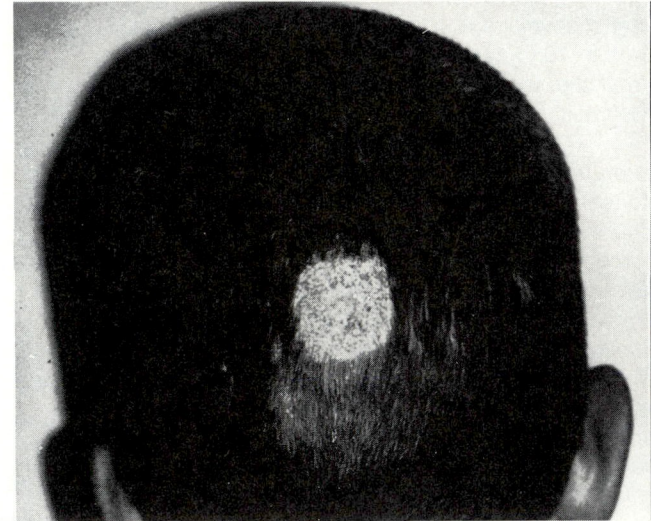
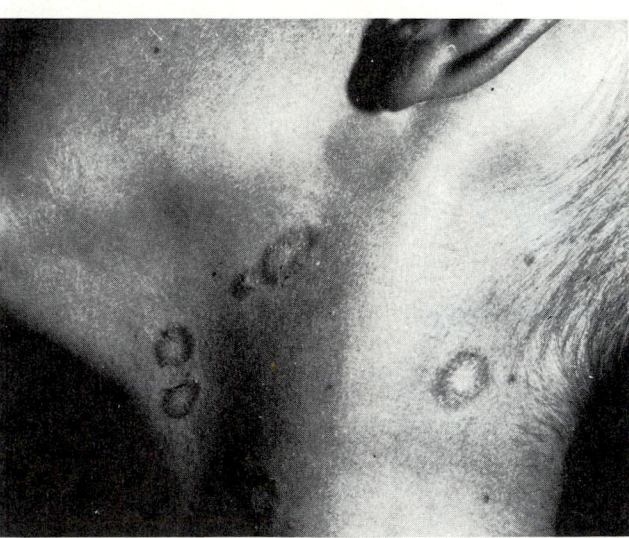

Fig. 39-2 **A,** Tinea capitis. **B,** Tinea corporis. (From Stewart, WD, Danto, JL, and Maddin, S: Dermatology; diagnosis and treatment of cutaneous disorders, ed 4, St. Louis, 1978, The CV Mosby Co.)

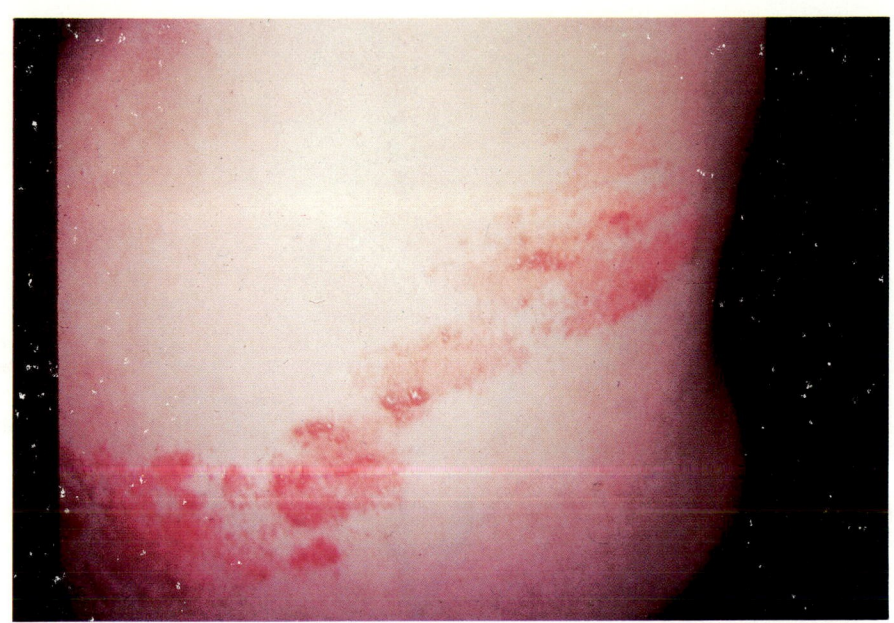

PLATE 1 Herpes zoster.

(Courtesy David Bickers, M.D., Cleveland, Ohio.)

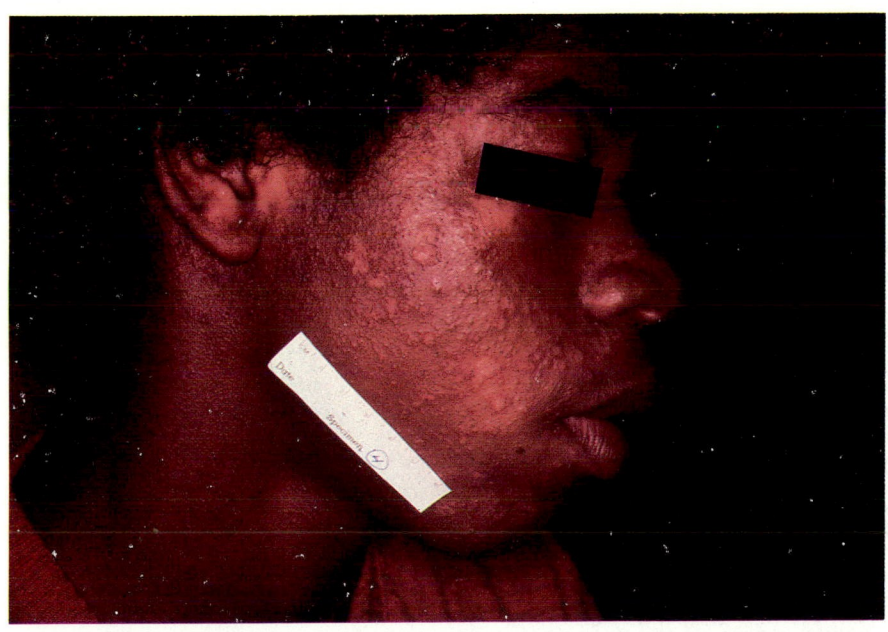

PLATE 2 Contact dermatitis from hair preparations.

(Courtesy David Bickers, M.D., Cleveland, Ohio.)

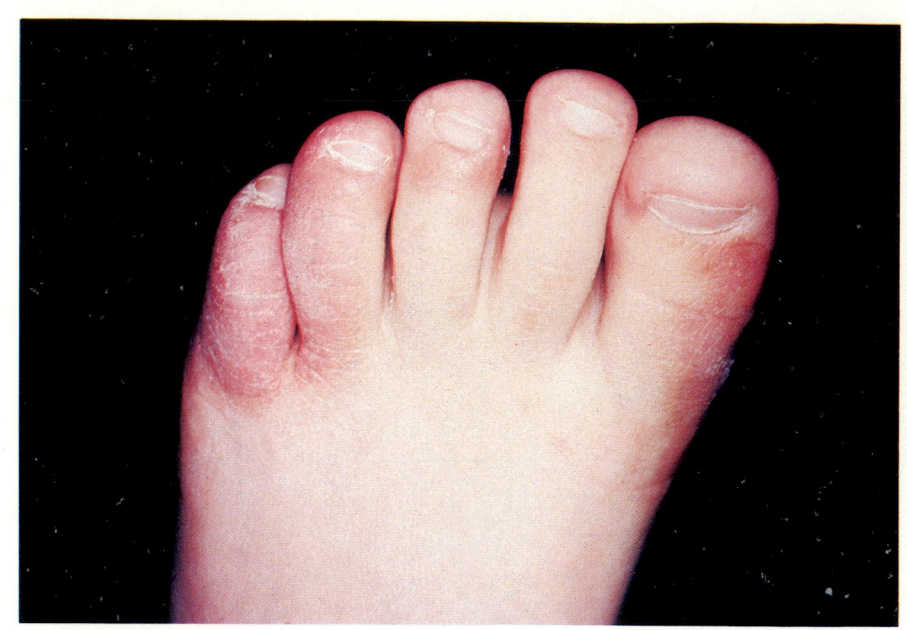

PLATE 3   Dermatitis from shoes.
(Courtesy David Bickers, M.D., Cleveland, Ohio.)

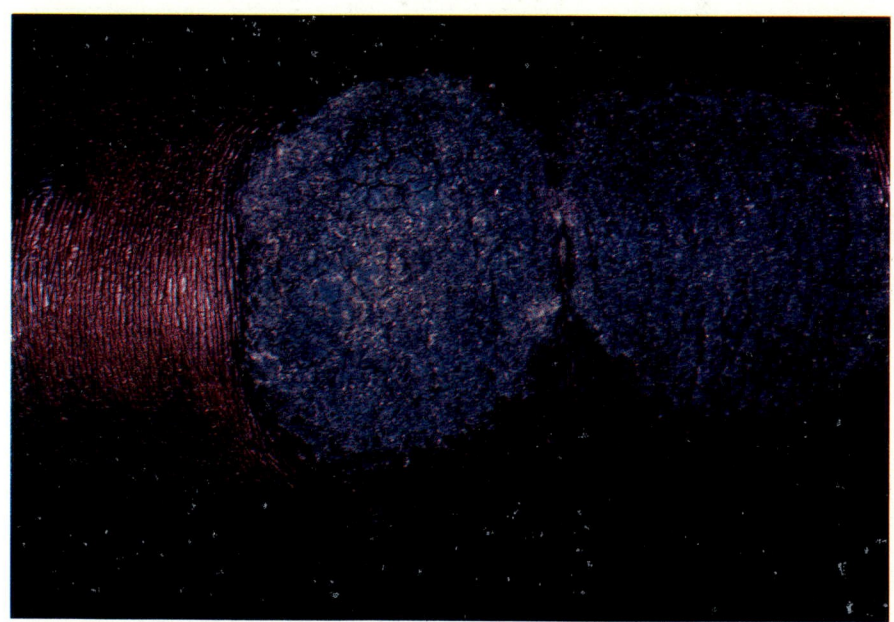

PLATE 4   Scaling lesions of psoriasis.
(Courtesy David Bickers, M.D., Cleveland, Ohio.)

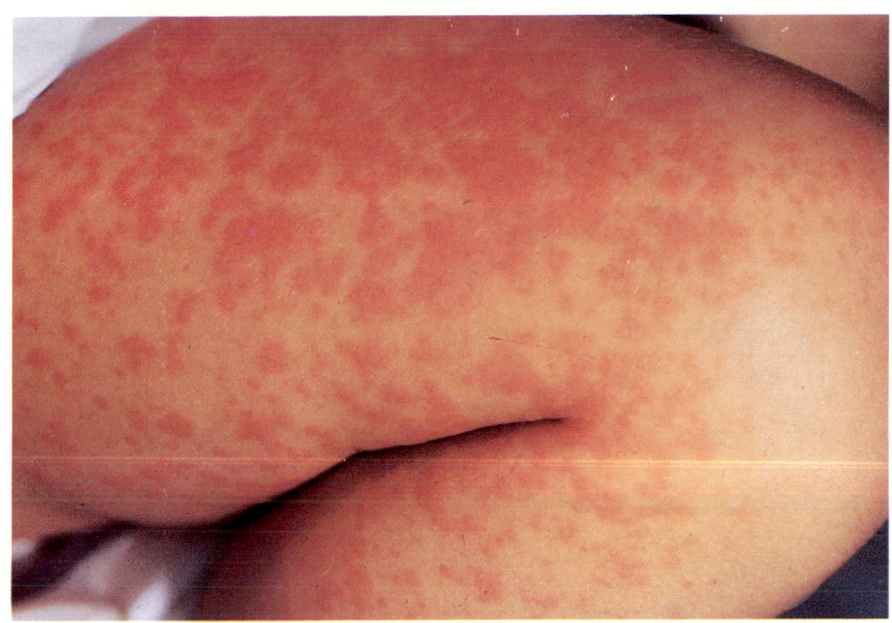

PLATE 5 Maculopapular rash resulting from a drug allergy.
(Courtesy David Bickers, M.D., Cleveland, Ohio.)

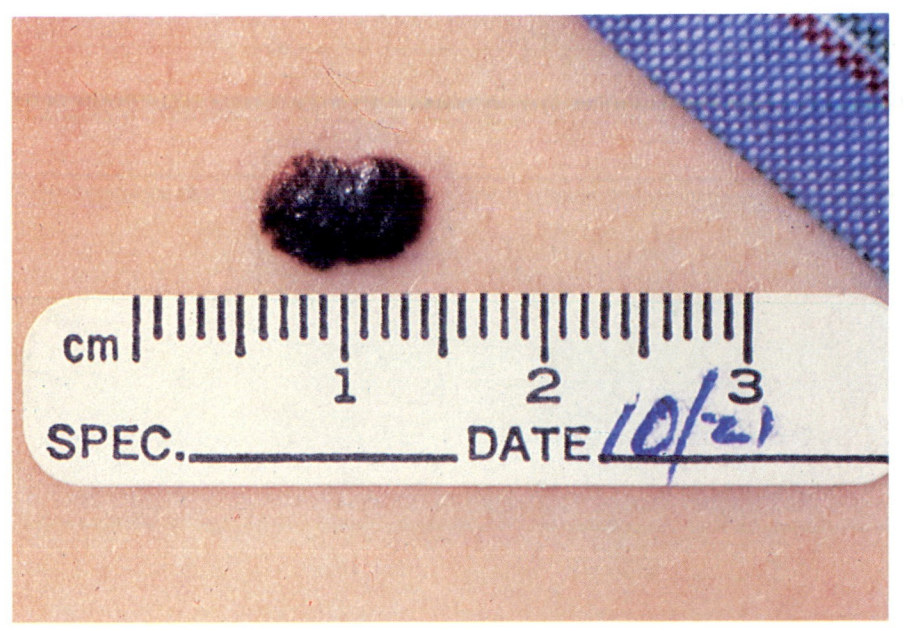

PLATE 6 Malignant melanoma.
(Courtesy David Bickers, M.D., Cleveland, Ohio.)

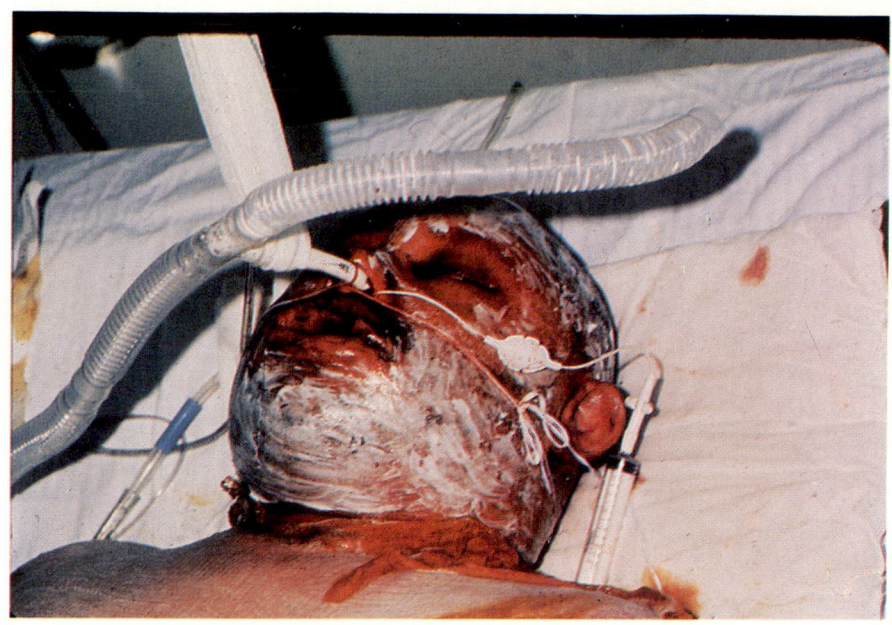

PLATE 7 Endotracheal intubation for patient with severe edema 5 hours postburn.

(Courtesy Burn Center, Cleveland Metropolitan General Hospital.)

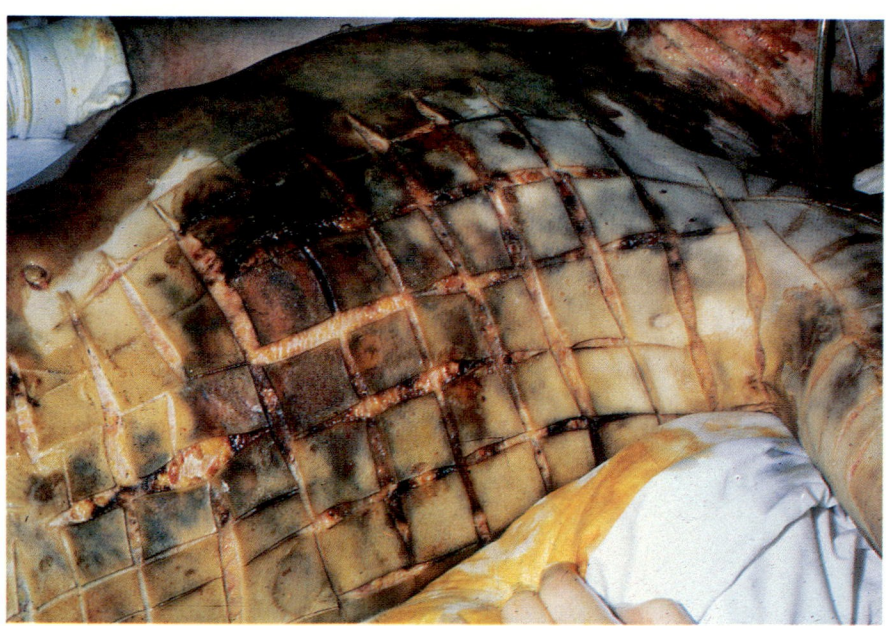

PLATE 8 Grid escharotomy used to alleviate circulatory and pulmonary constriction.

(Courtesy Burn Center, Cleveland Metropolitan General Hospital.)

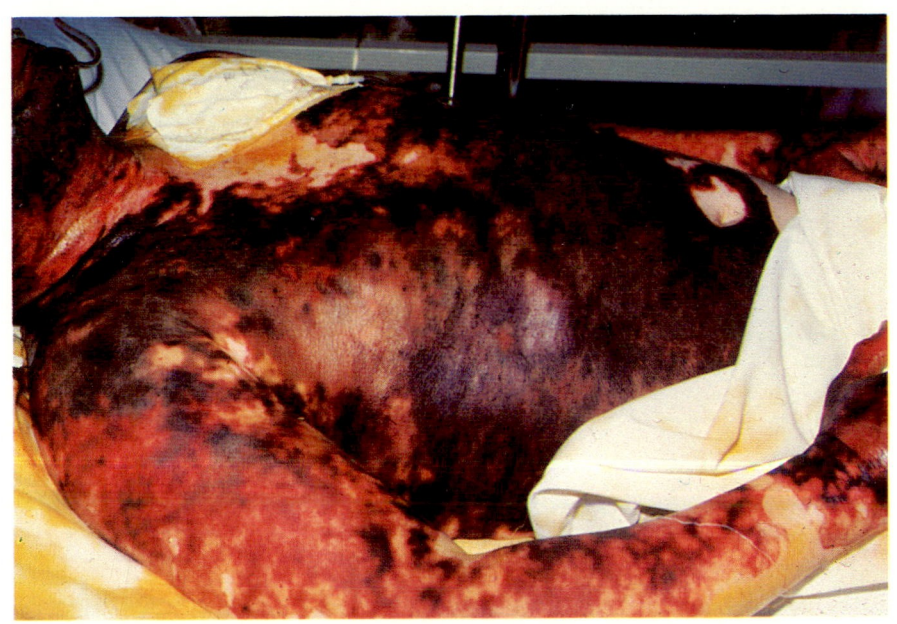

PLATE 9   Postburn *Pseudomonas* infection.

(Courtesy Burn Center, Cleveland Metropolitan General Hospital.)

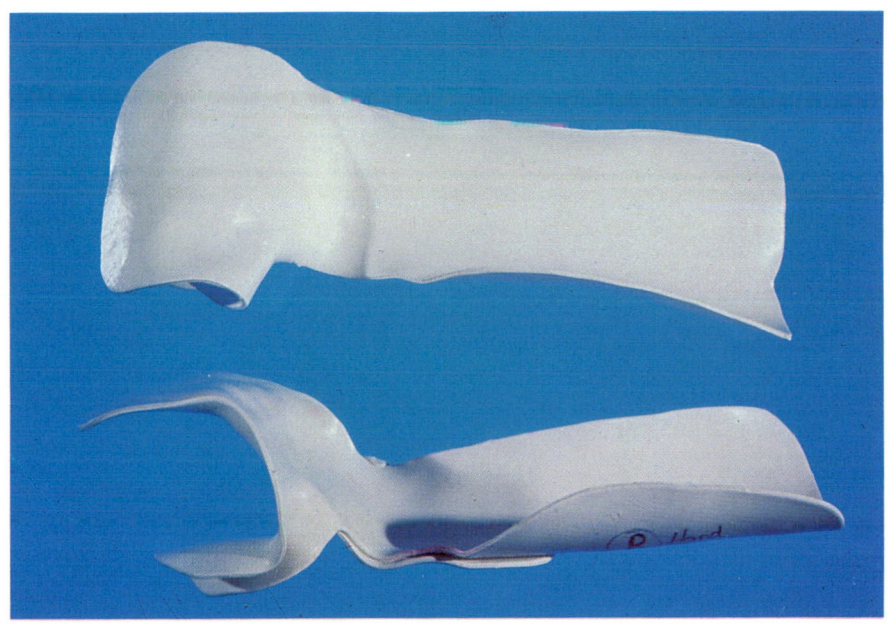

PLATE 10   Hand splints for burns.

(Courtesy Burn Center, Cleveland Metropolitan General Hospital.)

mellitus, other endocrine diseases, and immunosuppressed conditions. Oral candidiasis may be the first sign of AIDS or AIDS-related complex (ARC).[29]

The more common fungal infections are the dermatophytoses (tinea). Tinea *capitis* (Fig. 39-2) (inappropriately called ringworm of the scalp) is transmitted readily under crowded conditions where poor hygiene exists. Minor scalp trauma facilitates implantation of the spores; hence the infection can be spread by contaminated barber's instruments, combs, or sharp brushes. Tinea *cruris* (jock itch) occurs frequently in men, especially those who have tinea pedis and those who frequently wear athletic supporters or tight shorts, but it is being seen more frequently in women who wear tight pantyhose or slacks.

The most common dermatophytosis is tinea *pedis,* or athlete's foot. There are many misconceptions about prevention and treatment of athlete's foot (see box below).

Facts about athlete's foot

1. It is seen mostly in young men.
2. Walking barefoot in gymnasiums or around swimming pools does not necessarily lead to infection.
3. Prophylactic foot baths are ineffective.
4. Wearing white socks does not affect the course of infection.
5. Susceptible persons will acquire athlete's foot regardless of their activities.

It is often confused with other foot eruptions, such as contact dermatitis, psoriasis, or simple intertrigo (chronic bacterial infection of the areas between the toes, or intertriginous areas). Factors that may lessen infection include wearing sandal-type shoes or going barefoot (to decrease tissue moisture) and using good foot hygiene including washing the feet frequently and drying well between the toes.

■ PARASITIC INFESTATIONS

Parasites may live on the body or clothing (lice) or burrow under the skin (itch mite), causing inflammations of the skin (Table 39-5).

Lice obtain their nutrition by sucking blood from the skin. They leave their eggs on the skin surface attached to hair shafts, and this results in the transference from person to person. Control and treatment of pediculosis (lice infestation) can be hampered by persons of all incomes who refuse to admit that the lice exist among family members.

Scabies is highly prevalent during periods of overcrowding, such as that seen in Europe during World War II or in other war-torn areas. During the 1950s and 1960s the incidence of scabies decreased, but since the 1970s there has been a rise in the incidence of scabies worldwide. The reason for the pandemic is unknown and is thought to be multifactorial, including poverty, sexual promiscuity, increased worldwide travel, and ecologic changes.[48]

The itch mite penetrates the skin and lays eggs; the larvae mature in 10 days and move to the skin surface, where the female is impregnated; then the cycle is repeated. The incubation period varies, but often a long period elapses before symptoms are noted. Scabies occurs among all age groups and socioeconomic levels.

Table 39-5 Parasitic infestations

Type	Description	Signs and symptoms	Medical therapy
Pediculosis			
Head lice	Attach to hair shaft and lay eggs (nits); transmitted by direct contact	Itching of scalp, excoriation of skin, and secondary infection from scratching	Topical application of lindane (Kwell, Scabene), malathion (Prioderm), or pyrethrin (RID) by shampoo, lotion, or cream; combing with fine-toothed comb to remove nits
Body lice	Found in seams of underclothing; transmitted by direct contact, clothing, linens	Same as for head lice	Topical application of lindane or malathion by lotion or cream
Pubic lice	Resembles a tiny crab; nits are visible in pubic hair; transmitted by sexual contact, bed linen, towels	Same as for head lice	Same as for body lice
Scabies	Female itch mite burrows under skin and lays eggs; transmitted by prolonged contact	Severe itching; wavy brownish, thread-like lines seen mostly on hands, arms, and body folds and genitalia; secondary infections	Lindane (Kwell, Scabene), crotamiton (Eurax), or 4%/8% sulfur in petroleum

Assessment

Subjective data from persons with inflammations of the skin are centered on the extent of *itching* and *pain*. Data are collected concerning the site, intensity, duration, and methods found to be helpful in alleviation of the discomfort. Data are also collected concerning the person's knowledge of the type of infection, measures to control spread, and prescribed treatments to be carried out at home.

The skin is routinely assessed during physical inspection and whenever there is patient contact, such as while providing hygiene care, comfort measures, or prescribed treatments. Changes in previous lesions or occurrence of new lesions are reported.

Data analysis: nursing diagnoses

Nursing diagnoses are determined from assessment of patient data. Possible nursing diagnoses for the person with an inflammatory skin disorder may include, but are not limited to, the following:

Diagnostic title	Possible etiologies
Knowledge deficit	Lack of exposure or recall, information misinterpretation
Pain: itching	Skin lesions

Planning: expected patient outcomes

Expected patient outcomes for the person with an inflammatory skin disorder may include, but are not limited to, the following:
1. The patient states feeling comfortable.
2. The patient can describe measures to prevent spread.
3. The patient can describe prescribed treatment measures.
4. The patient can describe plans for medical follow-up for severe inflammatory disorders.

Implementation

ASSISTING WITH ACHIEVEMENT OF THERAPEUTIC GOALS

Inflammatory skin disorders are treated primarily by cleaning the lesions, then applying a topical medication. If pruritus or discomfort is present, antipruritic agents or analgesics may be prescribed. The nursing care of persons with bacterial, viral, or fungal inflammations, or with parasitic infestations are summarized in the box on p. 1387.

☐ Topical medications

Topical medications can be prepared in a variety of bases (Table 39-6). *Powders* are effective in reducing friction and moisture in intertriginous areas. The powders are first sprinkled into the hand, then applied to the skin to avoid releasing excess powder into the air and causing irritation to the mucous membrane. Powders are used sparingly to prevent caking and are not used on wet surfaces because this leads to caking. Cornstarch is *not* suggested, because it encourages growth of yeast, bacteria, and funguses.

Lotions must be shaken well because the insoluble powder may settle out. Lotions with a water or alcohol base are applied by patting gently. (Alcohol increases the cooling effect of the lotion.) A gauze pledget may be used to apply extremely thin lotions. Lotions with an oily base are applied thinly and evenly with the palm of the hand. A small area of skin is often tested to determine whether the cream or lotion will be tolerated over the entire body. The topical medication is applied to a small area (silver dollar size) on the person's forearm. The time and exact location of the trial are recorded, and the skin response to the trial medication is observed after 24 hours.

Ointments do not usually leave an oily residue on the skin unless they have a petrolatum base. A nonporous covering such as plastic should not be used over an ointment unless so prescribed, because the heat retention may increase percutaneous absorption of the medication.

Ointments may be applied with gloved hands or with the bare palm, depending on the type of ointment used. If a dressing is to be applied, the ointment may be spread on the dressing with a tongue blade before application to the skin. Anthralin may be caustic to normal skin, so gloves should be worn. Crude coal tar is always applied in firm, long, downward strokes to prevent folliculitis, because tar is an irritant. Creams, as opposed to ointments, may be rubbed in.

☐ Wet dermatologic dressings

Wet dressings are used frequently over various lesions for cooling, drying, antipruritic, vasoconstricting, or debriding effects. Plain tap water or physiologic saline solution may be used or medications may be added. An astringent effect may be obtained with the use of Burow's solution.

The type of dressing material used for a wet dressing should not have a cotton filling, because cotton leaves particles and a residue on the skin, which may cause irritation. Several layers of fine mesh gauze are ideal, and roller gauze or Kerlix may be used for extremities. A face mask may be designed by cutting openings for the eyes, nose, and mouth from several thicknesses of gauze. At home, muslin-type cotton material such as clean old sheets may be used; the materials need not be sterilized but are washed or discarded every 24 hours.

The best effects of wet dressings are obtained by several treatment periods spaced over the waking hours (see the box on p. 1385). The solution is applied at room temperature to prevent the marked vasoconstriction with subsequent vasodilation that occurs with cold solutions. Although the dressings can be kept wet by adding solution, this usually leads to excessive dripping.

Table 39-6   Comparison of vehicles for topical medications

Type	Base	Effect
Powder	Dry	Drying by absorbing moisture; cooling by evaporating moisture
Lotion	Powder suspended in water or oil	Protective, cleansing, cooling, antipruritic effect depending on drug and base used
Creams and ointments	Emulsions of oil and water	Occlusive covering over skin to prolong contact of medication with skin, good skin penetration, warming effect
Paste	≥50% powder in ointment base	Holds medication for longer period of time with slower skin penetration

---

Application of dermatologic wet dressings

1. Prepare solution to apply at room temperature. Sterility is not required.
2. Soak dressing thoroughly in solution.
3. Protect bed or clothing with towel or bath blanket.
4. Wring out dressing (should be wet but not dripping).
5. Apply dressings in smooth layers (two to four layers); wrap fingers and toes separately; wrap joints so that they can bend.
6. Remove, soak, and reapply dressings every 3 to 5 minutes.
7. Continue treatment for 20 to 30 minutes.
8. Pat skin dry.

Common causes of itching

Dry skin
Skin irritants: plastic or glass fibers, wool, plant products
Insects
Drug reactions
Psychogenic reactions
Skin diseases: inflammations, dermatitis
Infectious diseases
Systemic diseases: obstructive biliary disease, uremia, diabetes mellitus
Neoplasia: Hodgkin's disease, leukemia, lymphoma

■ PROMOTING COMFORT

Pain with skin inflammations is usually minimal except in selected situations such as herpes zoster. In general, aspirin or acetaminophen usually suffice as analgesics, and the application of wet dressings and topical medications usually relieves most discomfort from pain.

☐ Relief of pruritus

Pruritus (itching) is a major discomfort, to one extent or another, with skin inflammations.

☐ *Pathophysiology of pruritus*

Pruritus is a cutaneous symptom that provokes the desire to scratch and is an underlying symptom of many disorders. It is a modified form of pain but is less tolerable. It occurs only in the skin, certain mucous membranes, and the eyes. The areas most sensitive to itching are the nostrils, mucocutaneous junction, external ear canal, and perineum.

One of the most common causes of pruritus is dry skin, sometimes occurring as a result of excessive bathing, particularly with bubble bath, which has a drying effect.

Other causes of pruritus are listed in the box above. Factors that can intensify itching include vasodilation, tissue anoxia, and stasis of circulation.

Pruritus leads to the motor response of scratching. Persons with very intense itching may excoriate the skin severely by digging deeply into the skin with their fingernails when trying to alleviate the itch. Persons with generalized itching may be observed to be in almost constant motion—twisting, rubbing, and scratching.

☐ *General management for relief of pruritus*

1. Apply cold to cause vasoconstriction.
2. Avoid soaps and detergents with dry skin; use a bath oil.
3. Hydrate in a tepid bath followed by application of an emollient lotion.
4. Use cool, light, nonrestrictive clothing or bedclothes.
5. Keep nails trimmed to avoid skin excoriation from scratching.
6. Keep the room cool (about 20° C, or 68° to 70° F) and increase the humidity (30% to 40%).

Table 39-7 Preparations commonly used for baths or soaks

Substance	Effect	Suggested actions
Colloids: oatmeal, cornstarch, soybean powder	Antipruritic, drying	Tub surfaces become very slippery; support person to prevent falls
Potassium permanganate	Antifungal, drying, deodorizing	Strain pulverized tablet through cheesecloth to prevent irritation; stains surfaces and linens
Burow's solution (aluminum acetate)	Antibacterial, drying	Commonly used for soaks
Sulfur bath suspension	Antibacterial	Rinse body with tepid water after bath to remove residual sulfur particles
Tar preparations	Antipruritic, moisturizing	Do not use soap with tar baths
Bath oils: Alpha-Keri, Jeri-Bath, Domol	Antipruritic, moisturizing	Tub surfaces may become slippery

---

Guidelines for baths and soaks

1. The water temperature should be of comfort to patient—usually 32° to 38° C (90° to 100° F).
2. Medication should be completely dissolved while tub is filled.
3. The soak should last 20 to 30 minutes.
4. Persons are assisted out of the water when oils are added, to prevent slipping.
5. A rubber mat will help prevent slipping.
6. Skin is *patted* dry, not rubbed, to avoid skin irritation.
7. Creams or ointments are applied immediately after the bath to retain moisture.
8. After a medicated bath, pour 1 cup bleach into used tub water; let stand 5 minutes; wipe sides and bottom of tub; drain tub and clean as usual.

□ *Baths and soaks*

Tub baths or soaks to a specific part of the body are soothing and antipruritic and are an effective means of rehydrating the skin. Substances may be added to the bath for special therapeutic effects (Table 39-7). Guidelines for baths and soaks are listed in the box above.

■ TEACHING

□ Prevention of spread

Bacterial infections and parasitic infestations may spread to other persons, particularly caregivers and family members, if precautions are not instituted.

For *staphylococcal* infections in hospitalized patients, wound isolation procedures are instituted until drainage subsides. Hands must be washed thoroughly after contact with the patient. Gloves are usually worn when changing dressings.

It is not uncommon for entire families to have some type of staphylococcal infection after one member has had a boil. Teaching includes the following:

1. All family members should bathe and shampoo daily with bacteriostatic soap while infection lasts.
2. Razor blades are discarded after use.
3. Separate bath linens are used by each family member.
4. Bath linens are changed daily while infection lasts.
5. Contaminated wound supplies are discarded in two sealed plastic bags.

With *parasitic* infestations, all family members should take one treatment to prevent spread. Clothing, linen, and towels are washed, then dried in an automatic dryer or ironed after line drying, or are dry cleaned. Garments that have been stored for 1 month will not be infested. No special precautions are needed for other objects, because parasites do not live long away from the host.

When caring for persons with *herpetic* lesions, the Centers for Disease Control (CDC) recommends the use of drainage and secretion precautions (see Chapter 11) until all lesions are crusted. Finger infection (herpetic whitlow, Table 39-3) may result from contact with the herpes simplex virus. To help prevent a disseminated infection, strict isolation precautions are used for protection of the immunocompromised person with a localized herpes zoster infection.

□ Self-help skills

Many persons with skin inflammations will be carrying out treatments at home and, therefore, may need teaching about therapeutic measures. Written instructions are more likely to be followed correctly. Points to stress in teaching include the following:

1. Use medication only as prescribed.
2. Avoid harsh rubbing of the skin.
3. Avoid nonporous covering over dressing unless ordered.

Nursing care of the patient with inflammatory skin disorders

Bacterial infections

1. Cleanse skin well with soap and water or with hexachlorophene.
2. Use wet compresses to apply heat or as a medium for medication (for example, Burow's solution).
3. Apply prescribed antibiotic topical medication.
4. Elevate an extremity with cellulitis.
5. Teach family members how to prevent spread of staphylococcal infections:
   a. Avoidance of contamination from drainage
   b. Cleansing practices
   c. Disposal of contaminated articles

Viral inflammations

1. Assist with relief of pain and pruritus:
   a. Loose clothing to minimize contact
   b. Analgesics as prescribed
   c. Warm moist compresses
   d. Spirits of camphor or camphorated lip ice to oral lesions of herpes simplex
   e. Neuralgia after herpes zoster:
      (1) Analgesics as prescribed (narcotics are usually avoided)
      (2) Tranquilizers and sedatives as prescribed
      (3) Ethyl chloride spray for possible temporary relief
      (4) Other forms of pain relief measures (see Chapter 12) that might be helpful
   f. Calamine lotion over vesicular areas to relieve itching

Fungal inflammations

1. Promote dryness of affected area:
   a. Area dried well after washing
   b. Powders applied lightly to prevent maceration and caking
   c. Clean loose-fitting clothing for aeration
   d. For athlete's foot, cotton socks, changed at least daily; sandal-type shoes when possible
2. Promote healing:
   a. Prescribed topical medication
   b. Need for continuation of treatment for prescribed time (may be weeks or months)

Parasitic infestations

1. Wash area well before treatment.
2. Remove nits with a fine-toothed comb.
3. Apply a *thin* layer of prescribed lotion or cream.
4. Shampoo, shower, or bathe thoroughly after 24 hours to remove medication.
5. If eyelashes are involved, remove nits and apply petroleum jelly to smother lice.
6. Give analgesics or antipruritic agents as necessary.
7. Teach prevention of spread to all family members:
   a. Machine wash clothing and bed linens
   b. Dry clothing and linens in dryer or iron after line drying
   c. Dry clean clothing that cannot be washed
   d. Treat all family members if one is infested

---

4. Dissolve completely all solid medications added to baths and soaks.
5. Apply lotions and powders in thin layers.
6. Use old clean sheets, if desired, for wet dressings.

⌗ Evaluation

Evaluation is based on expected patient outcomes. Questions to ask may include the following: Is the person comfortable? Does the person know how to care for the lesions at home?

■ ACNE VULGARIS

Acne vulgaris is a common skin disorder seen mostly in adolescents, although it may also occur in adults. The cause of acne is still unknown but is thought to be multifactorial. Some causes that have been proposed are free fatty acids, endocrine effects, stress, heredity, and infection. Diet has been essentially ruled out as a causative factor. The disorder is more quiescent in summer months.

■ Prevention

Actions that contribute to plugging of the pilosebaceous follicles are to be avoided.

1. Keep hair and hands away from face.
2. Shampoo hair and scalp frequently.
3. Wear loose clothing and avoid tight collars.
4. Keep skin clean; avoid greasy, oil-based cosmetics.
5. Avoid any foods that appear to cause acne flare-ups.

■ Pathophysiology

At puberty sebaceous glands undergo enlargement from androgen stimulation. When sebum is released it passes through the follicular canal, where it is combined with sebaceous gland cell fragments, epidermal cells, and bacteria. The sebum and debris may become plugged in the hair follicle (Fig. 39-3) to form an open comedo (blackhead) if it is at the surface, or a closed comedo (whitehead) if it is below the surface. The dark color of the blackhead is melanin, not dirt, and results from passage of melanin from the adjoining epidermal cells.

Inflammatory lesions apparently develop from escape of sebum into the dermis; the sebum then serves as an irritant, causing an inflammatory reaction. Free fatty acids may also be an irritant in the follicle itself.

Acne occurs mostly on the face and neck, upper chest, and back, although the upper arms, buttocks, and thighs may also be involved. Comedones are the first visible signs, and the skin is characteristically oily. The inflammatory lesions include papules, pustules, nodules, and cysts. Superficial lesions usually heal without scarring, whereas large lesions often result in scarring. The typical scar resembles an old volcano (ice-pick scar); however, many other sizes and shapes may result, depending on the depth and extent of the inflammatory lesions.

■ Interventions

The major medical therapy for acne is with drug therapy, particularly topical application (see the box below). Comedones may be removed with a comedo extractor. Disfiguring scars may be removed by dermabrasion (p. 1402).

Counseling and teaching are the major nursing therapies. Stress appears to be one of the causative factors; therefore, the person may be helped by identifying and coping with stressors (Chapter 7). Acne can be a stressor, producing facial disfigurements and sometimes leading to behavior that is hostile, aggressive, and anxious, as well as shy and withdrawn. Psychologic counseling is often desirable. Teaching the person with acne includes the following:

1. General skin care
   a. Keep skin clean; wash face two to three times daily.
   b. Use a medicated soap/cleanser (see the box below) or agent prescribed by physician.

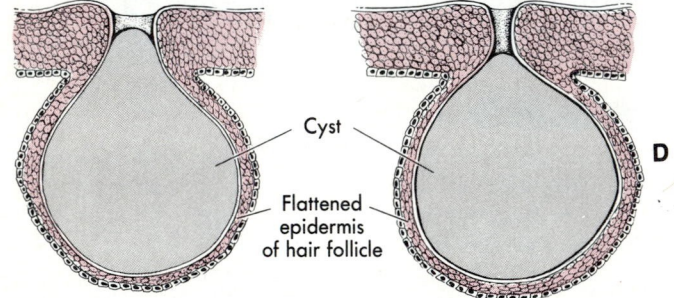

Fig. 39-3 Formation of lesions in acne vulgaris. **A,** Open comedo (blackhead), early stage. **B,** Closed comedo (whitehead), early stage. **C,** Cyst formation in open comedo, advanced stage. **D,** Cyst formation in closed comedo, advanced stage. (From Dermatology and skin care by JH Parrish. Copyright © 1975 by McGraw-Hill Book Co. Used with the permission of McGraw-Hill Book Co.)

Drug therapy for acne vulgaris

Topical therapy

Benzoyl peroxide
Vitamin A acid (tretinoin)
Topical antibiotics (erythromycin, tetracycline)
Sulfur-zinc lotion

Systemic therapy

Isotretinoin (Accutane)
Systemic antibiotics (tetracycline)
Estrogens for females (if needed)

Intralesional therapy

Corticosteroids

Selected cleansers/soaps useful for acne

Acnaveen
Acne-aid detergent soap
Acne cleansing soap
Epi-Clear
Fostex cake
Ionax foam
Neutrogena
Seba-Nil

c. Avoid vigorous rubbing of the skin.

d. Use cosmetics that are water based rather than cream based and avoid those that contain wax esters.

e. Never leave cosmetics on face at night.

2. During therapy

a. Follow the prescribed therapy even when immediate improvement is not noted for 2 to 3 weeks.

b. Expect skin desquamation during therapy.

c. Avoid using self-remedies during therapy.

d. Remove cosmetics before applying topical medications.

e. Avoid exposure to direct sunlight if using tretinoin or taking tetracycline (photosensitivity).

f. Avoid pregnancy if taking Accutane (possibility of birth defects).

■ DERMATITIS

Dermatitis, a superficial inflammation of the skin, refers to several different conditions resulting in the same type of lesions (Table 39-8). The term *eczema* is often used synonymously with dermatitis but frequently refers to the chronic type.

■ Pathophysiology

Contact dermatitis may result from irritation of the skin from the substance itself (*irritant contact dermatitis*) (see Plates 2 and 3) or from a hypersensitivity immune reaction from contact with a *specific* antigen (*allergic contact dermatitis*) (Table 39-9). The sensitizing allergen may reach the site by direct contact; by indirect contact such as transmission by animals, from one part of the body to the other, by the hands, or on clothing; or by the air such as in smoke.

Atopic dermatitis is hereditary hypersensitivity of the skin that lowers the threshold to pruritus so that minor stimuli cause intense itching. Exacerbating factors include sudden changes in temperature or humidity; exercise; psychologic stress; fibers such as wool, fur, or nylon; detergents; and perfumes. There is a marked tendency toward vasoconstriction of superficial blood vessels, and the skin blanches readily. Adults with eczema often have had atopic dermatitis during infancy and adolescence.

Persons with atopic dermatitis are highly susceptible to viral infections, especially herpes, and to bacterial infections such as those caused by *Staphylococcus* or beta hemolytic *Streptococcus*. There is also an increased incidence of fungal infections such as tinea.

■ Assessment

■ SUBJECTIVE DATA

When acute lesions from contact dermatitis or exacerbation of eczema occur, it is important to identify the causative factors in order to avoid further contacts or to change, if possible, any exacerbating factor. Data to collect initially include the following:

1. Knowledge of causative factors and method of contact

2. Possible contacts with irritants in the home, at work, or during recreational activities

3. History of recurrent infections (possible decreased immune response)

4. New drug prescriptions, especially penicillin or sulfanilamide

5. Increase in stress noted by patient

Table 39-8 Types of dermatitis

Type	Cause	Signs and symptoms	Medical therapy
Contact	External agents: irritants (mechanical, chemical, biologic) or allergens	Site and pattern of lesions depend on exposure pattern; erythema, local edema, vesicles, then oozing, crusting and scaling; pruritus Chronic: skin becomes brownish and thickened	Weeping uninfected lesions: wet dressings with Burow's solution; topical steroids; systemic antibiotics when infection present
Atopic	Hypersensitivity reaction, hereditary	Pruritus; lesions similar to contact dermatitis; become localized in adults to antecubital and popliteal areas, behind ears, under chin	Same as above
Stasis	Decreased circulation in legs	Skin reddened and edematous, pruritus, infection from excoriations with scratching	Elevation of legs; wet compresses for weeping lesions
Seborrheic (dandruff)	Unknown	Erythematous scaly lesions of scalp, face, ears, chest, or back	Selsun Blue shampoo for scalp; topical steroids for severe lesions

Table 39-9 Common causes of contact dermatitis of different areas

Area	Cause
Face	Cosmetics, hair sprays, hair dyes, airborne contactants
Earlobes	Nickel
Ears	
Pinnae	Photosensitizers
Canals	Medications
Eyelids	Cosmetics, airborne sensitizers, transfer by hands
Nose (bridge)	Metal or plastic spectacle supports
Lips and perioral area	Toothpaste, lipstick
Neck	Perfumes, clothing (especially wool)
Axillae	Deodorants, clothing, perfumes
Scapular area	Nickel in clasps on straps
Breasts	Elastic and other brassiere material
Waist	Elastic
Perianal area	Dibucaine (Nupercaine) and other medications, excessive use of cleansers
Arms and legs	Poison ivy and other plants
Wrists	Nickel, etc. in watchbands
Hands	Detergents and other cleansers, gloves
Feet	Medication for "athlete's foot," shoes

From Moschela, SL, Pillsbury, DM, and Hurley, HJ: Dermatology, Philadelphia, 1975, WB Saunders Co.

6. Alleviating factors (physician or self-prescribed)
7. Extent of pruritus and alleviating factors

■ OBJECTIVE DATA

The lesions are inspected daily for changes and presence of infections. Obsevations are also made concerning the extent of scratching of the lesions by the patient.

■ DIAGNOSTIC TESTS

Hypersensitivity to specific antigens can be tested in vivo by skin tests or by the use test (Chapter 38). In skin testing, the antigens are administered to the skin either through intradermal, scratch or patch tests, or an allergen may be instilled in the eye.

Data analysis: nursing diagnoses

Nursing diagnoses are determined from assessment of patient data. Possible nursing diagnoses for the person with dermatitis may include, but are not limited to, the following:

Diagnostic title	Possible etiologies
Knowledge deficit	Lack of exposure/recall, information misinterpretation
Pain: itching	Skin lesions

Planning: expected patient outcomes

Expected patient outcomes for the person with dermatitis may include, but are not limited to, the following:
1. The patient states itching is decreased.
2. The patient can describe:
   a. Causative agents (if known), source of the agent, and method of control
   b. Measures to prevent further contact
   c. Problems of self-treatment
   d. Treatment measures to be carried out at home

Implementation

■ ASSISTING WITH ACHIEVEMENT OF THERAPEUTIC GOALS

□ Promoting healing of lesions

Weeping infected lesions respond rapidly to wet dressings with Burow's solution (p. 1384) for 20 minutes four times daily. Crusts and scales are not removed but are allowed to drop off naturally as the skin heals.

The major form of *topical* therapy consists of corticosteroid cream or ointment. Fluorinated corticosteroids may be used for localized lesions in adults but are *never used on the face*. An occlusion wrap over the steroid in adults may enhance the steroid effect but may lead to folliculitis. The occlusion wrap consists of a nonpermeable covering, such as plastic wrap, over the dressing; it is only applied when prescribed by the physician.

Teaching for the patient with dermatitis

1. Nature of the causative agent (if known) and method of contact; avoidance of agent
2. Avoidance of extremes of heat and cold
3. Avoidance of dry skin:
   a. No harsh soaps and detergents (use a mild soap such as Ivory)
   b. Soak in bath water (oil may be added) for 20 to 30 minutes
   c. Steroid cream directly after bath
4. Avoidance of wool, nylon, or fur fibers on sensitized skin
5. Use of gloves if necessary to handle irritant or allergenic substance
6. Limiting of strenuous exercise, especially in hot weather (leads to itching)
7. Exposure of affected areas to sunlight (improves condition)
8. Dangers of self-treatment (may lead to delay in healing and increase in infected lesions or to increased absorption through denuded skin areas)
9. Avoidance of other persons with infections (for those with atopic dermatitis)

■ PROMOTING COMFORT

The focus of care is relief of the pruritus in order to break the itch-scratch cycle that leads to lesions and discomfort. Measures to promote relief of itching are described on p. 1385. Application of the wet dressings and topical steroids helps to reduce the itching. Colloidal baths may be helpful. Sedation and tranquilizers are used judiciously to help decrease itching but not induce sleepiness.

■ TEACHING

The more the person knows about the condition and what will affect it, the better the person can prevent further contacts and enhance recovery. Teaching includes avoidance of exacerbating factors, positive effects of sunlight, and dangers of self-treatment (see the box above).

■ Evaluation

Evaluation is based on expected patient outcomes. Questions to ask may include the following: Is itching decreased? Does the person know how to care for the skin at home and how to prevent further recurrence?

■ SCALING PAPULAR DISORDERS

Papulosquamous disorders are characterized by papular lesions with scaling borders. The most common of these is *psoriasis* (Table 39-10). There are no precipitating factors for psoriasis, but some persons may develop exacerbations after climatic changes, stress, trauma, or infection. Pregnant women often see a remission of symptoms.

■ Pathophysiology of psoriasis

The turnover time for normal skin is 28 days. After the cells in the basal layer of the skin divide, it normally takes them 14 days to reach the stratum corneum (outer skin layer) and an additional 14 days for the cells to be sloughed off. In psoriasis the time is accelerated to 4 to 7 days. Much of the scaling (see Plate 4) seen in psoriasis is rapid shedding of the cells; treatment is therefore based on slowing the mitotic activity.

■ Assessment

Subjective data include the following:
1. Knowledge about the disease
2. Measures used for control at home
3. Concerns about appearance
4. Usual recreational and social activities
Objective data include observations regarding changes in the lesions.

■ Data analysis: nursing diagnoses

Nursing diagnoses are determined from assessment of patient data. Possible nursing diagnoses for the person with psoriasis may include, but are not limited to, the following:

Diagnostic title	Possible etiologies
Body image disturbance	Change in body appearance
Knowledge deficit	Lack of exposure/recall, information misinterpretation

■ Planning: expected patient outcomes

Expected patient outcomes for the person with psoriasis may include, but are not limited to, the following:
1. The person can describe the nature of the disorder (noncurable, recurrence of symptoms).
2. The person can describe problems with self-medication.
3. The person can describe the prescribed treatment program.
4. The person can describe plans for socialization with others.

Table 39-10 Types of papulosquamous disorders

Type	Characteristic	Signs and symptoms	Medical therapy
Psoriasis	Common hereditary chronic disorder; not infectious or contagious; has periods of exacerbation	Elevated, erythematous, sharply circumscribed, scaling plaques; occur mostly on scalp, elbows, and knees; mild pruritus; nails become yellowed and pitted	Wet dressings with acute flare ups; topical steroids with occlusive wraps; PUVA therapy; coal tar therapy followed by ultraviolet light
Pityriasis rosea	Common skin disorder in young adults, especially women; not contagious; lasts 6 to 8 weeks, rarely recurs	Starts with single lesion; oval, thin scaly border, yellowish center; multiple lesions appear later; pruritus	Topical steroids; systemic steroids in severe cases
Lichen planus	Common skin disorder; may resolve in 6 to 18 months or become chronic	Shiny flat-topped papules on flexor surfaces of wrists, ankles, trunk, and mucous membranes; severe pruritus; nails become distorted	Topical steroids with occlusive wrap; intralesional or systemic steroids, PUVA therapy

---

NURSING CARE PLAN

Person with psoriasis

DATA: Mrs. Lee, age 35, was referred to a psoriasis day-care center for a 6-day Goeckerman regimen therapy (crude tar with exposure to ultraviolet light). Mrs. Lee told the nurse that she recently sent away for a new ointment that was supposed to cure her psoriasis, but the lesions began to flare up and itching increased. She also said that her husband has been urging her to go out with him more to social events, but her arms and legs have "looked so bad" that she has not wanted others to see her until she is better.

Nursing diagnosis: Body image disturbance: related to lesions on arms and legs

Expected patient outcomes	Nursing interventions	Rationale
Patient states plans to go out socially with husband	Help Mrs. Lee identify her positive attributes Discuss with Mrs. Lee types of clothing that could hide the more obvious lesions	Awareness of positive attributes helps to increase self-esteem Hiding the lesions may help her feel better about herself and increase her desire to interact with others

Nursing diagnosis: Knowledge deficit related to information misinterpretation

Expected patient outcomes	Nursing interventions	Rationale
Patient describes chronicity of psoriasis and plans to follow only prescribed treatment	Review her understanding of the nature of psoriasis Explain the lack of cure for psoriasis and problems with self-treatment Suggest she discuss with physician lotions or ointments to use after her present treatment when lesions itch or flare up Review with her how to apply ointments	Lesions may fade with treatment only to recur. Self-treatment products are often ineffective and costly Ointment is more effective if spread in thin layer over plaques

▚ Implementation

■ ASSISTING WITH ACHIEVEMENT OF THERAPEUTIC GOALS

Although there are several therapeutic regimens for psoriasis (Table 39-11), the more common treatments are steroids under occlusive wraps, crude tar therapy, and PUVA therapy.

☐ Application of occlusive wrap

Occlusive wraps are usually prescribed over topical steroid therapy for psoriasis. Plastic wrap or plastic bags may be used to cover large areas. The bags should not be rapidly flammable. If large areas must be covered for home therapy, a plastic exercise body suit can be worn, particularly for overnight therapy.

☐ Crude tar therapy

Coal tar preparations may be applied as a topical medication, as a bath (Balnetar), or in combination with ultraviolet light (UVA). In the latter case the tar preparation is applied 12 hours before the UVA treatment. Estar Gel or Fototar are applied to the affected area for 5 minutes, then the excess is removed by patting with tissue to minimize staining. Areas treated with coal tar preparation should be protected from direct sunlight for at least 24 hours after application of the tar product. Folliculitis may result from coal tar therapy.

Table 39-11 Psoriasis therapy

Type	Action	Comments
Bland emollients (petrolatum, mineral oil)	Hydration of skin	Use for mild lesions Facilitates scale removal
Keratolytics (salicylic acid, ammoniated mercury)	Hydration and softening of skin Antimitotic	Avoid using on face Cover with occlusive wraps May cause skin maceration and folliculitis Not applied to irritated skin
Corticosteroids	Antimitotic Antiinflammatory	Topical use for most lesions; cover with occlusive wraps; may cause folliculitis Intralesional use for plaques Rarely given systemically May produce rebound psoriasis when withdrawn
Coal tar preparations	Action unknown Have keratolytic, antipruritic, and photosensitizing effects	May develop folliculitis with long-term use Avoid direct sunlight for 24 hours after use Avoid use on face Stains skin, hair, and clothing Available as cream, lotion, gel, solution, and shampoo May be used with ultraviolet light therapy (Goeckerman routine)
Anthralin products	Antimitotic Inhibits enzyme metabolism	May cause skin irritation Not applied to open skin areas Petrolatum is used to protect normal skin during therapy Wear gloves during application; stains skin, hair, and clothing Avoid using on face
Photochemotherapy with ultraviolet light	Inhibition of DNA synthesis	May cause pruritus, erythema, vesicles, flare-up of lesions, transient nausea May be carcinogenic for light-skinned persons or those previously exposed to x-ray therapy Avoid direct sunlight for 12 to 24 hours after ingestion of Psoralen
Methotrexate	Antimitotic Inhibition of DNA synthesis	For severe lesions not amenable to other treatment Given orally unless nausea is present Requires close monitoring of hematologic, renal, and liver functioning
Synthetic retinoids	Corrects abnormal cell differentiation	Experimental Side effects: pruritus, lip edema, sore mouth, thirst, fragile skin, peeling of palms and soles[22] May be used with anthralin or ultraviolet therapies

□ PUVA therapy

PUVA therapy consists of a combination of orally administered methoxsalen (Psoralen) and long-wave ultraviolet light (UVA), hence the name. Methoxsalen is a photosensitizing agent. The person is exposed to UVA 2 hours after ingestion of the methoxsalen. Some side effects of PUVA therapy include pruritus, erythema, localized blistering, a moderate flare-up of psoriasis, and transient nausea. Because the skin remains photosensitive until methoxsalen is excreted, persons receiving this treatment are warned to avoid exposure to the sun for at least 8 hours after ingestion of the medication.

■ COUNSELING AND TEACHING

Because the lesions are commonly found on visible skin areas, persons with psoriasis are faced with a socially disabling disease. They may need help in identifying and coping with their feelings and with changes that may occur in their life-style. Arms and legs can be covered with clothing if the person is sensitive about appearance. Social contacts are encouraged.

Lesions may fade with treatment, only to recur eventually in the same area or elsewhere. The disease is not curable and may wax and wane continuously. Persons who are not aware of this may lose confidence in the physician and seek a quick cure. Because psoriasis is so common and so stubborn in response to treatment, manufacturers of patent remedies find a lucrative field for their products among persons with the disease. Self-treatment may lead to considerable expense for worthless products, increased discomfort, and delay in treatment of acute episodes. Persons with psoriasis are encouraged to consult a dermatologist as needed.

⊞ Evaluation

Evaluation is based on expected patient outcomes. Questions to ask may include the following: Does the person know the nature of the disease (incurable)? Does the person plan to follow medical therapy (rather than self-treatment) when exacerbation occurs? Is the person planning social activities with others?

■ SKIN REACTIONS FROM SYSTEMIC DISEASES

Changes in the skin may result from systemic conditions, most commonly dermatitis medicamentosa, erythema multiforme, and discoid lupus erythematosus.

■ Dermatitis medicamentosa

Skin lesions may result from toxic, metabolic, or allergic reactions to drugs (Table 39-12). Many of the reactions are hypersensitivity immune reactions and include fever, malaise, and vasculitis in addition to skin changes. The rash is often a bright red color, semiconfluent, maculopapular (see Plate 5), generalized, and bilateral. It can appear at any time, but the onset is usually sudden. Hypersensitivity occurs early when previous sensitization has taken place.

Persons are asked when admitted to the hospital if they have any known allergies. For drug allergies, a sticker indicating the drug is placed on every physician's order sheet to alert the physician or nurse not to order or give the drug to the patient. Sudden skin changes in patients receiving medications are brought to the physician's attention.

Teaching of the patient may include the suggestion that the patient wear a Medic-Alert bracelet specifying the drug to which the patient is allergic so that the drug is not administered unknowingly in an emergency situation. Persons who are taking drugs that cause photosensitivity reactions are advised to avoid direct exposure to sunlight.

■ Erythema multiforme

Erythema multiforme is a skin condition believed to occur secondary to an underlying systemic disease such as an infection. The skin eruption is characterized by red to purple macules, papules, and vesicles and may be preceded by fever, chest pain, and arthralgia. The treatment is to seek out the underlying cause and eliminate it if possible. Local treatment includes baths, soaks, and dressings. If the lesions appear in the mouth, special mouth care is indicated, including irrigations with warm salt solution.

■ Discoid lupus erythematosus

Lupus erythematosus occurs in two forms, systemic (SLE) (see Chapter 22) and discoid (DLE). DLE is a chronic, relatively benign skin condition seen in young adults, rarely after age 50 years. Precipitating factors include physical trauma and stress. There is no cure for DLE.

The lesions of DLE are well demarcated and erythematous, have a characteristic scaly border with an atrophied center, and vary in size. The most common sites are the cheeks (butterfly pattern), scalp, and chest, although other parts of the body may also be involved. In addition to the skin lesions the person may have leukopenia, an increased sedimentation rate, positive response to rheumatoid factor test and serologic test for syphilis (STS), and a low titer of antinuclear factors.

Preventive measures include avoiding physical trauma, such as by using protective lotions to prevent sunburn and wearing warm clothing to protect against cold and wind. If stress is a precipitating factor, measures to reduce stress (see Chapter 7) can be instituted. Palliative measures include topical steroid therapy under occlusive wraps or intralesional steroid therapy.

■ TUMORS OF THE SKIN

Tumors of the skin may be benign, premalignant, or malignant (Table 39-13).

Table 39-12   Skin reactions to common medications

Reaction	Medication
Erythematous rash	Antibiotics, sulfonamides, thiazide diuretics, barbiturates, phenylbutazone
Purpura (ecchymosis, petechiae)	Thiazides, sulfonamides, barbiturates, anticoagulants
Mucocutaneous lesions (vesicles, bullae, ulcers)	Sulfonamides, penicillin, barbiturates, phenylbutazone
Urticaria	Penicillin, salicylates
Photosensitivity	Phenothiazines, thiazides, tetracycline, griseofulvin, sulfonamides, chlorpromazine, nalidixic acid

Table 39-13   Tumors of the skin

Tumor	Description	Medical therapy
Keratoses		
Corns	Thickened skin lesion with a center core that thickens inwardly	Corrective shoes; felt pad with a center hole for relief of pressure
Callus	Thickened horny skin layer in circumscribed lesions often seen on plantar surface of foot	Well-fitting shoes, moleskin and padding; scraping with emery board; salicylic acid plasters
Seborrheic keratosis	Benign tumors; resemble large, darkened, greasy warts	Do not require treatment; may be removed by curettage and electrodessication or cryotherapy
Actinic keratosis (senile, solar)	Benign round or irregular tumors; red-brown to gray in color, with a dry scaly appearance; 25% may become malignant	Removal by curettage and electrodessication or by cryotherapy
Premalignant		
Leukoplakia	Thickened white or reddish patch on mucous membrane of mouth or vagina; may develop into invasive squamous cell carcinoma	Small lesions removed by electrodessication; large lesions excised
Pigmented nevi (mole)	Circumscribed pigmented papules; brown moles with hair or evenly colored dark moles are usually benign	Excised for cosmetic reasons or if sudden change in size or color, or bleeding
Malignant		
Squamous cell carcinoma	Malignant tumor of surface epidermis; starts as a firm nodule, becomes indurated with an inflammatory base; may metastasize if on lip or ear (Fig. 39-4)	Removal by surgical excision, curettage with electrodessication, irradiation, or chemosurgery
Basal cell carcinoma	Malignant tumor primarily over hairy areas; tumors have a translucent appearance with indurated center; may be ulcerated with crusting; grow slowly and rarely metastasize	Same as above
Malignant melanoma	Most serious but relatively uncommon skin cancer; lesions vary in appearance and rate of growth; often have irregular pigmentation; metastasize frequently; early diagnosis leads to more favorable prognosis	Total wide excision with skin grafts to cover defects in many cases; chemotherapy, immunotherapy

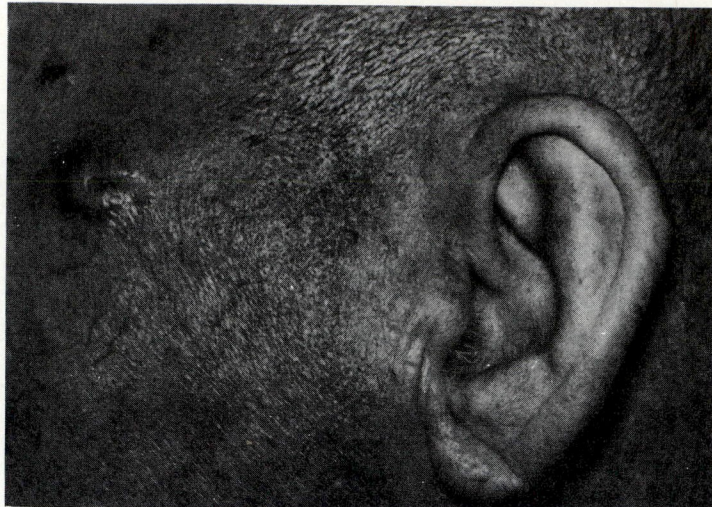

Fig. 39-4 Squamous cell carcinoma in infratemporal area, one of the commonest sites for this tumor. (From Stewart, WD, Danto, JL, and Maddin, S: Dermatology; diagnosis and treatment of cutaneous disorders, ed 4, St. Louis, 1978, The CV Mosby Co.)

■ Pathophysiology

The term *keratosis* refers to any cornification or growth of the horny layer of the skin; keratoses are benign growths. Corns and calluses result from pressure or friction from poorly fitting shoes, faulty weight-bearing, or with neuropathies such as diabetic neuropathy. Seborrheic keratoses are commonly seen in older persons. Actinic keratoses result from exposure of the skin to irradiation, primarily solar. They are noted most often on exposed skin areas of persons who work outdoors and on older persons. Light-skinned persons are more vulnerable to skin changes from irradiation. Actinic keratoses may develop into squamous cell carcinomas.

The term *premalignant* does *not* imply that all such lesions become malignant; it does imply that the tendency to become malignant exists. Leukoplakia develop in the mucous membranes of the mouth or vagina; red patches (erythroleukoplakia) have a higher malignancy potential than white patches. External irritants, such as poorly fitting dentures, cheek biting, and pipe or cigarette smoking, appear to have an etiologic relationship to oral leukoplakia. Chronic maceration, friction, and senile atrophy may lead to leukoplakia of the vagina. Pigmented nevi are commonly seen in all persons. Benign moles have an even color.

Malignant tumors, with the exception of some tumors such as malignant melanoma, are often of less serious consequence than malignant tumors elsewhere in the body. Skin carcinomas appear mostly on exposed skin or at areas of chronic irritation. Squamous cell carcinomas that develop on hair-bearing skin rarely metastasize, but lesions of the lip or ear frequently metastasize to regional lymph nodes. Basal cell carcinomas grow slowly and rarely metastasize, but untreated tumors can become locally invasive with severe tissue destruction, infection, and hemorrhage.

■ Preventive measures

Protection of the skin from excessive solar radiation and early detection of lesions are important preventive measures. Persons who are exposed frequently to direct sunlight should use protective lotions and other protective measures, such as hats. Fair-skinned persons should use a number 15 sun screen lotion for protection of direct solar rays.

Because pigmented moles may become malignant, persons are taught to report the following changes to the physician:

1. Development of a ring of new pigment around the base of a mole
2. Development of uneven pigmentation
3. Sudden growth in size
4. Loss of hair in a mole
5. Bleeding in a mole

■ Surgical removal

Skin tumors are removed by excision followed by suturing, curettage, electrosurgery, or chemosurgery.

■ CURETTAGE

The curet is a spoon-shaped instrument with sharp edges and is used in a downward scraping motion across a lesion (Fig. 39-5). A local anesthetic is usually first injected around the lesion. Curettage is usually followed by electrodessication to stop the bleeding.

■ ELECTRODESSICATION

In electrodessication an electric current is used to coagulate the tissue and curtail capillary bleeding. It may

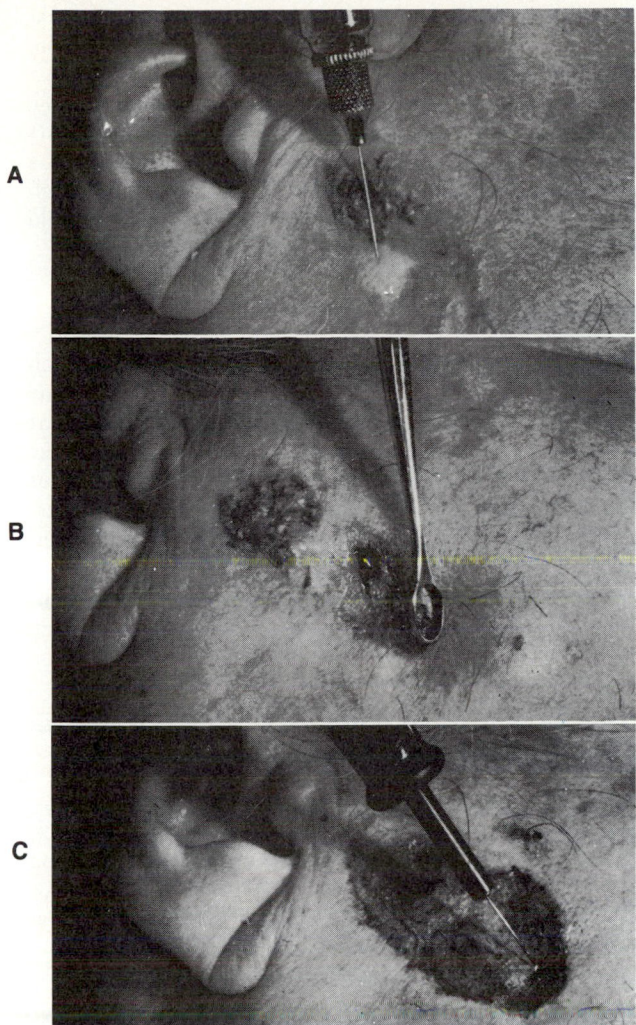

Fig. 39-5 **A,** Infiltration with local anesthetic. **B,** Curettage. **C,** Electrodesiccation for hemostasis. (From Stewart, WD, Danto, JL, and Maddin, S: Dermatology: diagnosis and treatment of cutaneous disorders, ed 4, St. Louis, 1978, The CV Mosby Co.)

also be used to cut tissue under local anesthesia. After most electrosurgical procedures the wound is left exposed to air dry. Dressings may be used if the area is subject to frequent trauma or rubbing or if oozing is present. The wound may be wiped with 70% alcohol to hasten drying. A hemostatic nonocclusive dressing may be made by covering the wound with Gelfoam powder and Micropore tape.

CHEMOSURGERY

Chemosurgery involves the application of a chemical to destroy cells for removal. Chemosurgery for malignant skin tumors usually consists of application of a dressing with a fixative paste such as zinc chloride and then removal of the dressing with some tissue fixed to it (the Mohs sur-

gery). Reapplication is often necessary until all malignant tissue has been removed. Chemosurgery is used only for tumors without well-defined borders.

Cryosurgery is the rapid freezing of tissue with substances such as carbon dioxide snow or liquid nitrogen. The rapid freezing causes formation of intracellular ice, which destroys the cell membranes and produces cell dehydration. Cryosurgery is frequently used for removal of warts and keloids as well as removal of skin tumors (benign and malignant).

Although cryosurgery is not usually painful, a tingling pain occurs when the freezing substance is applied and may be uncomfortable to some persons, particularly if multiple lesions are treated. Local anesthesia may be necessary. Analgesics may be helpful during thawing.

Tissue necrosis may not be evident until 24 hours after cryosurgery. A clear or hemorrhagic bulla forms during the first day, but inflammatory reactions and bleeding are unusual. A serous exudate occurs during the first week, followed by eschar, or crust, formation. The crust drops off in 3 to 4 weeks as the underlying tissue heals. Scarring usually results. Hypopigmentation may occur because melanocytes are highly vulnerable to freezing.

Malignant melanoma

Melanomas differ from the other types of skin cancers because of the higher incidence of metastasis and mortality. Most deaths from skin cancer result from melanomas. The incidence of melanomas in the United States has been increasing in recent years, probably because of increased exposure to the sun.

There are various types of melanomas. Two thirds of the melanomas are *superficial spreading* melanomas, which grow slowly and are slightly elevated, irregularly shaped, notched lesions with variations in color (blue, black, brown, pink, gray) (see Plate 6). Less frequently seen (15%) are the *nodular* melanomas, which are blueberry shaped with variations in color from blue-black to rose-gray. The nodular melanomas grow and metastasize more quickly than other forms. The patient's prognosis is based on the depth of invasion within the skin. The more superficial the growth the better the prognosis. Melanomas on the trunk have a poorer prognosis than those on the extremities.

Although melanomas cannot be prevented, all questionable moles should be examined by a physician so that early treatment can be instituted if malignancy is diagnosed. Suspect moles are those that change in color or appearance, grow suddenly, itch, or ulcerate. Persons at high risk include those with fair skin and those with familial history of melanomas.

The person who has a newly diagnosed melanoma is usually very anxious and requires considerable emotional support. The nursing approach consists of emphatic listening and promoting hope without giving false reassurance. The importance of immediate therapy is stressed because it enhances the prognosis. Surgery often involves a wide lesion, and skin grafting may be necessary. Regional lymph nodes are frequently dissected. Chemotherapy and immunotherapy are reserved for metastatic disease.

■ Kaposi's sarcoma

Kaposi's sarcoma was a rare malignant disorder in older men in the United States until recently, although it was endemic in young black men of equatorial Africa. The disorder is now seen with increasing frequency as one of the opportunistic disorders occurring in conjunction with acquired immunodeficiency syndrome (AIDS), especially in homosexual men.

Persons with Kaposi's sarcoma develop discrete, red, purple, or dark plaques or nodules scattered widely over the body on the skin and mucous membranes. Some lesions may regress spontaneously. The disorder is slowly progressive and successful treatment of the sarcoma, unfortunately, does not affect survival. Many persons die of an associated opportunistic infection.

Treatment is primarily for cosmetic and psychologic reasons. Individual lesions may be excised, but because lesions are usually numerous, therapy consists mainly of radiotherapy for accessible tumors or chemotherapy (vinblastine) given intralesionally or intravenously.[29]

■ SKIN DISORDERS IN BLACKS

The reported incidence of dermatologic disorders varies among different races. Persons with black skin rarely have skin disorders that are affected by solar irradiation, because the pigment of black skin screens out the sun's rays.

Pigmentary changes more commonly result from dermatologic disorders in blacks because of the greater amount of melanin present. *Hyperpigmentation* is commonly seen after acne vulgaris, skin eruptions caused by drugs, lichen simplex chronicus, and pityriasis rosea. *Hypopigmentation* may result from atopic dermatitis and tinea. Some dermatologic disorders that are unique to blacks include traumatic alopecia and pseudofolliculitis barbae. Keloids are common.

■ Traumatic alopecia

Hair shafts in blacks are highly susceptible to breakage, and hair loss may result from some hair care practices such as tight hair curlers, corn-row braiding, hot combing, or the use of picks. Wetting or "softening" the hair before the use of a pick may help prevent trauma to the hair. The hair usually grows back when the specific practice is discontinued.

■ Pseudofolliculitis barbae

Hair follicles in blacks are curved rather than straight; therefore, the hair curls back as it grows. After shaving, the sharpened point of the hair shaft (especially if a straight razor has been used) acts like a hook and reenters the skin, causing an inflammatory response. The most commonly affected areas include the chin and upper anterior neck. The legs and axilla may also develop pseudofolliculitis from shaving.

The lesions consist of papules and pustules, with some postinflammatory hyperpigmentation. Treatment consists of growing a beard or shaving with a safety razor set at a coarse setting. As the beard is growing, a brush or rough washcloth may be used to dislodge ingrowing hairs. A mild depilatory may be used in place of shaving.

■ Keloids

Although keloids are seen in all races, they are much more prevalent in blacks. Keloids are hard, raised, shiny growths of collagen tissue that usually originate from a scar and then grow beyond the wound, often with clawlike projections. Keloids occur most often in young adults but may require many years to reach full growth. Highly susceptible areas for keloid growth include the sternum, mandible, ear, and neck. Keloids may recur after simple excision; therefore surgery is often followed by intralesional steroid therapy, radiation therapy, or electron beam therapy.

■ PLASTIC SURGERY

Plastic surgery is concerned with correction or reconstruction of deformities of body structures either present at birth or resulting from disease or trauma. Purposes of the surgery include restoration of function and improvement in appearance. Types of plastic surgery are listed below:

Skin grafting
Cosmetic surgery
    Removal of skin marks
        Dermabrasion
        Medical tatooing
    Fat removal (liposuction)
    Nose straightening (rhinoplasty)
    Face lifting (rhytidoplasty)
    Breast reconstruction (mammoplasty)

■ General care of the person having plastic surgery

■ PREPARATION FOR SURGERY

It is believed that any plastic surgery for an obvious defect is justified if it helps people feel they have a better chance for positive recognition. The plastic surgeon may reshape a nose or repair a deformed hand so that an emotionally stable person will have more assurance. It is foolish to assume, however, that reconstructive surgery alone will correct a basic personality problem. Some people blame an apparently trivial physical defect for a long series of failures in their lives when the major defect lies within their personalities. Because of this possibility, the person is usually studied before surgery is planned. It is necessary to know what the person expects the surgery to accomplish before the physician can decide whether such expectations are realistic and if surgery should be performed.

Before surgery the surgeon will tell the patient what probably can be done and what changes are possible. It is important to know what the patient has been told so that misunderstandings and misinterpretations can be avoided. Preparation is necessary for the normal appearance of skin grafts and reconstructed tissue immediately after surgery. Postoperative tissue reaction may distort normal contours, suture lines may be reddened, and the color of the newly transplanted skin may differ somewhat from that of surrounding skin. The appearance of the surgical area changes as the edema decreases and the suture line becomes less reddened and indurated. The scar will be less noticeable 6 months after surgery than at 6 days or 6 weeks postoperatively.

The patient who is scheduled for plastic surgery may have extensive scarring and deformity and may be exceedingly sensitive to scrutiny. On the other hand, the patient may have little apparent deformity, and it may be difficult to understand why the patient wishes to have surgery. The nurse cannot know what the disfigurement means to the individual and should avoid judgment concerning the necessity of surgery.

Many plastic surgeries are now performed on an outpatient basis at a specialized plastic surgery clinic. Procedures that require extensive grafting usually require hospitalization.

■ MAINTAINING PSYCHOLOGIC COMFORT

Plastic surgery raises many of the same concerns of other surgeries. Specific concerns may include the following.
1. Economic
   a. Possible long hospitalization and convalescence for skin grafting
   b. Elective cosmetic surgery may not be covered by medical insurance
2. Physical discomfort
3. Physical appearance in postoperative period
4. Final outcome of surgery

These concerns may result in anxiety and mild depression during the first few days after surgery.[6] Empathic communication by the nurse helps the patient identify and deal with concerns.

■ Skin grafting

Skin grafting consists of replacing damaged skin with healthy skin to prevent unsightly scars.

■ GRAFT SOURCES

Skin for grafting may be obtained from various sources (see the box above). The most suitable form is the *autograft*, because it does not provoke an immune response with rejection of the graft. *Homografts* (which are temporary) may be necessary if the patient's condition is poor and if large

---

Graft sources

Autograft	Tissue moved from one part of the body to another
Homograft	Tissue transplanted from another person
Heterograft	Tissue transplanted from another species

---

and if large areas must be covered, as with burns. The survival time of homografts varies from a few days to a number of weeks. Depending on the tissue used and the recipient site, the transplanted tissue will then die and slough or be absorbed and replaced by the host's own developing tissues. *Heterografts,* which are rejected quickly by the recipient, are used only in special cases, such as when homografts are not available and covering of the wound is essential.

■ TYPES OF GRAFTS

Plastic surgery may be performed by means of *free grafting,* which consists of cutting tissue from one part of the body and moving it directly to another part. It may also be done by leaving one end of the graft attached to the body to provide a blood supply for the graft until blood vessels form at the new place of attachment (*flap graft*).

The surgeon selects skin for grafting that is similar in texture and thickness to that which has been lost, and studies the normal lines of the skin and its elasticity to avoid noticeable scars. Scar tissue contracts with time, and in normal circumstances this is good because it produces a complete closure of the line of injury. However, in some cases scar tissue may contract in such a way that surrounding tissues are pulled out of normal contour, and distortion may result.

□ Free grafts

Free grafts are the most commonly used skin grafts. There are several types of free grafts, each with its advantages and limitations (Table 39-14). Split-thickness grafts consist of epidermis and varying thicknesses of the dermis. Full-thickness grafts include the entire dermis and epidermis (Fig. 39-1). The most widely used type is the intermediate or thick split-thickness graft. This can be cut into large pieces with a dermatome set to ensure a uniform thickness of the graft, and these can then be cut into smaller pieces to match the area to be grafted.

Meshed grafts are either thin or intermediate split-thickness grafts that have been placed through a perforating

Table 39-14 Various types of skin grafts

Type of graft	Description	Use	Comments
Free grafts			
Split-thickness: thin	Epidermis and thin layer of dermis (0.25 to 0.30 mm)	Burns	Becomes vascularized quickly Survives transplantation readily Donor sites heal quickly Poor cosmetic results Considerable postgraft contraction Does not withstand trauma
Split-thickness: intermediate or thick	Epidermis and thicker layer of dermis (0.40 to 0.45 or 0.55 to 0.60 mm)	Widely used over large wounds	Less contraction Better cosmetic results Epithelialization of donor site occurs completely but more slowly
Full-thickness	Epidermis and all of dermis	For small areas where matching skin color and texture is important	Best cosmetic results No contraction Donor site must be sutured (no epithelialization) Limited donor sites Lowest transplantation survival
Flap grafts	Skin and subcutaneous tissue; one end remains attached to donor site for vascularization	Large areas of defect; over avascular areas	More complex, requires greater skill Bulky May introduce hair into nonhairy areas
Free flap grafts	Skin, subcutaneous tissue and major blood vessel transferred to recipient site; donor blood vessel anastomosed to recipient blood vessel (microsurgery)	Over bony areas or areas requiring large amounts of tissue (breast reconstruction, head and neck defects, deep decubiti)	Blood flow established immediately; less contraction; more normal skin appearance, but may not match; may introduce hair into nonhairy areas

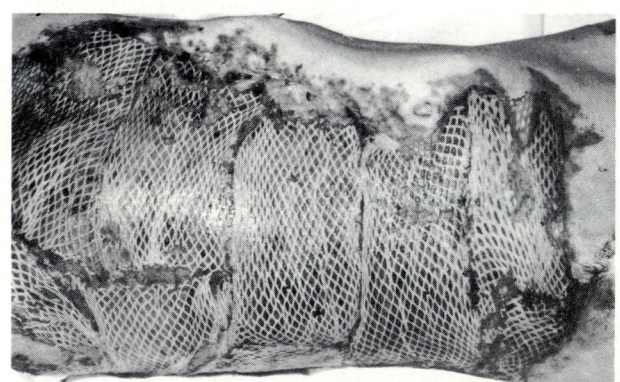

Fig. 39-6 Mesh graft covering full-thickness burn. (Courtesy Burn Unit, Cook County Hospital, Chicago.)

machine that creates a mesh. Meshed grafts are elastic and can be used to cover larger areas than the original size (Fig. 39-6). They also conform more easily to irregular surfaces and can be placed over less clean bases than regular split-thickness grafts. Cosmetic appearance is poor. Meshed grafts are used frequently to cover large burned areas.

Full-thickness grafts, for survival, must develop their own blood supply (which takes 2 weeks). If the graft dies, the skin is irretrievably lost to the body, because regeneration of skin at the donor site is not possible.

☐ **Flap grafts**

Flap grafts are used to cover larger defects than can be covered by free grafts. Flap grafts are made by cutting along three sides of a flap (two long and one short side). There are basically two major types of flap grafts. The *transposed* graft is slid over to a nearby skin area to be covered and is sutured in place. The *tube pedicle* graft is formed by suturing the long sides of the graft together to form a tube and then suturing the end to another area of the body. An intermediary site may be used, such as the forearm, in a two-step procedure, to permit moving the tube to a farther site on the body. After the graft has taken, the original site is freed and the graft is sutured to the recipient site.

Island flaps are narrow strips of neurovascular tissue from which the skin has been removed. The flap is transferred to a distant site through a tunnel made *under* the skin. The only scars that remain are at the donor and recipient sites.

☐ Free flap grafts

Development of microsurgical techniques has permitted the use of free flaps (Table 39-14). A large amount of tissue can be moved because blood flow is reestablished at the new site by anastomosing the donor blood vessel with a recipient site blood vessel. Some free flaps contain functional nerves that can be reattached to permit sensation at the recipient site. Surgery often takes from 4 to 12 hours. Significant peripheral disease and diabetes mellitus are contraindications for surgery.

■ CARE OF THE PERSON WITH A SKIN GRAFT

Four conditions are necessary for a graft to survive:
1. Adequate vascularization of the recipient site
2. Constant contact with the underlying tissue
3. Immobilization
4. Freedom from infection

Anything that comes between the undersurface of the graft and the recipient area, such as a discharge caused by infection, excess serous fluid, or blood, will float the graft away from close contact and may cause it to die. To prevent floating, some surgeons insert drains at strategic spots along the edges of the graft, or a small catheter is inserted on the edge of the graft under the recipient skin and attached to suction to remove the fluid.

The area is inspected frequently to see if the skin is adhering to the underlying tissue. If fluid collects under the skin graft, it is removed by aspiration with a sterile

---

Nursing care of patients with skin grafts

Preoperative care

1. Recipient site:
   a. Apply warm soaks and compresses under aseptic conditions (as prescribed).
   b. Apply prescribed topical antibiotics.
2. Donor site: cleanse with germicidal soap as prescribed, usually the night before and the morning of surgery.

Postoperative care of recipient site

1. Elevate graft site when possible.
2. Protect graft site from pressure and motion (for example, place graft site uppermost, use cradle over bed).
3. Instruct patient not to lie on dressing.
4. Apply warm moist compresses, if prescribed:
   a. Wash hands before changing dressings.
   b. Use meticulous aseptic technique.
   c. Warm compresses to no more than 40.5° C (105°F).
5. Compresses may sometimes be covered with a sterile petroleum jelly dressing and moistened by gently directing fluid from sterile syringe under edge of dressing.
6. Report any signs of hematoma or fluid collection under graft.

Postoperative care of donor site

1. Keep donor site covered for 24 to 48 hours until serum dries.
2. Apply heat lamp with caution (denuded skin is sensitive) to hasten drying.
3. Use a bed cradle, if appropriate, to allow more air circulation.
4. Leave fine-mesh gauze, which is adherent to donor site, in place until it drops off (usually within 3 weeks).
5. Trim loose edges of mesh gauze as it loosens with healing.
6. Give analgesics as necessary for discomfort.

Postoperative care after flap grafts

1. Support body parts placed in awkward position from immobilization of flap graft.
2. Assess graft as possible for circulatory insufficiency (sharp color demarcation, decreased temperature).
3. Maintain aseptic technique to prevent infection.
4. Assist patient to be as self-sufficient as possible with activities of daily living.
5. If hospitalization is prolonged, help patient plan diversionary activities.

Teaching the patient with a skin graft

1. Keep surface of healed graft moistened daily with a skin lotion for 6 to 12 months. (Grafted skin does not sweat; it dries and cracks easily.)
2. Protect grafted skin from direct sunlight with a sunscreen lotion for at least 6 months.
3. Wear a strong elastic stocking for 4 to 6 months with grafts on lower extremities.
4. Report changes in the graft (hematoma, fluid collection) to physician.

---

needle and syringe or the fluid is rolled to the wound edge with a sterile applicator.

A wide variety of materials are used as dressings. The choice depends on the kind of graft and the surgeon's preference. Petrolatum, Adaptic gauze, or Telfa dressings are often selected. Often the graft is covered with a piece of coarse mesh gauze anchored to the adjacent skin edges with an elastic bandage to give firm, gentle pressure and to immobilize the area. The first dressing may be covered with a compress of sterile normal saline solution. Because the compress is moist, it fits the contour of the wound better. Continuous pressure is necessary to keep the graft adherent to the recipient bed, but pressure should not be so firm as to cause death of the graft.

Inner dressings on the recipient site are usually changed by the surgeon 1 to 2 days after surgery, and it is usually possible to know then whether the result of the operation is satisfactory (see the box on p. 1401).

Before patients with skin grafts are discharged, they need to know how to care for the recipient and donor sites at home until healing has occurred (see the box at left).

■ Cosmetic surgery

■ REMOVAL OF SKIN MARKINGS

Disfiguring marks of the skin may be removed by abrasive action (dermabrasion) or by changing the color through medical tattooing. Both procedures are painful.

Either local or general anesthesia is used for *dermabrasion*, which may be performed on an inpatient or outpatient basis. The skin is abraded with a wire brush or diamond fraise (Fig. 39-7). There is postoperative swelling, discomfort, crusting, and erythema, which may persist for several weeks. The procedure may be done in stages. A Telfa dressing with antiseptic solution and a pressure dressing are usually applied, although the area may be left uncovered if oozing is slight.

Medical tatooing is performed on an ambulatory basis; no anesthesia is used, although a sedative may be prescribed to be taken 1 hour before surgery. The procedure is done in several stages; pigment is impregnated into the skin with a tattooing needle. The skin is left exposed to air to dry and crust. An ice bag may be applied to relieve postoperative discomfort.

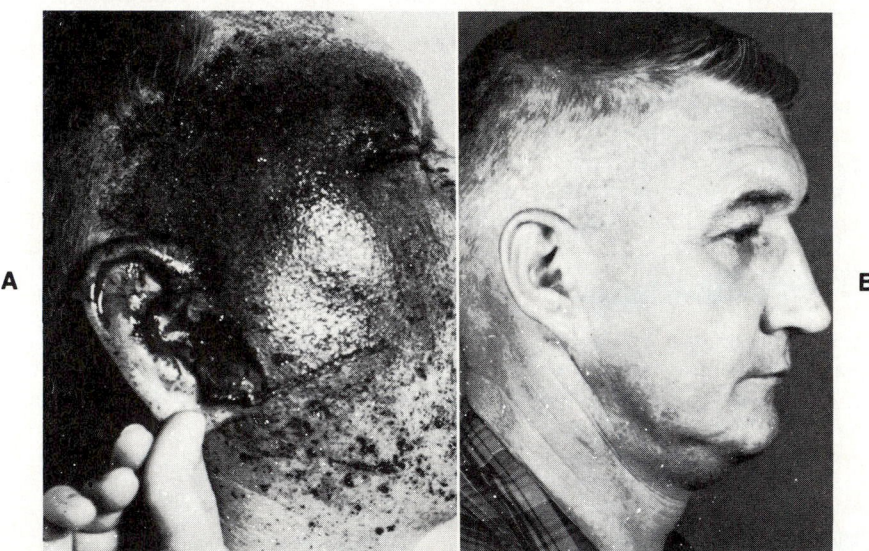

Fig. 39-7 **A,** Meticulous cleansing and dermabrasion were required to remove impregnated bits of galvanized metal. **B,** Postoperative view of patient 17 years after dermabrasion. (From Saunders, WH, and others: Nursing care in eye, ear, nose, and throat disorders, ed 4, St. Louis, 1979, The CV Mosby Co.)

LIPOSUCTION

Some persons develop excess fatty tissue in areas such as the abdomen, hips ("saddle bags"), thighs, upper arms, or posterior neck ("buffalo hump"). If these persons are of normal weight but have selected areas of excess fat, they may be candidates for liposuction.

Liposuction can be performed by ambulatory surgery. A long, hollow, blunt-tipped cannula is inserted through a small incision and is tunneled through the fat under the skin. The loosened fat is then removed through the cannula by suction. Local anesthetics can be used for small single areas, although general anesthetics may be required for large or multiple areas.

After surgery, the area is taped with an elastic bandage for a period of 1 to 2 weeks. The patient's activity is limited for 48 hours. Nonaspirin analgesics may be taken for discomfort. Complications, though relatively few, may include bleeding or infection. Initially the skin may be dimpled or hard, but it eventually softens and smooths out.

RHINOPLASTY

Reconstructive surgery of the nose can be done either to correct an anatomic problem (Chapter 23) or for cosmetic reasons (Fig. 39-8). A local anesthetic is usually used. The incision is usually made at the end of the nose inside the nostril so that it is not conspicuous. A nasal packing is inserted for 24 to 48 hours; the patient is cautioned not to sniff or blow the nose after the packing is removed, to prevent bleeding. A nasal splint may be applied for protection.

There will be ecchymosis (bruising) and swelling around the eyes and nose for 10 to 14 days after surgery; ice compresses and an ice bag may be used to hasten fluid reabsorption. The patient must anticipate waiting several weeks before evaluating the final result of surgery.

RHYTIDOPLASTY

For face lifting, an incision is made at the hairline, and excess skin is separated from its underlying tissue and

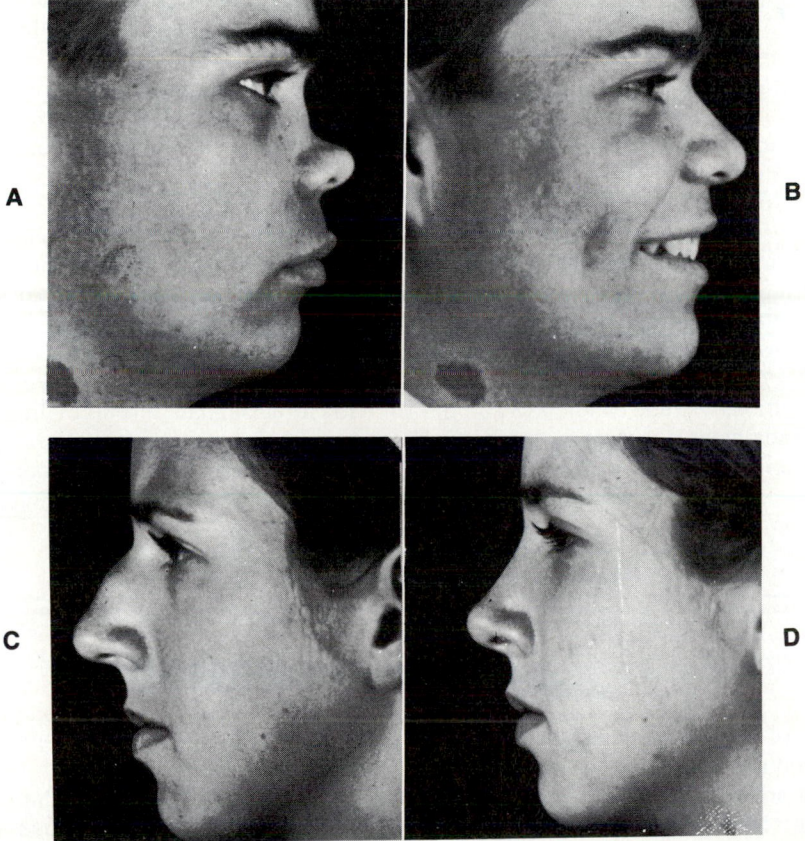

Fig. 39-8 **A,** Saddle nose after nasal infection at 8 years of age. **B,** It is repaired with Silastic nasal implant. **C** and **D,** Nasal convexity and chin retrusion repaired by combined rhinoplasty and chin augmentation. (From Saunders, WH, and others: Nursing care in eye, ear, nose, and throat disorders, ed 4, St. Louis, 1979, The CV Mosby Co.)

removed. The remaining skin is pulled up and sutured at the hairline, thus removing wrinkles and giving firmness and smoothness to the face. A gentle pressure dressing is then applied and left in place for 24 to 48 hours. The patient frequently needs medication for pain in the postoperative period because of the extent to which the tissue has been undermined. The surgery may be repeated at a later date.

■ MAMMOPLASTY

Reconstructive breast surgery may be done to replace breast tissued removed by surgery (Chapter 36) or to improve the appearance of the breasts. Some women with conspicuously large and pendulous breasts may wish to have then reduced in size. Large breasts are embarrassing to some women and make it difficult for them to participate in sports, maintain good posture, and buy clothes that fit. Such women often respond to reconstructive surgery remarkably well. Cosmetic surgery of the breast may also be done to make unusually small breasts larger. A variety of plastic materials may be used for this procedure (see Chapter 36).

■ SUMMARY

1. Skin disorders that produce marked visual disfigurement may result in alterations in body image and self-esteem.
2. Bacterial skin infections include folliculitis (infections of the hair follicle), furuncles (deep folliculitis), carbuncles (cluster of furuncles), or cellulitis (diffuse infection of skin and subcutaneous tissue); treatment includes warm soaks or hot moist dressings, and topical or systemic antibiotics.
3. Viral skin inflammations include herpes simplex, herpes zoster, and warts; treatment is primarily symptomatic.
4. Fungal skin inflammations include candidiasis and the dermatophytoses (tinea capitis, corporis, cruris, and pedis); treatment includes topical or oral antifungal drugs.

5. Parasitic infestations include those by lice or scabies mite; treatment includes a topical pediculocide/scabicide such as lindane.
6. Topical medications may be prepared as powders, lotions, creams, ointment, or paste.
7. Wet dermatologic dressings are given for cooling astringent, antipruritic, vasoconstricting, or debriding effects; the best effects are obtained by several treatments spaced over several hours.
8. Dermatologic baths and soaks are given for soothing, antipruritic, astringent, or medicinal effects; medication should be completely dissolved in the water, and creams or ointments are applied immediately after the bath.
9. Dermatitis may result from contact with irritants, as an atopic (hypersensitivity) reaction, from stasis of circulation in the legs, or from unknown cause (dandruff). Dressings moistened with Burow's solution and topical steroids may be used for uninfected weeping lesions, and antibiotics may be used for infected lesions.
10. The most common papulosquamous disorder is psoriasis, a chronic condition resulting from rapid cell mitosis. Exacerbations of psoriasis may be treated with occlusive wraps over topical steroid therapy; crude tar therapy, alone or in combination with ultraviolet light; or PUVA therapy.
11. Drugs that may cause photosensitivity reactions include phenothiazines, thiazides, tetracycline, griseofulvin, sulfonamide, nalidixic acid, and chlorpromazine; persons taking these drugs should avoid direct sunlight.
12. Nonmalignant skin lesions are primarily keratoses (corns, calluses, seborrheic keratosis, actinic keratosis) that are characterized by overgrowth and thickening of the epithelium; actinic keratoses result from solar irradiation and may become squamous cell carcinomas.
13. Premalignant lesions include leukoplakia (white or red patches), which may develop into invasive squamous cell carcinoma, and pigmented moles, which may develop into melanoma. Moles that change appearance

---

Putting knowledge to practice

■ Examine the skin of three of your patients. How do they differ? Describe any lesions in terms of color, shape, size (be specific), and distribution.

■ Imagine that you are a school nurse in an affluent community. You have discovered that several children have pediculosis (lice): Discuss with your classmates problems that you might expect. Discuss approaches you could use that would be most effective in eradicating the pediculosis.

■ Go to a drugstore and examine the products advertised for psoriasis. Estimate the yearly cost of using some of these drugs on a regular basis.

in color, size, loss of hair, or bleeding should be reported to the physician.

14. Squamous cell carcinoma, which may metastasize, and basal cell carcinoma, which rarely metastasizes, may be removed by surgical excision and curettage with electrodessication, irradiation, or chemosurgery.

15. Malignant melanomas have a high incidence of metastasis and mortality; they are treated by radical excision, chemotherapy, and immunotherapy.

16. Free grafts (split-thickness, full-thickness) are sections of epidermis and dermis that are taken from a donor area and transplanted to a distant area. Flap grafts include subcutaneous tissue, and one end remains attached to the donor site. Free flap grafts contain skin, subcutaneous tissue, and a major blood vessel, which are transplanted to a distant site with anastomosis of the blood vessel with a recipient vessel.

17. Care of the person with a graft includes (1) applying firm dressings, to maintain graft contact with the underlying tissue; (2) preventing collection of fluid under the graft, to protect against separation of the graft; (3) protecting the graft site from excess pressure and motion, to promote vascularization and prevent separation; and (4) using aseptic technique, to prevent infection.

18. Cosmetic surgery includes dermabrasion or medical tattooing to remove skin markings, liposuction to remove excess abdominal fat, face lifting (rhytidoplasty), and reconstructive surgery of the nose (rhinoplasty) and breast (mammoplasty).

REFERENCES AND SELECTED READINGS
Contemporary

1. *Acres, C, and Kraft, ER: Skin transplantation, Am J Nurs 81:1466-1467, 1981.
2. *Anders, JE, and Leach, EE: Sun versus skin, Am J Nurs 83:1015-1020, 1983.
3. Anderson, TF: Psoriasis, Med Clin North Am 66:769-793, 1982.
4. *Baj, PA: Liposuction: new wave plastic surgery, Am J Nurs 84:892-893, 1984.
5. *Baroni, JL: Herpetic whitlow, Am J Nurs 84:60-61, 1984.
6. Barratt, GE, and others: Skin grafts: physiology and clinical considerations, Otolaryngol Clin North Am 17(2):335-351, 1984.
7. Belfer, ML, and others: Appearance and the influence of reconstructive surgery on body image, Clin Plast Surg 9:307-315, 1982.
8. *Berliner, H: Aging skin, Pt 1, Am J Nurs 86:1138-1141, 1986.
9. *Berliner, H: Aging skin, Pt 2, Am J Nurs 86:1259-1261, 1986.
9a. Buxton, PK: ABC of dermatology: treatment of eczema and inflammatory dermatoses, Brit Med J 295:1112-1114, 1987.

10. *Chouinard, F: Be a skeptic while caring for post-op flaps, Plast Surg Nurs 3(2):44, 1983.
11. *Cohen, BE, and Aaronson, S: Microvascular reconstructive surgery: free tissue transfer, AORN J 38:602-629, 1983.
12. *Conlee, D: Put a new face on your care of cosmetic surgery patients, Nurs 81 11(11):90-95, 1981.
13. *Crawfort, E, and others: Mohs chemosurgery: day surgery for cutaneous malignancies, AORN J 43:464-468, 1986.
14. Dolsky, RL, Newman, J, and Fetzek JR: Liposuction: history, techniques, and complications, Dermatol Clin 5:313-334, 1987.
15. Douglas, RG, Jr: Antiviral drugs, Med Clin North Am 67(5):1163-1171, 1983.
16. Estes, SA: Diagnosis and management of scabies, Med Clin North Am 66(4):955-963, 1982.
17. *Fraser, MC, and McGuire, DB: Skin cancer's early warning system, Am J Nurs 84:1232-1236, 1984.
18. Grazer, FM, and Klingbell, JR: Body image: a surgical perspective, St. Louis, 1980, The CV Mosby Co.
19. Greany, D, and Goldsmith, HS: Cutaneous melanoma: diagnosis and surgical intervention, AORN J 42:43-49, 1985.
20. Habif, TP: Clinical dermatology: a color guide to diagnosis and treatment, St. Louis, 1985, The CV Mosby Co.
21. Harber, LC, and Whitman, GB: Photosensitivity: classification, Dermatol Clin 4:167-170, 1986.
22. *Hazards of topical therapy, Am J Nurs 84:1506-1507, 1984.
23. *Heckel, P: Teaching patients to cope with psoriasis: the unshared disease, Nurs 81 11(6):49-51, 1981.
24. *Hutton, B, and Hutton, J: Living with a facial prosthesis, Am J Nurs 84:50-52, 1984.
25. Jackson, R, and Laughlin, S: Electrosurgery, Dermatol Clin 2:233-244, 1984.
26. Kaye, D, and Rose, LF: Fundamentals of internal medicine, St. Louis, 1983, The CV Mosby Co.
27. Kleinsmith, D, and Perricone, NV: Common skin problems in the elderly, Dermatol. Clin 4:485-499, 1986.
28. Kotler, R: Cosmetic facial surgery, JAMA 249:523-525, 1983.
29. Krupp, MA, Schroeder, SA, and Tierney, LM, Jr: Current medical diagnosis and treatment 1987, Norwalk, Conn, 1987, Appleton & Lange.
30. Kuflek, EG, Lubritz, RR, and Torre, D: Cryosurgery, Dermatol Clin 2:319-332, 1984.
31. *Mangieri, D: Saving your elderly patient's skin, Nurs 82 12(10):44-45, 1982.
32. *McKay, M: Topical dermatologic therapy, Primary Care, 10(3):513-524, 1983.
32a. Nicol, NH: Atopic dermatitis: the (wet) wrap up, Am J Nurs 87:1560-1563, 1987.
33. Olsen, TG: Therapy of acne, Med Clin North Am 66(4):851-871, 1982.
34. Pathak, MA: Sunscreens: topical and systemic approaches for prevention of acute and chronic sun-induced skin reactions, Dermatol Clin 4:321-334, 1986.
35. Pillsbury, DM: A manual of dermatology, ed 2, Philadelphia, 1980, WB Saunders Co.
36. *Prigel, CL: How to spot melanoma, Nursing '87 17(6):60-62, 1987.

*References preceded by an asterisk are particularly well suited for student reading.

37. Rakel, RE, editor: Conn's current therapy 1986, Philadelphia, 1984, WB Saunders Co.

38. *Roy, DJ: Caring for the self-esteem of the cosmetic patient, Plast Surg Nurs 6:138-141, 1986.

39. *Schaal, PG, and Slemenda, MB: Nurses' response to transplants, AORN J 30:42-45, 1984.

40. Schaefer, DG, and Wolf, JE: Common dermatologic disorders, Clin Plast Surg 14:201-208, 1987.

41. *Schulmeister, L: Screening for skin cancer: a necessary part of your assessment routine, Nurs 81 11(10):74-78, 1981.

42. Stahl, S, Hamilton, S, and Spira, M: Surgical treatment of acne scars, Clin Plast Surg 14:261-276, 1987.

42a. *Stern, C: Melanoma: the most lethal skin cancer, RN 50(7):12-14, 1987.

43. Toback, AC, and Anders, JE: Phototoxicity from systemic agents, Dermatol Clin 4:223-229, 1986.

44. Way, LW: Current surgical diagnosis and treatment, ed 7, Los Altos, Calif, 1986, Lange Medical Publications.

45. Weinstein, GD, and Voorhees, JJ, editors: Symposium on psoriasis, Dermatol Clin 2:355-516, 1984.

46. Wyngaarden, JB, and Smith, LH: Textbook of medicine, ed. 17, Philadelphia, 1985, WB Saunders Co.

Classic

47. *Black skin problems, Am J Nurs 79:1092-1094, 1979.

48. Orkin, M, and Maibach, HI: Scabies, a current pandemic, Postgrad Med 66:533-62, 1979.

40

The Patient with Burns

DEBORAH GOLDENBERG KLEIN

CHAPTER OBJECTIVES

After studying this chapter, the student should be able to:

- Differentiate between partial-thickness and full-thickness burns.
- Describe the pathophysiologic changes that occur during the three stages following major burns.
- Describe the emergency care for major burns and the initial inpatient therapy.
- Describe interventions for replacing body fluids, preventing infection, promoting nutrition and mobility, and providing emotional support.
- Identify teaching needs of the patient with burns.

Burn injuries are in many respects the worst of all tragedies an individual can experience. With an intensive burn there is an overwhelming insult to the patient physically and psychologically, and it is catastrophic in cost and suffering to the family involved.

Approximately 300,000 people suffer thermal injury each year in the United States. Of these victims, 200,000 are admitted to hospitals, and 15,000 die as a direct result of the burn injury. Burns are caused by dry or moist heat, chemical exposure, electrical currents, and radiation. The most common cause of burns is fire with an estimate of 7,500 deaths, 310,000 injuries, and $13.6 billion in property losses yearly. Because of the systemic effects of the burn injury, psychologic implications, and prolonged hospitalization, comprehensive nursing care is required during the acute and long-term recovery phases.

■ PREVENTION AND HEALTH EDUCATION

Nurses can help prevent accidental burns by participating in health education programs that stress both fire prevention and the consequences of fires, such as burns, deformities, and death. Nurses can promote legislation that would control hazardous practices and make working and living environments safer. Community health nurses are in an unusually advantageous position to recognize unsafe practices in the home and to help families develop safe habits of living.

Approximately 80% of accidental burns occur in the home and are primarily caused by ignorance, carelessness, and the curiosity of *children.* Infants and children are the most common victims of fires in and about the home. A large number of children have been burned to death or permanently disabled or disfigured by fireworks. Legislation in many states now prohibits the sale of fireworks, but violations of the law and accidents still occur. Approximately 1000 serious burns occur each year from fireworks.

A high incidence of burn injuries affecting *adults* are related to accidents while cooking, smoking, or otherwise using matches. Burns commonly occur when the person is distracted while cooking or falls asleep while smoking. Activities that persons were engaged in when they caught on fire in their homes are shown in Table 40-1.

Each year brings increased demand for careful inspection and regulation of places in which the ill and infirm are housed. Aged persons frequently are housed in old and poorly equipped structures, and many of them have been victims of fire. Nurses can bring necessary pressures to bear to ensure adequate protection and planned evacuation if a fire occurs. The American Burn Association suggests

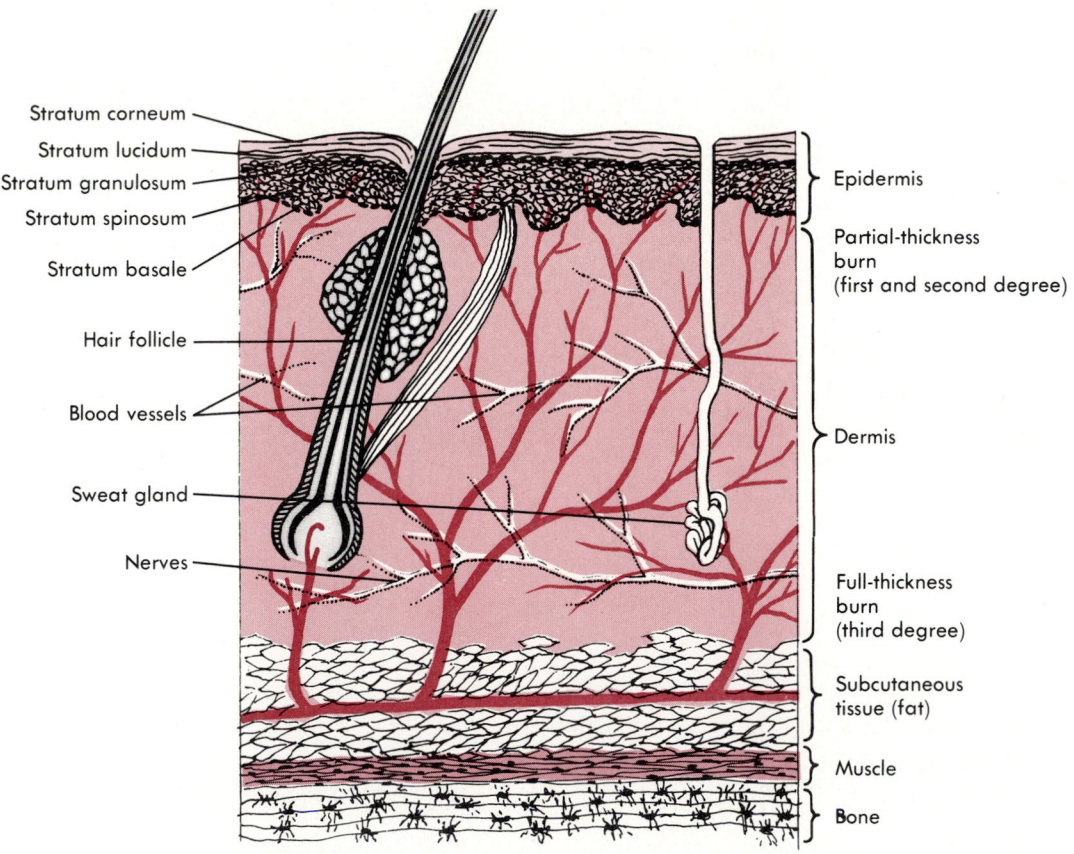

Fig. 40-1   Levels of human skin involved in burns.

that all health facilities conduct one mock evacuation drill each year.[3] Attention is being focused on places where large numbers of people congregate. Laws require that doors in public buildings are hinged to swing outward, that draperies and decorations be fireproof, and that stairways with special fire doors be used in new apartment buildings and hotels. Smoke detectors and sprinkler systems are also required in new buildings and residential health care facilities. Nurses working in institutions need to encourage and participate in fire prevention programs.

Rigid enforcement of laws requiring that industrial products be labeled when known to be flammable and that new products be tested carefully for their flammable qualities before being placed on the market is further evidence of government efforts to protect the public from accident by fire. Industry can be made safer by constant vigilance by management in cooperation with fire safety officers and health care professionals in identifying hazards and implementing a safety program. All chemicals should be labeled, and antidotes should be identified and available. A core of every work force should be well versed in emergency treatment of all types of burns for the protection of every employee.

Recent statistics indicate a rise in the number of chemical injuries as a result of "homemade" solutions for cleaning and home remodeling.

Sunburn should be cautioned against, because even a relatively mild burn of a large part of the body can cause change of fluid distribution and kidney damage. Camp nurses should keep this in mind in their educational programs for children and camp counselors. Many effective sunscreen products are available and should be used in times of exposure.

■ CLASSIFICATION OF BURNS

Traditionally, burns have been classified as first, second, or third degree. The terms *first, second,* and *third degree* are not descriptive of the injury, because they are based only on the visual characteristics of the burn wound. The injury of a burn extends beyond what can be seen. A more accurate description is *partial-* and *full-thickness,* which graphically describes the burn and indicates depth and severity of the tissue injury (Fig. 40-1).

Partial-thickness burns are characterized by destruction in varying depths from the epidermis (outer layer of skin) to the dermis (middle layer of skin). Partial-thickness burns of the skin involve a part of the epidermis and dermis. The depth of tissue injury is described further as *superficial* partial-thickness, which involves only the epidermis, and *deep* partial-thickness, which involves the entire epidermis and part of the dermis. Partial-thickness burns are likely to be painful because nerve endings have been injured and exposed. They have the ability to heal because a portion of the epithelial cells has not been destroyed. During the healing phase, dryness and itching are common and are caused by increased vascularization of sebaceous glands, reduction of secretions, and decreased perspiration.

Table 40-1 Activities of persons burned by fire

Activity	Number	Percent
Playing with matches/lighter	175	11.3*
Smoking	152	10.0
Using matches/lighter	116	7.5
Falling asleep while smoking	100	6.4
Reaching across stove	86	5.5
Sleeping	77	5.0
Standing too close to stove	64	4.1
Leaning against stove	47	3.0

From Flammable fabric investigations, Washington, DC, 1973, Department of Health, Education, and Welfare, Food and Drug Administration, Bureau of Product Safety, FY66-FY72.
*Percent based on 1554 cases in which activity is known.

The presence of blisters often indicates a deep partial-thickness injury. The blisters may increase in size as the result of continuous exudation and collection of tissue fluid.

Full-thickness burns include destruction of the epidermis and the entire dermis, as well as possible damage to the subcutaneous layer, muscle, and bone. Nerve endings are destroyed, resulting in a painless wound. *Eschar,* a leathery covering composed of denatured protein, may form as the result of surface dehydration. Black networks of coagulated capillaries may be seen. Full-thickness burns require skin grafting because the destroyed tissue is unable to epithelialize. Often a deep partial-thickness burn may convert to a full-thickness burn because of infection, trauma, or decreased blood supply.

■ PATHOPHYSIOLOGY OF SEVERE BURNS

As a result of burns, normal skin function is diminished, resulting in physiologic alterations. These include (1) loss of protective barriers against infection, (2) escape of body fluids, (3) lack of temperature control, (4) destroyed sweat and sebaceous glands, and (5) decrease in the number of sensory receptors. The severity of these alterations will depend on the extent of the burn and the depth to which damage has occurred.

Increased knowledge of the physiologic changes that occur during severe burns has led to the saving of many lives. There are two stages that occur following severe burns: the immediate hypovolemic stage and the diuretic stage. Fig. 40-2 presents an overview of the pathophysiologic changes seen in a severe burn.

■ Hypovolemic stage

The hypovolemic stage begins at the time of burn injury and lasts for the first 48 to 72 hours. It is characterized by a *rapid shift of fluid* from the vascular compartments into

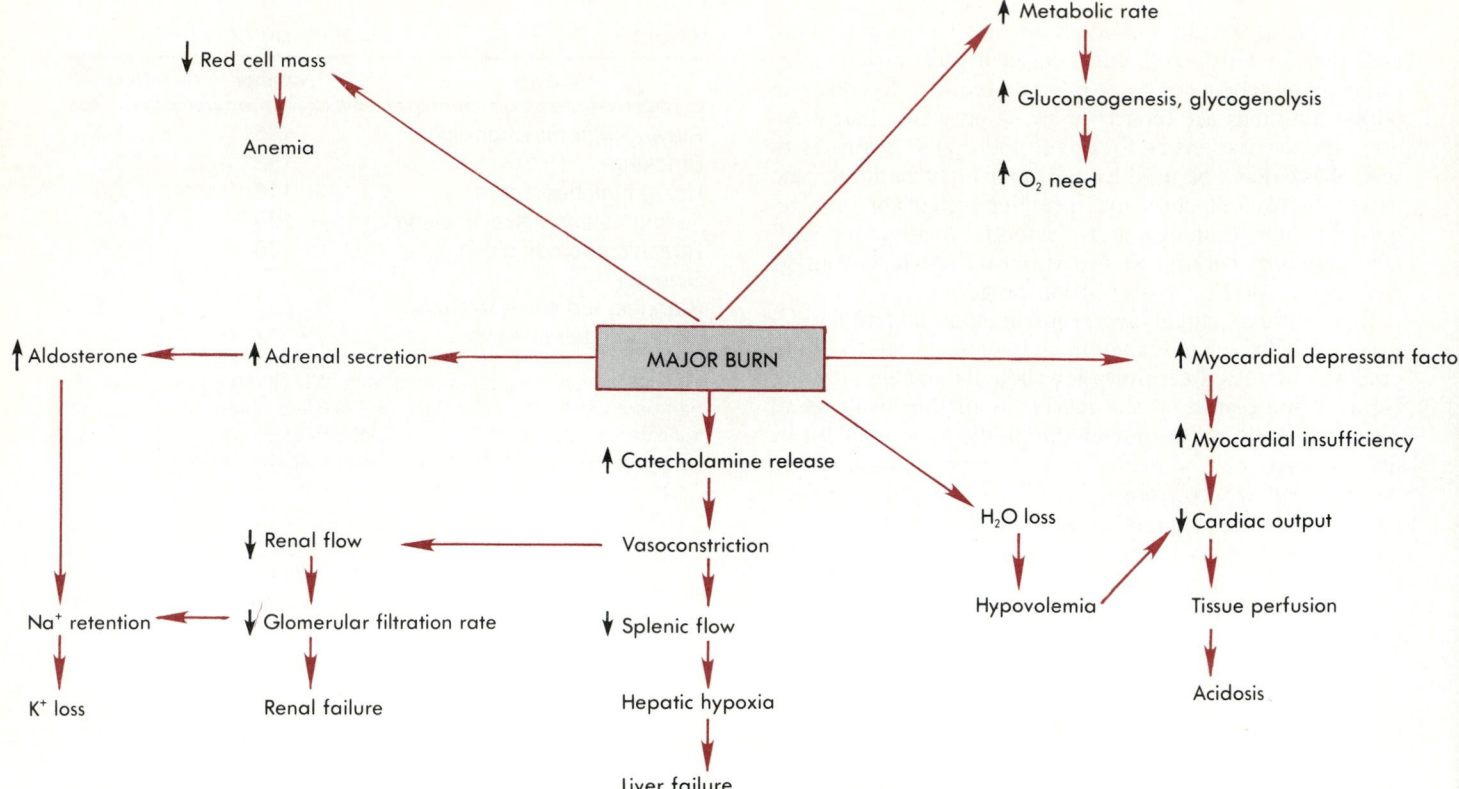

Fig. 40-2 Overview of pathophysiology of a major burn.

the interstitial spaces. When tissues are burned, vasodilation, increased capillary permeability, and changes in the permeability of tissue cells in and around the burn area occur. As a result, abnormally large amounts of extracellular fluid (ECF), sodium chloride, and protein pass through the burned area either to cause blister formation and local edema or to escape through the open wound.

Visible fluid loss makes up only a small part of the fluid lost from the circulating blood and other essential fluid compartments. Most of the fluid loss occurs deep in the wound, where the fluid extravasates into the deeper tissues. Burns occurring in highly vascular areas such as muscle tissue or the face are believed to cause a greater fluid shift than comparable burns occurring on other parts of the body. Fully half of the extracellular fluid of the body can shift from its normal distribution to the site of a severe burn. *Hypovolemic shock* occurs, and there is a tremendous drop in blood pressure and inadequate blood flow through the kidneys, which in turn leads to further shock and anuria. Death occurs within a short time if treatment is either not given promptly or is inadequate. These changes are summarized in Fig. 40-3.

As a result of these fluid shifts, *dehydration* of nondamaged tissue cells may occur. Initially, more fluids and sodium are lost from the capillaries than is protein. This increases the capillary osmotic pressure, leading to dehy-

dration with pronounced *edema* in the burned area. As protein continues to be lost into the burned area because of the increased capillary permeability, *hypoproteinemia* results. The increased amount of protein in the tissue spaces leads to edema. Proteins may be lost through the open wounds. The lymphatic system, which normally functions to remove increased tissue fluid, becomes overloaded and inefficient, thus contributing to edema. Nitrogen is lost through the kidney from catabolism, leading to significant negative nitrogen balance. Blood urea nitrogen (BUN) is elevated when *oliguria* is present.

With loss of fluid from the vascular system, *hemoconcentration* occurs and the hematocrit rises. Blood flow becomes sluggish in the burned area and cellular nutrition decreases. Large numbers of red blood cells become trapped in the burned area and are hemolyzed. Renal damage and hematuria may occur as a result of reduced blood volume and passage of the end products of the hemolyzed cells through the glomeruli. The decreased renal blood flow leads to oliguria.

Electrolyte imbalances also occur. *Hyperkalemia* (elevated serum potassium) results from the release of potassium from damaged tissue cells and red blood cells and from decreased urinary output. Hyperkalemia may lead to heart block and ventricular failure. Potassium may be encouraged to move back into the cells by the administration

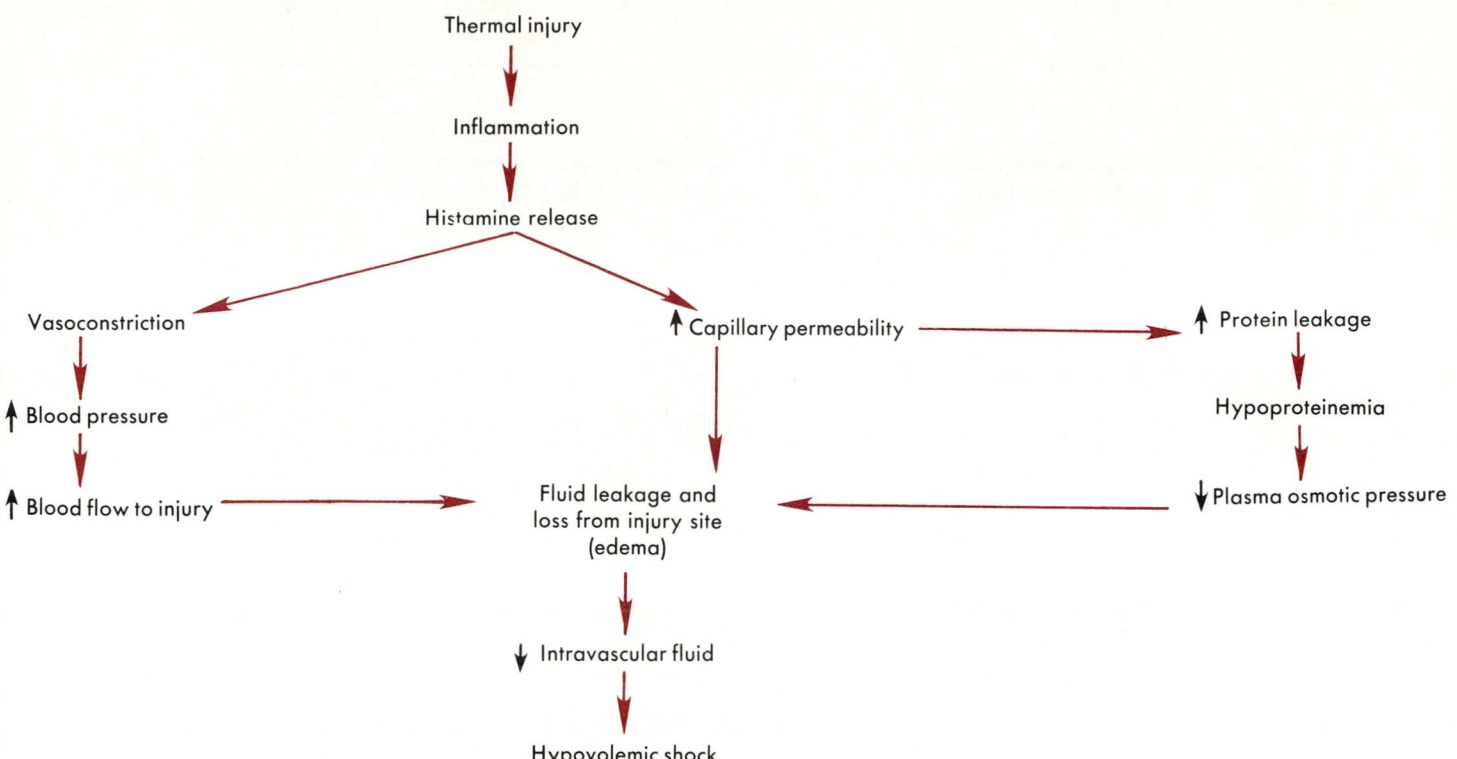

Fig. 40-3 Flow diagram of fluid shifts resulting in hypovolemic shock.

of insulin, because potassium is transported back into the cells along with glucose. Sodium is retained by the body as a result of the endocrine response to stress. Aldosterone is increased, leading to increased sodium reabsorption by the kidney. However, sodium quickly passes into the interstitial spaces of the burned area with the fluid shift. Despite the increased amount of sodium in the body, most of the sodium is trapped in the edema fluid and a *serum sodium deficit* occurs. Inadequate tissue perfusion results in anaerobic metabolism and the acid end products are retained because of the decreased kidney function. *Metabolic acidosis* may then occur.

Respiratory distress may result from upper airway obstruction or the effects of hypovolemic shock. Upper airway obstruction is caused by inhalation of noxious agents or super heated air, causing irritation of the airway, laryngeal edema, and potential obstruction.

■ Diuretic stage

Return of vascular integrity begins in approximately 12 hours and rapidly progresses at 18 to 24 hours following the initial burn injury. Although full capillary integrity may not be restored for a number of days, for clinical purposes it may be considered restored at 24 hours. The diuretic phase begins at about 48 to 72 hours after the burn injury as capillary membrane integrity returns and edema fluid shifts back from the interstitial spaces into the intravascular space. Blood volume increases, leading to increased renal blood flow and *diuresis* unless renal damage has occurred. Serum electrolyte and hematocrit levels will be decreased because of *hemodilution*. *Fluid overload* may occur as a result of the increase in intravascular volume. The patient's vital signs, breath sounds, and urinary output are used to determine the amount of intravenous fluid replacement. Dehydration may occur if rapid urinary output depletes the intravascular reserve. A sodium deficit continues because of the loss of sodium through the burn wound and from an increase in urinary output. *Hypokalemia* (lowered serum potassium) results from potassium moving back into the cells or being excreted in the urine. Protein continues to be lost from the wounds. *Metabolic acidosis* remains a possibility because of the loss of sodium bicarbonate in the urine and the increase in fat metabolism secondary to a decrease in carbohydrate intake.

Following the period of fluid shifts, the patient remains acutely ill. This period is characterized by *anemia* and *malnutrition*. Anemia develops from the loss of red blood cells. Negative nitrogen balance begins at the onset of the burn and is the result of tissue destruction, protein loss, and the stress response. It continues throughout the acute period because of continued loss of protein from the wound, tissue catabolism from immobility, and decreased protein intake. Special attention to the nutrition of the patient is important during this time. Increased metabolism from loss of water and heat from the wound, loss of fluid during

Table 40-2 Physiologic changes with burns

Change	Hypovolemic stage		Diuretic stage	
	Mechanism	Result	Mechanism	Result
Extracellular fluid shift	Vascular to interstitial	Hemoconcentration Edema at burn site	Interstitial to vascular	Hemodilution
Renal function	Decreased renal blood flow from decreased blood pressure and decreased cardiac output	Oliguria	Increased renal blood flow from increased blood volume	Diuresis
Sodium level	Na⁺ reabsorped by kidneys *but* Na⁺ lost in exudate and trapped in edema fluid	Sodium deficit	Na⁺ loss with diuresis (becomes normal in 1 week)	Sodium deficit
Potassium level	K⁺ released as result of tissue and red blood cell injury; decreased K⁺ excretion from decreased renal function	Hyperkalemia	K⁺ moves back into cells; K⁺ lost by diuresis (begins 4-5 days after the burn)	Hypokalemia
Protein level	Protein lost into tissues by increased capillary permeability	Hypoproteinemia	Loss of protein during continued catabolism	Hypoproteinemia
Nitrogen balance	Tissue catabolism; protein loss in tissues; more nitrogen lost than taken in	Negative nitrogen balance	Tissue catabolism, protein loss, immobility	Negative nitrogen balance
Acid base balance	Anaerobic metabolism from decreased tissue perfusion; increased acid end products; decreased renal function (causing retention of acid end products); loss of serum bicarbonate	Metabolic acidosis	Sodium bicarbonate lost in diuresis; hypermetabolism with increased metabolic end products	Metabolic acidosis
Stress response	Occurs because of trauma	Decreased renal blood flow	Occurs because of prolonged nature of injury and psychologic threat to self	Stress ulcers

diuresis, and catabolism during tissue breakdown all lead to *weight loss.*

The differences in changes between the hypovolemic and diuretic stages are summarized in Table 40-2.

■ PERIODS OF TREATMENT

Three periods of treatment can be identified in the care of the seriously burned patient. These are the emergent, the acute, and the rehabilitative periods.

The *emergent period* refers to the first 48 or 72 hours postburn when the patient is admitted, the severity of the injury is determined, and first aid and wound care are given. The *acute period* of treatment begins at the end of the emergent period and lasts until all of the full-thickness wounds are covered with skin grafts or partial thickness-wounds are healed. The *rehabilitation period* focuses on returning the patient to a useful place in society. There

are two areas of concern during this phase: (1) the restoration of function over joint surfaces that were scarred, and (2) the emotional assistance that the patient and family will need. The rehabilitaton of the patient actually begins during early hospitalization and is addressed throughout the hospitalization. After discharge, the patient may require emotional assistance and counseling, and many readmissions may be necessary for reconstructive surgical procedures.

■ Comprehensive team approach

Comprehensive care of the burn patient can best be provided by a multidisciplinary team approach. The physician, nurse, social workers, physical and occupational therapists, teacher (if a school-age child), registered dietitian, vocational counselor, and others all work together to address the needs of the patient. The nurse's role in the team is to coordinate the interactions of the various

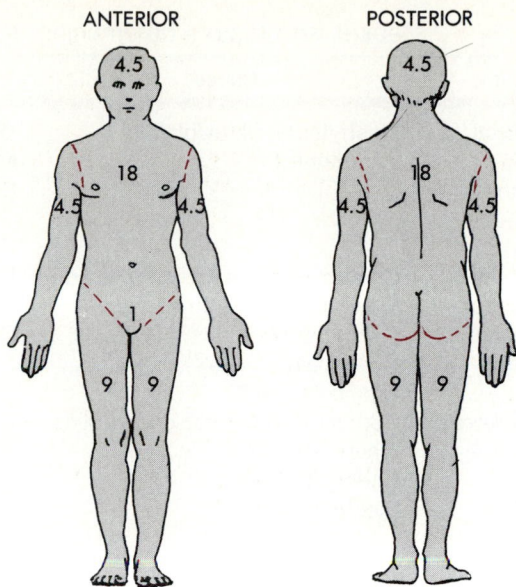

Fig. 40-4   Rule of nines.

Classification of severity of burns

Major burn injuries

Greater than 25% BSA (greater than 20% in children under 10 years and adults over 40 years of age)

Greater than 10% BSA, full-thickness

Involvement of face, eyes, ears, hands, feet, perineum

Electrical burns

Burns complicated by inhalation injury or major trauma

Burns in patients with preexisting disease (diabetes, congestive heart failure, or chronic renal failure)

Moderate burn injuries

15% to 25% BSA in adults, partial-thickness (10% to 20% BSA in children under 10 years and adults over 40 years of age)

Less than 10% BSA full-thickness

Burns with no concurrent injury

Burns in patients with no preexisting disease

Minor burn injuries

Less than 15% BSA in adults (10% in children or the elderly)

Less than 2% BSA full-thickness injury

Burns in patients with no preexisting disease

disciplines and to incorporate the team's suggestions and approaches into an effective plan of care.

■ Emergent period

The emergent period of therapy is defined as the time required to resolve the immediate problems resulting from the burn injury. First aid measures are directed toward treating the systemic response to trauma, concurrent injuries, and the burn wound.

▦ ASSESSMENT

Assessment of the person who has sustained a severe burn depends on the severity of the burn injury.

□ Subjective data

Information is obtained from either the burn victim or other persons. Data should include the following:

1. How the burn injury occurred
2. When the burn injury occurred
3. Duration of contact with the burning agent
4. Location (enclosed area suggests possibility of smoke inhalation and/or carbon monoxide poisoning)

5. Presence of an explosion (suggests possibility of other injuries)

The state of health and age of the burn victim are important factors that may modify treatment. The elderly and very young have a higher mortality than do young adults with the same percentage burn. Preexisting endocrine, pulmonary, cardiovascular, or renal disease or medication history will decrease the person's ability to cope with severe burns. The nurse has the responsibility to learn as much as possible about the patient, including preburn weight, from relatives and friends.

□ Objective data

Burns may be categorized as major, moderate, or minor and on the basis of the size of the burn and the presence of complicating factors (see the box above, left).

□ Assessing the severity of the burn injury
□ *Size and depth of burn*

For adults, the *rule of nines* is used in determining the size of the burn. The percentage of body surface burned is estimated by using charts that depict anterior and posterior drawings of the body. In adults, the body is divided into areas equal to multiples of 9% (Fig. 40-4). In clinical practice, the burned area is shaded in on the drawings, and the amount of body surface burned is calculated from the shaded areas. Calculations are modified for infants and children under 10 years of age because of their relatively larger head and smaller bodies (see pediatric textbooks for these figures). The depth of the burn injury is determined by appearance, color, and sensation (Table 40-3).

□ *Age of victim*

The severity of a burn also depends on the age of the victim. Infants under 2 years of age and adults over 60

Table 40-3 Causes and factors determining depth of burn injury

Depth	Cause	Appearance	Color	Sensation
Superficial partial-thickness (first degree)	Flash flame, ultraviolet light (sunburn)	Dry, no blisters Minimal or no edema Blanches with fingertip pressure and refills when pressure removed	Increased redness	Painful
Deep partial-thickness (second degree)	Contact with hot liquids or solids Flash flame to clothing Direct flame Chemicals Ultraviolet light	Large, moist blisters that will increase in size Blanches with fingertip pressure and refills when pressure removed	Mottled with dull, white, tan, pink, or cherry red areas	Very painful
Full-thickness (third degree)	Contact with hot liquids or solids Flame Chemicals Electrical contact	Dry with leathery eschar Charred vessels visible under eschar Blisters rare but thin walled blisters that do not increase in size may be present No blanching with pressure	White, charred, dark tan Black Red	Little or no pain Hair easily pulls out

years of age have a higher mortality than persons in other age groups with a similar size injury. Infants have a weak antibody response to infection and in older victims the serious burn may aggravate the degenerative processes or exacerbate a preexisting health problem.

□ **Body part involved**

The body part involved is an important factor in evaluating the severity of a burn. Injuries that involve cosmetic and functional areas of the body warrant a prognosis of long-term morbidity or mortality. A burn of the face, hands, and feet will require extensive and meticulous care. A burn of the head, neck, and chest may also involve injury to the respiratory tract and result in severe respiratory difficulty. Burns of the perineum are difficult to manage because of the high incidence of infection. The circumferential or encircling burn of a limb, the neck, or the chest has serious consequences. This type of burn will cause constrictive contraction of the skin and produce a tourniquet effect that may impair breathing and/or circulation. The anatomic part of the body burned must be considered when estimating the severity of the burn: a 3% burn of the anterior surface of the thigh will probably not be as serious as a 3% burn of the neck, face, or perineal area.

□ **Burning agent**

The identification of the causative agent is of prime importance because the nature of the agent has a direct effect on prognosis and treatment.

Thermal burns are the most common and occur as the result of the transfer of energy from a heat source to the body (flame, hot surfaces, sunburn, hot metals, and hot grease). Thermal injury caused by a flame or fire results in a dry burn that can be much deeper than is visually apparent. The flame is a highly concentrated heat that affects a localized area and burns deeply. In contrast, scald injuries, or moist burns, are caused by steam or boiling water, which conducts heat to a larger, widespread area (Fig. 40-5).

Chemical burns, commonly seen in industry, are caused by strong acids or alkali, such as hydrochloric acid and lye (Table 40-4). Household chemical burns frequently occur from accidental exposure to drain cleaners, paint removers, and disinfectants. Burns to the eye occur when a chemical splashes onto the face, and burns to the upper gastrointestinal tract occur when a noxious chemical is ingested.

Electrical burns are caused by electrical sparks and arcs or by an electrical current passing directly through the body. Tissue with the highest water content has the least resistance to electrical current and, consequently, suffers the most damage. Blood, muscles, skin, tendons, fat, and bones are affected in a decreasing order of resistance. Tissue damage may appear minor at the entrance and exit points, making electrical burns difficult to evaluate. The visual damage is referred to as the "tip of the iceberg" and does not reflect underlying tissue destruction generated by the passage of electrical current through the body. Victims of electrical burns must be checked frequently for signs and symptoms of hemorrhage, intestinal perforations, and cardiac arrhythmias. The passage of current through the body may cause cardiac arrest at the time of injury.

□ **Medical history**

Identification of known and unknown disorders may prevent fatal complications in the burn victim. A prior illness, such as diabetes or renal failure, may become acute during the postburn phase. The physiologic stress seen with the burn may exacerbate a latent disease process or worsen the process if it is active and thus increase mortality.

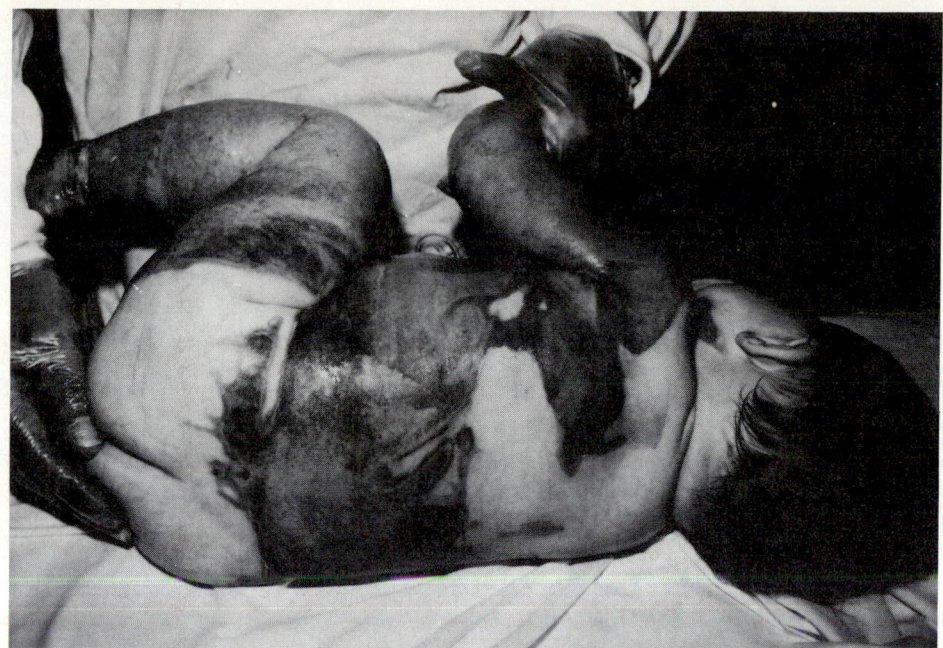

Fig. 40-5 Toddler with scald burn that resulted from being placed in a tub of water that was too hot. (Courtesy of Burn Center, Cleveland Metropolitan General Hospital/Highland View Hospital, Cleveland, Ohio.)

Table 40-4 Agents associated with chemical burns

Chemical agent	Common use	Characteristics	Systemic effects	Agents to remove or dilute chemicals
Oxidizing agents				
Chromic acid	Metal cleansing	Ulcerates, blisters		Water lavage
Potassium perman-ganate	Disinfectant, bleach, deo-dorizers	Thick, brownish purple eschar		Water lavage
				Eggwhite solution
Sodium hypochlorite (Clorox)	Disinfectant, bleach, deo-dorizers	Local irritation, inflam-mation		Water lavage
				Milk
				Eggwhite
				Starch
				Paste
Corrosive agents				
Phenol	Deodorizers; sanitizers; disinfectants; manufac-ture of plastics, dyes, fertilizers, explosives	Soft white eschar, brown stain when eschar removed, mild to no pain	Minor exposure: tachy-cardia arrhythmias	Copious water la-vage
				Polyethelene glycol solution
				Vegetable oil
			Significant exposure: CNS depression, hypothermia, cardiac depression, respira-tory depression	Lavage with water to debride particles
Phosphorus (white)	Manufacture of explo-sives, insecticides, ro-dent poisons, fertilizers	Necrotic with yellow-ish color	Nephrotoxicity	Lavage with 1% copper sulfate $(CuSO_4)$,
		Garlic odor	Hepatic necrosis	Cover with castor oil
		Glows in dark		
		Painful		

Continued.

Table 40-4 Agents associated with chemical burns—cont'd

Chemical agent	Common use	Characteristics	Systemic effects	Agents to remove or dilute chemicals
Pure sodium lye KOH NaOH NH_4OH LiOH $Ba_2(OH)_3$ $Ca(OH)_3$	Cleaning agents (washing powders, drain cleaners, paint removers), urine sugar reagent tablets, Portland cement	Soft gelatinous, brown eschar		Lye; water lavage Pure sodium; oil immersion
Protoplasmic poisons				
Salt-formers Tungstic Picric Sulfasalicyclic Tannic Trichloracetic Cresylic Acetate Formic	Industrial	Thin, hard eschar	Hepatic necrosis Nephrotoxicity	Water lavage
Metabolic competitor/inhibitor Oxalic acid	Industrial	Chalky white ulcers	Hypocalcemia	Large volume calcium salts Copious water lavage Intravenous calcium
Hydrofluoric acid	Etching of glass	Painful, deep ulcerations	Hypocalcemia	Water lavage Subcutaneous calcium to area Subcutaneous magnesium sulfate

---

Factors determining severity of burns

Size of burn
Depth of burn
Age of victim
Body part involved
Burning agent
History of cardiac, pulmonary, renal, or hepatic disease
Injuries sustained at time of burn

Diabetes and chronic obstructive pulmonary disease (COPD) may be aggravated. A patient with arteriosclerotic heart disease may develop a myocardial infarction.

Factors determining the severity of burns are listed in the box above.

▶ DATA ANALYSIS: NURSING DIAGNOSES

Nursing diagnoses are determined from assessment of patient data. Possible nursing diagnoses for the person with burns may include, but are not limited to, the following:

Diagnostic title	Possible etiologies
Ineffective airway clearance	Laryngeal edema, obstruction, secretions
Anxiety	Threat to self-concept, threat of death, threat/change in health status
Fluid volume deficit (1)	Movement of fluid from intravascular to interstitial space (hypovolemic stage), evaporation
Fluid volume deficit (2)	Movement of fluid from interstitial to intravascular space (diuretic stage)
Hypothermia	Environmental exposure of burn wounds

Diagnostic title	Possible etiologies
Potential for infection	Loss of protection created by damage to skin
Pain	Exposed nerve endings from burn injury, trauma
Impaired skin integrity	Loss of skin from burn injury
Altered renal, cerebral, cardiopulmonary, gastrointestinal, peripheral tissue perfusion	Hypovolemia (hypovolemic stage), hypervolemia (diuretic stage)

PLANNING: EXPECTED PATIENT OUTCOMES

Expected patient outcomes for the person with burns may include, but are not limited to, the following:

1. Patient maintains patent airway, adequate ventilation and oxygenation.
2. Patient exhibits control of anxiety.
3. Patient experiences minimal pain.
4. Optimal fluid and electrolyte balance is regained.
5. Patient's body temperature is normal.
6. Patient is free of pathogenic organisms.
7. No further skin loss occurs.
8. Vital organs have adequate perfusion.

IMPLEMENTATION

Assisting with airway management

Persons who are burned on the face and neck or those who have inhaled flame, steam, or smoke should be observed closely for signs or laryngeal edema and airway obstruction. Data indicating potential or existing airway injury are outlined in the box below.

Adequate ventilation and oxygenation may be possible on room air, however, when any inhalation injury has oc-

---

Factors determining inhalation injury and/or potential airway obstruction

Burns to face and neck
Singed hairs, nasal hair, beard, eyelids or eyelashes
Intraoral charcoal, especially on teeth and gums
Respiratory distress
Brassy cough
Hoarseness
Copious sputum production
Carbonaceous sputum
Burn injury occurred in a closed space
Smell of smoke on victim's clothes or on victim

---

curred it is best to give oxygen. If the victim is in respiratory distress or has a suspected inhalation injury, intubation may be necessary.

Prehospital care

At the scene of a burn injury, the first action is to remove the victim from the hazardous environment. The length of exposure to the causative agent is directly related to the severity of the injury.

The three most common causative agents for burn injury are fire, chemicals, and electricity. In the case of fire, flames should be extinguished, flammable or hot material removed from the victim, and the victim and rescuer removed from the unventilated or hazardous surroundings. If clothing is on fire, the victim's first reacton is to run, which only fans the flame. The best intervention is to stop the person and roll him or her in a blanket, coat, sheet, or towel on the ground to exclude oxygen and thereby put out the fire. The rule is stop, drop, and roll. The victim should never stand because this will cause the flame and smoke to engulf the facial area, possibly igniting the hair and causing an inhalation injury. Any water source can be used to extinguish flames.

First aid for burn wounds

Once all flame is extinguished, clothing, jewelry, and debris are carefully removed, avoiding removal of clothing that adheres to the burned area. Any clothing removed should be saved for possible analysis of flammability. The wounds are covered with dressings dampened with normal saline to ease the pain, reduce edema, and prevent evaporation of body water. The patient is entirely wrapped in a dry cover to prevent heat loss. Ice should never be used because sudden vasoconstriction causes severe shifting of fluids. Although sterile dressings are preferred, clean, nonsterile dressings can be used because all dressings will be removed at the medical facility. Oils, salves, and ointments should never be used on burns because they hamper treatment at the medical facility.

The severity of *chemical burns* is directly proportional to the length of exposure. Chemicals cause deep burns over a rather limited area. The chemical should be identified and treatment initiated quickly. The first priority is removal of the chemical agent. This is accomplished by copious flushing with water for as long as 20 to 30 minutes to ensure complete removal of the chemical. Although specific chemical agents have known antidotes, it is best to flood the exposed area with water to ensure removal of the chemical and transport the victim to the nearest medical facility. Burns occurring around the eyes should be lavaged continuously with copious amounts of cool, clean water for up to 30 minutes.

Electrical burns pose a special hazard to the victim because the total body surface area of the burn is not always apparent and is often internal. Dysrhythmias and neurological dysfunction are common in such exposure. Extreme care must be taken in removing the patient from the electrical source to prevent a similar injury to the rescuer.

□ *Pain relief*

Pain in extensive burns is best controlled by gentle and minimal handling and by the application of dressings that exclude air from the burned surfaces. The degree of pain is usually inversely proportional to the depth of the burn injury—full-thickness burns are usually painless because nerve endings have been destroyed.

In small partial-thickness burns, cool (not cold) compresses on the burn site may provide some relief as long as the victim is kept warm. Ice packs are contraindicated because they may cause further skin injury and hypothermia.

□ *Transport*

Burns are often more severe than they first appear to be. Therefore, all persons with burns, even if the burns appear to be superficial, should be seen by a physician. The hospital or burn center should be notified before a severely burned victim is transported so that preparation can be made for arrival.

For obviously small burns, fluids may be given by mouth with caution. Large burns are accompanied by decreased peristalsis; therefore, nothing should be given by mouth. Patients with large burns or smoke inhalation may vomit, and particular attention must be given to preventing them from aspirating vomitus.

According to the 1985 American Burn Association Directory, 178 hospitals in the United States reported the presence of a specialized burn care service. Of these 178 hospitals, only 140 reported that they had a special burn unit. These burn units are located throughout the United States in major medical centers in or near urban areas. The American Burn Association estimates that there are 70,000 annual acute inpatient burn admissions in the United States. Only about 21,000 (or 30%) of these patients are cared for in specialized units. The American Burn Association publishes a list of specialized burn care services every year.

The initial care for major burns is summarized in the box at top, right.

□ **Emergency room management**

Rapid and efficient care is essential in the emergency room management of the burn victim. If respiratory distress is present, an airway is established. Prophylactic intubation is initiated if heat or smoke has been inhaled, or if the head, neck, or face is involved. Inhalation injuries are best managed with controlled ventilation because swelling of the upper airway can rapidly cause obstruction (Plate 7). Endotracheal intubation is preferred over a tracheostomy. Edema of the respiratory passages frequently subsides within a few days after the injury; therefore, surgery of the airway should be avoided. Depending on the severity of symptoms, emergency treatment may include oxygen, suctioning, and postural drainage.

After an airway has been established, support of circulation is addressed. Burn injuries cause tremendous losses of fluid through the wound as well as into the burn wound and adjacent tissues in the form of edema. Fluid

---

Initial care for major burns

1. Remove victim from source of burn.
2. Douse with water and remove nonadherent, smoldering clothing.
3. If chemical burn, carefully remove clothing and flush wound with large amounts of water.
4. If electrical burn and victim is still in contact with electrical source, do *not* touch victim. Remove electrical source with dry nonconductive object (rope).
5. Establish patent airway and assess for inhalation injury. Give oxygen if available.
6. Assess and initiate treatment for injuries requiring immediate attention.
7. Remove tight-fitting jewelry or clothing.
8. Cover burn with moist sterile or clean cover.
9. Cover victim with warm dry cover to prevent heat loss.
10. Transport victim to nearest medical facility.

---

loss is best replaced through two large-caliber peripheral intravenous catheters. However, if the burn is large, or complicated by inhalation injuries or preexisting disease, one peripheral line and one central line (for central venous pressure measurement) is preferred. To prevent the introduction of infection, the lines are inserted through unburned areas. An indwelling Foley catheter is inserted to adequately monitor urine output. Hourly urine output measurements are used as a guide to the adequacy of fluid (plasma volume) replacement.

Almost every patient who is burned over more than 15% body surface area (BSA) develops thirst and an ileus. Oral fluids will not pass beyond the stomach and they create a threat of regurgitation and aspiration. A nasogastric tube is inserted and the stomach is kept empty by suction to prevent gastric distention.

□ *Managing pain*

Morphine sulfate is the drug of choice for pain relief and is given intravenously in small increments. A morphine sulfate drip can be used (15 mg in 250 ml D5W) and titrated to the patient's pain. The intravenous route is used because of inadequate absorption at peripheral sites. No medication of any kind should be given intramuscularly or subcutaneously because it may pool and be absorbed later when cardiac output and blood pressure improve. Large doses of sedatives and analgesics are avoided because of the danger of respiratory depression and the potential masking of other symptoms.

Tetanus prophylaxis is initiated in the emergency department. Tetanus toxoid is administered if the patient has been previously immunized but has not received tetanus toxoid in the preceding 5 years. If prior tetanus immuni-

---

Initial treatment of major burns in the emergency room

1. Establish airway.
2. Initiate fluid therapy by intravenous catheters.
3. Insert indwelling foley catheter for hourly urine measurement.
4. Insert nasogastric tube to remove stomach contents and prevent gastric distention.
5. Insert central intravenous catheter, if appropriate.
6. Manage pain by intravenous narcotics in small, frequent doses.
7. Provide tetanus prophylaxis.

Indications for fluid resuscitation

Burns greater than 20% BSA in adults
Burns greater than 10% BSA in children
Patient older than 65 or younger than 2 years of age
Patient with preexisting disease that would reduce normal compensatory responses to minor hypovolemia (cardiac or pulmonary disease, diabetes)

---

zation is not documented, a dose of human tetanus—immune globulin (TIGH) is administered and an active tetanus immunization program begun.

The treatment of major burns in the emergency room is summarized in the box above.

□ *Replacing body fluids*

Replacing fluids and electrolytes is an essential part of the treatment of the burn victim and is instituted as soon as the severity of the burn and the patient's condition is known. Ideally, fluid therapy is started within an hour after a severe burn to prevent hypovolemic shock. Insertion of two large-caliber peripheral catheters or one large-caliber central venous catheter and one large-caliber peripheral catheter permits the rapid administration of fluids and electrolytes.

Fluids administered during the first 48 hours are given to maintain circulating blood volume. Additional fluids and electrolytes are added to replace losses from vomiting or from nasogastric drainage. Three types of fluid are considered in calculating the needs of the patient: (1) colloids, including plasma and plasma expanders such as Dextran, (2) electrolytes, such as physiologic solution of sodium chloride, Ringer's solution, Hartmann's solution, or Tyrode's solution, and (3) nonelectrolyte fluids, such as distilled water with 5% glucose. Medical authorities do not agree about the proportion of colloids and electrolyte fluids needed. Several formulas are described in the medical literature to guide physicians in determining the type and amount of fluids to be administered based on the patient's weight, age, and the percentage of the body burned.[29] The present trend is to administer balanced salt solutions (for example, lactated Ringer's), water, and plasma and to use whole blood only if a large number of red blood cells are destroyed or if anemia develops. Colloids are not used in the first 24 hours because capillary changes in the wound allow protein-rich fluid to leak into the interstitial space, augmenting edema formation. Indications for the use of fluids are summarized in the box at top, right.

According to the crystalloid resuscitation formula, fluids are administered in three time periods of eight hours each. In the first three 8-hour periods (24 hours) Ringer's lactate solution (RL) or Hartmann's solution is administered according to the following formula:

$$4 \text{ ml RL} \times \text{weight (kg)} \times \% \text{ BSA burned} = \text{ml RL for 24 hr}$$

Because blood volume falls most rapidly and edema increases fastest in the first eight hours, intravenous replacement must be at a rapid rate. One half of the total amount calculated is given in the first 8 hours after the injury. The time is calculated from the *time of injury*, not from the time emergency care was started. In the second 8-hour period, one fourth of the total amount of calculated Ringer's lactate solution is given, and in the third 8-hour period, the remaining one fourth is given.

Patients may complain of moderate to severe thirst during this period. Frequent oral hygiene may alleviate patient discomfort. If oral fluids are permitted, accurate recording of intake is important. Unlimited oral intake and failure to measure and record it may result in water intoxication.

During the second 24 hours postburn, one half to two thirds of the initial 24-hour volume will be required. It is also during this second 24-hour period that colloid solutions are used to replace intravascular volume once capillary permeability significantly decreases.

During fluid resuscitation, adequate volume is assessed by monitoring mental status, vital signs, peripheral perfusion, body weight, and urine output. A 15% to 20% weight gain in the first 72 hours of resuscitation is anticipated. Important laboratory tests are serum and urine electrolytes, serum and urine osmolality, and hematocrit. Hourly urine output is generally the most reliable index of adequate fluid replacement. Fluid should be titrated to ensure an output of 30 to 50 ml/hr in the adult and 0.5 to 1 ml/kg/hr in the child. A drop in urine output below 30 ml/hr may indicate insufficient fluid replacement. The most common reasons for this are that the calculated amount of fluid is behind schedule or the severity of the burn has been underestimated. The urine is observed for color and checked for the presence of blood. The physician is notified if hematuria or a positive Hemastix reaction is present.

Signs of adequate resuscitation

Clear sensorium	
Pulse	< 120 beats/minute
Urine output	30 to 50 ml/hr (adult)
	0.5 to 1 ml/kg/hr
	(child)
Systolic blood pressure	100 mm Hg
Central venous pressure	5 to 10 mm Hg
Pulmonary artery end-diastolic pressure	5 to 15 mm Hg
Blood pH normal range	7.35 to 7.45

Criteria that indicate adequate fluid resuscitation are pulse rate of 120/min or less in the adult, central venous pressure in low to normal range, pulmonary artery end-diastolic pressure (PAEDP) in low to normal range, and mental alertness (see a summary in the box above).

After the first 48 to 72 hours, the patient enters the *diuretic phase* as edema reabsorption occurs. The urinary output increases dramatically, and it is no longer a reliable guide to fluid needs. Fluid needs are assessed by measuring serum and urine electrolyte levels, and replacement is based on individual assessment using 5% dextrose and water. If dehydration occurs from diuresis, fluid replacement therapy is continued until blood volume is stabilized. Potassium may be added to the intravenous fluid because of potassium losses through the urine. The patient is monitored closely for signs of water intoxication or pulmonary edema.

☐ *Wound care*

Care of the burn wound can be delayed until all first aid measures have been initiated. Wound care should be carried out carefully and with as little discomfort to the patient as possible. One of the most important factors to be considered is that the patient has lost the ability to withstand infection in the area where the skin is damaged or destroyed. The goals of the initial wound care are as follows:

1. Cleanse the wound to eliminate or decrease the dead tissue and debris that serve as the media for bacterial growth
2. Prevent further destruction of viable skin
3. Provide for patient comfort

During the admission procedure, the burn wound and the entire body are washed to remove dirt and debris as well as loose, dead tissue on the burned areas. Detergents (Dreft) or antiseptic preparations such as povidine-iodine (Betadine) are effective cleansing agents. Gentle cleansing with gauze squares is effective in removing dead tissue without causing further tissue damage.

All hair in and around the burn wound is shaved and wiped away because hair attracts and shelters bacteria. Singed hair is clipped short to avoid bacterial contamination of the wound.

Firm, intact blisters are left undisturbed because they are a natural, protective, pain-free dressing. If the blisters are broken and the epidermis is separated, loose tissue must be debrided.

Maintenance of body temperature is a critical factor during cleansing, because the severely burned patient has lost some of the ability to regulate body temperature. The environment must be heat controlled and kept warmer than usual. Drafts should be eliminated. A heat lamp or warming lights should be available. Prolonged exposure to air should be avoided. Exposed areas of the body should be covered with sterile sheets and blankets while other areas of the burn are being cleansed.

After the wound is cleaned and before a dressing is applied, cultures of the wound are obtained. Prophylactic systemic antibiotics are usually not indicated. However, wound cultures are obtained to determine which organisms are present in the wounds at the time of admission.

Photographs are taken on admission and at intervals during the patient's hospitalization. They provide a record of the appearance of the burn wound on admission, before the application of topical therapy, and during the healing process.

An early complication of thermal injury is the constricting effect of a *circumferential eschar* of the trunk or extremitites. Eschar is a crust or scab that forms over a burn wound. Edema forming rapidly under the constricting eschar of a full-thickness wound on the arms or legs will produce enough pressure to cause occlusion of venous and arterial circulation and may result in *ischemic necrosis*, especially if unburned areas are distal to the constrictive eschar. Circumferential burns of the neck and chest not only occlude circulation but also may result in pressure on the trachea or rib cage, causing respiratory distress. Frequent observations of chest excursions in addition to respiratory rate are necessary to determine whether respiratory restriction is developing. Peripheral pulses are checked every 15 minutes to ensure uninterrupted vascular flow to all extremities.

Treatment of constrictive eschar is by an escharotomy. The eschar is surgically cut linearly or into squares to alleviate stricture (Plate 8). This is a painless procedure in a full-thickness burn because the nerve endings have already been damaged.

☐ *Emotional support*

Patients with significant burn injuries have received a profound insult to their body and self-image. They are fearful and anxious about possible scarring and disfigurement. They are also aware that they may not survive, and this increases feelings of fear and helplessness. The shock and pain of the accident, the chaos and rush to the hospital, the unknown surroundings and people all itensify the emotional stress.

The nurse is the member of the burn team who spends the most time with the patient and has a considerable influence on the patient's psychologic adjustment. Interventions that can be employed to reassure the patient and alleviate anxiety include the following:

1. Identify self to patient
2. Orient patient to the surroundings
3. Describe the reasons for physical symptoms (skin loss, pain, cold)
4. Explain the equipment and procedures to be used in treatment.

⊞ EVALUATION

Evaluation is based on the expected patient outcomes. Questions to ask may include the following:

1. Does the patient demonstrate any respiratory distress?
2. Is the patient experiencing pain?
3. Is the patient in optimal fluid and electrolyte balance?
4. Is the patient anxious or fearful?
5. Is the patient free of infection?

■ Acute period

The acute period of treatment begins at the end of the emergent period and lasts until the burn wound is healed. The length of this period varies. If the burn is a partial-thickness injury, the acute period extends 10 to 20 days; if the burn is a full-thickness injury over a large percentage of the body requiring surgery for skin grafting, the acute period can last for months.

The nursing care of patients during the acute period of burns is complex. Analysis of data may lead to the identification of numerous nursing diagnoses.

During the acute period there are two main principles of management: (1) treatment of the burn wound, and (2) avoidance, detection, and treatment of complications. The most common complications are infection (septicemia, pneumonia), renal disease, and heart failure.

⊞ ASSESSMENT

☐ Subjective data

Burn patients are often frightened and anxious about their injury and the associated treatments. These responses can be compounded by the intensive care unit (ICU) environment.

Burn patients experience both physical and psychologic pain. Physical pain is usually focused on specific activities such as wound cleansing and debridement, dressing changes, and physical therapy. The patient may react to physical pain in three ways: (1) by ignoring it, (2) by accepting it, or (3) by overreacting to it. The nurse should not judge whether or not the patient is feeling real pain; the nurse must instead assess the patient's reaction to pain and intervene appropriately.

☐ Objective data

The nurse must perform a thorough head-to-toe assessment of the burn patient every shift. Data should include mental status, vital signs, breath sounds, bowel sounds, dietary intake, motor ability, intake and output, weight pattern, circulatory assessment, and observation of burn wounds, grafts, and donor site. Purulent drainage, abnormal color, foul odor, redness or swelling in surrounding normal skin, or presence of healing should be noted. Changes in these parameters from shift to shift or from day to day make further investigation necessary.

Metabolism is increased following moderate to severe burns as a result of stress, fluid loss, fever, infection, increased metabolism, and immobility. Wound healing may be prolonged if adequate nutritional support is not initiated on admission. A nutritional assessment is performed during the first days following burn injury and includes anthropometric measurements (to determine actual weight loss compared to ideal weight), serum electrolytes, liver function test, and urinalysis.

➡ DATA ANALYSIS: NURSING DIAGNOSES

Nursing diagnoses are determined from assessment of patient data. Possible nursing diagnoses for the person with burns may include, but are not limited to, the following:

Diagnostic title	Possible etiologies
Anxiety	Threat to self-concept, threat/change in health status/role functioning, situational crisis
Fear	Long-term illness, death, pain, treatment, life-style changes
Hypothermia	Environmental exposure of burn wounds
Potential for infection	Decreased nutrition, burn wound treatment (dressings, surgery)
Knowledge deficit	Unfamiliarity with routines
Altered nutrition: less than body requirements	Increased metabolic needs
Pain	Treatment of burn wounds (dressings, surgery)
Impaired skin integrity	Burn wounds
Social isolation	Alteration in physical appearance, physical isolation (wound/skin)

⊞ PLANNING: EXPECTED PATIENT OUTCOMES

Expected patient outcomes for the person with burns may include, but are not limited to, the following:

1. Patient will verbalize anxiety.
2. Patient obtains pain relief.
3. Patient is not fearful (establishes a trusting relationship with his or her primary nurse).
4. Patient is free of pathogenic organisms.

5. Patient verbalizes understanding of treatments and surgical procedures and participate appropriately in care.
6. Optimal nutritional status is achieved.
7. Wounds are clean, small, and open.
8. Majority of wounds are closed.
9. Patient is not withdrawn or depressed.
10. Body temperature is normal.

IMPLEMENTATION

☐ Assisting with psychologic support

The psychologic responses of the patient in the immediate postburn period are in response to a threat to survival. The fear of death is real as the patient senses the acuity of the situation by experiencing pain, disfigurement, isolation, and dependency from being attached to machines and monitors that maintain vital functions. A variety of behaviors may be seen during the acute and emergent phase (see Table 40-5 for a summary of emotional responses). Patients' reactions are determined by their personality, their degree of total adjustment to life, and the extent and location of their burns.

The nurse should support and encourage the patient to ease the patient's anxiety. Setting short-term, achievable goals will help motivate the patient. Providing the family with an explanation of the patient's needs will ease their fears and allow them to encourage the patient.

☐ Assisting with infection control

Infection control begins at the time the patient is admitted to the hospital and continues until healing is complete. Local and systemic infections (septicemia) are the most common complications of burns and are the major cause of death, particularly in burns covering more than 25% of the body. Initially autogenous sources are the primary sources of infection because of bacteria that survive in the hair follicles and sweat glands beneath the burned tissue. However, the patient is also susceptible to infection from exogenous sources.

The organisms that usually infect burns are *Staphylococcus aureus*, *Pseudomonas aerugenosa* (Plate 9), and the coliform bacilli. In recent years, there has been a high incidence of fungal infections resulting from the use of broad spectrum antibiotics. *Candida albicans*, which nor-

Table 40-5 Emotional responses to severe burns

Patient response	Definition	Behavior exhibited	Nursing approach
Denial	Inability to accept present condition (pain, disfigurement, events of burn accident, hospital environment); buffers impact of overwhelming physical and psychologic crisis	Level of comprehension and understanding in relation to degree of injury is distorted; denial of burn injury: states he or she is "fine"; avoids discussion of injury; may experience period of euphoria	Support patient: allow some degree of denial, but allay patient's fears without distorting truth
Flood reaction	Extreme agitation and concern over multiple issues in a disorganized fashion; problems that existed prior to the injury are exaggerated	Urgency to settle problems involving employment and finances; family may be gathered at patient's request to discuss patient's concerns	Support patient: orient patient to time and place
Paranoia	Suspicion of intended harm	Confusion; disorientation; lack of trust in caregiver	Acknowledge complaints or manifestations of fear; investigate all complaints; support patient: provide reality orientation
Regression	Adopting behavior of earlier life time-frame	Infantile, demanding, uncooperative behavior	Acknowledge inability to cope; provide structure: allow patient choice in some instances; reward appropriate behavior
Depression	Withdrawal into self; little or no recognition of external events	Lethargic, stuporous, apathetic, little or no response to painful stimuli	Support patient: encourage verbalization of frustrations; encourage activity within clinical limitations

mally is found in the gastrointestinal tract, accounts for the majority of the fungal infections. Cultures of the patient's nose, throat, wound, and unburned skin and also a punch biopsy may be taken on admission and at biweekly intervals to determine the presence of bacteria and their sensitivity to antibiotics.

To prevent the introduction of organisms into the wound, all persons who approach the patient should wear gowns, masks, caps, and gloves. Persons with upper respiratory infections should not be permitted near the patient. Surgical aseptic technique and sterile gloves are used when applying dressings. Hydrotherapy tanks and spray tables are used for aggressive cleansing of burn wounds and can be a source of infection. They need particular attention to prevent the spread of infection when the tanks are used by different patients. Care of the severely burned patient in special burn units can contribute to decreased infection because the environment is specifically geared to infection control. If the patient is cared for in a general hospital unit, a private room is essential and all equipment needed by the patient remains in the room. Reverse isolation precautions are initiated.

☐ Assisting with wound care

Eschar is the leathery covering of dead tissue and exudate that forms after the burn injury. It is conducive to bacterial growth because it contains dead tissue, moisture, and warmth. Cleansing and mechanical debridement are done daily to remove eschar. Washing and friction remove build-up of debris and help to support tissue regeneration.

Hydrotherapy is a painless method for removal of dressings and facilitates range of motion exercise with minimal energy expenditure and discomfort. The solution used in a hydrotherapy tank may be plain water, normal saline, or an electrolytically balanced solution. To minimize the chance of infection, the nurse should keep the procedure as clean as possible. Use of gowns, masks, gloves, and a plastic, disposable tub liner will decrease the chance of contamination between patients. Tubbing is usually performed once or twice daily and should not exceed 30 minutes to prevent exposure and chilling. Tubbing is started after the patient's vital signs and fluid balance have stabilized. The patient should not be tubbed if there are any sudden changes in body temperature, heart rate, blood pressure, or respiratory rate.

The current trend in wound cleansing is to use a spray table. The patient is placed on a special stretcher that has a drain and the person is showered with a hose. Patient comfort is enhanced because areas that are not being debrided can be kept covered.

☐ Assisting with therapeutic goals
☐ *Methods of treatment of burns*

Different methods of treating the burned area may be used, depending on the location of the burn, its size and depth, the facilities available, and the patient's response to therapy. One method may be replaced with another during the course of treatment.

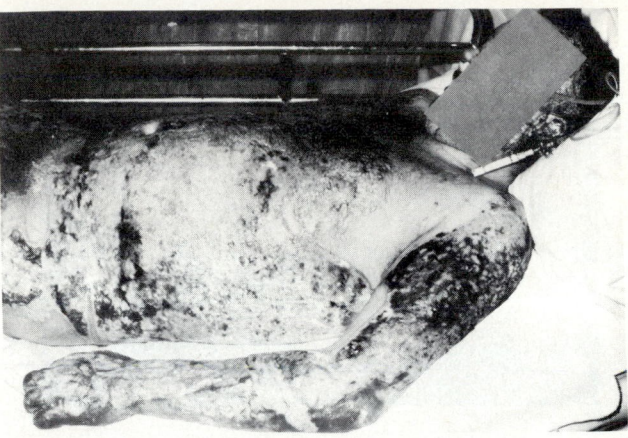

Fig. 40-6 *Severely burned man being treated by open method. (Courtesy Burn Center, Cleveland Metropolitan General/Highland View Hospital, Cleveland, Ohio.)*

OPEN OR EXPOSURE METHOD. The exposure method of treatment was accidently discovered to be effective in 1888 when, during a serious steamboat fire on the Mississippi River, those in attendance ran out of bandages and later observed that the neglected persons fared better than those who received more intensive local treatment.[37] Today the exposure method is used most often in the treatment of burns involving the face, neck, perineum, and broad areas of the trunk. The burned area is cleansed and exposed to air (Fig. 40-6). The exudate of a partial-thickness burn dries in 48 to 72 hours and forms a hard crust that protects the wound. Epithialization occurs beneath this crust and may be complete in 14 to 21 days. The crust then falls off spontaneously, leaving a healed, unscarred surface. The dead skin of a full-thickness burn is dehydrated and converted to black, leathery eschar in 48 to 72 hours. Loose eschar may be gradually removed through the use of hydrotherapy and debridement. Uninfected eschar acts as a protective covering. The danger of infection exists as bacteria proliferate beneath the eschar. Spontaneous separation, produced by bacterial action, occurs unless surgical debridement is performed first.

Isolation technique is essential when the exposure method is used. The nurse should wear a sterile gown and mask, and sterile linen may be used on the patient's bed. A cradle may be used on the patient's bed, because no clothing or bed clothes are allowed directly over burned areas. If the burn is extensive, a CircOlectric bed draped with a sheet is an ideal way to care for the patient (Fig. 40-7). The burned person can be kept from embarrassing exposure by wearing a halter and loin cloth. Lights or heat lamps may be used with caution to provide warmth. Advantages of the open method are that the wound is easily inspected and the patient has maximal freedom to perform exercises for the prevention of contracture and the improvement of circulation.

Patients having exposure treatment complain of pain and

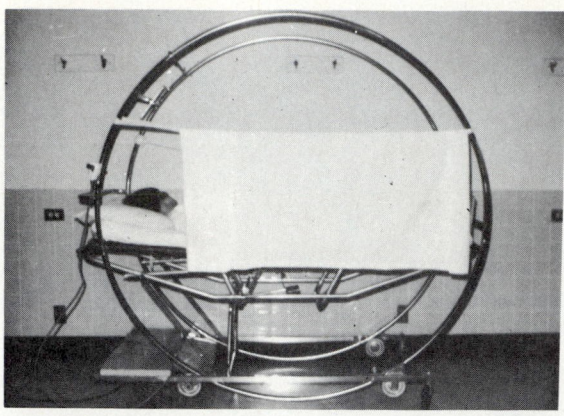

Fig. 40-7 Another exposure method of treating burns. A sheet is draped over CircOlectric bed so that burned areas are not touched. (Courtesy Burn Unit, Cook County Hospital, Chicago, Ill.)

chilling. Pain may be controlled by administering morphine sulfate, meperidine hydrochloride (Demerol), or salicylates as ordered. Discomfort can be decreased if drafts are avoided and the temperature of the room is kept at 24.4° C (85° F). Patients lose more heat from burned surfaces than from normal skin surfaces because the vascular bed that normally contracts and retains heat in the body is lost. The humidity of the room should also be controlled. A humidity of 40% to 50% is usually considered satisfactory. Portable electric humidifiers and dehumidifiers can be used to achieve and maintain this level.

SEMIOPEN METHOD. The semiopen wound care method consists of covering the wound with topical antimicrobial agents and a thin layer of gauze to help keep the agent in contact with the wound. This method permits the passage of wound exudate through the dressing without the loss of antimicrobial cream. The success of semiopen care depends on cleaning the wound once or twice a day, either at the bedside or in the hydrotherapy tank. Meticulous seimopen wound care speeds debridement, enhances the development of granulation tissue, and enables grafting sooner.

CLOSED METHOD. In the closed or occlusive method of burn treatment, the wounds are washed and the dressings are changed at least once a day, or in some instances once each shift. Commonly, the dressing consists of gauze impregnated with topical ointments and a gauze wrap. Counterpressure wrappings (elastic bandages) may be applied. When a dressing is in place, nursing observation includes monitoring for signs of impaired circulation (numbness, pain, and tingling) and for signs of infection (odor on dressings, elevated temperature, and elevated pulse rate).

APPLICATION OF TOPICAL AGENTS. The application of topical agents to the burn wound has helped decrease infection and hasten healing. They are effective because damage to blood vessels in the burn area prevents systemic antibiotics from reaching the burn wound. Antibiotics may be given prophylactically or may be withheld until an in-

fection occurs. The following is a description of some of the topical drugs currently in use for burn patients.

MAFENIDE

Mafenide (Sulfamylon) is a white cream containing sulfonamide. It is applied to the wound once or twice daily with a sterile gloved hand in a thin layer, just enough to cover the burn completely. The wound may be left open to air or a single layer of gauze may be used to hold the cream in place. The cream is removed from the wound, and active debriding is performed before the cream is reapplied.

Mafenide is known to inhibit carbonic anhydrase activity, especially in patients with burns of 40% or more of BSA. As a result, metabolic acidosis may occur. The patient is monitored for hyperventilation, which can result from attempts to balance the increased acid load. Other side effects include pain with application of the cream and an allergic rash. Mafenide inhibits epithelial proliferation; therefore, application should be stopped as soon as the wound is clean and there is evidence of healing.

SILVER SULFADIAZINE

Silver sulfadiazine (Silvadene) is a white cream with bactericidal action against many gram-negative and gram-positive bacteria, as well as against *Candida albicans*. It is applied directly to the wound once or twice daily on saturated gauze or with a sterile gloved hand. The wound may be covered with a dressing or left exposed. Silver sulfadiazine does not penetrate as readily as Mafenide acetate; however, patients do not complain of pain with its application.

The patient is observed for side effects common with sulfonamide drugs. The wound may develop a slimy, grayish appearance simulating an infection, despite negative cultures.[44] Silver sulfadiazine should not be used in patients with a history of kidney disease. No electrolyte imbalances are seen with its use; however, prolonged use may lead to toxic symptoms including nausea, vomiting, anemia, leukopenia, granulocytopenia, mental changes, oliguria, anuria, hematuria, jaundice, and skin rashes.

POVIDONE-IODINE

Povidone-iodine (Betadine) ointment is a reddish brown germicidal preparation of 10% povidone-iodine (1% available iodine) with broad-spectrum microbial action. It is applied three times daily. Povidone-iodine can be applied by (1) spreading it with a sterile gloved hand onto the burned surface or (2) impregnating a single-thickness gauze with the povidone-iodine and applying it to the burned surfaces and then spreading additional ointment on top of the gauze layer. Clothing and bedding need to be protected from staining. A dry, crusting wound may be seen as well as skin rashes in unaffected areas.

SILVER NITRATE

Although silver nitrate is being used less often than in the past, some physicians still prescribe it. In this treatment, thick gauze dressings are saturated with 0.5% so-

Table 40-6 Topical medications used in burn therapy

Topical medication	Advantages	Disadvantages
Mafenide acetate (Sulfamylon)	Bacteriostatic against gram-negative and gram-positive organisms Penetrates thick eschar	Metabolic acidosis Pain on application Allergic rash
Silver sulfadiazine (Silvadene)	Broad antimicrobial activity against gram-negative, gram-positive, and candida organisms No electrolyte imbalances Painless and somewhat soothing Not nephrotoxic	Repeated application may develop slimy, grayish appearance, simulating an infection despite negative cultures Prolonged use may cause skin rash and depress granulocyte formation
Povidone-iodine (Betadine)	Broad antimicrobial activity against gram-positive and gram-negative bacteria, fungi, yeasts, viruses, protozoa	Metabolic acidosis resulting from elevated serum iodine levels Stains clothing and linen Dry, crusting, scabbing wound Skin rash in unaffected area
Silver nitrate	Bacteriostatic effect Lessens pain and eliminates odor Reduces evaporative water loss from burns	Electrolyte imbalances Stains everything it comes into contact with Does not penetrate eschar Pain on application
Nitrofurazone (Furacin)	Inhibits enzymes necessary for bacterial metabolism Broad spectrum of activity Effective against *Staphylococcus aureus* Not absorbed systemically Low incidence of sensitivity	Contact dermatitis in unaffected skin Urine turns a reddish color
Gentamycin sulfate (Garamycin)	Broad antimicrobial activity Painless	Ototoxicity Nephrotoxicity Development of resistant bacterial strains
Neomycin	Broad antimicrobial activity Causes miscoding in the messenger RNA of bacterial cells	Serious toxic effects Ototoxicity Nephrotoxicity
Scarlet red	Nonantiseptic (applied to gauze soaked with oil-base red dye) Drying agent Applied to donor site Promotes epithelialization	No antimicrobial effects Stains and irritates skin Infection may develop beneath scarlet red gauze which may have systemic effects
Xeroform	Nonantiseptic Debrides and protects donor site Protects graft	Removal may be painful because it sometimes adheres to wound Neither antiseptic nor antimicrobial
Sodium hypochlorite (Dakin's Solution)	Chlorine-based solution that is bactericidal Aids in debriding wounds Aids cleaning and draining "soupy" wounds	Dissolves blood clots May inhibit clotting May irritate the skin
Sutilains Ointment (Travase)	Topical enzymatic agent Dissolves necrotic tissue by proteolytic action Facilitates removal of eschar and purulant drainage	Mild, transient pain on application Paresthesia, bleeding, dermatitis Dressing must be kept moist at all times

lution of silver nitrate. The dressings are kept wet so that the solution remains in constant contact with the burned surfaces. If the dressing is allowed to dry, the silver nitrate can concentrate and cause tissue destruction. These dressings retain moisture and heat and reduce evaporation. Proponents of this method of treatment believe that it reduces mortality, lessens pain, eliminates odors, and has a bacteriostatic effect. The dressings are removed every 12 to 24 hours, and the patient is placed in a bath of salt solution with the temperature carefully maintained at body temperature. When skin grafts are applied, silver nitrate dressings are placed over the grafts and donor sites on the first postoperative day. Because the silver nitrate is hypotonic, electrolytes are lost into the wound. Therefore, throughout treatment, frequent determinations of blood sodium levels are necessary, and sodium that is lost may need to be replaced. Everything that comes into contact with silver nitrate solution is stained black, so care should be taken when applying the solution to protect skin, clothing, furniture, walls, and floors.

The above treatments and other topical medications used in burn therapy are outlined in Table 40-6.

WOUND COVERINGS. The burn wound may be covered with dressings or grafts.

DRESSINGS

Large bulky dressings are rarely used today for large burns except in select instances because infection control is more difficult and partial-thickness burns may develop into full-thickness wounds. The purposes of applying some light covering include prevention of infection from exogenous sources, facilitation of debridement, maximal contact by topical agents, and prevention of fluid evaporation with loss of body heat. The type of dressing that is usually applied consists of a single layer of fine mesh gauze impregnated with a topical medication and held in place by a wrapping of a coarse gauze such as Kerlix.

The dressing change is usually a painful procedure requiring analgesics. Analgesics should be given 30 minutes before the procedure for maximal effectiveness. Most dressing changes are performed after tubbing to facilitate dressing removal and to lessen pain. Additional debridement of eschar and dead tissue may be performed before the new dressing is applied.

Wet dressings may be used with silver nitrate or normal saline applications. Normal saline is applied to clean granulation tissue or to new grafts to maintain moisture or is used with fine mesh gauze to provide for slight debridement. A single layer of fine mesh gauze is usually placed over the wound, covered with thick gauze pads to maintain moisture, and held in place with a gauze wrapping. The dressings must be kept wet. Plastic wrap should *not* be used to cover the dressings; this prevents fluid evaporation, causes increased heat at the wound site, and results in patient discomfort and increased tissue destruction and infection.

SKIN GRAFTS

Skin grafts are applied to cover the burn wound and speed healing, to prevent contractures, and to shorten con-

Table 40-7 Types of grafts

Graft	Source	Coverage
Autograft	Patient's own skin	Permanent
Homograft	Another of the same species (for example, cadaver skin obtained 6 to 24 hours after death)	Temporary
Heterograft	Another species (for example, pig skin)	Temporary
Synthetic substitute	Man-made substitute that has properties similar to skin	Temporary

valescence. Successful grafting reduces the patient's vulnerability to infection and prevents the loss of body heat and water vapor from the open wound. Grafting can also be done for cosmetic or functional purposes during the rehabilitative period. Most skin grafts are applied between the third and twenty-first day after the initial injury, depending on the depth and extent of the burn and the condition of the base.

Grafts are obtained from various sources (Table 40-7). An *autograft* is a graft of skin obtained from the patient's own body. A *homograft* is a graft of skin obtained from a cadaver 6 to 24 hours after death. A *heterograft* is a graft of skin obtained from other animals, such as a pig. Synthetic substitutes for skin are currently being investigated.

The latter three types of grafts afford only temporary coverage. Homografts may grow or "take," but in a matter of weeks it will be rejected by the body and sloughed. The advantage of a temporary graft is to reduce water, electrolyte, and protein loss at the burn surface. The covered wound is less painful and allows the patient freedom of movement. Temporary grafts are used until the patient is ready for autografts. Often autografting is delayed as a result of complications, such as pneumonia or gastric hemorrhage.

Split-thickness skin grafts are used most frequently in early stages of wound treatment (Fig. 40-8). The grafts include two upper layers of skin (epidermis) and part of the middle layer (dermis) but are not taken so deep as to prevent regeneration of the skin at the site from which they are taken (donor site). The grafts are removed with a dermatone blade from almost any unburned part of the body. The size of these grafts are determined by the sites available and the area to be covered. Grafts may be placed on the recipient bed by two methods—stamping and meshing. Stamping uses "postage stamp" grafts that are stamp-size pieces of donor skin applied over the recipient bed. It is generally done with a wound that is unclean, because it allows for drainage of excess debris. Meshing involves taking the sheet of skin after it is removed from the donor and feeding it into a meshing instrument which perforates the sheet with tiny slits. The meshing of the graft makes it more distensible so that it can be stretched to cover wider areas of the body surface (Fig. 40-9).

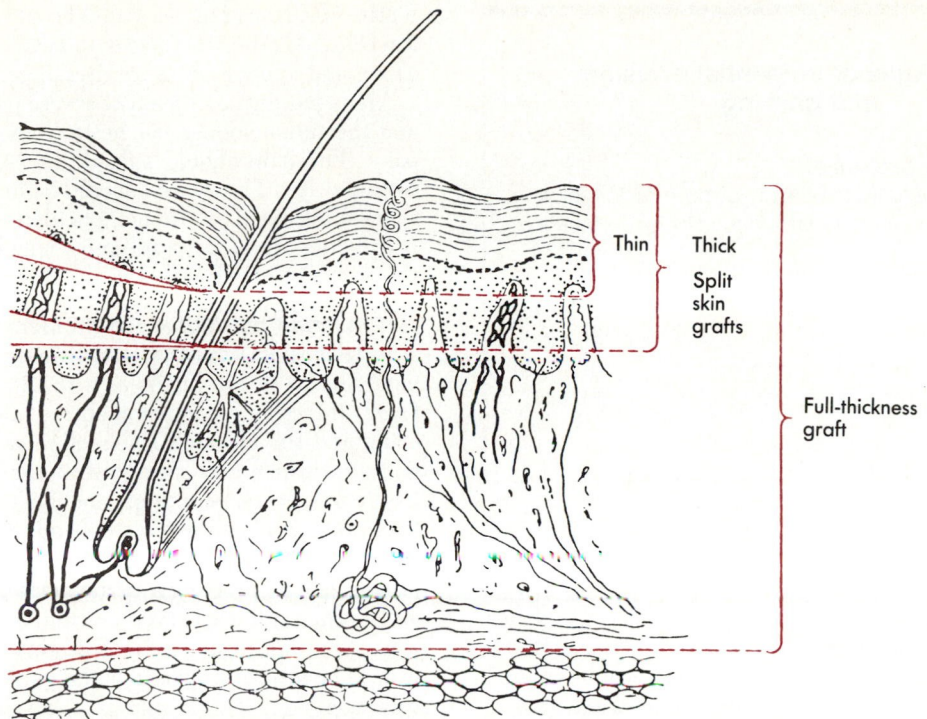

Fig. 40-8 Levels of the skin involved in thin and thick split skin grafts, and full-thickness grafts.

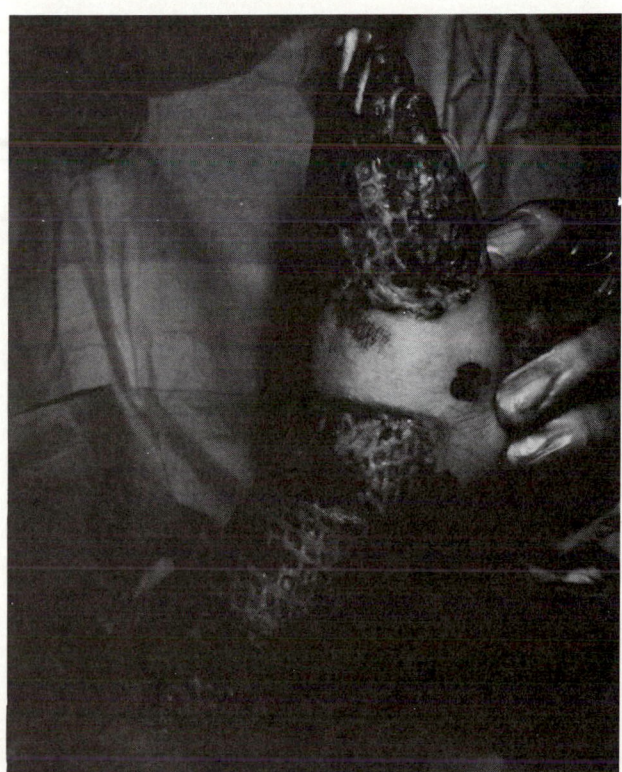

Fig. 40-9 Mesh graft covering a full-thickness burn 14 days after placement. (Courtesy Cleveland Metropolitan General/Highland View Hospital, Cleveland, Ohio.)

Full-thickness grafts are composed of layers of skin down to the subcutaneous tissue. They give a better cosmetic appearance than split-thickness grafts when healed and are used early in wound management and if there is a well-defined area of full-thickness burn. Areas that benefit from full-thickness grafts are the hands, neck, and face. Full-thickness grafts can also be used in rehabilitative stages to restore body function and to repair areas of released skin contractures.

Tangential excision and grafting is a surgical procedure where the necrotic tissue or eschar is excised down to viable tissue or fascia and immediately covered with autograft or skin substitute. The procedure is best performed between the second and fifth burn day. This technique is used with a well defined partial-thickness injury where deep epidermal cells remain intact for primary healing. Advantages of tangential excision and grafting are outlined in the box on p. 1428.

CARE OF GRAFT SITES

Graft sites require skilled nursing management. Autografts are delicate and should not be dislodged. The grafted area may be covered with a large, occlusive, bulky dressing to hold new skin securely in place. Splints may be applied in the operating room to provide immobilization and maintain position.

The dressing remains intact for 48 to 72 hours unless it is found to be purulent and has a strong odor. Dressings are moved slowly and carefully so as not to disturb the graft.

Advantages of tangential excision and grafting

Shortened hospitalization

Prevents potential conversion of burn to full-thickness by removing necrotic tissue before infection occurs

Definitive healing diminishes anxiety and lessens trauma to multiple graftings

Allows early grafting and early restoration of function

Scar formation reduced because of use of full-thickness graft

---

The donor site after grafting represents a wound similar to that of a partial-thickness injury. Care of the donor site is as important as care of the graft itself, because donor sites that fail to heal result in a net enlargement of the patient's open wound surface. Donor sites may be treated by a variety of methods. One method is covering the exposed surface with fine mesh gauze, Xeroform, or a synthetic dressing and leaving it exposed to the air. Exposing the donor site to a heat lamp also promotes healing because as the drainage from the wound dries, it serves as a pro-

tective covering (Fig. 40-10). The site usually heals within 2 weeks. Another method is to cover the site with sterile gauze and apply a pressure dressing.

Many patients complain of severe pain in the donor site, and the nurse should not hesitate to give medications for pain. The pain should subside in 24 to 48 hours as the wound dries. The wound should be inspected daily for any signs of infection (erythema, purulent drainage, foul odor). If infection develops, antibiotics may be administered and the wound treated with wet dressings.

□ *Providing nutritional requirements*

PATHOPHYSIOLOGY. Metabolism is increased following moderate to severe burns as a result of stress, fluid loss, fever, infection, hypercatabolism, and immobility. Shivering and the elevated levels of catecholamines, cortisol, and glucagon found shortly after thermal injury increase tissue oxygen consumption and heat production, deplete liver and muscle glycogen stores and fat deposits, and lead to a negative nitrogen balance and weight loss. Protein is broken down, providing amino acids for gluconeogenesis, and amino acids are prevented from incorporating into protein. The diminished rate of protein production prolongs wound healing and increases the patient's susceptibility to infection.

A burn patient remains catabolic until the caloric intake exceeds caloric expenditure. Hypermetabolism continues until the wounds are 90% healed[30] and homeostasis is restored. The patient's total energy and protein requirements

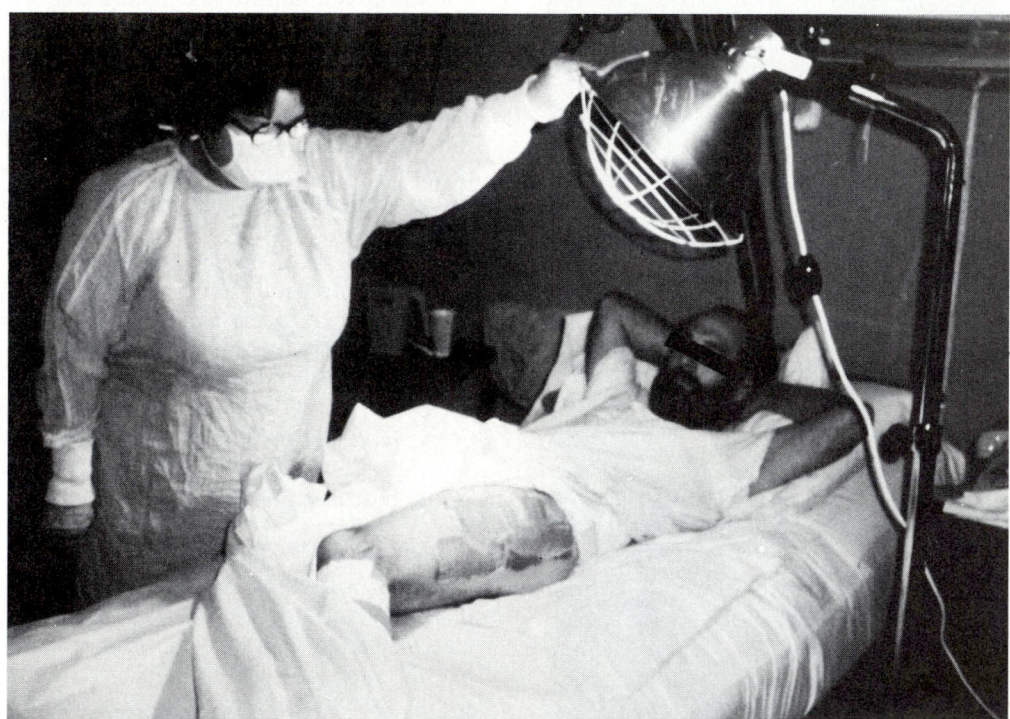

Fig. 40-10 Heat lamp used to dry donor site to promote epithelialization from deep layers and prevent infecton. (Courtesy Burn Center, Cleveland Metropolitan General/Highland View Hospital, Cleveland, Ohio.)

become those needed for normal homeostasis plus those required to offset the catabolic state and repair the injury.

GOALS OF NUTRITIONAL SUPPORT. Maintenance of a nutritional support program is critical to survival and is initiated on admission. The goals of the nutritional support program are to establish eating by the traditional route as soon as possible and to maintain sufficient calorie and protein intake to restore tissue loss. A team approach provides comprehensive input and integrates the efforts of the patient, physician, nurse, pharmacist, dietitian, and occupational and physical therapists.

The protein and caloric needs of the burned person are highly variable, depending on the extent and depth of injury and the patient's age, sex, preburn nutritional status, and preexisting diseases. The daily *protein* requirement is greater than normal as a result of the negative nitrogen balance. The normal daily protein requirement is 0.8 g/kg of body weight for the adult. The massive mobilization of protein after the burn injury increases the daily requirement by two to four times the amount required before the injury—approximately 1.5 to 3.2 g/kg of body weight. Protein is necessary for tissue repair and healing, not as a source of energy. Therefore, it is important to provide sufficient carbohydrate and fat calories to satisfy energy needs. An appreciable loss of *zinc* generally accompanies a protein and weight loss. Studies demonstrate that zinc deficiency impairs wound healing and recent data indicate that a zinc deficiency impairs cellular immunity.

The daily *caloric* requirement increases from a normal 1700 to 3000 calories to 3500 to 50,000 calories. Because the demand for calories increases with a major burn, appropriate vitamin therapy is essential. *Vitamins* and *minerals* are given at two to three times the recommended daily allowances established for normal healthy adults. Vitamin C promotes healing, and the daily requirement in the burn patient increases from a normal of 45 mg to 1 to 2 g. B complex vitamins are necessary for the metabolism of the increased protein and carbohydrate intake. Levels of vitamins A, E, K, and folic acid are monitored and supplemented as indicated. Serum levels of calcium, phosphate, and potassium are also monitored and therapeutic levels of iron must be maintained to prevent the ongoing threat of anemia associated with burn injury.

Weight loss and gain are monitored for evaluation of nutritional status. *Weight gain* occurs initially because of fluid retention; however, following diuresis there is a marked loss of weight. Severe *weight loss* is closely related to protein loss or the loss of body cell mass and the enormous amount of body fluid lost through the burn wound itself. As in other metabolic responses, weight loss depends on the extent of injury: the greater the burn, the greater the weight loss. The weight curve will level out at a point below the preburn weight, and weight gain does not begin until all the wound is nearly grafted.

The nutritional supplements given to the severely burned patient in the emergent period are aimed at stabilization and electrolyte balance to maintain stable cardiovascular function. Patients are initially supported with 5% or 10% dextrose solution.

FEEDING METHODS. Paralytic ileus or gastric dilation is frequently seen in severely burned patients as a result of the neuroendocrine response to stress, hypovolemia, or septicemia. This prevents enteral feeding until the gastrointestinal tract mobility is restored. Total parenteral nutrition (TPN) is indicated once fluid resuscitation is completed. TPN with supplemental fat solutions is used to provide calories.

Oral or tube feeding is the preferred method of providing adequate nutrition and is used as soon as possible. The enteral route is the most natural and convenient means of nutritional support. The burn patient will seldom consume more food from meals after the injury than before the injury; therefore, a combination of parenteral and enteral modes may be necessary to provide the enormous nutritional requirements. Dietary supplements that contain additional calories and protein can be provided by milkshakes which can be specially made by the hospital dietary department. Patients should be encouraged to drink supplements between meals.

Postburn lactose intolerance may occur in patients being tube fed. Signs of bloating, flatulence, cramps, and diarrhea may be seen. A modification of the strength and type of supplement may be necessary and starting the supplement at half or quarter strength, diluted with water, will often alleviate gastrointestinal complications.

Tube feeding provides a continous 24-hour infusion of a high-caloric, high-protein commercially prepared supplement. These supplements, containing 1 kcal/ml, are hypertonic, and because of the hypertonicity, diarrhea is common. The best means of administering tube feeding is a continuous, slow infusion through a small-diameter, soft, pliable tube inserted through the esophagus into the stomach or duodenum. Diarrhea, nausea, vomiting, and an uncomfortable feeling of fullness may be avoided with a slow, continuous infusion using an infusion pump to regulate the delivery. If diarrhea persists, a kaolin-pectin suspension (Kaopectate) or paregoric may be added to the feeding supplement or diphenoxylate HCl with atropine (Lomotil) may be prescribed.

The patient is advanced to a regular diet as quickly as possible. However, ingenuity by the nurses and dietitian is needed to motivate the patient to eat the food necessary to meet nutritional requirements. Relatives can suggest favorite foods. All dressing changes and treatments should be timed so they do not immediately precede meals. Milk shakes can supplement the patient's diet and can be taken more easily than solid foods.

Fecal impaction is a common problem in burn patients. Bulk foods and fruit juices must be stressed. Bulk-forming laxatives such as preparations of the psyllium seed (Metamucil) or a fecal softener such as dioctyl sodium sulfosuccinate (Colace) may be prescribed.

☐ *Pain management*

Psychologic pain may be induced or exaggerated because of loneliness. The patient's complaints of pain may be a call for attention that can be met by the presence and touch of the nurse providing care. Anxiety over anticipated

---

Nursing interventions that aid in minimizing pain during dressing changes

Provide analgesic medications 30 minutes before dressing change.

Provide clear explanations to gain patient's cooperation.

Handle burned areas gently.

Use sterile technique (infection causes increased pain).

Encourage patient to participate in treatment whenever possible.

Employ distracting techniques (radio, conversation) and relaxation techniques when appropriate.

---

procedures that may or may not be painful may cause a progressive increase in the degree of pain experienced.[32] Muscle tension related to fear and apprehension is known to lower the pain threshold. Sleep deprivation, a common occurrence in critical care units, can also make the patient less tolerant of pain. Self-hypnosis or relaxation exercises can be effective in altering the perception of either actual or anticipated discomfort and should be consistently reinforced by the team.[35] The box above outlines nursing interventions that can aid in minimizing pain during dressing changes. (See Chapter 10 for further information about pain and its management.)

EVALUATION

Evaluation is based on the expected outcomes. Questions to ask may include the following:
1. Is the patient able to respond to interventions to decrease anxiety?
2. Is the patient able to achieve pain relief?
3. Is infection present?
4. Can the patient verbalize an understanding of treatments and surgical procedure and participate appropriately in care?
5. Is the patient nutritionally depleted?
6. Is the burn wound healing?

■ Rehabilitation period

Rehabilitation begins at the time of admission. However, rehabilitation as the third stage of treatment begins when the patient's burn is reduced to less than 20% of BSA and the patient is capable of assuming some self-care activity. The principles of management are to return the patient to a productive place in society and accomplish functional and cosmetic reconstruction. It is important to remember that rehabilitation does not end when the patient is discharged;

it may take from 2 to 5 years after discharge for the patient to reach a maximal level of emotional and physical adjustment.

■ PREVENTING LIMITATIONS OF MOBILITY

As the survival rate of patients with large and deeper burns increases, so does the challenge to maintain optimal functioning and cosmetic results. Research indicates that the percentage of patients with joint limitations increases as the degree and extent of burn increases. Although these patients may be critically ill, their rehabilitative needs must be addressed immediately. A comprehensive program of positioning, splinting, exercise, ambulation, and activities of daily living (ADL) must begin on the first or second day after the burn injury and be carried through until after discharge. Any delays in initiating treatment will be detrimental to the patient's ultimate functional outcome. Contractures are among the most serious long-term complications of burns today. They result from muscle and joint stiffening, skin grafting, and prolonged bedrest. While the occupational and physical therapists are primarily responsible for addressing the patient's rehabilitation needs during all phases of the patient's recovery, the nurse is responsible for ensuring that all interventions are followed.

ASSESSMENT

☐ Subjective data

The patient must be helped to maintain range of joint motion to prevent scars from healing in positions that will result in deformity. Complaints of pain and pressure should not be overlooked, because damage may occur from an improperly applied splint or poor positioning. It is important that patients understand why ambulation or motion is necessary even though it may be painful.

The emotional impact of a severe burn is enormous. The psychologic scars last forever and affect the victim and family for the rest of their lives. The extent to which the family unit adapts depends on how the patient reacts to a new body image and feelings of self-worth.

The hospital environment and hospital personnel influence the adaptation process. In the immediate postburn period, the nurse is primarily concerned with physiologic survival of the patient. At the same time, the nurse must be able to identify psychologic problems and coping mechanisms of the patient and family.

☐ Objective data

The nurse is responsible for assessing the patient's response to positioning, splinting, exercise, and the ability of the patient and family to perform daily wound care after discharge. Correct positioning must be maintained to avoid the development of contractures. The splinted limb is assessed for adequate circulation, cyanosis, temperature, and the presence of pulses. Exercise, ADL, and ambulation must be continuously assessed for patient tolerance both physically and emotionally.

→ DATA ANALYSIS: NURSING DIAGNOSES

Nursing diagnoses are determined from assessment of patient data. Possible nursing diagnoses for the person with burns may include, but are not limited to, the following:

Diagnostic title	Possible etiologies
Activity intolerance	Immobility from splinting, generalized weakness, bed rest, pain
Anxiety	Change in health status/role functioning/socioeconomic status
Body image disturbance	Scarring, contractures, discoloration
Ineffective family coping	Inadequate or incorrect information or understanding, prolonged disability of significant person
Ineffective individual coping	Burn injury, personal vulnerability
Diversional activity deficit	Long-term hospitalization, frequent lengthy treatment
Fear	Long-term illness, surgery treatments, changes in life-style, pain, disfigurement, job security
Knowledge deficit	Wound/skin care, exercises, use of adaptive devices
Impaired physical mobility	Intolerance to activity, decreased strength and endurance, pain, severe anxiety
Pain	Increasing activity (exercise, ambulation, ADL)
Self-care deficit	Intolerance to activity, fatigue, pain/discomfort, severe anxiety

⌶ PLANNING: EXPECTED PATIENT OUTCOMES

Expected patient outcomes for the person with burns in the rehabilitation period may include, but are not limited to, the following:
1. Patient achieves activity tolerance consistent with desired levels.
2. Patient exhibits decreased anxiety.
3. Patient demonstrates a realistic concept of changes in body image and alterations required in daily activities.
4. Patient exhibits no pain.
5. Patient participates in diversional activities.
6. Patient verbalizes fears and participates in planned interventions that will decrease fears.
7. Patient is knowledgeable about self-care and follow-up.
8. Patient achieves optimal joint mobility.
9. Patient demonstrates ability to perform ADL.
10. Family demonstrates appropriate coping skills.

⌗ IMPLEMENTATION

☐ **Preventing contractures**
☐ *Therapeutic positioning*

Therapeutic positioning, or placing body parts in antideformity positions, is vital to the prevention of burn contractures. Frequent repositioning of the patient in bed (side lying, supine, prone) is done regularly during the day and night. Correct positioning varies, depending on the area of the body burned (Table 40-8). Positioning can be enhanced by placing patients on a Stryker frame, a Foster bed, a CircOlectric bed, or one of the many different types of flotation beds or mattresses currently available. These beds facilitate the use of the bedpan and urinal, permit change of position with a minimum of handling, and permit larger skin surfaces to remain free from body pressure than is possible when the patient lies on a regular mattress.

Table 40-8 Therapeutic positioning for the burn patient

Area burned	Description of position
Neck	No pillow
	Towel roll under cervical spine
	Neck splint
Shoulder	90 degrees abduction, neutral rotation
	Elbow splint may be used to aid in maintaining position
Axilla	Abduction with 10 to 15 degrees forward flexion and external rotation
	Support abducted arm by suspending from IV pole, or place on bedside table
	Axilla splint
Elbow	Extension
	Support extended arm on bedside table, foam trough
	Elbow splint
Hand	Hand splint
Dorsal surface	Flexion
Palmar surface	Hyperextension
Hip	Extension with neutral rotation
	Supine with lower extremity extended
	Prone lying (if medically appropriate)
	Trochanter roll
	Foam wedge along lateral aspect of thigh
	Knee or long leg splint
Knee	Extension
	Prone lying (if medically appropriate)
	Patient out of bed with lower extremities extended and elevated
	Knee splint
Ankle	Dorsiflexion
	Padded footboard with heels free of pressure
	Ankle splint

These special beds are particularly useful when both the back and front of the trunk, thighs, and legs have been burned. These beds also allow turning of the patient with a minimum of handling and thus help decrease pain.

Prolonged rest in semi-Fowler's position or with pillow pushing the head forward must be avoided even though many patients prefer this position because it enables them to see about the room better.

The bed can often be turned so that the patient can look about without having to assume positions that may lead to the formation of contractures. The bedside table may be changed from one side of the bed to the other at intervals.

□ Splints

Splints are used to prevent or correct contractures and to immobilize joints after grafting. They are custom made and often molded directly on the patient to ensure optimal conformity (Plate 10). It is the responsibility of the nurse to apply the splint properly and according to an established schedule. An improperly applied splint can promote contractures and lead to additional complications.

□ Exercises and ambulation

Exercises for prevention and correction of contractures are begun as soon as the patient's condition is stable. Active exercises are preferred, although active assistance and gentle pressure exercises may be more realistic. Supervision by a physical or occupational therapist is desirable. Exercises may be performed more easily in water and may be done along with dressing changes if the patient is able to tolerate the activity (Fig. 40-11). When burns are completely covered (by healing or by graft), exercises may be performed more easily in an occupational therapy or physical therapy department where the patient may benefit from a change in environment.

Ambulation decreases the risk of thromboemboli, promotes optimal ventilation, helps maintain range of motion and strength in the lower extremities, orients the patient to the environment, and provides a sense of functional independence. Mobilizing the patient requires a progressive approach in those patients with large burns who have less ability to tolerate activity. Initially the patient may need to be transferred with maximal assistance onto a stretcher chair and progress to a sitting position. Gradually the patient may progress to a standing pivot transfer into a nearby chair, and eventually ambulate with minimal assistance. Before getting out of bed, an elastic bandage support must be applied to the lower extremities to prevent venous stasis, edema, and orthostatic hypotension.

□ Promoting independence

One of the ultimate goals in the rehabilitation of a burn patient is to maintain or restore the patient's independence in performing ADL. The occupational therapist aids in this process by selecting activities that are appropriate to the patient's medical, physical, and mental status. Activities that the nurse can encourage are self-feeding, telephoning, reading mail, and assisting with grooming or burn wound management. The nurse must know what the patient is being taught by the physical and occupational therapist so that progress can be continued in the nursing unit.

After the initial period, the long healing process begins, accompanied by the realization of endless implications for the future. Burns on the face make adjustments difficult. Different kinds of fears include the following: pain, disfigurement, prolonged hospitalization, job security, change in life-style, and reactions of family and friends.

To the adolescent the thought of being different or conspicuous may be unbearable. If possible, the patient should see facial burns only after being prepared for the experience. Support and understanding will be needed in order for the patient to cope with what will be seen in the mirror. The patient will exhibit readiness by asking to look in the mirror. Interaction with other burn patients who are fur-

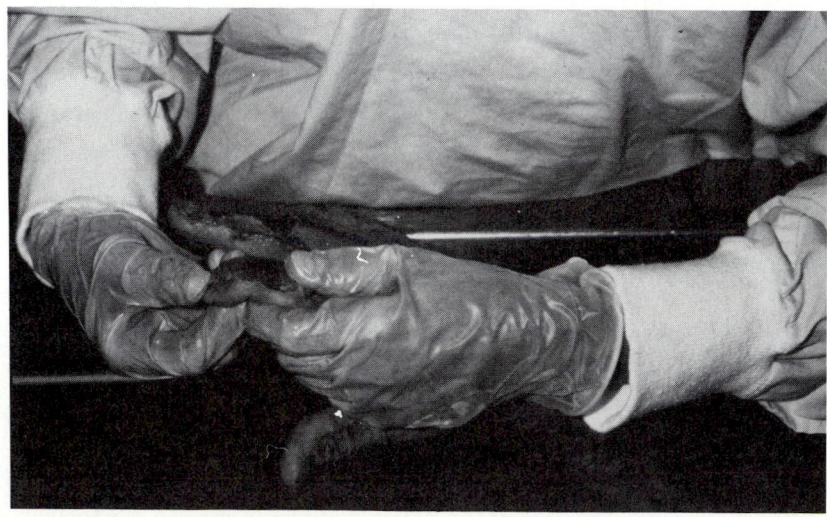

Fig. 40-11 Passive range of motion exercise during hydrotherapy. (Courtesy Cleveland Metropolitan General/Highland View Hospital, Cleveland, Ohio.)

ther along in their healing process may help the patient feel that recovery is possible. In some instances, the recovery is incredible, and although differences in skin pigmentation remain, the redness that accompanies healed burn wounds often fades considerably within a few months. Pigmentation problems are more acute for persons with brown or black skin. Their healed skin may be a different shade, freckled, or whitish in color.

☐ **Providing emotional support**

The patient should have the opportunity to talk about any concerns or fears. Some patients may discuss these with the nurse when they cannot express them to relatives, and the nurse must be prepared to listen and help the individual accept necessary changes in life-style. Almost every burn patient and family need the help of a social worker. The nurse should recognize this need and initiate

NURSING CARE PLAN

Person with burns

DATA: Mr. Smith is a 54-year-old businessman, married with two children. He fell asleep while smoking in bed. He woke up after several minutes to discover his bed on fire. He was admitted to the hospital with 25% of his body burned, including his anterior arms, chest, abdomen and scattered areas on his thighs. Six hours after admission he is receiving 40% oxygen through a face mask. Vital signs are as follows: heart rate 120, respiratory rate 30, blood pressure 140/80, temperature 38.8 C. Two peripheral IVs are placed, each running at 250 ml/hr. A Foley catheter has drained 50 ml the past hour. Mr. Smith has a productive cough of gray-tinged sputum and a hoarse voice. Breath sounds clear with coughing. His wounds had been cleansed with Dreft and normal saline and covered with a Silvadene dressing. He had complained of nausea and a nasogastric tube was inserted. Antacids were ordered to be administered every 2 hours via tube.

The nursing history identified the following:
1. He smokes 1½ packs/day; he has tried several times to quit.
2. The same day, his wife feared that he would fall asleep while smoking.
3. He owns his own business.

Nursing diagnosis: Ineffective airway clearance: related to laryngeal edema and irritation from smoke inhalation and history of cigarette smoking

Expected patient outcome	Nursing interventions	Rationale
Patient will maintain adequate ventilation and oxygenation	Assess and document rate, depth and ease of respirations; note type amount, color of sputum; observe patient's color	Increased respiratory effort, large amounts of tenacious, gray-tinged sputum and signs of tissue hypoxia indicate the need for endotracheal intubation
		Providing oxygen will increase oxygen supply to body tissues
	Provide respiratory treatment and medications as ordered (pulmonary drainage and clapping, incentive spirometer, bronchodilators)	Respiratory treatments will loosen and thin secretions and will allow patient to clear his own airway
	Turn patient every 2 hours	Change in position will help mobilize secretions

Collaborative nursing actions include those to prevent hypovolemia from, the movement of fluid from the intravascular to the interstitial compartment, to prevent respiratory distress, and to prevent gastrointestinal distress. Immediate reporting of the early signs of hypovolemia and/or respiratory distress may prevent serious effects (hypovolemic shock, respiratory failure). Nursing actions include monitoring for the following:
1. Signs of hypovolemia: increased heart rate, decreased urine output, decreased blood pressure, decreased sensorium
2. Signs of respiratory distress: increased respiratory rate, shortness of breath, change in patient's color, increased work of breathing, change in ABGs (decreasing pH, decreasing pO_2, increasing pCO_2)
3. Signs of gastrointestinal distress: low gastric pH, heme + nasogastric aspirate, absence of bowel sounds

Continued.

NURSING CARE PLAN

Persons with burns—cont'd

Nursing diagnosis: Potential fluid volume deficit

Expected patient outcome	Nursing intervention	Rationale
Patient will maintain optimal fluid balance	Provide patient with calculated IV fluids	Calculated IV fluids will prevent patient from developing hypovolemic shock
	Monitor and document output hourly	Any deficit or increase in fluid intake or output must be identified quickly to avoid complications of hypovolemia
	Assess patient for clinical signs of hypovolemia (decreased sensorium; changes in skin from pink to pale, from warm to cool)	These may be the first signs of hypovolemia
	Weigh patient daily; compare to preinjury weight	Weight is an accurate assessment of fluid balance

Nursing diagnosis: Pain: related to exposed nerve endings from burn injury

Expected patient outcome	Nursing interventions	Rationale
Patient will experience minimal pain	Provide patient with pain medication as ordered; administer 30 minutes before dressing changes (hydrotherapy and debridement); evaluate and document effectiveness	Decreasing pain will decrease patient's anxiety and increase his or her cooperation during dressing changes
	Assess need for other interventions that may decrease pain experience (use of the radio, relaxation therapy, hypnosis)	The pain experience is subjective; a variety of pain control techniques may decrease the pain experience
	Assess patient's pain history and response to pain	Information about past pain experiences will aid in planning techniques for pain control
	Educate patient about painful procedures and about techniques to reduce pain; encourage patient to participate in treatments whenever possible	Information and participation may help decrease the anxiety that is often seen with pain
	Use environmental comfort measures (speak in calm manner, keep patient warm)	Comfortable environment may decrease anxiety and pain

Nursing diagnosis: Anxiety

Expected patient outcome	Nursing interventions	Rationale
Patient will demonstrate control of anxiety	Gather information about patient's background, personality, and level of coping from friends, family, and patient (as appropriate)	Information will assist the nurse in planning interventions to decrease anxiety
	Offer patient and family simple explanations of his or her injury and treatments	Too much information may overwhelm patient and increase anxiety
	Assess patient's ability to cope with illness; consult with other services	Social services or pastoral care may be able to provide assistance to the patient

Continued.

NURSING CARE PLAN

Persons with burns—cont'd

Nursing diagnosis: Potential for infection: related to loss of skin from burn injury

Expected patient outcome	Nursing interventions	Rationale
Patient will be free of pathogenic organisms	Document initial appearance of the burn wound (color, dryness, odor)	Early changes in appearance of wound may be the first signs of infection
	Monitor for signs of infection (fever, altered sensorium, increased respiratory rate, foul odor from wound)	Early detection of infection will allow appropriate antibiotics to be prescribed before serious injury occurs
	Implement isolation procedures	To protect the patient from other organisms that may cause infection

Nursing diagnosis: Impaired skin integrity: related to burn injury

Expected patient outcome	Nursing interventions	Rationale
Patient will demonstrate viable healing tissue	Perform prescribed wound care (hydrotherapy and debridement); assess wound during each dressing change	Wound care procedures may change daily, depending on assessment of wound
	Assess need for equipment and supplies and have available before wound care	Adequate supplies should be ordered ahead of time to avoid the problem of discovering halfway through the dressing change that there are not enough supplies available

the referral. Visiting hours can be used to talk with relatives, who may be able to give information that will clarify the patient's needs and resources. This time also provides opportunity for the nurse to help relatives accept their loved one's change in appearance and to help them plan for the return of the loved one to the community.

☐ **Discharge teaching**

Before discharge, burn patients and their families have a great need for education so that they may take increasing responsibilities for their own care. Discharge teaching involves the entire burn team, and since rehabilitation is a gradual process, there should be ample time to plan the return home in every detail.

Early discharge planning accomplishes two goals. First, it helps solve problems early. For example, if the patient's house burned and needs to be repaired, the family may need to relocate. This could be done before the patient's discharge, thus preventing the added stress of moving after discharge. Second, early discharge planning emphasizes the future. If discharge is discussed, the patient and family will realize that recovery and a return home is possible.

Complete and comprehensive instructions followed by return demonstrations contribute to learning the necessary

---

Teaching priorities

Wound management
Signs and symptoms of complications
Use of pressure dressings
Exercises, splinting, and ADL
Methods of coping with resocialization

---

skills to be independent in self-care activities after discharge. Patients should not be discharged from the hospital until they can care for themselves physically, with assistance if necessary, and are prepared to meet the stresses involved in returning to their former living patterns.

Teaching priorities are summarized in the box above.

A major goal in discharge teaching is to prevent excessive scar formation by exercising, splinting, applying pressure dressings, and if necessary undergoing reconstructive surgery. A patient recovering from a major burn may need 12 to 18 months to achieve this goal.

Wound management instructions should include how to

Discharge instructions for the burn patient

We on the burn team are happy to see that you are able to go home. To ensure you the speediest possible recovery, it is important that you are able to care for yourself and recognize problems that may interfere with your complete recovery.

If any of the following occur, please call the hospital and ask for the burn clinic. The nurse will be able to assist you.

1. Healed area breaking open. Cover with clean dressing.
2. Formation of blisters.
3. Signs of infection:
   a. Fever, temperature over 37.2° C (99° F).
   b. Redness, pain, swelling, hardness, or warmth in or around wound or any other part of body.
   c. Increased or foul-smelling drainage from wound.
4. Problems with your Ace bandages or Jobst garment such as improper fit, formation of blisters, or opening of healed area underneath.

Your first clinic appointment will be on _____ . If a family member can come with you they can register for you and you may go to the burn clinic waiting room.

Skin care for healed burn

These are your guidelines for your daily skin care of a healed burn. When you do your skin care, this is the time to look at the involved areas and note if there are any changes that need to be reported.

1. Wash healed area every day with solution of 2 tbsp Dreft (or Ivory Snow) and water.
2. Wash gently with washcloth to remove dead skin.
3. Rinse skin well after washing.
4. Dry thoroughly.
5. Apply Nivea lightly twice a day and more frequently if the skin is dry and flaked.
6. Do not put Nivea on open areas.
7. You can purchase Nivea at your local drugstore.

Care for burn wound

These are your guidelines for the care of your burn wound. When you do your care, this is the time to look at the involved areas and note if there are any changes that need to be reported.

Procedure for burn wound care
1. Wash hands.
2. Remove dressing and dispose of in paper bag or wrap in newspaper.
3. Wash hands.
4. Wash open area with gauze using solution of Dreft (or Ivory Snow) and water. Add 1 tbsp Dreft to a basin of water; 2 tbsp Dreft, if you use the bathtub. Use a clean towel and washcloth with each dressing change.
5. Rinse skin well.
6. Wash hands.
7. Apply dressing as described below.
8. Wear gloves. Wash basin or bathtub with a disinfectant such as Lysol.
9. Wash hands.

Care of clothing

When you are discharged, you may find that healed burn areas are sensitive to harsh detergents, fabric softeners, and clothing dyes. If you are sensitive, we suggest the following:

1. Before use launder new clothing by machine or hand with Dreft or Ivory Snow.
2. Rinse clothes twice.
3. Do not use fabric softeners.
4. If you have open burns or a healed area that opens, wash all clothes separately from other family members.
5. Scarlet red ointment will permanently stain clothing.
6. If dyes used in clothing cause irritation, wear white articles.

Ace bandages

You have been taught to put on your own Ace bandages while in the hospital; but if you do have a problem with this, please notify the burn clinic. It is also important that you know how to care for them and understand problems that occur.

1. If they are too loose, they will be ineffective and must be rewrapped.
2. If they are too tight, they will cause discomfort, numbness, tingling, and puffiness and must be rewrapped.
3. They must be worn for a long period of time, probably 6-12 months to be effective, so please do not stop wearing them until your doctor tells you.
4. To care for your Ace bandages:
   a. Hand wash with Dreft or Ivory Snow in cold water.
   b. Towel dry.
   c. Lay flat or place over rod or clothesline.
   d. Do not use clothespins.

Jobst garment

You have been taught to put on your Jobst garment while in the hospital; but if you have a problem with this, please notify the burn clinic. It is also important that you know how to care for it and understand problems that can occur.

1. If it is too loose, it will be ineffective and you will require a new garment.
2. If it is too tight, it will cause discomfort, numbness, and tingling. Do not wear it if this occurs, but notify the burn clinic as soon as possible.
3. To care for your Jobst garment:
   a. Hand wash with Dreft or Ivory Snow in cold water.
   b. Towel dry.
   c. Lay flat or place over rod or clothesline.
   d. Do not use clothespins.

Courtesy Cleveland Metropolitan General/Highland View Hospital Department of Nursing Service, Cleveland, Ohio.

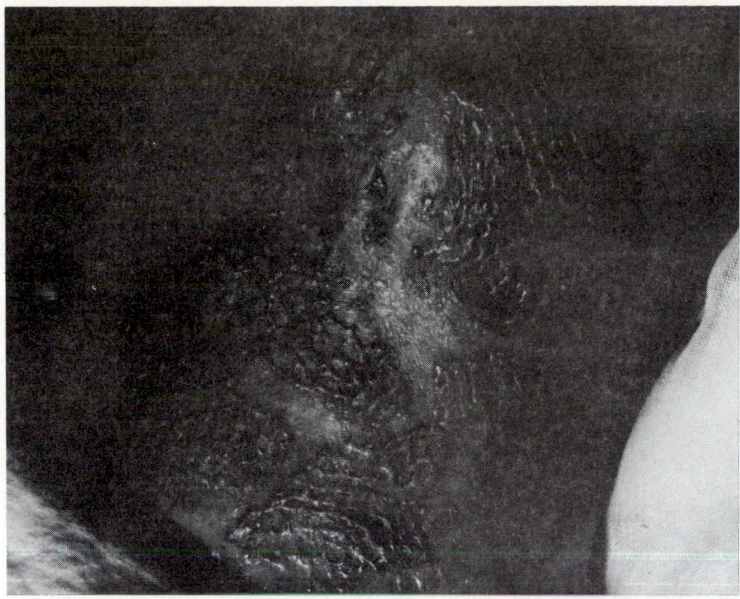

Fig. 40-12   Hypertrophic scarring over chest and abdomen. (Courtesy Cleveland Metropolitan General/Highland View Hospital, Cleveland, Ohio.)

care for the healed graft and nongrafted areas. Signs and symptoms of complications, including areas that may blister and break down, and signs of infection are also addressed. Written instructions should contain the name and phone number of a physician or nurse that the patient may call with questions or problems concerning follow-up care. (See Discharge instructions for the burn patient, p. 1436.) The Visiting Nurse Association may be of assistance in dressing the patient's wounds.

□ *Preventing scarring*

Any time a wound of connective tissue heals, hypertrophic scarring will occur unless the skin is adhered to the underlying structure, such as the palm of the hand. Hypertrophic scarring (Fig. 40-12) results from the overgrowth and overproduction of tissue. This occurs especially in areas of stress and movement, such as the hands, legs, and chest. The thickened, rigid scar that results may later cause contractures, especially over a joint.

It has been proved that the application of controlled, constant pressure to the surface of an immature scar will reduce the scar and leave a smooth, pliable tissue. If this pressure is applied to new, healthy tissue, hypertrophic scarring can be prevented (Fig. 40-13). The Jobst garment, a specially designed elastic woven material, provides tridimensional control. It is fitted to each patient and then custom made (Fig. 40-14). Until the garment is completed, ace bandages can be used for a pressure dressing.

Even though the pressure garment helps decrease the formation of thick, disfiguring scars, patient acceptance is a problem. The garment is uncomfortable, especially during hot weather. It must be tight enough to produce the 24 mm Hg of pressure required to exceed capillary pressure, reducing edema and scar formation. The patient must wear the garment 23 hours a day for 6 months to a year.

A plan for exercise and splinting must be established before discharge. To prevent scar contracture, daily therapy sessions may be necessary for several weeks or months. Assistive aids can be developed by the occupational therapist to help with ADL.

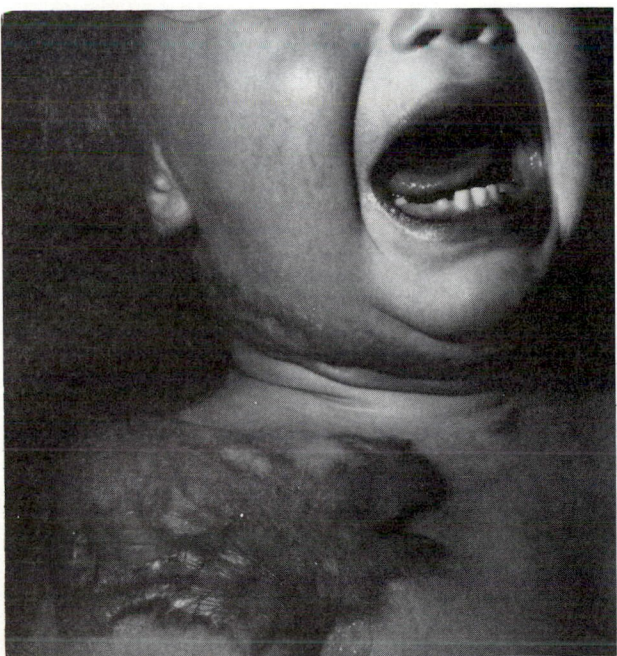

Fig. 40-13   Scar formation occurring from lack of pressure dressing application. (Courtesy Cleveland Metropolitan General/Highland View Hospital, Cleveland, Ohio.)

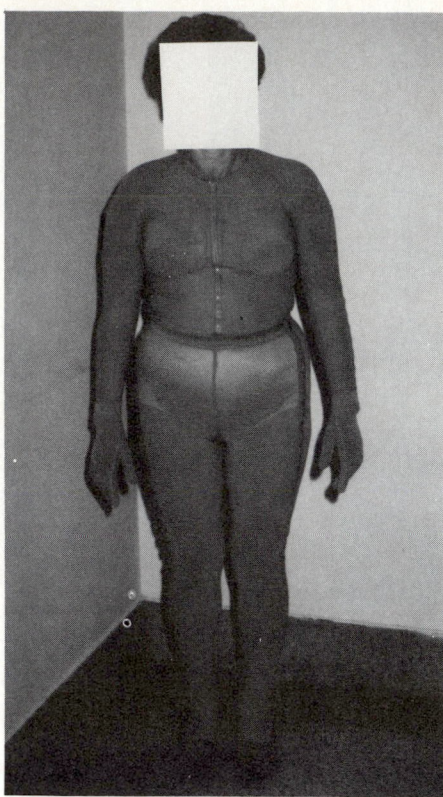

Fig. 40-14 Total body Jobst garment consisting of three separate pieces: jacket, pants, and gloves. (Courtesy Cleveland Metropolitan General/Highland View Hospital, Cleveland, Ohio.)

□ *Resocialization*

After discharge, the patient has to adjust to temporary or permanent function loss, cosmetic disfigurement, and the reactions of others. The ability to make these adjustments will depend on coping mechanisms before the burn, the severity and site of the burn, and the reactions of others. How well the patient is adapting to these changes can be evaluated during outpatient visits when the burn team and other personnel can discuss the patient's progress.

Follow-up care may not take place at the institution where the patient was hospitalized if the patient lives several hundred miles away. The burn team members may need to contact their counterparts in the patient's community to plan follow-up care. If possible, a member of the follow-up team should visit the patient in the hospital before discharge.

Job retraining may be necessary if the burn injury caused loss of joint function or other physical limitations that may prevent the patient from returning to a former job. The local office of State Labor and Industry Board can assign a vocational counselor to help the patient return to the work force. Even if retraining cannot begin for several months, contact with the vocational counselor and anticipation of retraining may help the patient look beyond immediate problems and think of the future.

✚ EVALUATION

Evaluation is based on the expected outcomes. Questions to ask may include the following:
1. Can the patient tolerate increasing activity as prescribed by the burn team?
2. Is the patient exhibiting a realistic concept of changes in body image?
3. Has the patient developed contractures?
4. Is the patient or family demonstrating appropriate coping skills?
5. Is the patient able to perform ADL?
6. Is the patient or family able to demonstrate correct dressing changes technique?

■ SUMMARY

1. The severity of a burn injury depends on the age of the victim, body part involved, burning agent, size and depth of the burn wound, and the victim's medical history.
2. The initial care for a burn includes removing the victim from the source of the burn and dousing the burn with water.
3. The initial systemic response to a burn is the shift of fluid from the intravascular to the interstitial space, creating hypovolemia. This is treated with a calculated dose of lactated Ringer's solution. After 48 to 72 hours

---

Putting knowledge to practice

- Differentiate between partial-thickness and full-thickness burns.
- Describe the pathophysiologic changes that occur during the emergent period.
- Describe the emergency care for major burns and the initial inpatient therapy.
- Write a nursing care plan which includes interventions for replacing body fluids, preventing infection, promoting nutrition and mobility, and providing emotional support.

the fluid shifts from the interstitial to the intravascular space and hypervolemia occurs.

4. Emotional support to the victim and victim's family is an important role for nurses.
5. Burn wounds must be assessed on a daily basis.
6. Correct splinting and positioning are the best methods for preventing contractures.
7. There is no way to predict how a burn wound will appear after healing.

REFERENCES AND SELECTED READINGS
Contemporary

1. *Abshagen, D: Topical agents and emergency care for minor burn injuries, J Emer Nurse 10:325-331, 1984.
2. Achaver, BM, editor: Management of the burned patient, Norwalk, Conn, 1987, Appleton & Lange.
3. American Burn Association, Guidelines for service standards and severity classifications in the treatment of burn injury, American College of Surgeons Bulletin 69:24-28, 1984.
4. *Dyer, C: Burn care in the emergent period, J Emerg Nurse 6:9-16, 1980.
5. *Finlayson, L: Emergent care of the burn patient, Crit Care Update 7:18-19, 22-23, 1980.
6. *Freeman, JW: Nursing care of the patient with a burn injury, Crit Care Nurse November/December:52-68, 1984.
7. *Gatson, SF, and Schumann, LL: Burn wound management, Crit Care Update 7:5-17, 1980.
8. Gordon, M: Manual of nursing diagnosis, New York, 1985, McGraw-Hill Book Co.
9. *Heidrich, B, Perry, S, and Amand, R: Nursing staff attitudes about burn pain, J Burn Care Rehab 2:259-261, 1981.
10. Hills, SW, and Birmingham, JJ: Burn care, Bethany, Conn, 1981, Flescher Publishing Co.
11. *Jacoby, FJ: Care of the massive burn wound, Crit Care Quart 7(3):44-53, 1984.
12. Jelenko, C: Burn shock, Top Emerg Med 3:69-74, 1981.
13. Kenner, CV: Burn injury. In Kenner, CV, Guzzetta, CE, Dossey, BM, editors: Critical care nursing: body-mind-spirit, Boston, 1981, Little, Brown & Co.
14. *Kenner, C, and Manning, S: Emergency care of the burn patient, Crit Care Update 7:24-27, 30-33, 1980.
15. *Kilbee, E: Burn pain management, Crit Care Quart 7(3): 54-62, 1984.
16. *King, MW: Nursing considerations of the burned patient during the emergent period, Heart Lung 11:353-363, 1982.
17. *Kinzie, Y, and Lau, C: What to do for the severely burned, RN 43(4):46-51, 104-110, 1980.
18. LeMaster, JE: Rehabilitation of the burn-injured patient. In Wachtel, TL, Kahn, V, and Frank, HA, editors: Current concepts in burn care, Rockville, Md, 1983, Aspen Systems Corp.
19. *Luterman, A, Adams, A, and Curreri, PW: Nutritional management of the burn patient, Crit Care Quart 7 (3):34-43, 1984.
20. *Marvin, JA: Planning home care for burn patients, Nurs 83 13(8):65-67, 1983.
21. *Nadel, E, and Kozerefski, PM: Rehabilitation of the critically ill burn patient, Crit Care Quart 7(3):19-33, 1984.
22. Ragiel, CA: The impact of critical injury on patient, family, and clinical systems, Crit Care Quart 7(3):73-78, 1984.
23. Rauscher, LA, and Ochs, GM: Prehospital care of the seriously burned patient. In Wachtel, TL, Kahn, V, and Frank, HA, editors: Current topics in burn care, Rockville, Maryland, 1983, Aspen Systems Corp.
24. *Robertson, KE, Cross, PJ, and Terry, JC: Burn care: the crucial first days, Am J Nurse 85(1):30-45, 1985.
25. Salisbury, RE, Newman, NM, and Dingeldein, GD, editors: Manual of burn therapeutics, Boston, 1983, Little, Brown & Co.
26. *Severely burned patients: anticipating their emotional needs, nursing grand rounds, Nurs 80 12(9):47-50, 1980.
27. Trunkey, DD: Transporting the critically burned patient, Top Emerg Med 3:21-24, 1981.
28. Wachtel, TL, Frank, HA, and Fortune, JB: Initial management of major burns. In Wachtel, TL, Kahn, V, and Frank, HA, editors: Current topics in burn care, Rockville, Md, 1983, Aspen Systems Corp.
29. Wachtel, TL, and Fortune, JB: Fluid resuscitation for burn shock. In Wachtel, TL, Kahn, V, and Frank, HA, editors: Current concepts in burn care, Rockville, Md, 1983, Aspen Systems Corp.
30. Wachtel, TL, Yen, M, and Fortune, JB: Nutritional support for burned patients. In Wachtel, TL, Kahn, V, and Frank, HA, editors: Current concepts in burn care, Rockville, Md, 1983, Aspen Systems Corp.
31. Walkenstein, MD: Comparison of burned patients' perception of pain with nurses' perception of patients' pain, J Burn Care Rehab 3:233-236, 1982.
32. *Wingate, E: Emergent burn care: a time for life-saving measures, Crit Care Update 10:49-54, 1983.

Classic

33. Andreason, NJC, Nayes, R Jr., and Hartford, CE, and others: Management of emotional reactions in seriously burned adults. NEJM 286:65-69, 1972.
34. Artz, CP, Moncrief, JA, and Pruitt, BA: Burns: a team approach, Philadelphia, 1979, WB Saunders Co.
35. Bernstein, NR: Emotional care of the facially burned and disfigured, Boston, 1976, Little, Brown & Co.
36. *Busby, HD: Nursing management of the acute burn patient and nursing management of optimal burn recovery, J Cont Educ Nurse 10:16-30, 1979.
37. Cockshott, WP: The history of the treatment of burns, Surg Gynecol Obstet 102:116-124, 1956.
38. Curreri, PW, and Luterman, A: Nutritional support of the burned patient, Surg Clin North Am 58:1151-1156, 1978.
39. Feller, I, and Archanbeault, C: Nursing the burned patient, Ann Arbor, Mich, 1973, Institute for Burn Medicine Press.
40. Feller, I, Jones, CA, and Richards, K: Emergent care of the burn victim, Ann Arbor, Mich 1977, Institute for Burn Medicine Press.
41. Hardy, JD, editor: Textbook of surgery: principles and practice, ed 5, Philadelphia, 1977, JB Lippincott Co.
42. *Jacoby, FG: Individualized burn wound dressings, Nurs '77 7(6):62-63, 1977.

---

*References preceded by an asterisk are particularly well suited for student reading.

43. Jacoby, FG: Nursing care of the patient with burns, ed 2, St. Louis, 1976, The CV Mosby Co.

44. Jelenko, C: Chemicals that "burn," J Trauma 14:65-72, 1974.

45. *Jones, CA, and Feller, I: Burns: avoiding and coping with complications before and after grafting, Nurs 77 7:72-81, 1977.

46. *Jones, CA, and Feller, I: Burns: The home stretch . . . rehabilitation, Nurs 77 7(12):54-57, 1977.

47. *Jones, CA, and Feller, I: Burns: what to do during the first crucial hours, Nurs 77 7(3):22-31, 1977.

48. *Marvin, J: Acute care of the burn patient, Crit Care Quart 1:25-35, 1978.

49. *Schumann, L, and Gatson, S: Common sense guide to topical burn therapy, Nurs 79 9(3):34-39, 1979.

50. Williams, BP: The problems and life-style of a severely burned man. In Bergersen, B, and others, editors: Current concepts in clinical nursing vol 2, St. Louis, 1969, The CV Mosby Co.

UNIT XI
Emergent and Critical Care

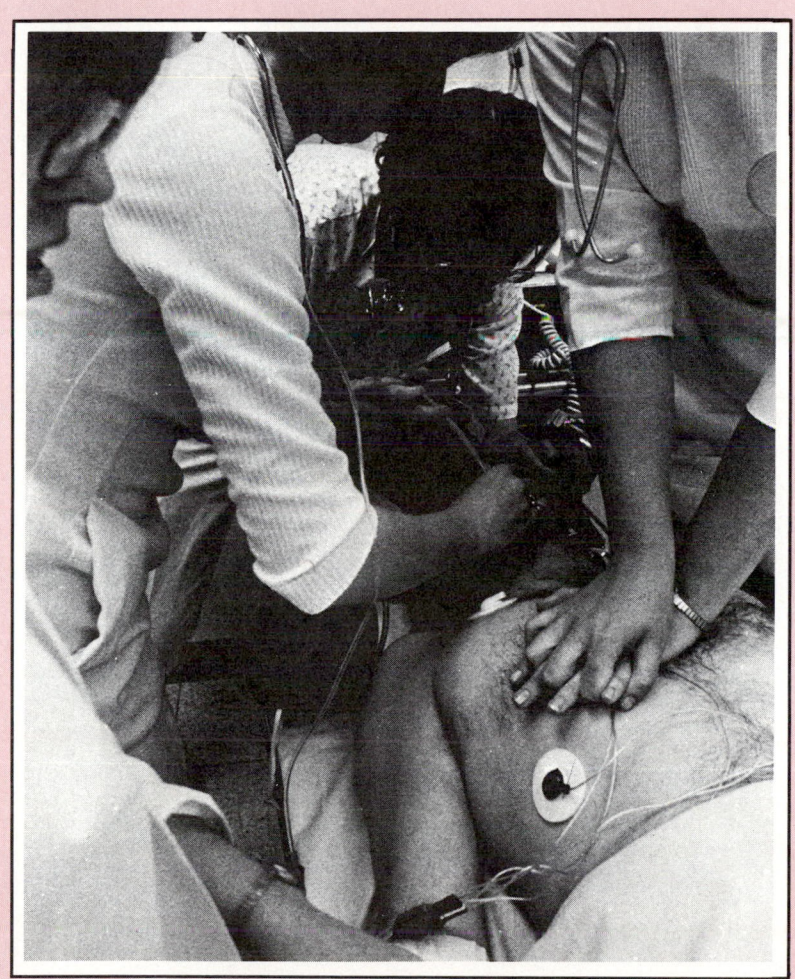

41

Problems Encountered in Emergencies and Disasters

BARBARA C. LONG

CHAPTER OBJECTIVES

After studying this chapter, the student should be able to:

- Describe preventive methods for accidents.

- Describe the nature of delivery of emergency care.

- Describe parameters of assessment of the injured or unconscious person.

- Identify principles of general management and specific care for accidental injuries or sudden illness (cardiac arrest, MI, near drowning, electrical injuries, poisoning, excess heat or cold, radiation, wounds, and fractures).

- Discuss the nature of rape and appropriate interventions.

- Describe the effects of disasters and appropriate roles of the nurse during disasters.

Nurses are frequently called on to provide emergency care in the community or in settings where medical help is not immediately available; therefore, all nurses need ot know the basics of emergency care. In this chapter major points are identified in the delivery of emergency care in the community, in assessment and intervention for common emergencies, and in principles of management in disasters.

■ PREVENTION OF ACCIDENTS

Accidents in the United States claim almost 100,000 lives each year, half from motor vehicle accidents. Accidents are the leading cause of death in persons younger than 45 years and are the third leading cause in those 45 to 64 years of age.

In terms of morbidity, approximately *60 million* persons, or about 30 of every 100, are injured in the United States every year. Billions of dollars are spent annually on medical expenses, property damage, and administrative costs related to accidents. Money lost from potential earnings or disability adds to this figure.

Accidents that result in injury or death involve human suffering that cannot be measured in dollars: pain, long-term rehabilitation, disabilities (temporary or permanent), loss and grief, and family disruption.

Accident prevention is a major public health goal, and both the Public Health Service and the American Public Health Association (APHA) actively promote accident prevention. Community groups can be helpful in investigating accident statistics in their local area and in disseminating information to encourage accident prevention. Nurses have an important role in accident prevention, both through their roles as professionals and as residents of a community. The influence of nurses can be extended in many areas because nurses are represented in schools, industry, community nursing programs, and hospitals.

■ Home

Accidents in and about the home are responsible for almost one fourth of all accidental deaths each year. Falls account for about half the number, and fires and poisoning for most of the remainder. Many aged persons who fall do so when walking from room to room. Some fall because of heavily waxed floors, loose rugs, poor lighting, scattered toys, and other conditions that could have been corrected (see the box at top, right). People fall from roofs, windows, high ladders, and steps; and are fatally burned or otherwise injured while using solvents and cleansing agents without proper knowledge of their hazards.

The number of electric appliances used in the home has increased the danger of electric shock and fire from overloaded circuits. Many persons die in fires caused by burning cigarette ashes dropped on furniture, rugs or discarded in waste containers, and by cigarettes that are dropped when the smoker falls asleep. Attention needs to be given to teaching homeowners to have older heating systems

---

**Home safety features
for elderly persons**

Floors	Large rugs and carpets anchored
	Small rugs with nonskid backing
	Avoidance of floor wax (unless nonskid)
Stairs	Uniform height
	Nonskid treads
	Risers marked with contrasting color
	Strong handrails
	Adequate lighting
Bathroom	Handrail in tub or shower
	Skidproof bath mat
	Treads in tub or on shower floor
	Seat in shower

---

checked periodically for gas leaks and other unsafe features. All persons in a household should be aware of what to do in the event of fire, and fire evacuation drills are encouraged. Homes should be equipped with smoke alarms in strategic places such as the kitchen, bedrooms, hallways, and basement.

Most accidental poisonings occur in children, but adults are also at risk. Nonpotable liquids should be kept in original containers, tightly capped, and *never* placed in a soft drink bottle, drinking glass, or cup. Medications should never be taken from unmarked or poorly marked bottles.

The community health nurse has an opportunity to assess safety hazards during home visits and to teach the family general accident prevention as well as specific measures for the safety of the ill person.

■ Community

Community action can best be effected by group action, but it often takes persistence to interest and stimulate group action. Parent-teacher associations, recreational associations, and religious and social groups are usually interested in accident control. Phases of accident prevention that should be of community interest include the following:
1. Teaching of accident prevention in public schools
2. Better control and inspection of homes for the aged and prisons
3. Rigid enforcement of driving regulations
4. Improvement of street lighting and traffic signals at busy intersections
5. Periodic inspection of all automobiles
6. Promotion of laws pertaining to fire proofing of buildings
7. Promotion of laws protecting the public from flammable clothing, potentially harmful toys, and similar items.

Safety measures to prevent falls of hospital patients

1. Handrails in hospital corridors
2. Armchairs rather than armless chairs
3. Chairs in bathrooms or showers
4. Call systems in bathrooms and lounges as well as in patients' rooms
5. Hi-Lo beds (placed in low position when patient ambulating)
6. Night lights in patient rooms (especially elderly patients).

Fire safety approaches

1. Close doors and windows of all patient rooms until evacuation is necessary.
2. General precautions
   a. Do not open a door that feels excessively hot
   b. Keep low as possible if air is hot and smoke-filled
   c. Use wet cloths around nose and mouth if air is hot (try not to inhale smoke or hot air).
3. If evacuation is advisable
   a. Patients closest to fire are evacuated to opposite end of corridor (horizontal evacuation)
   b. Downward evacuation is effected (when instructed) by *stairway* (never by elevator)
   c. Ambulatory patients are evacuated first; patients are led by hospital personnel, if possible.

■ Hospitals

Assessing the need for safety in the general environment and for the safety of specific patients, and taking measures to prevent injury are important functions of the nurse. The nurse can participate in policy making and safety monitoring through membership on hospital safety committees.

■ FALLS

Falls are the major cause of hospital-incurred injuries. Hospitalized persons are in unfamiliar surroundings with strange furniture and equipment, and may be weak for many reasons, or may become confused, all of which can contribute to falls. Elderly persons are at high risk for falls. All patients should be assessed for the potential of falling, and preventive measures should be instituted (see the box above).

The use of side rails is a nursing decision. Side rails should be kept raised for all unconscious patients. A confused patient may attempt to climb over the side rail and thus have farther to fall; a jacket restraint may be more useful in this situation.

Patients who are weak may need frequent reminders to seek assistance before ambulating. Some patients do not want to "bother the nurse" and attempt to walk to the bathroom unaided, especially at night. All patients should use supportive slippers; paper slippers can be a hazard.

■ FIRE

All hospitals and nursing homes must have established fire prevention routines, and all personnel must be familiar with these routines (see the box at top, right). Participation in fire drills should be taken seriously, and evaluation should follow each drill.

Fires usually occur from smoking or faulty electrical equipment. Because smoking is also hazardous to health, many hospitals restrict smoking in patients' rooms and in many public areas. If smoking is permitted, ashtrays should

be available and the patient and visitors instructed about not emptying them. If patients are careless smokers who may drop a cigarette or ash, their smoking should be monitored. Faulty electrical equipment should not be used. Any questions about smoke should be investigated and reported immediately. If a fire should occur, the nurse in charge who is most familiar with the patients' conditions should be in charge of any evacuation.

■ DELIVERY OF EMERGENCY CARE

■ Community

The National Safety Act of 1966 requires each county to appoint an emergency medical care committee. The effectiveness of these committees varies greatly, influenced to a large extent by citizen interest and political activity. Every community needs an organized emergency care system with support and input from community health organizations and community political elements.

Many communities have emergency medical technicians (EMTs) or paramedics to respond to emergency calls. EMTs have had preparation beyond basic first aid training but do not carry out invasive procedures. Paramedics have had more training than EMTs and can carry out such skills as starting intravenous fluids, giving medications, defibrillation, and intubation. The preparedness of personnel responding to emergency calls and the responsibilities that are legally permissible vary among states and communities within each state.

The American Heart Association has been instrumental in developing a program to educate large numbers of persons who are certified to administer cardiopulmonary resuscitation (CPR). This increases the possibility of a trained person being available to initiate resuscitation early in a larger number of emergency situations.

■ Hospitals

Hospital emergency rooms are often overloaded with persons seeking assistance for nonacute health problems. Newer approaches to delivery of both emergency and nonacute health care, such as urgent care centers in the community, have been initiated.

Many emergency departments have direct radio communication with rescue personnel in the community. Treatment can be initiated at the scene of the accident under medical direction and hospital personnel can be better prepared to receive the injured. This helps to eliminate some of the delays in initiation of care.

The role of the nurse in the emergency department has changed considerably in recent years as a result of the increased utilization of emergency departments by persons seeking medical attention and the increased sophistication of therapeutic management. Emergency department nurses are developing the following skills:

1. Assessment and triage (sorting patients to determine priority of medical attention)
2. Management of persons with high levels of anxiety
3. Specialized technical skills (initiating parenteral fluids, defibrillation, resuscitation, intubation, operating monitoring devices)
4. Interpreting selected laboratory findings and electrocardiograms and acting on these findings.

■ Legal aspects of emergency care

Nurses who intervene to assist victims in an emergency situation should be aware of the legal ramifications that can ensue as a result of their actions. Many states have enacted Good Samaritan laws in an effort to protect health personnel who aid accident victims. These laws vary in coverage among states as to the classes of people who are protected from liability, types of situations, geographic limits, and extent of immunity.

Good Samaritan laws serve to identify in statutory language those persons or situations that provide some degree of immunity from liability, many of which already exist by common law. Persons are judged as not liable unless they act willfully with gross negligence. Negligence is the key word. Damage must occur if negligence is to be proved, and the actions of the nurse must be the immediate cause of the damage.

"Reasonable care" provided by the nurse at the scene of an accident is usually judged as that care given by another similar nurse *under the prevailing situation*. Thus the care provided on a back road on a dark rainy night would not be judged the same as that given in an emergency room.

Nurses who work in hospital emergency departments need to be aware of legal implications of care provided in that setting, such as the care given to minors when parents are not present to give consent and actions that may be taken in helping police officers gather evidence.[8]

■ ASSESSMENT

When an emergency occurs or on arriving at the emergency scene, it is important to assess the situation, the patient, and the environment before initiating action. Some conclusions can be drawn from the immediate environment. If there is trauma to multiple victims, all should be assessed before any lifesaving interventions are initiated. Overt clues such as an automobile accident, report of falling, or ingestion of poison can give direction to probable

---

Head-to-toe assessment

Head and neck

Assess airway
Assess pupils
Examine ears, nose, mouth for bleeding, other drainage, foreign body
Palpate* cervical spine for pain (do not move head)
Examine head for bleeding, lacerations, contusions, depression of skull
Palpate jaw for fracture (pain, deformity)
Ask about stiffness of neck (if no history of trauma, assess movement)
Examine neck for distended neck veins, presence of tracheal stoma, tracheal deviation

Chest and spine

Observe chest movements for symmetry of expansion and character of respirations
Palpate clavicles for fracture (pain, deformity)
Examine chest for external injury
Palpate ribs for fracture (pain)
Palpate spine for point tenderness (do not move victim)

Abdomen and pelvis

Palpate pelvis for pain in groin when pressure applied over pelvis
Ask about abdominal pain
Examine abdomen for external injury, rigidity, distention, penetrating objects

Extremities

Examine for signs of external injury
Ask about pain in extremities
If no obvious injury, ask victim to move each limb
Test for sensation in each limb
Assess presence and strength of peripheral pulses

---

*All palpations should be carried out gently.

types of injuries. A complete head-to-toe assessment is carried out, if possible, before moving the victim so that additional injuries or conditions requiring intervention can be identified (see the box on p. 1446).

■ Data collection

A person who is not breathing, who has no palpable pulse, or who is hemorrhaging needs immediate assistance. Obtaining data to identify these circumstances is the first priority in assessment. This is sometimes referred to as the ABCs of emergency assessment (Airway, Breathing, Circulation) (see the box below). Assessing the general level of consciousness can be done as the nurse approaches the victim. If pulse and breathing are absent, CPR is initiated (p. 1450). Hemorrhage is treated by direct pressure to the wound.

Before starting the head-to-toe assessment, observe the following and assess those areas first:

1. Victim's general position
2. Obvious signs of deformities or asymmetry
3. Any purposeful movements
4. Signs or symptoms of pain or discomfort

During the overall assessment continue to monitor for changes in level of consciousness and respiratory status. Ask the victim or any relative or friends present to describe the preceding events; the presence of any medical conditions such as heart or lung disease, epilepsy, or diabetes; or any special medications taken by the victim that may have a bearing on the present situation.

If there is more than one person on the scene, the nurse or paramedic should remain with the victim while others are given directions to assess the environment for additional signs of danger and to call for any needed transportation.

■ Data analysis

■ RESPIRATIONS

The rate, depth, and character of respiration provide clues to the presence of ventilatory, central nervous system, or metabolic problems. Most trauma victims breathe a little faster than normal (18 to 24 breaths/min). If the person shows signs of respiratory effort (nasal flaring; suprasternal, intercostal, or substernal retractions), the airway may be partially obstructed. The type of sound accompanying respirations may indicate the degree and location of a partial obstruction. The following findings are suggestive of specific emergency care problems:

1. Rate
   a. Slow (<10 breaths/min): ventilatory or CNS problem
   b. Rapid (>26 breaths/min): hypoxia, acidosis, shock
2. Depth
   a. Shallow; shock, chest pain
   b. Deep: hypoxia, hypoglycemia, metabolic acidosis
3. Sound
   a. Inspiratory stridor: upper airway obstruction (above tracheal bifurcation)
   b. Expiratory wheezes or stridor: lower airway obstruction
4. Frothy, blood-tinged sputum: lung injury, pulmonary edema, pulmonary embolus

■ SHOCK

In persons who sustain major trauma or a major stressor to the system, such as myocardial infarction, shock usually develops (see Chapter 9). Signs of shock include restlessness, pale cold moist skin, rapid thready pulse, and rapid shallow respirations. Nausea and vomiting may occur. With anaphylactic shock the victim may complain of itching or burning of the skin, tightness in the chest, and difficulty in breathing. Wheals may develop on the skin, and the face and tongue may develop edema.

■ SENSATION

Pain may result from trauma if there is soft-tissue injury, fracture, or visceral damage. Pain may also occur with tissue anoxia, such as with obstruction of blood vessels or frostbite. Data obtained from the patient include location (region), severity, quality, onset and duration, and provoking factors. For a further discussion of pain, see Chapter 10.

Loss of sensation may result from injury to peripheral nerves or injury to nerves in the central nervous system. Peripheral nerve injuries may occur with fractures, lacerations, penetrating wounds, or dislocations. Loss of sensation concurrent with loss of movement and absence of

---

Priority assessment

Airway

Presence of respirations
Presence of foreign body, vomitus, loose dentures in mouth

Breathing

Respiration rate, depth, character
Use of accessory muscles for breathing
Tracheal deviation

Circulation

Presence of carotid pulse
Pulse rate, strength, rhythm
Presence of hemorrhage
Skin color, temperature, moisture

Level of consciousness

Response to voice and touch (or painful stimulus)
Pupillary response
If unconscious, presence of Medic-Alert tag

<table>
<tr><td colspan="2">

Possible causes of unconsciousness

1. Hypoxia (decreased oxygen to brain)
   a. Respiratory insufficiency
      (1) Airway obstruction from foreign body, secretions
      (2) Pneumothorax
      (3) Spinal cord injury
   b. Shock
      (1) Cardiogenic: cardiac arrest
      (2) Hypovolemic: hemorrhage
2. Metabolic (chemical brain depressants)
   a. Extrinsic
      (1) Drugs: alcohol, narcotics, barbiturates, antihistamines, tranquilizers
      (2) Poisons: carbon monoxide, carbon tetrachloride, hydrocarbons, methane gas
   b. Intrinsic
      (1) Ketones: diabetic ketoacidosis, starvation
      (2) Glucose: hypoglycemia, hyperglycemia
      (3) Ammonia: liver failure
      (4) Urea: kidney failure
      (5) Hormonal hypofunction: hypothyroidism, Addison's disease
      (6) Electrolyte imbalance: sodium, potassium, calcium, hydrogen ions
3. Brain pathologic conditions
   a. Trauma: concussion, brainstem contusion, intracranial hematoma
   b. Seizures: epilepsy, tumors, idiopathology
   c. Cerebrovascular accident: cerebral hemorrhage, thrombosis
   d. Tumors: benign, malignant
   e. Infections: meningitis, encephalitis
</td></tr>
</table>

Pupillary response in unconscious patients

Cause	Pupillary response
Shock or respiratory insufficiency	Equal, may be dilated
Drugs, chemicals	Equal, may be dilated or constricted
Intracranial hemorrhage, cerebrovascular accident	Usually unequal
Brain damage	Fixed, no response to light

matoma. Medical attention is urgent if an intracranial hematoma is suspected.

An unconscious person should be placed in a position that facilitates patency of the airway (side-lying position unless contraindicated) and the respiratory status constantly monitored.

■ OTHER DATA

Analysis of the data should include the following:
1. Type of injury or medical emergency that has probably occurred
2. Urgency of the need for medical attention
3. Availability of resources for carrying out necessary interventions
4. Availability of transportation
5. Time factor before medical attention can be obtained

local tissue or bone injury indicates central nervous system injury, for example, spinal cord injury or cerebral hemorrhage.

■ LEVEL OF CONSCIOUSNESS

Level of consciousness is assessed by determining whether the person responds immediately to voice and touch, responds only to painful stimuli, or does not respond. Unconsciousness may be due to many causes (see the box above). Pupillary response differs depending on the underlying problem (see the box at top, right).

If there has been trauma to the brain it is important to ascertain level of consciousness at different times. Temporary loss of consciousness followed by alertness and equal pupils usually indicates a concussion. If there is no skull fracture the patient is simply observed for 24 hours. *Alertness after injury followed by increasing loss of consciousness and unequal pupils* usually indicates an intracranial he-

■ GENERAL INTERVENTIONS

■ Principles of management

Some principles of management of injuries or sudden illnesses serve as guidelines for giving first aid:
1. Remain calm and think before acting.
2. Identify oneself as a nurse to victim and bystanders.
3. Do a rapid assessment for *priority* data (airway patency, breathing (respiration), and circulation (pulse).
4. Carry out *lifesaving* measures as indicated by the priority assessment.
5. Do a head-to-toe assessment before initiating *general* first aid measures.
6. Keep the victim lying down or in the position in which found (unless orthopnea is present), and protected from dampness and cold.
7. If victim is conscious, explain what is occurring; assure victim that help will be given.
8. Avoid unnecessary handling or moving of the victim; move the victim only if danger is present.

9. Do not give fluids if there is a possibility of abdominal injury or if anesthesia will be necessary within a short time.
10. Do not transport the victim until all first-aid measures have been carried out and appropriate transportation is available.

Lifesaving measures (described on succeeding pages) are carried out first when the initial assessment indicates the presence of breathing or circulatory difficulties. After breathing has been reestablished and excessive bleeding controlled, other interventions are carried out when the head-to-toe assessment is completed.

The victim is kept in a supine or sitting position, depending on symptoms, until all necessary interventions are carried out. Wounds are covered and fractures splinted before the victim is transported. Because shock is a possibility when major injuries occur, the victim should be protected from chilling. On a cold day, protection may be needed underneath the victim and sufficient covering to prevent loss of body heat but not to cause vasodilation. Fluids are given orally only to a conscious person showing signs of shock if there will be a considerable delay before medical care can be obtained and if abdominal injury is not present.

■ Psychologic support

People who experience trauma may have numerous anxieties. It is often easy to overlook the victim's need for emotional support when physiologic needs require immediate attention. Some patient concerns include the following:

Fear of pain
Fear of death
Fear of unknown
Disability
Loss of time from work
Cost of medical care

A calm, interested approach that conveys concern to the victim as a person is helpful. Giving information frequently during all phases of emergency care to both victim and family or friends will help them understand what is occurring and that help is being provided, thus decreasing some of the anxiety.

Varying levels of tolerance to stress are found in different individuals. Highly anxious persons may need someone to stay with them. At the scene of an accident a calm bystander can be helpful. Some hospitals provide selected volunteers for that purpose. All health personnel need to evaluate frequently their own effectiveness in assessing anxiety and in conveying understanding and emotional support to the victim and family during an emergency.

■ CARDIOPULMONARY PROBLEMS

For life to be maintained oxygen must be taken in by the lungs and pumped to the tissues; carbon dioxide must be returned from the tissues to the lungs and exhaled. Thus any obstruction that interferes with the diffusion of these gases, failure of the heart to pump, or inadequate blood to carry the oxygen to the tissues is a threat to life and demands immedaite emergency intervention. Airway patency, breathing facilitation, and circulation maintenance are the ABCs of emergency care and take first priority in assessment and intervention.

■ Airway obstruction and breathing difficulties

■ ASSESSMENT

Asphyxia occurs for various reasons (see the box below). Signs of asphyxia are related to the efforts made by the victim to take in air and to the decreasing oxygenation. These signs include the following:

1. Dyspnea
2. Use of accessory respiratory muscles (prominent neck muscles, intercostal rib retractions, nasal flaring)
3. Wheezing or stridor from air moving through narrowed passageways
4. Coarse rales (crackles) if fluid is present in alveoli
5. Skin pale (ashen in blacks)
6. Cyanosis (late sign)

■ INTERVENTION FOR ASPHYXIA

The first step in assisting a person who is having extreme difficulty in breathing is to position the person to ensure a maximal airway.

Causes of asphyxia

Inadequate oxygen in environment
Smoke
Toxic gases

Obstruction of air passages
Foreign bodies in airway
Tongue falling back in pharynx
Edema of respiratory tissue
Laryngospasm

Secretions in air passages
Near-drowning
Pulmonary edema

Interferences with respirations
Chest trauma
Depression of respiratory center (drugs)

Interferences with circulation
Electric shock
Myocardial infarction
Carbon monoxide poisoning

If the airway is obstructed by a *foreign body* the person may need assistance in its removal. The Heimlich abdominal thrust maneuver may be attempted (see the box below).

If the person is *unconscious* and the tongue is blocking the airway, and if there is no trauma suggesting a neck fracture, the neck is hyperextended (Fig. 41-2). This maneuver alone may be enough to open the airway.

If extension of the head and neck does not initiate breathing, artificial ventilation must be initiated immediately (see the box on p. 1451). Failure of the chest to rise with ventilation indicates that the airway is obstructed by a foreign body. Actions to be taken include the following:

1. Give four abdominal thrusts.
2. Check mouth quickly for dislodged foreign body; remove foreign body by sweeping a hooked finger across back of throat.

3. Repeat above maneuvers if normal breathing does not occur or chest expansion does not resume with artificial ventilation.

■ Cardiopulmonary resuscitation

Cardiopulmonary arrest is recognized by the cessation of breathing and circulation and signifies a state of clinical death. Immediate and definitive action must be instituted within 4 to 6 minutes after the arrest, or biologic death will occur.

Unresponsiveness, cessation of respirations, development of pallor and cyanosis, absence of heart sounds and blood pressure, loss of palpable pulse, and dilation of the pupils are present. (Pupillary response can be misleading in patients who are receiving drugs such as atropine or opium derivatives or in the presence of corneal pathologic conditions.) If a hospitalized patient is being monitored by means of an ECG machine or cardiac monitor, the elec-

---

Heimlich abdominal thrust maneuver

1. Stand behind victim.
2. Encircle arms around victim's waist (Fig. 41-1).
3. Place one fist between umbilicus and sternum with thumb against abdomen.
4. Place second hand over fist.
5. Press on abdomen with quick upward thrusts.

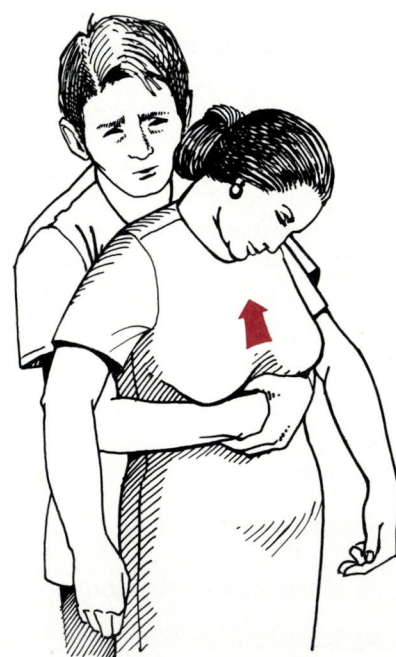

Fig. 41-1 Heimlich abdominal thrust maneuver. Rescuer places fist between umbilicus and xiphoid process with the thumb pressed against the abdomen. Pressure is applied upward.

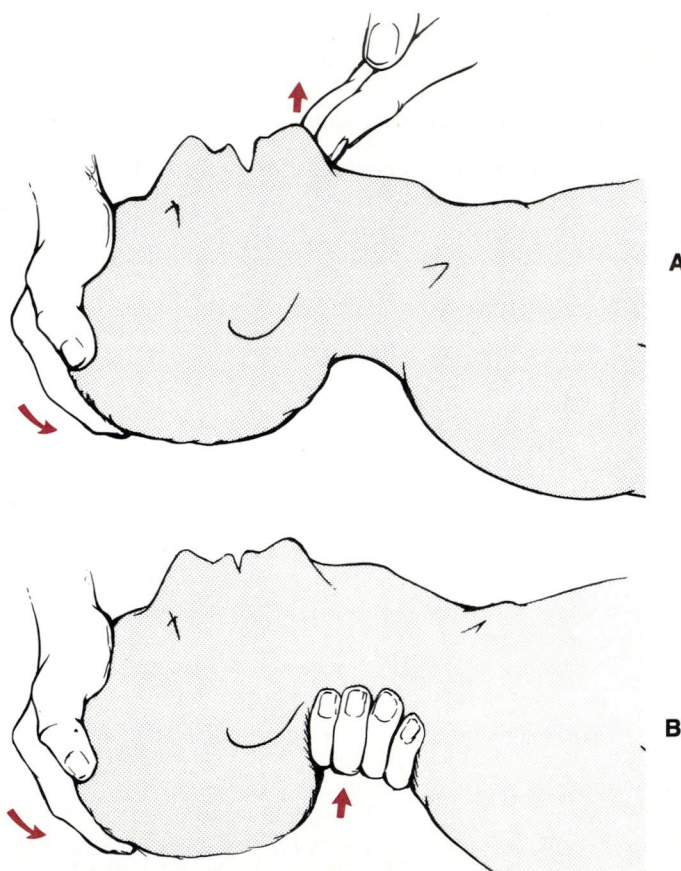

Fig. 41-2 Head tilt. **A,** Chin lift. Place one hand on forehead and tips of fingers of other hand under lower jaw near chin. Bring chin forward while pressing forehead down. **B,** Neck lift. Place one hand behind neck and other hand on forehead. Lift neck with one hand and tilt head backward by applying pressure to forehead. Method shown in **A** is preferred.

trocardiographic pattern of ventricular fibrillation or, less commonly, ventricular asystole will appear.

■ TECHNIQUES OF BASIC LIFE SUPPORT

Basic life support is an emergency procedure that consists of recognizing cardiopulmonary arrest and initiating proper CPR techniques to maintain life until the victim either recovers or is transported to a medical facility where advanced life support measures are available (Table 41-1). The sequence of CPR is listed below.

☐ Mouth-to-mouth ventilation

Mouth to mouth ventilation is performed as follows:
1. Maintain victim in head-tilt position.
2. Pinch nostrils.
3. Take a deep breath and place mouth around outside of victim's mouth, forming a tight seal.
4. Blow into victims mouth.
5. Adequate ventilation is demonstrated by:
   a. Rise and fall of chest (1 to 2 inches)
   b. Hearing and feeling air escape as victim passively exhales

Table 41-1 Life support measures in cardiac arrest

Findings	Action	ABCs of action
No response		
Absence of respirations; cyanosis; dilated pupils	Open airway	A—Open *Airway*
Respirations still absent	Initiate artificial ventilation	B—Restore *Breathing*
Carotid pulse not palpable	Initiate external cardiac compressions	C—Restore *Circulation*
ECG: ventricular fibrillation	Drug therapy; defibrillation	D—Provide *Definitive* treatment

---

Sequence of CPR in adults

Step 1: Assess level of consciousness
   1. Shake victim's shoulder and shout, "Are you OK?"
   2. If no response, summon help
   3. Place victim supine on *firm* surface.
Step 2: Open airway
   1. Hyperextend neck by head tilt or chin lift methods (Fig. 41-2)
   2. Place ear over victim's nose and mouth
      a. Look to see if chest is moving
      b. Listen for air escaping during exhalation
      c. Feel for air movement against face
   3. If patient is not breathing, proceed to step 3
Step 3: Initiate artificial ventilation
   1. Give two full mouth-to-mouth breaths each lasting 1 to 1½ seconds
Step 4: Assess circulation
   1. Palpate carotid pulse
   2. If carotid pulse not palpable, proceed to step 5
Step 5: Initiate external cardiac compressions
   1. If only one rescuer:
      a. Do 15 cardiac compressions at a rate of 80/min to 100/min
      b. Follow with two artificial ventilations
      c. Repeat sequence
   2. If two rescuers:
      a. One person does cardiac compressions, at a rate of 80/min to 100/min without pause
      b. Second rescuer ventilates victim quickly after every five compressions
   3. Palpate carotid pulse after four complete cycles to assess effectiveness, and subsequently every few minutes to check for return of spontaneous circulation. CPR is resumed with ventilation.

c. Feeling in own airway the resistance of victim's lungs expanding.

□ External cardiac compressions

External cardiac massage is the rhythmic compression of the heart between the lower half of the sternum and the thoracic vertebral column. This intermittent pressure compresses the heart, raises intrathoracic pressure, and produces an artificial pulsatile circulation. Correctly performed cardiac compressions can produce a peak systolic blood pressure of > 100 mm Hg, but the diastolic pressure is close to zero and the mean blood pressure in the carotid arteries is approximately 40 mm Hg, or one-fourth to one-third normal.

The technique for performing external cardiac compressions is as follows:

1. Position yourself close to victim's sternum.
2. Place heel of one hand on sternum two fingerwidths above tip of coccyx; and place second hand on top of first hand with fingers parallel and pointing away from body.
3. Position shoulders directly over victim's sternum.
4. Keep elbows locked in a straight position.
5. Depress lower sternum 1½ to 2 inches.
6. Keeping hands in position, release pressure on sternum to allow heart to fill.
7. Repeat, depressing and releasing sternum.
8. Perform compressions regularly and smoothly.

□ Precordial thump

The precordial thump is a quick blow delivered to the middle portion of the sternum. It is recommended only for *monitored* patients at the onset of ventricular tachycardia or asystole from heart block. It generates a small low-voltage stimulus in the heart. In an anoxic heart that is still beating the precordial thump could be hazardous because it may induce ventricular fibrillation.

■ CONTINUATION OF CPR

CPR should be stopped for no more than 5 seconds every 4 to 5 minutes to assess the return of spontaneous pulse and respiration. Rescuers should continue CPR until one of the following takes place:

1. Spontaneous circulation and ventilation return
2. Another rescuer takes over basic life support
3. Victim is transported to an emergency facility where qualified personnel assume the responsibility for CPR
4. Victim is pronounced dead by a physician
5. Rescuer is exhausted and unable to continue

■ IN-HOSPITAL CARDIAC ARREST

Many hospitals have prepared teams of personnel, including physicians, nurses, anesthesiologists, and technicians, who can be called to give immediate and complete care in the event of a cardiac arrest. Most hospitals have a specially equipped cart on which all necessary emergency items are available: ECG machine, suction device, oxygen, defibrillator, airway and Ambu or other breathing bag, laryngoscope, a variety of endotracheal tubes, cutdown set, fluids for intravenous administration, and tracheostomy set should this be necessary.

Medications usually administered during a cardiac arrest (Table 41-2) are generally available on the emergency cart. Supplementary oxygen is given after breathing resumes to treat the resultant hypoxemia. Oxygen is also given for other types of hypoxemia following trauma or stress such

Table 41-2 Medications commonly used for cardiac arrest

Medication	Use	Action
Atropine sulfate	Slow pulse following cardiac standstill	Accelerates heart rate
Bretylium tosylate (Bretylol)	Ventricular fibrillation, ventricular arrhythmias	Suppresses ventricular fibrillation and arrhythmias
Calcium chloride (10% solution)	Ventricular standstill	Increases myocardial contractility and conduction velocity
Dobutamine HCl (Dobutrex)	Refractory pump failure	Increases myocardial contractility
Epinephrine HCl (Adrenalin) 1:10,000 solution	Ventricular fibrillation	Positive inotropic (force of contractions) and chronotropic (regularity of beat) effect; peripheral vasoconstriction
Isoproterenol HCl (Isuprel)	Asystole, cardiovascular collapse	Positive inotropic and chronotropic effects that increase cardiac output
Metaraminol bitartrate (Aramine)	Shock	Potent vasopressor, increases peripheral resistance
Levarterenol bitartrate (Levophed)	Shock	Potent vasopressor, positive inotropic effect, increases peripheral resistance
Sodium bicarbonate (50 mEq)	Metabolic acidosis	Provides bicarbonate to return serum pH to normal
Lidocaine HCl (Xylocaine)	Arrhythmias	Shortens refractory period, suppresses automaticity of ectopic foci

as with smoke inhalation, carbon monoxide poisoning, near-drowning, myocardial infarction, or chest injuries.

■ COMPLICATIONS OF CPR

The most common complication of external cardiac massage is fracture of the ribs. This may occur in some individuals even though the technique of external cardiac compressions is performed correctly. Other complications that can occur despite correct CPR technique include fractured sternum, costochondral separation, lung contusions, and laceration of the liver. Any indication of labored respiration, paradoxical pulse, muffled heart sounds, tachycardia, decreased breath sounds, or drop in blood pressure is reported to the physician immediately.

■ Special cardiopulmonary problems

■ MYOCARDIAL INFARCTION

The person suspected of experiencing a myocardial infarction needs immediate attention. The greatest risk of mortality occurs within the first 2 hours after onset. If the heart ceases to beat, CPR is instituted immediately. The patient who is breathing may be more comfortable in a well-supported sitting position. Oxygen is given if available. A calm atmosphere is of utmost importance, and the patient should never be left alone; fear will add an additional stress to the already overburdened heart (see Chapter 25).

■ NEAR-DROWNING

Approximately 6000 people die from drowning in the United States every year, over half in home swimming pools. *Near-drowning* refers to asphyxiation or partial asphyxiation from a fluid medium, with the person either recovering spontaneously or resuscitated at least temporarily.[8] *Wet drowning* is the most common type and refers to asphyxiation from the aspiration of fluid into the lungs, inhaled as the person panics and gasps for breath. *Dry drowning* refers to asphyxiation from laryngospasm that prevents both air and water from entering the lungs. *Secondary drowning* is the recurrence of respiratory distress after recovery from the initial incident, and may occur a few minutes to several days later.

If the victim of near-drowning has ceased breathing, artificial ventilation is initiated as soon as possible, even before the victim has been completely removed from the water. Time should not be wasted trying to remove water from the lungs. If distention of the abdomen from *swallowed* water interferes with adequate ventilation, the victim can be rolled onto the stomach and lifted with pressure over the stomach to force the water out.

Persons who have experienced near-drowning should be observed closely for at least 24 hours, even if they indicate that they feel all right. Pulmonary edema can develop after several hours.

■ ELECTRICAL INJURIES

Electricity can cause injury in a number of ways:
1. Depression of respiratory center
2. Ventricular fibrillation (stimulation of heart at end of refractory period, even by low electric current)
3. Bone fractures and persistant muscle injury (from powerful muscle contractions)
4. Burns at entry and exit points

The extent of injury from electricity depends on the point in the heartbeat cycle that is stimulated by the electricity, the intensity of the current, and skin resistance. Moisture decreases skin resistance, so greater damage occurs when skin is moist from water or perspiration.

The victim must be removed from the source of electricity, with the rescuer being careful to avoid contact with the electric charge. CPR is started immediately if breathing and pulse are absent, and continued even when there is no evidence of response. Defibrillation is indicated for ventricular fibrillation.

■ Hemorrhage

■ PATHOPHYSIOLOGY

Considerable blood loss may result from external or internal bleeding (see the box below). Internal bleeding is more difficult to identify.

When a blood vessel is severed there is immediate contraction of the vessel wall, reducing the size of the opening and decreasing blood loss. Platelets begin to adhere to the roughened edges until a platelet plug is formed. A clot begins to form within 1 to 2 minutes. By 3 to 6 minutes the clot has filled the end of the blood vessel, blocking blood flow. Arteries have thick walls, and large arteries have musculature that can produce considerable vasospasms. Amputation of a leg, for example, may produce minimal bleeding. Veins and capillaries have thinner walls.

■ ASSESSMENT

External bleeding, if excessive, will saturate the clothing and be readily visible. If the person is wearing bulky outer

---

Causes of bleeding

External	Internal
Lacerations	Chest trauma
Crushing injuries	Abdominal trauma, for
Amputations	example, ruptured
Fractures	spleen
Nosebleeds	Trauma to thigh
	Esophageal varicies
	Peptic ulcers

garments, bleeding may be concealed. The examiner should run the hands quickly over the entire body under the outer clothing, being sure to check underneath the victim. Saturated clothing may need to be cut away so that the area of bleeding can be examined. The scalp is very vascular, and what appears to be considerable bleeding may result from a small scalp laceration.

Three types of bleeding may be observed:
1. Arterial bleeding: spurting bright red blood
2. Venous bleeding: continuous flow of darker blood
3. Capillary bleeding: oozing of blood

Internal bleeding may be difficult to identify. Bleeding into the thorax (hemothorax) may inhibit respirations, and chest pain may be present. Abdominal bleeding may be evidenced by rigidity of abdominal muscles and abdominal pain. Hemoptysis or hematemesis indicate pulmonary or gastrointestinal bleeding.

Shock occurs with severe internal or external bleeding. The victim is assessed for weak rapid pulse, slow shallow respirations, cold clammy skin, anxiety, restlessness, and thirst. The pupils are equal, may be dilated, and respond slowly to light.

■ INTERVENTION

Actions for control of *external* bleeding include the following:
1. Apply direct pressure over site of bleeding.
2. Apply pressure over a pressure point (Fig. 41-3) if bleeding cannot be controlled by direct pressure.
3. Use tourniquet *only* in selected situations (massive uncontrollable arterial bleeding):
   a. Use blood pressure cuff or wide triangular bandage folded six to eight times
   b. Do not cover or release tourniquet
   c. Attach a notation to patient giving location of tourniquet and time of application.

For suspected *internal* bleeding, keep the person lying down and protected from dampness and cold. Prevent further hypotension and seek immediate medical attention.

■ POISONING

Poisoning in adults occurs for various reasons:
1. Not checking medication labels (overdose or wrong medication)
2. Lack of knowledge (for example, taking alcohol and sedatives together)
3. Taking an excess amount in an attempt to obtain a desired effect
4. As a suicide attempt

■ Assessment

A *rapid* assessment is made to determine whether poisoning or overdose has occurred so that immediate action can be taken to prevent or diminish the effects of the poison or drug. It is important to identify clues that poisoning is a possibility and the type and quantity of the poisonous agent.

The conscious victim is questioned about the type and amount of substance taken or the nature of the poisoning. When the victim is unconscious, not much time should be spent looking for needle marks. Identification of the poison or drug can be facilitated by asking others to look for clues while you examine the victim. Empty containers, spilled fluids, open medication bottles, or syringes may provide needed information. *All* potential agents are gathered in their original containers and taken to the hospital with the victim. The physician may need to know the ingredients of the agent for those situations when an antidote is indicated.

■ Common accidental poisoning

Immediate action is necessary if poisoning is suspected; in some instances delay of a few minutes may make a difference between life and death. An *unconscious* victim

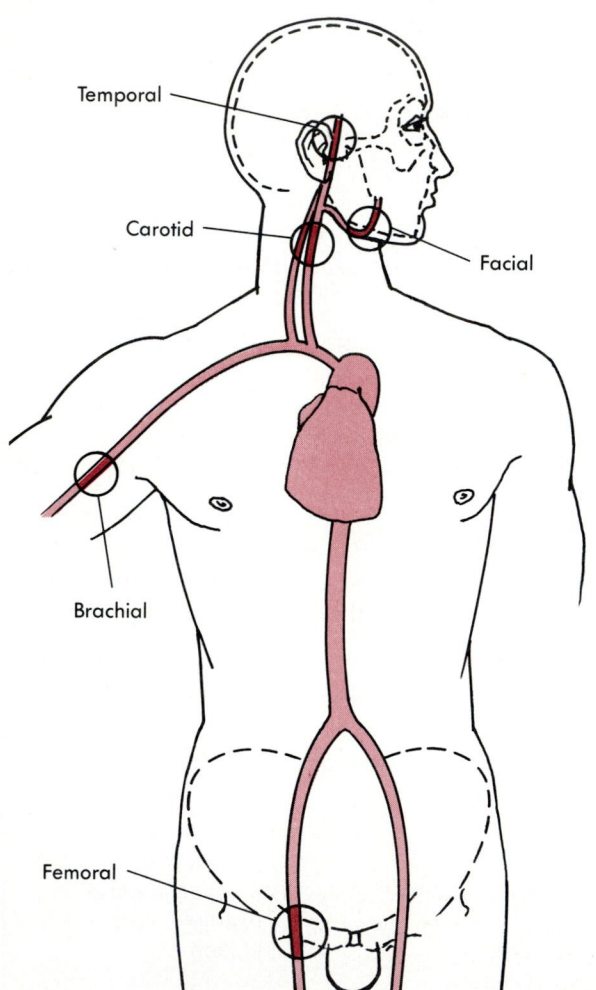

Temporal

Carotid

Facial

Brachial

Femoral

Fig. 41-3 Pressure points: locations at which large blood vessels may be compressed against bone to help control hemorrhage.

Table 41-3   Types of poisoning

Type	Examples	Therapy
Inhaled	Carbon monoxide, toxic gas	Remove victim from site to fresh air; give oxygen if available; give CPR if indicated; transport to medical center
Contact	Insecticides	Rinse skin with copious amounts of water
Ingested	Drugs, household chemicals, insecticides, lead	1. For noncaustic ingested substances, induce vomiting with syrup of ipecac a. 15 ml for adults b. May be repeated once in 20 minutes c. Follow with 1 to 2 full glasses of water 2. For drugs, follow vomiting with 30 to 50 gm activated charcoal in 60 to 90 ml water 3. For caustic substances a. Give nothing by mouth b. Seek immediate medical attention 4. In the emergency room, lavage may be used to eliminate agent
Injected	Insect bites, drugs	1. Bee stings: a. Remove stinger with scraping motion b. Apply ice c. A paste of sodium bicarbonate and water or weak solution of ammonia may be applied 2. Ticks a. Remove tick by applying turpentine or gasoline b. Apply ice after tick removed 3. Drugs: a. Take victim to medical center b. See Chapter 13 for discussion of substance abuse

must be transported *without delay* to the nearest medical facility.

If the victim is *conscious* identify the type, method, and estimated amount of poison or drug taken. Have someone call a physician immediately, if possible. Most large cities have poison control centers that maintain an extensive file on the most common substances and drugs. The telephone number is usually easily obtained from a list of emergency numbers in the front of the telephone directory.

Management consists of stopping absorption of the poisonous substance or drug. Poisonous substances can be inhaled, absorbed through the skin or mucous membranes, ingested, or injected. The type of intervention depends on the method by which the poison entered the system (Table 41-3).

If it is known exactly what poisonous substance or drug has been ingested, a specific antidote may be given in some cases by the physician. The use of a "universal antidote" has not proved effective.

■ Bacterial food poisoning

Food poisoning occurs more frequently than is reported, because the majority of persons recover quickly without treatment. The incidence of food poisoning from commercially prepared foods has become relatively uncommon in the United States, but food poisoning from home-cooked foods or improper handling of foods still occurs.

Prevention of food poisoning

1. Can low-acid foods (foods other than tomatoes or fruits) under pressure to prevent botulism.
2. Discard any can that bulges.
3. Avoid slow cooling of meat or poultry dishes.
4. Use a meat thermometer when cooking extremely large pieces of meat (especially pork).
5. Keep meats, fish, poultry, mayonnaise, and cream-filled foods refrigerated.

Bacteria such as *Staphylococcus aureus* or *Clostridium botulinum* can produce a toxin that acts as a poison, causing acute gastrointestinal tract upset. Because *S. aureus* toxin (the most common type) does not spread through the body, the symptoms are limited. The *C. botulinum* toxin does spread, and can be fatal (Table 41-4). *Salmonella* organisms introduced in food multiply in the intestines, causing acute gastrointestinal tract upset and infection.

Food poisoning is not caused by food that has spoiled or decomposed unless the food happens to contain disease-causing bacteria. Acute food poisoning can be prevented (see the box above).

Table 41-4 Bacterial food poisoning

Symptoms	Causative agent	Source	Comments
Nausea and vomiting, abdominal pain, lowered temperature, diarrhea is variable	*Staphylococcus aureus:* enterotoxin	Fish and meats (especially ham), dehydrated milk, unrefrigerated mayonnaise and cream-filled foods; skin and respiratory tract of food handlers	Mortality low Toxin heat stable Incubation 1 to 8 hours Symptoms last 8 to 24 hours Treatment: bed rest, fluids
Nausea and vomiting, diarrhea, abdominal pain, chills and fever, weakness	*Salmonella:* multiply in gut and produce toxin	Inadequately cooked eggs, poultry, meat (especially pork)	Mortality low Organism killed by heat Incubation 10 to 48 hours Symptoms last 2 to 5 days Treatment: bed rest, fluids (no antibiotics; they produce resistant strains)
Nausea and vomiting; double vision; flaccid paralysis of face, eyes, mouth, throat; dryness of skin, mouth, throat	*Clostridium botulinum:* exotoxin; spores germinate under anaerobic conditions and produce toxin	Improperly canned vegetables, meat (low-acid foods); spiced, smoked, vacuum-packed, or canned alkaline foods eaten without cooking	Mortality high Toxin heat labile Incubation 12 to 36 hours Death from respiratory failure

Table 41-5 Reactions to heat

Type	Cause	Signs and symptoms	Therapy
Heat cramps	Loss of sodium chloride in perspiration during strenuous exercise in hot weather	Severe cramps; pain in arms or legs	Salty fluids (for example, Gatorade) and food by mouth; extra water; rest in cool place
Heat exhaustion	Sodium and water depletion; fluids are replaced by some water, but inadequate salt	Vasomotor collapse: faintness, weakness; skin pale or ashen, cold moist	Recumbent position in cool environment; fluids, preferable with salt; transport to medical center if severe
Heat stroke (sunstroke)	Failure of perspiration regulating mechanism; prolonged exposure to heat, especially in elderly, obese, or unacclimatized person	Skin dry, hot flushed; faintness, dizziness; fever; unconsciousness	Reduce body temperature immediately by placing person in air-conditioned room; apply cool moist cloths, use fan; transport immediately to medical center
Burns	Direct heat, chemicals, electricity, radiation	First degree: erythema, pain Second degree: vesicles, pain Third degree: charred, coagulated, white skin	Apply cool water For specific care of severe burns, see Chapter 40

ENVIRONMENTAL INJURIES

Heat

Three types of general reactions to heat may occur (Table 41-5). *Heat cramps* can be prevented by taking extra salt and water before strenuous exercise in hot weather. The condition is self-limiting. *Heat exhaustion* is vasomotor collapse from the inability of the body to supply vessels adequately with sufficient fluid, usually from loss of sodium through perspiration. This usually occurs after vigorous exercise in hot weather, especially in the unacclimatized person.

Heatstroke is the most serious reaction to heat. It is caused by a failure of the perspiration regulating mechanism in the hypothalamus. It is typically seen during a heat wave, and elderly and obese persons are at high risk. The body retains heat rather than dissipating it through perspiration. Without treatment, most heatstroke victims die; the heat permanently damages the entire nervous system. Persons do not recover from heatstroke as quickly as from heat exhaustion, and may have faulty heat regulation for the rest of their lives. These individuals should avoid repeated long exposure to heat.

Cold

Excessive cold can lower body temperature, causing hypothermia, or can injure cells by direct exposure, causing frostbite.

HYPOTHERMIA

Hypothermia may result accidentally from exposure to cold weather. The extent of the cooling effect depends on the temperature and exposure time, the thermal conductivity of the environment, and the amount of air current present. Moisture is a good conductor, air is not. Wet clothing therefore contributes to increased cooling of the body. Several light layers of clothing to provide air insulation will keep a person warmer than one heavy layer. Air movement contributes to heat loss; thus lower environmental temperatures can be tolerated better in the absence of wind (windchill factor).

When the body is exposed to cold, shivering occurs to produce heat by increased metabolism. As the cold increases, shivering ceases and heat loss exceeds heat production. The individual becomes listless, apathetic, and sleepy and may become indifferent to the surroundings and not seek adequate protection. Pulse and respirations become slower as metabolism decreases. Freezing of the extremities, unconsciousness, and finally death result if help is not received.

The victim needs to be kept warm while being transferred to a medical facility. Wet clothing is removed immediately and warmed blankets applied. If a tub bath is given, the temperature should be approximately 40° to 42° C (104° to 108° F). Warmer temperatures can cause skin damage from the decreased circulation to the skin. Rubbing of the skin is to be avoided because this can also cause skin damage. Warm liquids may be given if the victim is conscious.

The person experiencing hypothermia is monitored closely during rewarming. Hypovolemic shock can occur from vasodilation. If fluids are given intravenously, overloading of the circulation is a potential complication. Vital signs are monitored for sudden changes. Cardiac monitoring may also be indicated for signs of ventricular fibrillation and cardiac arrest.

FROSTBITE

Cellular injury occurs with exposure to extreme cold. Cell water freezes, and the resulting ice crystals damage the cell. The degree of injury depends on the depth of freezing. Frostbite occurs most frequently in exposed areas such as the nose, cheeks, ears, and fingers and can be prevented by adequate covering with loose-fitting dry clothing. Toes are also susceptible because of dampness and tight pressure from shoes or boots. Persons with circulatory problems are more prone to develop frostbite.

Superficial frostbite is characterized by soft, whitened, or dull ashen skin that does not redden with pressure. The part can be rewarmed by contact with warm skin, covering, application of warm dry socks if toes are affected, or gently immersing the part in warm, not hot, water.

Deep frostbite is evidenced by hardness of the frozen tissue because of deep subcutaneous tissue injury. After thawing the skin becomes hyperemic and edematous with blister formation. The edema subsides in 24 to 48 hours, and tissue breakdown with necrosis results. The frozen part should be covered to warm it, and the victim should be taken to a medical center as soon as possible. Care is then similar to that for vascular disease of the extremities. Efforts are made to decrease the oxygen needs of the tissues while healing takes place, to improve blood supply by use of drugs, and to prevent infection of open lesions. Necrotic tissue may have to be debrided for healing to occur.

Radiation

Radiation injury is caused by exposure to gamma rays and neutrons from radioactive material. Persons can become contaminated directly from unshielded radioactive material, or indirectly by inhaling or swallowing particles of contaminated dust or smoke, or topically by skin contact. The amount of radiation that a person receives depends on various factors:

1. Strength of radiation source
2. Distance from the source
3. Duration of exposure
4. Area of the body exposed to the radiation source
5. Amount and type of shielding (see Chapter 12)

PREVENTION

Rescue workers who must remove a victim from an area of radioactivity need to protect themselves from radiation exposure. Because radioactive particles can be carried on dust, all skin areas must be covered and a filtering mask

Table 41-6 Effects of radiation on body systems

Organ or effect	Time to onset	Time to maximal effect	Total time from first dose to recovery	Dose required to cause injury (rad)	Major consequences
Cerebral syndrome	Few hours	1-2 days	Usually fatal	3000	Irreversible coma and cardio-vascular collapse
Hematologic syndrome					
Granulocyte depletion	1-2 weeks	4 weeks	6-8 weeks	200-400	Bacterial infection
Lymphocyte depletion	Few hours	1-2 days	4-8 weeks	200-400	Nonbacterial infection (virus, tuberculosis)
Platelet depletion	1-2 weeks	4 weeks	6-8 weeks	200-400	Bleeding
Gastrointestinal syndrome	3-4 days	6-7 days	2 weeks	600-2000	Fluid and electrolyte loss from mucosal sloughing
Skin lesions					
First-degree burn	Few hours	2-3 weeks	6-8 weeks	200	—
Second- or third-degree burn	Few days	1-2 weeks	8-12 weeks	1000	May need skin grafts
Hair loss	—	3 weeks	3-4 months	300	Permanent if greater than 700-800 rad
Sterility	—	Few days to few weeks	—	600-700	Permanent infertility
Hypothyroidism	—	Several years	—	Variable	Myxedema
Cataract	—	Several years	—	300-600	Visual loss
Leukemia	—	5-7 years	—	Unknown	Fatal
Solid tumors (thyroid, bone, breast, lung)	—	Many years	—	Unknown	Usually fatal, except thyroid tumors

From Kaye, D, and Rose, LF: Fundamentals of internal medicine, St. Louis, 1983, The CV Mosby Co.

worn by rescue workers after an explosion involving nuclear materials. The greater the duration of exposure, the greater the potential for injury; therefore the victim must be removed immediately to a less hazardous environment. Some of the basic principles of emergency care may have to be violated when there is danger of other explosions or when fires occur. The rescue worker should remove all contaminated clothing at the edge of the contaminated area, and any exposed skin areas are washed thoroughly. Rescue workers should take a shower as soon as possible as an additional preventive measure.

■ INTERVENTION

□ Local reactions

Radiation can cause a local inflammatory reaction of the skin, similar to a burn. The affected area may be washed gently with soap and water and a dry sterile dressing applied. Further treatment depends on the extent of injury. The person needs to know that continued observation of the skin is important for early detection of skin neoplasms.

□ Systemic reactions

Systemic reactions to ionizing radiation are primarily cerebral, hematologic, or gastrointestinal (Table 41-6). Cells that are rapidly dividing and differentiating (for example, blood cells and epithelial cells of the skin and gastrointestinal tract) are the most vulnerable. Loss of neutrophils predisposes the person to overwhelming bacterial infection, the loss of platelets results in bleeding. Loss of gastrointestinal epithelial cells leads to rapid fluid and electrolyte loss with severe dehydration and gastrointestinal bleeding. Radiation effects on slow turnover tissues, such as the eye or thyroid, may take several years to develop.

The cerebral syndrome usually results from massive exposure and includes progressive loss of consciousness followed by irreversible cardiovascular collapse.[27] Hematologic effects include decreased blood counts, petechiae, purpura, and bleeding from body orifices. Anorexia, nausea, and vomiting are commonly experienced from gastrointestinal injury. Recovery may be possible with active support of hematologic and gastrointestinal systems. Prolonged weakness, even during convalescence, is common.

The person with acute radiation syndrome is hospitalized. Early nausea and vomiting is usually self-limiting: sedatives and antiemetics may be helpful. Medical therapy is directed toward supportive care; that is, toward fluid and electrolyte replacement, nutrients (TPN may be necessary), and respiratory support as indicated. Various blood elements may be given for hematologic deficiencies. Bone marrow transplantation is frequently necessary. Prevention of infection, which takes high priority, consists of reverse isolation and prophylactic oral antimicrobial drugs. The same nursing care is required for the person with acute radiation syndrome as for the person receiving radiation therapy (see Chapter 12).

■ MUSCULOSKELETAL INJURIES

■ Wounds

Injury to soft tissue may result in open wounds, which damage the skin, or in closed wounds, which damage underlying tissue but leave the skin intact (Table 41-7).

Suturing of lacerations and incisions should be carried out within the first few hours after injury to obtain maximal healing with fewer complications or scarring. If the wound is grossly contaminated the decision may be made to delay suturing for a few days to permit thorough cleansing. Healing then occurs by tertiary intention.

Puncture wounds are particularly vulnerable to infection, and bacteria such as *Clostridium tetani,* which thrive without air, may infect these wounds. Because anaerobic bacterial infections are extremely serious, a physician should be consulted if the puncture was made by a dirty object.

Tetanus prophylaxis for contaminated wounds depends on the size of the wound and the person's previous tetanus immunization (Table 41-8). (See Chapter 11 for a discussion of active immunization with toxoid or passive immunization with immune serum globulin.) Tetanus (lockjaw) is highly fatal, and the only sure method of prevention is through immunization.

■ CHEST WOUNDS

Injuries to the chest may result in open chest wounds, fractured ribs, or injuries to the heart (cardiac tamponade) and lung (Table 41-9). These conditions are described in more detail elsewhere in the text.

Open wounds of the chest create a problem if there is intrusion into the pleural cavity. Air is drawn into the pleural space because of the existing negative pressure. The resultant positive pressure causes pneumothorax (collapse of the lung). A sucking noise is heard as the air is drawn in and respirations are impaired. Immediate action is indicated to cover the opening. A nonporous material must be used, because air can pass through a standard dressing or material. Plastic wrap, which is not only nonporous but tends to cling to the skin, is excellent. If a dressing is used it must be covered with petrolatum to create an air barrier. After the chest wound has been sealed, a pressure dressing is applied. Continual monitoring of respirations is indicated.

Persons with chest trauma are considered to have sustained serious injury until proved otherwise. Primary consideration in emergency management is maintenance of an open airway, breathing, and circulation. Oxygen is ad-

Table 41-7 Types of wounds

Type	Description	Therapy
Open wounds		
Abrasion	Scraping of skin surface (brush burn)	Wash well with soap and water; keep clean; no covering necessary
Laceration	Jagged cut through skin and underlying tissue	Wash well with soap and water; edges approximated by "butterfly" adhesive or by suturing
Incision	Straight cut through skin and underlying tissue by sharp knife	Same as for laceration
Puncture	Penetration of skin and underlying tissue by sharp-pointed object; skin quickly seals over when object is removed	Soak wound; encourage bleeding in small wound to wash out bacteria; monitor for signs of infection; tetanus prophylaxis
Stab	Form of puncture wound by large object such as a knife, stick, or piece of glass	Do not remove object; stabilize object to prevent further damage; control bleeding; seek immediate medical attention
Closed wound		
Contusion (bruise)	Injury by blunt object; blood vessels rupture, and blood seeps into tissue; edema from trauma to injured cells	Apply ice or cold compresses for 24 to 48 hours; analgesics for pain; rest injured part

ministered at high flow. Rapid transport after initial emergency measures is essential.

■ ABDOMINAL WOUNDS

Blows to the abdomen can rupture underlying organs. The spleen is often lacerated, and the intestines, liver, kidney, and bladder may also sustain injury. Symptoms may include abdominal pain and rigidity, nausea and vomiting, shock, and contusions on the abdominal wall. The victim may assume a position with knees drawn up toward the abdomen. If severe shock is present the use of antishock trousers (if available) is indicated before transport. The trousers extend from the ankle to below the lowest rib. After application the trousers are inflated to apply pressure on the lower half of the body, decreasing the size of the vascular system and redirecting blood flow to vital areas (Fig. 41-4).

Table 41-8 Tetanus prophylaxis following injury*

Booster date	Wound size	Prophylaxis
Within past 10 years	Small, moderate	0.5 ml toxoid†
	Severe or more than 24 hours old	0.5 ml toxoid
		250 units TIGH‡
More than 10 years ago or never	Small	0.5 ml toxoid (start series)
	Moderate	0.5 ml toxoid (start series)
		250 units TIGH
	Severe	0.5 ml toxoid (start series)
		500 units TIGH

*Recommended by the American College of Surgeons.
†Absorbed tetanus toxoid.
‡Tetanus immune globulin (human).

Table 41-9 Some major injuries affecting chest wall and pleural cavity

Injury	Cause	Signs and symptoms	Initial emergency care
Rib fracture	Blow to chest	Pain on inspiration; local tenderness	Transport
Flail chest	Ribs fractured in more than one place; chest wall becomes unstable	Paradoxical respirations; respiratory distress; chest pain	Apply external pressure: sandbags, pillow, your hand; give oxygen; transport with flail side down
Open pneumothorax (open sucking wound)	Penetrating trauma to chest; loss of negative intrathoracic pressure as air moves in and out of wound	Sucking sound on chest wall during inspiration; tracheal deviation	Cover wound with occlusive dressing during exhalation; give oxygen
Simple pneumothorax	Laceration of lung, hyperinflation (blast injuries, driving accidents), loss of negative intrathoracic pressure	Sudden onset of chest pain; decreased breath sounds of affected area; dyspnea, tachypnea	Semi-Fowler's or Fowler's position; give oxygen
Tension pneumothorax	Complication of other types of pneumothorax; air enters pleural cavity but cannot escape	Respiratory distress; paradoxical chest movements; neck vein distention; tracheal deviation to unaffected side	Maintain airway and breathing; give oxygen (needle thoracotomy by trained person)
Hemothorax	Blunt and penetrating chest injuries; injuries to major blood vessels and heart; blood collects in pleural cavity	Decreased breath sounds; dyspnea (cyanosis and signs of shock if severe)	Treat for shock; give oxygen

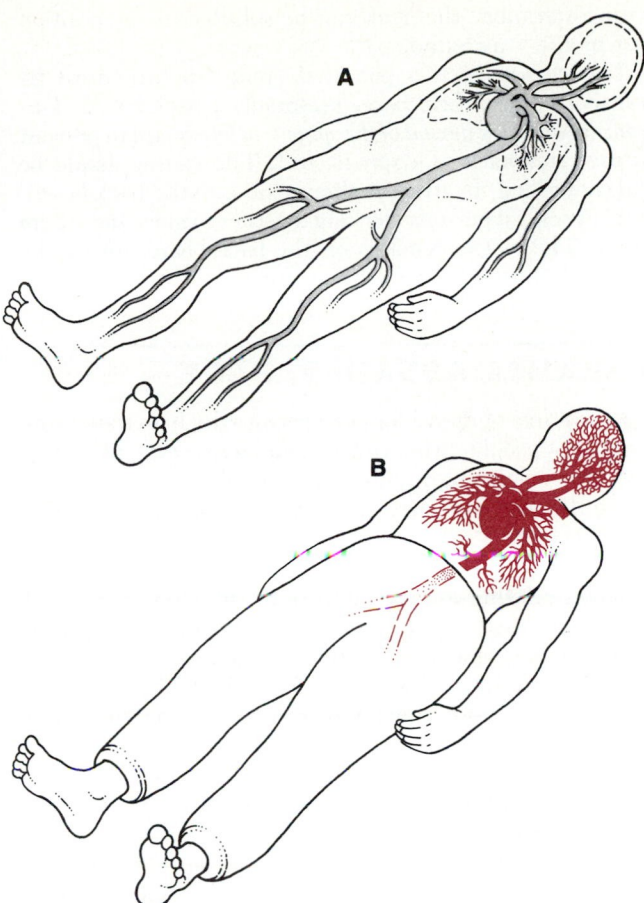

Fig. 41-4 In shock states, perfusion of vital organs is greatly enhanced by antishock trousers. **A,** Before application. **B,** After application. (From Budassi, S, and Barber, J: Emergency nursing: principles and practice, St. Louis, 1981, The CV Mosby Co.)

If there is an open wound evisceration may occur. If the abdominal organs are exposed to the air and become dry, necrosis can result. The abdominal organs lying outside the abdominal cavity should therefore be covered by a warm, moist, preferable sterile covering. If a sterile dressing is not available it is better to cover the organs with a clean moist cloth and risk infection than not to cover the organs and risk loss of tissue.

■ AMPUTATIONS

Traumatic amputations are treated as other wounds by controlling hemorrhage and applying pressure dressings. Severe bleeding does not always occur. The amount of bleeding is dependent on the extent of trauma that occurs; the greater the amount of trauma, such as the amputation of a limb by a crushing injury, the greater will be the amount of muscle spasm in the arterial walls. This causes the artery to contract, and bleeding is decreased. A limb or appendage that is severed cleanly by a sharp object such

as a knife will bleed more profusely. If a tourniquet is necessary it should be applied close to the site of the amputation to decrease potential injury to intervening tissue.

The amputated portion should be taken with the victim to the hospital because replantation is sometimes possible. The amputated part should be kept at about 5° C (40° F). It can be transported by placing the part in a dressing inside a plastic bag surrounded by ice. The part should not be placed against the ice. The amputated part should never be frozen, cleaned, disinfected, debrided, or perfused before transportation.

■ Fractures

Injury to the musculoskeletal system may result in fractures or dislocations of the bones, strained muscles, or torn ligaments (see Chapter 22 for a complete discussion of these injuries). Emergency care consists of assessment of injury and interventions to prevent further trauma until medical help is available.

■ ASSESSMENT

If pain is localized over a bone or joint it should be considered fractured until a definitive diagnosis is made. Obvious deformity can be either a dislocation (if at a joint) or a fracture. In a compound fracture the bone may protrude through the skin. The ability to move an extremity or digit does not negate a fracture, although the victim usually refrains from movement because of pain. Shock may occur with severe fractures, either from the stress of the trauma or from blood loss, such as the extravasation of blood in the thigh following injury.

Skull fractures may vary from a small linear fracture with few symptoms to severe depression of bone fragments into the brain. Basilar skull fractures may be accompanied by bleeding or draining serous fluid from the nose or ears or both. Fractures of facial bones may interfere with respiration if the air passages become blocked.

Pain or deformity at the *hip* can be caused by either a fracture or dislocation. The leg will be shortened in both instances but turned *outward* if there is a *fracture* and *inward* with a *dislocation*. Fractures of the extremities may be accompanied by loss of circulation or sensation if blood vessels or nerves are pinched by the bone fragment. Circulation distal to the fracture is assessed by observing skin color and presence of pulses. A neurologic check for sensation and circulatory system checks should be repeated after splinting and during transportation.

■ INTERVENTION

The general management of fractures is listed in the box on p. 1462.

□ Fracture of the spine

Any questionable injury to the head, neck, or back is treated as a fracture of the spine. The victim should not be moved when being examined for fracture of the spine

General management of fractures

1. Do not move patient before splinting a fracture (unless there is danger of fire, explosion, or radiation).
2. Cover open wound before splinting.
3. Support fractured bone and move it as little as possible while splinting.
4. Splint fracture in the position it is found.
5. In *severely angulated* fractures of the *shaft* of the extremity bone:
   a. Decrease muscle spasm and prevent damage to blood vessels by straightening severe angulation of bone shaft
   b. Place one hand just below fracture and other hand farther down extremity
   c. Apply gentle traction to straighten extremity
   d. Maintain traction until extremity is splinted
6. *Never* straighten deformities of a joint (shoulder, elbow, wrist, knee).
7. Apply splints to include joint above and below fracture.
8. Pad rigid splints (boards) for comfort.
9. Reinforce soft splints (pillows) with a rigid material such as a magazine or board.
10. If using air splint:
    a. Inflate only by mouth to a point where the thumb leaves a slight dent
    b. Keep fingers and toes free for assessment of circulation
11. Handle fractured part gently to prevent pain and shock.

(neck or back). The examiner slides a hand under the victim and checks for point tenderness along the length of the spine. Bruises on the head may indicate that a force has been exerted that could cause a neck fracture. Bruises on the shoulder, back, or abdomen are frequently seen with back fractures, but a spinal fracture can be present in the absence of any bruises. If the spinal cord has been damaged there may be loss of movement or sensation to the extremities.

Two problems can occur from a fractured spine: damage to the spinal cord and neurogenic shock. If the cervical spine is fractured there may be interference with respiration, and respirations must be continually monitored. The victim may use diaphragmatic breathing for a short period but be unable to sustain this. Artificial ventilation is more difficult in that the neck cannot be hyperextended because this can cause further injury to the spinal cord. The head can be extended by gentle traction and the jaw pulled forward to open the airway. Traction must be maintained until the neck can be supported in this position. *The neck should never be flexed, twisted, or hyperextended if a fracture is suspected.* If the victim is not having difficulty

with respiration, the neck can be splinted in the position in which it was found.

The person with a potential spine fracture must be transported on a firm base, preferably a back board. *Forward or backward flexion of the spine is to be avoided* to prevent further trauma to the spinal cord. The victim should be slid, not rolled, in straight alignment onto the back board. It takes several persons working together to move the victim safely. The victim remains on the back board during the initial diagnostic tests in the emergency room.

■ SEXUAL ASSAULT: RAPE

Rape is one of the violent crimes for which an increasing number of people, primarily women, are seeking help. Despite the increasing number of rapes reported, it is estimated that the incidence of unreported rape is from 200% to 300% higher.

It is difficult to obtain statistics concerning the sociologic variables relating to rape because of the large number of unreported cases. There are many misconceptions concerning rape; some *facts* include the following:

1. Rape occurs among persons of all social classes.
2. Rape is more commonly *reported* among the lower class.
3. Rape occurs mostly between persons of the same race.
4. A majority of rapes are committed by someone the victim knows.
5. Males, especially young boys, may also be rape victims; the attacker is usually another male.

Rape is a major problem in prisons in the United States. Some prison reform groups are actively addressing this problem, with the major emphasis on protecting the young and vulnerable from attack.

■ Rape crisis centers

Rape crisis centers are available in many large cities. These centers differ in their functions but usually provide one or more of the following:

1. Direct service to the rape victim
2. Service to professional agencies (health, law)
3. Community education

Service to health professionals and education of the community are efforts to help change the system for the rape victim.

The victim service consists of volunteers, many of whom have been raped themselves, who serve as victim advocates throughout the medical examination and police interview. Some form of follow-up service, such as counseling, may be available. Some rape crisis centers have volunteer attorneys who can offer the victim legal advice or representation.

■ Rape trauma syndrome

Rape is a traumatic event for the victim physically, psychologically, and socially. *Physical* force is often used; a weapon may be used either as a threat or to injure the victim, or the hands or fists may be used to beat the victim or threaten choking. Injury can also occur as the victim is attempting self-defense or is struggling on the ground or floor. The vagina and perineum may be injured by force used during the sexual attack, and the rectum may also be lacerated if anal sex has been attempted, more commonly in rape of males.

Psychologic trauma is usually severe; the rape victim is in a state of crisis. Fear is a dominant theme as the victim perceives the event as life threatening. Other feelings expressed by victims are depersonalization, shame degradation, defilement, violation, guilt, humiliation, and anger. The victim has not only been under threat of harm but has also been subjected in many instances to multiple sexual assaults, some natural, some perverted, by one or more persons. Fellatio (oral sex) is frequently demanded, and some rapists will urinate on the victim before leaving.

The person who has been raped goes through the same phases as any person facing a crisis situation. The initial phase is one of shock and disbelief. After the initial acute phase, there is a period of pseudoequilibrium when the victim rationalizes the event or attempts to suppress thoughts concerning the rape. Later there are periods of depression, phobic reactions, and nightmares.

The rape victim also experiences *sociologic* crisis. If the woman is married, marital relationships may be affected. If she is single she often fears repeated occurrences and may feel the need to move, especially if the attack occurred in her home or apartment. Decisions must be made concerning whom to tell about the incident, because loss of needed support of family and friends may occur. Job security or relationships with co-workers may be threatened. Sociologic problems take considerable time to resolve, but concerns related to these potential problems may occur in the initial emergency period.

■ Prevention and health care

All women need to know the measures they can take to help prevent rape from occurring (see the box at top, right). It would also be helpful if every woman learned methods of self-defense. Some communities introduce both issues of rape and self-defense into secondary school curricula. Many YWCAs teach classes in self-defense. Rape crisis centers can provide information on availability of classes in the community.

Persons who are raped may seek medical help directly or call the police, who will then take the victim for medical examination. Some victims fear reprisal by the rapist or are unwilling to let others know about the rape and therefore do not seek medical attention. Victims need to be encouraged to report the incident.

Many hospitals have developed protocols for care of the rape victim in the emergency department. If such a protocol does not exist, it behooves the nurses in the emergency department to work toward development of one. Rape crisis centers can be helpful in this regard. The protocol may include some of the following:

1. High priority in triage
2. Provision for privacy without leaving the victim alone

Rape preventive measures

Prevention of attack

Set house lights to go on and off by timer
Keep light on at all entrances
Place safety locks on windows and doors
Have key ready before reaching door of house or car
Look in car before entering
Insist on identification before letting a stranger in house; check identification with agency if suspicious
Do not list first name on mailbox or in telephone directory
Make arrangements with neighbor for needed assistance
Be alert when walking in street; walk in lighted areas
Walk down center of street if possible
Avoid lonely or enclosed areas

If attacked

Run toward a lighted house; yell, "Fire"
Spit in rapist's face; act bizarre; vomit
Rip off rapist's glasses
Step hard on his foot (instep)
Aim at eyes; try to gouge eyes, scrape face
Hit throat at Adam's apple (larynx)
Use fighting and screaming with caution; this may scare some rapists, encourage others
Try talking to avoid rape
Make close observations about rapist, car, location

---

3. Provision of a victim advocate (such as a woman from the rape crisis center)
4. Routines to ensure protection and comfort of the victim:
   a. Person(s) designated to have primary contact with the victim
   b. Authority of the primary contact person to make the decision of victim readiness for medical examination or police interview (if no life-threatening injury is present).

■ Assessment

■ SUBJECTIVE DATA

The victim will be asked many questions by the examiner to identify the type of assault and potential for injury. If the victim has been threatened she may have succumbed through fear, and this needs to be elicited. Victims often talk freely to the nurse about their feelings; their fears concerning injury, mutilation, or death at the time of assault; or present fears concerning pregnancy or sexually transmitted disease. Other feelings of degradation, feeling "dirty," shame, guilt, and so forth, may be expressed. Anger may be directed at the assailant or projected toward medical care personnel.

Data are collected related to pain or discomfort, either local at the site of assault or general and diffuse. The victim may complain of a sore throat if choking was used as a threat or after oral sex. Nausea may also be reported.

■ OBJECTIVE DATA

Objective behavioral signs are noted. Some women respond emotionally and cry, shake, laugh inappropriately, or are extremely restless. Other victims appear overtly calm and subdued, usually the impact of the experience hits them later.

A head-to-toe assessment for signs of physical trauma is usually carried out by the physician. The clothing will be inspected and described and is often requested by the police for evidence. Clothing should not be washed or discarded. Other data needed by the police usually include samples of the assailant's hair from combing of pubic hair and fingernail deposits for samples of the assailant's tissue.

■ TESTS

Papanicolaou smears of the vagina, mouth, or rectum and saline suspensions are done to test for the presence of sperm. An acid phosphatase test will demonstrate recency of intercourse. Tests will be inconclusive if the victim has bathed or douched since the rape. Tests for sexually transmitted disease are done at the initial visit to obtain baseline information for future comparison.

■ Intervention

■ EMOTIONAL SUPPORT

Most victims need to talk to someone who cares about what is happening to them and who is nonjudgmental. The nurse uses crisis intervention theory to decide how best to help the victim (see Chapter 7). Many hospitals have contacts with the rape crisis center, and the victim is given the choice of having a victim advocate from the center to be with her during the entire examination period, both medical and legal. Medical examinations or interviews by the police are not begun until the volunteer arrives.

Preparation for the physical examination is carried out in advance. Having a pelvic examination after a sexual assault can be a traumatic experience especially if the victim has never had a pelvic examination.

■ SEXUALITY

The victim has many concerns related to her sexuality. Time is needed to work through these concerns, and long-term counseling is helpful to many victims.

Concern about possible *pregnancy* depends on the circumstances: whether she is in the childbearing years, whether birth control is in effect at the time of sexual assault, and at what point in the menstrual period the rape occurs. If pregnancy is a possibility, contraceptive therapy is initiated immediately.

Concern about *sexually transmitted diseases* (STD) is common. Penicillin is given intramuscularly and probenecid is given orally as a preventive measure for STD after the initial examination. The person needs to know that medical follow-up is important and that she should be retested for STD in about 3 weeks unless symptoms occur before then. In addition, the woman may experience vaginal discharge, itching, and a burning sensation caused by an acute vaginal infection (vaginitis).

■ HOME DISCHARGE PLANS

The victim should not go home to an empty house or apartment. The volunteer from the rape crisis center, the social worker, or police can all facilitate arrangements for transportation to her home or to the home of family or friends. Frequently the victim goes to the police station after medical care is completed to follow up with the police report. The victim needs to know about the availability of follow-up medical services and counseling services. Some medical centers have psychiatrists who are especially interested in counseling rape victims.

■ DISASTERS

Disasters are sudden catastrophic events that disrupt patterns of life and in which there is possible loss of life and property in addition to multiple injuries. Disasters can be either natural phenomena or caused by people (see the box below).

Causes of disasters

Natural	**Man-made**
Air	*Transportation*
Tornado	Air
Hurricane	Land
Blizzard	Water
Land	*Fire*
Earthquake	Housing
Volcanic eruption	Forest
Avalanches	Explosion
Cave-in	
	Disease
Water	Epidemic
Floods: slow rising	
and flash floods	*Civil*
Tidal wave	Riot
	War (nuclear attack)

Table 41-10   Types of disasters

Type	Number of people	Cause
Multiple patients	<10	Multiple-vehicle accident, bus accident, bomb, explosion, fire
Multiple casualty	10 to 100	Airplane crash, riot, tornado, hurricane, minor earthquake
Mass casualty	>100	Severe hurricane, major earthquake, war bombing

■ Effect of disasters

The effects of disasters are multiple. People are killed or injured and separated from their families. Many become homeless. In mass casualty disasters (Table 41-10) confusion and chaos occur during the early stages. Panic rarely occurs, but when it does it is because the involved persons believe that escape routes are limited and may be closing off. Effective leadership and communication can usually prevent panic.

Transportation difficulties are created as streets and roads become clogged by persons trying to get away from the impact area or others trying to get in. Food and water supplies can become contaminated or nonexistent. Medical supplies may be inadequate to meet the sudden increased need. Utilities can become disrupted. Law enforcement is necessary to prevent looting and other civil disorders. Establishment of a communication system takes first priority to prevent chaos.

■ Roles of nurses in disasters

The actual role assumed by a given nurse at a disaster will depend on the abilities of the nurse and the specific situation. Nurses can participate in many ways. A nurse may be in a position of being the only health care provider in a given area and be responsible for giving initial first aid treatment or supervising the activities of others. Because of their education and experience, professional nurses can be especially helpful in aiding victims to cope with their emotional reactions to the disaster. Nurses may also be asked to serve at emergency morgues for support of families experiencing the loss of loved ones.

The American Red Cross, which assumes an active role during disasters along with governmental agencies, operates shelters for victims. They provide supplies and food as well as service personnel (shelter manager, nurses, physicians, food helpers). Nurses interested in serving during disasters at home or in other parts of the country may contact the local American Red Cross office. Other services provided by the American Red Cross include emergency services on an individual family basis and aid for recovery.

■ Prevention

Preparedness for disasters includes community planning to identify and, if possible, prevent disasters, and education of the public to minimize the number of casualties.

Community groups involved in disaster planning

Governmental	Political, law enforcement, fire department
Health	Hospitals, physicians, nurses, pharmacists, social workers
Official	American Red Cross
Nonofficial	Telephone company, parent-teacher organization, religious organization

---

■ COMMUNITY PLANNING

Most states have disaster service agencies, which are outgrowths of civil defense organizations. These agencies act as coordinating units for the local agencies. Every community should have a disaster planning group as part of the local emergency medical committee. There should be representation by all groups who will be active participants if a disaster occurs (see the box above). The disaster planning committee has the following functions and responsibilities:

1. Identifying the types of disasters that may occur in the local community
2. Organizing a disaster plan to be followed for different situations
3. Arranging for simulated drills to test the effectiveness of plans
4. Determining need for education or updating of necessary skills of participants

Nurses need to be active participants in the planning, implementation, and evaluation phases of community disaster preparedness.

During a disaster local hospitals become actively involved and need their own disaster plan to cope with the sudden influx of persons needing emergency care. Any time a large number of injured persons are in need of emergency care, hospital disaster plans are put into effect. Testing of hospital disaster plans at specified intervals by simulated drills is necessary for determining whether the plans are effective and what changes, if any, are needed.

■ PUBLIC EDUCATION

Public awareness of potential community disasters is needed for effective community preparedness. Disaster planning committees need support and participation of community members. Individuals need to know what they should do in the event of a disaster. Most radio and television stations regularly notify communities of potential disasters, give directions for preventive actions, and give methods of obtaining further information should the disaster occur. Because electricity may be cut off, battery-operated radios should be available in all homes for continued communication.

All homes should have an emergency food cabinet with sufficient nonperishable foods to meet nutritional needs for several days. Supplies are rotated with current supplies to prevent food from spoiling or becoming outdated.

■ Assessment

■ TRIAGE

There are essentially two different approaches to triage during a disaster. The *military* triage system, which may be initiated during a mass casualty disaster, is based on the philosophy of doing "the best for the most with the least by the fewest." Victims with injuries of such a magnitude that there is question of survival are given low priority for transportation. In this system the numbers of critically injured must greatly outnumber the health and transportation personnel available. Victims are reclassified as the emergency situation changes. Priority is then given to those victims with the greatest chance of survival.

The more commonly used *civilian* triage system is used with multiple patients or multiple casualties. Several victim-sorting methods can be used for triage, but essentially all methods give top priority to life-threatening injuries and low priority to minimal injuries (see the box below)

■ DISASTER SYNDROME

The behavior of victims after the impact of disaster can be characterized as progressing through phases of shock, awareness, euphoria, and anger. The victims are experiencing loss; therefore the phases are similar to those experienced by others during any kind of loss (grieving).

The *shock phase* may last only a few minutes or up to several hours after impact. The victim is dazed, unable to comprehend what is occurring, and cannot follow even simple directions. Persons prepared to function in emergencies are less apt to spend much time in the shock phase.

The *awareness phase* may last up to several days. Victims become aware of survival and try to help others, minimizing their own injuries or losses. During this stage guilt feelings may arise because others died and they survived. The victim is highly suggestible, can follow simple directions, but cannot carry out problem solving effectively.

The *euphoria phase* may last for several weeks. The victim feels a sense of brotherhood with the community and participates willingly in helping others with plans for recovery.

Before resolution, the victim may go through the "Why me?" or *anger phase* that occurs because of the experienced loss. The anger is often projected against helping persons who were not personally affected by the disaster. It is especially important for nurses who may be assisting victims during the recovery phase to understand that the anger is part of the loss experience. As the victim copes with the losses incurred by the disaster and life returns to more normal patterns, the anger will disappear.

Four-color coded triage system

0—Black: Dead

1—Red: Critical or life-threatening

These victims have a reasonable chance of survival only if they receive immediate treatment. Emergency treatment is initiated immediately and continued during transportation. This category includes victims with respiratory insufficiency, cardiac arrest, hemorrhage, and severe abdominal injury.

2—Yellow: Serious

These victims can wait for transportation after they receive initial emergency treatment. They include victims with immobilized closed fractures, soft-tissues injuries without hemorrhage, and burns on less than 40% of the body.

3—Green: Minimal

Victims in this category are ambulatory, have minor tissue injuries, and may be dazed. They can be treated by nonprofessionals and held for observation if necessary.

From Baker, FJ: Topics Emerg Med 1:49-157, 1979.

■ Intervention

■ EMERGENCY AID STATIONS

The number, size, and staffing of emergency aid stations depend on the type and extent of the disaster. One person in each aid station is designated for triage. One person must be designated the leader and is responsible for making decisions for maximal effectiveness of the unit. In the absence of a physician, a nurse assumes leadership of emergency care.

The types of injuries that occur will depend on the type of disaster. Common injuries and conditions requiring care include soft-tissue and bone injuries, respiratory insufficiency, cardiac arrest, and childbirth.

Victims are not transported until first aid care has been given, as in any emergency. If hemorrhage has not been controlled or fractures splinted, the victim may arrive at the medical center in shock that could have been prevented or minimized; surgical intervention will not take place until measures to treat shock are instituted and the patient's condition is stable. If first aid measures are instituted before transportation, the victim can be taken to surgery at the earliest opportunity. Records indicating all treatment given at an emergency aid center *must* accompany a victim who is referred or transported to a medical center or any other health care facility.

■ SHELTERS

Most shelters are set up in schools, which can house a large number of people. The role of the nurse in a shelter is to assess and provide for health needs of the shelter population. Some nursing functions include the following:

1. Isolating persons with suspected infectious diseases
2. Identifying persons with chronic illnesses and ascertaining whether prescribed drugs are available
3. Monitoring shelter occupants for signs of developing health problems
4. Identifying persons having problems coping with the disaster and providing emotional support and guidance as necessary
5. Making arrangements for care of pregnant women and infants
6. Assisting with necessary immunizations

Assessment of safety factors in the environment is also a nursing responsibility. The nurse is part of the shelter team and advises the shelter manager of any potential health hazards. The care of victims in a disaster is a team effort, and the nurse is an important member of this team.

■ ADAPTATION TO LOSS

Adaptation to loss after large-scale community disasters may differ from adaptation to losses under normal life situations because of the *lack of individual support* systems as a result of (1) death of usual support persons or (2) inability of usual support persons to provide help because of their own personal losses. There may also be a *loss of community support* systems resulting from the disaster.

Immediately following a disaster there is usually an immediate outpouring of material assistance and personnel services from people outside the community. This support diminishes with the passing of time, and the victims are often faced with having to work through their grief with less support than usual and sometimes with visual environmental reminders of loss. It is important that long-term counseling services be made available in these situations to people of all ages. Group therapy can be a useful method of providing support by helping the victim realize that he or she is not alone and that others understand what the victim is experiencing. Group therapy also aids in problem solving through group efforts.

■ SUMMARY

1. Accidents are the leading cause of death in persons less than 45 years of age and the third leading cause in those 45 to 65 years of age.
2. Accident prevention includes monitoring the home for hazards, equipping homes with smoke alarms, participating in fire drills, and using care while driving.
3. The difference between EMTs and paramedics is that the latter are prepared to carry out invasive procedures, such as starting IVs, defibrillation, and intubation.
4. Persons are not judged as liable unless they act willfully and with gross negligence. Reasonable care is judged on the basis of care given by someone with similar training and under the prevailing situation.
5. The parameters of priority assessment of the injured person are the ABCs (airway, breathing, circulation) and level of consciousness.
6. After the priority assessment, a head-to-toe assessment is made for signs of injury.
7. Shock usually develops in persons who sustain major trauma or a major stressor to the system.
8. Loss of consciousness following a period of alertness after a head injury may indicate an intracranial hematoma that requires immediate medical attention.
9. The sequence for providing care of an injured person is first the priority assessment with immediate lifesaving measures, followed by the head-to-toe assessment before carrying out general first-aid measures.
10. Keep an injured person lying down and protected from cold (but not heated); the person is not transported until all first aid measures have been carried out.
11. Asphyxia is indicated by dyspnea, adventitious sounds, use of accessory respiratory muscles, skin pallor, or eventually cyanosis.
12. Remove foreign bodies from the airway with the Heimlich maneuver if the person is unable to cough up object.
13. The sequence of CPR is to assess the level of consciousness, open the airway, initiate artificial ventilation, assess circulation, and initiate external cardiac compressions.
14. The precordial thump is only given for monitored pa-

Putting knowledge to practice

■ What is the most common cause of accidents in your community as noted in your newspapers?
■ What are some precautions taken in your hospital unit to prevent patient accidents? Are there any additional measures that could be taken?
■ What actions are taken in your hospital for the reporting of accidents within the hospital? What measures are taken to prevent further similar accidents?
■ Draw a diagram of your hospital unit, noting the location of exits, placement of fire extinguishers, and fire doors.
■ How are the personnel in your hospital alerted that a fire has occurred?
■ What precautions could you take in your life to avoid rape?
■ Examine the disaster plan for your hospital. As a nursing student, what actions should you take if the disaster plan were instituted? What actions would be expected if you were a staff nurse on your unit?

---

tients at the onset of ventricular tachycardia or asystole from heart block.

15. The person with a suspected myocardial infarction who is breathing should be placed in a comfortable, well-supported sitting position, given oxygen (if available), be cared for with a calm approach to minimize anxiety, and be transported to a hospital immediately.

15. Drowning may be caused by asphyxiation from the aspiration of fluid into the lungs or from laryngospasm that prevents both air and water from entering the lungs. Persons who have experienced near-drowning should be monitored closely for latent pulmonary edema for at least 24 hours.

16. The best method for stopping external bleeding is to place direct pressure on the bleeding vessel; tourniquets are used only for massive arterial bleeding that cannot be controlled by other means.

17. If poisoning is suspected in an unconscious person, the person should be transported immediately to the nearest medical facility.

18. For ingestion of noncaustic substances, give the conscious person syrup of ipecac followed by 1 or 2 glasses of water; if drugs have been ingested, follow the water with activated charcoal.

19. Heat exhaustion is a shocklike reaction to heat; place the person recumbent in a cool environment and provide salty fluids. Heat stroke results from inability to lose heat by perspiration; the skin is hot and dry and unconsciousness may occur. Heat stroke is more serious and requires immediate medical care.

20. Applying too much heat to persons overexposed to cold may lead to skin injury from the decreased circulation and hypovolemic shock from vasodilation.

21. The skin, gastrointestinal mucosa, and blood cells are the most sensitive tissues to radiation.

22. Pneumothorax may result from open chest wounds; a nonporous dressing is required to prevent air from entering the chest.

23. Suspected fractures must be splinted before the person is moved; severely angulated fractures of the shaft of

a long bone may be straightened by traction to prevent severe muscle spasms; deformities of a joint are *never* straightened.

24. Persons with a potential spine fracture are transported on a firm base avoiding spine flexion.

25. Persons who are raped experience physical, psychologic, and sociologic trauma.

26. Nurses participate during disasters by providing triage and first aid at emergency aid stations and hospitals, by providing health care at shelters, and by providing emotional support to persons at emergency morgues.

27. Victims of disasters experience grief and mourning reactions; long-term adaptation may be hampered by lack of usual support systems.

REFERENCES AND SELECTED READINGS*
Contemporary

1. American College of Surgeons, Committee on Trauma: Early care of the injured patient, ed 3, Philadelphia, 1982, WB Saunders Co.
2. *Bacot, EL, Jr: Community planning for disasters, Occup Health Nurs 32:310-311, 1984.
3. *Bailey, N: Emergency! First aid for factures, Nurs 82 12(11):72-81, 1982.
4. Bangs, CC: Hypothermia and frostbite, Emerg Med Clin North Am 2:563-577, 1984.
5. *Blauer, RE: Dealing with drownings: you can help keep the near-drowning victim alive, RN 48(5):41-42, 1985.
6. *Boyd, LT, Shurett, PH, and Coburn, C: Heat and heat-related illnesses, Am J Nurs 81:1298-1302, 1981.
7. *Bucanan, L: Emergency! First aid for spinal cord injury, Nurs 82 12(8):68-75, 1982.
8. Budassi, SA, and Barber, JM: Emergency nursing: principles and practice, ed 2, St. Louis, 1984, The CV Mosby Co.
9. *Burgess, AW: Rape trauma syndrome: a nursing diagnosis, Occup Health Nurs 33:405-406, 1985.

---

*References preceded by an asterisk are particularly well suited for student reading.

10. *Buschiazzo, L: What's new in CPR: Nurs 86 16(1):34-37, 1986.

11. Cain, HD: Flint's emergency treatment and management, ed 7, Philadelphia, 1985, WB Saunders Co.

12. Cosgriff, JG, Jr, and Anderson, D: The practice of emergency nursing, ed 2, Philadelphia, 1984, JB Lippincott Co.

13. *DeLapp, TD: Accidental hypothermia, Am J Nurs 83:62-67, 1983.

14. *DeLapp, TD: Taking the bite out of frostbite and other cold weather injuries, Am J Nurs 80:56-60, 1980.

15. DiNitto, D, and others: After rape: who should examine rape survivors, Am J Nurs 86:538-540, 1986.

16. Foley, T, Davies, M: Rape: nursing care of victims, St. Louis, 1983, The CV Mosby Co.

17. *Fritz, CP: Emergency! First aid for wounds, Nurs 82 12(10):68-75, 1982.

18. Garcia, LM: Disaster nursing: planning, assessment, and intervention, Rockville, Md, 1985, Aspen Systems, Inc.

19. *Gaston, SF, and Schumann, LL: Inhalation injury, smoke inhalation, Am J Nurs 80:94-97, 1980.

20. *Gray-Vickrey, MN: Education to prevent falls, Geriatr Nurs 5:179-183, 1984.

21. Henry, J, and Volans, G: ABC of poisoning: diagnosis, Br Med J 289:172-174, 1984.

22. Jacobs, LM, and Berrizbeitia, LD: Prehospital trauma care, Emerg Med Clin North Am 2:717-732, 1984.

23. *Jamison, DW: When emergency care is up to you, RN 50(4):26-31, 1987.

24. *Jankowski, CB: Radiation emergency, Am J Nurs 82:90-95, 1982.

25. *Johnson, LM: Giving a CPR form new life, Am J Nurs 86:60-61, 1986.

26. *Jones, MK: Fire! Am J Nurs 84:1368-1371, 1984.

27. Kaye, D, and Rose, LF: Fundamentals of internal medicine, St. Louis, 1983, The CV Mosby Co.

28. *King, RC: Dealing with poisonings, RN 47(12):48-48, 1984.

29. Krupp, MA, Schroeder, SA, and Tierney, LM: Current medical diagnosis and treatment 1987, Norwalk, Conn, 1987, Appleton & Lange.

30. *LaVoy, K: Dealing with hypothermia and frostbite, RN 48(1):53-56, 1985.

31. *Lee, G: Transport of the critically ill trauma patient, Nurs Clin North Am 21(4):741-749, 1986.

32. *Lenehan, GP: Emotional impact of trauma, Nurs Clin North Am 21(4):729-740, 1986.

33. *Maher, AB: Early assessment and management of musculoskeletal injuries, Nurs Clin North Am 21(4):717-727, 1986.

34. Martin, TG: Near-drowning and cold water immersion, Ann Emerg Med 13:263-273, 1984.

35. *Matheney, LL: Emergency! First aid for cardiopulmonary arrest, Nurs 82 12(6):34-45, 1982.

36. Matz, R: Hypothermia: mechanisms and countermeasures, Hosp Pract 21(2):45-48, 1986.

37. McGuigan, MA: Treatment of poisoning, Clin Symp 36(5):3-32, 1984.

38. *Moser, MY: When lightning strikes, Am J Nurs 86:802-803, 1986.

39. Newton, M, and other: General treatment of household poisoning, JEN 13(1):12-15, 1987.

40. Nicholson, DP: The immediate management of overdose, Med Clin North Am 67(6):1279-1291, 1983.

41. *Niggerman, EH: Near-drowning, Nurs 83 13(7):45, 1983.

42. *Nikas, DL: Resuscitation of patients with CNS trauma, Nurs Clin North Am 21(4):729-740, 1986.

43. Parker, JG: Emergency nursing: a guide to comprehensive care, New York, 1984, John Wiley & Sons, Inc.

44. *Parker, JG: Thoracic trauma: nursing assessment and management, Nurs Clin North Am 21(4):685-692, 1986.

45. *Rich, J: How to keep venom from endangering a victim's life and limb, Nurs 87 17(6):33, 1987.

46. *Rich, W, and Perchenbeger, M: Managing flail chest: a matter of maintaining breath and life, Nurs 81 11(12):26-31, 1981.

47. *Roderick, MA: Tetanus, Nurs 82 12(7):63, 1982.

48. *Scherer, P: ACLS guidelines: what nurses are saying about the drug changes, Am J Nurs 86:1352-1358, 1986.

49. *Shea, KG: Natural disaster: personal preparedness, AORN J 43:1226-1238, 1986.

50. Sheehy, SB, and Barber, J: Emergency nursing: principles and practice, ed 2, St. Louis, 1985, The CV Mosby Co.

50a. Sheehy, SA, Marvin JA, and Jimmerson, CL: Clinical trauma nursing: the first hour, St. Louis, 1988, The CV Mosby Co.

51. Skeet, M: Emergency procedures and first aid for nurses, St. Louis, 1981, The CV Mosby Co.

52. Standards and guidelines for cardiopulmonary resuscitation (CPR) and emergency cardiac care (ECC), JAMA 255:2905-2988, 1986.

53. *Sumner, SM, and Grau, PE: Emergency! first aid for choking, Nurs 82 12(7):40-49, 1982.

54. *Sumner, SM, and others: An update on BCLS standards, Nurs 86 16(11):48-49, 1986.

55. *Thompson, NA: Convert your assessment into a lifesaving care plan for the patient with abdominal trauma, Nurs 83 13(7):26-33, 1983.

55a. *Walz, JA: A simulated disaster drill, Am J Nurs 88:301-303, 1988.

56. Warner, C, editor: Emergency care: assessment and intervention, ed 3, St. Louis, 1982, The CV Mosby Co.

57. Way, LW: Current surgical diagnosis and treatment, ed 6, Los Altos, CA, 1983, Lange Medical Publications.

58. Welsh, MD: Acute radiation syndrome, DDDN 5(5):277-286, 1986.

42

Care of the Patient in a Critical Care Unit

MAURA HOPKINS

CHAPTER OBJECTIVES

After studying this chapter, the student should be able to:

- Describe the physical and psychologic environment of critical care units.

- Identify the types of data needed for the care of critically ill patients.

- Describe interventions to alleviate physiologic stressors (respiratory, cardiovascular, neurologic, renal, gastrointestinal, musculoskeletal/integumentary) which are specific to the critical care setting.

- Describe interventions to alleviate and prevent psychologic stressors for both the patient and the nurse.

When "respirator centers" were developed in isolated locations nationally to combat the polio epidemic of the 1950s, the expectation was that the concentration of highly skilled personnel along with sophisticated medical equipment would positively influence the victims' survival. In addition to providing treatment these centers were dedicated to research, education, and training. They were, perhaps, the earliest form of the modern day intensive care unit (ICU).

Through the evolution of the coronary intensive care unit of the 1960s to the current nationwide availability of single- and multipurpose critical care units the role of the nurse in the care of the critically ill patient has remained the focal point of the success of these units. With vigilant observation of the patient's ever-changing condition, the critical care nurse is uniquely able to identify and initiate appropriate therapies, maintain complex treatment regimens, and intervene to prevent life-threatening situations.

In the 1990s nurses will find themselves working in a wide array of adult and pediatric critical care environments. These may be multipurpose ICUs or units specially designated for patients with a common type of problem, such as medical, surgical, coronary, cardiovascular, neurologic/neurosurgical, pulmonary, renal transplant, neonatal, burn, and shock/trauma units. In all cases the goal of critical care nursing remains the same: to provide continuous, optimal nursing care to patients in life-threatening situations, remaining alert to the physiologic, psychologic, and social needs of the patient as an integrated being.

This chapter provides an overview of some of the common aspects of critical care nursing and the critical care environment. Effects of the critical care environment on patient, family, and staff are described. Assessment of the critically ill patient is followed by interventions designed to alleviate physical, psychologic, and social stressors experienced by critically ill patients.

The reader is referred to other sections of this text and to the chapter references for a more thorough discussion of the physiologic processes, nursing interventions, and techniques of caring for critically ill patients.

■ ENVIRONMENT IN THE CRITICAL CARE AREA

■ Physical environment

The critical care unit is designed, equipped, and staffed to meet the anticipated needs of patients in life-threatening situations. The physical layout is frequently a modified circular design around a central nurses' station, allowing for direct visualization of all patients at all times. Patients may be separated in individual cubicles or be situated in a large open area with curtains as partitions. The advantage of direct nurse-patient visualization may accompany the disadvantages of limited patient privacy and patient exposure to frequent crisis intervention.

Supplies and equipment in critical care areas are highly sophisticated and must be readily accessible for all patients

---

Equipment and resources commonly available within or near the ICU

Monitors

Cardiac
Hemodynamic (intraarterial, pulmonary artery, central venous)
Intracranial pressure
External arterial pressure
Respiratory/apnea
Oxygen saturation
Body temperature

General equipment

ECG machine
Defibrillator
Intubation equipment
Emergency medications
Oxygen therapy equipment
Arterial blood gas analyzer
Hyper-hypothermia machine
Fluoroscopy
Doppler flow detection device
Bed scale

Bedside equipment

Bed with removable headboard
Oxygen and manual ventilation device
Suction device
Intravenous infusion device

Support services

Pharmacy
Laboratory
Respiratory therapy
Radiology, including CAT, MRI, EEG
Dialysis
Chaplain
Social worker
Psychologist

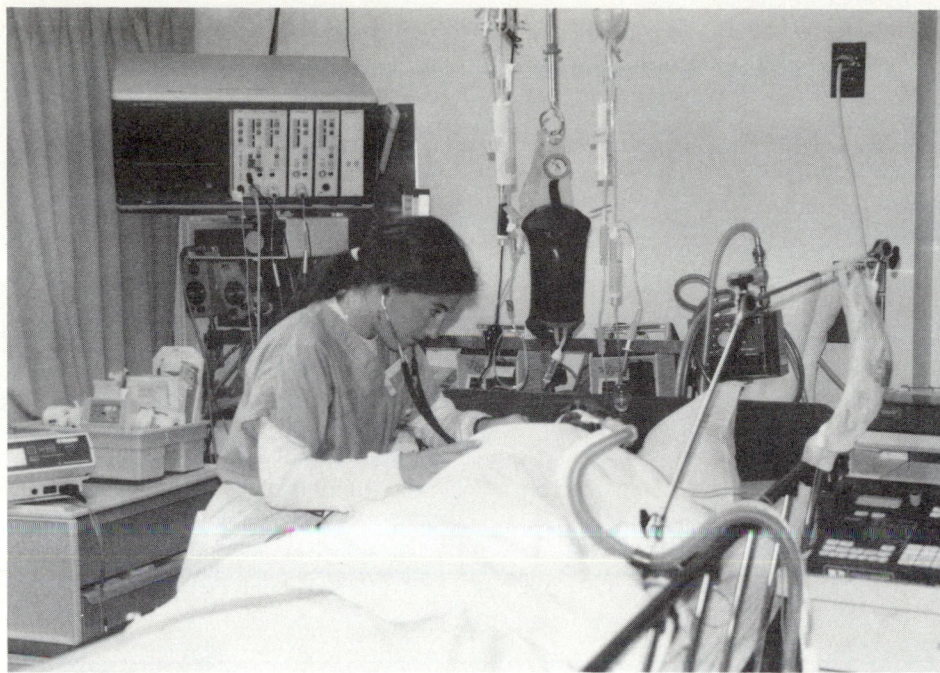

Fig. 42-1   Typical ICU unit.

(see the box on p. 1472) (Fig. 42-1). Certain pieces of equipment are in constant use at each bedside (for example, cardiac monitor, oxygen, suction equipment), and others must be available within seconds (defibrillator, ventilator, ECG machine, emergency medications). Existing hospital space has often been converted to ICU use, and as the need for more specialized and sophisticated ICU equipment grows the critical care environment often becomes overcrowded.

■ Psychologic environment: stress on patient and staff

In the critical care environment advanced forms of technology and medical and nursing therapeutics are used with patients in extended crisis. Although aware of the special nature of this care, the patient and family focus on its appearance: flashing lights; buzzing machines; painful procedures; a noisy, brightly lit, crowded, hyperactive environment permeated by vague fears. The stressors on the patient and family are immense, heightened by those very treatment modalities that may prove lifesaving.

The stress on nursing staff in the critical care area stems in part from very high expectations: advanced knowledge of physiology related to all body systems, astute observational and physical assessment skills, and the technical ability to operate the highly sophisticated equipment. Critical care nurses must have excellent communication skills to deal with the patient's and the family's psychologic and social needs, continually incorporating interventions that the nurse might be tempted to assign a low priority in a critical situation.

Both the patient and the nurse are bombarded by continuous stressors in the critical care environment (see the box on p. 1474). Low-level stress can be challenging and stimulating and may help to enhance creativity, production, and performance in any area. Continuous high-level stress can be devastating, both physically and psychologically. The patient's physiologic response to stress includes neural and hormonal activation that can cause stimulation of target organs (heart, blood vessels, GI tract) already compromised by illness or injury. (Review Chapter 7 on concepts of stress and adaptation for an indepth analysis of the effects of stress.) It is equally important for critical care nurses to understand how stress psychologically affects both the patient and family and to recognize that interactions will have to be modified to take this into account. In addition, nurses must be aware of their own stressors and the positive and negative effects of these stressors. They must safeguard their own physical and psychologic health and recognize how insufficient or ineffective coping mechanisms can lead to burnout.

Ethical considerations are taking an increasingly more prominent role in the day-to-day nursing care of critically ill patients. Nurses, as patient advocates, find themselves struggling to integrate their own sense of moral justice with those of the patient, family, medical staff, and others. The lack of "do not resuscitate" orders and the compulsion to aggressively treat patients with no chance of survival can cause nurses to question their role as independent professionals. Hospital ethics committees have fostered safe forums for discussion of differing viewpoints, and legal precedent is very slowly beginning to support the primacy of the patient's wishes.

Stressors on patients, families, and staff in the ICU

Patient/family

Unfamiliar environment, new faces
Noise, light levels
Interruption of sleep/wake cycles
Sensory deprivation/overload
Inaccessibility of family, friends
Lack of privacy
Lack of information/understanding of prognosis, care plan
Lack of information/understanding of policies, procedures
Anticipation of painful interventions
Confusion/disorientation related to physiologic factors
Impaired communication related to intubation
Observation of crisis intervention in other patients
Fear related to diagnosis
Fear of death

Staff

Expectations of self
Expectations of peers, supervisors
Intricate machinery and techniques
Closed, crowded work area
Constant contact with seriously ill, dying persons
Continual vigilance of multiple patients
Need for constant emergency readiness
Sustained high activity level
Limited breaks away from the high-stress unit
Limited communication with many patients related to intubation or altered level of consciousness
Limited opportunity to communicate with some families
Isolation from other nurses in the hospital
Ethical conflicts related to issues of resuscitation and use of life-maintenance equipment

---

The critical care unit is a powerful milieu that must be well understood by nurses who wish to take advantage of its environment to deliver truly comprehensive, patient-centered nursing care.

■ ASSESSMENT OF THE CRITICALLY ILL PATIENT

The nursing process is the same in critical care situations as in any other patient care setting. Management of critically ill patients requires establishing a data base, identifying real and potential problems, delineating priorities, defining outcome criteria, determining goals for intervention, executing the planned intervention, and modifying future goals and plans based on outcomes. Management of critically ill patients differs from management of other patients because of an ever-changing data base, a larger number of complex, interrelated problems, frequent reordering of priorities, and time limitations imposed by the rapidly changing condition of the patient.

The assessment process for the critically ill patient differs from the assessment of other patients only in terms of the number of supportive devices available to assist in data collection. The cardiac monitor, hemodynamic monitoring lines, and laboratory analyses provide data that must be incorporated into the total patient assessment. They are adjuncts to the direct observational data that the nurse gathers through careful history taking and physical examination. Monitored data is a useless string of unrelated facts and numbers until correlated to physical findings and integrated into a meaningful analysis by the critical care nurse.

■ Nursing history

There are three main sources from which critically ill patients come to an intensive care unit: direct admission, transfer from another patient care division in the same or a different hospital, and postoperatively after certain operations. The patient admitted directly to the ICU (for example, in the case of a myocardial infarction) will often be accompanied by family or friends. Both the patient and family members are useful in obtaining a thorough and accurate history of the current illness, past illnesses/hospitalizations, and a patient profile containing social information and usual coping strategies. Although at the time of admission emphasis is on alleviating physiologic threats to survival, one member of the health team may take the opportunity to concurrently interview family members so that crucial facts about the patient's history can immediately be used in patient care. Even in the critical care setting, accurate and thorough history taking is vital to intelligent, individualized care planning and intervention.

When the patient is received in transfer from another nursing division, either directly or after surgery, consultation between the transferring and receiving nursing staff is essential. The ICU nurses will benefit from the care plan developed by nurses who have had the opportunity to interact with the patient and family in a noncritical situation. Pertinent history, patient likes and dislikes, coping mechanisms, and family relations can all be relayed to the receiving nurses, enabling them to reduce the initial stress of the unfamiliar ICU environment. It is imperative that this type of pertinent history and care planning be shared among nurse colleagues to facilitate the patient's eventual recovery.

■ Physical examination

As with the assessment of any patient, history taking is followed by physical examination. The basic skills of inspection, palpation, percussion, and auscultation are used to elicit directly observed data from the patient. As in any other setting, explanations are given and patient cooperation is sought, even if the patient's comprehension of all that is said is questionable. (Refer to Chapter 3 on health assessment and to a physical assessment textbook for a thorough explanation on the use of these techniques.)

■ Monitored data

Nurses in all clinical settings use tools for isolated data collection from patients, for example, stethoscopes, sphygmomanometers, thermometers, and scales. Critical care nurses have the advantage of being able to use additional tools for continuous data collection, for example, cardiac monitors, hemodynamic pressure lines, and intracranial pressure monitoring devices. The explosion in critical care technology in the 1970s and 1980s is giving the critical care nurse amazing quantities of objective data with minimal time spent in system operation. Computerized monitoring systems are available that occupy less space and provide more capabilities than ever before. The most sophisticated of the "patient data management" systems take information from all the continuously monitored parameters (ECG, arrhythmias, pulmonary artery pressure, intraarterial pressure, central venous pressure, intracranial pressure, respiration and body temperature) and combine it with manually entered data such as body weight, height, intake and output, and times of drug administration, and prepare a wide array of hemodynamic calculations and patient response trends for analysis by critical care practitioners. Certain types of continuous monitoring devices are in widespread use in nearly all critical care environments.

■ CARDIAC MONITORING

Cardiac monitoring involves placement on the patient's chest of conductive electrodes that recognize the electrical activity of the heart and relay it to a video display screen. Before electrode placement the skin should be cleansed to remove debris and oils, then very lightly abraded to provide the best contact with the electrode. If necessary excessive hair is clipped. Pre-gelled electrodes are applied to the skin in standard three and five lead configurations depending on the leads to be monitored (Chapter 25). The electrodes are connected to the lead wires, then attached to a monitoring cable that is plugged into the bedside monitor. Both the actual appearance of the patient's ECG and the numeric representation of the heart rate are displayed on the monitor. Alarm limits are programmed by the nurse so that if the patient's heart rate rises above or falls below a safe range a tone sounds to alert the nurse.

In monitoring systems with computerized arrhythmia analysis the monitor also recognizes specific rhythm abnormalities such as single or paired premature ventricular contractions, bigeminal rhythms, runs of ventricular tachycardia, ventricular fibrillation, or asystole. Variations in the audio or visual display of the alarm can alert the nurse to the relative seriousness of the arrhythmia, even from a distance. Cardiac monitoring is a noninvasive procedure. With careful skin preparation, electrode placement, and daily inspection, the potential complication of electrode dermatitis can be prevented.

■ HEMODYNAMIC MONITORING

Hemodynamic monitoring refers to invasive monitoring of the arterial or vascular system via a continuous electronic monitoring device. Table 42-1 lists the normal values of pressures found in the cardiovascular system, many of which are measured via bedside monitoring.

□ Intraarterial monitoring

Intraarterial monitoring involves placement of a catheter into an artery, usually the radial or femoral artery. The catheter is connected to a high-pressure flush system normally filled with heparinized saline solution. The automatic flush, under pressure, delivers an average of 1 to 3 ml solution per hour through the catheter just to keep it patent. When an electronic transducer is connected to the system and attached to the bedside monitor a waveform appears on the monitor that represents the fluctuation of the patient's blood pressure in the catheterized artery. A numeric display of the arterial pressure also appears on the monitor; in most patients this direct intraarterial pressure correlates very closely to external cuff pressure measurements.

Intraarterial pressure monitoring also provides direct access to arterial blood, which can then be easily obtained without further needle punctures for various laboratory tests, including arterial blood gas analysis. However, intraarterial cannulation is not without its problems. Complications of intraarterial monitoring may include the following:

Bleeding
Thrombosis
Inflammation/infiltration
Infection
Air/particulate embolism
Paresthesias
Distal obstruction of the artery

Nursing responsibilities for intraarterial monitoring include the following:

1. Preliminary flush system and transducer set up
2. Assistance with insertion
3. Aseptic maintenance of the flush system and catheter insertion site
4. Maintenance of catheter patency with accurate waveform and pressure readings
5. Continuous patient observation to prevent the immediate life-threatening complication of hemorrhage

Table 42-1 Normal hemodynamic pressures

Area monitored	Type of measurement	Normal pressure (mm Hg)
Superior vena cava (SVC)	Mean	2 to 6 (3 to 10 cm H$_2$0)
Right atrium (RA)	Mean	2 to 6 (3 to 10 cm H$_2$0)
Right ventricle (RV)	Systolic	20 to 30
	Diastolic	0 to 5
	End diastolic	2 to 6
Pulmonary artery (PA)	Systolic	20 to 30
	Diastolic	10 to 20
	Mean	10 to 15
Pulmonary capillary wedge (PCW)	Mean	4 to 12
Left atrium (LA)	Mean	4 to 12
Left ventricle (LV)	Systolic	100 to 140
	Diastolic	0 to 5
Aorta (Ao)	Systolic	100 to 140
	Diastolic	60 to 80
	Mean	70 to 90

□ **Pulmonary artery monitoring**
□ *Multiple line catheter*

Pulmonary artery (Swan-Ganz) catheters are used to monitor cardiovascular function in critically ill patients. The catheter is inserted into the superior vena cava via the subclavian, internal jugular, or external jugular vein. The typical pulmonary artery catheter has several openings along its length, and is connected to a high-pressure heparinized flush solution, electronic transducer, and bedside monitor in the same fashion as an arterial line (Chapter 9). The catheter is threaded through the right atrium and right ventricle into the pulmonary artery, where the tip rests (see Fig. 25-29). When the small balloon at the catheter tip is inflated with approximately 1 ml of oxygen, the catheter floats with the blood flow from the pulmonary artery into a pulmonary capillary.

The pulmonary capillary wedge pressure (PCWP) is the same as the pressure in the left atrium because there are no valves to create a gradient between the pulmonary artery and the left atrium. During diastole, when the mitral valve is open, the PCWP represents the filling pressure of the left ventricle (barring mitral valve disease). The pulmonary artery catheter is useful in providing data on both left- and right-sided heart failure and cardiogenic shock (Chapter 25).

The tip of the catheter senses the pressure of the blood at its opening, and transmits a representative pressure waveform to the monitor screen, which in turn converts the waveform into a digital value. In this fashion the distinct waveform and pressure of the superior vena cava, right atrium, right ventricle, and pulmonary artery are visualized as the catheter is introduced.

By connecting the pulmonary artery catheter to a cardiac output computer the volume of cardiac output can be determined. A known quality of injectate (usually 10 ml of NS or D$_5$W) is injected into the right ventricle via the proximal injectate port of the catheter. Whether iced or at room temperature, the injectate is cooler than the surrounding blood that it mixes with in the ventricle. The blood plus injectate travel from the ventricle out into the pulmonary artery near the catheter tip. The computer registers the temperature change and calculates the volume of blood that was present to produce the change, and represents this as the cardiac output in liters of blood per minute. Table 42-2 lists the hemodynamic indices which can be calculated from monitored data.

Pulmonary artery pressures are obtained from the distal port when the catheter is not in the wedged position. Central venous pressures (CVP) are obtained from the proximal port, which may also be used for fluid and medication infusions. Some pulmonary artery catheters have two proximal ports to enhance the multipurpose nature of the catheter. Pulmonary artery catheters are replacing the widespread use of single lumen CVP lines in critical care units because of the information they provide on left-sided heart function (wedge pressure, cardiac output) that cannot be obtained from a single CVP line.

□ *Alternate approaches*

In some cardiovascular ICUs it is common practice to forego using the pulmonary artery catheter and to insert a single line directly into the left atrium during open-heart surgery, allowing direct monitoring of left-sided heart function. Other ICUs are now using a newer type of fiberoptic pulmonary artery catheter that is able to perform continuous monitoring. These special PA catheters have a fiber-optic tip that "reads" the oxygen content of the mixed

Table 42-2 Normal hemodynamic indices

Measurement	Formula	Normal range
Cardiac output (CO)	Heart rate $\times$ Stroke volume	4.0 to 8.0 L/min
Cardiac index (CI)	$\dfrac{\text{Cardiac output}}{\text{Body surface area}}$	2.5 to 4.0 L/min/m²
Stroke volume (SV)	$\dfrac{\text{Cardiac output}}{\text{Heart rate}}$	60 to 130 ml/beat
Stroke index (SI)	$\dfrac{\text{Stroke volume}}{\text{Body surface area}}$	35 to 70 ml/beat/m²
Mean arterial pressure (MAP)	2/3 Diastolic + 1/3 systolic pressure	70 to 90 mm Hg
Pulmonary vascular resistance (PVR)	Mean pulmonary artery pressure − mean pulmonary capillary wedge pressure ÷ cardiac output	<2 PVR units
Systemic vascular resistance (SVR)	$\dfrac{\text{Mean arterial pressure − central venous pressure (in mm Hg)} \times 80}{\text{Cardiac output}}$	900 to 1600 dynes/sec/cm⁻⁵

venous blood (SVO_2) in the pulmonary artery through spectrophotometry. Systemic oxygen saturation reflects the interplay of cardiac output, oxygen transport, and oxygen consumption. Changes in SVO_2 have been directly correlated with changes in cardiac index. Depending on the cause, a drop in SVO_2 may become apparent before other hemodynamic changes, allowing for faster clinical recognition and intervention. Additionally, because of the continuous monitoring, the direct impact on SVO_2 of such nursing interventions as turning, suctioning, and weighing the patient can easily be identified, and care plans modified accordingly. Because of the high correlation between changes in SVO_2 and changes in arterial oxygen saturation, costly arterial blood gas analyses can be reduced. Causes of decreased SVO_2 include the following:

Anemia
Low cardiac output
Arterial oxygen desaturation
Increased oxygen consumption

☐ *Risks of pulmonary artery monitoring*

As with intraarterial pressure monitoring, pulmonary artery monitoring is not without risk. Nursing responsibilities are similar to those for arterial catheters, with the addition of continuous waveform observation to detect inadvertent catheter tip migration. Complications of pulmonary artery (Swan-Ganz) monitoring include the following:

Arrhythmias
Infection
Intracardiac knotting
Thrombophlebitis
Balloon rupture with air embolism
Pulmonary artery rupture
Pulmonary infarction

■ **INTRACRANIAL PRESSURE MONITORING**

Intracranial pressure (ICP) is frequently monitored in critically ill patients who have or are suspected of having intracranial disease or secondary increases in intracranial pressure. A catheter placed through the skull into the subarachnoid or intraventricular space is connected to a fluid filled tube, transducer, and pressure monitor (see Chapter 19). The system is set up similarly to other types of hemodynamic pressure monitoring but does not use a continuous flush. The ICP wave is transmitted to the monitor screen and converted to a digital value.

Intracranial pressure monitoring allows continuous observation of the patient's response to therapies aimed at lowering intracranial pressure and immediately shows the patient's tolerance of nursing measures that can cause an unsafe rise in ICP (for example, turning, suctioning, changes in bed position). It also allows aspiration of cerebrospinal fluid for analysis or culturing or to relieve excess intracranial pressure unresponsive to other therapies. Nurses are responsible for obtaining accurate pressure measurements, analyzing trends and patient response to interventions, and preventing complications of monitoring. A scrupulous sterile technique is essential in handling the catheter or screw insertion site and all connections in the monitoring tubing system because of the direct avenue for microorganisms into the cerebrospinal fluid.

The preceeding are a few of the invasive monitoring techniques available to the critical care nurse for data collection. In all cases the nurse must be knowledgeable about maintaining these lines, about the normal appearance of the waveform associated with each line, of the usual procedures necessary to prevent complications, and of the signs and symptoms of actual complications. The risk to the patient from invasive monitoring lines is sig-

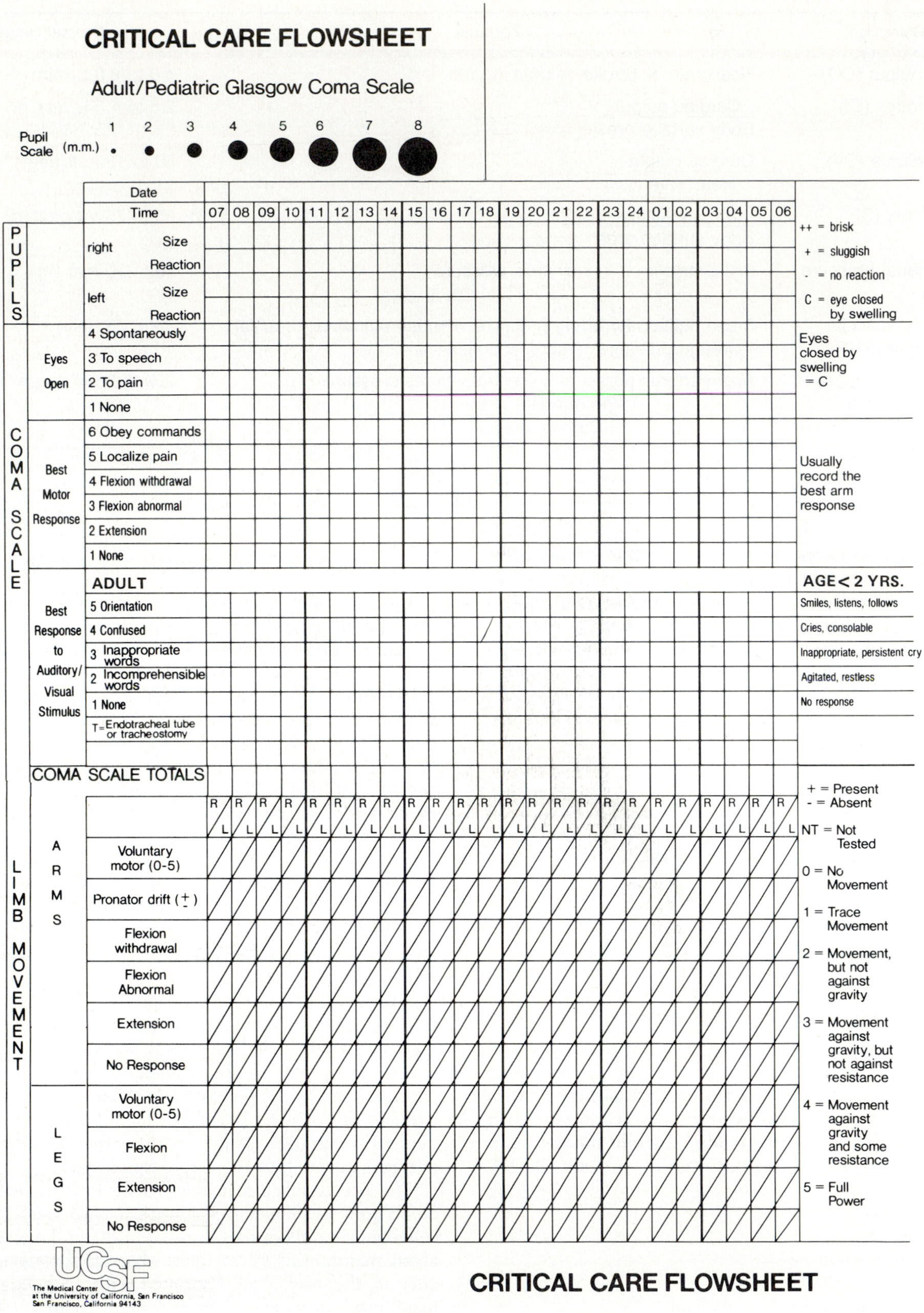

CRITICAL CARE FLOWSHEET

Adult/Pediatric Glasgow Coma Scale

Pupil Scale (m.m.) 1 2 3 4 5 6 7 8

		Date																									
		Time	07	08	09	10	11	12	13	14	15	16	17	18	19	20	21	22	23	24	01	02	03	04	05	06	
PUPILS	right	Size																									++ = brisk
		Reaction																									+ = sluggish
	left	Size																									- = no reaction
		Reaction																									C = eye closed by swelling
COMA SCALE	Eyes Open	4 Spontaneously																									Eyes closed by swelling = C
		3 To speech																									
		2 To pain																									
		1 None																									
	Best Motor Response	6 Obey commands																									
		5 Localize pain																									
		4 Flexion withdrawal																									Usually record the best arm response
		3 Flexion abnormal																									
		2 Extension																									
		1 None																									
	Best Response to Auditory/Visual Stimulus	**ADULT**																									**AGE < 2 YRS.**
		5 Orientation																									Smiles, listens, follows
		4 Confused																									Cries, consolable
		3 Inappropriate words																									Inappropriate, persistent cry
		2 Incomprehensible words																									Agitated, restless
		1 None																									No response
		T=Endotracheal tube or tracheostomy																									
COMA SCALE TOTALS																											
LIMB MOVEMENT	ARMS		R/L	R/L	R/L	R/L	R/L	R/L	R/L	R/L	R/L	R/L	R/L	R/L	R/L	R/L	R/L	R/L	R/L	R/L	R/L	R/L	R/L	R/L	R/L	R/L	+ = Present - = Absent
		Voluntary motor (0-5)																									NT = Not Tested
		Pronator drift (±)																									0 = No Movement
		Flexion withdrawal																									1 = Trace Movement
		Flexion Abnormal																									2 = Movement, but not against gravity
		Extension																									3 = Movement against gravity, but not against resistance
		No Response																									
	LEGS	Voluntary motor (0-5)																									4 = Movement against gravity and some resistance
		Flexion																									
		Extension																									5 = Full Power
		No Response																									

UCSF
The Medical Center at the University of California, San Francisco
San Francisco, California 94143

CRITICAL CARE FLOWSHEET

Fig. 42-2 Sample critical care flowsheet.

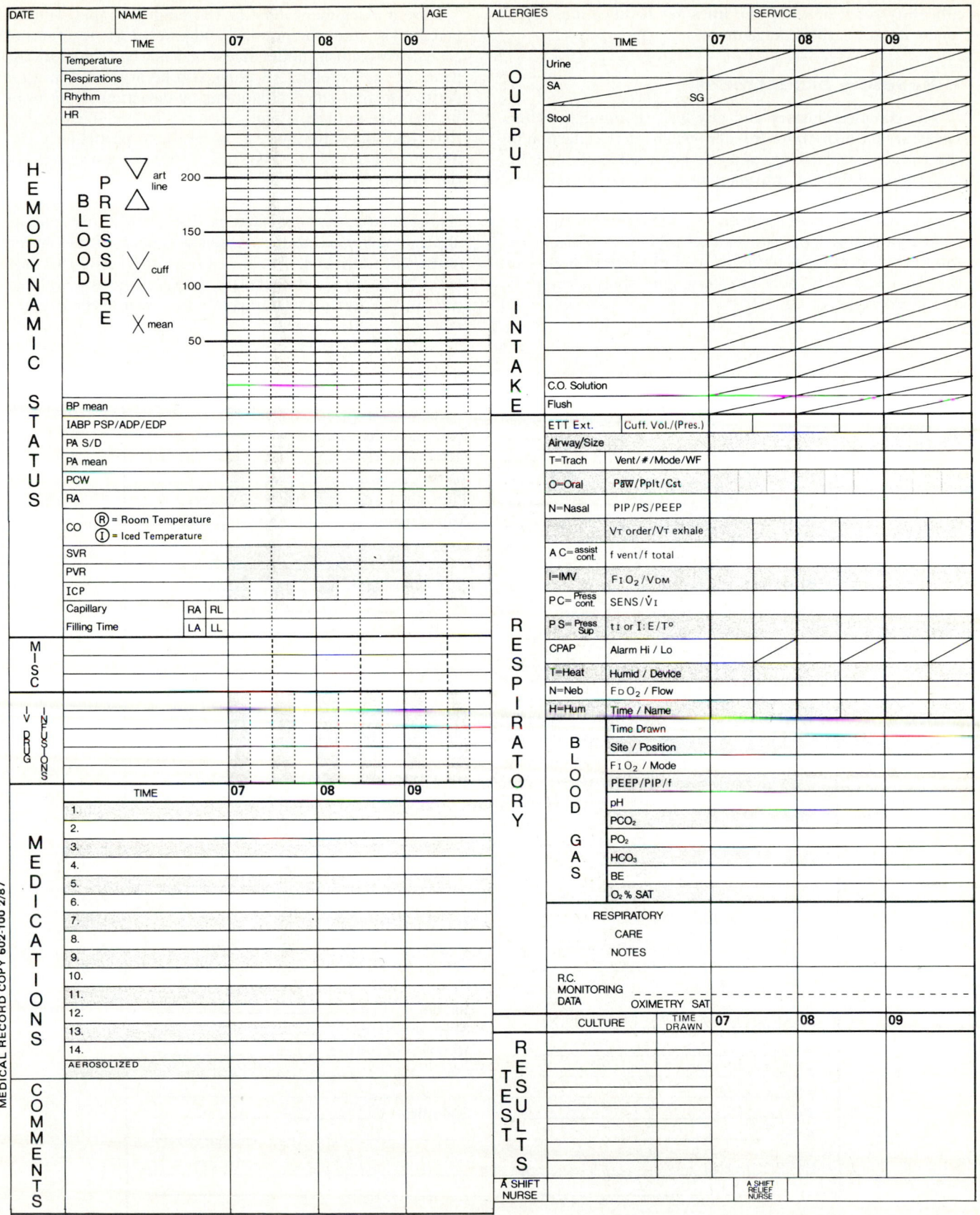

Fig. 42-2 cont'd Sample critical care flowsheet.

nificantly reduced when the lines are handled and cared for by knowledgeable personnel.

■ Baseline assessment

The complete history and physical examination is the necessary foundation for further ongoing data collection in the critical care setting, and the importance of accurate and thorough initial information cannot be overemphasized. But the multiple sources of data and the continually fluctuating stability of critically ill patients makes the constant reordering of priorities a necessity. The critical care nurse uses continuous observation of the patient to update the data base to be able to reformulate short-term goals and interventions.

Patient assessment must be thorough yet rapid. It must take into account the physical and psychologic reactions of an entire organism under stress and not be limited by the usual or the expected. It must also be organized and repetitive so that small alterations or deviations from prior findings are noticed. Finally, it must be individualized so that time and attention can be given to particularly significant aspects of the assessment without losing sight of the whole.

Many intensive care units utilize some form of a systems approach to patient assessment. Frequently this consists of a complete head-to-toe systems review at the beginning of the shift, at which time the nurse gathers an initial data base. More time and depth are spent on the systems that present the greatest real or potential threat to the patient.

CARDIOVASCULAR

Apical HR _____ ECG rhythm _____
BP _____ CVP _____ PAP _____ PCWP __
Pacer: Mode _____ Rate _____ MA _____
Heart sounds: _____
Skin color _____ Temp. _____
Peripheral R: R__ F__ P__ DP __
    pulses   L: R__ F__ P__ DP __
Specifics _____
_____
_____

NEUROLOGIC/PSYCHOLOGIC

LOC _____
Orientation _____
Affect _____
Pupils _____ ICP _____
Motor/sens. _____
Resp. to environment _____
_____
Social/emotional _____
_____
Specifics _____

RESPIRATORY

Rate _____ Quality _____
Breath   R _____
    sounds L _____
FIO_2 _____ Source _____
Mech. vent. TV __ Rate __ Mode _____
Chest tube(s) _____
Sputum _____ Cultures _____
Specifics _____
_____

GASTROINTESTINAL

Abdomen _____ Girth _____
Bowel sounds _____
NG_____ Stool _____
Nutrition _____
Incisions/drains/ostomies _____
Specifics _____
_____
_____

FLUIDS/ELECTROLYTES

Last labs done: _____ Time _____
Abnormals: _____
Labs needed _____
    Time _____
IVs infusing (sol., amt., rate, site)
#1 _____
#2 _____
#3 _____
#4 _____
#5 _____

GENITOURINARY

Urine: Amt. _____ Color _____
Appearance _____
S/A _____ S.G. _____ Voids _____
Catheter (type) _____
Skin condition _____
Renal function _____
_____
Specifics _____
_____

INTEGUMENT _____
_____

Fig. 42-3   ICU on-shift assessment worksheet.

When completed and documented the baseline systems assessment presents an accurate "status report" on the patient's condition and can be updated and compared to previous data. Throughout the rest of the shift, the nurse charts the progress as the patient's condition improves or deteriorates from the baseline, keeping track of vital parameters on an ongoing flow sheet, such as is seen in Fig. 42-2.

Fig. 42-3 shows the outline of a basic beginning of shift assessment guide, which includes the main items to be assessed under each body system. Routine parameters, individualized observations, and specific problems can be noted. The worksheet forms the outline of a repetitive assessment structure, which, once documented in the patient's record, makes information retrieval much easier.

After patient assessment is completed, nursing diagnoses are established and nursing care plans formulated. Nursing interventions for critically ill patients are based on these care plans.

Throughout this text nursing interventions have been described for care of the patient with a particular type of physiologic impairment. These are interventions intended to improve the patient's physiologic functioning before the impairment reaches the critical stage. In some critically ill patients many of these interventions have already been tried without success, and the patient's physiologic condition has deteriorated to the critical level, necessitating acute life-sustaining interventions. In other patients the initial illness is critical in itself (for example, acute myocardial infarction, severe trauma) and critical interventions are necessary immediately to sustain life.

The focus of the remaining three sections of this chapter is on physiologic, psychologic, and social interventions necessary for the individual who is critically ill.

■ INTERVENTIONS FOR THE CRITICALLY ILL PATIENT

■ Alleviation and prevention of physiologic and physical stressors

The ultimate goal of nursing intervention for any patient, regardless of the nature of the illness, is to promote, sustain, and restore optimum levels of physiologic, psychologic, and social functioning. However, in a critical care setting the immediate goal of ensuring a patient's survival initially determines the priorities for intervention; physiologic problems must be addressed first. Once life-threatening stressors have been alleviated, priorities are recorded and other problems can be addressed.

Physiologic priorities are determined by the degree of threat to the survival of the individual. Certain body systems are more prone to disorders that require intensive therapeutic interventions, and are frequently encountered in the critical care unit. These disorders are listed by system along with their specific interventions, as well as additional interventions necessary to prevent complications of therapy.

■ RESPIRATORY SYSTEM

The highest priority in caring for a critically ill individual is the maintenance of a patent airway and adequate ventilation.

☐ Acute respiratory failure

Acute respiratory failure may occur as a primary pulmonary deficit or as a result of a large number of other disorders that can affect the adequacy of ventilation or respiration. Crushing chest injuries, high-level spinal cord injury, neuromuscular diseases, extensive thoracic surgery, end-stage chronic obstructive pulmonary disease, sepsis, severe pneumonia, severe pulmonary edema, pulmonary embolus, congestive heart failure, and shock are just some disorders that may be exhibited by patients in respiratory failure requiring intensive care.

Interventions in respiratory failure are first directed at establishment of an unimpeded airway through endotracheal intubation via the nose or the mouth (see Chapter 24). Assisted ventilation may then be provided by a manual resuscitation device (Ambu or anesthesia bag), followed by continuous mechanical ventilation (Fig. 42-4). Mechanical ventilation devices are classified by the method through which air enters the lungs, that is, by either positive or negative pressure (see the box below). Mechanical ventilatory support mandates observation of the proper functioning of the equipment and assessment of the impact of the support on the patient's status (see Chapter 24).

Two methods of tracking the systemic effect of the patient's ventilatory status are common in ICUs. Arterial blood gas samples, drawn by direct arterial puncture or via an indwelling arterial line, are analyzed to reveal the patient's arterial pH, pCO_2, PaO_2, and O_2 saturation. A noninvasive transcutaneous oximeter (to measure oxygen saturation) or capnograph (to measure carbon dioxide) are

---

Types of mechanical ventilators

Positive pressure
Volume cycled

Bennett MA-1, MA-2, 7200
Bear
Ohio
Servo

Pressure cycled

Bennett PR-2
Bird

Negative pressure

Whole-body chamber (iron lung)
Chest cuirass, chest shell
Phrenic nerve stimulator
Direct diaphragm stimulator (investigational)

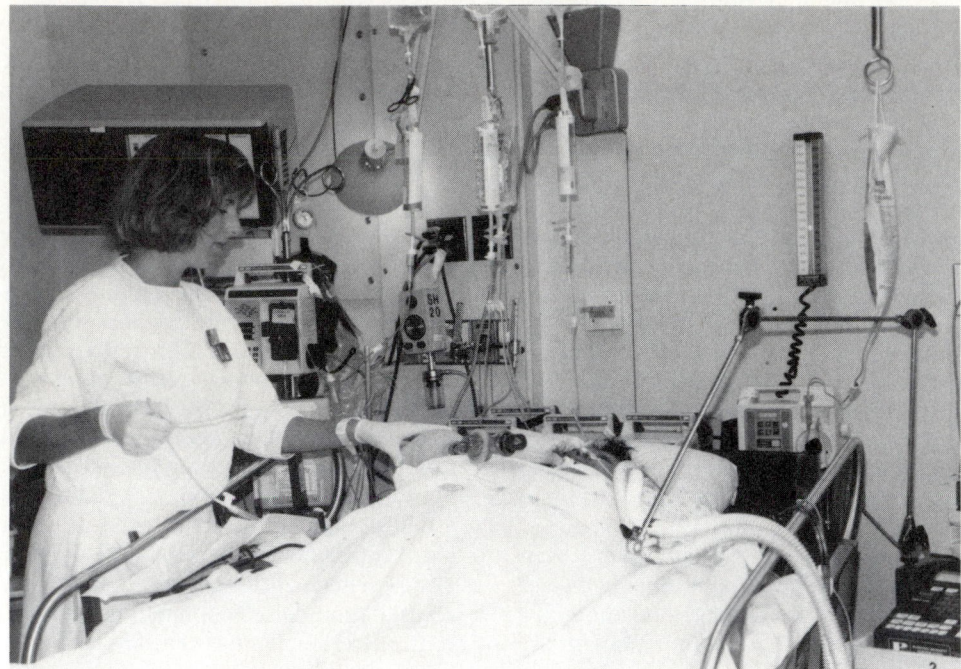

Fig. 42-4   Assisted ventilation in a critically ill patient.

also frequently used. The noninvasive devices use transcutaneous plethysmography to analyze the gas concentration in superficial capillary blood. Both direct and indirect methods are frequently used together. Once a relationship is established between the two methods, the risks and high cost of direct sampling can be minimized. Direct arterial sampling would then be indicated when there was an observed change in the surface saturation reading. Changes in mechanical ventilation therapy are usually based on the results of direct arterial sampling.

Mechanical ventilation is a complex therapy and poses major risks for the critically ill patient, including pneumothorax, atelectasis, decreased cardiac output (especially if positive-end expiratory pressure is used), gastrointestinal bleeding from a stress ulcer, and infection. Preventive interventions for the patient receiving mechanical ventilation include frequent assessment, position changes in bed, suctioning to remove secretions, intermittent deep ventilations (bagging or sighing), administration of antacids via nasogastric or gastrostomy tube, and scrupulous sterile technique in airway management to prevent a respiratory tract infection.

□   **Adult respiratory distress syndrome**

A particularly threatening respiratory complication that is prone to develop in critically ill patients is adult respiratory distress syndrome (ARDS). Also known as shock lung, wet lung, or post-pump lung, the predisposing factors for ARDS include a number of disorders seen in the critically ill: shock, trauma, disseminated intravascular coagulation (DIC), fat embolism, cardiopulmonary bypass, sepsis, cardiac arrest, and multiple blood transfusions.

Damage to the alveolar-capillary membrane and increased capillary permeability leads to pulmonary edema and diffuse microatelectasis. ARDS is characterized by severe dyspnea, hypoxemia, diminished lung compliance, and a significant ventilation-perfusion defect.

The primary intervention for ARDS is mechanical ventilation with the addition of positive-end expiratory pressure (PEEP). PEEP aids in reexpanding alveoli and preventing further alveolar collapse, thus improving oxygen transport. Nursing interventions for the patient with ARDS are the same as those for any patient with respiratory failure who is receiving mechanical ventilation, and require a very high degree of skill. (See Chapter 24 for further discussion of respiratory failure and ARDS.)

■ **CARDIOVASCULAR SYSTEM**

Cardiovascular problems requiring intensive patient care are so frequently encountered that many institutions have specific ICUs designed for the care of these patients (coronary care unit, postoperative cardiovascular unit). After support of ventilation, maintenance of cardiac function and systemic circulation is the highest priority in life-threatening situations. Disorders of the cardiovascular system that frequently require intensive observation and intervention include acute myocardial infarction, cardiogenic shock, congestive heart failure, open-heart surgery, and major vascular surgery.

□   **Drug therapy**

The first line of intervention in severe cardiovascular disorders frequently is *drug therapy* aimed at improving car-

Table 42-3   Intravenously administered cardiac and vasoactive drugs commonly used in ICU

Drug	Method	Clinical use
Atropine sulfate	IV push (diluted or undiluted in 10 ml sterile water)	Symptomatic bradyarrhythmias
Bretylium tosylate (Bretylol)	IV push, undiluted; may be followed by infusion	Ventricular fibrillation, ventricular tachycardia unresponsive to other agents such as lidocaine
Calcium chloride	IV push	Cardiac arrest, systemic hypocalcemia
Digoxin (Lanoxin)	IV push	Congestive heart failure, atrial fibrillation, paroxysmal atrial tachycardia
Dopamine hydrochloride (Intropin)	Diluted in infusion	Shock, hypotension (high dose); improve renal perfusion (low dose)
Dobutamine hydrochloride (Dobutrex)	Diluted in infusion	Low cardiac output states, cardiogenic shock
Epinephrine hydrochloride (Adrenalin)	IV bolus; intracardiac, intratracheal, IV infusion	Asystole, ventricular fibrillation, shock/hypotension, anaphylactic reactions
Isoproterenol hydrochloride (Isuprel)	IV infusion	Heart block, bradyarrhythmias, asystole, shock/hypotension
Lidocaine hydrochloride (Xylocaine)	IV bolus followed by IV infusion	To suppress ventricular arrhythmias or resistant seizure activity (low dose)
Morphine sulfate	IV bolus, IV infusion	Pulmonary edema, congestive heart failure, pain managament
Nitroglycerine (Nitro-Bid IV)	IV infusion	Hypertensive crisis, congestive heart failure associated with acute myocardial infarction, angina pectoris
Nitroprusside sodium (Nipride)	IV infusion	Hypertensive crisis, congestive heart failure
Norepinephrine (Levarterenol, Levophed)	IV infusion	Hypotension, shock
Propranolol (Inderal)	IV bolus	Supraventricular and ventricular tachyarrhythmias, angina pectoris
Sodium bicarbonate	IV bolus, IV infusion	Acidosis
Verapamil (Calan, Isoptin)	IV push	Paroxysmal supraventricular tachycardia

diac function until more definitive measures can be instituted. Cardioactive and vasoactive drugs most often administered in a critical care setting are listed in Table 42-3. These highly potent medications often have a very small margin between therapeutic doses and toxic levels, and the critical care nurse must use astute observational skills to monitor dose accuracy and its effect on the patient.

In addition to recording the patient's clinical response to the drug, the nurse will often be responsible for obtaining trough and peak blood samples before and after drug administration, thus tracking the drug's trough and peak levels. This is commonly done with digoxin and certain antiarrhythmics, as well as many antibiotics.

☐ Reducing myocardial work load

If medication dosage is insufficient to improve the patient's condition significantly, certain *invasive techniques* may be of some benefit. Temporary transvenous pacing of the heart may restore or enhance cardiac function until such time as a permanent pacemaker can be implanted. Intraaortic balloon counterpulsation (IABC) may be necessary for the patient who would benefit from temporary assistance in decreasing the work load on the myocardium (see the box at right). A balloon-tipped catheter is threaded

---

Indications and complications of IABC therapy

Indications

Cardiogenic shock with a reversible component
Low cardiac output states
Assist in removing patient from cardiopulmonary bypass
Unstable angina
Acute myocardial infarction
Drug-resistant lethal arrhythmias with ischemic cause

Complications

Ischemia of catheterized leg
Thrombus formation with eventual embolization
Infection
Aortic damage (aortic wall dissection, intimal laceration)
Balloon rupture with gas embolus (rare)

Measures to reduce myocardial work load

Enhance oxygenation	Supplemental oxygen
	Assisted ventilation
Decrease physical exertion	Bedrest
	Passive range of motion exercises
Decrease sympathetic stimulation	Reduced environmental stimuli (noise, light)
	Rest periods
	Information and reassurance to patient and family

into the aorta from a femoral artery; the balloon inflates during ventricular diastole to increase coronary artery filling and deflates just before ventricular systole to decrease afterload and improve left ventricular ejection. Care of the patient with IABC includes critical minute-to-minute assessment of the patient's physiologic response to IABC therapy and intervention to prevent complications (see Chapter 25).

Another advanced technique of myocardial support is the ventricular assist device (VAD). A relatively uncommon therapy, it is reserved for patients with severe left, right, or biventricular failure. It may be used to assist postoperative patients who cannot be weaned from cardiopulmonary bypass. VAD is now gaining more widespread use as a temporary support for end-stage patients awaiting cardiac transplantation. The technique involves implanting catheters into the atrium or ventricle to divert blood away from the ventricles into a roller pump located outside the body. The pump returns the blood directly to the aorta, thus bypassing the mitral or aortic valve and reducing the work load on the heart.

Prevention of physiologic stressors to the cardiovascular system is a continual priority of care for all ICU patients. Most preventive measures are aimed at myocardial work load reduction (see box above).

☐ Prevention of electrical microshock

Finally, in addition to decreasing myocardial work load the myocardium must also be protected from a particular hazard of the critical care environment, electrical microshock. The invasive monitoring and therapeutic interventions used in critically ill patients often create a direct pathway to the heart. Direct contact with stray or leaked current could prove fatal, particularly in critically ill patients whose resistance may be further decreased by other breaks in skin integrity and through electrolyte imbalances. Nursing staff in critical care areas are responsible for the safe and proper use of electrical equipment as well as for the implementation of appropriate electrical safety precautions.

■ NEUROLOGIC SYSTEM

Some neurologic disorders that may require intensive care during an acute phase of illness include the following:

1. Trauma: subdural or subarachnoid hemorrhage, cranial injuries
2. Intracranial neoplasms
3. Intracranial vascular anomalies: massive CVA, intracranial aneurysm rupture
4. Neuromuscular diseases that cause respiratory compromise: Guillain-Barrè syndrome, myasthenia gravis

Specialized neurologic interventions for critically ill patients are aimed at maintaining a homeokinetic state of brain metabolism and controlling elevations in intracranial pressure (see the box below). Intracranial monitoring (p. 1477) may be used to assess the extent of potentially dangerous rises in ICP. Meticulous insertion site and tubing care are essential to prevent the devastating complication of intracranial infection. Continuous observation by the critical care nurse is aimed at maintaining patency of the system and detecting changes in ICP.

Removal of cerebrospinal fluid is one method of controlling rising ICP. Other interventions include osmotic diuresis to remove excess brain tissue water and mechanical hyperventilation to artificially reduce circulating carbon dioxide (CO_2) levels. Lowered CO_2 levels will cause cerebral vasoconstriction, reducing the potential for progressive interstitial cerebral edema.

Efforts to lower the overall metabolism of the brain will reduce the brain's requirements for its natural substrates, oxygen and glucose. This is especially important when transport of these elements is impaired. Interventions to reduce brain metabolism include generalized hypothermia via a cooling mattress and induction of barbiturate coma. Caring for the artificially comatose patient requires the same attentive observations and extensive nursing interventions to prevent complications as are used in the

Nursing interventions to prevent increased ICP in critically ill patients

Maintain patent airway
Minimize arterial blood gas changes
Oxygenate patient before and after suctioning
Limit suctioning to 15 seconds
Elevate head of bed 30° (facilitates venous drainage without impeding arterial supply)
Maintain head and neck in straight alignment
Prevent overly tight tracheostomy ties
Prevent Valsalva maneuver
Assist patient in turning
Prevent coughing, sneezing, constipation
Monitor hydration status intake and output.

naturally comatose patient, with the addition of mechanical ventilation (see Chapter 19). In addition, complete neurologic assessment must be thoroughly performed at those times when sedation is withdrawn to evaluate patient progress. A lightened level of consciousness at those times necessitates sensitive communication with the patient, even though the ability to comprehend may not be apparent.

■ RENAL SYSTEM

Acute renal failure in the critically ill patient may result from a primary intrarenal cause, such as acute glomerulonephritis or acute cortical necrosis, or to a structural defect (see Chapter 32). It may be the result of directly nephrotoxic agents such as heavy metal poisoning or pharmacologic agents (for example, aminoglycoside antibiotics). But most commonly, acute renal failure in critically ill patients is the secondary result of any disorder that severely reduces cardiac output and renal perfusion, including cardiac arrest, left ventricular failure, or hemorrhage.

Interventions for the patient with renal failure are intended to provide the regulatory functions the kidneys can no longer maintain. The nurse keeps accurate daily weight and intake/output records so that only the exact amounts of body fluids lost plus a percentage for insensible loss, are replaced. Laboratory values are monitored carefully, with electrolyte intake limited and pharmacologic means of electrolyte removal utilized as necessary, for example, sodium polystyrene sulfonate (Kayexalate). Diuretics are given to increase marginal renal function. Nutrition is altered through restricted protein intake, because the body cannot appropriately excrete the nitrogen that is produced by amino acid breakdown. The nurse evaluates acid base balance, anticipating metabolic acidosis from the build up of acid metabolic wastes (carbonic and lactic acids). All other body systems are affected by the progression of acute renal failure, and continuous interventions are necessary to prevent altered acid base and electrolyte levels from impairing cardiovascular, respiratory, and neurologic function. Therefore the nurse is alert for such things as ECG changes indicative of increased myocardial irritability and altered contractility, changes in ventilatory pattern such as Kussmaul breathing and acidotic breath, and decreased level of consciousness, altered mentation, or unusual behavior.

As renal failure progresses, an early problem is significant fluid retention. A new intervention gaining popularity is continuous arteriovenous hemofiltration (CAVH). In CAVH a large artery and vein are cannulated, typically at the femoral site. Tubing primed with heparinized saline allows arterial-to-venous blood flow through a highly permeable hollow-filter fiber. The fiber separates plasma water and certain solutes from the blood, passing the ultrafiltrate into a collection bag while the blood returns to the patient. CAVH is a continuous process that uses the patient's blood pressure as the driving force; it is well tolerated even by unstable patients.

When renal failure has reached a level unresponsive to medical intervention, dialysis becomes necessary to mechanically remove the waste products of body metabolism. Hemodialysis, peritoneal dialysis, or CAVH may be initiated in the critically ill patient (see the box below).

■ GASTROINTESTINAL SYSTEM

The most common gastrointestinal problem seen in the critical care setting is *acute gastrointestinal bleeding*. This may be the initial sign in a newly admitted patient, or it may be a complication, such as a stress ulcer, in an already

---

Comparison of hemodialysis, peritoneal dialysis, and CAVH

Hemodialysis

Rapid, efficient correction of severe serum abnormalities
Short time required
Expensive
Requires highly technical equipment
Poorly tolerated by hemodynamically unstable patients
Risk of hemorrhage

Peritoneal dialysis

Well-tolerated even by very unstable patients
Inexpensive
Technologically simple
Must be performed over several hours or days
Cannot be performed after recent abdominal trauma or surgery
Risk of peritonitis

CAVH

Effective clearance of excess free water
Very well tolerated
Technologically simple to fairly complex
Retains most nutrients and protein-bound medications
Expense dependent upon filter complexity
Must be performed over several hours or days
Less effective clearance of nitrogen and creatinine
Filtration rate dependent upon blood pressure and tubing size and height of tube

critically ill person. Interventions, such as gastric lavage with saline solution and administration of antacid agents are intended to control bleeding until its cause and extent are determined. A Sengstaken-Blakemore tube may be used to provide direct compression of esophageal varices in order to tamponade a serious bleed (see Chapter 30). Administration of blood components and crystalloid fluids is initiated to reverse the hypovolemia of acute hemorrhage. Vasopressor medications cannot be administered to raise systemic blood pressure until the hypovolemic state is corrected. Once the patient's condition has stabilized sufficiently, endoscopic examination to determine the site of bleeding may be performed in the ICU. If indicated, surgical repair may follow.

The primary function of the gastrointestinal system is ingestion and digestion of liquid and solid nutrients. For many critically ill patients this process is interrupted for a lengthy period, during which either enteral or total parenteral nutrition (TPN) may be substituted. TPN solutions contain the essential protein, carbohydrates, and fat necessary to establish a catabolic state in which positive nitrogen balance is maintained. The critical care nurse assesses the adequacy of hydration, albumin level, electrolyte balance, and caloric intake. In addition, the nurse takes active measures to prevent the primary complication of TPN, infection.

Prevention of gastrointestinal complications such as stress ulcers in critically ill patients requires active interventions. Patients at highest risk include those who are receiving no food orally, who are receiving mechanical ventilation, have liver dysfunction, are receiving anticoagulants, and who have undergone any severe physiologic stress. In addition to the administration of local antacids and H_2 receptor antagonists (cimetidine), active interventions are required to reduce the psychologic stress inherent in the critical care environment.

■ MUSCULOSKELETAL/INTEGUMENTARY SYSTEM

Although few primary musculoskeletal problems necessitate intensive care, the majority of critically ill patients have severe restrictions placed on their mobility. Unstable hemodynamics, decreased blood flow, bedrest, weakness, and pain, as well as numerous therapeutic and monitoring devices, serve to significantly limit normal motion. Preserving function of weight-bearing muscles, maintaining joint mobility, and preserving continuous skin integrity are significant challenges to critical care nurses. All of the preventive and supportive nursing care techniques used in any patient with restricted mobility are appropriate in the ICU, including aggressive interventions to prevent skin breakdown with reduced-pressure beds (bead, air suspension, kinetic). Progress of the ICU patient to the highest level of activity within physiologic capabilities both facilitates continued improvement in physiologic function and visually reassures the patient of an improving condition.

One of the most serious potential complications of immobility is development of deep-vein thrombus, which can

---

Nursing interventions for prevention of pulmonary embolus

Elevation of lower extremities
Use of antiembolism stockings
Hourly active foot dorsiflexion
Active/resistive range of motion exercises
Observation for Homan's sign
Coughing and deep-breathing exercises
Administration of low-dose heparin as ordered
Inspection of intravenous sites with routine needle changes
Use of automatic sequential compression devices for lower extremities

---

embolize and travel to the lungs. *Pulmonary emboli* are found at autopsy in up to 60% of all individuals. Signs and symptoms of pulmonary embolism include dyspnea, pleuritic chest pain, fever, hemoptysis, tachycardia, and pleural friction rub. Preventive interventions can be instrumental in reducing the risk of serious complications (see the box above).

In the past decade the tremendous advances in treating immunocompromised patients has been matched only by the growth of therapeutic interventions which cause secondary immunosuppression. The number of critically ill patients who are compromised hosts increases daily, and routinely includes oncology, hematology, and organ transplant patients. Immunosuppression may be primary (AIDS, ARD, advanced systemic lupus erythematosis) or may be induced by the therapy for a particular disease state (leukemia, solid tissue tumors, bone marrow, or organ transplantation).

In many cases the immunosuppressed patient presents to the ICU in sepsis with accompanying hemodynamic instability and respiratory failure. Nursing interventions are directed at treating the shock state, supporting ventilation, and preventing further infection by scrupulous attention to isolation protocol.

Organ transplantation is an area in which critical care nurses can play a major role in helping to turn one family's tragedy into another family's hope. In 1986 there were over 10,000 kidney transplants, 2400 liver transplants, and over 4000 heart or heart/lung transplants. In addition, many patients received cornea, tissue, inner ear, and bone transplants. Both donors and recipients can be cared for in critical care units, and nursing interventions include both exquisite physiologic and psychologic support.

■ Alleviation and prevention of psychologic stressors

Despite the continuous attention that the critical care nurse must devote to the assessment of and intervention in physiologic derangements, the nurse must also focus attention on recognizing the psychologic stressors that confront the patient and family. The emotional discomfort and distress that the patient and family must endure will not only affect psychologic health but will have a direct impact on physical recovery as well.

The initial step in preventing or alleviating psychologic stress is to identify the patient's and family's perception of the critical event. Their perceptions will be affected by their individual personalities, cultural heritage, educational level, previous exposure to similar events, either positive or negative, and general level of familiarity with medical interventions and the hospital environment. Following are five specific interventions that nurses in any setting can implement to reduce the psychologic stress of illness on the family.

☐ Acknowledge, accept, and encourage patient and family to air feelings

Because the critically ill person is alienated from familiar surrounding and daily living patterns and is dependent on others to meet the most basic needs of survival, the patient becomes partially or totally isolated from usual support systems. Feelings of helplessness, powerlessness, loneliness, and depersonalization as well as disturbances in body image are common. Modes of expressing and therefore relieving the frustration, anger, hostility, fear, and depression generated by these feelings are limited by the physical constraints of the critical care environment.

Maintaining an atmosphere of openness and acceptance that encourages expression of feelings can help to provide patients with a means of coping. Talking with patients openly and honestly decreases feelings of depersonalization and anxiety and prevents isolation and alienation. Recognizing that anger and hostility are often indicative of fear, and that depression and withdrawal may mask signs of feelings of hopelessness, loneliness, powerlessness, or loss assist the nurse in accepting these feelings as normal and expected in this situation. Encouraging expression of feelings helps patients identify reasons for feeling or behaving in a way that may seem strange or wrong to them. At the same time it provides protection and permission to feel and act that way. Nurses or other health team members who are helping a patient to talk about feelings must be ready to accept whatever emotionally laden information might be expressed. Nonjudgmental recognition and acceptance of the patient's feelings will help to reinforce the patient's right to the feelings.

Patients who are intubated are unable to freely express their feelings even when alert and oriented, and therefore are particularly vulnerable to psychologic stressors. It is a natural tendency to communicate less with those who cannot talk easily and the nurse must guard against this. Keeping paper and pencil or a "magic slate" within the patient's reach and providing assistance when necessary will help to reduce the sense of isolation. However, such methods are not convenient for the expression of personal feelings or involved concerns. The nurse can recognize clues to the patient's emotional state by appearance and behavior and by knowing the types of concerns the patient is most likely to experience. The nurse can verbalize some potential concerns, allowing the patient to validate them as appropriate. Being empathetic with the patient and family conveys acceptance and understanding.

☐ Provide information about physical status, goals of treatment, and interventions

Because it is the patient's *perception* of stress and not the stressor itself that determines the patient's reaction to the illness and the environment, it is essential that the patient and family receive adequate information and simple explanations. Without explanations the critical care environment presents a mysterious and threatening array of noxious stimuli, which may be perceived as extremely unnatural and even magical. The high degree of technical sophistication increases the patient's feelings of vulnerability, and the patient may worry that the cardiac monitor is actually keeping the heart beating, that a blood transfusion indicates hemorrhaging, or that chest physiotherapy indicates pneumonia. A very common misconception of patients after coronary artery bypass is that "open heart" surgery involved cutting the heart wide open and sewing it back together again. Such a perception can lead to a drastic alteration in body image.

Much of what patients learn about their health problems depends on what is taught, both directly and indirectly, by the health care team. Patient teaching in critical care requires establishment of short-term goals. Pain, discomfort, weakness, anxiety, and transient confusion are some of the obstacles to learning that these patients experience. Despite these obstacles, patients and families need simple, repetitive explanations of all procedures and the purpose of each intervention, as well as an introduction to rehabilitation plans and health maintenance strategies. Patients may not understand or believe what they are told the first time, or anxiety and denial may prevent recollection of it. Reinterpretation and reiteration of diagnosis, prognosis, goals of treatment, types of intervention, and expectations of the patient and family may be continually necessary during the entire ICU stay. Keeping the patient and family apprised of the patient's current status as well as of changes in plans helps them to perceive the situation accurately, plan for the future realistically, and promotes cooperation by making them members of the health team.

☐ Encourage and support patient/family involvement in decision making and care

The essence of crisis intervention is to help individuals cope with a major life crisis such as a critical illness might precipitate. Critical care nursing in itself is far broader in scope and more future oriented than crisis intervention alone, but specific situations within the critical care setting may require the immediacy and limited focus of crisis intervention. At that time the patient and family are directed in establishing short-term goals and are given limited choice in acceptable responses. As the crisis situation stabilizes, even though it may be no less critical, the patient and family are given additional information and further

---

Interventions to minimize sensory deprivation/overload

Reduce noise level

Avoid excessive conversation
Avoid raising voice to talk to persons outside conversational range
Use carpeting where feasible
Avoid droning of continuous radio or TV; turn on or off at appropriate intervals
Locate nursing lounge away from patient care area

Maintain day/night orientation

Dim lights at night
Raise/lower shades or open/close window or curtains in normal day/night pattern
Reinforce progression of day in relation to specific events, such as meals

Maintain time orientation

Position large-numeral clocks in easy view
Provide wall calendars
Allow wristwatches for certain patients
Provide frequent reorientation to person, place, time

Promote rest and sleep

Schedule most exerting activities before rest period
Coordinate health team activities to provide periods of uninterrupted sleep
Minimize routine cleaning or stocking at night

Provide positive tactile stimuli

Touch or hold patient's hand during conversation
Use soothing physical contact as able (backrubs, face cleansings)
Encourage family to touch patient and hold hands despite dressings

Maintain personal/social integrity

Address patient by name, identify self by name
Provide full and complete information, explanations, and instructions
Avoid discussion over the patient; include the patient in rounds
Encourage visits by family and significant others
Allow important personal belongings at bedside

Reduce pain and discomfort

Administer analgesics appropriately to relieve pain
Reposition immobile patients every two hours
Prepare patients for all potentially uncomfortable or painful procedures

Maintain future orientation

Discuss transfer plans early with both patient and family
Initiate teaching regarding rehabilitation and health maintenance strategies as appropriate

---

responsibility in establishing mutual goals and choosing alternative responses. When the patient and family are knowledgeable about the goals of therapy and understand the patient's diagnosis, current status, and prognosis, they can be involved in many aspects of care planning and can make decisions consistent with the treatment regimen.

Involvement of the individuals who represent the patient's significant support system decreases their feelings of powerlessness, frustration, and anxiety. In addition, when these emotionally important figures, whether family or friends, understand and support the treatment goals and are involved in the patient's care, they are better able to sustain and expand this behavior after the patient leaves the ICU and the hospital. Even when a patient is unconscious, visits by key support figures who talk to and touch the patient may have positive, if unmeasurable, effects and help to decrease the family's feelings of helplessness.

An alert patient can be directly involved in establishing goals of treatment and care planning. One specific mechanism to increase the patient's feeling of personal control is to encourage involvement in structuring the daily schedule of activities. The knowledge that patient preferences are important to the nursing staff and that the person is viewed as capable of making decisions will support self-esteem and reinforce the centrality of the patient's role in recovery.

☐ Promote and maintain a sensory-regulated environment

The environment of the critical care unit is a major stressor with which both the patient and family must cope. (The many sources of external stress are outlined in the first section of this chapter.) In addition, disturbed thought processes and perceptual distortions are often likely to occur in patients receiving narcotics and sedatives, highly anxious patients, patients with multiple interrelated debilitating physical problems, patients with disturbed metabolic and respiratory function, patients deprived of sleep, and older patients. Reality reinforcement on a continuing basis is necessary for these individuals. Although some environmental factors cannot be altered, there are some specific interventions that the nurse can implement to provide a sensory regulated environment (see the box above).

☐ Prepare the patient and family for transfer from the ICU

Transfer from the critical care unit can represent a significant stress for some patients and their families. The critical care area with its sophisticated electronic equipment and attentive, highly-skilled staff represents security and protection. Patients know that transfer will be to an area where there are fewer nursing personnel per patient, less direct contact with nursing personnel, no automatic monitoring devices, and no direct observation of the bed from the nurses' station. Greater independence and higher levels of activity will be expected on the transfer unit, yet there will be the loss of support of the nursing staff who have come to know them. Patients may have conflicting feelings about the transfer as an indicator of physical improvement if they do not feel as well or as independent as they anticipated they would by transfer time.

The anxiety precipitated by the transfer can be prevented or reduced if the patient and family are taught to interpret particular signs and symptoms and are helped to understand the true purpose of equipment and routines. Signs that indicate progress need to be pointed out continuously, beginning when they first appear. Initiating the discussion of transfer plans with the patient and family as soon as the patient's condition begins to stabilize in the ICU will help them adjust to the idea and prepare for this eventuality. Transfer out of an ICU will frequently occur within several hours to one day after endotracheal extubation. Along with the projected time of transfer, the patient and family need to know what to expect on the new unit and what will be expected of them. Ideally, a nurse from the receiving unit should meet the patient and family prior to transfer. After transfer, visits from members of the ICU staff are helpful in conveying continued concern for the patient's welfare and in providing objective validation of continued progress. With careful planning and execution, transfer from the critical care unit can be a triumphant rather than a traumatic event.

■ Alleviation and prevention of social stressors

In the critical care setting the patient's physiologic needs often assume priority over psychologic needs, and the patient as a social being may be at risk of virtually being ignored. Limited visiting hours, the strange technical environment, and the aura of danger in the ICU isolates patients from their supportive family and friends and prevents them from assuming their usual social roles. For the most part, a person who is critically ill is narrowly viewed by staff primarily as a patient. The more significant roles of spouse, parent, child, lover, sibling, friend, or provider may go virtually unrecognized unless nursing staff initiate interventions to provide continuity in these relationships.

Such continuity is fostered through some of the same types of interventions that were used to reduce psychologic stress: increased visiting between patient and family; inclusion of family in discussions of disease process, prognosis, and care plans, and reporting by family of events and activities occurring in the other significant spheres of the patient's life. Relaying telephone messages between the patient and distant friends is one way of maintaining contact with the patient's external world.

One of the most effective and important ways to prevent disruption in relationships is to prepare the family or friends for their first visit with the patient in the ICU. The patient's physical appearance and the critical care environment should be explained thoroughly before the visitor enters. Visitors need to understand the patient's level of consciousness, ability to communicate, and ability to comprehend communication. They need to be made aware of the importance of their presence to the patient and the patient's need for their support. When the visitor approaches the bedside a staff member should remain with them to facilitate the initial interaction with the patient. At each subsequent visit the nurse caring for the patient meets with the significant others to answer questions and apprise them of the patient's progress.

In addition to supporting the maintenance of the patient's current roles and relationships the critical care nurse must also recognize the inevitability of actual role change for some patients and families during a critical illness. Roles of provider, decision maker, or employer/ employee may be altered, reversed, or eliminated. At this point some of the responsibilities of the patient need to be assumed by family and friends.

During the critical phase of illness the family members will be attempting to cope with precipitous role changes and may need assistance in working through problems that arise as family members and friends assume or fail to assume these additional responsibilities. The nurse needs to be aware of how problematic this time is and may need to help the family in requesting professional guidance, such as from a social worker, in assisting the family to reorganize themselves and their resources. The nurse may help the family appoint a temporary leader from among their ranks, one who could be requested to identify the wishes of the family as a whole and who could be contacted in the event of an emergency. The nurse may also help the family to plan visiting schedules that will meet the patient's needs without preventing the family members from maintaining their own responsibilities. It is a period of great emotional stress for both patient and family.

That emotional stress may eventually climax in the death of the critically ill patient. (The reader is referred to Chapter 15 for a complete discussion of dying and death.) The following are some suggestions for the critical care nurse caring for a dying patient:

1. Examine your own feelings about death.
2. Listen to assess the needs of the patient and family.
3. Remain available; be physically and emotionally present.
4. Help with administrative needs such as making telephone calls, obtaining release forms.
5. Provide reassurance of the patient's continued care, even if the patient is not to be resuscitated. Provide information.

6. Respect the person-family relationship, which existed long before the patient-hospital relationship.
7. Attempt to remain nonjudgmental about family or hospital issues.
8. Include the family in care.
9. Provide for patient and family privacy.
10. Provide the opportunity for the family to exercise religious or cultural traditions.
11. Use touch in caring for the patient and family.

The critical care environment is a dynamic milieu intended to maximize the application of critical interventions for the very ill. Knowledgeable nursing care is required to safeguard the patient from its potential hazards while promoting optimum patient outcomes.

■ SUMMARY

1. The physical layout of an ICU allows for direct observation of all patients at all times, yet provides for as much privacy as possible.
2. ICUs are stressful environments for the patient, family, and nurse. The patient and family are exposed to sensory overload by complex equipment, and experience anxieties and fears related to life-threatening situations.
3. The ICU nurse must have a sound knowledge base, astute observational and physical assessment skills, and excellent technical and communication skills.
4. The assessment process for the critically ill patient differs from management of other patients only in terms of the number of supportive devices available to assist in data collection.
5. Common types of monitored data in an ICU include cardiac monitoring, hemodynamic monitoring (intraarterial, pulmonary artery), and intracranial pressure monitoring.

6. The highest priority in caring for a critically ill person is the maintenance of a patent airway and adequate ventilation, followed by maintenance of cardiac function and systemic circulation.
7. Acute respiratory distress syndrome is prone to develop in critically ill patients; maintenance of respiration often requires mechanical ventilation devices.
8. Cardiovascular intervention includes drug therapy to improve cardiac function, measures to reduce myocardial work load, and prevention of electrical microshock. Intraaortic balloon counterpulsation (IABC) or a ventricular assist device (VAD) may be needed to reduce myocardial work load.
9. Neurologic interventions for the critically ill patient include preventing increased ICP and maintaining a homeokinetic state of brain metabolism.
10. Other types of major physical interventions relate to disturbances of kidney function, gastrointestinal bleeding, immunosuppression, and problems of immobility (especially threat of pulmonary embolism).
11. Nursing care of the patient in an ICU must include interventions to alleviate and prevent psychologic stressors; it is sometimes difficult to remember this important aspect of care when so much attention must be paid to monitoring parameters.
12. Interventions to relieve psychologic stressors include providing patients and families with opportunities to express feelings, providing necessary information, supporting decision making, maintaining a sensory-regulated environment, and preparing the patient and family for transfer from the ICU.
13. Interventions to alleviate and prevent social stressors for the patient and family include promoting patient/family relationships and decision making, preparing and supporting the family at their first ICU visit and subsequently as needed, and supporting realistic coping mechanisms.

REFERENCES AND SELECTED READINGS*
Contemporary

1. Aguilera, DC, and Messick, JM: Crisis intervention: theory and methodology, ed 4, St. Louis, 1982, The CV Mosby Co.
2. Alspach, JG, and Williams, SM: Core curriculum for critical care nursing, ed 3, Philadelphia, 1985, WB Saunders Co.
3. Baker, CF: Sensory overload and noise in the ICU: sources of environmental stress, CCQ 6(4):66-80, 1984.
4. *Brantigan, CO: Hemodynamic monitoring: interpreting values, Am J Nurs 82(1):86-89, 1982.
5. *Brewer, MJ: To sleep or not to sleep: the consequences of sleep deprivation, Crit Care Nurse 5(6):35-41, 1985.
6. Carnevale, FA: Transcutaneous O_2 monitoring: assessment techniques, DCCN 5(5):264-269, 1986.
7. Daily, EK, and Schroeder, JS: Techniques in bedside hemodynamic monitoring, ed 3, St. Louis, 1984, The CV Mosby Co.
8. Daley, L: The perceived immediate needs of families with relatives in the intensive care setting, Heart Lung 13(3):231-237, 1984.
9. Davidson, LJ, and Brown, S: Continuous SVO_2 monitoring: a tool for analyzing hemodynamic status, Heart Lung 15(3):287-292, 1986.
10. *Emmanuelson, KL, and Rosenlicht, JM: Handbook of critical care nursing, New York, 1986, Fleschner Publishing Co.
11. *Ensuring intensive care, Nursing 84 photobook series, Springhouse, Pa, 1984, Springhouse Corp.
12. *Gahart, BL: Intravenous medications, ed 4, St. Louis, 1985, The CV Mosby Co.
13. Griffin, JP: Nursing care of the immunocompromised patient in the ICU, Heart Lung 15(2):179-188, 1986.
14. Hammer, MC: The aged patient in the critical care setting, Focus Crit Care 10(6):22-29, 1983.
15. *Hoffman, LA: Airway management for the critically ill patient, Am J Nurs 87(1):39-53, 1987.
16. *Hook, SW: Intraaortic balloon pump techniques, DCCN 2(4):196-204, 1983.
17. Hudak, CM, Gallo, BM, and Lohr, T: Critical care nursing, a holistic approach, ed 4, Philadelphia, 1986, JB Lippincott Co.
18. *Jacquith, SM: Continuous measurement of SVO_2: clinical applications and advantages for critical care nursing, Crit Care Nurse 5(2):40-44, 1985.
19. Johanson, BC, and others: Standards for critical care, St. Louis, 1985, The CV Mosby Co.
20. Kemp, VH: The role of critical care nurses in the ethical decision-making process, DCCN 4(6):354-359, 1985.
21. Kenner, CV, Guzzetta, CE, and Dossey, BM: Critical care nursing: body, mind, spirit, ed 2, Boston, 1985, Little, Brown and Co.
22. Kinney, MR, editor: AACN's clinical reference for critical-care nursing, New York, 1981, McGraw-Hill Book Co.
23. Kleck, HG: ICU syndrome: onset, manifestations, treatment, stressors, and prevention, CCQ 6(4):21-28, 1984.
24. Leske, JS: Needs of relatives of critically ill patients: a follow-up, Heart Lung 15(2):89-93, 1986.
25. Millar, S, Sampson, LK, and Soukup, M: AACN procedure manual for critical care, Philadelphia, 1985, WB Saunders Co.
26. *Morra, L: Troubleshooting pulmonary artery catheters, RN 59(2):46-52, 1987.
27. *Mulford, E: Nursing perspectives for the patient receiving postoperative ventricular assistance in the critical care unit, Heart Lung 16(3):246-247, 1987.
28. *Murphy, P: When a nondeath death occurs: helping the family accept the reality of brain death, Nurs 16(7):34-39, 1986.
29. Ng, L, and Nuckols, OJ: Nursing management of the postoperative cardiac surgical patient in the critical care unit, Cardiovasc Clinics 16(3):211-233, 1986.
30. Quall, SJ: Comprehensive intraaortic balloon pumping, St. Louis, 1984, The CV Mosby Co.
31. *Robinet, K: Increased intracranial pressure: management with an intraventricular catheter, J Neurosurg Nurs 17(2):95-104, 1985.
32. *Smith, SL: Liver transplantation: implications for critical care nursing, Heart Lung 14(6):617-627, 1985.
33. *Stark, JL: How to succeed against acute renal failure, Nurs 82 12(7):26-33, 1982.
34. *Thornby, DC: Cardiac transplantation: nursing during the acute period, DCCN 2(4):212-224, 1983.
35. Winkelman, V: Hemofiltration: a new technique in critical care nursing, Heart Lung 14(3):265-271, 1985.

Classic

36. *Cassem, NH, Hackett, T, and Bascon, C: Reactions of coronary patients to the CCU nurse, Am J Nurs 70:312-319, 1970.
37. Hay, D, and Oken, D: The psychological stresses of intensive care nursing, Psychosom Med 34:117, 1972.
38. *Obier, K, and Haywood, LJ: Enhancing therapeutic communication with acutely ill patients, Heart Lung 2:49-53, 1973.
39. Roberts, SL: Behavioral concepts and the critically ill patient, Englewood Cliffs, NJ, 1976, Prentice-Hall, Inc.
40. Storlie, F: Patient teaching in critical care, New York, 1975, Appleton-Century-Crofts.

*References preceded by an asterisk are particularly well suited for student reading.

Appendixes

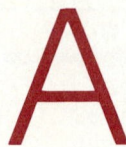

Normal Laboratory Values

■ Blood, plasma or serum values

Reference range

Determination	Conventional	SI
Acetoacetate plus acetone	0.3-2.0 mg/100 ml	3-20 mg/l
Aldolase	1.3-8.2 mU/ml	12-75 nmol · s^{-1}/l
Alpha amino nitrogen	3.0-5.5 mg/100 ml	2.1-3.9 mmol/l
Ammonia	80-110 μg/100 ml	47-65 μmol/l
Ascorbic acid	0.4-1.5 mg/100 ml	23-85 μmol/l
Barbiturate	0	0 μmol/l
	Coma level: phenobarbital, approximately 10 mg/100 ml; most other drugs, 1-3 mg per 100 ml	
Bilirubin (van den Bergh test)	One minute: 0.4 mg/100 ml	Up to 7 μmol/l
	Direct: 0.4 mg/100 ml	Up to 17 μmol/l
	Total: 1.0 mg/100 ml	
	Indirect is total minus direct	
Blood volume	8.5-9.0% of body weight in kg	80-85 ml/kg
Bromide	0	0 mmol/l
	Toxic level: 17 mEq/l	
Bromsulfalein (BSP)	Less than 5% retention 45 min after 5 mg/kg IV	<0.05 l
Calcium	8.5-10.5 mg/100 ml (slightly higher in children)	2.1-2.6 mmol/l
Carbon dioxide content	24-30 mEq/l	24-30 mmol/l
	20-26 mEq/l in infants (as HCO$_3^-$)	
Carbon monoxide	Symptoms with over 20% saturation	0 (1)
Carotenoids	0.8-4.0 μg/ml	1.5-7.4 μmol/l
Ceruloplasmin	27-37 mg/100 ml	1.8-2.5 μmol/l
Chloride	100-106 mEq/l	100-106 mmol/l
Cholinesterase (pseudocholinesterase)	0.5 pH U or more/h	0.5 or more arb. unit
	0.7 pH U or more/h for packed cells	
Copper	Total: 100-200 μg/100 ml	16-31 μmol/l
Creatine phosphokinase (CPK)	Female 5-35 mU/ml	0.08-0.58
	Male 5-55 mU/ml	μmol · s^{-1}/l
Creatinine	0.6-1.5 mg/100 ml	60-130 μmol/l

Modified from Kaye, DA, and Rose, LF: Fundamentals of internal medicine, St. Louis, 1983, The CV Mosby Co. Adapted by permission from the New England Journal of Medicine, Vol 302, pages 37-48, 1980.
Abbreviations used: SI, Système international d'Unités (The SI for the Health Professions, World Health Organization, Office of Publications, Geneva Switzerland, 1977); d, 24 hours; P, plasma; S, serum; B, blood; U, urine; l, liter; h, hour; and s, second.

Continued.

■ Blood, plasma or serum values—cont'd

Reference range—cont'd

Determination	Conventional	SI
Ethanol	0.3-0.4%, marked intoxication; 0.4-0.5%, alcoholic stupor; 0.5% or over, alcoholic coma	65-87 mol/l 87-109 mmol/l >109 mmol/l
Glucose	Fasting: 70-110 mg/100 ml	3.9-5.6 mmol/l
Iron	50-150 μg/100 ml (higher in males)	9.0-26.9 μmol/l
Iron-binding capacity	250-410 μg/100 ml	44.8-73.4 μmol/l
Lactic acid	0.6-1.8 mEq/l	0.6-1.8 mmol/l
Lactic dehydrogenase	60-120 U/ml	1.00-2.00 μmol · s^{-1}/l
Lead	50 μg/100 ml or less	Up to 2.4 μmol/l
Lipase	2 U/ml or less	Up to 2 arb. unit
Lipids		
Cholesterol	120-220 mg/100 ml	3.10-5.69 mmol/l
Cholesterol esters	60-75% of cholesterol	
Phospholipids	9-16 mg/100 ml as lipid phosphorus	2.9-5.2 mmol/l
Total fatty acids	190-420 mg/100 ml	1.9-4.2 g/l
Total lipids	450-1000 mg/100 ml	4.5-10.0 g/l
Triglycerides	40-150 mg/100 ml	0.4-1.5 g/l
Lithium	Toxic level 2 mEq/l	2 mmol/l
Magnesium	1.5-2.0 mEq/l	0.8-1.3 mmol/l
5'Nucleotidase	0.3-3.2 Bodansky U	30-290 nmol · s^{-1}/l
Osmolality	285-295 mOsm/kg water	285-295 mmol/kg
Oxygen saturation (arterial)	96-100%	0.96-1.00 l
P$_{CO_2}$	35-43 mm Hg	4.7-6.0 kPa
pH	7.35-7.45	Same
P$_{O_2}$	75-100 mm Hg (dependent on age) while breathing room air Above 500 mm Hg while on 100% O_2	10.0-13.3 kPa
Phenylalanine	0-2 mg/100 ml	0-120 μmol/l
Phenytoin (Dilantin)	Therapeutic level, 5-20 μg/ml	19.8-79.5 μmol/l
Phosphorus (inorganic)	3.0-4.5 mg/100 ml (infants in 1st year up to 6.0 (mg/100 ml)	1.0-1.5 mmol/l

■ Blood, plasma or serum values—cont'd

Reference range—cont'd

Determination	Conventional	SI
Potassium	3.5-5.0 mEq/l	3.5-5.0 mmol/l
Primidone (Mysoline)	Therapeutic level 4-12 μg/ml	18-55 μmol/l
Protein: Total	6.0-8.4 g/100 ml	60-84 g/l
Albumin	3.5-5.0 g/100 ml	35-50 g/l
Globulin	2.3-3.5 g/100 ml	23-35 g/l
Electrophoresis	*% of total protein*	*Of total protein*
Albumin	52-68	0.52-0.68
Globulin:		
Alpha$_1$	4.2-7.2	0.042-0.072
Alpha$_2$	6.8-12	0.068-0.12
Beta	9.3-15	0.093-0.15
Gamma	13-23	0.13-0.23
Pyruvic acid	0-0.11 mEq/l	0.011 mmol/l
Quinidine	Therapeutic: 1.5-3 μg/ml	4.6-9.2 μmol/l
	Toxic: 5-6 μg/ml	15.4-18.5 μmol/l
Salicylate:	0	
Therapeutic	20-25 mg/100 ml;25-30 mg/100 ml to age 10 yrs. 3 h post dose	1.4-1.8 mmol/l 1.8-2.2 mmol/l
Toxic	Over 30 mg/100 ml	Over 2.2 mmol/l
	Over 20 mg/100 ml after age 60	Over 1.5 mmol/l
Sodium	135-145 mEq/l	135-145 mmol/l
Sulfate	0.5-1.5 mg/100 ml	0.05-1.2 mmol/l
Sulfonamide	0 mg/100 ml	0 mmol/1
	Therapeutic: 5-15 mg/100 ml	
Transaminase (SGOT) (aspartate amino-transferase)	10-40 U/ml	0.08-0.32 μmol $\cdot$ s^{-1}/l
Urea nitrogen (BUN)	8-25 mg/100 ml	2.9-8.9 mmol/l
Uric acid	3.0-7.0 mg/100 m	0.13-0.42 mmol/l
Vitamin A	0.15-0.6 μg/ml	0.5-2.1 μmol/l
Vitamin A tolerance test	Rise to twice fasting level in 3 to 5 h	

■ Urine values

Reference range

Determination	Conventional	SI
Acetone plus acetoacetate (quantitative)	0	0 mg/l
Alpha amino nitrogen	64-199 mg/d; not over 1.5% of total nitrogen	4.6-14.2 mmol/d
Amylase	24-76 U/ml	24-76 arb. unit
Calcium	150 mg/d or less	3.8 or less mmol/d
Catecholamines	Epinephrine: under 20 µg/d	<55 nmol/d
	Norepinephrine: under 100 µg/d	<590 nmol/d
Copper	0-100 µg/d	0-1.6 µmol/d
Coproporphyrin	50-250 µg/d	80-380 nmol/d
	Children under 80 lb 0-75 µg/d	0-115 nmol/d
Creatine	Under 100 mg/d or less than 6% of creatinine. In pregnancy: up to 12%. In children under 1 yr.: may equal creatinine. In older children: up to 30% of creatinine	<0.75 mmol/d
Cystine or cysteine	0	0
Follicle-stimulating hormone:		
Follicular phase	5-20 IU/d	Same
Mid/cycle	15-60 IU/d	
Luteal phase	5-15 IU/d	
Menopausal	50-100 IU/d	
Men	5-25 IU/d	
Hemoglobin and myoglobin	0	
5-Hydroxyindole acetic acid	2-9 mg/d (women lower than men)	10-45 µmol/d
Lead	0.08 µg/ml or 120 µg or less/d	0.39 µmol/l or less
Phenolsulfonphthalein (PSP)	At least 25% excreted by 15 min; 40% by 30 min; 60% by 120 min.	0.25 l
Phosphorus (inorganic)	Varies with intake, average 1 g/d	32 mmol/d
Porphobilinogen	0	0
Protein:		
Quantitative	<150 mg/24 hr	<0.15 g/d

Steroids:

17-Ketosteroids (per day)	Age (yr)	Male (mg)	Female (mg)	Male (µmol/d)	Female (µmol/d)
	10	1-4	1-4	3-14	3-14
	20	6-21	4-16	21-73	14-56
	30	8-26	4-14	28-90	14-49
	50	5-18	3-9	17-62	10-31
	70	2-10	1-7	7-35	3-24

Determination	Conventional	SI
17-Hydroxysteroids	3-8 mg/d (women lower than men)	8-22 µmol/d as hydrocortisone
Sugar:		
Quantitative glucose	0	0 mmol/l
Identification of reducing substances		
Fructose	0	0 mmol/l
Pentose	0	0 mmol/l
Titratable acidity	20-40 mEq/d	21-40 mmol/d
Urobilinogen	Up to 1.0 Ehrlich U	To 1.0 arb. unit
Uroporphyrin	0	0 nmol/d
Vanilmandelic acid (VMA)	Up to 9 mg/24 hr	Up to 45 µmol/d

■ Special endocrine tests

Reference range

Determination	Conventional	SI
Steroid hormones		
Aldosterone	Excretion: 5-19 μg/24 h	14-53 nmol/d
Fasting, at rest, 210 mEq sodium diet	Supine: 48 ± 29 pg/ml	133 ± 80 pmol/l
	Upright: (2 h) 65 ± 23 pg/ml	180 ± 64 pmol/l
Fasting, at rest, 110 mEq sodium diet	Supine: 107 ± 45 pg/ml	279 ± 125 pmol/l
	Upright: (2 h) 239 ± 123 pg/ml	663 ± 341 pmol/l
Fasting, at rest, 10 mEq sodium diet	Supine: 175 ± 75 pg/ml	485 ± 208 pmol/l
	Upright: (2 h) 532 ± 228 pg/ml	1476 ± 632 pmol/l
Cortisol		
Fasting	8 a.m.: 5-25 μg/100 ml	0.14-0.69 μmol/l
At rest	8 p.m.: Below 10 μg/100 ml	0-0.28 μmol/l
20 U ACTH	4 h ACTH test: 30-45 μg/100 ml	0.83-1.24 μmol/l
Dexamethasone at midnight	Overnight suppression test: Below 5 μg/100 ml	<0.14 nmol/l
	Excretion: 20-70 μg/24 h	55-193 nmol/d
11-Deoxycortisol	Responsive: Over 7.5 μg/100 ml (after metrapone)	>0.22 μmol/l
Testosterone	Adult male: 300-1100 ng/100 ml	10.4-38.1 nmol/l
	Adolescent male: over 100 ng/100 ml	>3.5 nmol/l
	Females: 25-90 ng/100 ml	0.87-3.12 nmol/l
Unbound testosterone	Adult male: 3.06-24.0 ng/100 ml	106-832 pmol/l
	Adult female: 0.09-1.28 ng/100 ml	3.1-44.4 pmol/l
Polypeptide hormones		
Adrenocorticotropin (ACTH)	15-70 pg/ml	3.3-15.4 pmol/l
Calcitonin	Undetectable in normals	0
	>100 pg/ml in medullary carcinoma	>29.3 pmol/l
Growth hormone		
Fasting, at rest	Below 5 ng/ml	<233 pmol/l
After exercise	Children: Over 10 ng/ml	>465 pmol/l
	Male: Below 5 ng/ml	<233 pmol/l
	Female: Up to 30 ng/ml	0-1395 pmol/l
After glucose	Male: Below 5 ng/ml	<233 pmol/l
	Female: Below 10 ng/ml	0-465 pmol/l
Insulin		
Fasting	6-26 μU/ml	43-187 pmol/l
During hypoglycemia	Below 20 μU/ml	<144 pmol/l
After glucose	Up to 150 μU/ml	0-1078 pmol/l
Leuteinizing hormone	Male: 6 -18 mU/ml	6-18 u/l
Pre- or postovulatory	Female: 5-22 mU/ml	5-22 u/l
Midcycle peak	30-250 mU/ml	30-250 u/l
Parathyroid hormone	<10 μl equiv/ml	<10 ml equiv/l
Prolactin	2-15 ng/ml	0.08-6.0 nmol/l
Renin activity		
Normal diet	Supine:1.1 ± 0.8 ng/ml/h	0.9 ± 0.6 (nmol/l)h
	Upright: 1.9 ± 1.7 ng/ml/h	1.5 ± 1.3 (nmol/l)h
Low-sodium diet	Supine: 2.7 ± 1.8 ng/ml/h	2.1 ± 1.4 (nmol/l)h
	Upright: 6.6 ± 2.5 ng/ml/h	5.1 ± 1.9 (nmol/l)h
Low-sodium diet	Diuretics: 10.0 ± 3.7 ng/ml/h	7.7 ± 2.9 (nmol/l)h
Thyroid hormones		
Thyroid-stimulating-hormone (TSH)	0.5-3.5 μU/ml	0.5-3.5 mU/l
Thyroxine-binding globulin capacity	15-25 μg T_4/100 ml	193-322 nmol/l
Total tri-iodothyronine by radioimmunoassay (T_3)	70-190 ng/100 ml	1.08-2.92 nmol/l
Total thyroxine by RIA (T_4)	4-12 μg/100 ml	52-154 nmol/l
T_3 resin uptake	25-35%	0.25-0.35
Free thyroxine index (FT$_4$l)	1-4 ng/100 ml	12.8-51-2 pmol/l

■ Cerebrospinal fluid values

Reference range

Determination	Conventional	SI	Determination	Conventional	SI
Bilirubin	0	0 μmol/l	Glucose	50-75 mg/100 ml (30%-50% less than blood)	2.8-4.2
Chloride	120-130 mEq/l (20 mEq/l higher than serum)		Pressure (initial)	70-180 mm of water	mmol/l 70-80 arb. u.
Albumin	Mean: 29.5 mg/100 ml ±2 SD: 11-48 mg/ 100 ml	0.295 g/l ±2 SD: 0.11-0.48	Protein: Lumbar	15-45 mg/100 ml	0.15-0.45 g/l
IgG	Mean: 4.3 mg/100 ml ±2 SD: 0-8.6 mg/100 ml	0.043 g/l ±2 SD: 0-0.086	Cisternal Ventricular	15-25 mg/100 ml 5-15 mg/100 ml	0.15-0.25 g/l 0.05-0.15 g/l

■ Hematologic values

Reference range

Determination	Conventional	SI
Coagulation factors:		
Factor I (fibrinogen)	0.15-0.35 g/100 ml	4.0-10.0 μmol/l
Factor II (prothrombin)	60-140%	0.60-1.40
Factor V (accelerator globulin)	60-140%	0.60-1.40
Factor VII-X (proconvertin-Stuart)	70-130%	0.70-1.30
Factor X (Stuart factor)	70-130%	0.70-1.30
Factor VIII (antihemophilic globulin)	50-200%	0.50-2.0
Factor IX (plasma thromboplastic cofactor)	60-140%	0.60-1.40
Factor XI (plasma thromboplastic antecedent)	60-140%	0.60-1.40
Factor XII (Hageman factor)	60-140%	0.60-1.40
Coagulation screening tests:		
Bleeding time (Simplate)	3-9 min	180-540 s
Prothrombin time	Less than 2-s deviation from control	Less than 2-s deviation from control
Partial thromboplastin time (activated)	25-37 s	25-37 s
Whole-blood clot lysis	No clot lysis in 24 h	O/d
Fibrinolytic studies:		
Euglobin lysis	No lysis in 2 h	0 (in 2 h)
Fibrinogen split products:	Negative reaction at greater than 1:4 dilution	0 (at >1:4 dilution)
Thrombin time	Control ± 5 s	Control ± 5 s

■ **Hematologic values—cont'd**

Reference range—cont'd

Determination	Conventional	SI
"Complete" blood count:		
Hematocrit	Male: 45-52%	Male: 0.42-0.52
	Female: 37-48%	Female: 0.37-0.48
Hemoglobin	Male: 13-18 g/10 ml	Male: 8.1-11.2 mmole/l
	Female: 12-16 g/100 ml	Female: 7.4-9.9 mmol/l
Leukocyte count	4300-10,800/mm³	$4.3\text{-}10.8 \times 10^9/l$
Erythrocyte count	4.2-5.9 million/mm³	$4.2\text{-}5.9 \times 10^{12}/l$
Mean corpuscular volume (MCV)	80-94 μm³	80-94 fl
Mean corpuscular hemoglobin (MCH)	27-32 pg	1.7-2.0 fmol
Mean corpuscular hemoglobin concentration (MCHC)	32-36%	19-22.8 mmol/l
Erythrocyte sedimentation rate (Westergren method)	Male: 1-13 mm/h	Male: 1-13 mm/h
	Female: 1-20 mm/h	Female: 1-20 mm/h
Erythrocyte enzymes		
Glucose-6-phosphate dehydrogenase	5-15 U/gHb	5-15 U/g
Pyruvate kinase	13-17 U/gHb	13-17 U/g
Ferritin (serum)		
Iron deficiency	0-20 ng/ml	0-20 μg/l
Iron excess	Greater than 400 ng/l	>400 μg/l
Folic acid		
Normal	Greater than 1.9 ng/ml	>4.3 mmol/l
Borderline	1.0-1.9 ng/ml	2.3-4.3 mmol/l
Haptoglobin	100-300 mg/100 ml	1.0-3.0 g/l
Hemoglobin studies:		
Electrophoresis for A₂ hemoglobin	1.5-3.5%	0.015-0.035
Hemoglobin F (fetal hemoglobin)	Less than 2%	<0.02
Hemoglobin, met- and sulf-	0	0
Serum hemoglobin	2-3 mg/100 ml	1.2-1.9 μmol/l
Thermolabile hemoglobin	0	0
L.E. (lupus erythematosus) preparation:		
Heparin as anticoagulant	0	0
Defibrinated blood	0	0
Leukocyte alkaline phosphatase:		
Quantitative method	15-40 mg of phosphorus liberated/h/10¹⁰ cells	15-40 mg/h
Qualitative method	Males: 33-188 U	33-188 U
	Females (off contraceptive pill): 30-160 U	30-160 U
Muramidase	Serum, 3-7 μg/ml	3-7 mg/l
	Urine, 0.2 μg/ml	0.2 mg/l
Osmotic fragility of erythrocytes	Increased if hemolysis occurs in over 0.5% NaCl; decreased if hemolysis is incomplete in 0.3% NaCl	
Peroxide hemolysis	Less than 10%	<0.10
Platelet count	150,000-350,000/mm³	$150\text{-}350 \times 10^9/1$
Platelet function tests:		
Clot retraction	50-100%/2 hr	0.50-1.00/2 h
Platelet aggregation	Full response to ADP, epinephrine and collagen	1.0
Platelet factor 3	33-57 s	33-57 s
Reticulocyte count	0.5-1.5% red cells	0.005-0.15
Vitamin B₁₂	90-280 pg/ml (borderline: 70-90)	66-207 pmol/l (borderline: 52-66)

■ Miscellaneous values

Reference range

Determination	Conventional	SI
Autoantibodies in serum		
Thyroid colloid and microsomal antigens	Absent	
Stomach parietal cells	Absent	
Smooth muscle	Absent	
Kidney mitochondria	Absent	
Rabbit renal collecting ducts	Absent	
Cytoplasm of ova, theca cells, testicular interstitial cells	Absent	
Skeletal muscle	Absent	
Adrenal gland	Absent	
Carcinoembryonic antigen (CEA) in blood	0-2.5 ng/ml, 97% healthy nonsmokers	0-2.5 μg/l, 97% healthy nonsmokers
Cryoprecipitable proteins in blood	0	0 arb. unit
Digitoxin in serum	17 $\pm$ 6 ng/ml	22 $\pm$ 7.8 nmol/l
Digoxin in serum		
0.25 mg/d	1.2 $\pm$ 0.4 ng/ml	1.54 $\pm$ 0.5 nmol/l
0.5 mg/d	1.5 $\pm$ 0.4 ng/ml	1.92 $\pm$ 0.5 nmol/l
Duodenal drainage:		
pH	5.5-7.5	5.5-7.5
Amylase	Over 1200 U/total sample	>1.2 arb. u
Trypsin	Values from 35 to 160% "normal"	0.35-1.60
Viscosity	3 min or less	180 s or less
Gastric analysis	Basal:	
	Females 2.0 $\pm$ 1.8 mEq/h	0.6 $\pm$ 0.5
	Males 3.0 $\pm$ 2.0 mEq/h	0.8 $\pm$ 0.6 μmol/s
	Maximal: (after histalog or gastrin)	
	Females 16 $\pm$ 5 mEq/h	4.4 $\pm$ 1.4 μmol/s
	Males 23 $\pm$ 5 mEq/h	6.4 $\pm$ 1.4 μmol/s
Gastrin-I in blood	0-200 pg/ml	0-95 pmol/l
Immunologic tests		
Alpha-feto-globulin	Abnormal if present	
Alpha 1-antitrypsin	200-400 mg/100 ml	2.0-4.0 g/l
Antinuclear antibodies	Positive if detected with serum diluted 1:10	
Anti-DNA antibodies	Less than 15 units/ml	
Complement, total hemolytic	150-250 U/ml	
C3	Range 55-120 mg/100 ml	0.55-1.2 g/l
C4	Range 20-50 mg/100 ml	0.2-0.5 g/l

■ Miscellaneous values—cont'd

Reference range—cont'd

Determination	Conventional	SI
Immunoglobulins in blood:		
IgG	1140 mg/100 ml	11.4 g/l
	Range 540-1663	5.5-16.6 g/l
IgA	214 mg/100 ml	2.14 g/l
	Range 66-344	0.66-3.44 g/l
IgM	168 mg/100 ml	1.68 g/l
	Range 39-290	0.39-2.9 g/l
Viscosity	1.4-1.8 expressed as relative viscosity of serum compared to water	
Iontophoresis	Children: 0-40 mEq sodium/liter	0-40 mmol/l
	Adults: 0-60 mEq sodium/l	0-60 mmol/l
Propranolol (includes bioactive 4-OH metabolite) in serum 4h after last dose	100-300 ng/ml	386-1158 nmol/l
Stool fat	Less than 5 g in 24 h or less than 4% of measured fat intake in 3-d period	<5 g/d
Stool nitrogen	Less than 2 g/d or 10% of urinary nitrogen	<2 g/d
Synovial fluid:		
Glucose	Not less than 20 mg/100 ml lower than simultaneously drawn blood sugar	See blood glucose mmol/l
Mucin	Type 1 or 2	1-2 arb. u
	Grades as:	
	Type 1-tight clump	
	Type 2-soft clump	
	Type 3-soft clump that breaks up	
	Type 4-cloudy, no clump	
D-Xylose absorption	5-8 g/5 h in urine	33-53 mmol
	40 mg per 100 ml in blood 2 h after ingestion of 25 g of D-xylose	2.7 mmol/l

B

Abbreviations in Common Usage

ā	Before	CVA	Cerebrovascular accident
aa	Of each	CVA	Costovertebral angle
ac	Before meals	CVP	Central venous pressure
ad lib	As desired	Cx	Cervix
A/G ratio	Albumin/globulin ratio	Cysto	Cystoscopy
AK	Above knee	D/C	Discontinue
aPTT	Activated partial thromboplastin time	D & C	Dilation and curettage
A/R pulse	Apical/radial pulse	Diff	Differential white blood cell count
ARDS	Adult respiratory distress syndrome	DIP	Distal interphalangeal joint
ARV	Aortic valve replacement	DJD	Degenerative joint disease
ASHD	Arteriosclerotic heart disease	DM	Diabetes mellitus
ASCVD	Arteriosclerotic cardiovascular disease	DOA	Dead on arrival
BaE	Barium enema	DOE	Dyspnea on exertion
b.i.d.	Twice daily	DPT	Diphtheria, pertussis, tetanus toxoid
BFT	Biofeedback therapy	Dx	Diagnosis
BK	Below knee	ECG	Electrocardiogram
BMR	Basal metabolism rate	EEG	Electroencephalogram
BPH	Benign prostatic hypertrophy	EENT	Eye, ear, nose and throat
B.R.P.	Bathroom privileges	EMG	Electromyogram
BS	Bowel sounds	ENT	Ear, nose and throat
BSP	Bromsulphalein	ESR	Erythrocyte sedimentation rate
BUN	Blood urea nitrogen	FB	Foreign body
Bx	Biopsy	FBS	Fasting blood sugar
c̄	With	FH	Family history
CA	Cancer	FUO	Fever of unknown origin
CABG	Coronary artery bypass graft	FWB	Full weight bearing
CAD	Coronary artery disease	Fx	Fracture
CBC	Complete blood count	GI	Gastrointestinal
cc	Chief complaint	gtt	Drops
CCK	Cholecystokinin	GTT	Glucose tolerance test
C.D.	Constant drainage	GU	Genitourinary
CDC	Centers for Disease Control	h	Hour
CHF	Congestive heart failure	HAV	Hepatitis A virus
CNS	Central nervous system	HBV	Hepatitis B virus
c/O	Complained of	Hct	Hematocrit
COPD	Chronic obstructive pulmonary disease	HCTZ	Hydrochlorothiazide
CPK	Creatine phosphokinase	HCVD	Hypertensive cardiovascular disease
CPR	Cardiopulmonary resuscitation	HDL	High-density lipoproteins
C & S	Culture and sensitivities	Hgb	Hemoglobin
CSF	Cerebrospinal fluid	HMO	Health maintenance organization
CT	Computed tomography	HNP	Herniated nucleus pulposus

HPI	History of present illness	O.S.	Left eye
HTN	Hypertension	O.T.	Occupational therapy
h.s.	At bedtime	O.U.	Both eyes
Hwb	Hot water bottle	p̄	After
hx	History	P & A	Percussion and auscultation
IABP	Intraaortic balloon counterpulsation	PAEDP	Pulmonary artery end-diastolic pressure
ICP	Intracranial pressure	PAP	Pulmonary artery pressure
ICS	Intercostal space	PAP	Papanicolaou smear
ICU	Intensive care unit	PBI	Protein bound iodine
IDDM	Insulin-dependent diabetes mellitus	p.c.	After meals
IHSS	Idiopathic hypertrophic subaortic stenosis	PCWP	Pulmonary capillary wedge pressure
		P.D.	Postural drainage
IM	Intramuscular	PEEP	Positive end expiratory pressure
IMB	Intermenstrual bleeding	PERRLA	Pupils equal, round, reactive to light and accommodation
I & O	Intake and output		
IPPB	Intermittent positive pressure breathing	PFT	Pulmonary function test
ITP	Idiopathic thrombocytopenic purpura	Ph	Past history
IV	Intravenous	PI	Present illness
IVC	Intravenous cholangiogram	PIP	Proximal interphalangeal joint
IVP	Intravenous pyelogram	Plt	Platelet
LBP	Low back pain	PMI	Point of maximal impulse
LDH	Lactic dehydrogenase	PMNs	Polymorphonuclear leukocytes
LDL	Low-density lipoproteins	PMP	Past menstrual period
L.E. prep	Lupus erythematosus prep	PND	Paroxysmal nocturnal dyspnea
LLL	Left lower lobe	PNS	Peripheral nervous system
LLQ	Left lower quadrant	po	By mouth
LMD	Local medical doctor	POD	Postoperative day
LMP	Local medical physician	PPD	Postpartum day
LMP	Last menstrual period	PPD	Purified protein derivative
LOC	Level of consciousness	prn	According to necessity
LP	Lumbar puncture	Pro time	Prothrombin time
LVEDP	Left ventricular end-diastolic pressure	PSP	Phenosulphonphthalein
L & W	Living and well	PSRO	Professional standards review organization
lytes	Electrolytes		
(m)	Murmur	PT	Prothrombin time
MCH	Mean corpuscular hemoglobin	P.T.	Physical therapy
MCHC	Mean corpuscular hemoglobin concentration	PTA	Prior to admission
		PTT	Partial thromboplastin time
MCP	Metacarpopharangeal joint	PVC	Premature ventricular contraction
MCV	Mean corpuscular volume	PWB	Partial weight bearing
MGW	Magnesium, glycerin, and water enema enema	PZI	Protamine zinc insulin
		qd	Every day
MST	Mean survival time	qhs	At bedtime
MTP	Metacarpophalangeal joint	qod	Every other day
MVR	Mitral valve replacement	qid	Four times a day
MWB	Minimal weight bearing	qh	Every hour
NAD	No acute distress	qns	Quantity not sufficient
NIDDM	Noninsulin dependent diabetes mellitus	qoh	Every other hour
NMR	Nuclear magnetic resonance	qpr	At earliest convenience
NPH	Nonprotein Hagedorn (insulin)	qs	As much as necessary
NPN	Nonprotein nitrogen	RBC	Red blood cells
N.P.O.	Nothing by mouth	RLL	Right lower lobe
NVD	Neck vein distention	RLQ	Right lower quadrant
NWB	Nonweight bearing	R/O	Rule out
OD	Overdose	ROS	Review of symptoms
O.D.	Right eye	RSR	Regular sinus rhythm
OOB	Out of bed	Rx	Treatment
O.R.	Operating room	s̄	Without
ORIF	Open reduction internal fixation	SBE	Subacute bacterial endocarditis

sc	Subcutaneous		t.i.d.	Three times a day
Sed rate	Sedimentation rate		TKA	Total knee arthroplasty
SGOT	Serum glutamic oxidase transaminase		TKR	Total knee replacement
SGPT	Serum glutamic pyruvate transaminase		TM	Tympanic membrane
SLE	Systemic lupus erythematosus		TP	Total protein
SLR	Straight leg raising		TPN	Total parenteral nutrition (hyperalimentation)
SOB	Short of breath			
s.o.s.	Administer once if necessary		TSP	Total serum protein
S/P	Status post (occurred in past)		TSS	Toxic shock syndrome
SR	Systems review		TURP	Transurethral resection of prostate
SSE	Soapsuds enema		Tx	Traction
stat	At once		ung	Ointment
STD	Sexually transmitted disease		URI	Upper respiratory infection
STS	Serologic test for syphilis		US	Ultrasound
T_3	Triiodothyronine		UTI	Urinary tract infection
T_4	Thyroxine		UV	Ultraviolet
tab	Tablet		VC	Vital capacity
TBC	Tuberculosis		VDRL	Venereal disease research laboratory test
TBG	Thyroxine binding globulin		VNA	Visiting nurse association
TENS	Transcutaneous electrical nerve stimulator		VS	Vital signs
			wa	While awake
THA	Total hip arthroplasty		WBC	White blood count
THR	Total hip replacement		WNL	Within normal limits
TIA	Transient ischemic attacks			

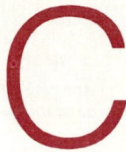

C

Recommended Daily Dietary Allowances, Revised 1980

Mean heights and weights and recommended energy intake

Category	Age (years)	Weight		Height		Energy needs (with range)		
		kg	lb	cm	in	kcal		MJ
Infants	0.0-0.5	6	13	60	24	kg × 115	(95-145)	kg × .48
	0.5-1.0	9	20	71	28	kg × 105	(80-135)	kg × .44
Children	1-3	13	29	90	35	1300	(900-1800)	5.5
	4-6	20	44	112	44	1700	(1300-2300)	7.1
	7-10	28	62	132	52	2400	(1650-3300)	10.1
Males	11-14	45	99	157	62	2700	(2000-3700)	11.3
	15-18	66	145	176	69	2800	(2100-3900)	11.8
	19-22	70	154	177	70	2900	(2500-3300)	12.2
	23-50	70	154	178	70	2700	(2300-3100)	11.3
	51-75	70	154	178	70	2400	(2000-2800)	10.1
	76+	70	154	178	70	2050	(1650-2450)	8.6
Females	11-14	46	101	157	62	2200	(1500-3000)	9.2
	15-18	55	120	163	64	2100	(1200-3000)	8.8
	19-22	55	120	163	64	2100	(1700-2500)	8.8
	23-50	55	120	163	64	2000	(1600-2400)	8.4
	51-75	55	120	163	64	1800	(1400-2200)	7.6
	76+	55	120	163	64	1600	(1200-2000)	6.7
Pregnancy						+300		
Lactation						+500		

From Recommended Dietary Allowances, Revised 1980. Food and Nutrition Board National Academy of Sciences–National Research Council, Washington, D.C..

The data in this table have been assembled from the observed median heights and weights of children together with desirable weights for adults for the mean heights of men (70 in) and women (64 in) between the ages of 18 and 34 years as surveyed in the U.S. population (HEW/NCHS data).

The energy allowances for the young adults are for men and women doing light work. The allowances for the two older age groups represent mean energy needs over these age spans, allowing for a 2% decrease in basal (resting) metabolic rate per decade and a reduction in activity of 200 kcal per day for men and women between 51 and 75 years, 500 kcal for men over 75 years, and 400 kcal for women over 75. The customary range of daily energy output is shown for adults in parentheses and is based on a variation in energy needs of ±400 kcal at any one age, emphasizing the wide range of energy intakes appropriate for any group of people.

Energy allowances for children through age 18 are based on median energy intakes of children these ages followed in longitudinal growth studies. The values in parentheses are 10th and 90th percentiles of energy intake, to indicate the range of energy consumption among children of these ages.

Recommended daily dietary allowances for growth

	Age (yr)	Weight		Height		Energy (kcal)	Protein (g)	Fat soluble vitamins			
								Vit. A		Vit. D (μg*)	Vit. E (mgαTE)
		kg	lb	cm	in			μg RE	IU		
Infants	Birth-0.5	6	13	60	24	kg × 115	kg × 2.2	420	1,400	10	3
	0.5-1	9	20	71	28	kg × 105	kg × 2.0	400	2,000	10	4
Children	1-3	13	29	90	35	1,300	23	400	2,000	10	5
	4-6	20	44	112	44	1,700	30	500	2,500	10	6
	7-10	28	62	132	52	2,400	34	700	3,300	10	7
Males	11-14	45	99	157	62	2,700	45	1,000	5,000	10	8
	15-18	66	145	176	69	2,800	56	1,000	5,000	10	10
Females	11-14	46	101	157	62	2,200	46	800	4,000	10	8
	15-18	55	120	163	64	2,100	46	800	4,000	10	8

*As cholecalciferol; 10 μg cholecalciferol = 400 IU vitamin D.

Daily dietary guide—the basic four food groups

Food group	Main nutrients	Daily amounts*
Milk		
Milk, cheese, ice cream, or other products made with whole or skimmed milk	Calcium Protein Riboflavin	Children under 9: 2-3 cups Children 9-12: 3 or more cups Teen-agers: 4 or more cups Adults: 2 or more cups Pregnant women: 3 or more cups Nursing mothers: 4 or more cups (1 cup = 8 oz fluid milk or designated milk equivalent†)
Meats		

Beef, veal, lamb, pork, poultry, fish, eggs	Protein Iron Thiamin	2 or more servings
		Count as 1 serving
		  2-3 oz of lean, boneless, cooked meat, poultry, or fish
		  2 eggs

Alternates: dry beans, dry peas, nuts, peanut butter	Niacin Riboflavin	1 cup cooked dry beans or peas 4 tbsp peanut butter
Vegetables and fruits		4 or more servings Count as 1 serving ½ cup of vegetable or fruit or a portion such as 1 medium apple, banana, orange, potato, or ½ a medium grapefruit, melon Include
	Vitamin A	A dark-green or deep-yellow vegetable or fruit rich in vitamin A at least every other day
	Vitamin C (ascorbic acid)	A citrus fruit or other fruit or vegetable rich in vitamin C daily
	Smaller amounts of other vitamins and minerals	Other vegetables and fruits including potatoes
Bread and cereals		4 or more servings of whole grain, enriched or restored Count as 1 serving
	Thiamin	1 slice of bread
	Niacin	1 oz (1 cup) ready to eat cereal, flake or puff varieties
	Riboflavin	½-¾ cup cooked cereal
	Iron	½-¾ cup cooked pastas (macaroni, spaghetti, noodles)
	Protein	Crackers: 5 saltines, 2 squares graham crackers

*Use additional amounts of these foods or added butter, margarine, oils, sugars, etc., as desired or needed.
†Milk equivalents: 1 oz cheddar cheese, 3 servings cottage cheese, 1 cup fluid skimmed milk, 1 cup buttermilk, ½ cup dry skimmed milk powder, 1 cup ice milk, 1⅔ cups ice cream, ½ cup evaporated milk.

	Water-soluble vitamins							Minerals					
Vit. C (mg)	Folacin (μg)	Niacin (mg)	Riboflavin (mg)	Thiamin (mg)	Vit. B_6 (mg)	Vit. B_{12} (μg)	Calcium (mg)	Phosphorus (mg)	Iodine (μg)	Iron (mg)	Magnesium (mg)	Zinc (mg)
35	30	6	0.4	0.3	0.3	0.5	360	240	40	10	50	3
35	45	8	0.6	0.5	0.6	1.5	540	360	50	15	70	5
45	100	9	0.8	0.7	0.9	2.0	800	800	70	15	150	10
45	200	11	1.0	0.9	1.3	2.5	800	800	90	10	200	10
45	300	16	1.4	1.2	1.6	3.0	800	800	120	10	250	10
50	400	18	1.6	1.4	1.8	3.0	1,200	1,200	150	18	350	15
60	400	18	1.7	1.4	2.0	3.0	1,200	1,200	150	18	400	15
50	400	15	1.3	1.1	1.8	3.0	1,200	1,200	150	18	300	15
60	400	14	1.3	1.1	2.0	3.0	1,200	1,200	150	18	300	15

Recommended daily dietary allowances of some selected nutrients for pregnancy and lactation

| | Nonpregnant girl | | Nonpregnant woman | Pregnancy | | | | Lactation (850 ml daily) | | | |
| | | | | | Girl | | Woman | | Girl | | Woman |
Nutrients	12-14 yr 47 kg (103 lb)	14-18 yr 55 kg (120 lb)	25 yr 58 kg (128 lb)	Added need	12-14 yr	14-18 yr	25 yr	Added need	12-14 yr	14-18 yr	25 yr
Calories	2,200	2,100	2,000	300	2,500	2,400	2,300	500	2,700	2,600	2,500
Protein (g)	46	46	44	30	76	76	74	20	66	68	64
Calcium (g)	1.2	1.2	0.8	0.4	1.6	1.6	1.2	0.4	1.6	1.6	1.2
Iron (mg)	18	18	18	‡	18+	18+	18+	‡	18+	18+	18+
Vitamin A (RE)*	800	800	800	200	1,000	1,000	1,000	400	1,200	1,200	1,200
Thiamin (mg)	1.1	1.1	1.0	0.4	1.5	1.5	1.4	0.5	1.6	1.6	1.5
Riboflavin (mg)	1.3	1.3	1.2	0.3	1.6	1.6	1.5	0.5	1.8	1.8	1.7
Niacin equivalent and tryptophan (mg)	15	14	13	2	17	16	15	5	20	19	18
Ascorbic acid (mg)	50	60	60	20	70	80	80	40	90	100	100
Vitamin D (μg)†	10	10	5	5	15	15	10	5	15	15	10

*Retinol equivalents.
†Cholecalciferol; 10 μg equals 400 IU vitamin D.
‡Required iron supplement 30-60 mg.

Index

A

Entries referring to tables are denoted by an
italic *t* following the page number. An italic
number indicates an illustration.

Ditropan; *see* Oxybutynin chloride (Ditropan)
Diuresis, osmotic, 123
Diuretic therapy
 for congestive heart failure, 799-800
 with hepatic dysfunction, 1021
Diuretics
 adverse effects on anesthesia or surgery
  from, 337t
 for balance disorders, 558
 for congestive heart failure, onset, duration, and side effects of, 800t
 in edema treatment, 125
 fluid and electrolyte imbalance from, 138t
  prevention of, 137
 for hypertension, action and effects of, 858t
 osmotic
  for craniocerebral trauma, 490
  for increased intracranial pressure, 437
 ototoxic, 551
Diuril; *see* Chlorothiazide (Diuril)
Diverticuli of bladder, 1159
Diverticulitis, 1092, *1093*
 bowel elimination pattern in, 1094
 diet and, 1094
 etiology, signs and symptoms, and therapy
  of, 1093t
 implementation in, 1097-1098
 pathophysiology of, 1092, 1094
 surgery for, 1100
Diverticulosis, 1094
Diverticulum, esophageal, 1060, *1060*
 etiology, signs and symptoms, and therapy
  of, 1059t
DNA; *see* Deoxyribonucleic acid (DNA)
Dobbhoff enteric tube, purpose and characteristics of, 1068t
Dobutamine (Dobutrex)
 for cardiac arrest, use and action of, 1452t
 in shock therapy, 162t
Dobutrex; *see* Dobutamine (Dobutrex)
DOCA; *see* Desoxycorticosterone (DOCA)
Dolobid; *see* Diflunisal (Dolobid)
Donovan bodies, 1297
Donovanosis
 assessment of, 1297
 epidemiology and etiology of, 1297
 implementation in, 1297
Dopamine
 as neurotransmitter, 405
 prolactin excess and, 951
 sexual response and, 1222
 in shock therapy, 162t
Doppler effect, 849, *849*
Dorsal column stimulator for pain relief, 179,
  180
Douching
 for inflammations, 1253
 recommendations about, 1285
Douglas, cul-de-sac of, 1240
Doxorubicin (Adriamycin)
 action and toxic effects of, 247t
 alopecia and, 251
 cardiac effects of, 253
 in chemotherapy of liver, 1019
 intravenous administration of, 248, 248t
Doxycycline for lymphogranuloma venereum,
  1296
Drainage
 after urologic surgery, 1167
 catheter, maintenance of system for, 1134
 chest; *see* Chest drainage
 gastric; *see* Nasogastric drainage
 nasogastric; *see* Nasogastric drainage

Drainage—cont'd
 postural
  contraindications to, 729
  with endotracheal tube, 743
  for patient with emphysema, 727, 727,
   728t, 729
  positions for, by area of lung, 728t
 urinary
  after prostate surgery, 1177
  for treating urinary incontinence, 1141-
   1142
 water-seal, after lung surgery, 703-704
Drainage/secretion precautions, 207-208
Drainage tubes after thoracic surgery, 708
Draining fistulas, preventing fluid and electrolyte imbalance from, 137
Drains, 377, 377t, 378
 insertion of, after surgery, 367
Dramamine; *see* Demenhydrinate (Dramamine)
Draping, sterile, 357-358
Dressings
 application of, after surgery, 367
 postoperative assessment of, 376
 with total parenteral nutrition, 90
 types of, 383
DRGs; *see* Diagnosis related groups (DRGs)
Drift, testing of, in increased intracranial
  pressure assessment, 435
Droperidol and fentanyl, administration, advantages, and disadvantages, 360t
Drowning, near, emergency treatment of,
  1453
Drug abuse, 276-286; *see also* specific drugs;
   Substance abuse
 assessment of, 283, 285
 counseling and teaching about, 286
 diagnostic test for assessing, 285
 evaluation of patient in, 286
 methadone maintenance in treatment of,
  285
 narcotic, adult respiratory distress syndrome and, 696
 nurses impaired by, 286
 nursing implementation in, 285-286
 residential communities in treatment of,
  285
 risk of disease with, 286
 in young adulthood, 62
Drug addiction; *see also* Addiction
 defined, 177, 276
Drug and Alcohol Nursing Association
  (DANA), 286
Drug dependence, defined, 177, 276
Drug habituation, defined, 276
Drug holiday, 464
Drug tolerance, defined, 177
Drug users, AIDS and, 1357
Drugs; *see also* Medications
 antiinflammatory, wound healing and,
  383
 aplastic anemia and, 869, 871
 for cancer pain, 255-256
 cell cycle nonspecific, 246
 cell cycle specific, 246
 chemotherapeutic, 246-247, 247t
 cytotoxic; *see* Chemotherapy
 excretion of, 1127
 hemolysis produced by, 875
 mind-altering
  effects of, 276t
  intoxication and withdrawal from, 284t
 nonsteroidal antiinflammatory; *see* Nonsteroidal antiinflammatory drugs

Drugs—cont'd
 over-the-counter
  alcohol contained in, 275
  caffeine content of, 278
 psychoactive, 277
 in shock therapy, 161, 161t-162t, 163
 with thrombocytopenic effects, 883
 types of, 276
 vesicant, administration of, 248, 248t
DTs; *see* Delirium tremens
Duck-bill prosthesis, 661
Duct of Wirsung, 995
Dulcolax; *see* Bisacodyl (Dulcolax)
Dumping syndrome
 after stomach surgery, 1083-1084
 symptoms and therapy of, 1084t
Duodenum, 1048
 peptic ulcer of, 1071, 1071t
  pathophysiology of, *1072*
Dupuytren's contracture
 assessment of, 595
 implementation in, 596
 pathophysiology of, 595
 patient evaluation in, 596
 patient outcomes in, 596
Dura mater, 414
Durabolin; *see* Nandrolone phenpropionate
  (Durabolin)
Dwarfism, 949t, 952
 from growth hormone deficit, 952
Dying
 choices about, 321
 chronicity of, 319
 defined, 314
 family and, 322-323
 home care during, 322
 mental capacity and, 317
 nursing diagnoses related to, 324
 nursing intervention during, 324-326
 paternalism and, 318
 patterns of, 320-321
 quality of life and, 317
 rights associated with, 315
 role of confidante in, 321
 stages and phases of, 319-320
 terminating or withholding treatment and,
  316
Dymelor; *see* Acetohexamide (Dymelor)
Dynamic equilibrium, defined, 6
Dyrenium; *see* Triamterene (Dyrenium)
Dyscrasias, plasma cell, 897
Dysesthesia, defined, 429
Dysmenorrhea, 1246-1247
 causes of, 1246
 dilation and curettage for, 1262
Dyspareunia, 67, 1230
 after menopause, 1243-1244
 with inflammatory disease of female reproductive tract, 1257
Dysphagia
 in esophageal disorders, 1061
 management of, 1061
Dyspnea
 with anemia, 869
 with congestive heart failure, 797
 with left ventricular failure, 794
 in mountain sickness, 669
 paroxysmal nocturnal, 794
 with pulmonary edema, 802
 as symptom of respiratory disorder, 671
Dysreflexia, autonomic, with spinal cord injury, 493-494, *494*
Dysrhythmias; *see also* Arrhythmias
 shock and, 147

ALSO AVAILABLE!

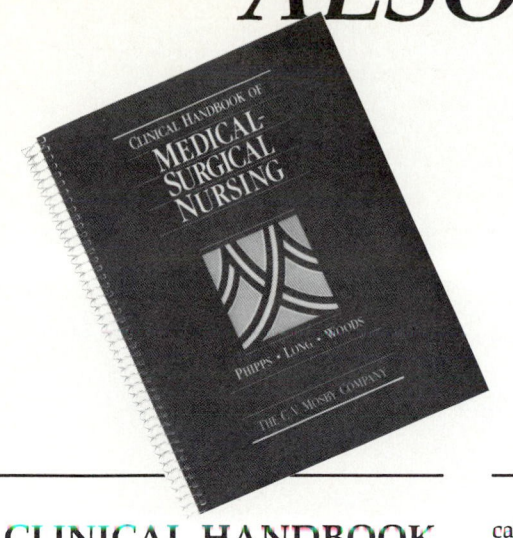

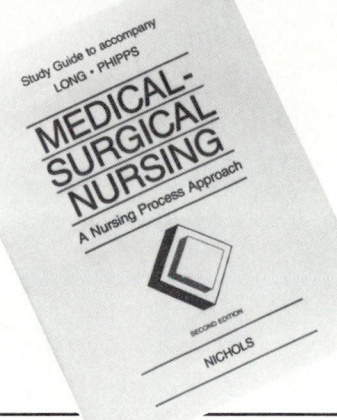

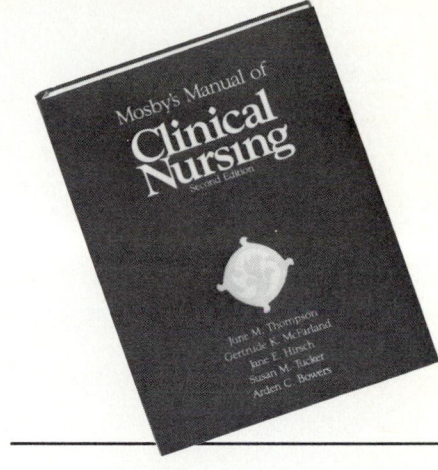

CLINICAL HANDBOOK OF MEDICAL-SURGICAL NURSING

By Wilma J. Phipps, Ph.D., R.N., F.A.A.N.; Barbara C. Long, R.N., M.S.N.; and Nancy F. Woods, Ph.D., R.N., F.A.A.N.; with 58 contributors.

(3850)

The **Clinical Handbook of Medical-Surgical Nursing** is an essential tool for the hospital setting. Wilma Phipps, Barbara Long, and Nancy Woods have put together a concise, spiral-bound, clinical guide that is easy to read and use. The book features approximately 275 common medical-surgical problems and diagnostic procedures. The chapter format will be easy for you to follow because it consistently utilizes the five-step nursing process for presenting nursing care information.

MEDICAL-SURGICAL NURSING: A Nursing Process Approach Study Guide

By Mary Sayer Nichols, R.N., M.S.N.

(5494)

If you're a student using ME**DICAL-SURGICAL NURSING: A Nursing Process Approach**, you will find invaluable assistance in the new *study guide.* The guide follows the chapter format of the book and helps you assimilate the enormous amount of material in a medi-

cal-surgical course, use your study time more productively, and prepare for both classroom and licensure examination. This guide includes:

- Chapter outlines from the parent text.
- Prerequisite and suggested readings -- specific page numbers from the parent text, as well as outside texts, references, and journal articles.
- Self assessment activities such as multiple choice questions, true-false, labeling, and charting to vary the learning mode within each chapter.
- Clinical applications in the form of case studies with questions that enable you to test your decision-making skills.
- Nursing care plans with fill-in-the-blank portions to guide you through the process of planning quality patient care.
- Supplemental activities such as classroom and/or outside activities to enhance your understanding of complex concepts.

MOSBY'S MANUAL OF CLINICAL NURSING Second Edition

By June M. Thompson, R.N., M.S.; Gertrude K. McFarland, R.N., D.N.Sc., F.A.A.N.; Jane E. Hirsch, R.N., M.S.; Susan M. Tucker, R.N., B.S.N.; and Arden C. Bowers, R.N., M.S.

(5157)

The first edition of **MOSBY'S MANUAL OF CLINICAL NURSING** was voted nursing's #1 most indispensible reference in an American Journal of Nursing poll, and the second edition is even better than the first. No student should be without this comprehensive reference for planning nursing care.

- Part I, "Clinical Nursing Practice," is organized by body systems and covers virtually every condition, disease, or disorder you are likely to encounter. Complete nursing care is presented for all medical conditions and medical interventions.
- **NEW!** Part II, "Diagnostic Procedures," contains nursing care associated with every significant diagnostic test. The tests are presented by category and are also alphabetically indexed for easy access.
- Part III, "Nursing Diagnoses," has all NANDA-accepted nursing diagnoses, including the 16 new diagnoses accepted at the Eighth NANDA Conference held in March 1988.
- Nursing care is concisely organized according to the nursing process. An assessment for each disease provides a checklist to ensure comprehensive nursing assessment.
- Comprehensive nursing interventions with rationales are linked to every possible nursing diagnosis for every disease to allow individualization of care.
- Patient teaching in the nursing care of each disease encourages you to build teaching interventions right into care plans.
- An evaluation section for each disease provides specific data to help determine when your nursing goals have been met or when they need to be revised.

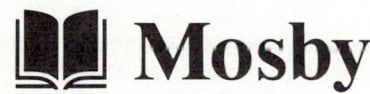 **Mosby**

You can experience Mosby's tradition of excellence first hand by ordering these helpful learning tools. To order these texts, ask your bookstore manager, or call **TOLL-FREE 800-221-7700, ext. 15A.** We look forward to hearing from you soon!

NURSING CARE PLANS